DAILY VALUES FOR FOOD LABELS

◆

The Daily Values are standard values developed by the Food and Drug Administration (FDA) for use on food labels. In creating the Daily Values, the FDA first established two sets of reference values. The first set, the Reference Daily Intakes (RDI), is for protein, vitamins, and minerals and reflect average allowances based on the RDA. The second set, the Daily Reference Values (DRV), is for nutrients and food components, such as fat and fiber, that do not have an established RDA but do have important relationships with health. Together, the RDI and DRV make up the Daily Values used on food labels (Chapter 2 provides more details).

Reference Daily Intakes (RDI)

Nutrient	Amount
Protein[a]	50 g
Thiamin	1.5 mg
Riboflavin	1.7 mg
Niacin	20 mg NE
Biotin	300 µg
Pantothenic acid	10 mg
Vitamin B_6	2 mg
Folate	400 µg
Vitamin B_{12}	6 µg
Vitamin C	60 mg
Vitamin A[b]	5000 IU
Vitamin D[b]	400 IU
Vitamin E[b]	30 IU
Vitamin K	80 µg
Calcium	1000 mg
Iron	18 mg
Zinc	15 mg
Iodine	150 µg
Copper	2 mg
Chromium	120 µg
Selenium	70 µg
Molybdenum	75 µg
Manganese	2 mg
Chloride	3400 mg

[a]The RDI for protein varies for different groups of people: pregnant women, 60 g; nursing mothers, 65 g; infants under 1 year, 14 g; children 1 to 4 years, 16 g.
[b]The RDI for fat-soluble vitamins are expressed in International Units (IU), an old system of measurement. The current RDA and tables of food composition use a more accurate system of measurement. Equivalent values are as follows: for vitamin A, 875 µg RE; for vitamin D, 10 µg; for vitamin E, 9 mg α-TE.

Daily Reference Values (DRV)

Food Component	DRV	Calculation
Fat	65 g	30% of kcalories
Saturated fat	20 g	10% of kcalories
Cholesterol	300 mg	Same regardless of kcalories
Carbohydrate (total)	300 g	60% of kcalories
Fiber	25 g	11.5 g per 1000 kcalories
Protein	50 g	10% of kcalories
Sodium	2400 mg	Same regardless of kcalories
Potassium	3500 mg	Same regardless of kcalories

Note: The DRV were established for adults and children over 4 years old. The values for energy-yielding nutrients are based on 2000 kcalories a day.

Glossary of Nutrient Measures

kcal: kcalories; a unit by which energy is measured (see Chapter 1).

g: grams; a unit of weight equivalent to about 0.03 ounces.

mg: milligrams; one-thousandth of a gram.

µg: micrograms; one-millionth of a gram.

mg NE: milligrams niacin equivalents; a measure of niacin activity (see Chapter 10).

mg α-TE: milligrams alpha-tocopherol equivalents; a measure of vitamin E activity (see Chapter 11).

µg RE: micrograms retinol equivalents; a measure of vitamin A activity (see Chapter 11).

IU: international units; an old measure of vitamin activity determined by biological methods (as opposed to new measures that are determined by direct chemical analysis).

www.wadsworth.com

wadsworth.com is the World Wide Web site for Wadsworth Publishing Company and is your direct source to dozens of online resources.

At *wadsworth.com* you can find out about supplements, demonstration software, and student resources. You can also send e-mail to many of our authors and preview new publications and exciting new technologies.

wadsworth.com
Changing the way the world learns®

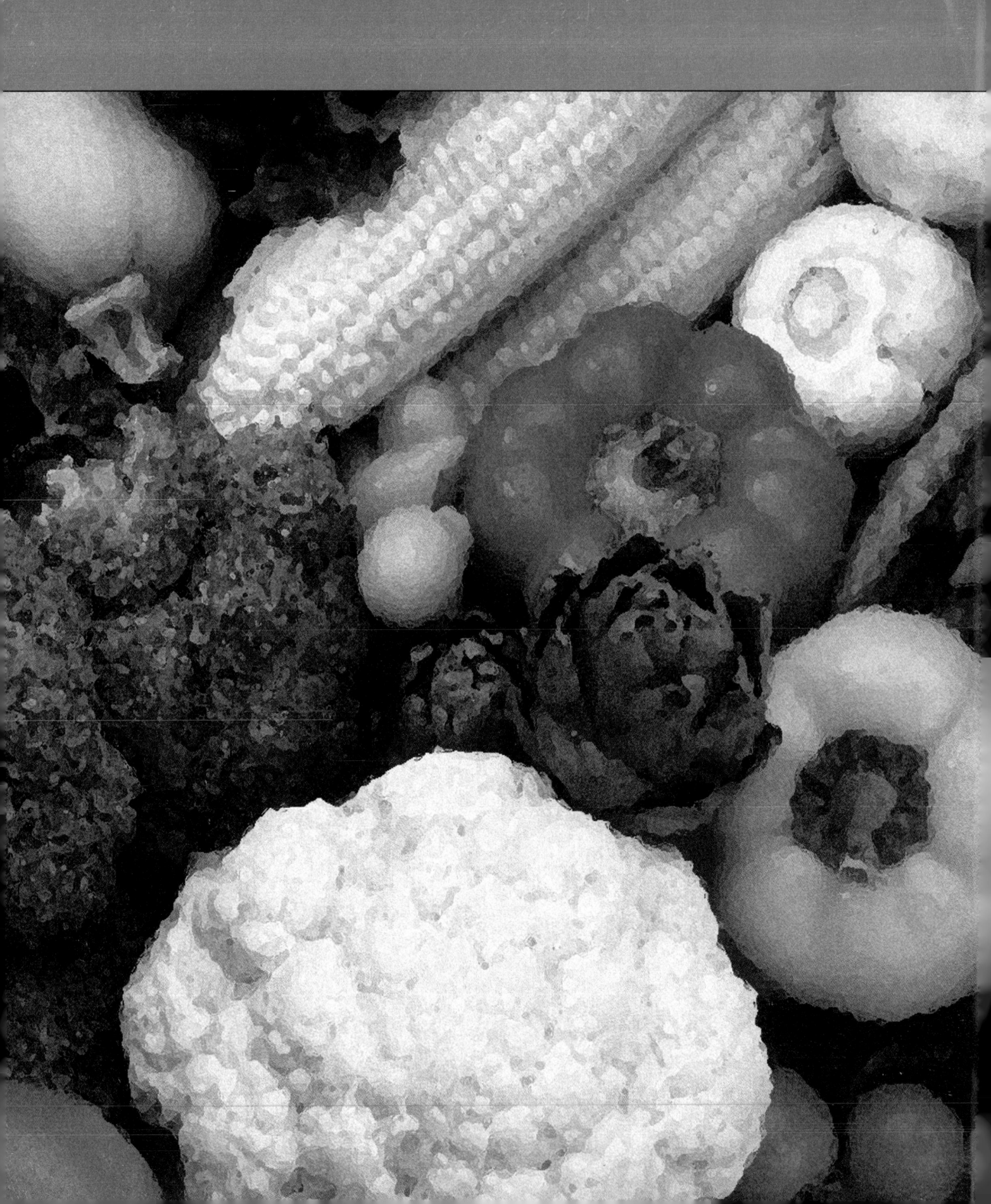

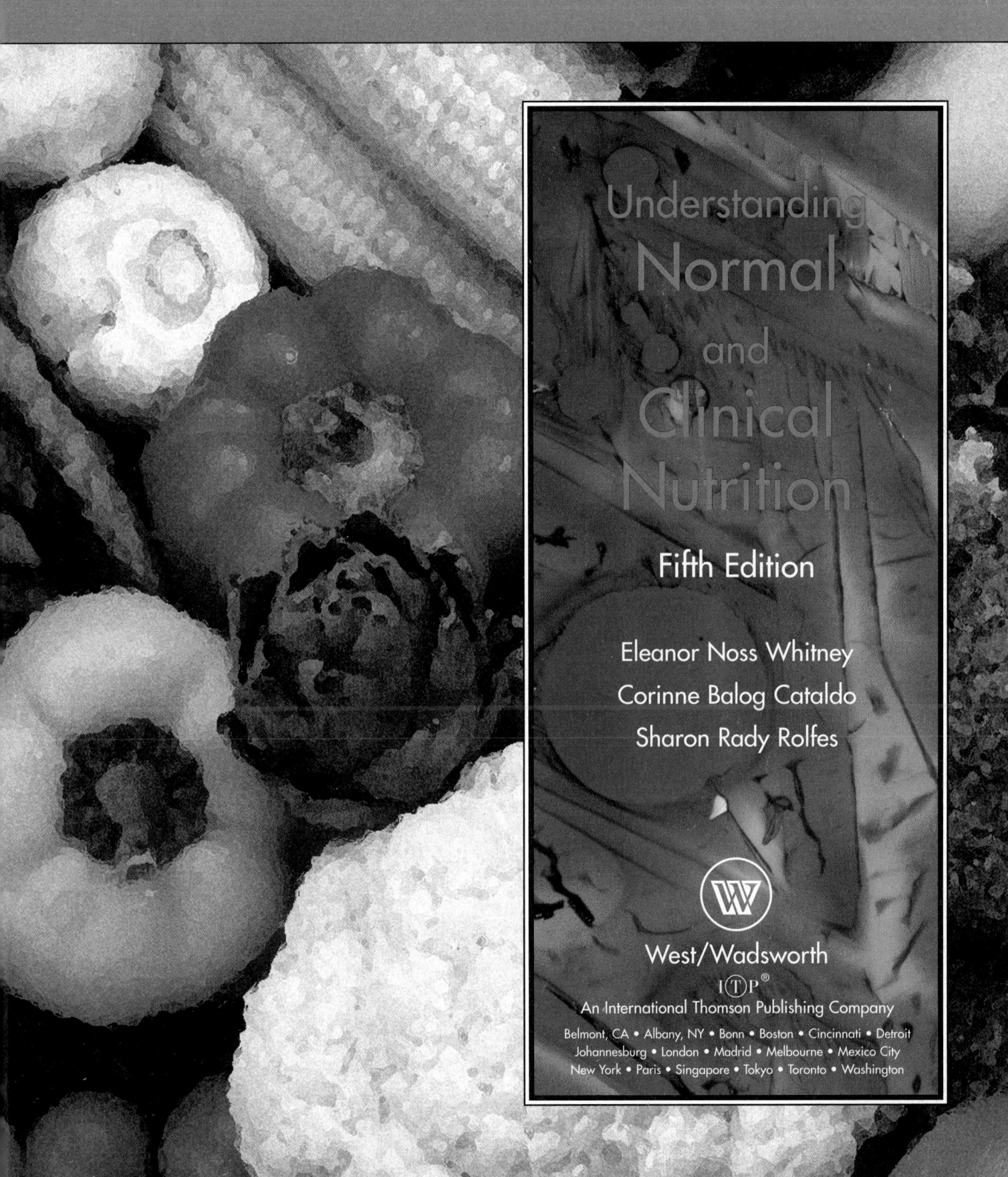

Understanding Normal and Clinical Nutrition

Fifth Edition

Eleanor Noss Whitney

Corinne Balog Cataldo

Sharon Rady Rolfes

West/Wadsworth

I(T)P®

An International Thomson Publishing Company

Belmont, CA • Albany, NY • Bonn • Boston • Cincinnati • Detroit
Johannesburg • London • Madrid • Melbourne • Mexico City
New York • Paris • Singapore • Tokyo • Toronto • Washington

Nutrition Publisher:	Peter Marshall
Associate Development Editor:	Laura Perkinson
Editorial Assistant:	Tangelique Williams
Marketing Manager:	Becky Tollerson
Project Editor:	Sandra Craig
Print Buyer:	Barbara Britton
Permissions Editor:	Peggy Meehan
Production Coordinator:	The Book Company
Text and Cover Design:	Janet Bollow
Cover Image:	Leptin, © Michael Davidson
Copy Editor:	Pat Lewis
Photo Research:	Photo Edit, Stephen Forsling
Illustrations:	J/B Woolsey and Associates, Todd Smith, Regina Hollistor, Impact Publications
Index:	Barbara Farabaugh
Compositor:	Parkwood Composition Service
Printer:	World Color Book Services/ Taunton

A Word about the Photomicrographs

The chapter opening photomicrographs by Michael Davidson at Florida State University were made of recrystallized vitamins and other nutrients using a variety of different techniques. Many vitamins can be imaged using the melt-recrystallization process where a few milligrams of the chemical are sandwiched between a microscope coverslip and slide, then heated until melted and allowed to slowly recrystallize. Alternately, for vitamin-salts that will not melt, the chemical is dissolved in a suitable solvent (water or alcohol) and a few microliters of solution are allowed to slowly evaporate between a microscope slide and coverslip. Upon recrystallization, the vitamins are viewed in a microscope using cross-polarized illumination where the crystallites diffract light depending both on the molecular orientation within the crystal and the crystal thickness. The colorful patterns illustrated in this text are a manifestation of both molecular orientation and crystal thickness.

COPYRIGHT © 1998 by Wadsworth Publishing Company

A Division of International Thomson Publishing Inc.

I(T)P® The ITP logo is a registered trademark under license.

Printed in the United States of America

3 4 5 6 7 8 9 10

For more information, contact Wadsworth Publishing Company, 10 Davis Drive, Belmont, CA 94002, or electronically at http://www.wadsworth.com/wadsworth.html

International Thomson Publishing Europe
Berkshire House 168-173
High Holborn
London, WC1V 7AA, England

International Thomson Editores
Campos Eliseos 385, Piso 7
Col. Polanco
11560 México D.F. México

Thomas Nelson Australia
102 Dodds Street
South Melbourne 3205
Victoria, Australia

International Thomson Publishing Asia
221 Henderson Road
#05-10 Henderson Building
Singapore 0315

Nelson Canada
1120 Birchmount Road
Scarborough, Ontario
Canada M1K 5G4

International Thomson Publishing Japan
Hirakawacho Kyowa Building, 3F
2-2-1 Hirakawacho
Chiyoda-ku, Tokyo 102, Japan

International Thomson Publishing GmbH
Königswinterer Strasse 418
53227 Bonn, Germany

International Thomson Publishing Southern Africa
Building 18, Constantia Park
240 Old Pretoria Road
Halfway House, 1685 South Africa

Library of Congress Cataloging-in-Publication Data

Whitney, Eleanor Noss.
  Understanding normal and clinical nutrition / Eleanor Noss Whitney, Corinne Balog Cataldo, Sharon Rady Rolfes.—5th ed.
    p. cm.
  Includes bibliographical references and index.
  ISBN 0-534-53334-5
  1. Nutrition.   2. Diet in disease.   3. Dietetics.   I. Cataldo, Corinne Balog.   II. Rolfes, Sharon Rady.   III. Title.
  [DNLM: 1. Nutrition. 2. Diet Therapy. QU 145 W618ua 1998]
QP141.W458   1998
613.2—dc21
DNLM/DLC
for Library of Congress   97–41398

Credits appear at the end of the book.

To ....

Lynn, Liza, and Sally,
all nurturers.
I am proud to call
all three my daughters.

Ellie

To ....

My son, Adam,
who has been a source
of happiness and pride,
a reminder of the promise
that the future holds,
and a wonderful person
to talk with.
Good luck as you enter
college and begin your life
as an adult.

Mom (Corkie)

To ....

My loving husband, Tom,
and
our delightful children,
Lyle and Marni.

Sharon

About the Authors

Eleanor Noss Whitney, Ph.D., received her B.A. in biology from Radcliffe College in 1960 and her Ph.D. in biology from Washington University, St. Louis, in 1970. Formerly on the faculty at Florida State University, and a dietitian registered with the American Dietetic Association, she now devotes full time to research, writing, and consulting. Her earlier publications include articles in *Science, Genetics,* and other journals. Her textbooks include *Understanding Nutrition, Nutrition Concepts and Controversies, Life Span Nutrition: Conception through Life, Nutrition and Diet Therapy,* and *Essential Life Choices* for college students and *Making Life Choices* for high school students. Her most intense interests currently include energy conservation, solar energy uses, alternatively fueled vehicles, and ecosystem restoration.

Corinne Balog Cataldo, M.M.Sc., R.D., C.N.S.D., received her B.S. in community health nutrition from Georgia State University in 1976 and her M.M.Sc. in clinical dietetics from Emory University in 1979. She has worked in private practice in Atlanta, as a clinical dietitian and metabolic support nutritionist at Georgia Baptist Medical Center in Atlanta, as a faculty member and dietetic internship coordinator at Emory University, and as a nutritionist with the Infant Formula Council. She has made numerous presentations, and in addition to this book, she has written a manual on tube feedings and the books *Nutrition and Diet Therapy, Nutrition for Health and Health Care,* and *Understanding Clinical Nutrition.* She is a certified nutrition support dietitian.

Sharon Rady Rolfes, M.S., R.D., received her B.S. in psychology and criminology in 1974 and her M.S. in nutrition and food science in 1982 from Florida State University. She is a founding member of Nutrition and Health Associates, an information resource center that maintains an ongoing bibliographic database that tracks research in over 1000 nutrition-related topics. Her other publications include the textbooks *Understanding Nutrition, Understanding Clinical Nutrition, Life Span Nutrition: Conception through Life,* and *Nutrition for Health and Health Care* and a multimedia CD-ROM called *Nutrition Interactive.* In addition to writing, she also lectures at universities and at professional conferences and serves as a consultant for various educational projects. She maintains a professional membership in the American Dietetic Association.

Contents in Brief

Preface xxi

Chapter 1   **An Overview of Nutrition**   1
HIGHLIGHT: Who Speaks on Nutrition?   29

Chapter 2   **Planning a Healthy Diet**   36
HIGHLIGHT: Ethnic Cuisines and Healthy Choices   63

Chapter 3   **Digestion, Absorption, and Transport**   71
HIGHLIGHT: Common Digestive Problems   94

Chapter 4   **The Carbohydrates: Sugars, Starch, and Fibers**   101
HIGHLIGHT: Alternatives to Sugar   133

Chapter 5   **The Lipids: Triglycerides, Phospholipids, and Sterols**   146
HIGHLIGHT: Alternatives to Fat   176

Chapter 6   **Protein: Amino Acids**   179
HIGHLIGHT: Vegetarian, Mediterranean, and Other
Meat-Restricted Foodways   209

Chapter 7   **Metabolism: Transformations and Interactions**   218
HIGHLIGHT: Alcohol and Nutrition   245

Chapter 8   **Energy Balance and Body Composition**   256
HIGHLIGHT: Fitness: Physical Activity and Nutrition   278

Chapter 9   **Weight Control: Overweight and Underweight**   287
HIGHLIGHT: Eating Disorders—Anorexia Nervosa and Bulimia
Nervosa   315

Chapter 10   **The Water-Soluble Vitamins: B Vitamins and
Vitamin C**   325
HIGHLIGHT: Vitamin and Mineral Supplements   366

Chapter 11   **The Fat-Soluble Vitamins: A, D, E, and K**   374
HIGHLIGHT: Antioxidant Nutrients and Nonnutrients in Disease
Prevention   400

Chapter 12   **Water and the Major Minerals**   408
HIGHLIGHT: Osteoporosis and Calcium   439

Chapter 13   **The Trace Minerals**   449
HIGHLIGHT: Our Children's Daily Lead   480

Chapter 14   **Consumer Concerns about Foods**   485
HIGHLIGHT: Consumer Concerns about Public Water   515

Contents in Brief

Chapter 15 ☀ **The Nutrition Care Process: Assessing Historical and Physical Data** 518
HIGHLIGHT: Diet and Health 539

Chapter 16 ☀ **The Nutrition Care Process: Assessing Anthropometric and Biochemical Data** 543
HIGHLIGHT: Nutrition and Diagnostic Tests 559

Chapter 17 ☀ **The Nutrition Care Process: Developing a Nutrition Care Plan** 561
HIGHLIGHT: The Team Approach 581

Chapter 18 ☀ **Life Cycle Nutrition: Pregnancy and Lactation** 584
HIGHLIGHT: Hunger and Global Environmental Problems 614

Chapter 19 ☀ **Life Cycle Nutrition: Infancy, Childhood, and Adolescence** 625
HIGHLIGHT: Childhood Obesity and the Early Development of Chronic Diseases 658

Chapter 20 ☀ **Life Cycle Nutrition: The Later Years** 665
HIGHLIGHT: Alternative Therapies 688

Chapter 21 ☀ **Nutrition and Disorders of the Upper GI Tract** 694
HIGHLIGHT: Living with Feeding Disabilities 716

Chapter 22 ☀ **Nutrition and Disorders of the Lower GI Tract** 722
HIGHLIGHT: Promoting Intestinal Adaptation 752

Chapter 23 ☀ **Enteral Nutrition** 755
HIGHLIGHT: Enteral Formulas: Who's Minding the Market? 779

Chapter 24 ☀ **Parenteral Nutrition** 782
HIGHLIGHT: Ethical Issues in Nutrition Care 797

Chapter 25 ☀ **Nutrition and Severe Stress** 803
HIGHLIGHT: Food and Foodservice in the Hospital 820

Chapter 26 ☀ **Nutrition and Disorders of the Liver and Biliary Tract** 825
HIGHLIGHT: Inborn Errors of Metabolism 839

Chapter 27 ☀ **Nutrition, Diabetes, and Hypoglycemia** 845
HIGHLIGHT: Living with Diabetes 877

Chapter 28 ☀ **Nutrition and Disorders of the Blood Vessels, Heart and Lungs** 881
HIGHLIGHT: Diet and Protection against CHD 905

Chapter 29 ☀ **Nutrition and Disorders of the Kidneys** 909
HIGHLIGHT: Kidney Stones—Treatments and Prevention 930

Chapter 30 ☀ **Nutrition and Wasting Disorders: Cancer and HIV Infections** 933
HIGHLIGHT: Cost-Conscious Health Care 959

Contents in Brief

Appendix A   Cells, Hormones, and Nerves

Appendix B   Basic Chemistry Concepts

Appendix C   Biochemical Structures and Pathways

Appendix D   Aids to Calculation

Appendix E   Nutrition Assessment: Supplemental Information

Appendix F   Nutrition Resources

Appendix G   United States: Recommendations and Exchanges

World Health Organization: Recommendations

Appendix H   Table of Food Composition

Appendix I   Canada: Recommendations, Choices, and Labels

Appendix J   Measures of Protein Quality

Appendix K   Enteral Formulas

Glossary

Index

Contents

Preface xxi

Chapter 1

An Overview of Nutrition   1

Food Choices   2
Introducing the Nutrients   4
   The Six Classes of Nutrients   4
   How to Think Metric   6
   The Energy-Yielding Nutrients   6
   How to Calculate the Energy Available from Foods   8
   The Vitamins   10
   The Minerals   10
   Water   10
The Science of Nutrition   11
   Nutrition Research   11
   Research Versus Rumors   14
Recommended Nutrient Intakes   14
   Recommended Dietary Allowances (RDA)   15
   Setting the RDA for Vitamins and Minerals   16
   Using the RDA   18
Nutrition Assessment   20
   Nutrition Assessment of Individuals   21
   Nutrition Assessment of Populations   23
Diet and Health   24
   Risk Factors   24
   Dietary Recommendations   26
   HIGHLIGHT ONE: Who Speaks on Nutrition?   29

Chapter 2

Planning a Healthy Diet   36

Principles and Guidelines   37
   Diet-Planning Principles   37
   Dietary Guidelines for Americans   39
Diet-Planning Guides   40
   Food Group Plans   40
   From Guidelines to Groceries   45
Food Labels   51
   The Ingredient List   52
   Serving Sizes   54
   Nutrition Facts   54
   The Daily Values   55

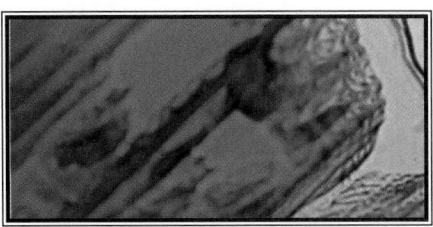

   How to Calculate Personal Daily Values   57
   Descriptive Terms   57
   Health Claims   58
   Consumer Education   61
   HIGHLIGHT TWO: Ethnic Cuisines and Healthy
      Choices   63

Chapter 3

Digestion, Absorption, and Transport   71

Digestion   72
   Anatomy of the Digestive Tract   72
   The Muscular Action of Digestion   76
   The Secretions of Digestion   78
   The Final Stage   80
Absorption   81
   Anatomy of the Absorptive System   83
   A Closer Look at the Intestinal Cells   83
The Circulatory Systems   86
   The Vascular System   86
   The Lymphatic System   90
Regulation of Digestion and Absorption   90
   Gastrointestinal Hormones and Nerve Pathways   90
   The System at Its Best   92
   HIGHLIGHT THREE: Common Digestive Problems   94

Chapter 4

The Carbohydrates: Sugars, Starch, and Fibers   101

The Chemist's View of Carbohydrates   102
The Simple Carbohydrates   103
   Monosaccharides   103
   Dissaccharides   105
The Complex Carbohydrates   107
   Glycogen   107
   Starch   108
   The Fibers   108

Contents

Digestion and Absorption of Carbohydrates   111
  The Processes of Digestion and Absorption   111
  Lactose Intolerance   115
Glucose in the Body   116
  A Preview of Carbohydrate Metabolism   116
  The Constancy of Blood Glucose   118
Health Effects and Recommended Intakes of Sugars   121
  Health Effects of Sugars   122
  Accusations against Sugars   125
  Recommended Intakes of Sugars   125
Health Effects and Recommended Intakes of Starch and
  Fibers   126
  Health Effects of Starch and Fibers   126
Recommended Intakes of Starch and Fiber   128
  HIGHLIGHT FOUR: Alternatives to Sugar   133

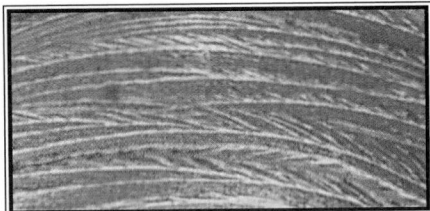

Chapter 5

The Lipids: Triglycerides, Phospholipids, and Sterols   146

The Chemist's View of Triglycerides and Fatty Acids   141
  The Fatty Acids   142
  Fats in Foods   145
  Roles of Triglycerides and Fatty Acids   148
  Essential Fatty Acids   148
The Chemist's View of Phospholipids and Sterols   151
  The Phospholipids   151
  The Sterols   152
Digestion, Absorption, and Transport of Lipids   154
  Lipid Digestion   154
  Lipid Absorption   157
  Lipid Transport   159
Lipids in the Body   160
  Triglycerides in the Blood   160
  A Preview of Lipid Metabolism   160
Health Effects and Recommended Intakes of Lipids   163
  Health Effects of Lipids   164
  Recommended Intakes of Fat   167

  How to Lower Fat Intake—by Food Group   168
  How to Calculate a Personal Daily Value for Fat   172
  HIGHLIGHT FIVE: Alternatives to Fat   176

Chapter 6

Protein: Amino Acids   179

The Chemist's View of Proteins   180
  Amino Acids   180
  Proteins   182
Digestion and Absorption of Protein   184
  The Process of Digestion   184
  The Process of Absorption   184
Proteins in the Body   186
  Protein Synthesis   186
  Roles of Proteins   188
  A Preview of Protein Metabolism   193
Protein in Foods   195
  Protein Quality   196
  Measures of Protein Quality   197
  Protein Regulations for Food Labels   198
Health Effects and Recommended Intakes of Protein   199
  Protein-Energy Malnutrition   199
  Health Effects of Protein   202
  Recommended Intakes of Protein   203
  How to Calculate Recommended Protein Intakes   204
  Protein and Amino Acid Supplements   205
  HIGHLIGHT SIX: Vegetarian, Mediterranean, and
    Other Meat-Restricted Foodways   209

Chapter 7

Metabolism: Transformations and Interactions   218

Chemical Reactions in the Body   219
Breaking Down Nutrients for Energy   224
  Glucose   224
  Glycerol and Fatty Acids   229
  Amino Acids   231
  The Final Steps of Catabolism   234
The Body's Energy Budget   238
  The Economics of Feasting   239
  The Transition from Feasting to Fasting   240
  The Economics of Fasting   240
  HIGHLIGHT SEVEN: Alcohol and Nutrition   245

Contents

Chapter 8

Energy Balance and Body Composition   256

Energy Balance   257
Energy In: The kCalories in Food   258
  Food Composition   258
  Food Intake   258
Energy Out: The kCalories the Body Spends   261
  Components of Energy Expenditure   262
  Estimating Energy Requirements   265
Body Weight, Body Composition, and Health   266
  How to Estimate Energy Output   267
  Defining Healthy Body Weight   268
  Body Weight and Its Standards   268
  Body Fat and Its Distribution   271
  Health Risks Associated with Body Weight and
    Body Fat   274
HIGHLIGHT EIGHT: Fitness: Physical Activity and
    Nutrition   278

Chapter 9

**Weight Control: Overweight and
    Underweight**   287

Causes of Obesity   288
  Fat Cell Development   288
  Genetics   289
  Fat Cell Metabolism   290
  Set-Point Theory   291
  Overeating   291
  Inactivity   291
Controversies in Obesity Treatment   292
Treatments of Obesity: Poor Choices   294
  Dangers of Weight Loss   294
  Pills, Procedures, and Other Possibilities   295
  *How to Identify Unsound Weight-Loss Schemes
    and Diets*   296
  Very-Low-kCalorie Diets   299
Treatments of Obesity: Good Choices   301
  Eating Plans   301
  Physical Activity   303
  Behavior and Attitude   305
  *How to Apply Behavior-Modification Strategies to
    Weight Loss*   308
Underweight   308
Problems of Underweight   309
Weight-Gain Strategies   310
HIGHLIGHT NINE: Eating Disorders—Anorexia
    Nervosa and Bulimia Nervosa   315

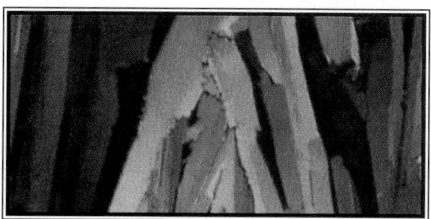

Chapter 10

**The Water-Soluble Vitamins: B Vitamins and
    Vitamin C**   325

The Vitamins—An Overview   326
The B Vitamins—As Individuals   328
  Thiamin   329
  Riboflavin   330
  How to Look to Foods for Single Nutrients   331
  Niacin   334
  How to Determine Niacin Intake   337
  Biotin   337
  Pantothenic Acid   339
  Vitamin B_6 340
  Folate   342
  How to Understand Dose Levels and Effects   343
  Vitamin B_{12} 347
  Vitamin Impostors   350
The B Vitamins–In Concert   352
  B Vitamin Interactions   354
  B Vitamin Deficiencies   354
  How to Distinguish Symptoms and Causes   355
  B Vitamin Toxicities   356
  B Vitamin Food Sources   356
Vitamin C   356
  Vitamin C Roles   357
  Vitamin C Recommendations   359
  Vitamin C Deficiency   359
  Vitamin C Toxicity   361
  Vitamin C Food Sources   362
HIGHLIGHT TEN: Vitamin and Mineral
    Supplements   366

Contents

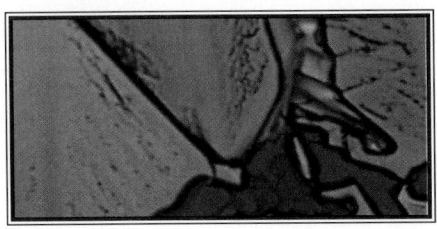

Chapter 11

The Fat-Soluble Vitamins: A, D, E, and K   374

Vitamin A and Beta-Carotene   375
 Roles in the Body   375
 Vitamin A Recommendations   380
 Vitamin A Deficiency   380
 Vitamin A Toxicity   383
 Vitamin A in Foods   384
Vitamin D   387
 Roles in the Body   387
 Vitamin D Deficiency   388
 Vitamin D Toxicity   388
 Vitamin D Recommendations and Sources   390
Vitamin E   391
 Vitamin E as an Antioxidant   391
 Vitamin E Deficiency   393
 Vitamin E Toxicity   393
 Vitamin E Recommendations   393
 Vitamin E in Foods   394
Vitamin K   394
 Vitamin K Deficiency   396
 Vitamin K Toxicity   396
 Vitamin K Recommendations and Sources   397
The Fat-Soluble Vitamins—In Summary   397
 HIGHLIGHT ELEVEN: Antioxidant Nutrients
  and Nonnutrients in Disease Prevention   400

Chapter 12

Water and the Major Minerals   408

Water and the Body Fluids   409
 Water Balance and Recommended Intakes   409
 Blood Volume and Blood Pressure   411
 Fluid and Electrolyte Balance   412
 Fluid and Electrolyte Imbalance   415
 Acid-Base Balance   416

The Minerals—An Overview   418
Sodium   419
 How to Cut Salt Intake   421
Chloride   423
Potassium   424
Calcium   426
 Calcium Roles in the Body   427
 Calcium Recommendations and Intakes   429
 Calcium Deficiency   432
Phosphorus   433
Magnesium   434
Sulfur   435
 HIGHLIGHT TWELVE: Osteoporosis and Calcium   439

Chapter 13

The Trace Minerals   449

The Trace Minerals—An Overview   450
Iron   451
 Iron Roles in the Body   451
 Iron Absorption and Metabolism   452
 How to Calculate Iron Absorbed from Meals   454
 Iron Deficiency   455
 Iron Toxicity   459
 Iron Recommendations and Intakes   460
 How to Estimate the Recommended Daily Intake
  of Iron   461
 Contamination and Supplemental Iron   461
Zinc   463
 Zinc Roles in the Body   463
 Zinc Absorption and Metabolism   464
 Zinc Deficiency   466
 Zinc Toxicity   466
 Zinc Recommendations and Intakes   468
 Contamination and Supplemental Zinc   468
Iodine   468
Selenium   471
Copper   472
Manganese   473
Fluoride   474
Chromium   475
Molybdenum   476
Other Trace Minerals   476
Closing Thoughts on the Nutrients   477
 HIGHLIGHT THIRTEEN: Our Children's Daily
  Lead   480

Contents

Chapter 14

Consumer Concerns about Foods 485

Food-Borne Illnesses 487
  Food-Borne Infections and Food Intoxications 487
  Food Hazards in the Marketplace 487
  How to Prevent Food-Borne Illnesses 490
  Food Safety in the Kitchen 492
  How to Achieve Food Safety while Traveling 494
Nutritional Adequacy of Foods and Diets 495
Environmental Contaminants 495
  Harmfulness of Environmental Contaminants 495
  Examples of Environmental Contaminants 495
Natural Toxicants in Foods 498
Pesticides 499
  How to Prepare Foods to Minimize Pesticide Residues 502
Food Additives 503
  Regulations Governing Additivies 503
  Intentional Food Additives 505
  Indirect Food Additives 507
  Hormones 509
  Radiation 510
  Food Biotechnology 511
  HIGHLIGHT FOURTEEN: Consumer Concerns about Public Water 515

Chapter 15

The Nutrition Care Process: Assessing Historical and Physical Data 518

The Nutrition Care Process 519
Assessing Nutrition Status 520
Historical Information 520
  Health History 522
  How to Conduct Successful Interviews 522
  Drug History 525
  Socioeconomic History 530
  Diet History 531
Physical Examinations 536
  HIGHLIGHT FIFTEEN: Diet and Health 539

Chapter 16

The Nutrition Care Process: Assessing Anthropometric and Biochemical Data 543

Anthropometric Measurements 544
  Measures of Growth and Development 544
  How to Quickly Estimate Ideal Body Weight 547
  Measures of Body Fat and Lean Tissue 548
  How to Estimate %IBW and %UBW 549
  Functional Measures of Nutrition Status 550
Biochemical Analyses 550
  Limitations of Biochemical Tests 551
  Biochemical Tests of Protein Status 551
  How to Calculate Total Lymphocyte Count 554
Nutrition Screening 555
  HIGHLIGHT SIXTEEN: Nutrition and Diagnostic Tests 559

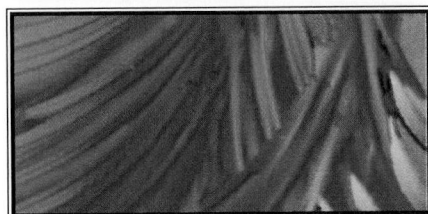

Chapter 17

The Nutrition Care Process: Developing a Nutrition Care Plan 561

Analyzing Assessment Data 562
  Nutrient Needs 562
  Nutrition Education Needs 562
The Nutrition Care Plan 563
  Implementing the Nutrition Care Plan 563
  Evaluating the Nutrition Care Plan 565
Medical Nutrition Therapy 565
Diet Planning 567
  Exchange Lists 570
  Diet Prescriptions Using Exchanges 572
Nutrition Education 575
Professional Communications 578
  Medical Records 578
  Other Communication Channels 579
  HIGHLIGHT SEVENTEEN: The Team Approach 581

Contents

Chapter 18

Life Cycle Nutrition: Pregnancy and Lactation 584

Growth and Development during Pregnancy 585
  Placental Development 585
  Fetal Growth and Development 585
  Critical Periods 586
Maternal Weight 588
  Weight for Height prior to Conception 588
  Weight Gain and Exercise during Pregnancy 589
Nutrition during Pregnancy 591
  Energy and Nutrient Needs during Pregnancy 591
  Common Nutrition-Related Concerns of
    Pregnancy 595
High-Risk and Low-Risk Pregnancies 596
  Malnutrition and Pregnancy 597
  Food Assistance Programs for Pregnant Women, Infants,
    and Children 597
  The Infant's Birthweight 598
  The Mother's Health Status 598
  Pregnancy in Adolescence 600
  Pregnancy in Older Women 601
  Fetal Alcohol Syndrome 604
  Other Practices Incompatible with Pregnancy 604
Nutrition during Lactation 606
  Breastfeeding: A Learned Behavior 606
  The Mother's Nutrient Needs 607
  Concerns of Breastfeeding Mothers 608
  HIGHLIGHT EIGHTEEN: Hunger and Global
    Environmental Problems 614

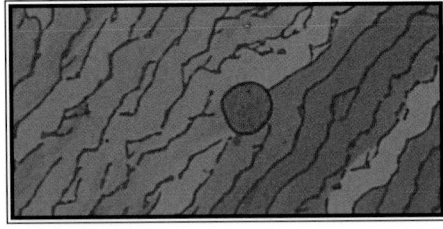

Chapter 19

Life Cycle Nutrition: Infancy, Childhood, and Adolescence 625

Nutrition during Infancy 626
  Energy and Nutrient Needs 626
  Breast Milk versus Infant Formula 627
  Breast Milk 629
  Infant Formula 631
  Special Needs of Preterm Infants 633
  Introducing First Foods 634
  Mealtimes with Infants 637
Nutrition during Childhood 638
  Energy and Nutrient Needs 638
  Hunger and Malnutrition in Children 640
  Nutrition, Hyperactivity, and "Hyper" Behavior 642
  Television and Children's Nutrition 644
  Adverse Reactions to Foods 644
  Mealtimes at Home 645
  Nutrition at School 648
  Food Assistance Programs for Children 649
Nutrition during Adolescence 650
  Growth and Development 650
  Energy and Nutrient Needs 651
  Food Choices and Health Habits 652
  Problems Adolescents Face 652
  HIGHLIGHT NINETEEN: Childhood Obesity and the
    Early Development of Chronic Diseases 658

Chapter 20

Life Cycle Nutrition: The Later Years 665

Nutrition and Longevity 666
  Observation of Elderly People 667
  Manipulation of Diet 667
The Aging Process 668
  Physiological Changes 669
  Other Changes 670
Nutrient Needs of Older Adults 671
  Water 671
  Energy Needs and Activity 671
  Vitamins and Minerals 673
  Supplements for Older Adults 675
Special Concerns of Older Adults 676
  Cataracts and Arthritis 676
  The Aging Brain 678
Food Choices and Eating Habits of Older Adults 681
  Nutrition Programs 681
  Meals for Singles 681
  Food Assistance Programs for Older Adults 683
  HIGHLIGHT TWENTY: Alternative Therapies 688

Contents

Chapter 21

Nutrition and Disorders of the Upper GI Tract   694

Disorders of the Mouth and Esophagus   695
 Difficulties Chewing   696
 Dysphagia   697
 How to Improve Acceptance of Pureed Diets   698
Disorders of the Stomach   699
 Indigestion and Reflux Esophagitis   699
 Nausea and Vomiting   702
 How to Prevent and Treat Reflux Esophagitis   702
 Gastritis   704
 How to Minimize Nausea   704
 Ulcers   705
 Gastric Surgery   706
 How to Adjust Meals to Prevent Dumping Syndrome   708
 HIGHLIGHT TWENTY-ONE: Living with Feeding Disabilities   716

Chapter 22

Nutrition and Disorders of the Lower GI Tract   722

Severe Diarrhea and Irritable Bowel Syndrome   724
 Diarrhea   724
 Irritable Bowel Syndrome   725
Nutrition Consequences of Malabsorption   727
 Fat Malabsorption   727
 How to Lessen the Symptoms of Irritable Bowel Syndrome   727
 Treatments for Fat Malabsorption   728
Malabsorption Syndromes   731
 Pancreatitis   731
 How to Improve Acceptance of Fat-Restricted Diets   731
 Cystic Fibrosis   733
 Crohn's Disease   736
 Malabsorption Caused by Bacterial Overgrowth   738
 Short-Bowel Syndrome   739
 Celiac Disease   741
Disorders of the Large Intestine   742
 Diverticular Disease of the Colon   742
 Ulcerative Colitis   744
 Resections of the Large Intestine   745

 HIGHLIGHT TWENTY-TWO: Promoting Intestinal Adaptation   752

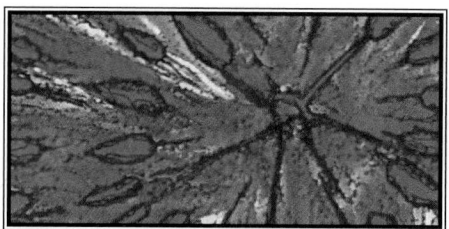

Chapter 23

Enteral Nutrition   755

Enteral Formulas   756
 How to Help Clients Meet Nutrient Needs with Ordinary Foods   757
 Types of Formulas   758
 Distinguishing Characteristics   758
 Formula Selection   760
 Enteral Formulas Provided Orally   761
 Tube Feedings   761
 How to Help Clients Accept Oral Formulas   762
 Feeding Tube Placement   763
 How to Help Clients Cope with Tube Feedings   766
 Formula Preparation   767
 Formula Administration   767
 Drug Administration through Feeding Tubes   769
 How to Plan a Tube-Feeding Schedule   769
Addressing Tube-Feeding Complications   771
 Failure to Achieve or Maintain Adequate Nutrition Status   771
 Diarrhea   774
 What to Chart   775
From Tube Feedings to Table Foods   775
 HIGHLIGHT TWENTY-THREE: Enteral Formulas: Who's Minding the Market?   779

Chapter 24

Parenteral Nutrition   782

Intravenous Nutrition   783
 Intravenous Solutions   783
 Types of Intravenous Feeding   784

Contents

How to Calculate the Nutrient Content of IV Solutions 785

Intravenous Nutrition Techniques 788
Insertion and Care of the Catheter 788
Administration of the TPN Solution 789
From Parenteral to Enteral Feedings 791
Specialized Nutrition Support at Home 793
The Basics of Home Programs 793
Home Enteral Nutrition 794
Home Parenteral Nutrition 794
HIGHLIGHT TWENTY-FOUR: Ethical Issues in Nutrition Care 797

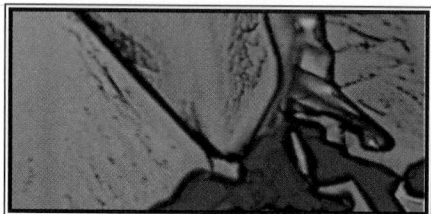

Chapter 25

Nutrition and Severe Stress   803

The Body's Response to Stress 804
Metabolic Responses to Severe Stress 804
Effects on Nutrition Status 807
Effects on GI Tract Immune Function 808
Secondary Effects of Stress and Illness on Nutrition Status 810
Nutrition Support during Stress 811
Nutrient Needs 811
How to Estimate Energy and Protein Needs Following Severe Stress 814
Delivering Nutrients during Stress 816
HIGHLIGHT TWENTY-FIVE: Food and Foodservice in the Hospital 820

Chapter 26

Nutrition and Disorders of the Liver and Biliary Tract   825

Fatty Liver and Hepatitis 827
Fatty Liver 827
Hepatitis 827
Cirrhosis 828
Consequences of Cirrhosis 829
Treatment of Cirrhosis 830
How to Adjust Diets for Liver Disease 831
Liver Transplantation 834
HIGHLIGHT TWENTY-SIX: Inborn Errors of Metabolism 839

Chapter 27

Nutrition, Diabetes, and Hypoglycemia   845

Diabetes Mellitus 846
Overview of Diabetes 846
Acute Complications of Diabetes 848
Chronic Complications of Diabetes 850
Screening for Diabetes 851
Treatment of Insulin-Dependent Diabetes Mellitus (IDDM) 851
Diet in IDDM 852
How to Plan a Diet for Diabetes using Exchange Lists 855
Physical Activity 856
Insulin and Insulin Analogs 858
Mastering Glucose Control 861
Managing Hyperglycemia 862
Managing Hypoglycemia 864
Children with Diabetes 865
Treatment of Noninsulin-Dependent Diabetes Mellitus (NIDDM) 865
Diet in NIDDM 866
Drug Therapy in NIDDM 867
Diabetes in Pregnancy and Later Life 868
Diabetes Management in Pregnancy 868
Diabetes Management in Later Life 870
Hypoglycemia 871
Reactive Hypoglycemia 871
Fasting Hypoglycemia 872
HIGHLIGHT TWENTY-SEVEN: Living with Diabetes 877

Chapter 28

Nutrition and Disorders of the Blood Vessels, Heart, and Lungs   881

Atherosclerosis 883
Consequences of Atherosclerosis 883
Risk Factors for CHD 883
How to Assess Your Heart Disease Risk 886

Contents

Prevention and Treatment of Atherosclerosis   887
Hypertension   889
Blood Pressure Regulation and Hypertension   890
Treatment of Hypertension   892
Heart Attacks, Heart Failure, and Strokes   894
Heart Attacks   894
Congestive Heart Failure   895
How to Manage Diets after a Myocardial Infarction (MI)   895
Strokes   897
How to Manage Diets for Congestive Heart Failure (CHF)   897
Disorders of the Lungs   898
Acute Respiratory Failure   898
Chronic Obstructive Pulmonary Disease (COPD)   900
HIGHLIGHT TWENTY-EIGHT: Diet and Protection against CHD   905

Chapter 29

Nutrition and Disorders of the Kidneys   909

The Nephrotic Syndrome   910
Consequences of Nephrotic Syndrome   911
Treatment of Nephrotic Syndrome   912
Acute Renal Failure   913
Consequences of Acute Renal Failure   914
How to Modify the Diet for Nephrotic Syndrome   914
Treatment of Acute Renal Failure   915
Chronic Renal Failure   916
Consequences of Chronic Renal Failure   917
Treatment of Chronic Renal Failure   920
How to Help Clients Comply with a Renal Diet   924
Kidney Transplants and Diet   925
HIGHLIGHT TWENTY-NINE: Kidney Stones—Treatments and Prevention   930

Chapter 30

Nutrition and Wasting Disorders: Cancer and HIV Infections   933

Cancer   934
How Cancer Develops   934
Dietary Guidelines to Reduce Cancer Risks   937
Nutrition Consequences of Cancer   938
Treatments for Cancer   940

Nutrition Support for People with Cancer   943
How to Help Clients Handle Food-Related Problems   946
Human Immunodeficiency Virus (HIV) Infection and Acquired Immune Deficiency Syndrome (AIDS)   948
How AIDS Develops   949
Treatments for HIV Infection   950
The HIV Wasting Syndrome   950
Nutrition Support for People with HIV Infection   953
HIGHLIGHT THIRTY: Cost-Conscious Health Care   959

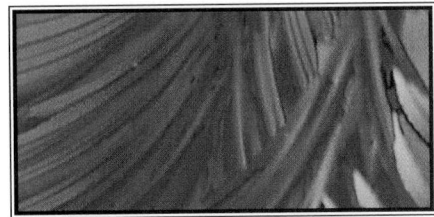

Appendixes

A   Cells, Hormones, and Nerves

B   Basic Chemistry Concepts

C   Biochemical Structures and Pathways

D   Aids to Calculation

E   Nutrition Assessment: Supplemental Information

F   Nutrition Resources

G   United States: Recommendations and Exchanges

World Health Organization: Recommendations

H   Table of Food Composition

I   Canada: Recommendations, Choices, and Labels

J   Measures of Protein Quality

K   Enteral Formulas

Contents

Glossary

Index

Recommended Dietary Allowances	*inside front cover, left*
Daily Values for Food Labels	*inside front cover, right*
Body Mass Index Tables	*inside back covers*

How-To Boxes

How to Think Metric 6–7
How to Calculate the Energy Available From Foods 8
How to Find Credible Sources of Nutrition Information 35
How to Calculate Personal Daily Values 57
How to Lower Fat Intake—by Food Group 168
How to Calculate a Personal Daily Value for Fat 172
How to Calculate Recommended Protein Intakes 204
How to Estimate Energy Output 267
How to Identify Unsound Weight-Loss Schemes and Diets 296
How to Apply Behavior-Modification Strategies to Weight Loss 308
How to Look to Foods for Single Nutrients 331
How to Determine Niacin Intake 337
How to Understand Dose Levels and Effects 343
How to Distinguish Symptoms and Causes 355
How to Cut Salt Intake 421
How to Calculate Iron Absorbed from Meals 454
How to Estimate the Recommended Daily Intake for Iron 461
How to Prevent Food-Borne Illnesses 490–491
How to Achieve Food Safety while Traveling 494
How to Prepare Foods to Minimize Pesticide Residues 502
How to Conduct Successful Interviews 522–523
How to Quickly Estimate Ideal Body Weight 547
How to Estimate %IBW and %UBW 549

How to Calculate the Total Lymphocyte Count 554
How to Identify Food Insecurity in a U.S. Household 615
How to Improve Acceptance of Pureed Diets 698
How to Prevent and Treat Reflux Esophagitis 702
How to Minimize Nausea 704
How to Adjust Meals to Prevent Dumping Syndrome 708
How to Lessen the Symptoms of Irritable Bowel Syndrome 727
How to Improve Acceptance of Fat-Restricted Diets 731
How to Help Clients Meet Nutrient Needs with Ordinary Foods 757
How to Help Clients Accept Oral Formulas 762
How to Help Clients Cope with Tube Feedings 766
How to Plan a Tube-Feeding Schedule 769
How to Calculate the Nutrient Content of IV Solutions 785
How to Estimate Energy and Protein Needs Following Severe Stress 814
How to Adjust Diets for Liver Disease 831
How to Plan a Diet for Diabetes Using Exchange Lists 855–856
How to Assess Your Heart Disease Risk 886
How to Manage Diets after a Myocardial Infarction (MI) 895
How to Manage Diets for Congestive Heart Failure (CHF) 897
How to Modify the Diet for Nephrotic Syndrome 914
How to Help Clients Comply with a Renal Diet 924
How to Help Clients Handle Food-Related Problems 946–947

Case Studies

Nutrition Assessment of a Computer Scientist Following a Car Accident 557
Computer Scientist with Car Accident Injuries 566
Accountant with Reflux Esophagitis 703
Commercial Artist Requiring Gastric Surgery 711
Homemaker with Pancreatitis 734
Child with Cystic Fibrosis 736
College Student with Crohn's Disease 738
Retired Schoolteacher with Diverticular Disease 745
Accountant with an Ileostomy 747

Graphics Designer Requiring Enteral Nutrition 777
Mail Carrier Requiring Parenteral Nutrition 793
Journalist with a Third-Degree Burn 817
Carpenter with Cirrhosis 835
Child with IDDM 866
Truck Driver with NIDDM 869
History Professor with Cardiovascular Disease 898
Store Manager with Acute Renal Failure 917
Child with Chronic Renal Failure 926
Retired Newscaster with Cancer 949
Travel Agent with HIV Infection 955

The goal of this fifth edition of *Understanding Normal and Clinical Nutrition* is to reveal the fascination of the science of nutrition and share the fun and excitement of nutrition with the reader. This text seeks not only to provide facts, but also to show readers how to apply these facts to their daily lives and to clinical practice. Every chapter has been substantially revised to reflect the many changes that have occurred in the field of nutrition and dietetics over the years.

This book presents the core information of an introductory nutrition course. Chapter 1 wastes no time in exploring why we eat the foods we do and continues with a brief overview of the nutrients, the science of nutrition, recommended nutrient intakes, assessment, and important relationships between diet and health. Chapter 2 describes diet-planning principles and food guides used to create diets that support good health and includes instructions on how to read a food label. In Chapter 3 readers follow the journey of digestion and absorption as the body transforms foods into nutrients. Chapters 4 through 6 describe carbohydrates, fats, and proteins—their chemistry, health effects, roles in the body, and places in the diet. Then Chapter 7 shows how the body derives energy from these three energy nutrients. Chapters 8 and 9 continue the story with a look at energy balance, the factors associated with overweight and underweight, and the benefits and dangers of weight loss and weight gain. Chapters 10 through 13 then describe the vitamins, the minerals, and water—their roles in the body, deficiency and toxicity symptoms, and sources. Chapter 14 completes the introductory lessons by addressing consumer concerns about the safety of the food and water supply.

The next three chapters weave the basic information into practical applications, describing ways health care professionals assess clients' nutrition status and then use this information to make plans for a client's nutrition care. Chapter 15 focuses on how health care professionals use information from clients' health, drug, socioeconomic, and diet histories and physical findings to help pinpoint nutrition problems. Chapter 16 then examines how anthropometric data and biochemical tests help complete the assessment process. Chapter 17 shows how health care professionals integrate assessment data into a plan that meets the client's nutrient and nutrition education needs.

The text continues with emphasis on conditions that alter nutrient needs. Chapters 18, 19, and 20 present the special needs of people throughout the life cycle: pregnancy and lactation; infancy, childhood, and adolescence; and the later years. The remaining chapters explore how diseases, their symptoms, and their treatments influence nutrient needs and how meeting those needs then affects recovery. The path of exploration follows the course that foods take as they are ingested, digested, metabolized, distributed, and excreted by the body. Thus Chapters 21 and 22 examine the upper and lower GI tract, and Chapters 23 and 24 describe special ways of feeding people who cannot eat conventional foods. Chapters 25 through 27 delve into disorders whose primary effects are on metabolism—severe stresses, liver disorders, and diabetes and hypoglycemia.

Chapter 28 looks at disorders of the heart and blood vessels, which affect the distribution of nutrients, and disorders of the lungs, which affect the distribution of oxygen to the cells that need it to make energy to fuel the body. Chapter 29 describes kidney disorders, which affect the excretion of nutrients. Finally, Chapter 30 examines cancer and HIV infections—disorders that often lead to wasting and have multiple effects on nutrition status.

To the person reading this text, it will be obvious that, like most sciences, nutrition possesses no absolute certainties. Nutrition scientists simply do not have all the answers; in some cases, we have not even asked all the questions. This is true in virtually all areas of nutrition; it is a young, growing science dating only from around the turn of the century. One of the missions of this text, beginning in Chapter 1, is to show readers how to ascertain the "facts"—a skill vital to developing sound clinical judgment.

Since the last edition of this text, the number of websites on the Internet has grown exponentially. The Internet offers endless opportunities to obtain high-quality information. Unfortunately, it also delivers an abundance of incomplete, misleading, or inaccurate information. Simply put: anyone can publish anything. To distinguish a credible and helpful source from all the others, users must adopt standards similar to those used for printed publications. They must consider whether the author's educational degrees, credentials, and affiliations qualify him or her to speak authoritatively on nutrition. They also need to determine whether the information is based on valid scientific research and note whether credible references are provided. Highlight 1 examines these issues in greater detail. To explore several credible nutrition websites on the Internet, start with a visit to our website:

http://www.wadsworth.com/nutrition

Highlights on current issues of interest alternate with the chapters. Each highlight provides readers with a brief look at a topic that relates to the companion chapter. New highlights in this edition explore healthy ethnic cuisines (including the Mediterranean diet), the roles of antioxidant nutrients and nonnutrients in disease prevention, nutrition and diagnostic tests, childhood obesity and its influence on the early development of chronic diseases, alternative therapies, foodservice in hospitals, and possible diet-related risk factors for atherosclerosis. The highlights on living with diabetes and cost-conscious health care have been significantly revised.

The appendixes are valuable references. Appendix A summarizes background information on the hormonal and nervous systems, complementing Appendixes B and C on basic chemistry, the chemical structures of nutrients, and the major metabolic pathways. Appendix D assists readers with calculations and conversions, and Appendix E provides additional information regarding nutrition assessments. Appendix F lists book and journal recommendations and addresses for many nutrition resources including dozens of Internet addresses. Appendix G presents the Recommended Dietary Allowances (1989 RDA), the nutrition-related priorities of Healthy People 2000, the United States Exchange System, and recommendations from the World Health Organization. Appendix H is a 2000-item food composition table created from the latest nutrient database assembled by ESHA Research, Inc., of Salem, Oregon. Appendix I presents detail. To explore several credible nutrition websites on the Internet, start with a visit to our website:

http://www.wadsworth.com/nutrition

We have tried to keep the number of notes to a minimum. Many statements that have appeared in previous editions with notes now appear without them, but every statement is backed by research, and the authors will supply references upon request. We have not provided a separate list of suggested readings, but have tried to include references that will provide readers with additional details or a good overview of the subject.

Preview of Text Elements

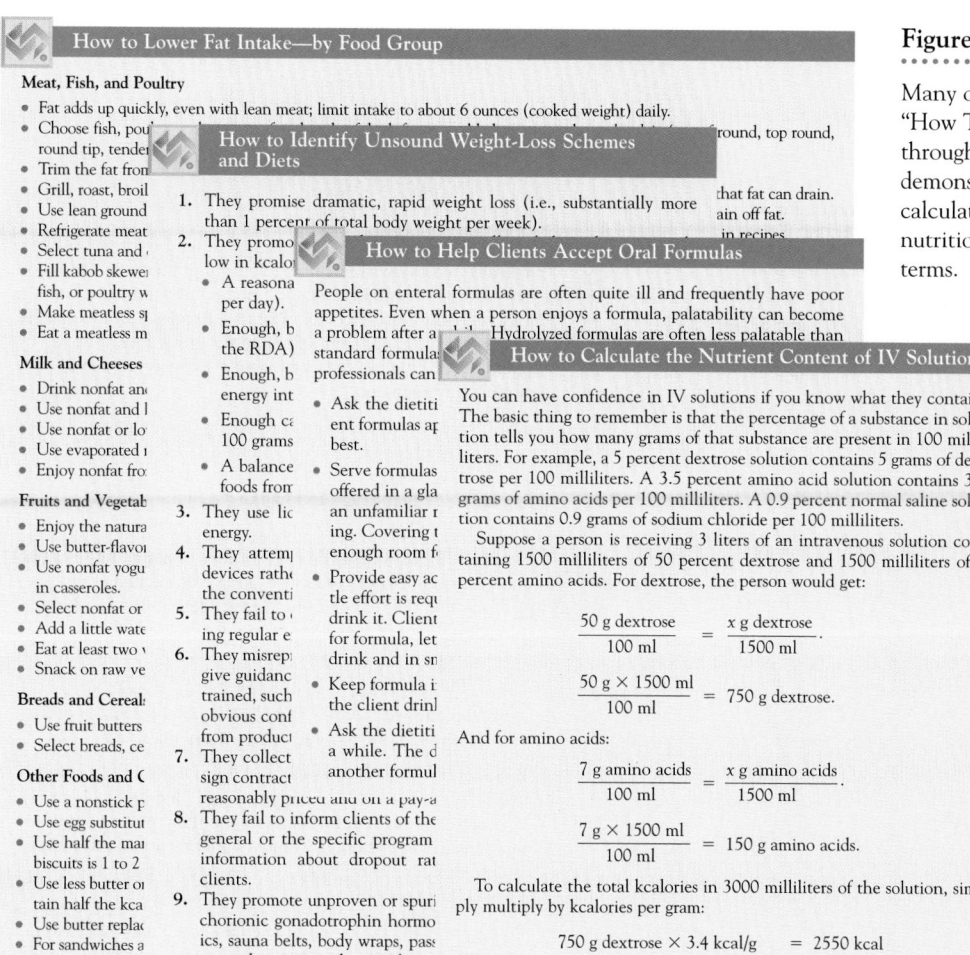

Figure A   How-To Boxes

Many of the chapters in this edition include "How To" skill boxes that guide readers through problem-solving tasks. These boxes demonstrate how to perform mathematical calculations or how to apply nutrition or nutrition-related information in practical terms.

Figure B Summary Paragraphs

New to this edition are summary paragraphs, marked with a thin blue bar in the margin. These paragraphs review the contents of the previous sections; in some chapters, such as those covering the vitamins and minerals, summaries appear in tables.

In summary, scientists learn about nutrition by conducting experiments that follow the protocol of scientific research. Researchers take care to establish similar control and experimental groups, large sample sizes, placebos, and blind treatments. Their findings must be reviewed and replicated by other scientists before being accepted as valid. These are a few of the characteristics of research that is well designed to study the actions of nutrients in the body. Such research has laid the foundation for quantifying how much of each nutrient the body needs.

Figure C Healthy People 2000

The early chapters of this edition present Healthy People 2000 nutrition-related priorities wherever their subjects are discussed (Appendix G presents them in full). Healthy People 2000 is a report developed by the U.S. Department of Health and Human Services that establishes national objectives in health promotion and disease prevention for the year 2000.

 HEALTHY PEOPLE 2000: Reduce overweight to a prevalence of no more than 20% among people aged 20 years and older and maintain prevalence at no more than 15% among adolescents aged 12 and 19 years.

Causes of Obesity

Excess body fat accumulates when people consistently take in more food energy than they spend. Why do they do this? Is it genetic? Environmental? Cultural? Behavioral? Socioeconomic? Psychological? Metabolic? All of these? Most likely, obesity has many interrelated causes; some experts in the field speak of many different *obesities*. Why an imbalance between energy intake and energy expenditure occurs is unclear; the next sections summarize possible explanations.

Figure D Nutrition Assessment Checklists

New to Chapters 21 through 30 are the nutrition assessment checklists. The checklists help readers determine the impact of various disorders on nutrition status by highlighting the medical, drug, nutrient intake, anthropometric, laboratory, and physical findings that are particularly relevant to a specific group of clients.

✓ Nutrition Assessment Checklist
For People Receiving Tube Feedings

 Medical Review the client's medical record for the information necessary to select the appropriate feeding site (gastric versus intestinal), insertion procedure (transnasal or enterostomy), and formula. The development of undesirable symptoms associated with the client's medical condition, therapy (especially drug), or formula selection requires prompt intervention.

 Drug Review the client's drug therapy for possible drug-nutrient interactions and GI side effects that may affect the client's tolerance for the tube feeding. If the feeding tube is used to deliver drugs, follow the precautions on pp. 769–771.

 Nutrient Intake Ensure that formula is being delivered as prescribed, and take corrective actions as needed (see p. 774). For clients beginning to eat, determine the degree to which nutrient needs are being met by table foods or formula taken orally, and reduce the volume of the tube feeding accordingly.

 Anthropometric Assess the client's weight daily to make sure that the client is meeting nutrition goals.

 Laboratory Monitor serum and urine lab values for signs of fluid and electrolyte imbalances and glucose intolerance. Check serum protein levels to ensure that they are improving or being maintained. When available, assess nitrogen balance to determine if the tube feeding is meeting the client's protein needs.

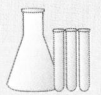 **Physical** Check gastric residual for signs of delayed gastric emptying to prevent GI complications and reduce the risk of aspiration. Check tube placement and gravity drip rate or infusion pump drip rate as needed (see Table 23–4). Assess blood pressure, temperature, pulse, and respiration every 4 hours. Look for physical signs of malnutrition or dehydration.

Study Questions

1. Which carbohydrates are described as simple, and which are complex?
2. Describe the structure of a monosaccharide and name the three monosaccharides important in nutrition. Name the three disaccharides commonly found in foods and their component monosaccharides. In what foods are these sugars found?
3. What happens in a condensation reaction? In a hydrolysis reaction?
4. Describe the structure of polysaccharides and name the ones important in nutrition. How are starch and glycogen similar, and how do they differ? How do the fibers differ from the other polysaccharides?
5. Describe carbohydrate digestion and absorption.

What role does fiber play in the process?
6. What are the possible fates of glucose in the body? What is the protein-sparing action of carbohydrate?
7. How does the body maintain blood glucose concentrations? What happens when it rises too high or falls too low?
8. What are the health effects of sugars? What are the dietary recommendations regarding concentrated sugar intakes?
9. What are the health effects of starches and fibers? What are the dietary recommendations regarding these complex carbohydrates?
10. What foods provide starches and fibers?

Figure E **Study Questions**

Each chapter closes with study questions. These offer readers the opportunity to review the major concepts presented in the chapter. Later chapters also include case studies and clinical applications.

Case Study   Truck Driver with NIDDM

Mr. Evans, a truck driver, was 52 years old when he was first diagnosed with NIDDM. He visited his physician after experiencing excessive thirst, excessive urination, and excessive appetite. Mr. Evans, who stands 5 feet 11 inches tall and currently weighs 200 pounds, experienced a 30-pound weight gain over the past two years. His fasting blood glucose is 235 milligrams per 100 milliliters. His fasting triglycerides and cholesterol are also elevated.

The diabetes health care team members have evaluated Mr. Evans's case. They are eager to help him achieve the first goal of diabetes management—to bring his blood glucose under control. The team has helped Mr. Evans plan a diet and physical activity program that considers the nature of his job and life on the road.

Mr. Evans is concerned about his health. He is worried that he may need insulin injections and overwhelmed by all the information presented to him over the past few days.

What are the differences between NIDDM and IDDM? Describe the factors in Mr. Evans's history that might have predisposed him to NIDDM. Can you explain to Mr. Evans why he will not need insulin injections at this time?

What will be the primary objective of the diet therapy for Mr. Evans? Determine Mr. Evans's desirable body weight, and describe two diet plans that might help him control both his blood glucose and his lipids. Select one of these diet plans and plan Mr. Evans's diet using the information in the box on pp. 855–856. Suggest some types of physical activities that might be appropriate for Mr. Evans. Remember that he travels frequently and needs a plan he can follow regularly. In what ways do diet and physical activity plans benefit clients with NIDDM?

What alternative treatments might Mr. Evans's physician consider if diet and physical activity fail to control his blood glucose?

Consider Mr. Evans's emotional health. How can the health care team help him during this difficult period?

Figure F **Case Studies**

Case studies guide readers in translating what they have learned about a disorder to a situation involving an actual client.

Clinical Applications

1. Using the box on pp. 855–856, plan a diet using the exchange lists for a sedentary woman with IDDM who is 5 feet 9 inches tall and weighs 160 pounds. Assume that the distribution of kcalories will be 55 percent from carbohydrate, 20 percent from protein, and 25 percent from fat. Round off kcalories to develop a sample diet pattern.
2. An important part of learning is being able to apply knowledge and guidelines to real-life situations. Using Table 27–5 as a guide, think about the possible remedies for either hyper- or hypoglycemia. Describe at least one situation when it might be preferable to alter the insulin dose and one situation when it might be preferable to alter the carbohydrate intake.
3. Take a trip to a pharmacy and price these items: blood glucose meter, test strips for the meter

selected, glucose test strips for use without a meter, lancets, insulin, and syringes. Determine the approximate cost of insulin injections for a person who uses 14 units of regular insulin and 26 units of NPH insulin daily (don't forget to include the cost of the syringes). Then estimate the cost of testing blood glucose four times daily. How does the cost of using a blood glucose meter compare to the cost of regular blood glucose test strips? How much do lancets add to the total daily cost? Consider how an external pump might affect the total cost of managing diabetes. How does the need for a balanced diet influence the cost of diabetes care? If intensive therapy requires more expenditures for insulin injections, blood glucose testing, and medical checkups than does traditional therapy, how might the added costs be justified?

Figure G **Clinical Applications**

Clinical applications may ask the reader to perform mathematical calculations, synthesize information from previous chapters, or demonstrate the impact of nutrition care on health care professionals or clients.

Figure H   Menus

Throughout these clinical nutrition discussions are sample menus and prescription pads. The sample menus show readers how the diet order translates into a typical day's meals.

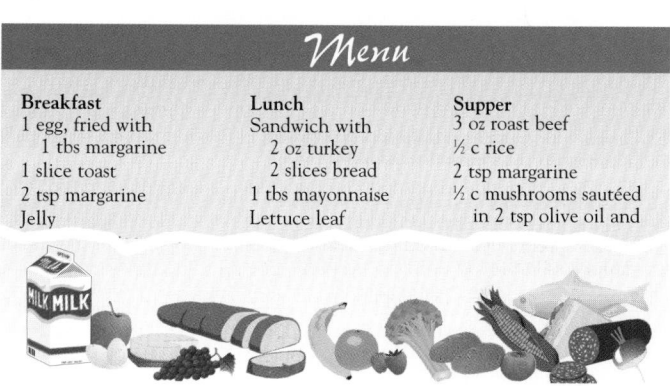

Menu

Breakfast
1 egg, fried with
   1 tbs margarine
1 slice toast
2 tsp margarine
Jelly

Lunch
Sandwich with
   2 oz turkey
   2 slices bread
1 tbs mayonnaise
Lettuce leaf

Supper
3 oz roast beef
½ c rice
2 tsp margarine
½ c mushrooms sautéed
   in 2 tsp olive oil and

Figure I   Prescription Pads

The prescription pads list the major classes of drugs used in the treatment of specific disorders and refer readers to a table in Appendix E that explains the timing of food intake with drug administration and lists common nutrition-related side effects.

Rx   PRESCRIPTION PAD

Drugs used in the treatment of cardiovascular disease may include:

- Anticoagulants (including aspirin)
- Antihypertensives
- Antilipemics
- Diuretics (isosorbide nitrate)
- Nitroglycerin (to ease angina)

See Appendix E for timing with meals and nutrition-related side effects.

What Is Available Along with the Textbook?

For the Student

DIET ANALYSIS PLUS SOFTWARE VERSION 3.0 (WINDOWS, DOS, OR MAC)

This software (based on award-winning ESHA Food Processor Software) calculates personal RDA or RNI (for Canadians) goal percentages for fats, carbohydrates and proteins. The software allows you to adjust for personal recommended kcaloric levels by factoring in exercises, and/or choosing a weight loss or weight gain plan. You may then compare your actual diet to these recommendations by entering the foods you eat for up to 7 days. A total of 4,000 foods are available via onscreen lookup, and up to 30 more foods (WIN and DOS versions only) may be added to personalize the database. See your results in spreadsheet and graphic formats. This is software that can be used for a lifetime.

NUTRITION INTERACTIVE CD-ROM

This CD-ROM includes animations, video, and interactive computer exercises which help to bring nutrition to life. For example, after having explored the workings of the digestive tract on the CD-ROM, you will be ready to test your knowledge of common GI problems by identifying their symptoms and preventive strategies. The 25 individual modules cover the body, metabolism, the energy nutrients, vitamins and minerals, fitness, diet choices, medical concerns, life span, health promotion and more.

STUDENT STUDY GUIDE

This study aid is designed to reinforce the key concepts that are presented in the text and to prepare students for exams. The study guide is three-hole punched and perforated, and makes a handy, easy-to-carry review tool!

The Student Study Guide contains:

Chapter Objectives define the essential concepts for each chapter.

Assignments provide study questions, terms to be defined, short answer questions, and problems to solve.

Sample Test Questions offer multiple-choice questions similar to questions instructors are likely to ask on exams.

Nursing Exam Review Questions (for chapters 15–17 and 21–30) review questions to help students prepare for the NCLEX-RN.

Discussions of Clinical Application Questions and Case Studies encourage students to apply knowledge gained from each chapter to hypothetical situations.

Answers to the chapter study questions, problems, and short-answer, sample test, and nursing exam review questions are found at the end of each chapter.

For the Instructor

- **ACETATE OVERHEADS** *or* **ELECTRONIC OVERHEADS*** include figures from the text along with enrichments from other sources.

- **SOFTWARE** includes Computerized Testing* and complimentary Diet Analysis Plus version 3.0 (Windows, DOS, or MAC). See "For the Student".

- **INSTRUCTOR'S MANUAL WITH TEST BANK**

- **CNN/WEST NUTRITION CHRONOLOG QUARTERLY*** (exclusive to West/Wadsworth) updates viewers four times per year on important issues in the nutrition field. Each video presents the best of CNN's broadcast coverage which ties into issues and concepts being explored in today's nutrition classrooms.

- **NUTRITION VIDEO LIBRARY*** includes selected videos on topics such as eating disorders, digestion, metabolism, and more!

- **NUTRITION RESOURCE CENTER** links you to other nutrition resources via www.wadsworth. com/nutrition

*Please check with your local ITP representative for qualification details.

Acknowledgments

To produce a book requires the coordinated efforts of a team of people—and, no doubt, each team member has another team of support people as well. We salute, with a big round of applause, everyone who has worked so diligently to ensure the quality of this book.

We thank Linda DeBruyne and Yvonne Jones for their valuable contributions to the fitness and hunger highlights, respectively, and Margaret Hedley for her assistance in keeping the Canadian information current. A million thank yous to Mary Ann Riveccio and Sally Mayo for their patient attention to manuscript preparation and a multitude of other daily tasks. Thanks also to Mary Ann Riveccio and Laura Perkinson for their help in securing permissions. We thank the many people who have prepared the ancillaries that accompany this text: Harry Sitren and Melaney Jones for writing and enhancing the Test Bank; Lori Turner, Melaney Jones, and Margaret Hedley for preparing the Instructor's Manual; and Lori Turner and Jana Kicklighter for preparing the Student Study Guide. A big thank you to Elizabeth Hands, Bob Geltz, and their staff at ESHA for their meticulous efforts in creating the food composition appendix, verifying the data in figures and tables, and developing the computerized data analysis program that accompanies this book. Our special thanks to the editorial team of Peter Marshall, Becky Tollerson, Jane Bass, Laura Perkinson, Sandra Craig, and Dusty Davidson for their conscientious coordination of reviews and production. We also thank John Woolsey and his associates for creating accurate and attractive artwork to complement our writing; Michael Davidson for transforming nutrients into outstanding works of art that grace the cover and chapter opening pages; Tom Harm and Tom Peterson for photographing foods beautifully; and Pat Lewis for copyediting thousands of pages of manuscript. To the many others involved in designing, indexing, typesetting, dummying, and marketing, we tip our hats in appreciation.

We are especially grateful to our associates, friends, and families for their continued encouragement and support. We also thank our many reviewers for their comments and contributions.

Reviewers of Understanding Normal and Clinical Nutrition

Sara Long Anderson,
Southern Illinois University at
Carbondale

Wayne Billon,
University of Southern Mississippi

M. Brian-Keber,
University of San Francisco

Eileen Monahan Chopnick,
Widener University School of
Nursing

Beth Clark,
University of Maine at Augusta

Colleen Duggan,
Johnson Community College

Carmen Edwards,
Midland College

Amelia C. Finan,
Anne Arundel Community College

Denise T. Garner,
York College of Pennsylvania

Judith Harr,
University of San Francisco

Irene Langille,
Southern Alberta Institute of
Technology

Dawna Torres Mughal,
Gannon University

Amy R. Pemberton,
Lamar University

Tonia Reinhard,
Wayne State University

Marilyn Tapia,
Montana State University at Billings

Connie B. Till,
Orangeburg-Calhoun Technical
College

We hope our informal, conversational writing style makes the study of nutrition an enjoyable experience. Nutrition is a fascinating subject, and we hope our enthusiasm for it comes through on every page.

Eleanor Noss Whitney
Corinne Balog Cataldo
Sharon Rady Rolfes
August 1997

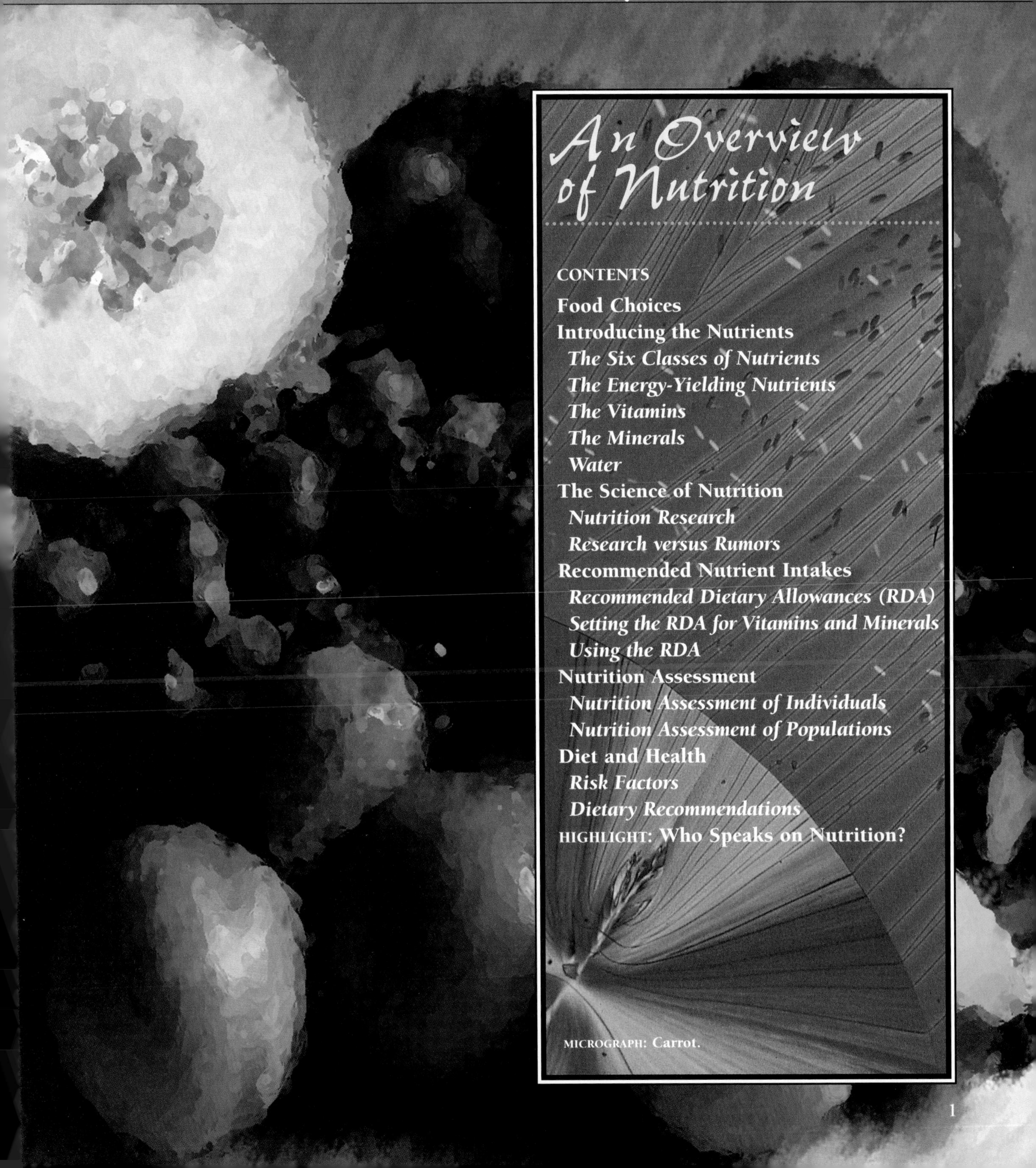

Chapter 1

An Overview of Nutrition

CONTENTS

Food Choices
Introducing the Nutrients
The Six Classes of Nutrients
The Energy-Yielding Nutrients
The Vitamins
The Minerals
Water
The Science of Nutrition
Nutrition Research
Research versus Rumors
Recommended Nutrient Intakes
Recommended Dietary Allowances (RDA)
Setting the RDA for Vitamins and Minerals
Using the RDA
Nutrition Assessment
Nutrition Assessment of Individuals
Nutrition Assessment of Populations
Diet and Health
Risk Factors
Dietary Recommendations
HIGHLIGHT: **Who Speaks on Nutrition?**

MICROGRAPH: **Carrot.**

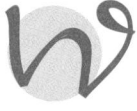elcome to the world of nutrition. Nutrition has played a significant role in your life, even from before your birth, although you may not always have been aware of it. And it will continue to affect you in major ways, depending on how you choose your foods.

Every day, several times a day, you make food choices that influence your body's health for better or worse. Each day's choices may benefit or harm your health only a little, but when these choices are repeated over years and decades, the rewards or consequences become major. That being the case, close attention to good nutrition now can bring health benefits later. Conversely, carelessness about nutrition from youth on can be a major contributor to many of today's most prevalent chronic diseases of later life, including heart disease and cancer. Of course, some people will become ill or die young no matter what choices they make, and others will live long lives despite making poor choices. For the large majority, however, the food choices they make each and every day will benefit or impair their health in proportion to the wisdom of those choices.

While most people realize that their food habits affect their health, they often choose foods for other reasons. After all, foods bring to the table a variety of pleasures, traditions, and associations as well as nourishment. The challenge, then, is to combine favorite foods and fun times with a nutritionally balanced diet.

In general, a **chronic** disease is one of long duration that progresses slowly. By comparison, an **acute** disease develops quickly, produces sharp symptoms, and runs a short course.

  acute = sharp
  chronos = time

diet: the foods and beverages a person eats and drinks.

Food Choices

People decide what to eat, when to eat, and even whether to eat in highly personal ways, often based on behavioral or social motives rather than on awareness of nutrition's importance to health. Fortunately, many different food choices can be healthy ones, but nutrition awareness helps to make them so.

Personal Preference   One reason people choose foods, of course, is that they like certain flavors. Two widely shared preferences are for the sweetness of sugar and the tang of salt. Other preferences might be for the hot peppers common in Mexican cooking or the curry spices of Indian cuisine. Some research suggests that genetics may influence people's food preferences.[1]

Habit   People sometimes select foods out of habit. They eat cereal every morning, for example, simply because they have always eaten cereal for breakfast. Eating a familiar food and not having to make any decisions can be comforting.

Ethnic Heritage or Tradition   Among the strongest influences on food choices are ethnic heritage and tradition. People eat the foods they grew up eating. Every country—and every region of a country—has its own typical foods and ways of combining foods into meals. Highlight 2 shows how people can make healthful food choices within their own ethnic cuisines.

Social Interactions   Food signifies friendliness. Meals are social events, and the sharing of food is part of hospitality. Social customs almost compel people to accept food or drink offered by a host or shared by a group. When your friends are going out for pizza or ice cream, how can you refuse to go along?

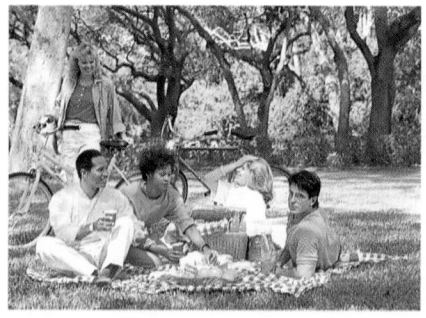

People enjoy companionship while eating.

Availability, Convenience, and Economy　People eat foods that are accessible, quick and easy to prepare, and within their financial means. Consumers today value convenience especially highly, as reflected in their choices of meals they can prepare quickly, recipes with few ingredients, and products they can cook in microwave ovens. Many people frequently eat out or have food delivered, which limits food choices to the selections on the restaurant's menu.

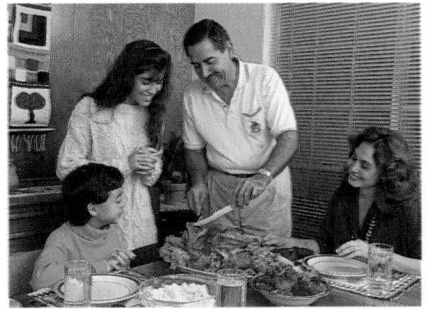

For many people, a special family dinner brings pleasant memories of the holidays.

Positive and Negative Associations　People tend to like foods with happy associations—such as hot dogs at ball games or turkey at Thanksgiving. By the same token, people can attach intense and unalterable dislikes to foods that they ate when they felt sick, or that were forced on them when they weren't hungry. Parents may teach their children to like and dislike certain foods by using those foods as rewards or punishments.

Sometimes foods are associated with certain uses.[2] For example, people may believe that peanut butter is for children, or that lobster is for the rich. Then, depending on whether they permit themselves to be childlike or to indulge in luxuries, they will choose to eat or refrain from eating those foods.

Emotional Comfort　Some people eat in response to emotional stimuli—for example, to relieve boredom or depression or to calm anxiety. A lonely person may choose to eat rather than to call a friend and risk rejection. A person who has returned home from an exciting evening out may unwind with a late-night snack. Eating in response to emotions can easily lead to overeating and obesity, but may be appropriate at times. For example, sharing food at times of bereavement serves both the giver's need to provide comfort and the receiver's need to be cared for and to interact with others, as well as to take nourishment.

Values　Food choices may reflect people's religious beliefs, political views, or environmental concerns. For example, many Christians forgo meat during Lent, the period prior to Easter, and Jewish law includes an extensive set of dietary rules. A political activist may boycott vegetables picked by migrant workers who have been exploited. People may buy vegetables from local farmers to save the fuel and environmental costs of foods shipped in from far away. Consumers may also select foods packaged in containers that can be reused or recycled.

Body Image　Sometimes men and women select certain foods and supplements that they believe will improve their physical appearances and avoid those they believe might be detrimental. Such decisions can be beneficial when based on sound nutrition and fitness knowledge, but undermine good health when based on faddism or carried to extremes.

Nutrition　Finally, of course, a valid reason to select certain foods is that they will benefit health. Nutritional and health values have become influential in many consumers' food choices, even when other forces are at work. A person may choose for social reasons to go out "for pizza" with friends, but once there, might eat only one slice with a large salad of fresh vegetables. Food manufacturers have responded to scientific findings linking health with nutrition by offering an abundant selection of health-promoting foods and beverages. Consumers welcome these new foods into their diets, provided that the foods are reasonably priced, clearly labeled, easy to find in the grocery store, and convenient to prepare. These foods must also taste good—as good as the traditional choices. Of course, a person need not eat any of these "special" foods to enjoy a healthy diet; ordinary foods, well chosen, serve just as well.

In summary, a person selects foods for a variety of reasons. Whatever those reasons may be, food choices influence health. Individual food selections neither make nor break a diet's healthfulness, but the balance of foods selected over time can make an important difference to health. For this reason, people are wise to allow nutrition knowledge to play a major role in their food decisions.

Introducing the Nutrients

Do you ever think of yourself as a collection of carefully arranged atoms, molecules, cells, tissues, and organs? Are you aware of the activity going on within your body even as you sit still? The atoms, molecules, and cells of your body continually move and change, even though the structures of your tissues and organs, and your external appearance, remain relatively constant.

Your skin, which seems to have covered you since your birth, is replaced entirely by new cells every seven years. The fat beneath your skin is not the same fat that was there a year ago. Your oldest red blood cell is only 120 days old, and the entire lining of your digestive tract is renewed every 3 days. To maintain your "self," you must continually replenish, from foods, the energy and the nutrients you deplete in maintaining your body.

THE SIX CLASSES OF NUTRIENTS

Amazingly, the body can derive all the energy, structural materials, and regulating agents that it needs from the foods we eat. The secret lies in the genetic information you inherited from your parents, which gives the instructions for assembling body structures from the nutrients in foods. As long as you give your body the energy and nutrients it needs in sufficient amounts, your genetic blueprints will direct that the pieces be put together and work according to the plan. This section introduces the nutrients that foods bring to the body and shows how they take part in the dynamic processes that keep people alive and well.

Composition of Foods   Chemical analysis of a food such as a tomato shows that it is composed primarily of water (95 percent). Most of the solid materials are the compounds carbohydrate, fat, and protein. If you could remove these materials, you would find a tiny residue of vitamins, minerals, and other compounds. Water, carbohydrate, fat, protein, vitamins, and some of the minerals found in foods are nutrients—substances the body uses for the growth, maintenance, and repair of its tissues. Other nutritionally important constituents of foods are the fibers—members of the carbohydrate family that also support good health.

Composition of the Body   A complete chemical analysis of your body would show that it is made of materials similar to those found in foods. A healthy 150-pound body contains about 90 pounds of water and about 30 pounds of fat. The

foods: products derived from plants or animals that can be taken into the body to yield nutrients for the maintenance of life and the growth and repair of tissues.

nutrients: substances obtained from food and used in the body to provide energy and structural materials and to regulate growth, maintenance, and repair of the body's tissues; nutrients may also reduce the risks of some chronic diseases.

The six classes of nutrients:
- Carbohydrate.
- Fat.
- Protein.
- Vitamins.
- Minerals.
- Water.

The human body, like foods, is composed largely of nutrients.

other 30 pounds are mostly compounds containing protein and carbohydrate and the major minerals of the bones. Vitamins, other minerals, and incidental extras constitute a fraction of a pound.

Chemical Composition of Nutrients   The simplest of the nutrients are the minerals. Each mineral is a chemical element, which means that its atoms are all alike. As a result, its identity never changes. Iron, for example, remains iron when a food is cooked, when a person eats the food, when iron becomes part of a red blood cell, when the cell is broken down, and when the iron is lost from the body by excretion. The next simplest nutrient is water, a compound made of two elements—hydrogen and oxygen. Minerals and water are inorganic nutrients—they contain no carbon.

The other four classes of nutrients (carbohydrate, fat, protein, and vitamins) are more complex. In addition to hydrogen and oxygen, they all contain carbon, an element that is found in all living things. They are therefore called organic compounds (meaning, literally, "alive"). Protein and some vitamins also contain nitrogen and may contain other elements as well (see Figure 1–1).

Essential Nutrients   The body can make some nutrients for itself. The body cannot make all the nutrients, however: some, it cannot make at all; and some, it makes in insufficient quantities to meet its needs. It must obtain these nutrients from foods. The nutrients that foods must supply are *essential nutrients*. When used to refer to nutrients, then, the word *essential* means more than just "necessary"; it means "needed from outside the body"—normally, from foods.

This book focuses mostly on the nutrients, but other constituents also occur in foods and in the body—alcohols, organic acids, pigments, additives, and others. Some are beneficial, some are neutral, and a few are harmful. Later sections of the book touch on these nonnutrients and their significance.

---

*This definition excludes coal, diamonds, and a few carbon-containing compounds that contain only a single carbon and no hydrogen, such as carbon dioxide (CO_2), calcium carbonate ($CaCO_3$), magnesium carbonate ($MgCO_3$), and sodium cyanide (NaCN).

element: a substance composed of atoms that are alike—for example, iron (Fe).

atom: the smallest component of an element that has all of the properties of the element.

compound: a substance composed of two or more different atoms—for example, water (H_2O).

inorganic: not containing carbon or pertaining to living things.
  in = not

organic: a substance or molecule containing carbon-carbon bonds or carbon-hydrogen bonds.* Some farmers call their produce "organic" if it was grown without manufactured fertilizers and pesticides, but by the definition given here, all foods are organic.

molecule: two or more atoms of the same or different elements joined by chemical bonds. Examples are molecules of the element oxygen, composed of two oxygen atoms (O_2), and molecules of the compound water, composed of two hydrogen atoms and one oxygen atom (H_2O).

essential nutrients: nutrients a person must obtain from food because the body cannot make them for itself in sufficient quantity to meet physiological needs; also called **indispensable nutrients.** About 40 nutrients are known to be essential for human beings.

nonnutrients: compounds in foods with no known nutritional value.

	Carbon	Hydrogen	Oxygen	Nitrogen	Minerals
Inorganic nutrients					
Minerals					✓
Water		✓	✓		
Organic nutrients					
Carbohydrates	✓	✓	✓		
Fats	✓	✓	✓		
Proteins[a]	✓	✓	✓	✓	
Vitamins[b]	✓	✓	✓		

[a]Proteins also contain the mineral sulfur.
[b]Some vitamins contain nitrogen; some contain minerals.

Figure 1–1

Elements in the Six Classes of Nutrients
Notice that organic nutrients contain carbon.

How to Think Metric

Like other scientists, nutrition scientists use metric units of measure. They measure food energy in kilocalories, people's height in centimeters, people's weight in kilograms, and the weights of foods and nutrients in grams, milligrams, or micrograms. For ease in using these measures, it helps to remember that the prefixes on the grams imply 1000. For example, a *kilogram* is 1000 grams; a *milligram* is ⅟₁₀₀₀ of a gram, and a *microgram* is ⅟₁₀₀₀ of a milligram.

Most food labels and many recipe books provide "dual measures," listing both household measures, such as cups, quarts, and teaspoons, and metric measures, such as milliliters, liters, and grams. This practice gives people a chance to gradually learn to "think metric."

A person might begin to "think metric" by simply observing the measure—by noticing the amount of soda in a 2-liter bottle, for example. Through such experiences, a person can become familiar with a measure without having to do any conversions.

Many members of the international scientific community have adopted a common system of measurement to facilitate communication—the International System of Units (SI). In addition to using metric measures, the SI establishes common units of measurement. For example, the SI unit for measuring food energy is the joule (not the kcalorie). A joule is the amount of energy expended when 1 kilogram is moved 1 meter by a force of 1 newton. The joule is thus a measure of *work* energy, whereas the kcalorie is a measure of *heat* energy. While many scientists and journals report their findings in kilojoules (kJ), many others, particularly those in the United States, use kcalories. To convert energy measures from kcalories to kilojoules, multiply by 4.2. For example, a 50-kcalorie cookie provides 210 kilojoules:

$$50 \text{ kcal} \times 4.2 = 210 \text{ kJ}.$$

Exact conversion factors for these and other units of measure are in Appendix D.

- **Volume: Liters (L)**

1 L = 1000 milliliters (mL).

0.95 L = 1 quart.

1 mL = 0.03 fluid ounces.

250 mL = 1 cup.

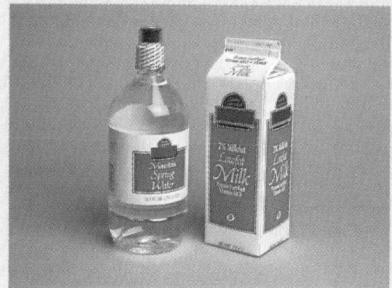

A liter of liquid is approximately one quart. (Four liters are only about 5 percent more than a gallon.)

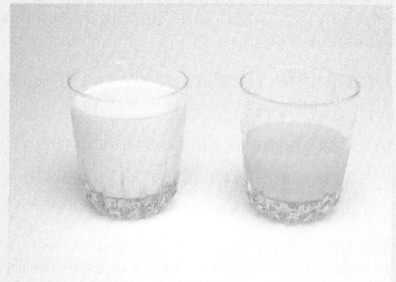

A half-cup of liquid is about 125 milliliters; one cup is about 250 milliliters.

THE ENERGY-YIELDING NUTRIENTS

energy: the capacity to do work. The energy in food is chemical energy. The body can convert this chemical energy to mechanical, electrical, or heat energy.

energy-yielding nutrients: the nutrients that break down to yield energy the body can use:
- Carbohydrate.
- Fat.
- Protein.

In the body, three of the organic nutrients are broken down to provide usable energy: carbohydrate, fat, and protein. In contrast, vitamins, minerals, and water do not yield energy in the human body.

Energy Measured in kCalories The energy released from the energy-yielding nutrients can be measured in calories—tiny units of energy so small that a single apple provides tens of thousands of them. To ease calculations, energy is expressed in 1000-calorie units known as kilocalories (shortened to kcalories, but commonly called "calories"). When you read in popular books or magazines that an apple provides "100 calories," understand that it means 100 kcalories. This

- **Weight: Grams (g)**

1 g = 1000 milligrams (mg).

1 g = 0.04 ounces (oz).

1 oz = 28.35 grams or ≈ 30 grams.

100 g ≈ 3 ½ ounces.

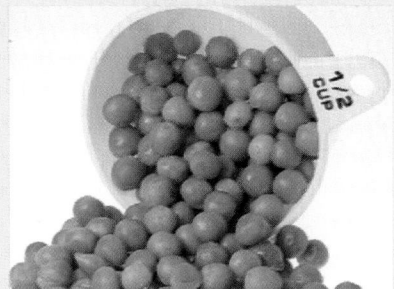

A half-cup of vegetables weighs about 100 grams.

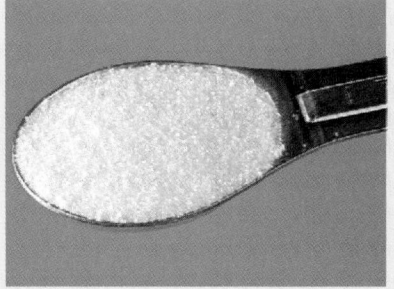

One teaspoon of dry granular powder such as salt or sugar weighs about 5 grams.

1 kilogram (kg) = 1000 grams.

1 kg = 2.2 pounds.

454 g = 1 pound.

A kilogram is slightly more than 2 pounds; conversely, a pound weighs about ½ kilogram.

- **Height: Meters (m)**

1 m = 100 centimeters (cm).

2.54 cm = 1 inch.

10 cm = 1 millimeter (mm).

1 mm = 0.04 inches.

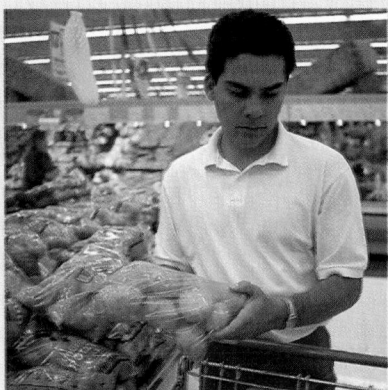

A 5-pound bag of potatoes weighs about 2 kilograms, and a 176-pound person weighs 80 kilograms.

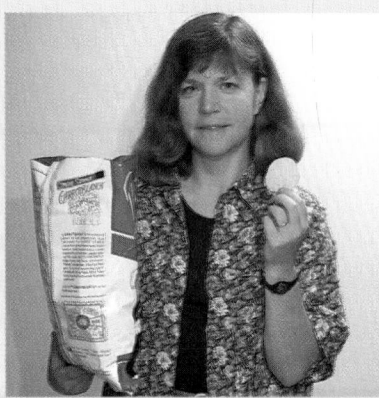

A person 5 feet 5 inches tall measures about 165 centimeters, and a rippled potato chip is about 1 millimeter thick.

book uses the term *kcalorie* and its abbreviation *kcal* throughout, as do other scientific books and journals. The accompanying box provides a few tips on how to "think metric."

A kcalorie is not a constituent of foods; it is a measure of the potential energy in foods. Thus to speak of the "kcalories" in a cookie is technically incorrect, just as to speak of the inches in a person is incorrect. It is correct to speak of the *energy* available from a food (and of the *height* of a person).

Energy in Foods   The energy content of a food depends on how much carbohydrate, fat, and protein it contains. When completely broken down in the body, a gram of carbohydrate yields about 4 kcalories of energy; a gram of protein

calorie: a unit by which energy is measured. Food energy is measured in kilocalories (1000 calories equal 1 kilocalorie), abbreviated kcalories or kcal. A capitalized version is also sometimes used: Calories. One kcalorie is the amount of heat necessary to raise the temperature of 1 kilogram (kg) of water 1°C.

How to Calculate the Energy Available from Foods

To calculate the energy available from a food, multiply the number of grams of carbohydrate, protein, and fat by 4, 4, and 9, respectively. Then add the results together. For example, 1 slice of bread with 1 tablespoon of peanut butter on it contains 16 grams carbohydrate, 7 grams protein, and 9 grams fat:

$$16 \text{ g carbohydrate} \times 4 \text{ kcal/g} = 64 \text{ kcal.}$$
$$7 \text{ g protein} \times 4 \text{ kcal/g} = 28 \text{ kcal.}$$
$$9 \text{ g fat} \times 9 \text{ kcal/g} = 81 \text{ kcal.}$$
$$\text{Total} = 173 \text{ kcal.}$$

From this information, you can calculate the percentage of kcalories each of the energy nutrients contributes to the total. To determine the percentage of kcalories from fat, for example, divide the 81 fat kcalories by the total 173 kcalories:

$$81 \div 173 = 0.468 \text{ (rounded to 0.47).}$$

Then multiply by 100 to get the percentage:

$$0.47 \times 100 = 47\%.$$

Health recommendations that urge people to limit fat intake to 30 percent of kcalories refer to the day's total energy intake, not to individual foods. Still, if the proportion of fat in each food choice throughout a day exceeds 30 percent of kcalories, then the day's total surely will too. Knowing that this snack provides 47 percent of its kcalories from fat alerts a person to the need to make lower-fat selections at other times that day.

1 g carbohydrate = 4 kcal.
1 g protein = 4 kcal.
1 g fat = 9 kcal.
1 g alcohol = 7 kcal.

also yields 4 kcalories; and a gram of fat yields 9 kcalories.* The accompanying box explains how to calculate the energy available from foods.

One other substance contributes food energy: alcohol. Alcohol is not considered a nutrient because it interferes with the growth, maintenance, and repair of the body, but it does yield energy when metabolized in the body.[†]

Most foods contain all three energy-yielding nutrients, as well as water, vitamins, minerals, and other substances. Thus it is inaccurate to identify foods with their predominant nutrients—for example, to speak of meat as a protein or of bread as a carbohydrate. Meat and bread are *foods* rich in these nutrients. Meat contains water, fat, vitamins, and minerals as well as protein. Bread contains water, a trace of fat, a little protein, and some vitamins and minerals in addition to its carbohydrate. Only a few foods are exceptions to this rule, the common ones being sugar (pure carbohydrate) and oil (essentially pure fat).

Energy in the Body The body uses the energy-yielding nutrients to fuel its metabolic and physical activities. All the energy used to keep the heart beating, the brain thinking, and the legs walking comes from energy-yielding nutrients.

---

*For those using kilojoules: 1 g carbohydrate = 17 kJ; 1 g protein = 17 kJ; 1 g fat = 37 kJ.

[†]For those using kilojoules: 1 g alcohol = 29 kJ. For those using milliliters: 1 mL alcohol = 5.6 kcal.

When the body metabolizes the energy-yielding nutrients, the bonds between their atoms break. As the bonds break, they release energy in a controlled version of the process by which wood burns in a fire. When wood burns, it releases heat (energy), steam (water), some carbon and minerals as carbon dioxide and other oxides, and some carbon and minerals as ash. During the body's metabolism of nutrients, some of the energy from food is released as heat just as in the burning of wood, but some is used to send electrical impulses through the brain and nerves, to synthesize body compounds, and to move muscles. Thus the energy from food supports every activity from quiet thought to vigorous sports. To support this metabolism, you continually inhale oxygen and exhale carbon dioxide made by combining oxygen with the carbons of the foods you have eaten. You also excrete the hydrogens of foods, combined with oxygen, as water in your urine and vapor as you breathe. Thus food fuels all of life's activities.

The processes by which nutrients are broken down to yield energy or rearranged into body structures are known as *metabolism* (defined and described further in Chapter 7).

If the body has an excess of any of the three energy-yielding nutrients, it rearranges them (and the energy they contain) into carbohydrate and fat storage compounds, to be drawn upon between meals and overnight when fresh energy supplies run low. If you take in more energy than you expend, especially when the excess energy is from foods rich in fat, you gain weight as body fat.

When taken in excess of energy need, alcohol, too, can be converted to body fat and stored. However, when alcohol contributes a substantial portion of the energy in a person's diet, the harm it does extends far beyond the problems of adding fat to the body. (Highlight 7 is devoted to alcohol and nutrition.)

During energy metabolism, the carbon atoms combine with oxygen to yield carbon dioxide; the hydrogen atoms combine with oxygen to yield water.

The body's use (metabolism) of the energy-yielding nutrients can be summarized as follows. Carbohydrate, fat, and protein from foods are broken down to simpler compounds. The process yields energy and smaller molecules. The energy may:

- Escape as heat.
- Help build new compounds (and some energy may be stored in them).
- Help move the body (do work).

The smaller molecules may:

- Serve as building blocks for new compounds (fat, muscle, or other tissues).
- Be excreted as waste materials.

Other Roles of Energy-Yielding Nutrients   In addition to providing energy, carbohydrate, fat, and protein provide the raw materials for building the body's tissues and regulating its many activities. In fact, protein's role as a fuel source is relatively minor compared with both the other two nutrients and its other roles. Proteins are found in structures such as the muscles and skin and help to regulate activities such as digestion and energy production.

Chapters 4, 5, and 6 provide more details about carbohydrate, fat, and protein. Chapter 4 includes the fibers in its discussion of the carbohydrates. Most fibers are carbohydrates, but unlike the carbohydrates, the fibers yield little or no energy. In fact, fibers pass through the body largely undigested. Fibers are important to health because they exercise the digestive tract muscles and carry potentially harmful substances out of the body, helping to lower the risks of heart disease and cancer. Fibers also provide bulk, which makes them filling, a characteristic that benefits weight control. Chapter 7 presents an introductory lesson on metabolism and sets

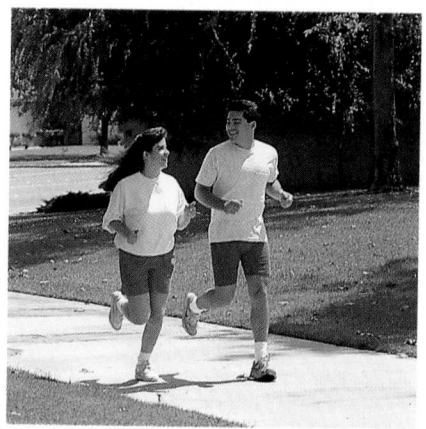

The energy to run a mile or read a book comes from the carbohydrate, fat, and protein in foods.

the stage for understanding energy balance and weight control (Chapters 8 and 9) and nutrition's role in exercise (Highlight 8).

THE VITAMINS

vitamins: organic, essential nutrients required in small amounts by the body for health. The water-soluble vitamins are vitamin C and the eight B vitamins: thiamin, riboflavin, niacin, vitamins B_6 and B_{12}, folate, biotin, and pantothenic acid. The fat-soluble vitamins are vitamins A, D, E, and K. The water-soluble vitamins are the subject of Chapter 10 and the fat-soluble vitamins, of Chapter 11.

Like the first three classes of nutrients (carbohydrate, fat, and protein), the vitamins are vital to life, organic, and available in food. They differ, however, in that the body does not extract usable energy from vitamins; rather, it uses them as helpers in metabolic processes.

Vitamins can function only if they are intact, but because they are complex organic molecules, they are vulnerable to destruction by heat, light, and chemical agents. This is why the body handles them carefully, and why nutrition-wise cooks do too. The strategies of cooking foods at moderate temperatures, in or over small amounts of water, and for short times all help to preserve the vitamins.

There are 13 different vitamins, each with its own special roles to play. One vitamin enables the eyes to see in dim light, another helps protect the lungs from air pollution, and still another helps make the sex hormones—among other things. When you cut yourself, one vitamin helps stop the bleeding and another helps repair the skin. Vitamins busily help replace old red blood cells and the lining of the digestive tract. Almost every action in the body requires the assistance of vitamins.

THE MINERALS

minerals: inorganic elements; some minerals are essential nutrients required in small amounts. The major minerals are calcium, phosphorus, potassium, sodium, chloride, magnesium, and sulfur. The trace minerals are iron, iodine, zinc, chromium, selenium, fluoride, molybdenum, copper, and manganese. Chapters 12 and 13 are devoted to the major and trace minerals, respectively.

The problems caused by one of the contaminant minerals, lead, are detailed in Highlight 13.

In contrast to the vitamins, which are organic compounds, the minerals are pure inorganic elements. That means the minerals occur in the simplest of chemical forms, as atoms of a single element. Some minerals may be put together into orderly arrays in such structures as bones and teeth. Some minerals are found in the fluids of the body and influence the properties of those fluids. Whatever their roles, minerals are not metabolized, nor do they yield energy.

Some 16 minerals are known to be essential in human nutrition; others are still being studied to determine whether they play significant roles in the human body. Still other minerals are important because they are *not* nutrients, but toxic environmental contaminants, which may displace nutrient minerals from their workplaces in the body, disrupting body functions.

Because they are indestructible, minerals in foods need not be handled with the special care that vitamins need. Minerals can, however, be bound by substances that make it hard for the body to absorb them. They can also be lost during food refining processes or dissolve into water during cooking and then be discarded.

WATER

Water, indispensable and abundant, provides the environment in which nearly all the body's activities are conducted. It participates in many metabolic reactions and supplies the medium for transporting vital materials to cells and waste products away from them. Water is discussed fully in Chapter 12, but it is mentioned in every chapter. If you watch for it, you cannot help but be impressed by water's participation in all life processes.

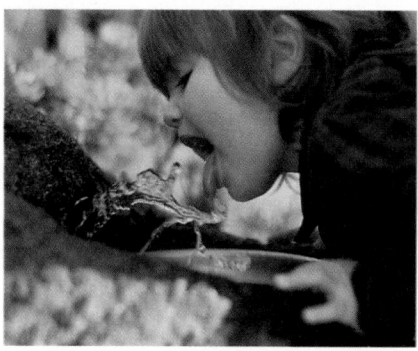

Water itself is an essential nutrient and naturally contains many minerals, which give it flavor.

To sum up, foods provide energy and nutrients—substances that support the growth, maintenance, and repair of the body's tissue. Three nutrients (carbohydrate, fat, and protein) provide the major materials for building the body's tissues and yield energy for the body's use or storage. Energy is measured in kcalories. The other three (vitamins, minerals, and water) facilitate a variety of activities in the body. Without exaggeration, nutrients provide the physical basis for nearly all that we are and all that we do.

The Science of Nutrition

The science of nutrition is the study of the nutrients in foods and the body's handling of those nutrients. As sciences go, nutrition is a young one. To put its age in perspective, if the 3-million-year history of the human race were compressed into 24 hours, then scientific discoveries began about 12 seconds ago, and nutrition as an organized science emerged only during the last 3 to 6 seconds.[3] As you can see from the size of this book, though, much has happened in nutrition's short life. This section introduces the research methods scientists have used in uncovering the wonders of the nutrients.

science of nutrition: the study of the nutrients in foods and of the body's handling of them (including ingestion, digestion, absorption, transport, metabolism, interaction, storage, and excretion). A broader definition includes the study of the environment and of human behavior as it relates to food.

NUTRITION RESEARCH

Research always begins with a question. For example, "what foods or nutrients might protect against the common cold?" In search of an answer, scientists make educated guesses (hypotheses) and then systematically conduct research studies to test each hypothesis. Examples of some types of research studies follow:

- *Epidemiological studies* observe how much and what kinds of foods a group of people eat and how healthy those people are. Such findings bring to light factors that might influence the incidence of a disease in various populations.

- *Case-control studies* compare people who do and do not have a given condition such as a disease, closely matching them in age, occupation, and other key variables so that differences in other factors will stand out. Differences then appear that may account for the condition in the group that has it.

- *Animal studies* might feed specific nutrients or diets to animals and then observe any changes in health. Such studies test possible disease causes and treatments in a laboratory where all conditions can be controlled.

- *Human intervention (or clinical) trials* ask people to adopt a new behavior (for example, eat a citrus fruit, take a vitamin C supplement, or exercise daily). These trials help determine the effects such measures have on the development or prevention of disease. Each type of study has advantages and disadvantages. Findings must be interpreted with an awareness of the study's limitations. (See Highlight 1 for a discussion on evaluating research findings.)

In attempting to discover whether a nutrient relieves symptoms or cures a disease, all research tries to answer the same kinds of questions. Research on vitamin C and the common cold illustrates particularly well what those questions are.

Controls In most studies on the efficacy of vitamin C, researchers divide people into two groups. One group (the experimental group) receives a vitamin C supplement, and the other (the control group) does not. Researchers follow both groups to determine whether the vitamin C group has fewer or shorter colds

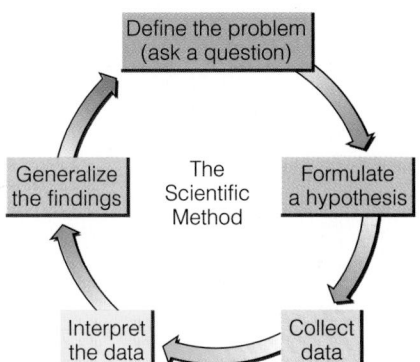

In conducting research, scientists follow these steps, which define the scientific method.

Glossary of Research Terms

blind experiment: an experiment in which the subjects do not know whether they are members of the experimental group or the control group.

control group: a group of individuals similar in all possible respects to the experimental group except for the treatment. Ideally, the control group receives a placebo while the experimental group receives a real treatment.

correlation (CORE-ee-LAY-shun): the simultaneous increase, decrease, or change of two variables. If A increases as B increases, or if A decreases as B decreases, the correlation is positive. (This does not mean that A causes B or vice versa.) If A increases as B decreases, or if A decreases as B increases, the correlation is negative. (This does not mean that A prevents B or vice versa.) Some third factor may account for both A and B.

double-blind experiment: an experiment in which neither the subjects nor the researchers know which subjects are members of the experimental group and which are serving as control subjects, until after the experiment is over.

experimental group: a group of individuals similar in all possible respects to the control group except for the treatment. The experimental group receives the real treatment.

peer review: a process in which a panel of scientists rigorously evaluates a research study to assure that the scientific method was followed.

placebo (pla-SEE-bo): an inert, harmless medication given to provide comfort and hope; a sham treatment used in controlled research studies.

placebo effect: the healing effect that faith in medicine, even inert medicine, often has.

randomization (RAN-dom-ih-ZAY-shun): a process of choosing the members of the experimental and control groups without bias.

replication (REP-lee-KAY-shun): repeating an experiment and getting the same results. The skeptical scientist, on hearing of a new, exciting finding, will ask, "Has it been replicated yet?" If it hasn't, the scientist will withhold judgment regarding the finding's validity.

validity (va-LID-ih-tee): having the quality of being founded on fact or evidence.

variable: a factor that changes. A variable may depend on another variable (for example, a child's height depends on his age), or it may be independent (for example, a child's height does not depend on the color of her eyes). Sometimes both variables correlate with a third variable (a child's height and eye color both depend on genetics).

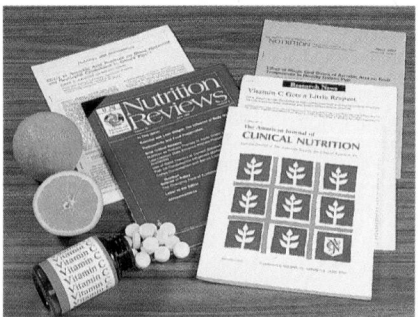

Knowledge about the nutrients and their effects on health comes from scientific study.

than the control group. A number of pitfalls are inherent in an experiment of this kind and must be avoided.

First, the two groups of people must be similar in all respects (except that one group receives vitamin C). Similarity of the experimental and control groups is accomplished by randomization, a process of choosing the members from the same population by throws of the dice or some other method involving chance.

Importantly, both groups must have the same track record with respect to colds to rule out the possibility that an observed difference might have occurred anyway. If group A would have caught twice as many colds as group B anyway, then the fact that group B happened to receive the treatment proves nothing.

In experiments involving a nutrient, the diets of both groups must also be similar, especially with respect to that nutrient. If those in group B were receiving less vitamin C from their diet, this might cancel the effects of the supplement.

Sample Size   To ensure that chance variation between the two groups does not influence the results, the groups must be large. If one member of a group of five people catches a bad cold by chance, he will pull the whole group's average toward bad colds; but if one member of a group of 500 catches a bad cold, she will not unduly affect the group average. Statistical methods are used to determine whether differences between groups of various sizes support a hypothesis or are insignificant.

Placebos   If people take vitamin C for colds and *believe* it will cure them, their chances of recovery are improved. Taking anything believed to be beneficial hastens recovery in about half of all cases. This phenomenon, the effect of faith on healing, is known as the placebo effect. In experiments designed to determine vitamin C's effect on colds, this mind-body effect must be rigorously controlled. Severity of symptoms is often a subjective measure, and people who believe they are being treated may report less severe symptoms.

One way experimenters control for the placebo effect is to give pills to all participants; some pills contain vitamin C, and others of similar appearance and taste contain an inactive ingredient (placebos). This way, the effects of faith will work equally in both groups. It is not necessary to convince all subjects that they are receiving vitamin C, but the extent of belief or unbelief must be the same in both groups. A study conducted under these conditions is called a blind experiment—that is, the subjects do not know (are blind to) whether they are members of the experimental group (receiving treatment) or the control group (receiving the placebo).

Double Blind   The experimenters, too, must not know which subjects are in which group. Being fallible human beings and having an emotional investment in a successful outcome, researchers might interpret and record results with a bias in the expected direction. To prevent such distortions, the pills given to the subjects are coded by a third party, who does not reveal to the experimenters which subjects were which until all results have been recorded quantitatively.

Correlations and Causes   Research often examines the relationships between two or more variables—for example, daily vitamin C intake and the number of colds. Findings sometimes suggest no correlation between the two variables (regardless of the amount of vitamin C eaten, the number of colds remains the same). Other times, studies find either a positive correlation (the more vitamin C, the more colds) or a negative correlation (the more vitamin C, the fewer colds). Correlational evidence proves only that two variables are associated, not that one is the cause of the other. People often jump to conclusions when they learn of correlations, but the conclusions are often wrong. To prove that A causes B, scientists have to find evidence of the *mechanism*—that is, to catch A in the act of causing B, so to speak. Furthermore, other scientists must confirm or disprove the findings through replication before the results are accepted into the body of nutrition knowledge. Before the findings are published, they are subjected to peer review—a process whereby a panel of scientists evaluates the study to confirm that it followed standard scientific methods.

RESEARCH VERSUS RUMORS

In discussing these subtleties of experimental design, our intent is to show you what a far cry scientific validity is from the experience of your neighbor Mary (sample size, one; no control group), who says she takes vitamin C when she feels a cold coming on and "it works every time." She knows what she is taking, she has faith in its efficacy, and she tends not to notice when it doesn't work. Before concluding that an experiment has shown that a nutrient cures a disease or alleviates a symptom, ask these questions:

- Was there similarity between the control group and the experimental group?
- Was the sample size large enough to rule out chance variation?
- Was a placebo effectively administered (blind)?
- Was the experiment double blind?

In summary, scientists learn about nutrition by conducting experiments that follow the protocol of scientific research. Researchers take care to establish similar control and experimental groups, large sample sizes, placebos, and blind treatments. Their findings must be reviewed and replicated by other scientists before being accepted as valid. These are a few of the characteristics of research that is well designed to study the actions of nutrients in the body. Such research has laid the foundation for quantifying how much of each nutrient the body needs.

Recommended Nutrient Intakes

If nutrition experts could define all the dietary factors a person needs to support good health, they ideally would:

1. Estimate the amount of food energy the person needs to consume and the amount of physical activity the person needs to engage in to balance that energy intake.
2. Distribute the three energy-yielding nutrients so that the person receives:
   a. enough protein to meet protein needs, and
   b. sufficient carbohydrate and fat to fill the remainder of the energy allowance, balanced in the way that supports health best.
3. Estimate how much water and fiber will support health optimally.
4. Estimate the minimum and maximum amounts of each vitamin and mineral consistent with health.
5. Set upper limits for intakes of dietary constituents that are harmful in large amounts (salt, fat, and alcohol are familiar examples).

That is what the experts have done, and their dietary recommendations are presented in this section.

Two national committees take responsibility for defining the amounts of dietary factors that best support health. These committees are selected by the National Academy of Sciences and subject to approval by the National Research Council. The Committee on Dietary Allowances concerns itself primarily with maintaining health and focuses on energy and nutrient needs; the Committee on Diet and Health pays particular attention to reducing the risks of chronic diseases and focuses on dietary inadequacies and excesses.

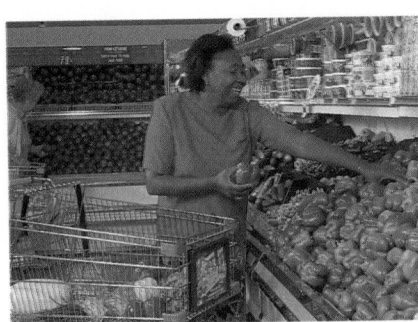

When people shop for foods, they are buying nutrients.

RECOMMENDED DIETARY ALLOWANCES (RDA)

The Committee on Dietary Allowances produces the set of nutrient standards known as the Recommended Dietary Allowances (RDA). A summary table of the RDA appears on the inside front cover (left) of this book; Appendix G presents additional RDA tables. At least 40 different nations and international organizations have published standards similar to the RDA.

The Committee on Dietary Allowances consists of highly qualified scientists. They base their estimates of nutrient needs on careful examination and interpretation of scientific evidence. Every few years, the committee reviews and revises the RDA as needed. For each new edition, committee members reexamine the data, concepts, and assumptions that underlie the RDA; restudy their own prior reasoning; and record how they have arrived at their recommendations.[4]

Developing the RDA is a huge task. Parts of it have occupied the committee's attention since the early 1940s. RDA have been established for energy and for nutrients for which deficiencies are known to occur. These recommendations change only a little from one revision to the next. For nutrients that are abundant in the diet, estimated minimum requirements have been set. For other nutrients that are less well studied, Estimated Safe and Adequate Dietary Intakes (ESADDI) are given. The next paragraphs discuss specific aspects of the RDA.

Energy RDA   Each person's food energy *intake* must equal the energy *expended*, if the person is to maintain body weight. In recommending energy intakes, the Committee on Dietary Allowances reviewed research on thousands of individuals and derived *averages* for each of several age-sex groups. The committee finally arrived at a *single average number of kcalories* spent per day for each group—2900 kcalories, for example, for males 19 to 24 years of age.

Of course, tremendous variation surrounds this number. Males aged 19 to 24 come in all shapes and sizes and participate in all kinds of activities. The average energy recommendation is directly applicable to only a few individuals, but it serves as a ballpark figure; it gives a sense of how many kcalories are reasonable for this group.

The committee has not established an RDA for the output side of the energy balance equation—that is, how much energy people should expend. In deriving an RDA for energy intake, the Committee on Dietary Allowances assumes most people engage in light-to-moderate activity. The committee does say that people should balance energy intake with expenditure and that those who need to lose weight should increase energy expenditure rather than reduce energy intake. The more physical activity a person engages in, the more fit the person becomes, and the more food the person can eat without gaining weight. A person who can eat more food can obtain more nutrients, and this also supports health.

Protein RDA   For protein, recommendations are based on body weight. The protein RDA is high, unlike the energy RDA, so it covers most people's needs.*

Recommended Dietary Allowances (RDA): the amounts of selected nutrients considered adequate to meet the known nutrient needs of practically all healthy people.

The RDA are based on scientific knowledge and are prepared by a committee of the Food and Nutrition Board (FNB) of the National Academy of Sciences (NAS).

The Canadian equivalent of the RDA is the Recommended Nutrient Intakes (RNI); see Appendix I.

RDA set for :
- Energy.
- Protein.
- Vitamins (A, D, E, K, C, thiamin, riboflavin, niacin, B_6, folate, B_{12}).
- Minerals (calcium, phosphorus, magnesium, iron, zinc, iodine, selenium).

Estimated minimum requirements set for:
- Sodium, potassium, chloride.

ESADDI set for:
- Vitamins (biotin, pantothenic acid).
- Minerals (copper, manganese, fluoride, chromium, molybdenum).

See inside front cover and Appendix G for details.

Chapters 8 and 9 revisit the energy RDA and show how to estimate your individual energy requirements and how to control your energy intake to meet your needs.

---

*The *average* daily requirement for protein is 0.6 grams per kilogram of body weight; the RDA is set at 0.8 grams per kilogram to meet the needs of 97.5 percent of the population—see Chapter 6.

No RDA for Carbohydrate and Fat The amount of protein recommended represents a relatively small percentage of a person's energy allowance; the remainder comes from carbohydrate and fat. No RDA for carbohydrate and fat is given, but the general guideline is that more than half of daily energy should come from carbohydrate, and no more than one-third should come from fat.

Water Recommendation The bigger and more active a person is, the more water the person needs. Water recommendations are tied directly to energy expenditures as described in Chapter 12. Generally, most people need at least six to eight 8-ounce glasses of water or liquids a day.

Fiber Recommendation There is no RDA for fiber. Instead, the Committee on Dietary Allowances recommends that people obtain sufficient fiber from fruits, vegetables, legumes, and whole-grain products, which provide vitamins, minerals, and water as well as fiber.

SETTING THE RDA FOR VITAMINS AND MINERALS

In contrast to some of the foregoing dietary constituents, many of the vitamins and minerals have specific recommended allowances in the main RDA table (inside front cover, left). They have been well studied and restudied for decades.

Estimating a Minimal Requirement To set vitamin and mineral recommendations, the Committee on Dietary Allowances reviews and selects the most valid studies of deficiency states, of the body's nutrient stores and their depletion, of nutrient intakes of apparently healthy people, and of findings from animal research. From this information, the committee estimates an *average requirement* for each nutrient—an amount that appears sufficient to maintain body processes *for a population.* When people consistently obtain a *deficient* intake (one that is less than the requirement), their nutrient stores decline, and over time this decline leads to deficiency symptoms.

Examining all the available data, the committee finds that each person's body is unique and has its own set of requirements. For example, Mr. A might need 40 units of the nutrient each day to prevent deficiency; Ms. B might need 35; Mr. C, 57. A look at enough individuals might reveal that their requirements fall into a symmetrical distribution (as shown in Figure 1–2), with most near the midpoint and only a few at the extremes.

Establishing a Generous Recommendation Then, to set the RDA, the committee must decide what intake to recommend for everybody. Should the RDA reflect the average requirement (shown in Figure 1–2 as 45 units)? The average requirement for each nutrient is probably closest to everyone's need, assuming the distribution shown in Figure 1–2. (Actually, the data for most nutrients other than protein have a distribution that is much less symmetrical.) But if people consumed exactly the average requirement of a given nutrient each day, half of the population would develop deficiencies of that nutrient; in Figure 1–2, Mr. C would be among them.

In this example, a reasonable choice for an RDA for everybody might be 63 units a day (see Figure 1–2). Such a point can be calculated mathematically so that it covers about 98 percent of a population. Even those whose needs were

requirement: the amount of a nutrient that will maintain normal biochemical and physiological functions and prevent the development of specific deficiency signs; distinguished from the RDA, which is a recommended and generous allowance that provides for variability among individuals.

deficient: the amount of a nutrient below which *almost all healthy people* can be expected, over time, to experience deficiency symptoms.

Each of the 120 squares shown here represents a person. Some people require only a small amount of the nutrient, and some require a lot, but most fall somewhere near the middle. The text discusses three of these people: Mr. A, Ms. B, and Mr. C.

The RDA for nutrients is set well above the average requirement. It covers about 98% of the population.

Figure 1–2

Setting the RDA for a Nutrient

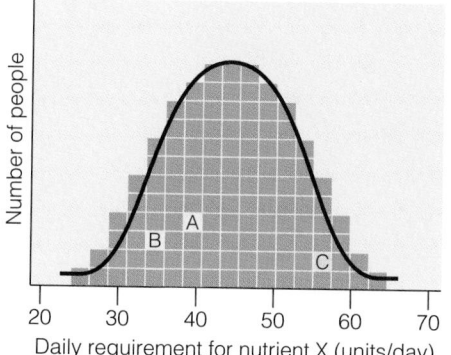

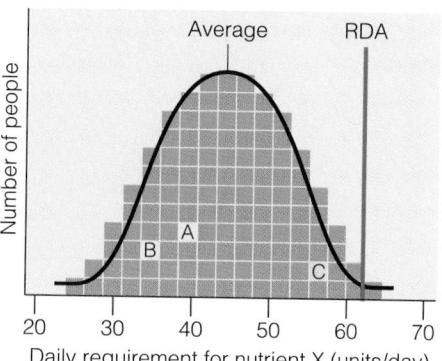

higher than the average would be covered. Relatively few people's requirements would exceed the RDA, and even then, they wouldn't exceed by much.

Committee members make this kind of judgment in setting the RDA for each vitamin and mineral. They set it well above the average requirement determined from the best available information. For these reasons, people cannot use the RDA as their own individual requirements, but they can be reasonably sure that the RDA probably cover their needs adequately.

The RDA for protein, vitamins, and minerals are generous, and although the recommendations do not necessarily cover every individual for every nutrient, people's intakes should not exceed the RDA by much. People's tolerances for high doses of nutrients vary, and somewhere above the RDA there is an *upper safe* level beyond which some nutrients can be toxic. It is naive to think of the RDA as minimum amounts. A more accurate view is to see a person's nutrient needs as falling within a range, with marginal and danger zones both below and above it (see Figure 1–3). This consideration can be seen especially clearly in the RDA tables that state recommended intakes in terms of "safe and adequate" ranges, "safe" meaning "not too high" and "adequate" meaning "not too low."

Energy and Nutrient RDA Compared   Figure 1–4 illustrates a contrast between the RDA for energy and the RDA for nutrients. The RDA for energy is set at the mean of the population's known requirements. In the case of energy, more than the need is as bad for health as less because excess energy leads to obesity, and deficient energy causes undernutrition. In contrast, in the case of vitamins and minerals, small amounts above the daily requirement do no harm, whereas amounts below the requirement lead to deficiencies. Their RDA are set near the top end of the range of the population's known requirements, so that as many people as possible will meet their needs given the RDA.

The preceding discussion has covered most of the goals listed at the start (p. 14)—setting recommended intakes for energy, energy-yielding nutrients, water, fiber,

upper safe: the amount of a nutrient that appears safe for *most healthy people* and beyond which there is concern that some people will experience toxicity symptoms.

Figure 1–3

Naive versus Accurate View of Nutrient Needs

The RDA for a given nutrient represents a point within a range of appropriate and reasonable intakes that lies between toxicity and deficiency. The recommendation is high enough to provide reserves in times of short-term dietary inadequacies, but not so high as to approach toxicity. Nutrient intakes above or below this range might be equally harmful.

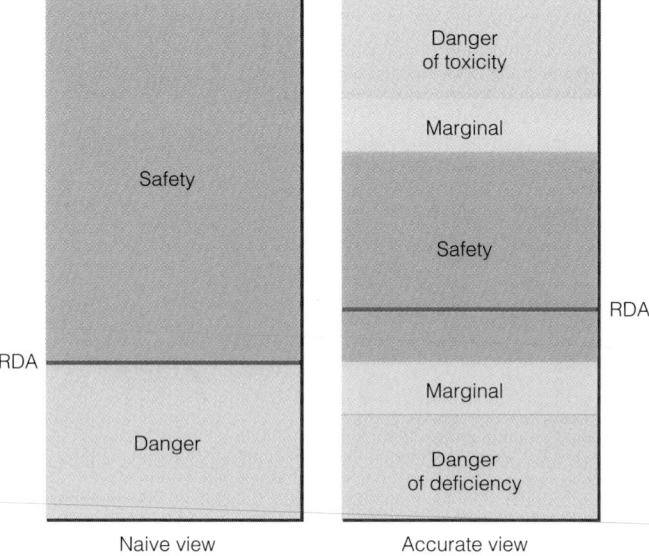

and vitamins and minerals. Energy and these nutrients represent the primary focus of the Committee on Dietary Allowances. The remaining dietary constituents (salt, fat, alcohol, and others) differ from these, in that deficiencies are not a risk, but excesses threaten health. This aspect of diet is the province of the Committee on Diet and Health and other agencies and is discussed further at the end of this chapter.

USING THE RDA

Although the intent of the RDA may seem simple enough, they are the subject of much misunderstanding and controversy. Perhaps the following facts will help

Figure 1–4

The Nutrient RDA and the Energy RDA Compared

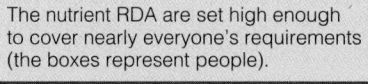

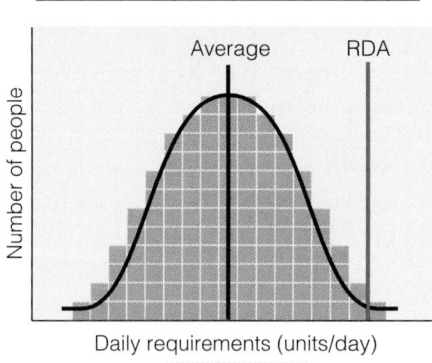

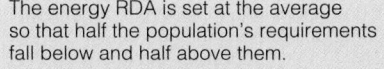

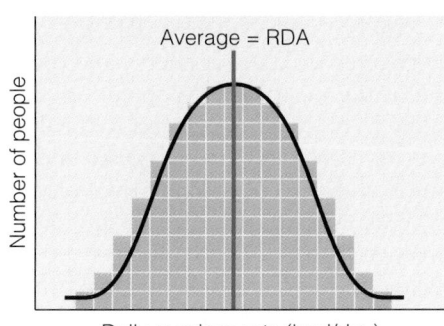

put the RDA in perspective. First, the RDA serve as estimates of adequate energy and nutrient intakes for *healthy* people. They do not apply to people with health problems who may require supplemented or restricted intakes.

Second, the RDA are safe and adequate *recommendations* that include a generous margin of safety. They are not minimum requirements, nor are they necessarily optimal intakes for all individuals.

Third, the RDA are intended to be met through diets composed of a variety of *foods*. Because foods contain mixtures of nutrients, they deliver more than just those nutrients named in the RDA table. Excess intakes of vitamins and minerals are unlikely when their sources are foods rather than supplements.

Fourth, the RDA apply to *average daily intakes*. To try to meet the RDA for every nutrient every day is difficult and unnecessary. The length of time over which a person's intake can deviate from the average without risk of deficiency or overdose varies; for most nutrients, it is best to try to achieve the average intakes recommended by the RDA within three days or so.

Fifth, the RDA are most appropriately used to develop and evaluate nutrition programs for *populations* such as schoolchildren or military personnel. The RDA can be used to estimate the risks of deficiencies for an individual only if the person's intakes are determined and averaged over a sufficient length of time.[5] After all, the recommended intakes do meet the needs of essentially all members of a healthy population, so by definition, they apply to individuals within that population. To use the RDA this way, though, an individual must compare the RDA with the *typical* intake, and not just with an arbitrary day's intake.

With these understandings, researchers use the RDA as a yardstick to assess the adequacy of diets—for example, in nutrition surveys. Diet planners use them as guidelines in planning and evaluating diets for groups of people—for example, the children in school districts. Dietitians working in social service programs use the RDA to establish criteria for foods delivered by food assistance programs. The Food and Drug Administration (FDA) uses the RDA as guidelines for the labeling of foods, and the food industry uses them to develop new food products.

Revising the RDA The RDA are not etched on stone tablets. They are revised periodically as convincing new evidence becomes available. Since the first edition in 1943, the RDA have been the authoritative standard for the nutrient needs of people in the United States.[6] In general, the current edition shares many similarities with previous editions. The RDA have served their purpose of protecting against nutrient deficiencies. Over the past several decades, deficiencies have not been reported in groups of people who were receiving the RDA. Clearly, the safety margins used in setting the nutrient RDA do indeed cover practically all people, just as they claim to do.

The Food and Nutrition Board now faces the challenge of redefining the RDA's goal beyond preventing nutrient deficiencies to include supporting optimal health and preventing chronic diseases.[7] Plans for the next edition of the RDA call for it to address "the potential roles of nutrients and other food constituents in reducing chronic disease risk."[8] Suggestions being considered for the next revision include:[9]

- Providing several sets of RDA (one for health, one for disease prevention, another for disease treatment).
- Providing a range of values to accommodate people's diverse needs.

Beginning in 1997, the revised recommendations are called Dietary Reference Intakes.

- Using the most current RDA for food labels (labels now use the 1968 edition).
- Establishing RDA for nutrients and nonnutrients such as fiber, cholesterol, and beta-carotene (a relative of vitamin A) that influence health.
- Addressing the needs of elderly people and other nutritionally vulnerable subgroups such as minority populations and smokers.
- Changing the name from *dietary* to *nutrient* allowances in recognition that in some circumstances, desired intakes may not be possible from foods alone.

Unlike past revisions, the next edition of the RDA is likely to exhibit more differences from previous editions than similarities. It is appropriate that the RDA continue to evolve.

Comparing the RDA with Other Recommendations Other recommendations work similarly to the RDA. For example, like the RDA, recommendations of the international agencies FAO and WHO are considered sufficient for the maintenance of health in nearly all people. These recommendations differ from the RDA, however, in that they serve populations worldwide and are based on different judgment factors. For example, the FAO/WHO recommendations consider that people worldwide are generally smaller and more active than people in the United States. Nevertheless, the recommendations of all nations and agencies fall within the same range.

To recap, the RDA represent intakes of selected nutrients considered adequate to meet the needs of practically all healthy people. The energy RDA is set at the average of people's needs so as to discourage overconsumption of food energy. The RDA for protein, vitamins, and minerals, on the other hand, are set well above the average so as to cover the needs of most healthy people. The RDA are commonly used to assess the adequacy of diets.

FAO: the Food and Agriculture Organization (of the United Nations).

WHO: the World Health Organization.

Nutrient recommendations from FAO/WHO are provided in Appendix G.

Nutrition Assessment

What happens when a person doesn't get enough of a nutrient or energy or gets too much? If the deficiency or excess is significant over time, the person exhibits signs of malnutrition. With a deficiency of energy, the person may display the symptoms of undernutrition by becoming extremely thin, losing muscle tissue, and becoming prone to infection and disease. With a deficiency of a nutrient, the person may experience skin rashes, depression, hair loss, bleeding gums, muscle spasms, night blindness, or other symptoms. With an excess of energy, the person may become obese and vulnerable to diseases associated with overnutrition such as diabetes, heart disease, and cancer. With a sudden nutrient overdose, the person may experience hot flashes, yellowing skin, paralysis, a rapid heart rate, low blood pressure, or other symptoms.

Malnutrition symptoms are easy to miss. They resemble the symptoms of other diseases: diarrhea, skin rashes, pain, and the like. But a person who has learned how to read the signs can tell when these conditions are caused by malnutrition and can take steps to correct it. Dietitians have developed assessment techniques to detect malnutrition. This discussion presents the basics of nutrition assessment; many more details are offered in Chapters 15 and 16 and in Appendix E.

malnutrition: any condition caused by excess or deficient food energy or nutrient intake or by an imbalance of nutrients.
  mal = bad

undernutrition: deficiency of energy or nutrients.

overnutrition: excess energy or nutrients.

NUTRITION ASSESSMENT OF INDIVIDUALS

To prepare a nutrition assessment, the assessor, usually a registered dietitian or a physician trained in clinical nutrition, uses:

- Historical information.
- Anthropometric data.
- Physical examinations.
- Laboratory tests.

Each of these methods involves collecting data in various ways and interpreting each finding in relation to the others in order to create a total picture.

Historical Information   One step in evaluating nutrition status is to obtain information about a person's history with respect to health status, socioeconomic status, drug use, and diet. The health history may reveal a disease that interferes with the person's ability to eat or the body's use of nutrients. Socioeconomic circumstances may show a financial inability to buy foods or inadequate kitchen facilities in which to prepare them. A drug history may highlight possible drug-nutrient interactions that lead to nutrient deficiencies. A diet history can indicate whether the diet may be under- or oversupplying nutrients or energy.

To take a diet history, the assessor collects and analyzes data about the foods a person eats. The data may be collected by recording the foods the person has eaten over a period of 24 hours, three days, or a week or more or by asking what foods the person typically eats and how much of each. The days in a record have to be fairly typical of the person's diet, and the record has to pay special attention to portion sizes. To determine the amounts of nutrients consumed, the assessor usually enters the foods and their portion sizes into a computer using a diet analysis program. Alternatively, this step can be done manually by looking up each food in a table of food composition such as Appendix H in this book. Then the assessor compares the calculated nutrient intakes with recommended intakes such as the RDA.

An estimate of energy and nutrient intakes from a diet history, combined with other sources of information, can help confirm or rule out the *possibility* of suspected nutrition problems. A sufficient intake of a nutrient does not guarantee adequate nutrition status for an individual, and an insufficient intake does not always indicate a deficiency, but such findings warn of possible problems.

Anthropometric Data   A second technique that may help reveal nutrition problems is the taking of measures such as height and weight. The assessor compares measurements taken on an individual with standards specific for sex and age or with previous measures on the same individual.

Measurements taken periodically and compared with previous measurements reveal patterns and indicate trends in a person's overall nutrition status; they provide little information about the status of specific nutrients. Measurements out of line with expectations may reveal such problems as growth failure in children, wasting or swelling of body tissue in adults, and obesity—conditions that may reflect nutrient deficiencies or excesses.

nutrition assessment: a comprehensive approach, completed by a registered dietitian, to defining nutrition status that uses health, socioeconomic, drug, and diet histories; anthropometric measurements; physical examinations; and laboratory tests.

A *registered dietitian* is a college-educated food and nutrition specialist who is qualified to evaluate people's nutritional health and needs. See Highlight 1 for more on what constitutes a nutrition expert.

Chapter 15 describes the tools used to obtain food intake data: the 24-hour recall, usual intake record, food frequency checklist, and food record.

anthropometric (AN-throw-poe-MET-rick): relating to measurement of the physical characteristics of the body, such as height and weight.
anthropos = human
metric = measuring

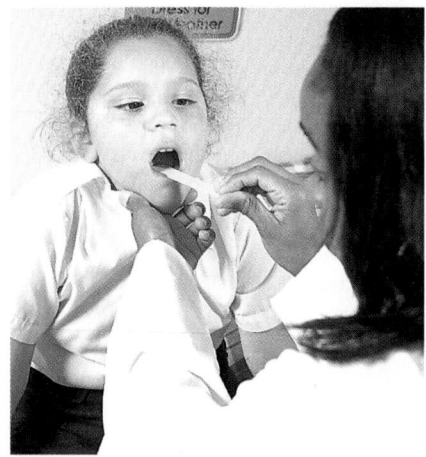

A peek inside the mouth provides clues to a person's nutrition status.

overt (oh-VERT): out in the open and easy to observe.

   ouvrir = to open

primary deficiency: a nutrient deficiency caused by inadequate dietary intake of a nutrient.

secondary deficiency: a nutrient deficiency caused by something other than diet, such as a disease condition that reduces absorption, accelerates use, hastens excretion, or destroys the nutrient.

Physical Examinations   A third nutrition assessment technique is a physical examination that looks for clues to poor nutrition status. Every part of the body that can be inspected can offer such clues: the hair, eyes, skin, posture, tongue, fingernails, and others. The examination requires skill, for many physical signs can reflect more than one nutrient deficiency or toxicity or even nonnutrition conditions. Like the other assessment techniques, a physical examination does not by itself point to firm conclusions. Instead, it reveals possible nutrient imbalances for other assessment techniques to confirm or confirms data collected from other assessment measures.

Laboratory Tests   A fourth way to detect a developing deficiency, imbalance, or toxicity state is to take samples of body tissues or fluids (blood or urine), analyze them in the laboratory, and compare the results with normal values for a similar population. A goal of nutrition assessment is to uncover early signs of malnutrition before symptoms appear. Laboratory tests are useful this way and can also confirm suspicions raised by other assessment methods.

Iron, for Example   The mineral iron can be used to illustrate the stages in the development of a nutrient deficiency and the assessment techniques useful in detecting them. The overt, or outward, signs of an iron deficiency appear at the end of a long sequence of events. Figure 1–5 describes what happens in the body as a nutrient deficiency progresses and shows how assessment methods can reveal those changes.

First, too little iron gets into the body—either because iron is lacking in the person's food (a primary deficiency) or because the person's body doesn't absorb or use iron normally (a secondary deficiency). A diet history provides clues to primary deficiencies; a health history provides clues to secondary deficiencies.

Figure 1–5

Stages in the Development of a Nutrient Deficiency

Internal changes precede outward signs of deficiencies. As a corollary, signs of sickness need not appear before a person takes corrective measures. Tests can either reveal the presence of problems in the early stages or confirm that nutrient stores are adequate.

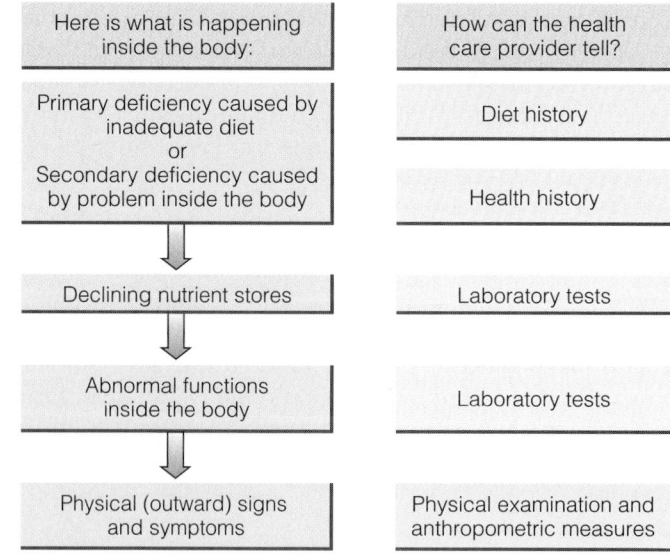

Then the body begins to use up its stores of iron. At this stage, the deficiency might be described as subclinical. It exists as a covert condition and might be detected by laboratory tests, but outward signs have not yet appeared.

Finally, iron stores are exhausted. Now, the body cannot make enough iron-containing red blood cells to replace those that are aging and dying. The red blood cells normally carry oxygen to all the body's tissues. When iron is lacking, fewer red blood cells are made, the new ones are pale and small, and every part of the body feels the effects of an oxygen shortage. Now, the overt symptoms of deficiency appear—weakness, fatigue, pallor, and headaches, reflecting the iron-deficient state of the blood. Physical examination would reveal these symptoms.

Thus reviewing dietary data may suggest a nutrition problem in its earliest stages. Laboratory tests may detect it before it becomes overt, whereas physical examination picks up on the problem only after it is causing symptoms.

> HEALTHY PEOPLE 2000: Increase to at least 75% the proportion of primary care providers who provide nutrition assessment and counseling and/or referral to qualified nutritionists or dietitians.

NUTRITION ASSESSMENT OF POPULATIONS

To assess a population's nutrition status, researchers conduct surveys using techniques similar to those used on individuals. One kind of survey—a food consumption survey—determines the kinds and amounts of foods people eat. Then researchers calculate the energy and nutrients in the foods and compare the amounts consumed with a standard such as the RDA. An example of this type of survey is the Nationwide Food Consumption Survey (NFCS). Information for the third NFCS (1994–1996) was gathered from 15,000 people using food intake records for two nonconsecutive days.

Another kind of survey—a nutrition status survey—examines the people themselves, using nutrition assessment methods. The National Health and Nutrition Examination Survey (NHANES) is an example of a nutrition status survey. The third NHANES (1988–1996) gathered information from between 40,000 and 70,000 people using diet histories, anthropometric measurements, physical examinations, and laboratory tests. The data provide information on several nutrition-related conditions, such as growth retardation, heart disease, and nutrient deficiencies. Both the NFCS and the NHANES oversample high-risk groups (low-income families, infants and children, and the elderly) in order to glean an accurate estimate of their health and nutrition status.

Until 1990, findings from the nation's many nutrition surveys, including these two largest ones, were almost impossible to compare and synthesize into a single cohesive report. Then the National Nutrition Monitoring and Related Research Act was enacted to coordinate the many nutrition-related activities that had been underway within 22 different federal agencies. The law mandated that the U.S. Department of Agriculture (USDA) and the Department of Health and Human Services (DHHS) establish and implement a Ten-Year Comprehensive Plan for nutrition monitoring and related research.[11]

The resulting wealth of information can be used for a variety of purposes. For example, Congress uses this information to establish public policy on nutrition education, food assistance programs, and the regulation of the food supply. Scientists use the information to establish research priorities. All major reports that

subclinical deficiency: a deficiency in the early stages, before the outward signs have appeared.

covert (KOH-vert): hidden, as if under covers.

couvrir = to cover

The Healthy People 2000 report sets national objectives in health promotion and disease prevention for the year 2000.[10] The 21 nutrition-related priorities are listed in Appendix G and appear in the text where their subjects are discussed.

food consumption survey: a survey that measures the amounts and kinds of foods people consume (using diet histories), estimates the nutrient intakes, and compares them with a standard such as the RDA.

nutrition status survey: a survey that evaluates people's nutrition status using diet histories, anthropometric measures, physical examinations, and laboratory tests.

examine the contribution of diet and nutrition status to the health of the people of the United States depend on information collected and coordinated by this national program.* These data provided the basis for the mid-decade report on Healthy People 2000 that shows we are not meeting many of our health goals; in fact, we are not even heading in the right direction for some goals, such as reducing the prevalence of overweight in this country.[12]

To review, people become malnourished when they get too little or too much energy or nutrients. To detect malnutrition in individuals, health care professionals use nutrition assessment techniques. Assessments gather data from historical information, anthropometric measures, physical examinations, and laboratory tests. Assessment methods are also used in surveys to measure people's food consumption and to evaluate the nutrition status of populations.

Diet and Health

Diet has always played a vital role in supporting health. Early nutrition research focused on identifying the nutrients in foods that would prevent such common diseases as rickets and scurvy, the vitamin D– and vitamin C–deficiency diseases. More recently, with nutrient deficiencies no longer a major threat, nutrition research has focused on diseases associated with energy and nutrient excesses. Today, overconsumption of foods—especially foods high in fats—is a major health concern for people in the United States.[13]

Figure 1–6 shows the ten leading causes of illness and death in the United States. These "causes" are stated as if single conditions such as heart disease caused death, but most chronic diseases arise from multiple factors over many years. A person who died of heart failure may have had preexisting conditions such as overweight and high blood pressure, may have been a cigarette smoker, and may have spent years eating a high-fat diet and getting too little exercise.

Of course, not all people who die of heart disease fit this description, nor do all people with these characteristics die of heart disease. People who are overweight might die from the complications of diabetes instead, or those who smoke might die of cancer. They might even die from something totally unrelated to any of these factors, such as an automobile accident. Still, statistical studies have shown that certain conditions and behaviors are linked to certain diseases.

RISK FACTORS

Factors that increase or reduce the *risk* of developing chronic diseases are identified by analyzing statistical data. A strong association between a risk factor and a disease means that when the factor is present, the *likelihood* of developing the

chronic diseases: degenerative diseases characterized by deterioration of the body organs; also called chronic, **noncommunicable diseases (NCD)**. Examples include heart disease, cancer, and diabetes.

risk factors: factors associated with an elevated frequency of a disease but not proven to be causal.

---

*Such reports include:
- *Recommended Dietary Allowances.*
- *Healthy People 2000: National Health Promotion and Disease Prevention Objectives.*
- *Diet and Health: Implications for Reducing Chronic Disease Risks.*
- *Surgeon General's Report on Nutrition and Health.*
- *Dietary Guidelines for Americans.*

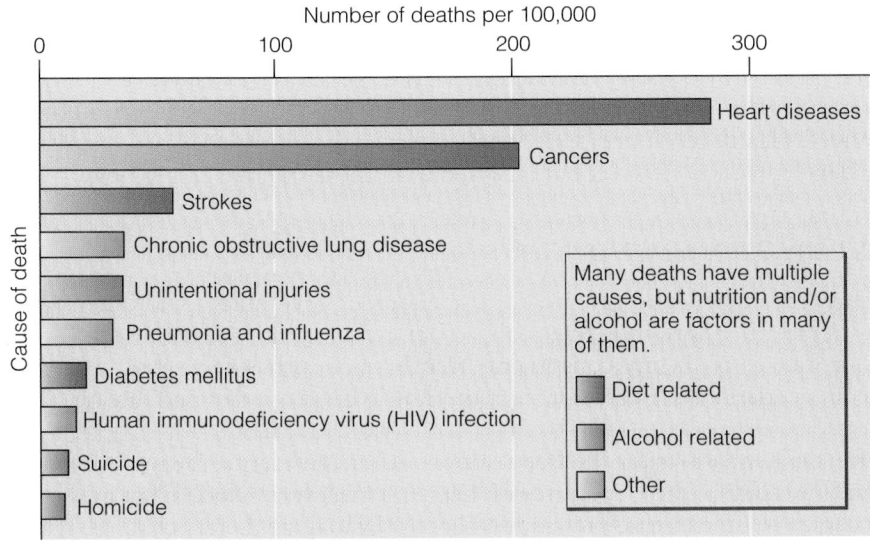

Number of deaths per 100,000

Heart diseases
Cancers
Strokes
Chronic obstructive lung disease
Unintentional injuries
Pneumonia and influenza
Diabetes mellitus
Human immunodeficiency virus (HIV) infection
Suicide
Homicide

Cause of death

Many deaths have multiple causes, but nutrition and/or alcohol are factors in many of them.

☐ Diet related
☐ Alcohol related
☐ Other

Figure 1–6

The Ten Leading Causes of Illness and Death in the United States
Diet influences the development of several chronic diseases—notably, heart disease, some types of cancer, stroke, and diabetes. Taken together, these four diseases account for about two-thirds of the nation's 2 million deaths each year.
Source: National Center for Health Statistics, *Monthly Vital Statistics Report,* October 1994.

disease is great. It does not mean that all people with the risk factor will develop the disease. Similarly, a lack of risk factors does not guarantee freedom from a given disease. On the average, though, the more risk factors in a person's life, the greater that person's chances of developing the disease. Conversely, the fewer risk factors in a person's life, the better the chances for good health.

Risk Factors Persist   Risk factors tend to persist over time. Without intervention, a young adult with high blood pressure will most likely continue to have high blood pressure as an older adult, for example. To minimize the damage, then, early intervention is most effective.

Risk Factors Cluster   Risk factors also tend to cluster. For example, a person who is overweight is likely to be physically inactive, to have high blood pressure, and to have high blood cholesterol—all risk factors associated with heart disease. Intervention that focuses on one risk factor often benefits the others as well. For example, physical activity can help reduce weight. Then both physical activity and weight loss will help to lower blood pressure and blood cholesterol.

Risk Factors in Perspective   Many people live well into their later years. Today's average life expectancy is a record high of 75.5 years.[14] Whether those years are burdened by poor health depends, in part, on personal behaviors.

An estimated half of all deaths each year can be attributed to specific risk factors, many of which reflect personal behaviors.[15] The most prominent factor contributing to death in the United States is tobacco use, followed by diet and activity patterns and alcohol use (see Table 1–1). The 1988 *Surgeon General's Report* concluded that for the two out of three Americans who do not smoke or drink alcohol excessively, the one choice that can influence long-term health prospects more than any other is diet.[16]

Some risk factors, such as smoking, dietary habits, physical activity, and alcohol consumption, are personal behaviors that can be changed. Decisions to not

Table 1–1

Actual Causes of Death in the United States (1990)

Cause	Percentage of Total Deaths
Tobacco	19
Diet/activity	14
Alcohol	5
Microbial agents	4
Toxic agents	3
Firearms	2
Sexual behavior	1
Motor vehicles	1
Illicit drugs	<1
Total	50

Source: J. M. McGinnis and W. H. Foege, Actual causes of death in the United States, *Journal of the American Medical Association* 270 (1993): 2207–2212.

smoke, to eat a well-balanced diet, to engage in regular physical activity, and to drink alcohol in moderation (if at all) improve the likelihood that a person will enjoy good health. Other risk factors, such as genetics, sex, and age, also play important roles in the development of chronic diseases, but they cannot be changed. Health recommendations acknowledge the influence of such factors on the development of disease, but must focus on those that are changeable.

DIETARY RECOMMENDATIONS

Dietary recommendations represent the efforts of government and other agencies to meet the last of the five goals set out earlier (p. 14): to define upper limits for intakes of dietary constituents that harm health when eaten in excess. Recommendations are based on current knowledge about diet and disease.

Several agencies have published similar sets of recommendations, which differ only slightly in detail. The *Diet, Nutrition, and Prevention of Chronic Diseases* report from WHO is presented in Appendix G.

Recommendations for the Population   After considering the results of more than 7000 studies, the Committee on Diet and Health concluded that most people can gain some disease-prevention benefits by making dietary changes.[17] The *Diet and Health* recommendations are intended to be used together with the RDA in planning diets (see Table 1–2).[18] The RDA are aimed at maintaining health and provide guidelines for energy and nutrient intakes. The *Diet and Health* recommendations are aimed at reducing disease risks and describe the kinds of foods people should include, limit, or avoid. They also address weight maintenance and exercise and pinpoint trouble areas surrounding specific nutrients. Like the *Diet and Health* report, the *Nutrition Recommendations for Canadians* report makes recommendations that will supply enough nutrients, while reducing the risk of chronic disease (see Table 1–3).

Several of the *Diet and Health* recommendations are aimed at weight control: cut fat, add complex carbohydrates, and balance food intake with activity. Obesity is common in this country, and it is linked with most of the chronic diseases that threaten life. The problems of overweight people multiply when medical problems develop. For example, overweight people readily develop diabetes, which is often accompanied by high blood pressure and high blood cholesterol. Such a combination of problems may require only one treatment: lose the excess weight by adopting a healthful diet combined with regular exercise.

Recommendations that urge all people to make dietary changes believed to forestall or prevent diseases are taking a preventive or population approach. Alternatively, recommendations that urge dietary changes only for people who are known to need them are taking a medical or individual approach.

The *Diet and Health* recommendations are aimed at the general population in the hope that all people at all levels of risk may benefit. Such a strategy is similar to national efforts to vaccinate to prevent polio, fluoridate water to prevent dental caries, and fortify grains to prevent iron deficiency.

Recommendations for Individuals   People's hereditary susceptibility to diseases and their responsiveness to dietary measures vary. Unlike nutrient-deficiency diseases, which develop when nutrients are lacking and disappear when the nutrients are provided, chronic diseases are neither caused nor prevented by diet alone. Many people have followed dietary advice and developed heart disease or cancer anyway; others have ignored all advice and lived long and healthy lives. For many people, though, diet does influence the time of onset and course of some chronic diseases, and many health care professionals urge dietary measures as part of a disease-prevention strategy. The recommendations were established for "the potential public health benefit, and the likelihood of minimal risk."[19]

Table 1–2

Diet and Health Recommendations

- Reduce total *fat* intake to 30 percent or less of kcalories. Reduce saturated fatty acid intake to less than 10 percent of kcalories and the intake of cholesterol to less than 300 milligrams daily.
- Increase intake of starches and other *complex carbohydrates*.
- Maintain *protein* intake at moderate levels.
- Balance food intake and physical activity to maintain appropriate *body weight*.
- For those who drink *alcoholic beverages*, limit consumption to the equivalent of less than 1 ounce of pure alcohol in a single day. Pregnant women should avoid alcoholic beverages.
- Limit total daily intake of *salt* (sodium chloride) to 6 grams or less.
- Maintain adequate *calcium* intake.
- Avoid taking dietary *supplements* in excess of the RDA in any one day.
- Maintain an optimal intake of *fluoride*, particularly during the years of primary and secondary tooth formation and growth.

Note: Italics added to highlight the areas of concern.
Source: Adapted from the Committee on Diet and Health, *Diet and Health: Implications for Reducing Chronic Disease Risk* (Washington, D.C.: National Academy Press, 1989).

Table 1–3

Nutrition Recommendations for Canadians

- The Canadian diet should provide energy consistent with the maintenance of *body weight* within the recommended range.
- The Canadian diet should include *essential nutrients* in amounts recommended.
- The Canadian diet should include no more than 30 percent of energy as *fat* (33 grams/1000 kcalories or 39 grams/5000 kilojoules) and no more than 10 percent as saturated fat (11 grams/1000 kcalories or 13 grams/5000 kilojoules).
- The Canadian diet should provide 55 percent of energy as *carbohydrate* (138 grams/1000 kcalories or 165 grams/5000 kilojoules) from a variety of sources.
- The *sodium* content of the Canadian diet should be reduced.
- The Canadian diet should include no more than 5 percent of total energy as *alcohol*, or two drinks daily, whichever is less.
- The Canadian diet should contain no more *caffeine* than the equivalent of four regular cups of coffee per day.
- Community water supplies containing less than 1 milligram per liter should be *fluoridated* to that level.

Note: Italics added to highlight areas of concern.
Source: Health and Welfare Canada, *Nutrition Recommendations: The Report of the Scientific Review Committee* (Ottawa: Canadian Government Publishing Centre, 1990).

To determine whether dietary recommendations are important to you personally, look at your family history to see which diseases are common to your relatives. In addition, examine your personal history, taking note of your blood pressure, blood test results, and lifestyle habits such as smoking.

In conclusion, diet is one of several factors that can influence the development of chronic diseases. To have the greatest impact possible, dietary recommendations are aimed at the entire population, and not just at the individuals who might benefit most. Recommendations focus on weight control and urge people to limit fat, increase complex carbohydrates, and balance food intake with activity.

The next several chapters will provide many more details about the nutrients and how they support health. Whenever appropriate, they will show how diet influences each of today's major diseases. The *Diet and Health* recommendations will appear again and again, as each nutrient's relationships with health are explored. Most people who follow the recommendations will benefit and can enjoy good health into their later years.

Study Questions

These questions will help you review the chapter.

1. Give several reasons (and examples) why people make the food choices that they do.
2. What is a nutrient? Name the six classes of nutrients found in foods. What is an essential nutrient?
3. Which nutrients are inorganic, and which are organic? Discuss the significance of that distinction.
4. Which nutrients yield energy, and how much energy do they yield per gram? How is energy measured?
5. Describe how alcohol resembles nutrients. Why is alcohol not considered a nutrient?
6. What is the science of nutrition? Describe the types of research studies and methods used in acquiring nutrition information.
7. Explain how variables may be correlational but not causal.
8. What factors must be included in the full definition of a healthy diet? Which are covered by the RDA?
9. What are the RDA? Who develops the RDA? To whom do they apply? How are they used? In your description, address the issues of whether the RDA represent minimum requirements, whether the RDA need to be met daily, and whether the RDA apply to individuals.
10. What judgment factors are involved in setting the energy and nutrient intake recommendations?
11. What balance of energy-yielding nutrients is recommended to meet energy needs?
12. What happens when people get either too little or too much energy or nutrients? Define malnutrition, undernutrition, and overnutrition. Describe the four methods used to detect energy and nutrient deficiencies and excesses.
13. What methods are used in nutrition surveys? What kinds of information can these surveys provide?
14. Describe the differences between the population approach and the individual approach to making dietary recommendations. Which approach do today's dietary recommendations take?
15. What recommendations are made in the *Diet and Health* report?

Notes

1. G. A. Falciglia and P. A. Norton, Evidence for a genetic influence on preference for some foods, *Journal of the American Dietetic Association* 94 (1994): 154–158.
2. I. M. Parraga, Determinants of food consumption, *Journal of the American Dietetic Association* 90 (1990): 661–663.
3. A. E. Harper, 1990 Atwater lecture—The science and the practice of nutrition: Reflections and directions, *American Journal of Clinical Nutrition* 53 (1991): 413–420.
4. Committee on Dietary Allowances, *Recommended Dietary Allowances,* 10th ed. (Washington, D.C.: National Academy Press, 1989).
5. Committee on Dietary Allowances, 1989, pp. 8–9.
6. P. Lachance and L. Langseth, The RDA concept: Time for a change? *Nutrition Reviews* 52 (1994): 266–270.
7. L. J. Machlin and H. E. Sauberlich, New views on the function and health effects of vitamins, *Nutrition Today,* January/February 1994, pp. 25–29.
8. How should the Recommended Dietary Allowances be revised? A concept paper from the Food and Nutrition Board, (Washington, D.C.: National Academy Press, 1994).
9. ADA testifies on need for revised RDAs, *Journal of the American Dietetic Association* 93 (1993): 864.
10. *Healthy People 2000: National Health Promotion and Disease Prevention Objectives* (Washington, D.C.: U.S. Department of Health and Human Services, 1990).
11. Ten-year comprehensive plan for the national nutrition monitoring and related research program, *Federal Register,* June 11, 1993.
12. J. M. McGinnis and P. R. Lee, *Healthy People 2000* at mid decade, *Journal of the American Medical Association* 273 (1995): 1123–1129.
13. *The Surgeon General's Report on Nutrition and Health: Summary and Recommendations,* DHHS (PHS) publication no. 88–50211 (Washington, D.C.: Government Printing Office, 1988).
14. National Center for Health Statistics, Monthly vital statistics report, August 1993.
15. J. M. McGinnis and W. H. Foege, Actual causes of death in the United States, *Journal of the American Medical Association* 270 (1993): 2207–2212.
16. *The Surgeon General's Report,* 1988.
17. Committee on Diet and Health, *Diet and Health: Implications for Reducing Chronic Disease Risk* (Washington, D.C.: National Academy Press, 1989).
18. Committee on Dietary Allowances, 1989, p. 9.
19. Committee on Diet and Health, 1989, pp. 665–710.

Who Speaks on Nutrition?

People are bombarded by nutrition news as they read newspapers, turn the pages of magazines, talk with friends, and watch television. Today, more than ever before, people want to know what nutrition news they can believe and safely use. They want to know how best to take care of themselves. Some people seek miracles: tricks to help them lose weight, foods to forestall aging, and supplements to prevent baldness. People's heightened interests in nutrition and health translate into billions of dollars spent on services and products peddled by both legitimate and fraudulent businesses. While consumers who obtain legitimate health care can improve their health, those enticed into scams may lose their health, their savings, or both. Unfortunately, fraudulent health care, most of it related to nutrition, rings cash registers to the tune of $25 billion annually.[1] Ironically, nutrition quackery prevents people from attaining the health they are searching for by giving them false hope and delaying effective strategies.

Science and quackery may be easy to tell apart at the extremes, but an abundance of nutrition information lies between the extremes. How can people distinguish valid nutrition information from misinformation? One excellent approach is to notice who is purveying the information. If an instructor at the gym praises a high-protein diet, or the author of a magazine article recommends eating three pineapples a day to lose weight, or a health-store clerk suggests an amino acid supplement, should you believe these peo-

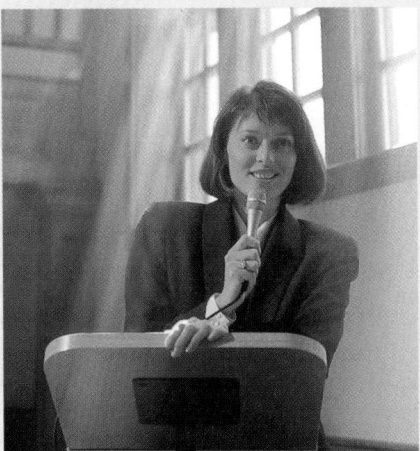

The quality of nutrition information depends on the provider's knowledge and credentials.

ple? What qualifies them to give nutrition advice? When you are confused or need sound dietary advice, whom should you ask?

IDENTIFYING NUTRITION EXPERTS

Most people turn to their physicians for dietary advice. Physicians are expected to know all about health-related matters—but are they the best sources of accurate and current information on *nutrition*? Only about one-fourth of all medical schools in the United States require students to take even one nutrition course.[2] Students attending these classes receive an average of 20 hours of nutrition instruction—an amount they themselves consider inadequate.[3] (By comparison, most students reading this text are taking a nutrition class that provides an average of 45 hours of instruction.) Many experts call for nutrition to play a much larger role in the medical curriculum, but they acknowl-

edge that the curriculum already carries a heavy burden. They prefer to integrate nutrition into already-existing courses such as biochemistry, microbiology, and physiology. Then clinical dietetics could be presented in the same way clinical pharmacology is taught, and community dietetics could be incorporated into public health courses.[4]

In 1990, Congress passed a law mandating that:

> Students enrolled in United States medical schools and physicians practicing in the United States [must] have access to adequate training in the field of nutrition and its relationship to human health.[5]

Plans are in the works to make nutrition education a standard course in medical schools. The American Dietetic Association (ADA) supports the inclusion of nutrition education as an essential component at all levels of medical education.[6] Furthermore, the ADA asserts that standardized nutrition education should be included in the curricula for all health care professionals: physician's assistants, dental hygienists, physical and occupational therapists, social workers, and all others who provide services directly to clients.[7] When these professionals have command of reliable nutrition information, then all the people they serve will also be better informed.

Most physicians appreciate the connections between health and nutrition. Those who have specialized in clinical nutrition are especially well qualified to speak on the subject. Membership in the American Society for Clinical Nutrition, whose journal is cited many times throughout this text, is another sign

Glossary

accredited: approved; in the case of medical centers or universities, certified by an agency recognized by the U.S. Department of Education.

American Dietetic Association (ADA): the professional organization of dietitians in the United States. The Canadian equivalent is the Dietitians of Canada (DC), which operates similarly.

correspondence school: a school that offers courses and degrees by mail. Some correspondence schools are accredited; others are *diploma mills*.

dietetic technician registered (DTR): a person with an associate's degree and training in nutrition, food science, and diet planning who works under the guidance of an RD (registered dietitian).

dietitian: a person trained in nutrition, food science, and diet planning. See also *registered dietitian*.

DTR: see *dietetic technician registered*.

fraud or quackery: the promotion, for financial gain, of devices, treatments, services, plans, or products (including diets and supplements) that alter or claim to alter a human condition without proof of safety or effectiveness. (The word *quackery* comes from the term *quacksalver*, meaning a person who quacks loudly about a miracle product—a lotion or a salve.)

license to practice: permission under state or federal law, granted on meeting specified criteria, to use a certain title (such as dietitian) and offer certain services. Licensed dietitians may use the initials LD after their names.

misinformation: false or misleading information.

nutritionist: a person who specializes in the study of nutrition. Some nutritionists are registered dietitians, whereas others are self-described experts whose training is questionable. In states with responsible legislation, the term applies only to people who have MS or PhD degrees from properly accredited institutions.

public health nutritionist: a dietitian who specializes in public health nutrition.

RD: see *registered dietitian*.

registered dietitian (RD): a dietitian who has graduated from a university or college after completing a program of dietetics that has been accredited by the American Dietetic Association (or Dietitians of Canada), has served in an internship or coordinated program to practice the necessary skills, has passed the association's registration examination, and maintains competency through continuing education. Many states require licensing for practicing dietitians.

registration: listing; with respect to health professionals, listing with a professional organization that requires specific course work, experience, and passing of an examination.

ADA;* and maintain up-to-date knowledge by participating in required continuing education activities: attending seminars, taking courses, or writing professional papers. Meeting these established criteria certifies that a dietitian is a true nutrition authority.

Dietitians perform a multitude of duties in many settings in most communities.[†] They work in the food industry, in pharmaceutical companies, in home health agencies, in long-term care institutions, in private practice, in public health departments, in research centers, in education settings, in fitness centers, and in hospitals.

Dietitians can assume a number of different job responsibilities depending on their work settings and positions.[8] In hospitals, administrative dietitians manage the food-service system; clinical dietitians provide client care (see Table H1–1); and nutrition support team dietitians coordinate nutrition care with other health care professionals. In the food industry, dietitians conduct research, develop products, and market services.

Public health dietitians who work in government-funded agencies play a key role in delivering nutrition services to people in the community.[9] Among their many roles, public health nutritionists

of nutrition knowledge. Still, few physicians have the time or experience to develop diet plans and provide detailed diet instructions for clients. Often physicians wisely refer their clients to qualified nutrition experts—registered dietitians (RD).

A registered dietitian has the educational background necessary to deliver reliable nutrition advice and care. To become an RD, a person must earn an undergraduate degree requiring some 60 or so semester hours in nutrition and food science; complete a year's clinical internship or the equivalent; pass a national examination administered over five competency areas by the

*The five content areas included on the registration examination for dietitians are nutrition services, foodservice systems, management, education and communication, and evaluation and standards. L. C. Webb and J. O. Maillet, The development of test specifications for the registration examinations, *Journal of the American Dietetic Association* 90 (1990): 1134–1135.

†To find a registered dietitian in your area, call the American Dietetic Association hotline: (800) 366–1655.

Table H1–1

● ● ● ● ● ● ● ● ● ● ● ● ●

Responsibilities of a Clinical Dietitian

- Assesses clients' nutrition status.
- Determines clients' nutrient requirements.
- Monitors clients' nutrient intakes.
- Develops, implements, and evaluates clients' nutrition care plans.
- Counsels clients to cope with unique diet plans.
- Teaches clients and their families about nutrition and diet plans.
- Provides training for other dietitians, nurses, interns, and dietetics students.
- Serves as liaison between clients and the foodservice department.
- Communicates with physicians, nurses, pharmacists, and other health care professionals about clients' progress, needs, and treatments. (Highlight 17 describes the team approach and some of the responsibilities of health care team members.)
- Participates in professional activities to enhance knowledge and skill.

help plan, coordinate, and evaluate food assistance programs; act as consultants to other agencies; manage finances; and much more.[10] Those with advanced degrees in public health are well placed for employment in this vast field.

In some facilities, dietetic technicians assist registered dietitians in both administrative and clinical responsibilities. A dietetic technician has been educated and trained to work under the guidance of a registered dietitian.

Other dietary employees may include clerks, aides, cooks, porters, and other assistants. These dietary employees do not have extensive formal training in nutrition, and their ability to provide accurate information may be limited.

IDENTIFYING FAKE CREDENTIALS

In contrast to registered dietitians, thousands of people possess fake nutrition degrees and claim to be nutrition counselors, nutritionists, or "dietists." These and other such titles may sound meaningful, but most of these people lack the established credentials and training of the ADA-sanctioned dietitian. If you look closely, you can see signs of their fake expertise.

Take, for example, a nutrition expert's educational background. The minimal standards of education for a dietitian specify a bachelor of science (BS) degree in food science and human nutrition or related fields from an accredited college or university. Such a degree generally requires four to five years of study. In contrast, a fake nutrition expert may display a degree from a six-month correspondence course. Such a degree simply falls short.* In some cases, schools posing as legitimate correspondence schools offer even less—they sell certificates to anyone who pays the fees. To obtain these "degrees," a candi-

date need not read any books or pass any examinations.†

To guard educational quality, an accrediting agency recognized by the U.S. Department of Education (DOE) certifies that certain schools meet criteria established to ensure that an institution provides complete and accurate schooling. Unfortunately, fake nutrition degrees are available from schools "accredited" by more than 30 phony accrediting agencies.**

To dramatize the ease with which anyone can obtain a fake nutrition degree, one writer enrolled in a correspondence course for a fee of $82. She made every attempt to fail, intentionally answering all examination questions incorrectly. Even so, she received a "nutritionist" certificate at the end of the course. The "school" explained that it was sure she must have just misread the test.

In a similar stunt, Ms. Sassafras Herbert was named a "professional member" of a professional association. For her efforts, Sassafras has received a wallet card and is listed in a sort of fake *Who's Who* in nutrition that is distributed at health fairs and trade shows nationwide. Sassafras is a poodle; her master,

---

*To find out whether a correspondence school is accredited, write the Distance Education and Training Council, Accrediting Commission, 1601 Eighteenth Street, N.W., Washington, D.C. 20009, or call (202) 234–5100.

†To find out whether a school is properly accredited for a dietetics degree, write the American Dietetic Association, Division of Education and Research, 216 West Jackson Boulevard, Chicago, IL 60606, or call (312) 899–4870.

**The American Council on Education publishes a directory of accredited institutions, professionally accredited programs, and candidates for accreditation in *Accredited Institutions of Postsecondary Education Programs Candidates* (available from many libraries). For additional information, write the Council on Postsecondary Accreditation, One Dupont Circle, Suite 305, Washington, D.C. 20036, or call (202) 452–1433.

Victor Herbert, MD, paid $50 to prove that she could be awarded these honors merely by sending in her name. Mr. Charlie Herbert, who is also a professional member of such an organization, is a cat.

Some states allow anyone to use the titles *dietitian* or *nutritionist*, but others have responded to the need for professional regulation. Some states allow only RDs or people with certain graduate degrees to call themselves dietitians. Many states now provide a further guarantee: the license to practice.[11] Licensing provides a way to identify people who have met minimal standards of education and experience.

By knowing what qualifies someone to speak on nutrition, consumers can determine whether that person's advice might be harmful or helpful. Don't be afraid to ask for credentials. Does the instructor at the spa have a degree in nutrition from an accredited university? Is the author of the magazine article an RD or otherwise qualified to write on nutrition? Have you seen the health-store clerk's license to practice as a dietitian? If not, seek a better-qualified source. After all, your health depends on it.

IDENTIFYING VALID INFORMATION

Where do nutrition experts get their information? As Chapter 1 explained, nutrition is a science; that is, it derives information from scientific research.

Researchers conduct experiments and then record and analyze their results, exercising caution in their interpretation of the findings. For example, in an epidemiological study, scientists may use a specific segment of the population—say, men 50 to 60 years old. When the

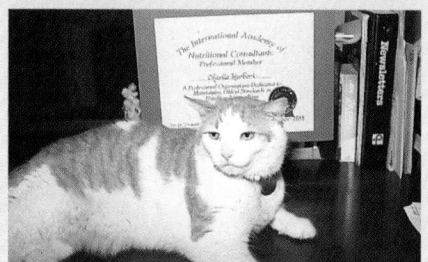

Charlie displays his professional credentials.

scientists draw conclusions, they are careful not to generalize the findings to all people. Similarly, scientists performing research studies using animals are cautious in applying their findings to human beings. Conclusions from any one research study are always tentative and take into account findings from studies conducted by other scientists as well. As evidence accumulates, scientists gain confidence about making recommendations that affect people's health and lives. Still, their statements are worded cautiously, as in "A diet high in fruits and vegetables *may* protect against some cancers."

Quite often, as they approach an answer to one research question, scientists raise several more questions, so future research projects are never lacking. Further scientific investigation then seeks to answer questions such as "What substance or substances within fruits and vegetables provide protection?" If those substances turn out to be the vitamins A and C found so abundantly in fresh produce, then, "how much vitamin A and C is needed to offer protection?" "How do these vitamins protect against cancer?" "Is it their action as antioxidant nutrients?" "If not, might it be another action or even another substance that accounts for the protection fruits and vegetables provide against

cancer?" (Highlight 11 explores the answers to these questions and reviews recent research on antioxidant nutrients and disease.)

The findings from a research study are submitted to a board of reviewers composed of other scientists who rigorously evaluate the study to assure that the scientific method was followed—a process known as peer review. The reviewers critique the study's hypothesis, methodology, statistical significance, and conclusions (Table H1–2 describes the parts of a research article). If the reviewers consider the conclusions to be well supported by the evidence, they endorse the work for publication in a scientific journal where others can read it. The readers can then evaluate the study and assess the findings in light of knowledge gleaned from other studies. Figure H1–1 (on p. 34) provides examples of reliable nutrition information.

Even when a new finding is published, it is still only preliminary, and not very meaningful by itself. Other scientists will need to confirm or disprove the findings through replication. To be accepted into the body of nutrition knowledge, a finding must stand up to rigorous, repeated testing in experiments performed by several different researchers. What we "know" in nutrition results from years of replicating study findings.

With each report from scientists, the field of nutrition changes a little—each finding contributes another piece to the whole body of knowledge. People who know how science works understand that single findings, like single frames in a movie, are just small parts of a larger story. Over years, the picture of what is "true" in nutrition gradually changes, and modifications in recommendations then follow.[12]

Table H1–2
. . . .

Parts of a Research Article

- *Abstract*. The abstract provides a brief overview of the article.
- *Introduction*. The introduction clearly states the purpose of the current study by proposing a hypothesis and provides a comprehensive review of the literature.
- *Review of literature*. The review reveals all that science has uncovered on the subject to date.
- *Methodology*. The methodology section defines key terms and describes the instruments and procedures used in conducting the study.
- *Results*. The results report the findings and may include tables and figures that summarize the information.
- *Conclusions*. The conclusions drawn are those supported by the data and reflect the original purpose as stated in the introduction. Usually, they answer a few questions and raise several more.
- *References*. The references reflect the investigator's knowledge of the subject and should include an extensive list of relevant studies (including key studies several years old as well as current ones).

Instead of eating 4 servings of fruits and vegetables as recommended by the old Four Food Group plan, people are now encouraged to eat 2 to 4 servings of fruits and 3 to 5 servings of vegetables as suggested by the current Daily Food Guide (presented in Chapter 2).

There is much to learn about the effects of foods and nutrients on the body. The media, hungry for the latest news, often report scientific findings prematurely—without benefit of the careful interpretation, replication, and review that evaluate the findings. As a result, the public receives news quickly, but not always in perspective. Oftentimes findings from studies seem to contradict one another, and consumers feel frustrated and betrayed, when, in fact, this is simply the normal course of science at work. Science is constantly building on an already-existing foundation of knowledge.

People who do not understand how science operates may become distrustful as they try to learn nutrition from current news reports: "How am I supposed to know what to eat when the scientists themselves don't know?" General background knowledge about the science of nutrition is the best foundation a person can have for judging the validity of new nutrition information. (Congratulations on your decision to take this course.)

Because science is a step-by-step, information-gathering and testing process, old research still has value. A hypothesis first advanced in 1960 that stands up to decades of validation has real strength. When it comes to scientific information, "new" does not necessarily mean "improved." In fact, any science report based on all new references is suspect, for truly strong research is based on a body of work conducted over many years. This is why, even in books published just this year, you will see references to old reports. Some studies have become classics: they were exciting when they first appeared, and they have stood up to the test of time.

IDENTIFYING QUACKS

Nutrition is a hot topic and scattered among the valid research findings are thousands of unfounded claims. How can a person identify nutrition quackery? Once upon a time, quacks rode into town in wooden wagons hawking snake oil for 50 cents a bottle to "cure what ails you," but those days are gone. Today's purveyors manipulate consumers in less obvious ways. Fraudulent claims may *sound* logical, but they lack the research support found in nutrition science. The following techniques can alert consumers to quackery and misinformation:[13]

- Quacks use anecdotes, case histories, testimonials, and subjective evidence to support their claims.
- Quacks promise quick, dramatic, miraculous cures.
- Quacks use pseudo-medical terms and jargon, which lend a false legitimacy to the claim, confuse the client, and camouflage the lack of substance.
- Quacks display fake credentials.
- Quacks contend that most health problems are caused by poor nutrition and therefore can be corrected with proper nutrition.
- Quacks claim that "natural" vitamins are better than synthetic ones.
- Quacks sometimes recommend eating products derived from animal tissues to rejuvenate the counterpart in a human being.
- Quacks belittle medicine, science, and government regulations, offering "alternatives" that have not been proven safe or effective.

Figure H1–1
. . . .

Sources of Reliable Nutrition Information

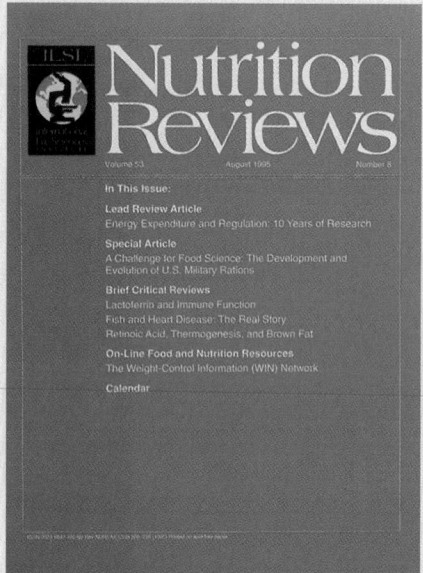

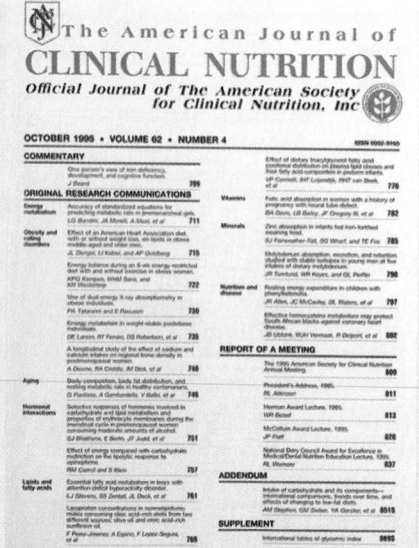

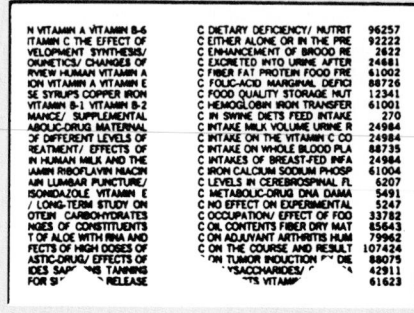

Reviews

Articles that examine all the major work on a subject are published in review journals like *Nutrition Reviews*. These articles provide references to all of the original work reviewed.

Journals

Articles that present all the details of the methods, results, and conclusions of a particular study are published in journals like the *American Journal of Clinical Nutrition*.

Indexes

An index of abstracts directs you to many research articles on a given subject. This index from *Biological Abstracts* lists recently published works on vitamin C.

- Quacks believe that products from health-food stores are better than those from regular grocery stores.
- Quacks oppose public health strategies such as fluoridating the water supply or vaccinating children against infectious diseases.
- Quacks claim that food processing and storage destroy all nutrients.
- Quacks depict food additives as poisons responsible for a variety of problems—from misbehavior to murder.
- Quacks insist that stress and other conditions raise nutrient needs higher than can be met by foods alone.

- Quacks make claims that people want to hear but that are too good to be true—such as that vitamin and mineral supplements will prevent cancer.
- Quacks use hair analysis and other unproven diagnostic tests to detect "alleged" nutrient deficiencies.
- Quacks profit from the sales of the products they are advocating.
- Quacks claim sugar is a poison.
- Quacks diagnose "nutrient deficiencies" by computerized questionnaires.
- Quacks advocate restrictive fad diets for a variety of health conditions.

- Quacks portray physicians as money-grabbing, incompetent misfits who are not to be trusted.

In short, quackery respects neither science nor honesty in its pursuit of ill-gotten gains.

In summary, when you hear nutrition news, consider its source. Ask yourself these two questions: Is the person purveying the information qualified to speak on nutrition? Is the information based on valid scientific research? To check an "expert's" qualifications, first look for the degrees and credentials listed by the person's name (such as MS, PhD, RD, or MD). Then find out

How to Find Credible Sources of Nutrition Information

Government health agencies, volunteer health agencies, consumer groups, and professional health organizations provide consumers with reliable health and nutrition information. Credible sources of nutrition information include:

- Government health agencies such as the Federal Trade Commission (FTC), the U.S. Department of Health and Human Services (DHHS), the Food and Drug Administration (FDA), and the U.S. Department of Agriculture (USDA).
- Local agencies such as the County Cooperative Extension Service.
- Nutrition and food science departments at a university or community college.
- Volunteer health agencies such as the American Cancer Society, the American Diabetes Association, and the American Heart Association.
- Reputable consumer groups such as the Better Business Bureau, the Consumers Union, the American Council on Science and Health, and the National Council Against Health Fraud.
- Professional health organizations such as the American Dietetic Association, the Society for Nutrition Education, and the American Medical Association.
- Journals such as the *American Journal of Clinical Nutrition*, *Journal of the American Dietetic Association*, and *Nutrition Reviews*.

Appendix F provides addresses for these and other organizations.

Source: Adapted from Position of The American Dietetic Association: Food and nutrition misinformation, *Journal of the American Dietetic Association* 95 (1995): 705–707.

about the reputation of the institution that awarded each degree. Call and ask your state's health-licensing agency if dietitians are licensed in your state and (if so) if the person giving you dietary advice has met licensing criteria. If not, find someone better qualified, for your health is your most precious asset.

NOTES

1. M. E. Shils, Separating food facts and myths, in *The Mount Sinai School of Medicine Complete Book of Nutrition*, eds. V. Herbert and G. J. Subak-Sharpe (New York: St. Martin's Press, 1990), pp. 21–29.

2. M. E. Shils, National Dairy Council award for excellence in medical and dental nutrition education lecture, 1994: Nutrition education in medical schools—The prospect before us, *American Journal of Clinical Nutrition* 60 (1994): 631–638.

3. A. G. Swanson, 1990 ASCN Nutrition educators' symposium and information exchange: Nutrition sciences in medical-student education, *American Journal of Clinical Nutrition* 53 (1991): 587–588.

4. D. S. McLaren, Nutrition in medical schools: A case of mistaken identity, *American Journal of Clinical Nutrition* 59 (1994): 960–963.

5. National Nutrition Monitoring and Related Research Act of 1990, public law 101–445, as quoted in C. H. Halstead, Toward standardized training of physicians in clinical nutrition, *American Journal of Clinical Nutrition* 56 (1992): 1–3.

6. Position of The American Dietetic Association: Nutrition—An essential component of medical education, *Journal of the American Dietetic Association* 94 (1994): 555–557.

7. Position of The American Dietetic Association: Nutrition education of health professionals, *Journal of the American Dietetic Association* 91 (1991): 611–613.

8. M. T. Kane and coauthors, Role delineation for dietetic practitioners: Empirical results, *Journal of the American Dietetic Association* 90 (1990): 1124–1133.

9. M. C. Egan, Public health nutrition: A historical perspective, *Journal of the American Dietetic Association* 94 (1994): 298–302.

10. B. Haughton and J. Shaw, Functional roles of today's public health nutritionist, *Journal of the American Dietetic Association* 92 (1992): 1218–1222.

11. Licensure of dietitians and nutritionists: Update on state laws, *Journal of the American Dietetic Association* 94 (1994): 974.

12. K. McNutt, Where truth comes from, *Nutrition Today*, March/April 1994, pp. 43–48.

13. Adapted with permission from Thirty ways to spot quacks and pushers, in S. Barrett and V. Herbert, *The Vitamin Pushers: How the "Health Food" Industry Is Selling America a Bill of Goods* (Amherst, N.Y.: Prometheus Books, 1994), pp. 15–35.

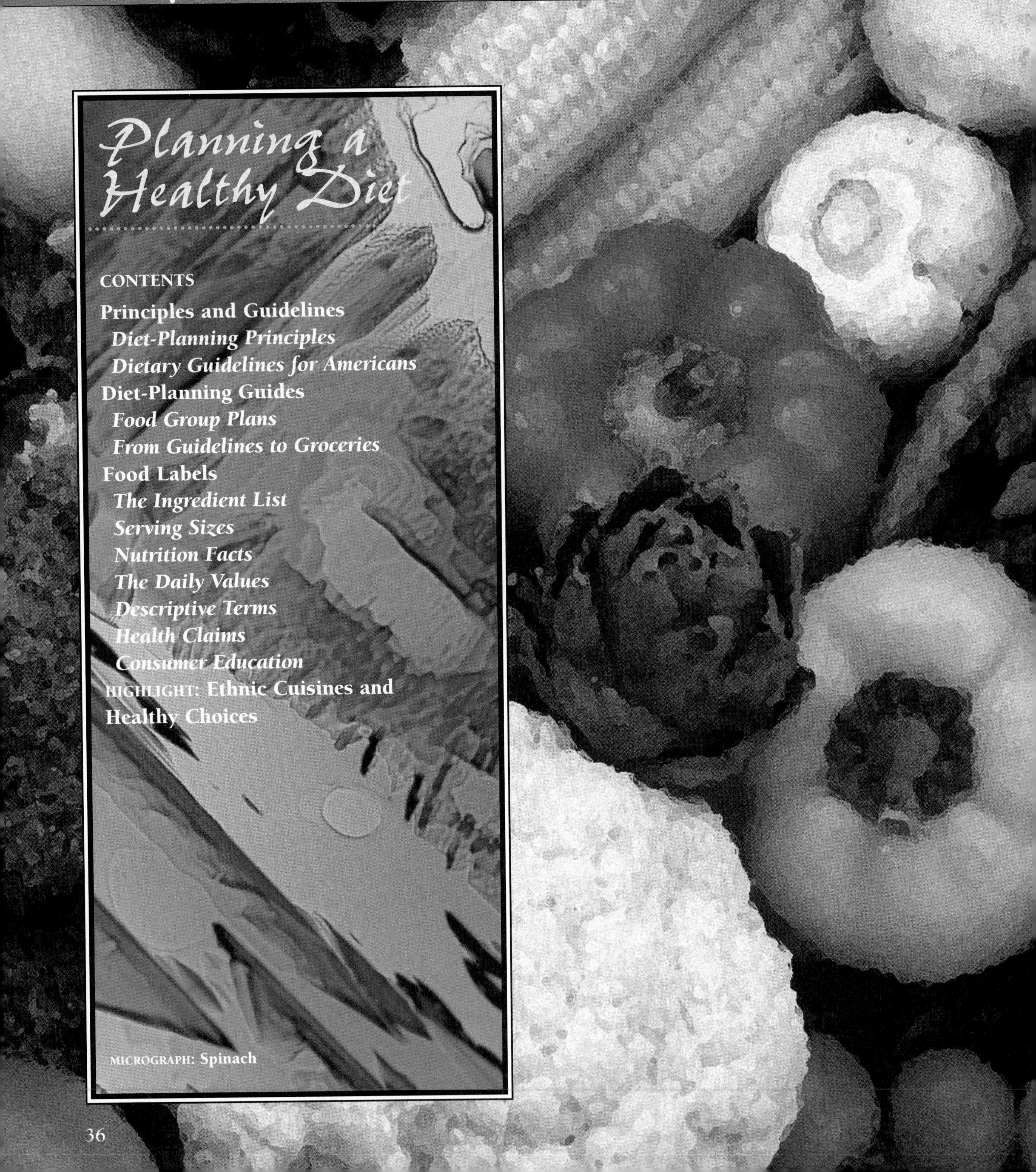

Chapter 2

Planning a Healthy Diet

CONTENTS

Principles and Guidelines
Diet-Planning Principles
Dietary Guidelines for Americans
Diet-Planning Guides
Food Group Plans
From Guidelines to Groceries
Food Labels
The Ingredient List
Serving Sizes
Nutrition Facts
The Daily Values
Descriptive Terms
Health Claims
Consumer Education
HIGHLIGHT: **Ethnic Cuisines and Healthy Choices**

MICROGRAPH: **Spinach**

Chapter 1 explained that the body's many activities are supported by the array of nutrients delivered by the foods people eat. Food choices made over years influence the body's health, and consistently poor choices increase the risks of developing chronic diseases. This chapter attempts to show how a person can select from the tens of thousands of foods available to create a diet that supports health. In a way, the task sounds simple: just select foods that will provide all the needed nutrients. On learning that an adult needs 60 milligrams of vitamin C a day, an enthusiastic novice might buy an orange. To get the needed milligram of thiamin, the person might add ten slices of bread. This approach quickly runs into trouble, though. Faced with the need for 40-odd nutrients, a person who selected one type of food for each nutrient would soon have a basket of 40 different foods, and thousands too many kcalories to eat in a day. Fortunately, most foods provide several nutrients, so one trick for wise diet planning is to select a combination of foods that deliver a full array of nutrients. This chapter begins with an introduction of the diet-planning principles and dietary guidelines that assist people in selecting foods that will deliver nutrients without excess energy.

Principles and Guidelines

How well you nourish yourself does not depend on the selection of any one food. Instead it depends on the selection of many different foods at numerous meals, over days, months, and years. Diet-planning principles and dietary guidelines are key concepts to keep in mind whenever you are selecting foods—whether shopping at the grocery store, choosing from a restaurant menu, or preparing a home-cooked meal.

DIET-PLANNING PRINCIPLES

Diet planners have developed several ways to select foods. Whatever plan or combination of plans they use, though, they keep in mind the six basic diet-planning principles listed in the margin.

Adequacy The RDA discussion in Chapter 1 was all about dietary adequacy. An adequate diet provides sufficient energy and enough of all the nutrients to meet the needs of healthy people. Take the essential nutrient iron, for example. Each day the body loses some iron, so people have to replace it by eating foods that contain iron. A person whose diet fails to provide enough iron-rich foods may develop the symptoms of iron-deficiency anemia: the person may feel weak, tired, and listless; have frequent headaches; and find that even the smallest amount of muscular work brings disabling fatigue. To prevent these deficiency symptoms, diet planners include foods that supply adequate iron. The same is true for all the other essential nutrients introduced in Chapter 1.

Balance The essential minerals calcium and iron, taken together, illustrate the importance of dietary balance. Meats, fish, and poultry are rich in iron but poor in calcium. Similarly, milk and milk products are rich in calcium but poor in iron. In fact, milk (except breast milk) and milk products are so low in iron that overuse of these foods can actually lead to iron-deficiency anemia by

Diet-planning principles:
- **A**dequacy.
- **B**alance.
- **k**Calorie (energy) control.
- **N**utrient **D**ensity.
- **M**oderation.
- **V**ariety.

adequacy (dietary): providing all the essential nutrients, fiber, and energy in amounts sufficient to maintain health.

balance (dietary): providing foods of a number of types in proportion to each other, such that foods rich in some nutrients do not crowd out the diet foods that are rich in other nutrients.

displacing iron-rich foods from the diet. Yet milk is the single most nutritious food for infants and can be an important source of calcium for people of all ages.

The art of balancing the diet involves using enough—but not too much—of each type of food. Use some meat or meat alternates for iron; use some milk and milk products for calcium; and save some space for other foods, too, since a diet consisting of milk and meat alone would not be adequate. For the other nutrients, people need vegetables, fruits, and grains.

kCalorie (Energy) Control   Clearly, the task of designing an adequate, balanced diet requires some thought and skillful planning. Even more thought and skill are required to create an adequate, balanced diet without overeating. The discussion of weight control in Chapter 9 examines this issue in more detail, but the key to controlling energy intake is to select foods of high nutrient density.

Nutrient Density   To eat well without overeating, select foods that deliver the most nutrients for the least food energy. Consider foods containing calcium, for example. You can get about 300 milligrams of calcium from either 1½ ounces of cheddar cheese or 8 ounces of nonfat milk, but the cheese contributes about twice as much food energy as the milk. The nonfat milk, then, is twice as calcium dense as the cheddar cheese; it offers the same amount of calcium for half the energy intake. Both foods are excellent choices for adequacy's sake alone, but to achieve adequacy while controlling kcalories, the nonfat milk is the better choice.

Just like a person who has to pay for rent, food, clothes, and tuition on a tight budget, a person whose energy allowance is limited has to obtain iron, calcium, and all the other essential nutrients on a tight energy budget. To succeed, the person has to get many nutrients for each kcalorie "dollar." In the cola and watermelon example in the margin, both provide about the same number of kcalories, but the watermelon delivers many more nutrients. A person who makes nutrient-dense choices such as fruit over cola can meet daily nutrient needs on a lower energy budget.

Moderation   Foods rich in fat and sugar provide enjoyment and energy, but relatively few nutrients. In addition, they promote weight gain when eaten in excess. A person practicing moderation would eat such foods only on occasion and would regularly select foods low in fat and sugar, a practice that automatically improves nutrient density. Returning to the example of cheddar cheese and nonfat milk, the nonfat milk not only offers the same amount of calcium for less energy, but it contains far less fat than the cheese.

Variety   A diet may have all of the virtues just described and still lack variety, if a person eats the same foods day after day. People should select foods from each of the food groups daily. Diets that omit several food groups are associated with an increased risk of mortality.[1] Furthermore, people should vary their choices within each food group from day to day for several reasons. First, different foods within the same group contain different arrays of nutrients. Among the fruits, for example, strawberries are especially rich in vitamin C while cantaloupes are rich in vitamin A. Second, no food is guaranteed entirely free of substances that, in excess, could be harmful. The strawberries might contain trace amounts of one contaminant, the cantaloupes another. By alternating fruit

---

Balance in the diet helps to ensure adequacy.

kcalorie (energy) control: management of food energy intake.

nutrient density: a measure of the nutrients a food provides relative to the energy it provides. The more nutrients and the fewer kcalories, the higher the nutrient density.

Nutrient density promotes adequacy and kcalorie control.

moderation: in relation to dietary intake, providing enough but not too much of a substance.

Moderation contributes to adequacy, balance, and kcalorie control.

variety (dietary): eating a wide selection of foods within and among the major food groups (the opposite of monotony).

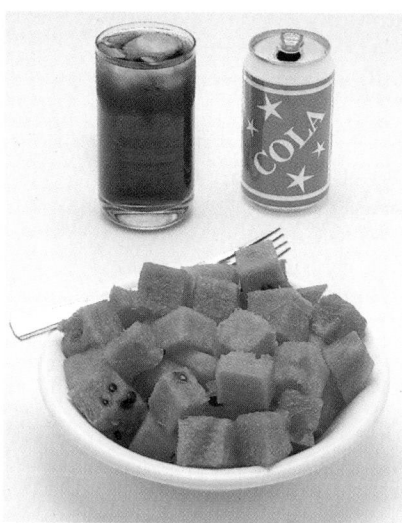

This cola and bowl of watermelon illustrate nutrient density. Each provides about 150 kcalories, but the watermelon offers a little protein, some vitamins, minerals, and fiber along with the energy; the cola beverage offers only "empty" kcalories. Watermelon, or any fruit for that matter, is more nutrient dense than cola beverages.

choices, a person will ingest very little of either contaminant. (Contamination of foods is the subject of Chapter 14.) Stated another way, variety within the diet helps ensure dilution of contaminants. Third, as the adage goes, variety is the spice of life. Even if a person eats beans frequently, the person can choose pinto beans in Mexican chili today, garbanzo beans in Greek salad tomorrow, and baked beans with barbecued chicken on the weekend. Eating nutritious meals need never be boring.

DIETARY GUIDELINES FOR AMERICANS

The *Dietary Guidelines for Americans* coordinate the health recommendations introduced in Chapter 1 with the diet-planning principles just presented. For example, they combine the recommendation to "increase intake of starches and complex carbohydrates" with the principle of variety, offering the practical advice to "choose a diet with plenty of grain products, vegetables, and fruits." In general, the *Dietary Guidelines* answer the question, What should an individual eat to stay healthy?

Table 2–1 presents the 1995 *Dietary Guidelines.* The first two guidelines encourage people to eat a variety of foods to get the nutrients needed to support good health and to balance food intake with physical activity in order to maintain or improve body weight. The next two guidelines urge a shift in the balance of energy nutrients: they encourage people to increase their carbohydrate intakes and reduce their fat intakes by choosing a diet that is abundant in grains, vegetables, and fruits and low in fat, saturated fat, and cholesterol. The last three guidelines recommend a diet moderate in sugars, salt and sodium, and alcoholic beverages for those who partake. Together, these seven guidelines point the way toward better health. Table 2–2 presents *Canada's Guidelines for Healthy Eating.*

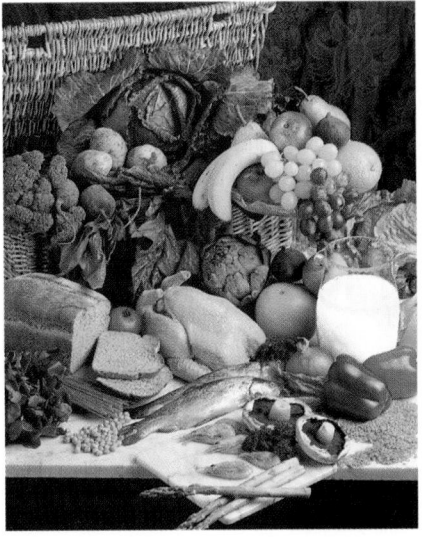

To ensure an adequate and balanced diet, eat a variety of foods daily, choosing different foods from each group.

Table 2–1

Dietary Guidelines for Americans

- Eat a variety of foods.
- Balance the food you eat with physical activity; maintain or improve your weight.
- Choose a diet with plenty of grain products, vegetables, and fruits.
- Choose a diet low in fat, saturated fat, and cholesterol.
- Choose a diet moderate in sugars.
- Choose a diet moderate in salt and sodium.
- If you drink alcoholic beverages, do so in moderation.

Note: These guidelines are designed for healthy people over two years old.
Source: The *Dietary Guidelines for Americans* are developed by the U.S. Department of Agriculture and the U.S. Department of Health and Human Services.

Table 2–2

Canada's Guidelines for Healthy Eating

- Enjoy a variety of foods.
- Emphasize cereals, breads, other grain products, vegetables, and fruits.
- Choose lower-fat dairy products, leaner meats, and foods prepared with little or no fat.
- Achieve and maintain a healthy body weight by enjoying regular physical activity and healthy eating.
- Limit salt, alcohol, and caffeine.

Source: These guidelines derive from *Action Towards Healthy Eating: The Report of the Communications/Implementation Committee* and *Nutrition Recommendations . . . . A Call for Action: Summary Report of the Scientific Review Committee and the Communications/Implementation Committee,* which are available from Branch Publications Unit, Health Services and Promotion Branch, Department of Health and Welfare, 5th Floor, Jeanne Mance Building, Ottawa, Ontario K1A 1B4.

HEALTHY PEOPLE 2000: Increase to at least 90% the proportion of restaurants and institutional foodservice operations that offer identifiable low-fat, low-kcalorie food choices, consistent with the *Dietary Guidelines for Americans*.

To sum up, a well-planned diet delivers adequate nutrients, a balanced array of nutrients, and an appropriate amount of energy. It is based on nutrient-dense foods, moderate in substances that can be detrimental to health, and varied in its selections. The *Dietary Guidelines* apply these principles, offering practical advice on how to eat for good health.

Diet-Planning Guides

To plan a diet that achieves all of the dietary ideals just outlined, a planner needs not only knowledge but tools. Food group plans are one of the most widely used tools for diet planning.

FOOD GROUP PLANS

food group plans: diet-planning tools that sort foods of similar origin and nutrient content into groups and then specify that people should eat certain numbers of servings from each group.

The Daily Food Guide replaced the old Four Food Group Plan and is illustrated as the Food Guide Pyramid.

Five food groups:
- Breads, cereals, and other grain products.
- Vegetables.
- Fruits.
- Meat, poultry, fish, and alternates.
- Milk, cheese, and yogurt.

Food group plans build a diet from clusters of foods that are similar in origin and nutrient content. One such cluster is the milk group, which includes milk, cheese, and yogurt. Another cluster is the grains: breads, cereals, rice, and pasta. Each food group may include dozens of different items. No two items are identical, but they can be arranged into families of foods with similar nutrient compositions. Thus each group represents a set of nutrients that differs from the nutrients supplied by the other groups. Selecting foods from each of the groups eases the task of creating a balanced diet.

Daily Food Guide   Figure 2–1 (pp. 42–43) presents the USDA's Daily Food Guide, a food group plan that assigns foods to five major food groups. The figure lists the most notable nutrients of each group, the foods within each group categorized by nutrient density, the number of servings recommended, and the serving sizes. It also includes an illustration of the USDA's Food Guide Pyramid, a pictorial description of the Daily Food Guide.

Notable Nutrients   The beauty of the Daily Food Guide lies in its simplicity and flexibility. For example, a person can substitute cheese for milk because both supply the key nutrients for the milk group. A person following a food group plan receives not only the nutrients each group is noted for, but small amounts of other nutrients as well. For example, milk, cheese, and yogurt are notable for their calcium, protein, and riboflavin, but they also provide other nutrients. In contrast, a drink concocted from sugar, water, calcium, protein, and riboflavin lacks this nutrient richness, although a label featuring these ingredients might make the drink appear to resemble milk. Milk, cheese, and yogurt are foundation foods; synthetic drinks are not.

Miscellaneous Foods   Some foods—such as the synthetic drink just mentioned—do not fit into any of the food groups. Foods that are high in fat, sugar, or alcohol provide energy, but too few nutrients to hold a significant place in the diet. Such foods should be used sparingly and only after basic nutrient needs have

Milk "beverages" or "drinks" may taste delicious, but they lack the nutrient richness of real milk products.

been met by the foundation foods. Examples of "miscellaneous" foods include salad dressings, jams, and alcoholic beverages.

Nutrient Density   The Daily Food Guide provides a strong foundation for a healthy diet, but it fails to specify food energy intakes. Large fat and energy differences exist within a single food group—for example, between nonfat milk and ice cream, fish and hot dogs, green beans and french fries, apples and avocados, or bread and biscuits—yet according to the Daily Food Guide, any of these substitutions would be acceptable. People who have low energy allowances are advised to select the most nutrient-dense foods within each group, whereas people with high energy needs may select some of the less nutrient-dense, higher-kcalorie foods. Notice that Figure 2–1 provides a key indicating which foods *within each group* are high, moderate, or low nutrient density choices.

Recommended Servings   As mentioned earlier, all food groups are important, and people should make selections from each group daily. The recommended numbers of daily servings are:

- 6 to 11 servings of breads and cereals.
- 3 to 5 servings of vegetables.
- 2 to 4 servings of fruits.
- 2 to 3 servings of meats and meat alternates.
- 2 servings of milk and milk products. (Women who are pregnant or breast-feeding and teenagers are advised to have 3 servings, and teenagers who are pregnant or breastfeeding should have 4.)

The lower number of servings from each group provides about the right amount of food energy for sedentary women and older adults. The middle of the range is appropriate for most children, teenage girls, active women, and sedentary men. The upper end meets the needs of teenage boys, active men, and very active women. Table 2–3 provides estimated kcalorie amounts for each of these three levels. Physical activity raises a person's energy allowance and permits the person to eat more foods, or higher-kcalorie foods, to supply needed nutrients without gaining unwanted weight.

Serving Sizes   What counts as a serving? The answer differs for each food group and for various foods within a group. Furthermore, serving sizes may not represent the amounts people actually put on their plates. Figure 2–1 provides the serving sizes for standard foods within each group. For example, ½ cup of cooked rice is considered one serving. So, 1 cup of rice counts as 2 of the recommended 6 to 11 daily servings from the bread group. Similarly, ¼ cup counts as ½ serving.

Food Guide Pyramid   The Food Guide Pyramid is a graphic depiction of the Daily Food Guide (see Figure 2–1 again). The illustration was designed to depict variety, moderation, and also proportions: the size of each section represents the number of daily servings recommended. The broad base at the bottom conveys the message that grains should be abundant and form the foundation of a healthy diet. Fruits and vegetables appear at the next level, showing that they have a less prominent, but still important, place in the diet. Meats and milks appear in a

Table 2–3

Sample Diet Plans for Different Levels of Energy Intake

Food Group	Servings		
Bread	6	9	11
Vegetable	3	4	5
Fruit	2	3	4
Milk[a]	2–3[a]	2–3[a]	2–3[a]
Meat[b]	5	6	7
kCalories	1600	2200	2800

Note: The 1600-kcalorie plan assumes a total of 53 grams of fat and allows 6 teaspoons of added sugar. The 2200-kcalorie plan assumes a total of 73 grams of fat and allows 12 teaspoons of added sugar. The 2800-kcalorie plan assumes a total of 93 grams of fat and allows 18 teaspoons of added sugar.
[a]Women who are pregnant or breastfeeding, teenagers, and young adults to age 24 need 3 servings.
[b]Meat group amounts are in total ounces.

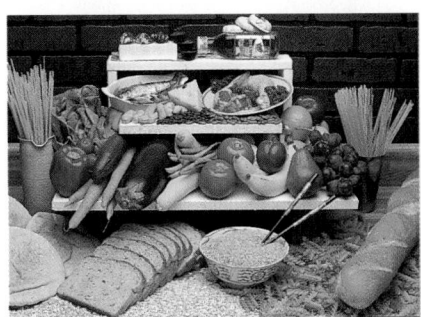

Each of the five major food groups appears in the pyramid in proportion to the number of daily servings recommended.

Figure 2–1

The Daily Food Guide

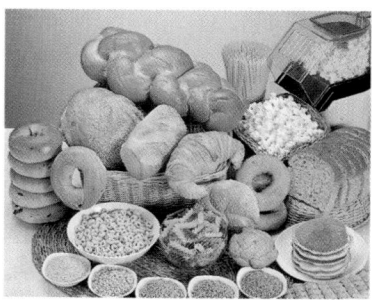

Breads, Cereals, and Other Grain Products

These foods are notable for their contributions of complex carbohydrates, riboflavin, thiamin, niacin, iron, protein, magnesium, and fiber.

6 to 11 servings per day.

Serving = 1 slice bread; ½ c cooked cereal, rice, or pasta; 1 oz ready-to-eat cereal; ½ bun, bagel, or English muffin; 1 small roll, biscuit, or muffin; 3 to 4 small or 2 large crackers.

♦ Whole grains (wheat, oats, barley, millet, rye, bulgur), enriched breads, rolls, tortillas, cereals, bagels, rice, pastas (macaroni, spaghetti), air-popped corn.
◊ Pancakes, muffins, cornbread, crackers, cookies, biscuits, presweetened cereals, granola, taco shells, waffles.
♦ Croissants, fried rice, doughnuts, pastries, cakes, pies.

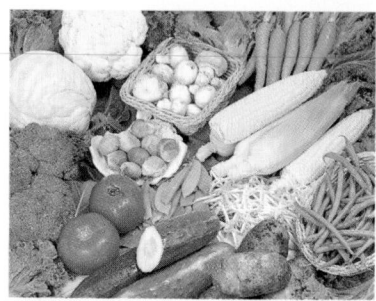

Vegetables

These foods are notable for their contributions of vitamin A, vitamin C, folate, potassium, magnesium, and fiber, and for their lack of fat and cholesterol.

3 to 5 servings per day (use dark green, leafy vegetables and legumes several times a week).

Serving = ½ c cooked or raw vegetables; 1 c leafy raw vegetables; ½ c cooked legumes; ¼ c vegetable juice.

♦ Bean sprouts, broccoli, brussels sprouts, cabbage, carrots, cauliflower, corn, cucumbers, green beans, green peas, leafy greens (spinach, mustard, and collard greens), legumes, lettuce, mushrooms, potatoes, tomatoes, winter squash.
◊ Candied sweet potatoes.
♦ French fries, tempura vegetables, scalloped potatoes, potato salad.

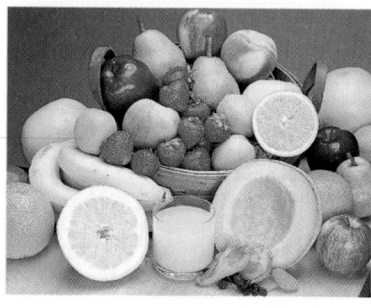

Fruits

These foods are notable for their contributions of vitamin A, vitamin C, potassium, and fiber, and for their lack of sodium, fat, and cholesterol.

2 to 4 servings per day.

Serving = typical portion (such as 1 medium apple, banana, or orange, ½ grapefruit, 1 melon wedge); ¾ c juice; ½ c berries; ½ c diced, cooked, or canned fruit; ¼ c dried fruit.

♦ Apricots, cantaloupe, grapefruit, oranges, orange juice, peaches, strawberries, apples, bananas, pears; unsweetened juices.
◊ Canned or frozen fruit (in syrup); sweetened juices.
♦ Dried fruit, coconut, avocados.

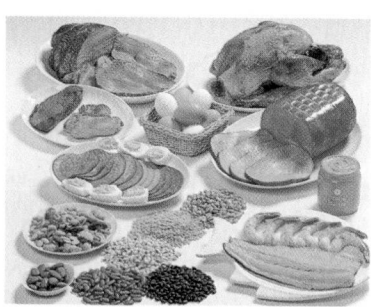

Meat, Poultry, Fish, and Alternates

These foods are notable for their contributions of protein, phosphorus, vitamin B_6, vitamin B_{12}, zinc, magnesium, iron, niacin, and thiamin.

2 to 3 servings per day.

Servings = 2 to 3 oz lean, cooked meat, poultry, or fish (total 5 to 7 oz per day); count 1 egg, ½ c cooked legumes, 4 oz tofu, or 2 tbs nuts, seeds, or peanut butter as 1 oz meat (or about ⅓ serving).

♦ Poultry (light meat, no skin), fish, shellfish, legumes, egg whites.
◊ Lean meat (fat-trimmed beef, lamb, pork); poultry (dark meat, no skin); ham; refried beans; whole eggs, tofu, tempeh.
♦ Hot dogs, luncheon meats, ground beef, peanut butter, nuts, sausage, bacon, fried fish or poultry, duck.

Key:
♦ Foods generally highest in nutrient density (good first choice).
◊ Foods moderate in nutrient density (reasonable second choice).
♦ Foods lowest in nutrient density (limit selections).

Milk, Cheese, and Yogurt

These foods are notable for their contributions of calcium, riboflavin, protein, vitamin B_{12}, and, when fortified, vitamin D and vitamin A.

2 servings per day.

3 servings per day for teenagers and young adults, pregnant/lactating women, women past menopause.

4 servings per day for pregnant/lactating teenagers.

Serving = 1 c milk or yogurt; 2 oz process cheese food; 1½ oz cheese.

♦ Nonfat and 1% low-fat milk (and nonfat products such as buttermilk, cottage cheese, cheese, yogurt); fortified soy milk.

♦ 2% low-fat milk (and low-fat products such as yogurt, cheese, cottage cheese); chocolate milk; sherbet; ice milk.

♦ Whole milk (and whole-milk products such as cheese, yogurt); custard; milk shakes; ice cream.

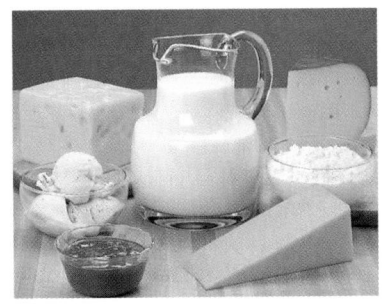

Fats, Sweets, and Alcoholic Beverages

These foods are notable for their contributions of sugar, fat, alcohol, and food energy. No servings are suggested because these foods provide few nutrients. Note that some of the following items, for example, doughnuts, are high in both sugar and fat. Alcoholic beverages are not classed as foods; they contribute few nutrients, but do provide food energy and so are included in this miscellaneous group. Miscellaneous foods not high in kcalories, such as spices, herbs, coffee, tea, and diet soft drinks, can be used freely.

♦ Foods high in fat include margarine, salad dressing, oils, mayonnaise, sour cream, cream cheese, butter, gravy, sauces, potato chips, chocolate bars.

♦ Foods high in sugar include cakes, pies, cookies, doughnuts, sweet rolls, candy, soft drinks, fruit drinks, jelly, syrup, gelatin, desserts, sugar, and honey.

♦ Alcoholic beverages include wine, beer, and liquor.

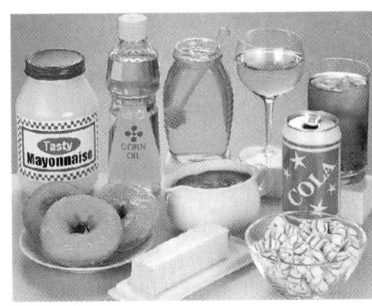

Note: Serve children at least the lower number of servings from each group, but in smaller amounts (for example, ¼ to ⅓ cup rice). Children should receive the equivalent of 2 cups of milk each day, but again in smaller quantities per serving (for example, 4 half-cup portions). Pregnant women may require additional servings of fruits, vegetables, meats, and breads to meet their higher needs for energy, vitamins, and minerals.

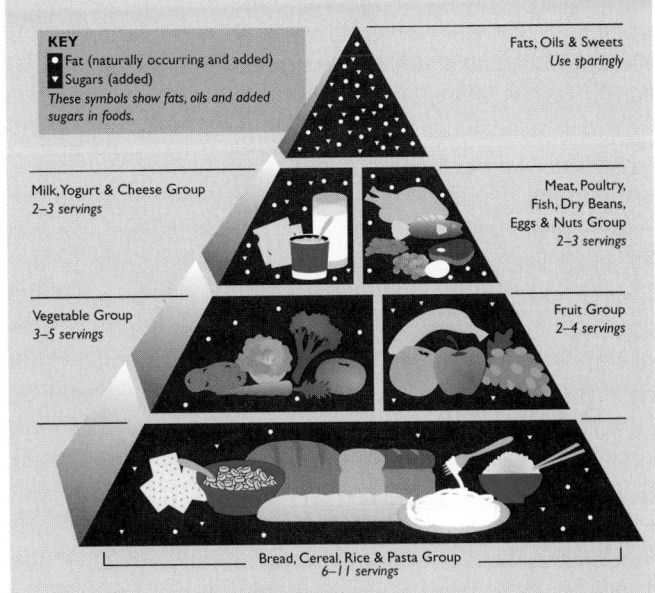

Food Guide Pyramid

A Guide to Daily Food Choices

The breadth of the base shows that grains (breads, cereals, rice, and pasta) deserve most emphasis in the diet. The tip is smallest: use fats, oils, and sweets sparingly.

smaller band near the top. A few servings of each can contribute valuable nutrients, such as protein, vitamins, and minerals, without too much fat and cholesterol. Fats, oils, and sweets occupy the tiny apex, indicating that they should be used sparingly.

Alcoholic beverages do not appear in the pyramid, but they too should be limited. Items such as spices, coffee, tea, and diet soft drinks provide few, if any, nutrients, but can add flavor and pleasure to meals when used judiciously.

Icons of tiny dots and triangles are sprinkled over the food groups, representing naturally occurring and added fats and added sugars, respectively. These icons are meant to remind users that specific foods within the various groups are high in fats, sugars, or both, and so should be eaten in moderation.

The Daily Food Guide plan and Food Guide Pyramid emphasize grains, fruits, and vegetables—all plant foods. Some 75 percent of a day's servings should come from these three groups. This strategy helps all people obtain complex carbohydrates, fiber, vitamins, and minerals with little fat. It also eases diet planning for vegetarians.

Highlight 6 defines vegetarian terms and provides more information on vegetarian diets.

legumes (leg-GYOOMS, LEG-yooms): plants of the bean and pea family. Bacteria in the root nodules of legumes "fix" nitrogen by trapping nitrogen from the air into the soil and then making it a part of the protein in the beans. Thus legumes are rich in high-quality protein compared with other plant-derived foods. Ultimately, the plant leaves more nitrogen in the soil than it takes out (sparing the land). Farmers sometimes plow under legume plants to fertilize the soil.

Vegetarian Food Guide   Vegetarian diets rely mainly on plant foods: grains, vegetables, legumes, fruits, seeds, and nuts. Some vegetarian diets include eggs, milk products, or both. People who do not eat meats or milk products can still use the Daily Food Guide to create an adequate diet.[2] The food groups are similar, and the number of servings remain the same. Vegetarians select *meat alternates* from the meat group—foods such as legumes, seeds, nuts, tofu, and for those who eat them, eggs. Legumes help to supply the iron that meats usually provide, and vegetable selections need to include at least one cup of dark leafy greens for additional iron. Vegetarians who do not drink cow's milk can use soy "milk"—a product made from soybeans that provides similar nutrients if it has been fortified with calcium, vitamin D, and vitamin B_{12}.

Ethnic Food Guides   The Daily Food Guide and Food Guide Pyramid can easily be adapted to include foods from different cultures.[3] For example, a Mexican-American guide would include tortillas in the bread group, jicama in the vegetable group, and guava in the fruit group.

Perceptions and Actual Intakes   The Daily Food Guide and Food Guide Pyramid were developed to help people choose a balanced and healthful diet. Are we selecting foods that reflect the recommendations of the pyramid? According to one survey, many adults *think* they are, when, in fact, they are eating too many fats, sweets, and oils and too little from most of the other food groups.[4] In a sense, our pyramids are top heavy and "tumbling." They need more support from the bread, vegetable, fruit, milk, and meat groups to build a balanced diet.

Canada's Food Guide   Canada's Food Guide to Healthy Eating, shown in Figure 2–2 (pp. 46–47), gives detailed information for selecting foods to meet the nutritional needs of all Canadians four years of age and older. Like the U.S. Daily Food Guide, Canada's Food Guide takes a total diet approach, rather than emphasizing a single food, meal, or day's meals and snacks.

The rainbow side of the Food Guide shows the four food groups with pictorial examples of foods in each group. Key statements advise consumers about

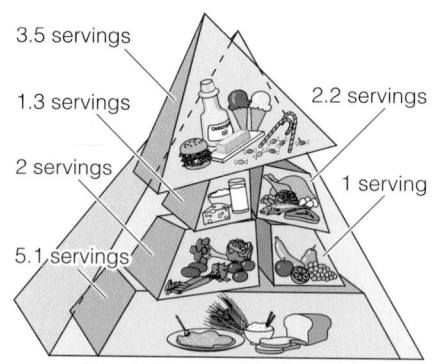

3.5 servings

1.3 servings

2.2 servings

2 servings

1 serving

5.1 servings

Actual Consumption Pyramid

Compared with recommendations, actual consumption resembles a precariously built or "tumbling" pyramid.

selecting foods generally from all the groups, and more specifically within each group. The bar side shows the number of servings recommended for each group and the serving sizes for some foods.

FROM GUIDELINES TO GROCERIES

Dietary recommendations emphasize foods low in fat such as grains, fruits, vegetables, lean meats, fish, poultry, and low-fat milk products. Only you can design such a diet for yourself, but how do you begin? Start with the foods you enjoy eating. Then try to make improvements, little by little. When shopping, think of the food groups, and choose nutrient-dense foods within each group.

Breads, Cereals, and Other Grain Products   When shopping for grain products, you will find them described as *refined, enriched,* or *whole grain* (see the accompanying glossary). These terms refer to the milling process and the making of products, and they have different nutrition implications. Refined foods may have lost many nutrients during processing; enriched products may have had some nutrients added back; and whole-grain products may be rich in all nutrients found in the original grain (see Figure 2–3 on p. 48).

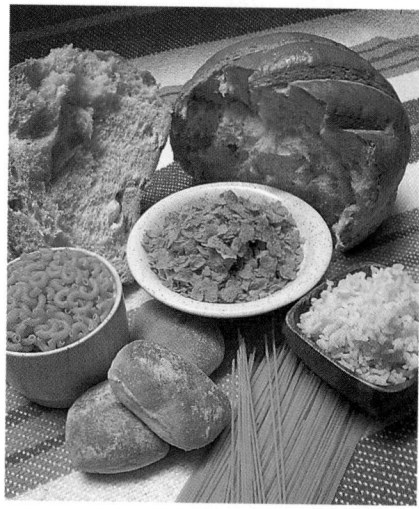

With its many grains (including wheat, rye, oats, corn, and rice) and types of foods (such as pastas, breads, and cereals), this group does more than its share for variety.

Glossary of Grain Terms

bran: the protective coating around the kernel similar in function to the shell of a nut; rich in nutrients and fiber.

endosperm (EN-doe-sperm): the bulk of the edible part of the kernel containing starch and proteins.

enriched: the addition of nutrients to a food to meet a specified standard; often used interchangeably with *fortified*. In the case of refined bread or cereal, four nutrients have been added: thiamin, niacin, and riboflavin in amounts approximately equivalent to, or higher than, those originally present, and iron in amounts to alleviate the prevalence of iron-deficiency anemia.

germ: the nutrient-rich inner part of a grain. The germ is the seed that grows into a wheat plant, so it is especially rich in vitamins and minerals to support new life.

gluten (GLOO-ten): an elastic protein found in wheat and other grains that gives dough its structure and cohesiveness.

husk: the outer, inedible part of a grain; also called the *chaff.*

refined: the process by which the coarse parts of a food are removed. When wheat is refined into flour, the bran, germ, and husk are removed, leaving only the endosperm.

unbleached flour: a tan-colored endosperm flour with texture and nutritive qualities that approximate those of regular white flour.

wheat flour: any flour made from wheat, including white flour; wheat flour has been refined whereas *whole-wheat flour* has not.

white flour: an endosperm flour that has been refined and bleached for maximum softness and whiteness.

whole grain: a grain milled in its entirety (all but the husk), not refined.

whole-wheat flour: flour made from whole-wheat kernels; a whole-grain flour.

Figure 2–2 Canada's Food Guide to Healthy Eating

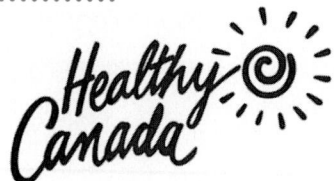

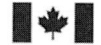

Healthy Canada
Health and Welfare Canada
Santé et Bien-être social Canada
CANADA'S
Food Guide
TO HEALTHY EATING
Enjoy a variety of foods from each group every day.
Choose lower-fat foods more often.
YOGOURT 2.2%
0.1%
SKIM MILK CHEESE
EVAP MILK
POWDER
2%
SKIM
TOFU
Grain Products
Choose whole grain and enriched products more often.
Vegetables & Fruit
Choose dark green and orange vegetables and orange fruit more often.
Milk Products
Choose lower-fat milk products more often.
Meat & Alternatives
Choose leaner meats, poultry and fish, as well as dried peas, beans and lentils more often.

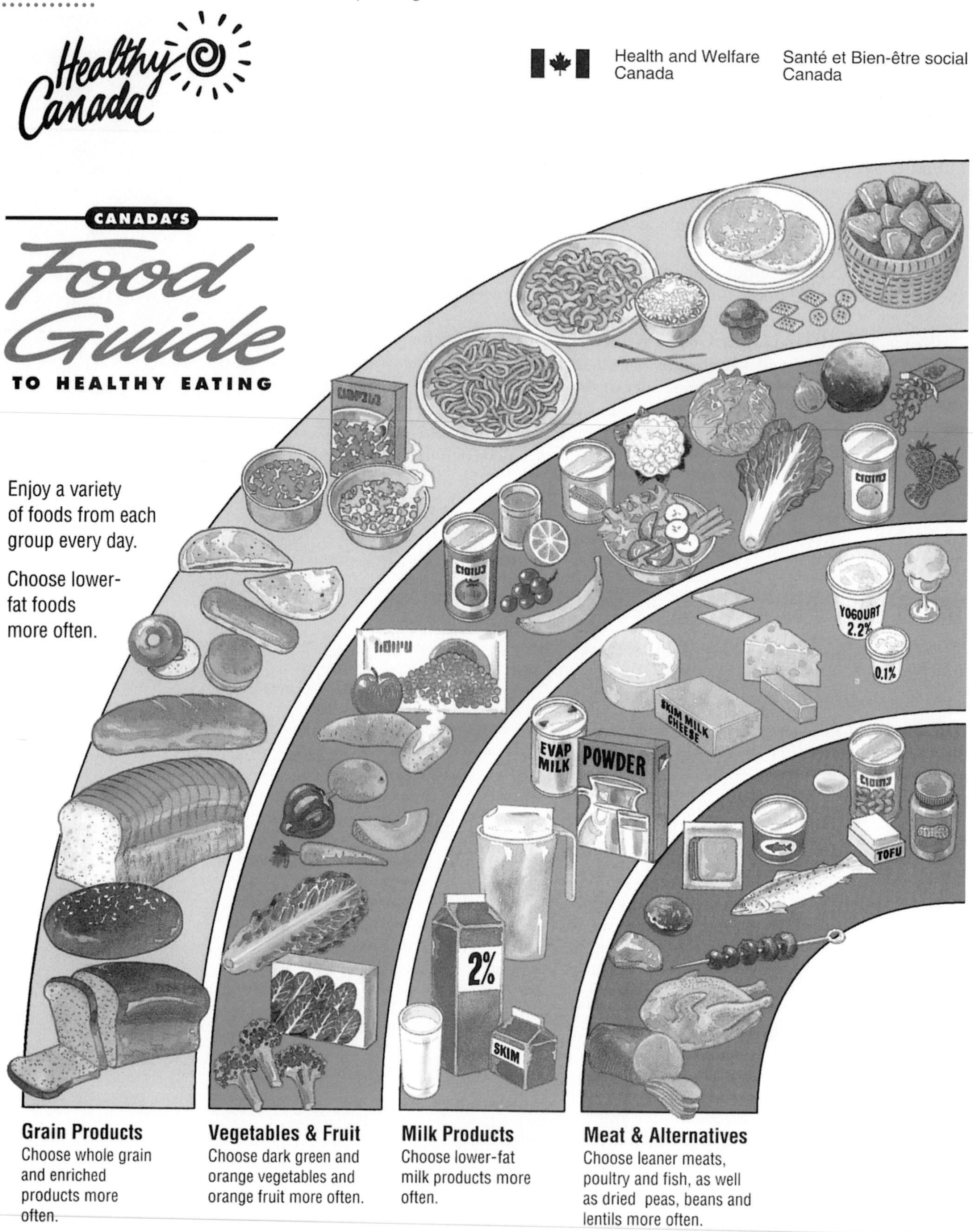

CANADA'S Food Guide TO HEALTHY EATING
FOR PEOPLE FOUR YEARS AND OVER

Different People Need Different Amounts of Food

The amount of food you need every day from the 4 food groups and other foods depends on your age, body size, activity level, whether you are male or female and if you are pregnant or breast-feeding. That's why the Food Guide gives a lower and higher number of servings for each food group. For example, young children can choose the lower number of servings, while male teenagers can go to the higher number. Most other people can choose servings somewhere in between.

Grain Products
5-12 SERVINGS PER DAY

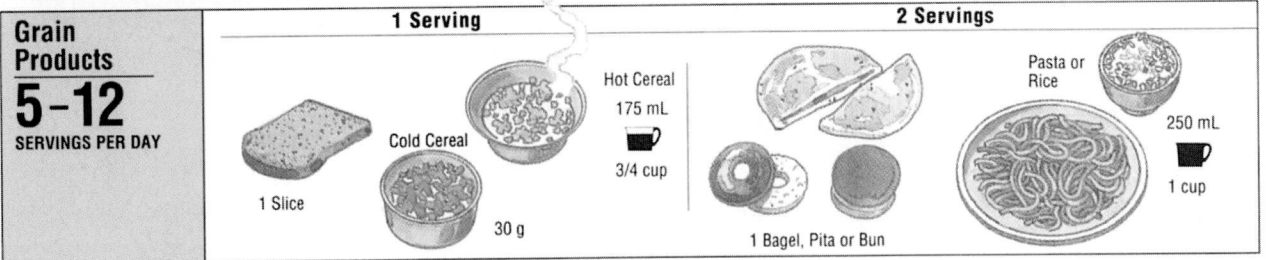

1 Serving
- 1 Slice
- Cold Cereal 30 g
- Hot Cereal 175 mL 3/4 cup

2 Servings
- 1 Bagel, Pita or Bun
- Pasta or Rice 250 mL 1 cup

Vegetables & Fruit
5-10 SERVINGS PER DAY

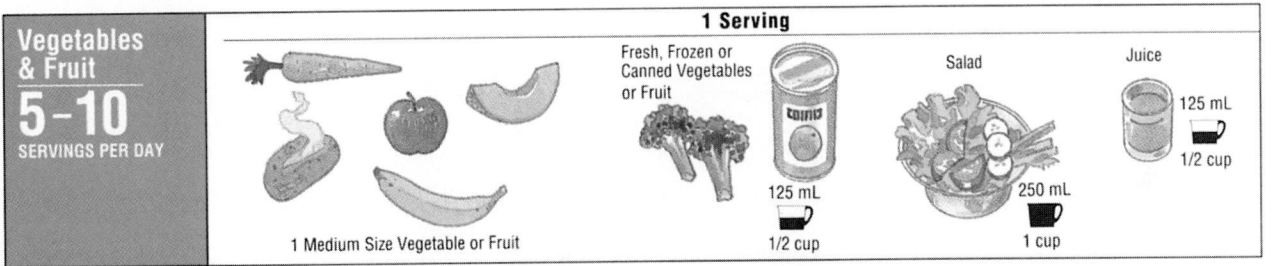

1 Serving
- 1 Medium Size Vegetable or Fruit
- Fresh, Frozen or Canned Vegetables or Fruit 125 mL 1/2 cup
- Salad 250 mL 1 cup
- Juice 125 mL 1/2 cup

Milk Products
SERVINGS PER DAY
Children 4–9 years: 2–3
Youth 10–16 years: 3–4
Adults: 2–4
Pregnant & Breast-feeding Women: 3–4

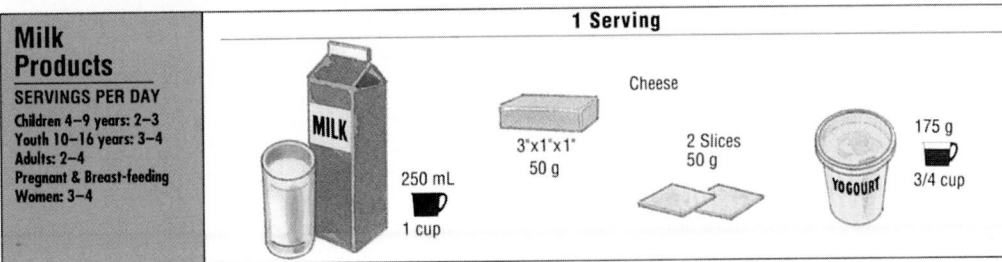

1 Serving
- MILK 250 mL 1 cup
- Cheese 3"x1"x1" 50 g
- 2 Slices 50 g
- YOGOURT 175 g 3/4 cup

Other Foods

Taste and enjoyment can also come from other foods and beverages that are not part of the 4 food groups. Some of these foods are higher in fat or Calories, so use these foods in moderation.

Meat & Alternatives
2-3 SERVINGS PER DAY

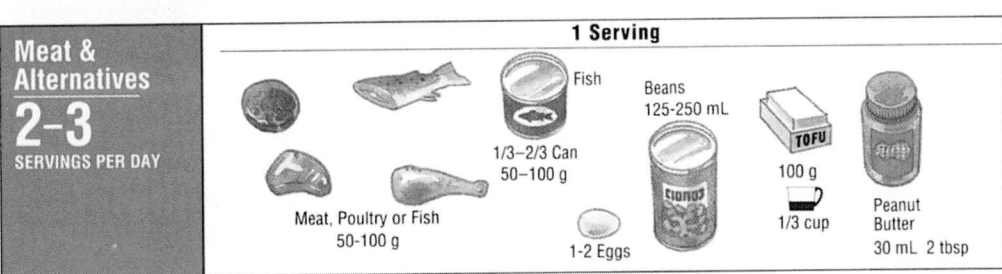

1 Serving
- Meat, Poultry or Fish 50-100 g
- Fish 1/3–2/3 Can 50–100 g
- 1-2 Eggs
- Beans 125-250 mL
- TOFU 100 g 1/3 cup
- Peanut Butter 30 mL 2 tbsp

Enjoy eating well, being active and feeling good about yourself. That's VITALIT⟋

Figure 2–3

A Wheat Plant
The milling process breaks wheat kernels into their parts, shown here.

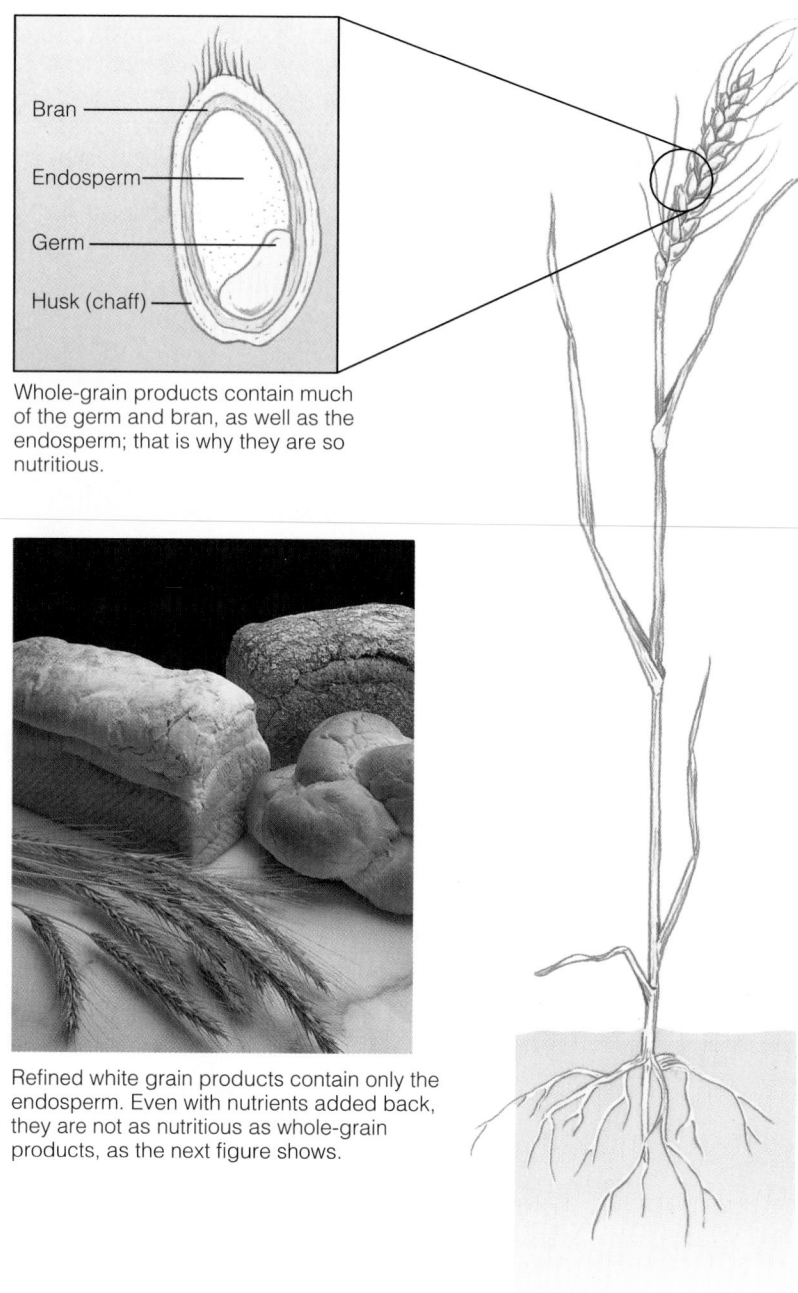

Bran
Endosperm
Germ
Husk (chaff)

Whole-grain products contain much of the germ and bran, as well as the endosperm; that is why they are so nutritious.

Refined white grain products contain only the endosperm. Even with nutrients added back, they are not as nutritious as whole-grain products, as the next figure shows.

When it became a common practice to refine the wheat flour used for bread by milling it and throwing away the bran and the germ, consumers suffered a tragic loss of many nutrients. As a consequence, legislation was passed in the early 1940s requiring that all grain products that cross state lines be enriched with iron, thiamin, riboflavin, and niacin.[5] Enrichment restores these nutrients to the levels present in the original whole wheat and actually raises thiamin and especially riboflavin to higher levels. Most grain products that have been refined, such as rice, wheat pastas like macaroni and spaghetti, and cereals (both cooked and ready-to-eat types), have subsequently been enriched, and their labels say so.

Enrichment doesn't make a slice of bread rich in these added nutrients, but people who eat several slices a day obtain significantly more of these nutrients than they would from unenriched white bread. To a great extent, the enrichment of white flour helps to prevent deficiencies of these four nutrients, but it fails to compensate for losses of many other nutrients and fiber. As Figure 2–4 shows, whole-grain items still outshine the enriched ones. Only *whole-grain* flour contains all of the nutritive portions of the grain.

Whole-grain products, such as brown rice or oatmeal, not only provide more nutrients and fiber, but do not contain the added salt and sugar of flavored, processed rice or sweetened cereals. So, when grocery shopping, choose whole-grain breads and cereals often.

Speaking of cereals, ready-to-eat breakfast cereals lead the list of the most highly fortified foods on the market. Like an enriched food, a *fortified* food has had nutrients added during processing, but in a fortified food, the added nutrients may not have been present in the original product. Some breakfast cereals made from refined flour and fortified with high doses of vitamins and minerals are actually more like supplements disguised as cereals than they are like whole

fortified: the addition to a food of nutrients that were either not originally present or present in insignificant amounts. Fortification can be used to correct or prevent a widespread nutrient deficiency, to balance the total nutrient profile of a food, or to restore nutrients lost in processing.

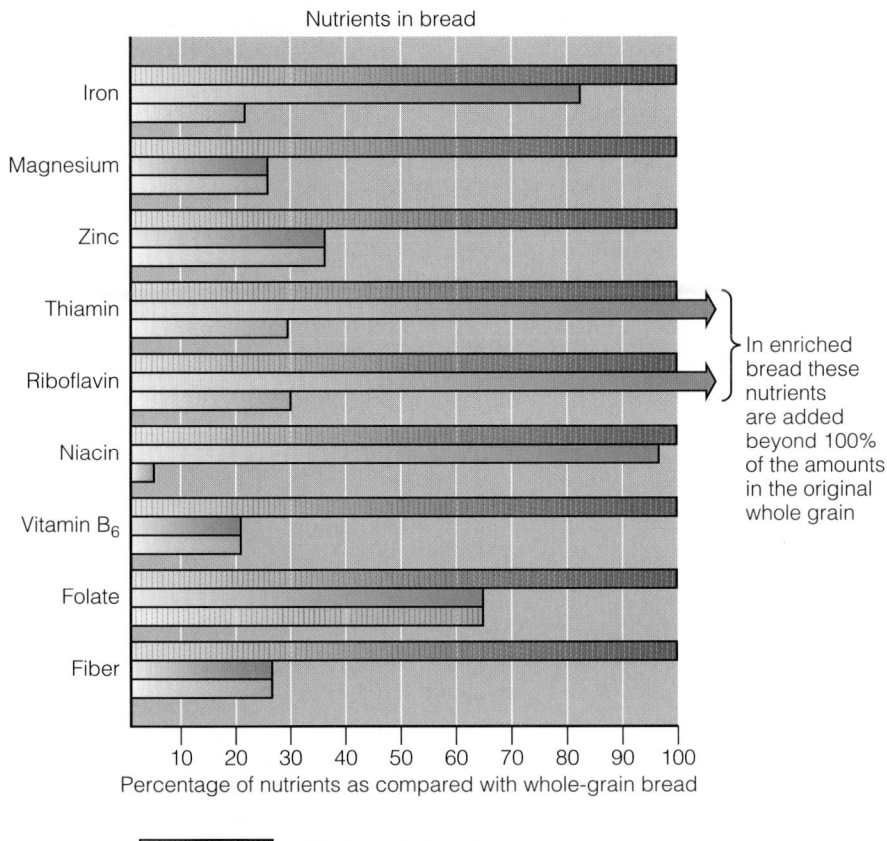

Nutrients in bread

In enriched bread these nutrients are added beyond 100% of the amounts in the original whole grain

Percentage of nutrients as compared with whole-grain bread

= Whole-grain bread
= Enriched white bread
= Unenriched white bread

Figure 2–4

Nutrients in Bread

Whole-grain bread is more nutritious than other breads, even enriched bread. For iron, thiamin, riboflavin, and niacin, enriched bread provides about the same quantities as whole-grain bread and significantly more than unenriched bread. For fiber and the other nutrients (both those shown here and those not shown), enriched bread provides less than whole-grain bread.

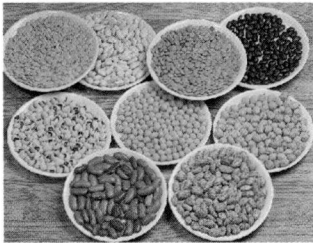

Combining legumes with foods from other food groups creates delicious meals.

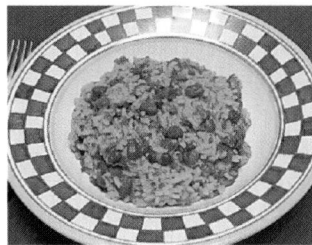

Add rice to red beans for a hearty meal.

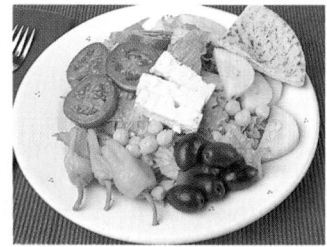

Enjoy a Greek salad topped with garbanzo beans for a little ethnic diversity.

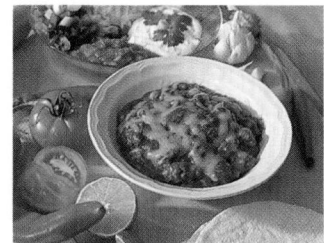

A bit of meat and lots of spices turn kidney beans into chili con carne.

grains. They may be nutritious—with respect to the nutrients added—but they still may fail to convey the full spectrum of nutrients that a whole-grain food or a mixture of such foods might provide.

Vegetables Choose fresh vegetables, especially green and yellow-orange vegetables like spinach, broccoli, and sweet potatoes. Cooked or raw, vegetables are good sources of vitamins, minerals, and fiber. Frozen and canned vegetables without added salt are acceptable alternatives to fresh. To control fat, energy, and sodium intakes, limit butter, salad dressings, and salt on vegetables.

Fruit Choose fresh fruits often, especially citrus fruits and yellow-orange fruits like cantaloupes and apricots. Fruits supply valuable vitamins, minerals, and fibers. They add flavors, colors, and textures to meals, and their natural sweetness makes them enjoyable as snacks or desserts.

Fruit juices are healthy beverages, but contain little dietary fiber compared with whole fruits. Whole fruits satisfy the appetite better than juices and are a better selection for people who need to limit food energy intakes. Juices, on the other hand, are a good choice for people who need extra food energy. Frozen, dried, and canned fruits without added sugar are acceptable alternatives to fresh. Be aware that sweetened fruit "drinks" or "ades" contain mostly water, sugar, and a little juice for flavor. Some may have been fortified with vitamin C, but lack any other significant nutritional value.

Legumes include:
- Black beans.
- Black-eyed peas.
- Garbanzo beans.
- Great northern beans.
- Kidney beans.
- Lentils.
- Navy beans.
- Peanuts.
- Pinto beans.
- Soybeans.
- Split peas.

Legumes Choose often from the legumes (beans and peas such as pinto beans, split peas, lima beans, and black beans). They are available fresh, frozen, dried, or canned. Whether you buy legumes ready to eat or incorporate them into a recipe, use them often as they are an economical, low-fat, nutrient- and fiber-rich food choice.

Percent kCalories Fat in Selected Meats

• Ground beef		
Regular		66%
Lean		57%
Extra lean		54%
• Ground turkey		51%
• Ground round		
(lean and trimmed)		27%

Meat, Fish, and Poultry Meat, fish, and poultry provide essential minerals, such as iron and zinc, and abundant B vitamins as well as protein. To buy and prepare these foods without excess energy, fat, and sodium takes skill. Choose fish, poultry, and lean meats when shopping in the meat department. Lean cuts of beef and pork are named "round" or "loin" (as in top round or pork tenderloin). As a guide, "prime" and "choice" cuts generally have more fat than "select" cuts. Restaurants usually serve prime cuts. Ground beef, even "lean" ground beef, derives most of its food energy from fat as the accompanying table shows. Have the butcher trim and grind a lean round steak instead.

Weigh meat after it is cooked and the bones and fat are removed. In general, 4 ounces of raw meat is equal to about 3 ounces of cooked meat. Some examples of 3-ounce portions of meat include 1 medium pork chop, ½ chicken breast, or 1 steak or hamburger about the size of a deck of cards. To keep fat intake down, bake, roast, broil, grill, or braise meats (but do not fry them in fat); remove the skin from poultry; trim visible fat before cooking; and drain fat after cooking.

Milk Shoppers will find fortified foods in the dairy case. Examples are milk, to which vitamins A and D have been added, and soy milk, to which calcium, vitamin D, and vitamin B$_{12}$ have been added. In addition, shoppers may find imitation foods (such as cheeses) and food substitutes. As food technology advances, many such foods offer low-fat alternatives. For example, egg substitutes help people who want to reduce their fat and cholesterol intakes. Highlight 5 gives other examples.

When shopping, choose low-fat or nonfat milk, yogurt, and cheeses. They are important sources of calcium, but can provide too much sodium and fat if selections are not made with care.

In summary, food group plans select from different families of similar foods to provide adequacy, balance, and variety in the diet. They make it easier to plan a diet that includes abundant grains, vegetables, legumes, and fruits and moderate amounts of meats and milk products. In making any food choice, remember to view the food in the context of your total diet. It is the combination of many different foods that provides the abundance of nutrients so essential to a healthy diet.

Quick and easy estimate:
- 3 oz meat is about the size of a deck of cards.
- ¼ lb (4 oz) hamburger patty, uncooked, is about 3 oz, cooked.

Chapter 5 offers many additional strategies for lowering fat intake.

imitation food: a food that substitutes for and resembles another food, but is nutritionally inferior to it with respect to vitamin, mineral, or protein content. If the substitute is not inferior to the food it resembles and if it provides an accurate name for itself, it need not be labeled "imitation."

substitute food: a food that is designed to replace another.

Food Labels

Many consumers want to eat less fat, saturated fat, cholesterol, and sodium and more complex carbohydrates and dietary fiber. Until recently, however, grocery shoppers found foods without nutrition labels or labels without enough useful information. The Nutrition Labeling and Education Act of 1990 brought sweeping changes to the regulations that define what is required on a food label.[6] The Food and Drug Administration (FDA) and the U.S. Department of Agriculture (USDA) designed the new requirements so that labels would provide consumers with useful information about the foods they eat, and especially about how individual foods fit into their daily diets. (Chapter 14 provides more information on how federal agencies monitor our food system.)

A major objective of the changes was to ensure that labels would appear on virtually all foods and would provide consistent nutrition information. A few foods need not carry nutrition labels: those contributing few nutrients, such as plain coffee, tea, and spices; those produced by small businesses; and those prepared and sold in the same establishment. Producers of some of these items, however, are voluntarily using labels. Even producers and marketers of nonpackaged items are encouraged to voluntarily present nutrient information, either in brochures or on signs posted at the point of purchase. The FDA provides guidelines and oversees this voluntary nutrition information program for the 20 most

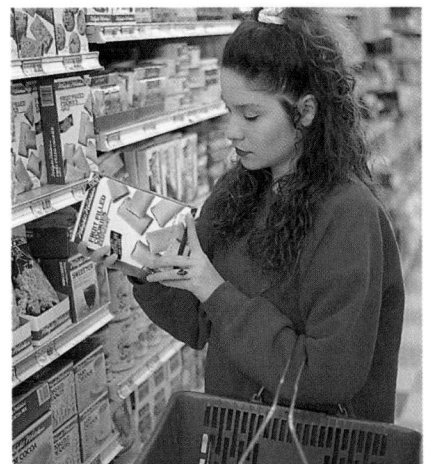

Consumers read food labels to learn about nutrition and its possible connections with health.

Posters in the produce department present nutrition information for nonpackaged items such as raw fruits and vegetables.

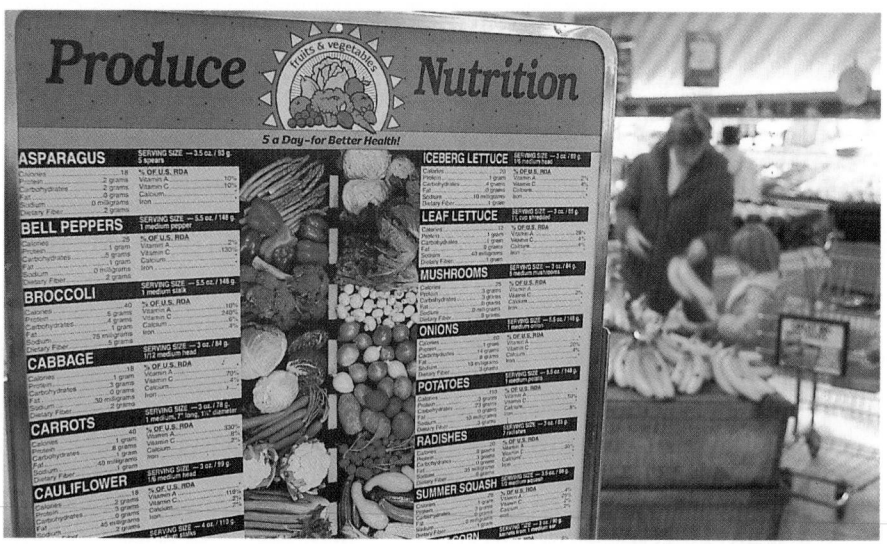

frequently eaten fresh fruits, vegetables, and seafoods (see Table 2–4). The USDA monitors a similar program for 45 major cuts of meat and poultry. Thus essentially all foods are now covered, and as a result, consumers can garner much more useful information in the grocery store than ever before.

 HEALTHY PEOPLE 2000: Achieve useful and informative nutrition labeling for virtually all processed foods and at least 40% of fresh meats, poultry, fish, fruits, vegetables, baked goods, and ready-to-eat carry-away foods.

According to law, every food label must prominently display and express in ordinary words:

- The common or usual name of the product.
- The name and address of the manufacturer, packer, or distributor.
- The net contents in terms of weight, measure, or count.
- The ingredients in descending order of predominance by weight.
- The serving size and number of servings per container.
- The quantities of specified nutrients and food constituents.

The information in the first three items is useful, of course, but it is the last three items that tell consumers about the nutritional value of a product. Many manufacturers supply additional nutrition information upon request. Appendix F lists addresses for several food corporations.

THE INGREDIENT LIST

In the past, a few foods, such as mayonnaise and bread, were exempt from listing ingredients. Instead, manufacturers were required simply to comply with standards of identity that specified the exact ingredients allowed in the products. Now all foods must list all ingredients on the label. Ingredients are listed in descending order of predominance by weight.

Table 2–4

Most Frequently Eaten Raw Fruits, Vegetables, and Seafood

The FDA's voluntary nutrition labeling program applies to the 20 most frequently consumed members of each category: raw fruits, vegetables, and seafood. They are listed here in descending order of consumption.

Fruits	Vegetables	Seafood
Bananas	Potatoes	Shrimp
Apples	Iceberg lettuce	Cod
Watermelons	Tomatoes	Pollock
Oranges	Onions	Catfish
Cantaloupes	Carrots	Scallops
Grapes	Celery	Salmon
Grapefruits	Corn	Flounder
Strawberries	Broccoli	Sole
Peaches	Cabbage	Oysters
Pears	Cucumbers	Orange roughy
Nectarines	Bell peppers	Mackerel
Honeydew melons	Cauliflower	Ocean perch
Plums	Leaf lettuce	Rockfish
Avocados	Sweet potatoes	Whiting
Lemons	Mushrooms	Clams
Pineapples	Green onions	Haddock
Tangerines	Green beans	Blue crabs
Cherries	Radishes	Rainbow trout
Kiwi fruit	Summer squash	Halibut
Limes	Asparagus	Lobster

By knowing that the first ingredient named is the one that predominates by weight, consumers who read ingredient lists can glean much information. Compare these products, for example:

- An orange powder that contains "sugar, citric acid, orange flavor . . ." versus a juice that contains "water, tomato concentrate, concentrated juices of carrots, celery . . . ."
- A cereal that contains "puffed milled corn, sugar, corn syrup, molasses, salt . . ." versus one that contains "100 percent rolled oats."
- A canned fruit that contains "sugar, apples, water" versus one that contains simply "apples, water."

In each comparison, consumers can tell that the second product is the more nutrient dense.

The FDA considered—and rejected—a proposal to group sweeteners together in the ingredient list and declare them in the order of predominance appropriate for their *sum*. The agency reasoned that consumers can find the quantity of total sugars on the "nutrition facts" panel of a label and that this information is more valuable than determining from the ingredient list whether the combined weight of the sugar, corn syrup, and molasses exceeds that of puffed milled corn, for example.

The mandate to list *all* ingredients means that manufacturers must now list all the additives they have used. Such information is particularly useful to people who suffer adverse reactions to specific ingredients such as the milk protein casein or the flavor enhancer MSG (monosodium glutamate).

SERVING SIZES

Table 2–5

Household and Metric Measures

- 1 teaspoon (tsp) = 5 milliliters (ml)
- 1 tablespoon (tbs) = 15 ml
- 1 cup (c) = 240 ml
- 1 fluid ounce (fl oz) = 30 ml
- 1 ounce (oz) = 28 grams (g)

Because labels present nutrient information per serving, they must identify the size of a serving. The FDA has established specific serving sizes that reflect amounts that people customarily consume and requires that all labels for a given product use the same serving size. For example, the serving size for all ice creams is a half-cup and for all beverages, 8 fluid ounces. This facilitates comparison shopping. Consumers can see at a glance whether one brand or another has more or fewer kcalories or grams of fat. Standard serving sizes are expressed in both common household measures, such as cups, and metric measures, such as milliliters, to accommodate users of both types of measures (see Table 2–5).

NUTRITION FACTS

An easy way to recognize a new label is to look for the words "Nutrition Facts" (old labels read "Nutrition Information"). In addition to the serving size and the servings per container, the "Nutrition Facts" panel on a label shows quantities of energy (in kcalories), of fat (in both kcalories and grams), and of certain other nutrients (in grams or milligrams) in a serving:

- Total food energy (kcalories).
- Food energy from fat (kcalories).
- Total fat (grams).
- Saturated fat (grams).
- Cholesterol (milligrams).
- Sodium (milligrams).
- Total carbohydrate, including starch, sugar, and fiber (grams).
- Dietary fiber (grams).
- Sugars (grams).
- Protein (grams).

In addition, labels must present nutrient content information as compared with a standard for the following vitamins and minerals:

- Vitamin A.
- Vitamin C.
- Iron.
- Calcium.

Comparing nutrient amounts against a standard helps make them meaningful to label readers. A label reader might wonder, for example, whether 1 milligram of iron or calcium is a little or a lot. Well, the standard value for iron is 18 milligrams, so 1 milligram of iron is enough to take notice of: it is over 5 percent.

But compared with the standard value for calcium, 1 milligram of calcium is essentially nothing.

It would be nice for consumers if food labels could express each food's nutrient contents as a percentage of each individual's recommended intakes. Unfortunately, though, recommended intakes, such as the RDA, are not the same for everybody; they depend on age and sex. Manufacturers can't know who will be reading the label—an 8-year-old boy, a 70-year-old woman, or a pregnant teenage girl. Label makers do the best they can with this variability, though: they use one set of standard values to represent the needs of a "typical consumer." These standard values, developed by the FDA for use on food labels, are called the Daily Values.

THE DAILY VALUES

In creating the Daily Values, the FDA first established two sets of reference values: Reference Daily Intakes (RDI) and Daily Reference Values (DRV). These two sets of standards are "behind the scenes" characters only; they do not appear as such on labels but are used to determine the Daily Values. The following paragraphs explain each set individually before describing the Daily Values information found on labels.

Reference Daily Intakes (RDI)   The first set of standards, the Reference Daily Intakes (RDI), are for protein, some vitamins, and some minerals. They are based on the RDA and represent intakes to achieve. For example, the RDI for iron is 18 milligrams—an amount to aim for daily. (The RDI replace an earlier set of label standards, the U.S. RDA, in name only: except for protein, the RDI values are the same as the old U.S. RDA, which were based on the 1968 edition of the RDA.) Most labels use the RDI developed for adults and children four years old and older (see Table 2–6); foods designed for certain groups (such as cereals for infants) must use the RDI developed specifically for that group.

Daily Reference Values (DRV)   The second set of standard values, the Daily Reference Values (DRV), are for nutrients and food components, such as fat and fiber, that have important relationships with health, but no RDA. The DRV are based on scientific evidence and reflect current dietary recommendations. For example, several agencies have consistently recommended that fat intake be limited to 30 percent of total energy intake. The DRV represent some intakes to achieve, as for complex carbohydrates, and some to limit, as for cholesterol (see Table 2–7).

The FDA decided to use 2000 kcalories as a standard for energy intake in calculating the DRV for energy-yielding nutrients. A 2000-kcalorie diet is considered about right for moderately active women, teenage girls, and sedentary men. Older adults, children, and sedentary women may need fewer kcalories. Large labels list, at the bottom, Daily Values for both a 2000-kcalorie and a 2500-kcalorie diet, but the "% Daily Value" column on all labels applies only to a 2000-kcalorie diet. A 2500-kcalorie diet is considered about right for many men, teenage boys, and active women. People who are exceptionally active may need still higher kcalorie intakes. Labels may also provide a reminder of the kcalories in a gram of carbohydrate, fat, and protein below the Daily Value information.

Table 2–6

Reference Daily Intakes (RDI)

Nutrient	Amount
Protein[a]	50 g
Thiamin	1.5 mg
Riboflavin	1.7 mg
Niacin	20 mg NE
Biotin	300 µg
Pantothenic acid	10 mg
Vitamin B_6	2 mg
Folate	400 µg
Vitamin B_{12}	6 µg
Vitamin C	60 mg
Vitamin A[b]	5000 IU
Vitamin D[b]	400 IU
Vitamin E[b]	30 IU
Vitamin K	80 µg
Calcium	1000 mg
Iron	18 mg
Zinc	15 mg
Iodine	150 µg
Copper	2 mg
Chromium	120 µg
Selenium	70 µg
Molybdenum	75 µg
Manganese	2 mg
Chloride	3400 mg

[a]The RDI for protein varies for different groups of people: pregnant women, 60 g; nursing mothers, 65 g; infants under 1 year, 14 g; children 1 to 4 years, 16 g.
[b]The RDI for fat-soluble vitamins are expressed in International Units (IU), an old system of measurement. The current RDA and tables of food composition use a more accurate system of measurement. Equivalent values are as follows: for vitamin A, 875 µg RE; for vitamin D, 10 µg; for vitamin E, 9 mg α-TE.

Reference Daily Intakes (RDI): a set of standards for protein, vitamins, and minerals used on food labels as part of the Daily Values; previously known as the U.S. RDA.

Daily Reference Values (DRV): a set of standards for nutrients and food components (such as fat and fiber) that have important relationships with health; used on food labels as part of the Daily Values.

Table 2–7
Daily Reference Values (DRV)

Food Component	DRV	Calculation
Fat	65 g	30% of kcalories
Saturated fat	20 g	10% of kcalories
Cholesterol	300 mg	Same regardless of kcalories
Carbohydrate (total)	300 g	60% of kcalories
Fiber	25 g	11.5 g per 1000 kcalories
Protein	50 g	10% of kcalories
Sodium	2400 mg	Same regardless of kcalories
Potassium	3500 mg	Same regardless of kcalories

Note: The DRV were established for adults and children over four years old. The values for energy-yielding nutrients are based on 2000 kcalories a day.

Daily Values (DV): reference values developed by the FDA specifically for use on food labels. The Daily Values represent two sets of standards: Reference Daily Intakes (RDI) and Daily Reference Values (DRV).

The Two Combined: Daily Values   The FDA strongly believes that the RDI and DRV serve different purposes and prefers to treat them separately. For example, the RDI serve as standards for federal food assistance programs, whereas the DRV do not. But the FDA also recognizes the need to use only one set of values on labels to limit consumer confusion. Hence the Daily Values, which include both the RDI and the DRV and cover all the nutrients that labels list.

Percent Daily Values   Labels present nutrient information in two ways—in quantities (such as grams) and as percentages of Daily Values. The "% Daily Value" column provides a ballpark estimate of how individual foods contribute to the total diet. It compares key nutrients in a serving of food with the daily goals of a person consuming 2000 kcalories. A person who consumes 2000 kcalories a day can simply add up all the "% Daily Values" for a particular nutrient to see if the day's diet fits with recommendations. If the "% Daily Values" total 100 percent, then recommendations are met.

People who require more or less than 2000 kcalories daily must do some calculations to see how foods compare with their personal nutrition goals. They can use the last column in the DRV table shown in Table 2–7 or the suggestions presented in the accompanying box.

Consumers can use Daily Values to evaluate the contributions of individual foods to their daily diets and health goals. Such information helps consumers see easily whether a food contributes "a little" or "a lot" of a nutrient. For example, the "% Daily Value" column on a label of macaroni and cheese may say 20 percent for fat. This tells the consumer that each serving of this food contains about 20 percent of the day's allotted 65 grams of fat. That leaves about 80 percent available for other foods to contribute. A person consuming 2000 kcalories a day could simply keep track of the percentages of Daily Values from foods eaten in a day and try not to exceed 100 percent. To determine whether a particular food was a wise choice, a consumer would need to consider the other foods to be eaten during the day.

Daily Values make it easy to compare foods. For example, a consumer might discover that frozen macaroni and cheese has a Daily Value for fat of 20 percent,

How to Calculate Personal Daily Values

The Daily Values on food labels are designed for a 2000-kcalorie intake, but you can calculate a personal set of Daily Values based on your energy allowance. Consider a person with a 1500-kcalorie intake, for example. To calculate a daily goal for fat, multiply energy intake by 30 percent:

$$1500 \text{ kcal} \times 0.30 \text{ kcal from fat} = 450 \text{ kcal from fat.}$$

The "kcalories from fat" are listed on food labels, so a person could then add all the "kcalories from fat" values for a day, using 450 as a goal. A person who preferred to count grams of fat could divide this 450 kcalories from fat by 9 kcalories per gram to determine the goal in grams:

$$450 \text{ kcal from fat} \div 9 \text{ kcal/g} = 50 \text{ g fat.}$$

Alternatively, a person could calculate that 1500 kcalories is 75 percent of 2000 kcalories:

$$1500 \text{ kcal} \div 2000 \text{ kcal} = 0.75.$$

$$0.75 \times 100 = 75\%.$$

Then, instead of trying to achieve 100 percent of the Daily Value, a person consuming 1500 kcalories would aim for 75 percent. Similarly, a person consuming 2800 kcalories would aim for 140 percent:

$$2800 \text{ kcal} \div 2000 \text{ kcal} = 1.40 \text{ or } 140\%.$$

whereas macaroni and cheese prepared from a boxed mix has a Daily Value of 15 percent. By comparing labels, consumers who are concerned about their fat intakes will be able to make informed decisions.

With an understanding of the Daily Values, consumers can extract a lot of information from a nutrition label. Labels provide different amounts of information based on their package size. Figure 2–5 highlights key information areas on a large food label; Figure 2–6 presents the abbreviated versions that small packages can use.

DESCRIPTIVE TERMS

The FDA specifies what words a label may use to describe a product and what those words mean. See Table 2–8 (on p. 60) for definitions of such terms as "free" (as in fat-free), "low" (as in low-sodium), "high" (as in high-fiber), "light" or "lite," and "more" and "less."

The FDA's definitions also state the conditions under which each term can be used. For example, in addition to having less than 2 milligrams of cholesterol, a "cholesterol-free" product may not contain more than 2 grams of saturated fat per serving. The term "fresh" can be used only for raw food; the descriptive term "freshly" (baked or prepared) can be used only if the food has been recently made and has not been frozen, heated, processed, or chemically preserved.

Figure 2–5

An Example of a Large Food Label

◆ The name and address of the manufacturer

◆ The product name

◆ Descriptive terms if the product meets specified criteria

◆ The weight or measure

◆ Approved health claims stated in terms of the total diet

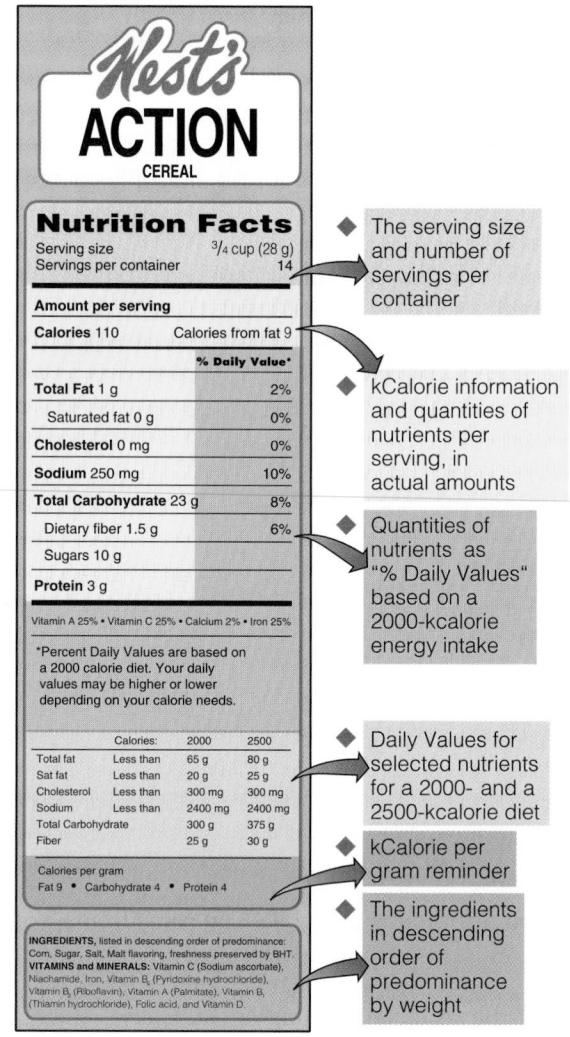

◆ The serving size and number of servings per container

◆ kCalorie information and quantities of nutrients per serving, in actual amounts

◆ Quantities of nutrients as "% Daily Values" based on a 2000-kcalorie energy intake

◆ Daily Values for selected nutrients for a 2000- and a 2500-kcalorie diet

◆ kCalorie per gram reminder

◆ The ingredients in descending order of predominance by weight

Some descriptions *imply* that a food contains, or does not contain, a nutrient. Implied claims are prohibited unless they meet specified criteria. For example, a claim that a product "contains no oil" *implies* that the food contains no fat. If the product is truly fat-free, then it may make the no-oil claim, but if it contains another source of fat, such as butter, it may not.

HEALTH CLAIMS

health claim: any statement that characterizes the relationship between any nutrient or other substance in a food and a disease or health-related condition.

Health claims describe an association between a specific nutrient or food substance and a specific health problem. They are permitted only in cases where scientifically valid links between diet and health have been clearly established. The FDA has approved several health claims based on specified criteria, including:

Figure 2–6

Examples of Small Food Labels

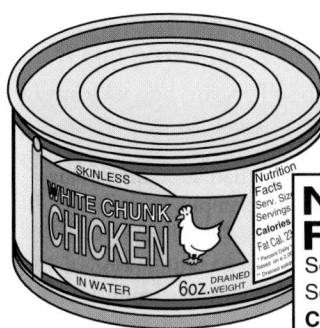

A container with fewer than 40 square inches of surface area can present fewer facts in this format.

Nutrition Facts

Serv. Size ⅓ cup (85g)**
Servings 2
Calories 111
Fat Cal. 23

*Percent Daily Values (DV) are based on a 2000 calorie diet.

** Drained solids only

Amount/serving		%DV*	Amount/serving		%DV*
Total Fat	3g	5%	**Total Carb.**	0g	0%
Sat. Fat	1g	5%	Fiber	0g	0%
Cholest.	60mg	20%	Sugars	0g	
Sodium	200mg	8%	**Protein**	21g	

Vitamin A 0% • Vitamin C 0% • Calcium 0% • Iron 2%

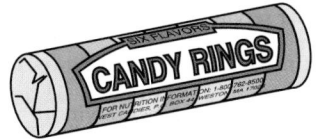

Packages with fewer than 12 square inches of surface area need not carry nutrition information, but they must provide an address or telephone number for obtaining information.

- The nutrient or food substance must be related to a disease or health condition for which most people or a specific group of people, such as the elderly, are at risk.

- The claim is supported by scientific evidence from well-designed studies conducted with recognized scientific procedures and principles.

Health claims on products must emphasize the importance of the total diet and not exaggerate the role of a particular food or diet in disease prevention. No one food possesses magical healing powers, and manufacturers must take care not to distort the roles of their products in promoting health.

Claims must be honest and balanced. For example, health claims can say that foods high in calcium "may" or "might" reduce the risk of osteoporosis. Claims must also explain that diseases develop in response to many factors. They may even mention beneficial factors, such as exercise. For example, a health claim may state that "Development of cancer depends on many factors. A diet low in total fat may reduce the risk of some cancers." The health claim is true, it acknowledges that diet is among many factors influencing disease development, and it is phrased in terms of total diet, not in terms of the particular product. The following relationships for health claims on labels have been authorized:

Health claims on supplement labels are presented in Highlight 10.

- *Calcium and osteoporosis.* Foods or supplements must be high in calcium (at least 20 percent of the RDI) and contain no more phosphorus than calcium.

- *Sodium and hypertension (high blood pressure).* Foods must qualify as "low sodium" (see Table 2–8)."

- *Dietary saturated fat and cholesterol and risk of coronary heart disease.* Foods must

Study Questions

1. Name the diet-planning principles and briefly describe how each principle helps in diet planning.
2. What recommendations appear in the *Dietary Guidelines for Americans?* How do they compare with the *Diet and Health* recommendations introduced in Chapter 1?
3. Name the five food groups in the Daily Food Guide and identify several foods typical of each group. Explain how such plans group foods and what diet-planning principles the plans best accommodate. How are food group plans used, and what are some of their strengths and weaknesses?
4. Review the *Dietary Guidelines*. What types of grocery selections would you make to achieve those recommendations?
5. What information can you expect to find on a food label? How can this information help you choose between two similar products?
6. What are the Daily Values? How can they help you meet health recommendations?
7. What health claims have been approved by the FDA for use on labels? What criteria must all health claims meet?

Notes

1. A. K. Kant and coauthors, Dietary diversity and subsequent mortality in the First National Health and Nutrition Examination Survey Epidemiological Follow-up Study, *American Journal of Clinical Nutrition* 57 (1993): 434–440.
2. Position of The American Dietetic Association: Vegetarian diets, *Journal of the American Dietetic Association* 93 (1993): 1317–1319.
3. C. Achterberg, E. McDonnell, and R. Bagby, How to put the Food Guide Pyramid into practice, *Journal of the American Dietetic Association* 94 (1994): 1030–1035.
4. National Live Stock and Meat Board, *Eating in America Today: A Dietary Pattern and Intake Report,* 1994.
5. W. H. Sebrell, A fiftieth anniversary—Cereal enrichment, *Nutrition Today,* January/February 1992, pp. 20–21.
6. The information on food labels reflects the final regulations as published in the *Federal Register,* January 6, 1993, subsequent amendments, and a special report published in *FDA Consumer,* May 1993.
7. Position of The American Dietetic Association: Nutrition and health information on nutrition labels, *Journal of the American Dietetic Association* 90 (1990): 583–585.

Ethnic Cuisines and Healthy Choices

$\mathcal{D}$o some foodways support health better than others? This highlight presents a few of the many ethnic foodways to show how basic diet-planning principles can apply to many different cuisines (the glossary on p. 64 defines foodways, cuisines, and related terms). A look at the traditional foods of other countries is a delightful way to learn about the world's people and is especially useful to those who advise others on nutrition. A counselor who is familiar with the cultural and religious traditions that influence a person's food choices is better able to make suggestions that fit into the person's life.[1]

Every country, and in fact every region of a country, has its own typical foods and ways of combining them into meals. Ethnic foods have become an integral part of the "American diet," expanding the number of foods available and thus helping people to achieve variety in their diets. While variety helps to ensure nutrient adequacy, only moderation can control energy and fat intakes, and these are the keys to reducing the risks of chronic diseases. How can people enjoy ethnic meals and still limit their energy and fat intakes? Keep this question in mind as you read the following sections.

NORTHERN EUROPEAN INFLUENCE

An evening meal of hearty roast beef, mashed potatoes, boiled cabbage, and bread, with fruit pie for dessert, is typical of cuisines of Germany, England, and Ireland. Such

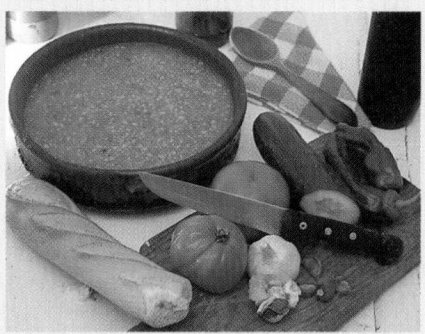

Low-fat ethnic foods, such as gazpacho, have become such common restaurant fare that we often forget their origins.

meals are served for countless dinners across the United States, too, and variations on this plan are numerous. Even a Thanksgiving turkey dinner with all the trimmings follows this pattern.

Traditionally, people have filled their plates with meat and served starches and vegetables on the side. Today's health advice, however, encourages people to load their plates with tasty grains and vegetables and to limit meat to 2- to 3-ounce portions. This way, the meal provides plenty of carbohydrate and fiber, adequate protein, and not too much fat.

Another familiar meal that derives from northern Europe is the bacon and eggs breakfast. The English serve it with baked beans; in the United States, northerners select potatoes and southerners choose grits. The legumes offer a fiber advantage. More fruit and a lower-fat meat choice would improve the breakfast further.

Every eating style has advantages and drawbacks. The northern European style ensures adequate protein and all the other nutrients associated with meat. It delivers a lot of fat, though, and is short on fiber and the vitamins and minerals associated with fruits and vegetables. For better health, people who eat this way need to reduce portions of meats and added fats and choose more whole grains, fruits, and vegetables.

French cuisine is among the world's most popular foodways. The French expertly combine butter, cream, eggs, herbs, and wine into classic sauces. They prepare pastries filled with seafood, cheese, or meats and covered with rich sauces for a main dish or wrapped around sweetened fruits and creams for dessert. These choices are extraordinarily high in fat, but typical serving sizes are small. Eating French food can be healthful when a person follows the suggestion to "keep it simple." The country cuisine of southern France along the Mediterranean Sea offers equally wonderful options: elegant clear soups; steamed and poached seafood; lean meats, legumes, and vegetables seasoned with lemon, herbs, or wine; fruit; and huge loaves of french bread.

The notion that red wine protects the French and others of the Mediterranean region against heart disease, while not proved, may have some validity. Studies do show low rates of heart disease in populations that drink moderate amounts of wine (red or white) with meals. Other correlations have not been ruled out, though, and correlations are not causes. Furthermore, any advantage of cardiovascular protection may be offset by other health problems. French people have a higher incidence of stomach and

cuisine (kwi-ZEEN): style of cooking or preparing food.

ethnic diets: foodways and cuisines typical of national origins, cultural heritages, or geographic locations.

foodways: the sum of the food habits, customs, beliefs, and preferences of a culture.

kosher (KOE-sure): foods prepared according to Jewish dietary laws.

esophagus cancer than people in the United States, and they suffer high rates of liver disease as a direct result of high alcohol intakes. Still, the French have heart disease rates lower than U.S. rates despite a similar fat intake.

The French have clearly influenced the bayou regions of Louisiana, and so have the African-American ancestors of the present population there. The settlers in southern Louisiana adapted their heritages to the local food supply, creating the Cajun style of cooking that is now popular across the nation. Many Cajun dishes are based on a roux made by browning flour and salt with oil. Cajun dishes include spicy stews (gumbo, jambalaya), sausages, hot pepper sauce, red beans and rice, seafood, and dirty rice (rice made brown with chopped chicken livers and seasonings). Many people enjoy Cajun coffee brewed with chicory root and a sugared doughnut known as a beignet (pronounced ben-YAY).

Nutritionists agree with enthusiastic diners that red beans and rice is a classic dish—full of flavor from expert use of spices and abundant in carbohydrate, protein, and fiber, while low in fat. A jambalaya (stew) of seafood (crawfish, shrimp, and fish), tomatoes, vegetables, and rice seasoned with a little strong-flavored sausage is packed with vitamins and minerals, adequate in protein, rich

in carbohydrate, and usually low in fat. With a careful eye on the fat during food preparation and a limit on the beignets, people eating Cajun style can easily achieve the goals embodied in the *Dietary Guidelines*.

MEDITERRANEAN DIETS AND HEART HEALTH

Coastal populations that share the bounty of the Mediterranean waters may also share some important health advantages. Mediterranean people die less frequently of heart disease and certain cancers than do people of northern Europe and North America.[2] While popular sources report the marvels of "the Mediterranean diet," scientists who have attempted to define that diet or its health benefits have run into problems.[3] One problem is that many countries border the Mediterranean Sea: Italy, Spain, Portugal, France, Greece, Syria, Lebanon, Israel, Turkey, Egypt, Algeria, and more. Consequently, there is no single "Mediterranean diet." Also, some of the data backing claims about causes of death in Mediterranean countries were collected in the 1960s, when the majority of people still consumed traditional diets. Even with these limitations, the links between Mediterranean diets and health are worth pondering, and Highlight 6 reviews some of the findings of recent research.

Today's Greek and Italian cuisines stem from some of the world's most ancient foodways.[4] Ancient Greeks and Romans ate mostly grain foods such as breads and cakes, along with seeds including lentils and beans, fish and other seafoods, goat cheese, vegetables, and fruits (especially grapes and figs). They ate meat on special occasions only and drank wine diluted half-and-half with water. Their favored cooking fat was oil pressed from olives; butter was shunned as a "food of barbarians." In modern U.S. terms, the ancient Greek and Roman diets fit fairly well into the Daily Food Guide pattern. Unfortunately, no one knows much about the causes of death in those days, but the average life span was only about 40 years or so. So many people died of childhood diseases, in war, in childbirth, or from infectious diseases that few lived long enough to develop heart disease or cancer.

Today, Greeks are known for a robust cuisine that includes whole broiled fish and other seafoods; roasts and stews of vegetables such as eggplant with lamb, chicken, or beef; and the flavors of fresh lemons, garlic, and herbs (dill, mint, and parsley); and, always, olives and their oil, which lavishly season many dishes.[5] Traditional Greek salads contain no lettuce but combine chunks of tomato, peppers, cucumbers, onions, a salty cheese (feta), anchovies, and cured ripe olives with a tangy olive oil and lemon dressing. Stuffed grape leaves may be topped by a famous Greek soup of eggs and lemon juice. Gyros (pronounced YEE-roce, meaning "a circle" in Greek) is a high-fat, highly seasoned meat that is roasted over open flames as it slowly turns on a spit. When cooked, the gyros is thinly sliced, dressed with yogurt and cucumber, and served in a pita (pocket) bread. As for Greek desserts, pastries (baklava) soaked with butter and honey and layered with nuts are traditional at celebrations. Because of their intense sweetness, small servings of these desserts are usually satisfying.

The Greek diet provides a startling 42 percent of its kcalories from fat, mostly from olive oil and olives.[6] Yet people living in Greece have a lower incidence of cardiovascular disease than northern Europeans and North Americans and enjoy one of the longest life expectancies worldwide (1986 data), despite the tendency of many Greeks to carry excess body fat.[7] These facts have led some to suggest that a diet similar to that of Greece might be healthier and easier to follow than the limited fat diet recommended in the United States for heart health (Highlight 6 revisits this topic).[8]

Like Greece, Italy relies on the Mediterranean Sea for seafoods, but its cuisine is perhaps best known for its pastas. Italian cuisines—and pastas—differ from north to south. Generally, northern pastas are egg based and usually ribbon shaped or stuffed like dumplings (tortellini). Northern Italians eat their pasta with plenty of meat, butter, cheese, eggs, and cream. In the southern regions, the diet is more "Mediterranean" in character; wheat pastas are made without eggs, shaped more like macaroni, and served with vegetables such as artichokes, eggplants, peppers, and tomatoes. Beans appear on the table more often than meat, and all dishes are seasoned with olive oil, not butter. Unlike the Greeks, southern Ital-

ians keep total fat intakes relatively low.[9] Death rates from heart disease are low among natives of Italy (and neighboring Spain), so health experts are reluctant to suggest "improvements" for their diets.[10]

While heart disease rates may be low in Mediterranean countries, no one can explain why the incidence of stroke is almost double that of the United States. If diet is credited for heart health, shouldn't it also be blamed for stroke?

Also, while the link between diet and heart disease is strong, no one knows what part of the diet might be beneficial. Some think using olive oil instead of butter or shortening is the key factor, while others point to the protective effects of both nutrients and nonnutrients found in vegetables, seafoods, or seasonings.[11] They say that while fat may play a role, an antioxidant effect from constituents of plant foods is probably more important in defending the heart. (More about antioxidants appears in Highlight 11.)

A valid question is whether Mediterranean people may be naturally resistant to heart disease, but this seems not to be the case. People who move from one place to another and adopt the dietary habits of the new locale have heart disease rates typical of people native to that area.[12] Mediterranean populations are, however, more physically active than those in the United States and Canada. They also consume more fruits and vegetables, less meat and animal fat, more olive oil, and more of each day's kcalories early in the day. The effects of meal timing on heart disease risk may be important. A small but significant improvement in blood lipids has been observed in people who eat frequent small meals

each day, rather than the standard larger meals.[13] Many aspects of life affect heart health.

WEST AFRICAN FOODS IN THE DEEP SOUTH

Peanut *butter* is considered an American food, invented by the agricultural scientist George Washington Carver, but peanuts are native to South America. They were spread by Portuguese explorers to Africa, where peanuts and peanut paste became staple foods and were brought to U.S. soil by African slaves. Many southern specialties, such as boiled peanuts, okra, and black-eyed (cow) peas, are of African origin. Today's rural southern cuisine varies little between African Americans and people of European descent.

Southern cuisine provides ample vitamins and minerals from a variety of vegetables: sweet potatoes, collards and other leafy greens, okra, tomatoes, meats, and corn. Unfortunately, many of these traditional vegetable dishes are flavored with salted pork, smoked bacon and its fat, or lard, or they are fried in shortening. Fried green tomatoes, a southern specialty, have been dredged in spicy cornmeal and then deep-fried. Many southerners enjoy large servings of high-fat, high-salt meats, such as fried chicken, fatty pork cuts or sausages, and spareribs, greatly overemphasizing protein and fat in the diet while slighting whole grains, fruits, and vegetables. Biscuits, a favored bread, are made with almost as much shortening as flour and are often served with butter or fat-rich gravy. Southern families take pride in their recipes for pecan pie, a pastry shell filled with butter, syrup, and nuts.

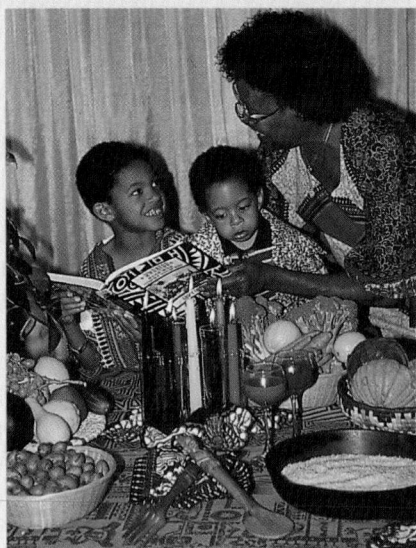

Ethnic meals and family gatherings nourish the spirit as well as the body.

Such a high-fat diet is associated with many health problems, including obesity, heart disease, and stroke. The southeastern United States has the dubious distinction of being the nation's Stroke Belt because of its high incidence of cardiovascular disease. People indulging in traditional southern cuisine need to keep moderation in mind if they are to maintain their health. The trick to choosing health-promoting rural southern food is to limit the fatty, salty meats and vegetables, biscuits, and gravies. Instead select low-fat meats; prepare sweet potatoes, greens, and other vegetables without fat and salt; and eat beans, rice, and cornbread with nonfat seasonings and spreads.

NATIVE AMERICAN DIETS

Over the last 200 years, Native Americans have seen unprecedented changes in their foodways. Hunter-gatherer and agricultural lifestyles have given way to a mod-ern culture relying on fast foods, alcohol, abundant high-fat meats, and dairy products. For Native Americans, the effects of these changes on health have been overwhelmingly negative.

The Pima Indians of central Arizona are a well-studied example of a group that has experienced the effects of a "modernized" diet. Until the 1930s, the Pima diet consisted of wild and cultivated desert legumes, cactus leaves and fruit, fish, venison (deer meat), small seeds, mesquite pods, acorns, and corn.[14] Then, a change began. The Pima largely replaced their traditional wild foods, which had become scarce, with modern ones such as wheat flour, lard, sugar, coffee, and ready-to-eat cereals that were easily obtained. The result has been tragic: the Pima now suffer the highest per capita rate of diabetes known among any people in the world.[15] Likewise, the Sioux Indians rarely suffered heart disease when consuming their traditional diets, but now suffer one of the highest known rates of heart and artery disease.

Both the Pima and the Sioux changed not only their diets, but also their highly active lifestyles. Modern-day Pima and Sioux no longer hunt game on the windswept plains, toil in the fields, or cook over stone fireplaces as their ancestors did. Like others in the United States, they now drive to supermarkets to purchase convenience foods and cook them in microwave ovens. The Sioux also traded their traditional ceremonial pipes for daily cigarette smoking, a habit that is especially damaging to the heart.

While changed diets and lifestyles have almost certainly contributed to the declines in health, disease rates and risk factors differ greatly among tribes, despite a uni-versal adoption of modern foods and television watching.[16] Genetic, as well as environmental, factors must account for these differences.

Native diets are not perfect. They may not provide adequate amounts of some nutrients, and availability of foods depends on such unpredictable factors as weather changes and herd movements. While modern foods are usually safe and sanitary, Native Alaskans eating traditional foods suffer more botulism (a deadly food poisoning described in Chapter 14) than any other group worldwide. Modern descendants changed the ancient methods of preserving meat, fish, and blubber (fat) in slight but critical ways that encourage the growth of the bacteria that cause botulism.[17] The point is that all diets, even those that have supported human beings through many centuries, have drawbacks. Still, by studying them, scientists are beginning to believe that when Native Americans consumed their original high-fiber, low-fat native foods, their hearts and bodies benefited.

MEXICAN ETHNIC FOODS

Mexican restaurants in the United States typically offer beautiful plates of complex food mixtures—tortillas filled with meats and cheeses, some fried and crisp and others baked and soft, along with flavored rice, refried beans, sour cream, guacamole (avocado sauce), and salsa (tomato sauce). These foods are of Mexican origin, but Mexican families typically eat them only on special occasions, not as daily fare. A typical Mexican lunch or dinner is rather simple, consisting of a stew of beans, meat, rice, and potatoes served with tortillas or bread, tomato salsa, and lettuce salad or

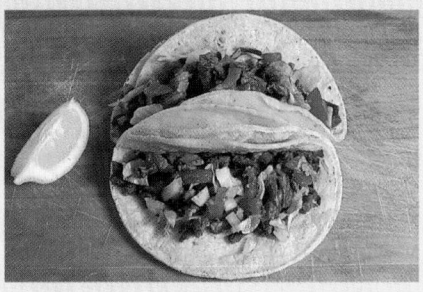

Tortillas filled with lean beef and fresh vegetables are a welcome alternative to sandwiches.

cooked vegetables.[18] A Mexican breakfast might include tortillas and eggs with a beverage.

If carefully chosen, the foods from both taco stands and fancier Mexican restaurants can make valuable contributions to the diet. Many traditional Mexican dishes, even the fast-food type, provide beans in abundance. Beans are high in nutrient density and fiber while low in fat (although some restaurants prepare the refried variety with lard). Soft corn tortillas filled with beans, lettuce, and salsa with a side order of rice are high in nutrient density. Without careful selection, though, Mexican foods can be extraordinarily high in fat, such as a fried tortilla shell filled with high-fat ground beef and topped with cheese and sour cream.

For a healthy special-occasion Mexican meal, use sour cream lightly, and skip the fried varieties of stuffed tortillas. Try instead a low-fat dish called fajita—lean meats, marinated and sizzled on a grill, wrapped in soft tortillas with chili salsa toppings. Salsa (made of chopped tomatoes, onions, and hot peppers) is rich in vitamins and zest but adds no fat to a meal. As for guacamole, even though avocados are high in fat, they add interest and flavor to a meal, and the type of fat avocados contain is not implicated in disease causation. Their high fat content does mean that people who tend to gain weight easily should eat avocados in small quantities on infrequent occasions.

THE CHINESE ADVANTAGE

Tried and true, the diet of China has supported the health of its people for thousands of years. China's foodways reflect the efficiency that is essential in a country where the population density is more than 1000 people per acre, yet only 10 percent of the land can be used to grow food. China has over a billion people, and 75 percent of them are involved in agriculture. Contrast these figures with the United States: population density, 113 per acre; land in farms, about 50 percent; population, 250 million; farmers, 1 to 2 percent.

There seems to be little malnutrition or obesity in China, even though the people consume 20 percent more food energy each day than we do.[19] On the whole, Chinese people eating traditional foods consume three times the fiber of people eating the American way, take in about half the fat, and have blood cholesterol values about half of what they are in the United States.[20] Only 4 out of every 100,000 men in China die of heart disease each year compared with 67 in the United States. Chinese living in China also suffer much less cancer of the colon and rectum than do Chinese Americans who have adopted a Western diet.[21] It seems worthwhile to study the fine points of a diet so conservative of resources yet so superbly supportive of health—not to convince everyone to eat Chinese meals three times a day, but to illustrate the governing principles that can be applied to foods of all origins.

Typical Chinese meals do not follow the meat-vegetable-starch pattern of northern Europe that is common in much of the United States today. Instead, the vegetables and meats are cooked together. The total amount of meat (or fish or egg) in a Chinese dish is small by Western standards; meals center on a staple starch food—every diner has a dish of rice and chooses other foods from serving dishes according to appetite. The Chinese also usually drink soup or tea throughout each meal, which slows dining to a relaxing pace.

Vegetables and fruits provide tremendous variety, and subtle flavors in main dishes come largely from fat-free seasonings and sauces such as ginger root, scallions, rice wine, garlic, soy, hoisin, oyster, bean, and plum. Most sauces add tasty flavors but little fat unlike our gravies, butter, or sour cream. The Chinese mode of cooking in a wok requires just a tablespoon or two of oil for an entire dish. Chinese dishes do, however, tend to be high in sodium. Diners can enjoy low-sodium meals if they are prepared without salt or monosodium glutamate (MSG) and with judicious use of soy sauce.

Cooking foods the Chinese way tends to preserve nutrients. All food is cut into bite-sized pieces before cooking, so cooking is quick and destroys few nutrients. No cooking water is thrown away, so nutrients are not lost that way either. The water in which the rice is cooked soaks back into the rice, so the rice retains its nutrients.

The Chinese diet and cooking techniques are also land-efficient, as they must be in view of the scarcity of agricultural land and fuels. Nearly

67

all of the food energy comes from plants rather than animals. A million kcalories in wheat or rice can be produced on less than 1 acre of land; a million kcalories in beef require 17 acres. In a world that is often wasteful of fuel and land, the Chinese way of eating offers a model to all nations.

Some Chinese dishes do have nutrition drawbacks, though. In China, deep-fried foods are eaten only seldom, but Chinese restaurants in this country often feature these and other high-fat items. Another drawback is the inclusion of salted, fermented pickles, which have been linked to a high incidence of digestive tract cancers. Chinese restaurants in the United States rarely serve these fermented items because they tend not to appeal to Western tastes.

THE CHANGING JAPANESE DIET

Traditional Japanese cuisine bears similarities to the Chinese diet. Grains such as rice or millet form the bulk of most traditional Japanese meals. Vegetables and fruits are next in prominence, and seafood, eggs, poultry, and meats play a supporting role. For a favored traditional snack, a Japanese commuter might stop by a "noodle house" for a bowl of noodles (somen) in a clear, seasoned broth—a dish of Chinese origin. A Japanese delicacy popular in the United States is sushi— vinegar-flavored rice holding bits of colorful vegetables and seafood, wrapped in seaweed and served with horseradish or seasoned soy sauce. In the United States, the word *sushi* has come to mean "raw fish," which may be an ingredient, but sushi actually refers to vinegared rice, and many types of sushi are made with

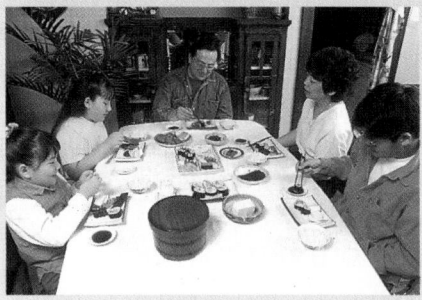

Foodways and cuisines of all cultures can support heart health when dietary fat is limited.

cooked ingredients. Sushi delights diners visually, as do most traditional Japanese foods. In Japan, the visual imagery created on the plate is at least as important as the taste of the food.

Since the 1950s, Japan has transformed itself from a wartorn, still largely traditional country struggling to feed its population to an industrial and economic world leader. Today, Japan's cuisine reflects the "hurry-up" lifestyle of a nation buzzing with mass communications media, high incomes, and high expenses. Time-consuming, home-cooked traditional dishes, though still favored in restaurants, have proved impractical for the two-income family of the 1990s.

In a land where rice once occupied center stage at every meal, meats, breads, and milk products now dominate. Meat consumption in Japan has jumped more than ten-fold since the 1940s.[22] Egg intakes rose more than sixfold in the same period. Vegetable intakes have fallen precipitously, and margarine intakes have more than doubled. Japanese families choose microwavable frozen entrees; instant noodle and curry mixes; precooked hamburgers and fried shrimp. Ice cream has replaced fruit as the preferred dessert, and instant coffee is replac-

ing tea. High-fat snacks from hamburger places, southern fried chicken restaurants, and doughnut shops have shoved low-fat noodle houses into the background.

The health implications of such changes are turning out to be two-sided. Deaths in Japan have declined as modern sanitation and immunizations have brought infectious diseases under control, but a steady increase in heart attacks and strokes is now reversing this trend. Japanese men who grew up consuming a "Western" diet are more likely to suffer from diabetes than are men who grew up on a traditional Japanese diet, and diabetes is a risk factor for heart disease.[23] On the other side, the new diet provides much more protein than a traditional rice-based diet, and extra protein during the growing years has enabled the younger generation to grow taller and stronger than any generation before them.[24] In general, Japan still enjoys a lower overall rate of heart disease than many other nations, but new choices present new risks.

People in the United States who wish to dine in the Japanese style can freely choose from traditional dishes, being wary only of a few battered and deep-fried meats and vegetables (tempuras). A traditional Japanese chef may toss together a mixture of mushrooms, carrots, and bamboo shoots with bits of seafood or meat; season it with fat-free (but salty) soy sauce; add sesame seeds; and serve it with a large portion of rice. Shrimp in rice-cake soup features a clear broth, mushrooms, shrimp, and spinach and is served with rice cakes (mochi). A fish-and-noodle casserole might combine a lean fish fillet and broth seasoned with sugar, soy sauce, and mirin (a syrupy rice wine) with a big bowl of thick noodles. Beware of any restaurant that claims to serve traditional Japanese meals but centers the meals around large portions of meat. Today's Japanese diners may consume such meals, but they are not traditional cuisine, and they incur the same warnings that accompany northern European foodways.

RELIGIOUS DIETARY TRADITIONS

A discussion of ethnic foodways would be incomplete without mentioning foodways practiced by religious groups. According to many religions, ritual and ceremony surrounding food can provide nourishment for the spirit as well as for the body. Like national groups, religious groups derive their distinct identity in part from special foodways.

The Jewish laws set forth an extensive set of dietary rules. Many people, on hearing the word *kosher,* think of foods such as pickles, bagels and lox, corned beef, or matzoh crackers. Kosher is not a cuisine, however, but rather a set of restrictions that Orthodox Jews place on the selection and preparation of animal-derived foods. Jews from Eastern Europe, Germany, the former Soviet Union, the Middle East, or India eat different foods, but the kosher rules apply to all.[25]

Religious commitment is the sole intent of those who keep kosher. Occasionally, someone suggests that the laws of kosher originated for reasons of health—that kosher food was "clean" and therefore kept people safe from food-borne illnesses, but the rules of kosher offer no special benefits to health. These rules permit Orthodox Jews to eat beef but not pork, fish but not shellfish, and they dictate special handling methods for permitted foods.

Because blood is forbidden as food, kosher rules govern methods of animal slaughter, cuts that may be eaten, and preparation rituals.

Kosher law prohibits Jews from consuming milk and meat in the same meal. This law leads some kosher cooks to replace milk with nondairy creamer in meals that include meat. Nutritionally, however, creams do not resemble milk, and they are high in saturated fat. A better choice is to use soy "milk" products formulated to resemble the nutrient and cooking qualities of milk products.

Like other cuisines, Jewish cuisines and kosher foods can be evaluated according to dietary standards. A meal might be improved by reducing the schmaltz (chicken fat) used in cooking or by frying latke (potato pancakes) in nonstick pans rather than in oil. Bagels with lox (a form of salmon) and nonfat cream cheese are an excellent breakfast choice—bagels are naturally low in fat, and lox is rich in fish oils thought to be protective against the development of heart disease. A person dining on European Jewish cuisine might limit meat to the 2- to 3-ounce serving sizes recommended by the Daily Food Guide and fill in with grains, legumes, fruits, and vegetables.

Food symbolism abounds in most other religions as well. During certain days of Lent, the period prior to Easter, many Christians eat only vegetarian dishes, giving up meat until Easter dinner. Eastern Orthodox Christians observe many fast days on which they consume no animal products at all. The Mormon faith allows no alcohol, coffee, or tea. Many Seventh-Day Adventists consume no meat, but eat eggs and milk products; they also shun alcohol, coffee, and tea. Their doctrine

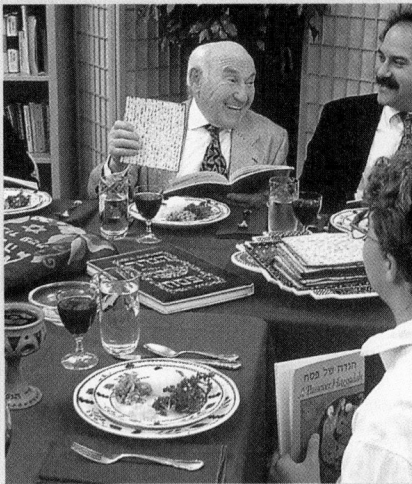

Many religions include foods in their ceremonies.

advises them to avoid strong spices such as mustard or pepper and discourages between-meal snacks. Other faiths, such as Islam, Hinduism, and Buddhism, prohibit some dietary practices while promoting others.

As you can see by now, consumers can apply the diet-planning principles introduced in Chapter 2 to any ethnic foodway. It is not the ethnic cuisine itself, but the diner's habitual selections from the many traditional choices that determine whether a diet will benefit health. Whatever the cuisine, consumers must learn to balance all foods in a way that provides adequate nourishment without excess.*

---

*The American Diabetes Association and the American Dietetic Association offer a series of booklets on the ethnic and regional food practices of dozens of foodways. These booklets describe food practices, customs, and holidays; present meals modified according to nutrition recommendations; provide exchange lists, food composition values, and glossaries for ethnic foods; and list additional resources. See Appendix F for addresses.

NOTES

1. K. P. Sucher and P. G. Kittler, Nutrition isn't color blind, *Journal of the American Dietetic Association* 91 (1991): 297–299.

2. F. Berrino and P. Muti, Mediterranean diet and cancer, *European Journal of Clinical Nutrition* 43 (1989): 49–55.

3. A. Ferro-Luzzi and S. Sette, The Mediterranean diet: An attempt to define its present and past composition, *European Journal of Clinical Nutrition* 43 (1989): 13–29.

4. J. C. Waterlow, Diet of the classical period of Greece and Rome, *European Journal of Clinical Nutrition* 43 (1989): 3–12.

5. D. Kromhout and coauthors, Food consumption patterns in the 1960s in seven countries, *American Journal of Clinical Nutrition* 49 (1989): 889–894.

6. A. Trichopoulou, Correspondence, *New England Journal of Medicine* 327 (1992): 53.

7. World Health Organization, Life expectancy, number of survivors, and chances per 1000 of eventually dying from specified causes, at selected ages, by sex, latest available year, in *World Health Statistics Annual* (Geneva: World Health Organization, 1989), pp. 158–163.

8. F. M. Sacks and W. W. Willet, More on chewing the fat, *New England Journal of Medicine* 325 (1991): 1740–1742.

9. Ferro-Luzzi and Sette, 1989.

10. L. Masana and coauthors, The Mediterranean-type diet: Is there a need for further modification? *American Journal of Clinical Nutrition* 53 (1991): 886–889.

11. W. P. T. James, G. G. Duthie, and K. W. J. Whale, The Mediterranean diet: Protective or simply nontoxic? *European Journal of Clinical Nutrition* 43 (1989): 31–41.

12. Committee on Diet and Health, *Diet and Health: Implications for Reducing Chronic Disease Risk* (Washington, D.C.: National Academy Press, 1989), pp. 177–178.

13. L. M. Arnold and coauthors, Effect of isoenergetic intake of three or nine meals on plasma lipoproteins and glucose metabolism, *American Journal of Clinical Nutrition* 57 (1993): 446–451.

14. J. C. Brand and coauthors, Plasma glucose and insulin responses to traditional Pima Indian meals, *American Journal of Clinical Nutrition* 51 (1990): 416–420.

15. B. A. Swinburn, Deterioration in carbohydrate metabolism and lipoprotein changes induced by modern, high-fat diet in Pima Indians and Caucasians, *Journal of Clinical Endocrinology and Metabolism* 73 (1991): 156–165.

16. R. Fabsitz, Administrator of the Strong Heart Study, as quoted by K. A. Fackelmann, *Science News* 142 (1992): 168–170.

17. M. Segal, Native food preparation fosters botulism, *FDA Consumer*, January/February 1992, pp. 23–26.

18. S. J. Algert and T. H. Ellison, Mexican American food practices, customs, and holidays, *Ethnic and Regional Food Practices* (series) (Chicago and Alexandria, Va.: American Dietetic Association and American Diabetes Association, 1989).

19. L. Roberts, Diet and health in China, *Science* 240 (1988): 27.

20. Roberts, 1988.

21. A. S. Whittemore and coauthors, Diet, physical activity, and colorectal cancer among Chinese in North America and China, *Journal of the National Cancer Institute* 82 (1990): 915–926.

22. M. Motoko, Eating is a solitary pastime, *Japan Quarterly* 36 (1989): 207–210.

23. E. H. Tsunehara, D. L. Leonetti, and W. Y. Fujimoto, Diet of second-generation Japanese-American men with and without noninsulin-dependent diabetes, *American Journal of Clinical Nutrition* 52 (1990): 731–738.

24. E. A. Martin and V. A. Beal, *Roberts' Nutrition Work with Children*, 4th ed. (Chicago: University of Chicago Press, 1978) presents details of these classic findings.

25. C. Higgins and H. S. Warshaw, Jewish food practices, customs, and holidays, *Ethnic and Regional Food Practices* (series) (Chicago and Alexandria, Va.: American Dietetic Association and American Diabetes Association, 1989).

Chapter 3

Digestion, Absorption, and Transport

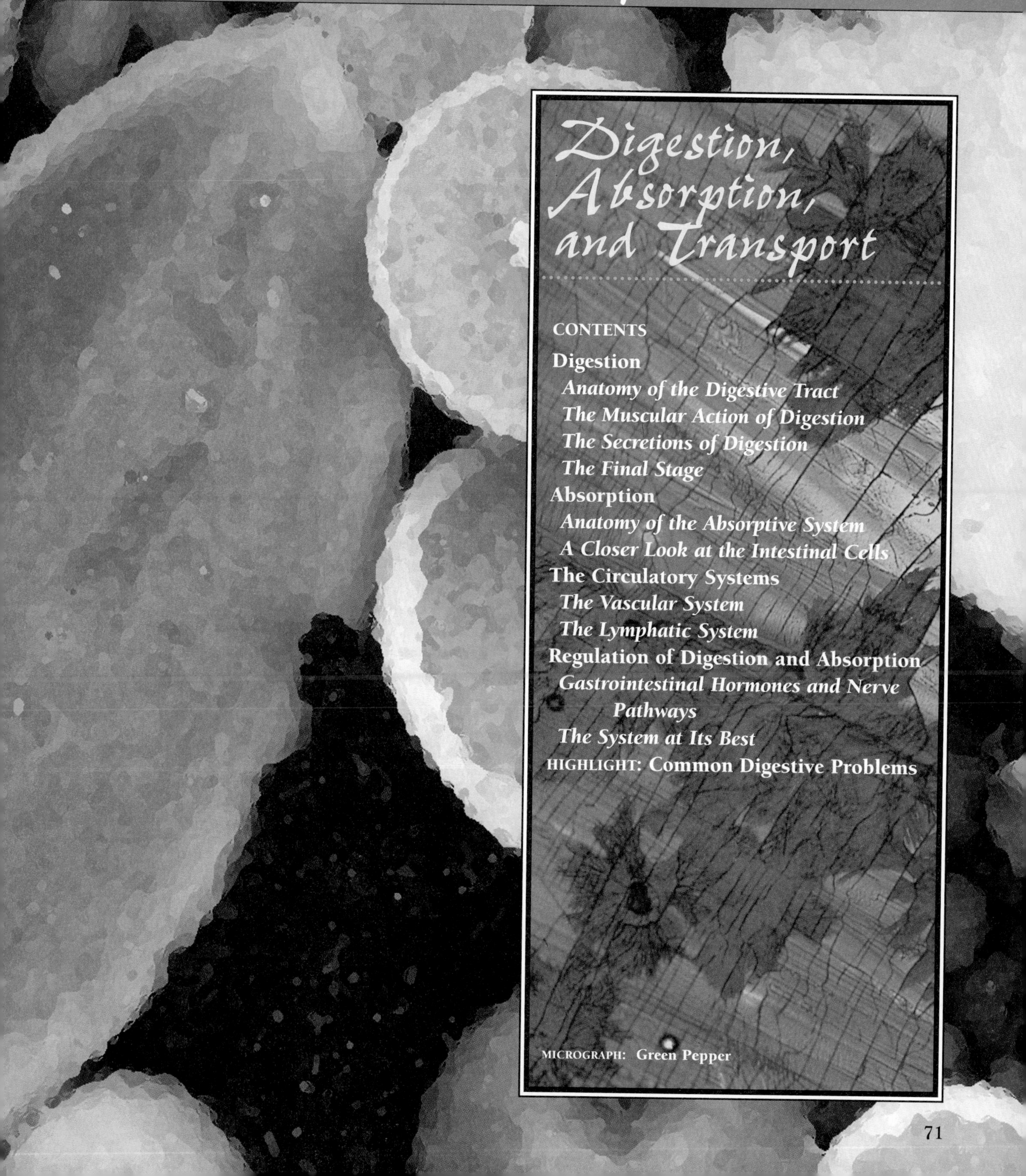

CONTENTS

Digestion
Anatomy of the Digestive Tract
The Muscular Action of Digestion
The Secretions of Digestion
The Final Stage
Absorption
Anatomy of the Absorptive System
A Closer Look at the Intestinal Cells
The Circulatory Systems
The Vascular System
The Lymphatic System
Regulation of Digestion and Absorption
Gastrointestinal Hormones and Nerve
Pathways
The System at Its Best
HIGHLIGHT: Common Digestive Problems

MICROGRAPH: **Green Pepper**

*H*ave you ever wondered what happens to the food you eat after you swallow it? Or how your body extracts nutrients from food? Have you ever marveled how it all just seems to happen? This chapter takes you on the journey that transforms the foods you eat into the nutrients featured in the later chapters. Then it follows the nutrients as they travel through the intestinal cells and into the body to do their work. This introduction presents a general overview of the processes common to all nutrients; later chapters discuss the specifics of digesting and absorbing individual nutrients.

Digestion

digestion: the process by which food is broken down into absorbable units.

The digestive tract is the body's ingenious way of getting the nutrients ready for absorption, and it solves many problems for you without any conscious effort on your part. Consider these problems:

1. Human beings breathe, eat, and drink through their mouths. Air taken in through the mouth must go to the lungs; food and liquid must go to the stomach. The throat must be arranged so that swallowing and breathing don't interfere with each other.
2. Below the lungs lies the diaphragm, a dome of muscle that separates the upper half of the major body cavity from the lower half. Food must pass through this wall to reach the stomach.
3. To move through the system, food must be lubricated with water. Too much water would form a liquid that would flow too rapidly; too little water would form a paste too dry and compact to move at all. The amount of water must be regulated to keep the intestinal contents at the right consistency to move smoothly along.
4. When the digestive enzymes are breaking food down, they need it in finely divided form, suspended in enough water so that every particle is accessible. Once digestion is complete and the needed nutrients have been absorbed out of the tract into the body, the system must excrete the residue that remains, but excreting all the water along with the solid residue would be both wasteful and messy. Some water should be withdrawn, leaving a paste just solid enough to be smooth and easy to pass.
5. The materials within the tract should be kept moving, slowly but steadily, at a pace that permits all reactions to reach completion.
6. The enzymes of the digestive tract are designed to digest carbohydrate, fat, and protein. The walls of the tract, composed of living cells, are also made of carbohydrate, fat, and protein. These cells need protection against the action of the powerful digestive juices that they secrete.
7. Once waste matter has reached the end of the tract, it must be excreted, but it would be inconvenient and embarrassing if this function occurred continuously. Provision must be made for periodic, voluntary evacuation.

The following sections show how the body elegantly and efficiently handles these problems.

ANATOMY OF THE DIGESTIVE TRACT

GI tract: the gastrointestinal tract or digestive tract; the principal organs are the stomach and intestines.

gastro = stomach

The gastrointestinal (GI) tract is a flexible muscular tube from the mouth, through the esophagus, stomach, small intestine, large intestine, and rectum to the anus. Figure 3–1 (on p. 74) traces the path followed by food from one end to the other, and the glossary (on p. 75) defines GI anatomy terms. In a sense, the human body surrounds the GI tract. Only when a nutrient or other substance penetrates the GI tract's wall does it enter the body proper; many nonnutritive materials pass through the GI tract without being digested or absorbed.

Mouth   The process of digestion begins in the mouth. As you chew, your teeth crush large pieces of food into smaller ones, and fluids blend with these pieces to ease swallowing. Fluids also help dissolve the food so that you can taste it; only particles in solution can react with taste buds. The tongue not only allows you to taste food, but to move food around the mouth, facilitating chewing and swallowing. When you swallow a mouthful of food, it first slides across your epiglottis, bypassing the entrance to your lungs. This is the body's solution to problem 1: the epiglottis closes off your air passages so that you don't choke when you swallow. After a mouthful of food has been swallowed, it is called a bolus.

Choking is discussed on p. 94.
bolus (BOH-lus): a portion; with respect to food, the amount swallowed at one time.

Esophagus to the Stomach   Next, the bolus slides down the esophagus, which conducts it through the diaphragm (problem 2) to the stomach. The stomach cells produce secretions both to break down food particles and to protect themselves from being broken down (problem 6). The cardiac sphincter at the entrance to the stomach closes behind the bolus so that it can't slip back into the esophagus (problem 5). The stomach retains the bolus for a while in its upper portion. Little by little, the stomach transfers the food to its lower portion, adds juices to it, and grinds it to a semiliquid mass called chyme. Then, bit by bit, the stomach releases the chyme through the pyloric sphincter, which opens into the small intestine and then closes behind the chyme.

chyme (KIME): the semiliquid mass of partly digested food expelled by the stomach into the duodenum.
chymos = juice

Small Intestine   At the top of the small intestine, the chyme bypasses the opening from the common bile duct, which is dripping fluids (problem 3) into the small intestine from two organs outside the GI tract—the gallbladder and the pancreas. The chyme travels on down the small intestine through its three segments—the duodenum, the jejunum, and the ileum—almost 10 feet of tubing coiled within the abdomen.[1]

Large Intestine (Colon)   Having traveled the length of the small intestine, the chyme arrives at another sphincter (problem 5 again): the ileocecal valve, at the beginning of the large intestine (colon) in the lower right-hand side of the abdomen. As the chyme enters the colon, it passes another opening. Had it slipped into this opening, it would have ended up in the appendix, a blind sac about the size of your little finger. The chyme bypasses this opening, however, and travels along the large intestine up the right-hand side of the abdomen, across the front to the left-hand side, down to the lower left-hand side, and finally below the other folds of the intestines to the back side of the body, above the rectum.

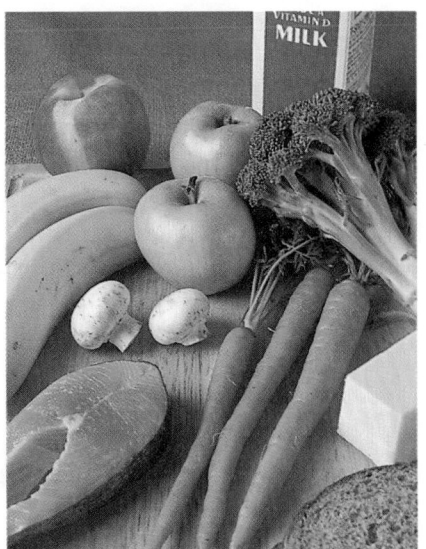

Rectum   During the chyme's passage to the rectum, the colon withdraws water from it, leaving semisolid waste (problem 4). The strong muscles of the rectum hold back this waste until it is time to defecate. Then the rectal muscles relax (problem 7), and the last sphincter in the system, the anus, opens to allow passage of the waste.

The process of digestion transforms all kinds of *foods* into *nutrients*.

Figure 3–1

The Gastrointestinal Tract

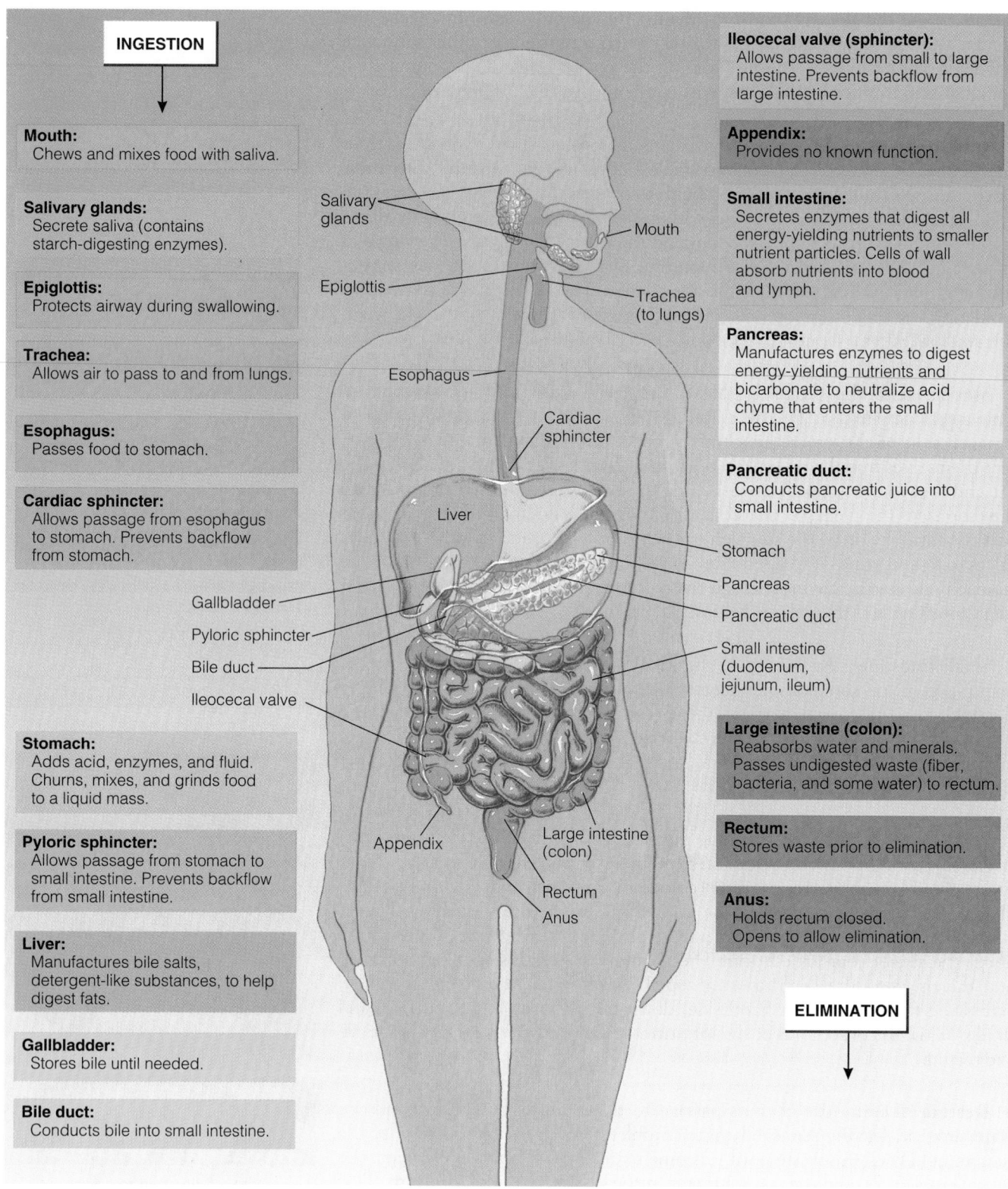

INGESTION

Mouth:
Chews and mixes food with saliva.

Salivary glands:
Secrete saliva (contains starch-digesting enzymes).

Epiglottis:
Protects airway during swallowing.

Trachea:
Allows air to pass to and from lungs.

Esophagus:
Passes food to stomach.

Cardiac sphincter:
Allows passage from esophagus to stomach. Prevents backflow from stomach.

Stomach:
Adds acid, enzymes, and fluid. Churns, mixes, and grinds food to a liquid mass.

Pyloric sphincter:
Allows passage from stomach to small intestine. Prevents backflow from small intestine.

Liver:
Manufactures bile salts, detergent-like substances, to help digest fats.

Gallbladder:
Stores bile until needed.

Bile duct:
Conducts bile into small intestine.

Ileocecal valve (sphincter):
Allows passage from small to large intestine. Prevents backflow from large intestine.

Appendix:
Provides no known function.

Small intestine:
Secretes enzymes that digest all energy-yielding nutrients to smaller nutrient particles. Cells of wall absorb nutrients into blood and lymph.

Pancreas:
Manufactures enzymes to digest energy-yielding nutrients and bicarbonate to neutralize acid chyme that enters the small intestine.

Pancreatic duct:
Conducts pancreatic juice into small intestine.

Large intestine (colon):
Reabsorbs water and minerals. Passes undigested waste (fiber, bacteria, and some water) to rectum.

Rectum:
Stores waste prior to elimination.

Anus:
Holds rectum closed. Opens to allow elimination.

ELIMINATION

Salivary glands

Mouth

Epiglottis

Trachea (to lungs)

Esophagus

Cardiac sphincter

Liver

Gallbladder

Pyloric sphincter

Bile duct

Ileocecal valve

Appendix

Stomach

Pancreas

Pancreatic duct

Small intestine (duodenum, jejunum, ileum)

Large intestine (colon)

Rectum

Anus

Glossary of GI Anatomy Terms

These terms are listed in order from start to end of the digestive tract.

epiglottis (epp-ee-GLOTT-iss): cartilage in the throat that guards the entrance to the trachea and prevents fluid or food from entering it when a person swallows.
epi = upon (over)
glottis = back of tongue

trachea (TRAKE-ee-uh): the windpipe; the passageway from the mouth and nose to the lungs.

esophagus (e-SOFF-uh-gus): the food pipe; the conduit from the mouth to the stomach.

cardiac sphincter (CARD-ee-ack SFINK-ter): the sphincter muscle at the junction between the esophagus and the stomach; also called the *lower esophageal sphincter* or the *gastroesophageal sphincter*.
cardiac = the heart

sphincter: a circular muscle surrounding, and able to close, a body opening.
sphincter = band (binder)

stomach: a muscular, elastic, saclike portion of the digestive tract that grinds and churns swallowed food, mixing it with acid and enzymes to form chyme.

pyloric (pie-LORE-ic) **sphincter**: the circular muscle that separates the stomach from the small intestine and regulates the flow of partially digested food into the small intestine (also called **pylorus** or **pyloric valve**).
pylorus = gatekeeper

liver: the organ that manufactures bile and is the first to receive nutrients from the intestines. The liver's many other functions are described in Chapter 7.

gallbladder: the organ that stores and concentrates bile. When it receives the signal that fat is present in the duodenum, the gallbladder contracts and squirts bile through the bile duct into the duodenum.

pancreas: a gland that secretes digestive enzymes and juices into the duodenum.

small intestine: a 10-foot length of small-diameter intestine that is the major site of digestion of food and absorption of nutrients; its segments are the duodenum, jejunum, and ileum.

duodenum (doo-oh-DEEN-um, doo-ODD-num): the top portion of the small intestine (about "12 fingers' breadth" long in ancient terminology).
duodecim = twelve

jejunum (je-JOON-um): the first two-fifths of the small intestine beyond the duodenum.

ileum (ILL-ee-um): the last segment of the small intestine.

ileocecal (ill-ee-oh-SEEK-ul) **valve**: the sphincter separating the small and large intestines.

large intestine or colon (COAL-un): the lower portion of intestine that completes the digestive process; its segments are the ascending colon, the transverse colon, the descending colon, and the sigmoid colon.
sigmoid = shaped like an **S** (sigma in Greek)

appendix: a narrow blind sac extending from the beginning of the colon; a vestigial organ with no known function.

rectum: the muscular terminal part of the intestine, extending from the sigmoid colon to the anus.

anus (AY-nus): the terminal sphincter of the GI tract.

To sum up, food follows the path shown in Figure 3–1. Food enters the mouth and travels past the epiglottis, down the esophagus and through the cardiac sphincter to the stomach, then through the pyloric sphincter to the small intestine (duodenum, with entrance from the gallbladder and pancreas; then jejunum; then ileum), on through the ileocecal valve to the large intestine, past the appendix to the rectum, ending at the anus. Considering all that happens on the way, the route is remarkably simple.

THE MUSCULAR ACTION OF DIGESTION

The first step in the reduction of food to a liquid takes place in the mouth, where chewing, the addition of saliva, and the action of the tongue reduce the food to a coarse mash. Then you swallow, and thereafter, you are generally unaware of all the activity that follows. As is the case with so much else that happens in the body, the muscles of the digestive tract meet internal needs without your having to exert any conscious effort. They keep things moving at just the right pace, slow enough to get the job done and fast enough to make progress.

The ability of the GI tract muscles to move is called their motility.

Peristalsis   Peristalsis begins when the bolus enters the esophagus. The entire GI tract is ringed with circular muscles that can squeeze it tightly. Surrounding these rings of muscle are longitudinal muscles. When the rings tighten and the long muscles relax, the tube is constricted. When the rings relax and the long muscles tighten, the tube bulges. These actions follow each other continuously and push the intestinal contents along (problem 5). (If you have ever watched a lump of food pass along the body of a snake, you have a good picture of how these muscles work.)

peristalsis (peri-STALL-sis): wavelike muscular contractions of the GI tract that push its contents along.
    peri = around
    stellein = wrap

The waves of contraction ripple along the GI tract at varying rates and intensities depending on the part of the GI tract and on whether food is present. For example, waves occur three times per minute in the stomach, but speed up to ten times per minute when chyme reaches the small intestine. When you have just eaten a meal, the waves are slow and continuous; when the GI tract is empty, the intestine is quiet except for periodic bursts of powerful rhythmic waves. Peristalsis, along with the sphincter muscles that surround the tract at key places, keeps things moving along (see Figure 3–2).

Stomach Action   The stomach has the thickest walls and strongest muscles of all the GI tract organs. In addition to the circular and longitudinal muscles, it has a third layer of diagonal muscles that also alternately contract and relax. These three sets of muscles work to force the chyme downward, but the pyloric sphincter usually remains tightly closed, preventing the chyme from passing into the duodenum. As a result, the chyme is churned and forced down, hits the pyloric sphincter, and remains in the stomach. Meanwhile, the stomach wall releases juices. When the chyme is completely liquefied, the pyloric sphincter opens briefly, about three times a minute, to allow small portions of chyme through. At this point, the chyme no longer resembles food in the least.

segmentation (SEG-men-TAY-shun): a periodic squeezing or partitioning of the intestine at intervals along its length by its circular muscles.

Segmentation   The intestines not only push, but also periodically squeeze their contents—as if a string tied around the intestines were being pulled gently. This motion, called segmentation, momentarily forces the intestinal contents back a few inches, mixing them and promoting close contact with the digestive juices and the absorbing cells of the intestinal walls before letting the contents move slowly along (see Figure 3–2).

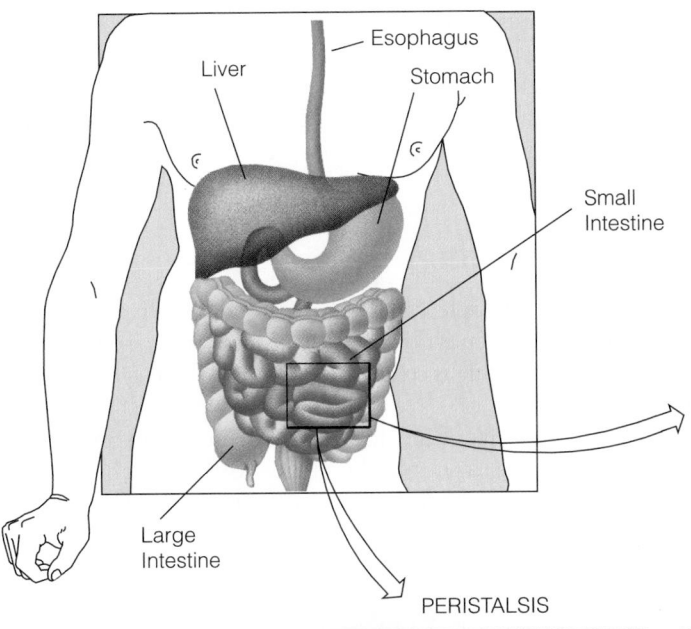

Figure 3–2

Peristalsis and Segmentation

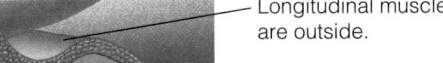

Esophagus

Liver

Stomach

Small
Intestine

Large
Intestine

Longitudinal muscles
are outside.

Circular muscles are
inside.

The small intestine has two
muscle layers that work
together in peristalsis
and segmentation.

PERISTALSIS

SEGMENTATON

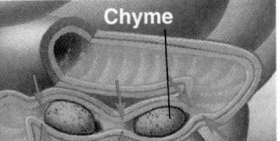

The inner circular muscles
contract, tightening
the tube and pushing the
food forward in the intestine.

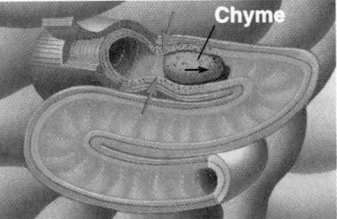

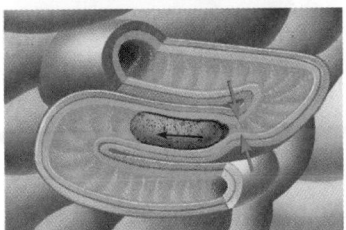

Circular muscles contract,
creating segments within
the intestine.

When the circular muscles
relax the outer longitudinal
muscles contract, and
the intestinal tube is loose.

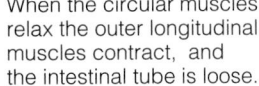

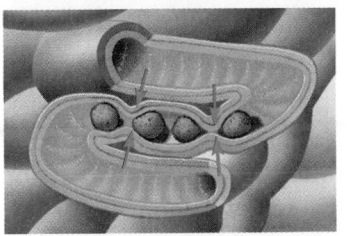

As each set of circular
muscles relaxes and
contracts, the chyme is
broken up and mixed with
digestive juices.

As the circular and
longitudinal muscles tighten
and relax, the chyme
moves ahead of the
constriction.

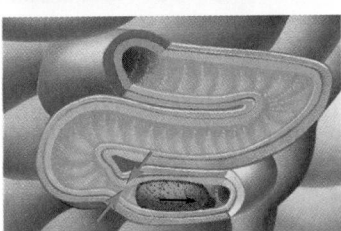

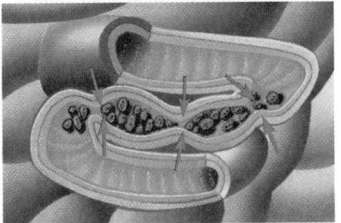

These alternating
contractions, occuring
12 to 16 times per minute,
continue to mix the chyme
and bring the nutrients
into contact with the
intestinal lining
for absorption.

Sphincter Contractions Four major sphincter muscles divide the GI tract into its principal divisions. At the bottom of the esophagus, the cardiac sphincter prevents reflux of the stomach contents. At the bottom of the stomach, the pyloric sphincter, which stays closed most of the time, holds the bolus in the stomach long enough so that it can be thoroughly mixed with gastric juice and

reflux: a backward flow.
re = back
flux = flow

liquefied. It also prevents the intestinal contents from backing up into the stomach. At the end of the small intestine, the ileocecal valve performs a similar function, emptying the contents of the small intestine into the large intestine. Finally, the tightness of the rectal muscle is a kind of safety device; together with the anus, it prevents elimination until you choose to perform it voluntarily (problem 7).

THE SECRETIONS OF DIGESTION

Remember from Chapter 1 how people can eat differently yet have essentially the same body composition? It all comes down to the process of digestion, of rendering food—whatever kind of food it is to start with—into the basic units that make up the nutrients.

To break down food to small units of nutrients that the body can absorb, five different organs produce secretions: the salivary glands, the stomach, the pancreas, the liver (via the gallbladder), and the small intestine. (The glossary below identifies some of the digestive glands and their secretions.) These secretions enter the GI tract at various points along the way, bringing an abundance of water and a variety of enzymes.

gland: a cell or group of cells that secretes materials for special uses in the body. Glands may be exocrine (EKS-oh-crin) glands, secreting their materials "out" (into the digestive tract or onto the surface of the skin), or endocrine (EN-doe-crin) glands, secreting their materials "in" (into the blood).

exo = outside
endo = inside
krine = to separate

Glossary of Digestive Glands and Their Secretions

These terms are listed in order from start to end of the digestive tract.

salivary glands: exocrine glands that secrete saliva into the mouth.

saliva: the secretion of the salivary glands; its principal enzyme begins carbohydrate digestion.

gastric glands: exocrine glands in the stomach wall that secrete gastric juice into the stomach.

gastro = stomach

gastric juice: the digestive secretion of the gastric glands of the stomach.

hydrochloric acid: an acid composed of hydrogen and chloride atoms (HCl). The gastric glands normally produce this acid.

mucus (MYOO-cuss): a slippery substance secreted by goblet cells of the GI lining (and other body linings) that protects the cells from exposure to digestive juices (and other destructive agents). The lining of the GI tract with its coat of mucus is a mucous membrane. (The noun is mucus; the adjective is mucous.)

bile: an emulsifier that prepares fats and oils for digestion; an exocrine secretion made by the liver, stored in the gallbladder, and released into the small intestine when needed.

emulsifier (ee-MUL-sih-fire): a substance with both water-soluble and fat-soluble portions that promotes the mixing of oils and fats in a watery solution.

pancreatic (pank-ree-AT-ic) **juice:** the exocrine secretion of the pancreas, containing enzymes for the digestion of carbohydrate, fat, and protein as well as bicarbonate, a neutralizing agent. The juice flows from the pancreas into the small intestine through the pancreatic duct. (The pancreas also has an endocrine function, the secretion of insulin and other hormones.)

bicarbonate: an alkaline secretion of the pancreas, part of the pancreatic juice. (Bicarbonate also occurs widely in all cell fluids.)

Glossary of Digestive Enzymes

digestive enzymes: proteins found in digestive juices that act on food substances, causing them to break down into simpler compounds.

-ase (ACE): a word ending denoting an enzyme. Enzymes are often identified by the place they come from and the compounds they work on; *gastric lipase*, for example is a stomach enzyme that acts on lipids, whereas *pancreatic lipase* comes from the pancreas (and also works on lipids).

carbohydrase (KAR-boe-HIGH-drase): an enzyme that hydrolyzes carbohydrates.

hydrolysis (high-DROL-ih-sis): a chemical reaction in which a major reactant is split into two products, with the addition of a hydrogen atom (H) to one and a hydroxyl group (OH) to the other (from water, H_2O).
  hydro = water
  lysis = breaking

lipase (LYE-pase): an enzyme that hydrolyzes lipids (fats).

protease (PRO-tee-ase): an enzyme that hydrolyzes proteins.

All enzymes and some hormones are proteins, but an enzyme is not a hormone. Enzymes facilitate the making and breaking of bonds in chemical reactions; hormones act as chemical messengers, sometimes regulating enzyme action.

Enzymes are formally introduced in Chapter 6, but for now, a simple definition will suffice. An enzyme is a giant protein molecule that facilitates a chemical reaction—making a molecule from smaller parts, breaking a molecule into smaller parts, changing the arrangement of a molecule, or exchanging parts of molecules. As a catalyst, the enzyme itself remains unchanged. The enzymes involved in digestion facilitate a chemical reaction known as hydrolysis—the addition of water (hydro) to break (lysis) a molecule into smaller pieces. The glossary above identifies some of the digestive enzymes and defines related terms.

Saliva The salivary glands squirt just enough saliva to moisten each mouthful of food so that it can pass easily down the esophagus (problem 3). The saliva contains water, salts, and enzymes that initiate the digestion of carbohydrates. In fact, you can taste the change if you hold a piece of starchy food like a cracker in your mouth for a few minutes without swallowing it—the cracker begins tasting sweeter as the enzyme acts on it. Saliva also protects the tooth surfaces and the linings of the mouth, esophagus, and stomach from attack by substances that might harm them.

Gastric Juice Cells in the stomach secrete gastric juice, a mixture of water, enzymes, and hydrocholoric acid. The acid is so strong that it causes the sensation of heartburn if it chances to reflux into the esophagus. Highlight 3, following this chapter, discusses heartburn and other common digestive problems.

The strong acidity of the stomach prevents bacterial growth and kills most bacteria that enter the body with food. It would destroy the cells of the stomach as well, but for their natural defenses. To protect themselves from gastric juice, the goblet cells of the stomach wall secrete mucus, a thick, slippery, white substance that coats the cells, protecting them from the acid and enzymes that might otherwise harm them.

Figure 3–3 shows how the strength of acids is measured—in pH units. Note that the acidity of gastric juice registers below "2" on the pH scale—stronger than vinegar. The stomach enzymes work most efficiently in the stomach's strong acid, but

catalyst (CAT-uh-list): a compound that facilitates chemical reactions without itself being changed in the process.

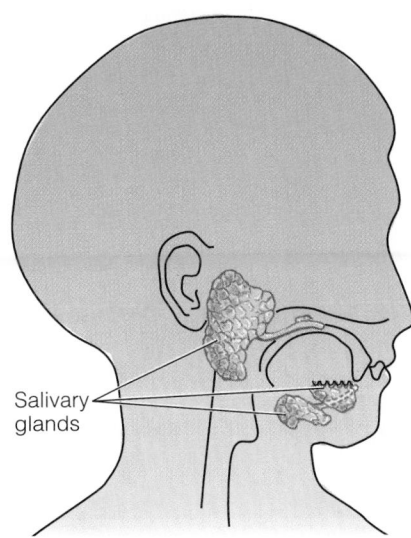

The salivary glands secrete saliva into the mouth and begin the digestive process. Given the short time food is in the mouth, salivary enzymes contribute little to digestion.

goblet cells: cells of the GI tract (and lungs) that secrete mucus.

Figure 3–3

The pH Scale

A substance's acidity or alkalinity is measured in pH units. The pH is the negative logarithm of the hydrogen ion concentration. Each increment presents a tenfold increase in concentration of hydrogen particles. For example, a pH of 2 is 1000 times stronger than a pH of 5.

pH's of common substances:

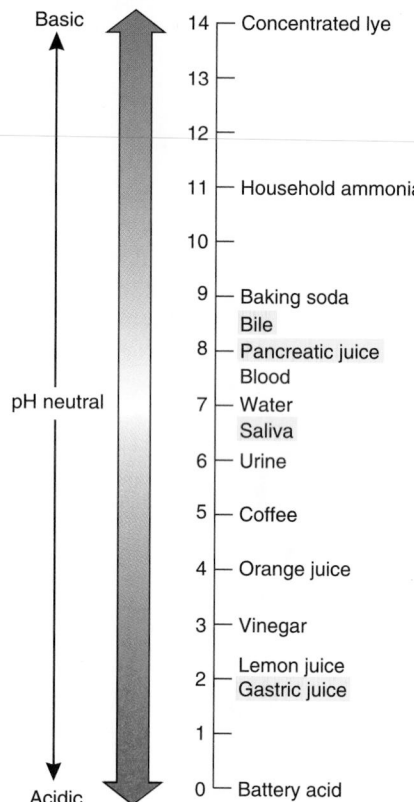

pH: the unit of measure expressing a substance's acidity or alkalinity (Chapter 12 and Appendix B provide a more detailed definition).

The bacterial inhabitants of the GI tract are known as the intestinal flora.

flora = plant growth

---

the salivary enzymes, which are swallowed with food, do not work in acid this strong. Consequently, the salivary digestion of carbohydrate gradually ceases as the stomach acid penetrates each newly swallowed bolus of food. In fact, salivary enzymes become just other proteins to be digested, and carbohydrate digestion waits to resume in the next digestive organ, the small intestine.

The major digestive event in the stomach is the partial breakdown (hydrolysis) of proteins. There, the acid helps to uncoil proteins, making them available for digestion. Both an enzyme and the stomach acid itself act as catalysts for this reaction. Minor events are the digestion of a very little fat by a gastric lipase; the breakdown of some carbohydrate by gastric acid; and the attachment of a protein carrier to vitamin B_{12}.

Pancreatic Juice and Intestinal Enzymes By the time food leaves the stomach, digestion of all three energy nutrients has begun, and the action gains momentum in the small intestine. There, the pancreas and liver contribute additional digestive juices by way of ducts leading into the duodenum. The pancreatic juice contains enzymes that act on all three energy nutrients, and the cells of the intestinal wall also possess digestive enzymes on their surfaces.

In addition to enzymes, the pancreatic juice contains sodium bicarbonate, which is basic or alkaline—the opposite of the stomach's acid (review Figure 3–3). The pancreatic juice thus neutralizes the acid chyme arriving in the small intestine from the stomach. From this point on, the chyme remains at a neutral or slightly alkaline pH. The enzymes of both the intestine and the pancreas work best in this environment.

Bile Bile also flows into the duodenum. The liver continuously secretes bile, which is then concentrated and stored in the gallbladder, which squirts the bile into the duodenum when fat arrives there. Bile is not an enzyme, but an emulsifier that brings fats into suspension in water so that enzymes can break them down into their component parts. Thanks to all these secretions, the three energy-yielding nutrients are digested in the small intestine (see Table 3–1 for a summary of digestive secretions and their actions).

Protective Factors Both the small and the large intestine, being neutral in pH, permit the growth of bacteria. In fact, a healthy intestinal tract supports a thriving bacterial population that normally does the body no harm and may actually do some good. Bacteria in the GI tract produce a couple of vitamins, including a significant amount of vitamin K, although the amount is insufficient to meet the body's total need for that vitamin.[2]

Provided that the normal intestinal flora are thriving, infectious bacteria have a hard time getting established and launching an attack on the system. Diet is one of several factors that influence the bacterial population and its environment.[3] In addition, secretions from the GI tract—saliva, mucus, gastric acid, and digestive enzymes—not only help with digestion, but also defend against foreign invaders. The GI tract also maintains several different kinds of defending cells that confer specific immunity against intestinal diseases.

THE FINAL STAGE

The story of how digestion prepares food for absorption is now nearly complete. The three energy-yielding nutrients—carbohydrate, fat, and protein—have been

Table 3–1

Summary of Digestive Secretions

Organ or Gland	Target Organ	Secretion	Action
Salivary glands	Mouth	Saliva	Fluid eases swallowing; salivary enzyme breaks down carbohydrate.
Gastric glands	Stomach	Gastric juice	Fluid mixes with bolus; hydrochloric acid uncoils proteins; enzymes break down proteins; mucus protects stomach cells.
Pancreas	Small intestine	Pancreatic juice	Bicarbonate neutralizes acidic gastric juices; pancreatic enzymes break down carbohydrates, fats, and proteins.
Liver	Gallbladder	Bile	Bile stored until needed.
Gallbladder	Small intestine	Bile	Bile emulsifies fat into small particles that enzymes can attack.
Intestinal glands	Small intestine	Intestinal juice	Intestinal enzymes break down carbohydrate and protein fragments; mucus protects the intestinal wall.

disassembled to basic building blocks and are ready to be absorbed. Most of the other nutrients—vitamins, minerals, and water—need no such disassembly; they are absorbed as they are. Undigested residues, such as some fibers, are not absorbed, but continue through the digestive tract, providing a semisolid mass that helps exercise the muscles and keep them strong enough to perform peristalsis efficiently. Fiber also retains water, accounting for the stools' pasty consistency, and carries some bile acids, some minerals, and some additives and contaminants with it out of the body.

The process of absorbing the nutrients into the body presents its own problems, to be discussed in the next section. For the moment, assume that the digested nutrients simply are absorbed from the GI tract as soon as they are ready. Most are gone by the time the contents of the GI tract reach the end of the small intestine. Little remains but water, a few dissolved salts and body secretions, and undigested materials such as fiber. These enter the large intestine (colon).

In the colon, intestinal bacteria degrade some of the fiber to simpler compounds, while the colon itself retrieves all materials that the body is designed to recycle—water and dissolved salts. The waste that is finally excreted has little or nothing of value left in it. The body has extracted all that it can use from the food. Figure 3–4 (on p. 82) summarizes digestion by following a sandwich through the GI tract and into the body.

Some vitamins and minerals are slightly altered during digestion as later chapters explain.

Chapter 4 discusses fiber in more detail.

stools: waste matter discharged from the colon; also called *feces* (FEE-seez).

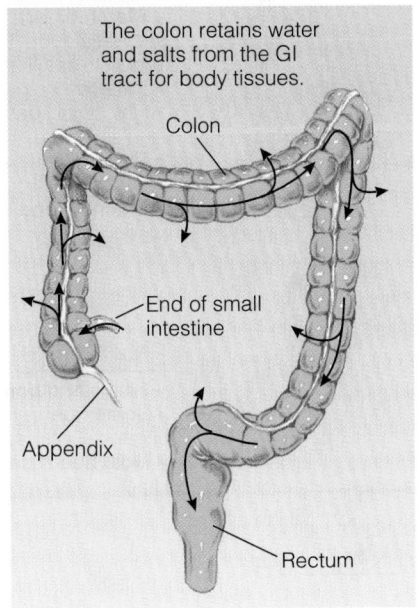

The colon retains water and salts from the GI tract for body tissues.

Colon

End of small intestine

Appendix

Rectum

The colon reabsorbs water and salts.

Absorption

Problem: Given an elaborate production in which 1000 actors are on stage at once, provide a means by which all can exit simultaneously. This is the problem of absorption. Within three or four hours after you have eaten a dinner of beans and rice (or spinach lasagna, or steak and potatoes) with vegetable, salad, beverage, and dessert, your body must find a way to absorb—one by one—some two

Figure 3–4

The Digestive Fate of a Sandwich

To review the digestive processes and enzymes, follow a peanut butter and banana sandwich on whole-wheat, sesame seed bread through the GI tract.

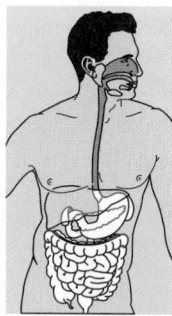

MOUTH: CHEWING AND SWALLOWING, WITH LITTLE DIGESTION

- **Carbohydrate** digestion begins as the salivary enzyme starts to break down the starch from bread and peanut butter.
- **Fiber** covering on the sesame seeds is crushed by the teeth, which exposes the nutrients inside the seeds to the upcoming digestive enzymes.

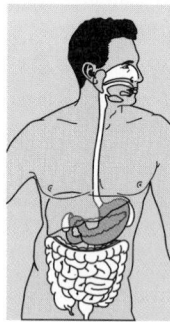

STOMACH: COLLECTING AND CHURNING, WITH SOME DIGESTION

- **Carbohydrate** digestion continues until the mashed sandwich has been mixed with the gastric juices; the stomach acid of the gastric juices inactivates the salivary enzyme.
- **Proteins** from the bread, seeds, and peanut butter begin to uncoil when they mix with the gastric acid, making them available to the gastric protease enzymes that begin to digest proteins.
- **Fat** from the peanut butter forms a separate layer on top of the watery mixture.

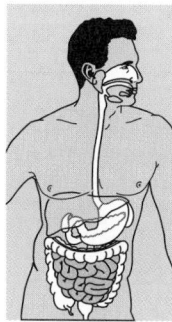

SMALL INTESTINE: DIGESTING AND ABSORBING

- **Sugars** from the banana require so little digestion that they begin to traverse the intestinal cells immediately on contact.
- **Starch** digestion picks up when the pancreas sends pancreatic enzymes to the small intestine via the pancreatic duct. Enzymes on the surfaces of the small intestinal cells complete the process of breaking down starch into small fragments that can be absorbed through the intestinal cell walls and into the blood.
- **Fat** from the peanut butter and seeds is emulsified with the watery digestive fluids by bile. Now the pancreatic and intestinal lipases can begin to break down the fat to smaller fragments that can be absorbed through the cells of the small intestinal wall and into the lymph.
- **Protein** digestion depends on the pancreatic and intestinal proteases. Small fragments of protein are liberated and absorbed through the cells of the small intestinal wall and into the blood.
- **Vitamins and minerals** are absorbed.

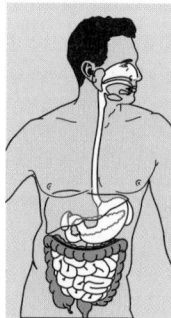

LARGE INTESTINE: REABSORBING AND ELIMINATING

- **Fluids and some minerals** are absorbed.
- **Some fibers** from the seeds, whole-wheat bread, peanut butter, and banana are partly digested by the bacteria living there, and some of these products are absorbed.
- **Most fibers** pass through the large intestine and are excreted as feces; some fat, cholesterol, and minerals bind to fiber and are also excreted.

hundred thousand million, million, million molecules derived from carbohydrate digestion; a comparable number of molecules derived from protein and fat digestion; and many vitamin and mineral molecules as well.

For the stage production, the manager might design multiple wings that the actors could crowd into, a dozen at a time. A mechanical genius might somehow design conveyor-belt wings that would actively sweep up the actors as they approached. The absorptive system is no such fantasy; the lowly "gut" is actually one of the most elegantly designed organ systems in the body. In 10 feet of small intestine, it provides a surface area equivalent to a quarter of a football field, which engulfs and absorbs the nutrient molecules. To remove the molecules rapidly and provide room for more to be absorbed, a rush of circulating blood continuously washes the underside of this surface, carrying the absorbed nutrients away to the liver and other parts of the body.

absorption: the taking up of nutrients into the intestinal cells.

ANATOMY OF THE ABSORPTIVE SYSTEM

The inner surface of the small intestine looks smooth and slippery, but viewed through a microscope, it turns out to be wrinkled into hundreds of folds. Each fold, in turn, is contoured into thousands of nipplelike projections, as numerous as the hairs on velvet fabric. These small intestinal projections are the villi. A single villus, magnified still more, turns out to be composed of hundreds of cells, each covered with its own microscopic hairs, the microvilli (see Figure 3–5 on p. 84). In the crevices between the villi lie the crypts—tubular glands that secrete the intestinal juices into the small intestine.

The villi are in constant motion. Each villus is lined by a thin sheet of muscle, so it can wave, squirm, and wriggle like the tentacles of a sea anemone. Any nutrient molecule small enough to be absorbed is trapped among the microvilli that coat the cells and then drawn into the cells. Some partially digested nutrients are caught in the microvilli, digested further by enzymes there, and then absorbed into the cells. Figure 3–6 (on p. 85) describes how nutrients are absorbed by diffusion, facilitated diffusion, or active transport.

The body's two transport systems—the bloodstream and the lymphatic system—supply vessels to each villus, as shown in Figure 3–5. When a nutrient molecule has crossed the cell of a villus, it may enter either the lymph or the blood, but before following nutrients through the body, we must look more closely at the digestive cells themselves.

villi (VILL-ee, VILL-eye): fingerlike projections from the folds of the small intestine; singular **villus.**

microvilli (MY-cro-VILL-ee, MY-cro-VILL-eye): tiny, hairlike projections on each cell of every villus that can trap nutrient particles and transport them into the cells; singular **microvillus.**

crypts: tubular glands that lie between the intestinal villi and secrete intestinal juices into the small intestine.

A CLOSER LOOK AT THE INTESTINAL CELLS

One of the beauties of the digestive tract is that it is selective. Materials that are nutritive for the body are broken down into particles that can be assimilated into the bloodstream. Most of the materials that are not nutritive are left undigested and pass out the other end of the digestive tract. The cells of the villi are among the most amazing in the body, for they recognize and select the nutrients the body needs and regulate their absorption. A close look at these cells is worthwhile, because it will help to explode a common misconception about nutrition: that you have to do anything to ensure that your digestive tract does its job. Nothing could be further from the truth.

The problem of food contaminants, which may be absorbed defenselessly by the body, is the subject of Chapter 14.

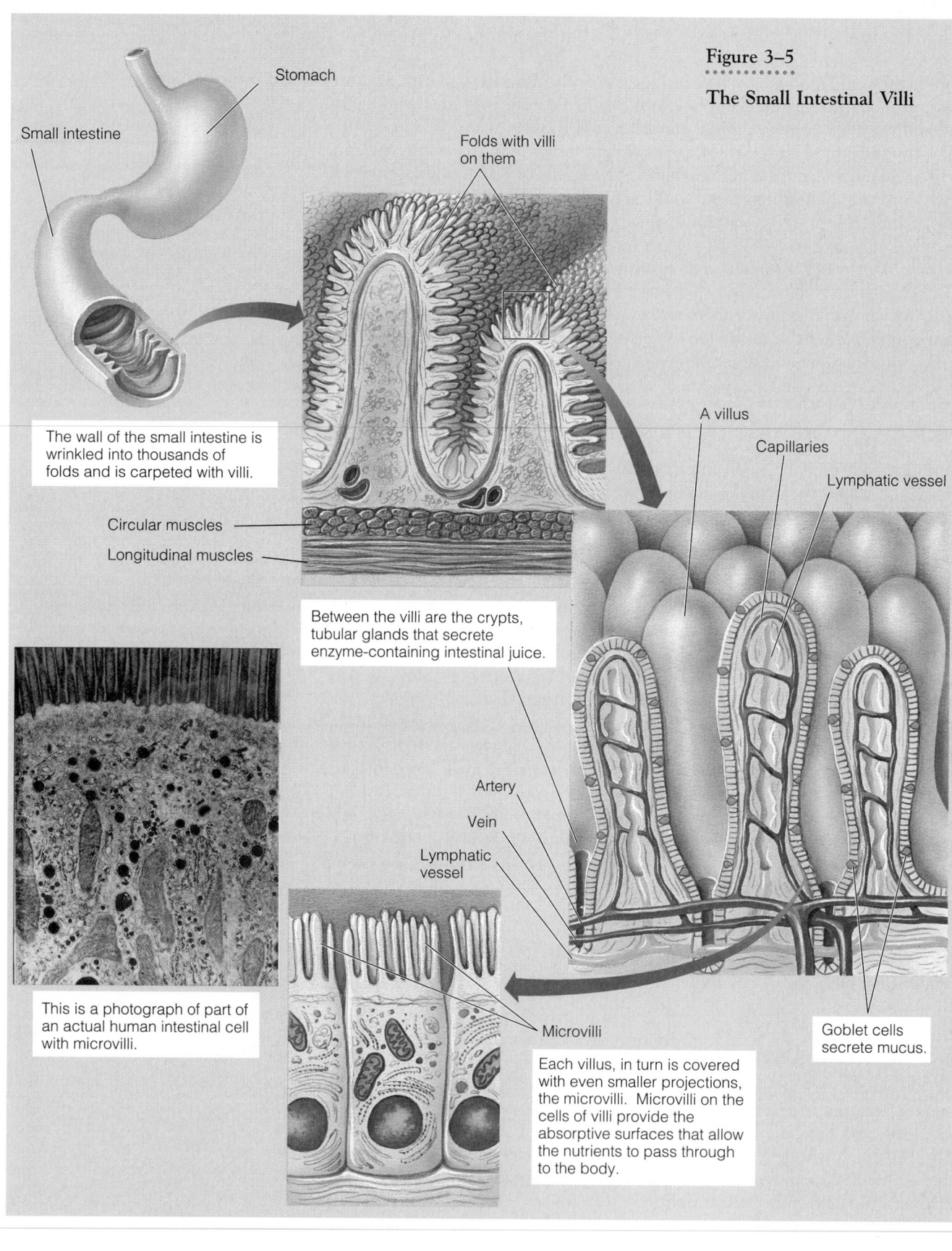

Figure 3–5

The Small Intestinal Villi

Stomach

Small intestine

Folds with villi on them

The wall of the small intestine is wrinkled into thousands of folds and is carpeted with villi.

Circular muscles

Longitudinal muscles

A villus

Capillaries

Lymphatic vessel

Between the villi are the crypts, tubular glands that secrete enzyme-containing intestinal juice.

Artery

Vein

Lymphatic vessel

This is a photograph of part of an actual human intestinal cell with microvilli.

Microvilli

Goblet cells secrete mucus.

Each villus, in turn is covered with even smaller projections, the microvilli. Microvilli on the cells of villi provide the absorptive surfaces that allow the nutrients to pass through to the body.

Figure 3–6

Absorption of Nutrients

Absorption of nutrients into intestinal cells typically occurs by diffusion, facilitated diffusion, or active transport.

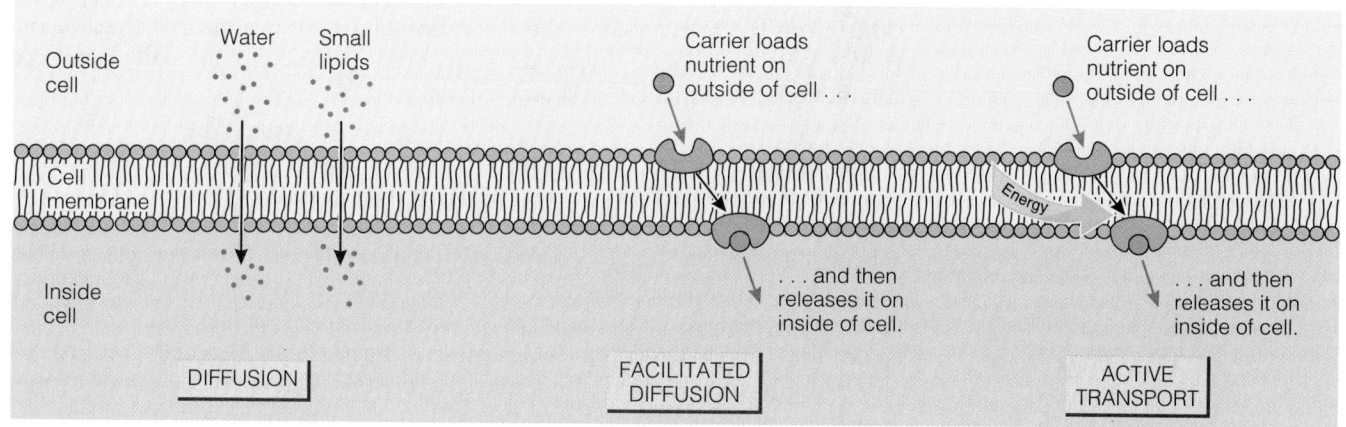

Some nutrients, such as water and small lipids, cross into intestinal cells freely.

Some nutrients, such as the water-soluble vitamins, need a specific carrier to transport them from one side of the cell membrane to the other. (Alternatively, facilitated diffusion may occur when the carrier changes the cell membrane in such a way that the nutrients can pass through.)

Some nutrients, such as glucose and amino acids, must be absorbed actively. These nutrients move against a concentration gradient, which requires energy.

The Cells' Capabilities   As already described, each cell of a villus is coated with thousands of microvilli, which project from the cell's membrane (review Figure 3–5). In these microvilli and in the membrane lie hundreds of different kinds of enzymes and "pumps," which recognize and act on different nutrients. Descriptions of specific enzymes and "pumps" for each nutrient are presented in the following chapters where appropriate, but the point here is that the cells are equipped to handle all kinds and combinations of foods and nutrients.

Specialization in the GI Tract   A further refinement of the system is that the cells of successive portions of the intestinal tract are specialized to absorb different nutrients. The nutrients that are ready for absorption early are absorbed near the top of the tract; those that take longer to be digested are absorbed farther down. The rate at which digested nutrients travel through the GI tract is finely adjusted to maximize their availability to the appropriate absorptive segments of the tract. Medical and health professionals who deal with digestion learn the specialized absorptive functions of different parts of the GI tract so that if one part becomes dysfunctional, the diet can be adjusted accordingly.

The Myth of "Food Combining"   The idea that people should not eat certain food combinations (for example, fruit and meat) at the same meal, because the digestive system cannot handle more than one task at a time, is a myth. The art of "food combining" (which actually emphasizes "food separating") is based on this idea, and it represents faulty logic and a gross underestimation of the body's capabilities. If a person ate only fruit, the carbohydrate enzymes for digestion and carriers for absorption would be extremely busy while those for protein and fat sat idle. In fact, the contrary is often true; foods eaten together can enhance each other's use by the body. For example, vitamin C in a pineapple or other citrus fruit can enhance the absorption of iron from a meal of chicken and rice or other iron-containing foods. Many other instances of mutually beneficial interactions are presented in later chapters.

Preparing Nutrients for Transport   Once inside the intestinal cells, the products of digestion must be released for transport to the rest of the body. The water-soluble nutrients (including the smaller products of fat digestion) are released directly into the bloodstream via the capillaries. The larger fats and the fat-soluble vitamins are insoluble in water, however, and blood is mostly water. The intestinal cells assemble many of the products of fat digestion into larger molecules. These larger molecules cluster together, and special proteins are inserted into their surfaces, forming chylomicrons. These chylomicrons cannot pass into the capillaries and are released into the lymphatic system instead; the chylomicrons move through the lymph and later enter the bloodstream at a point near the heart.

Chylomicrons (kye-lo-MY-cronz) are described in Chapter 5.

The Circulatory Systems

Once a nutrient has entered the bloodstream, it may be transported to any part of the body and thus become available to any of the cells, from the tips of the toes to the roots of the hair. The circulatory systems are arranged to deliver nutrients wherever they are needed.

THE VASCULAR SYSTEM

The vascular, or blood circulatory, system is a closed system of vessels through which blood flows continuously in a figure eight, with the heart serving as a pump at the crossover point (see Figure 3–7). As the blood circulates through this system, it picks up and delivers materials as needed.

All the body tissues derive oxygen and nutrients from the blood and deposit carbon dioxide and other wastes into it. The lungs exchange carbon dioxide (which leaves the blood to be exhaled) and oxygen (which enters the blood to be delivered to all cells). The digestive system supplies the nutrients to be picked up. In the kidneys, wastes other than carbon dioxide are filtered out of the blood to be excreted in the urine (see Figure 3–8 on p. 88).

Blood leaving the right side of the heart circulates by way of arteries into the lung capillaries and then back through veins to the left side of the heart. The left side of the heart then pumps the blood out through arteries to all systems of the body. The blood circulates in the capillaries, where it exchanges material with the cells, and then collects into veins, which return it again to the right side of the heart. In short, blood travels this simple route:

- Heart to arteries to capillaries to veins to heart.

artery: a vessel that carries blood away from the heart.

capillary (CAP-ill-ary): a small vessel that branches from an artery. Capillaries connect arteries to veins. Exchange of oxygen, nutrients, and waste materials takes place across capillary walls.

vein: a vessel that carries blood back to the heart.

Figure 3–7

The Vascular System

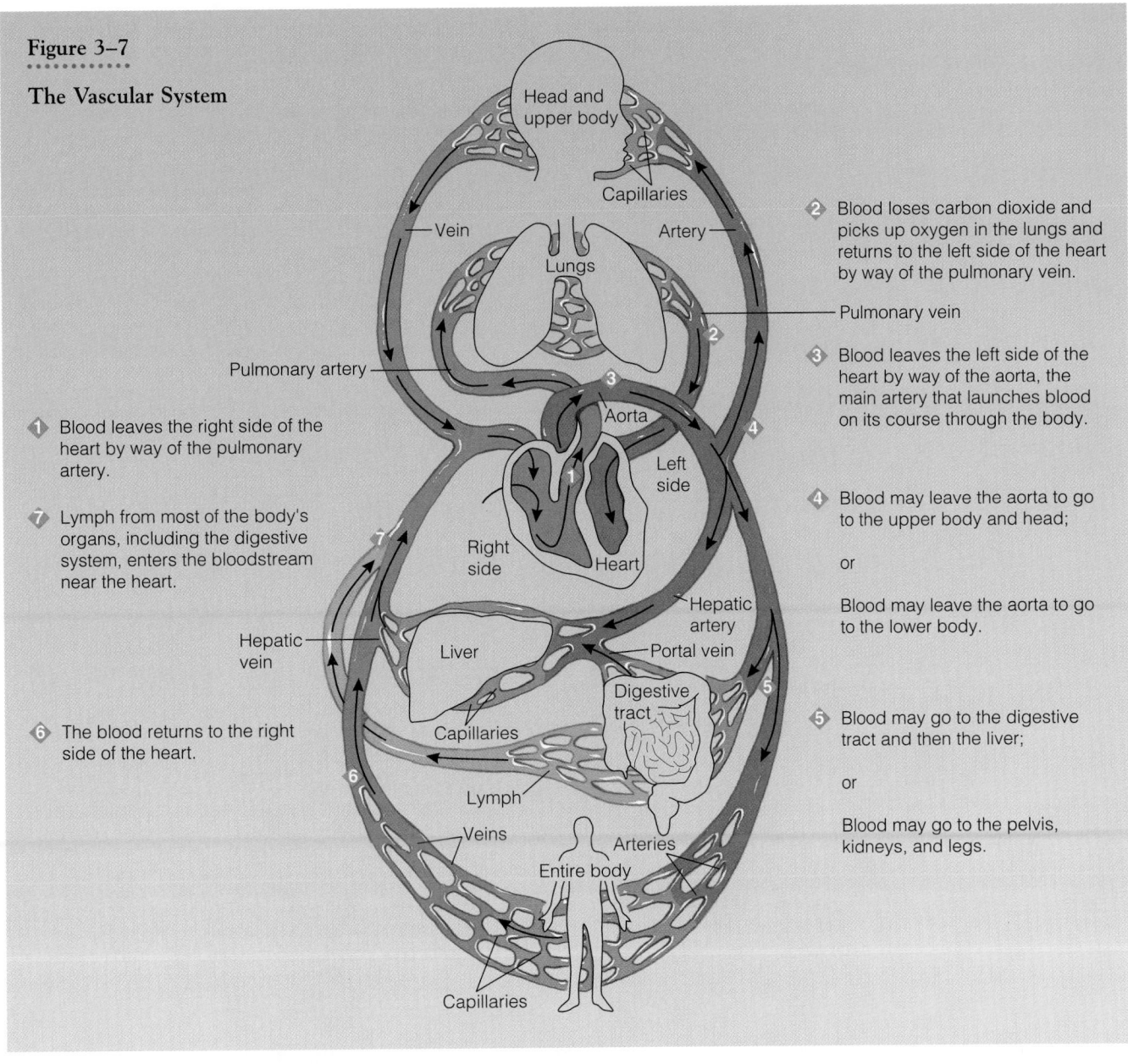

1 Blood leaves the right side of the heart by way of the pulmonary artery.

7 Lymph from most of the body's organs, including the digestive system, enters the bloodstream near the heart.

6 The blood returns to the right side of the heart.

2 Blood loses carbon dioxide and picks up oxygen in the lungs and returns to the left side of the heart by way of the pulmonary vein.

3 Blood leaves the left side of the heart by way of the aorta, the main artery that launches blood on its course through the body.

4 Blood may leave the aorta to go to the upper body and head;

or

Blood may leave the aorta to go to the lower body.

5 Blood may go to the digestive tract and then the liver;

or

Blood may go to the pelvis, kidneys, and legs.

The routing of the blood past the digestive system has a special feature. The blood is carried to the digestive system (as to all organs) by way of an artery, which (as in all organs) branches into capillaries to reach every cell. Blood leaving the digestive system, however, goes by way of a vein, not back to the heart, but to another organ—the liver. This vein *again* branches into *capillaries*, so that every cell of the liver also has access to the blood carried by the vein. Blood leaving the liver then *again* collects into a vein, which returns to the heart.

The vein that collects blood from the GI tract and conducts it to capillaries in the liver is the portal vein.

portal = gateway

The vein that collects blood from the liver capillaries and returns it to the heart is the hepatic vein.

hepatic = liver

Figure 3–8

A Nephron, One of the Kidney's Many Functioning Units

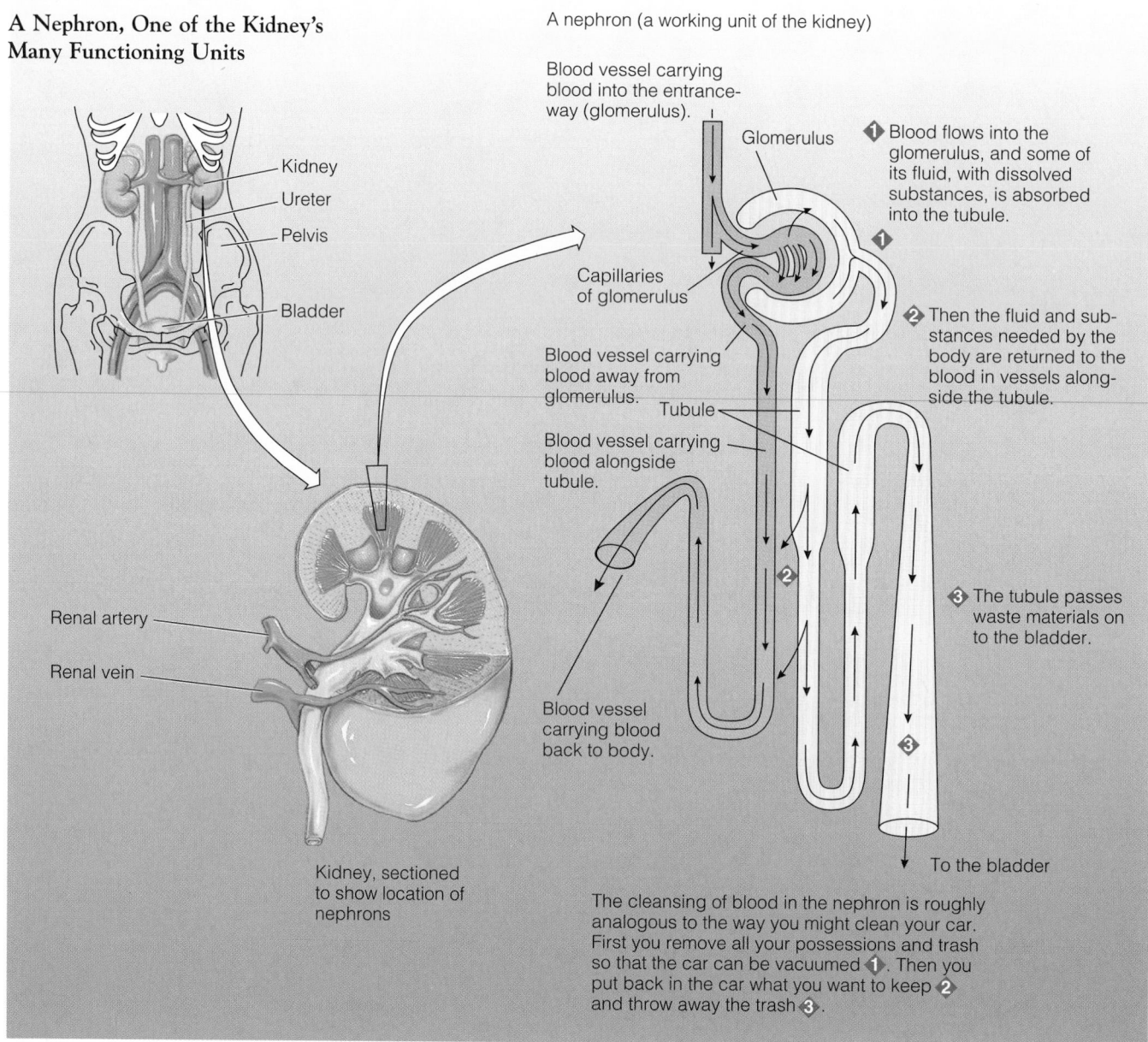

A nephron (a working unit of the kidney)

Blood vessel carrying blood into the entranceway (glomerulus).

Glomerulus

❶ Blood flows into the glomerulus, and some of its fluid, with dissolved substances, is absorbed into the tubule.

❶

Capillaries of glomerulus

❷ Then the fluid and substances needed by the body are returned to the blood in vessels alongside the tubule.

Blood vessel carrying blood away from glomerulus.

Tubule

Blood vessel carrying blood alongside tubule.

❷

❸ The tubule passes waste materials on to the bladder.

Kidney

Ureter

Pelvis

Bladder

Renal artery

Renal vein

Blood vessel carrying blood back to body.

❸

To the bladder

Kidney, sectioned to show location of nephrons

The cleansing of blood in the nephron is roughly analogous to the way you might clean your car. First you remove all your possessions and trash so that the car can be vacuumed ❶. Then you put back in the car what you want to keep ❷ and throw away the trash ❸.

The route is:

- Heart to arteries to capillaries (in intestines) to vein to capillaries (in liver) to vein to heart.

An anatomist studying this system knows there must be a reason for this special arrangement. The liver is placed in the circulation at this point so that it will have the first chance at the materials absorbed from the GI tract. In fact, the

Figure 3–9

The Liver

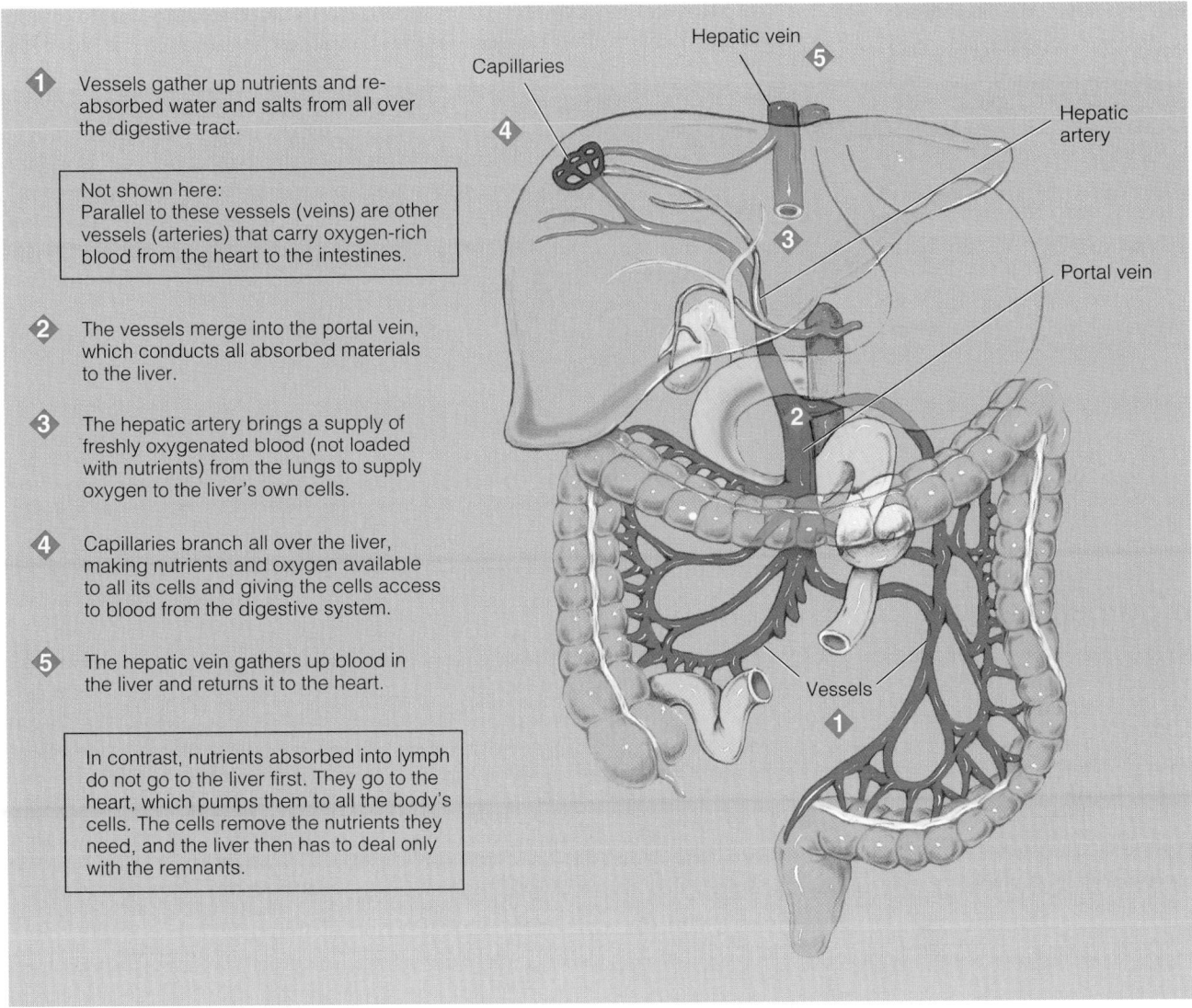

1. Vessels gather up nutrients and re-absorbed water and salts from all over the digestive tract.

   Not shown here:
   Parallel to these vessels (veins) are other vessels (arteries) that carry oxygen-rich blood from the heart to the intestines.

2. The vessels merge into the portal vein, which conducts all absorbed materials to the liver.

3. The hepatic artery brings a supply of freshly oxygenated blood (not loaded with nutrients) from the lungs to supply oxygen to the liver's own cells.

4. Capillaries branch all over the liver, making nutrients and oxygen available to all its cells and giving the cells access to blood from the digestive system.

5. The hepatic vein gathers up blood in the liver and returns it to the heart.

   In contrast, nutrients absorbed into lymph do not go to the liver first. They go to the heart, which pumps them to all the body's cells. The cells remove the nutrients they need, and the liver then has to deal only with the remnants.

Hepatic vein

Capillaries

Hepatic artery

Portal vein

Vessels

liver has many jobs to do in preparing the absorbed nutrients for use by the body. It is the body's major metabolic organ.

You might guess that, in addition, the liver stands as gatekeeper to waylay intruders that might otherwise harm the heart or brain. Perhaps this is why, when people ingest poisons that succeed in passing the first barrier (the intestinal cells), the liver quite often suffers the damage—from the hepatitis virus, from drugs such as barbiturates or alcohol, from poisons, and from contaminants such as mercury. Perhaps, in fact, you have been undervaluing your liver, not knowing what heroic tasks it quietly performs for you. Figure 3–9 shows the liver's key position in nutrient transport.

lymphatic (lim-FAT-ic) system: a loosely organized system of vessels and ducts that convey fluids toward the heart; the GI part of the lymphatic system carries the products of digestion into the bloodstream.

lymph (LIMF): a clear yellowish fluid that resembles blood without the red blood cells; lymph from the GI tract transports fat and fat-soluble vitamins to the bloodstream via lymphatic vessels.

The duct that conveys lymph toward the heart is the thoracic (thor-ASS-ic) duct. The subclavian vein connects this duct with the right upper chamber of the heart, providing a passageway by which lymph can be returned to the vascular system.

THE LYMPHATIC SYSTEM

The lymphatic system provides a one-way route for fluid from the tissue spaces to enter the blood. Lymph fluid circulates between the cells of the body and collects into tiny vessels. Lymph is almost identical to blood except that it contains no red blood cells or platelets, because they cannot escape through the blood vessel walls.

The lymphatic system has no pump; instead, lymph is squeezed from one portion of the body to another like water in a sponge, as muscles contract and create pressure here and there. Ultimately, much of the lymph collects in a large duct behind the heart. This duct terminates in a vein that conducts the lymph toward the heart. Thus materials from the GI tract that enter lymphatic vessels (large fats and fat-soluble vitamins) ultimately enter the blood circulatory system, circulating through arteries, capillaries, and veins like the other nutrients, with a notable exception—they bypass the liver at first.

Once inside the vascular system, the nutrients can travel freely to any destination and can be taken into cells and used as needed. What becomes of them is described in later chapters.

Regulation of Digestion and Absorption

homeostasis (HOME-ee-oh-STAY-sis): the maintenance of constant internal conditions (such as blood chemistry, temperature, and blood pressure) by the body's control systems. A homeostatic system is constantly reacting to external forces so as to maintain limits set by the body's needs.
   homeo = the same
   stasis = staying

Factors influencing GI function:
• Physical immaturity.
• Aging.
• Illness.
• Nutrition.

There is nothing random about digestion and absorption; they are coordinated in every detail. The ability of the digestive tract to handle its ever-changing contents routinely illustrates an important physiological principle that governs the way all living things function—the principle of homeostasis. Simply stated, conditions have to stay about the same for an organism to survive; if they deviate too far from the norm, the organism must "do something" to bring them back to normal. The body's regulation of digestion is one example of homeostatic regulation. The body also regulates its temperature, its blood pressure, and all other aspects of its blood chemistry in similar ways.

The following paragraphs describe the regulation of digestion and absorption in healthy adults, but many factors can influence normal GI function. For example, peristalsis and sphincter action are poorly coordinated in newborns, and so infants tend to "spit up" during the first several months of life. Older adults often experience constipation, in part because the intestinal wall loses strength and elasticity with age, which slows GI motility. Diseases can also interfere with digestion and absorption and often lead to malnutrition. Lack of nourishment, in general, and lack of certain dietary constituents such as fiber, in particular, alter the structure and function of GI cells. Quite simply, GI tract health depends on food.

hormones: chemical messengers. Hormones are secreted by a variety of glands in response to altered conditions in the body. Each hormone travels to one or more specific target tissues or organs, where it elicits a specific response to restore normal conditions. In general, a gastrointestinal hormone is called an enterogastrone (EN-ter-oh-GAS-trone).*

GASTROINTESTINAL HORMONES AND NERVE PATHWAYS

Two intricate and sensitive systems coordinate all the digestive and absorptive processes: the hormonal (or endocrine) system and the nervous system. The contents of the GI tract either stimulate or inhibit digestive secretions by way of

*The term *enterogastrone* refers specifically to any hormone that inhibits gastric secretions, including secretin, cholecystokinin (CCK), and gastric-inhibitory peptide; more broadly, the term refers to any hormone released from the intestine.

messages that are carried from one section of the GI tract to another by both hormones and nerve pathways.

Notice that the kinds of regulation that will be described are all examples of *feedback* mechanisms. A certain condition demands a response. The response changes that condition, and the change then cuts off the response. Thus the system is self-corrective. Examples follow.

The stomach normally maintains a pH between 1.5 and 1.7. How does it stay that way? One of the regulators of the stomach pH is the hormone gastrin, secreted by cells in the stomach wall. The entrance of food into the stomach stimulates these cells to release gastrin, which, in turn, stimulates other stomach glands to secrete the components of hydrocholoric acid. When pH 1.5 is reached, the acid itself turns off the gastrin-producing cells, so that they stop releasing the hormone. Once the hormone stimulus has ceased, the glands stop producing hydrochloric acid. Thus the system adjusts itself.

Another regulator consists of nerve receptors in the stomach wall. These receptors respond to the presence of food and stimulate both the gastric glands to secrete juices and the muscles to contract. As the stomach empties, the receptors are no longer stimulated, the flow of juices slows, and the stomach quiets down.

The pyloric sphincter opens to let out a little chyme, then closes again. How does it know when to open and close? When the pyloric sphincter relaxes, acidic chyme slips through. The cells of the pyloric muscle on the intestinal side sense the acid, causing the pyloric sphincter to close tightly. Only after the chyme has been neutralized by pancreatic bicarbonate and the medium surrounding the pyloric sphincter has become alkaline can the muscle relax again. This process ensures that the chyme will be released slowly enough to be neutralized as it flows through the small intestine. This is important, because the small intestine has less of a mucous coating than the stomach does and so is not as well protected from acid.

As the chyme enters the intestine, the pancreas adds bicarbonate to it, so that the intestinal contents always remain at a slightly alkaline pH. How does the pancreas know how much to add? The presence of chyme stimulates the cells of the duodenum wall to release the hormone secretin into the blood. As this hormone circulates through the pancreas, it stimulates the pancreas to release its bicarbonate-rich juices. Thus, whenever the duodenum signals that acidic chyme is present, the pancreas responds by sending bicarbonate to neutralize it. When the need has been met, the secretin cells of the duodenal wall are no longer stimulated to release the hormone, the hormone no longer flows through the blood, the pancreas no longer receives the message, and it stops sending pancreatic juice. Nerves also regulate pancreatic secretions.

Pancreatic secretions contain a mixture of enzymes to digest carbohydrate, fat, and protein. How does the pancreas know how much of each type of enzyme to provide? This is one of the most interesting questions physiologists have asked. The question awaits final answer, but clearly the pancreas does know, somehow, what its owner has been eating, and it secretes enzyme mixtures tailored to deal with the food mixtures that have been arriving lately (over the last several days). Enzyme activity changes proportionately in response to the amounts of carbohydrate, fat, and protein in the diet.[4] If a person has been eating mostly carbohydrates, the pancreas makes and secretes mostly carbohydrases; if the person's diet has been high in fat, the pancreas produces more lipases; and so forth. Presumably, hormones from the GI tract, secreted in response to meals, keep the pancreas

Appendix A presents a brief summary of the body's hormonal system and nervous system.

gastrin: a hormone secreted by cells in the stomach wall. Target organ: the stomach. Response: secretion of gastric juice.

secretin (see-CREET-in): a hormone produced by cells in the duodenum wall. Target organ: the pancreas. Response: secretion of bicarbonate-rich pancreatic juice.

informed as to its digestive tasks. The day or two lag between the time a person's diet changes and the time digestion of the new diet becomes efficient explains why dietary changes can "upset digestion" and should be made gradually.

When fat is present in the intestine, the gallbladder contracts to squirt bile into the intestine to emulsify the fat. How does the gallbladder get the message that fat is present? Fat in the intestine stimulates cells of the intestinal wall to release the hormone cholecystokinin (CCK). This hormone, traveling by way of the blood to the gallbladder, stimulates it to contract, releasing bile into the small intestine. Once the fat in the intestine is emulsified and enzymes have begun to work on it, the fat no longer provokes release of the hormone, and the message to contract is canceled.

Fat takes longer to digest than carbohydrate does. When fat is present, intestinal motility slows to allow time for its digestion. How does the intestine know when to slow down? Cholecystokinin and gastric-inhibitory peptide slow GI tract motility. By slowing the digestive process, fat helps to maintain a pace that will allow all reactions to reach completion. Gastric-inhibitory peptide also inhibits gastric acid secretion. Hormonal and nervous mechanisms like these account for much of the body's ability to adapt to changing conditions.

Once a person has started to learn the answers to questions like these, it may be hard to stop. Some people devote their whole lives to the study of physiology. For now, however, these few examples will be enough to illustrate how all the processes throughout the digestive system are precisely and automatically regulated without any conscious effort.

THE SYSTEM AT ITS BEST

This chapter has described the anatomy of the digestive tract on several levels: the sequence of digestive organs, the cells and structures of the villi, and the selective machinery of the cell membranes. The intricate architecture of the GI tract makes it sensitive and responsive to conditions in its environment. Knowing what the optimal conditions are will help you to promote the best functioning of the system.

One indispensable condition is good health of the digestive tract itself. This health is affected by such lifestyle factors as sleep, physical activity, and state of mind. Adequate sleep allows for repair, maintenance of tissue, and removal of wastes that might impair efficient functioning. Activity promotes healthy muscle tone. Mental state profoundly affects digestion and absorption through the activity of regulatory nerves and hormones; for healthy digestion, you should be relaxed and tranquil at mealtimes.

Another factor is the kind of meals you eat. Among the characteristics of meals that promote optimal absorption of nutrients are those mentioned in Chapter 2: balance, moderation, variety, and adequacy. Balance and moderation require having neither too much nor too little of anything. For example, too much fat is harmful, but some fat is needed to slow down intestinal motility, permitting time for absorption of some of the nutrients that are slow to be absorbed.

Variety is important for many reasons, but partly because some food constituents interfere with nutrient absorption. For example, some compounds that occur in whole-grain cereals, certain leafy green vegetables, and legumes bind with minerals, so, to some extent, the minerals in those foods may become "unavailable." This does not mean that these high-fiber foods are undesirable;

cholecystokinin (coal-ee-sis-toe-KINE-in), or CCK: a hormone produced by cells of the intestinal wall. Target organ: the gallbladder. Response: release of bile and slowing of GI motility.

gastric-inhibitory peptide: a hormone produced by the intestine. Target organ: the stomach. Response: slowing of the secretion of gastric juices and of GI motility.

To become part of your body, food must first be digested and absorbed.

they are rightly prized for their nutrient contributions. It does mean, though, that people who use cereals, leafy greens, and legumes to the exclusion of other foods may be obtaining fewer minerals from their diets than they would if they were to vary their choices. They might want to exercise moderation in their use of these high-fiber foods.

As for adequacy—in a sense, this entire book is about dietary adequacy. But here, at the end of this chapter, is a good place to underline the interdependence of the nutrients. It could almost be said that every nutrient depends on every other. All the nutrients work together and are all present in the cells of a healthy digestive tract. To maintain health and promote the functions of the GI tract, you should make balance, moderation, variety, and adequacy features of every day's menus.

Study Questions

1. Describe the problems involved with digesting food and the solutions offered by the human body.
2. Describe the path food follows as it travels through the digestive system. Summarize the muscular actions that take place along the way.
3. Name five organs that secrete digestive juices. How do the juices and enzymes facilitate digestion?
4. Describe the problems involved with absorbing nutrients and the solutions offered by the small intestine.

5. How is blood routed through the digestive system? Which nutrients enter the bloodstream directly? Which are first absorbed into the lymph?
6. Describe how the body coordinates and regulates the processes of digestion and absorption.
7. How does the composition of the diet influence the functioning of the GI tract?
8. What steps can you take to help your GI tract function at its best?

Notes

1. The length of the small intestine in living adults is almost 2½ times shorter than at death, when muscles are relaxed and elongated. W. F. Ganong, *Review of Medical Physiology*, (Norwalk, Conn.: Appleton & Lange, 1993), pp. 438–465; E. A. Shaffer, Disgestive system, physiology, and biochemistry, in *Encyclopedia of Human Biology* (San Diego: Academic Press, 1991), p. 76.
2. Committee on Dietary Allowances, *Recommended Dietary Allowances,* 10th ed. (Washington, D.C.: National Academy Press, 1989), pp. 108–109.

3. M. B. Roberfroid and coauthors, Colonic microflora: Nutrition and health, *Nutrition Reviews* 53 (1995): 127–130; D. Kelly, R. Begbie, and T. P. King, Nutritional influences on interactions between bacteria and the small intestinal musoca, *Nutrition Research Reviews* 7 (1994): 233–257.
4. P. M. Brannon, Adaptation of the exocrine pancreas to diet, *Annual Review of Nutrition* 10 (1990): 85–105.

Common Digestive Problems

The facts of anatomy and physiology presented in Chapter 3 permit easy understanding of some common situations. Everyone, at one time or another, has to deal with choking on food, vomiting, diarrhea, constipation, belching, gas, and heartburn; and everyone is familiar with ulcers (the glossary on p. 96 defines these terms).

CHOKING ON FOOD

When someone chokes on food, it is because the food has slipped into the air passage and cut off breathing (see Figure H3–1). Food can lodge so securely in the trachea that it cuts off all air. No sound can be made, because the larynx is in the trachea and makes sounds only when air is pushed across it.

The choking scenario might read like this. A person is dining in a restaurant with friends. A chunk of food, usually meat, becomes lodged in his trachea so firmly that he cannot make a sound. Often he chooses to suffer alone rather than "make a scene in public." If he tries to communicate distress to his friends, he must depend on pantomime. The friends are bewildered by his antics and become terribly worried when the victim "faints" after a few minutes without air. They call for an ambulance. By the time the victim arrives at the hospital, however, he is dead from suffocation.

To help a person who is choking, first ask this critical question: "Can you make any sound at all?" If the victim makes a sound, relax. You have time to continue with your questioning to see what you can do

to help; you are not going to have to make a quick decision. But whatever you do, don't hit him on the back—the particle may become lodged more firmly in his air passage. If the victim cannot make a sound, follow the procedures described in Figure H3–2. You would do well to take a life-saving course and practice these techniques, for you will have no time for hesitation once you are called on to perform this death-defying act.

Almost any food can cause choking, although some are cited more often than others: tough meats, hot dogs, nuts, grapes, carrots, hard candies, popcorn, and peanut butter. These foods are particularly difficult for young children to safely chew and swallow. Each year, more than 300 children in the United States

choke to death. Always remain alert to the dangers of choking whenever young children are eating. To prevent choking, cut food into small pieces, chew thoroughly before swallowing, don't talk or laugh with food in your mouth, and don't eat when breathing hard.

VOMITING

Another common digestive mishap is vomiting. Vomiting can be a symptom of many different diseases or may arise in any situation that upsets the body's equilibrium, such as air or sea travel. For whatever reason, the waves of peristalsis reverse direction, and the contents of the stomach are propelled up through the esophagus to the mouth and expelled.

Figure H3–1

Normal Swallowing and Choking

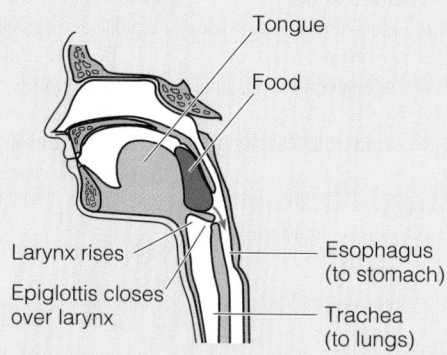
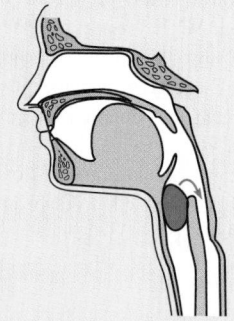

Tongue
Food
Larynx rises
Epiglottis closes over larynx
Esophagus (to stomach)
Trachea (to lungs)

Swallowing. The epiglottis closes over the larynx, blocking entrance to the lungs via the trachea. The red arrow shows that food is heading down the esophagus normally.

Choking. A choking person cannot speak or gasp because food lodged in the trachea blocks the passage of air. The red arrow points to where the food should have gone to prevent choking.

- If the choking victim is an infant, lay her face down on your lap with her head firmly supported and held lower than her body.

Figure H3–2
. . . .

First Aid for Choking

Sources: Adapted from Committee on Pediatric Emergency Medicine, First aid for the choking child, *Pediatrics* 92 (1993): 477–479; H. J. Heimlich and M. H. Uhley, The Heimlich maneuver, *Clinical Symposia* 31 (1979): 1–32; H. J. Heimlich, Self-application of the Heimlich maneuver, *New England Journal of Medicine* 318 (1988): 714–715.

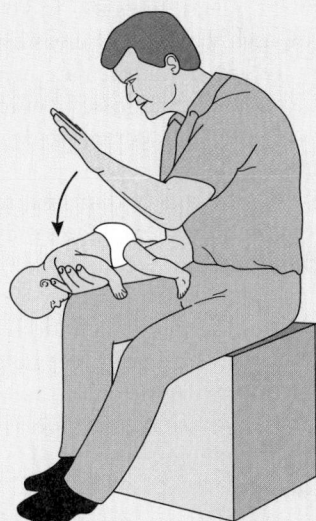

Administer five blows rapidly with the heel of your hand high between her shoulder blades.

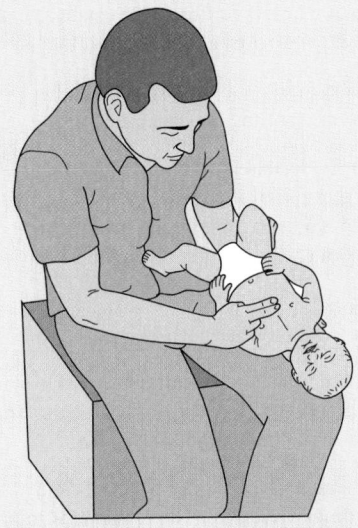

If that doesn't work, turn her over and deliver five quick downward thrusts over her sternum using two fingers.

- If the choking victim is an older child or adult, the strategy most likely to succeed is abdominal thrusts, sometimes called the Heimlich maneuver.

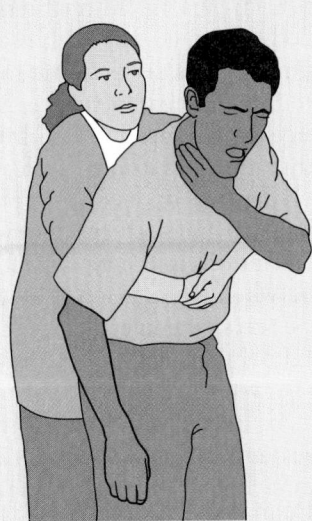

Stand behind the victim, and wrap your arms around him. Place the thumb side of one fist snugly against his body, slightly above the navel and below the rib cage. Grasp your fist with your other hand and give him a sudden strong hug inward and upward. Repeat thrusts as necessary.

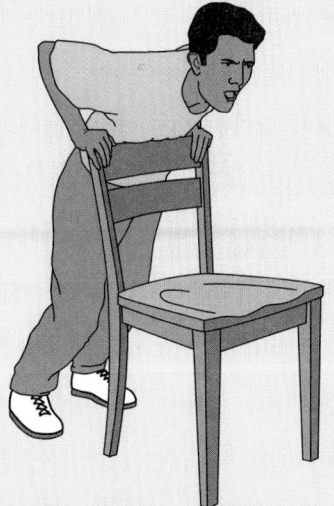

To self-administer first aid, place the thumb side of one fist slightly above the navel and below the rib cage, grasp the fist with your other hand, and then press inward and upward with a quick motion. If this is unsuccessful, quickly press your upper abdomen over any firm surface such as the back of a chair, a countertop, or a railing.

- If all else fails, open the mouth by grasping both the tongue and lower jaw and lifting. Then, and only if you can see the object, use your finger to sweep it out and begin rescue breathing.

If vomiting continues long enough or is severe enough, the reverse peristalsis will extend beyond the stomach and carry the contents of the duodenum, with its green bile salts, into the stomach and then up the esophagus. Although certainly unpleasant and wearying for the nauseated person, vomiting such as this is no cause for alarm. Vomiting is one of the body's adaptive mechanisms to rid itself of something irritating. The best advice is to rest and drink small amounts of fluids as tolerated until the nausea subsides.

Vomiting can be serious, however, when large quantities of fluid are lost from the GI tract, causing dehydration. A physician's care may be needed in those cases. With massive fluid loss from the GI tract, all of the body's other fluids redistribute themselves so that, eventually, fluid is taken from every cell of the body. Leaving the cells with the fluid are salts that are absolutely essential to the life of the cells, and they must be replaced, which is difficult while the vomiting continues. Intravenous feedings of saline and glucose are frequently necessary while the physician is diagnosing the cause of the vomiting and instituting corrective therapy.

In an infant, vomiting is likely to become serious early in its course, and a physician should be contacted

95

Glossary

belch: the expulsion of gas from the stomach through the mouth.

colonic irrigation: the popular, but potentially harmful practice of "washing" the large intestine with a powerful enema machine.

constipation: the condition of having painful or difficult bowel movements (elapsed time between movements is not relevant).

defecate (DEF-uh-cate): to move the bowels and eliminate waste.
defaecare = to remove dregs

diarrhea: the frequent passage of watery bowel movements.

heartburn: a burning sensation in the chest area caused by backflow of stomach acid into the esophagus.

Heimlich maneuver: a technique for removing an object from the trachea of a choking person (see Figure H3–2).

hemorrhoids: painful swelling of the veins surrounding the rectum.

hiccups: repeated cough-like sounds and jerks that are produced when an involuntary spasm of the diaphragm muscle sucks air down the windpipe; also spelled *hiccoughs*.

larynx: the voice box (see Figure H3–1).

peptic ulcer: an erosion in the mucous membrane of either the stomach (a gastric ulcer) or the duodenum (a duodenal ulcer).

ulcer: an erosion in the topmost, and sometimes underlying, layers of cells in an area. See also *peptic ulcer*.

vomiting: expulsion of the contents of the stomach up through the esophagus to the mouth.

considerable fluid and salt losses, but the composition of the fluids is different. Stomach fluids lost in vomiting are highly acidic, whereas intestinal fluids lost in diarrhea are nearly neutral. When fluid losses require medical attention, correct replacement is crucial.

For short bouts of diarrhea, rest and drink fluids to replace losses. If diarrhea continues, call for help. A medical evaluation is needed to identify and correct the underlying problem.[1] For an infant, get help promptly, for diarrhea may quickly lead to dehydration so severe as to require emergency medical treatment.

CONSTIPATION

Unlike diarrhea, constipation is generally not a cause for immediate concern. Each person's GI tract responds to food in its own way, with its own rhythm. Food is digested and the waste becomes ready for excretion in a predictable number of hours. Each GI tract thus has its own cycle, which depends on its owner's physical makeup and such environmental considerations as the type of food eaten, when it was eaten, and when the person's schedule allows time to defecate. Even when several days pass between movements, a person is not constipated, as long as these movements take place without discomfort. But if a movement is passed with difficulty, discomfort, or pain, then the person is constipated. The time that has elapsed since the previous bowel movement is irrelevant.

Often a person's lifestyle may cause constipation. If a person receives the signal to defecate and ignores it, the signal may not return for several hours. In the meantime,

soon after onset. Infants have more fluid between their body cells than adults do, so more fluid can move readily into the digestive tract and be lost from the body. Consequently, the body water of infants becomes depleted and their body salt balance upset faster than in adults.

Self-induced vomiting, such as occurs in bulimia, also has serious consequences. (Bulimia nervosa is the subject of Highlight 9.) In addition to fluid and salt imbalances, repeated vomiting can cause irritation and infection of the pharynx, esophagus, and salivary glands; erosion of the teeth; and dental caries. The esophagus may rupture or tear, as may the stomach. Sometimes the eyes become red from pressure during vomiting. Bulimic behavior

reflects underlying problems that require intervention.

Projectile vomiting is also serious. The contents of the stomach are expelled with such force that they leave the mouth in a wide arc like a bullet leaving a gun. This type of vomiting requires immediate medical attention.

DIARRHEA

Diarrhea is characterized by frequent, loose, watery stools. This sort of stool indicates that the intestinal contents have moved too quickly through the intestines for fluid absorption to take place, or that water has been drawn from the cells lining the intestinal tract and added to the food residue. Like vomiting, diarrhea can lead to

water continues to be withdrawn from the fecal matter, so that when the person does defecate, the bowel movement is dry and hard.

Careful review of daily habits may reveal the causes of the constipation. Being too busy to respond to the defecation signal is a common complaint. In that case, a person's daily regimen may need to be revised to allow time to have a bowel movement when the body sends its signal. One possibility is to go to bed earlier in order to rise earlier, allowing ample time for a leisurely breakfast and a movement.

Another cause of constipation is lack of physical activity.[2] In today's society many people drive cars or ride buses to work, stand at assembly lines or sit behind desks, and then sit in front of television sets in the evening. Increasing physical activity may require some rearrangement of one's lifestyle. People can work out in spas or health clubs; more simply, they can just park their cars a distance from the office and walk the extra blocks, or they can walk up several flights of stairs a day rather than taking the elevator. Such activity will improve the muscle tone, not just of the outer body, but also of the digestive tract.

Although constipation usually reflects lifestyle habits, in some cases it may be a side effect of medication or may reflect a medical problem such as tumors that are obstructing the passage of waste. If discomfort is associated with passing fecal matter, a physician's help should be sought to rule out disease. Once this has been done, dietary or other measures for correction can be considered.

One dietary measure that may be appropriate is to increase dietary fiber. Some fibers—those found in cereal products—help to prevent constipation by increasing fecal mass. In the GI tract, fiber attracts water, creating soft, bulky stools that stimulate bowel contractions to push the contents along. These contractions strengthen the intestinal muscles. The improved muscle tone, together with the water content of the stools, eases elimination, reducing the pressure in the rectal veins and helping to prevent hemorrhoids. Although the major impact of dietary fiber is on the colon, fiber acts as a bulking agent all along the intestine. Chapter 4 provides more information on fiber's role in maintaining a healthy colon and reducing the risks of colon cancer and diverticulosis.

Drinking plenty of water in conjunction with eating high-fiber foods also helps with constipation. The increased bulk physically stimulates the upper GI tract, promoting peristalsis throughout.

Eating prunes can also be helpful. Prunes are high in fiber and also contain a laxative substance.* If a morning defecation is desired, a person can drink prune juice at bedtime; if the evening is preferred, the person can drink prune juice with breakfast.

Adding fat to the diet can relieve some constipation by stimulating the hormone cholecystokinin, which summons bile into the duodenum. Bile's high salt content draws water from the intestinal wall, which stimulates peristalsis and softens the fecal matter.

These suggested changes in lifestyle or diet should correct chronic constipation without the

---

*This substance is dihydroxyphenyl isatin.

use of laxatives, enemas, or mineral oil, although television commercials often try to persuade people otherwise. One of the fallacies often perpetrated by television commercials is that one person's successful use of a product is a good recommendation for others to use that product.

As a matter of fact, even diet changes that relieve constipation for one person may increase the constipation of another. For instance, increasing fiber intake stimulates peristalsis and helps the person with a sluggish colon. Some people, though, have a spastic type of constipation, in which peristalsis promotes strong contractions that close off a segment of the colon and prevent passage; for these people, increasing fiber intake would be exactly the wrong thing to do.

A person who seems to need products such as laxatives should seek a physician's opinion. Advice from friends or alternative medicine practitioners may cause more harm than good. One potentially harmful but currently popular practice that is being promoted by some alternative medicine practitioners is colonic irrigation—the internal washing of the large intestine with a powerful enema machine. Such an extreme cleansing is not only unnecessary, but the force of the machine can rupture the intestine. Less extreme practices can cause problems, too. Frequent use of laxatives and enemas can lead to dependency; can upset the body's fluid, salt, and mineral balances; and, in the case of mineral oil, can interfere with the absorption of fat-soluble vitamins. (Mineral oil dissolves the vitamins, but is not itself absorbed; instead, it leaves the body, carrying the vitamins with it.)

BELCHING AND GAS

Many people complain of problems that they attribute to excessive gas. For some, belching is the complaint. Others blame intestinal gas for abdominal discomforts and embarrassment. Most people believe that the problems occur after they eat certain foods. This may be the case with intestinal gas, but belching results from swallowing air. The best advice for belching seems to be to eat slowly, chew thoroughly, and relax while eating.

Everyone swallows a little bit of air with each mouthful of food, but people who eat too fast may swallow too much air and then have to belch. Ill-fitting dentures, carbonated beverages, and chewing gum can also contribute to the swallowing of air with resultant belching. Occasionally, belching can be a sign of a more serious disorder, such as gallbladder pain, colonic distress, or an impending obstruction of a coronary blood vessel.

People who eat or drink too fast may also trigger hiccups, the repeated spasms that produce a cough-like sound and jerky movement. Normally, hiccups soon subside and are of no medical significance, but they can be bothersome. The most effective cure is to hold the breath for as long as possible, which helps to relieve the spasms of the diaphragm.

Little is known about intestinal gas, but techniques for collecting gas directly from the abdomen have allowed researchers to gain some knowledge. While expelling gas can be a humiliating experience, it is quite normal. (People experiencing painful bloating from malabsorption diseases, however, require medical treatment.) Healthy people expel several hundred milliliters of gas several times a day. Almost all (99 percent) of the gases expelled—nitrogen, oxygen, hydrogen, methane, and carbon dioxide—are odorless. The remaining "volatile" gases are the infamous ones.

Foods that produce gas usually must be determined individually. The most common offenders are foods rich in the carbohydrates—sugars, starches, and fibers. When partially digested carbohydrates reach the large intestine, bacteria digest them, giving off gas as a by-product. People can test foods suspected of forming gas by omitting them individually for a trial period and seeing if there is any improvement.

One aspect of gas may offer an important medical opportunity. An association observed in methane-producing people may help in the early diagnosis of colon cancer. Twice as many people with colon cancer produce methane as members of the general population. Methane-producing people may have a high risk of cancer because the changes in acid balance associated with methane production may favor cancer formation.[3] In addition, researchers believe that methane production increases in response to the presence of the tumor.[4]

HEARTBURN AND "ACID INDIGESTION"

Almost everyone has experienced heartburn at one time or another, usually after a meal. Heartburn is the painful sensation a person feels when the cardiac sphincter fails to prevent the stomach contents from refluxing into the esophagus. This may happen if a person eats or drinks too much (or both): back-pressure from the stomach forces food up into the esophagus. Tight clothing and even changes of position (lying down, bending over) can cause it, too, as can some medications and smoking. A defect of the cardiac sphincter itself is a possible, but less likely cause.

If the heartburn is not caused by an anatomical defect, treatment is fairly simple. Tips for people suffering from heartburn include the following:

- Eat small meals.
- Drink liquids one hour before or one hour after meals.
- Refrain from lying down or bending over and from wearing tight-fitting clothing, particularly after a meal.
- Lose weight, if overweight.
- Elevate the head of the bed by 4 to 6 inches.
- Avoid food, beverages, and medicines that seem to aggravate the heartburn.
- Refrain from smoking cigarettes.

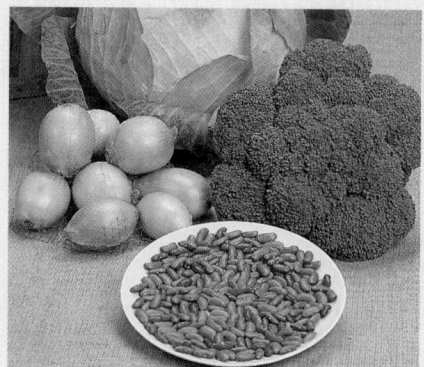

Beans, broccoli, cabbage, and onions produce gas in many people. People troubled by gas need to determine which foods bother them and then eat those foods in moderation.

Use antacids infrequently for occasional heartburn; they may mask or cause problems if used regularly. Chewing gum may bring relief of symptoms by increasing the flow of saliva, which helps in re-swallowing the esophageal contents.

As far as "acid indigestion" is concerned, recall from Chapter 3 that the strong acidity of the stomach is a desirable condition—television commercials for antacids notwithstanding. People who overeat or eat too quickly are likely to suffer from indigestion. The muscular reaction of the stomach to unchewed lumps or to being overfilled may be so violent that it causes regurgitation (reverse peristalsis). When this happens, overeaters may taste the stomach acid and feel pain. Responding to television commercials, they may take antacids to neutralize the "acid indigestion."

Antacids will provide quick relief, but they are not appropriate therapy for the stomach's discomfort. An antacid places a demand on the stomach to secrete more acid to counteract the neutralizer and enable the digestive enzymes to do their work. So the person still ends up with acid in the stomach, but the stomach has had to work against the antacid to produce it.

Antacids are designed to help relieve the acute symptoms from abnormal conditions, such as the pain felt by an ulcer patient whose stomach or duodenal lining has been attacked by acid. The person who overeats or swallows unchewed food needs to sit upright until the unhappy stomach has had a chance to cope with the problem it faces. Then, to avoid such misery in the

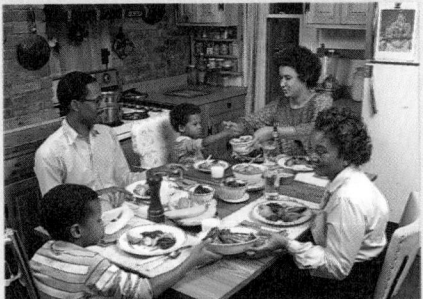

Taking the time to enjoy a meal can enhance people's physical and emotional health.

future, the person needs to learn to eat less at a sitting, chew food more thoroughly, and eat it more slowly.

ULCERS

Ulcers of the stomach (gastric ulcers) or duodenum (duodenal ulcers) are another common digestive problem. (The term *peptic ulcer* includes both types.) An ulcer is an erosion of the top layer of cells from an area, such as the wall of the stomach or duodenum. This erosion leaves the underlying layers of cells unprotected and exposed to gastric juices. The erosion may proceed until the gastric juices reach the capillaries that feed the area, leading to bleeding, and reach the nerves, causing pain. If the erosion penetrates all the way through the GI lining, a life-threatening infection can develop.

Some people naively believe that an ulcer is caused by the secretion of stomach acid, but this is not the case—at least not at first. The stomach lining in a healthy person is well protected by its mucous coat. What, then, causes ulcers to form?

Three major causes of ulcers have been identified: bacterial infection, the use of certain anti-inflammatory

drugs, and disorders that cause excessive gastric acid secretion.[5]* The treatment of ulcers aims at relieving pain, healing the ulcer, and minimizing the likelihood of recurrence. Drug therapy plays the primary role in the treatment; the specific type of drug depends on the cause of the ulcer. The most widely used treatment regimen includes the mineral bismuth and two other antimicrobial drugs.[6] Other drugs may be used to neutralize gastric acidity, reduce gastric acid secretion, or otherwise protect the stomach and duodenal wall from the eroding effect of gastric acid. The same treatment regimen is used for both gastric and duodenal ulcers.

Diet therapy once played a major role in ulcer treatment, but it no longer does. Current practice is simply to treat for infection, eliminate any food that routinely causes indigestion or pain, and avoid coffee and caffeine- and alcohol-containing beverages. Both regular and decaffeinated coffee stimulate stomach acid secretion and so aggravate *existing* ulcers.

Many of the common GI problems presented here reflect hurried lifestyles. For this reason, many of their remedies require that people slow down: take the time to eat slowly; chew food thoroughly to prevent choking, heartburn, and acid indigestion; take the time to rest until vomiting and diarrhea subside; and take the time to heed the urge to defecate. In addition,

---

*The bacterial infection frequently associated with ulcers is caused by *Helicobacter pylori*. The drugs associated with ulcers are nonsteroidal anti-inflammatory agents such as ibuprofen and naproxen.

learn how to handle life's day-to-day problems and challenges without overreacting and becoming upset; learn how to relax, to get enough sleep, and to enjoy life. Remember, "what's eating you" may cause more GI distress than what you eat.

NOTES

1. M. Donowitz, F. T. Kokke, and R. Saidi, Evaluation of patients with chronic diarrhea, *New England Journal of Medicine* 332 (1995): 725–729.

2. R. S. Sandler, M. C. Jordan, and B. J. Shelton, Demographic and dietary determinants of constipation in the US population, *American Journal of Public Health* 80 (1990): 185–189.

3. J. A. Flick and J. A. Perman, Nonabsorbed carbohydrate: Effect on fecal pH in methane-excreting and nonexcreting individuals, *American Journal of Clinical Nutrition* 49 (1989): 1252–1257.

4. J. M. Pique, Methane production and colon cancer, *Gastroenterology* 87 (1987): 601–605.

5. D. Y. Graham, *Helicobacter pylori*: Its epidemiology and its role in duodenal ulcer disease, *Journal of Gastroenterology and Hepatology* 6 (1991): 105–113.

6. D. Y. Graham, Treatment of peptic ulcers caused by *Helicobacter pylori*, *New England Journal of Medicine* 328 (1993): 349–350.

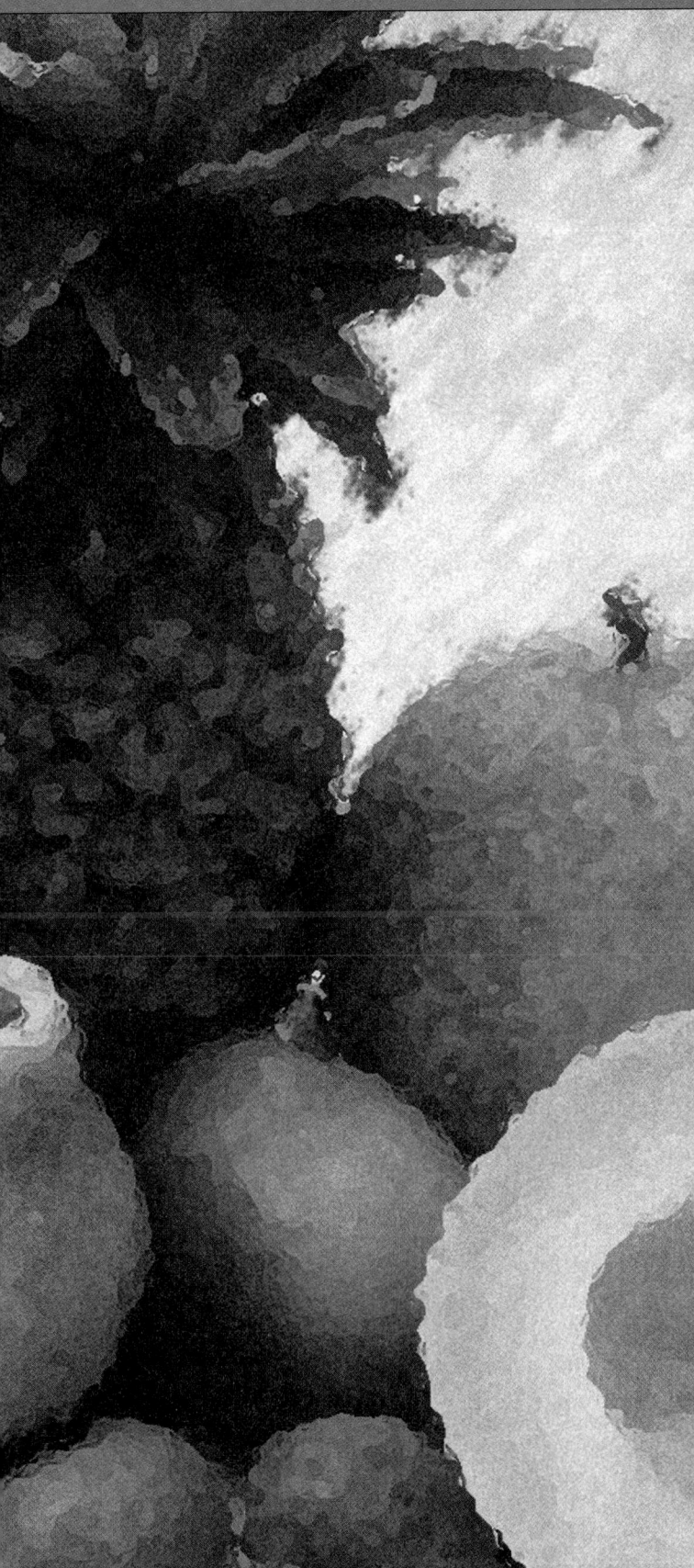

Chapter 4

The Carbohydrates: Sugars, Starch, and Fibers

CONTENTS

The Chemist's View of Carbohydrates
The Simple Carbohydrates
Monosaccharides
Disaccharides
The Complex Carbohydrates
Glycogen
Starch
The Fibers
Digestion and Absorption of Carbohydrates
The Processes of Digestion and Absorption
Lactose Intolerance
Glucose in the Body
A Preview of Carbohydrate Metabolism
The Constancy of Blood Glucose
Health Effects and Recommended Intakes
        of Sugars
Health Effects of Sugars
Accusations against Sugars
Recommended Intakes of Sugars
Health Effects and Recommended Intakes
        of Starch and Fibers
Health Effects of Starch and Fibers
Recommended Intakes of Starch and Fiber
HIGHLIGHT: Alternatives to Sugar

MICROGRAPH: Fructose, the sugar of fruits

A student, quietly studying a textbook, is seldom aware that within his brain cells, billions of glucose molecules are splitting each second to provide the energy that permits him to learn. Yet glucose provides nearly all of the energy the human brain uses daily. Similarly, a marathon runner, bursting across the finish line in an explosion of sweat and triumph, seldom gives thanks to the glycogen fuel her muscles have devoured to help her finish the race. Yet, together, glucose and its storage form glycogen provide about half of all the energy human nerves, muscles, and other body tissues use. The other half of the body's energy comes mostly from fat.

People don't eat glucose and glycogen directly; they eat foods rich in carbohydrates. Then their bodies convert the carbohydrates mostly into glucose for immediate energy and into glycogen for reserve energy.

Carbohydrates contribute so much to the bulk of most foods that many people mistakenly think of them as "fattening" and avoid them when trying to lose weight. Actually, such a strategy may be counterproductive. People can better control body weight by selecting high-carbohydrate, high-fiber foods and limiting fat-rich foods. All unrefined plant foods—vegetables, fruits, legumes, and grains—provide ample carbohydrate and fiber with little or no fat. (Milk also contains carbohydrates. So do shellfish and organ meats such as liver, but only a little.)

Table 4–1 offers a preview of the dietary carbohydrate family, which includes the simple carbohydrates (the sugars) and the complex carbohydrates (the starches and fibers). All of the carbohydrates are made of simple sugars; they are *complex* when they have more than two simple sugars in a molecule. The simple carbohydrates are those that chemists describe as:

- Monosaccharides—single sugars.
- Disaccharides—sugars composed of pairs of monosaccharides.

The complex carbohydrates are:

- Polysaccharides—large molecules composed of chains of monosaccharides.

The Chemist's View of Carbohydrates

To understand the structure of carbohydrates, look at the units of which they are made. The sugars most important in nutrition are the monosaccharides known as 6-carbon sugars, or hexoses. Each contains 6 carbon atoms, 12 hydrogens, and 6 oxygens (written in shorthand as $C_6H_{12}O_6$).

Each atom can form a certain number of chemical bonds with other atoms:

- Carbon atoms can form four bonds.
- Nitrogen atoms, three.
- Oxygen atoms, two.
- Hydrogen atoms, only one.

Chemists represent the bonds as lines between the chemical symbols (such as C, N, O, and H) that stand for the atoms (see Figure 4–1).

Atoms form molecules in ways that satisfy the bonding requirements of each atom. Figure 4–1 shows the structure of ethyl alcohol, the active ingredient of alcoholic beverages, as an example. The two carbons each have four bonds represented by lines; the oxygen has two; and each hydrogen has one bond con-

Table 4–1

The Carbohydrate Family

Simple Carbohydrates (sugars)

- Monosaccharides
  Glucose
  Fructose
  Galactose
- Disaccharides
  Sucrose
  Lactose
  Maltose

Complex Carbohydrates[a]

- Starch (polysaccharides)
- Fibers (nonstarch polysaccharides)
  Soluble
  Insoluble

[a]Glycogen is a complex carbohydrate (a polysaccharide), but not a *dietary* source of carbohydrate.

carbohydrates: compounds composed of carbon, oxygen, and hydrogen arranged as monosaccharides or multiples of monosaccharides.
carbo = carbon (C)
hydrate = with water (H_2O)

simple carbohydrates (sugars): monosaccharides and disaccharides.

complex carbohydrates (starches and fibers): polysaccharides composed of straight or branched chains of monosaccharides.

Most of the monosaccharides important in nutrition are hexoses, simple sugars with six atoms of carbon and the formula $C_6H_{12}O_6$.
hex = six

Figure 4–1

Atoms and Their Bonds

The four main types of atoms found in nutrients are hydrogen, oxygen, nitrogen, and carbon. Appendix B presents basic chemistry terms and relationships.

Each atom has a characteristic number of bonds it can form with other atoms.

Ethyl alcohol, a simple molecule showing bonding.

necting it to other atoms. An accurate drawing of a chemical structure must obey these rules because the laws of nature demand it.

To quickly recap, the carbohydrates are made of carbon (C), oxygen (O), and hydrogen (H). Each of these atoms can form a specified number of chemical bonds: carbon forms four, oxygen forms two, and hydrogen forms one.

The Simple Carbohydrates

The following list of the six sugars most important in nutrition symbolizes them as hexagons and pentagons of different colors. The shapes reflect their chemical structures as drawn on paper. Three are single sugars or monosaccharides:

- Glucose.
- Fructose.*
- Galactose.†

Three are double sugars or disaccharides:

- Maltose (glucose + glucose).
- Sucrose (glucose + fructose).
- Lactose (glucose + galactose).

See Appendix C for the complete chemical structures of the sugars.

monosaccharide (mon-oh-SACK-uh-ride): a carbohydrate of the general formula $C_nH_{2n}O_n$ that consists of a single ring.
  mono = one
  saccharide = sugar

MONOSACCHARIDES

The three monosaccharides important in nutrition all have the same numbers and kinds of atoms, but in different arrangements. These chemical differences account for the differing sweetness of the monosaccharides. A pinch of purified glucose on the tongue gives only a mild sweet flavor and galactose hardly tastes sweet at all, but fructose is as intensely sweet as honey and, in fact, is the sugar primarily responsible for honey's sweetness.

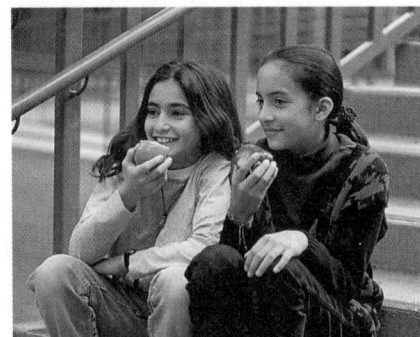

Fruits package their simple sugars with fibers, vitamins, and minerals, making them a sweet and healthy snack.

---

*Fructose is shown as a pentagon, but it does have 6 carbon atoms. The ring contains 4 carbons and an oxygen; 2 carbons stick out from the ring (see Figure 4–4).

†Galactose occurs only as a part of lactose.

Figure 4–2

Chemical Structure of Glucose

On paper, the structure of glucose has to be drawn flat, but in nature the five carbons and oxygen are roughly in a plane. The atoms attached to the ring carbons extend above and below the plane.

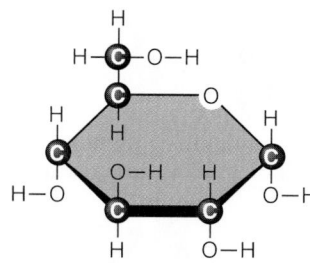

glucose: a monosaccharide; sometimes known as blood sugar or dextrose.

ose = carbohydrate

⬡ = glucose

Glucose Chemically, glucose is a larger and more complicated molecule than ethyl alcohol, but it obeys the same rules of chemistry: each carbon atom has four bonds; each oxygen, two bonds; and each hydrogen, one bond. Figure 4–2 illustrates the chemical structure of a glucose molecule.

The diagram of a glucose molecule shows all the relationships between the parts and proves simple on examination, but chemists have adopted even simpler ways to depict chemical structures. Figure 4–3 shows that a chemical structure can combine or omit a number of letters without losing the information it conveys.

The significance of glucose to nutrition is tremendous. Glucose is one of the two sugars in every disaccharide and is the unit from which the polysaccharides are made almost exclusively. One of these polysaccharides, starch, is the chief energy food of the world's people; another, glycogen, is a major storage form of energy in the body. Glucose will therefore reappear frequently throughout this chapter and all those that follow.

Figure 4–3 Simplified Diagrams of Glucose

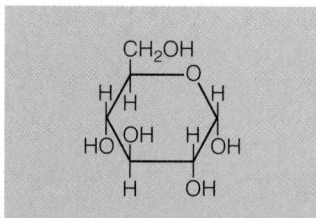

The carbons at the corners are not shown, and the formula CH₂OH stands for the structure in Figure 4–2.

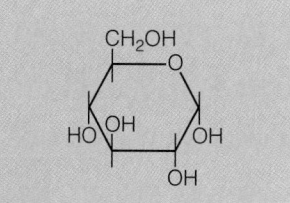

Now the single hydrogens are not shown, but lines still extend upward or downward from the ring to show where they belong. You can easily reconstruct the complete structure, with all its details, from such a diagram by putting a C for carbon at each corner of the hexagon and an H for hydrogen at the end of each single line. This is the traditional chemical shorthand used for glucose.

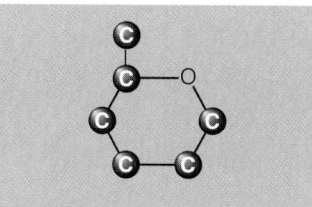

Another way to look at glucose is to notice that its six carbon atoms are all connected.

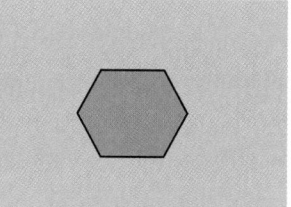

For convenience, in this and other illustrations throughout this book, glucose is represented as a blue hexagon.

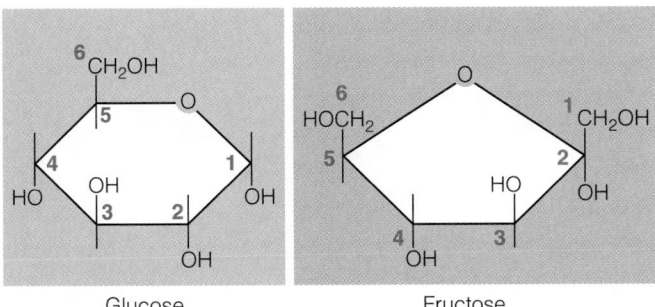

Figure 4–4

Two Monosaccharides: Glucose and Fructose

Can you see the similarities? If you learned the rules in Figure 4–3, you will be able to "see" 6 carbons (numbered), 12 hydrogens, and 6 oxygens in both these compounds.

Fructose   Fructose is the sweetest of the sugars. Curiously, fructose has exactly the same chemical *formula* as glucose—$C_6H_{12}O_6$—but its *structure* differs (see Figure 4–4). The arrangement of the atoms in fructose stimulates the taste buds on the tongue to produce the sweet sensation. Fructose occurs naturally in fruits and honey; food manufacturers also use it in products sweetened with high-fructose corn syrup (HFCS), a corn product used as an additive.

fructose: a monosaccharide; sometimes known as fruit sugar or levulose, fructose is found abundantly in fruits, honey, and saps.
fruct = fruit
⬟ = fructose

Galactose   Seldom occurring free in nature, galactose binds with another monosaccharide to form the sugar in milk. Galactose has the same numbers and kinds of atoms as glucose and fructose, but in yet another arrangement. Figure 4–5 shows galactose beside a molecule of glucose for comparison.

galactose: a monosaccharide; part of the disaccharide lactose.
⬡ = galactose

DISACCHARIDES

The disaccharides are pairs of the three sugars just discussed. Glucose occurs in all three; the second member of the pair is either fructose, galactose, or another glucose. These carbohydrates and all the other energy nutrients are put together and taken apart by similar chemical reactions.

disaccharide: a pair of monosaccharides linked together.
di = two

Condensation   To make a disaccharide, a chemical reaction known as condensation links two monosaccharides together (see Figure 4–6). A hydroxyl (OH) group from one monosaccharide and a hydrogen atom (H) from the other combine to create a molecule of water (H_2O). The two originally separate monosaccharides link together with a single oxygen (O).

condensation: a chemical reaction in which two reactants combine to yield a larger product.

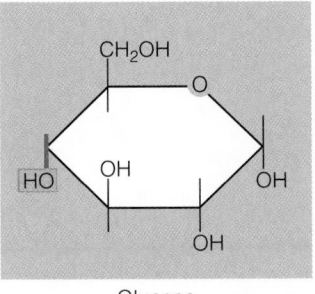

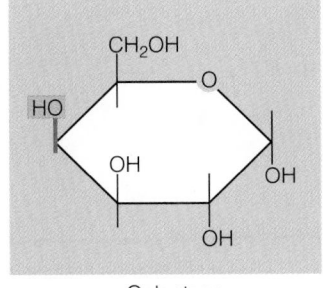

Figure 4–5

Two Monosaccharides: Glucose and Galactose

Notice the similarities and the difference.

Figure 4–6

Condensation of Two Monosaccharides to Form a Disaccharide

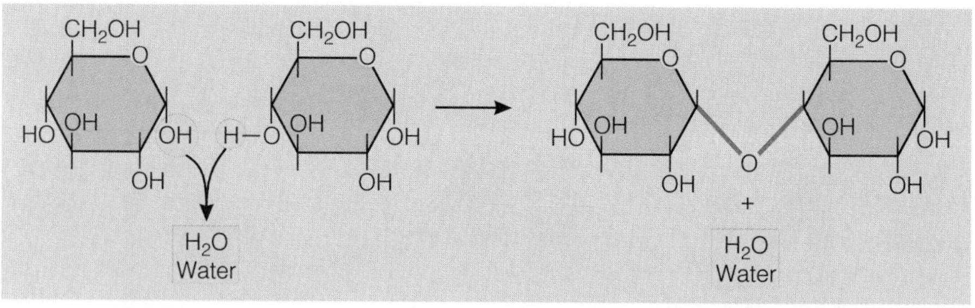

Glucose + glucose

An OH group from one glucose and an H atom from another glucose combine to create a molecule of H_2O.

Maltose

The two glucose molecules bond together with a single O atom to form the disaccharide maltose.

Reminder: A *hydrolysis* reaction splits a major reactant into two products, with H added to one and OH to the other (from water).

maltose: a disaccharide composed of two glucose units; sometimes known as malt sugar.

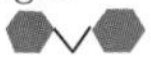

⬣◡⬡ = maltose

sucrose: a disaccharide composed of glucose and fructose; commonly known as table sugar, beet sugar, or cane sugar. Sucrose also occurs in many fruits and some vegetables and grains.

sucro = sugar

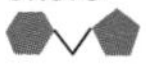

⬣◡⬠ = sucrose

Hydrolysis To break a disaccharide in two, a chemical reaction known as hydrolysis occurs (see Figure 4–7). A molecule of water splits to provide the H and OH needed to complete the resulting monosaccharides. Hydrolysis reactions commonly occur during digestion.

Maltose The disaccharide maltose consists of two glucose units. Maltose is produced whenever starch breaks down—as happens in plants when seeds germinate and in human beings during carbohydrate digestion. It also occurs during the fermentation process that yields alcohol. Maltose is only a minor constituent of a few foods.

Sucrose Fructose and glucose together form sucrose, or table sugar, the most familiar of the sugars. Because the fructose is in a position accessible to the taste receptors, sucrose tastes sweet, accounting for some of the natural sweetness of fruits, vegetables, and grains. To make table sugar, sucrose is refined from the juices of sugarcane and sugar beets, then granulated. Depending on the extent to which it is refined, the product becomes the brown, white, and powdered sugars available at grocery stores.

Figure 4–7

Hydrolysis of a Disaccharide
Hydrolysis occurs during digestion.

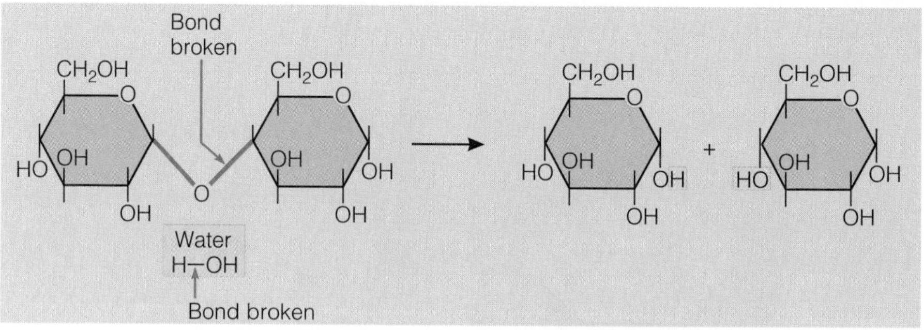

Maltose

Glucose + glucose

The disaccharide maltose splits into two glucose molecules with H added to one and OH to the other (from water).

Lactose   The combination of galactose and glucose makes the disaccharide lactose, the principal carbohydrate of milk. Known as milk sugar, lactose contributes about 5 percent of milk's weight. Depending on the milk's fat content, lactose contributes 30 to 50 percent of milk's energy.

In summary, then, six major simple carbohydrates, or sugars, are important in nutrition. The three monosaccharides (glucose, fructose, and galactose) all have the same chemical formula ($C_6H_{12}O_6$), but their structures differ. The three disaccharides (sucrose, lactose, and maltose) are pairs of monosaccharides. The sugars derive primarily from plants, except for lactose and its component galactose, which come from milk and milk products. Two monosaccharides can be linked together by a condensation reaction to form a disaccharide and water. A disaccharide, in turn, can be broken into its two monosaccharides by a hydrolysis reaction using water.

lactose: a disaccharide composed of glucose and galactose; commonly known as milk sugar.

lact = milk

◆◡⬡ = lactose

The Complex Carbohydrates

The simple carbohydrates are the sugars just mentioned: glucose, fructose, and galactose, either singly or paired with glucose. In contrast, the complex carbohydrates contain many glucose units and a few other monosaccharides strung together as polysaccharides. Three are important in nutrition: glycogen, starch, and the fibers.

Glycogen is a storage form of energy in the animal body; starch plays that role in plants; and the fibers of plants serve as structural elements in stems, trunks, roots, leaves, and skins. Both glycogen and starch are built of glucose units, but they are linked together differently. The fibers are composed of a variety of monosaccharides and other carbohydrate derivatives.

polysaccharide: many monosaccharides linked together.

poly = many
saccharide = sugar

GLYCOGEN

Glycogen is found only to a limited extent in meats and not at all in plants.* For this reason, glycogen is not a significant food source of carbohydrate, but it does perform an important role in the body. It is the form in which the human body stores much of its glucose. Glycogen consists of many glucose molecules linked together in highly branched chains (see the left side of Figure 4–8). This arrangement permits rapid hydrolysis. When the hormonal message "Release energy" arrives at the storage sites in a liver or muscle cell, enzymes respond by attacking all the many branches of each glycogen simultaneously, making a surge of fuel available.†

glycogen (GLY-co-gen): an animal polysaccharide composed of glucose; it is manufactured and stored in the liver and muscles as a storage form of glucose. Glycogen is not a significant food source of carbohydrate and is not counted as one of the complex carbohydrates in foods.

glyco = glucose
gen = gives rise to

---

*Glycogen in animal muscles rapidly hydrolyzes after slaughter.

†Normally, only the liver can return glucose *directly* from glycogen to the blood; muscle cells use glycogen internally to produce glucose. Muscle cells can restore the blood glucose level *indirectly*, however: when muscles oxidize glucose without oxygen for energy, they release a breakdown product (lactic acid) into the blood, which the liver can pick up and reconvert to glucose. The return of glucose via this pathway is called the Cori cycle, and it accounts for 15 percent or more of blood glucose. L. J. Hoffer, Cori cycle contribution to plasma glucose appearance in man, *Journal of Parenteral and Enteral Nutrition* 14 (1990): 646–648.

Figure 4–8

Glycogen and Starch Molecules Compared (Small Segments)

Notice that the more highly branched the structure, the greater the number of ends from which glucose can be released. (These units would have to be magnified millions of times to appear at the size shown in this figure. For details of the chemical structures, see Appendix C.)

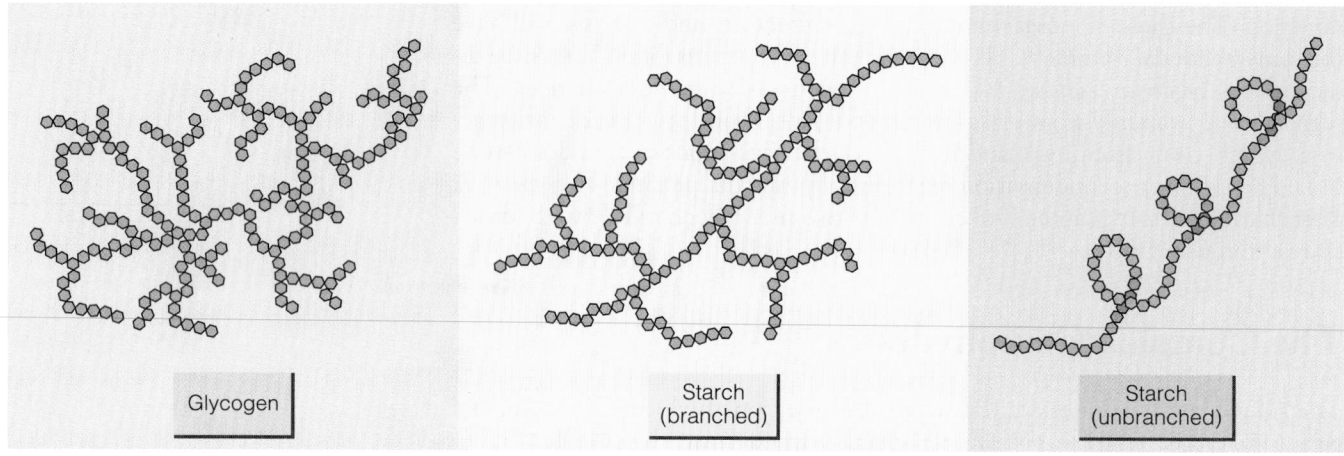

| Glycogen | Starch (branched) | Starch (unbranched) |

A glycogen molecule contains hundreds of glucose units in long, highly branched chains.

A starch molecule contains hundreds of glucose molecules in either occasionally branched chains or unbranched chains.

starch: a plant polysaccharide composed of glucose that is digestible by human beings. For the structures of starch's two forms, amylose (straight chain) and amylopectin (branched chain), see Appendix C.

Starch and sugar are called available carbohydrates because human digestive enzymes make them available to the body. In contrast, fibers are called unavailable carbohydrates because human digestive enzymes cannot break their bonds.

fiber: a general term denoting in plant foods the *nonstarch polysaccharides* that are not digested by *human* digestive enzymes, although some are digested by GI tract bacteria; fibers include cellulose, hemicelluloses, pectins, gums, and mucilages and the nonpolysaccharides lignins, cutins, and tannins.

STARCH

Just as the human body stores glucose as glycogen, plant cells store glucose as starch—long, unbranched or branched chains of hundreds or thousands of glucose molecules linked together (see the middle and right side of Figure 4–8). These giant molecules are packed side by side in grains such as wheat or rice, in tubers such as potatoes, and in legumes such as peas and beans. A cubic inch of food may contain as many as a million starch molecules.

In a plant such as a potato, starch stores the glucose needed to support the plant's first growth. When you eat the plant, your body hydrolyzes the starch to glucose and uses the glucose for its own energy purposes. Together with the sugars, then, starch is considered to be an available carbohydrate.

All starchy foods come from plants. Grains are the richest food source of starch, providing much of the food energy for people all over the world—rice in Asia; wheat in Canada, the United States, and Europe; corn in much of Central and South America; and millet, rye, barley, and oats elsewhere. The legumes are another important source of starch, as well as of dietary fibers and protein. Tubers, such as potatoes, yams, and the cassava of many non-Western societies, are another major source of starch.

THE FIBERS

Fibers are the structural parts of plants and thus are found in all plant-derived foods—vegetables, fruits, grains, and legumes. Most are polysaccharides, but starch is not one of them; in fact, fibers are often described as nonstarch poly-

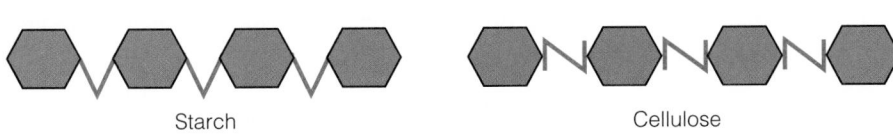

Starch

Cellulose

Figure 4–9

Starch and Cellulose Molecules Compared (Small Segments)
The bonds that link the glucose units together in cellulose are different from the bonds in starch (and glycogen). Human enzymes cannot digest cellulose. See Appendix C for chemical structures and descriptions of linkages.

saccharides. Nonstarch polysaccharides include cellulose, hemicelluloses, pectins, gums, and mucilages. Fibers also include some nonpolysaccharides such as lignins, cutins, and tannins.*

Even though most are polysaccharides, fibers differ from starch in that the bonds between their monosaccharide units cannot be broken down by human digestive enzymes. The bacteria of the GI tract can break some fibers down, however, and this is important to digestion and to health.

Each of the fibers has a different structure. Most contain monosaccharides, but differ in the types they contain and in the bonds that link the monosaccharides to each other. These differences produce diverse health effects.

Cellulose   Cellulose is the primary constituent of plant cell walls and therefore occurs in all vegetables, fruits, and legumes. Like starch, cellulose is composed of glucose units connected in long chains. Unlike starch, however, the chains do not branch, and the bonds holding the glucose units together resist digestion by human enzymes (see Figure 4–9).

Hemicelluloses   The hemicelluloses are the main constituent of cereal fibers. They are composed of various monosaccharide backbones with branching side chains of monosaccharides.† The many backbones and side chains make the hemicelluloses a diverse group; some are soluble, while others are insoluble.

Pectins   All pectins consist of a backbone derived from carbohydrate with side chains of various monosaccharides. Commonly found in vegetables and fruits (especially citrus fruits and apples), pectins may be isolated and used by the food industry to thicken jelly, keep salad dressing from separating, and otherwise control texture and consistency. Pectins can perform these functions because they readily form gels in water.

---

*The terms *crude fiber*, *neutral-detergent fiber*, and *dietary fiber* reflect different methodologies used to estimate the fiber contents of foods; they do not identify different types of fiber. The structure of cellulose is shown in Appendix C; the other polysaccharide fibers are similar, but differ slightly in their bonding. Besides glucose, their component sugars may include rhamnose, arabinose, and others. As for the lignins, they are polymers of several dozen molecules of phenol (an organic alcohol), with strong internal bonds that make them impervious to digestive enzymes.

†In hemicelluloses, the most common backbone monosaccharides are xylose, mannose, and galactose; the common side chains are arabinose, glucuronic acid, and galactose (see Appendix C for structures).

Gums and Mucilages   When cut, the branch of a plant secretes gums from the site of the injury. Like the other fibers, gums are composed of various monosaccharides and their derivatives. Gums such as *gum arabic* are used as additives by the food industry. Mucilages are similar to gums in structure; they include *guar* and *carrageenan*, which are added to foods as stabilizers.

Lignin   This *nonpolysaccharide* fiber has a three-dimensional structure that gives it strength. Because of its toughness, few of the foods that people eat contain much lignin. It occurs in the woody parts of vegetables such as carrots or the small seeds of fruits such as strawberries.

Other Classifications of Fibers   Scientists classify fibers in several ways. The previous paragraphs classified them according to their chemical properties. Fibers can also be classified according to their solubility. The effects of fibers on the body do not neatly divide along the lines of solubility, but some generalizations of significance to health can be made.

Soluble fibers:
- Gums.
- Pectins.
- Some hemicelluloses.
- Mucilages.

In general, soluble fibers occur in higher concentrations in fruits, oats, barley, and legumes. In the body, soluble fibers:

- Delay the stomach's emptying and the transit of chyme through the intestines.
- Delay glucose absorption.
- Lower blood cholesterol.[1]

Insoluble fibers:
- Cellulose.
- Many hemicelluloses.
- Lignins.

In general, insoluble fibers are found in higher concentrations in vegetables, wheat, and cereals. In the body, insoluble fibers:

- Accelerate the transit of chyme through the intestines.
- Increase fecal weight.
- Slow starch breakdown and delay glucose absorption into the blood.

In the body, *both* soluble and insoluble fibers:

- Influence transit time and nutrient absorption in the GI tract.
- Are partially fermented by microorganisms in the digestive tract to fragments that the body can use.*

Table 4–2 summarizes these fiber facts. Such generalizations are useful, but exceptions occur. For example, insoluble rice bran also lowers blood cholesterol, and the soluble fiber psyllium effectively promotes bowel movements.[2]

Some researchers classify fibers according to other physical properties that affect GI function and nutrient absorption. Physical properties of fibers include:

- *Water-holding capacity*—the capacity to capture water like a sponge, swelling and increasing the bulk of the intestines' contents.
- *Viscosity*—the capacity to form viscous, gel-like solutions.
- *Cation-exchange capacity*—the ability to bind minerals.
- *Bile-binding capacity*—the ability to bind bile.
- *Fermentability*—the extent to which bacteria can ferment them in the digestive tract.

---

*Dietary fibers are fermented by colon bacteria to short-chain fatty acids, which are absorbed and metabolized by the GI mucosa and liver.

Table 4–2

Fibers: Their Sources, Actions, and Structures

	Soluble Fibers	Insoluble Fibers
Food sources	Fruits (apples, citrus), oats, barley, legumes	Wheat bran, whole-grain breads and cereals, vegetables
Action in the body	Delay GI transit. Delay glucose absorption. Lower blood cholesterol.	Accelerate GI transit. Increase fecal weight. Slow starch hydrolysis. Delay glucose absorption.
Type of fiber	Gums, pectins, some hemicelluloses, mucilages	Cellulose, many hemicelluloses, lignins

Clearly, the fibers are a diverse group of compounds. Like a basket of threads of various colors and sizes, they can be used for many different projects depending on the interests of the craftsperson selecting them.[3]

A compound not classed as a fiber but often found with it in foods is phytic acid. Most dietary phytic acid comes from seeds such as the cereal grains. A person on a high-fiber diet may lose minerals that become bound to phytic acid and are excreted with it. (In plant seeds, phytic acid may store these minerals and hold them in plant tissue during germination.) The nutrition consequences of such mineral losses are described in Chapters 12 and 13.

In summary, the complex carbohydrates are the polysaccharides (chains of monosaccharides): glycogen, starch, and fibers. Both glycogen and starch are storage forms of glucose—glycogen in the body, and starch in plants—and both yield energy for human use. The fibers also contain glucose (and other monosaccharides), but their bonds cannot be broken by human digestive enzymes, so they yield little, if any, energy.

phytic acid: a nonnutrient component of plant seeds; also called **phytate** (FYE-tate). Phytic acid occurs in the husks of grains, legumes, and seeds and is capable of binding minerals such as zinc, iron, calcium, magnesium, and copper in insoluble complexes in the intestine, which the body excretes unused.

Digestion and Absorption of Carbohydrates

The ultimate goal of digestion and absorption of sugars and starch is to render all available carbohydrates into small compounds that the body can absorb and use—chiefly glucose. The large starch molecules require extensive breakdown; the disaccharides need only to be split once. The splitting of the larger carbohydrates begins in the mouth; the final splitting and absorption occur in the small intestine; and conversion to a common energy currency (glucose) is the task of the liver. The details follow.

THE PROCESSES OF DIGESTION AND ABSORPTION

Figure 4–10 traces the digestion of carbohydrates through the GI tract. When a person eats foods containing starch, enzymes hydrolyze the long chains to shorter chains, the short chains to disaccharides, and, finally, the disaccharides to monosaccharides. This process begins in the mouth.

The short chains of glucose units that result from the breakdown of starch are known as **dextrins**. The word sometimes appears on food labels because dextrins can be used as thickening agents in foods.

Figure 4–10

Carbohydrate Digestion in the GI Tract

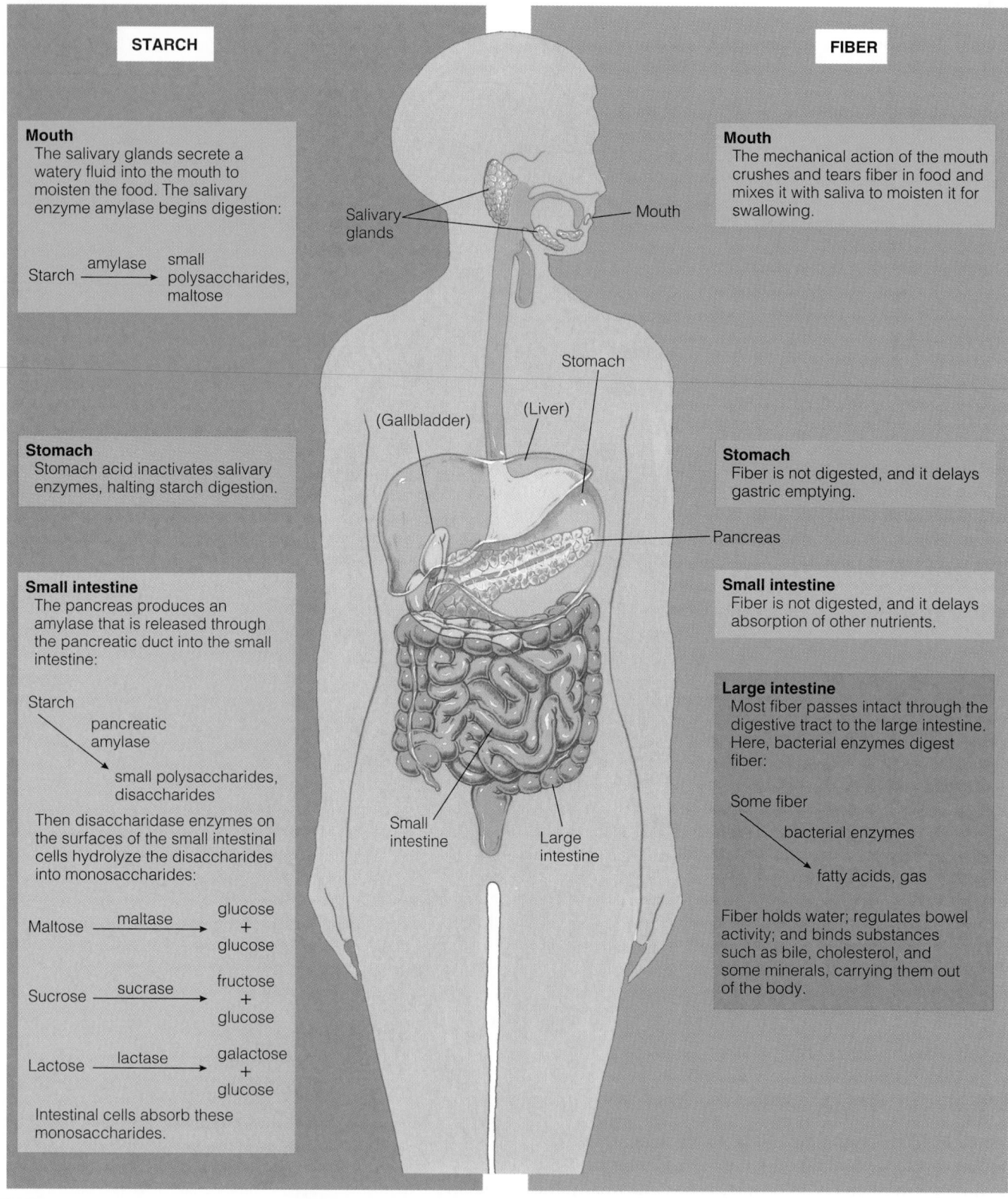

STARCH

Mouth
The salivary glands secrete a watery fluid into the mouth to moisten the food. The salivary enzyme amylase begins digestion:

Starch $\xrightarrow{\text{amylase}}$ small polysaccharides, maltose

Stomach
Stomach acid inactivates salivary enzymes, halting starch digestion.

Small intestine
The pancreas produces an amylase that is released through the pancreatic duct into the small intestine:

Starch
$\xrightarrow{\text{pancreatic amylase}}$
small polysaccharides, disaccharides

Then disaccharidase enzymes on the surfaces of the small intestinal cells hydrolyze the disaccharides into monosaccharides:

Maltose $\xrightarrow{\text{maltase}}$ glucose + glucose

Sucrose $\xrightarrow{\text{sucrase}}$ fructose + glucose

Lactose $\xrightarrow{\text{lactase}}$ galactose + glucose

Intestinal cells absorb these monosaccharides.

FIBER

Mouth
The mechanical action of the mouth crushes and tears fiber in food and mixes it with saliva to moisten it for swallowing.

Stomach
Fiber is not digested, and it delays gastric emptying.

Small intestine
Fiber is not digested, and it delays absorption of other nutrients.

Large intestine
Most fiber passes intact through the digestive tract to the large intestine. Here, bacterial enzymes digest fiber:

Some fiber
$\xrightarrow{\text{bacterial enzymes}}$
fatty acids, gas

Fiber holds water; regulates bowel activity; and binds substances such as bile, cholesterol, and some minerals, carrying them out of the body.

Salivary glands

Mouth

(Gallbladder)

(Liver)

Stomach

Pancreas

Small intestine

Large intestine

In the Mouth   In the mouth, vigorous chewing of high-fiber foods slows eating and stimulates the flow of saliva. The salivary enzyme amylase starts to work, hydrolyzing starch to shorter polysaccharides and to maltose. Because food is in the mouth for only a short time, very little digestion takes place there.

amylase (AM-ih-lace): an enzyme that hydrolyzes amylose (a form of starch). Amylase is a carbohydrase, an enzyme that breaks down carbohydrates.

Reminder: A *bolus* is a portion of food swallowed at one time.

In the Stomach   The swallowed bolus mixes with the stomach's acid and protein-digesting enzymes, and these digest the salivary enzyme amylase. Thus amylase is removed from the scene before its job of starch digestion is completed. To a small extent, the stomach's acid continues breaking starch down, but its juices contain no enzymes to digest carbohydrate. Fibers tend to linger in the stomach, delaying gastric emptying. This provides a feeling of fullness and satiety. Carbohydrate digestion speeds up again in the small intestine.

In the Small Intestine   The small intestine carries out most of the work of carbohydrate digestion. A major carbohydrate-digesting enzyme, pancreatic amylase, enters the intestine via the pancreatic duct and continues breaking down the polysaccharides to shorter glucose chains and disaccharides. The final step takes place on the outer membranes of the intestinal cells. There, specific enzymes dismantle specific disaccharides:

- Maltase breaks maltose into 2 glucose molecules.
- Sucrase breaks sucrose into 1 glucose and 1 fructose molecule.
- Lactase breaks lactose into 1 glucose and 1 galactose molecule.

maltase: an enzyme that hydrolyzes maltose.

sucrase: an enzyme that hydrolyzes sucrose.

lactase: an enzyme that hydrolyzes lactose.

At this point, all disaccharides contribute at least one glucose molecule to the body. Other monosaccharides can eventually become glucose after being processed in the liver, as explained later.

Fibers delay the absorption of carbohydrates and fats in the small intestine, conferring benefits on health that a later section describes further. In addition, fibers in the intestines can bind with minerals there. This prevents the minerals' absorption and presents a risk of deficiency, but the risk is minimal when fiber intake is reasonable and mineral intake adequate.

In the Large Intestine   Within one to four hours after a meal, all the sugars and most of the starches have been digested. Only a small fraction of the starches and the indigestible fibers remain in the digestive tract.[4]

Most of the fibers' actions occur in the large intestine. There, fibers attract water, which softens the stools for passage without straining. Also, bacteria in the human digestive tract ferment fibers—that is, they digest fibers in the absence of oxygen. This process generates water, gas, and short-chain fatty acids (described in Chapter 5).* The short-chain fatty acids are absorbed in the colon and yield energy when metabolized. Metabolism of short-chain fatty acids occurs in both the intestinal mucosa and the liver.[5] Food fibers, therefore, do contribute some energy, depending on the extent to which they are broken down and absorbed. The energy contribution can rise to as much as 15 percent of daily food energy intake on a high-fiber diet.

Starch that is not absorbed in the small intestine of healthy people is known as **resistant starch**.

---

*The short-chain fatty acids produced by GI bacteria are primarily acetic acid, propionic acid, and butyric acid.

Figure 4–11

Absorption of Monosaccharides

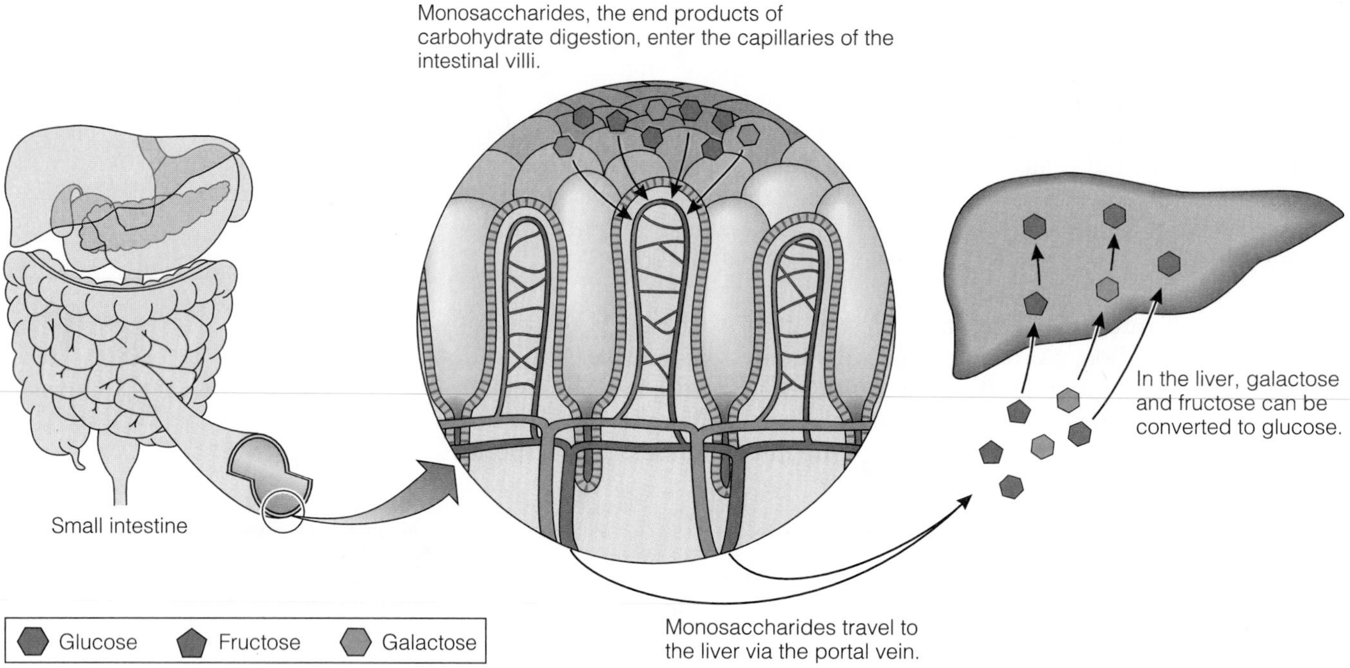

Monosaccharides, the end products of carbohydrate digestion, enter the capillaries of the intestinal villi.

Small intestine

| ⬡ Glucose | ⬠ Fructose | ⬡ Galactose |

In the liver, galactose and fructose can be converted to glucose.

Monosaccharides travel to the liver via the portal vein.

Absorption into the Bloodstream   Glucose is unique in that it can be absorbed to some extent through the lining of the mouth, but for the most part, all nutrient absorption takes place in the small intestine. The monosaccharides traverse the cells lining the small intestine by active transport and are washed away in the circulating blood.*

The blood then circulates through the liver, whose cells take up fructose and galactose and convert them to other compounds, most often to glucose, as shown in Figure 4–11. Thus all disaccharides not only provide at least one glucose molecule directly, but they also can provide another one indirectly—through the conversion of fructose and galactose to glucose. (The body does not use fructose and glucose in exactly the same ways, but for purposes of this book, they are treated as being metabolically identical.)

This description of the way the body receives carbohydrate should help explode a myth perpetrated by advertisers of high-sugar foods and beverages. They describe sugar as "quick energy" and imply that when you need quick energy, you should reach for a candy bar and a cola beverage. Clearly, though, the best pick-me-ups are not concentrated sugars. Sugars do offer energy, but so does any other food containing carbohydrate. Why not have a delicious peanut butter and banana sandwich, a tall, cool glass of milk, and a fresh, juicy orange as a pick-me-up?

*Fructose is absorbed by facilitated diffusion (see Figure 3–6 on p. 85).

LACTOSE INTOLERANCE

Normally, the enzyme lactase ensures that the disaccharide lactose found in milk is both digested and absorbed efficiently. Lactase levels are highest immediately after birth, as befits an infant whose first and only food for a while will be milk.[6] In the great majority of the world's populations, lactase activity declines dramatically during childhood and adolescence to about 5 to 10 percent of the activity at birth.[7] Only a relatively small percentage (about 30 percent) of the people in the world retain enough lactase to digest and absorb lactose efficiently throughout adult life.

Symptoms   When more lactose is consumed than the available lactase can handle, lactose molecules remain in the intestine undigested, attracting water and causing bloating, abdominal discomfort, and diarrhea—the symptoms of lactose intolerance. The undigested lactose becomes food for intestinal bacteria, which multiply and produce irritating acid and gas, further contributing to the discomfort and diarrhea.

Causes   As mentioned, lactase activity commonly declines with age. Lactase deficiency may also develop when the intestinal villi are damaged by disease, certain medicines, prolonged diarrhea, or malnutrition; this can lead to temporary or permanent lactose malabsorption, depending on the extent of the intestinal damage. In extremely rare cases, an infant is simply born with a lactase deficiency.

Prevalence   The prevalence of lactose intolerance varies widely among ethnic groups, indicating that the trait is genetically determined.[8] The prevalence of lactose intolerance is lowest among Scandinavians and other Northern Europeans and highest among native North Americans and Southeast Asians.

Dietary Changes   Managing lactose intolerance requires some dietary changes, although total elimination of milk products is usually not necessary. Excluding all milk products from the diet can lead to nutrient deficiencies, for milk is a major source of several nutrients, notably the mineral calcium and the B vitamin riboflavin. Fortunately, many people with lactose intolerance can consume small amounts of milk products, especially if they take them with other foods in meals.[9] In some cases, people can increase their tolerance by gradually increasing the amounts of milk products they consume; they may become able to tolerate as much as a cup of milk a day.[10] A change in the GI bacteria, not the reappearance of the missing enzyme, accounts for the ability to adapt to milk products.

In many cases, lactose-intolerant people can tolerate fermented milk products such as yogurt and acidophilus milk. The bacteria in these products digest lactose for their own use, leaving these foods relatively low in lactose. Hard cheeses and cottage cheese are often well tolerated because most of the lactose is removed with the whey during manufacturing. Lactose continues to diminish as the cheese ages.

Many lactose-intolerant people use commercially prepared milk products that have been treated with an enzyme that breaks down the lactose. Alternatively, they take enzyme tablets with meals or add enzyme drops to their milk. The

lactose intolerance: a condition that results from inability to digest the milk sugar lactose; characterized by bloating, gas, abdominal discomfort, and diarrhea. Lactose intolerance differs from milk allergy, which is caused by an immune reaction to the protein in milk.

lactase deficiency: a lack of the enzyme required to digest the disaccharide lactose into its component monosaccharides (glucose and galactose).

Estimated prevalence of lactose intolerance:

>80% Asian Americans.
 80% Native Americans.
 75% African Americans.
 70% Mediterranean peoples.
 60% Inuits.
 50% Hispanics.
 20% Caucasians.
<10% Northern Europeans.

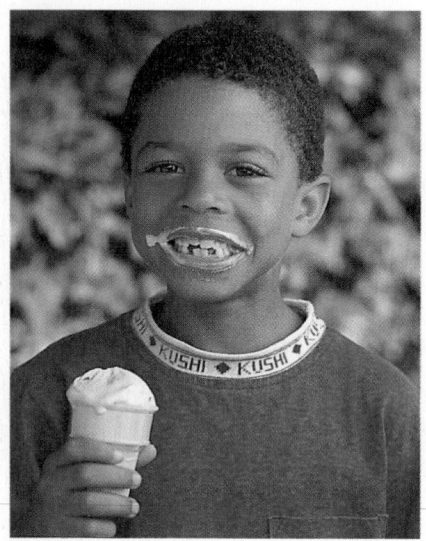

Many people who are lactose intolerant cannot enjoy ice cream without GI distress.

enzyme hydrolyzes much of the lactose in milk to glucose and galactose, which lactose-intolerant people can absorb without ill effects. Most healthy adults with lactose intolerance can drink milk when the lactose content has been reduced by 50 percent.[11]

Because people's tolerance to lactose varies widely, lactose-restricted diets must be highly individualized. Each case differs. A completely lactose-free diet can be difficult because lactose appears not only in milk and milk products but also as an ingredient in many nondairy foods such as breads, cereals, breakfast drinks, salad dressings, and cake mixes. People on strict lactose-free diets need to read labels and avoid foods that include milk, milk solids, whey (milk liquid), and casein (milk protein, which may contain traces of lactose). They also need to check all drugs with the pharmacist because 20 percent of prescription drugs and 5 percent of over-the-counter drugs contain lactose as a filler.

People who consume few or no milk products must take care to meet riboflavin and calcium needs. Later chapters on the vitamins and minerals offer help with finding good nonmilk sources of these nutrients.

To summarize the digestion and absorption of carbohydrates, the body breaks down starches into disaccharides and disaccharides into monosaccharides, and then converts monosaccharides mostly to glucose to fuel the cells' work. The fibers help to regulate the passage of food through the GI system, but contribute only a little energy. Lactose intolerance is a common condition that occurs when there is insufficient lactase to digest the disaccharide lactose found in milk and milk products. Symptoms include GI distress. Because treatment requires limiting milk intake, other calcium-rich substitutes must be included in the diet.

Glucose in the Body

The primary role of the available carbohydrates in human nutrition is to supply the body's cells with glucose to deliver the indispensable commodity, energy. Starch contributes most to the body's glucose supply, but as explained earlier, any of the sugars can also be converted to glucose.

Glucose plays the central role in carbohydrate metabolism. The next two sections provide an overview first of the pathways glucose can follow in the body and then of the ways the body regulates those pathways.

A PREVIEW OF CARBOHYDRATE METABOLISM

This brief discussion provides just enough information about carbohydrate metabolism to illustrate that the body needs and uses glucose as a chief energy nutrient. Chapter 7 provides a full description of how all of the energy-yielding nutrients—carbohydrate, fat, and protein—contain energy and how the body metabolizes these molecules to free that energy for its use.

Storing Glucose as Glycogen The liver stores and releases glucose as needed. During times of plenty, liver cells combine excess glucose molecules into long, branching chains of glycogen. The liver stores one-third of the body's total glycogen. When blood glucose falls, the liver cells dismantle the glycogen into single molecules of glucose and release them into the bloodstream. Thus glucose can supply energy to the central nervous system and other organs regardless of whether the person has eaten recently. Muscle cells can also store glucose as glycogen (the other two-thirds), but they hoard most of their own supply, using it just for themselves during exercise.

Glycogen holds water and therefore is rather bulky. The body can store only enough glycogen to provide energy for relatively short periods of time—during exercise, a few hours' worth at most. For its long-term energy reserves, for use over days or weeks of food deprivation, the body employs its unlimited, water-free fuel, fat, as Chapter 5 describes.

Using Glucose for Energy   Glucose fuels the work of most of the body's cells. Inside a cell, enzymes break glucose in half. These halves can be put back together to make glucose, or they can be further broken down into smaller fragments (never again to be reassembled to form glucose). The small fragments can yield energy when broken down completely to carbon dioxide and water, or they can be reassembled, but only into units of body fat.

To keep providing glucose to meet the body's energy needs, a person has to eat dietary carbohydrate frequently, for as mentioned, glycogen stores last only for hours, not for days. People do not always attend faithfully to their bodies' carbohydrate needs, yet they survive. How do they manage without glucose from dietary carbohydrate? Do they simply draw energy from the other two energy-yielding nutrients, fat and protein? They do draw energy, but not simply.

Making Glucose from Protein   Body protein can be converted to glucose to some extent, but protein has jobs of its own that no other nutrient can do. Body fat cannot be converted to glucose to any significant extent, and although fat breakdown can yield energy for many of the body's cells "as is," glucose does some jobs that fat cannot normally do—for example, glucose provides energy for brain cells, other nerve cells, and developing red blood cells.

Thus, when a person does not replenish depleted glycogen stores by eating carbohydrate, body proteins are dismantled to make glucose to fuel these special cells. The conversion of protein to glucose is called gluconeogenesis—literally, the making of new glucose. Only adequate dietary carbohydrate can prevent this use of protein for energy, and this role of carbohydrate is known as its protein-sparing action.

Making Ketone Bodies from Fat Fragments   Without sufficient glucose, the body also changes its way of using fat. Normally, when fat breaks down to provide energy, glucose is also present, and the two fuels are metabolized together. Fat fragments combine with glucose fragments, and the combined molecules then break down completely. Without glucose, fat fragments do not break down completely but combine with each other, forming ketone bodies. Muscles and other tissues can use ketone bodies for energy, but when their production exceeds their use, they accumulate in the blood, causing ketosis, a condition that disturbs the body's normal acid-base balance, as described in Chapter 7.

To ensure complete sparing of body protein and prevent ketosis requires 50 to 100 grams of carbohydrate a day.[12] Dietary recommendations urge people to select abundantly from carbohydrate-rich foods to provide for this allowance and considerably more.

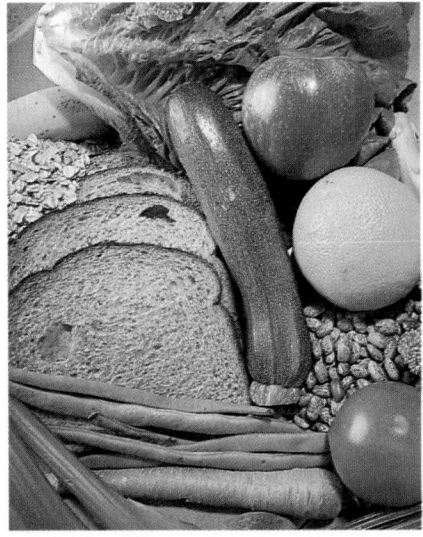

The carbohydrates of grains, vegetables, fruits, and legumes supply most of the energy in a healthful diet.

gluconeogenesis (gloo-co-nee-oh-GEN-ih-sis): the making of glucose from a noncarbohydrate source (described in more detail in Chapter 7).

  gluco = glucose
  neo = new
  genesis = making

protein-sparing action: the action of carbohydrate (and fat) in providing energy that allows protein to be used for other purposes.

ketone (KEE-tone) **bodies:** the product of the incomplete breakdown of fat when glucose is not available in the cells.

ketosis (kee-TOE-sis): an undesirably high concentration of ketone bodies in the blood and urine.

acid-base balance: the equilibrium in the body between acid and base concentrations; see Chapter 12.

Converting Glucose to Fat   Given more carbohydrate than it needs, the body uses glucose to meet its energy needs, fills its glycogen stores to capacity, and may still have some left over. To store the extra glucose, the liver breaks it (and energy-containing fragments from protein or fat, too) into smaller molecules and puts them together into the more permanent energy-storage compound—fat. Then the fat travels to the fatty tissues of the body for storage. Unlike the liver cells, which can store only about half a day's worth of glycogen, fat cells can store unlimited quantities of fat.

Even though excess carbohydrate can be converted to fat and stored, this is a minor pathway.[13] The amount of fat being made from carbohydrate at any given time is less than the amount of fat being used for energy. Body fat comes mainly from dietary fat.[14] A balanced diet high in complex carbohydrates actually helps control body weight. Most carbohydrate-rich foods are so bulky and naturally so low in fat that when large quantities are eaten, they tend to crowd fat out of the diet. Since carbohydrate is less energy dense than fat (with only 4 kcalories to the gram compared with fat's 9), eating a diet high in carbohydrate usually tends to *reduce* energy intake. Thus abundant dietary carbohydrate combined with little dietary fat supports weight control.

THE CONSTANCY OF BLOOD GLUCOSE

Every body cell depends on glucose for its fuel to some extent, and ordinarily, the cells of the brain and the rest of the nervous system depend *primarily* on glucose for their energy. The activities of these cells never cease, and they do not have the ability to store glucose. Day and night they continually draw on the supply of glucose in the fluid surrounding them. To maintain the supply, a steady stream of blood moves past these cells bringing more glucose from either the intestines (food) or the liver (glycogen).

Reminder: *Homeostasis* is the maintenance of constant internal conditions by the body's control systems.

Normal blood glucose: 80 to 120 mg/dL.

Maintaining Glucose Homeostasis   To function optimally, the body must maintain blood glucose within limits that permit the cells to nourish themselves. If blood glucose falls below normal, the person may become dizzy and weak; if it rises above normal, the person may become confused and have difficulty breathing. Left untreated, fluctuations to the extremes—either high or low—can be fatal.

insulin (IN-suh-lin): a hormone secreted by special cells in the pancreas in response to (among other things) increased blood glucose concentration. The primary role of insulin is to control the transport of glucose from the bloodstream into the cells.

glucagon (GLOO-ka-gon): a hormone that is secreted by special cells in the pancreas in response to low blood glucose concentration and elicits release of glucose from storage.

The Regulating Hormones   Blood glucose homeostasis is regulated primarily by two hormones: insulin, which moves glucose from the blood into the cells, and glucagon, which brings glucose out of storage when necessary. Figure 4–12 depicts these hormonal regulators at work.

After a meal, as blood glucose rises, special cells of the pancreas respond by secreting insulin into the blood.* As the circulating insulin contacts the receptors on the body's other cells, the receptors respond by ushering glucose from the blood into the cells. Most of the cells take only the glucose they can use for energy right away, but the liver and muscle cells can assemble the small glucose units into long, branching chains of glycogen for storage. The liver cells can also convert glucose to fat for export to other cells. Thus high blood glucose returns

---

*The *beta* (BAY-tuh) *cells,* one of several types of cells in the pancreas, secrete insulin in response to elevated blood glucose concentration.

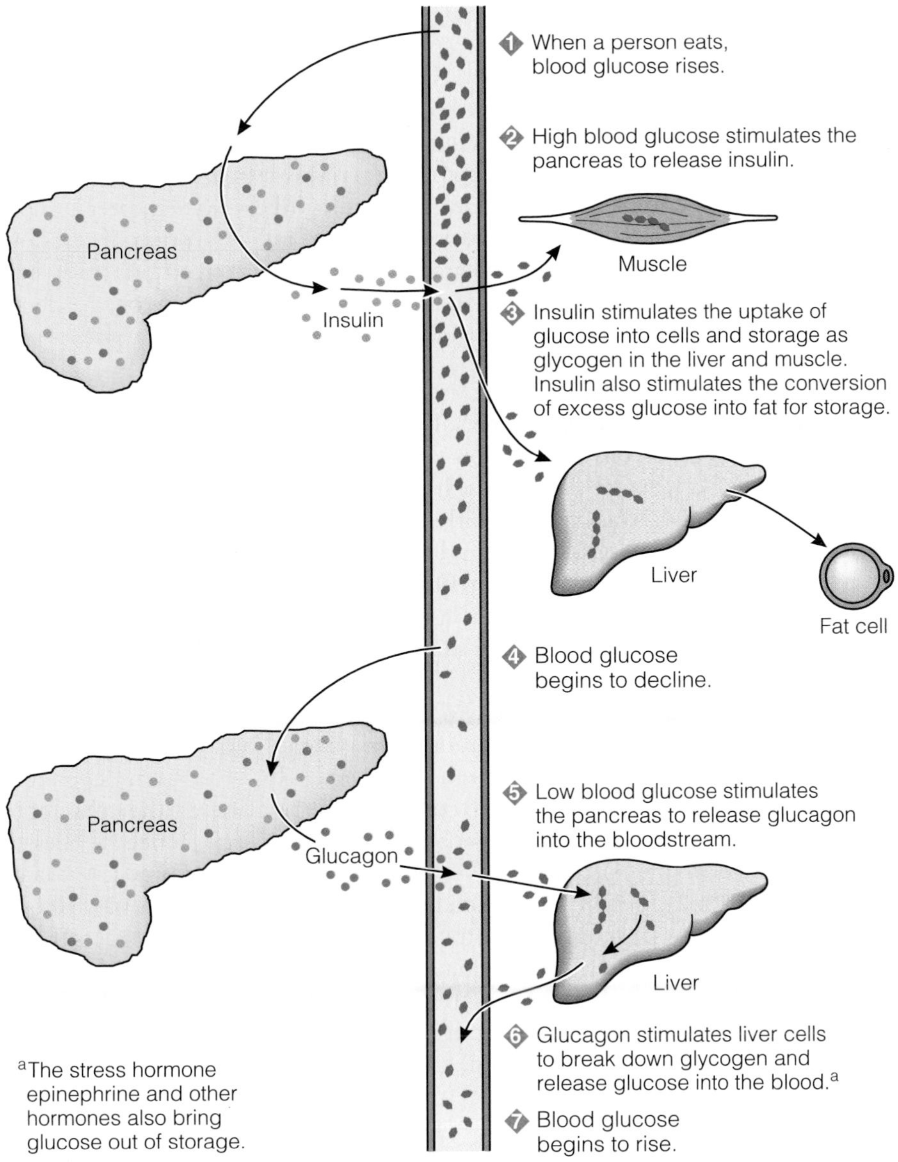

Figure 4–12

Maintaining Blood Glucose Homeostasis

❶ When a person eats, blood glucose rises.

❷ High blood glucose stimulates the pancreas to release insulin.

Muscle

Pancreas

Insulin

❸ Insulin stimulates the uptake of glucose into cells and storage as glycogen in the liver and muscle. Insulin also stimulates the conversion of excess glucose into fat for storage.

Liver

Fat cell

❹ Blood glucose begins to decline.

❺ Low blood glucose stimulates the pancreas to release glucagon into the bloodstream.

Pancreas

Glucagon

Liver

❻ Glucagon stimulates liver cells to break down glycogen and release glucose into the blood.[a]

❼ Blood glucose begins to rise.

[a]The stress hormone epinephrine and other hormones also bring glucose out of storage.

to normal as excess glucose is stored as glycogen (which can be converted back to glucose) and fat (which cannot be).

When blood glucose falls (as occurs between meals), other special cells of the pancreas respond by secreting glucagon into the blood.* Glucagon raises blood glucose by signaling the liver to dismantle its glycogen stores and release glucose into the blood for use by all the other body cells.

Another hormone that calls glucose from the liver cells is the "fight-or-flight" hormone, epinephrine. Epinephrine acts quickly when a person experiences stress, ensuring that all the body cells have energy fuel in emergencies. Like glucagon, epinephrine works to return glucose to the blood from liver glycogen.

epinephrine (EP-ih-NEFF-rin): a hormone of the adrenal gland that modulates the stress response; formerly called *adrenaline*.

---

*Glucagon is produced by the *alpha cells* of the pancreas.

hypoglycemia: an abnormally low blood glucose concentration.

insulin-dependent diabetes mellitus (IDDM): the less common type of diabetes in which the person produces no insulin at all; also known as type I diabetes or juvenile-onset diabetes (because it frequently develops in childhood), although some cases arise in adulthood.

noninsulin-dependent diabetes mellitus (NIDDM): the more common type of diabetes in which the fat cells resist insulin; also called type II diabetes or adult-onset diabetes. NIDDM is usually milder than IDDM and progresses more slowly.

glycemic (gligh-SEEM-ic) effect: a measure of the extent to which a food, as compared with pure glucose, raises the blood glucose concentration and elicits an insulin response.

Popular articles sometimes describe eating many small meals and snacks throughout the day as grazing.

Balancing within the Normal Range   The maintenance of normal blood glucose thus ordinarily depends on two processes. When blood glucose falls too low, food can readily replenish it, or in the absence of food, glucagon can signal the liver to break down glycogen stores. When blood glucose rises too high, insulin can signal the cells to take in glucose for energy. Eating balanced meals helps the body maintain a happy medium between the extremes. Balanced meals provide abundant complex carbohydrates, including fibers, some protein, and a little fat. The fibers and fat slow down the digestion and absorption of carbohydrate, so that glucose enters the blood gradually, providing a steady, ongoing supply. Dietary protein elicits the secretion of glucagon, whose effects oppose those of insulin, helping to maintain blood glucose within the normal range.[15]

Falling outside the Normal Range   This influence of foods on blood glucose has given rise to the oversimplification that foods *govern* blood glucose concentrations. Foods do not; the body does. In some people, however, blood glucose regulation fails. When this happens, either of two conditions can result: diabetes or hypoglycemia. People with these conditions can often use special diet patterns to help maintain their blood glucose within a normal range.

In diabetes, blood glucose remains high after a meal because insulin is either inadequate or ineffective. Thus while *blood* glucose is central to diabetes, *dietary* carbohydrates do not cause diabetes.

In insulin-dependent diabetes (IDDM), which is the less common type of diabetes, the pancreas fails to make insulin; researchers hold genetics, toxins, a virus, and a disordered immune system responsible. In noninsulin-dependent diabetes (NIDDM), which is the more common type of diabetes, the cells fail to respond to insulin; this condition tends to occur as a consequence of obesity. Because obesity can precipitate NIDDM, the best preventive measure is to maintain a healthy body weight. Recommendations for those who have diabetes encourage a diet low in fat and rich in complex carbohydrates and fibers. Concentrated sweets are not strictly excluded from the diabetic diet as they once were, but can be eaten in limited amounts with meals as part of a healthy diet.[16] The many environmental, genetic, and metabolic factors surrounding diabetes and its associated problems receive full attention in Chapter 27.

The Glycemic Effect   The term *glycemic effect* describes the effect of food on blood glucose: how quickly glucose is absorbed after a person eats, how high blood glucose rises, and how quickly it returns to normal. Slow absorption, a modest rise in blood glucose, and a smooth return to normal are considered desirable; fast absorption, a surge in blood glucose, and an overreaction that forces glucose below normal are undesirable. Different foods have different effects on blood glucose depending on a number of factors working together, and the effect is not always what a person might expect.[17] Ice cream, for example, is a high-sugar food, but it produces less of a response than potatoes, a high-starch food.

Most relevant to real life, a food's glycemic effect differs depending on whether it is eaten alone or as part of a mixed meal. In addition, eating small meals frequently spreads glucose absorption across the day and thus offers the same metabolic advantages as do foods with a low glycemic effect.[18]

The rate of glucose absorption is particularly important to people with diabetes, who may benefit from avoiding foods that produce too great a rise, or too sudden a fall, in blood glucose. Indeed, some studies have shown that taking the glycemic effect into account in meal planning is a practical way to improve glucose control.[19] Overall, though, meal planning should focus on total carbohydrate intake rather than the source of carbohydrate.[20]

To sum up, dietary carbohydrates provide glucose that can be used by the cells for energy, stored by the liver and muscle as glycogen, or converted into fat if intakes exceed needs. All of the body's cells depend on glucose; those of the central nervous system are especially dependent on it. Without glucose, the body is forced to break down its protein tissues to make glucose and to alter its metabolism to make ketone bodies from fats. Blood glucose regulation depends primarily on two pancreatic hormones: insulin to remove glucose from the blood into the cells when levels are high and glucagon to free glucose from glycogen stores and release it into the blood when levels are low.

Health Effects and Recommended Intakes of Sugars

Ever since people first discovered honey and dates, they have enjoyed the sweetness of sugars. In the United States, the natural sugars of milk, fruits, vegetables, and grains account for about half of the sugar intake; the other half consists of sugars that have been refined and added to foods for a variety of purposes. Added sugars assume various names: sucrose, invert sugar, corn sugar, corn syrups and solids, high-fructose corn syrup, and honey (see the glossary on p. 122).

The use of sweeteners in food manufacturing has risen steadily over the past two decades, reaching a record high of 139 pounds per person per year (see Figure 4–13). This estimate represents all sweeteners used in the marketing

As an additive, sugar:
- Enhances flavor.
- Supplies texture and color to baked goods.
- Provides fuel for fermentation, causing bread to rise or producing alcohol.
- Acts as a bulking agent in ice cream and baked goods.
- Acts as a preservative in jams.
- Balances the acidity of tomato- and vinegar-based products.

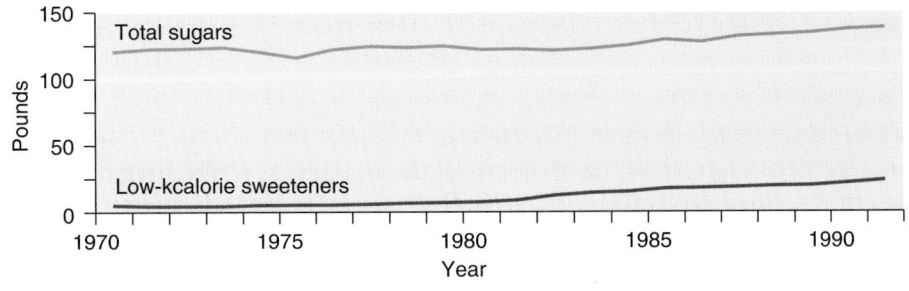

Figure 4–13

Use of Sweeteners

Source: U.S. Department of Agriculture, Economic Research Service, Commodity Economics Division.

Total per capita use of sugars increased 15 percent from 1971 to 1991. In that same time, use of low-kcalorie sweeteners increased approximately 10 percent.

These data do not represent the amount of sugars actually consumed; instead, they represent the total disappearance of sweeteners into the marketing system divided by the total U.S. population. Estimates based on dietary intake indicate that the average consumption of refined sugar is less than half of the per capita estimate.

Glossary of Sugars

brown sugar: refined white sugar crystals to which manufacturers have added molasses syrup with natural flavor and color; 91 to 96 percent pure sucrose.

confectioners' sugar: finely powdered sucrose; 99.9 percent pure.

corn sweeteners: corn syrup and sugars derived from corn.

corn syrup: a syrup produced by the action of enzymes on cornstarch; contains mostly glucose. See also *high-fructose corn syrup (HFCS).*

dextrose: an older name for glucose.

granulated sugar: crystalline sucrose; 99.9 percent pure.

high-fructose corn syrup (HFCS): a corn-syrup sweetener made especially for use in processed foods and beverages, where it is the predominant sweetener. HFCS is mostly fructose; glucose makes up the balance.

honey: sugar (mostly sucrose) formed from nectar gathered by bees. An enzyme splits the sucrose into glucose and fructose. Composition and flavor vary, but honey always contains a mixture of sucrose, fructose, and glucose.

invert sugar: a mixture of glucose and fructose formed by the hydrolysis of sucrose in a chemical process; sold only in liquid form and sweeter than sucrose. Invert sugar is used as a food additive to help preserve freshness and prevent shrinkage.

levulose: an older name for fructose.

maple sugar: a sugar (mostly sucrose) purified from the concentrated sap of the sugar maple tree.

molasses: the thick brown syrup produced during sugar refining. Molasses retains residual sugar and other by-products and a few minerals; blackstrap molasses contains significant amounts of calcium and iron—the iron comes from the *machinery* used to process the sugar.

raw sugar: the first crop of crystals harvested during sugar processing. Raw sugar cannot be sold in the United States because it contains too much filth (dirt, insect fragments, and the like). Sugar sold as "raw sugar" domestically has actually gone through over half of the refining steps.

turbinado (ter-bih-NOD-oh) **sugar:** sugar produced using the same refining process as white sugar, but without the bleaching and anti-caking treatment; traces of molasses give turbinado its sandy color.

white sugar: pure sucrose or "table sugar," produced by dissolving, concentrating, and recrystallizing raw sugar.

---

system, including sugar lost or wasted, such as in the brine of sweet pickles or in jams or bakery goods that spoil before they are eaten. It also includes sugar used in pet foods and in fermentation. Estimates of *intake* indicate that on the average, each person consumes about 45 pounds of added sugar per year.[21] As a percentage of daily energy intake, this amount is roughly equivalent to current recommendations that sugar contribute no more than about 10 percent of energy intake.

HEALTH EFFECTS OF SUGARS

In moderate amounts (similar to current consumption levels), sugars add pleasure to meals without harming health. In excess, however, they can be detrimental in two ways. One, sugars can contribute to nutrient deficiencies by supplying energy (kcalories) without providing nutrients, and so dietary guidelines caution people against eating large quantities. Two, sugars contribute to tooth decay, and so dietary guidelines caution people against eating frequent snacks containing sugars and starches.

Nutrient Deficiencies   Foods that contain lots of added sugar deliver energy without other nutrients—they are empty-kcalorie foods. By comparison, starch comes packaged in foods with protein, vitamins, and minerals.

A person spending 200 kcalories of a day's energy allowance on a 16-ounce cola gets nothing of value for those kcaloric "dollars." In contrast, a person using 200 kcalories on three slices of whole-wheat bread gets 9 grams of protein plus several of the B vitamins with those kcalories. For the person who wants something sweet, perhaps a reasonable compromise would be to have two slices of bread with a teaspoon of jam on each. The amount of sugar a person can afford depends on how many kcalories are available beyond those needed to deliver indispensable vitamins and minerals.

With careful food selections, a person can obtain all the needed nutrients within an allowance of about 1500 kcalories. Some people have more generous energy allowances with which to "purchase" nutrients. For example, an active teenage boy may need as many as 4000 kcalories to get all the energy he needs. If he eats mostly nutritious foods, then the "empty kcalories" of cola beverages are probably an acceptable addition to his diet. On the other hand, an inactive older woman who can use fewer than 1500 kcalories a day cannot afford any but the most nutrient-dense foods.

Some people believe that because honey is a natural food, it is nutritious—or, at least, more nutritious than sugar. A look at their chemical structures reveals the truth. Honey, like table sugar, contains glucose and fructose. The primary difference is that in table sugar the two monosaccharides are bonded together, whereas in honey some of them are free. Whether a person eats monosaccharides individually, as in honey, or linked together, as in table sugar, they end up the same way in the body: as glucose and fructose.

Honey does contain a few vitamins and minerals, but not many, as Table 4–3 (on p. 124) shows. Honey is denser than crystalline sugar, too, so it provides more energy per spoon.

This is not to say that all sugar sources are alike, for some are more nutritious than others. Consider a fruit, say, an orange. The fruit may give you the same amounts of fructose and glucose and the same number of kcalories as a dose of sugar or honey, but the packaging is more valuable nutritionally. The fruit's sugars arrive in the body diluted in a large volume of water, packaged in fiber, and mixed with valuable minerals and vitamins.

As these comparisons illustrate, the really significant difference between sugar sources is not between "natural" honey and "purified" sugar but between concentrated sweets and the dilute, naturally occurring sugars that sweeten foods. You can suspect an exaggerated nutrition claim when you hear the assertion that one product is more nutritious than another because it contains honey.

Sugar can contribute to nutrient deficiencies only by displacing nutrients. The appropriate attitude to take is not that sugar is "bad" and must be avoided, but that nutritious foods must come first. If the nutritious foods end up crowding

empty-kcalorie food: a popular term used to denote foods that contribute energy but lack protein, vitamins, and minerals. Empty-kcalorie foods are *low–nutrient density foods.* The most notorious empty-kcalorie foods are sugar, fat, and alcohol.

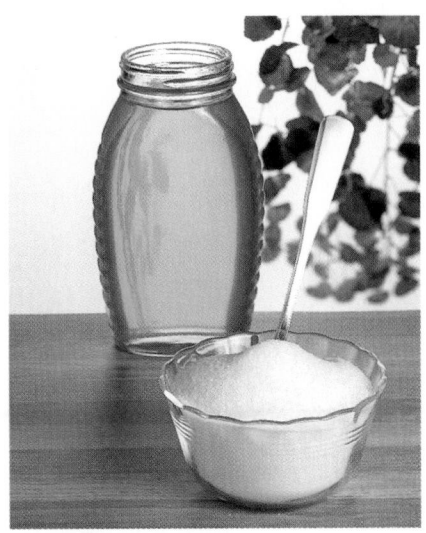

1 tsp honey = 22 kcal.
1 tsp sugar = 16 kcal.

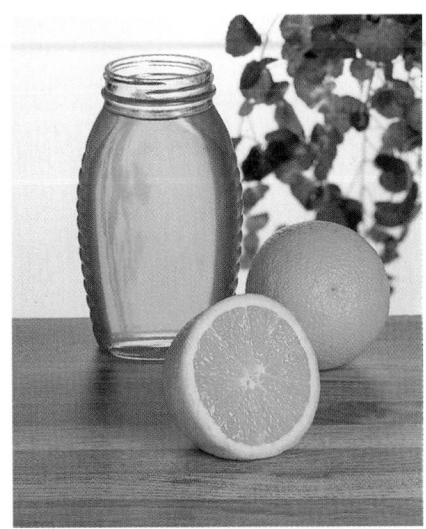

You receive the same sugars from an orange as from honey, but the packaging makes a big nutrition difference.

Table 4–3

Sample Nutrients in Sugars and Other Foods

The indicated portion of any of these foods provides approximately 100 kcalories. Notice that for a similar number of kcalories and grams of carbohydrates, milk, legumes, fruits, vegetables, and grains offer more of the other nutrients than do the sugars.

	Size of 100 kcal Portion	Carbohydrate (g)	Protein (g)	Calcium (mg)	Iron (mg)	Vitamin A (µg RE)	Vitamin C (mg)
Foods							
Milk, 1% low-fat	1 c	12	8	300	0.1	144	2
Kidney beans	½ c	20	7	30	1.6	0	2
Apricots	6	24	2	30	1.1	554	22
Bread, whole wheat	1½ slices	20	4	30	1.9	0	0
Broccoli, cooked	2 c	20	12	188	2.2	696	148
Sugars							
Sugar, white	2 tbs	24	0	trace	trace	0	0
Molasses, blackstrap	2½ tbs	28	0	343	12.6	0	0.1
Cola beverage	1 c	26	0	6	trace	0	0
Honey	1½ tbs	26	trace	2	0.2	0	trace

dental caries: decay of teeth.

caries = rottenness

To prevent dental caries:
- Eat sugary foods with meals.
- Limit between-meal snacks containing sugars and starches.
- Brush and floss teeth regularly.
- If brushing and flossing are not possible, at least rinse with water.

plaque, dental: a gummy mass of bacteria that grows on teeth and can lead to dental caries and gum disease.

sugar out of the diet, that is fine—but not the other way around. As always, the goals to seek are balance, variety, and moderation.

Dental Caries   Both sugars and starches begin breaking down to sugars in the mouth and so can contribute to tooth decay. Bacteria in the mouth ferment the sugars and in the process produce an acid that dissolves tooth enamel. People can eat sugar without this happening, though, for much depends on how long acid-yielding foods stay in the mouth. Sticky foods stay on tooth surfaces longer and keep yielding acid longer than foods that are readily cleared from the mouth. For that reason, sugar consumed quickly in a soft drink, for example, is less likely to cause dental caries than sugar in a pastry. By the same token, the sugar in sticky foods such as dried fruits is more detrimental than its quantity alone would suggest.

Another concern is how often people eat sugar. Bacteria produce acid for 20 to 30 minutes after each exposure. If a person eats three pieces of candy at one time, the teeth will be exposed to approximately 30 minutes of acid destruction. But, if the person eats three pieces at half-hour intervals, the time of exposure increases to 90 minutes. Likewise, slowly sipping a sugary soft drink may be more harmful than drinking quickly and clearing the mouth of sugar. Nonsugary foods can help remove sugar from tooth surfaces; hence, it is better to eat sugar with meals than between meals.

The development of caries depends on several factors: the bacteria that reside in the plaque, the saliva that cleanses the mouth, the minerals that form the teeth, and the foods that remain after swallowing.[22] For most people, good oral hygiene and a well-balanced diet will prevent dental caries. In short, sugars cause dental caries, but they require a cooperating victim to do so.

ACCUSATIONS AGAINST SUGARS

Sugars have been blamed for a variety of other problems. The following paragraphs evaluate some of these accusations.

Accusation: Sugar Causes Obesity Population studies show that obesity rises as sugar consumption increases, but sugar is not the sole cause. Foods high in added sugars are usually high in fat, too, so that whenever sugar intake increases, total energy and fat intakes do, too. Simultaneously, physical activity often declines. Obesity also occurs where sugar intakes are low. In some instances, obese people eat less sugar than thin people.[23] Thus sugar can contribute to obesity but does not cause obesity by itself—and obesity can occur without it.

Accusation: Sugar Causes Heart Diseases Researchers agree that unusually high doses of refined sugar can alter blood lipids to promote heart disease. This effect is most dramatic in "carbohydrate-sensitive" individuals—people who respond to sucrose with abnormally high insulin secretion, which promotes the making of excess fat. For most people, though, moderate sugar intakes do *not* influence the risk of heart disease. To keep these findings in perspective, consider that heart disease correlates most closely with factors that have nothing to do with nutrition, such as smoking and genetics. Among dietary risk factors, several—such as total fats, saturated fats, cholesterol, and obesity—have much stronger associations with heart disease than do sugar intakes.

Accusation: Sugar Causes Misbehavior in Children and Criminal Behavior in Adults Sugar has been blamed for the misbehaviors of hyperactive children, delinquent adolescents, and lawbreaking adults. Such speculations have been based on personal stories and have not been confirmed by scientific research.[24] No scientific evidence supports a relationship between sugar and hyperactivity or other misbehaviors. Chapter 19 provides accurate information on diet and children's behavior.

RECOMMENDED INTAKES OF SUGARS

The *Dietary Guidelines* urge people to use sugars only in moderation. Other recommendations specify that sugars should occupy only 10 percent or less of the day's total energy intake. A person consuming 2000 kcalories a day, then, should receive no more than 200 kcalories (that is, 50 grams or less) from concentrated sugars.

Food labels list the total grams of sugar a food provides. This total reflects both added sugars and those occurring naturally in foods. A food is likely to be high in sugars if its ingredient list starts with any of the sugars named in the glossary on p. 122 or if it includes several of them.

In summary, as currently consumed, sugars pose no major health threat except for an increased risk of dental caries. Excessive intakes may displace needed nutri-

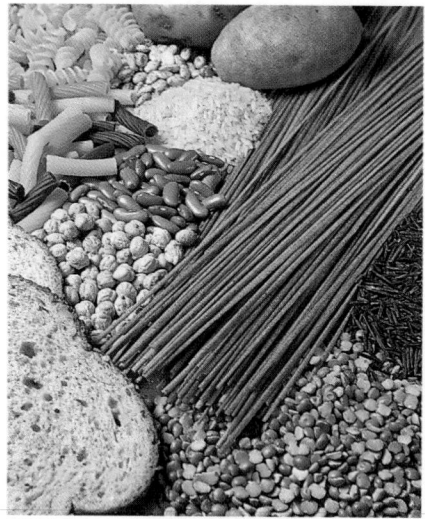

Foods rich in starch and fiber offer many health benefits.

ents and fiber; when accompanied by fat, sugars may be associated with obesity. If on these grounds a person decides to limit daily sugar intake, it is important to recognize that not all sugars need to be restricted, just *concentrated* sweets, which are relatively empty of other nutrients and high in kcalories. Sugars that occur naturally in fruits, vegetables, and milk are acceptable.

Health Effects and Recommended Intakes of Starch and Fibers

Carbohydrates and fats are the two major sources of energy in the diet. When one is high, the other is usually low—and vice versa. The average fat intake in the United States is high compared with health recommendations. To lower fat intake and improve the balance between these two energy nutrients, people need to replace fatty foods with vegetables, legumes, fruits, and grain products—foods noted for their complex carbohydrates.

HEALTH EFFECTS OF STARCH AND FIBERS

In addition to starch and dietary fibers, vegetables, legumes, fruits, and grains supply valuable vitamins and minerals and little or no fat. The following paragraphs describe some of the health benefits of diets rich in complex carbohydrates.

Weight Control   Foods rich in complex carbohydrates tend to be low in fat and simple sugars and can therefore promote weight loss by providing less food energy per bite. They also provide satiety and delay hunger. In addition, fiber-rich foods slow the rate at which food leaves the stomach and draw water into the GI tract, prolonging the satiety enjoyed from carbohydrate-rich meals. Several studies have found that people who eat a high-carbohydrate breakfast take in fewer kcalories at later meals and snacks than people who eat low-fiber or high-fat breakfasts.[25]

Many weight-loss products on the market today contain bulk-inducing fibers such as methylcellulose, but buying pure fiber compounds like this is neither necessary nor advisable. To use fiber in a weight-loss plan, select fresh fruits, vegetables, legumes, and whole-grain foods. High-fiber foods not only add bulk to the diet, but are economical and nutritious. (A note of caution, though: on baked goods, read the label—those popular large bran muffins are high in fat, and many items, of course, contain added sugar.)

The role of animal fat and cholesterol in heart disease is discussed in Chapter 5. The role of vegetable proteins in heart disease is discussed in Chapter 6.

Heart Disease   High-carbohydrate diets are associated with low blood cholesterol and a low risk of heart disease.[26] Sorting out the exact reasons why can be difficult. Such diets are low in animal fat and cholesterol and high in soluble fibers and vegetable proteins—all factors associated with a lower risk of heart disease.

Foods rich in soluble fibers (such as oat bran, barley, and legumes) lower blood cholesterol by binding with bile, the emulsifier that otherwise would assist with fat and cholesterol absorption.[27] With less bile available, less fat and cholesterol are absorbed and blood cholesterol declines. Then the liver makes more bile from cholesterol to compensate for the bile bound to fiber and excreted in the

GI tract.[28] This reduces blood cholesterol further. The products of fiber digestion, once absorbed, also inhibit cholesterol synthesis.

Several researchers have speculated that fiber also exerts an indirect cholesterol-lowering effect by displacing fats in the diet.[29] Even when dietary fat is low, however, research shows that high intakes of soluble fibers exert a separate and significant cholesterol-lowering effect.[30]

Cancer   A high-carbohydrate diet, especially one that includes plenty of green and yellow vegetables and citrus fruits, protects against some types of cancer. Again, it is unclear whether the protection derives from the fiber or the vitamins.

Populations consuming high-fiber diets generally have lower rates of colon cancer than similar populations consuming low-fiber diets. Fiber may help prevent colon cancer by diluting, binding, and rapidly removing potentially cancer-causing agents from the colon. Alternatively, the protective effect may be due to the fermentation of resistant starch and fiber in the colon, which lowers the pH. A decreased pH in the colon is associated with decreased colon cancer risks.[31]

The role antioxidant vitamins and nutrients play in cancer prevention is discussed in Highlight 11.

Diabetes   Populations eating high-carbohydrate diets often have low rates of diabetes, most likely because such diets are low in fat. High-carbohydrate, low-fat diets help control weight, and this is the most effective way to prevent the most common type of diabetes (NIDDM). Furthermore, when soluble fibers trap nutrients and delay their exit from the stomach, glucose absorption is slowed, and this helps to prevent the glucose surge and rebound that seem to be associated with diabetes onset.

Diabetes is the topic of Chapter 27.

GI Health   Dietary fibers enhance the health of the large intestine. Their short-chain fatty acid products promote salt absorption and help maintain mucosal integrity. The healthier the intestinal walls, the better they can block absorption of unwanted constituents, such as bacteria. Fibers enlarge the stools, easing passage, and they speed up transit time; up to a point, transit time depends on stool weight. Insoluble fibers such as cellulose (as in cereal brans, fruits, and vegetables) are most important in this regard. Their undigested residue, together with the microbial growth they stimulate, enlarges the stools, helping to alleviate or prevent constipation. Fibers also stimulate microbial digestion of absorbable products.

Taken with ample fluids, fibers help to prevent several GI disorders. Large, soft stools ease elimination for the rectal muscles and reduce the pressure in the lower bowel, making it less likely that rectal veins will swell (hemorrhoids). Fiber prevents compaction of the intestinal contents, which could obstruct the appendix and permit bacteria to invade and infect it (appendicitis). In addition, fiber stimulates the GI tract muscles so that they retain their strength and resist bulging out into pouches known as diverticula (illustrated in Figure 4–14 on p. 128).

Harmful Effects of Excessive Fiber Intake   Despite fiber's benefits to health, research indicates that a diet high in fiber also has a few drawbacks. A person who has a small capacity and eats mostly high-fiber foods may not be able to take in enough food energy or nutrients. The malnourished, the elderly, and children adhering to all-plant diets are especially vulnerable to this problem.

diverticula (dye-ver-TIC-you-la): a sac or pouch that develops in the weakened areas of the intestinal wall (like bulges in an inner tube where the tire wall is weak). The term diverticulosis (DYE-ver-tic-you-LOH-sis) describes the condition of having diverticula. The danger of diverticulosis is that it can give rise to diverticulitis (DYE-ver-tic-you-LYE-tis), in which the pockets become infected or inflamed and may rupture. About one in every six people in Western countries develops diverticulosis in middle or later life.

divertir = to turn aside

osis = condition

itis = infection or inflammation

Figure 4–14

Diverticula

Outpocketings of intestinal linings that balloon through weakened intestinal wall muscles are known as diverticula. Diverticula may develop anywhere along the GI tract, but are most common in the colon.

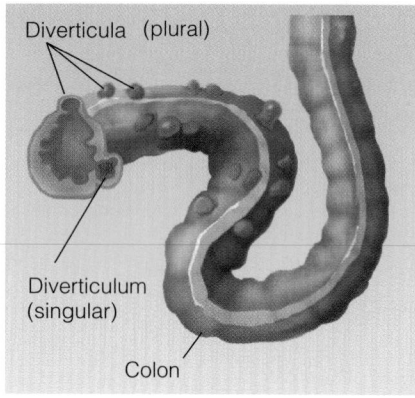

Diverticula (plural)

Diverticulum (singular)

Colon

Quick and easy estimate: To attain 55 to 60% of energy from carbohydrate, look for 14 to 15 g of carbohydrate for each 100 kcal of food.

Chapter 2 described how whole-grain products retain many nutrients that are commonly lost during processing (see Figure 2–4 on p. 49).

Launching suddenly into a high-fiber diet can cause temporary bouts of abdominal discomfort, gas, and diarrhea and, more seriously, can obstruct the GI tract. To prevent such complications, a person adopting a high-fiber diet is advised to:

- Increase fiber intake gradually over several weeks to give the GI tract time to adapt.
- Drink lots of fluids to soften the fiber as it moves through the GI tract.
- Select fiber-rich foods from a variety of sources—fruits, vegetables, legumes, and whole-grain breads and cereals.

By speeding the transit of foods through the GI tract, excess fiber can limit the absorption of some nutrients. Also, insoluble fibers can bind to minerals and interfere with their absorption. When mineral intake is adequate, however, a reasonable intake of high-fiber foods does not seem to compromise mineral balance.

Clearly, fiber is like all the nutrients in that "more" is only "better" up to a point. Too much is no better than too little. Again, the key words are balance, moderation, and variety.

RECOMMENDED INTAKES OF STARCH AND FIBER

The Committee on Dietary Allowances has not established a specific RDA for carbohydrates, but it does suggest that carbohydrates should provide more than half the energy requirement.[32] Most nutrition experts suggest that 55 to 60 percent of total energy should be from carbohydrate to support long-term health. A person consuming 2000 kcalories a day should therefore have 1100 to 1200 kcalories of carbohydrate, or about 275 to 300 grams. The FDA used this guideline in establishing a Daily Value for carbohydrate of 300 grams per day or 60 percent of kcalories. For most people, this means increasing total carbohydrate intake. To this end, the *Dietary Guidelines* and the *Diet and Health* report both suggest a diet with plenty of vegetables, fruits, and grain products.

HEALTHY PEOPLE 2000: Increase complex carbohydrate and fiber-containing foods in the diets of adults to five or more daily servings for vegetables (including legumes) and fruits and to six or more daily servings for grain products.

The Committee on Dietary Allowances has not established a fiber RDA; instead, the committee suggests the same foods just mentioned: fruits, vegetables, legumes, and whole-grain cereals, which also provide minerals and vitamins.[33] The *Dietary Guidelines* and the *Diet and Health* report make similar suggestions. The FDA set a Daily Value for fiber at 25 grams or 11.5 grams per 1000-kcalorie energy intake. The American Dietetic Association suggests 20 to 35 grams of dietary fiber daily, which is about two times higher than the average intake in the United States.[34] An effective way to add fiber while cutting fat is to substitute plant sources of proteins (legumes) for animal sources (meats). Table 4–4 presents a listing of fiber sources.

Choose Wisely In selecting high-fiber foods, keep in mind the principle of variety. The fibers in some foods lower cholesterol, those in other foods help pro-

Table 4–4

Fiber in Selected Foods

Bread, Cereal, Rice, and Pasta Group

Whole-grain products provide about 2 grams of fiber per serving:

- 1 slice whole-wheat, pumpernickel, rye bread.
- 1 oz ready-to-eat bran cereal.
- ½ c cooked barley, bulgur, grits, oatmeal.

Vegetable Group

Most vegetables contain 2 to 3 grams of fiber per serving:

- 1 c raw bean sprouts.
- ½ c cooked broccoli, brussels sprouts, cabbage, carrots, cauliflower, collards, corn, eggplant, green beans, green peas, kale, mushrooms, okra, parsnips, potatoes, pumpkin, spinach, sweet potatoes, swiss chard, winter squash.
- ½ c chopped raw carrots, peppers.

Fruit Group

Fresh, frozen, and dried fruits have about 2 grams of fiber per serving:

- 1 medium apple, banana, kiwi, nectarine, orange, pear.
- ½ c applesauce, blackberries, blueberries, raspberries, strawberries.
- Fruit juices contain very little fiber.

Legumes

Many legumes provide about 8 grams of fiber per serving:

- ½ c cooked baked beans, black beans, black-eyed peas, kidney beans, navy beans, pinto beans.

Some legumes provide about 5 grams of fiber per serving:

- ½ c cooked garbanzo beans, great northern beans, lentils, lima beans, split peas.

Note: Appendix H provides fiber grams for over 2000 foods.

Adequate fiber:
- Fosters weight control.
- Lowers blood cholesterol.
- Helps prevent colon cancer.
- Helps prevent and control diabetes.
- Helps prevent and alleviate hemorrhoids.
- Helps prevent appendicitis.
- Helps prevent diverticulosis.

Excess fiber:
- Displaces energy- and nutrient-dense foods.
- Causes intestinal discomfort and distention.
- Interferes with mineral absorption.

mote GI tract health. The FDA authorizes two health claims on food labels concerning fiber: one is for "fruits, vegetables, and grain products that contain fiber, particularly soluble fiber, and risk of coronary heart disease," and the other is for "fiber-containing grain products, fruits, and vegetables and cancer." Another more general health claim addresses "fruits and vegetables and cancer." Chapter 2 describes the criteria foods must meet to bear these health claims.

A diet following the Daily Food Guide plan, which includes 3 to 5 vegetable servings, 2 to 4 fruit servings, and 6 to 11 bread servings daily, can easily supply the recommended amount of carbohydrates and fiber. To help estimate carbohydrate and energy intakes accurately, the list in the margin shows what concentrated sweets are equivalent to 1 teaspoon of white sugar. These sugars all provide *about* 5 grams of carbohydrate and *about* 20 kcalories per teaspoon. Some are lower (16 kcalories for table sugar), while others are higher (22 kcalories for

1 tsp white sugar =
- 1 tsp brown sugar.
- 1 tsp candy.
- 1 tsp corn sweetener or corn syrup.
- 1 tsp honey.
- 1 tsp jam or jelly.
- 1 tsp maple sugar or maple syrup.
- 1 tsp molasses.
- 1½ oz carbonated soda.
- 1 tbs catsup.

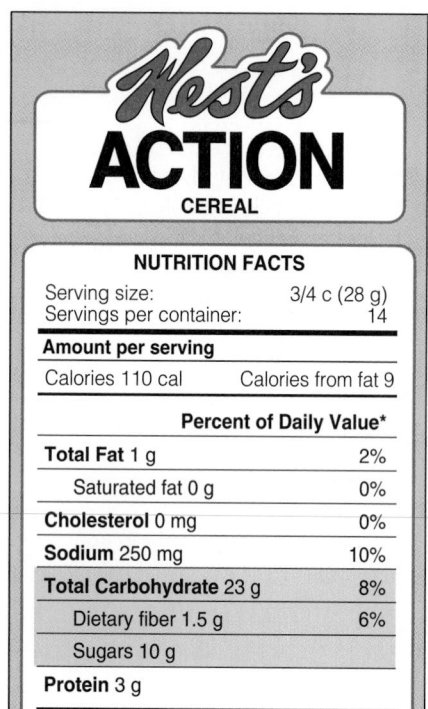

NUTRITION FACTS

Serving size:	3/4 c (28 g)
Servings per container:	14

Amount per serving

Calories 110 cal	Calories from fat 9

Percent of Daily Value*

Total Fat 1 g	2%
Saturated fat 0 g	0%
Cholesterol 0 mg	0%
Sodium 250 mg	10%
Total Carbohydrate 23 g	8%
Dietary fiber 1.5 g	6%
Sugars 10 g	
Protein 3 g	

honey), but a 20-kcalorie average is an acceptable approximation. For a person who uses catsup liberally, it may help to remember that 1 tablespoon of catsup supplies about 1 teaspoon of sugar.

Read Food Labels   Food labels list the amount, in grams, of total carbohydrate—including starch, fibers, and sugars—per serving. Fiber grams are also listed separately, as are the grams of sugars. (With this information, you can calculate starch grams by subtracting the grams of fibers and sugars from the total carbohydrate.) Sugars reflect both added sugars and those that occur naturally in foods. Total carbohydrate and dietary fiber are also expressed as "% Daily Values" for a person consuming 2000 kcalories; there is no Daily Value for sugars.

Clearly, a diet rich in complex carbohydrates—starches and fibers—supports efforts to control body weight and prevent heart disease, cancer, diabetes, and GI disorders.[35] For these reasons, recommendations urge people to eat plenty of grains, vegetables, legumes, and fruits—enough to provide 55 to 60 percent of the daily energy intake from carbohydrate.

In today's world, there is one other reason why plant foods high in starch and natural sugars are a better choice than animal foods or foods high in concentrated sweets. In general, the energy and resources required to grow and process plant foods are less, and the health benefits greater.

Study Questions

1. Which carbohydrates are described as simple, and which are complex?
2. Describe the structure of a monosaccharide and name the three monosaccharides important in nutrition. Name the three disaccharides commonly found in foods and their component monosaccharides. In what foods are these sugars found?
3. What happens in a condensation reaction? In a hydrolysis reaction?
4. Describe the structure of polysaccharides and name the ones important in nutrition. How are starch and glycogen similar, and how do they differ? How do the fibers differ from the other polysaccharides?
5. Describe carbohydrate digestion and absorption.

What role does fiber play in the process?
6. What are the possible fates of glucose in the body? What is the protein-sparing action of carbohydrate?
7. How does the body maintain blood glucose concentrations? What happens when it rises too high or falls too low?
8. What are the health effects of sugars? What are the dietary recommendations regarding concentrated sugar intakes?
9. What are the health effects of starches and fibers? What are the dietary recommendations regarding these complex carbohydrates?
10. What foods provide starches and fibers?

Notes

1. S. R. Glore and coauthors, Soluble fiber and serum lipids: A literature review, *Journal of the American Dietetic Association* 94 (1994): 425–436.
2. M. Kestin and coauthors, Comparative effects of three cereal brans on plasma lipids, blood pressure, and glucose metabo-

lism in mildly hypercholesterolemic men, *American Journal of Clinical Nutrition* 52 (1990): 661–666; J. K. C. Chan and V. Wypyszyk, A forgotten natural dietary fiber: Psyllium mucilloid, *Cereal Foods World* 33 (1988): 921–922.
3. J. L. Slavin, Dietary fiber: Mechanisms or magic on disease

prevention? *Nutrition Today*, November/December 1990, pp. 6–10.

4. G. Annison and D. L. Topping, Nutritional role of resistant starch: Chemical structure vs physiological function, *Annual Review of Nutrition* 14 (1994): 297–320; N. Asp, Nutritional classification and analysis of food carbohydrates, *American Journal of Clinical Nutrition* 59 (1994): 679S–681S.

5. M. I. McBurney and P. J. van Soest, Structure-function relationships: Lessons from other species, in *The Large Intestine: Physiology, Pathophysiology, and Diseases*, eds. S. F. Phillips, J. H. Pemberton, and R. G. Shorter (New York: Raven Press, 1991), pp. 37–50.

6. J. M. Saavedra and J. A. Perman, Current concepts in lactose malabsorption and intolerance, *Annual Review of Nutrition* 9 (1989): 475–502.

7. S. Auriechio and G. Semenza, Late-onset hypolactasia and persistent high lactose activity in humans, in *Sugars in Nutrition*, eds. M. Gracey, N. Kretchmer, and E. Rossi (New York: Raven Press, 1991).

8. G. Flatz, Genetics of lactose digestion in humans, in *Advances in Human Genetics*, eds., H. Harris and K. Hirschhorn (New York: Plenum Press, 1987), pp. 1–77; Committee on Nutrition, Practical significance of lactose intolerance in children: Supplement, *Pediatrics* 86 (1990): 643–644.

9. S. R. Hertzler, B. L. Huynh, and D. A. Savaiano, How much lactose is low lactose? *Journal of the American Dietetic Association* 96 (1996): 243–246.

10. Committee on Nutrition, 1990; A. O. Johnson and coauthors, Adaptation of lactose maldigesters to continued milk intakes, *American Journal of Clinical Nutrition* 58 (1993): 879–881; F. L. Suarez, D. A. Savaiano, and M. D. Levitt, A comparison of symptoms after the consumption of milk or lactose-hydrolyzed milk by people with self-reported severe lactose intolerance, *New England Journal of Medicine* 333 (1995): 1–4.

11. J. C. Brand and S. Holt, Relative effectiveness of milks with reduced amounts of lactose in alleviating milk intolerance, *American Journal of Clinical Nutrition* 54 (1991): 148–151.

12. Committee on Dietary Allowances, *Recommended Dietary Allowances*, 10th ed. (Washington, D.C.: National Academy Press, 1989), p. 41.

13. E. Jéquier, Carbohydrates as a source of energy, *American Journal of Clinical Nutrition* (supplement) 59 (1994): 682S–685S.

14. J. Hirsch, Role and benefits of carbohydrate in the diet: Key issues for future dietary guidelines, *American Journal of Clinical Nutrition* 61 (1995): 996S–1000S.

15. S. A. Westphal, M. C. Gannon, and F. Q. Nuttall, Metabolic response to glucose ingested with various amounts of protein, *American Journal of Clinical Nutrition* 52 (1990): 267–272.

16. B. Vessby, Dietary carbohydrates in diabetes, *American Journal of Clinical Nutrition* (supplement) 59 (1994): 742S–746S.

17. T. M. S. Wolever and J. B. Miller, Sugars and blood glucose control, *American Journal of Clinical Nutrition* 62 (1995): 212S–227S; I. Björck and coauthors, Food properties affecting the digestion and absorption of carbohydrates, *American Journal of Clinical Nutrition* (supplement) 59 (1994): 699S–705S.

18. D. J. A. Jenkins and coauthors, Low glycemic index: Lente carbohydrates and physiological effects of altered food frequency, *American Journal of Clinical Nutrition* (supplement) 59 (1994): 706S–709S.

19. J. C. B. Miller, Importance of glycemic index in diabetes, *American Journal of Clinical Nutrition* (supplement) 59 (1994): 747S–752S.

20. Position statement: Nutrition recommendations and principles for people with diabetes mellitus, *Diabetes Care* 17 (1994): 519–522.

21. W. H. Glinsmann and Y. K. Park, Perspective on the 1986 Food and Drug Administration Assessment of Carbohydrate Sweeteners: Uniform definitions and recommendations for future assessments, *American Journal of Clinical Nutrition* 62 (1995): 161S–169S.

22. J. M. Navia, Carbohydrates and dental health, *American Journal of Clinical Nutrition* (supplement) 59 (1994): 719S–727S.

23. C. J. Lewis and coauthors, Nutrient intakes and body weights of persons consuming high and moderate levels of added sugars, *Journal of the American Dietetic Association* 92 (1992): 708–713.

24. M. L. Wolraich and coauthors, Effects of diets high in sucrose or aspartame on the behavior and cognitive performance of children, *New England Journal of Medicine* 330 (1994): 301–307; D. A. Gans, Sucrose and unusual childhood behavior, *Nutrition Today*, May/June 1991, pp. 8–14; J. A. Bachorowski and coauthors, Sucrose and delinquency: Behavioral assessment, *Pediatrics* 86 (1990): 244–253.

25. J. E. Blundell, S. Green, and V. Burley, Carbohydrates and human appetite, *American Journal of Clinical Nutrition* 59 (1994): 728S–734S; A. S. Levine and coauthors, Effect of breakfast cereals on short-term food intake, *American Journal of Clinical Nutrition* 50 (1989): 1303–1307; L. Lissner and coauthors, Dietary fat and the regulation of energy intake in human subjects, *American Journal of Clinical Nutrition* 46 (1987): 886–892.

26. A. S. Truswell, Food carbohydrates and plasma lipids—An update, *American Journal of Clinical Nutrition* 59 (1994): 710S–718S.

27. G. H. McIntosh and coauthors, Barley and wheat foods: Influence on plasma cholesterol concentrations in hypercholesterolemic men, *American Journal of Clinical Nutrition* 53 (1991): 1205–1209; Kestin and coauthors, 1990; J. W. Anderson and coauthors, Serum lipid response of hypercholesterolemic men to single and divided doses of canned beans, *American Journal of Clinical Nutrition* 51 (1990): 1013–1019; L. P. Bell and coauthors, Cholesterol-lowering effects of soluble-fiber cereals as part of a prudent diet for patients with mild to moderate hypercholesterolemia, *American Journal of Clinical Nutrition* 52 (1990): 1020–1026; J. W. Anderson and N. J. Gustafson, Hypocholesterolemic effects of oat and bean products, *American Journal of Clinical Nutrition* 48 (1988): 749–753.

28. Y. A. Kesaniemi, S. Tarpila, and T. A. Miettinen, Low vs high

dietary fiber and serum, biliary, and fecal lipids in middle-aged men, *American Journal of Clinical Nutrition* 51 (1990): 1007–1112.

29. J. F. Swain and coauthors, Comparison of the effects of oat bran and low-fiber wheat on serum lipoprotein levels and blood pressure, *New England Journal of Medicine* 322 (1990): 147–152; W. Denmark-Wahnefried, J. Bowering, and P. S. Cohen, Reduced serum cholesterol with dietary change using fat-modified and oat bran supplemented diets, *Journal of the American Dietetic Association* 90 (1990): 223–229.

30. D. J. A. Jenkins and coauthors, Effect on blood lipids of very high intakes of fiber in diets low in saturated fat and cholesterol, *New England Journal of Medicine* 329 (1993): 21–26.

31. I. P. Munster and coauthors, Effect of resistant starch on breath-hydrogen and methane excretion in healthy volunteers, *American Journal of Clinical Nutrition* 59 (1994): 626–630.

32. Committee on Dietary Allowances, 1989, p. 41.

33. Committee on Dietary Allowances, 1989, p. 42.

34. Position of The American Dietetic Association: Health implications of dietary fiber, *Journal of the American Dietetic Association* 93 (1993): 1446–1447.

35. J. W. Anderson, B. M. Smith, and N. J. Gustafson, Health benefits and practical aspects of high-fiber diets, *American Journal of Clinical Nutrition* 59 (1994): 1242S–1247S.

Alternatives to Sugar

People who want to limit their use of sugar may encounter two sets of alternative sweeteners. One set, the artificial sweeteners, provide virtually no energy and are sometimes referred to as nonnutritive sweeteners. The other set, the sugar alcohols, yield energy and are sometimes referred to as nutritive sweeteners. The artificial sweeteners are sugar substitutes; the sugar alcohols are sugar relatives. The glossary on p. 135 presents the most common members of both groups.

ARTIFICIAL SWEETENERS

Artificial sweeteners permit people to keep their sugar and energy intakes down, yet still enjoy the delicious sweet tastes of their favorite foods and beverages. The Food and Drug Administration (FDA) has approved the use of three artificial sweeteners—saccharin, aspartame, and acesulfame potassium (acesulfame-K). Saccharin holds the honor of being the oldest artificial sweetener, having been around since before 1900. Aspartame was approved by the FDA in 1981 and currently dominates the world market for artificial sweeteners. Acesulfame-K is the "new kid on the block," having received FDA approval in 1988. Three others have petitioned the FDA and are awaiting approval—alitame, cyclamate, and sucralose. Table H4–1 provides general details about each of these sweeteners.

Both saccharin and acesulfame-K present the body with no chemical compounds to deal with and pass through the digestive system unchanged. In contrast, the body does digest aspartame, receiving

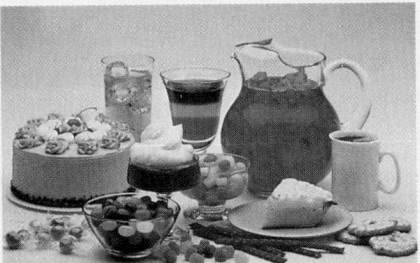

People wanting to limit their sugar intake can find a variety of foods and beverages made with artificial sweeteners.

tiny quantities of nutrients and other compounds. Aspartame is, in fact, *technically* classified as a nutritive sweetener because it yields tiny amounts of energy, but for all practical purposes, that energy is negligible.

Some consumers have challenged the safety of using artificial sweeteners. Considering that all compounds are toxic at some dose, it is little surprise that large doses of artificial sweeteners (or their components or metabolic by-products) have toxic effects. The question to ask is whether their ingestion is safe for human beings in quantities people normally use (and potentially abuse). The answer is yes, except in the special case described for aspartame later.

The Safety of Saccharin

Saccharin, used for over 100 years in the United States, is currently used by some 50 million people—primarily in soft drinks, secondarily as a tabletop sweetener. Saccharin is rapidly excreted in the urine and does not accumulate in the body.

Questions about saccharin's safety surfaced in 1977, when experiments suggested that large doses of saccharin increased the risk of bladder cancer in rats. The FDA proposed banning saccharin as a result. Public outcry in favor of saccharin was so loud, however, that Congress imposed a moratorium on the ban—a moratorium that was repeatedly extended until 1991, when the FDA withdrew its proposal to ban saccharin.[1] Products containing saccharin must still carry the warning label, "use of this product may be hazardous to your health. This product contains saccharin, which has been determined to cause cancer in laboratory animals."

Does saccharin cause cancer? The largest population study to date, involving 9000 men and women, showed overall that saccharin use did not raise the risk of cancer. Among certain small groups of the population, however, such as those who both smoked heavily and used saccharin, the risk of bladder cancer was slightly greater. Other studies involving more than 5000 people with bladder cancer showed no association between bladder cancer and saccharin use.[2] Common sense dictates that consuming large amounts of any substance is probably not wise, but at current, moderate intake levels, saccharin is assumed to be safe for most people. It has been approved for use in more than 90 countries.

The Safety of Aspartame

Aspartame is one of the most studied of all food additives; extensive animal and human studies docu-

133

Figure H4–1

Structure of Aspartame

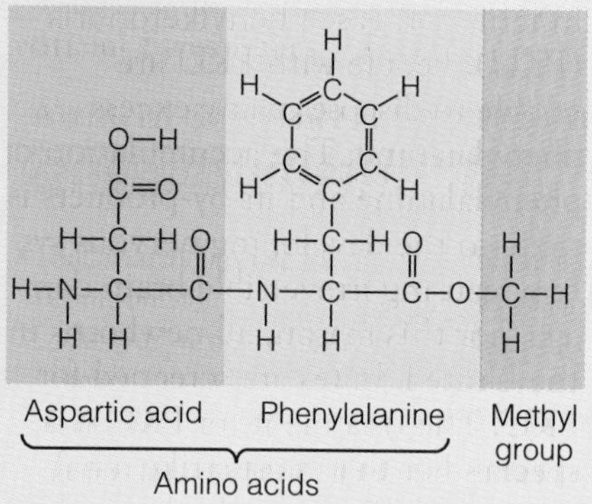

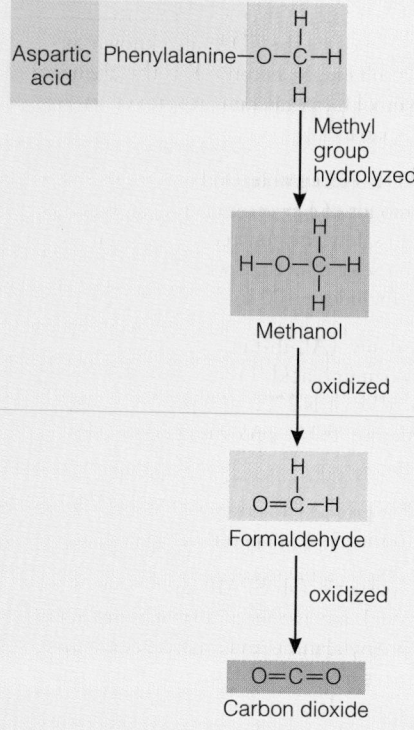

Aspartic acid Phenylalanine Methyl group

Amino acids

---

reason to be concerned about the products it yields in the body? During metabolism, the methyl group momentarily becomes methyl alcohol (methanol)—a potentially toxic compound (see Figure H4–2). Then enzymes convert methanol to formaldehyde, another toxic compound. Finally, formaldehyde is broken down to carbon dioxide. Before aspartame could be approved for public use, the quantities of these products generated during metabolism had to be determined; they were found to fall below the threshold at which they would cause harm. In fact, ounce for ounce, tomato juice yields six times as much methanol as a diet soda.[5]

Finally, aspartame breaks down to diketopiperazine, or DKP for short. Long-term studies using animals have directly tested this product and eliminated it as a source of concern.

Still another concern was over the effect aspartame use might have on the brain. Experiments with rats, monkeys, and human beings were performed, and none showed any cause for concern. In the monkey study, infant monkeys were given up to 3000 milligrams of aspartame per

kilogram of body weight for nine months, and the researchers found no ill effects on growth, development, health, or behavior either during the test or on the withdrawal of aspartame. The conclusion reached was that aspartame is safe except for people with PKU. Some 500 individual complaints received after its approval were reviewed by the Centers for Disease Control, which concluded that some individuals may exhibit vague, but not dangerous, symptoms due to unusual sensitivity to aspartame, but that the product is generally safe. Like saccharin, aspartame has been approved for use in more than 90 countries.

The Safety of Acesulfame-K

The FDA approved acesulfame-K in 1988 after reviewing more than 90 safety studies conducted over 15 years. Some consumer groups believe that acesulfame-K causes tumors in rats and should not have been approved by the FDA. The FDA counters that the tumors were not caused by the sweetener, but were typical of those commonly found in rat studies.

The Safety of Alitame, Cyclamate, and Sucralose

FDA approval for alitame, cyclamate, and sucralose is still pending. To date, no safety issues have been raised for alitame or sucralose. Cyclamate, on the other hand, has been battling safety issues for 50 years. Approved by the FDA in 1949, cyclamate was banned in 1969 principally on the basis of one study indicating that it caused bladder cancer in rats.

Figure H4–2

Metabolism of Aspartame

Aspartic acid Phenylalanine—O—C—H

Methyl group hydrolyzed

H—O—C—H
Methanol

oxidized

O=C—H
Formaldehyde

oxidized

O=C=O
Carbon dioxide

The National Research Council has reviewed dozens of studies on cyclamate and concluded that neither cyclamate nor its metabolites cause cancer. The council did, however, recommend further research to determine the risks for heavy or long-term use. Although cyclamate does not initiate cancer, it may promote cancer development once started. The FDA has no policy on substances that enhance the cancer-causing activities of other substances. Consequently, the FDA is unlikely to approve cyclamate soon, if at all. Agencies in more than 50 other countries, including Canada, have approved cyclamate.

Acceptable Daily Intake

The FDA has established an Acceptable Daily Intake (ADI) for artificial sweeteners. The ADI represents the level of consumption that, if maintained every day throughout a person's life, would still be considered safe by a wide margin.

For example, the ADI for aspartame is 50 milligrams per kilogram of body weight. That is, the FDA approved aspartame based on the assumption that no one would consume more than 50 milligrams per kilogram of body weight in a day. This maximum daily intake is indeed a lot: for a 150-pound adult, it adds up to 97 packets of Equal or 20 cans of soft drinks sweetened only with aspartame. The company that produces aspartame estimates that if all the sugar and saccharin in the U.S. diet were replaced with aspartame, 1 percent of the population would be consuming the FDA maximum. Most people who use aspartame consume less than 5 milligrams per kilogram of body weight per day.[6] A five-year-old child who drinks four glasses of aspartame-sweetened beverages on a hot day and has five servings of other products with aspartame that day (such as pudding, chewing gum, cereal, gelatin, and frozen desserts) takes in the FDA maximum level. Although this presents no proven hazard, it seems wise to offer children other foods so as not to exceed the limit. Table H4–2 lists the average amounts of aspartame in some common foods.

For persons choosing to use artificial sweeteners, the American Dietetic Association wisely advises that they be used in moderation and only as part of a well-balanced nutritious diet.[7] The dietary principles of both moderation and variety are useful in reducing the possible risks associated with any food.

Artificial Sweeteners and Weight Control

Many people eat and drink products sweetened with artificial sweeteners to help them control weight. Does this work? Ironically, a few studies have reported that intense sweeteners, such as aspartame, may stimulate appetite, which could lead to weight gain. Contradicting these reports, most studies find either no change or a decline in feelings of hunger and conclude that most people using the sweeteners don't seem to increase their food intakes.[8] Adding to the confusion, some studies report reduced food intakes and weight losses when people eat or drink artificially sweetened products.[9]

In studying the effects of artificial sweeteners on food intake and body weight, different researchers ask different questions and take different approaches in searching for the answers. It matters, for example, whether the people used in the study were of a healthy weight or obese, and whether they were on weight-loss diets or not. Motivations for using sweeteners differ, too, and this influences a person's actions. For example, a person might drink a low-kcalorie beverage now so as to be able to eat a high-kcalorie food later. This person's energy intake might stay the same or increase. On the other hand, a person trying to control food energy intake might use the artificial sweetener and then still choose a low-kcalorie food in place of the high-kcalorie option. This would reduce the person's energy intake.

In designing experiments on artificial sweeteners, researchers have to distinguish between the effects of sweetness and the effects of a particular substance. If a person wants to eat again shortly after eating an artificially sweetened snack, is that because the sweet taste (of all sweeteners, including sugars) stimulates appetite? Or is it because the artificial sweetener itself stimulates appetite? Research must also distinguish between the effects of food energy and the effects of the substance. If a person is hungrier after eating an artificially sweetened food than after a sugar-sweetened product, is that because less food energy was available to satisfy hunger? Or is it because the artificial sweetener itself triggers hunger? Furthermore, if appetite is stimulated and a person feels hungry, does that actually lead to increased food intake?

One recent study tried to answer these questions by feeding normal-weight people one of four cheese samples for breakfast and then measuring their food intake at later meals throughout the day.[10] Two of the samples provided 700 kcalories:

Table H4–2

Aspartame Contents of Selected Foods

Food	Aspartame (mg)
12 oz diet soft drink	170
8 oz powdered drink	100
8 oz sugar-free fruit yogurt	124
4 oz gelatin dessert	80
1 packet sweetener	35

one contained sucrose, and the other aspartame with enough starch to equalize the kcalories. The other two samples provided 300 kcalories: one was plain and the other contained aspartame. Those who ate the lower-kcalorie breakfast, regardless of sweetness, were hungrier later. They also ate more at lunch (100 kcalories on average), although not enough to fully compensate for the 400-kcalorie difference between the breakfasts. Because energy intake at later meals was similar, those who ate the 700-kcalorie breakfasts had higher total energy intakes.

Overall it seems that artificial sweeteners alone do not stimulate appetite but that low-kcalorie intakes may leave people hungry, so that they compensate at later meals. Whether a person compensates for the energy reduction either partially or fully depends on several factors, including the person's characteristics. Using artificial sweeteners will not automatically lower energy intake; to control energy intake successfully, a person will need to make informed diet and activity decisions throughout the day (as Chapter 9 explains).

SUGAR ALCOHOLS

Some "sugar-free" dietary products such as hard candies, sugarless gums, jams, and jellies contain the sugar alcohols—mannitol, sorbitol, xylitol, and maltitol. They claim to be "sugar-free" on their labels, but in this case, "sugar-free" does not mean they are free of kcalories. Sugar alcohols occur naturally in fruits and vegetables; they are also used by manufacturers as a low-energy bulk ingredient in many products.[11] Sugar alcohols provide energy, although the exact kcalorie value has not been determined.[12] The FDA uses 4 kcalories per gram as a standard, but some research indicates that the value may be only 2.5 to 3.5 kcalories per gram. Table H4–3 presents a general description of each of the sugar alcohols.

Sugar alcohols evoke a low glycemic response. The body absorbs sugar alcohols slowly; consequently, they are slower to enter the bloodstream than other sugars. Side effects such as gas, abdominal discomfort, and diarrhea, however, make them less attractive than the artificial sweeteners. For this reason, labeling regulations require foods to state that "Excess consumption may have a laxative effect" if reasonable consumption could result in the daily ingestion of 50 grams of a sugar alcohol.

The real benefit of using sugar alcohols is that they do not contribute as much to dental caries as sugar does. Bacteria in the mouth cannot metabolize sugar alcohols as rapidly as sugar. They are therefore valuable in chewing gums, breath mints, and other products that people keep in their mouths for a while.

The sugar alcohols, like the artificial sweeteners, can occupy a place in the diet, and provided they are used in moderation, they will do no harm. In fact, they can help, both by providing an alternative to sugar for people with diabetes and by inhibiting caries-causing bacteria. People may find it appropriate to use all three sweeteners at times: the artificial kind, the sugar alcohols, and sugar itself.

Table H4–3

Sugar Alcohols

Sugar Alcohols	Sweetness Compared with Sucrose	Advantages	Disadvantages
Sorbitol	One-half as sweet	Opposes dental caries; controls browning, stability, and moisture loss in foods	Abdominal cramps, gas, diarrhea
Mannitol	Three-fourths as sweet		Abdominal cramps, gas, diarrhea
Maltitol	Three-fourths as sweet	Opposes dental caries	Expensive
Xylitol	Equivalent	Opposes dental caries; may assist in weight control	Diarrhea

NOTES

1. Withdrawal of certain pre-1986 proposed rules: Final actions, *Federal Register* 56 (1991): 67422.

2. Position of The American Dietetic Association: Use of nutritive and nonnutritive sweeteners, *Journal of the American Dietetic Association* 93 (1993): 816–821.

3. Position of The American Dietetic Association, 1993.

4. Position of The American Dietetic Association, 1993.

5. H. H. Butchko and F. N. Kotsonis, Acceptable intake vs actual intake: The aspartame example, *Journal of American College of Nutrition* 10 (1991): 258–266.

6. Butchko and Kotsonis, 1991.

7. Position of The American Dietetic Association, 1993.

8. D. J. Canty and M. M. Chan, Effects of consumption of caloric vs noncaloric sweet drinks on indices of hunger and food consumption in normal adults, *American Journal of Clinical Nutrition* 53 (1991): 1159–1164; B. J. Rolls, Effects of intense sweeteners on hunger, food intake, and body weight: A review, *American Journal of Clinical Nutrition* 53 (1991): 872–878; L. A. Chen and E. S. Parham, College students' use of high-intensity sweeteners is not consistently associated with sugar consumption, *Journal of the American Dietetic Association* 91 (1991): 686–690.

9. M. G. Tordoff and A. M. Alleva, Effect of drinking soda sweetened with aspartame or high-fructose corn syrup on food intake and body weight, *American Journal of Clinical Nutrition* 51 (1990): 963–969.

10. A. Drewnowski and coauthors, Comparing the effects of aspartame and sucrose on motivational ratings, taste preferences, and energy intake in humans, *American Journal of Clinical Nutrition* 59 (1994): 338–345.

11. F. R. J. Bonet, Undigestible sugars in food products, *American Journal of Clinical Nutrition* 59 (1994): 763S–769S.

12. Position of The American Dietetic Association, 1993.

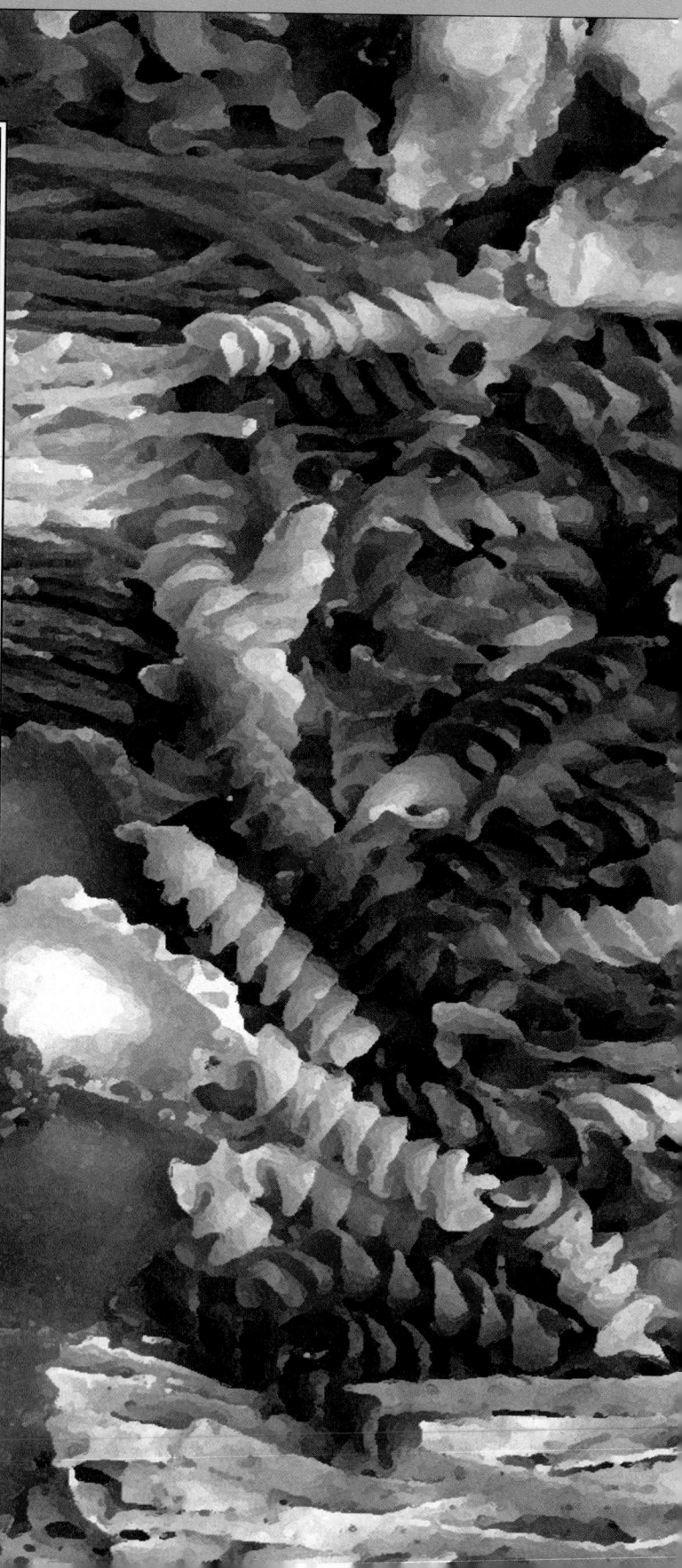

Chapter 5

The Lipids: Triglycerides, Phospholipids, and Sterols

CONTENTS

The Chemist's View of Triglycerides and Fatty Acids
The Fatty Acids
Fats in Foods
Roles of Triglycerides and Fatty Acids
Essential Fatty Acids
The Chemist's View of Phospholipids and Sterols
The Phospholipids
The Sterols
Digestion, Absorption, and Transport of Lipids
Lipid Digestion
Lipid Absorption
Lipid Transport
Lipids in the Body
Triglycerides in the Blood
A Preview of Lipid Metabolism
Health Effects and Recommended Intakes of Lipids
Health Effects of Lipids
Recommended Intakes of Fat
HIGHLIGHT: Alternatives to Fats

MICROGRAPH: Oleic acid the fatty acid of olive oil.

Most people are surprised to learn that fat has some virtues. It is only when people consume either too much or too little of it that ill health follows. It is true, though, that in our society of abundance, people are likely to encounter too much fat.

Fat is actually a subset of the class of nutrients known as lipids, but the term *fat* is often used to refer to all the lipids. Table 5–1 offers a preview of the lipid family, which includes triglycerides (fats and oils), phospholipids, and sterols, all important to nutrition. The triglycerides provide the body with a continuous fuel supply, keep it warm, and protect it from mechanical shock; their component fatty acids serve as starting materials for important hormonal regulators. The phospholipids and sterols contribute to the cells' structures, and the sterol cholesterol serves as the raw material for some hormones, vitamin D, and bile.

In foods, triglycerides carry with them the four fat-soluble vitamins—A, D, E, and K—together with many of the compounds that give foods their flavor, tenderness, and palatability. Fat is responsible for the delicious aromas associated with sizzling bacon and hamburgers on the grill, onions being sautéed, or vegetables in a stir-fry. Of course, these wonderful aromas lure people into eating too much from time to time. Studies have found that obese people have a strong preference for fat, but have not revealed whether the preference or the obesity comes first.[1]

When people speak of fats and oils, they are usually speaking of triglycerides. The triglycerides predominate, both in foods and in the body.

The Chemist's View of Triglycerides and Fatty Acids

Like carbohydrates, triglycerides are composed of carbon, hydrogen, and oxygen. However, triglycerides have many more carbons and hydrogens in proportion to their oxygens, and so can supply more energy per gram (Chapter 7 provides details).

For people who think more easily in words than in chemical symbols, this *preview* of the upcoming chemistry may be helpful. The following paragraphs and diagrams demonstrate that:

1. Every triglyceride contains one molecule of glycerol (see Figure 5–1) and three fatty acids (basically chains of carbon atoms).
2. Fatty acids may be 4 to 24 (even numbers of) carbons long, the 18-carbon ones being the most common in foods and especially noteworthy in nutrition.
3. Fatty acids may also be saturated or unsaturated. The latter may have one or more points of unsaturation (may be mono- or polyunsaturated).
4. Polyunsaturated fatty acids of special importance in nutrition are the ones whose *first* point of unsaturation is next to the third carbon (known as omega-3 fatty acids) or next to the sixth carbon (omega-6), when counting from the methyl end (CH_3) of the carbon chain.
5. The 18-carbon fatty acids that fit this description are linolenic acid (omega-3) and linoleic acid (omega-6). Each is the primary member of a "family" of longer-chain fatty acids that regulate blood pressure, clotting, and other body functions important to health.

Table 5–1

The Lipid Family

Triglycerides (fats and oils)
• Glycerol (1 per triglyceride)
• Fatty acids (3 per triglyceride)
Saturated
Monounsaturated
Polyunsaturated
Omega-6
Omega-3
Phospholipids (such as lecithin)
Sterols (such as cholesterol)

fat: the lipids in foods or body fat, both of which are composed mostly of triglycerides.

lipids: a family of compounds that includes triglycerides (fats and oils), phospholipids, and sterols.

Of the lipids in foods, 95% are fats and oils (triglycerides), and 5% are other lipids (phospholipids and sterols). Of the lipids stored in the body, 99% are triglycerides.

triglycerides (try-GLISS-er-rides): the chief form of fat in the diet and the major storage form of fat in the body; composed of a molecule of glycerol with three fatty acids attached; also called **triacylglycerols** (try-ay-seel-GLISS-er-ols).

tri = three
glyceride = a compound of glycerol
acyl = a carbon chain

glycerol (GLISS-er-ol): an alcohol composed of a three-carbon chain, which can serve as the backbone for a triglyceride.

ol = alcohol

Figure 5–1

Glycerol

Notice that glycerol has three OH groups to which three fatty acids can attach to form a triglyceride.

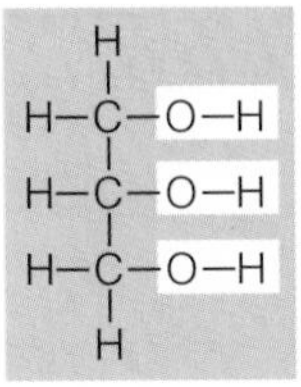

THE FATTY ACIDS

fatty acid: an organic compound composed of a carbon chain with hydrogens attached and an acid group (COOH) at one end. The COOH group of an organic acid can be represented this way:

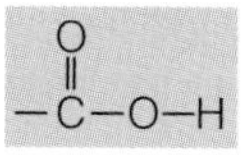

$$\begin{matrix} & O \\ & \parallel \\ -C&-O-H \end{matrix}$$

Notice that this structure meets the requirement that C must have four bonds and O two. To accomplish this, O and C form a double bond.

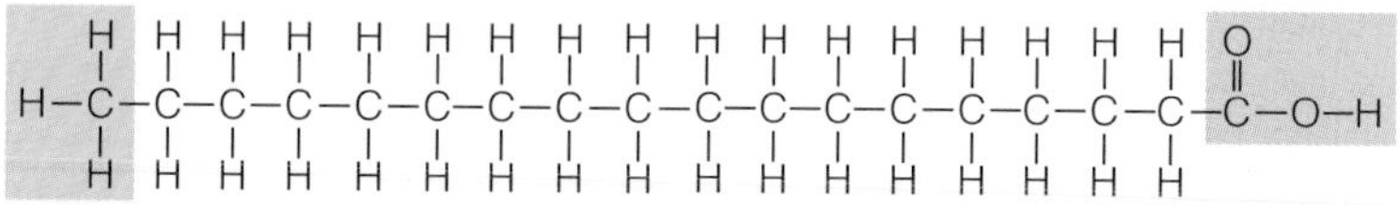

Stearic acid, an 18-carbon saturated fatty acid.

A fatty acid is an organic acid—a chain of carbon atoms with hydrogens attached—that has an acid group (COOH) at one end and a methyl group (CH$_3$) at the other end. The organic acid shown in Figure 5–2 is acetic acid, the compound that gives vinegar its sour taste. Acetic acid is the simplest such acid, with a "chain" only two carbon atoms long.

The Carbon Chain   Most naturally occurring fatty acids contain even numbers of carbons in their chains—up to 24 carbons in length. This discussion begins with the 18-carbon fatty acids, which are abundant in our food supply. Stearic acid is the simplest of the 18-carbon fatty acids; the bonds between its carbons are all alike:

(As you can see, stearic acid is 18 carbons long and each atom meets the rules of chemical bonding described in Chapter 4.) A fatty acid like stearic acid that contains only single bonds between its carbon atoms is a saturated fatty acid. The following structure also depicts stearic acid, but in a simpler way, with each "corner" on the zigzag line representing a carbon atom with two attached hydrogens:

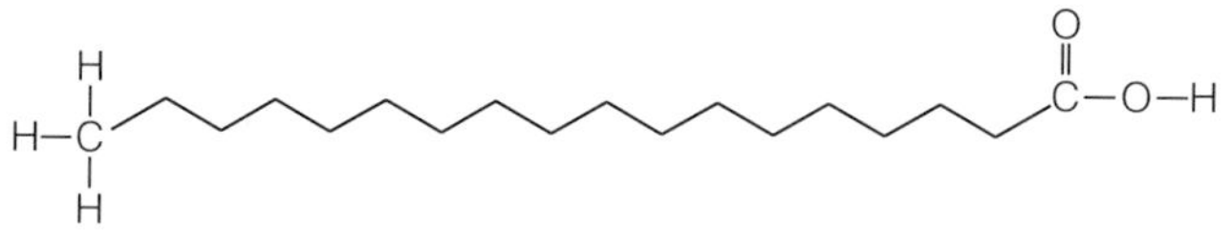

Stearic acid (simplified structure).

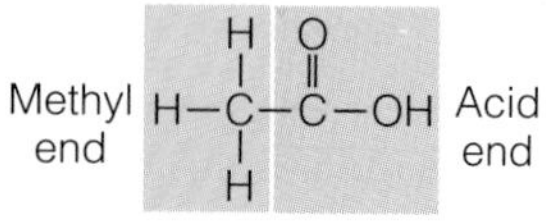

Triglyceride Formation   Few fatty acids occur free in foods or in the body. Most often, they are incorporated into triglycerides. To make a triglyceride, three fatty acids are attached to a glycerol molecule by condensation reactions (see Figure 5–3 on p. 143). Each condensation reaction combines a hydrogen atom (H) from the glycerol and a hydroxyl (OH) group from a fatty acid, forming a molecule of water (H$_2$O) and leaving a bond between the other two molecules.

Figure 5–2

Acetic Acid

Acetic acid is a two-carbon organic acid.

point of unsaturation: the double bond of a fatty acid, where hydrogen atoms can easily be added to the structure.

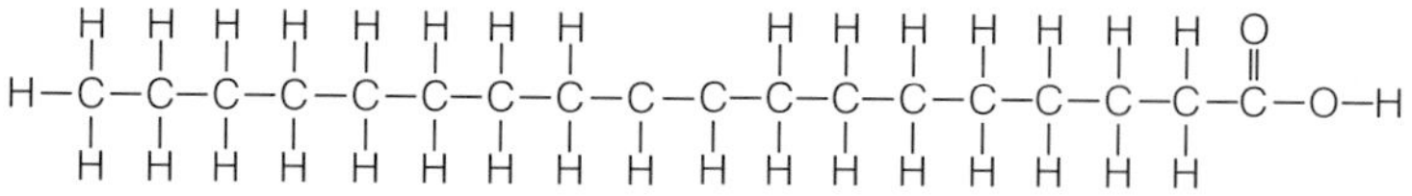

Degree of Saturation   The glossary on p. 144 defines the terms that describe fatty acids. The triglyceride shown in Figure 5–3 is a saturated fat because all three fatty acids are saturated fatty acids—that is, fully loaded with hydrogen atoms. If hydrogens were missing, there would be points of unsaturation where the carbons would have to form double bonds with one another. The result would be an unsaturated, or even a polyunsaturated, fat. Consider stearic acid once more. If two hydrogens were missing from the middle of the carbon chain, the structure that remained might be:

An impossible chemical structure.

Such a compound cannot exist, however, because two of the carbons have only three bonds each, and nature requires that every carbon have four bonds.

Figure 5–3

Condensation of Glycerol and Fatty Acids to Form a Triglyceride

To make a fat (triglyceride), three fatty acids attach to glycerol in condensation reactions:

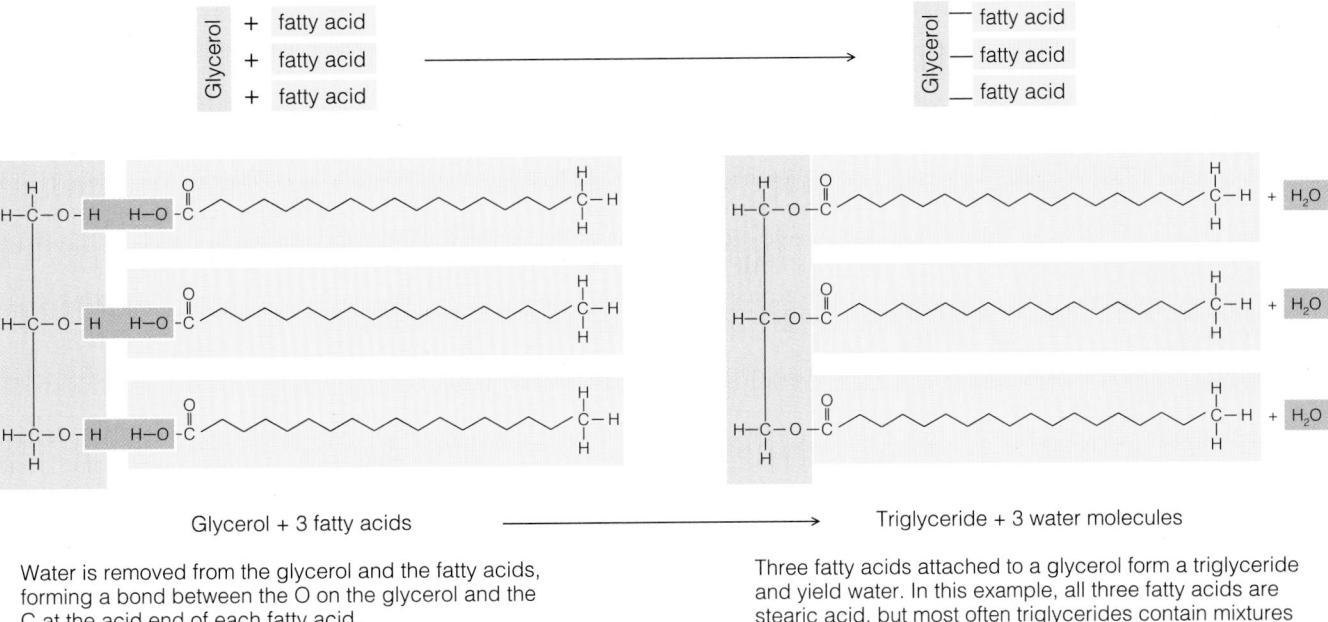

Glycerol + 3 fatty acids   →   Triglyceride + 3 water molecules

Water is removed from the glycerol and the fatty acids, forming a bond between the O on the glycerol and the C at the acid end of each fatty acid.

Three fatty acids attached to a glycerol form a triglyceride and yield water. In this example, all three fatty acids are stearic acid, but most often triglycerides contain mixtures of fatty acids.

The two carbons therefore form a double bond:

Oleic acid, an 18-carbon monounsaturated fatty acid.

The same structure drawn more simply looks like this:*

Oleic acid (simplified structure).

A fatty acid like this—with two hydrogens missing and a double bond—is an *uns*aturated fatty acid. This one is the 18-carbon *mono*unsaturated fatty acid oleic acid, which is abundant in the triglycerides of olive oil.

A *poly*unsaturated fat contains triglycerides whose fatty acids have two or more carbon-to-carbon double bonds. The best known of these is linoleic acid,

linoleic acid (lin-oh-LAY-ick): an essential fatty acid with 18 carbons and two double bonds (18:2).

---

*Remember that each "corner" on the zigzag line represents a carbon atom with two attached hydrogens. In addition, the actual shape bends at the double bonds and rotates around single bonds. These molecules, although drawn straight on paper, are constantly twisting and bending. At any given moment, they may be coiled, horseshoe shaped, or straight.

Glossary of Fatty Acids

These terms are listed in order from the most saturated to the most unsaturated.

saturated fatty acid: a fatty acid carrying the maximum possible number of hydrogen atoms—for example, stearic acid. A saturated fat is composed of triglycerides in which all or virtually all of the fatty acids are saturated.

unsaturated fatty acid: a fatty acid that lacks hydrogen atoms and has at least one double bond between carbons (includes monounsaturated and polyunsaturated fatty acids). An unsaturated fat is composed of triglycerides in which some of the fatty acids are unsaturated.

monounsaturated fatty acid: a fatty acid

that lacks two hydrogen atoms and has one double bond between carbons—for example, oleic acid.

mono = one

polyunsaturated fatty acid (PUFA): a fatty acid that lacks four or more hydrogen atoms and has two or more double bonds between carbons—for example, linoleic acid (two double bonds) and linolenic acid (three double bonds). A polyunsaturated fat is composed of triglycerides containing a high percentage of PUFA.

poly = many

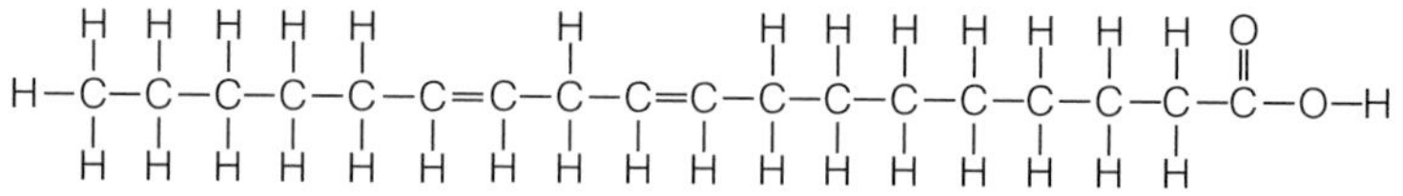

Linoleic acid, an 18-carbon polyunsaturated fatty acid.

the 18-carbon fatty acid common in vegetable oils. Linoleic acid lacks four hydrogens and has two double bonds:

Drawn more simply, linoleic acid looks like this:

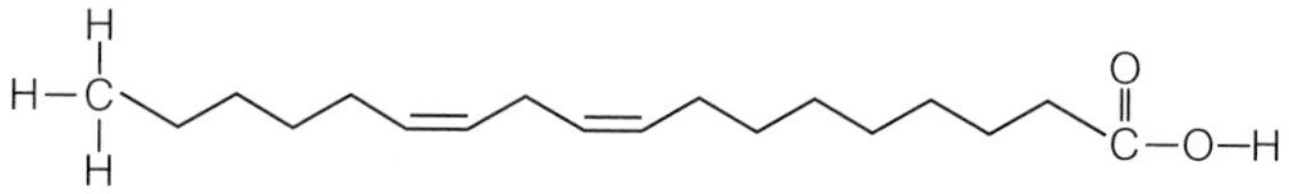

Linoleic acid (simplified structure).

linolenic acid (lin-oh-LEN-ick): an essential fatty acid with 18 carbons and three double bonds (18:3).

A fourth 18-carbon fatty acid is linolenic acid, which has three double bonds (see Table 5–2).

Having looked at four of the most common fatty acids in foods, one can predict what the others will look like. They vary only in their degrees of unsaturation

Table 5–2

18-Carbon Fatty Acids

Name	Notation[a]	Number of Double Bonds	Saturation
Stearic acid	18:0	0	Saturated
Oleic acid	18:1	1	Monounsaturated
Linoleic acid	18:2	2	Polyunsaturated
Linolenic acid	18:3	3	Polyunsaturated

[a]Chemists use a shorthand notation to describe fatty acids. The first number indicates the number of carbon atoms; the second, the number of double bonds.

Figure 5–4

A Mixed Triglyceride

fatty acid (18-C saturated)

Glycerol

fatty acid (18-C monounsaturated)

fatty acid (18-C polyunsaturated)

This mixed triglyceride includes a saturated fatty acid, a monounsaturated fatty acid, and a polyunsaturated fatty acid.

Another way to show the chemical structure of a triglyceride is to draw the second fatty acid to the left of the glycerol.

and the lengths of their chains. The long-chain (12- to 24-carbon) fatty acids of meats and fish are most common in the diet. Smaller amounts of medium-chain (6- to 10-carbon) and short-chain (less-than-6-carbon) fatty acids also occur, primarily in dairy products.

Tables C–1 and C–2 in Appendix C provide the names, chain length, and sources of fatty acids commonly found in foods.

To sum up to this point, dietary fats and oils are mostly (95 percent) triglycerides: glycerol backbones with three fatty acids attached. Fats that are fully loaded with hydrogens are saturated; fats that are missing hydrogens and therefore have double bonds are unsaturated (monounsaturated and polyunsaturated). The degree of unsaturation of fats affects health, as a later section in this chapter explains. The vast majority of triglycerides contain mixtures of more than one type of fatty acid. Figure 5–4 provides an example. The fatty acid compositions of some typical dietary fats are shown in Figure 5–5, and Appendix H provides the fat and fatty acid contents of many other foods.

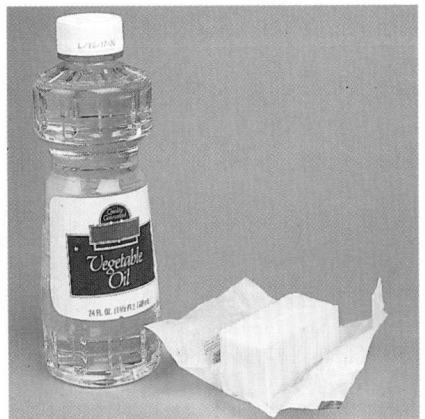

At room temperature, unsaturated fats (such as those found in vegetable oils) are usually liquid, whereas saturated fats (such as those found in butter) are solid.

FATS IN FOODS

The degree of saturation influences the firmness of fats at room temperature. Generally speaking, the polyunsaturated vegetable oils are liquid and the more

Figure 5–5

Comparison of Dietary Fats

Most fats are a mixture of saturated, monounsaturated, and polyunsaturated fatty acids. See pp. 148–150 for information on omega-6 (ω6) and omega-3 (ω3) fatty acids.

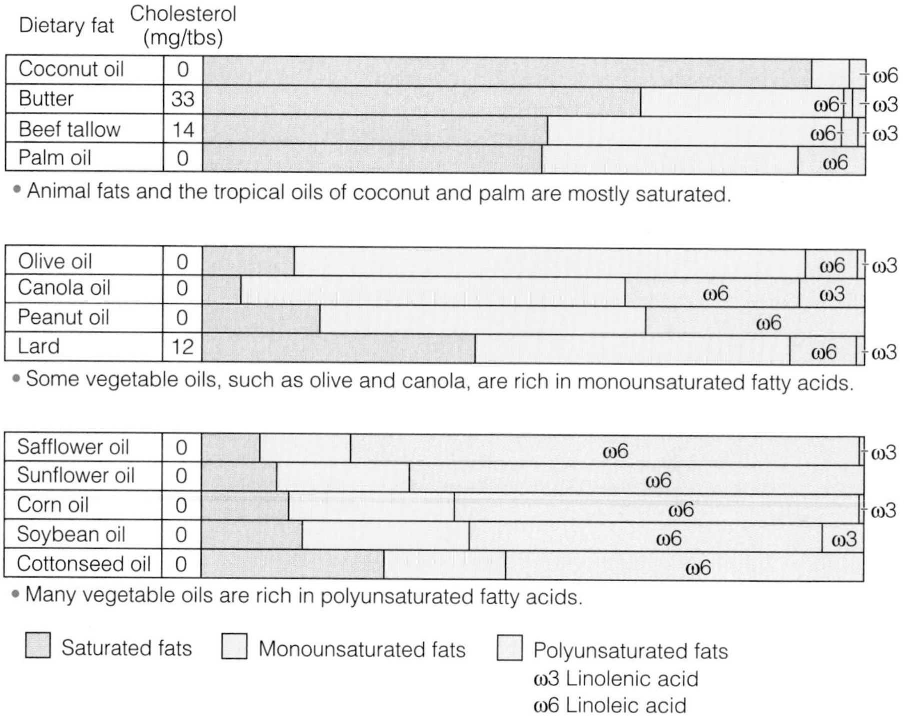

Dietary fat	Cholesterol (mg/tbs)			
Coconut oil	0			ω6
Butter	33		ω6	ω3
Beef tallow	14		ω6	ω3
Palm oil	0		ω6	

• Animal fats and the tropical oils of coconut and palm are mostly saturated.

Olive oil	0		ω6	ω3
Canola oil	0	ω6	ω3	
Peanut oil	0	ω6		
Lard	12		ω6	ω3

• Some vegetable oils, such as olive and canola, are rich in monounsaturated fatty acids.

Safflower oil	0	ω6	ω3
Sunflower oil	0	ω6	
Corn oil	0	ω6	ω3
Soybean oil	0	ω6	ω3
Cottonseed oil	0	ω6	

• Many vegetable oils are rich in polyunsaturated fatty acids.

☐ Saturated fats ☐ Monounsaturated fats ☐ Polyunsaturated fats
ω3 Linolenic acid
ω6 Linoleic acid

Sources: The Lipid Handbook, ed. F. D. Gunstone (London: Chapman and Hall, 1986) and USDA data, as cited by the Malaysian Palm Oil Promotion Council in material distributed by Edelman Public Relations, 1420 K Street, NW, Washington, D.C. 20005 in undated materials received in 1991; J. B. Reeves and J. L. Weihrauch, *Composition of Foods, Agriculture Handbook No. 8–1* (Washington, D.C.: USDA, 1979) as cited by Procter & Gamble in copyrighted material provided as a professional service, 1992.

The food industry often refers to palm and coconut oils as the "tropical oils."

oxidation (OK-see-day-shun): the process of a substance combining with oxygen.

antioxidant: a compound that protects others from oxidation by being oxidized itself; Highlight 11 provides more details.

saturated animal fats are harder at room temperature (review Figure 5–5). Butter is harder than margarine because butter is more saturated than margarine; this is why people limiting their intakes of saturated fats use margarine. Not all vegetable oils are polyunsaturated, however. Palm and coconut oils are saturated even though they are of vegetable origin; they are firmer than most vegetable oils because of their saturation, but softer than most animal fats because of their short carbon chains (only 10 and 12 carbons long, respectively). Generally, the longer the carbon chain, the more liquid the fat is at room temperature.

Processed Fat Saturation also influences stability. All fats can become rancid when exposed to oxygen. Polyunsaturated fatty acids spoil most readily because their double bonds are unstable. The oxidation of unsaturated fats yields a variety of products that smell and taste rancid; saturated fats are more resistant to oxidation and thus less likely to become rancid. Other types of spoilage can occur due to microbial growth.

Manufacturers can protect fat-containing products against rancidity in three ways—none of them perfect. First, products may be sealed air-tight and refrigerated—an expensive and inconvenient storage system. Second, manufacturers may add antioxidants to compete for the oxygen and thus protect the oil (examples are the additives BHA and BHT and vitamins C and E); the advantages and disadvantages of antioxidants in food processing are presented in Chapter 14. Third, manufacturers may saturate some or all of the points of unsaturation by adding hydrogen molecules—a process known as partial or complete hydrogenation.

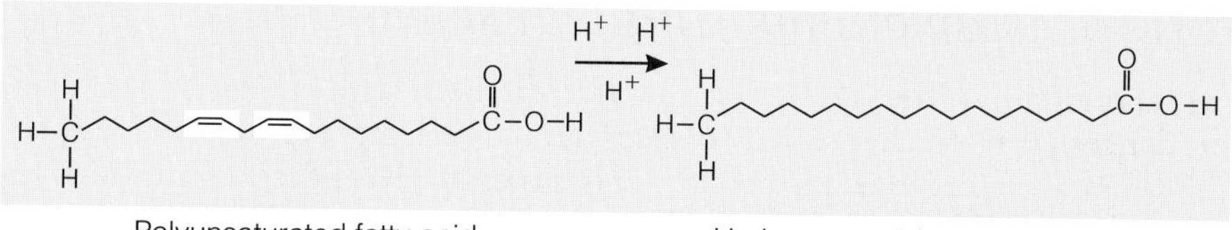

Figure 5–6

Hydrogenation

Hydrogenation yields a product that is more saturated, more spreadable, and more resistant to oxidation.

Polyunsaturated fatty acid   Hydrogenated (saturated) fatty acid

Double bonds carry a slightly negative charge and readily accept positively charged hydrogen atoms, creating a saturated fatty acid.

Hydrogenation of Fats The process of hydrogenation offers two advantages: it protects against oxidation (thereby prolonging shelf life) and alters the texture of foods. When partially hydrogenated, vegetable oils become spreadable margarine. Hydrogenated fats make pie crusts flaky and puddings creamy. A disadvantage is that hydrogenation makes polyunsaturated fats more saturated (see Figure 5–6). Consequently, any health advantages of using polyunsaturated fats instead of saturated fats are lost in hydrogenation.

Formation of *Trans*-Fatty Acids Another disadvantage of hydrogenation has to do with some of the molecules that remain unsaturated after processing. Some of these molecules change shape from *cis* to *trans*. In nature, most unsaturated fatty acids are *cis*-fatty acids—meaning that the hydrogens next to the double bonds are on the same side of the carbon chain. Only a few (notably those found in milk and butter) are *trans*-fatty acids—meaning that the hydrogens next to the double bonds are on opposite sides of the carbon chain (see Figure 5–7). These arrangements result in different configurations for the fatty acids, and the differences affect function.

People's intakes of *trans*-fatty acids from food products have risen in recent years as manufacturers have increased their use of partially hydrogenated vegetable oils.[2] A food that lists partially hydrogenated oils among its first three ingredients usually contains substantial amounts of *trans*-fatty acids, as well as some saturated fat. The relationship between *trans*-fatty acids and heart disease has been the subject of much recent research, as a later section describes.

hydrogenation (high-dro-gen-AY-shun): a chemical process by which hydrogens are added to monounsaturated or polyunsaturated fats to reduce the number of double bonds, making the fats more saturated (solid) and more resistant to oxidation (protecting against rancidity). Hydrogenation produces *trans*-fatty acids.

trans-fatty acids: fatty acids with an unusual configuration around the double bond.

Major sources of *trans*-fatty acids:
- Margarine (the hard stick type).
- Cakes, cookies, doughnuts, crackers.
- Snack chips.
- Meat and dairy products.
- Peanut butter.
- Fried foods.

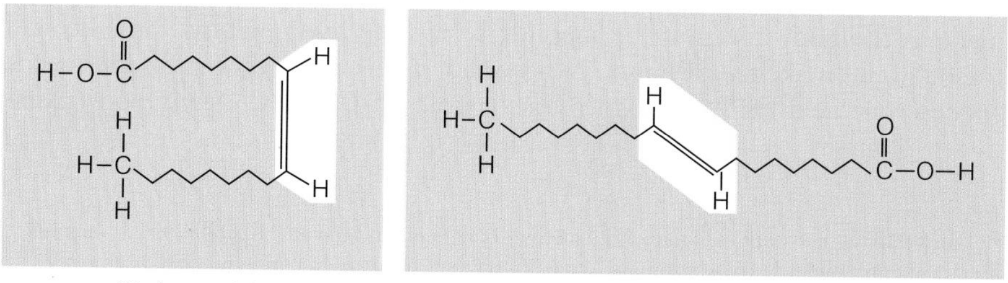

Cis-fatty acid

A *cis*-fatty acid has its hydrogens on the same side of the double bond; *cis* molecules fold back into a U-like formation. Most unsaturated fatty acids in foods are *cis*.

Trans-fatty acid

A *trans*-fatty acid has its hydrogens on the opposite sides of the double bond; *trans* molecules are more linear. The *trans* form typically occurs in partially hydrogenated foods when hydrogen atoms shift around some double bonds and change the configuration from *cis* to *trans*.

Figure 5–7

Cis- and *Trans*-Fatty Acids Compared

Manufacturers rarely use total hydrogenation; most often a fat is partially hydrogenated, yielding a *trans*-monounsaturated fatty acid. This example shows the *cis* configuration for oleic acid and its corresponding *trans* configuration (elaidic acid).

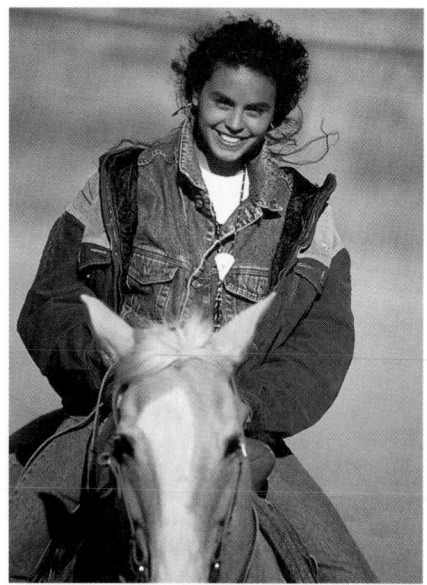

Thanks to the body's fat pads, a horseback ride causes no serious damage to internal organs.

Triglycerides in the body:
• Provide energy.
• Insulate against temperature extremes.
• Protect organs against shock.
• Help the body use carbohydrate and protein efficiently.

essential fatty acids: fatty acids needed by the body, but not made by the body in amounts sufficient to meet physiological needs.

eicosanoids (eye-COSS-uh-noyds): derivatives of fatty acids; hormonelike compounds that regulate blood pressure, clotting, and other body functions. They include *prostaglandins*, *thromboxanes*, and *leukotrienes*.

omega: the last letter of the Greek alphabet (ω), used by chemists to refer to the position of the endmost double bond in a fatty acid.

omega-6 fatty acid: a polyunsaturated fatty acid in which the first double bond is six carbons from the methyl (CH_3) end of the carbon chain.

arachidonic (a-RACK-ih-DON-ic) **acid:** an omega-6 polyunsaturated fatty acid with 20 carbons and four double bonds (20:4); synthesized from linoleic acid.

ROLES OF TRIGLYCERIDES AND FATTY ACIDS

First and foremost, the triglycerides provide the body with energy. When a person dances all night, her stored triglycerides provide the fuel to keep her moving; when a person loses his appetite, his stored triglycerides fuel much of his body's work until he can eat again. Stored fat supports many of life's activities.

Stored fat also insulates the body. Fat is a poor conductor of heat; the layer of fat beneath the skin helps keep the body warm. Fat pads also serve as shock absorbers, supporting and cushioning the vital organs.

Fat also helps the body use its two other energy nutrients—carbohydrate and protein—efficiently. Fat fragments combine with glucose fragments in the release of energy, and fat helps spare protein, providing energy so that protein can be used for other important tasks.

ESSENTIAL FATTY ACIDS

The human body can make all but two fatty acids—linoleic acid and linolenic acid. Because these two fatty acids are indispensable to body function, they must be supplied by the diet. They are therefore called essential fatty acids. The body uses these essential fatty acids to maintain the structural parts of cell membranes and to make many hormonelike substances known as eicosanoids. Eicosanoids help regulate blood pressure, blood clot formation, blood lipids, and the immune response to injury and infection.[3]

Linoleic acid and linolenic acid are the 18-carbon members of the two omega families mentioned in the introductory remarks.* Figure 5–8 (on p. 149) shows the structures of these two omega families.

Linoleic Acid, an Omega-6 Fatty Acid Linoleic acid is the primary member of the omega-6 family. Given linoleic acid, the body can make other members of the omega-6 family—such as the 20-carbon polyunsaturated fatty acid, arachidonic acid. Should a linoleic acid deficiency develop, arachidonic acid, and all the other fatty acids that derive from linoleic acid, would also become essential and would have to be obtained from the diet. Normally, vegetable oils and meats supply enough omega-6 fatty acids to meet the body's needs.

Linolenic Acid, an Omega-3 Fatty Acid Linolenic acid is the primary member of the omega-3 family.[†] Like linoleic acid, this 18-carbon acid cannot be made in the body and must be supplied by foods. Given dietary linolenic acid, the body can make the 20- and 22-carbon members of the omega-3 series, eicosapentaenoic acid (EPA) and docosahexaenoic acid (DHA). Many body tissues

---

*A fatty acid has two ends, designated the methyl (CH_3) end and the acid (COOH) end. Chemists usually number the carbons beginning at the acid end, but make an exception for polyunsaturated fatty acids. Because the body lengthens fatty acid chains by adding carbons at the acid end of the chain, these numbers would change as the chains grew longer. Chemists therefore number the carbons beginning at the methyl end, which eases the task of keeping track of fatty acids: when an omega-3 fatty acid is lengthened, the derivative is also an omega-3 fatty acid.

[†]This omega-3 linolenic acid is known as alpha-linolenic acid and is the fatty acid referred to in this discussion. Another fatty acid, also with 18 carbons and three double bonds, belongs to the omega-6 family and is known as gamma-linolenic acid.

Omega carbon

H
H—C—H
H

3

O
‖
C—O—H

Methyl end

Acid end

Linolenic acid, an omega-3 fatty acid

Omega carbon

H
H—C—H
H

6

O
‖
C—O—H

Methyl end

Acid end

Linoleic acid, an omega-6 fatty acid

Figure 5–8

Structural Formulas for Omega-3 and Omega-6 Fatty Acids

The omega number indicates the position of the first double bond in a fatty acid, counting from the methyl (CH_3) end. Thus an omega-3 fatty acid's first double bond occurs three carbons from the methyl end, and an omega-6 fatty acid's first double bond occurs six carbons from the methyl end. The members of a given family may have different lengths and different numbers of double bonds, but the first double bond occurs at the same point in all of them.

---

contain EPA and DHA; they make up a large proportion of the communicating membranes of the brain, and so their availability is necessary for normal brain development.[4] EPA and DHA are also active in the retina of the eye.[5] These omega-3 fatty acids are essential for normal growth and development, and they may play an important role in the prevention and treatment of heart disease, hypertension, arthritis, and cancer.[6]

A Comment on Essentiality   A simple definition of an essential nutrient has already been given: a nutrient that the body cannot make, or cannot make in sufficient quantities to meet its physiological needs. In the case of fatty acids, though, the body can make some fatty acids only if others are available. Also, some may be essential only for growth or for disease prevention.

The cells do not possess the enzymes to make any of the omega-6 or omega-3 fatty acids from scratch; nor can they convert an omega-6 fatty acid to an omega-3 fatty acid or vice versa. They *can* start with the 18-carbon member of a series and make the longer fatty acids of that series by forming double bonds (desaturation) and lengthening the chain two carbons at a time (elongation). This is a slow process because the two families compete for the same enzymes. Therefore the most effective way to maintain body supplies of these polyunsaturated fatty acids is to obtain them directly from foods.

Polyunsaturated Fats in Foods   A balanced diet that includes grains, seeds, nuts, leafy vegetables (or small amounts of vegetable oils), and fish supplies all the omega-6 and omega-3 fatty acids in abundance. Table 5–3 lists the chief dietary sources of the omega fatty acids.

When dietary intakes exceed the body's immediate needs, the body stores the omega-3 fatty acids EPA and DHA.[7] Most North Americans, however, do not eat enough fish to store any extra EPA and DHA. (Optimal omega-3 intake is estimated to be about 1 to 1.5 grams a day; current intake in the United States is about one-tenth of that.) They do, however, receive plenty of the omega-6

omega-3 fatty acid: a polyunsaturated fatty acid in which the first double bond is three carbons away from the methyl (CH_3) end of the carbon chain.

eicosapentaenoic (EYE-cossa-PENTA-ee-NO-ic) **acid (EPA):** an omega-3 polyunsaturated fatty acid with 20 carbons and five double bonds (20:5); synthesized from linolenic acid.

docosahexaenoic (DOE-cossa-HEXA-ee-NO-ic) **acid (DHA):** an omega-3 polyunsaturated fatty acid with 22 carbons and six double bonds (22:6); synthesized from linolenic acid.

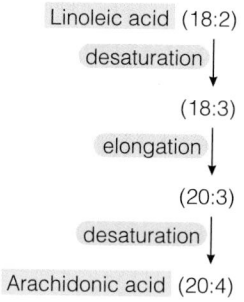

Linoleic acid (18:2)

desaturation ↓

(18:3)

elongation ↓

(20:3)

desaturation ↓

Arachidonic acid (20:4)

Note: The first number indicates the number of carbons and the second, the number of double bonds. Similar reactions occur when the body makes EPA and DHA from linolenic acid.

Table 5–3

Sources of Omega Fatty Acids

Omega-6	
Linoleic acid	Leafy vegetables, seeds, nuts, grains, vegetable oils (corn, safflower, soybean, cottonseed, sesame, sunflower)
Arachidonic acid	Meats (or can be made from linoleic acid)
Omega-3	
Linolenic acid	Fats and oils (canola, soybean, walnut, wheat germ, margarine and shortening made from canola and soybean oil)
	Nuts and seeds (butternuts, walnuts, soybean kernels)
	Vegetables (soybeans)
EPA and DHA	Human milk
	Shellfish and fish[a] (mackerel, tuna, salmon, bluefish, mullet, sturgeon, menhaden, anchovy, herring, trout, sardines)
	(or can be made from linolenic acid)

[a]These fish provide at least 1 gram of omega-3 fatty acids in 100 grams of fish (3.5 ounces); the fish oil content of each species varies with the season and site of harvest.

fatty acids. A comparison with the fish-eating people of Greenland is illuminating. Greenlanders have higher energy intakes and a higher percentage of kcalories from omega-3 fatty acids. North Americans have lower energy intakes and a higher percentage of kcalories from omega-6 fatty acids; indeed, they eat about twice as many omega-6 and half as many omega-3 fatty acids as Greenlanders do. Researchers have speculated that this difference may explain why the heart attack rate in North America is so much higher than in Greenland. It also explains why the people in Greenland have prolonged bleeding times and a high incidence of stroke. Such findings highlight the importance of dietary balance. Ideally, the ratio between these two lipid families in the diet is 4 to 10 grams of omega-6 fatty acids to 1 gram of omega-3 fatty acids.[8]

Fatty Acid Deficiencies   Essential fatty acids should make up at least 3 percent of the day's energy intake. Deficiencies of these polyunsaturated fatty acids cause growth retardation, reproductive failure, skin lesions, kidney and liver disorders, and subtle neurological and visual problems. There is no need to panic, though; most diets meet minimum requirements more than adequately.[9] Deficiencies have historically developed only in infants and young children fed non-fat milk and low-fat diets or in hospital clients fed formulas that provided no polyunsaturated fatty acids for long times.

In summary, the lipids important in nutrition, commonly called simply *fat,* are of three classes: triglycerides, phospholipids, and sterols. The triglycerides are by far the predominant class both in foods and in the body. They are energy-dense, important energy-storage compounds. Each triglyceride contains three fatty acids, which may be long, medium, or short chain; may be saturated, monounsaturated, or polyunsaturated; and if the latter, may be members of the omega-3 or omega-6 families of fatty acids. Linoleic acid (18 carbons, omega-6) and linolenic acid (18 carbons, omega-3) are essential nutrients; the essentiality of other polyunsaturated fatty acids is debated.

Fatty acid saturation affects fats' cooking qualities, their storage properties, and their contributions to people's susceptibility to heart disease and cancer. Hydrogenation, which makes polyunsaturates more saturated, gives rise to some *trans*-fatty acids, altered fatty acids that may exert adverse health effects. Small amounts of fats are necessary to support health, carry fat-soluble vitamins, and spare protein; deficiencies are unlikely.

The Chemist's View of Phospholipids and Sterols

The preceding pages have been devoted to one of the three classes of lipids, the triglycerides, and their component parts, the fatty acids. The other two classes of lipids, the phospholipids and sterols, make up only 5 percent of the lipids in the diet, but they are nevertheless interesting and important.

THE PHOSPHOLIPIDS

The best-known phospholipids are the lecithins. Each lecithin has a backbone of glycerol with two of its three attachment sites occupied by fatty acids like those in triglycerides. The third site is occupied by a phosphate group and a molecule of choline. The fatty acids make phospholipids soluble in fat; the phosphate-containing group enables them to dissolve in water. Such versatility enables the food industry to use phospholipids as emulsifiers, mixing fats with water in such products as mayonnaise and candy bars. A diagram of a lecithin molecule is shown in Figure 5–9.

phospholipid: a compound similar to a triglyceride but having choline (or another nitrogen-containing compound) and a phosphate group (a phosphorus-containing salt) in place of one of the fatty acids.

lecithin (LESS-uh-thin): one of the phospholipids; a compound of glycerol to which are attached two fatty acids, a phosphate group, and a choline molecule. Both nature and the food industry use lecithin as an emulsifier to combine two ingredients that do not ordinarily mix, such as water and oil.

Reminder: An *emulsifier* promotes the mixing of two substances, such as oil and water, that are not mutually soluble.

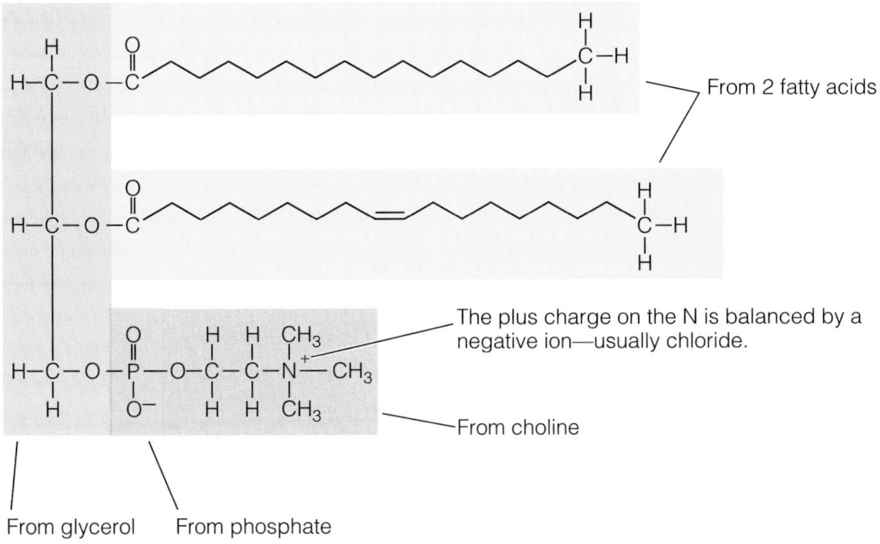

Figure 5–9

A Lecithin

This is one of the lecithins. Other lecithins have different fatty acids at the upper two positions. Notice that a molecule of lecithin is similar to a triglyceride but contains only two fatty acids. The third position is occupied by a phosphate group and a molecule of choline.

choline (KOH-leen): a nitrogen-containing compound found in plant and animal tissues as part of lecithin and other phospholipids.

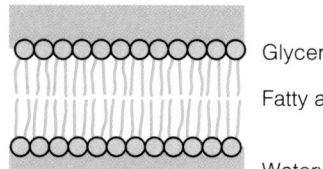

Glycerol heads

Fatty acid tails

Watery fluid

A cell membrane is made of phospholipids assembled into an orderly formation called a bilayer. The fatty acid "tails" orient themselves away from the watery fluid inside and outside of the cell. The glycerol and phosphate "heads" are attracted to the watery fluid.

Reminder: The word ending *-ase* denotes an enzyme. Hence, lecithinase is an enzyme that works on lecithin.

sterol: a compound composed of C, H, and O atoms arranged in rings, like those of cholesterol, with any of a variety of side chains attached.

cholesterol: one of the sterols.

Phospholipids in Foods   In addition to the phospholipids used by the food industry as emulsifiers, phospholipids are also found in foods naturally. The richest food sources of lecithin are eggs, liver, soybeans, wheat germ, and peanuts.

Roles of Phospholipids   The lecithins and other phospholipids are important constituents of cell membranes. Because phospholipids can dissolve in both water and fat, they can help lipids move back and forth across the lipid-containing cell membranes into the watery fluids on both sides. They thus allow fat-soluble substances, including vitamins and hormones, to pass easily in and out of cells. The phospholipids also act as emulsifiers in the body, helping to keep fats suspended in the blood and body fluids.

Lecithin periodically receives attention in the popular press. Its fans claim that it is a major constituent of cell membranes (true), that all cells depend on the integrity of their membranes (true), and that consumers must therefore take lecithin supplements (false). The liver makes from scratch all the lecithin a person needs. As for lecithin taken as a supplement, the digestive enzyme lecithinase in the intestine hydrolyzes most of it before it passes into the body fluids, so little lecithin reaches the body tissues intact. In other words, the lecithins are *not essential nutrients*; they are just another lipid. Like all the other lipids, they contribute 9 kcalories per gram to the body's energy economy—an unexpected "bonus" many people taking lecithin supplements fail to realize. Labels on lecithin supplements suggest a 7-gram daily dosage, which can add 6½ pounds a year to body weight. Furthermore, large doses of lecithin may cause GI distress, sweating, salivation, and loss of appetite. Perhaps these symptoms are beneficial because they may warn people to stop self-dosing with lecithin.

THE STEROLS

The sterols are lipid compounds with a multiple-ring structure. The most famous sterol is cholesterol; Figure 5–10 shows its chemical structure. All sterols have the same multiple-ring structure, but each has different side groups attached.

Sterols in Foods   Both plant and animal foods contain sterols, but only animal foods contain cholesterol: meats, eggs, fish, poultry, and dairy products. Organ meats, such as liver and kidneys, and eggs, are richest in cholesterol; cheeses and meats have less. Shellfish contain many sterols, but much less cholesterol than has been thought in the past. Table 5–4 lists the cholesterol contents of selected foods. Many more foods, with their cholesterol contents, appear in Appendix H.

Figure 5–10

Cholesterol

The fat-soluble vitamin D is synthesized from cholesterol; notice the similarities. Notice, too, how different cholesterol is from the triglycerides and phospholipids.

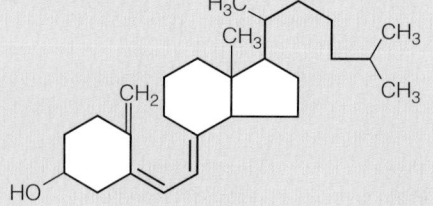

Cholesterol   Vitamin D₃

Table 5–4

Approximate Amounts of Cholesterol in Common Foods

Foods	Cholesterol (mg)
Grains, vegetables, fruits	0
Milks (1 c serving)	
Whole milk and yogurt	30–35
Low-fat milk and yogurt	15–20
Nonfat milk and buttermilk	5–10
Cheeses (1 oz serving)	25–30
Ice cream (½ c serving)	30
Pudding (½ c serving)	15
Butter (1 tsp)	10
Margarine, all vegetable (1 tsp)	0
Creams (1 tsp)	10–20
Meats (3 oz serving)	
Veal cutlet	100
Beef steak, chicken, lamb chop, pork chop	70–85
Hot dog	45
Organ meats (3 oz serving)	
Brains	1696
Liver	410
Kidneys	329
Egg yolk	213
Egg white	0
Seafood (3 oz serving)	
Shrimp	165
Lobster, clams, fish fillets, oysters	50–60

Note: Only foods of animal origin contain cholesterol.
Source: Food Processor computer diet analysis program, ESHA, Salem, OR 97302.

Eggs contain just over 200 milligrams of cholesterol each, all of it in the yolks. A person on a strict low-cholesterol diet must curtail the use of egg yolks, and food manufacturers have produced several nonfat, no-cholesterol egg substitutes. For most people trying to lower blood cholesterol, however, limiting saturated fat is more effective than limiting cholesterol intake. Eggs are a valuable part of the diet because they are inexpensive, useful in cooking, and a source of high-quality protein. The American Heart Association approves an intake of up to four eggs a week.

Some people, confused about the distinction between dietary and blood cholesterol, have asked which foods contain the "good" cholesterol. "Good" cholesterol is not a type of cholesterol found in foods, but refers to the way the body transports cholesterol in the blood, as explained later (pp. 159–160).

Roles of Sterols Many vitally important body compounds are sterols. Among them are bile, the sex hormones (such as testosterone), the adrenal hormones (such as cortisol), and vitamin D, as well as cholesterol itself. Cholesterol in the body can serve as the starting material for synthesis of these compounds or as a structural component of cell membranes; more than nine-tenths of all the body's cholesterol resides in the cells. Despite popular impressions to the con-

Cholesterol that is made in the body is **endogenous** (en-DODGE-eh-nus), whereas cholesterol from outside the body (from foods) is **exogenous** (eks-ODGE-eh-nus).

> *endo* = within
> *gen* = arising
> *exo* = outside (the body)

Reminder: Eating many small meals and snacks throughout the day is sometimes called *grazing*.

atherosclerosis (ath-er-oh-scler-OH-sis): a type of artery disease characterized by accumulations of lipid-containing material on the inner walls of the arteries (see Chapter 28).

> *athero* = porridge or soft
> *scleros* = hard
> *osis* = condition

hydrophobic: a term referring to water-fearing, or non-water-soluble, substances; also known as **lipophilic** (fat loving).

> *hydro* = water
> *phobia* = fear
> *lipo* = lipid
> *phile* = friend

hydrophilic: a term referring to water-loving, or water-soluble, substances.

monoglyceride: a molecule of glycerol with one fatty acid attached. A molecule of glycerol with two fatty acids attached is a **diglyceride**.

Reminder: An enzyme that hydrolyzes lipids is called a *lipase*.

trary, therefore, cholesterol is not a villain lurking in some evil foods—it is a compound the body makes and uses. Your liver is manufacturing cholesterol now, as you read. At the rate of perhaps 5×10^{16} (50,000,000,000,000,000) molecules per second (800 to 1500 milligrams per day), the liver contributes much more cholesterol to the body's total than does the diet. The liver can use fragments derived from carbohydrate, protein, or fat as the starting material from which to make cholesterol.

Cholesterol synthesis depends on the availability of the raw materials, the extent of bile production, and the presence of regulating hormones such as insulin. When insulin concentrations remain low, as occurs when people eat many small meals, cholesterol synthesis slows. Spreading total food intake over many meals and snacks a day without an increase in energy intake is a relatively easy and effective way to lower blood cholesterol.[10]

Cholesterol's harmful effects in the body occur when it forms deposits in the artery walls. These deposits lead to atherosclerosis, a disease that causes heart attacks and strokes.

In summary, phospholipids, including lecithin, have a unique chemical structure that allows them to be soluble in both water and fat. In the body, phospholipids are part of cell membranes; the food industry uses phospholipids as emulsifiers. Sterols, including cholesterol, have a multiple-ring structure that differs from the other lipids. Sterols in the body include bile, vitamin D, and the sex hormones. Only animal-derived foods contain cholesterol.

Digestion, Absorption, and Transport of Lipids

Each day, the GI tract receives, on the average, 50 to 100 grams of triglycerides, 4 to 8 grams of phospholipids, and 300 to 450 milligrams of cholesterol. The body faces a challenge in digesting and absorbing these lipids: getting at them.

Fats carry no net charge and are neutral. They are hydrophobic—that is, they tend to separate from water—whereas the enzymes for digesting fats are hydrophilic. Since the watery fluids of the GI tract tend to settle at the bottom of the stomach while the dietary fats tend to float on top, the fats start out separated from their enzymes. The following paragraphs describe how the body mixes the fats into the watery fluids and then digests them.

LIPID DIGESTION

The goal of fat digestion is to dismantle triglycerides into small molecules that the body can absorb and use—namely, monoglycerides, fatty acids, and glycerol. Figure 5–11 traces the digestion of triglycerides through the GI tract.

In the Mouth   Fat digestion starts off slowly in the mouth, with some hard fats beginning to melt when they reach body temperature. The salivary glands at the base of the tongue release a lipase enzyme that plays a small role in fat digestion in adults and an active role in infants. In infants, this enzyme efficiently digests the short- and medium-chain fatty acids found in milk.[11]

In the Stomach   In the stomach, fat floats as a layer above the other components of swallowed food. As a result, little fat digestion takes place.

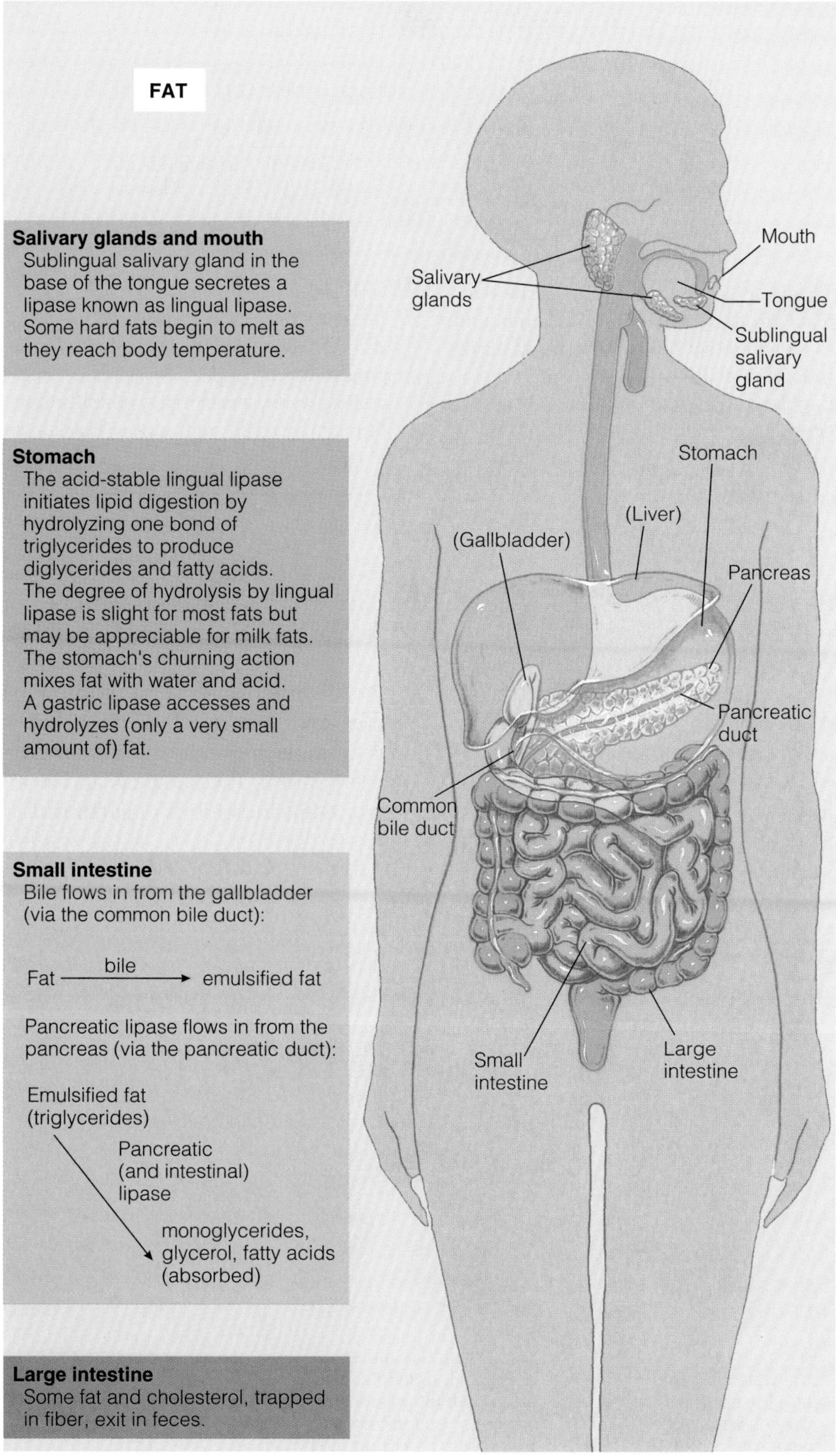

Figure 5–11

Triglyceride Digestion in the GI Tract

FAT

Salivary glands and mouth
Sublingual salivary gland in the base of the tongue secretes a lipase known as lingual lipase. Some hard fats begin to melt as they reach body temperature.

Stomach
The acid-stable lingual lipase initiates lipid digestion by hydrolyzing one bond of triglycerides to produce diglycerides and fatty acids. The degree of hydrolysis by lingual lipase is slight for most fats but may be appreciable for milk fats. The stomach's churning action mixes fat with water and acid. A gastric lipase accesses and hydrolyzes (only a very small amount of) fat.

Small intestine
Bile flows in from the gallbladder (via the common bile duct):

Fat $\xrightarrow{\text{bile}}$ emulsified fat

Pancreatic lipase flows in from the pancreas (via the pancreatic duct):

Emulsified fat (triglycerides)
$\xrightarrow{\text{Pancreatic (and intestinal) lipase}}$
monoglycerides, glycerol, fatty acids (absorbed)

Large intestine
Some fat and cholesterol, trapped in fiber, exit in feces.

Labels: Mouth, Tongue, Salivary glands, Sublingual salivary gland, Stomach, (Liver), (Gallbladder), Pancreas, Pancreatic duct, Common bile duct, Small intestine, Large intestine

Figure 5–12

A Bile Acid

Bile acid made from cholesterol

$$HO \quad CH_3$$
$$CH-CH_2-CH_2-C-NH-CH_2-COOH$$
$$O$$

HO OH
H

Bound to an amino acid

This is one of several bile acids the liver makes from cholesterol. It is then bound to an amino acid to improve its ability to form micelles, spherical complexes that carry fatty acids into the intestinal cells during digestion. Most bile acids occur as bile salts, usually in association with sodium, but sometimes with potassium or calcium. In addition to bile acids and bile salts, bile contains cholesterol, phospholipids (especially lecithin), antibodies, water, electrolytes, and bilirubin (a pigment resulting from the breakdown of heme).

Reminder: Fat in the intestine triggers the release of the hormone *cholecystokinin* (CCK), which signals the gallbladder to send bile.

Reminder: *Bile* is an emulsifier, as are lecithins and other phospholipids. An *emulsifier* promotes the mixing of oils and fats in a watery solution.

In the Small Intestine   When fat enters the small intestine, the hormone cholecystokinin (CCK) signals the gallbladder to release its stores of bile, an emulsifier. (The liver manufactures bile acids from cholesterol, and the gallbladder stores the bile until it is needed.)

At one end of each bile acid are side chains of amino acids (units of protein) that are attracted to water, and at the other end is a sterol portion that is attracted to fat (see Figure 5–12). Bile draws fat molecules into the surrounding watery fluids. There, the fats meet lipase enzymes from the pancreas and small intestine and are fully digested. The process of emulsification is diagrammed in Figure 5–13.

Figure 5–13

Emulsification of Fat by Bile
Detergents are emulsifiers and work the same way, which is why they are effective in removing grease spots from clothes. Molecule by molecule, the grease is dissolved out of the spot and suspended in the water, where it can be rinsed away.

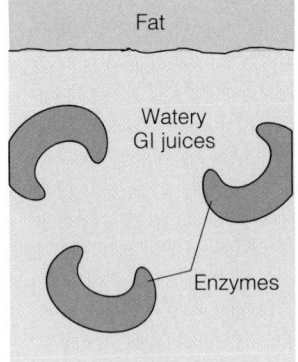

In the stomach, the fat and watery GI juices tend to separate. The enzymes are in the water and can't get at the fat.

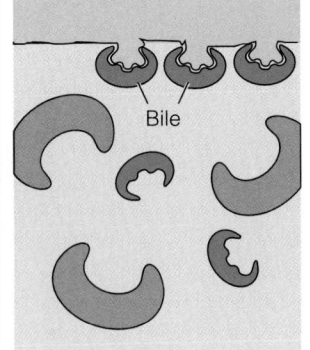

When fat enters the small intestine, the gallbladder secretes bile. Bile has an affinity for both fat and water, so it can bring the fat into solution in the water.

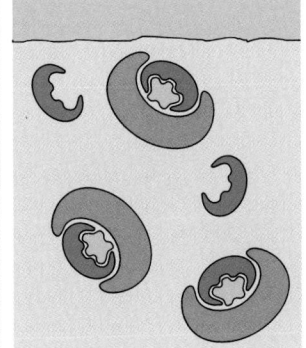

After emulsification, the fat is mixed in the water solution, so the enzymes have access to it.

Figure 5–14

Digestion (Hydrolysis) of a Triglyceride

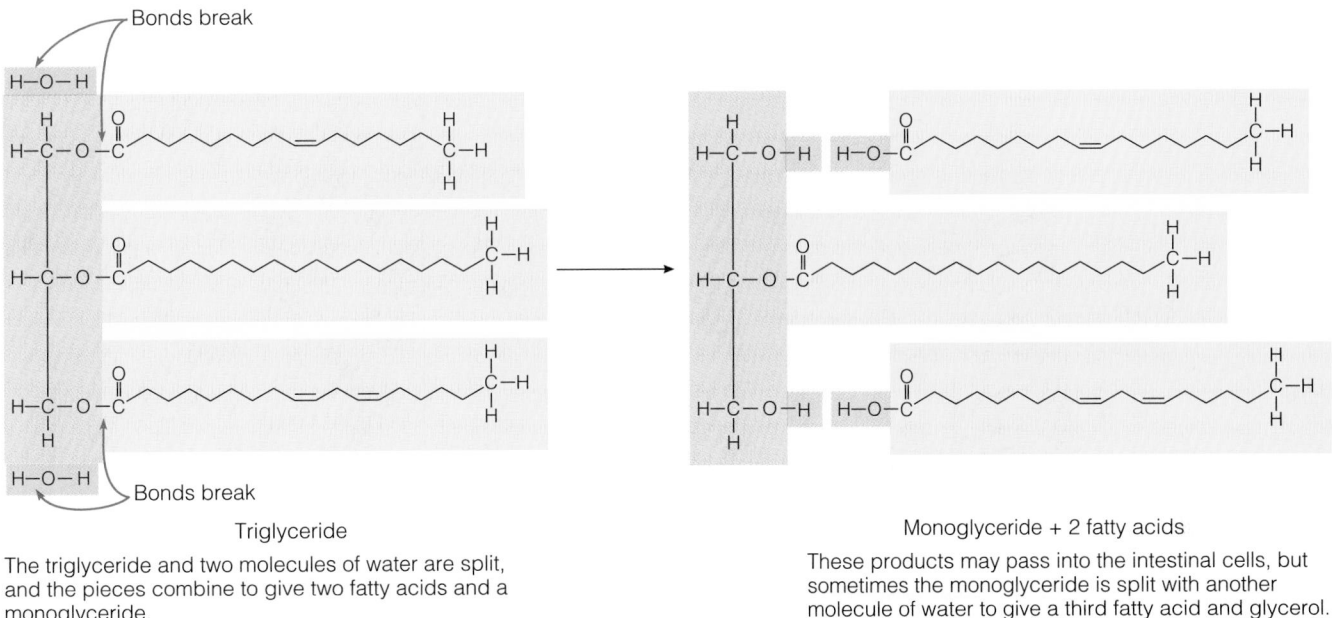

Triglyceride

The triglyceride and two molecules of water are split, and the pieces combine to give two fatty acids and a monoglyceride.

Monoglyceride + 2 fatty acids

These products may pass into the intestinal cells, but sometimes the monoglyceride is split with another molecule of water to give a third fatty acid and glycerol. Fatty acids, monoglycerides, and glycerol are absorbed into intestinal cells.

Most of the hydrolysis of triglycerides occurs in the small intestine. The major fat-digesting enzymes are pancreatic lipases; some intestinal lipases are also active. These enzymes remove one, then the other, of each tryglyceride's outer fatty acids, leaving a monoglyceride. Occasionally, enzymes remove all three fatty acids, leaving a free molecule of glycerol. The process of hydrolysis is shown in Figure 5–14.

Phospholipids are digested similarly—that is, their fatty acids are removed by hydrolysis. The two fatty acids and the remaining phospholipid fragment are then absorbed. Sterols can be absorbed as is; if any fatty acids are attached, they are first hydrolyzed off.

Bile's Routes   After bile has entered the intestine and emulsified fat, it has two possible destinations, illustrated in Figure 5–15. For one, bile can be reabsorbed from the intestine and recycled. The other possibility is that some of the bile can be trapped by dietary fibers in the large intestine and carried out of the body with the feces. Because it takes cholesterol to make bile, the excretion of bile effectively reduces elevated blood cholesterol. The fibers most effective at lowering blood cholesterol this way are the soluble pectins and gums commonly found in fruits, oats, and legumes.

LIPID ABSORPTION

Figure 5–16 illustrates the absorption of lipids. Small units of digested fats (glycerol and short- and medium-chain fatty acids) can diffuse easily into the intesti-

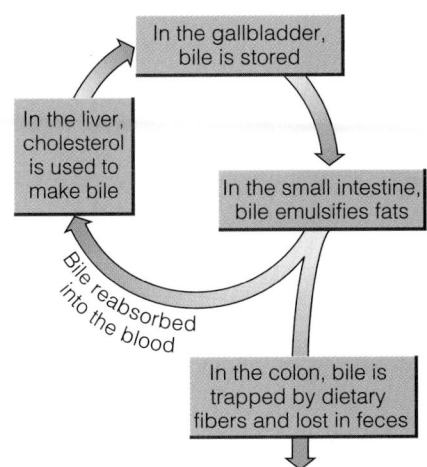

Figure 5–15

Enterohepatic Circulation

The recycling of cholesterol and bile through the intestine and liver is known as the enterohepatic circulation of bile.

enteron = intestine

hepat = liver

Figure 5–16

Absorption and Transport of Lipids

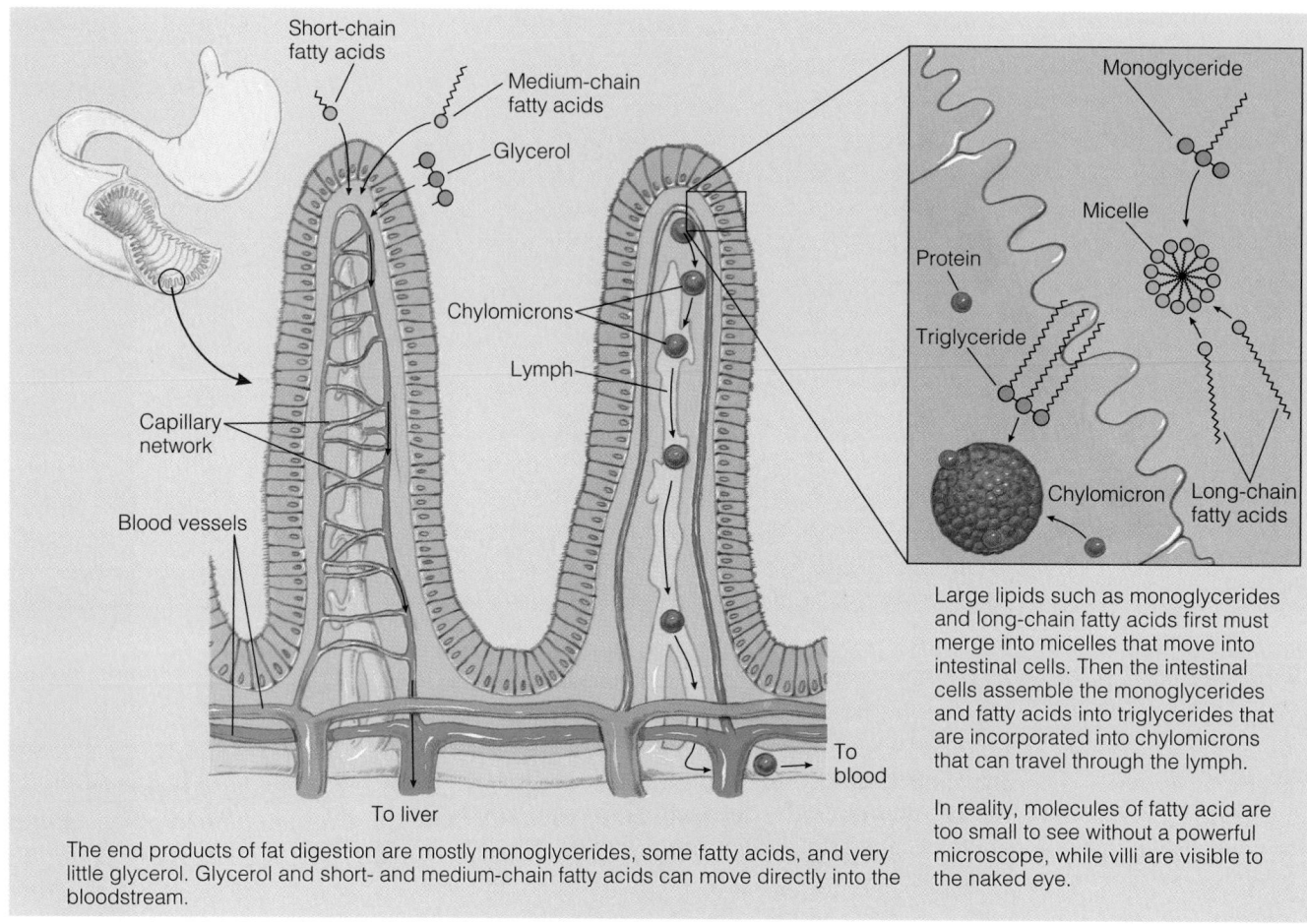

Large lipids such as monoglycerides and long-chain fatty acids first must merge into micelles that move into intestinal cells. Then the intestinal cells assemble the monoglycerides and fatty acids into triglycerides that are incorporated into chylomicrons that can travel through the lymph.

In reality, molecules of fatty acid are too small to see without a powerful microscope, while villi are visible to the naked eye.

The end products of fat digestion are mostly monoglycerides, some fatty acids, and very little glycerol. Glycerol and short- and medium-chain fatty acids can move directly into the bloodstream.

micelles (MY-cells): tiny spherical complexes that arise during fat digestion; each carries about 20 fatty acids and/or monoglycerides into intestinal cells.

Absorbed directly into blood:
• Glycerol.
• Short-chain fatty acids.
• Medium-chain fatty acids.

Merge into micelles, move into the intestinal cells, and made into triglycerides:
• Long-chain fatty acids.
• Monoglycerides.

Assembled into chylomicrons, absorbed into lymph, then into blood:
• Triglycerides.   • Phospholipids.
• Cholesterol.

nal cells; they are absorbed directly into the bloodstream. Larger units (the monoglycerides and long-chain fatty acids) merge into spherical complexes, known as micelles, which are so small that they can fit between the tiny, hairlike microvilli of a single intestinal cell. (Emulsified fat particles are 100 times larger in diameter and contain tens of thousands of molecules.) The micelles easily diffuse into the intestinal cells. Once inside, the monoglycerides and long-chain fatty acids are reassembled into new triglycerides.

Within the intestinal cells, the newly made triglycerides and the other large lipids (cholesterol and phospholipids) are packed into transport vehicles known as chylomicrons. The intestinal cells then release the chylomicrons into the lymphatic system. The chylomicrons glide through the lymph until they reach a point of entry into the bloodstream at the thoracic duct near the heart. The blood can then carry these lipids to the rest of the body. The margin summarizes the absorption of lipids.

LIPID TRANSPORT

The chylomicrons are only one of several clusters of lipids and proteins that are used as transport vehicles for fats. As a group, these vehicles are known as lipoproteins, and they solve the body's problem of transporting fatty materials through the watery medium of the bloodstream. The body makes four main types of lipoproteins, distinguished by their size and density.* Each type contains different kinds of special proteins and carries different amounts of the various lipids.

Chylomicrons The chylomicrons are the largest and least dense of the lipoproteins. They transport *diet*-derived lipids (mostly triglycerides) from the intestine to the rest of the body. Cells all over the body remove lipids from the chylomicrons as they pass by, so the chylomicrons get smaller and smaller. Within 14 hours after absorption, little is left of them but protein remnants and a few odds and ends of lipid. Special protein receptors on the membranes of the liver cells recognize and remove these remnants from the blood.[12] Once the liver cells have collected the chylomicron remnants, they dismantle them.

VLDL Meanwhile, the liver cells are synthesizing other lipids to be shipped out to other parts of the body. The liver cells pick up fatty acids arriving in the blood and use them to make cholesterol, other fatty acids, and other compounds. At the same time, the liver cells may be making lipids from carbohydrates, proteins, or alcohol. The liver is the most active site of lipid synthesis. Ultimately, the lipids made in the liver are shipped to other parts of the body and packaged with proteins as very-low-density lipoproteins (VLDL).

As the VLDL travel through the body, cells remove triglycerides, causing the VLDL to shrink. As they lose triglycerides, the VLDL gather cholesterol from other lipoproteins circulating through the bloodstream and eventually become low-density lipoproteins (LDL).† This exchange explains why LDL contain few triglycerides but are loaded with cholesterol.

LDL The LDL circulate throughout the body, making their contents available to the cells of all tissues—muscle, including the heart muscle; fat stores; the mammary glands; and others. The cells take triglycerides from the LDL; they also collect cholesterol and phospholipids to build new membranes, to make hormones or other compounds, or to store for later use. Special LDL receptors on the liver cells play a crucial role in the control of blood cholesterol concentrations by removing LDL from circulation.

HDL Fat cells may release glycerol, fatty acids, cholesterol, and phospholipids to the blood. The liver makes high-density lipoprotein (HDL) packages to

lipoproteins (LIP-oh-PRO-teenz): clusters of lipids associated with proteins that serve as transport vehicles for lipids in the lymph and blood.

chylomicrons (kye-lo-MY-cronz): the class of lipoproteins that transport lipids from the intestinal cells into the body.

VLDL (very-low-density lipoprotein): the type of lipoprotein made primarily by liver cells to transport lipids to various tissues in the body; composed primarily of triglycerides.

LDL (low-density lipoprotein): the type of lipoprotein derived from very-low-density lipoproteins (VLDL) as cells remove triglycerides from them; composed primarily of cholesterol.

HDL (high-density lipoprotein): the type of lipoprotein that transports cholesterol back to the liver from peripheral cells; composed primarily of protein.

---

*The lipoproteins are distinguished by density because the chemist uses this feature to separate them in the laboratory. The chemist layers a blood sample below a thick fluid in a test tube and spins the tube in a centrifuge. The most buoyant particles (highest in lipids) rise to the top, and the densest particles (highest in proteins) remain at the bottom. Lipoproteins with a low protein-to-lipid ratio have a low density; those with a high protein-to-lipid ratio have a high density.

†Before becoming LDL, the VLDL are first transformed into intermediate-density lipoproteins (IDL), sometimes called VLDL remnants. Some IDL may be picked up by the liver and rapidly broken down; those IDL that remain in circulation pick up cholesterol and become LDL. Researchers debate whether IDL are simply transitional particles or a separate class of lipoproteins.

carry cholesterol and phospholipids from the cells back to the liver for recycling or disposal.

In summary, all four types of lipoproteins carry all classes of lipids (triglycerides, phospholipids, and cholesterol), but the chylomicrons are the largest and the highest in triglycerides; VLDL are smaller and are about half triglycerides; LDL are smaller still and are high in cholesterol; and HDL are the smallest and are rich in protein. Figure 5–17 (on p. 161) shows the relative sizes and compositions of the lipoproteins.

The distinction between LDL and HDL has implications for the health of the heart and blood vessels. The blood cholesterol linked to heart disease is LDL cholesterol. HDL also carry cholesterol, but elevated HDL represent cholesterol returning from the arteries to the liver for breakdown and excretion. High LDL cholesterol is associated with a high risk of heart attack, whereas high HDL cholesterol seems to have a protective effect.[13] This is why some people refer to LDL as "bad," and HDL as "good," cholesterol. Keep in mind, though, that there is only *one* kind of cholesterol, and that the differences between LDL and HDL reflect the *proportions* of lipids and proteins within them—not the type of cholesterol. The margin lists factors that influence LDL and HDL, and Chapter 28 provides many more details.

Lipids in the Body

The blood carries lipids to various sites around the body. Once they arrive at their destinations, the lipids can get to work providing energy, insulating against temperature extremes, protecting against shock, and building cell structures. This section provides an overview first of the triglycerides in the blood and then of the metabolic pathways triglycerides can follow within the body's cells.

TRIGLYCERIDES IN THE BLOOD

The body's cells use both glucose and fat to fuel their activities. The energy to make a muscle contract, including the heart muscle, is supplied mostly from fat, so the blood must continuously deliver a supply of triglycerides—either from the intestines where foods have provided fat or from the adipose tissue where fat has been stored. Either way, triglycerides are always circulating in the blood.

A PREVIEW OF LIPID METABOLISM

The blood delivers its cargo of triglycerides to the cells for their use. This discussion provides a preview of how the cells store and release energy from fat; Chapter 7 provides many more details.

Storing Fat as Fat   The triglycerides, familiar as the fat in foods and as body fat, serve the body primarily as a source of fuel. Fat provides more than twice the energy of carbohydrate and protein, making it an extremely efficient storage form of energy. The body's storage space for energy is virtually unlimited, thanks to the special cells of the adipose tissue. Unlike most body cells, which can store

To help you remember, think of elevated **H**DL as **H**ealthy and elevated **L**DL as **L**ess healthy.

Factors that improve the LDL-to-HDL ratio:
- Weight control.
- Monounsaturated or polyunsaturated, instead of saturated, fatty acids in the diet.
- Soluble fibers (see Chapter 4).
- Antioxidants (see Highlight 11).
- Moderate alcohol consumption.
- Physical activity.

adipose (ADD-ih-poce) **tissue:** the body's fat tissue, which consists of masses of fat-storing cells.

Figure 5–17

Sizes and Compositions of the Lipoproteins

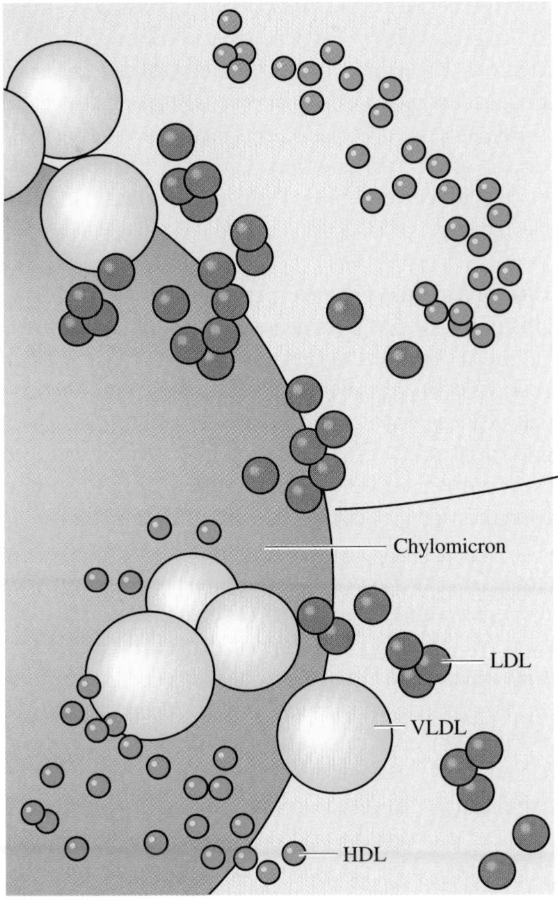

Phospholipid

Protein

Cholesterol

Triglyceride

Chylomicron

LDL

VLDL

HDL

This solar system of lipoproteins shows their relative sizes. Notice how large the fat-filled chylomicron is compared with the others and how the others get progressively smaller as their proportion of fat declines and protein increases.

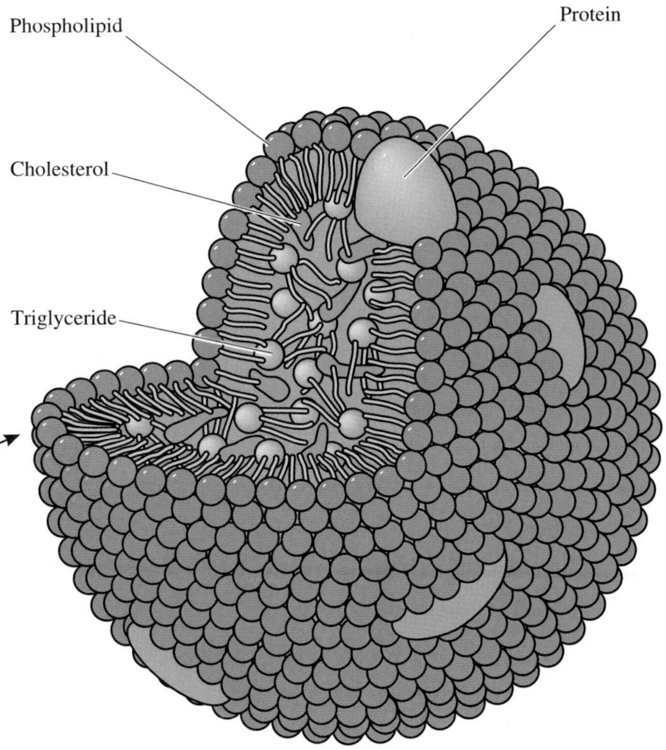

A typical lipoprotein contains an interior of triglycerides and cholesterol surrounded by phospholipids. The phospholipids' fatty acid "tails" point toward the interior, where the lipids are. Proteins near the outer ends of the phospholipids cover the structure. This arrangement of hydrophobic molecules on the inside and hydrophilic molecules on the outside allows lipids to travel through the watery fluids of the blood.

Chylomicrons contain so little protein and so much triglyceride that they are the lowest in density.

Very-low-density lipoproteins (VLDL) are half triglycerides, accounting for their low density.

Low-density lipoproteins (LDL) are half cholesterol, accounting for their implication in heart disease.

High-density lipoproteins (HDL) are half protein, accounting for their high density.

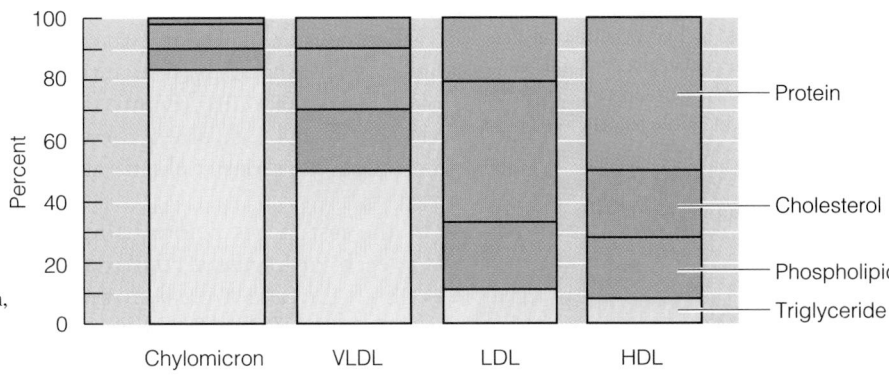

Protein

Cholesterol

Phospholipid

Triglyceride

Figure 5–18

An Adipose Cell

An adipose, or fat, cell seems to expand almost indefinitely. The more fat it stores, the larger it grows.

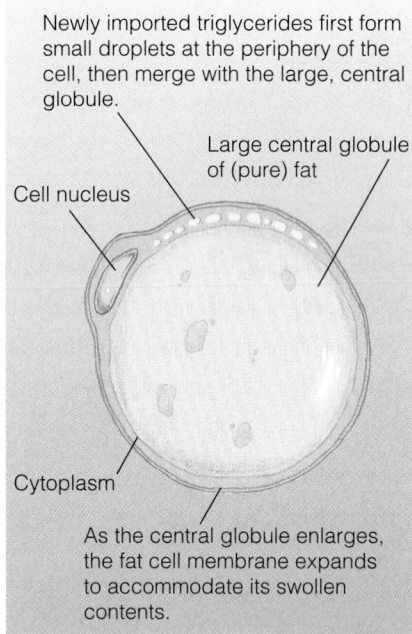

Newly imported triglycerides first form small droplets at the periphery of the cell, then merge with the large, central globule.

Large central globule of (pure) fat

Cell nucleus

Cytoplasm

As the central globule enlarges, the fat cell membrane expands to accommodate its swollen contents.

lipoprotein lipase (LPL): an enzyme mounted on the surface of fat cells (and other cells) that hydrolyzes triglycerides passing by in the bloodstream and directs their parts into the cells, where they can be metabolized or reassembled for storage.

hormone-sensitive lipase: an enzyme inside adipose cells that responds to the body's need for fuel by hydrolyzing triglycerides so that their parts (glycerol and fatty acids) escape into the general circulation and thus become available to other cells as fuel. The signals to which this enzyme responds include epinephrine and glucagon, which oppose insulin (see Chapter 4).

Reminder: When fat is metabolized in the absence of carbohydrate, *ketone bodies* are formed.

only limited amounts of fat, the fat cells of the adipose tissue readily take up and store fat. An adipose cell is depicted in Figure 5–18.

Adipose cells have a special enzyme on their surfaces—lipoprotein lipase (LPL)—that captures circulating triglycerides from lipoproteins passing by after meals. This enzyme hydrolyzes the triglycerides to fatty acids and monoglycerides and passes these products into the cells' interiors. Inside the cells, other enzymes reassemble the pieces into triglycerides again for storage. Triglycerides pack tightly together within adipose cells, storing a lot of energy in a relatively small space. Adipose cells always store fat after meals, when a heavy traffic of chylomicrons and VLDL loaded with triglycerides passes by; they release it later when the blood cargo needs replenishing.

Making Fat from Carbohydrate or Protein   Earlier, Figure 5–3 showed how the body can make triglycerides from glycerol and fatty acids. Fatty acids, in turn, can be made from two-carbon fragments derived from any nutrient. (This is why most fatty acid carbon chains come in even numbers.) Thus glucose can be converted to body fat: enzymes break glucose into two-carbon fragments and then combine them to make long-chain fatty acids. Enzymes can also convert some of the components of protein (certain amino acids) to fatty acids. The food source from which the body most easily makes fat for storage, though, is fat itself.

Efficiency of Making Fat from Fat   To convert food fats to body fat, the body simply absorbs the parts and puts them (or others) together again in storage. It requires very little energy to do this. By comparison, to convert dietary carbohydrate to body fat, the body must first break starches into disaccharides and then into monosaccharides, absorb the monosaccharides, then dismantle glucose, and reassemble many of the fragments into fatty acid chains. Each conversion requires energy. Thus it costs less (energetically) to store dietary fat as body fat than to convert and store dietary carbohydrate as body fat. Whether fat is stored at all depends more on total energy intake and on how much fat is eaten than on how much carbohydrate is eaten. The message is clear: to limit fat storage in the body, limit fat intake from foods. Chapter 8 discusses energy balance in more detail.

Using Fat for Energy   Unlike the liver's glycogen stores, the body's fat stores have virtually unlimited capacity, and fat supplies 60 percent of the body's ongoing energy needs during rest.[14] During exercise or prolonged periods of food deprivation, fat stores may make an even greater contribution to energy needs.

When cells demand energy, an enzyme (hormone-sensitive lipase) inside the adipose cells responds by dismantling stored triglycerides and releasing the glycerol and fatty acids directly into the blood. Energy-hungry cells anywhere in the body can then break down these components into small fragments and take them through a series of chemical reactions to yield energy, carbon dioxide, and water.

In the last stages before being completely oxidized to carbon dioxide and water, each fat fragment combines with a fragment from the breakdown of glucose. Body fat cannot break down completely unless carbohydrate is simultaneously present. Without carbohydrate, ketosis will develop, as mentioned in Chapter 4.

A person who fasts (drinking only water) will rapidly metabolize body fat. A pound of body fat provides 3500 kcalories, so you might think a fasting person who expends 2000 kcalories a day could lose more than half a pound of body fat each day.* Actually, the person has to obtain some energy from lean tissue because the brain, nervous system, and red blood cells need glucose, which fat cannot supply. Also, as mentioned, fat itself needs glucose to break down completely. Even on a total fast, a person cannot lose more than half a pound of pure fat per day. Still, in conditions of enforced starvation—say, during a siege or a famine—a fatter person can survive longer than a thinner person thanks to this energy reserve.

Although fat provides energy during a fast, it can provide only very little glucose to give energy to the brain and nerves. Only the small glycerol molecule can be converted to glucose; fatty acids cannot be. After prolonged glucose deprivation, brain and nerve cells develop the ability to derive about two-thirds of their energy from the ketone bodies that the body makes from fat without carbohydrate. Ketone bodies cannot sustain life by themselves, however. As Chapter 7 explains, fasting for too long will cause death, even if the person still has ample body fat.

In summary, the body makes special arrangements to digest, absorb, transport, store, and use lipids. It provides the emulsifier bile to make them accessible to the fat-digesting lipases that dismantle triglycerides, mostly to monoglycerides, for absorption by the intestinal cells. The intestinal cells assemble freshly absorbed lipids into chylomicrons, lipid packages with protein escorts, for transport so that cells all over the body may select needed lipids from them. The liver also packages lipids and proteins into other lipoproteins—VLDL, LDL, and HDL—for transport around the body. Cells, especially fat cells, select and store triglycerides from these lipoproteins for later use as an energy fuel and assimilate other lipids such as cholesterol into their membranes. Unneeded lipids are returned to the liver for disposal. High LDL (which are high in cholesterol) portend a high risk of heart disease; high HDL (which are returning lipids for disposal) signify a low risk.

The body can easily store unlimited amounts of fat if excesses are available, and this body fat is used for energy when needed. The liver can also convert excess carbohydrate and protein into fat. Fat breakdown requires simultaneous carbohydrate breakdown for maximum efficiency; without carbohydrate, fats break down to ketone bodies producing ketosis.

Health Effects and Recommended Intakes of Lipids

Of all the nutrients, fat is most often linked with chronic diseases. A high-fat diet raises the risks of heart disease, some types of cancer, and obesity. Fortunately, the same recommendation can help with all of these health problems: eat less fat.

1 lb body fat = 3500 kcal.

The small contribution that fat can make to the body's glucose supply is detailed in Chapter 7.

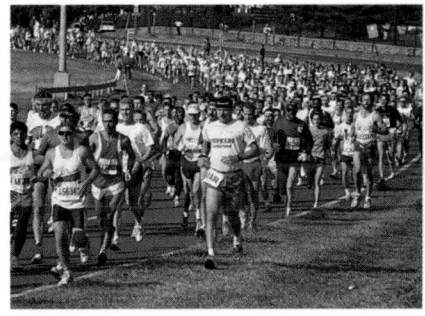
Fat supplies most of the energy in a long-distance run.

---

*The reader who knows that 1 pound = 454 grams and that 1 gram of fat = 9 kcalories may wonder why a pound of body fat does not equal 9×454 kcalories. The reason is that body fat contains some cell water and other materials; it is not quite pure fat.

blood lipid profile: results of blood tests that reveal a person's total cholesterol, triglycerides, and various lipoproteins.

Desirable blood lipid profile:
- Total cholesterol: <200 mg/dL.
- LDL cholesterol: <130 mg/dL.
- HDL cholesterol: >35 mg/dL.
- Triglycerides: <200 mg/dL.

cardiovascular disease (CVD): a general term for all diseases of the heart and blood vessels. Atherosclerosis is the main cause of CVD. When the arteries that carry blood to the heart muscle become occluded, the heart suffers damage known as **coronary heart disease (CHD)**.

　cardio = heart
　vascular = blood vessels

Other risk factors for heart disease include smoking, high blood pressure, diabetes, family history, sex, race, and obesity. Chapter 28 provides many more details about these risk factors, the development of heart disease, and dietary recommendations.

Hearing a physician say, "Your blood lipid profile looks fine," is reassuring. The blood lipid profile reveals the concentrations of various lipids in the blood, notably triglycerides and cholesterol, and their lipoprotein carriers (VLDL, LDL, and HDL). This information alerts people to their disease risks and their need to change eating habits.

Heart Disease　Most people realize that elevated blood cholesterol is a major risk factor for cardiovascular disease.* Cholesterol accumulates in the arteries, restricting blood flow and raising blood pressure. The consequences are deadly; in fact, heart disease is the nation's number one killer of adults. Blood cholesterol is often used to predict the likelihood of a person's suffering a heart attack or stroke; the higher the cholesterol, the earlier and more likely the tragedy.

Commercials advertise products that are low in cholesterol, and magazine articles tell readers how to cut the cholesterol in their favorite recipes. What most people don't realize, though, is that *food* cholesterol does not raise *blood* cholesterol as dramatically as *saturated fat* does.

Risks from Saturated Fats　Recall that LDL cholesterol raises the risk of heart disease. LDL concentrations respond to both the total amount and the type of fat in the diet. Most often implicated in raising LDL cholesterol are the saturated fats, although not all saturated fats have the same cholesterol-raising effect.[15] Most notable among the saturated fatty acids that raise blood cholesterol are lauric, myristic, and palmitic acids (12, 14, and 16 carbons, respectively). In contrast, stearic acid (18 carbons) does not seem to raise blood cholesterol.[16] Common sources of stearic acid are beef (tallow) and milk chocolate (cocoa butter).

Effects of Polyunsaturated and Monounsaturated Fats　In general, polyunsaturated fatty acids lower LDL cholesterol, and monounsaturated fatty acids have little or no independent effect.[17] Dietary cholesterol's influence on blood cholesterol is relatively minor.

Also of interest are the effects these fats have on the "good" HDL cholesterol. Some research suggests that polyunsaturated fats tend to lower both HDL and LDL, whereas monounsaturated fats raise HDL, thus improving the blood lipid profile.[18] Other research finds that both polyunsaturated and monounsaturated fatty acids lower both LDL and HDL.[19]

Risks from *Trans*-Fatty Acids　In the body, *trans*-fatty acids—even the monounsaturated ones—alter blood cholesterol the same way as some saturated fats do: they raise LDL and lower HDL cholesterol, although not to the same extent.[20] Recent epidemiological studies have linked dietary *trans*-fatty acids to heart disease risk,[21] but a study examining *trans*-fatty acids in adipose tissue found no correlation.[22] Clearly, this is an area of active research that is not yet ready for the evening news.

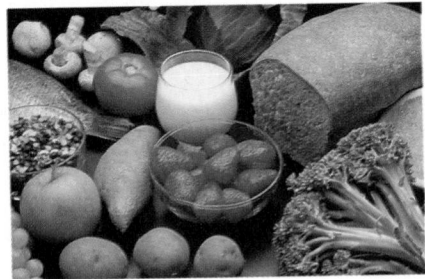

Enjoy low-fat foods for good heart health.

*The concentration of cholesterol is similar in *blood*, *plasma*, and *serum*; this book uses the term *blood* cholesterol. Plasma is blood with the cells removed; serum is plasma with the clotting factors also removed.

Reports on *trans*-fatty acids have raised consumer doubts about whether margarine is, after all, a better choice than butter for heart health. The American Heart Association has stated that because butter is rich in both saturated fat and cholesterol and because margarine is made from vegetable fat with no dietary cholesterol, margarine is still preferable to butter.[23] Others disagree, claiming the occasional use of butter is preferable to the use of products containing *trans*-fatty acids.[24] In addition to strict limits on *trans*-fatty acid use, some experts are calling for food labels to state the *trans*-fatty acid amounts in foods.[25]

The exact amount of *trans*-fatty acids in the diet is unknown, but it is lower than saturated fat intake.[26] If consumers limit their consumption of all types of fat, their *trans*-fatty acid intakes will most likely remain the same or decline.[27] The American Dietetic Association considers that current intakes are not harmful and that health risks from saturated fatty acids far outweigh those from *trans*-fatty acids.[28]

Benefits from Omega-3 Fatty Acids   Research on the omega-3 polyunsaturated fatty acids has spotlighted the unique effects of different types of fat on blood cholesterol and heart disease. Inuit peoples of Alaska and Greenland enjoy relative freedom from heart disease despite high-energy, high-fat, high-cholesterol diets. Why? Their foods derive primarily from marine animals and are rich in omega-3 fatty acids, particularly EPA and DHA. Research reveals that a diet rich in fish oils can lower blood cholesterol, just as a low-fat, low-saturated fat diet can.[29] (The research compared a diet with 2 percent of daily intake from fish oils with a diet of 25 percent total fat, 5 percent saturated.) A diet with both attributes produces an optimal lipid profile. In addition to improving blood lipids, fish oils prevent blood clots and may also lower blood pressure, especially in people with hypertension or atherosclerosis.[30]

Data from Japan seem to confirm that a diet low in fat and high in fish benefits health. The Japanese diet today has become westernized with few Japanese people eating the large quantities of rice and fish their ancestors ate. These dietary changes have been accompanied by health consequences: higher rates of cardiovascular disease and cancer.[31]

Cancer   The evidence linking dietary fats with cancer is less conclusive than for heart disease, but it does suggest an association between total fat and some types of cancers. Dietary fat seems not to *initiate* cancer development but to *promote* cancer once it has arisen. Some epidemiological studies suggest a relationship between specific cancers and saturated fats or dietary fat from animal sources (which is mostly saturated). Thus health advice to reduce cancer risks parallels that given to reduce heart disease risks: reduce total fat, especially saturated fat, intake.

Animal studies confirm that high-fat diets promote cancer development.[32] The data, however, are not fully consistent with evidence from epidemiological studies, most likely because the animals are fed extremely large amounts of specific fats—much higher than people typically eat. Animal studies suggest that *polyunsaturated fats* from vegetable oils (mostly omega-6 fatty acids) are more likely to promote cancer than are saturated fats. On the other hand, polyunsaturated fats from fish oils (mostly omega-3 fatty acids) are likely to delay cancer development and reduce the rate of growth and the size and number of tumors.[33] Research indicates that the omega-6 linoleic acid promotes tumor activity

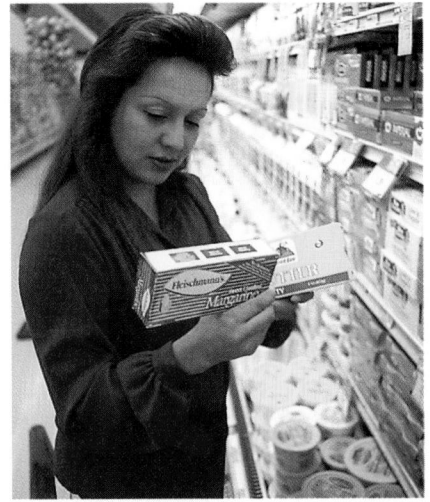

Whether you decide to use butter or margarine, remember to use them sparingly.

Chapter 28 presents many more details on the action of omega-3 fatty acids in preventing heart disease.

hypertension: high blood pressure; defined further in Chapter 28.

Other risk factors for cancer include smoking, alcohol, and environmental contaminants. Chapter 30 provides many more details about these risk factors and the development of cancer.

through the synthesis of prostaglandins derived from arachidonic acid and that omega-3 fatty acids inhibit that metabolism.[34]

The relationship between dietary fat and the risk of cancer differs for various types of cancers. In the case of breast cancer, some studies suggest little or no association between dietary fat and cancer.[35] Others find that total *energy* intake is a better predictor than percentage of kcalories from fat.[36] In the case of prostate cancer, there does appear to be a strong association with fat.[37] Research suggests that this association is due primarily to the saturated fat from meats; fat from milk or fish is not implicated in cancer risk.

Obesity   As the photos in Figure 5–19 show, fat accounts for a lot of the energy in foods, and removing the fat from foods cuts energy intake dramatically. Fat contributes twice as many kcalories per gram as either carbohydrate or protein. Consequently, people who eat high-fat diets tend to exceed their energy needs and gain weight.

Furthermore, people who eat high-fat diets tend to store body fat efficiently.[38] Some studies suggest that dietary fat influences body fat independently of total

Remember, fat is a more concentrated energy source than the other energy nutrients: 1 g carbohydrate or protein = 4 kcal, but 1 g fat = 9 kcal.

Figure 5–19

Cutting Fat Cuts kCalories

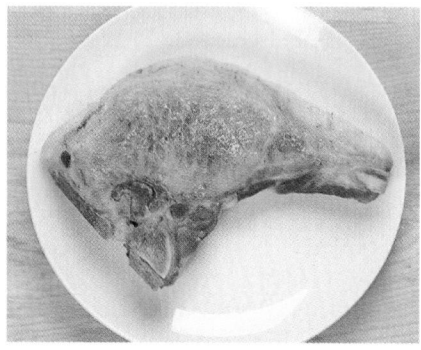

Pork chop with a half-inch of fat (275 kcal and 19 g fat).

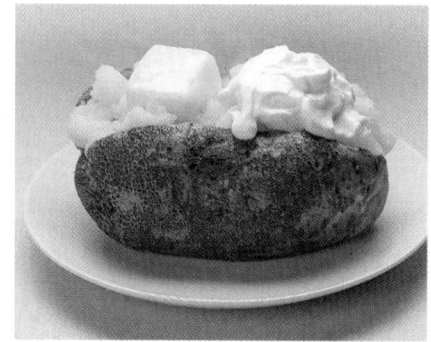

Potato with 1 tbs butter and 1 tbs sour cream (350 kcal and 14 g fat).

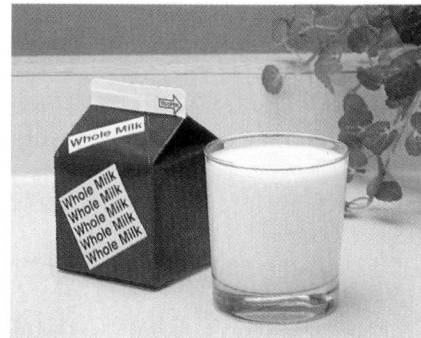

Whole milk, 1 c (150 kcal and 8 g fat).

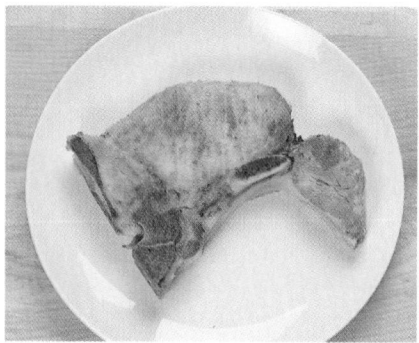

Pork chop with fat trimmed off (165 kcal and 8 g fat).

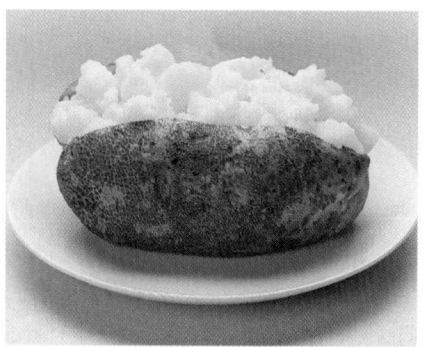

Plain potato (220 kcal and <1 g fat).

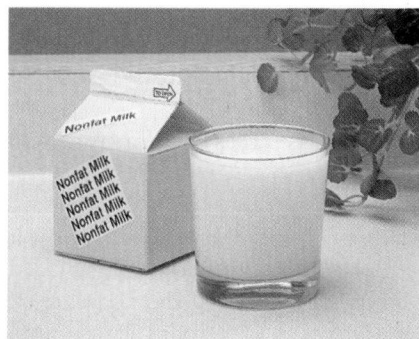

Nonfat milk, 1 c (90 kcal and 1 g fat).

energy intake; that is, people who eat high-fat diets have more body fat than their energy intakes would predict.[39] For satisfying hunger and controlling appetite, low-fat, high-carbohydrate foods are most appropriate.[40]

Don't Overdo Fat Restriction   Although it is very difficult to do, some people actually manage to eat too little fat—to their detriment. Among them are people with eating disorders, described in Highlight 9. As a practical guideline, it is wise to include the equivalent of at least a teaspoon of fat in every meal—a little peanut butter on toast or mayonnaise on tuna, for example. Parents should not restrict the fat intakes of their infants and young children; dietary recommendations that limit fat were developed for healthy people over age two.

RECOMMENDED INTAKES OF FAT

The Committee on Dietary Allowances has not established an RDA for fat, but the Committee on Diet and Health makes the following recommendations:

- Reduce total fat intake to 30 percent or less of energy intake.
- Reduce saturated fat intake to less than 10 percent of energy intake.
- Reduce cholesterol intake to less than 300 milligrams daily.

A person consuming 2000 kcalories a day should therefore have 600 kcalories or less from fat (roughly 65 grams). Of those fat kcalories, only 200 should come from saturated fats (roughly 22 grams).

HEALTHY PEOPLE 2000: Reduce dietary fat intake to an average of 30% of energy or less and average saturated fat intake to less than 10% of energy among people aged two years and older.

To meet dietary fat recommendations, many people have reduced their fat intakes. Fat intake peaked at 42 percent of daily kcalories in the late 1950s and has fallen steadily ever since.[41] The most recent surveys report that adults in the United States receive about 34 percent of their total energy from fat, with saturated fat contributing about 12 percent of the total.[42] The average cholesterol intake in the United States is 300 to 450 milligrams a day.[43]

Reduce Total Fat Intake   Triglycerides are abundant in all fats and oils. They also accompany protein in foods derived from animals, such as meat, fish, poultry, and eggs, and carbohydrate in foods derived from plants, such as avocados and coconuts.

To reduce dietary fat, eliminate fat as a seasoning and in cooking; remove the fat from high-fat foods; replace high-fat foods with low-fat alternatives; and emphasize grains, fruits, and vegetables. The accompanying box provides additional tips for reducing fat in the diet, food group by food group.

Reduce Saturated Fat Intake   Fats from animal sources are the main sources of saturated fats in most people's diets. Some vegetable fats (coconut and palm) and hydrogenated fats provide smaller amounts of saturated fats. Selecting lean meats and nonfat milk products helps to lower saturated fat intake.

Meat, Fish, and Poultry

- Fat adds up quickly, even with lean meat; limit intake to about 6 ounces (cooked weight) daily.
- Choose fish, poultry, or lean cuts of pork or beef; look for unmarbled cuts named *round* or *loin* (eye of round, top round, round tip, tenderloin, sirloin, and top loin).
- Trim the fat from pork and beef; remove the skin from poultry.
- Grill, roast, broil, bake, stir-fry, stew, or braise meats; don't fry. When possible, place meat on a rack so that fat can drain.
- Use lean ground turkey or lean ground beef in recipes; brown ground meats without added fat, then drain off fat.
- Refrigerate meat pan drippings and broth; when it solidifies, remove the fat and use the defatted broth in recipes.
- Select tuna and other canned meats packed in water; rinse oil-packed items with hot water to remove much of the fat.
- Fill kabob skewers with lots of vegetables and slivers of meat; create main dishes and casseroles by combining a little meat, fish, or poultry with a lot of pasta, rice, or vegetables.
- Make meatless spaghetti sauces and casseroles; use legumes often.
- Eat a meatless meal or two daily.

Milk and Cheeses

- Drink nonfat and low-fat milk instead of whole milk.
- Use nonfat and low-fat cheeses (such as part-skim ricotta and low-fat mozzarella) instead of regular cheeses.
- Use nonfat or low-fat yogurt or fat-free sour cream instead of regular sour cream.
- Use evaporated nonfat milk instead of cream.
- Enjoy nonfat frozen yogurt, sherbet, or ice milk instead of ice cream.

Fruits and Vegetables

- Enjoy the natural flavor of steamed vegetables for dinner and fruits for dessert.
- Use butter-flavored granules on vegetables instead of butter or margarine.
- Use nonfat yogurt or nonfat salad dressing instead of sour cream, cheese, mayonnaise, or other sauces on vegetables and in casseroles.
- Select nonfat or low-fat salad dressings, or use herbs, lemon juice, and spices instead of regular salad dressing.
- Add a little water to thick, bottled salad dressing to dilute the amount of fat each serving provides.
- Eat at least two vegetables (in addition to a salad) with dinner.
- Snack on raw vegetables or fruits instead of high-fat items like potato chips.

Breads and Cereals

- Use fruit butters or jellies on bread instead of butter or margarine.
- Select breads, cereals, and crackers that are low in fat (for example, bagels instead of croissants).

Other Foods and Cooking Tips

- Use a nonstick pan or coat the pan lightly with vegetable oil.
- Use egg substitutes in recipes instead of whole eggs or use 2 egg whites in place of each whole egg.
- Use half the margarine, butter, or oil called for in a recipe. (The minimum amount of fat for muffins, quick breads, and biscuits is 1 to 2 tablespoons per cup of flour; for cakes and cookies, 2 tablespoons per cup.)
- Use less butter or margarine. Select the whipped types of butter, margarine, or cream cheese for use at the table; they contain half the kcalories of the regular types.
- Use butter replacers instead of butter.
- For sandwiches and salads, use spicy mustard, nonfat salad dressing, lemon juice, flavored vinegar, salsa or the nonfat versions instead of regular mayonnaise, salad dressing, or sour cream.
- Use wine; lemon, orange, or tomato juice; herbs; spices; fruits; or broth instead of butter, margarine, or oil when cooking.
- Stir-fry in a small amount of oil; add moisture and flavor with broth, tomato juice, or wine.
- Use variety to enhance enjoyment of the meal: vary colors, textures, and temperatures—hot cooked versus cool raw foods—and use garnishes to complement food.

Reduce Cholesterol Intake   Recall that cholesterol is found only in animal products. Consequently, eating less fat from meat, eggs, and milk products will also help lower dietary cholesterol intake (as well as total and saturated fat intakes).

Balance Omega-3 and Omega-6 Intakes   The Committee on Dietary Allowances has not established an RDA for omega-3 and omega-6 fatty acids, but recommends that future committees consider the possibility.[44] The 1990 Canadian RNI include specific amounts for both omega-3 and omega-6 fatty acids.* Many researchers believe the body's requirements depend on an optimal ratio; that is, that more omega-3 fatty acids are not necessarily better, but that an appropriate balance between the two omega families may be crucial.[45] A ratio of about 1 to 4 (omega-3 to omega-6 fatty acids) has been suggested as appropriate.

To obtain the right balance between omega-3 and omega-6 fatty acids, most people need to eat more fish and less vegetable oil. Eating fish instead of meat two or three meals a week supports heart health, especially when combined with physical activity.[46] Even one fish meal a week may be enough to make a difference.[47] The fish may not even need to be rich in omega-3 fatty acids; one study found that farm-raised catfish (which is relatively low in omega-3 fatty acids) improves lipid profiles similarly to wild Alaskan salmon.[48] Fish provides many minerals (except iron) and vitamins and is leaner than most other animal-protein sources. In an effort to improve health, people are well advised to eat fish periodically.

Fish oil should come from fish, not from supplements. Fish oil supplements are not recommended for a number of reasons.† Perhaps most importantly, the scientific evidence on their safety and effectiveness is not conclusive.[49] Also, high intakes of fish oil increase bleeding time, interfere with wound healing, worsen diabetes, and impair immune function.[50] Fish oil supplements are made from fish skins and livers, which may contain other environmental contaminants. Fish oils also naturally contain high levels of the two most potentially toxic vitamins, A and D. Lastly, supplements are expensive; money is better spent on foods that can provide a full array of nutrients.

Select Lean Meats and Nonfat Milks   Many foods that contain fat, saturated fat, and cholesterol—such as meats, milk, cheese, and eggs—also provide high-quality protein and valuable vitamins and minerals. They can be included in a healthy diet if a person selects lean and nonfat products and prepares them using the suggestions outlined in the box on p. 168.

Eat Plenty of Vegetables, Fruits, and Grains   Choosing vegetables, fruits, cereals, and legumes also helps lower fat intake. Vegetables and fruits contain no fat, and most grains contain only trace amounts. Some grain *products* such as fried taco shells, croissants, and granola cereal are high in fat, though, so consumers need to read product labels.

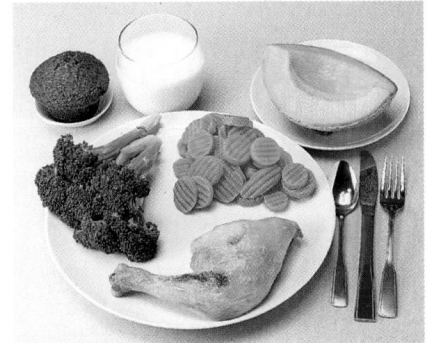

Even well-balanced, healthy meals provide some fat. In this meal, no butter is used and the beverage is nonfat milk, but 30 percent of the kcalories come from fat.

---

*For omega-3 fatty acids, the RNI is 0.5 percent of total energy or 0.55 grams per 1000 kcalories; for omega-6 fatty acids, the RNI is 3 percent of total energy or 3.3 grams per 1000 kcalories.

†In Canada, fish oil supplements require a physician's prescription.

Because a low-fat diet is usually rich in vegetables, fruits, cereals, and legumes, it offers abundant vitamin C, folate, vitamin A, and dietary fiber—all important in supporting health. Consequently such a diet protects against disease in two ways, reducing fat and increasing nutrients.[51]

Use Fats and Oils Sparingly   Practice moderation when using oils and fats such as butter, margarine, mayonnaise, and salad dressings. These foods offer much fat and little nourishment.

Look for Invisible Fat   It can be surprising how much *invisible* fat some foods contain. Any *fried* food contains abundant fat: potato chips, french fries, fried wontons, and fried fish. Many *baked* goods, too, are high in fat: pie crusts, pastries, biscuits, cornbread, doughnuts, sweet rolls, cookies, and cakes. Most chocolate bars contain more fat energy than sugar energy. Even cream-of-mushroom soup prepared with water derives 66 percent of its energy from fat. Abundant fat lurks on salad bars, too, not only in the dressings, but also in the potato salad, the macaroni salad, the coleslaw, and the marinated beans that are mixed with oil-based dressings. Keep invisible fats in mind when making food selections.

Some fat is easy to see: *visible fat,* such as butter, the oil in salad dressing, and the fat trimmed from meat. Other fat is less apparent: *invisible fat,* such as the fat that "marbles" a steak or is hidden in foods like nuts, cheese, crackers, avocados, olives, fried foods, bakery items, and chocolate.

Choose Wisely   The *Dietary Guidelines* urge people to choose a diet low in fat, saturated fat, and cholesterol. A diet following the Daily Food Guide plan can support this goal if selections are made carefully. Only by following such a plan and making low-fat choices consistently can the goals of the *Diet and Health* recommendations be met.

Consumers are finding more low-fat food choices available than ever before. In many cases, they are familiar foods presented now with less fat. Leaner animals are raised for meat, and cuts of meat are often trimmed of fat more closely than in the past. In the dairy case, nonfat and reduced-fat milk, yogurt, cheeses, and sour cream offer healthy alternatives to their higher-fat counterparts. Many processed foods such as salad dressings, crackers, chips, and cookies are now available with little or no fat. Such choices make low-fat eating easy. A simple switch to nonfat salad dressing can bring the average fat intake for women down from 37 to 34 percent of total kcalories.[52] Every little fat-saving step helps a person get closer to the 30 percent goal.

Many fat-free foods have been developed using familiar nutrients. Milk and egg proteins or carbohydrate derivatives, for example, are heated, acidified, or blended to simulate the properties of fat. Highlight 5 examines some of these new alternatives to fat.

 HEALTHY PEOPLE 2000: Increase to at least 5000 brand items the number of processed food products that are reduced in fat and saturated fat.

Read Food Labels   Labels list total fat, saturated fat, and cholesterol contents of foods in addition to fat kcalories per serving. (Labels do not provide information on *trans*-fatty acids; if the ingredients list includes hydrogenated oils, though, you know the food contains *trans*-fatty acids—you just don't know how much.) Because each package provides information for a single serving and serving sizes are standardized, consumers can easily compare similar products. Total

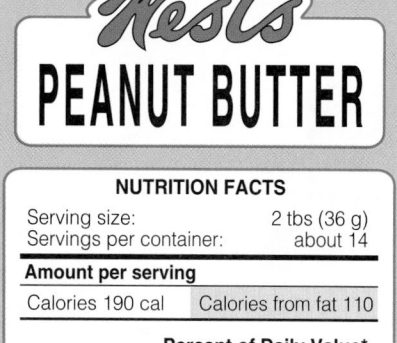

Hest's
PEANUT BUTTER

NUTRITION FACTS

Serving size:	2 tbs (36 g)
Servings per container:	about 14

Amount per serving

Calories 190 cal	Calories from fat 110

Percent of Daily Value*

Total Fat 12 g	18%
Saturated fat 2.5 g	13%
Cholesterol 0 mg	0%
Sodium 150 mg	6%
Total Carbohydrate 14 g	5%
Dietary fiber 2 g	8%
Sugars 5 g	
Protein 8 g	

The Lipids: Triglycerides, Phospholipids, and Sterols **171**

fat, saturated fat, and cholesterol are also expressed as "% Daily Values" for a person consuming 2000 kcalories. People who are consuming more or less than 2000 kcalories daily can calculate their personal Daily Value for fat as described in the box on p. 172.

Be aware that the "% Daily Value" for fat is not the same as "% kcalories from fat." Consider, for example, a piece of lemon meringue pie that provides 140 kcalories and 12 grams of fat. Because the Daily Value for fat is 65 grams for a 2000-kcalorie intake, 12 grams represents about 18 percent, or almost one-fifth, of the day's fat allowance (the pie's "% Daily Value" is 18). Uninformed consumers may mistakenly believe that this food meets the guideline to limit fat to "30 percent kcalories," but it doesn't—for two reasons. First, the pie's 12 grams of fat contribute 108 of the 140 kcalories, for a total of 77 percent kcalories from fat. Second, the "30 percent kcalories from fat" guideline applies to a day's total intake, not to an individual food. (Of course, if every selection throughout the day exceeds 30 percent kcalories from fat, you can be certain that the day's total intake does, too.)

Because recommendations apply to average daily intakes and not to individual food items, food labels do not provide the percent kcalories from fat. Still, you can get an idea of whether a particular food is high or low in fat. To quickly compare recommendations with the fat content of a food, use the rule of thumb that 3 grams of fat (27 kcalories of fat) represent about 30 percent of the kcalories in 100 kcalories of food. Alternatively, you can multiply the grams of fat in a serving by 30 and then compare that number to the kcalories.[53] If it is less, then the food has less than 30 percent kcalories from fat.

The FDA authorizes two health claims on labels concerning fat: one for "dietary saturated fat and cholesterol and risk of coronary heart disease" and one for "dietary fat and cancer." To make these claims, foods must meet specified criteria, as described in Chapter 2.

In summary, health authorities single out high fat intakes as a major flaw in the North American diet: excess fat contributes to heart disease, cancer, obesity, and other health problems. High blood LDL cholesterol, specifically, poses a risk of heart disease, and high intakes of saturated fat contribute most to high LDL. Cholesterol itself, in foods, presents much less of a risk; *trans*-fatty acids' effects are not yet clear from research. Omega-3 fatty acids appear to be protective, especially if consumed in a 1-to-4 ratio with omega-6 fatty acids. High fat diets also accelerate (but do not initiate) cancer development. Health authorities recommend limiting total fat to 30 percent or less of energy intake; saturated fat to one-third of total fat, or 10 percent of energy intake; and cholesterol to less than 300 milligrams a day. They also recommend consuming relatively more polyunsaturates, particularly omega-3 fatty acids, than in the past from foods such as fish, not from supplements. Many purchasing and cooking strategies can help bring these goals within reach, and the new food labels make it easier to select foods consistent with these guidelines.

If people were to make only one change in their diets, they would be wise to limit their intakes of total fat, which would control their energy intake as well. A second change might be to specifically limit saturated fat. Chances are good that if total fat and saturated fat meet recommendations, then cholesterol intake will, too. Many guidelines suggest these changes in that order of priority: low in fat, saturated fat, and cholesterol.

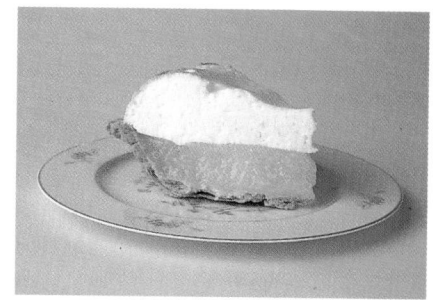

% Daily Value:
- 12 g ÷ 65 g = 0.18 × 100 = 18%.

% kCalories from Fat:
- 12 g × 9 kcal/g = 108 kcal.
  108 kcal ÷ 140 kcal = 77%.

How to Calculate a Personal Daily Value for Fat

The % Daily Value for fat on food labels is based on 65 grams. To know that you've met recommendations, you can either count grams until you reach 65, or add the "% Daily Values" until you reach 100 percent—if your energy intake is 2000 kcalories a day. If your energy intake is more or less, there are a couple of options.

You can calculate your personal daily fat allowance in grams. Multiply your total energy intake by 30 percent, then divide by 9. Suppose your energy intake is 1800 kcalories per day and your goal is 30 percent kcalories from fat:

$$1800 \text{ total kcal} \times 0.30 \text{ from fat} = 540 \text{ fat kcal.}$$

$$540 \text{ fat kcal} \div 9 \text{ kcal/g} = 60 \text{ g fat.}$$

Another way to calculate your personal fat allowance is to cross out the last digit of your energy intake and divide by 3.[a] For example, 1800 kcalories becomes 180; then you divide by 3:

$$180 \div 3 = 60 \text{ g fat/day.}$$

(In familiar measures, 60 grams of fat is about the same as ⅔ stick of butter or ¼ cup of oil.)

The accompanying table shows the numbers of grams of fat allowed per day for various energy intakes. With one of these numbers in mind, you can quickly evaluate the number of fat grams in foods you are considering eating.

Recommended Grams of Fat for Different Energy Intakes

Energy (kcal/day)	30 Percent kCalories	Fat (g/day)
1200	360	40
1500	450	50
1800	540	60
1900 (RDA for women 51 years and over)	570	63
2000 (Daily Value for food labels)	600	65
2200 (RDA for women 19 to 50 years old)	660	73
2300 (RDA for men 51 years and over)	690	77
2600	780	87
2900 (RDA for men 19 to 50 years old)	870	97
3000	900	100

[a]K. McNutt, Fat traps, tips, and tricks, *Nutrition Today*, May/June 1992, pp. 47–49.

Quick and easy estimates:
- A food is low in fat if it has:
  ≤3 g fat in 100 kcal food.
- A food is low in fat if:
  g fat × 30 < kcal.

Lowering fat intake can be difficult, though, because fats make foods taste delicious. To maintain good health, must a person give up all high-fat foods forever—never again to eat marbled steak, hollandaise sauce, or gooey chocolate cake? Not at all. These foods bring pleasure to a meal and can be enjoyed as part of a healthy diet when eaten in small quantities on occasion, but it is true that they are not everyday foods. The key word for fat is not deprivation, but moderation: appreciate the energy and enjoyment that fat provides, but take care not to exceed your needs.

Study Questions

1. Name the three classes of lipids found in the body and in foods. What features do fats bring to foods? What are some of their functions in the body?
2. Describe the structure of a triglyceride. What are the differences between saturated, unsaturated, monounsaturated, and polyunsaturated fats?
3. What two features distinguish fatty acids from each other?
4. What does hydrogenation do to fats? What are *trans*-fatty acids, and how do they influence heart disease?
5. What does the term *omega* mean with respect to fatty acids? Describe the roles of the omega fatty acids in disease prevention.
6. Which of the fatty acids are essential? Name their chief dietary sources.
7. How do phospholipids differ from triglycerides in structure? How does cholesterol differ? How do these differences in structure affect function?
8. Trace the steps in fat digestion, absorption, and transport.
9. What do lipoproteins do? What are the differences among the chylomicrons, VLDL, LDL, and HDL?
10. What roles does cholesterol play in the body?
11. Describe the routes cholesterol takes in the body.
12. What roles do the triglycerides and phospholipids perform in the body?
13. How does excessive fat intake influence health? What factors influence LDL, HDL, and total blood cholesterol?
14. What are the dietary recommendations regarding fat and cholesterol intake? List ways to reduce intake.
15. What is the Daily Value for fat (for a 2000-kcalorie diet)? What does this number represent?

Notes

1. D. J. Mela and D. A. Sacchetti, Sensory preferences for fat: Relationships with diet and body composition, *American Journal of Clinical Nutrition* 53 (1991): 908–915.
2. J. E. Hunter and T. H. Applewhite, Reassessment of *trans* fatty acid availability in the US diet, *American Journal of Clinical Nutrition* 54 (1991): 363–369; M. G. Enig and coauthors, Isomeric *trans* fatty acids in the U.S. diet, *Journal of the American College of Nutrition* 9 (1990): 471–486.
3. C. A. Drevon, Marine oils and their effects, *Nutrition Reviews* 50 (1992): 38–45.
4. M. A. Crawford, The role of essential fatty acids in neural development: Implications for perinatal nutrition, *American Journal of Clinical Nutrition* 57 (1993): 703S–710S; J. A. Nettleton, Are n-3 fatty acids essential nutrients for fetal and infant development? *Journal of the American Dietetic Association* 93 (1993): 58–64.
5. W. E. Connor, M. Neuringer, and S. Reisbick, Essential fatty acids: The importance of n-3 fatty acids in the retina and brain, *Nutrition Reviews* 50 (1992): II21–II29.
6. A. P. Simopoulos, Omega-3 fatty acids in health and disease and in growth and development, *American Journal of Clinical Nutrition* 54 (1991): 438–463.
7. D. S. Lin and W. E. Connor, Are the n-3 fatty acids from dietary fish oil deposited in the triglyceride stores of adipose tissue? *American Journal of Clinical Nutrition* 51 (1990): 535–539.
8. Scientific Review Committee, *Nutrition Recommendations: The Report of the Scientific Review Committee, 1990* (Ottawa: Canadian Government Publishing Centre, 1990), p. 45; P. J. Nestel, Polyunsaturated fatty acids (n-3, n-6), *American Journal of Clinical Nutrition* 45 (1987): 1161–1167; M. Neuringer, G. J. Anderson, and W. E. Connor, The essentiality of N-3 fatty acids for the development and function of the retina and brain, *Annual Review of Nutrition* 8 (1988): 517–541.
9. J. A. Nettleton, ω-3 Fatty acids: Comparison of plant and seafood sources in human nutrition, *Journal of the American Dietetic Association* 91 (1991): 331–337; J. E. Hunter, n-3 Fatty acids from vegetable oils, *American Journal of Clinical Nutrition* 51 (1990): 809–814; Committee on Dietary Allowances, *Recommended Dietary Allowances*, 10th ed. (Washington, D.C.: National Academy Press, 1989), pp. 47–48.
10. L. M. Arnold and coauthors, Effect of isoenergetic intake of three or nine meals on plasma lipoproteins and glucose metabolism, *American Journal of Clinical Nutrition* 57 (1993): 446–451; P. J. H. Jones, C. A. Leitch, and R. A Pederson, Meal-frequency effects on plasma hormone concentrations and cholesterol synthesis in humans, *American Journal of Clinical Nutrition* 57 (1993): 868–874; D. J. A. Jenkins and coau-

thors, Nibbling versus gorging: Metabolic advantages of increased meal frequency, *New England Journal of Medicine* 321 (1989): 929–934.

11. M. Hamosh, *Lingual and Gastric Lipases: Their Role in Fat Digestion* (Boston: CRC Press, 1990).

12. R. Havel, McCollum Award Lecture, 1993: Triglyceride-rich lipoproteins and atherosclerosis—New perspectives, *American Journal of Clinical Nutrition* 59 (1994): 795–799.

13. NIH Consensus Conference, Triglyceride, high-density lipoprotein, and coronary heart disease, *Journal of the American Medical Association* 269 (1993): 505–510; M. J. Stampfer and coauthors, A prospective study of cholesterol, apolipoproteins, and the risk of myocardial infarction, *New England Journal of Medicine* 325 (1991): 373–381.

14. J. L. Groff, S. S. Gropper, and S. M. Hunt, *Advanced Nutrition and Human Metabolism* (St. Paul, Minn.: West, 1995), pp. 466–483.

15. R. P. Mensink, Effects of the individual saturated fatty acids on serum lipid and lipoprotein concentrations, *American Journal of Clinical Nutrition* (supplement) 57 (1993): 711S–714S.

16. S. M. Grundy, Influence of stearic acid on cholesterol metabolism relative to other long-chain fatty acids, *American Journal of Clinical Nutrition* 60 (1994): 986S–990S.

17. B. V. Howard and coauthors, Polyunsaturated fatty acids result in greater cholesterol lowering and less triacylglycerol elevation than do monounsaturated fatty acids in a dose-response comparison in a multiracial study group, *American Journal of Clinical Nutrition* 62 (1995): 392–402; M. B. Katan, P. L. Zock, and R. P. Mensink, Effects of fats and fatty acids on blood lipids in humans: An overview, *American Journal of Clinical Nutrition* 60 (1994): 1017S–1022S; D. M. Hegsted and coauthors, Dietary fat and serum lipids: An evaluation of the experimental data, *American Journal of Clinical Nutrition* 57 (1993): 875–883.

18. Katan, Zock, and Mensink, 1994; P. Mata and coauthors, Effects of long-term monounsaturated- vs polyunsaturated-enriched diets on lipoproteins in healthy men and women, *American Journal of Clinical Nutrition* 55 (1992): 846–850.

19. M. C. Nydahl, I. B. Gustafsson, and B. Vessby, Lipid-lowering diets enriched with monounsaturated or polyunsaturated fatty acids but low in saturated fatty acids have similar effects on serum lipid concentrations in hyperlipidemic patients, *American Journal of Clinical Nutrition* 59 (1994): 115–122.

20. M. B. Katan, and P. L. Zock, *Trans* fatty acids and their effects on lipoproteins in humans, *Annual Review of Nutrition* 15 (1995): 473–493; A. H. Lichtenstein, *Trans* fatty acids and hydrogenated fat—What do we know? *Nutrition Today,* 30 (1995): 102–107; J. T. Judd and coauthors, Dietary *trans* fatty acids: Effects on plasma lipids and lipoproteins of healthy men and women, *American Journal of Clinical Nutrition* 59 (1994): 861–868; R. Troisi, W. C. Willett, and S. T. Weiss, *Trans*-fatty acid intake in relation to serum lipid concentrations in adult men, *American Journal of Clinical Nutrition* 56 (1992): 1019–1024.

21. A. Ascherio and coauthors, *Trans*-fatty acids intake and risk of myocardial infarction, *Circulation* 89 (1994): 94–101;

W. C. Willett and coauthors, Intake of *trans* fatty acids and risk of coronary heart disease among women, *Lancet* 341 (1993): 581–585.

22. L. C. Hudgins, J. Hirsch, and E. A. Emken, Correlation of isomeric fatty acids in human adipose tissue with clinical risk factors for cardiovascular disease, *American Journal of Clinical Nutrition* 53 (1991): 474–482.

23. American Heart Association, Nutrition Advisory Committee, *News Release,* Trans fatty acids, May 13, 1994.

24. W. C. Willett and A. Ascherio, *Trans* fatty acids: Are the effects only marginal? *American Journal of Public Health* 84 (1994): 722–724.

25. A. P. Simopoulos and coauthors, Conferences, symposia, and reports—The 1st Congress of the International Society for the Study of Fatty Acids and Lipids (ISSFAL): Fatty acids and lipids from cell biology to human disease, *Nutrition Today,* July/August 1994, pp. 24–27; Willett and Ascherio, 1994; M. B. Katan, European researcher calls for reconsideration of *trans* fatty acids, *Journal of the American Dietetic Association* 94 (1994): 1097–1098.

26. A. Lichtenstein, *Trans* fatty acids, blood lipids, and cardiovascular risk: Where do we stand? *Nutrition Reviews* 51 (1993): 340–343.

27. American Dietetic Association, *News Release,* Evidence inconclusive on trans fatty acids, May 16, 1994.

28. Editor's note (in response to Katan, 1994), *Journal of the American Dietetic Association* 94 (1994): 1097–1098.

29. A Nordöy and coauthors, Individual effects of dietary saturated fatty acids and fish oil on plasma lipids and lipoproteins in normal men, *American Journal of Clinical Nutrition* 57 (1993): 634–639.

30. M. C. Morris, F. Sacks, and B. Rosner, Does fish oil lower blood pressure? A meta-analysis of controlled trials, *Circulation* 88 (1993): 523–533; L. J. Appel and coauthors, Does supplementation of diet with 'fish oil' reduce blood pressure? A meta-analysis of controlled clinical trials, *Archives of Internal Medicine* 153 (1993): 1429–1438.

31. Y. Goto, Changing trends in dietary habits and cardiovascular disease in Japan: An overview, *Nutrition Reviews* 50 (1992): 398–401.

32. K. K. Carroll, Dietary fats and cancer, *American Journal of Clinical Nutrition* 53 (1991): 1064S–1067S.

33. M. Anti and coauthors, Effect of ω-3 fatty acids on rectal mucosal cell proliferation in subjects at risk for colon cancer, *Gastroenterology* 103 (1992): 883–891; Simopoulos, 1991; L. A. Sauer, R. T. Dauchy, and A. S. Hurtubise, Effects of omega-6 and omega-3 fatty acids on rate of ^{3}H-thymidine incorporation in hepatoma, *FASEB Journal* 4 (1990): A508; D. Magrane and M. Philley, Effects of dietary corn oil and menhaden oil on rat mammary tumorigenesis and PGE$_2$ levels, *FASEB Journal* 4 (1990): A1176.

34. R. A. Karmali, Fatty acid metabolism and biochemical mechanisms in cancer, in *Health Effects of Dietary Fatty Acids,* ed. G. J. Nelson (Champaign, Ill.: American Oil Chemists' Society, 1991), pp. 150–156.

35. L. H. Kushi and coauthors, Dietary fat and postmenopausal

breast cancer, *Journal of the National Cancer Institute* 84 (1992): 1092–1099; W. C. Willett and coauthors, Dietary fat and fiber in relation to risk of breast cancer: An 8-year follow-up, *Journal of the American Medical Association* 628 (1992): 2037–2044.

36. E. Barrett-Connor and N. J. Friedlander, Dietary fat, calories, and the risk of breast cancer in postmenopausal women: A prospective population-based study, *Journal of the American College of Nutrition* 12 (1993): 390–399.

37. K. J. Pienta and P. S. Esper, Is dietary fat a risk factor for prostate cancer? *Journal of the National Cancer Institute* 85 (1993): 1538–1540; E. Giovannuci and coauthors, A prospective study of dietary fat and risk of prostate cancer, *Journal of the National Cancer Institute* 85 (1993): 1571–1579.

38. C. Bennett and coauthors, Short-term effects of dietary-fat ingestion on energy expenditure and nutrient balance, *American Journal of Clinical Nutrition* 55 (1992): 1071–1077.

39. T. E. Prewitt and coauthors, Changes in body weight, body composition, and energy intakes in women fed high- and low-fat diets, *American Journal of Clinical Nutrition* 54 (1991): 304–310.

40. B. J. Rolls, Carbohydrates, fats, and satiety, *American Journal of Clinical Nutrition* 61 (1995): 960S–967S.

41. A. M. Stephen and N. J. Wald, Trends in individual consumption of dietary fat in the United States, 1920–1984, *American Journal of Clinical Nutrition* 52 (1990): 457–469.

42. Daily dietary fat and total food-energy intakes—Third National Health and Nutrition Examination Survey, Phase 1, 1988–91, *Morbidity and Mortality Weekly Report* 43 (1994): 116–117, 123–125.

43. C. L. Johnson and coauthors, Declining serum total cholesterol levels among US adults, *Journal of the American Medical Association* 269 (1993): 3002–3008.

44. Committee on Dietary Allowances, 1989, p. 48.

45. M. D. Boudreau and coauthors, Lack of dose response by dietary n-3 fatty acids at a constant ratio of n-3 to n-6 fatty acids in suppressing eicosanoid biosynthesis from arachidonic acid, *American Journal of Clinical Nutrition* 54 (1991): 111–117.

46. Simopoulos, 1991; K. N. Seidelin, B. Myrup, and B. Fischer-Hansen, n-3 fatty acids in adipose tissue and coronary artery disease are inversely related, *American Journal of Clinical Nutrition* 55 (1992): 1117–1119.

47. A. Ascherio and coauthors, Dietary intake of marine n-3 fatty acids, fish intake, and the risk of coronary disease among men, *New England Journal of Medicine* 332 (1995): 977–982; K. H. Bönaa, K. S. Bjerve, and A. Nordöy, Habitual fish consumption, plasma phospholipid fatty acids, and serum lipids: The Tromsö Study, *American Journal of Clinical Nutrition* 55 (1992): 1126–1134.

48. D. K. Tidwell and coauthors, Comparison of the effects of adding fish high or low in n-3 fatty acids to a diet conforming to the Dietary Guidelines for Americans, *Journal of the American Dietetic Association* 93 (1993): 1124–1128.

49. Fish oil supplements, *FDA Consumer*, October 1990, p. 32.

50. S. J. Bhathena and coauthors, Effects of ω-3 fatty acids and vitamin E on hormones involved in carbohydrate and lipid metabolism in men, *American Journal of Clinical Nutrition* 54 (1991): 684–688; K. L. Fritsche, S. C. Huang, and M. Misfeldt, Fish oil and immune function (letter), *Nutrition Reviews* 51 (1993): 24; H. Flaten and coauthors, Fish-oil concentrate: Effects on variables related to cardiovascular disease, *American Journal of Clinical Nutrition* 52 (1990): 300–306.

51. A. F. Subar and coauthors, US dietary patterns associated with fat intake: The 1987 National Health Interview Survey, *American Journal of Public Health* 84 (1994): 359–366.

52. M. Hudnall, M. G. Hermann-Zaidins, and J. S. Stern, Fat replacements: Helpful or not? *Journal of the American Dietetic Association* 92 (1992): 1330–1331.

53. D. Green-Burgeson, Calculating fat the easy way, *Journal of the American Dietetic Association* 94 (1994): 256.

Alternatives to Fat

As people learn more and more about the health consequences of high-fat diets, they want to lower their fat intake, but they'd rather not give up their favorite foods. As the adage goes, they want to have their cake and eat it, too—both figuratively and literally. Fat replacements offer an easy way to lower fat intake, while enjoying many foods that were once high in fat. Skeptics say that people will use these artificial fats the same way they use artificial sweeteners: in *addition* to fats rather than *instead* of fats, but preliminary reports indicate that people who use fat substitutes do eat less fat. They compensate with more carbohydrate, however, so that their total energy intakes remain constant.[1] Still, even if energy intakes remain steady, eating carbohydrate in place of fat improves blood lipids and helps to shift body composition toward the lean.

Food chemists have been working for decades on ways to reduce the fat in foods. Juggling the needs of the human body, the taste perceptions of consumers, and the requirements of food preparation is a complex task. For the body, products must contribute little food energy, must be nontoxic and completely excreted, and must not rob the body of valuable fat-soluble nutrients. To satisfy consumers, products must be attractive, feel right in the mouth, and have the right flavor. Food manufacturers need a compound that remains stable while meeting a product's requirements for temperature, moisture, and texture. That's a tall order, but it looks as though food chemists are mastering the task. Today shoppers can select from thousands of

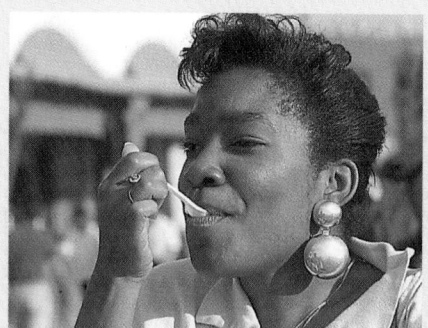

Low-fat and nonfat foods offer as much flavor and enjoyment as their high-fat counterparts—for less fat and fewer kcalories.

new reduced-fat products. Many bakery goods, cheeses, frozen desserts, and other products are available that offer less than half a gram of fat in a serving.

Some techniques for reducing food fat are quite simple. For example, manufacturers can lower fat by adding water or whipping in air. They use nonfat milk in creamy desserts and lean meats in frozen entrees. Sometimes they simply prepare the products differently. For example, fat-free potato chips are now baked instead of fried.

Some new products contain common food ingredients such as carbohydrates or proteins that replicate the texture of fat. Many of these products lack the sensation of richness provided by the fatty ingredients they replace. Innovative technologies are attempting to solve this problem by imitating the experience of eating fat—the creaminess as well as the taste—without the kcalories.[2] The many laboratories working to develop artificial fats are currently testing some 20 possible fat substitutes, most of them based on either carbohydrate, protein, or fat.

OATRIM AND OTHER CARBOHYDRATE-BASED FAT REPLACEMENTS

Several fat replacements are based on carbohydrate derivatives such as dextrins, modified food starches, and gums. One such product is maltodextrin, a carbohydrate derived from corn. When sprinkled on hot, moist foods such as baked potatoes, this product melts, providing a flavor similar to that of butter or margarine.

Another carbohydrate-based fat replacement is Oatrim, which is derived from oat fiber. Oatrim was developed by the U.S. Department of Agriculture to both reduce fat intake and lower blood cholesterol. An added advantage is that it provides satiety.

Most carbohydrate-based fat replacements are heat stable and can be used in baking, but not in frying. They mimic the texture and feel of fat by forming gels in foods such as margarines, frozen desserts, and salad dressings.

Because these carbohydrate derivatives are common dietary substances, companies can ask the FDA to approve them as generally recognized as safe (GRAS) substances. In fact, manufacturers have used these carbohydrate-based compounds for years as thickeners and stabilizers. The body digests and absorbs these substances, so they contribute some energy, although significantly less than fat's 9 kcalories per gram.

SIMPLESSE AND OTHER PROTEIN-BASED FAT REPLACEMENTS

Perhaps the best-known protein-based fat replacement is Simplesse. The FDA declared Simplesse safe for

use in ice cream and frozen desserts in 1990. Simplesse is made from either egg white or milk proteins processed into mistlike particles that feel and taste like fat. Because the components of Simplesse are common in foods, safety studies have not been required.

Simplesse cannot be used for frying or baking because it gels when heated and loses its creaminess. It works fine on hot foods, though; for example, it makes a good imitation butter spread for toast or a sour cream–type topping for a baked potato. Simplesse is not available for home use.

Simplesse creates the *perception* of fat without all the kcalories. In the body, Simplesse is digested and absorbed, contributing 1 to 2 kcalories per gram—a substantial reduction from fat's 9 kcalories per gram. Substituting Simplesse for fat reduces the energy values of some foods dramatically. In some cases, though, such as fat-free ice cream, so much sugar is added that the kcalorie count of a fat-free product may be as high as in the original (see Table H5–1). Replacing both the fat and sugar in a product is difficult to do, because both contribute to flavor, texture, and stability. Substituting Simplesse for fat, however, does reduce a food's fat and cholesterol content appreciably.

Some people, such as those who are allergic or sensitive to egg or milk proteins, may have to avoid Simplesse. (New regulations require a product's label to identify the source of its protein in the ingredient list.) People on protein-restricted diets may have to consult with their dietitians before including Simplesse in their diets, although its use is not expected to raise protein intake by more than 2 grams daily. Companies have developed other protein-

Table H5–1

Fat Content of Regular Foods and Foods Prepared with Fat Replacements

Food	Fat (g)	Cholesterol (mg)	Energy (kcal)
Ice cream			
Super premium (½ c)	19	97	274
Regular (½ c)	7	30	135
Ice milk (½ c)	3	9	92
Frozen dessert			
Made with Simplesse (½ c)	<1	14	120
Made with Oatrim (½ c)	1	4	135
Butter (1 tsp)	4	11	36
Margarine (1 tsp)	4	0	34
Maltodextrin sprinkles (½ tsp)	<1	0	3
French fries			
Fried in vegetable oil	12.3	0	227
Fried in 75% olestra blend	3.1	0	144
Chicken			
Fried in vegetable oil	14.6	0	252
Fried in 75% olestra blend	8.6	0	198
Onion rings			
Fried in vegetable oil	19.5	0	315
Fried in 75% olestra blend	4.9	0	184

Note: Equivalent serving sizes were compared; in the case of butter and margarine, ½ teaspoon of sprinkles was compared with 1 teaspoon butter or margarine as per label directions.

Sources: Oatrim: A potential fat substitute, *Nutrition Today*, July/August 1990, p. 4; M. Segal, Fat substitutes: A taste of the future? *FDA Consumer*, December 1990, pp. 25–27; J. E. Shields and E. Young, Fat in fast foods—Evolving changes, *Nutrition Today*, March/April 1990, pp. 32–35.

derived products similar to Simplesse but have yet to petition the FDA for approval.

OLESTRA AND OTHER FAT-BASED FAT REPLACEMENTS

In January 1996, the FDA approved a fake fat known as olestra for use in snack foods.[3] Olestra is the first artificial fat to reach the market that can withstand the heat needed to fry foods such as potato chips or cheese puffs. Manufactured under the trade name Olean (pronounced oh-LEEN), olestra will soon appear in snack foods such as potato chips, crackers, and tortilla chips.

Olestra's chemical structure is similar to that of a regular fat (a triglyceride) but with important differences. A triglyceride is composed of a glycerol molecule with three fatty acids attached, whereas olestra is made of a sucrose molecule with six to eight fatty acids attached. Enzymes in the digestive tract cannot break the bonds of olestra, so unlike sucrose or fatty acids, olestra passes through the system unabsorbed. As you will see, this characteristic is responsible for both the triumphs and the troubles of this nonfat fat.

Because olestra contains several of the fatty acids common to shortening and cooking oils, it shares many physical properties with them such as appearance, color, taste, heat stability, and shelf life. Consequently, olestra looks, feels, and tastes like dietary fat and can be used in frying, cooking, and baking. Best of all, olestra performs like a fat without losing flavor, adding kcalories, or raising blood lipids. Potato chips made with olestra deliver half the kcalories of regular chips and none of the fat. Does this sound too good to be true? It may be.

The FDA's evaluation of olestra's safety answered two questions. First, is olestra toxic? Second, does it affect either nutrient absorption or the health of the digestive tract?

Regarding possible toxicity, there is little controversy. Research on both animals and human beings supports the safety of olestra as a partial replacement for dietary fats and oils.[4] Studies on animals have reported no evidence of either cancer or birth defects caused by olestra.

Olestra's effects on nutrient absorption and digestive tract health, on the other hand, raise serious concerns.[5] One of the positive attributes of fats is that they carry the fat-soluble vitamins A, D, E, and K with them into the body. When olestra passes through the digestive tract unabsorbed, it binds with some of these vitamins and carries them out of the body, robbing the person of these valuable nutrients. To compensate for these losses, the FDA has required the manufacturer to fortify olestra with vitamins A, D, E, and K. Saturating olestra with these vitamins blocks its ability to bind with the vitamins from other foods.

Olestra also sweeps other fat-soluble substances through the digestive system. Among those lost are the carotenoids, the colorful pigments found in fruits and vegetables. Carotenoids act as antioxidants and may be important in protecting against a variety of diseases, including heart disease, some cancers, and macular degeneration (an eye disorder that causes blurry vision and blindness). Because the relationships between carotenoids and disease prevention have not yet been proved, the FDA has required the manufacturer to conduct long-term studies on whether carotenoid losses due to olestra use will impair health. Should this prove to be a problem, fortifying products is not a likely solution. If you consider that there are hundreds of carotenoids commonly found in foods and then think of the hundreds of noncarotenoid substances that may also be beneficial to health, you will quickly realize that fortification is not feasible. The FDA will review olestra's status when new research findings become available.

Consumers may not perceive any immediate ill effects of a diet depleted of its fat-soluble vitamins and carotenoids, but they will surely notice the digestive distress that sometimes accompanies olestra consumption: cramps, gas, bloating, and diarrhea. People eating as little as two ounces of olestra-containing potato chips may experience "fecal urgency" (the immediate need for a bathroom) and "anal leakage" (resulting in stained underwear). The FDA considers these symptoms "unpleasant," but not "medically significant." Whether consumers will agree and accept such "annoyances" in exchange for a bag of fat-free chips with lunch remains an unanswered multimillion dollar question.

In approving olestra, the FDA has required foods made with olestra to carry a label warning that "olestra may cause abdominal cramping and loose stools" and that it "inhibits the absorption of some vitamins and other nutrients." Those who read food labels may hesitate to purchase products with these warnings; others may not even notice the warnings.

Will people become slimmer by munching on chips and cookies made with artificial fats? Or will they simply feel free to eat more chips and cookies? After all, fat-free foods still deliver kcalories. Decades ago, consumers hailed the arrival of artificial sweeteners as a weight-loss wonder, but in reality, kcalories saved by using artificial sweeteners were readily replaced by kcalories from other foods.

Fat substitutes are not magic, of course; they cannot make people eat healthy diets. What they can do, though, is offer a low-fat alternative to the high-fat foods that bring flavor and pleasure to meals and snacks. Used wisely, they can help consumers achieve their dietary goals.[6]

NOTES

1. L. L. Birch and coauthors, Effects of a nonenergy fat substitute on children's energy and macronutrient intake, *American Journal of Clinical Nutrition* 58 (1993): 326–333; R. W. Foltin and coauthors, Caloric, but not macronutrient, compensation by humans for required-eating occasions with meals and snack varying in fat and carbohydrate, *American Journal of Clinical Nutrition* 55 (1992): 331–342; B. J. Rolls and coauthors, Effects of olestra, a noncaloric fat substitute, on daily energy and fat intakes in lean men, *American Journal of Clinical Nutrition* 56 (1992): 84–92.
2. A. Drewnowski, Sensory properties of fats and fat replacements, *Nutrition Reviews* 50 (1992): II17–II20.
3. Olestra: Approved with special labeling, *FDA Consumer*, April 1996, p. 11.
4. K. L. Skare, J. A. Skare, and E. O. Thompson, Evaluation of olestra in short-term genotoxic assays, *Food and Chemical Toxicology* 28 (1990): 69–73.
5. H. Blackburn, Olestra and the FDA, *New England Journal of Medicine* 334 (1996): 984–986.
6. Position of The American Dietetic Association: Fat replacements, *Journal of the American Dietetic Association* 91 (1991): 1285–1288.

Chapter 6

Protein: Amino Acids

CONTENTS

The Chemist's View of Proteins
  Amino Acids
  Proteins
Digestion and Absorption of Protein
  The Process of Digestion
  The Process of Absorption
Proteins in the Body
  Protein Synthesis
  Roles of Proteins
   A Preview of Protein Metabolism
Protein in Foods
  Protein Quality
  Measures of Protein Quality
  Protein Regulations for Food Labels
Health Effects and Recommended
      Intakes of Protein
  Protein-Energy Malnutrition
  Health Effects of Protein
  Recommened Intakes of Protein
  Protein and Amino Acid Supplements
HIGHLIGHT: Vegetarian, Mediterranean,
and Other Meat-Restricted Foodways

MICROGRAPH: **Hemoglobin, the body's oxygen-carrying protein**

eople commonly associate protein with strength and meat with protein. Consequently, they eat steak to build their muscles, but their thinking is only partly correct. Protein is a vital structural and working substance in all cells, not just muscle cells. Meat is a good source of protein, but so are milk, eggs, legumes, and many grains and vegetables. People who overvalue protein may overemphasize meat in their diets, sometimes at the expense of other, equally important nutrients and foods. Protein is important, but it is only one of the nutrients needed to maintain the body's health.

The Chemist's View of Proteins

Chemically, proteins contain the same atoms as carbohydrates and lipids—carbon, hydrogen, and oxygen—but proteins also contain nitrogen atoms. These nitrogen atoms give the name *amino* (nitrogen containing) to the amino acids— the links in the chains of proteins. Also, proteins assume extraordinary and unique shapes, which enable them to play their vital roles in the body.

AMINO ACIDS

All amino acids have the same basic structure—a central carbon atom with a hydrogen (H), an amino group (NH_2), and an acid group (COOH) attached to it. Carbon atoms need to form four bonds, though, so a fourth attachment is necessary, and it is this fourth site that distinguishes each amino acid from the others. Attached to the carbon atom at the fourth bond is a distinct atom, or group of atoms, known as the *side group* or *side chain* (see Figure 6–1).

Unique Side Groups   The side groups on amino acids vary from one amino acid to the next, making proteins more complex than either carbohydrates or lipids. A polysaccharide (starch, for example) may be several thousand units long, but every unit is a glucose molecule just like all the others. A protein, on the other hand, is made up of about 20 different amino acids, each with a different side group. Table 6–1 lists the amino acids most common in proteins.*

The simplest amino acid, glycine, has a hydrogen atom as its side group. A slightly more complex amino acid, alanine, has an extra carbon with three hydrogen atoms. Other amino acids have more complex side groups (see Figure 6–2 for examples). Thus, although all amino acids share a common structure, they differ in size, shape, electrical charge, and other characteristics because of differences in these side groups.

Nonessential Amino Acids   The body can synthesize more than half of the amino acids for itself, if it is given nitrogen to form the amino group and fragments

proteins: compounds composed of carbon, hydrogen, oxygen, and nitrogen atoms, arranged into amino acids linked in a chain. Some amino acids also contain sulfur atoms.

amino (a-MEEN-oh) **acids:** building blocks of proteins; each contains an amino group, an acid group, a hydrogen atom, and a distinctive side group attached to a central carbon atom.

   amino = containing nitrogen

Reminder:
- H forms 1 bond.
- O forms 2 bonds.
- N forms 3 bonds.
- C forms 4 bonds.

Figure 6–1

Amino Acid Structure

All amino acids have a carbon (known as the alpha-carbon), with an amino group (NH_2), an acid group (COOH), a hydrogen (H), and a side group attached. The side group is a unique chemical structure that differentiates one amino acid from another.

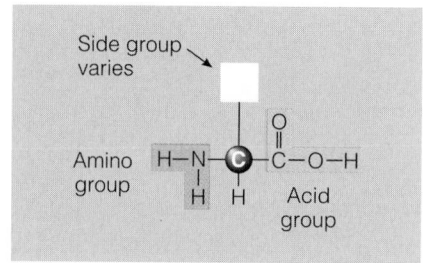

*Amino acids sometimes occur in related forms (for example, proline can acquire an OH group to become hydroxyproline; two cysteines in a protein chain can bind to make cystine). Besides the 20 common amino acids, which can all be components of proteins, others occur individually (for example, taurine and ornithine). Chemists can make still others. This text presents (in Appendix C) the chemical structures of the 20 amino acids most common in proteins, as in Nomenclature policy: Abbreviated designations of amino acids, *Journal of Nutrition* 117 (1987): 15.

Table 6–1

Amino Acids

Proteins are made up of about 20 common amino acids. The first column lists the *essential* amino acids (those the body cannot make—that must be provided in the diet).

Essential Amino Acids		Nonessential Amino Acids	
Histidine	(HISS-tuh-deen)	Alanine	(AL-ah-neen)
Isoleucine	(eye-so-LOO-seen)	Arginine	(ARJ-ih-neen)
Leucine	(LOO-seen)	Asparagine	(ah-SPAR-ah-geen)
Lysine	(LYE-seen)	Aspartic acid	(ah-SPAR-tic acid)
Methionine	(meh-THIGH-oh-neen)	Cysteine	(SIS-teh-een)
Phenylalanine	(fen-il-AL-ah-neen)	Glutamic acid	(GLU-tam-ic acid)
Threonine	(THREE-oh-neen)	Glutamine	(GLU-tah-meen)
Tryptophan	(TRIP-toe-fan,	Glycine	(GLY-seen)
	TRIP-toe-fane)	Proline	(PRO-leen)
Valine	(VAY-leen)	Serine	(SEER-een)
		Tyrosine	(TIE-roe-seen)

Note: In special cases, some nonessential amino acids may become conditionally essential (see the text).

from carbohydrate and fat to form the rest of the structure. Proteins in foods usually deliver these amino acids, but it is not essential that they do so.

Essential Amino Acids   There are nine amino acids that the body either cannot make at all or cannot make in sufficient quantity to meet its needs. These nine amino acids must be supplied by the diet; they are essential.

Conditionally Essential Amino Acids   Sometimes a nonessential amino acid becomes essential under special circumstances. For example, the body normally makes tyrosine (a nonessential amino acid) from the essential amino acid phenylalanine. But if the diet fails to supply enough phenylalanine, or if the body cannot make the conversion for some reason (as happens in the inherited disease phenylketonuria, which is discussed in Highlight 26), then tyrosine becomes *conditionally* essential.

essential amino acids: amino acids that the body cannot synthesize in amounts sufficient to meet physiological needs (see Table 6–1). Some researchers refer to essential amino acids as indispensable and to nonessential amino acids as dispensable.

conditionally essential amino acid: an amino acid that is normally nonessential, but must be supplied by the diet in special circumstances when the need for it exceeds the body's ability to produce it.

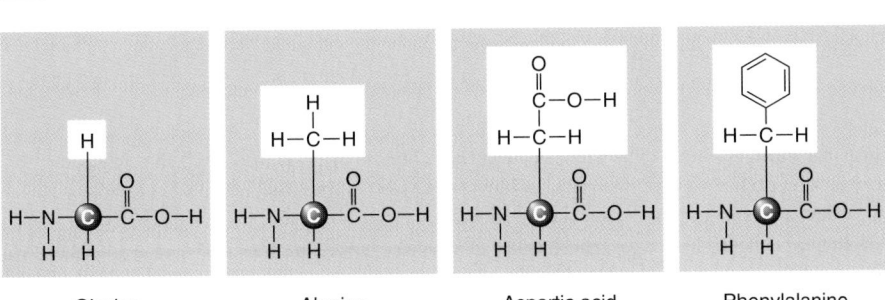

Glycine   Alanine   Aspartic acid   Phenylalanine

Figure 6–2

Examples of Amino Acids

Note that all amino acids have a common chemical structure but that each has a different side chain.

Figure 6–3

Condensation of Two Amino Acids to Form a Dipeptide

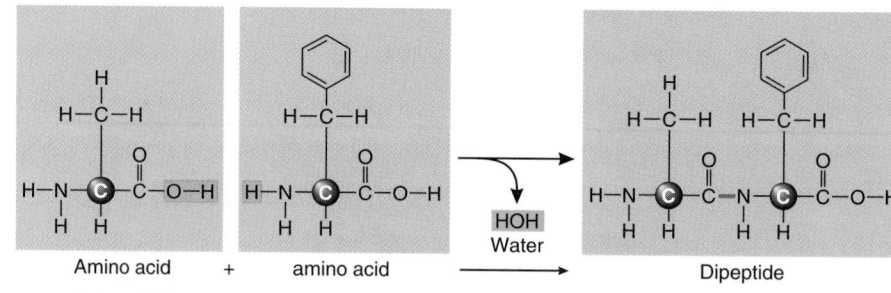

Amino acid   +   amino acid   →   Dipeptide

An OH group from the acid end of one amino acid and an H atom from the amino group of another join to form a molecule of water.

A peptide bond (highlighted in red) forms between the two amino acids, creating a dipeptide.

---

peptide bond: a bond that connects the acid end of one amino acid with the amino end of another, forming a link in a protein chain.

dipeptide: two amino acids bonded together.

> *di* = two
> *peptide* = amino acid

tripeptide: three amino acids bonded together.

> *tri* = three

polypeptide: many (ten or more) amino acids bonded together. An intermediate string of four to nine amino acids is an oligopeptide.

> *poly* = many
> *oligo* = few

PROTEINS

Cells link amino acids end-to-end in a virtually infinite variety of sequences to form thousands of different proteins. Each link connecting one amino acid with another is a peptide bond.

Amino Acid Chains   Condensation reactions create the bonds between amino acids, just as they combine monosaccharides to form disaccharides, and fatty acids with glycerol to form triglycerides.* Two amino acids bonded together form a dipeptide (see Figure 6–3). By another such reaction, a third amino acid can be added to the chain to form a tripeptide. As additional amino acids join the chain, a polypeptide is formed. Most proteins are a few dozen to several hundred amino acids long. Figure 6–4 provides an example—insulin.

---

*Later in this chapter, Figure 6–6 shows how each protein's sequence is dictated by the genetic code in DNA, and the text describes how the sequence shapes the protein.

Figure 6–4

Amino Acid Sequence of Human Insulin

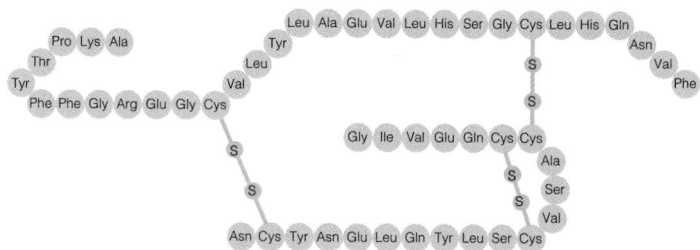

Human insulin is a relatively small protein that consists of 51 amino acids in two short polypeptide chains. (For amino acid abbreviations, see Appendix C.) Two bridges link the two chains. A third bridge spans a section within the short chain.

Known as disulfide bridges, these links always involve the amino acid cysteine (cys), whose side group contains sulfur. Cysteines connect to each other when bonds form between these side groups.

Amino Acid Sequences   If a person could step onto a carbohydrate molecule like starch and walk along it, the first stepping stone would be a glucose. The next stepping stone would also be a glucose, and it would be followed by a glucose, and yet another glucose. But if a person were to walk along a polypeptide chain, each stepping stone would be one of 20-odd different amino acids. The first stepping stone might be the amino acid methionine. The second might be an alanine. The third might be a glycine, and the fourth a tryptophan, and so on. Walking along another polypeptide path, a person might step on a phenylalanine, then a valine, and a glutamine. In other words, amino acid sequences within proteins vary.

The amino acids can act somewhat like the letters in an alphabet. If you only had the letter G, you could write an unvarying string of Gs: G–G–G–G–G–G–G. But with 20 different letters available, you could create poems, songs, or novels. The 20 amino acids can be linked together in an even greater variety of sequences than are possible for letters in a word or words in a sentence. Thus the variety of possible sequences for polypeptide chains is tremendous.

Protein Shapes   Polypeptide chains twist into complex, tangled shapes. Each amino acid has a unique chemical character that attracts it to, or repels it from, the surrounding fluids and other amino acids. Some amino acid side chains carry electrical charges that are attracted to water molecules (they are hydrophilic). Other side chains are neutral and are repelled by water (they are hydrophobic). As amino acids are strung together to make a polypeptide, the chain folds so that its charged hydrophilic side chains are on the outer surface near water; the neutral hydrophobic groups tuck themselves inside, away from water. The intricate, coiled shape the polypeptide finally assumes gives it maximum stability in the body's watery fluids.

Reminder: Substances that are attracted to water are *hydrophilic*; those that are repelled by water are *hydrophobic*.

Protein Functions   The different shapes of proteins enable them to perform various tasks in the body. Some form hollow balls that can carry and store materials within them, and some, such as those of tendons, are more than ten times as long as they are wide, forming strong, rodlike structures. Some polypeptides may be functioning proteins as they are; others may need to associate with other polypeptides to form larger working complexes. Some proteins require minerals to activate them. One molecule of hemoglobin—the large, globular protein molecule that, by the billions, packs the red blood cells and carries oxygen—is made of four associated polypeptide chains, each holding the mineral iron.

hemoglobin: the globular protein of the red blood cells that carries oxygen from the lungs to the cells throughout the body.
  hemo = blood
  globin = globular protein

Protein Denaturation   When proteins are subjected to heat, acid, or other conditions that disturb their stability, they undergo denaturation—that is, they uncoil and lose their shapes and, consequently, their functions. Past a certain point, denaturation is irreversible. Familiar examples of denaturation include the hardening of an egg when it is cooked, the curdling of milk when acid is added, and the stiffening of egg whites when they are whipped.

denaturation: the change in a protein's shape brought about by heat, acid, base, alcohol, heavy metals, or other agents.

In summary, proteins are made of some 20 different amino acids, 9 of which the body cannot make (they are essential). Cells synthesize each protein that they need by stringing together amino acids in a distinctive sequence.

Digestion and Absorption of Protein

Proteins in foods do not become body proteins, but supply the amino acids from which the body makes its own proteins. When a person eats foods containing protein, enzymes break the long polypeptide strands into shorter strands, the short strands into tripeptides and dipeptides, and, finally, the tripeptides and dipeptides into amino acids.

THE PROCESS OF DIGESTION

Figure 6–5 illustrates the digestion of protein through the GI tract. Proteins are crushed and moistened in the mouth, but the real action begins in the stomach.

In the Stomach In the stomach, hydrochloric acid uncoils (denatures) each protein's tangled strands so that digestive enzymes can attack the peptide bonds. The hydrochloric acid also converts the inactive form of the enzyme pepsinogen to its active form pepsin. Pepsin cleaves proteins—large polypeptides—into smaller polypeptides and some amino acids.

In the Small Intestine When polypeptides enter the small intestine, pancreatic and intestinal proteases hydrolyze them further into short peptide chains (oligopeptides), tripeptides, dipeptides, and amino acids. Figure 6–5 includes the details of digestive enzyme action for dietary protein. A number of distinct carriers transport these protein pieces into the intestinal cells.

THE PROCESS OF ABSORPTION

The cells of the small intestine absorb amino acids and have peptidase enzymes on their surfaces that split most of the dipeptides and tripeptides into single amino acids. A few dipeptides, tripeptides, and even larger molecules sometimes escape digestion and cross the digestive tract wall to enter the bloodstream.

Some nutrition faddists fail to realize that most proteins are broken down to amino acids before absorption. They urge consumers to "Eat enzyme A. It will help you digest your food." Or "Don't eat food B. It contains enzyme C, which will digest cells in your body." In reality, though, enzymes in foods are digested, just as all proteins are. Only the digestive enzymes, whose design prevents them from being denatured or digested, can work in such an environment.

Another misconception is that eating predigested proteins (amino acid supplements) saves the body from having to digest proteins and keeps the digestive system from "overworking." Such a belief grossly underestimates the body's abilities. As a matter of fact, the digestive system handles whole proteins *better* than predigested ones because it dismantles and absorbs the amino acids at rates that are optimal for the body's use.[1] (The last section of this chapter discusses amino acid supplements further.)

In short, via digestion facilitated mostly by the stomach's acid and enzymes, the body first denatures dietary proteins, then cleaves them into polypeptides, then oligo-, tri-, and dipeptides, and some amino acids. Intestinal enzymes split these

---

Reminder: An enzyme that hydrolyzes protein is a *protease*.

The inactive form of an enzyme is called a **proenzyme**.
  pro = before

pepsin: a gastric protease. Pepsin is secreted in an inactive form, **pepsinogen**, which is activated by stomach acid.

peptidase: a digestive enzyme that hydrolyzes peptide bonds. *Tripeptidases* cleave tripeptides; *dipeptidases* cleave dipeptides. *Endopeptidases* cleave peptide bonds *within* the chain to create smaller fragments, whereas *exopeptidases* cleave bonds at the *ends* to release free amino acids.

Figure 6–5

Protein Digestion in the GI Tract

Protein Digestive Enzymes

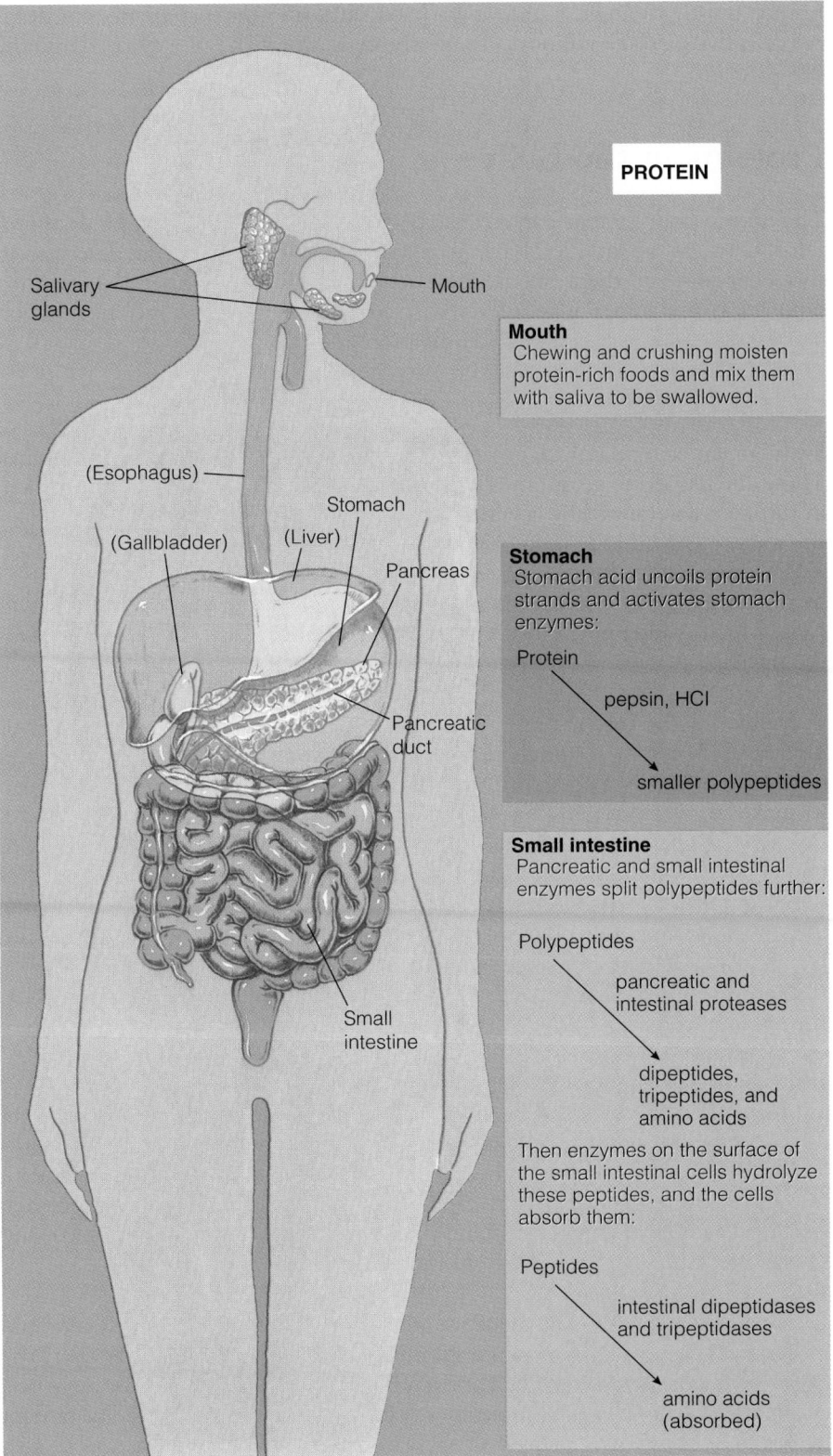

PROTEIN

Mouth
Chewing and crushing moisten protein-rich foods and mix them with saliva to be swallowed.

Stomach
Stomach acid uncoils protein strands and activates stomach enzymes:

Protein

pepsin, HCl

smaller polypeptides

Small intestine
Pancreatic and small intestinal enzymes split polypeptides further:

Polypeptides

pancreatic and intestinal proteases

dipeptides, tripeptides, and amino acids

Then enzymes on the surface of the small intestinal cells hydrolyze these peptides, and the cells absorb them:

Peptides

intestinal dipeptidases and tripeptidases

amino acids (absorbed)

In the Stomach:

HCl
- Denatures protein structure.
- Activates pepsinogen to pepsin.

Pepsin
- Cleaves proteins to smaller poly-peptides and some free amino acids.
- Inhibits pepsinogen synthesis.

In the Small Intestine:

Enteropeptidase[a]
- Converts pancreatic trypsinogen to trypsin.

Trypsin
- Converts pancreatic chymotryp-sinogen to chymotrypsin.
- Converts pancreatic procarboxy-peptidases to carboxypeptidases.
- Inhibits trypsinogen synthesis.
- Cleaves peptide bonds next to the amino acids lysine and arginine.

Chymotrypsin
- Cleaves peptide bonds next to the amino acids phenylalanine, tyro-sine, tryptophan, methionine, asparagine, and histidine.

Elastase and collagenase
- Cleave polypeptides into smaller polypeptides and tripeptides.

Carboxypeptidases
- Cleave amino acids from the acid (carboxyl) ends of polypeptides.

Aminopeptidases
- Cleave amino acids from the amino ends of small polypeptides (oligopeptides).

Tripeptidases
- Cleave tripeptides to dipeptides and amino acids.

[a]Enteropeptidase was formerly known as *enterokinase.*

further, mostly to single amino acids. Then carriers in the membranes of intestinal cells transport the amino acids into the cells, where they are released into the bloodstream.

Proteins in the Body

The human body contains an estimated 10,000 to 50,000 different kinds of proteins. Of these, about 1000 have been studied. Only about 10 are described in this chapter—but these should be enough to illustrate proteins' versatility, uniqueness, and importance. As you will see, each protein has a specific function and that function is determined during protein synthesis.

PROTEIN SYNTHESIS

Each human being is unique because of minute differences in the body's proteins. These differences are determined by the amino acid sequences of proteins, which, in turn, are determined by genetics. The following paragraphs describe in words the ways cells synthesize proteins; Figure 6–6 provides a pictorial description.

The instructions for making every protein in a person's body are transmitted by way of the genetic information received at conception. This body of knowledge, which is filed in the DNA within the nucleus of every cell, never leaves the nucleus.

Delivering the Instructions   To inform a cell of the sequence of amino acids for a needed protein, a stretch of DNA serves as a template for making a strand of RNA that carries a code, listing in order the amino acids that will be needed to make a given protein. Known as messenger RNA, this molecule escapes through the nuclear membrane. Messenger RNA seeks out and attaches itself to one of the ribosomes (a protein-making machine, which is itself composed of RNA and protein). Thus situated, messenger RNA presents its list, specifying the sequence in which the amino acids are to line up to make a strand of protein.

Lining Up the Amino Acids   Other forms of RNA, called transfer RNA, collect amino acids from the cell fluid and bring them to the messenger. Each of the 20 amino acids has a specific transfer RNA. Thousands of transfer RNA, each carrying its amino acid, cluster around the ribosomes, awaiting their turn to unload. When the messenger's list calls for a specific amino acid, the transfer RNA carrying that amino acid moves into position. Then the next loaded transfer RNA moves into place and then the next and the next. Thus the amino acids line up in the sequence that is called for, and enzymes bind them together. Finally, the completed protein strand is released, the messenger is degraded, and the transfer RNA are freed to return for another load of amino acids.

Sequencing Errors   The sequence of amino acids in each protein determines its configuration, which supports a specific function. If a genetic error alters the amino acid sequence of a protein, or if a mistake is made in copying the sequence, an altered protein will result, sometimes with dramatic consequences. The protein hemoglobin offers one example of such a genetic variation. In a person with sickle-cell anemia, two of hemoglobin's four polypeptide chains (described earlier

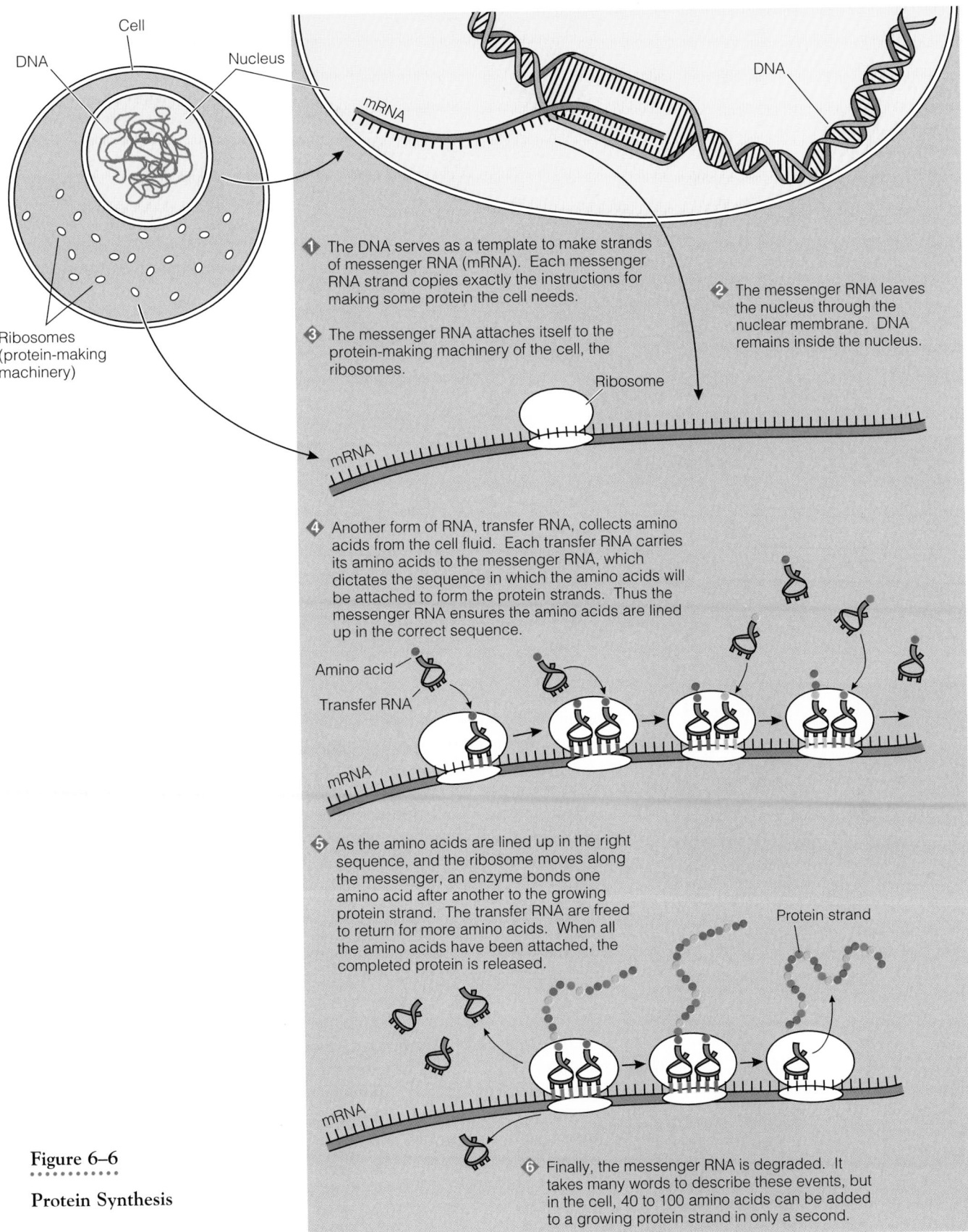

Cell

DNA

Nucleus

mRNA

DNA

Ribosomes
(protein-making
machinery)

1 The DNA serves as a template to make strands of messenger RNA (mRNA). Each messenger RNA strand copies exactly the instructions for making some protein the cell needs.

2 The messenger RNA leaves the nucleus through the nuclear membrane. DNA remains inside the nucleus.

3 The messenger RNA attaches itself to the protein-making machinery of the cell, the ribosomes.

Ribosome

mRNA

4 Another form of RNA, transfer RNA, collects amino acids from the cell fluid. Each transfer RNA carries its amino acids to the messenger RNA, which dictates the sequence in which the amino acids will be attached to form the protein strands. Thus the messenger RNA ensures the amino acids are lined up in the correct sequence.

Amino acid

Transfer RNA

mRNA

5 As the amino acids are lined up in the right sequence, and the ribosome moves along the messenger, an enzyme bonds one amino acid after another to the growing protein strand. The transfer RNA are freed to return for more amino acids. When all the amino acids have been attached, the completed protein is released.

Protein strand

mRNA

6 Finally, the messenger RNA is degraded. It takes many words to describe these events, but in the cell, 40 to 100 amino acids can be added to a growing protein strand in only a second.

Figure 6–6

Protein Synthesis

Figure 6–7

Normal Red Blood Cells Compared with Sickle Cells

Normally, red blood cells are disc-shaped; in the inherited disorder sickle-cell anemia, red blood cells are sickle- or crescent-shaped. This alteration in shape occurs because valine replaces glutamic acid in the amino acid sequence of hemoglobin's polypeptide chain. As a result of this one amino acid's being in the wrong place, the hemoglobin has a diminished capacity to carry oxygen.

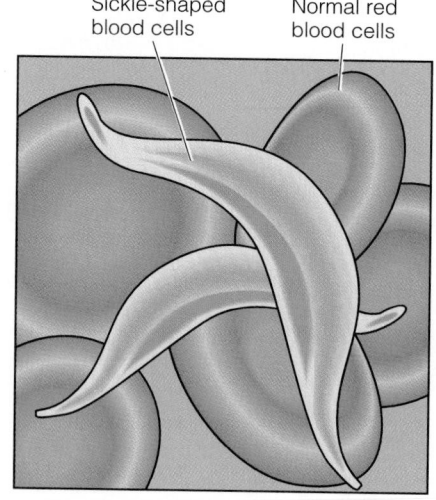

Sickle-shaped blood cells   Normal red blood cells

Amino acid sequence of normal hemoglobin:

Val — His — Leu — Thr — Pro — Glu — Glu

Amino acid sequence of sickle-cell hemoglobin:

Val — His — Leu — Thr — Pro — Val — Glu

sickle-cell anemia: a hereditary form of anemia characterized by abnormal sickle- or crescent-shaped red blood cells. Sickled cells interfere with oxygen transport and blood flow. Symptoms include hemolytic anemia (red blood cells burst), fever, and severe pain in the joints and abdomen; they are precipitated by dehydration and insufficient oxygen (as may occur at high altitudes).

Note: Anemia is not a disease, but a symptom of various diseases. In the case of sickle-cell anemia, a defect in the hemoglobin molecule changes the shape of the red blood cells. Later chapters describe how vitamin and mineral deficiencies change the size and color of the red blood cells. In all cases, the abnormal blood cells are unable to meet the body's oxygen demands.

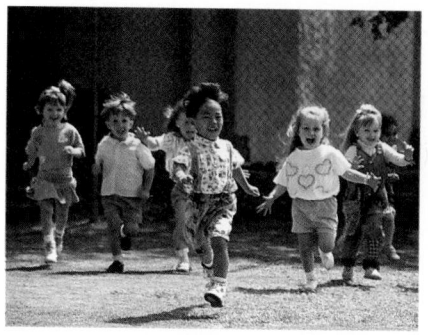

Growing children end each day with more bone, blood, muscle, and skin cells than they had at the beginning of the day.

collagen: the protein material from which connective tissues such as scars, tendons, ligaments, and the foundations of bones and teeth are made.

matrix (MAY-tricks): the basic substance that gives form to a developing structure; in the body, the formative cells from which teeth and bones grow.

on p. 183) have the normal sequence of amino acids, but the other two chains do not—they have the amino acid valine in a position that is normally occupied by glutamic acid (see Figure 6–7). This single alteration in the amino acid sequence changes the character and shape of the protein so much that hemoglobin loses its ability to carry oxygen effectively. The red blood cells filled with this abnormal hemoglobin stiffen into elongated sickle, or crescent, shapes instead of maintaining their normal pliable disc shape—hence the name, sickle-cell anemia. Sickle-cell anemia causes many medical problems and can be fatal.

ROLES OF PROTEINS

Whenever the body is growing, repairing, or replacing tissue, proteins are involved. Sometimes their role is to facilitate or to regulate; other times it is to become part of a structure. Yes, versatility is a key feature of proteins.

As Building Materials   From the moment of conception, as the body grows, it uses proteins as building blocks. For example, to build a bone or a tooth, cells first lay down a matrix of the protein collagen and then fill it with crystals of calcium, phosphorus, fluoride, and other minerals.

The protein collagen is also the material of ligaments and tendons and the strengthening glue between the cells of the artery walls that enables the arteries to withstand the pressure of the blood surging through them with each heartbeat. Also made of collagen are scars that knit the separated parts of torn tissues together.

As old skin cells fall off, new cells made largely of protein grow from underneath to compensate. Cells in the deeper skin layers synthesize new proteins to go into hair and fingernails. GI tract cells are replaced every three days. Both inside and outside, then, the body constantly deposits protein into new cells that replace those that have been lost.

As Enzymes   Digestive enzymes have appeared in every chapter since Chapter 3, but digestion is only one of the many processes enzymes facilitate. Enzymes not only break down substances, they also build substances and transform one substance into another. Figure 6–8 diagrams a synthesis reaction.

An analogy may help to clarify the role of enzymes. Enzymes are comparable to the clergy and judges who make and dissolve marriages. When a minister marries two people, they become a couple, with a new bond between them. They are joined together—but the minister remains unchanged. The minister represents synthetase enzymes that make large compounds from smaller ones. One minister can perform thousands of marriage ceremonies, just as one enzyme can perform billions of synthetic reactions.

Similarly, a judge who lets married couples separate may decree many divorces before retiring or dying. The judge represents enzymes that hydrolyze larger compounds to smaller ones; for example, the digestive enzymes. The point is that, like the minister and the judge, enzymes themselves are not altered by the reactions they facilitate. They are catalysts, permitting reactions to occur more quickly and efficiently than if substances depended on chance encounters alone.

The chemical structures in the margin and the paragraphs that follow provide an example of enzyme action. This single biochemical pathway illustrates how one compound encounters an enzyme, is converted to another compound that encounters another enzyme, and so forth until the final product is entirely different from the starting material. The details are offered only to give you insight into the kinds of processes that take place in the daily lives of the body's cells.

In the breakdown of glucose (a 6-carbon compound), enzymes add two phosphate groups, alter the arrangement of the atoms, and then split the molecule in half, leaving two 3-carbon compounds. One of these is compound A and the other is converted to compound A, so the two halves derived from glucose follow the same path from that point on.

enzymes: proteins that facilitate chemical reactions without being changed in the process; protein catalysts.

The breakdown of large molecules into smaller ones is known as *catabolism*; the synthesis of small molecules into larger ones is known as *anabolism*. These two types of reactions receive further attention in Chapter 7.

synthetase (SIN-the-tase): an enzyme that enables two or more substances to form a more complex structure.

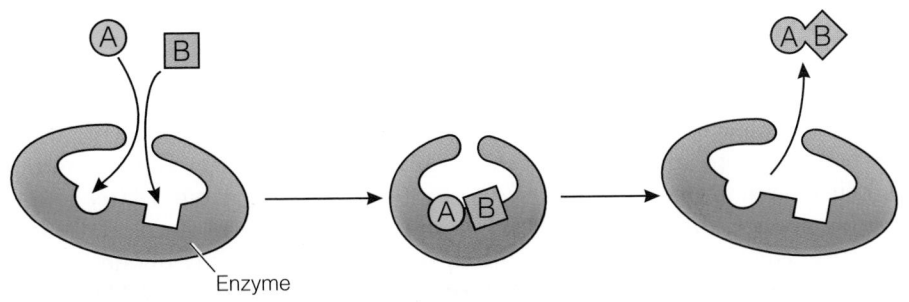

Enzyme

Two separate compounds, A and B, are attracted to the enzyme's active site, making a reaction likely.

The enzyme forms a complex with A and B.

The enzyme is unchanged, but A and B have formed a new compound, AB.

Figure 6–8

Enzyme Action

Each enzyme facilitates a specific chemical reaction. In this diagram, an enzyme enables two compounds to make a more complex structure, but the enzyme itself remains unchanged.

Compound A

Compound B

Compound C

Compound D

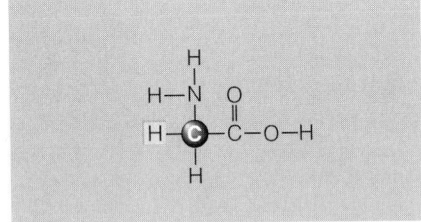

Compound E

fluid and electrolyte balance: maintenance of the proper types and amounts of fluid and minerals in each compartment of the body fluids (see also Chapter 12).

Compound A floats around until it encounters an enzyme that recognizes it. This enzyme removes hydrogens from molecules of compound A. Without hydrogens, carbon and oxygen must form a double bond; thus compound B is created. Compound B is released from this enzyme and encounters another enzyme that removes an oxygen and substitutes an amino group in its place; the result is compound C. The next enzyme removes the phosphate group and replaces it with a hydrogen, leaving compound D.

The characteristics of compound D become apparent upon close examination and may not surprise some readers, but this example takes the process one step further before revealing the identity of compound D. Another enzyme, whose function is to remove CH_2OH groups from molecules, forms compound E.

Compound E appeared earlier in this chapter. It has an amino group at one end, an acid group at the other, and a central carbon carrying two hydrogen atoms. It is the amino acid glycine (introduced in Figure 6–2).

Amazing! The cellular machinery started with a molecule of glucose (a derivative of dietary carbohydrate), made one small change after another, and transformed it into an amino acid (a member of the protein family). The lesson of this sequence of events is that the body can use glucose and nitrogen-containing compounds to make many of the amino acids needed to build body proteins. The nonessential amino acid glycine is just one example. Compound D, which precedes glycine on the pathway, is another example: the nonessential amino acid serine. Thus, among the thousands of tasks that enzymes perform, they even manufacture many of the nonessential amino acids they themselves are made of.

Perhaps you have realized by now that the protein story is circular. To follow the circle in nutrition, start with a person eating food proteins. The proteins are broken down by proteins (digestive enzymes) into amino acids. The amino acids enter the body cells, where proteins (synthetases) link them into long chains whose sequences are specified by DNA. The chains twist and fold forming proteins, some of which are enzymes. Some enzymes break apart compounds; others put compounds together. Day by day, in billions of reactions, these processes repeat themselves, and life goes on. Only living systems work with such self-renewal. A car cannot make another car; a toaster cannot fix another toaster. Only living creatures and the parts they are composed of—the cells—can duplicate and repair themselves.

As Hormones Cells can switch their protein machinery on or off in response to the body's needs. Often hormones do the switching, with marvelous precision. The body's many hormones are messenger molecules, and some hormones are proteins. Various glands in the body release hormones in response to changes in the internal environment. The blood carries the hormones to their target tissues, where they elicit the appropriate responses to restore normal conditions.

The hormone insulin provides a familiar example. When blood glucose rises, the pancreas steps up its release of insulin. Insulin stimulates the cells' transport proteins to pump glucose into the cells faster than it can leak out. (After acting on the message, the cells destroy the insulin.) Then, as blood glucose falls, the pancreas reduces its insulin output. Many other proteins act as hormones, maintaining the distribution of hundreds of substances in the body (see Table 6–2).

As Regulators of Fluid and Electrolyte Balance Proteins help to maintain the body's fluid and electrolyte balance. As Figure 6–9 shows, the body's fluids

Table 6–2

Examples of Hormones and Their Actions

Hormones	Actions
Growth hormone	Promotes growth.
Insulin and glucagon	Regulate blood glucose (see Chapter 4).
Thyroxin	Regulates the body's metabolic rate (see Chapter 8).
Calcitonin and parathormone	Regulate blood calcium (see Chapter 12).
Antidiuretic hormone	Regulates fluid and electrolyte balance (see Chapter 12).

Note: Hormones are chemical messengers that are secreted by endocrine glands in response to altered conditions in the body. Each travels to one or more specific target tissues or organs, where it elicits a specific response. For descriptions of many hormones important in nutrition, see Appendix A.

Figure 6–9

One Cell and Its Associated Fluids

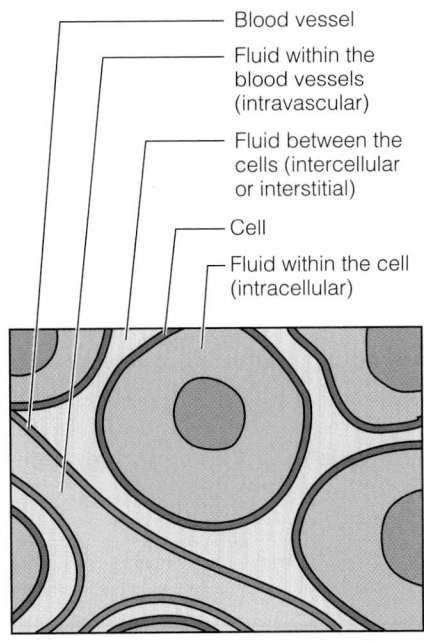

Minerals also help regulate fluid distribution; Chapter 12 provides more details.

edema (eh-DEEM-uh): the swelling of body tissue caused by excessive amounts of fluid in the interstitial spaces; seen in protein deficiency (among other conditions).

are contained inside the blood vessels (intravascular), within the cells (intracellular), and surrounding the cells (intercellular). Fluids can flow freely between these compartments, but the cells can't move fluids directly. They can manufacture proteins, though. Being large, proteins cannot pass freely across membranes; they are trapped on one side where they attract water. By making and keeping proteins, cells can retain fluids. Similarly, the cells can ship proteins out into the blood and intercellular spaces to maintain the fluid volume there. Should this system fail, too much fluid would collect outside the cells, causing edema.

Not only the quantity, but also the composition of body fluids depends on proteins. Special transport proteins maintain equilibrium in the surrounding fluids by moving molecules into and out of cells. Most of these proteins reside in cell membranes and act as "pumps," picking up compounds on one side of the membrane and depositing them on the other. In doing so, transport proteins enable cells to take up and release substances as needed. Each transport protein is specific for a certain compound or group of related compounds. Figure 6–10 illustrates how a membrane-bound transport protein maintains the sodium and potassium concentrations in the fluids inside and outside of the cells. The balance of these two electrolytes is critical to neural transmissions and muscle contractions; any disturbance triggers a major medical emergency. Such imbalances can cause irregular heartbeats, muscular weakness, kidney failure, and even death.

As Acid-Base Regulators   Proteins also help to maintain the balance between acids and bases within the body fluids. Normal body processes continually produce acids and bases, which the blood carries to the kidneys and lungs for excretion. The challenge is to do this without upsetting the blood's acid-base balance.

In an acid solution, hydrogen ions abound; the more hydrogen ions, the more concentrated the acid. Proteins, which have negative charges on their surfaces, attract hydrogen ions, which have positive charges. By accepting and releasing hydrogen ions, proteins act as buffers, maintaining the acid-base balance of the blood and body fluids.

The blood's acid-base balance is tightly controlled. The extremes of acidosis and alkalosis lead to coma and death, largely because they denature working pro-

acids: compounds that release hydrogen ions in a solution.

bases: compounds that accept hydrogen ions in a solution.

Reminder: The *acid-base balance* is the equilibrium between acid and base concentrations in the blood and body fluids.

buffers: compounds that help keep a solution's acidity or alkalinity constant.

acidosis (assi-DOE-sis): above-normal acidity in the blood and body fluids.

alkalosis (alka-LOE-sis): above-normal alkalinity (base) in the blood and body fluids.

Figure 6–10

Transport Proteins

A transport protein within a cell membrane picks up substances on one side of the membrane and carries them to the other side without leaving the membrane. The substances being transported here are sodium and potassium. Maintaining a high concentration of potassium and a low concentration of sodium within the cells requires energy.

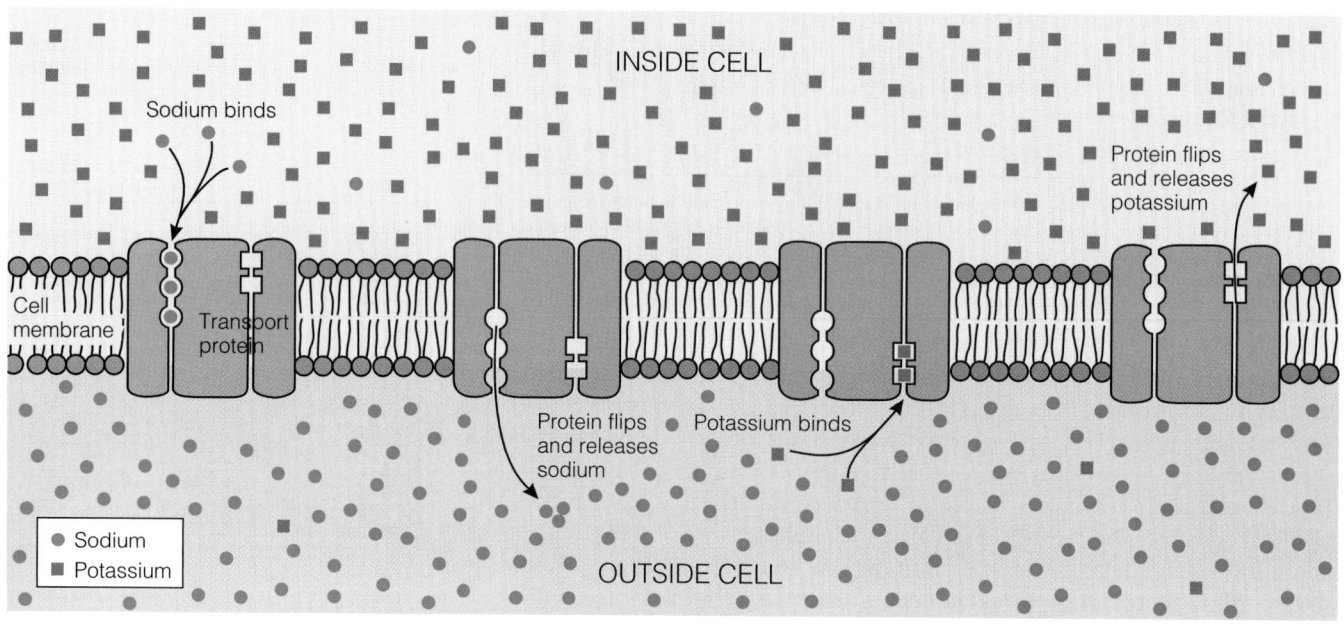

INSIDE CELL

Sodium binds

Protein flips and releases potassium

Cell membrane

Transport protein

Protein flips and releases sodium

Potassium binds

● Sodium
■ Potassium

OUTSIDE CELL

The protein residing in the cells of the intestinal wall is ferritin; the carrier protein, transferrin; the storage protein, ferritin again; the red blood cell protein, hemoglobin; and the muscle cell protein, myoglobin.

teins. Disturbing a protein's shape renders it useless. To give just one example, hemoglobin, when denatured, loses its capacity to carry oxygen.

As Transporters Some transport proteins are not attached to membranes, but move about in the body fluids, carrying nutrients and other molecules. The protein hemoglobin carries oxygen from the lungs to the cells. The lipoproteins transport lipids around the body. Special proteins carry vitamins and minerals.

The transport of the mineral iron provides an especially good illustration of these proteins' specificity and precision. When iron enters an intestinal cell, it is captured by a protein that will not let go unless the body needs iron. Before leaving the cell to enter the bloodstream, iron is attached to a carrier protein. The carrier, in turn, can pass iron on to a storage protein in the bone marrow or other tissues, which will hold it until it is needed. Then, when it is needed, iron is incorporated into proteins in the red blood cells and muscles that assist in oxygen transport and use.

As Antibodies Proteins also defend the body against disease. A virus—whether it is one that causes flu, smallpox, measles, or the common cold—enters the cells and multiplies there. One virus may produce 100 replicas of itself within an hour or so. Each replica can then burst out and invade 100 different cells, soon yielding 10,000 virus particles, which invade 10,000 cells. Left free to do their worst, they will soon overwhelm the body with disease.

Fortunately, when the body detects invaders, it manufactures antibodies, giant protein molecules designed specifically to combat them. The antibodies work so swiftly and efficiently that in a normal, healthy individual, most diseases never have a chance to get started. Without sufficient protein, though, the body cannot maintain its resistance to disease.

Each antibody is designed to destroy just one invader. Once the body has manufactured antibodies against a particular antigen (such as the measles virus), it remembers how to make them. Consequently, the next time the body encounters that same invader, it will produce antibodies even more quickly. In other words, it develops a molecular memory, known as immunity.

Other Roles   As mentioned earlier, proteins form integral parts of most body structures such as skin, muscles, and bones. They also participate in some of the body's most amazing activities such as blood clotting and vision. When a tissue is injured, a rapid chain of events leads to the production of fibrin, a stringy, insoluble mass of protein fibers that forms a clot from liquid blood. Later, more slowly, the protein collagen forms a scar to replace the clot and permanently heal the cut. The light-sensitive pigments in the cells of the retina are molecules of the protein opsin. Opsin responds to light by changing its shape, thus initiating the nerve impulses that convey the sense of sight to higher brain centers.

The protein functions discussed here are summarized in Table 6–3. They are only a few of the many roles proteins play, but they convey some sense of the immense variety of proteins and their importance in the body.

A PREVIEW OF PROTEIN METABOLISM

This section previews protein metabolism; Chapter 7 provides a full description. Cells have several metabolic options, depending on their amino acid needs.

antibodies: large proteins of the blood and body fluids, produced by the immune system in response to the invasion of the body by foreign molecules (usually proteins called *antigens*); antibodies combine with and inactivate the foreign invaders, thus protecting the body.

antigen: a substance that elicits the formation of antibodies or an inflammation reaction from the immune system. A bacterium, a virus, a toxin, and a protein in food that causes allergy are all examples of foreign antigens.

immunity: the body's ability to recognize and eliminate foreign invaders; see Chapter 25.

Table 6–3

Summary of Proteins' Functions

- *Growth and maintenance*. Proteins form integral parts of most body structures such as skin, tendons, membranes, muscles, organs, and bones. As such, they support the growth and repair of body tissues.
- *Enzymes*. Proteins facilitate chemical reactions.
- *Hormones*. Proteins regulate body processes. (Some, but not all, hormones are made of protein.)
- *Antibodies*. Proteins inactivate foreign invaders, thus protecting the body against diseases.
- *Fluid and electrolyte balance*. Proteins help to maintain the fluid volume and the composition of body fluids.
- *Acid-base balance*. Proteins help maintain the acid-base balance of body fluids by acting as buffers.
- *Transportation*. Proteins transport substances, such as lipids, vitamins, minerals, and oxygen, around the body.
- *Energy*. Proteins provide some fuel for the body's energy needs.

protein turnover: the degradation and synthesis of endogenous protein.

endogenous protein: the protein in the body. In contrast, protein in foods is exogenous protein.

   endo = within
   gen = arising
   exo = outside (the body)

nitrogen balance: the amount of nitrogen consumed (N in) as compared with the amount of nitrogen excreted (N out) in a given period of time.*

Nitrogen equilibrium (zero nitrogen balance): N in = N out.
Positive nitrogen balance: N in > N out.
Negative nitrogen balance: N in < N out.

Protein Turnover Within each cell, proteins are constantly being made and broken down. When proteins break down, they free amino acids to join the general circulation. Some of these amino acids may be promptly recycled into other proteins; others may be stripped of their nitrogen and used for energy. Together the constant synthesis and degradation of body proteins are known as protein turnover;[2] and the protein that participates in this flux is called endogenous protein.

Nitrogen Balance If the body maintains the same *amount* of protein in its tissues from day to day, it is in nitrogen balance. If the body adds protein, it is in positive nitrogen balance; if it loses protein, it is in negative nitrogen balance.

Normally, healthy adults receive enough protein to meet their needs, and they dispose of any excess. Their nitrogen intake equals their nitrogen output, and they are said to be in zero nitrogen balance, or nitrogen equilibrium. Growing infants and children, pregnant women, and people recovering from protein deficiency or illness are in positive nitrogen balance: their nitrogen intake exceeds their nitrogen output. They are building protein tissues—adding new blood, bone, skin, and muscle cells to their bodies. In contrast, people who are starving or suffering other severe stresses such as burns, injuries, infections, and fever are in negative nitrogen balance: nitrogen output exceeds nitrogen intake. During these times, the body loses protein as it breaks down body proteins for energy.

Using Amino Acids to Make Proteins or Nonessential Amino Acids Cells can assemble amino acids into the proteins they need to do their work. If a particular nonessential amino acid is not readily available, cells can dismantle another amino acid and combine the amino group with carbon fragments from glucose to make the needed one. If an essential amino acid is missing, the body may break down some of its own proteins to obtain it.

Using Amino Acids to Make Other Compounds Cells can also use amino acids to make other compounds. For example, the amino acid tyrosine is used to make the neurotransmitters norepinephrine and epinephrine, which relay nervous system messages throughout the body. Tyrosine can also be made into the pigment melanin, which is responsible for brown hair, eye, and skin color, or into the hormone thyroxin, which helps to regulate the metabolic rate. For another example, the amino acid tryptophan serves as a precursor for the neurotransmitter serotonin and the vitamin niacin.

neurotransmitters: chemicals that are released at the end of a nerve cell when a nerve impulse arrives there; they diffuse across the gap to the next cell and alter the membrane of that second cell to either inhibit or excite it.

Using Amino Acids for Energy Even though amino acids are needed to do the work that only they can perform—build vital proteins—they will be sacrificed to provide energy and glucose if need be. Without energy, cells die; without glucose, the brain and nervous system falter. When glucose or fatty acids are limited, cells are forced to use amino acids for energy and glucose. The body does not make a specialized storage form of protein as it does for carbohydrate and fat. Glucose is stored as glycogen and fat as triglycerides, but protein in the body is available only

---

*The genetic materials DNA and RNA contain nitrogen, but the quantity is insignificant compared with the amount in protein. The average amino acid weighs about 6.25 times as much as the nitrogen it contains, so scientists can estimate the amount of protein in a sample of food, body tissue, or other material by multiplying the weight of the nitrogen in it by 6.25.

as the working and structural components of the tissues. When the need arises, the body dismantles its tissue proteins and uses them for energy.[3] Thus, over time, energy deprivation (starvation) always incurs wasting of lean body tissue as well as fat loss. An adequate intake of carbohydrates and fats spares amino acids from being used for energy and allows them to perform their unique roles.

Deaminating Amino Acids When amino acids are broken down (as occurs when they are to be used in energy production), they are first deaminated—stripped of their nitrogen-containing amino groups. Deamination produces ammonia, which the cells release into the bloodstream. The liver picks up the ammonia, converts it into urea (a less toxic compound), and returns the urea to the blood. The kidneys filter urea out of the blood; thus the amino nitrogen ends up in the urine. Urea is produced from both exogenous and endogenous amino acids. The remaining carbon fragments may enter a number of metabolic pathways—for example, they may be used to make fat.

Using Amino Acids to Make Fat If a person eats more protein than the body needs, the amino acids are deaminated, the nitrogen is excreted, and the remaining carbon fragments are converted to fat and stored for later use.* In this way, valuable, expensive, protein-rich foods can contribute to obesity.

To summarize, proteins serve the body as building blocks in the growth and repair of tissues; as enzymes in metabolism; as hormones; as regulators of the body's fluid balances; as transporters; as antibodies; and in many other ways (see Table 6–3). In the process, the proteins themselves are constantly being synthesized and broken down as needed. The body's assimilation of amino acids into proteins and release of amino acids via protein degradation and excretion can be tracked by measuring nitrogen balance, which should be positive during growth and steady in adulthood. An energy deficit or an inadequate protein intake may force the body to use amino acids as fuel, causing negative nitrogen balance. Protein eaten in excess of need is degraded and stored as body fat.

Reminder: The making of glucose from noncarbohydrate sources such as amino acids is *gluconeogenesis*. The action of carbohydrate and fat in providing enough energy to allow amino acids to be used to build body proteins is known as the *protein-sparing action* of carbohydrate and fat.

deamination: removal of the amino (NH_2) group from a compound such as an amino acid.

Urea metabolism is described in Chapter 7.

Protein in Foods

In the United States, where nutritious foods are abundant, people eat protein in such large quantities that even if its amino acid balance is not perfect, they receive all the amino acids they need. Where people eat only marginal amounts of protein-rich foods, however, the quality of the protein becomes crucial to their health. Hence, the protein quality of the diet is of great concern when making nutrition recommendations in countries where malnutrition is widespread.

---

*Chemists sometimes classify amino acids according to the destinations of their carbon fragments after deamination. If the fragment leads to the production of glucose, the amino acid is called "glucogenic"; if it leads to the formation of ketone bodies, fat, and sterols, the amino acid is called "ketogenic." There is no sharp distinction between glucogenic and ketogenic amino acids, however. A few are both; most are considered glucogenic; only one (leucine) is clearly ketogenic. E. M. N. Hamilton and S. A. S. Gropper, *The Biochemistry of Human Nutrition—A Desk Reference* (St. Paul, Minn.: West, 1987), pp. 116–117.

PROTEIN QUALITY

Food proteins that provide an unbalanced assortment of amino acids, so that the body cannot make full use of them, are poor-quality proteins. In countries where food is scarce, or where the people receive marginal or inadequate amounts of protein, the quality of the dietary protein determines, in large part, how well the children grow and how well the adults maintain their health.

limiting amino acid: the essential amino acid found in the shortest supply relative to the amounts needed for protein synthesis in the body. Four amino acids are most likely to be limiting:
- Lysine.
- Methionine (plus cysteine).
- Threonine.
- Tryptophan.

Limiting Amino Acids   To make proteins, a cell must have all the needed amino acids available simultaneously. The liver can produce any nonessential amino acid that may be in short supply so that the cells can continue linking amino acids into protein strands. If an essential amino acid is missing, though, a cell must dismantle its own proteins to obtain it. Therefore, to prevent protein breakdown, dietary protein must supply at least the nine essential amino acids plus enough nitrogen-containing amino groups and energy for the synthesis of the others. If the diet supplies too little of any essential amino acid, protein synthesis will be limited. The body makes complete proteins only; if one amino acid is missing, the others cannot form a "partial" protein. The body has no storage site for extra amino acids and is forced to either waste them or use them for another purpose. An essential amino acid supplied in less than the amount needed to support protein synthesis is called a *limiting* amino acid.

complete protein: a dietary protein containing all the amino acids essential in human nutrition in amounts adequate for human use.

complementary proteins: two or more proteins whose amino acid assortments complement each other in such a way that the essential amino acids missing from one are supplied by the other.

mutual supplementation: the strategy of combining two protein foods in a meal so that each food provides the essential amino acid(s) lacking in the other. Mutual supplementation is the dietary strategy that brings complementary proteins together in a meal.

Complete Protein   A complete dietary protein contains all the essential amino acids in relatively the same amounts as human beings require; it may or may not contain all the nonessential amino acids. Generally, proteins derived from animals (meat, fish, poultry, cheese, eggs, and milk) are complete, although gelatin is an exception (it lacks tryptophan and cannot support growth and health as a diet's sole protein). Proteins from plants (vegetables, grains, and legumes) have more diverse amino acid patterns, and some tend to be limiting in one or more essential amino acids. Some plant proteins (for example, corn protein) are notoriously incomplete. Others (for example, soy protein) are complete.[4]

Complementary Proteins   In general, plant proteins are of lower quality than animal proteins, and plants also offer less protein per unit (either weight or measure) of food. For this reason, many vegetarians combine plant-protein foods with different but complementary amino acid patterns to obtain the full array of essential amino acids in their diets. This strategy is called mutual supplementa-

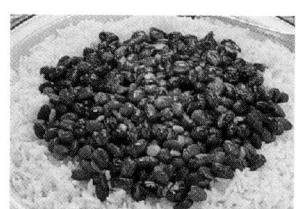

Black beans and rice, a favorite Hispanic combination, together provide a full array of amino acids.

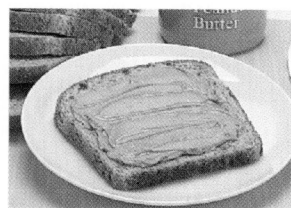

Another simple example of mutual supplementation: peanut butter on wheat bread, a North American tradition.

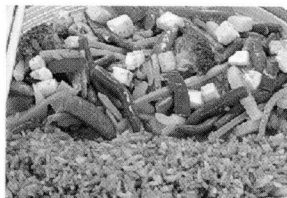

Tofu and stir-fried vegetables with rice offer the proteins of legumes, vegetables, and grains.

tion, and it yields complementary proteins that contain all the essential amino acids in quantities sufficient to support health. The protein quality of the combination is greater than for either food alone.

Many people have long believed that mutual supplementation at every meal was critical to protein nutrition. For most healthy vegetarians, though, it is not necessary to balance amino acids at each meal when protein intake is varied and energy intake is sufficient.[5] Vegetarians can receive all the amino acids they need over the course of a day, if they eat a variety of grains, legumes, seeds, nuts, and vegetables. Protein deficiency will develop, however, when fruits and certain vegetables make up the core of the diet, severely limiting the *quantity* and *quality* of protein. Highlight 6 shows how to plan a nutritious vegetarian diet.

Digestibility   Ideally, a protein is both complete and easily digestible, so that enough amino acids are available for protein synthesis. Such a protein is a high-quality protein. Digestibility depends on a protein's configuration, other foods eaten with it, and reactions that influence the release of amino acids.

Reference Protein   One of the most complete and digestible proteins is egg protein. Until the early 1990s, egg protein was used as the standard for measuring protein quality; it was assigned a value of 100, and the quality of other food proteins was determined based on how they compared with egg. Such a standard is called a reference protein. Now, the Food and Agriculture Organization (FAO) of the United Nations and the World Health Organization (WHO) have established a new standard for the reference protein: the essential amino acid requirements of preschool-age children.

MEASURES OF PROTEIN QUALITY

Researchers have developed several methods for evaluating the quality of food proteins. The object of all of these methods is to identify high-quality proteins—that is, proteins that contain all of the essential amino acids in relatively the same proportion as human beings require. Proteins that are low in an essential amino acid cannot, by themselves, support protein synthesis. The following paragraphs briefly describe these measures; Appendix J provides more detail.

Amino Acid Scoring   The simplest way to evaluate a food protein's quality is to determine its amino acid composition and compare it with a reference protein. Scientists can easily identify the limiting amino acid—it is the one that falls shortest compared with the reference. If the test protein's limiting amino acid is 70 percent of the amount found in the reference protein, it receives a chemical score of 70. Such calculations fail to estimate digestibility, however.

Biological Value   The biological value (BV) of a protein measures its efficiency in supporting the body's needs. Scientists feed a given food protein to experimental animals as the sole protein in their diet and measure the animals' retention and loss of nitrogen. The more nitrogen retained, the higher the protein quality. (Recall that when an essential amino acid is missing, protein synthesis stops, and the remaining amino acids are deaminated and the nitrogen excreted.)

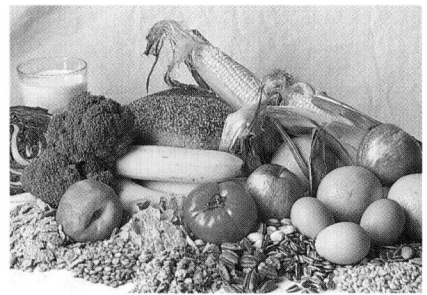

Vegetarians obtain their protein from legumes, nuts, whole grains, vegetables, and, in some cases, eggs and milk products.

protein digestibility: a measure of the amount of amino acids absorbed from a given protein intake.

high-quality protein: an easily digestible, complete protein.

reference protein: a standard against which to measure the quality of other proteins.

amino acid scoring: a method of evaluating protein quality by comparing a test protein's amino acid pattern with that of a reference protein; sometimes called **chemical scoring.**

biological value (BV): the amount of protein nitrogen that is retained for growth and maintenance, expressed as a percentage of the protein nitrogen that has been digested and absorbed; a measure of protein quality.

BV of proteins:
- Egg 100
- Fish 75
- Milk 93
- Corn 72
- Beef 75

Biological value is expressed as a percentage of the absorbed nitrogen that is retained. For egg protein, the BV is 100 (all the absorbed protein is retained); the margin lists the BV of a few other proteins. Supplied in adequate quantity, a protein with a BV of 70 or greater can support human growth as long as energy intake is adequate.

net protein utilization (NPU): the amount of protein nitrogen that is retained from a given amount of protein nitrogen eaten; a measure of protein quality.

Net Protein Utilization Like BV, net protein utilization (NPU) measures nitrogen retention. Instead of measuring retention of absorbed nitrogen (as in BV), NPU measures retention of food nitrogen.

protein efficiency ratio (PER): a measure of protein quality assessed by determining how well a given protein supports weight gain in growing rats; used to establish the protein quality for infant formulas and baby foods.

Protein Efficiency Ratio The protein efficiency ratio (PER) measures the weight gain of a growing animal and compares it to the animal's protein intake. Until recently, PER was generally accepted as the official method used in the United States and Canada to assess protein quality.

protein digestibility–corrected amino acid score (PDCAAS): a measure of protein quality assessed by comparing the amino acid balance of a food protein with the amino acid requirements of preschool-age children and then correcting for the true digestibility of the protein; recommended by the FAO/WHO and used to establish protein quality of foods for Daily Value percentages on food labels.

PDCAAS The protein digestibility–corrected amino acid score or PDCAAS method compares the amino acid contents of a protein with human amino acid requirements and corrects for digestibility.[6] The protein's amino acid profile is determined as described earlier ("Amino Acid Scoring"), and then it is compared against the amino acid requirements of preschool-age children. This comparison reveals the most limiting amino acid. The rationale behind using the requirements of this age group is that if a protein will effectively support a young child's growth and development, then it will meet or exceed the requirements of older children and adults. Thus the PDCAAS method evaluates dietary protein quality for all age groups except infants. (The PER method described earlier is used to evaluate proteins for infants.)

To arrive at the PDCAAS, the amino acid score is multiplied by the food's protein digestibility percentage. Because the digestibility of many foods is similar in human beings and in rats, values for protein digestibility in rats are commonly used. Appendix J provides an example of how to calculate the PDCAAS, and Table 6–4 lists the PDCAAS values of selected foods.

Table 6–4

PDCAAS Values of Selected Foods

Casein (milk protein)	1.00
Egg white	1.00
Soybean (isolate)	.99
Beef	.92
Pea flour	.69
Kidney beans (canned)	.68
Chick peas (canned)	.66
Pinto beans (canned)	.63
Rolled oats	.57
Lentils (canned)	.52
Peanut meal	.52
Whole wheat	.40

Note: 1.0 is the maximum PDCAAS a food protein can receive.

PROTEIN REGULATIONS FOR FOOD LABELS

The PDCAAS method has been integrated into the new labeling regulations of the Food and Drug Administration (FDA).[7] The FDA determined that the PDCAAS method assesses protein quality more precisely for people over age one than the PER, which was used previously for labeling purposes. The PER method using casein as a standard has been retained to measure protein quality for infant formulas and baby foods.

All food labels must state the *quantity* of protein in gram amounts. The "% Daily Value" for protein is not mandatory on all labels, but is required whenever a food makes a protein claim or is intended for consumption by children under four years old.* Whenever the Daily Value percentage is declared, researchers must factor the quantity of the protein determined by using the PDCAAS method. Thus the "% Daily Value" for protein reflects both quantity and quality.

---

*For labeling purposes, the RDI (Reference Daily Intakes) for protein are as follows: for infants, 14 grams; for children under age 4, 16 grams; for older children and adults, 50 grams; for pregnant women, 60 grams; and for lactating women, 65 grams.

The quality of protein is of great importance in dealing with malnutrition worldwide. In the United States and Canada, protein deficiency is not common, but protein quality does play a crucial role in the growth of infants and the health of older adults. Protein quality becomes more important as consumers shift from a diet based on meat to a diet based on grains, vegetables, and fruits as recommended by the Daily Food Guide. All things considered, the best guarantee of amino acid adequacy is to eat mixtures of foods containing protein from a variety of sources in the presence of adequate amounts of vitamins, minerals, fiber, and energy. Protein quality scores of individual foods deserve little emphasis.

Health Effects and Recommended Intakes of Protein

No nutrient has been more intensely scrutinized than protein. As you know by now, it is indispensable to life. And it should come as no surprise that protein deficiency can have devastating effects on people's health. But like the other nutrients, protein in excess can also be harmful. This section examines the health effects and recommended intakes of protein.

PROTEIN-ENERGY MALNUTRITION

When people are deprived of protein, energy, or both, the result is protein-energy malnutrition (PEM). Although PEM touches many adult lives, it most often strikes early in childhood. It is the most widespread form of malnutrition in the world today, afflicting over 500 million children.[8] Most of the 40,000 children who die each day are malnourished.

Inadequate food intake leads to poor growth in children and to weight loss and wasting in adults. Children who are thin for their height may be suffering from acute PEM (recent severe food deprivation), whereas children who are short for their age have experienced chronic PEM (long-term food deprivation). Poor growth due to PEM is easy to overlook because a small child may look quite normal, but it is the most common sign of malnutrition.

PEM is most prevalent in Africa, Central America, South America, the Middle East, and East and Southeast Asia. In the United States, homeless people and those living in substandard housing in inner cities and rural areas have been diagnosed with PEM.[9] In addition to those living in poverty, elderly people who live alone and adults who are addicted to drugs and alcohol are frequently victims of PEM.[10] Adult PEM is also seen in people hospitalized with infections such as AIDS or tuberculosis; infections deplete body proteins, demand extra energy, induce nutrient losses, and alter metabolic pathways. PEM is also common in those suffering from the eating disorder anorexia nervosa. Prevention emphasizes frequent, nutrient-dense, energy-dense meals and, equally important, resolution of the underlying causes of PEM—poverty, infections, and illness.

Classifying PEM Researchers have long believed that PEM occurs in two forms: marasmus and kwashiorkor, which differ in their clinical features (see Table 6–5). The child with marasmus looks emaciated, whereas the child with kwashiorkor looks swollen, particularly in the belly. Historically, marasmus was

protein-energy malnutrition (PEM), also called **protein-kcalorie malnutrition (PCM)**: a deficiency of both protein and energy; the world's most widespread malnutrition problem, including kwashiorkor, marasmus, and instances in which they overlap.

acute PEM: protein-energy malnutrition caused by recent severe food restriction; characterized in children by thinness for height (wasting).

chronic PEM: protein-energy malnutrition caused by long-term food deprivation; characterized in children by short height for age (stunting).

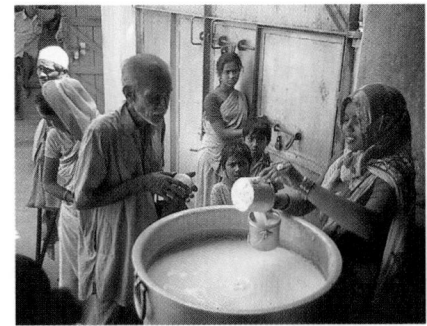

Donated food saves some people from starvation, but it is usually insufficient to meet nutrient needs or even to provide a full belly for every person who is hungry.

Table 6–5

Features of Marasmus and Kwashiorkor in Children

Separating PEM into two classifications oversimplifies the condition, but at the extremes, marasmus and kwashiorkor exhibit marked differences. Marasmus-kwashiorkor mix presents symptoms common to both marasmus and kwashiorkor. In all cases, children are likely to develop diarrhea, infections, and multiple nutrient deficiencies.

Marasmus	Kwashiorkor
Infancy (less than 2 yr)	Older infants and young children (1 to 3 yr)
Severe deprivation, or impaired absorption, of protein, energy, vitamins, and minerals	Inadequate protein intake or, more commonly, infections
Develops slowly; chronic PEM	Rapid onset; acute PEM
Severe weight loss	Some weight loss
Severe muscle wasting, with fat	Some muscle wasting, with retention of some body fat
Growth: <60% weight-for-age	Growth: 60 to 80% weight-for-age
No detectable edema	Edema
No fatty liver	Enlarged fatty liver
Anxiety, apathy	Apathy, misery, irritability, sadness
Good appetite possible	Anorexia
Hair is sparse, thin, and dry; easily pulled out	Hair is dry and brittle; easily pulled out; changes color; becomes straight
Skin is dry, thin, and easily wrinkles	Skin develops lesions

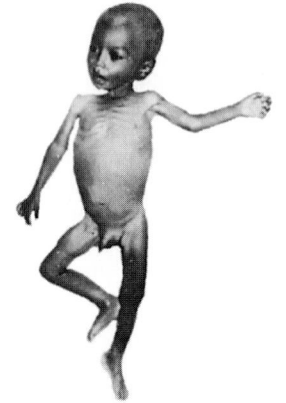

A child suffering the severe wasting of marasmus.

thought to be caused by a lack of energy, with protein deficiency an indirect result. Kwashiorkor was thought to be caused by an inadequate amount or quality of protein in the presence of adequate energy. In reality, though, marasmus reflects a severe deprivation of food over a long time (chronic PEM) and therefore is caused by an inadequate energy *and* protein intake (and by inadequate vitamins and minerals as well). By comparison, kwashiorkor typically reflects a more sudden and recent deprivation of food (acute PEM). It too has probably been mischaracterized, because diets that are adequate in energy are rarely deficient in protein.[11] Some researchers maintain that marasmus and kwashiorkor are two stages of the same disease. Others suggest that kwashiorkor develops when malnourished children eat moldy grains.[12] Researchers continue to question the exact causes of kwashiorkor, but clearly, protein deficiency appears to be one of several factors involved. Most likely, dietary imbalances, multiple infections, parasitic diseases, and toxins together influence the development of kwashiorkor.[13] The following paragraphs describe three clinical syndromes—marasmus, kwashiorkor, and the combination of the two.

Marasmus Marasmus occurs most commonly in children from 6 to 18 months of age in all the overpopulated urban slums of the world. Children in impoverished nations simply do not have enough to eat and subsist on diluted cereal drinks that supply scant energy and protein of low quality; such food can barely sustain life, much less support growth. Consequently, marasmic children look like old people—just skin and bones.

marasmus (ma-RAZ-mus): a form of PEM that results from a severe deprivation, or impaired absorption, of energy, protein, vitamins, and minerals.

Without adequate nutrition, muscles, including the heart, waste and weaken. Because the brain normally grows to almost its full adult size within the first two years of life, marasmus impairs brain development and learning ability. Reduced synthesis of key hormones slows metabolism and lowers body temperature. There is little or no fat under the skin to insulate against cold. Hospital workers find that children with marasmus need to be wrapped up and kept warm. They also need love because they have often been deprived of parental attention as well as food.

The starving child faces this threat to life by engaging in as little activity as possible—not even crying for food. The body musters all its forces to meet the crisis, so it cuts down on any expenditure of protein not needed for the heart, lungs, and brain to function. Growth ceases; the child is no larger at age four than at age two. Digestive enzymes are in short supply, the GI tract lining deteriorates, and absorption fails. The child can't assimilate what little food is eaten.

Kwashiorkor Kwashiorkor was originally a Ghanaian word meaning "the evil spirit that infects the first child when the second child is born." When a mother who has been nursing her first child bears a second child, she weans the first child and puts the second one on the breast. The first child, suddenly switched from nutrient-dense, protein-rich breast milk to a starchy, protein-poor cereal, soon begins to sicken and die. Kwashiorkor typically sets in between 18 months and two years.

Kwashiorkor usually develops rapidly as a result of protein deficiency or, more commonly, is precipitated by an illness such as measles or other infection.[14] As mentioned, some researchers believe that kwashiorkor and marasmus are two stages of the same disease. They point out that kwashiorkor and marasmus often exist side by side in the same community that consumes the same diet. They note that a child who has marasmus can later develop kwashiorkor. Some research indicates that marasmus represents the body's adaptation to starvation, and that kwashiorkor develops when adaptation fails.

Another possibility is that kwashiorkor may be a form of food poisoning superimposed on malnutrition. One supporting piece of evidence is that kwashiorkor seems to appear only in rainy, tropical communities. Many temperate regions have experienced widespread famine, yet have not had kwashiorkor. Another clue is that under hot, humid conditions, a common mold, *Aspergillus flavus*, produces aflatoxin, a toxin that inhibits protein synthesis. When malnourished children are forced to eat moldy grain for lack of other foods, their weakened bodies cannot defend against the toxin.

The loss of weight and body fat is usually not as severe in kwashiorkor as in marasmus, but there may be some muscle wasting. Proteins and hormones that previously maintained fluid balance diminish, and fluid leaks into the interstitial spaces. The child's limbs and face become swollen with edema, a distinguishing feature of kwashiorkor. The belly bulges with a fatty liver, caused by lack of the protein carriers that transport fat out of the liver. The fatty liver lacks enzymes to clear poisons from the body, so their toxic effects are prolonged. Without sufficient tyrosine to make melanin, the child's hair loses its color; inadequate protein synthesis leaves the skin patchy and scaly, often with sores that fail to heal.

Marasmus-Kwashiorkor Mix The combination of marasmus and kwashiorkor is characterized by the edema of kwashiorkor with the wasting of marasmus. Most often, the child is suffering the effects of both malnutrition and infections.

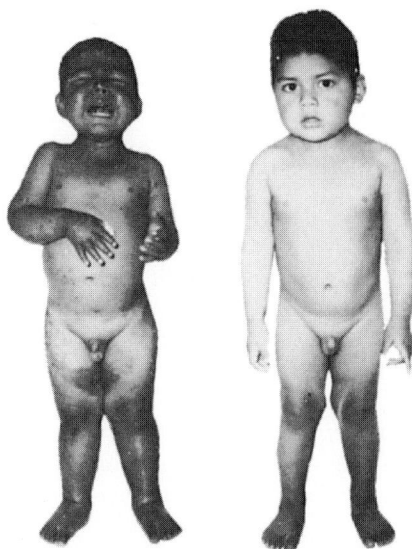

At left, a child swollen with the characteristic edema of kwashiorkor. At right, the same child after nutritional therapy.

kwashiorkor (kwash-ee-OR-core, kwash-ee-or-CORE): a form of PEM that results from either inadequate protein intake or, more commonly, from infections.

aflatoxin: potent cancer-causing toxin produced by the mold *Aspergillus flavus* that infects grains and peanuts. The USDA tests grains and peanuts grown in this country for aflatoxin contamination.

Reminder: *Edema* is the swelling of body tissue caused by excessive fluid in the interstitial spaces, seen in protein deficiency (among other conditions).

Chapter 25 describes the relationships between PEM and severe stress; Chapter 16 presents assessment of protein status.

dysentery (DISS-en-terry): an infection of the digestive tract that causes diarrhea.

Infections In PEM, antibodies to fight off invading bacteria are degraded to provide amino acids for other uses, leaving the malnourished child vulnerable to infections. Blood proteins, including hemoglobin, are no longer synthesized, so the child becomes anemic and weak. Dysentery, an infection of the digestive tract, causes diarrhea, further depleting the body of nutrients. In the marasmic child, once infection sets in, kwashiorkor often follows.[15]

The combination of infections, fever, electrolyte imbalances, and anemia often leads to heart failure and occasionally sudden death. Infections combined with malnutrition are responsible for two-thirds of the deaths of young children in developing countries.[16] Measles, which might make a healthy child sick for a week or two, kills a child with PEM within two or three days.

Reminder: The term *electrolyte balance* refers to the proper concentrations of salts within the body fluids (see Chapter 12 for details).

Rehabilitation If caught in time, the life of a starving child may be saved by careful nutrition therapy. Diarrhea will have depleted the body's potassium and disturbed other electrolyte balances. Careful correction of fluid and electrolyte imbalances usually raises the blood pressure and strengthens the heartbeat. After the first 24 to 48 hours, protein and food energy may be given in small quantities, gradually increasing intakes as tolerated.

Experts assure us that we possess the knowledge, technology, and resources to end hunger. Programs that have involved the local people in the process of identifying problems and devising solutions have met with some success. But until those who have the food, technology, and resources make fighting hunger a priority, the war on hunger will not be won (see Highlight 18 for more on hunger).

HEALTH EFFECTS OF PROTEIN

While many of the world's people struggle to obtain enough food energy and protein, in developed countries both are so abundant that problems of excess are seen. Overconsumption of protein offers no benefits and may pose health risks.

The relationships between protein and chronic diseases are not clearly evident. Population studies have difficulty determining whether diseases correlate with animal proteins or with their accompanying saturated fats. Studies that rely on data from vegetarians must sort out the many lifestyle factors, other than a "no-meat diet," that might explain relationships between protein and health.

Heart Disease As mentioned, foods rich in animal protein tend to be rich in saturated fats. Consequently, it is not surprising to find a correlation between animal-protein intake and heart disease, although no independent effect has been demonstrated. On the other hand, substituting soy protein for animal protein lowers blood cholesterol, especially in those with high blood cholesterol.[17]

Recent research suggests that the amino acid homocysteine may be an independent risk factor for heart disease.[18] When compared with others, men with elevated homocysteine were three times as likely to have heart attacks.[19] Researchers do not yet know what role homocysteine plays in heart disease, nor do they understand what raises homocysteine in the blood. Elevated homocysteine is associated with suboptimal concentrations of B vitamins and can usually be corrected with vitamin B_{12}, vitamin B_6, and folate supplements.[20] Whether such treatments will reduce the risk of heart attacks remains unknown.

Cancer   As in heart disease, the effects of protein and fats cannot be easily separated. Some studies have found a link between high-meat diets and colon cancer. Population studies suggest a correlation between high intakes of animal proteins and some types of cancer (notably, cancer of the colon, breast, pancreas, and prostate). One recent study has reported an increase in the risk of kidney cancer with a high consumption of red meat and high-protein foods.[21] A high protein intake increases the work of the kidneys, and excretion of the end products of protein metabolism depends, in part, on an adequate fluid intake and healthy kidneys.

Adult Bone Loss (Osteoporosis)   Do high protein intakes accelerate bone loss? Calcium excretion rises as protein intake increases; furthermore, calcium excretion appears to rise with intakes of animal-derived proteins, but not with plant-derived proteins.[22] Whether excess protein may deplete the bones of their chief minerals depends largely upon the ratio of calcium to protein intakes.[23] An ideal ratio has not been established, but a woman whose intake meets the RDA for both nutrients has a calcium-to-protein ratio of 16 to 1 (milligrams to grams). For most women in the United States, however, average calcium intakes are lower and protein intakes are higher, yielding a 9-to-1 ratio, which may produce calcium losses that compromise bone health.[24] In contrast, moderate increases in physical activity and calcium intake may protect against such losses.[25]

Weight Control   Protein-rich foods are often fat-rich foods that contribute to obesity with its accompanying health risks. Weight-loss gimmicks that encourage a high-protein diet are rarely useful; overweight people have better success with diets that provide adequate protein, minimal fat, and ample energy from carbohydrates. The higher a person's intake of protein-rich foods such as meat and milk, the more likely that fruits, vegetables, and grains will be crowded out, making the diet inadequate in other nutrients.

RECOMMENDED INTAKES OF PROTEIN

As mentioned earlier, the body continuously breaks down and loses its proteins and cannot store amino acids. To replace protein, the body needs dietary protein for two reasons: first, food protein is the only source of the *essential* amino acids; and second, it is the only practical source of *nitrogen* with which to build the nonessential amino acids and other nitrogen-containing compounds.

The *Diet and Health* report recommends that people's fat intakes should contribute 30 percent or less of total food energy, and carbohydrate, 55 percent or more—which leaves about 15 percent for protein. Current intakes in the United States and Canada, though higher than recommendations, do not seem to be high enough to cause harm. The *Diet and Health* report advises people to maintain moderate protein intakes—between the RDA and twice the RDA.

Protein RDA   The protein RDA for healthy adults is 0.8 grams per kilogram of appropriate body weight per day. For infants and children, the RDA is higher. When compared to total energy intake, however, the protein RDA for infants and children is similar to that of adults as Table 6–6 shows. The RDA generously covers the needs for replacing worn-out tissue, so it increases for larger people; it also covers the needs for building new tissue during growth, so it increases for

Other risk factors for adult bone loss (osteoporosis) are sex, age, and race, as Highlight 12 explains.

Table 6–6

Protein RDA as a Percentage of Energy RDA

When expressed as a percentage of energy intake, the protein requirement represents about 10 percent of the energy RDA.

Age (yr)	Protein RDA (g/kg)	Protein RDA (in kCalories) as a Percentage of Energy RDA (%)
0 to ½	2.2	8.0
½ to 1	1.6	6.5
1 to 3	1.2	4.9
4 to 6	1.1	5.3
7 to 10	1.0	5.6
Males		
11 to 14	1.0	7.2
15 to 18	0.9	7.9
19 to 24	0.8	8.0
25 to 50	0.8	8.7
51 +	0.8	11.0
Females		
11 to 14	1.0	8.4
15 to 18	0.8	8.0
19 to 24	0.8	8.4
25 to 50	0.8	9.1
51 +	0.8	10.5

How to Calculate Recommended Protein Intakes

To figure your protein RDA:

- Look up the appropriate weight for a person of your height (inside back cover). If your present weight falls within that range, use it for the following calculations. If your present weight falls outside the range, use the midpoint of the acceptable weight range as your reference weight.

- Convert pounds to kilograms, if necessary (pounds divided by 2.2 equals kilograms).

- Multiply kilograms by 0.8 to get your RDA in grams per day. (Males 18 years old and younger, multiply by 0.9.) Example:

$$\text{Weight} = 150 \text{ lb.}$$
$$150 \text{ lb} \div 2.2 \text{ lb/kg} = 68 \text{ kg (rounded off).}$$
$$68 \text{ kg} \times 0.8 \text{ g/kg} = 54 \text{ g protein (rounded off).}$$

The special protein needs of people who are ill are described in later chapters.

Protein recommendations for athletes are presented in Highlight 8.

children and pregnant women. The accompanying box shows how to calculate your RDA for protein.

In setting the RDA, the committee assumes that people are healthy and do not have unusual metabolic needs for protein; that the protein eaten will be of mixed quality; and that the body will use the protein about as efficiently as it uses reference proteins. In addition, the committee assumes that the protein is consumed along with sufficient carbohydrate and fat to provide adequate energy and that other nutrients in the diet are adequate.

Adequate Energy Note the qualification "adequate energy" in the preceding statement, and consider what happens if energy intake falls short of needs. An intake of 50 grams of protein, which is equal to 200 kcalories, provides about 10 percent of the total energy from protein, if the person receives 2000 kcalories a day. But if the person cuts energy intake drastically—to, say 800 kcalories a day—then an intake of 200 kcalories from protein is suddenly 25 percent of the total; yet it's still the same number of grams. The protein intake is reasonable, but the energy intake is not; the low energy intake will force the body to use the protein to meet energy needs rather than to replace lost body protein. Similarly, if the person's energy intake is high—say, 4000 kcalories—the 50-gram protein intake will represent only 5 percent of the total, yet it *still* is a reasonable protein intake. Again, the energy intake is unreasonable for most people, but in this case, it will permit the protein to be used to meet the body's needs.

Be careful when judging a protein intake as a percentage of energy. Always ascertain the number of grams as well, and compare it with the RDA or another standard stated in grams. A recommendation stated as a percentage of energy intake is useful only if the energy intake is within reason.

Protein in Abundance Many people tend to overvalue protein, perhaps because they have been so impressed with its many critical roles in the body. They think they need *lots* of protein, when, in fact, they are already receiving plenty. Even athletes typically don't need to increase their protein intakes. Most people in developed countries such as the United States and Canada receive much more protein than they need. This is not surprising considering the abundance of food eaten and the central role meats hold in the diet. A single ounce of meat delivers about 7 grams of protein, so one 8-ounce serving of meat alone supplies more than the RDA for an average-sized person. Besides meat, well-fed people eat many other nutritious foods, many of which also contain protein.

To illustrate how easy it is to overconsume protein, consider the *minimum* recommended servings for the Daily Food Guide. Six servings from the bread, cereal, rice, and pasta group provide about 18 grams of protein; 3 servings of vegetables deliver about 6 grams; 2 servings of milk offer 16 grams; and 2 servings of meat contain about 35 grams. This totals 75 grams of protein—higher than recommendations for most people.

Just think how much more protein people receive when they eat additional servings. No wonder most people in the United States and Canada get more protein than they need. If they have an adequate *food* intake, they have a more-than-adequate protein intake. The key diet-planning principle to emphasize for protein is moderation. Even though most people receive plenty of protein, some feel compelled to take supplements as well, as the next section describes.

PROTEIN AND AMINO ACID SUPPLEMENTS

Health food stores and popular magazine articles advertise a wide variety of protein supplements, and people take these supplements for many different reasons, all of them unfounded. Athletes take them to build muscle. Dieters take them to spare their bodies' protein while losing weight. Women take them to strengthen their fingernails. People take individual amino acids, too—to cure herpes, to make themselves sleep better, to lose weight, and to relieve pain and depression.* Like many other magic solutions to health problems, protein and amino acid supplements don't work these miracles, and they can be harmful.

Muscle work builds muscle; protein supplements do not, and athletes do not need them. Instead, athletes need a well-balanced diet that provides sufficient dietary protein and adequate food energy. Food energy spares body protein; carbohydrate and fat serve this purpose equally well, and carbohydrate is safer. Fingernails are not affected by protein supplements, provided the diet is adequate. Normal, healthy people never need protein supplements.

Furthermore, protein supplements are expensive, less completely digested than protein-rich foods, and, when used as replacements for such foods, often downright dangerous. The "liquid protein" diet, advocated some years ago for weight loss, caused deaths in many users; even some physician-supervised protein-sparing fasts based on liquid protein have caused abnormal heart rhythms. The FDA warns that their use as a total diet without medical supervision "may cause serious illness or death."

Single amino acids do not occur naturally in foods and offer no benefit to the body; in fact, they can be harmful.[26] The body was not designed to handle the high concentrations and unusual combinations of amino acids found in supple-

Highlight 8 discusses athletes' nutrition needs further.

Use of amino acids as dietary supplements is inappropriate, especially for:[27]
- All women of childbearing age.
- Pregnant or lactating women.
- Infants, children, and adolescents.
- Elderly people.
- People with inborn errors of metabolism that affect their bodies' handling of amino acids.
- Smokers.
- People on low-protein diets.
- People with chronic or acute mental or physical illnesses who take amino acids without medical supervision.

_____

*Canada allows single amino acid supplements to be sold only as drugs or as food additives.

ments.[28] An excess of one amino acid can create such a demand for a carrier that it prevents the absorption of another amino acid, creating a deficiency. Those amino acids winning the competition enter in excess, creating the possibility of a toxicity. Toxicity of single amino acids in animal studies raises concerns about their use in human beings.[29] Anyone considering taking amino acid supplements should check with a physician first.

In two cases, recommendations for single amino acid supplements have led to widespread public use—lysine to prevent or relieve the infections that cause herpes cold sores on the mouth or genital organs, and tryptophan to relieve pain, depression, and insomnia. In both cases, enthusiastic popular reports and careful scientific experiments are at odds. Lysine does not relieve or cure herpes infections, and if long-term use helps prevent them, it does so only in some individuals and with unknown associated risks.

Tryptophan does have some interesting effects with respect to pain and sleep, but its use for these purposes is still experimental. More than 1500 people who elected to take tryptophan supplements developed a rare blood disorder known as eosinophilia-myalgia syndrome (EMS). EMS is characterized by severe muscle pain, extremely high fever, and, in over three dozen cases, death. Treatment usually involves physical therapy and low doses of corticosteroids to relieve symptoms temporarily. Some evidence suggests that changes in procedures at a major Japanese tryptophan processing plant may have introduced contaminants that caused the disease.[30] Later research suggests multiple factors were involved, and the exact causes of EMS remain unknown. The FDA issued a recall of all products containing tryptophan.*

It is safest to obtain lysine, tryptophan, and all other amino acids in protein foods, eaten with carbohydrate to facilitate their use in the body. With all that we know about science, it is hard to improve on nature.

In summary, protein is indispensable to life and growth. Deficiencies arise from both energy-poor and protein-poor diets and lead to the devastating diseases of marasmus and kwashiorkor. Together these diseases are known as PEM (protein-energy malnutrition), the major form of malnutrition causing infections and death in children worldwide. Excesses of food energy and protein are also harmful. Optimally, the diet will be adequate in energy from carbohydrate and fat and will deliver 0.8 grams of protein per kilogram of normal body weight each day. U.S. and Canadian diets are typically more than adequate in this respect, and protein or amino acid supplements are superfluous.

Study Questions

1. How does the chemical structure of proteins differ from the structures of carbohydrates and fats?
2. Describe the structure of amino acids, and explain how their sequence in proteins affects the proteins' shapes. What are essential amino acids?
3. Describe protein digestion and absorption.
4. Describe protein synthesis.
5. Describe some of the roles proteins play in the human body.
6. What are enzymes? What roles do they play in chemical reactions? Describe the differences between enzymes and hormones.

7. How does the body use amino acids? What is deamination?
8. What factors affect the quality of dietary protein? What is a complete protein?
9. How can vegetarians meet their protein needs without eating meat?
10. What are the health consequences of ingesting inadequate protein and energy? Describe marasmus and kwashiorkor. How can the two conditions be distinguished, and in what ways do they overlap?

11. How might protein excess, or the type of protein eaten, influence health?
12. What factors are considered in establishing recommended protein intakes? Define nitrogen balance. What conditions are associated with zero, positive, and negative balance?
13. What are the benefits and risks of taking protein and amino acid supplements?

Notes

1. *Report of the Expert Advisory Committee on Amino Acids* (Ottawa: Health and Welfare Canada, 1990), p. 9.
2. J. C. Waterlow, Whole-body protein turnover in humans—Past, present, and future, *Annual Review of Nutrition* 15 (1995): 57–92.
3. V. R. Young and J. S. Marchini, Mechanisms and nutritional significance of metabolic responses to altered intakes of protein and amino acids, with reference to nutritional adaptation in humans, *American Journal of Clinical Nutrition* 51 (1990): 270–289.
4. V. R. Young, Soy protein in relation to human protein and amino acid nutrition, *Journal of the American Dietetic Association* 91 (1991): 828–835; J. W. Erdman and E. J. Fordyce, Soy products and the human diet, *American Journal of Clinical Nutrition* 49 (1989): 725–737.
5. V. R. Young and P. L. Pellett, Plant proteins in relation to human protein and amino acid nutrition, *American Journal of Clinical Nutrition* 59 (1994): 1203S–1212S; Position of The American Dietetic Association: Vegetarian diets, *Journal of the American Dietetic Association* 93 (1993): 1317–1319.
6. Protein quality evaluation, Report of the Joint FAO/WHO Expert Consultation, FAO Food and Nutrition Paper 51 (Rome: Food and Agriculture Organization of the United Nations, 1991); G. Sarwar and F. E. McDonough, Evaluation of protein digestibility–corrected amino acid score method for assessing protein quality of foods, *Journal of the Association of Official Analytical Chemists* 73 (1990): 347–356.
7. E. C. Henley, Food and Drug Administration's proposed labeling rules for protein, *Journal of the American Dietetic Association* 92 (1992): 293–296; V. R. Young and P. L. Pellett, Protein evaluation, amino acid scoring and the Food and Drug Administration's proposed food labeling regulation, *Journal of Nutrition* 121 (1991): 145–150.
8. M. C. Latham, Protein-energy malnutrition, in *Present Knowledge in Nutrition*, 6th ed., ed. M. L. Brown (Washington, D.C.: International Life Sciences Institute—Nutrition Foundation, 1990), pp. 39–46.
9. J. Wolgemuth and coauthors, Wasting malnutrition and inadequate nutrient intakes identified in a multiethnic homeless population, *Journal of the American Dietetic Association* 92 (1992): 834–839; E. Luder and coauthors, Health and nutrition survey in a group of urban homeless adults, *Journal of the American Dietetic Association* 90 (1990): 1387–1392.
10. B. Torún and F. Chew, Protein-energy malnutrition, in *Modern Nutrition in Health and Disease*, 8th ed., eds., M. E. Shils, J. A. Olson, and M. Shike (Philadelphia: Lea & Febiger, 1994), pp. 950–976.
11. C. Gopalan, The contribution of nutrition research to the control of undernutrition: The Indian experience, *Annual Review of Nutrition* 12 (1992): 1–17.
12. R. G. Hendrickse, Kwashiorkor: The hypothesis that incriminates aflatoxins, *Pediatrics* 88 (1991): 376–379.
13. D. B. Jelliffe and E. F. P. Jelliffe, Causation of kwashiorkor: Toward a multifactorial consensus, *Pediatrics* 90 (1992): 110–112.
14. J. C. Waterlow, Childhood malnutrition in developing nations: Looking back and looking forward, *Annual Review of Nutrition* 14 (1994): 1–19.
15. L. Lewinter-Suskind and coauthors, The malnourished child, in *Textbook of Pediatric Nutrition*, 2nd ed., eds., R. M. Suskind and L. Lewinter-Suskind (New York: Raven Press, 1993), pp. 127–140.
16. R. K. Chandra, 1990 McCollum Award Lecture: Nutrition and immunity: Lessons from the past and new insights into the future, *American Journal of Clinical Nutrition* 53 (1991): 1087–1101.
17. J. W. Anderson, B. M. Johnstone, and M. E. Cook-Newell, Meta-analysis of the effects of soy protein intake on serum lipids, *New England Journal of Medicine* 333 (1995): 276–282; K. K. Carroll, Review of clinical studies on cholesterol lowering response to soy protein, *Journal of the American Dietetic Association* 91 (1991): 820–827; K. Widhalm and coauthors, Effect of soy protein diet versus standard low fat, low cholesterol diet on lipid and lipoprotein levels in children with familial or polygenic hypercholesterolemia, *Journal of Pediatrics* 123 (1993): 30–34.
18. K. S. McCully, Micronutrients, homocysteine metabolism, and atherosclerosis, in *Micronutrients in Health and in Disease*

Prevention, eds. A. Bendich and C. E. Butterworth, Jr. (New York: Marcel Dekker, 1991), pp. 69–93; J. Selhub and coauthors, Association between plasma homocysteine concentrations and extracranial carotid-artery stenosis, *New England Journal of Medicine* 332 (1995): 286–291; M. J. Stampfer and M. R. Malinow, Can lowering homocysteine levels reduce cardiovascular risk? *New England Journal of Medicine* 332 (1995): 328–329; J. B. Ubbink, Vitamin nutrition status and homocysteine: An atherogenic risk factor, *Nutrition Reviews* 52 (1994): 383–393.

19. M. J. Stampfer and coauthors, A prospective study of plasma homocyst(e)ine and risk of myocardial infarction in U.S. physicians, *Journal of the American Medical Association* 268 (1992): 877–881.

20. N. Pancharuniti and coauthors, Plasma homocyst(e)ine, folate, and vitamin B-12 concentrations and risk for early-onset coronary artery disease, *American Journal of Clinical Nutrition* 59 (1994): 940–948; J. B. Ubbink and coauthors, Vitamin B-12, vitamin B-6, and folate nutritional status in men with hyperhomocysteinemia, *American Journal of Clinical Nutrition* 57 (1993): 47–53; J. Selhub and coauthors, Vitamin status and intake as primary determinants of homocysteinemia in an elderly population, *Journal of the American Medical Association* 270 (1993): 2693–2698.

21. W. H. Chow and coauthors, Protein intake and risk of renal cell cancer, *Journal of the National Cancer Institute* 86 (1994): 1131–1139.

22. J. Hu and coauthors, Dietary intakes and urinary excretion of calcium and acids: A cross-sectional study of women in China, *American Journal of Clinical Nutrition* 58 (1993): 398–406.

23. Committee on Dietary Allowances, *Recommended Dietary Allowances,* 10th ed. (Washington, D.C.: National Academy Press, 1989), pp. 72–73; C. D. Arnaud and S. D. Sanchez, The role of calcium in osteoporosis, *Annual Review of Nutrition* 10 (1990): 397–414; R. P. Heaney, Protein intake and the calcium economy, *Journal of the American Dietetic Association* 93 (1993): 1259–1260.

24. J. A. Metz, J. J. B. Anderson, and P. N. Gallagher, Intakes of calcium, phosphorus, and protein, and physical activity level are related to radial bone mass in young adult women, *American Journal of Clinical Nutrition* 58 (1993): 537–542; Heaney, 1993.

25. R. R. Recker and coauthors, Bone gain in young adult women, *Journal of the American Medical Association* 268 (1992): 2403–2408.

26. V. Herbert, L-Tryptophan: A mediocolegal case against over-the-counter marketing of supplements of amino acids, *Nutrition Today,* March/April 1992, pp. 27–30.

27. S. A. Anderson and D. J. Raiten, eds., *Safety of Amino Acids Used as Supplements* (Bethesda, Md.: Federation of American Societies for Experimental Biology, 1992).

28. H. N. Christensen, Amino acid nutrition: A two-step absorptive process, *Nutrition Reviews* 51 (1993): 95–100.

29. *Report of the Expert Advisory Committee on Amino Acids,* 1990, p. 9.

30. D. J. Clauw and P. Katz, Treatment of the eosinophilia-myalgia syndrome, *New England Journal of Medicine* 323 (1990): 417–418; E. A. Belongia, A. N. Myeno, and M. T. Osterholm, The eosinophilia-myalgia syndrome and tryptophan, *Annual Review of Nutrition* 12 (1992): 235–256.

Vegetarian, Mediterranean, and Other Meat-Restricted Foodways

The waiter presents this evening's specials: a fresh spinach salad topped with mandarin oranges, raisins, and sunflower seeds, served with a bowl of pasta smothered in a mushroom and tomato sauce and topped with grated parmesan cheese. Then this one: a salad made of chopped parsley, scallions, celery, and tomatoes mixed with bulgar wheat and dressed with olive oil and lemon juice, served with a spinach and feta cheese pie. Do these meals sound good to you? Or is something missing . . . a pork chop or ribeye, perhaps?

Would vegetarian fare be acceptable to you some of the time? Most of the time? Ever? Perhaps it is helpful to recognize that dietary choices fall among a continuum—from one end, where people eat no meat or foods of animal origin, to the other end, where they eat generous quantities daily. Meat's place in the diet has been the subject of much research and controversy, as this highlight will reveal. One of the missions of this highlight, in fact, is to identify the *range* of meat intakes most compatible with health.

People who choose to exclude meat and other animal-derived foods from their diets today do so for many of the same reasons the Greek philosopher Pythagoras cited in the sixth century B.C.: physical health, ecological responsibility, and philosophical concerns. They might also cite world hunger issues, economic reasons, ethical concerns, or religious beliefs as motivating factors.

Vegetarians generally are categorized, not by their motivations, but

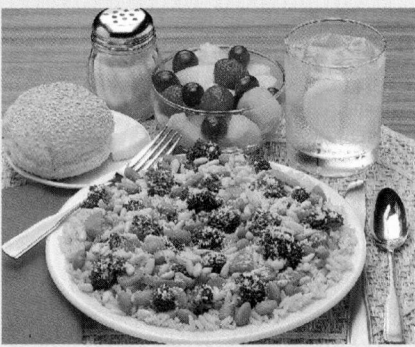

A balanced meal need not include meat to be nutritious.

by the foods they choose not to eat (see the glossary on p. 210). Some exclude red meat only; some also avoid chicken or fish; others also exclude eggs; and still others choose not to drink milk or eat milk products as well. As you will see, though, the foods a person *excludes* are not nearly as important as the foods a person *includes* in the diet. Most vegetarian diets include a variety of grains, vegetables, legumes, and fruits, which offer abundant complex carbohydrates and fibers, an assortment of vitamins and minerals, and little fat—characteristics that reflect current dietary recommendations aimed at reducing obesity and the risks of several chronic diseases such as hypertension, heart disease, and cancer. Vegetarian diets that are well planned can offer sound nutrition and health benefits to adults.[1]

This highlight first looks at the health benefits and potential problems of vegetarian diets and then shows how to plan a well-balanced vegetarian diet. It closes with a description of the Mediterranean

diet—an ethnic pattern of eating that includes very little meat and exceeds current dietary recommendations for fat and alcohol, yet still seems to support good health.

HEALTH BENEFITS OF VEGETARIAN DIETS

Research on the health impacts of vegetarianism would be relatively easy if vegetarians differed from other people only in not eating meat. Many vegetarians, however, have adopted lifestyles that differ from those of meat eaters in many other ways. Compared with others, vegetarians are more likely to practice healthy habits: they typically maintain a healthy weight, use no tobacco or illicit drugs, use alcohol in moderation (if at all), and are physically active. Researchers must account for the effects of these lifestyle differences before they can pick out what aspects of health correlate just with diet. Even then, *correlations* are merely statements of what health factors *go with* the vegetarian diet; they do not show what health effects may be *caused by* the diet. Without more evidence, conclusions are only tentative. Still, with all these qualifications, research findings are intriguing. They seem to suggest that vegetarian diets offer some health benefits.

Weight Control

In general, vegetarians maintain a healthier body weight than nonvegetarians. Since obesity impairs health in a number of ways, this gives vegetarians a health advantage.

Glossary

lactovegetarians: people who include milk and milk products, but exclude meat, poultry, fish, seafood, and eggs from their diets.

   lacto = milk

lacto-ovo-vegetarians: people who include milk, milk products, and eggs, but exclude meat, poultry, fish, and seafood from their diets.

   ovo = egg

macrobiotic diets: extremely restrictive diets limited to a few cereals and fluids; based on metaphysical beliefs and not on nutrition.

meat replacement: products formulated to look and taste like meat, fish, or poultry; usually made of textured vegetable protein.

omnivores: people who have no formal restriction on the eating of any foods.

   omni = all
   vores = to eat

semivegetarians: people who include some, but not all, groups of animal-derived foods in their diets; they usually exclude red meat, but may occasionally include poultry, fish, and seafood; sometimes called **partial vegetarians.**

tempeh (TEM-pay)**:** a fermented soybean food, rich in protein and fiber.

textured vegetable protein: processed soybean protein used in vegetarian products such as soy burgers.

tofu (TOE-foo)**:** a curd made from soybeans, rich in protein and often fortified with calcium; used in many Asian and vegetarian dishes in place of meat.

vegans (VAY-guns or VEJ-ans)**:** people who exclude all animal-derived foods (including meat, poultry, fish, eggs, and dairy products) from their diets; also called **pure vegetarians, strict vegetarians,** or **total vegetarians.**

vegetarians: a general term used to describe people who exclude meat, poultry, fish, or other animal-derived foods from their diets.

Blood Pressure

Appropriate body weight helps to maintain a healthy blood pressure, as does a diet low in total fat and saturated fat and high in fiber, fruits, and vegetables.[2] In one group of volunteers, blood pressure declined during the period when they ate a vegetarian diet and rose again when they resumed eating meat.[3] Lifestyle factors also seem to influence blood pressure: smoking and alcohol intake raise blood pressure, and exercise lowers it.

Coronary Artery Disease

Fewer vegetarians than meat eaters suffer from diseases of the heart and arteries. The dietary factors most directly related to coronary artery disease is saturated fat, and in general, vegetarian diets are lower in total fat, saturated fat, and cholesterol than typical meat-based diets. Vegetarian diets are also higher in dietary fiber, another factor that helps control blood lipids.

When vegetarians are fed meat, which contains saturated fat, their blood lipid profiles change for the worse; when meat eaters are fed a low-fat vegetarian diet, their lipid profiles improve. In fact, one study reversed severe coronary artery disease without drugs by implementing a low-fat vegetarian diet, stress management, physical activity, and a no-smoking plan.[4] Another study compared two low-fat diets—one vegetarian and the other containing lean meats—and found that both diets lowered blood cholesterol, but the vegetarian diet's effects were greater.[5] People who eat meat can lower their blood cholesterol by keeping their intake to a minimum.[6] For example, one study found that semivegetarians who ate one to three servings of meat per week had blood lipids between the low blood lipids of vegetarians and the higher lipids of nonvegetarians.[7]

Cancer

Seventh-Day Adventists, a religious group whose foodways center on a lacto-ovo-vegetarian diet, have a significantly lower mortality rate from cancer than the rest of the population, even after all the cancers attributed to smoking and alcohol are discounted.[8] Their low cancer rates may be due to their vegetarian diets; evidence is overwhelming that high intakes of fruits and vegetables reduce the risks of cancer.[9]

Some scientific findings indicate that vegetarian diets are not only associated with lower cancer mortality in general, but with lower incidence of cancer at specific sites as well, most notably, colon cancer.[10] People with colon cancer seem to eat more meat, more saturated fat, and less fiber than others without cancer. High-protein, high-fat, low-fiber diets create an environment in the human colon that promotes the development of cancer in some people.[11]

In general, then, adults who eat vegetarian diets can reduce their risks of several chronic diseases, including obesity, high blood pressure, heart disease, and cancer. But there is nothing mysterious about the vegetarian diet; it simply includes ample fruits, vegetables, whole grains, and legumes—foods that are higher in fiber, richer in certain vitamins and minerals, and lower in fats than meat-based diets. Some people find it easier to meet today's dietary recommendations for health by following a vegetarian diet than by eating meals with meat. A meat eater can gain some of the same advantages by limiting meat intake to the recommended 5 to 7 ounces daily and selecting lean cuts, as well as including abundant grains, fruits, and vegetables.

Conversely, both vegetarian and meat-based diets can be detrimental to health when overloaded with fat. A vegetarian who dines on cheddar cheese, butter sauces, sour cream, and deep-fried vegetables invites the same health hazards as the person who overeats high-fat meats. And both diets, if not properly balanced, can lack nutrients. Poorly planned vegetarian diets typically lack iron, zinc, calcium, vitamin B_{12}, and vitamin D; without planning, the meat eater's diet may lack vitamin A, vitamin C, folate, and fiber, among others.

PROBLEMS ASSOCIATED WITH VEGETARIAN DIETS

The negative health aspects of any diet, including vegetarian diets, reflect poor diet planning. Careful attention to energy intake and specific problem nutrients can ensure adequacy. Diet planning during pregnancy, lactation, infancy, childhood, and illness, in particular, must provide for the increases in energy and nutrients needed during those times—when the consequences of poor nutrition can be great.

Adequacy of Most Vegetarian Diets

Vegetarians who include milk products and eggs have few nutrient-deficiency concerns. Such diets can adequately support the growth of children.

Inadequacy of Strict Vegetarian Diets

Achieving adequate energy and nutrient intakes may be difficult for the vegan who excludes all animal products, and particularly for growing children and pregnant and lactating women. Foods of plant origin generally offer much less energy per bite than foods of animal origin; while a diet that delivers a lot of food with relatively little energy may be advantageous for many adults, it can be detrimental for children who need energy-dense foods for growth. Vegan diets can fail to provide sufficient energy to support the growth of a child within a quantity of food small enough for the child to eat. A child's small stomach can hold only so much food, and a vegan child may feel full before eating enough to meet nutrient and energy needs. A vegan child's diet should emphasize cereals, legumes, and nuts to meet protein and energy needs in a small volume. Meat, which contains abundant protein, iron, and food energy in less bulk, supports the growth of children more efficiently. Compared with meat-eating children, vegan children tend to be smaller in height and lighter in weight; their low energy intakes can impair growth.[12]

When vegan children get their protein only from plant foods, they may need protein intakes higher than the RDA for normal growth and health. The standard protein recommendations may be inadequate to support the growth of vegan children, but specific recommendations have not been established.[13]

Approximately 2 out of every 15 households include one or more members who are vegetarians. These people number some 12 million nationwide, representing an eightfold increase over the past two decades.[14] Those who plan their diets carefully easily obtain all the nutrients they need to support good health.

VEGETARIAN DIET PLANNING

The vegetarian has the same meal-planning task as any other person—using a variety of foods that will deliver all the needed nutrients within an energy allowance that maintains a healthy body weight. An added challenge is to do so with fewer foods.

Well-planned vegetarian meals can provide adequate amounts of all the nutrients a person needs for good health. Vegetarians can follow the Daily Food Guide presented in Chapter 2 with a few modifications (see Table H6–1). Those who include milk products and eggs can follow the regular plan, using legumes and products made from them, such as peanut butter, tempeh, and tofu, in place of meat. Those who do not use milk can use soy milk fortified with calcium, vitamin D, and vitamin B_{12}. Vegetarian adults should include at least one cup of dark green vegetables daily to help meet iron needs and legumes to help meet zinc needs. In general, these tactics ensure adequate intakes of the main nutrients

Table H6–1

Daily Food Guide for Vegetarians

Food Group	Suggested Daily Servings	Serving Sizes
Breads, cereals and other grain products	6 or more	1 slice bread ½ bun, bagel, or English muffin ½ c cooked cereal, rice, or pasta 1 oz dry cereal
Vegetables	4 or more[a]	½ c cooked or 1 c raw
Fruits	3 or more	1 piece fresh fruit ¾ c fruit juice ½ c canned or cooked fruit
Legumes and other meat alternates	2 to 3	½ c cooked beans 4 oz tofu or tempeh 8 oz soy milk 2 tbs nuts or seeds (these tend to be high in fat, so use sparingly) 1 egg or 2 egg whites
Milk and milk products	2 to 3[b]	1 c low-fat or nonfat milk 1 c low-fat or nonfat yogurt 1½ oz low-fat cheese

[a]Include 1 cup of dark green vegetables daily to help meet iron requirements.
[b]People who do not use milk or milk products: use soy milk fortified with calcium, vitamin D, and vitamin B_{12}.
Source: Adapted with permission from Position of The American Dietetic Association: Vegetarian diets, *Journal of the American Dietetic Association* 93 (1993): 1318.

vegetarian diets might otherwise lack: iron, zinc, calcium, vitamin B_{12}, and vitamin D. In contrast, most vegetarians easily obtain large quantities of the nutrients that are abundant in plant foods: thiamin, riboflavin, folate, and vitamins B_6, C, A, and E.

Protein

Protein is not the problem it was once thought to be for vegetarian diets. People who use animal-derived foods such as milk and eggs receive high-quality proteins and are unlikely to develop protein deficiencies. Even those who eat only plant-derived foods are unlikely to develop protein deficiencies provided that energy intakes are adequate and the protein sources varied.[15] The proteins of whole grains, legumes, seeds, nuts, and vegetables can provide adequate amounts of all the amino acids. An advantage of many vegetarian protein foods is that they are generally lower in saturated fat than meats and are often higher in fiber and richer in some vitamins and minerals.

To ease meal preparation, vegetarians sometimes use meat replacements made of textured vegetable protein (soy protein). These foods are formulated to look and taste like meat, fish, or poultry. Many of these products are designed to match the known nutrient contents of animal-protein foods, but sometimes they fall short. A wise vegetarian does not rely on these products too heavily, but learns to use a variety of whole foods instead. Vegetarians may also use soybeans in the form of bean curds, or tofu, to bolster protein intake.

Iron

Getting enough iron can be a problem even for meat eaters, and those who eat no meat must pay special attention to their iron intake. The iron in plant foods such as legumes, dark green leafy vegetables, iron-fortified cereals, and whole-grain breads and cereals is not readily absorbed. Iron absorption is enhanced by vitamin C, though, and vegetarians typically eat many vitamin C–rich fruits and vegetables, so that they suffer no more iron-deficiency anemia than other people do.[16]

Zinc

Zinc is similar to iron in that meat is its richest food source and zinc from plant sources is not well absorbed. In addition, soy, which is commonly used as a meat alternate, interferes with zinc absorption. Nevertheless, most vegetarian adults are not zinc deficient.[17] Perhaps the best advice to vegetarians regarding zinc is to eat a variety of nutrient-dense foods; include grains, nuts, and legumes such as black-eyed peas, pinto beans, and kidney beans; and maintain an adequate energy intake. For vegetarians who include seafood, oysters, crabmeat, and shrimp are rich in zinc.

Calcium

The calcium intakes of lactovegetarians are similar to those of the general population, but people who use no milk risk deficiency. Careful planners select calcium-rich foods, such as calcium-fortified juices or soy milk, in ample quantities regularly. This is especially important for children. Soy formulas for infants are fortified with calcium and can be used in cooking, even for adults. Other good calcium sources include calcium-set tofu, some legumes, some green vegetables such as broccoli and turnip greens, some nuts such as almonds, and certain seeds such as sesame seeds.[18]* The choices should be varied because binders in some plant foods may limit absorption.

Vitamin B₁₂

The requirement for vitamin B_{12} is small, but this vitamin is found only in animal-derived foods. Fermented plant products such as tempeh, made from soybeans, may contain some vitamin B_{12} from the bacteria that did the fermenting, but unfortunately, much of the vitamin B_{12} found in these products may be an inactive form.[19] Vegans must rely on vitamin B_{12}-fortified sources (such as soy milk or breakfast cereals) or vitamin B_{12} supplements to ensure against deficiency.[20]

Vitamin D

For people who do not use vitamin D–fortified milk and who do not receive enough exposure to sunlight to synthesize adequate vitamin D, supplements may be warranted.[21] This is particularly important for children and older adults. In northern climates during winter months, young children on vegan diets can readily develop rickets, the vitamin D–deficiency disease.[22]

As you can see, vegetarianism is not a religion like Buddhism or Hinduism, but merely an eating plan that selects plant foods to deliver needed nutrients. The quality of the diet depends not on whether it includes meat, but on whether the food choices are nutritionally sound. Health experts would quickly add that one should also limit intakes of substances such as fat and alcohol that are harmful in excess—and vegetarians in this country typically do. Interestingly, the Mediterranean diet—a predominantly vegetarian diet with an ethnic flair—breaks these rules on moderation, yet still seems to have health advantages.

AN ALMOST-VEGETARIAN DIET: THE MEDITERRANEAN DIET

The Mediterranean diet is based on the traditional eating habits of people in a region of the world where the incidence of chronic disease is low and life expectancy is high.[23]*

Each of the many countries that border the Mediterranean Sea has its own culture, traditions, and dietary habits, but similarities are also evident.[24] The people dine on crusty breads, grains, potatoes, and pasta; a variety of vegetables; feta and mozzarella cheeses and yogurt; and ripe fruit.[25] They eat some fish and poultry, a few eggs, and very little meat.

Their principal source of fat is olive oil, and they typically drink wine with meals. Consequently, traditional Mediterranean diets are:[26]

- Low in saturated fat.
- Rich in monounsaturated fat.
- Rich in carbohydrate and fiber.
- Rich in nutrients and nonnutrients that support good health.

Furthermore, because processed foods are used modestly in these countries, intakes of salt, refined sugars, and *trans*-fatty acids are low.[27] All in all, the Mediterranean diet has been gaining a reputation for its health benefits as well as its delicious flavors.

The Mediterranean Diet Pyramid

A few nutrition experts were so impressed with the Mediterranean diet and its health benefits that they created a renegade food pyramid.* Like the official USDA Food Guide Pyramid introduced in Chapter 2, their pyramid is based on breads,

---

*Calcium salts are often added during processing to coagulate the tofu.

*Much of the early research (late 1950s and early 1960s) focused on men living in farming communities on the Greek island of Crete.

*The Mediterranean diet pyramid was developed by the Harvard School of Public Health, the European office of the World Health Organization, and the Oldways Preservation & Trust in Boston.

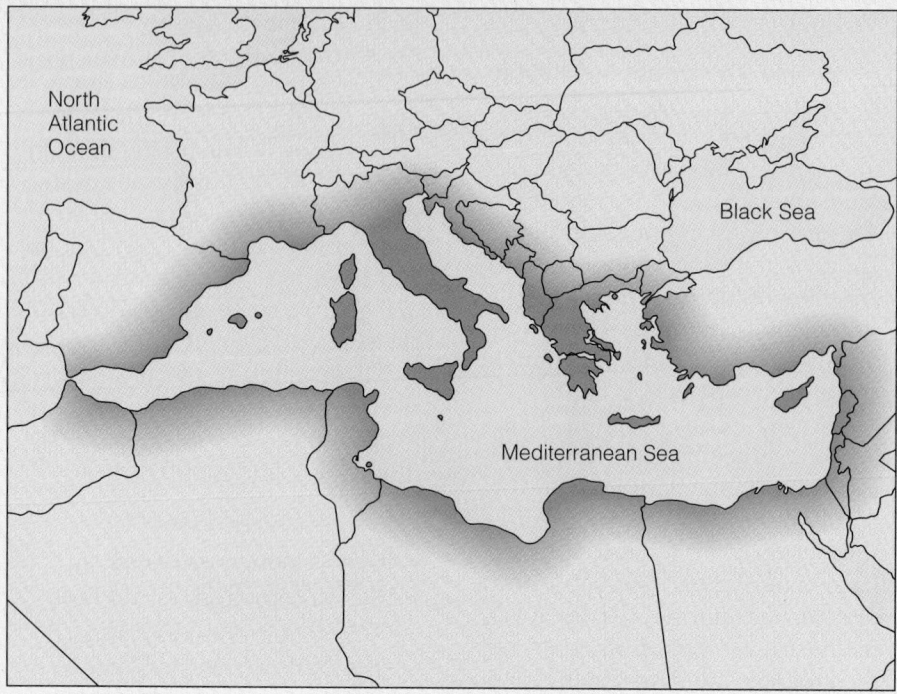

The people of the Mediterranean area (see area shaded in dark green) eat plenty of fruits, vegetables, legumes, and grains; some dairy products, fish, and poultry; and very little red meat. Olive oil is their principal source of dietary fat.

cereals, rice, pasta, and other grains, and it places vegetables and fruits on the next level up. The Mediterranean pyramid introduces a small difference at this level in that it includes legumes with the vegetable group instead of with the meats, but greater differences become apparent farther up the pyramid. Olive oil sits just above the fruits, vegetables, and legumes, with cheese and yogurt above that; these foods are to be included daily. Fish, poultry, eggs, and sweets come next and are to be eaten a few times per week. Lean red meats sit at the tip of the pyramid, to be eaten only a few times per month. Figure H6–1 compares the two pyramids.

This Mediterranean pyramid contradicts many diet and health

recommendations and is worth examining because it raises interesting issues. For example, although current dietary recommendations restrict fat to no more than 30 percent of daily kcalories, the traditional Mediterranean diet can deliver as much as 40 percent of a day's kcalories from fat. The Mediterranean plan does not restrict total fat, but it does limit *animal* fat—a distinction not made in the USDA plan. People following the USDA plan get most of their fat from red meat, poultry, eggs, milk, yogurt, and cheese; consequently much of their fat is saturated fat. Those following the Mediterranean plan use olive oil abundantly, and so receive most of their fat as monounsaturated veg-

etable oil. Their limited consumption of dairy products and meats provides less than 10 percent of their kcalories from saturated fats—a goal both plans agree on, but the USDA plan typically fails to meet.

The distinctions between types of fat have implications for chronic diseases, as Chapter 5 points out. The monounsaturated fats of olive oil and canola oil and the omega-3 polyunsaturated fats of fish may actually benefit heart health; in contrast, most, but not all, saturated fats are detrimental. Substituting unsaturated fats such as olive oil for saturated fats or *trans*-fatty acids improves blood lipids and reduces the risks of cardiovascular disease.[28] In addition to its beneficial fatty acid composition (high in monounsaturated and low in saturated fatty acids), olive oil contains vitamin E and other antioxidant compounds that protect against heart disease. These distinctions in types of fat are not evident in the USDA pyramid and dietary recommendations. People are simply advised to cut back on all fat so that they will cut back on saturated fat—the real culprit.

Many Mediterranean people drink wine with each meal, and the Mediterranean pyramid includes wine in moderation. Moderate alcohol consumption reduces the risk of cardiovascular disease and seems to be compatible with a healthy lifestyle.[29] The USDA pyramid does not address alcoholic beverages directly, but most diet and health recommendations advise people to drink alcoholic beverages in moderation, if at all.

Perhaps the hallmark of the Mediterranean diet is its abundance of vegetables, fruits, legumes, and whole grains—foods associated with lower risks of cardiovascular disease

Figure H6–1
. . . .

Food Pyramids Compared

Mediterranean Diet Pyramid

This pyramid is based on the dietary traditions of Crete around 1960, structured in light of current nutrition research.

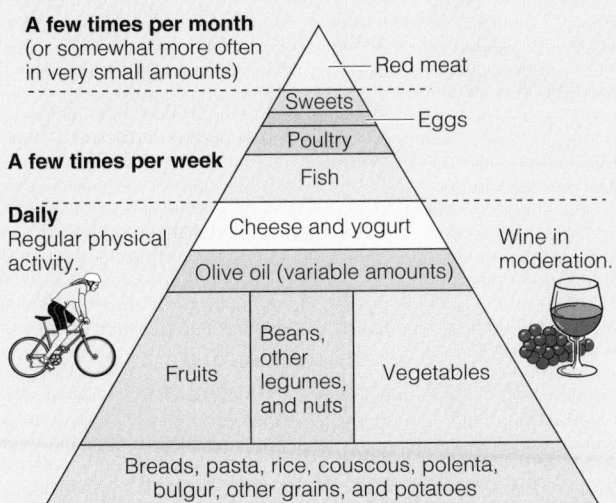

A few times per month
(or somewhat more often
in very small amounts)
— Red meat
— Sweets
— Eggs
A few times per week
— Poultry
— Fish

Daily
Regular physical
activity.
— Cheese and yogurt
— Olive oil (variable amounts)
Wine in
moderation.

Fruits | Beans, other legumes, and nuts | Vegetables

Breads, pasta, rice, couscous, polenta,
bulgur, other grains, and potatoes

USDA Pyramid

This pyramid is based on the dietary guidelines established in 1992 by the U.S. Department of Agriculture.

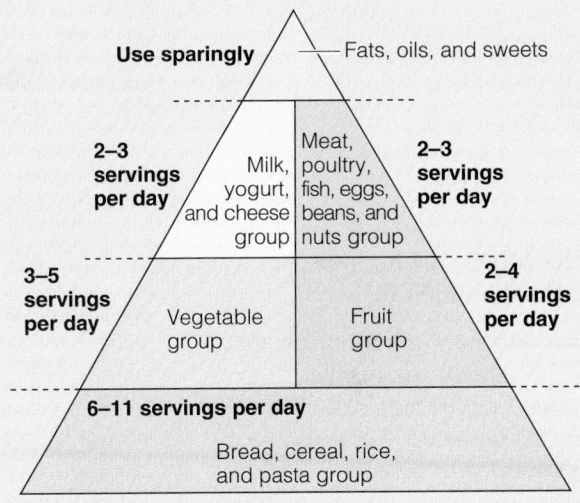

Use sparingly — Fats, oils, and sweets

**2–3
servings
per day** — Milk, yogurt, and cheese group

Meat, poultry, fish, eggs, beans, and nuts group — **2–3
servings
per day**

**3–5
servings
per day** — Vegetable group | Fruit group — **2–4
servings
per day**

6–11 servings per day

Bread, cereal, rice,
and pasta group

Sources: 1994 Oldways Preservation & Exchange Trust, U.S. Department of Agriculture.

and cancer.[30] The protective effects of these plant-derived foods are attributed not only to their lack of fat, but also to their abundance of nutrients and nonnutritents, many of which act as antioxidants (see Highlight 11).[31]

Some Concerns about the Mediterranean Plan

Critics of the Mediterranean Plan have expressed concerns that it may be inadequate in calcium and iron—two problem nutrients for many people, especially women. Because these nutrients are typically lacking in many people's diets, it seems unwise to restrict calcium selections to cheeses and yogurt and iron-rich meat consumption to a few times a month.

An Implication of the Mediterranean Plan: Limit Meat

Is it appropriate to suggest that people in the United States should adopt Mediterranean eating habits and begin indulging in olive oil and wine? Not really, for at least two reasons. First, diet is not the only, or even the most important, factor implicated in heart disease, as Chapter 28 points out. Many other differences between the lifestyles of the people living in the Mediterranean and those living here could account for the differences in life expectancy and disease risks. Furthermore, as

Highlight 2 pointed out, all ethnic food patterns have pros and cons. Perhaps the most important suggestion to be taken from the Mediterranean Plan is to focus more on grains, vegetables, and fruits, and less on meats. The average daily consumption of meat in the United States is more than half a pound per person per *day*; in the Mediterranean region, it is about half a pound per person per *week*. The difference in meat intake, and therefore in saturated fat intake, is significant.

In general, at most, two 3-ounce servings of meat per day are needed.[32] This amount of meat alone provides most of a person's daily recommended protein intake—and other foods together

215

can provide a similar amount. Some researchers argue that this much meat eaten daily is not compatible with good health; if any meat is eaten, they suggest it should be eaten infrequently and in small portions.[33] With the evidence pointing to the health advantages of a meat-restricted diet, perhaps between 0 and 6 ounces of meat daily would best serve the needs of most people; the USDA pyramid suggests 5 to 7 ounces of meat, poultry, or fish a day.

PYRAMIDS—OFFICIAL AND OTHERWISE

What about this renegade pyramid? It seems almost sacrilegious to oppose the government's official word on nutrition, but it can be enlightening to take a peek at the politics involved in developing such recommendations.

For more than a century, government agencies have issued statements advising consumers about food choices. Dietary guidelines may originally have been developed purely for the public good, but now they underlie national policy in many areas. They are used to define curricula for nutrition education, establish regulations for food labels, develop new food products, regulate institutional foodservices, provide commodity foods, and create school menus. And because the guidelines encourage people to eat more of some foods and less of others, they exert a profound effect on food purchases. Inevitably, therefore, politics has become involved in the dietary guidelines.

Food producers did not complain when early dietary recommendations urged people to "Eat more" of their products to help prevent nutrient deficiencies. However, when

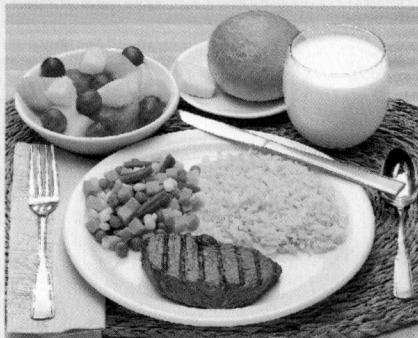

Two meat servings of the size depicted here represent the maximum daily meat intake suggested by the Daily Food Guide as health promoting.

recommendations began to urge people to "Eat less" of some products to help prevent chronic diseases, food producers became aroused. Now, lobbyists representing the food industry scurry about Capitol Hill trying to protect their interests and influence national policies that affect dietary intakes. Their efforts have been successful.

The influence of the meat industry on government policy makers provides a notable example.[34] In 1977, a dietary goal was to "Decrease consumption of meat." The "Eat less" guideline was changed in 1980 to "Choose lean meat." By 1990 the recommendation was stated even more favorably, "Have two or three servings, with a daily total of about 6 ounces." By 1992, when the pyramid was created, the daily total had been revised to "5 to 7 ounces." The design of the pyramid itself was delayed by a year and cost an additional million dollars, in large part because of protests from the meat industry.

The preceding paragraph was not written to pick on the meat industry. Lobbyists representing the dairy industry, the egg industry, the sugar industry, and every other food man-

ufacturer try to influence dietary recommendations. The point is that people outside the world of nutrition science profoundly influence our nation's diet. Shifting our diet towards a healthier plan would require major changes in the agricultural and food manufacturing policies and practices of this nation.[35] One wonders what the government's nutrition advice would be if it were untainted by politics.

Having learned some of the relationships between diet and health, many people may discover that their strategies for planning meals need to change. In the past, they decided what cut of beef, ham, pork, lamb, poultry, or fish to prepare and then filled in the menu with an accompanying "starch" (potato, rice, or noodles), salad or other vegetable, and bread. Now, they fill their dinner plates with legumes, grains, vegetables, and fruits. Then they add small quantities of milk products, eggs, lean meat, fish, or poultry.

For the most part, it seems that nonmeat and low-meat diets can both support good health. Keep in mind, too, that diet is only one factor influencing health. Whatever a diet consists of, its context is also important: no smoking; alcohol consumption in moderation, if at all; regular physical activity; adequate rest; and medical attention when needed all contribute to a healthy life. Establishing these healthy habits early in life seems to be the most important step one can take to reduce the risks of later diseases.[36]

NOTES

1. Position of The American Dietetic Association: Vegetarian diets, *Journal of the American*

Dietetic Association 93 (1993): 1317–1319.

2. L. J. Beilin, Vegetarian and other complex diets, fats, fiber, and hypertension, *American Journal of Clinical Nutrition* 59 (1994): 1130S–1135S.

3. L. J. Beilin and coauthors, Vegetarian diet and blood pressure levels: Incidental or causal association? *American Journal of Clinical Nutrition* 48 (1988): 806–810.

4. D. Ornish and coauthors, Can lifestyle changes reverse coronary heart disease? *Lancet* 336 (1990): 129–133.

5. M. Kestin and coauthors, Cardiovascular disease risk factors in free-living men: Comparison of two prudent diets, one based on lacto-ovovegetarianism and the other allowing meat, *American Journal of Clinical Nutrition* 50 (1989): 280–287.

6. S. A. Morgan, A. J. Sinclair, and K. O'Dea, Effect on serum lipids of addition of safflower oil or olive oil to very-low-fat diets rich in lean beef, *Journal of the American Dietetic Association* 93 (1993): 644–648.

7. C. L. Melby, M. L. Toohey, and J. Cebrick, Blood pressure and blood lipids among vegetarian, semivegetarian, and nonvegetarian African Americans, *American Journal of Clinical Nutrition* 59 (1994): 103–109.

8. P. K. Mills and coauthors, Cancer incidence among California Seventh-Day Adventists, 1976–1982, *American Journal of Clinical Nutrition* 59 (1994): 1136S–1142S.

9. W. C. Willett, Micronutrients and cancer risk, *American Journal of Clinical Nutrition* 59 (1994): 1162S–1165S.

10. R. Frentzel-Beyme and J. Chang-Claude, Vegetarian diets and colon cancer: The German experience, *American Journal of Clinical Nutrition* 59 (1994): 1143S–1152S.

11. M. I. McBurney, P. J. Van Soest, and J. L. Jeraci, Colonic carcinogenesis: The microbial feast or famine mechanism, *Nutrition and Cancer* 10 (1987): 23–28.

12. T. A. B. Sanders and S. Reddy, Vegetarian diets and children, *American Journal of Clinical Nutrition* 59 (1994): 1176S–1181S.

13. P. B. Acosta, Availability of essential amino acids and nitrogen in vegan diets, *American Journal of Clinical Nutrition* 48 (1988): 868–874.

14. P. K. Johnson, Preface to the Second International Congress on Vegetarian Nutrition, *American Journal of Clinical Nutrition* (supplement) 59 (1994): vii.

15. V. R. Young and P. L. Pellett, Plant proteins in relation to human protein and amino acid nutrition, *American Journal of Clinical Nutrition* 59 (1994): 1203S–1212S; Position of The American Dietetic Association, 1993.

16. W. J. Craig, Iron status of vegetarians, *American Journal of Clinical Nutrition* 59 (1994): 1233S–1237S.

17. R. J. Gibson, Content and bioavailability of trace elements in vegetarian diets, *American Journal of Clinical Nutrition* 59 (1994): 1223S–1232S.

18. C. M. Weaver and K. L. Plawecki, Dietary calcium: Adequacy of a vegetarian diet, *American Journal of Clinical Nutrition* 59 (1994): 1238S–1241S.

19. V. Herbert, Vitamin B-12: Plant sources, requirements, and assay, *American Journal of Clinical Nutrition* 48 (1988): 852–858.

20. D. R. Miller and coauthors, Vitamin B-12 status in a macrobiotic community, *American Journal of Clinical Nutrition* 53 (1991): 524–529.

21. C. Lamberg-Allardt and coauthors, Low serum 25-hydroxyvitamin D concentrations and secondary hyperparathyroidism in middle-aged white strict vegetarians, *American Journal of Clinical Nutrition* 58 (1993): 684–689.

22. P. C. Dagnelie, High prevalence of rickets in infants on macrobiotic diets, *American Journal of Clinical Nutrition* 51 (1990): 202–208.

23. A. Keys, Mediterranean diet and public health: Personal reflections, *American Journal of Clinical Nutrition* 61 (1995): 1321S–1323S.

24. E. Helsing, Traditional diets and disease patterns of Mediterranean, circa 1960, *American Journal of Clinical Nutrition* 61 (1995): 1329S–1337S.

25. W. C. Willett and coauthors, Mediterranean diet pyramid: A cultural model of healthy eating, *American Journal of Clinical Nutrition* 61 (1995): 1402S–1406S.

26. A. P. Simopoulos, The Mediterranean Food Guide—Greek column rather than an Egyptian Pyramid, *Nutrition Today* 30 (1995): 54–61.

27. W. P. T. James, Nutrition science and policy research: Implications for Mediterranean diets, *American Journal of Clinical Nutrition* 61 (1995): 1324S–1328S.

28. M. B. Katan, P. L. Zock, and R. P. Mensink, Dietary oils, serum lipoproteins, and coronary heart disease, *American Journal of Clinical Nutrition* 61 (1995): 1368S–1373S.

29. E. B. Rimm and R. C. Ellison, Alcohol in the Mediterranean diet, *American Journal of Clinical Nutrition* 61 (1995): 1378S–1382S.

30. A. Tavani and C. LaVecchia, Fruit and vegetable consumption and cancer risk in a Mediterranean population, *American Journal of Clinical Nutrition* (1995): 1374S–1377S; L. H. Kushi, E. B. Lenart, and W. C. Willett, Health implications of Mediterranean diets in light of contemporary knowledge. 1. Plant foods and dairy products, *American Journal of Clinical Nutrition* 61 (1995): 1407S–1415S.

31. W. P. T. James, G. G. Duthie, and K. W. J. Wahle, The Mediterranean diet: Protective or simply non-toxic? *European Journal of Clinical Nutrition* (supplement 2) 43 (1989): 31–41.

32. Members of the Committee on Diet and Health as quoted in *The Nation's Health*, a newsletter published by the American Public Health Association, April 1989, p. 15.

33. L. H. Kushi, E. B. Lenart, and W. C. Willett, Health implications of Mediterranean diets in light of contemporary knowledge. 2. Meat, wine, fats, and oils, *American Journal of Clinical Nutrition* 61 (1995): 1416S–1427S.

34. M. Nestle, Editorial: The politics of dietary guidance—A new opportunity, *American Journal of Public Health* 84 (1994): 713–715.

35. P. O'Brien, Dietary shifts and implications for US agriculture, *American Journal of Clinical Nutrition* 61 (1995): 1390S–1396S.

36. V. Fønnebø, The healthy Seventh-day Adventist lifestyle: What is the Norwegian experience? *American Journal of Clinical Nutrition* 59 (1994): 1124S–1129S.

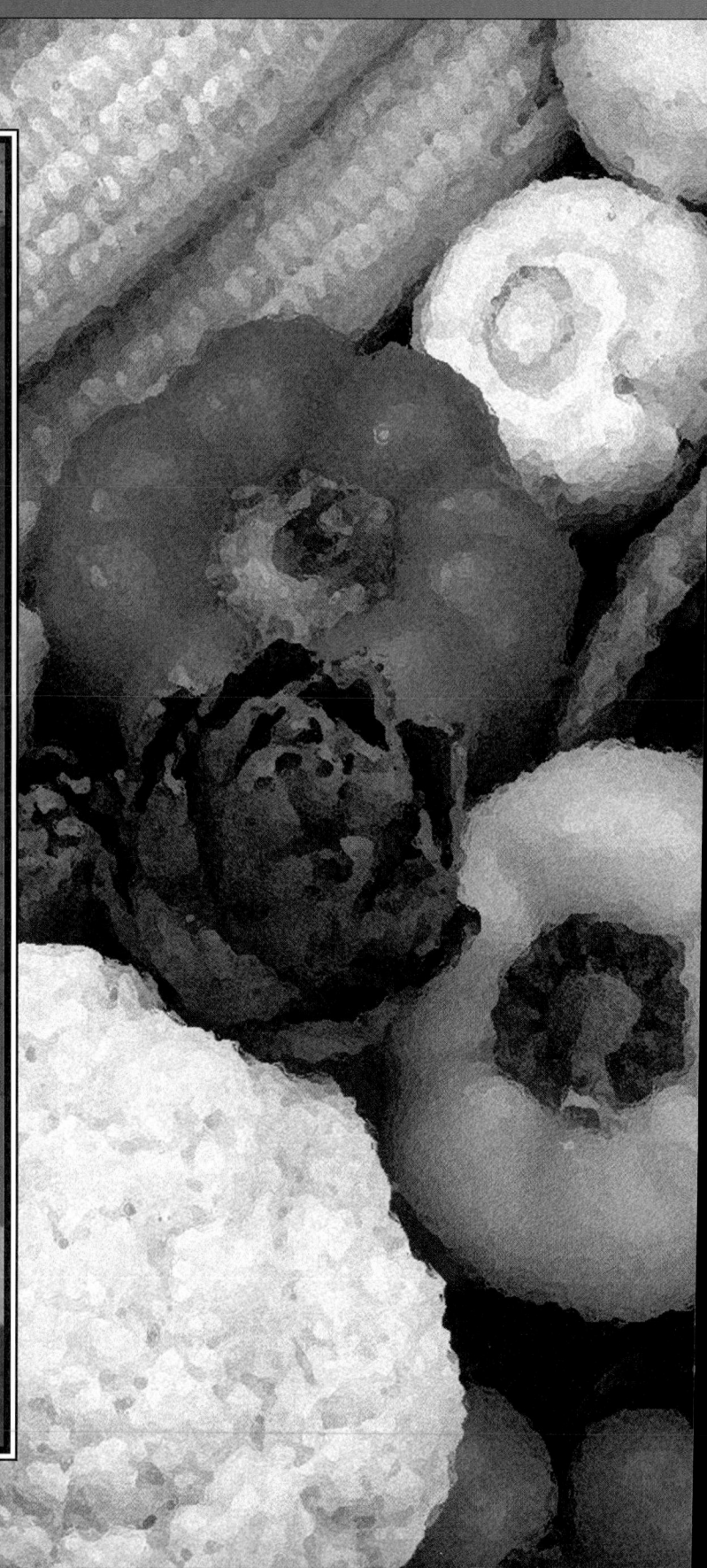

Chapter 7

Metabolism: Transformations and Interactions

CONTENTS

Chemical Reactions in the Body

Breaking Down Nutrients for Energy

Glucose

Glycerol and Fatty Acids

Amino Acids

The Final Steps of Catabolism

The Body's Energy Budget

The Economics of Feasting

The Transition from Feasting to Fasting

The Economics of Fasting

HIGHLIGHT: **Alcohol and Nutrition**

MICROGRAPH: Acetyl CoA, the cross-roads compound of energy metabolism

e are all solar creatures. Almost all living things depend on the sun's energy. Plants rely directly on the sun to provide the light energy that drives the reactions of photosynthesis—the process by which plants make carbohydrate from carbon dioxide and water using the energy from sunlight. That energy from the sun is captured in the energy that holds atoms together—the energy of chemical bonds. We humans, and all other animals, use the sun indirectly, for we cannot photosynthesize. We depend on plants, or on animals that eat plants, for the food that gives us our energy-yielding nutrients.

This chapter describes the processes in the human body that *release* energy from the chemical bonds in nutrients. In so doing, it lays the groundwork for understanding many of the daily realities examined in later chapters. Energy derived from the metabolism of nutrients enables people to ride bicycles, compose music, and do everything else they do. An excess of food energy makes people fat, though most people do not understand how it does this. Nor do most people understand exactly how physical activity speeds up energy use and fat loss. By studying metabolism, readers who are interested in losing weight will discover which foods contribute most to body fat and which to select when trying to lose weight safely. Physically active readers will discover which foods best support endurance activities and which to select when trying to build lean body mass.

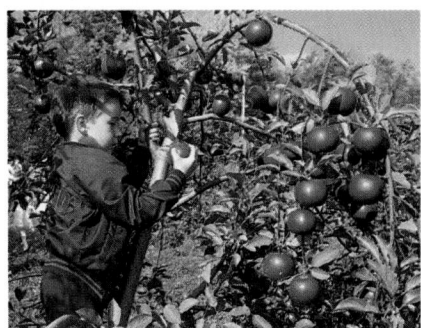

We receive energy from the sun by way of the foods we eat.

photosynthesis: the process by which green plants make carbohydrates from carbon dioxide and water using the green pigment chlorophyll to trap the sun's energy.
  photo = light
  synthesis = put together (making)

Chemical Reactions in the Body

Earlier chapters have already introduced some of the body's chemical reactions: examples are the making and breaking of the bonds in carbohydrates, lipids, and proteins. The sum of these and all the other chemical reactions that go on in living cells is known as metabolism; and *energy* metabolism includes all the ways the body obtains and spends energy from food.

Chapters 4, 5, and 6 laid the groundwork for the study of metabolism; a brief review may be helpful. During digestion, the body breaks down the three energy-yielding nutrients—carbohydrates, fats, and proteins—into four basic units that can be absorbed into the blood:

- From carbohydrates—glucose.
- From fats—glycerol and fatty acids.
- From proteins—amino acids.

Amino acids are not primarily energy nutrients, but they can flow into energy pathways if needed or if eaten in excess, so they are included.

Look for these four basic units to appear again and again in the metabolic reactions described in this chapter. Alcohol also enters many of the metabolic pathways; Highlight 7 focuses on how alcohol disrupts metabolism and how the body handles it.

Building Reactions—Anabolism The cells can use the basic units of energy-yielding nutrients to build body compounds. Glucose units may be joined together to make glycogen chains. Glycerol and fatty acids may be assembled into triglycerides. Amino acids may be linked together to make proteins. Each of these reactions starts with small, simple compounds and uses them as building

Appendix B provides an overview of basic chemistry concepts.

metabolism: the sum total of all the chemical reactions that go on in living cells; **energy metabolism** includes all the reactions by which the body obtains and spends the energy from food.
  meta = among
  bole = change

anabolism (an-ABB-o-lism): reactions in which small molecules are put together to build larger ones. Anabolic reactions require energy.
  ana = up

Figure 7–1

Anabolic and Catabolic Reactions Compared

Note: You need not memorize a color code to understand the figures in this chapter but you may find it helpful to know that blue is used for carbohydrates, yellow for fats, and red for proteins.

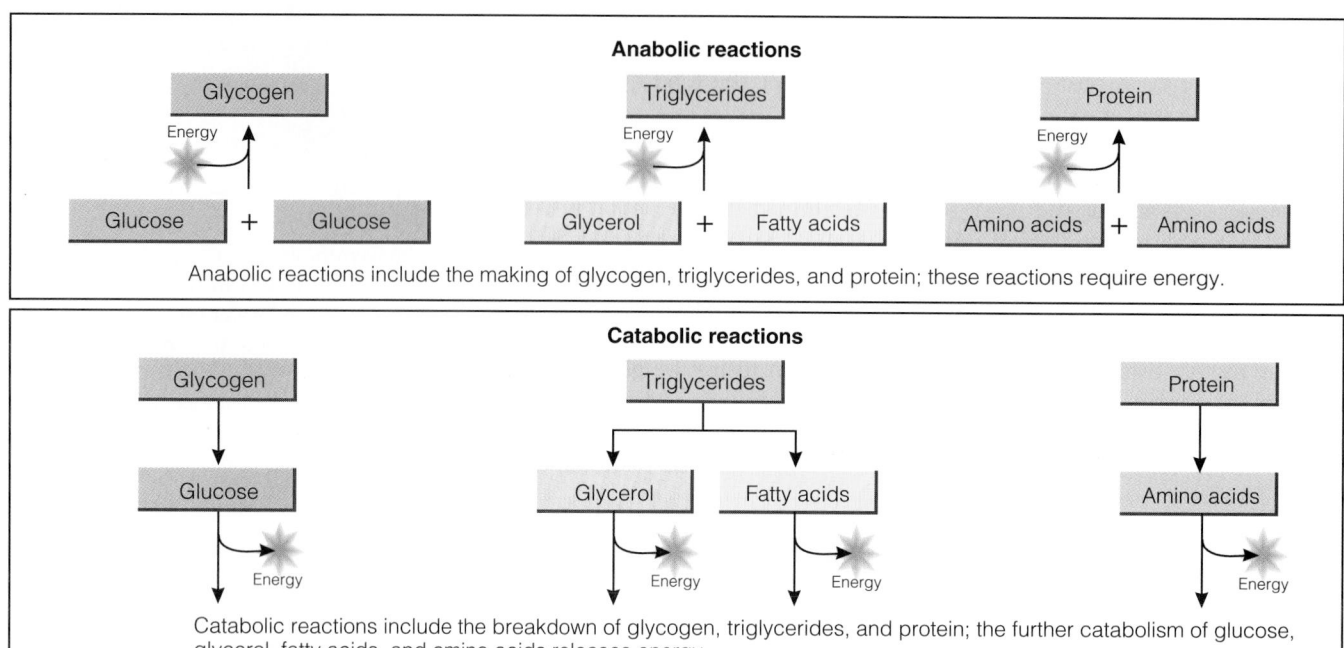

Anabolic reactions

Glycogen	Triglycerides	Protein
Energy	Energy	Energy
Glucose + Glucose	Glycerol + Fatty acids	Amino acids + Amino acids

Anabolic reactions include the making of glycogen, triglycerides, and protein; these reactions require energy.

Catabolic reactions

Glycogen	Triglycerides	Protein
Glucose	Glycerol Fatty acids	Amino acids
Energy	Energy Energy	Energy

Catabolic reactions include the breakdown of glycogen, triglycerides, and protein; the further catabolism of glucose, glycerol, fatty acids, and amino acids releases energy.

blocks to form larger, more complex structures. Such reactions involve doing work and so require energy. The building up of body compounds is known as anabolism; this book represents anabolic reactions, wherever possible, with "up" arrows in chemical diagrams (such as those shown in Figure 7–1).

catabolism (ca-TAB-o-lism): reactions in which large molecules are broken down to smaller ones. Catabolic reactions usually release energy.

  kata = down

Breakdown Reactions—Catabolism The breaking down of body compounds is known as catabolism; catabolic reactions usually release energy and are represented, wherever possible, by "down" arrows in chemical diagrams (as in Figure 7–1). Catabolic reactions include the breakdown of glycogen to glucose, of triglycerides to fatty acids and glycerol, and of protein to amino acids. When the body needs energy, it breaks down any or all of these four basic units into even smaller units, as described later.

The Transfer of Energy in Reactions When a chemical bond breaks, energy can be released as heat, captured in another chemical bond, or both. Often, as one compound is broken apart, some of the energy is released as heat, and some is used to put together another compound. Such reactions, in which the breakdown of one compound provides energy for the building of another, are known as coupled reactions.

coupled reactions: pairs of chemical reactions in which energy released from the breakdown of one compound is used to create a bond in the formation of another compound.

The energy released during catabolism is often captured by go-between molecules that can easily transfer that energy to other compounds. These molecules are sometimes called the body's "common energy currency," or "high-energy compounds." One such compound is ATP (adenosine triphosphate). The breakdown of energy-nutrient molecules is coupled to the making of many ATP molecules, which capture much of the released energy in their bonds.

ATP, as its name indicates, contains three phosphate groups. The energy in the phosphate bonds is greater than the energy in most other chemical bonds. When energy is needed, hydrolysis readily breaks the high-energy bonds between ATP's phosphate groups, splitting off one or two of them and releasing their energy. These reactions, in turn, are coupled to other reactions that use that energy. Thus the body uses ATP to transfer the energy produced during catabolic reactions to power its anabolic reactions. Figure 7–2 explains how the body uses ATP to carry its energy currency, build body structures, do other work, or generate heat, as needed.

ATP (adenosine triphosphate): a common high-energy compound composed of a purine (adenine), a sugar (ribose), and three phosphate groups.

ATP = A–P~P~P.

(Each ~ denotes a "high-energy" bond.)

Reminder: *Hydrolysis* is the process by which a molecule is broken apart with the addition of water.

Before ATP use:

Glucose and fat have broken down, and some of their energy has been used to attach phosphate groups to molecules of adenosine diphosphate (ADP), building ATP.[a]

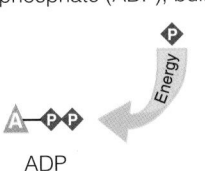

ADP

Enzymes are present that can hydrolyze ATP.

Enzyme

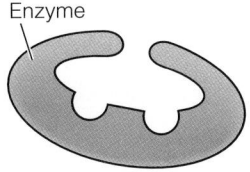

Building blocks are available to build compounds.[b]

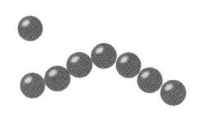

During ATP use:

The enzyme hydrolyzes ATP, splitting off a phosphate group. Energy is released.

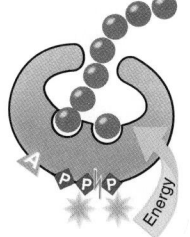

The enzyme uses that energy to attach a building block to a growing molecule.[c]

After ATP use:

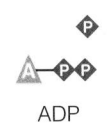

ADP

ADP and a phosphate group remain. More energy from nutrients will be required to regenerate ATP.

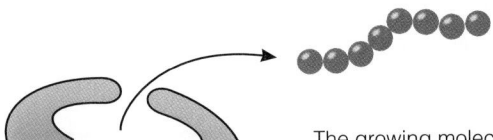

The enzyme complex is now ready to work again.

The growing molecule is now longer.

Figure 7–2

ATP (Adenosine Triphosphate), One of the Body's Quick-Energy Molecules

[a]ADP (adenosine diphosphate) is lower in energy than ATP; AMP (adenosine monophosphate) is even lower.

[b]Compounds that ATP energy might be used to build include glycogen, fat, proteins, and hormones, among others.

[c]In all such reactions, half or more of the total original energy is lost as heat, accounting for the temperature-raising effect of metabolism. ATP can also break apart without doing work and release all of its energy as heat if needed.

Appendix A presents a brief summary of the structure and function of the cell.

Reminder: An *enzyme* is a special protein that serves as a catalyst for a chemical reaction and is not altered in the process.

coenzymes: small organic molecules that work with enzymes to facilitate the enzymes' activity. Many coenzymes have B vitamins as part of their structures (Figure 10–1 in Chapter 10 illustrates coenzyme action).

   co = with

The Site of Reactions—Cells   The body's metabolic work is going on all the time within all the cells. Figure 7–3 illustrates a typical cell and shows where the major reactions of energy production take place. The type and extent of metabolic activity vary depending on the type of cell, but of all the body's cells, the liver cells are the most versatile and metabolically active. Table 7–1 offers insights into the liver's work.

The Helpers in Reactions—Enzymes and Coenzymes   Metabolic reactions almost always require enzymes to facilitate their action. In some cases, the enzymes need assistants to help them. Enzyme helpers are called coenzymes.

Coenzymes are small organic molecules that associate closely with most enzymes, but are not proteins themselves. The relationships between coenzymes and enzymes differ in detail, but one thing is true of all: without its coenzyme, an enzyme cannot function. Some of the B vitamins serve as coenzymes to the enzymes that release energy from glucose, glycerol, fatty acids, and amino acids. These B vitamin coenzymes stand alongside the metabolic pathways, so to speak, and help to keep the disassembly lines moving. Chapter 10 provides more details on the coenzyme actions of the B vitamins.

With these introductory remarks in mind, it is time to enter a cell and follow the various paths that glucose, glycerol, fatty acids, and amino acids take to yield

Figure 7–3

A Typical Cell (Simplified Diagram)

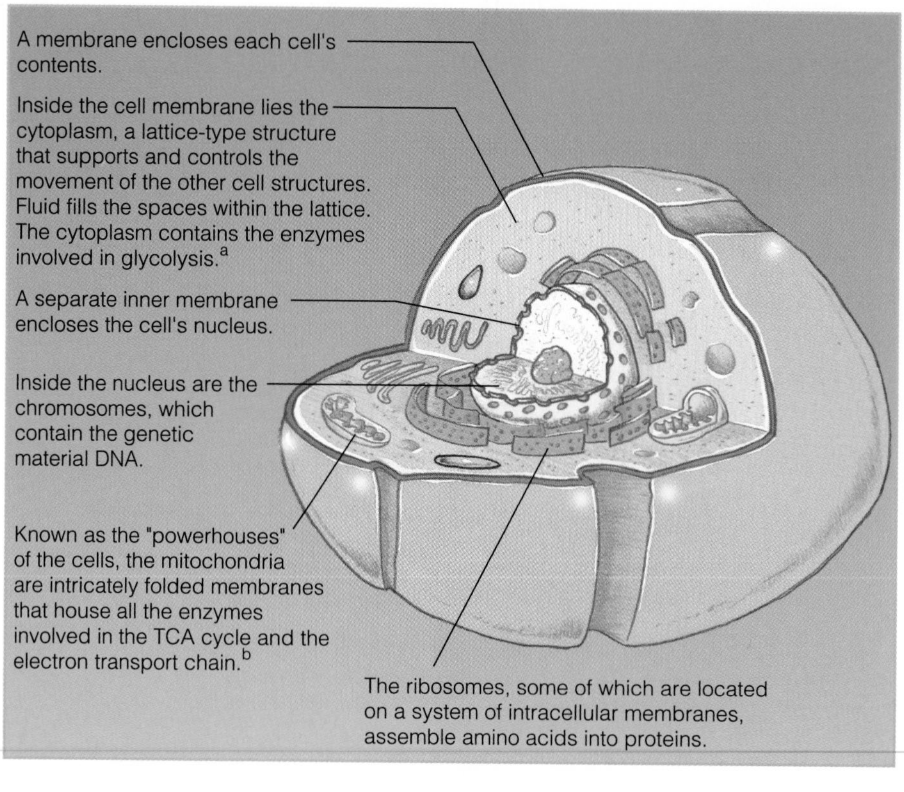

A membrane encloses each cell's contents.

Inside the cell membrane lies the cytoplasm, a lattice-type structure that supports and controls the movement of the other cell structures. Fluid fills the spaces within the lattice. The cytoplasm contains the enzymes involved in glycolysis.[a]

A separate inner membrane encloses the cell's nucleus.

Inside the nucleus are the chromosomes, which contain the genetic material DNA.

Known as the "powerhouses" of the cells, the mitochondria are intricately folded membranes that house all the enzymes involved in the TCA cycle and the electron transport chain.[b]

The ribosomes, some of which are located on a system of intracellular membranes, assemble amino acids into proteins.

[a]Glycolysis is described on pp. 224–225.
[b]The TCA cycle and electron transport chain are described on p. 235.

energy. As you will see, each starts down a different path, but they all reach a common destination. At a certain point, they lose their individuality and most of their options—during catabolism all roads lead to energy.

Table 7–1

Metabolic Work of the Liver

The liver is the most active processing center in the body. When nutrients enter the body, the liver receives them first; then it metabolizes, packages, stores, or ships them out for use by other organs. When alcohol, drugs, or poisons enter the body, they are also sent directly to the liver; here they are detoxified and their by-products shipped out for excretion. An enthusiastic anatomy and physiology professor once remarked that given the many vital activities of the liver, we should express our feelings for others by saying, "I love you with all my liver," instead of with all my heart. Granted, this declaration lacks romance, but it makes a valid point. Here are just *some* of the many jobs performed by the liver.

Carbohydrates:

- Converts fructose and galactose to glucose.
- Makes and stores glycogen.
- Breaks down glycogen and releases glucose.
- Breaks down glucose for energy when needed.
- Makes glucose from amino acids and glycerol when needed.

Lipids:

- Builds and breaks down triglycerides, phospholipids, and cholesterol as needed.
- Breaks down fatty acids for energy when needed.
- Packages extra lipids in lipoproteins for transport to other body organs.
- Manufactures bile to send to the gallbladder for use in fat digestion.
- Makes ketone bodies when necessary.

Proteins:

- Manufactures nonessential amino acids that are in short supply.
- Removes from circulation amino acids that are present in excess of need and deaminates them or converts them to other amino acids.
- Removes ammonia from the blood and converts it to urea to be sent to the kidneys for excretion.
- Makes other nitrogen-containing compounds the body needs (such as bases used in DNA and RNA).
- Makes plasma proteins such as clotting factors.

Other:

- Detoxifies alcohol, other drugs, and poisons; prepares waste products for excretion.
- Helps dismantle old red blood cells and captures the iron for recycling.
- Stores most vitamins and many minerals.
- Forms lymph.

To renew your appreciation for this remarkable organ, you might want to review Figure 3–9 on p. 89.

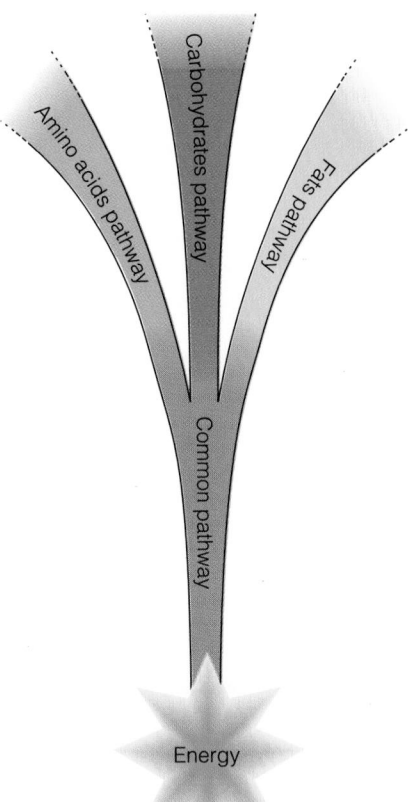

This simple overview introduces the metabolism that is presented in the upcoming text and detailed in Figure 7–18.

Breaking Down Nutrients for Energy

Glucose, glycerol, fatty acids, and amino acids are the basic units derived from food, but a molecule of each of these compounds is made of still smaller units, the atoms—carbons, nitrogens, oxygens, and hydrogens. During catabolism, the body separates these atoms from one another. To follow this action, recall how many carbons are in the "backbones" of these compounds.

- Glucose has 6 carbons:

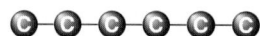

- Glycerol has 3 carbons:

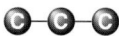

- A fatty acid usually has an even number of carbons, commonly 18 carbons or more:

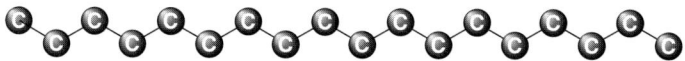

- An amino acid has 2, 3, or more carbons with a nitrogen attached:*

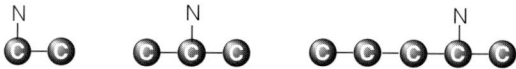

Full chemical structures and reactions appear both in the earlier chapters and in Appendix C; this chapter diagrams the reactions using just the compounds' carbon and nitrogen backbones.

What happens to these compounds inside cells can best be understood by starting with glucose. Two new names appear—pyruvate (a 3-carbon structure) and acetyl CoA (a 2-carbon structure with a coenzyme attached)—and the rest of the story falls into place around them. A major point to notice in the following discussion is that all compounds that can be converted to pyruvate can be used to make glucose. Compounds that are converted directly to acetyl CoA cannot make glucose, however.

GLUCOSE

The first pathway glucose takes on its way to yield energy is called glycolysis (glucose splitting).[†] Figure 7–4 shows a simplified drawing of glycolysis, which actually involves several steps and several enzymes (see Appendix C for details). Along the way, the 6-carbon glucose is split in half, forming two 3-carbon compounds. These 3-carbon compounds continue along the pathway until they are converted to pyruvate. Thus the net yield of one glucose molecule is two pyruvate

---

pyruvate (PIE-roo-vate): pyruvic acid, a 3-carbon compound that, in metabolism, can be derived from glucose, certain amino acids, or glycerol. The term *pyruvate* means a salt of *pyruvic acid*. (Throughout this book, the ending *-ate* is used interchangeably with *-ic acid*; for our purposes they mean the same thing.)

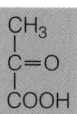

acetyl CoA (ASS-eh-teel, or ah-SEET-il, coh-AY): a 2-carbon compound (acetate, or acetic acid, shown in Figure 5–2 on p. 142) to which a molecule of CoA is attached.

CoA (coh-AY): coenzyme A; the coenzyme derived from the B vitamin pantothenic acid and central to the energy metabolism of nutrients.

---

*The figures in this chapter usually show amino acids as compounds of 2, 3, or 5 carbons arranged in a straight line, but in reality amino acids may contain other numbers of carbons and assume other structural shapes (see Appendix C).

[†]Glycolysis takes place in the cytoplasm of the cell (see Figure 7–3).

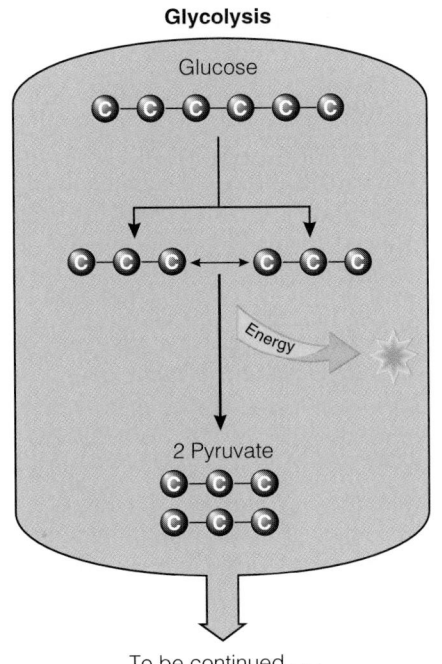

Glycolysis

Glucose

2 Pyruvate

To be continued . . .

The 6-carbon compound glucose is split into two interchangeable 3-carbon compounds that are converted to pyruvate in a series of reactions.

All of the other monosaccharides can enter the pathway at various points.

Glycolysis ends with the production of pyruvate (unless there is a shortage of oxygen, in which case pyruvate is converted to lactic acid, as a later section of the text describes).

Figure 7–4

Glycolysis: Glucose-to-Pyruvate Pathway (Anaerobic)

Glucose splits to two 3-carbon compounds that become pyruvate. The pathway is called glycolysis (glucose splitting) and may occur in anaerobic conditions (does not require oxygen).

---

molecules. If they continue breaking down, both pyruvate molecules will release much of their energy to form ATP molecules and some of their energy as heat.

Glucose-to-Pyruvate, and Back Again   After splitting glucose to pyruvate, a cell can make glucose again from pyruvate in a process similar to the reversal of glycolysis. Making glucose requires energy, however, and a few different enzymes. Still, glucose is retrievable from pyruvate, so the arrows between glucose and pyruvate are shown pointing up as well as down.

Glucose-to-Pyruvate, an Anaerobic Pathway   To start the process of splitting glucose to pyruvate, the cell must use a little energy, but it then produces more energy than it had to invest initially.* No oxygen has been required thus far—that is, glycolysis is an anaerobic pathway. More energy can be released by taking pyruvate through additional metabolic reactions, but oxygen is needed for these reactions (they are aerobic).†

Pyruvate-to-Acetyl CoA   If the cell needs energy and oxygen is available, it removes a carbon group (COOH) from pyruvate to produce acetyl CoA. The carbon group from pyruvate becomes carbon dioxide, which is released into the blood, circulated to the lungs, and breathed out. The remaining 2-carbon compound bonds with a molecule of CoA, becoming acetyl CoA. Figure 7–5 diagrams the pyruvate-to-acetyl CoA reaction.

glycolysis (gligh-COLL-ih-sis): the metabolic breakdown of glucose to pyruvate. Glycolysis does not require oxygen (anaerobic).
   glyco = glucose
   lysis = breakdown

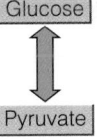

anaerobic (AN-air-ROE-bic): not requiring oxygen.
   an = not

aerobic (air-ROE-bic): requiring oxygen.

---

*The cell uses 2 ATP to begin the breakdown of glucose to pyruvate, but then gains 4 ATP for a net gain of 2 ATP.

†With sufficient oxygen, pyruvate molecules enter the mitochondria of the cell (see Figure 7–3) where they will be converted to acetyl CoA.

Figure 7–5

Pyruvate-to-Acetyl CoA (Aerobic)

Each pyruvate loses a carbon as carbon dioxide and picks up a molecule of CoA, becoming acetyl CoA. The arrow goes only one way (down), because the step is not reversible. Result (from 1 glucose): 2 carbon dioxide and 2 acetyl CoA.

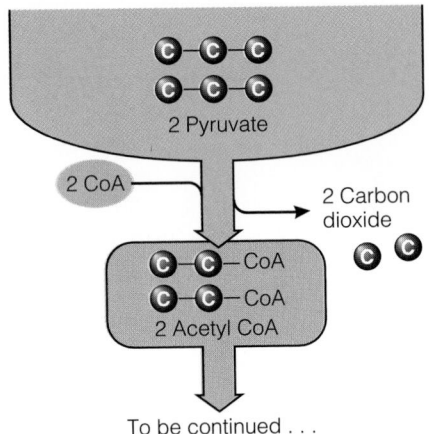

To be continued . . .

lactic acid: an acid produced from pyruvate during anaerobic metabolism.

Cori cycle: the path from muscle glycogen to glucose to pyruvate to lactic acid (which travels to the liver) to glucose (which can travel back to the muscle) to glycogen; named after the scientist who elucidated this pathway.

Glucose Retrieval via the Cori Cycle   Alternatively, when less oxygen is available, pyruvate is converted to lactic acid. This anaerobic reaction occurs to a limited extent even at rest, but increases dramatically during high-intensity exercise—that is, whenever exertion exceeds the capacity of the heart and lungs to clear carbon dioxide from the muscles. With limited oxygen available and limited carbon dioxide clearance, lactic acid accumulates in muscles, causing burning pain and fatigue. (To relieve this pain, relax the muscles frequently so that the circulating blood can carry the lactic acid away to the liver.) The liver can convert lactic acid to glucose, a recycling process that is called the Cori cycle.

Muscles' Needs for Oxygen   The role of oxygen in metabolism is worth noticing, for it helps make many things understandable. As you breathe oxygen into your lungs, the oxygen is attached to a carrier (hemoglobin) in your red blood cells that delivers it to the cells, making oxygen available for energy metabolism. You know you need to breathe harder when you are using energy faster (exercising), but you may not have realized why. Energy nutrients are being broken down to provide that energy, and oxygen is always ultimately involved in the process. As just mentioned, oxygen combines with the carbons of glucose to form carbon dioxide; later sections will describe how oxygen combines with the hydrogens to form water.

Highlight 8 provides an overview of the body's use of the energy nutrients to fuel physical activity, but the facts just presented offer a sneak preview. The first pathway in glucose metabolism (glycolysis) yields some energy without oxygen (it is anaerobic), but the later pathways require oxygen (they are aerobic). Aerobic metabolism yields by far the *most energy* and so is crucial for endurance activities.

Pyruvate-to-Acetyl CoA, an Irreversible Step   The step from pyruvate to acetyl CoA is metabolically irreversible: a cell cannot retrieve the shed carbons from carbon dioxide to remake pyruvate, and then glucose. It is a one-way step and is therefore shown with only a "down" arrow in Figure 7–6. Notice that acetyl CoA can be used as a building block for fatty acids, but it cannot be used to remake glucose.

Acetyl CoA-to-Carbon Dioxide: The TCA Cycle   Once made, acetyl CoA has the option of taking different metabolic paths, depending on the cell's needs. If the cell needs energy, acetyl CoA may proceed through a series of reactions

Figure 7–6

The Paths of Pyruvate and Acetyl CoA

Pyruvate and acetyl CoA may follow several reversible paths, but the path from pyruvate to acetyl CoA is irreversible.

Amino acids that can be used to make glucose are called *glucogenic*; amino acids that are converted to acetyl CoA are called *ketogenic*.

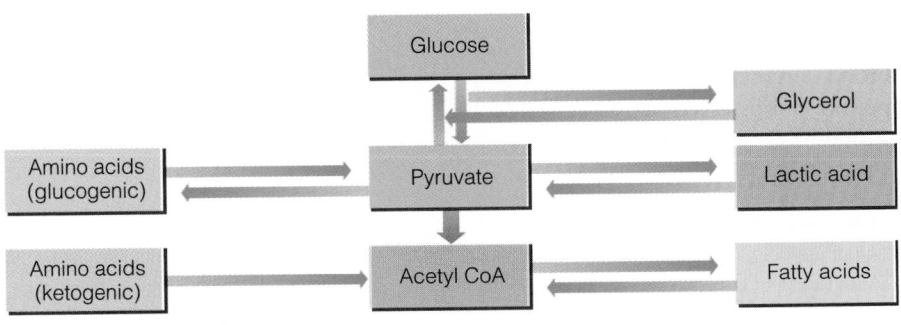

known as the TCA cycle. The TCA cycle converts the 2-carbon acetyl CoA to two carbon dioxide molecules and frees its coenzyme (CoA) to be reused (see Figure 7–7). In the process, much more energy is made available than during glycolysis (more details are given later).

Acetyl CoA-to-Fat   If energy is not needed, acetyl CoA will not enter the TCA cycle, but will be used to make fatty acids instead. This explains how carbohydrate, eaten in excess of the body's needs, can lead to fat deposition. As you will see, fat or protein eaten in excess of immediate energy needs can take the same pathway to body fat.

Figure 7–8 (on p. 228) combines Figures 7–4, 7–5, and 7–7 and shows the whole sequence of steps in glucose breakdown. In summary, the main steps in the catabolism of glucose are:

Glucose
    to
        pyruvate
            to
                acetyl CoA
                    to
                        carbon dioxide.

Keep in mind that glucose can be retrieved only from pyruvate or compounds

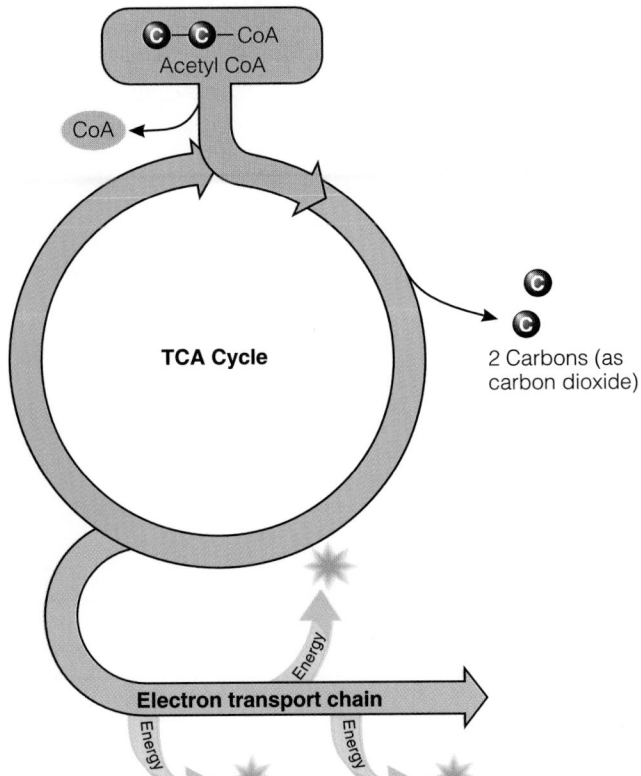

TCA Cycle

2 Carbons (as carbon dioxide)

Electron transport chain

Energy

Figure 7–7

The Breakdown of Acetyl CoA
The complete oxidation of acetyl CoA is accomplished through the reactions of the **TCA** (tricarboxylic acid) **cycle,** or **Krebs cycle** (named for the biochemist who elucidated them), and the **electron transport chain.** In the TCA cycle, the acetyl CoA carbons are converted to carbon dioxide. Each CoA returns to pick up another acetate (coming from glucose, lipids, or protein).

The net result is that acetyl CoA splits, the carbons combine with oxygen, and the energy originally in the acetyl CoA is stored in ATP and similar compounds, thus becoming available for the body's use. Chapter 10 describes how the B vitamin coenzymes participate in these metabolic pathways. For more details, see the text and Appendix C.

Figure 7–8

Glucose-to-Energy Pathway

Through these processes, energy from glucose is made available to do the cells' work. Ultimately, glucose is completely disassembled to single-carbon fragments, and the fragments are combined with oxygen to form carbon dioxide. Much of the energy released is trapped and stored in ATP. Details of the TCA cycle and the electron transport chain are shown later and in Appendix C.

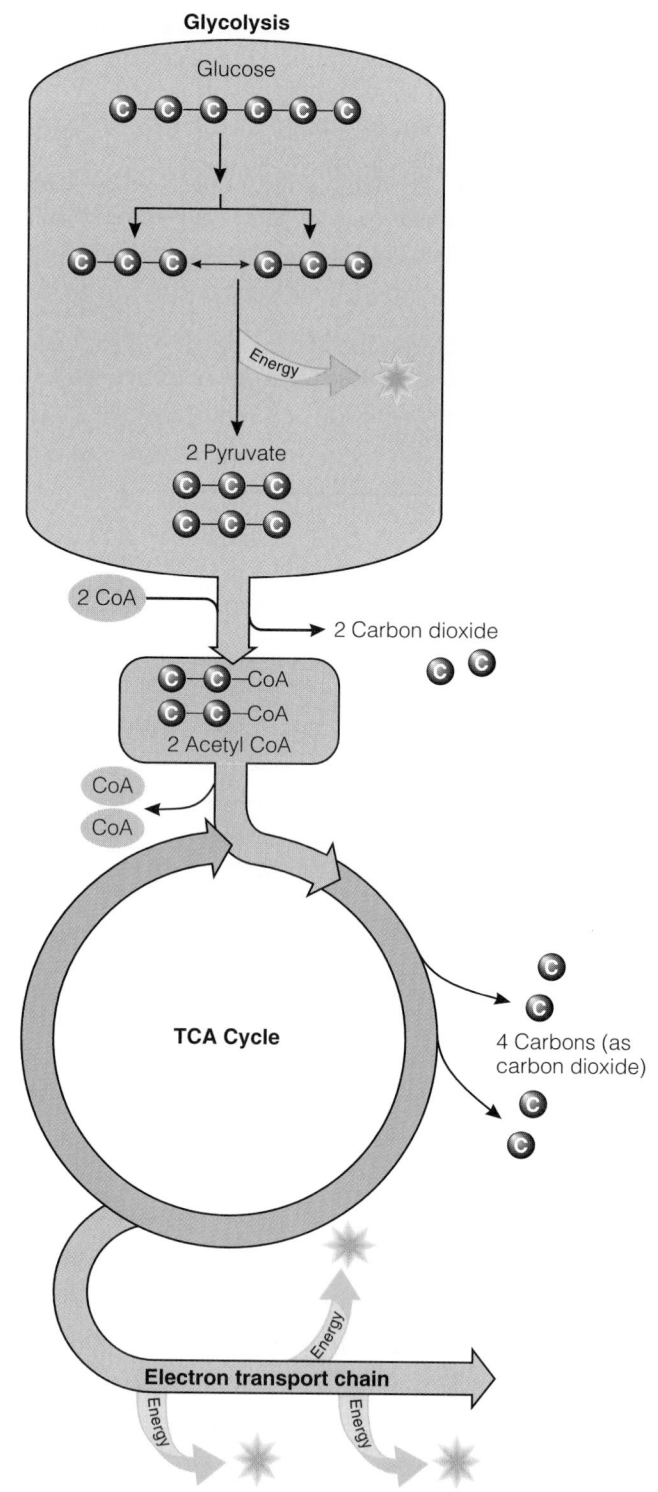

earlier in the pathway. Once the commitment to acetyl CoA is made, glucose is not retrievable; acetyl CoA can go on to carbon dioxide, fat, or other compounds but not back to glucose.

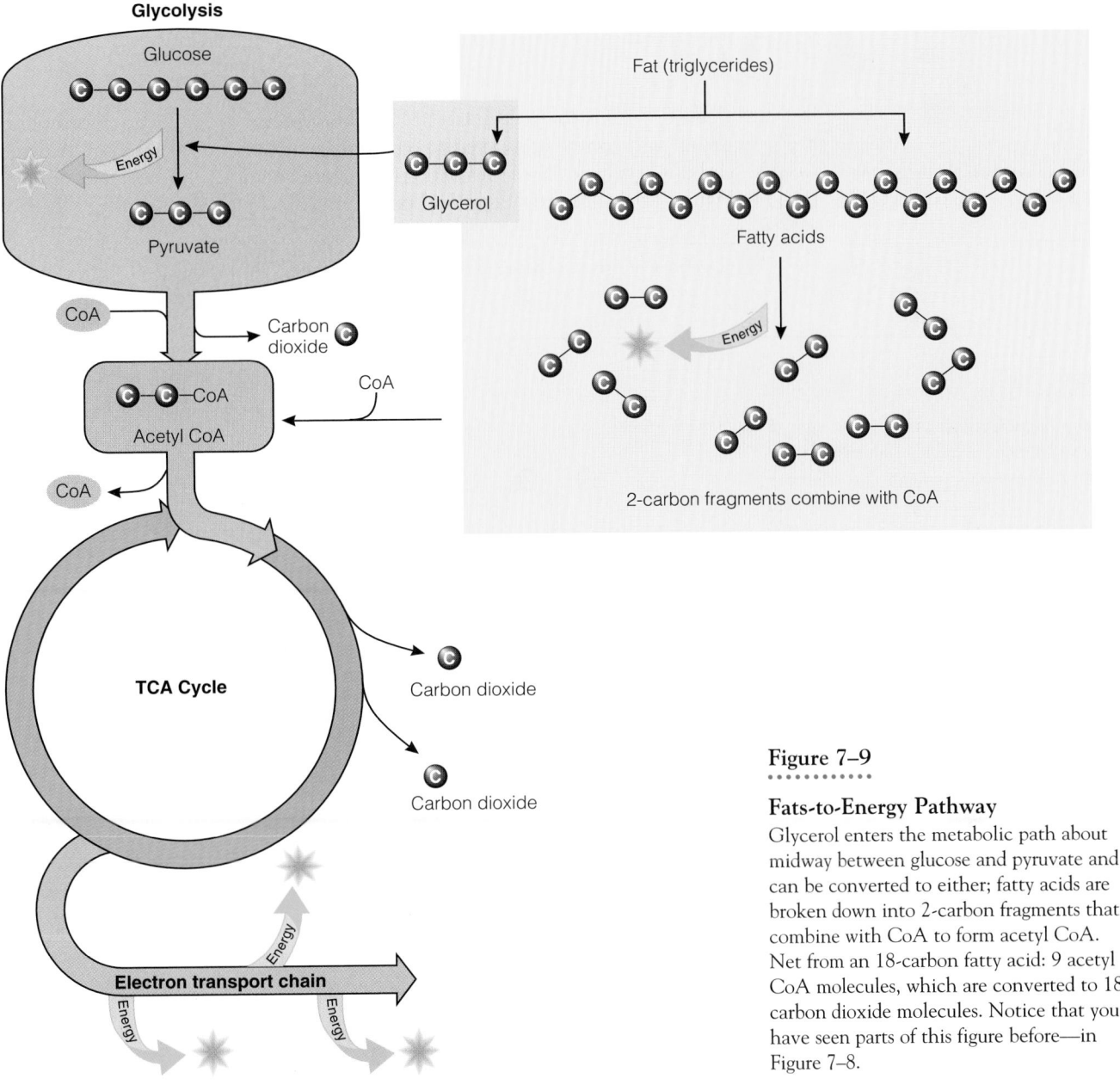

Figure 7–9

Fats-to-Energy Pathway

Glycerol enters the metabolic path about midway between glucose and pyruvate and can be converted to either; fatty acids are broken down into 2-carbon fragments that combine with CoA to form acetyl CoA. Net from an 18-carbon fatty acid: 9 acetyl CoA molecules, which are converted to 18 carbon dioxide molecules. Notice that you have seen parts of this figure before—in Figure 7–8.

GLYCEROL AND FATTY ACIDS

Once glucose breakdown is understood, fat and protein breakdown are easily learned, for all three share a common metabolic pathway. Recall that triglycerides can break down to glycerol and fatty acids. Figure 7–9 repeats the pathway that glucose follows and shows how glycerol and fatty acids enter into it.

Glycerol-to-Pyruvate Glycerol (a 3-carbon compound like pyruvate, but with a different arrangement of H and OH on the C) is easily converted to

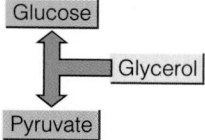

fatty acid oxidation: the metabolic breakdown of fatty acids to acetyl CoA.

another 3-carbon compound. This compound may go either "up" the pathway to form glucose or "down" to form pyruvate and acetyl CoA and, finally, carbon dioxide.

Fatty Acids-to-Acetyl CoA   Unlike glycerol, which is a 3-carbon compound that can be converted to 3-carbon pyruvate, fatty acids are taken apart 2 carbons at a time in a series of aerobic reactions known as fatty acid oxidation.* Figure 7–10 illustrates fatty acid oxidation and shows that in the process, each

---

*Oxidation of fatty acids occurs in the mitochondria of the cells (see Figure 7–3).

Figure 7–10

Fatty Acid Oxidation

During oxidation, fatty acids are taken apart to 2-carbon fragments that combine with CoA to make acetyl CoA. Fatty acid oxidation is a series of aerobic reactions.

The fatty acid is first activated by coenzyme A.

A little energy is released each time a carbon-carbon bond is cleaved.

Another CoA joins the chain, and the bond at the second carbon (the beta-carbon) weakens. Acetyl CoA splits off, leaving a fatty acid that is two carbons shorter.

The shorter fatty acid enters the pathway and the cycle repeats. The molecules of acetyl CoA enter the TCA cycle, yielding abundant energy.

16-C fatty acid

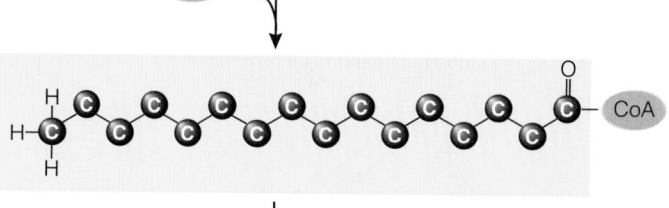

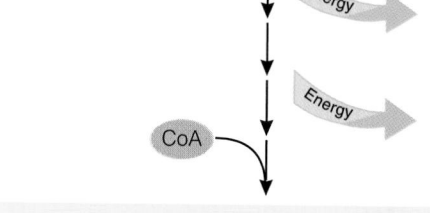

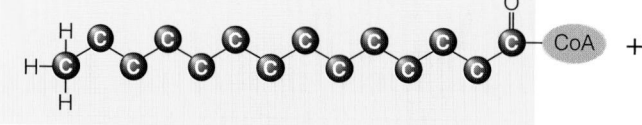

Net result from a 16-C fatty acid:	14-C fatty acid CoA	+	1 acetyl CoA
Cycle repeats, leaving:	12-C fatty acid CoA	+	2 acetyl CoA
Cycle repeats, leaving:	10-C fatty acid CoA	+	3 acetyl CoA
Cycle repeats, leaving:	8-C fatty acid CoA	+	4 acetyl CoA
Cycle repeats, leaving:	6-C fatty acid CoA	+	5 acetyl CoA
Cycle repeats, leaving:	4-C fatty acid CoA	+	6 acetyl CoA
Cycle repeats, leaving:	2-C fatty acid CoA*	+	7 acetyl CoA

*Notice that 2-C fatty acid CoA = acetyl CoA, so that the final yield from a 16-C fatty acid is 8 acetyl CoA.

2–carbon fragment splits off and combines with a molecule of CoA to make acetyl CoA. Each acetyl CoA then enters the TCA cycle in the same manner as acetyl CoA from glucose does (review Figure 7–9). A little energy is released each time a 2-carbon fragment breaks off from a fatty acid during oxidation, but when these 2-carbon units enter the TCA cycle as acetyl CoA, they yield nearly three times as much energy. If the cell does not need energy, the acetyl CoA molecules will combine with each other to make body fat, in the same way acetyl CoA produced from excess carbohydrate does.

Glucose Not Retrievable from Fatty Acids   Cells can make glucose from pyruvate and other 3-carbon compounds, as mentioned earlier, but they cannot make glucose from the 2-carbon fragments of fatty acids. In chemical diagrams, the arrow between pyruvate and acetyl CoA always points only one way—down—and fatty acid fragments enter the metabolic path below this arrow (review Figure 7–6). Thus fatty acids cannot be used to make glucose.

The significance of this is that fat, for the most part, normally cannot provide energy for red blood cells or the brain and nervous system, which require glucose as fuel. Remember that almost all dietary fats are triglycerides, and that triglycerides contain only one small molecule of glycerol (3 carbons) with three fatty acids. The glycerol can yield glucose, but that represents only 3 of the 50 or so carbon atoms in the molecule—about 5 percent of its weight (see Figure 7–11). Thus fat is an insignificant source of glucose; about 95 percent of fat cannot be converted to glucose.

Reminder: The making of glucose from the glycerol of triglycerides (or from amino acids) is *gluconeogenesis*. About 5% of fat (the glycerol portion of a triglyceride) and most amino acids can be converted to glucose.

AMINO ACIDS

The preceding two sections have shown how the breakdown of carbohydrate and fat provides energy for the body's use. One energy-yielding nutrient remains: protein or, rather, the amino acids of protein.

Amino Acid Catabolism   If amino acids are needed for energy, or if they are consumed in excess of the need to synthesize protein, they enter the metabolic pathway as shown in Figure 7–12 (on p. 232). First, amino acids are deaminated (that is, they lose their nitrogen as described in the next section), and then they are catabolized in a variety of ways. Some amino acids can be converted to pyruvate; others are converted to acetyl CoA; and still others enter the TCA cycle directly as compounds other than acetyl CoA.

Reminder: *Deamination* is the reaction that removes the nitrogen-containing amino group from an amino acid.

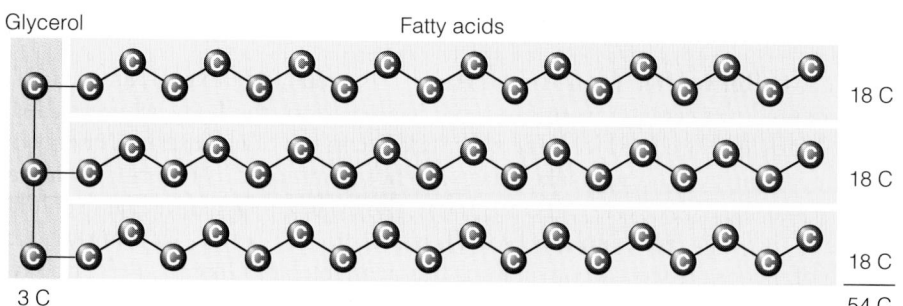

Glycerol   Fatty acids

18 C

18 C

18 C

3 C   54 C

Figure 7–11

The Carbons of a Typical Triglyceride

A typical triglyceride contains only one small molecule of glycerol (3 C), but has three fatty acids (each about 18 C on the average, or about 54 C). Only the glycerol portion of a triglyceride can yield glucose.

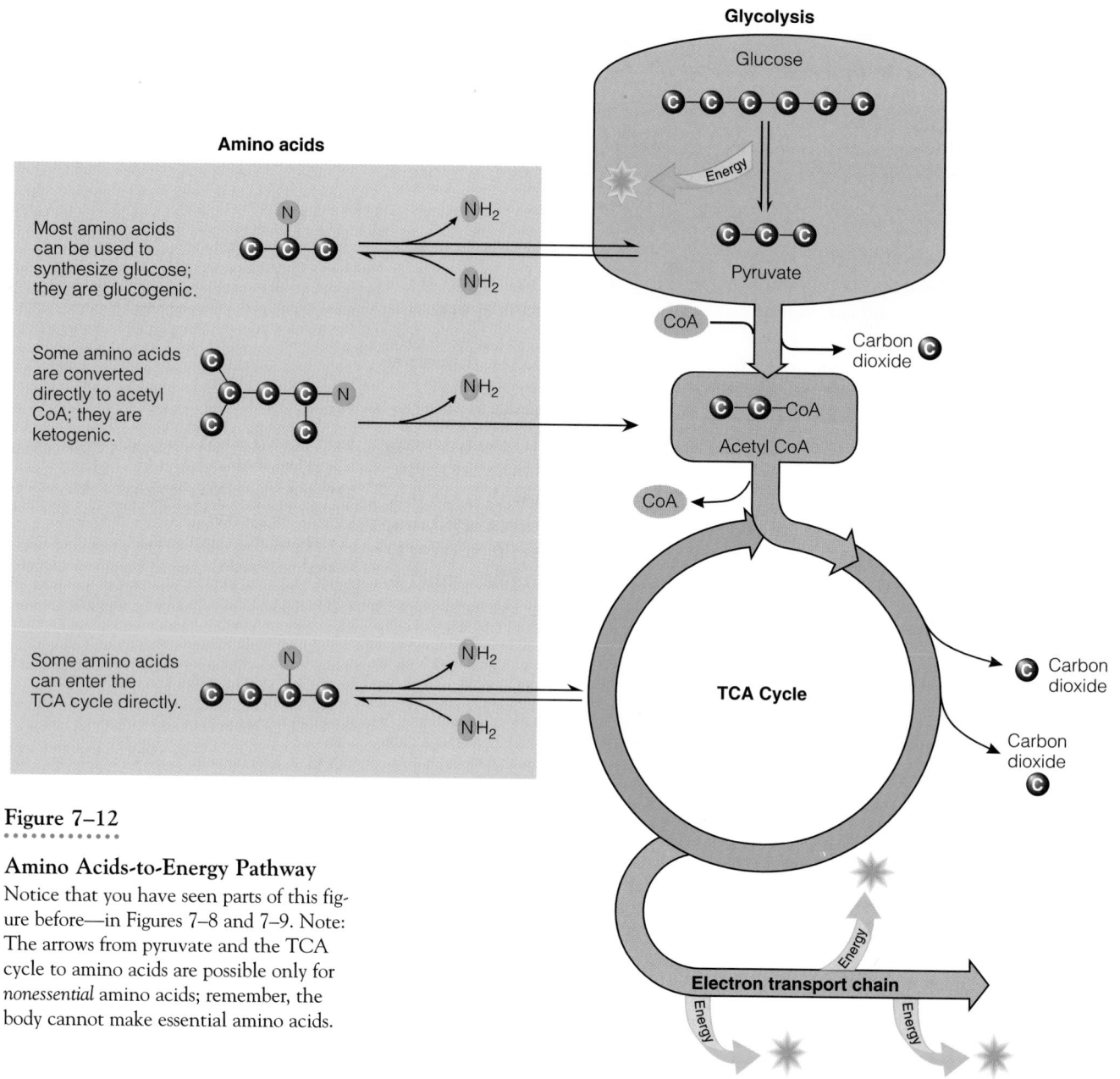

Figure 7–12

Amino Acids-to-Energy Pathway

Notice that you have seen parts of this figure before—in Figures 7–8 and 7–9. Note: The arrows from pyruvate and the TCA cycle to amino acids are possible only for *nonessential* amino acids; remember, the body cannot make essential amino acids.

Glucose Retrievable from Amino Acids   As you might expect, amino acids that are used to make pyruvate can provide glucose for the body, whereas those amino acids that are used to make acetyl CoA can provide additional energy or make body fat but cannot make glucose. Those amino acids entering as intermediates to the TCA cycle can continue in the cycle and generate energy; alternatively, they can generate glucose. Thus protein, unlike fat, is a fairly good source of glucose when carbohydrate is not available; and like fat and carbohydrate, it is converted to body fat when consumed beyond the body's needs.

A key to understanding these metabolic pathways is learning which fuels can be converted to glucose and which cannot. The parts of protein and fat that can be converted to pyruvate *can* provide glucose for the body, whereas the parts that are converted to acetyl CoA *cannot* provide glucose, but can readily provide fat. You must have glucose to fuel your brain's activities, and if you don't obtain it from food, your body will devour its own lean tissue to provide it. Therefore, to keep this from happening, you need to supply fuels that can provide glucose—primarily carbohydrate. If you offer your body only fat, which delivers mostly acetyl CoA, you put your body in the position of having to break down protein tissue for glucose. If you offer your body only protein, you put your body in the position of having to convert protein to glucose. Clearly, the best diet supplies some protein, some fat, and abundant carbohydrate.

Amino Acids-to-Fat Once amino acids have been converted to acetyl CoA, if energy is not needed, fatty acids are made and stored as triglycerides in adipose tissue. (Recall from Chapter 6 that the body cannot store surplus amino acids as such; it has to convert them to other compounds.) Thus protein can also add to fat stores if eaten in excess.

People who eat huge portions of meat and other protein-rich foods may wonder why they have weight problems. Not only does the fat in those foods lead to fat storage; the protein can, too, when energy intake exceeds energy needs. Many fad weight-loss diets encourage high protein intakes based on the false assumption that protein builds only muscle, not fat.

Deamination When amino acids are metabolized for energy or used to make fat, they must be deaminated first. Two products result from deamination. One is, of course, the structure without its amino group—often a keto acid (see Figure 7–13). The other product is ammonia, a toxic compound chemically identical to the strong-smelling ammonia in bottled cleaning solutions. Ammonia is a base, and if the body produces larger quantities than it can handle, the blood's critical acid-base balance becomes upset.

Transamination As the discussion of protein in Chapter 6 pointed out, only some amino acids are essential; others can be made in the body, given a source of nitrogen. The body does this by transferring an amino group from one amino

Reminder: Diet and health recommendations advise that daily energy intake provide:
- 55–60% carbohydrate.
- ≤ 30% fat.
- 10–15% protein.

Products of deamination:
- Keto acid.
- Ammonia.

keto acid: an organic acid that contains a carbonyl group (C=O).

ammonia: a compound with the chemical formula NH_3; produced during the deamination of amino acids.

transamination: the transfer of an amino group from one amino acid to a keto acid, producing a new nonessential amino acid and a new keto acid.

The deamination of an amino acid produces ammonia (NH_3) and a keto acid:

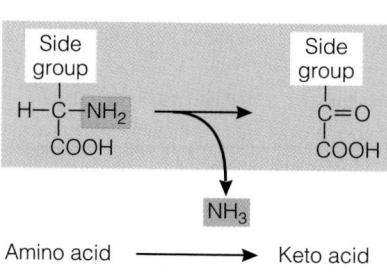

Given a source of NH_3, the body can make nonessential amino acids from keto acids:

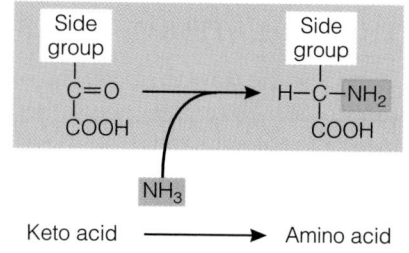

Figure 7–13

Keto Acids

Figure 7–14

Transamination to Make a Nonessential Amino Acid

The body can transfer amino groups from an amino acid to a keto acid, forming a new nonessential amino acid and a new keto acid.

Transamination reactions require the vitamin B_6 coenzyme.

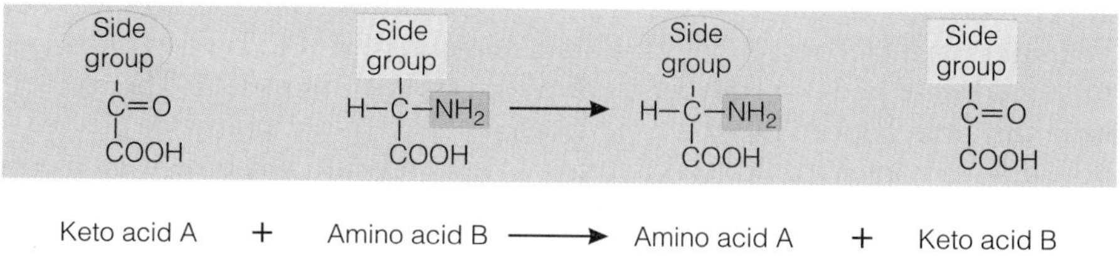

Keto acid A   +   Amino acid B   ⟶   Amino acid A   +   Keto acid B

acid to its corresponding keto acid, producing a new amino acid and a new keto acid, as shown in Figure 7–14. Through many such reactions, involving many different keto acids, the liver cells can synthesize the nonessential amino acids.

Ammonia-to-Urea in the Liver   The liver continuously produces small amounts of ammonia in deamination reactions. Some of this ammonia provides the nitrogen needed for the synthesis of nonessential amino acids. The liver quickly combines any unused ammonia with carbon dioxide to make urea, a much less toxic compound (see Figure 7–15). The diagram greatly oversimplifies the reactions; details are shown in Appendix C.

Urea Excreted via the Kidneys   Liver cells release urea into the blood, where it circulates until it passes through the kidneys (see Figure 7–16 on the next page). The kidneys then remove urea from the blood for excretion in the urine. Normally, the liver efficiently scoops up all the ammonia, makes urea from it, and releases the urea into the blood; then the kidneys clear all the urea from the blood. This division of labor allows easy diagnosis of diseases of both organs. If the liver is sick, blood ammonia will be high; if the kidneys are sick, blood urea will be high.

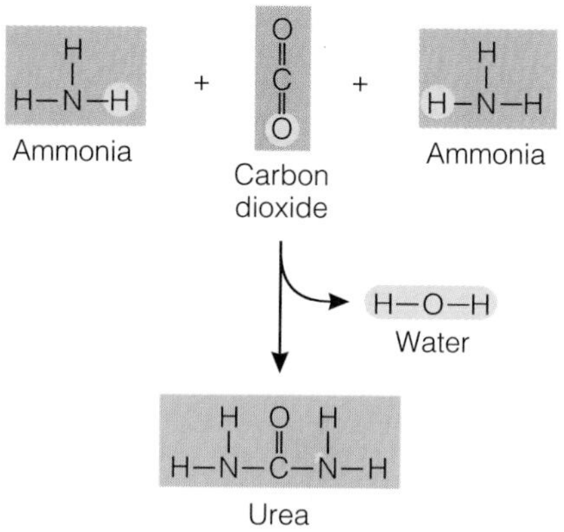

Water Needed to Excrete Urea   Urea is the body's principal vehicle for excreting unused nitrogen, and the amount produced increases with protein intake. To keep urea in solution, the body needs water. For this reason, a person who regularly consumes a high-protein diet (say, 100 grams a day or more) must drink more water than usual; without extra water, the person risks an accumulation of urea in the blood. In fact, the weight loss from water loss makes high-protein diets *appear* to be effective, but water loss, of course, is of no value to the person who wants to lose body fat.

THE FINAL STEPS OF CATABOLISM

To review the ways the body can use the energy-yielding nutrients, see Table 7–2 (on p. 236). To obtain energy, the body uses glucose and fatty acids as its primary fuels, although it can use amino acids to provide energy if need be. To make glucose, the body can use all carbohydrates and most amino acids, but can convert only 5 percent of fat (the glycerol portion) to glucose. To make body proteins,

urea (you-REE-uh): the principal nitrogen-excretion product of metabolism. Two ammonia fragments are combined with carbon dioxide to form urea.

Figure 7–15

Urea Synthesis

When amino nitrogen is stripped from amino acids, ammonia is produced. The liver detoxifies ammonia before releasing it into the bloodstream by combining it with another waste product, carbon dioxide, to produce urea. See Appendix C for details.

the body needs amino acids. It can use glucose to make some amino acids when nitrogen is available; it cannot use fats to make body proteins. Finally, when energy is consumed beyond the body's needs, the body can convert all three energy-yielding nutrients to fat for storage.

The TCA Cycle   To this point the discussion has followed each of the energy-yielding nutrients to the point where acetyl CoA enters the TCA cycle.* The TCA cycle serves as a busy traffic center through which these 2-carbon acetyl CoA molecules pass on their way to carbon dioxide, releasing their energy to other compounds as they go.

The TCA cycle is called a cycle, but that doesn't mean it regenerates acetyl CoA. Acetyl CoA goes one way only—to carbon dioxide and water, releasing energy as it goes. The TCA cycle is a circular path, though, in the sense that a 4-carbon carbohydrate-like compound does cycle around and around.† This compound picks up acetyl CoA (a 2-carbon compound), drops off one carbon (as carbon dioxide), then another carbon (as carbon dioxide), and returns to pick up another acetyl CoA. As for the acetyl CoA, its carbons go only one way—to carbon dioxide (see Appendix C for additional details).

As acetyl CoA molecules break down to carbon dioxide and water, hydrogen atoms with their electrons are removed from the compounds in the cycle. Coenzymes of the B vitamins niacin and riboflavin receive the hydrogens and their electrons and transfer them to the electron transport chain.

The Electron Transport Chain   The electron transport chain (ETC) consists of a series of proteins that serve as electron "carriers." These carriers are mounted in sequence on a membrane inside the energy-generating organelles within the cell known as mitochondria (review Figure 7–3). As each carrier receives electrons, it releases a little energy and passes the electrons on to the next carrier. While some of the energy is released as heat, much of it is captured in the bonds of ATP molecules. These electron-transferring molecules continue passing electrons and giving up energy until, at the end of the chain, any usable energy has been captured in the body's ATP molecules. The last step is to donate the low-energy electrons with their hydrogen atoms (H) to oxygen (O), forming water (H_2O), from which the body cannot extract any more energy. Everyone knows that breathing oxygen is essential to life—now you understand why. Figure 7–17 provides a simple diagram of the process; see Appendix C for details.

---

*The TCA cycle reactions take place in the mitochondria of the cell (see Figure 7–3).

†Actually, the 4-carbon compound does not cycle around as the same structure throughout; instead it travels through a series of reactions. On picking up acetyl CoA, it becomes a 6-carbon compound. On dropping off carbon dioxide, it becomes a 5- and then a 4-carbon compound. Each reaction changes the structure slightly until finally the original 4-carbon compound forms again and picks up another acetyl CoA, starting the series of reactions over again.

The carbons that enter the cycle in acetyl CoA may not be the ones that are given off as carbon dioxide. In one of the steps of the cycle, a 6-carbon compound of the cycle becomes symmetrical, both ends being identical. Thereafter it loses carbons to carbon dioxide at one end or the other. Thus only half of the carbons from acetyl CoA are given off as carbon dioxide in any one turn of the cycle; the other half become part of the compound that returns to pick up another acetyl CoA. It is true to say, though, that for each acetyl CoA that enters the TCA cycle, 2 carbons are given off as carbon dioxide. It is also true that with each turn of the cycle the energy equivalent of one acetyl CoA is released.

Figure 7–16

Urea Excretion

The liver and kidneys both play a role in disposing of excess nitrogen. Can you see why the person with liver disease has high blood ammonia, while the person with kidney disease has high blood urea? (Figure 3–8 provides details of how the kidneys work.)

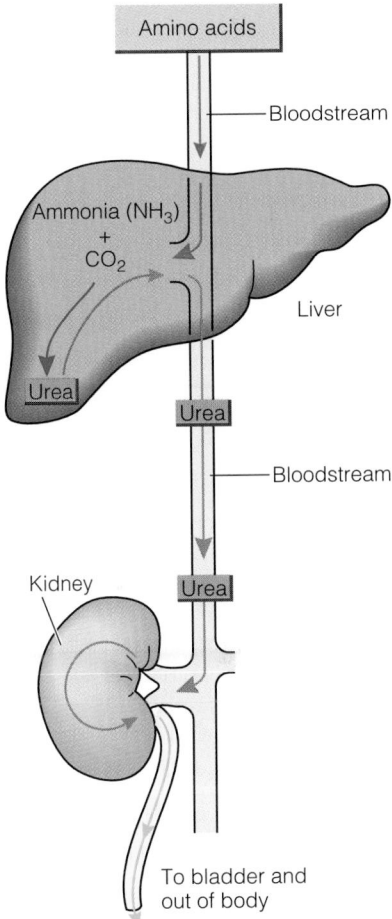

Table 7–2

Summary of Energy-Yielding Nutrient Metabolism

Nutrient	Yields Energy	Can Yield Glucose	Can Yield Amino Acids and Body Proteins	Can Yield Fat Stores
Carbohydrates (glucose)	Yes	Yes	Yes—when nitrogen is available, can yield *nonessential* amino acids	Yes
Lipids (triglycerides)	Yes	No—glycerol provides minimal amount	No	Yes
Proteins (amino acids)	Yes—if needed	Yes—when carbohydrate is unavailable	Yes	Yes

The TCA cycle and the ETC are both aerobic processes. They represent the body's most efficient means of capturing the energy from nutrients and transferring it into the bonds of ATP.

Summary   All the details this chapter has presented so far are combined in Figure 7–18. After a balanced meal, the body handles the nutrients as shown. The digestion of *carbohydrate* yields glucose; some is stored as glycogen, and some

Figure 7–17

Electron Transport Chain

An important concept to remember is that an electron is not a fixed amount of energy. The electrons that bond the H to the B vitamin coenzyme have a relatively large amount of energy. In the series of reactions that follow, they lose this energy in small amounts, until at the end they are attached (with H) to oxygen (O) to make water (H_2O). In some of the steps, the energy they lose is captured into ATP in coupled reactions. Appendix C provides a more detailed explanation.

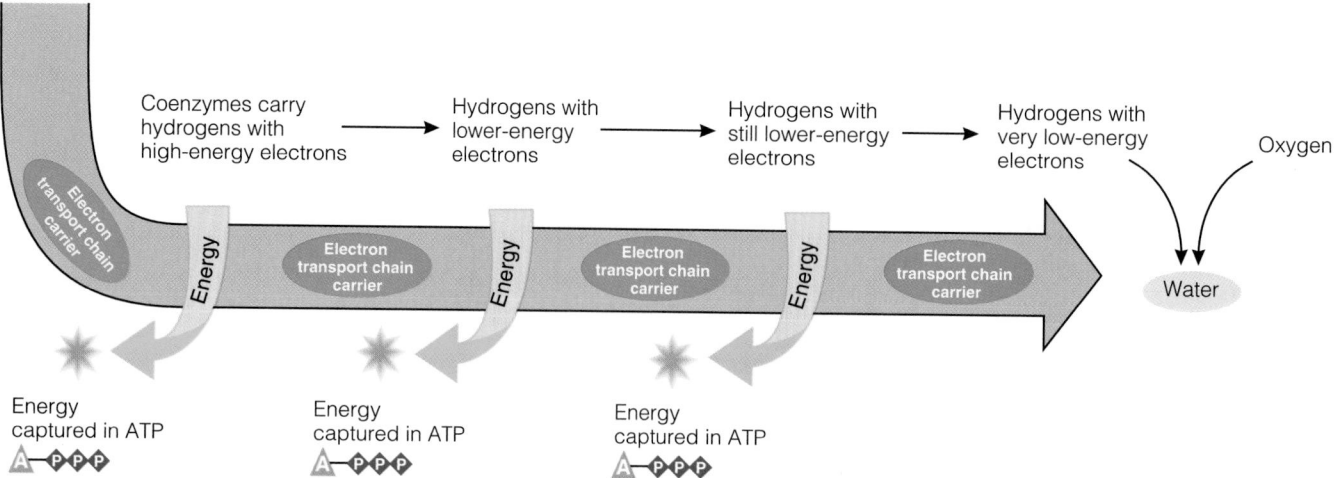

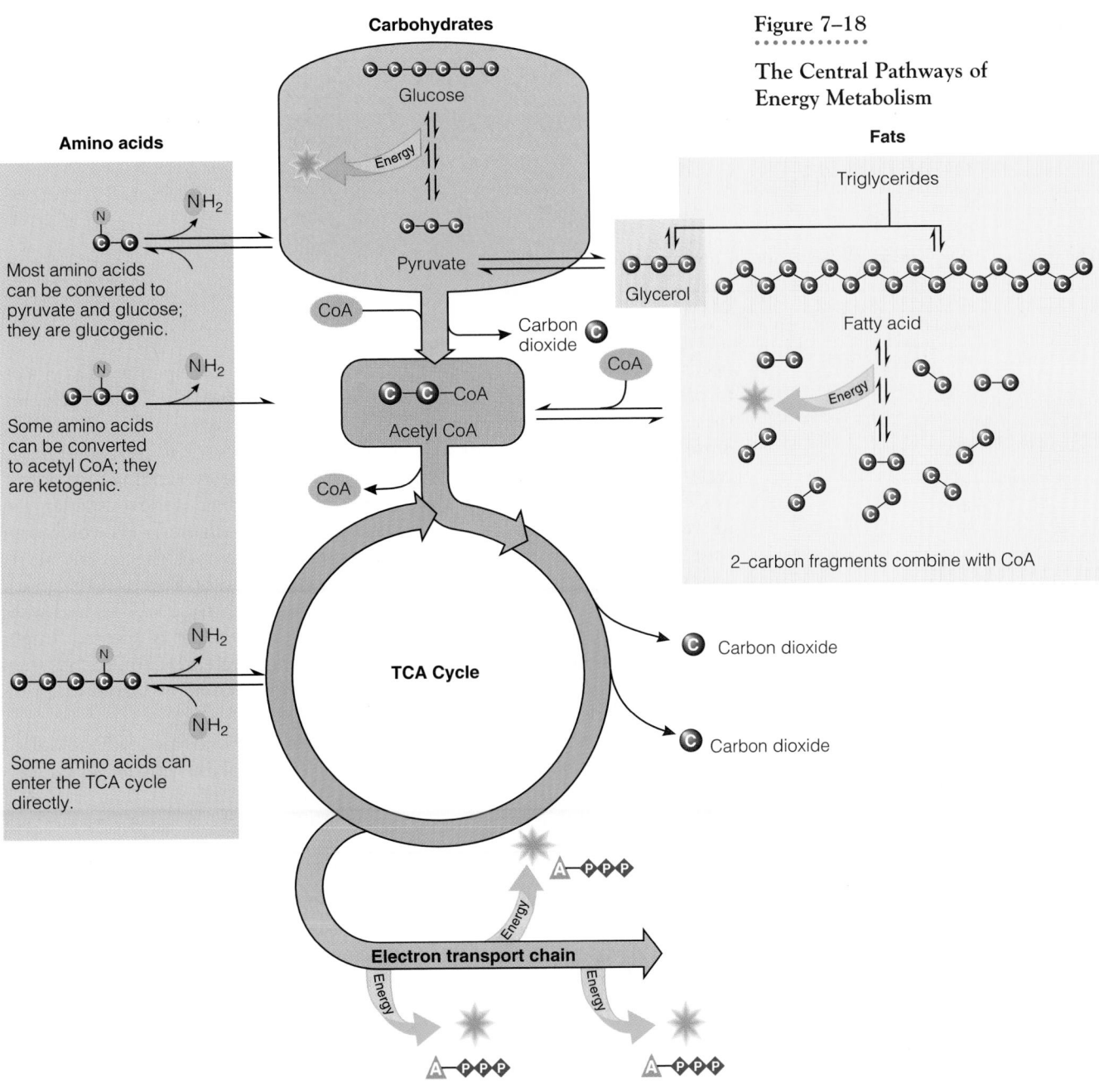

Carbohydrates

Amino acids

Most amino acids can be converted to pyruvate and glucose; they are glucogenic.

Some amino acids can be converted to acetyl CoA; they are ketogenic.

Some amino acids can enter the TCA cycle directly.

Glucose

Energy

Pyruvate

CoA

Carbon dioxide

Acetyl CoA

CoA

CoA

TCA Cycle

Carbon dioxide

Carbon dioxide

Electron transport chain

Energy

Energy

Energy

Figure 7–18

The Central Pathways of Energy Metabolism

Fats

Triglycerides

Glycerol

Fatty acid

Energy

2–carbon fragments combine with CoA

is taken into the brain and other cells and broken down to pyruvate and acetyl CoA to provide energy. The acetyl CoA can then enter the TCA cycle and ETC to provide more energy. The digestion of *fat* yields glycerol and fatty acids; some are reassembled and stored as fat, and others are broken down to acetyl CoA, enter the TCA cycle and ETC, and provide energy. The digestion of *protein* yields amino acids, some of which are used to build body protein. If there is a surplus, however, or if not enough carbohydrate and fat are available to meet energy

Figure 7–19
. . . .

Chemical Structures of a Fatty Acid and Glucose Compared

Fatty acid

Glucose

The structure shown here for glucose is not the ring structure shown in Chapter 4, but an alternative way of drawing its chemical structure.

needs, some amino acids are broken down through the same pathways as glucose to provide energy. Other amino acids enter directly into the TCA cycle, and these, too, can be broken down to yield energy. In summary, although carbohydrate, fat, and protein enter the TCA cycle by different routes, the energy-generating pathways that follow are common to all energy-yielding nutrients.

Of the various energy-containing compounds, fat provides the most energy for its weight. The reason this is so may be apparent from Figure 7–19, which compares a fatty acid molecule with a glucose molecule. Notice that nearly all the bonds in a fatty acid molecule are between carbons and hydrogens. Oxygen can be added to all of them (forming carbon dioxide with the carbons, and water with the hydrogens). As this happens, the energy in the fat is released. In glucose, on the other hand, an oxygen is already bonded to each carbon; thus there is less potential for oxidation, and less energy will become available when the remaining bonds are broken.

Because fat contains many hydrogen atoms and its bonds are readily oxidized, it generates abundant ATP during oxidation. This explains why fat yields more kcalories per gram than carbohydrate or protein. (Remember that each ATP holds energy and that kcalories measure energy; thus the more ATP generated, the more kcalories have been collected.) The more hydrogens a molecule of a fuel nutrient contains, the more ATP it will produce upon oxidation. For example, one glucose molecule with 12 hydrogen atoms will yield 38 ATP when completely oxidized. In comparison, one 16-carbon fatty acid molecule with 32 hydrogen atoms will yield 129 ATP when completely oxidized. Gram for gram, fat can pack much more energy than either of the other two energy-yielding nutrients, making it the body's preferred form of energy storage.

The Body's Energy Budget
. . . .

The average person takes in close to a million kcalories a year and expends more than 99 percent of them, maintaining a stable weight for years on end. This remarkable achievement, which many people manage without even thinking about it, could be called the economy of maintenance. The body's energy budget is balanced. Some people, however, eat too much and get fat; others eat too little and get thin. The metabolic details have already been described; the next sections will review them from the perspective of the body fat gained or lost. The possible reasons why people eat too much or too little are explored in Chapter 8.

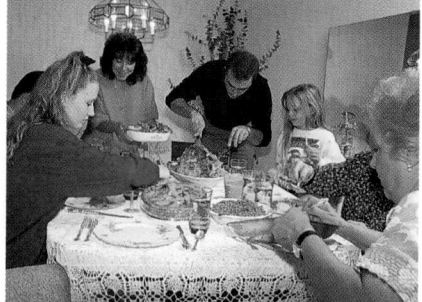

People can enjoy bountiful meals such as this without storing body fat, provided that they spend as much energy as they take in.

THE ECONOMICS OF FEASTING

Figure 7–20 shows how metabolism favors fat formation when a person eats too much of any energy-yielding nutrient. Carbohydrate, fat, and protein can all enlarge the body's fat stores.

Surplus Carbohydrate Surplus carbohydrate (glucose) is first stored as glycogen, but there is a limit to the capacity of the glycogen-storing cells. Once glycogen stores are filled, the overflow is routed to fat (part A of the figure). Fat cells enlarge as they fill with fat, and they seem to be able to multiply indefinitely. Thus excess carbohydrate can contribute to obesity.

Surplus Fat Surplus dietary fat moves efficiently into the body's fat stores. It may break down to fragments such as acetyl CoA, but if energy flow is already

Figure 7–20

How Carbohydrate, Fat, and Protein, Eaten in Excess, Contribute to Body Fat

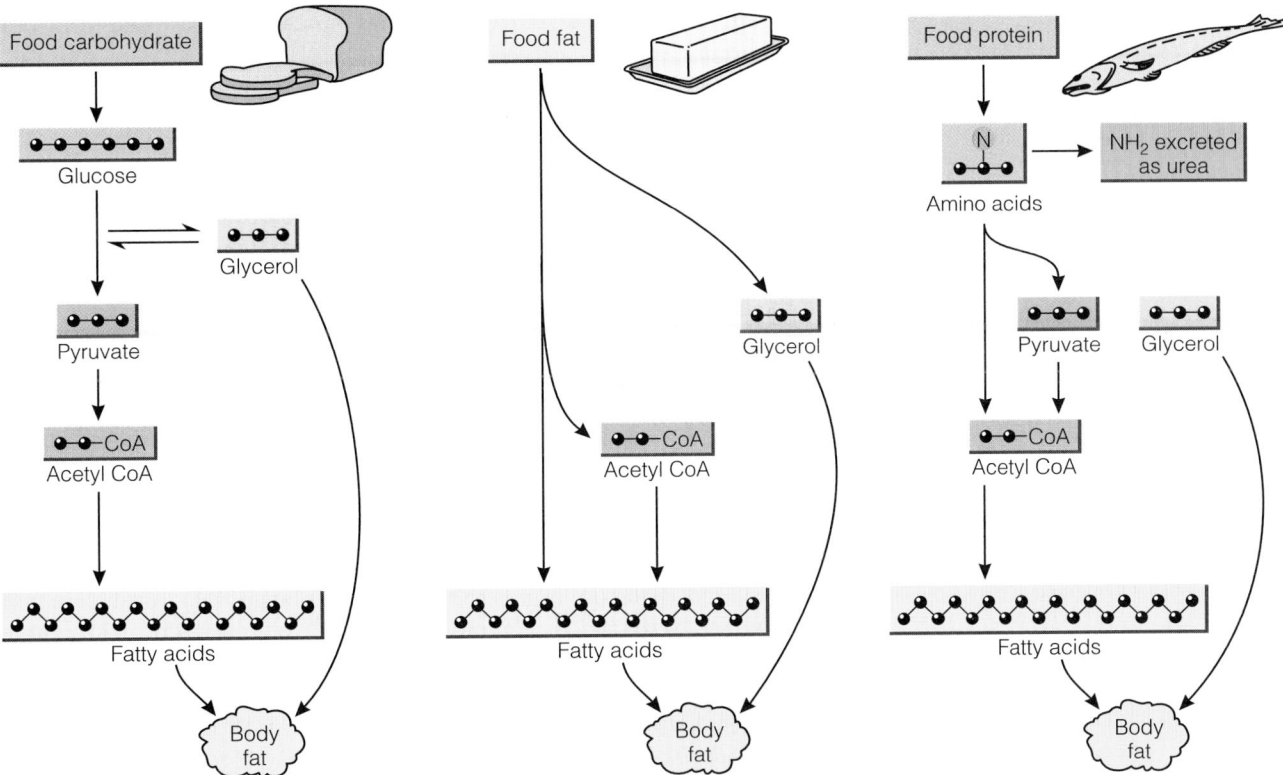

A. Carbohydrate, eaten in excess of need, is broken down to pyruvate and acetyl CoA; acetyl CoA molecules are then assembled into fatty acids, combined with glycerol, and stored as body fat.

B. Fat, eaten in excess of need, is either stored directly or broken down to glycerol and acetyl CoA, and then built up into different fat molecules.

C. Protein is broken down to amino acids. These, if not used to build body protein, are deaminated, and the nitrogen is excreted as urea; some carbon skeletons are converted to pyruvate and acetyl CoA and then to fat.

rapid enough to meet the demand, these fragments will not break down further. Instead, they will be routed to the assembly of triglycerides and stored in the fat cells (part B of Figure 7–20).

Surplus Protein   Finally, surplus protein encounters the same fate (part C of Figure 7–20). If not needed to build body protein or to meet present energy needs, amino acids will be deaminated and their carbon skeletons converted through the intermediates, pyruvate and acetyl CoA, to triglycerides. Thus amino acids, too, expand the fat cells and add to body weight.

THE TRANSITION FROM FEASTING TO FASTING

After a meal, glucose, glycerol, and fatty acids from foods are either used or stored. Later, as the body shifts from a fed state to a fasting one, it begins drawing energy out of storage. Glycogen and fat are released from storage to provide more glucose, glycerol, and fatty acids to produce energy.

Energy is needed all the time. Even when a person is asleep and totally relaxed, the cells of many organs are hard at work. In fact, this work—the cells' work that maintains all life processes without any conscious effort—represents about two-thirds to three-fourths of the total energy a person spends in a day. The small remainder is the work that a person's muscles perform voluntarily during waking hours.

The body's top priority is to meet the cells' needs for energy, and it normally does this by periodic refueling—that is, by eating. When food is not available, the body turns to its own tissues for other fuel sources. If people choose not to eat, we say they are fasting; if they have no choice, we say they are starving. The body makes no such distinction. In either case, the body is forced to switch to a wasting metabolism, drawing on its reserves of carbohydrate and fat and, within a day or so, on its vital protein tissues as well. Figure 7–21 shows the metabolic pathways operating in the body as it shifts from feasting (part A) to fasting (parts B and C).

Reminder: The action of carbohydrate and fat in providing energy that allows protein to be used for other purposes is called protein-sparing action.

THE ECONOMICS OF FASTING

As Figure 7–21 shows, during fasting, all paths lead to energy—fuel must be delivered to every cell. As the fast begins, glucose from the liver's stored glycogen and fatty acids from the body's stored fat are both flowing into cells, then breaking down to yield acetyl CoA, and delivering energy to power the cells' work.* Several hours later, however, most of the glucose is used up—liver glycogen is exhausted and blood glucose begins to fall. The liver begins making glucose from lactic acid formed by red blood cells and muscles and from the amino acid alanine. Low blood glucose serves as a signal to promote further fat breakdown.

Glucose Needed for the Brain   At this point, most of the cells are depending on fatty acids to continue providing their fuel. But red blood cells and the cells of the nervous system need glucose. Glucose is their major energy fuel, and even when other energy fuels are available, glucose must be present to permit the energy-metabolizing machinery of the nervous system to work. Normally, the brain and nerve cells consume about two-thirds of the total *glucose* used each

---

*The muscles' stored glycogen provides glucose only for the muscle in which the glycogen is stored.

Figure 7–21

Feasting and Fasting

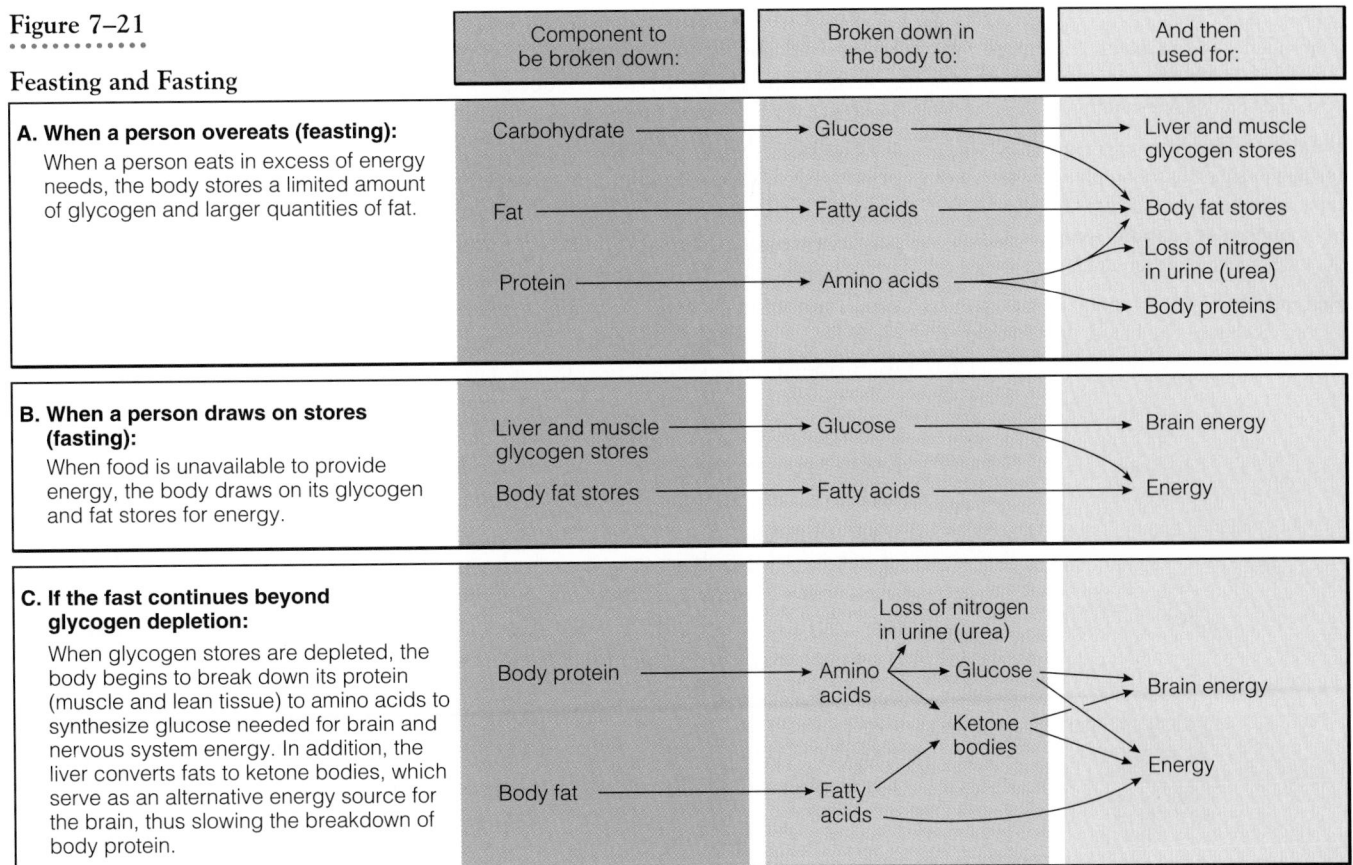

	Component to be broken down:	Broken down in the body to:	And then used for:
A. When a person overeats (feasting): When a person eats in excess of energy needs, the body stores a limited amount of glycogen and larger quantities of fat.	Carbohydrate → Fat → Protein →	Glucose Fatty acids Amino acids	Liver and muscle glycogen stores Body fat stores Loss of nitrogen in urine (urea) Body proteins
B. When a person draws on stores (fasting): When food is unavailable to provide energy, the body draws on its glycogen and fat stores for energy.	Liver and muscle glycogen stores Body fat stores →	Glucose Fatty acids	Brain energy Energy
C. If the fast continues beyond glycogen depletion: When glycogen stores are depleted, the body begins to break down its protein (muscle and lean tissue) to amino acids to synthesize glucose needed for brain and nervous system energy. In addition, the liver converts fats to ketone bodies, which serve as an alternative energy source for the brain, thus slowing the breakdown of body protein.	Body protein → Body fat →	Loss of nitrogen in urine (urea) Amino acids → Glucose Ketone bodies Fatty acids	Brain energy Energy

day—about 400 to 600 kcalories. About one-fifth of the *energy* the body uses when it is at rest is used for the brain.

Protein Called on to Meet Glucose Needs The red blood cells' and brain's special requirements for glucose pose a problem for the fasting body. The body can use its stores of fat, which may be quite generous, to furnish most of its cells with energy, but the brain and nerves prefer energy in the form of glucose. For this reason, body protein tissues such as muscle and liver always break down to some extent during fasting. Amino acids that yield pyruvate can be used to make glucose; and to obtain them, body proteins must be broken down. The amino acids that can't be used to make glucose are used as an energy source for other body cells.

Fat's Small Glucose Contribution from Glycerol The breakdown of body protein is an expensive way to obtain glucose. In the first few days of a fast, body protein provides about 90 percent of the needed glucose; glycerol, about 10 percent. If body protein loss were to continue at this rate, death would ensue within three weeks, regardless of the quantity of fat a person had stored. Fortunately, fat breakdown also increases with fasting—in fact, fat breakdown almost doubles, providing energy for other body cells and glycerol for glucose production.[1]

Reminder: *Condensation* is the process by which two molecules are joined together with the removal of water.

Reminder: The group of ketones that are formed during the incomplete oxidation of fatty acids are *ketone bodies*. A *ketone* is a compound that contains a carbonyl group (C=O) between other carbons.

Reminder: The combination of elevated ketone bodies in the blood (ketonemia) and in the urine (ketonuria) is *ketosis*.

The Shift to Ketosis   As the fast continues, the body finds a way to use its fat to fuel the brain. It adapts by condensing together acetyl CoA fragments derived from fatty acids to produce an alternate energy source, ketone bodies (see Figure 7–22). Normally produced and used only in small quantities, ketone bodies can provide fuel for some brain cells. Ketone body production rises until, after about 10 days of fasting, it is meeting much of the nervous system's energy needs.[2] Still, many areas of the brain rely exclusively on glucose, and body protein continues to be sacrificed to produce it.

When ketone bodies contain a COOH (acid) group, they are called keto acids. Small amounts of keto acids are a normal part of the blood chemistry; but when their concentration rises, the pH of the blood declines and ketone bodies spill into the urine. This is ketosis, and it is a sign that the body's chemistry is going awry.

Suppression of Appetite   The starvation that produces ketosis also causes loss of appetite. Researchers have theorized that having no appetite is an advantage to a person without access to food, because the search for food would be a waste of energy. When the person finds food and eats again, the body shifts out of ketosis, the hunger center gets the message that food is again available, and the appetite returns. This chain of events has served as justification for weight-loss routines that induce ketosis, such as fasting and low-carbohydrate diets. However, any kind of food restriction, with or without ketosis, leads a person to adapt by losing appetite. A well-balanced low-kcalorie diet can induce the same effect. Therefore ketosis-producing diets offer no special advantage in terms of appetite suppression, and because ketosis can disrupt the body's acid-base balance, other weight-loss regimens are preferred to ketogenic diets.

Figure 7–22

Ketone Body Formation

❶ The first step in the formation of ketone bodies is the condensation of two molecules of acetyl CoA and the removal of the CoA to form a compound that is converted to the first ketone body.

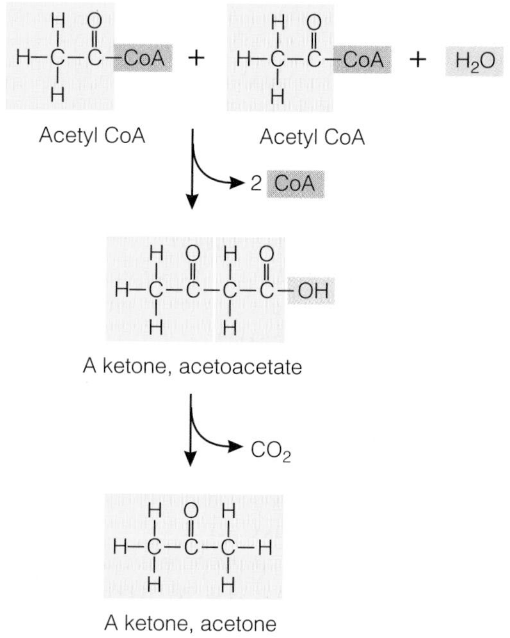

Acetyl CoA   Acetyl CoA

2 CoA

A ketone, acetoacetate

❷ This ketone body may lose a molecule of carbon dioxide to become another ketone.

CO_2

A ketone, acetone

❸ Or, the acetoacetate may add two hydrogens, becoming another ketone body (beta-hydroxybutyrate). See Appendix C for more details.

Slowing of Metabolism   In any case, while the body is shifting to the use of ketone bodies, it simultaneously reduces its energy output and conserves both its fat and lean tissue. As the lean (protein-containing) organ tissues shrink in mass, they perform less metabolic work, reducing energy expenditures. As the muscles waste, they can do less work and so demand less energy, reducing expenditures further. The hormones of fasting slow metabolism even further in the effort to conserve lean body mass for as long as possible. Because of the slowed metabolism, the loss of fat falls to a bare minimum—less, in fact, than the fat that would be lost on a low-kcalorie diet. Thus, although *weight* loss during fasting may be quite dramatic, *fat* loss may be less than when at least some food is eaten.

Symptoms of Starvation   The adaptations just described—slowing of energy output and reduction in fat loss—occur in the starving child, the hungry homeless adult, the fasting religious person, the person with anorexia nervosa, and the malnourished hospital client. Such adaptations help to prolong their lives and explain the physical symptoms of energy deprivation: wasting, slowed metabolism, lowered body temperature, and reduced resistance to disease.

The body's adaptations to fasting are sufficient to maintain life for a long time. Mental alertness need not be diminished, and even physical energy may remain unimpaired for a surprisingly long time. Still, fasting presents hazards. The same alterations in metabolism occur on a low-carbohydrate diet.

The Low-Carbohydrate Diet   An economy similar to that of fasting prevails when a person consumes a low-carbohydrate diet. Once the body's available glycogen reserves are spent, the only significant remaining source of glucose is protein. The low-carbohydrate diet usually provides some protein from food, but some is still taken from body tissue. The onset of ketosis signals that this wasting process has begun.

People are attracted to the low-carbohydrate diet because it brings a dramatic weight loss within the first few days. They would be disillusioned if they realized that much of this weight loss is a loss of glycogen and protein together with large quantities of water and important minerals. A dieter who boasts of losing 7 pounds in two days on a low-carbohydrate diet must be unaware that *at best*, a pound or two is fat, and 5 or 6 pounds are lean tissue, water, and minerals. Once the dieter begins to eat a balanced diet, the body will avidly devour and retain these needed materials, and the weight will zoom back, quite often to higher than the starting point.

These facts offer a warning: beware of quick-weight-loss schemes. Learn to distinguish between loss of *fat* and loss of *weight*.

> Low-carbohydrate dieting = living on dietary protein and fat and on body protein and fat almost exclusively.

The Protein-Sparing Fast   A variant on fasting is the technique of ingesting only protein. The hope is that the protein will spare lean tissue and that the person will break down body fat at a maximal rate to meet other energy needs. The protein does spare the lean tissues to some extent, but then it is used to provide glucose, just as dietary carbohydrate would be.

Protein formulas (liquid and powdered) were popular weight-loss regimens during the late 1970s—until serious health risks, including deaths, emerged. Since then products have been reformulated to contain high-quality protein, carbohydrates, some fat, vitamins, and minerals. In addition, such formulas are sold only to doctors or hospitals for supervised use and must carry a "Protein Diet Warning" on their labels.[3] Even with more complete formulas, such weight-loss

> Protein-sparing fasting = living on dietary protein and on body protein and fat.

regimens present serious health risks and need to be carefully monitored. In addition to the health risks, protein fasts have a poor long-term success rate; most people regain the lost weight. Thus the protein-sparing fast has to be judged at best a moderate success and at worst a failure.

The term *protein sparing* has been used in another situation. Hospital clients enduring severe physical stresses such as cancer or major surgery also lose body protein. This is especially likely, and especially dangerous, if they are simultaneously fighting infection, which prevents the body from going into ketosis. Physicians make every effort to prevent the loss of vital lean tissue by supplying amino acids as well as glucose in some form—through a vein if the client can't eat. The effort to provide protein-sparing *therapy* for prevention of malnutrition should not be confused with the protein-sparing *fast* for weight loss.

This chapter has probed the intricate details of metabolism at the level of the cells, exploring the transformations of nutrients to energy and to storage compounds. Several chapters and highlights to come build on this information. The highlight that follows this chapter shows how alcohol disrupts normal metabolism. Chapter 8 describes how a person's intake and expenditure of energy is reflected in body composition. Highlight 8 revisits metabolism to show how it supports the work of physically active people and how athletes can best apply that information in their choices of foods to eat. Chapter 9 examines the consequences of unbalanced energy budgets—overweight and underweight—and what to do about them. And Chapter 10 shows the vital roles the B vitamins play as coenzymes assisting all the metabolic pathways described here.

We are all solar creatures, indeed. The sun's energy sparks every move that we make, and our beautifully designed bodies make use of it in astonishing ways.

Study Questions

1. Define metabolism, anabolism, and catabolism; give an example of each.
2. Name one of the body's quick-energy molecules, and describe how is it used.
3. What are coenzymes, and what service do they provide in metabolism?
4. Name the four basic units, derived from foods, used by the body in metabolic transformations. How many carbons are in the "backbones" of each?
5. Summarize the main steps in the metabolism of glucose, glycerol, fatty acids, and amino acids.
6. Define aerobic and anaerobic metabolism. How does insufficient oxygen influence metabolism?
7. How does the body dispose of excess nitrogen?
8. Describe how a surplus of the three energy nutrients contributes to body fat stores.
9. What adaptations does the body make during a fast? What are ketone bodies? Define ketosis.
10. Distinguish between a loss of *fat* and a loss of *weight,* and describe how both might happen.

Notes

1. M. G. Carlson, W. L. Snead, and P. J. Campbell, Fuel and energy metabolism in fasting humans, *American Journal of Clinical Nutrition* 60 (1994): 29–36.
2. M. C. Linder, Nutrition and metabolism of proteins, in *Nutrition Biochemistry and Metabolism,* ed. M. C. Linder (New York: Elsevier, 1991), pp. 87–109.
3. M. Segal, A sometime solution to a weighty problem, *FDA Consumer,* April 1990, pp. 11–15.

Alcohol and Nutrition

S ocial gatherings offer opportunities for people to share conversation, food, and drink. Among the beverages available are those that contain alcohol, and people must choose whether to drink them. Most people who drink manage their relationships with alcohol relatively safely.[1] Unfortunately, some 18 million people in the United States abuse alcohol to the point that their personal relationships, work, and health become impaired. With the understanding of metabolism gained from Chapter 7, you are in a position to understand how the body handles alcohol, how alcohol affects metabolism, and how alcohol can impair health.

ALCOHOL IN BEVERAGES

To the chemist, *alcohol* refers to a class of organic compounds containing hydroxyl (OH) groups. The glycerol to which fatty acids are attached in triglycerides is an example of an alcohol to a chemist. But to most people, *alcohol* refers to the intoxicating ingredient in beer, wine, and hard liquor (distilled spirits). The chemist's name for this particular alcohol is *ethyl alcohol,* or *ethanol.* Glycerol has 3 carbons with 3 hydroxyl groups attached; ethanol has only 2 carbons and 1 hydroxyl group (see Figure H7–1). The remainder of this highlight talks about the particular alcohol, ethanol, but refers to it simply as *alcohol.*

Alcohols affect living things profoundly, partly because they act as lipid solvents. Their ability to dissolve lipids out of cell membranes

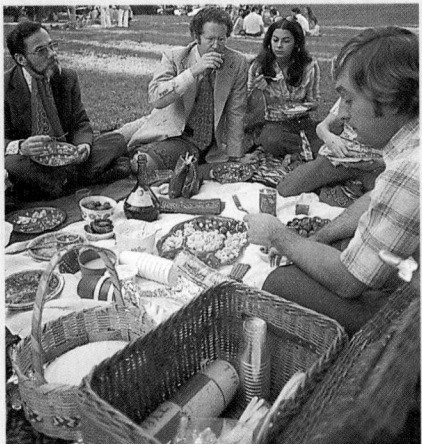

Shared conversations and meals sometimes include alcoholic beverages.

allows them to penetrate rapidly into cells, destroying cell structures and thereby killing the cells. For this reason, most alcohols are toxic, or poisonous, in relatively small amounts; by the same token, because they kill microbial cells, they are useful as disinfectants.

Ethanol is less toxic than the other alcohols. Sufficiently diluted

---

Figure H7–1

Two Alcohols: Glycerol and Ethanol

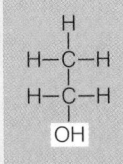

Glycerol is the alcohol used to make triglycerides.

Ethanol is the alcohol in beer, wine, and distilled spirits.

and taken in small enough doses, its action in the brain produces euphoria—a pleasing effect that people seek—not with zero risk, but with a low enough risk (if the doses are low enough) to be tolerable. Used to achieve this effect, alcohol is a drug—that is, a substance that modifies body functions. Like all drugs, alcohol offers both benefits and hazards. It must be used with caution, if used at all.

Alcohol arises naturally from carbohydrates when certain microorganisms metabolize them in the absence of oxygen—an anaerobic process called fermentation (the glossary on p. 246 defines fermentation and other alcohol-related terms). Since all plants contain carbohydrate, all can serve as the starting material for fermentation.

People have consumed wine, beer, and other fermented beverages for more than 5000 years. Different societies use different plants to produce alcoholic beverages; the most familiar are grapes and other berries (used to make wine), apples (fermented, or hard, cider), and grains (beer and various distilled liquors). Wines, ciders, and beers are ready for use after fermentation, whereas the liquors undergo further distilling to concentrate the alcohol. Thus grain mashes can be distilled further to yield the whiskeys—bourbon (at least half from corn), rye (from rye), scotch (from barley), vodka (from wheat, rye, corn, or potatoes), rum (from cane products such as molasses), and brandy (from wine). Distilled liquors are often served with mixers such as carbonated beverages or fruit juices (cocktails) or

Glossary

acetaldehyde (ass-et-AL-duh-hide): an intermediate in alcohol metabolism.

alcohol: a class of organic compounds containing hydroxyl (OH) groups.

alcohol dehydrogenase: an enzyme that converts ethanol to acetaldehyde. The MEOS also oxidizes alcohol (see MEOS).

antidiuretic hormone (ADH): a hormone produced by the pituitary gland in response to dehydration (or a high sodium concentration in the blood); it stimulates the kidneys to reabsorb more water and therefore to excrete less. This ADH should not be confused with the enzyme alcohol dehydrogenase, which is sometimes also abbreviated ADH.

beer: an alcoholic beverage brewed by fermenting malt and hops.

cirrhosis (seer-OH-sis): advanced liver disease in which liver cells turn orange, die, and harden, permanently losing their function; often associated with alcoholism.
    cirrhos = an orange

distilled liquor: an alcoholic beverage made by fermenting and distilling grains; sometimes called distilled spirits or hard liquor.

drink: a dose of any alcoholic beverage that delivers ½ oz of pure ethanol:
- 4 to 5 oz of wine.
- 10 oz of wine cooler.
- 12 oz of beer.
- 1¼ oz of hard liquor (80 proof whiskey, scotch, rum, or vodka).

drug: a substance that can modify one or more of the body's functions.

ethanol: a particular type of alcohol found in beer, wine, and distilled spirits; also called ethyl alcohol (see Figure H7–1). Ethanol is the most widely used—and abused—drug in our society. It is also the only legal, nonprescription drug that produces euphoria.

euphoria (you-FORE-eh-uh): a feeling of great well-being, which people often seek through the use of drugs such as alcohol.
    eu = good
    phoria = bearing

fatty liver: an early stage of liver deterioration seen in several diseases, including kwashiorkor and alcoholic liver disease. Fatty liver is characterized by an accumulation of fat in the liver cells.

fermentation: the oxidation of carbohydrate in the absence of atmospheric oxygen, a process that yields alcohol as an end product.

fibrosis (fye-BROH-sis): an intermediate stage of liver deterioration seen in several diseases, including viral hepatitis and alcoholic liver disease. In fibrosis, the liver cells lose their function and assume the characteristics of connective tissue cells (fibers).

gout (GOWT): a painful condition in which uric acid crystals form in the joints.

MEOS (microsomal ethanol-oxidizing system): a system of enzymes in the liver that oxidize not only alcohol, but also several classes of drugs. (The microsomes are tiny particles of membranes with associated enzymes that can be collected from broken-up cells.)
    micro = tiny
    soma = body

moderation: in relation to alcohol consumption, not more than two drinks a day for the average-sized man and not more than one drink a day for the average-sized woman.

NAD (nicotinamide adenine dinucleotide): the main coenzyme form of the vitamin niacin; its reduced form is NADH.

narcotic (nor-KOT-ic): any drug that dulls the senses, induces sleep, and becomes addictive with prolonged use.

proof: a way of stating the percentage of alcohol in distilled liquor. Liquor that is 100 proof is 50% alcohol; 90 proof is 45%, and so forth.

wine: an alcoholic beverage made by fermenting grape juice.

---

flavored with herbs and spices to make liqueurs or after-dinner drinks.

Beer, wine, and liquor deliver different amounts of alcohol. The amount of alcohol in distilled liquor is stated as proof: distilled liquor of 100 proof is 50 percent alcohol, 80 proof liquor is 40 percent alcohol, and so forth. Regular wine (at 8 to 14 percent) and beer (at 4 to 6 percent) have less alcohol. (Some fortified wines and beers have more alcohol.)

Taken in moderation, alcohol can be compatible with good health. The term moderation is important in describing alcohol use. How many drinks constitute moderate use, and how much is "a drink"? First, a drink is any alcoholic beverage that delivers ½ ounce of pure ethanol:

- 4 to 5 ounces of wine.
- 10 ounces of wine cooler.
- 12 ounces of beer.
- 1¼ ounce of distilled liquor (80 proof whiskey, scotch, rum, or vodka).

Second, it is impossible to name an

exact amount of alcohol per day that is appropriate for everyone because people have different tolerances to alcohol. Authorities have attempted to set limits that are acceptable for most healthy people. An accepted definition of moderation is not more than two drinks a day for the average-sized man and not more than one drink a day for the average-sized woman. Notice that this advice is stated as a maximum, not as an average; seven drinks one night a week would not be considered moderate, even though one a day would be. Doubtless some people could consume slightly more; others could not handle nearly so much without risk. The amount a person can drink safely is highly individual, depending on genetics, health condition, sex, weight, age, and family history.

ALCOHOL IN THE BODY

From the moment an alcoholic beverage enters the body, it is treated as if it has special privileges. Unlike foods, which require time for digestion, alcohol needs no digestion and is quickly absorbed. About 20 percent is absorbed directly across the walls of an empty stomach and can reach the brain within a minute. Consequently, a person can immediately feel euphoric when drinking, especially on an empty stomach.

When the stomach is full of food, alcohol has less chance of touching the walls and diffusing through, so its influence on the brain is slightly delayed. This information leads to a practical tip: eat snacks when drinking alcoholic beverages. Carbohydrate snacks slow alcohol absorption and high-fat snacks slow peristalsis, keeping the alcohol in the stomach longer. Salty snacks make a person

thirsty; to quench thirst, drink water instead of more alcohol.

The stomach begins to break down alcohol with its alcohol dehydrogenase enzyme. This action can reduce the amount of alcohol entering the blood by about 20 percent. Research shows that women produce less of this stomach enzyme than men, which partially explains why women become more intoxicated on less alcohol than men.[2] Women absorb about one-third more alcohol than men of the same size who drink the same amount of alcohol.

Alcohol is rapidly absorbed in the duodenum. From this point on, alcohol receives VIP (Very Important Person) treatment: it gets absorbed and metabolized before most nutrients.

ALCOHOL ARRIVES IN THE LIVER

The capillaries of the digestive tract merge into veins that carry the alcohol-laden blood to the liver. These veins branch and rebranch into capillaries that touch every liver cell. Liver cells are the only cells in the body that can make enough of the enzyme alcohol dehydrogenase to oxidize alcohol at an appreciable rate. The routing of blood through the liver cells gives them the chance to dispose of some alcohol before it moves on.

Alcohol affects every organ of the body, but the most dramatic evidence of its disruptive behavior appears in the liver. If liver cells could talk, they would describe the alcohol of intoxicating beverages as demanding, egocentric, and disruptive of the liver's efficient way of running its business. For example, liver cells normally prefer fatty acids

as their fuel, and they like to package excess fatty acids into triglycerides and ship them out to other tissues. When alcohol is present, however, the liver cells are forced to metabolize alcohol and let the fatty acids accumulate, sometimes in huge stockpiles. Alcohol metabolism also permanently changes liver cell structure, which impairs the liver's ability to metabolize fats.[3] This explains why heavy drinkers develop fatty livers.

The liver can process about ½ ounce *ethanol* per hour (the amount in a typical drink), depending on the person's body size, previous drinking experience, food intake, and general health. This maximum rate of alcohol breakdown is set by the amount of alcohol dehydrogenase available. If more alcohol arrives at the liver than the enzymes can handle, the extra alcohol travels to all parts of the body, circulating again and again until liver enzymes are finally available to process it. Another practical tip derives from this information: drink slowly enough to allow the liver to keep up—no more than 1 drink per hour.

The amount of alcohol dehydrogenase enzyme present in the liver varies with individuals, depending on the genes they have inherited and on how recently they have eaten. Fasting for as little as a day forces the body to degrade its proteins, including the alcohol-processing enzyme, and this can slow the rate of alcohol metabolism by half. Drinking on an empty stomach thus causes the drinker to feel the effects more promptly for two reasons: rapid absorption and slowed breakdown. By maintaining higher blood alcohol concentrations for longer times, alcohol can anesthetize the brain more completely.

The alcohol dehydrogenase enzyme breaks down alcohol by removing hydrogens in two steps. (Figure H7–2 provides a simplified diagram of alcohol metabolism; Appendix C provides the chemical details.) In the first step, alcohol dehydrogenase oxidizes alcohol to acetaldehyde. High concentrations of acetaldehyde in the brain and other tissues are responsible for many of the punishing effects of alcohol abuse.

In the second step, a related enzyme, acetaldehyde dehydrogenase, oxidizes the acetaldehyde to acetyl CoA, the "crossroads" compound that can enter the TCA cycle to generate energy. These reactions produce hydrogen ions (acid). The B vitamin niacin (in its role as the coenzyme known as NAD) helpfully picks up these hydrogen ions (becoming NADH). Thus, whenever the body breaks down alcohol, NAD diminishes and NADH accumulates.

ALCOHOL DISRUPTS THE LIVER

During alcohol metabolism, NAD becomes unavailable for the multitude of other vital body processes for which it is required, including glycolysis, the TCA cycle, and the electron transport chain. Its presence is sorely missed in these energy pathways because it is the chief carrier of the hydrogens that travel with their electrons along the electron transport chain. Without NAD, the energy pathway is blocked. Traffic either backs up, or an alternate route is taken. Such changes in the normal flow from glucose to energy have striking physical consequences.

Figure H7–2

Alcohol Metabolism

The conversion of alcohol to acetyl CoA requires the B vitamin niacin in its role as NAD. When the enzymes oxidize alcohol, they remove H atoms and attach them to NAD. Thus NAD is used up, and NADH accumulates. (Note: More accurately, NAD^+ is converted to $NADH + H^+$. For simplicity's sake, the process has been described here as if one hydrogen were added to NAD, but, in reality, two are added.)

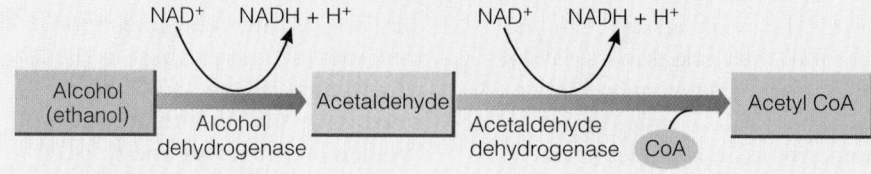

For one, the accumulation of hydrogen ions during alcohol metabolism shifts the body's acid-base balance toward acid. For another, the accumulation of NADH slows the TCA cycle, so pyruvate and acetyl CoA build up.

Excess acetyl CoA then takes the route to fatty acid synthesis (as Figure H7–3 illustrates), and fat clogs the liver.

As you might expect, a liver clogged with fat cannot function properly. Liver cells become less effi-

Figure H7–3

Alternate Route for Acetyl CoA: To Fat

Acetyl CoA molecules are blocked from getting into the TCA cycle by the high level of NADH. Instead of being used for energy, the acetyl CoA molecules become building blocks for fatty acids.

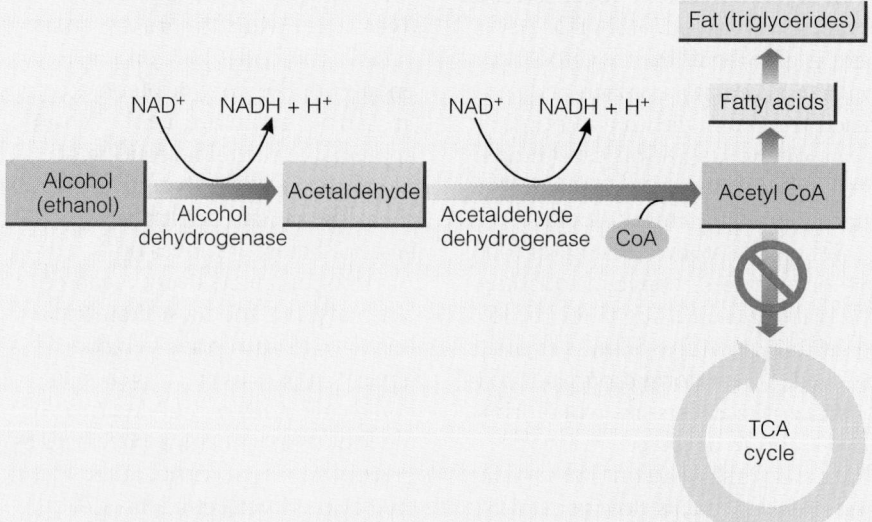

cient at performing a number of tasks. Much of this inefficiency impairs a person's nutritional health in ways that cannot be corrected by diet alone. For example, the liver has difficulty activating vitamin D, as well as producing and releasing bile. To overcome such problems, a person needs to stop drinking alcohol.

The synthesis of fatty acids accelerates with exposure to alcohol. Fat accumulation can be seen in the liver after a single night of heavy drinking. Fatty liver, the first stage of liver deterioration seen in heavy drinkers, interferes with the distribution of nutrients and oxygen to the liver cells. If the condition lasts long enough, the liver cells will die and form fibrous scar tissue—the second stage of liver deterioration, called fibrosis. Some liver cells can regenerate with good nutrition and abstinence from alcohol, but in the most advanced stage, cirrhosis, damage is the least reversible.

The fatty liver has difficulty generating glucose from protein. The lack of glucose together with the overabundance of acetyl CoA sets the stage for ketosis. The body uses the acetyl CoA to make ketone bodies, which push the acid-base balance further toward acid.

Excess NADH also promotes the making of lactic acid from pyruvate. The conversion of pyruvate to lactic acid uses the hydrogens from NADH and restores some NAD, but a lactic acid buildup has serious consequences of its own—it adds still further to the body's acid burden and interferes with the excretion of another acid, uric acid, causing goutlike symptoms.

Alcohol alters both amino acid and protein metabolism. Synthesis of proteins important in the immune system slows down, weakening the body's defenses against infection. Protein deficiency can develop, both from the depression of protein synthesis and from a poor diet. Normally, the cells would at least use the amino acids that a person happened to eat, but the drinker's liver deaminates the amino acids and uses the carbon fragments to make fat or ketones. Eating well does not protect the drinker from protein depletion; a person has to stop drinking alcohol.

The liver's VIP treatment of alcohol affects its handling of drugs as well as nutrients. In addition to the dehydrogenase enzyme already described, the liver possesses an enzyme system that metabolizes *both* alcohol and several types of other drugs. Called the MEOS (microsomal ethanol-oxidizing system), this system handles about one-fifth of the total alcohol a person consumes. At high blood alcohol concentrations, however, or if repeatedly exposed to alcohol, the MEOS grows larger.

As a person's blood alcohol rises, alcohol competes with—and wins out over—other drugs whose metabolism relies on the MEOS. If a person drinks and uses another drug at the same time, the drug will be metabolized more slowly and will therefore exert greater effects. The MEOS is busy disposing of alcohol, so the drug cannot be handled until later; the dose may build up so that its effects are greatly amplified—sometimes to the point of being fatal.

In contrast, once a heavy drinker stops drinking and alcohol is no longer competing with other drugs, the enlarged MEOS metabolizes drugs much faster than before. As a result, determining the correct dosages of medications can be confusing and tricky. The physician who prescribes sedatives every four hours, for example, unaware that the person has recently gone from being a heavy drinker to an abstainer, expects the MEOS to dispose of the drug at a certain predicted rate. The MEOS is adapted to metabolizing large quantities of alcohol, though, so it metabolizes the drug extra fast. The drug's effects wear off unexpectedly fast, leaving the client undersedated. Imagine the doctor's alarm should a patient wake up on the table during an operation! A skilled anesthesiologist always asks clients about their drinking patterns before putting them to sleep.

This discussion has emphasized the major way that the blood is cleared of alcohol—metabolism by the liver—but there is another way. About 10 percent of the alcohol leaves the body through the breath and in the urine. This is the basis for the breath and urine tests for drunkenness. The amounts of alcohol in the breath and in the urine are in proportion to the amount still in the bloodstream and brain. In nearly all states, legal drunkenness is set at 0.10 percent or less, reflecting the relationship between alcohol use and industrial and traffic accidents.

ALCOHOL ARRIVES IN THE BRAIN

Alcohol is a narcotic. People used it for centuries as an anesthetic because it can deaden pain. But alcohol was a poor anesthetic because one could never be sure how much a person would need and

Chapter 8

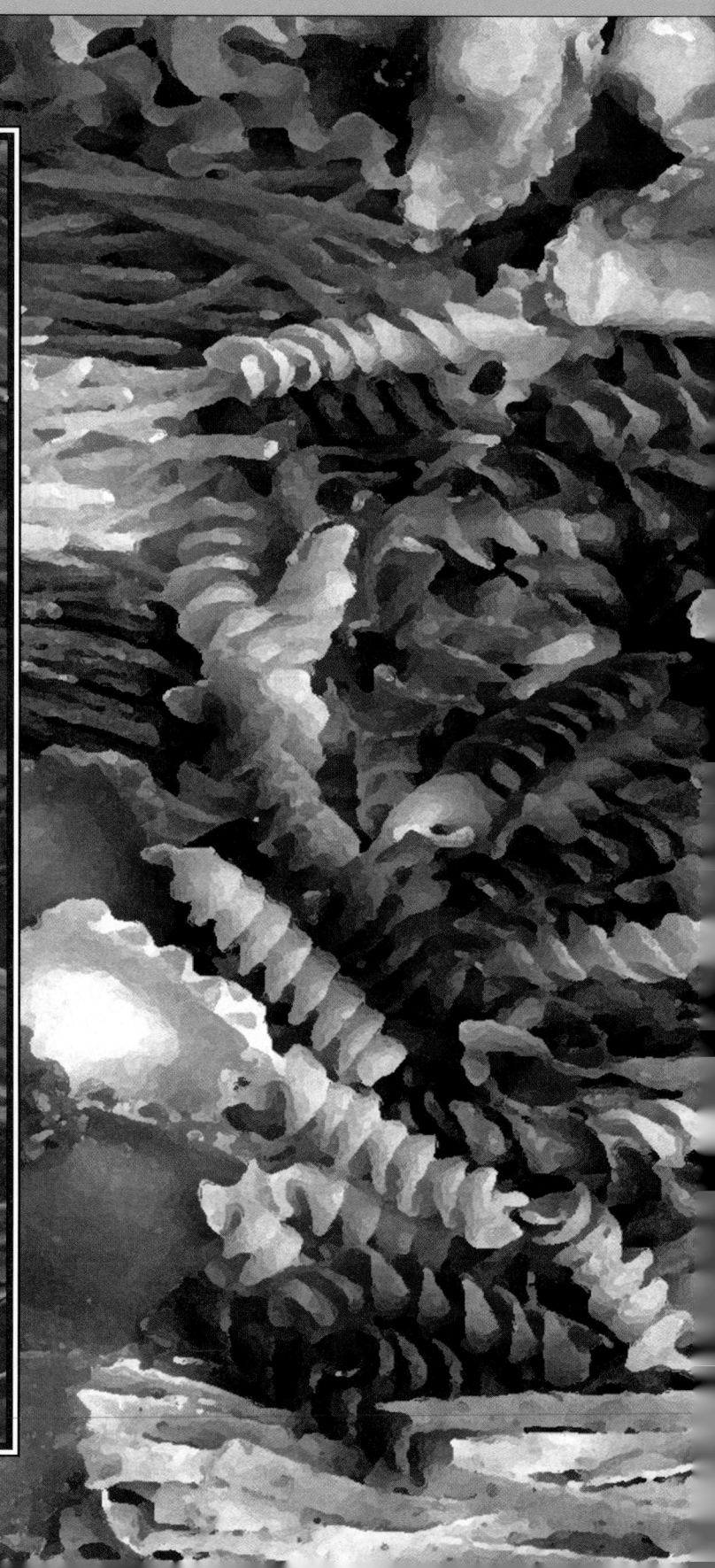

Energy Balance and Body Composition

CONTENTS

Energy Balance
Energy In: The kCalories in Food
  Food Composition
  Food Intake
Energy Out: The kCalories the Body Spends
  Components of Energy Expenditure
  Estimating Energy Requirements
Body Weight, Body Composition, and Health
  Defining Healthy Body Weight
  Body Weight and Its Standards
  Body Fat and Its Distribution
  Health Risks Associated with Body Weight and Body Fat
HIGHLIGHT: **Fitness—Physical Activity and Nutrition**

MICROGRAPH: Adenosine triphosphate, the body's common energy currency

*t*he body's remarkable machinery can cope with many extremes of diet. As you have seen, it can convert both carbohydrate (glucose) and protein (amino acids) to fat. To some extent, it can convert amino acids to glucose. To a very limited extent, it can even convert fat (the glycerol portion) to glucose. But a grossly unbalanced diet imposes hardships on the body. If energy intake is too low or if too little carbohydrate or protein is supplied, the body must degrade its own lean tissue to meet its glucose and protein needs. If energy intake is too high or if fat is oversupplied, the body stores fat.

Overfatness and underweight both result from unbalanced energy budgets. The simple picture is as follows. Overfat people have consumed more food energy than they have spent and have banked the surplus in their body fat. To reduce fat reserves, overfat people need to spend more energy than they take in from food. In contrast, underweight people have consumed too little food energy to support their bodies' activities and so have depleted their bodies' fat stores and possibly their lean tissues as well. To gain weight, they need to take in more food energy than they expend. As you will see, though, the details of the body's weight regulation are quite complex. This chapter describes energy balance and body composition and examines the problems associated with having too much or too little body fat; the next chapter presents strategies toward resolving these problems.

The term *overfat* refers to an excess of body fat, which is not necessarily the same as *overweight*, as a later section of the chapter explains.

Energy Balance

People spend energy continuously and eat periodically to refuel. Ideally, their food intakes cover their energy needs without too much excess. Excess energy is stored as fat, and stored fat is used for energy between meals. The amount of body fat a person deposits in, or withdraws from, "savings" on any given day depends on the energy balance for that day—the amount consumed (energy in) versus the amount expended (energy out). When a person is maintaining weight, energy in equals energy out.

Most people maintain a steady energy balance over time. On any given day, they may eat a little more or a little less than usual, and their weight may go up or down a pound or two, but for the most part, they stay in balance. When the balance shifts, their weight changes.

A pound of body fat stores about 3500 kcalories. It stands to reason that a person who eats 3500 extra kcalories should gain a pound, and that a person who cuts 3500 kcalories should lose a pound, but this does not always happen. When a person overeats, much of the excess energy is stored, but some energy is spent to maintain the heavier body.[1] Furthermore, people seem to gain more body fat when they eat extra fat kcalories than when they eat extra carbohydrate kcalories, and they seem to lose body fat most efficiently when they limit kcalories specifically from fat.[2] Whether a person chooses extra potatoes or extra butter may make a great difference to body weight and body composition.

A reasonable rate of weight loss for overweight people is ½ to 1 pound a week. Even for obese people, a reasonable weight-loss rate is only 1 percent of body weight per week.[3] Such a gradual loss is more likely to stay off than rapid weight losses and can be achieved with a reasonable energy intake of about 10 kcalories per pound of body weight. If food energy is restricted too severely, dieters lose

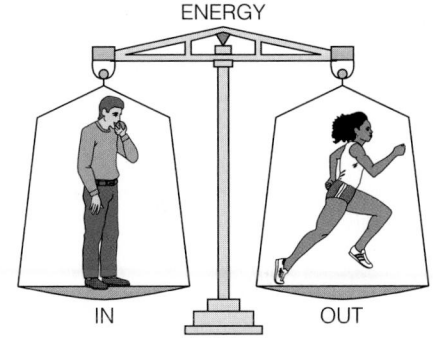

When energy in balances with energy out, a person's body weight is stable.

1 lb body fat = 3500 kcal.
Body fat, or adipose tissue, is composed of a mixture of mostly fat, some protein, and water. A pound of body fat (454 g) is approximately 87% fat, or (454 × 0.87) 395 g, and 395 g × 9 kcal/g = 3555 kcal.

Energy intake for weight loss:
    10 kcal/lb body weight.

As Chapter 12 explains, water constitutes about 60% of an adult's body weight. Consequently, retention or loss of water influences body weight.

lean tissue and may not receive enough nutrients. In addition, restrictive eating may set in motion the unhealthy cycle of restrictive dieting and binge eating.

Besides, quick changes in weight are not just changes in fat. Weight gained or lost rapidly includes some fat, large amounts of fluid, and some lean tissues such as muscles and bone minerals. Even over the long term, the composition of weight gained or lost is normally about 75 percent fat and 25 percent lean. During starvation, losses of fat and lean are about equal. Invariably, though, *fat* gains and losses are gradual. The next two sections introduce the two sides of the energy-balance equation: energy in and energy out.

Energy In: The kCalories in Food

Foods and beverages are the "energy in" part of the energy-balance equation. How much energy a person receives depends on how much the person eats and drinks and on the composition of the foods and beverages.

FOOD COMPOSITION

bomb calorimeter (KAL-oh-RIM-eh-ter): an instrument that measures the *heat* energy released when foods are burned, thus providing an estimate of the potential energy of foods.

calor = heat

metron = measure

Reminder: A *kcalorie* is a unit of *heat* energy. One kcalorie is the amount of heat necessary to raise the temperature of 1 kg of water 1°C.

Food energy values can be determined by:
- Direct calorimetry, which measures the amount of heat released.
- Indirect calorimetry, which measures the amount of oxygen consumed.

The number of kcalories that the human body derives from a food, as contrasted with the number of kcalories determined by calorimetry, is the physiological fuel value.

Reminder:
- 1 g carbohydrate = 4 kcal.
- 1 g fat = 9 kcal.
- 1 g protein = 4 kcal.
- 1 g alcohol = 7 kcal.

To find out how many kcalories a food provides, a laboratory scientist can burn the food in a bomb calorimeter (see Figure 8–1). When the food burns, the chemical bonds between the carbon and hydrogen atoms break, releasing energy in the form of heat. The amount of heat given off provides a *direct* measure of the food's energy value (remember that kcalories are units of heat energy). In addition to releasing heat, these reactions generate carbon dioxide and water—just as the body's cells do when they metabolize the energy-yielding nutrients in a controlled version of this same process. When the food burns and the chemical bonds break, the carbons (C) and hydrogens (H) combine with oxygen (O) to form carbon dioxide (CO_2) and water (H_2O). The amount of oxygen consumed gives an *indirect* measure of the amount of energy released.

A bomb calorimeter measures the available energy in foods but overstates the amount of energy that the human body derives from foods. The body is less efficient than a calorimeter and cannot metabolize all of a food's energy-yielding nutrients all the way to carbon dioxide and water. Researchers who use calorimetry can correct for this discrepancy mathematically to make useful tables of the energy values of foods (such as Appendix H). These values are reasonable estimates, but do not reflect the *precise* amount of energy a person will derive from the foods consumed.

The energy values of foods can also be computed from the amounts of carbohydrate, fat, and protein (and alcohol, if present) in the foods.* For example, a food containing 8 grams protein, 12 grams carbohydrate, and 5 grams fat would provide 32 protein kcalories, 48 carbohydrate kcalories, and 45 fat kcalories, for a total of 125 kcalories.

FOOD INTAKE

To achieve energy balance, the body must meet its needs without storing too much or too little energy. Somehow the body must decide how often and how

*Some of the food energy values in the table of food composition in Appendix H were derived by bomb calorimetry, and many were calculated from their energy-yielding nutrient contents.

much to eat—when to start eating and when to stop. Eating is a complex behavior controlled by a variety of psychosocial, metabolic, and physiological factors.[4] The hypothalamus appears to be the control center, integrating messages about energy intake, expenditure, and storage from other parts of the brain and from the mouth, GI tract, and liver.

Short-Term Controls   Some of these messages influence immediate food intake, controlling the size and frequency of meals. For example, the hunger message influences how much food will be eaten at one meal and how fast a person might eat. Palatability is also important: more is likely to be eaten when a meal is appetizing. Then satiety comes into play: receptors in the GI tract detect nutrients and signal satiety after each meal.[5] These receptors also influence when the next meal will be eaten.

Hunger   People typically eat meals at roughly four-hour intervals; the stomach is ideally designed to handle periodic batches of food. Four hours after a meal, most, if not all, of the food has left the stomach and been absorbed by the intestine. When the stomach is empty, the hunger message is delivered to initiate eating. Most normal-weight people do not feel like eating until the stomach is either empty, or almost so. Even then, feelings of satiety may have disappeared quite a while before a person feels hungry. Hunger is also triggered by gastric contraction, the absence of nutrients in the small intestine, and GI hormones.

The body seems to be able to adapt its hunger response to accommodate changes in energy intake. People who restrict their energy intakes may feel pangs of hunger for the first few days, but these sensations diminish with time. After the body has adapted to a lower energy intake, eating a large, energy-rich meal makes the person feel uncomfortable. People can adapt to eating excessive amounts of food as well. Some research suggests that repeated binge eating enlarges the stomach's capacity.[6] Consequently the person may experience less satiety after a normal meal, setting the stage for another binge.

Receptors in the GI tract also adapt and change their responses depending on whether nutrient intake has been high or low. One study found that after two weeks on a high-fat diet, the digestion and absorption of a high-fat meal were accelerated.[7] The GI tract had adapted to handle this increase in fat intake efficiently, thus conserving energy. Such findings have interesting implications for the development of obesity.

Appetite   Like hunger, appetite initiates eating, but it differs from hunger in being psychological (a learned response to food), whereas hunger is physiological (an inborn instinct). The two do not always coincide. A person may experience appetite without hunger, for example, when presented with a hot piece of homemade apple pie after having eaten a large Thanksgiving dinner. In contrast, a person may feel hungry but have no appetite for food when faced with a stressful situation or illness; in such circumstances eating becomes a chore. Figure 8–2 lists factors thought to be involved in hunger and appetite.

Satiety   Most normal-weight people stop eating when they feel full or satisfied. Satiety occurs in response to gastric distention, nutrients in the small intestine, and GI hormones. Gastric distention can make a person feel too uncomfortable to eat, but it cannot by itself provide the comfortable sensation of satiety, which depends

Figure 8–1

Bomb Calorimeter

When food is burned, the chemical bonds between the carbons and hydrogens are broken, and energy is released in the form of heat. The amount of heat generated provides a direct measure of the amount of energy stored in the food's chemical bonds.

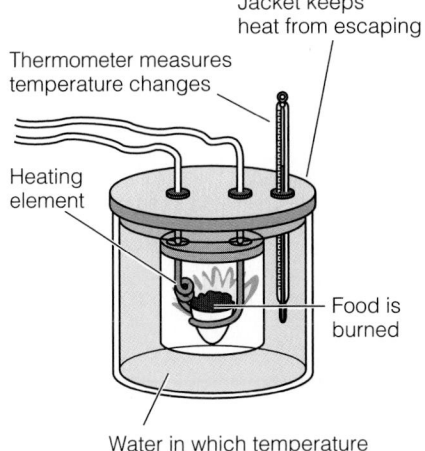

Jacket keeps heat from escaping

Thermometer measures temperature changes

Heating element

Food is burned

Water in which temperature increase from burning food is measured

palatability: pleasing taste. When tasting foods, the tongue presses them against the *palate* (PAL-ut), or roof of the mouth.

hunger: the physiological need to eat, experienced as a drive to obtain food; an unpleasant sensation.

appetite: the psychological desire to eat or an interest in food; a positive sensation that accompanies the sight, smell, or thought of food.

satiety (sah-TIE-eh-tee): the feeling of satisfaction and fullness that food brings. *sate* = to fill

Figure 8–2

Hunger and Appetite

This is a partial list of the factors thought to affect hunger and appetite.

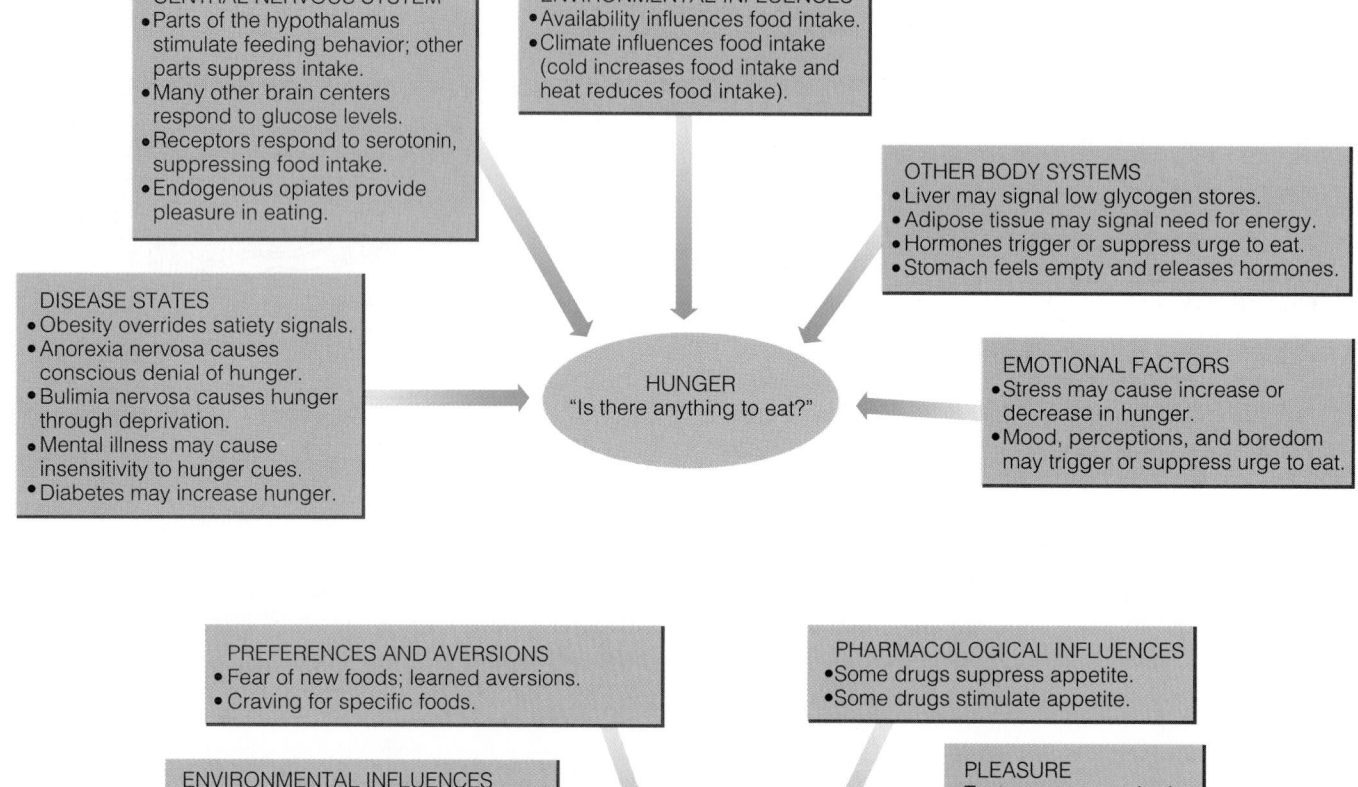

CENTRAL NERVOUS SYSTEM
- Parts of the hypothalamus stimulate feeding behavior; other parts suppress intake.
- Many other brain centers respond to glucose levels.
- Receptors respond to serotonin, suppressing food intake.
- Endogenous opiates provide pleasure in eating.

ENVIRONMENTAL INFLUENCES
- Availability influences food intake.
- Climate influences food intake (cold increases food intake and heat reduces food intake).

OTHER BODY SYSTEMS
- Liver may signal low glycogen stores.
- Adipose tissue may signal need for energy.
- Hormones trigger or suppress urge to eat.
- Stomach feels empty and releases hormones.

DISEASE STATES
- Obesity overrides satiety signals.
- Anorexia nervosa causes conscious denial of hunger.
- Bulimia nervosa causes hunger through deprivation.
- Mental illness may cause insensitivity to hunger cues.
- Diabetes may increase hunger.

HUNGER
"Is there anything to eat?"

EMOTIONAL FACTORS
- Stress may cause increase or decrease in hunger.
- Mood, perceptions, and boredom may trigger or suppress urge to eat.

PREFERENCES AND AVERSIONS
- Fear of new foods; learned aversions.
- Craving for specific foods.

PHARMACOLOGICAL INFLUENCES
- Some drugs suppress appetite.
- Some drugs stimulate appetite.

ENVIRONMENTAL INFLUENCES
- Temperature—people prefer hot foods in winter and cold foods in summer.

PLEASURE
- Taste, texture, and odor suppress or stimulate appetite.

SOCIAL INFLUENCES
- Culture determines which foods are acceptable.
- Religions sometimes determine which foods are acceptable.
- Social pressure may influence personal choices.

INBORN APPETITES
- Thirst encourages drinking water.
- Salt preference encourages eating salty foods.
- Sweet preference encourages eating sweet foods.

METABOLIC INFLUENCES
- Energy requirements encourage sufficient intake.
- Neurotransmitters regulate appetite signals.
- Hormones regulate appetite signals.

APPETITE
"What do I want to eat?"

DISEASE INFLUENCES
- AIDS reduces appetite.
- Obesity may increase taste sensitivity.
- Cancer and its therapies reduce appetite.

Source: Adapted from T. W. Castonguay and coauthors, Hunger and appetite: Old concept/new distinctions, *Nutrition Reviews* 41 (1983): 101–110.

on nutrients in the small intestine. Foods rich in carbohydrates and fibers delay the absorption of nutrients and extend the duration of satiety.[8] Nutrients in the small intestine also trigger the release of GI hormones (such as cholecystokinin) and the stimulation of nerves, sending messages about food intake to the hypothalamus. Eating in response to social schedules instead of hunger may override satiety, however, and contribute to overeating.[9]

Overriding Hunger and Satiety Signals Eating is intimately connected to emotional needs such as the primitive fear of starvation and the infant's association of food with mother love. Not surprisingly, eating can be triggered by signals other than hunger, even when food is not needed. Some people experience food cravings when they are bored or anxious.[10] In fact, they may eat in response to any kind of stress, negative or positive. (What do I do when I'm grieving? Eat. What do I do when I'm celebrating? Eat!) Some people respond to external stimuli such as the time of day ("It's time to eat") or the availability, sight, and taste of food ("I'd love a piece of chocolate even though I am stuffed!"). Being presented with a variety of foods stimulates eating; people eating one food until satisfied may begin eating enthusiastically again when given a fresh selection of different foods. Such behavior can easily lead to weight gain.

Eating can also be suppressed by signals other than satiety, even when a person is hungry. People with the eating disorder anorexia nervosa, for example, use tremendous discipline to ignore the pangs of hunger. Some people simply cannot eat during times of stress, negative or positive. (I'm too sad to eat. I'm too excited to eat!) Why some people overeat in response to stress and others cannot eat at all remains a bit of a mystery. Factors that appear to be involved include how the person perceives the stress and whether normal eating behaviors are restrained.

Long-Term Controls Other types of messages influence longer-term food intakes. Such is the case with metabolic signals from nutrients and hormones, which reflect the overall balance between energy intake and energy needs over spans of several days. Some metabolic signals, such as those arising in a pregnant woman or an athlete, may influence food intake for several months.

In summary, a mixture of signals governs people's eating behavior. Hunger, appetite, and satiety each result from stimuli generated by the nervous and hormonal systems. Superimposed on these are complex factors involving emotions, habit, and other aspects of human functioning that are poorly understood.

Energy Out: The kCalories the Body Spends

The body converts the energy of food to the energy currency of ATP molecules with about 50 percent efficiency, radiating the rest as heat. Then, when ATP energy is used to do work, again about 50 percent is lost as heat. Thus the overall efficiency of the human body in converting food energy to work is 25 percent; the other 75 percent is released as heat. The work itself, as it is done, generates heat as well, so that a body's total heat production reflects the amount of energy it is spending.

The body's generation of heat is known as thermogenesis, and it can be measured to determine the amount of energy expended. This measurement of heat output is known as *direct calorimetry*. Alternatively, a person's energy expenditure can be calculated by *indirect calorimetry*, which involves measuring the amount of oxygen consumed and carbon dioxide expelled.

Eating in response to arousal is called **stress eating**.

The theory that some people eat in response to such external factors as the presence of food or the time of day rather than to such internal factors as hunger is known as the **external cue theory**.

thermogenesis: the generation of heat; used in physiology and nutrition studies as an index of how much energy the body is spending. The total energy a body spends reflects three main categories of thermogenesis:
- Basal thermogenesis (metabolism).
- Exercise-induced thermogenesis (physical activity).
- Diet-induced thermogenesis (thermic effect of food).

A fourth category is sometimes involved:
- Adaptive thermogenesis (energy of adaptation).

direct calorimetry (cal-o-RIM-uh-tree): the measurement of energy output as heat energy.

indirect calorimetry: the estimation of energy output from measures of the amount of oxygen used and carbon dioxide eliminated.

COMPONENTS OF ENERGY EXPENDITURE

People spend energy when they are physically active, of course, but they also spend energy when they are resting quietly. In fact, quiet metabolic activities account for the lion's share of most people's energy expenditures, as Figure 8–3 shows.

Basal Metabolism   At least two-thirds of the energy the average person spends in a day supports the body's metabolic activities. Metabolic activities maintain the body temperature and keep the lungs inhaling and exhaling air, the bone marrow making new red blood cells, the heart beating 100,000 times a day, the kidneys filtering wastes—in short, they support all the basic processes of life.

The basal metabolic rate (BMR) is the rate at which the body spends energy for these maintenance activities. The rate may vary dramatically from person to person and may vary for the same individual with a change in circumstances or physical condition.[11] The rate is slowest when a person is sleeping undisturbed, but it is usually measured in a room with a comfortable temperature when the person is lying still after a restful sleep and is not digesting any food.

In general, the more a person weighs, the more *total* energy is required, but the amount of energy *per pound* of body weight may be lower. For example, an adult's BMR might be 1500 kcalories and an infant's only 500, but compared with their body weights, the infant's BMR is more than twice as fast. Similarly, a normal-weight adult may have a metabolic rate one and a half times that of an obese adult when compared to body weight.

Table 8–1 summarizes the factors that raise and lower the BMR. For the most part, the BMR is highest in people with considerable lean body mass (growing children, physically active people, pregnant women, and males). One way to increase the BMR then is to participate in endurance and strength-building activities regularly to maximize lean body tissue.[12] The BMR is also high in people who are tall and so have a large surface area for their weight, in people with fever or under stress, and in people with highly active thyroid glands.

The BMR declines during adulthood as lean body mass diminishes. This change in body composition occurs, in part, because some hormones that influence metabolism become more, or less, active as a person ages. Voluntary activity tends to be reduced as well, bringing the average decline in energy expenditure to

basal metabolism: the energy needed to maintain life when a body is at complete rest after a 12-hour fast (to exclude the thermic effect of the previous meal).

basal metabolic rate (BMR): the rate of energy use for metabolism under basal conditions, usually expressed as kcalories per kilogram body weight per hour. (Table 8–3 on p. 265 provides equations for estimating BMR.)

A similar measure of energy output is the resting energy expenditure (REE). The REE measure is usually less precise than the BMR because the criteria for rest and fasting are less strict, but the difference is usually less than 10% and can be discounted for most purposes.

Figure 8–3

Components of Energy Expenditure

The amount of energy spent in a day differs for each individual, but in general, basal metabolism is the largest component of energy expenditure (60 to 65%), and the thermic effect of food is the smallest (only 10%). The amount spent in voluntary physical activities has the greatest variability, depending on a person's activity patterns.

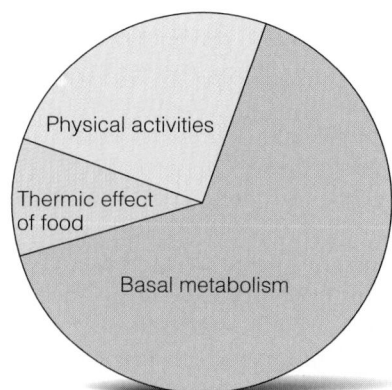

Table 8–1

Factors That Affect the BMR

Factor	Effect on BMR
Age	Lean body mass diminishes with age, slowing the BMR.[a]
Height	In tall, thin people, the BMR is higher.[b]
Growth	In children and pregnant women, the BMR is higher.
Body composition	The more lean tissue, the higher the BMR (which is why males usually have a higher BMR than females). The more fat tissue, the lower the BMR.
Fever	Fever raises the BMR.[c]
Stresses	Stresses (including many diseases and certain drugs) raise the BMR.
Environmental temperature	Both heat and cold raise the BMR.
Fasting/starvation	Fasting/starvation lowers the BMR.[d]
Malnutrition	Malnutrition lowers the BMR.
Hormones	The thyroid hormone thyroxin, for example, can speed up or slow down the BMR.[e]
Smoking	Nicotine increases energy expenditure.
Caffeine	Caffeine increases energy expenditure.
Sleep	BMR is lowest when sleeping.

[a]The BMR begins to decrease in early adulthood (after growth and development cease) at a rate of about 2 percent/decade. A reduction in voluntary activity as well brings the total decline in energy expenditure to 5 percent/decade.

[b]If two people weigh the same, the taller, thinner person will have the faster metabolic rate, reflecting the greater skin surface, through which heat is lost by radiation, in proportion to the body's volume (see margin drawing).

[c]Fever raises the BMR by 7 percent for each degree Fahrenheit.

[d]Prolonged starvation reduces the total amount of metabolically active lean tissue in the body, although the decline occurs sooner and to a greater extent than body losses alone can explain. More likely, the neural and hormonal changes that accompany fasting are responsible for changes in the BMR.

[e]The thyroid gland releases hormones that travel to the cells and influence cellular metabolism. Thyroid hormone activity can speed up or slow down the rate of metabolism by as much as 50 percent.

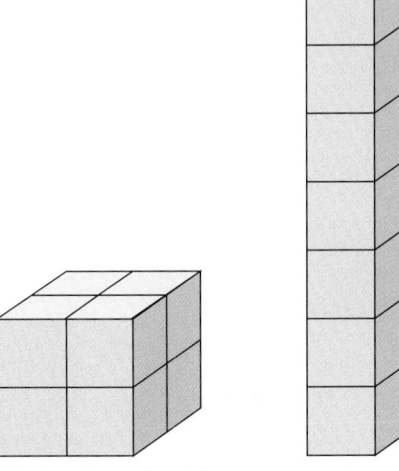

Notice that each of these structures is made of 8 blocks. They weigh the same, but they are arranged differently. If you were to count the sides of these structures, you would see that the short, wide one has 24 sides and the tall, thin one has 34. Because the tall, thin structure has a greater surface area, it will lose more heat (expend more energy) than the short, wide one. Similarly, two people of different heights might weigh the same, but the taller, thin one will have a higher BMR (expending more energy) because of the greater skin surface.

about 5 percent per decade.[13] This decline in the BMR that occurs when a person reduces voluntary activity reflects the loss of lean body mass and may be prevented with ongoing physical activity. The BMR also slows down during fasting and malnutrition.[14]

Physical Activity The second component of a person's energy output is physical activity: voluntary movement of the skeletal muscles and support systems. Physical activity is the most variable component of energy expenditure. Consequently, its influence on both weight gain and weight loss can be significant.[15]

During physical activity, the muscles need extra energy to move, and the heart and lungs need extra energy to deliver nutrients and oxygen and dispose of wastes. The amount of energy needed for any activity, whether playing tennis or studying for an exam, depends on three factors: muscle mass, body weight, and

voluntary activities: the component of a person's daily energy expenditure that involves conscious and deliberate muscular work—walking, lifting, climbing, or other physical activity. In contrast, **involuntary activities** occur independently, without conscious will or knowledge—heart beating, lungs breathing, glands secreting, GI tract muscles contracting, and other activities critical to maintaining life.

activity. The larger the muscle mass required and the heavier the weight of the body part being moved, the more energy is spent. Table 8–2 gives average energy expenditures for people of different body weights engaged in various activities

Table 8–2

Energy Spent on Various Activities

Activity	kCal/lb/min[a]	kCalories per Minute at Different Body Weights				
		110 lb	125 lb	150 lb	175 lb	200 lb
Aerobic dance (vigorous)	.062	6.8	7.8	9.3	10.9	12.4
Basketball (vigorous, full court)	.097	10.7	12.1	14.6	17.0	19.4
Bicycling						
13 mph	.045	5.0	5.6	6.8	7.9	9.0
15 mph	.049	5.4	6.1	7.4	8.6	9.8
17 mph	.057	6.3	7.1	8.6	10.0	11.4
19 mph	.076	8.4	9.5	11.4	13.3	15.2
21 mph	.090	9.9	11.3	13.5	15.8	18.0
23 mph	.109	12.0	13.6	16.4	19.0	21.8
25 mph	.139	15.3	17.4	20.9	24.3	27.8
Cross-country skiing						
8 mph	.104	11.4	13.0	15.6	18.2	20.8
Golf (carrying clubs)	.045	5.0	5.6	6.8	7.9	9.0
Handball	.078	8.6	9.8	11.7	13.7	15.6
Horseback riding (trot)	.052	5.7	6.5	7.8	9.1	10.4
Rowing (vigorous)	.097	10.7	12.1	14.6	17.0	19.4
Running						
5 mph	.061	6.7	7.6	9.2	10.7	12.2
6 mph	.074	8.1	9.2	11.1	13.0	14.8
7.5 mph	.094	10.3	11.8	14.1	16.4	18.8
9 mph	.103	11.3	12.9	15.5	18.0	20.6
10 mph	.114	12.5	14.3	17.1	20.0	22.9
11 mph	.131	14.4	16.4	19.7	22.9	26.2
Soccer (vigorous)	.097	10.7	12.1	14.6	17.0	19.4
Studying	.011	1.2	1.4	1.7	1.9	2.2
Swimming						
20 yd/min	.032	3.5	4.0	4.8	5.6	6.4
45 yd/min	.058	6.4	7.3	8.7	10.2	11.6
50 yd/min	.070	7.7	8.8	10.5	12.3	14.0
Table tennis (skilled)	.045	5.0	5.6	6.8	7.9	9.0
Tennis (beginner)	.032	3.5	4.0	4.8	5.6	6.4
Walking (brisk pace)						
3.5 mph	.035	3.9	4.4	5.2	6.1	7.0
4.5 mph	.048	5.3	6.0	7.2	8.4	9.6

[a]To calculate kcalories spent per minute of activity for your own body weight, multiply kcal/lb/min by your exact weight and then multiply that number by the number of minutes spent in the activity. For example, if you weigh 142 pounds, and you want to know how many kcalories you spent doing 30 minutes of vigorous aerobic dance: 0.062 × 142 = 8.8 kcalories per minute; 8.8 × 30 (minutes) = 264 total kcalories spent.

Sources: Values for swimming, bicycling, and running have been adapted with permission of Ross Products Division, Abbott Labs, Columbus, Ohio 43216, from G. P. Town and K. B. Wheeler, Nutrition concerns for the endurance athlete, *Dietetic Currents* 13 (1986): 7–12. Copyright 1986 Ross Laboratories. Values for all other activities have been adapted with permission from Consumer Reports Books, 1983. *Physical Fitness for Practically Everybody: The Consumer's Union Report on Exercise.* Copyright 1983 by Consumers Union of U.S. Inc., Yonkers, NY 10703–1057.

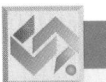

and shows that a heavy person usually uses more energy per minute to perform a task than a light person does. The activity's duration, frequency, and intensity also influence energy cost: the longer, the more frequent, and the more intense the activity, the more kcalories spent per minute.

Thermic Effect of Food   The body uses some energy to process food. When a person eats, the GI tract muscles speed up their rhythmic contractions, and the cells that manufacture and secrete digestive juices begin their tasks. This acceleration of activity produces heat and is known as the thermic effect of food (TEF).

The thermic effect of food is proportional to the food energy taken in and is usually estimated at 10 percent of energy intake. Thus a person who ingests 2000 kcalories in a day probably spends about 200 kcalories on the thermic effect of food. Because the thermic effect of food reflects the body's digestion and absorption activities, it is influenced by factors such as meal size, frequency, and composition; in general, the thermic effect of food is greater for high-carbohydrate foods than for high-fat foods and for a meal eaten all at once rather than spread out over a couple of hours.[16] For most purposes, however, the thermic effect of food can be ignored because its contribution to total energy output is smaller than the probable errors involved in estimating overall energy intake and output.

Adaptive Thermogenesis   Some additional energy is spent when a person must adapt to dramatically changed circumstances (adaptive thermogenesis). When the body has to adapt to physical conditioning, cold, overfeeding, starvation, trauma, or other types of stress, it has extra work to do, building the tissues and producing the enzymes and hormones necessary to cope with the demand. In some circumstances this energy makes a considerable difference in the total energy spent. Because this component of energy expenditure is so variable and specific to individuals, the Committee on Dietary Allowances does not include it when calculating energy requirements.

ESTIMATING ENERGY REQUIREMENTS

In calculating the energy RDA, the Committee on Dietary Allowances considered the following components of energy expenditure:

- Energy spent on basal metabolism.
- Energy spent on physical activities.
- Energy spent on digesting and metabolizing food.

These three components vary, depending on a person's age, sex, body size, heredity, state of health, and other factors. The committee first estimated energy spent on basal metabolism for each age-sex group. Then the committee added increments for physical activity, assuming the average person would be lightly to moderately active. Finally, it added increments for the influence of food, assuming that each person would meet energy needs by eating a mixed diet of ordinary foods.

To estimate energy spent on basal metabolism, the committee used an equation that considers age, sex, and weight as shown in Table 8–3. (The box on p. 267 shows a sample calculation.)

Highlight 8 describes how the activity's duration, frequency, and intensity also influence the body's fuel mix of carbohydrate and fat.

thermic effect of food (TEF): an estimation of the energy required to process food (digest, absorb, transport, metabolize, and store ingested nutrients); also called *diet-induced thermogenesis (DIT)*, the *specific dynamic effect (SDE)* of food, or the *specific dynamic activity (SDA)* of food.

adaptive thermogenesis: adjustments in energy expenditure related to changes in environment such as cold and to physiological events such as overfeeding, trauma, and changes in hormone status.

Table 8–3

Equations for Estimating BMR from Body Weight

Sex and Age (yr)	Equation to Derive BMR in kCal/day
Males	
0–3	$(60.9 \times wt^a) - 54$
3–10	$(22.7 \times wt) + 495$
10–18	$(17.5 \times wt) + 651$
18–30	$(15.3 \times wt) + 679$
30–60	$(11.6 \times wt) + 879$
>60	$(13.5 \times wt) + 487$
Females	
0–3	$(61.0 \times wt) - 51$
3–10	$(22.5 \times wt) + 499$
10–18	$(12.2 \times wt) + 746$
18–30	$(14.7 \times wt) + 496$
30–60	$(8.7 \times wt) + 829$
>60	$(10.5 \times wt) + 596$

^{a}Weight expressed in kilograms.

Source: Reprinted with permission from *Recommended Dietary Allowances*, 10th edition. Copyright 1989 by National Academy of Sciences. Published by the National Academy Press, Washington, D.C.

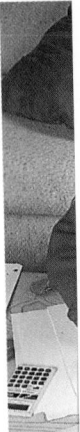

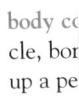

It feels
tired, b
or two

body co
cle, bor
up a pe

Table
• • • • • •
Estima

Lev Int
Ver
Ligh
Mo
Hea
Exc

Sour
lishe

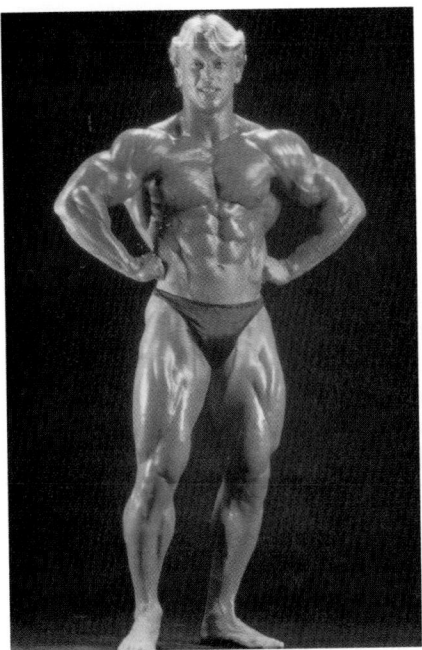

At 5 feet 7½ inches and 200 pounds, Andreas Cahling would be considered over*weight* by most weight-for-height standards, but he is clearly not over*fat*. In fact, his body fat is only 10 percent.

frame size: the size of a person's bones and musculature. Appendix E describes how to take measures to estimate body frame size and provides tables of standards used in assessment.

overweight: body weight above some standard of acceptable weight that is usually defined in relation to height (such as the weight-for-height tables).

underweight: body weight below some standard of acceptable weight that is usually defined in relation to height (such as the weight-for-height tables).

The 1983 Metropolitan Height and Weight table appears in Appendix E.

Weight gains and losses tell us nothing about how the body's composition may have changed, yet that is the measure most people use to judge their "fatness." For many people, overweight means overfat. This is not always the case, though. Athletes with dense bones and well-developed muscles may be overweight by an arbitrary standard such as weight-for-height tables, but have little body fat. Conversely, inactive people may seem to have acceptable weights, when, in fact, they may have too much body fat.

DEFINING HEALTHY BODY WEIGHT

How much should a person weigh? How can a person know if her weight is appropriate for her height and age? How can a person know if his weight is jeopardizing his health? Such questions seem so simple, yet even the experts can't agree on the answers. Most often, they try to identify the weights associated with lowest mortality.[17] With this in mind, healthy body weight is defined by three criteria:[18]

- A weight within the suggested range for height and age, as shown in Table 8–5.
- A fat distribution pattern that is associated with a low risk of illness or death.
- Freedom from all medical conditions that would suggest a need for weight loss.

People who meet all of these criteria may not gain any health advantage by changing their weights. Those who mistakenly think of themselves as overweight even though they meet these criteria for healthy weight may need to revise their self-image. Such people may still want to improve their eating and exercise habits, but they should do so to reap the rewards of being physically fit, not for the sake of weight loss. Anyone who does not meet all of the above criteria may want to consult with a health care professional, who should carefully consider each criterion in relation to the others.[19] The rest of the chapter examines these three criteria in more detail.

BODY WEIGHT AND ITS STANDARDS

Health care professionals often compare people's weights with standard weight-for-height tables, such as the table issued by the Metropolitan Life Insurance Company in 1983, which specifies weights for height, sex, and frame size. Normally, the assessor uses the midpont of the weight range for a person of a given height and assumes a medium build. If the person's actual weight is 10 to 20 percent above that, then the person is considered overweight; if 20 percent or more above the standard, the person is obese; and if 10 percent below the standard, the person is underweight.

Changing Weight Standards　Standards for desirable weights have steadily increased over the past 35 years. In 1990, the U.S. government issued a set of suggested weights (shown in Table 8–5) that were more permissive than the Metropolitan Life standards of 1983—and those in turn were more generous than the company's previous standards issued in 1959.

Disagreements over Standards　Authorities argued over which weight standards were most appropriate. Some criticized, and some praised, the 1990 standards because they allowed people ages 35 and older to be heavier and to gain weight as they aged.[20] Some approved, and some disapproved, of the 1990 weight tables for not specifying recommendations by sex; the tables simply stated

Table 8–5

Suggested Weights for Adults

Height[a]	1990 Guidelines				Height[a]	1995 Guidelines	
	Weight (lb)[a]					Weight (lb)[a]	
	19 TO 34 YEARS		35 YEARS AND OVER			ADULTS OF ALL AGES	
	MIDPOINT	RANGE	MIDPOINT	RANGE		MIDPOINT	RANGE
					4′10″	105	91–119
					4′11″	109	94–124
5′0″	112	97–128	123	108–138	5′0″	112	97–128
5′1″	116	101–132	127	111–143	5′1″	116	101–132
5′2″	120	104–137	131	115–148	5′2″	120	103–137
5′3″	124	107–141	135	119–152	5′3″	124	107–141
5′4″	128	111–146	140	122–157	5′4″	128	111-146
5′5″	132	114–150	144	126–162	5′5″	132	114–150
5′6″	136	118–155	148	130–167	5′6″	136	118–155
5′7″	140	121–160	153	134–172	5′7″	140	121–160
5′8″	144	125–164	158	138–178	5′8″	144	125–164
5′9″	149	129–169	162	142–183	5′9″	149	129–169
5′10″	153	132–174	167	146–188	5′10″	153	132–174
5′11″	157	136–179	172	151–194	5′11″	157	136–179
6′0″	162	140–184	177	155–199	6′0″	162	140–184
6′1″	166	144–189	182	159–205	6′1″	166	148–195
6′2″	171	148–195	187	164–210	6′2″	171	148–195
6′3″	176	152–200	192	168–216	6′3″	176	152–200
6′4″	180	156–205	197	173–222	6′4″	180	156–205
6′5″	185	160–211	202	177–228	6′5″	185	160–211
6′6″	190	164–216	208	182–234	6′6″	190	164–216

Note: The higher weights in the ranges generally apply to men, who tend to have more muscle and bone; the lower weights more often apply to women, who have less muscle and bone. The higher weights for people aged 35 and older reflects recent research that seems to indicate that people can carry a little more weight as they grow older without added risk to health.
[a]Without shoes or clothes.

Sources: Nutrition and Your Health: Dietary Guidelines for Americans, 3rd ed. (Washington, D.C.: Government Printing Office, 1990); *Report of the Dietary Guidelines Advisory Committee on the Dietary Guidelines for Americans, 1995.*

that higher weights in the ranges generally apply to men and lower weights more often apply to women. Fueling the debate are findings that higher weights within the normal range may increase cardiovascular disease risks in women.[21]

Changing Weight Standards—Again   By 1995, the proposed dietary guidelines had discarded the 1990 position that allowed weight gain with age; the 1995 suggested weight standards for all adults are the same as those isued in 1990 for young adults (see Table 8–5). As the 1995 guidelines explain, "health risks due to excess weight appear to be same for older as for younger adults."

As long as there have been tables of recommended weights, debates have raged over their validity and usefulness. The Metropolitan tables were not unanimously

body mass index (BMI): an index of a person's weight in relation to height, determined by dividing the weight (in kilograms) by the square of the height (in meters).

Appendix E presents a nomogram that permits people to scan for their BMI rather than calculating it. The inside back cover shows weight ranges for various heights using the BMI to define underweight, acceptable weight, overweight, and obesity.

- BMI <20 = underweight.
- BMI 20 to 25 = normal.
- BMI 25 to 30 = overweight.
- BMI >30 = obese.

accepted either. They were criticized for grouping all adults together without considering that appropriate weights may vary with age. Furthermore, recommended weights were based on insurance data, which underrepresent the lower socioeconomic class, minorities, and the elderly. Insurance-based weight-for-height tables are specifically inadequate for identifying the weights most closely associated with minimal health risks.

Body Mass Index   Many health professionals prefer to use a standard derived by manipulating the height and weight measures mathematically—the body mass index (BMI):

$$BMI = \frac{weight\ (kg).}{height\ (m)^2}$$

A person who takes measurements in pounds and inches can convert them to metric units or can use this modified equation:[22]*

$$BMI = \frac{weight\ (lb) \times 705.}{height\ (in)^2}$$

Overweight may then be defined by a BMI between 25 and 30 and obesity as a BMI above 30.[23] The average BMI of adults in the United States is 26.3.[24] Figure 8–4 presents visual images associated with various BMI values.

A person whose BMI reflects an unacceptable health risk can choose a desired BMI and then calculate an appropriate body weight for it by using Table 8–6. For

---

*The conversion factor 705 was selected because it is a whole number that is relatively easy to remember; it does overestimate BMI by 0.06 percent, however, and some experts have suggested that 703 might be a better value.

Figure 8–4

Silhouettes and BMI

Source: Reprinted from material of the Canadian Dietetic Association.

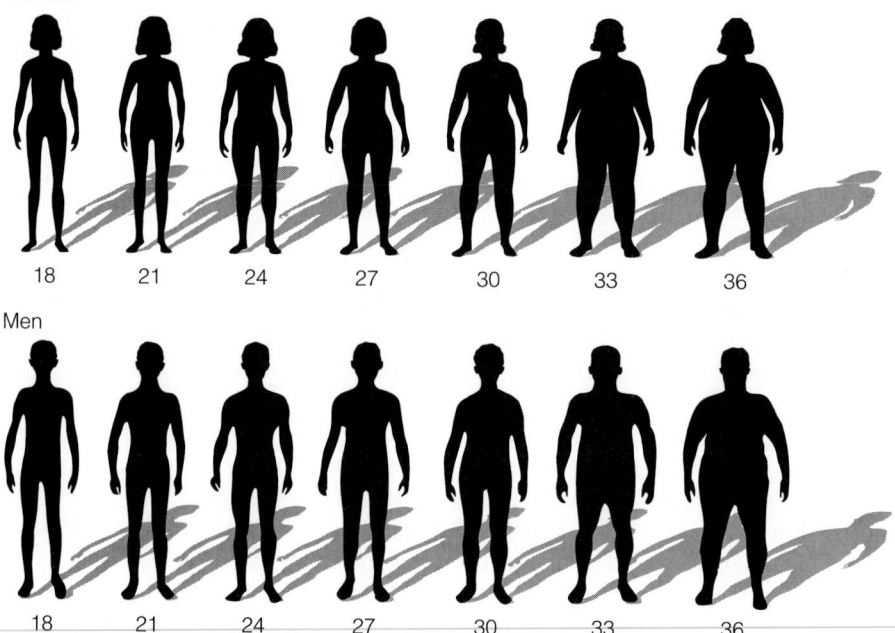

example, a person who is 5 feet 5 inches tall and weighs 165 pounds has a BMI of 27.5. To reach a BMI of 24, the person would need to weigh about 145 pounds (24 ÷ 0.166). Such a calculation can help a person to determine realistic weight goals using health risks as a guide.

Weight measures are inexpensive, easy to take, and highly accurate. Unfortunately, they fail to reveal two valuable pieces of information in assessing disease risk: how much of the weight is fat and where the fat is located.

BODY FAT AND ITS DISTRIBUTION

The ideal amount of body fat depends partly on the person. A normal-weight man may have from 10 to 25 percent body fat; a woman, because of her greater quantity of indispensable fat, 18 to 32 percent.

Some People Need Less   For many athletes, a lower percentage of body fat may be ideal—just enough fat to provide fuel, insulate and protect the body, assist in nerve impulse transmissions, and support normal hormone activity, but not so much as to burden the muscles with excess weight to carry. For athletes, then, ideal body fat might be 5 to 10 percent for men and 15 to 20 percent for women.[25] (You may want to review the photo of Andreas Cahling on p. 268 to appreciate what 10 percent body fat looks like.)

Some People Need More   For an Alaskan fisherman, a higher percentage of body fat is probably beneficial because fat provides an insulating blanket to prevent excessive loss of body heat in cold climates. A woman starting a pregnancy needs sufficient body fat to support conception and fetal growth. Below a certain

Table 8–6

Weight Needed for a Certain BMI

To obtain the weight needed for a certain BMI, divide the desired BMI by the height factor appropriate for your height.

Height	Height Factor	Height	Height Factor	Height	Height Factor
4'7"	0.232	5'3"	0.177	5'11"	0.139
4'8"	0.224	5'4"	0.172	6'0"	0.136
4'9"	0.216	5'5"	0.166	6'1"	0.132
4'10"	0.209	5'6"	0.161	6'2"	0.128
4'11"	0.202	5'7"	0.157	6'3"	0.125
5'0"	0.195	5'8"	0.152	6'4"	0.122
5'1"	0.189	5'9"	0.148	6'5"	0.119
5'2"	0.183	5'10"	0.143	6'6"	0.116

Source: R. P. Abernathy, Body mass index: Determination and use. Copyright the American Dietetic Association. Reprinted by permission from *Journal of the American Dietetic Association* 91 (1991): 843.

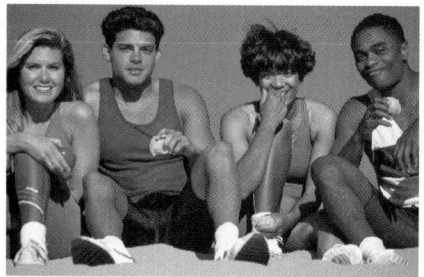

A healthy body contains enough lean tissue to support health and the right amount of fat to meet body needs.

threshold for body fat, hormone synthesis falters, and individuals may become infertile, develop depression, experience abnormal hunger regulation, or become unable to keep warm. These thresholds differ for each function and for each individual; much remains to be learned about them.

The Criterion of Health   In asking what is ideal, people often mistakenly turn to fashion for the answer. Keep in mind that fashion is fickle; body shapes that society values change with time and have little in common with health. Fashion models whose careers depend on body shape often develop eating disorders.

Clearly, the most important criterion for determining how much a person should weigh and how much body fat a person needs is health. Ideally, a person has enough fat to meet basic needs but not so much as to incur health risks. Researchers find health problems develop when body fat exceeds 22 percent in young men, 25 percent in older men, 32 percent in younger women, and 35 percent in older women; these are the values used to define obesity, and age 40 is the dividing line.[26]

intra-abdominal fat: fat stored within the abdominal cavity in association with the internal abdominal organs, as opposed to the fat stored directly under the skin (subcutaneous fat).

central obesity: excess fat around the trunk of the body; also called abdominal fat or upper-body fat.

Fat Distribution   The distribution of fat on the body may be more critical than fatness alone. Intra-abdominal fat that is stored around the organs of the abdomen presents a greater risk to health than fat elsewhere on the body and increases the risk of premature death.[27] This distribution of fat is referred to as central obesity or upper-body fat and, independently of total body fat, is associated with increased risks of heart disease, stroke, diabetes, hypertension, and some types of cancer.[28]

Abdominal fat is common in women past menopause and even more common in men. Even when total body fat is similar, men have more abdominal fat than either premenopausal or postmenopausal women.[29] Interestingly, people with central obesity smoke more and drink alcohol more than the average. A smoker may weigh less than the average nonsmoker, but the smoker's central obesity may be greater, leading researchers to think that smoking may directly affect fat distribution.[30] Exercise, in contrast, correlates negatively with central obesity.

Popular articles sometimes call bodies with upper-body fat "apples" and those with lower-body fat, "pears." Researchers sometimes refer to upper-body fat as "android" (manlike) obesity and to lower-body fat as "gynoid" (womanlike) obesity.

Fat around the hips and thighs, sometimes referred to as lower-body fat, is most common in women in their reproductive years and seems relatively harmless. In fact, people who are overweight, but who do not have excessive fat around the abdomen "seem robust" and less susceptible to health problems than overweight people with central obesity; theirs is a benign obesity.[31]

Exactly how abdominal fat influences disease development remains unknown. Researchers are studying the links between abdominal fat stores, blood lipids, blood pressure, and glucose metabolism. Abdominal fat seems to be more active than lower-body fat. When mobilized, abdominal fat goes directly to the liver rather than emptying into the general circulation, as other fat does. The liver then packages this fat into VLDL, and these become LDL, the lipoprotein most implicated in heart disease. As blood lipids rise, the nervous system responds by releasing hormones and neurotransmitters that accelerate the heart rate and raise the blood pressure, aggravating heart problems and hypertension. Fat metabolism interferes with the liver's ability to clear insulin from the bloodstream.[32] As a consequence, blood glucose and insulin levels remain elevated, setting the stage for diabetes.

Fatfold Measures   Health care professionals use several techniques to estimate body fat and its distribution. Fatfold measures provide a good estimate of total body fat and a fair assessment of the fat's location.[33] About half of the fat in the body lies directly beneath the skin, so the thickness of this subcutaneous fat reflects total body fat. On some parts of the body, such as the back and the back of the arm over the triceps muscle, this fat is loosely attached; a skilled assessor can measure its thickness and then compare the measurement with standards (see Appendix E).

If a person gains body fat, the fatfold increases proportionately; if the person loses fat, it decreases. Measures taken from central-body sites (around the abdomen) better reflect changes in fatness than those taken from upper sites (arm and back).

A major limitation of the fatfold test is that fat may be thicker under the skin in one area than in another. This limitation can be overcome by taking fatfold measurements at three or more different places on the body (including both central- and lower-body sites) and comparing each measurement with standards for that site. Most often, however, the triceps fatfold measurement alone is used because it is easily accessible.

Fatfold measurements correlate directly with the risk of heart disease.[34] They assess central obesity and its associated risks better than do weight measures such as the BMI.

Waist-to-Hip Ratio   Another valuable indicator of fat distribution is the waist-to-hip ratio: the waist circumference divided by the hip circumference. Many clinicians use the waist-to-hip method to assess abdominal obesity, but this ratio may not be appropriate for women, older people, and some racial or ethnic groups.[35] Furthermore, it may not be useful in assessing *changes* in body fat. When people lose weight, they readily lose fat from the abdominal region, most likely because it is metabolically more active than lower-body fat. But while the fat distribution changes with weight loss, the waist-to-hip ratio seems to remain fairly stable.[36]

Other Measures of Body Composition   Other techniques for estimating body fat include hydrodensitometry and bioelectrical impedance analysis. To estimate body density using hydrodensitometry, the person is weighed twice—first on land and then again when submerged under water. The difference between the person's actual weight and underwater weight provides a measure of the body's volume. A mathematical equation using two measurements (volume and actual weight) allows the assessor to calculate body density, from which the percentage of body fat can be estimated. Underwater weighing usually generates a good estimate of body fat and is useful in research, although the technique has drawbacks: it requires bulky, expensive, and nonportable equipment. Furthermore, submerging some people (especially those who are very young, very old, ill, or fearful) underwater is not always practical.

To measure body fat using the bioelectrical impedance technique, a very-low-intensity electrical current is briefly sent through the body by way of electrodes placed on the wrist and ankle. Since electrolyte-containing fluids, which readily conduct an electrical current, are found primarily in lean body tissues, the leaner

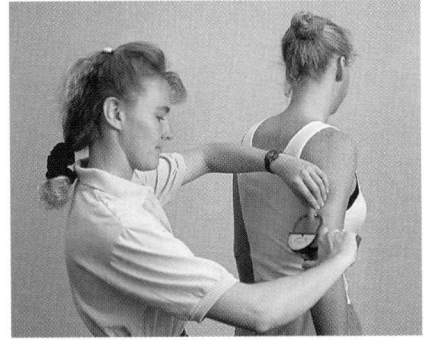

Obtaining an accurate fatfold measure requires training in the use of a caliper that has been calibrated.

fatfold measure: a clinical estimate of total body fatness in which the thickness of a fold of skin on the back of the arm (over the triceps muscle), below the shoulder blade (subscapular), or in other places is measured with a caliper. (The older, less preferred, term is **skinfold test**.)

To calculate the waist-to-hip ratio, divide the waistline measurement by the hip measurement. For example, a woman with a 28-inch waist and 38-inch hips would have a ratio of:

$$28 \div 38 = 0.74.$$

In general, women with a ratio of 0.80 or greater and men with a ratio of 0.95 or greater are at high risk of obesity-related health problems.

hydrodensitometry (HI-dro-DEN-see-TOM-eh-tree): a method of measuring body density in which the person is first weighed and then submerged in water.

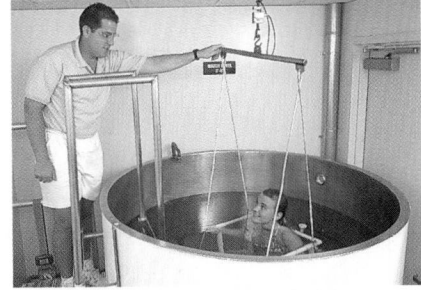

Researchers may use hydrodensitometry to estimate the percentage of body fat.

bioelectrical impedance: a method for estimating body fat using low-intensity electrical current.

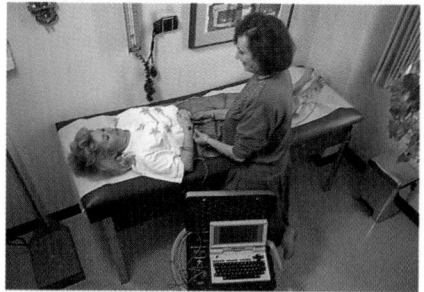

Bioelectrical impedance provides a simple and painless way to estimate body fat.

the person, the less resistance to the current. The measurement of electrical resistance is then used in a mathematical equation to estimate the percentage of body fat.

In addition to anthropometric measures, energy expended in leisure-time physical activities can be used to predict body density and body fat.[37] An increase in activity correlates with an increase in body density and a decrease in body fat. Appendix E provides more details and includes many of the tables and charts routinely used in assessment procedures.*

HEALTH RISKS ASSOCIATED WITH BODY WEIGHT AND BODY FAT

BMI values correlate with disease risks.[38] Most people with a BMI between 20 and 25 have few health risks; risks increase as BMI falls below 20 or rises above 25, indicating that both too little and too much body fat impair health.[39] Factors such as blood pressure or smoking habits raise risks independently of BMI.

Similarly, epidemiological data show a J-shaped relationship between body weights and mortality (see Figure 8–5).[40] People who are underweight or extremely overweight carry high risks of early deaths; people whose weights fall within the acceptable to slightly overweight range live longest.

Health Risks of Underweight It has long been known that thin people die first during a siege or a famine. Overly thin people are also at a disadvantage in the hospital, where they sometimes receive little, if any, food so that they can undergo tests or surgery. Underweight also increases the risk for any person fighting a wasting disease such as cancer, especially when accompanied by undernutrition. A person without adequate nutrient and energy reserves will have a particularly tough battle against such medical stresses. In fact, many people with cancer die, not from the cancer itself, but from malnutrition. Underweight women become infertile, and those who do conceive may give birth to unhealthy infants. An underweight woman can improve her chances of having a healthy infant by gaining weight prior to conception, during pregnancy, or both. For all these reasons, underweight people are urged to gain some body fat as an energy reserve and to acquire protective amounts of all the nutrients that can be stored.

Figure 8–5

Body Mass Index and Mortality

Both underweight and overweight present risks of a premature death. This J-shaped curve describes the relationship between body mass index (BMI) and mortality and shows that optimal BMI is between 21 and 25 (some researchers extend this range from 19 to 27).

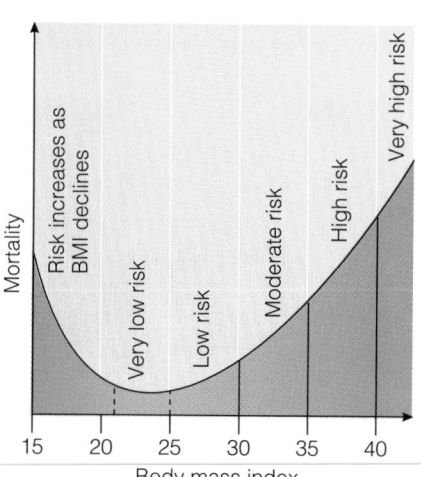

Health Risks of Overweight As for excessive body fat, the health risks are so many that it has been declared a disease: obesity.[41] Among the health risks of obesity are diabetes, hypertension, cardiovascular disease, sleep apnea (abnormal ceasing of breathing during sleep), osteoarthritis, abdominal hernias, some cancers, varicose veins, gout, gallbladder disease, arthritis, respiratory problems (including Pickwickian syndrome, a breathing blockage linked with sudden death), liver malfunction, complications in pregnancy and surgery, flat feet, and even a high accident rate. The costs of these obesity-related illnesses were estimated at more than $39 billion in 1986.[42] The costs in terms of lives is also great. Mortality increases as excess weight increases; people with a BMI greater than 35 are twice as likely to die prematurely as others.[43]

---

*Researchers sometimes estimate body composition using these methods: total body water, radioactive potassium count, dual-energy X-ray absorptiometry, near-infrared spectrophotometry, ultrasound, computed tomography, and magnetic resonance imaging. Each has advantages and disadvantages with respect to cost, technical difficulty, and precision of estimating body fat (see Appendix E for a comparison).

Cardiovascular Disease   The relationship between obesity and cardiovascular disease risk is strong, with links to both blood cholesterol and blood pressure. Central obesity may raise the risk of heart disease as much as the leading three risk factors (high blood cholesterol, hypertension, and smoking) do.[44] Weight loss is effective in preventing and treating hypertension in overweight people.[45] Of course, lean and normal-weight people may also have high blood pressure, and hypertension is just as dangerous in lean people as it is in obese people.

Cardiovascular disease risk factors associated with obesity:
- High LDL cholesterol.
- Low HDL cholesterol.
- High blood pressure (hypertension).
- Diabetes.

Chapter 28 provides many more details.

Diabetes   Diabetes (NIDDM) is three times more likely to develop in an obese person than in a nonobese person. Furthermore, the diabetic person often has central obesity. Central-body fat cells appear to be larger and more insulin-resistant than lower-body fat cells, and insulin resistance is a major risk factor for the development of NIDDM.[46] For those who are overweight, weight loss is effective in improving glucose tolerance and insulin resistance.

Reminder: *NIDDM* refers to noninsulin-dependent diabetes, the most common form of diabetes in which the body's cells fail to respond to insulin (insulin resistance).

Cancer   The risk of cancer increases with body weight, but researchers do not fully understand the relationship. One possible explanation may be that obese people have elevated levels of hormones that could influence cancer development. For example, adipose tissue is the major site of estrogen synthesis in women, obese women have elevated levels of estrogen, and estrogen has been implicated in the development of cancers of the female reproductive system. These cancers account for half of all cancers in women.[47]

In summary, controversy surrounds the setting of standards for body weight. The standard currently considered most valid as an index of health is based on the body mass index (BMI) and rises with advancing age. The weight appropriate for an individual depends largely on factors specific to that individual, including body fat distribution, family health history, occupation, and current health status. At the extremes, overweight and underweight carry clear risks to health, and the attempt to correct them is worthwhile.

Excess body fat is implicated in many of today's chronic diseases. Most health authorities urge people to achieve and maintain a healthy weight, yet they are baffled by the question why people become fat. For some reason, people who are overweight consume more food energy than they use each day and store that energy as fat—their energy budget is unbalanced. The highlight that follows shows how physical activity influences energy balance and body composition.

Study Questions

1. What are the consequences of an unbalanced energy budget?
2. Define hunger, appetite, and satiety and describe how each influences food intake.
3. Describe each component of energy expenditure. What factors influence each? How can energy expenditure be estimated?
4. Distinguish between body weight and body composition. What assessment techniques are used to measure each?
5. What problems are involved in defining "ideal" body weight?
6. What is central obesity, and what is its relationship to disease?
7. What risks are associated with excess body weight and excess body fat?

Notes

1. A. Tremblay and coauthors, Overfeeding and energy expenditures in humans, *American Journal of Clinical Nutrition* 56 (1992): 857–862.

2. M. Shah and R. W. Jeffery, Is obesity due to overeating and underactivity, or to a defective metabolic rate? A review, *Annals of Behavioral Medicine* 13 (1991): 73–81.

3. A. J. Stunkard, Address presented at the North American Association for the Study of Obesity and Emory University School of Medicine conference on Obesity Update: Pathophysiology, Clinical Consequences, and Therapeutic Options, Atlanta, Georgia, August 31–September 2, 1992.

4. N. Read, S. French, and K. Cunningham, The role of the gut in regulating food intake in man, *Nutrition Reviews* 52 (1994): 1–10; P. Norton, G. Falciglia, and D. Gist, Physiologic control of food intake by neural and chemical mechanisms, *Journal of the American Dietetic Association* 93 (1993): 450–454.

5. D. J. Shide and coauthors, Accurate energy compensation for intragastric and oral nutrients in lean males, *American Journal of Clinical Nutrition* 61 (1995): 754–764.

6. A. Geliebter and coauthors, Gastric capacity, gastric emptying, and test-meal intake in normal and bulimic women, *American Journal of Clinical Nutrition* 56 (1992): 656–661.

7. K. M. Cunningham and coauthors, Gastrointestinal adaptation to diets of differing fat composition in human volunteers, *Gut* 32 (1991): 483–486.

8. A. Raben and coauthors, Decreased postprandial thermogenesis and fat oxidation but increased fullness after a high-fiber meal compared with a low-fiber meal, *American Journal of Clinical Nutrition* 59 (1994): 1386–1394; J. E. Blundell, S. Green, and V. Burley, Carbohydrates and human appetite, *American Journal of Clinical Nutrition* 59 (1994): 728S–734S; W. H. Turnbull, J. Walton, and A. R. Leeds, Acute effects of mycoprotein on subsequent energy intake and appetite variables, *American Journal of Clinical Nutrition* 58 (1993): 507–512; S. J. French and N. W. Read, Effect of guar gum on hunger and satiety after meals of differing fat content: Relationship with gastric emptying, *American Journal of Clinical Nutrition* 59 (1994): 87–91.

9. J. Rodin, Determinants of food intake regulation in obesity, in *Obesity*, eds. P. Björntorp and B. N. Brodoff (Philadelphia: J. B. Lippincott, 1992), pp. 220–230.

10. A. J. Hill, C. F. Weaver, and J. E. Blundell, Food craving, dietary restraint and mood, *Appetite* 17 (1991): 187–197.

11. L. O. Schulz and D. A. Schoeller, A compilation of total daily energy expenditures and body weights in healthy adults, *American Journal of Clinical Nutrition* 60 (1994): 676–681.

12. T. J. Horton and C. A. Geissler, Effect of habitual exercise on daily energy expenditure and metabolic rate during standardized activity, *American Journal of Clinical Nutrition* 59 (1994): 13–19.

13. W. J. Carter, Macronutrient requirements for elderly persons, in *Geriatric Nutrition: The Health Professional's Handbook*, ed. R. Chernoff (Gaithersburg, Md.: Aspen Publishers, 1991), pp. 11–24.

14. S. Krug-Wispé, Nutritional assessment, in *Handbook of Pediatric Nutrition*, eds. P. M. Queen and C. E. Lang (Gaithersburg, Md.: Aspen Publishers, 1991), pp. 26–76; J. C. Waterlow, Childhood malnutrition in developing nations: Looking back and looking forward, *Annual Review of Nutrition* 14 (1994): 1–19.

15. A. C. King and D. L. Tribble, The role of exercise in weight regulation in nonathletes, *Sports Medicine* 11 (1991): 331–349.

16. R. S. Schwartz and coauthors, The thermic effect of carbohydrate versus fat feeding in man, *Metabolism* 34 (1985): 285–293; M. M. Tai, P. Castillo, and F. X. Pi-Sunyer, Meal size and frequency: Effect on the thermic effect of food, *American Journal of Clinical Nutrition* 54 (1991): 783–787.

17. R. F. Kushner, Body weight and mortality, *Nutrition Reviews* 51 (1993): 127–136.

18. U.S. Department of Agriculture and U.S. Department of Health and Human Services, Home and Garden Bulletin No. 232, *Nutrition and Your Health: Dietary Guidelines for Americans*, 3rd ed. (Washington, D.C.: Government Printing Office, 1990).

19. C. W. Callaway, New weight guidelines for Americans, *American Journal of Clinical Nutrition* 54 (1991): 171–172.

20. W. C. Willett and coauthors, New weight guidelines for Americans: Justified or injudicious? *American Journal of Clinical Nutrition* 53 (1991): 1102–1103; Callaway, 1991; G. A. Bray and R. L. Atkinson, New weight guidelines for Americans, *American Journal of Clinical Nutrition* 55 (1992): 481–483; R. B. Abernathy, New weight guidelines for Americans, *American Journal of Clinical Nutrition* 56 (1992): 1066–1067.

21. W. C. Willett and coauthors, Weight, weight change, and coronary heart disease in women, *Journal of the American Medical Association*, 273 (1995): 461–465.

22. S. H. Stensland and S. Margolis, Simplifying the calculation of body mass index for quick reference, *Journal of the American Dietetic Association* 90 (1990): 856.

23. Committee on Diet and Health, *Diet and Health: Implications for Reducing Chronic Disease Risk* (Washington, D.C.: National Academy Press, 1989), pp. 99–135.

24. R. J. Kuczmarski and coauthors, Increasing prevalence of overweight among US adults, *Journal of the American Medical Association* 272 (1994): 205–211.

25. T. G. Lohman, Body composition assessment in sports medicine, *Sports Medicine Digest*, September 1990, pp. 1–2.

26. G. A. Bray, An approach to the classification and evaluation of obesity, in *Obesity*, eds. P. Björntorp and B. N. Brodoff (Philadelphia: J. B. Lippincott, 1992), pp. 294–308; G. A. Bray, Definition and characterization of obesity, an address presented at the North American Association for the

Study of Obesity and Emory University School of Medicine conference on Obesity Update: Pathophysiology, Clinical Consequences, and Therapeutic Options, Atlanta, Georgia, August 31–September 2, 1992.

27. P. Björntorp, Regional adiposity, in *Obesity*, eds. P. Björntorp and B. N. Brodoff (Philadelphia: J. B. Lippincott, 1992), pp. 579–586.

28. M. Zamboni and coauthors, Obesity and regional body-fat distribution in men: Separate and joint relationships to glucose tolerance and plasma lipoproteins, *Amerian Journal of Clinical Nutrition*, 60 (1994): 682–687; E. M. Emery and coauthors, A review of the association between abdominal fat distribution, health outcome measures, and modifiable risk factors, *American Journal of Health Promotion* 7 (1993): 342–353; F. X. Pi-Sunyer, Health implications of obesity, *American Journal of Clinical Nutrition* 53 (1991): 1595S–1603S.

29. S. Lemieux and coauthors, Sex differences in the relation of visceral adipose tissue accumulation to total body fatness, *American Journal of Clinical Nutrition* 58 (1993): 463–467; C. J. Ley, B. Lees, and J. C. Stevenson, Sex- and menopause-associated changes in body-fat distribution, *American Journal of Clinical Nutrition* 55 (1992): 950–954.

30. R. J. Troisi, Cigarette smoking, dietary intake, and physical activity: Effects on body fat distribution—The Normative Aging study, *American Journal of Clinical Nutrition* 53 (1991): 1104–1111.

31. Björntorp, 1992.

32. Björntorp, 1992.

33. C. Orphanidou and coauthors, Accuracy of subcutaneous fat measurement: Comparison of skinfold calipers, ultrasound, and computed tomography, *Journal of the American Dietetic Association* 94 (1994): 855–858.

34. R. P. Donahue and coauthors, Central obesity and coronary heart disease in men, *Lancet*, April 11, 1987, pp. 821–824.

35. J. B. Croft, Waist-to-hip ratio in a biracial population: Measurement, implications, and cautions for using guidelines to define high risk for cardiovascular disease, *Journal of the American Dietetic Association* 95 (1995): 60–64.

36. K. van der Kooy and coauthors, Waist-hip ratio is a poor predictor of changes in visceral fat, *American Journal of Clinical Nutrition* 57 (1993): 327–333; M. Zamboni and coauthors, Effect of weight loss on regional body fat distribution in premenopausal women, *American Journal of Clinical Nutrition* 58 (1993): 29–34.

37. A. W. Gardner and E. T. Poehlman, Physical activity is a significant predictor of body density in women, *American Journal of Clinical Nutrition* 57 (1993): 8–14.

38. G. A. Bray, Pathophysiology of obesity, *American Journal of Clinical Nutrition* 55 (1992): 488S–494S.

39. Committee on Diet and Health, 1989, pp. 563–592.

40. T. B. VanItallie, Body weight, morbidity, and longevity, in *Obesity*, eds. P. Björntorp and B. N. Brodoff (Philadelphia: J. B. Lippincott, 1992), pp. 361–369.

41. Pi-Sunyer, 1991.

42. G. A. Colditz, Economic costs of obesity, *American Journal of Clinical Nutrition* 55 (1992): 503S–507S.

43. L. V. Sjöström, Mortality of severely obese subjects, *American Journal of Clinical Nutrition* 55 (1992): 516S–523S.

44. C. Bouchard, G. A. Bray, and V. S. Hubbard, Basic and clinical aspects of regional fat distribution, *American Journal of Clinical Nutrition* 52 (1990): 946–950.

45. J. Wylie-Rosett and coauthors, Trial of Antihypertensive Intervention and Management: Greater efficacy with weight reduction than with a sodium-potassium intervention, *Journal of the American Dietetic Association* 93 (1993): 408–415; S. A. Corrigan and coauthors, Weight reduction in the prevention and treatment of hypertension: A review of representative clinical trials, *American Journal of Health Promotion* 5 (1991): 208–214.

46. S. Lillioja and coauthors, Insulin resistance and insulin secretory dysfunction as precursors of non-insulin-dependent diabetes mellitus: Prospective Studies of Pima Indians, *New England Journal of Medicine* 329 (1993): 1988–1992.

47. A. P. Simopoulos, Characteristics of obesity, in *Obesity*, eds. P. Björntorp and B. N. Brodoff (Philadelphia: J. B. Lippincott, 1992), pp. 308–319.

Fitness—Physical Activity and Nutrition

Extensive evidence confirms that regular physical activity promotes health and prevents disease.[1] Still, despite an increasing awareness of the health benefits that physical activity confers, more than 75 percent of adults in the United States are either irregularly active or completely inactive.[2] Physical inactivity is linked to the major degenerative diseases—heart disease, cancer, stroke, diabetes, and hypertension—that are the primary killers of adults in developed countries.[3]

People don't have to run marathons to reap the health rewards of physical activity. In fact, people who are extremely inactive stand to gain the greatest health benefits by engaging in regular, moderate-intensity, endurance-type activity.[4]

For health's sake, the American College of Sports Medicine (ACSM) specifies that people should spend an accumulated minimum of 30 minutes in some sort of physical activity on most days of each week.[5] Eight minutes spent climbing up stairs, another 10 spent pulling weeds, and 12 more spent walking the dog all contribute to the day's total. The types and amounts of physical activity needed to promote *fitness*, however, may differ from those needed to obtain *health* benefits (see Table H8–1).[6] The guidelines for developing fitness may be optimal, though, because improving fitness provides additional health benefits (the glossary on p. 282 defines fitness and related terms.

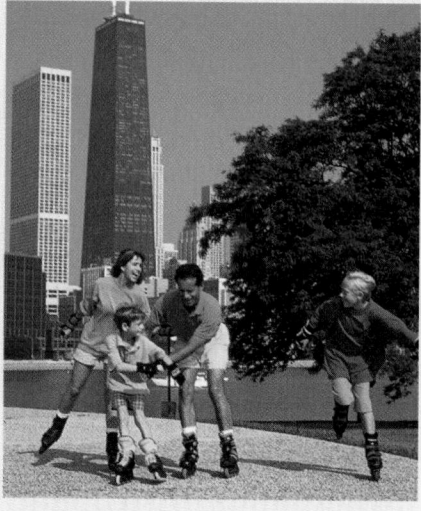

Physical activity helps you look good, feel good, and have fun, and it brings many long-term health benefits as well.

FITNESS AND PHYSICAL ACTIVITY

Fitness depends on a certain minimum amount of regular physical activity. Physical activity leads to fitness, and fitness, in turn, makes activity easy, a beneficial cycle. Activity and fitness are so closely connected that this highlight makes no distinction between them. The benefits of fitness are the benefits of physical activity, and vice versa (see Table H8–2). As a person becomes physically fit, the health of the entire body improves.

The opposite of a physically active life is a sedentary life, which means literally "sitting down a lot." Today's world fosters inactivity by providing people with escalators, cars, and other labor-saving devices. As people go through life exerting minimal physical effort, they become weak and unfit and begin to

Table H8–1

Physical Activity Guidelines

Guidelines for developing and maintaining *physical fitness*:
- **Frequency of activity:** three to five days per week.
- **Intensity of activity:** 50 to 90% of maximum heart rate.
- **Duration of activity:** 20 to 60 minutes of continuous activity.
- **Mode of activity:** any activity that uses large muscle groups.
- **Resistance activity:** strength training of moderate intensity at least two times per week.

Guidelines for obtaining *health* benefits:
- **Frequency of activity:** every day.
- **Intensity of activity:** any level (can be minimal).
- **Duration of activity:** at least 30 minutes total of activity (can be intermittent).
- **Mode of activity:** any activity.

Note: Duration and intensity are inversely related. To obtain similar fitness benefits, a person may exercise either at a low intensity for a long duration or at a high intensity for a short duration. For example, a person may choose to walk briskly for 40 to 50 minutes (lower intensity and longer duration) or to jog for 20 to 30 minutes (higher intensity and shorter duration).

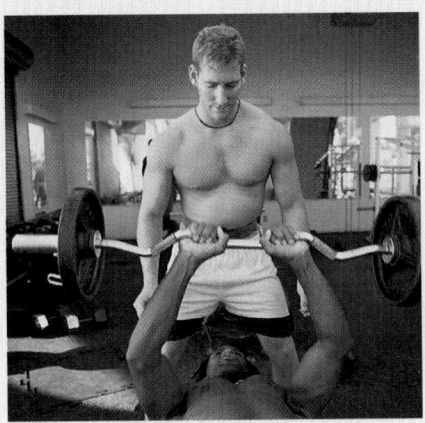

Split-second surges of power as in the heave of a barbell or the jump of a basketball player involve *anaerobic* work.

feel unwell. Without activity, muscles diminish in size and lose strength, a response called atrophy. Conversely, muscles gain size and strength after being made to work repeatedly, a response called hypertrophy.

A balanced fitness program includes both aerobic activities to improve cardiorespiratory fitness and anaerobic activities to develop muscle strength and endurance. As later sections of this highlight explain, these two types of activities use different fuels and bear heavily on what foods best support your chosen activities.

Anaerobic activity is associated with strength, agility, and split-second surges of power. The jump of the basketball player, the slam of the tennis serve, the heave of the weight lifter at the barbells, and the blast of the fullback through the opposing line are all anaerobic work. Such high-intensity, short-duration activities depend mostly on the breakdown of glucose without oxygen for their energy.

Endurance activities of low intensity and long duration depend more on fat to provide energy aerobically. The ability to continue swimming to the shore, to keep on hiking to the top of the mountain, or to continue pedaling all the way home reflects aerobic capacity. Such training requires the heart and lungs to work hard for a sustained period to deliver oxygen to the muscle

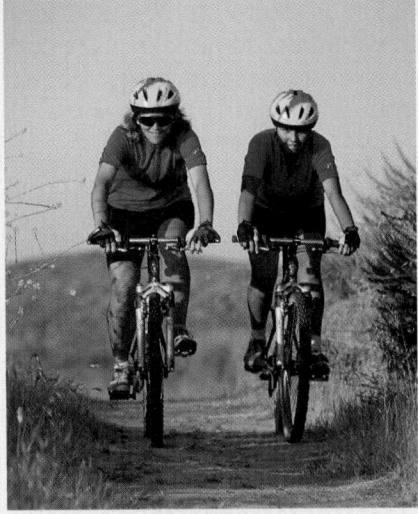

Sustained muscular efforts as in a long-distance bike ride or cross-country run involve *aerobic* work.

cells. Aerobic workouts improve the health of the heart and circulatory system, on which all other body systems depend. Training enhances the ability of the heart, lungs, and blood to deliver oxygen to, and remove waste from, the body's cells.

Physical activity, appropriately pursued, brings positive rewards: good health, long life, and freedom from disease. Pursued in excess, however, intense physical activity combined with poor eating habits can undermine health, as Highlight 9 explains.

ENERGY SYSTEMS, FUELS, AND NUTRIENTS TO SUPPORT ACTIVITY

Nutrition and physical activity go hand in hand. Activity demands carbohydrate and fat as fuel, protein to build and maintain lean tissues, vitamins and minerals to support both

Table H8–2
....

Benefits of Fitness (Summary)

- Sound, beneficial rest and sleep.
- Improved nutritional health.
- Reduced fatness and increased lean body tissue.
- Improved resistance to colds, other infectious diseases, and cancer.
- Reduced risk of heart and blood vessel disease, diabetes, and other diseases.
- Reduced probability of accidents; fewer and less severe injuries.
- Reduced incidence and severity of anxiety and depression.
- Freedom from drug (including alcohol) abuse.
- Improved self-image and self-confidence.
- Better learning ability.
- Greater interpersonal, social, and spiritual strengths.
- Improved quality of life in the later years.
- Longer life.

energy metabolism and tissue building, and water to help distribute the fuels and to dissipate the resulting heat and wastes. This section describes how nutrition supports a person who decides to get up and go.

To meet the demands of physical activity, the muscles generate energy from glucose, fatty acids, and, to a small extent, amino acids. During rest, the body derives slightly more than half of its energy from fatty acids and most of the rest from carbohydrate, along with a small percentage from amino acids. How much of which fuels are used during physical activity depends on an interplay among the fuels available from the diet, the intensity and duration of the activity, and the degree to which the body is conditioned to perform that activity. The following paragraphs examine each of the energy-yielding nutrients individually, but keep in mind that muscles never use just one single fuel. One fuel may predominate at a given time, but the other two will still be active.

Glucose Use during Physical Activity

During exertion, the muscles use both the glucose released from the liver into the bloodstream and their own private glycogen stores to fuel their work. The more glycogen the muscles store, the longer the stores will last during physical activity.

Diet How much carbohydrate a person eats influences how much glycogen is stored, which in turn influences performance. When glycogen is depleted, the muscles become fatigued.

A classic study compared fuel use during activity among three groups of runners on different diets. For several days before testing, one group consumed a normal mixed diet, a second group consumed a high-carbohydrate diet, and the third group consumed a no-carbohydrate diet. As Figure H8–1 shows, the high-carbohydrate diet allowed the runners to keep going longer before exhaustion. This study and many

others that followed have confirmed that high-carbohydrate diets enhance endurance by enlarging glycogen stores.[7]

Intensity of Activity The most intense activities—the kind that make it difficult "to catch your breath," such as a quarter-mile run—use glycogen quickly. Glycogen depletion usually occurs within two hours from the onset of intense activity. Other, less intense activities, such as jogging, during which breathing is steady and easy, use glycogen more slowly.

During *moderate* physical activity, the lungs and circulatory system have no trouble keeping up with the muscles' need for oxygen. The individual breathes easily, and the heart beats steadily—the activity is aerobic. The muscles derive their energy from both glucose and fatty acids. By depending partly on fatty acids, moderate aerobic activity conserves glycogen. Table H8–3 shows how fuel use changes according to the intensity of the activity.

Figure H8–1

The Effect of Diet on Physical Endurance

A high-carbohydrate diet can increase an athlete's endurance. In this study, the fat and protein diet provided 94 percent of kcalories from fat and 6 percent from protein; the normal mixed diet provided 55 percent of kcalories from carbohydrate; and the high-carbohydrate diet provided 83 percent of kcalories from carbohydrate.

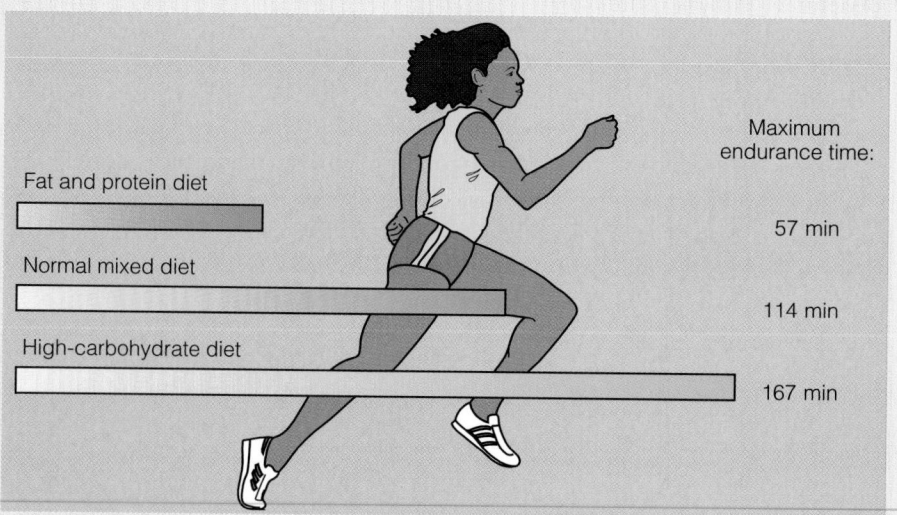

Fat and protein diet

Normal mixed diet

High-carbohydrate diet

Maximum endurance time:

57 min

114 min

167 min

Table H8–3

Fuels Used for Activities of Different Intensities and Durations

Activity Intensity	Activity Duration	Preferred Fuel Source	Oxygen Needed?	Activity Example
Extreme	Less than 30 sec	ATP (immediate availability)	No	100-yard dash, shot put
Very high	30 sec to 3 min	Carbohydrate	No (anaerobic)	¼-mile run at maximal speed
High	3 min to 20 min	Mostly carbohydrate (and some fat)	Yes (aerobic)	Cycling, swimming, or running
Moderate	More than 20 min	Mostly fat (and some carbohydrate)	Yes (aerobic)	Hiking

During *intense* activity—whenever a person exercises at a rate that exceeds the capacity of the heart and lungs to supply oxygen to the muscles—aerobic metabolism is not sufficient to meet energy needs. Instead, the muscles must draw more heavily on glucose, which they can use anaerobically, breaking it down to pyruvate and producing some energy without requiring oxygen. (See Chapter 7 for a review of carbohydrate metabolism.)

Lactic Acid When the rate of activity exceeds the ability to provide enough oxygen, the accumulating pyruvate molecules are converted to lactic acid in an anaerobic process. At low intensities, lactic acid is readily cleared from the blood, but at higher intensities, lactic acid accumulates. Muscle cells cannot accommodate much lactic acid; they release it, and it travels in the blood to the liver where enzymes convert it back into glucose. Glucose can then return to the muscles to fuel additional activity.

Duration of Activity Within the first 20 minutes or so of moderate activity, a person uses mostly glycogen for fuel. After 20 minutes, a

person who continues exercising moderately (mostly aerobically) begins to use less and less glycogen and more and more fat for fuel (review Table H8–3). Still, glycogen use continues, and if the activity lasts long enough and is intense enough, muscle and liver glycogen stores will be depleted.

Glucose Depletion When glycogen depletion hits, continued exertion is almost impossible. Marathon runners refer to this point of glucose exhaustion as "hitting the wall." To avoid such debilitation, endurance athletes try to maintain their blood glucose for as long as they can by:

- Eating a high-carbohydrate diet (approximately 8 grams of carbohydrate per kilogram of body

---

*Percentage of energy intake is meaningful only when total energy intake is known. Consider that at high energy intakes (say, 5000 kcalories/day), even a moderate carbohydrate diet (40 percent of energy intake) supplies 500 grams of carbohydrate—enough for a 137-pound athlete in heavy training. By comparison, at a moderate energy intake (2000 kcalories/day), a high carbohydrate intake (70 percent of energy intake) supplies 350 grams—plenty of carbohydrate for most people, but not enough for athletes in heavy training.

weight or about 70 percent of energy intake) regularly.*
- Training the muscles to store as much glycogen as possible.
- Taking glucose (usually in diluted fruit juice or other sweet beverages) periodically during activity that lasts for an hour or more.
- Eating high-carbohydrate foods within 15 minutes *after* physical activity.

Carbohydrate Loading Some athletes use a technique called carbohydrate loading to trick their muscles into storing extra glycogen before a competition. Ideally, the athlete in training eats a high-carbohydrate diet regularly. During the first 4 days of the week before competition, the athlete trains moderately hard (1 to 2 hours per day) and eats a diet that is moderate in carbohydrate. During the 3 days before competition, the athlete gradually cuts back on activity and eats a very-high-carbohydrate diet. Carbohydrate loading can benefit an athlete who must keep going for 90 minutes or longer. Those who exercise for shorter times simply need a regular high-carbohydrate diet. In a hot climate, extra glycogen confers an additional advantage: as glycogen breaks down, it

Glossary of Fitness Terms

atrophy (AT-ro-fee): of muscles, a decrease in size because of disuse, undernutrition, or wasting diseases.

carbohydrate loading: a regimen of exhaustive exercise followed by the consumption of a high-carbohydrate diet that enables muscles to store glycogen beyond their normal capacity; also called glycogen loading or glycogen supercompensation.

fitness: the characteristics that enable the body to perform physical activity; more broadly, the ability to meet routine physical demands with enough reserve energy to rise to a sudden challenge; or the body's ability to withstand stress of all kinds.

heat stroke: the dangerous accumulation of body heat with accompanying loss of body fluid.

hyperthermia: an above-normal body temperature.

hypertrophy (high-PER-tro-fee): of muscles, growing larger; an increase in size in response to use.

hypothermia: a below-normal body temperature.

moderate exercise: activity that can be sustained comfortably for 60 minutes or so.

muscle endurance: the ability of a muscle to contract repeatedly without becoming exhausted.

muscle strength: the ability of muscles to work against resistance.

sedentary: physically inactive (literally, "sitting down a lot").

---

releases water, which helps to meet the athlete's fluid needs.

Training   Muscle cells that repeatedly deplete their glycogen through hard work adapt to store greater amounts of glycogen to support that work. Conditioned muscles also rely less on glycogen and more on fat for energy, so that glycogen breakdown occurs more slowly in trained than in untrained individuals at a given work intensity.

Fat Use during Physical Activity

An active person who eats a fat-rich diet with little carbohydrate will burn more fat during activity, but will sacrifice performance, as Figure H8–1 showed. Since even physically active people can suffer heart attacks and strokes, every reliable source speaks out against high-fat diets for active people.

In contrast to *dietary* fat, *body* fat stores are of tremendous importance during physical activity. Unlike glycogen stores, which are limited, body fat stores can fuel hours of activity without depletion, as long as the activity is not too intense.

Duration of Activity   Early in an activity, the fat cells begin breaking down their stored triglycerides and liberating fatty acids into the blood. After about 20 minutes of sustained moderate activity, fat becomes the major fuel in energy production.

Intensity of Activity   In general, as the intensity increases, fat makes less and less of a contribution to the mix of fuels used. Remember that fat can be broken down for energy only by aerobic metabolism. For fat to fuel activity, then, oxygen must be abundantly available. If a person is breathing easily during activity, the muscles are getting all the oxygen they need and are able to use more fat in the fuel mixture.

Training   It is training—repeated aerobic activity—that permits the body to draw heavily on fat for fuel. Just 20 minutes or more of aerobic activity, three or more times each week, stimulates even the untrained body to adapt by packing its cells with more fat-metabolizing enzymes and by improving the ability of the heart and lungs to deliver oxygen.

Recommended Intensities and Durations   Health care professionals frequently advise people who want to control their body weight and lose fat to engage in activities of low-to-moderate intensity for a long duration, such as an hour-long fast-paced walk. The reasoning behind such advice is that people exercising at low-to-moderate intensity are likely to stick with their exercise programs for longer times and are less likely to injure themselves. In addition, some research suggests that the longer the duration of activity, the greater the contribution fat will make to the fuel mixture, and consequently, the more body fat will be lost—but this is controversial.[8]

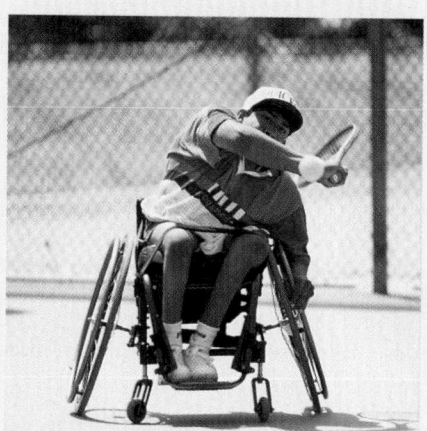

Abundant energy from the breakdown of fat can come only from aerobic metabolism.

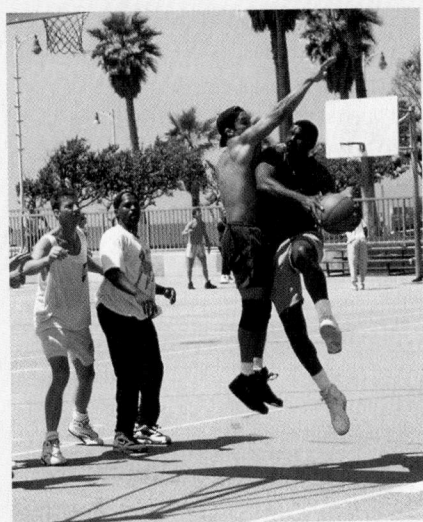

The key to regular physical activity is finding an activity that you enjoy.

Choosing an Activity The intensity and type of physical activity that are best for one person may not be good for another. The intensity to choose depends on your present fitness: work so as to breathe fast, but not so fast as to incur an oxygen debt. A rule of thumb is that you should be breathing easily enough to talk but not sing. If you can sing, pick up the pace; if you have to huff and puff to talk, slow down. If you have been sedentary for the past few years, the activity intensity that will initially make you breathe slightly fast will differ dramatically from the intensity at which a fit person will breathe slightly fast.

The type of physical activity that is best for you depends, too, on what you want to achieve and what you enjoy doing. If you are looking for health benefits, such as reducing your disease risks and lowering your blood cholesterol, then you might want to spend at least 30 minutes each day doing some kind of physical activity. If you are looking to lose weight and improve body com-

position, then choose an activity that you can sustain for 45 minutes or more at least 3 days a week. Choose an activity you enjoy: some people love walking, others prefer to dance or ride a bike. If you want to be stronger and firmer, lift weights or do calisthenics. And remember, muscle is more metabolically active than body fat, so the more muscle you have, the more energy you'll burn.

Table H8–3 summarized the fuel uses discussed so far, but did not include the third energy-yielding nutrient, protein, because protein is not a major fuel for exercise. Protein does provide some energy, however, and more importantly, it provides the structural material of muscle tissue, so it is important to active people.

Protein Use during Physical Activity—and between Times

Physically active people use protein just as other people do—to build muscle and other lean tissue structures and, to some extent, to fuel activity. The body does handle protein differently during activity than during rest, however.

Muscle Building and Fuel Synthesis of body proteins is suppressed during activity and for several hours afterward. In the hours following this period, though, protein synthesis accelerates beyond normal resting levels.

During active muscle-building phases of training, an athlete may add between ¼ ounce and 1 ounce (between 7 and 28 grams) of body protein to existing muscle mass each day. This increase occurs only during periods of *building*—not times of maintenance—when the athlete exercises at high intensities. Not

only do athletes retain more protein in their muscles, they also use more protein as fuel: muscles speed up their use of amino acids for energy during physical activity, just as they speed up their use of fat and carbohydrate.[9] Still, protein contributes at most about 10 percent of the total fuel used, both during activity and during rest. The most active people of all, endurance athletes, use up enormous amounts of all energy fuels, including protein, during performance, but such athletes also eat more food and therefore usually consume enough protein.

Diet People who consume diets adequate in energy and rich in *carbohydrate* use less protein than those who eat protein- and fat-rich diets. Recall that carbohydrates spare proteins from being broken down to make glucose when needed. Since physical activity requires glucose, a diet lacking in carbohydrate necessitates the conversion of amino acids to glucose. So does a diet high in fat, because fatty acids can never provide glucose.

Intensity and Duration of Activity The intensity and duration of activity affect the way the body uses protein. Endurance athletes who train for over an hour a day, engaging in aerobic activity of moderate intensity and long duration, may deplete their glycogen stores by the end of their workouts and become somewhat more dependent on body protein for energy. The protein needs of bodybuilders and weight lifters are slightly higher than those of sedentary people, but not as high as some recommendations and certainly not as high as the protein intakes many bodybuilders consume.

Training In addition to diet and the intensity and duration of the activity, training also influences a person's use of protein during physical activity. Predictably, the higher the degree of training, the less protein a person uses during an activity.

Protein Recommendations All active people, and especially those who work like athletes, probably need a little more protein than do sedentary people: 1.0 to 1.5 grams of protein per kilogram of body weight each day.[10] Endurance athletes use more protein for fuel than power athletes do, and they retain some, especially in the muscles used for their sport. Power athletes use less protein for fuel but still use some, and retain much more. Therefore, *all* athletes in training should attend to protein needs, but should back up the protein with ample carbohydrate. Otherwise, they will burn off as fuel the very protein that they wish to retain in muscle.

Vitamins and Minerals to Support Activity

Many of the vitamins and minerals assist in releasing energy from fuels and in transporting oxygen. This knowledge has led many people to believe, mistakenly, that vitamin and mineral *supplements* offer physically active people both health benefits and athletic advantages. (Highlight 10 includes a discussion of supplements for athletes.) In general, active people who eat enough nutrient-dense foods to meet energy needs also meet their vitamin and mineral needs. After all, active people eat more food; it stands to reason that with the right choices, they'll get more nutrients.

Fluids to Support Activity

Water is a crucial nutrient for everyone, especially those engaged in physical activity. During physical activity, water losses via sweat and vapor are significant, and dehydration becomes a threat. Dehydration's first symptom is fatigue: a water loss of even 1 to 2 percent of body weight can reduce a person's capacity to do muscular work. At about 7 percent water loss, a person is likely to collapse.[11]

Hyperthermia Working muscles produce heat, and the body cools itself by sweating. Each liter of sweat dissipates almost 600 kcalories of heat, preventing a rise in body temperature of almost 10°C. In hot, humid weather, sweat doesn't evaporate well because the surrounding air is already laden with water. Without sweat evaporation, little cooling takes place in the body. In such conditions, active people must take precautions to prevent heat stroke: drink enough fluid before and during the activity, rest in the shade when tired, and wear lightweight clothing that allows evaporation. The symptoms of heat stroke include headache, nausea, dizziness, clumsiness, stumbling, excessive or insufficient sweating, and confusion or other mental changes. If you ever experience any of these symptoms, stop your activity, sip fluids, seek shade, and ask for help. Heat stroke can be fatal, young people often die of it, and these symptoms demand attention.

Hypothermia In cold weather, *hypothermia* or low body temperature, can pose as serious a threat as heat stroke does in hot weather. Inexperienced, slow runners partici-

pating in long races on cold or wet, chilly days are especially vulnerable to hypothermia. Early symptoms of hypothermia include shivering and euphoria. As body temperature continues to fall, shivering may stop, and weakness, disorientation, and apathy may occur. Each of these symptoms can impair a person's ability to act against a further drop in body temperature. Even in cold weather, however, the active body still sweats and still needs fluids. The fluids should be warm or at room temperature to help protect against hypothermia.

Fluid Replacement via Hydration Endurance athletes can easily lose 1.5 liters or more of fluid during *each hour* of activity. To prepare for fluid losses, a person must hydrate before activity. To replace fluid losses, the person must rehydrate during and after activity. (Table H8–4 presents one schedule of hydration for physical activity.)

What is the best fluid for an exercising body? For noncompetitive, everyday active people, plain,

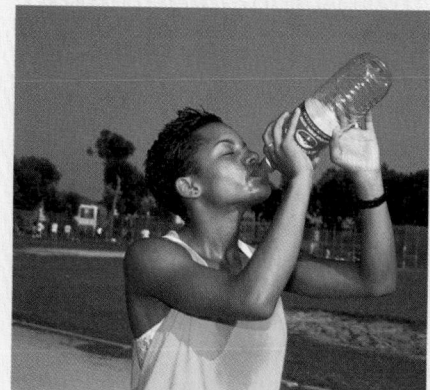

To prevent dehydration and the fatigue that accompanies it, drink plenty of liquids before, during, and after physical activity.

Table H8–4

Hydration Schedule for Physical Activity

Water recommendation: 1.0 to 1.5 mL/kcal expended (1 mL = 0.03 fluid oz).
Easy estimation: ½ c/100 kcal.

When to Drink	Approximate Amount of Fluid
2 hr before exercise	3 c
10 to 15 min before exercise	2 c
Every 15 min during exercise	1 c
After exercise	2 c

Source: D. C. Nieman, *Fitness and Sports Medicine: An Introduction* (Palo Alto, Calif.: Bull Publishing, 1990), p. 234.

cool water is recommended, especially in warm weather, for two reasons: it rapidly leaves the digestive tract to enter the tissues where it is needed, and it cools the body from the inside out. For trained endurance athletes who exercise for an hour or more, sports drinks may provide a slight advantage over water. Fluid ingestion during the event has the dual purposes of replenishing water lost through sweating and providing a source of carbohydrate to supplement the body's limited glycogen stores. Carbohydrate depletion brings on fatigue in the athlete, but as already mentioned, fluid loss and the accompanying buildup of body heat can be life-threatening. Thus the first priority for endurance athletes should be to replace fluids.[12]

DIETS FOR PHYSICALLY ACTIVE PEOPLE

No one diet best supports physical performance. Active people who choose foods within the framework of the diet-planning principles pre-sented in Chapter 2 can design many excellent diets.

Choosing a Diet to Support Fitness

First, remember that water is depleted more rapidly than any other nutrient. A diet to support fitness must provide water, energy, and all the other nutrients. A diet that is high in carbohydrate (60 percent of total kcalories or more), low in fat (25 percent or less), and adequate in protein (12 to 15 percent) ensures full glycogen and other nutrient stores.

Athletes who train exhaustively for endurance events may want to aim for somewhat higher carbohydrate intakes. Beyond these specific concerns of total energy, protein, and carbohydrate, the diet most beneficial to athletic performance is remarkably similar to the diet recommended for most people.

Meals Before and After Competition

No single food improves speed, strength, or skill in competitive

events. Still, a competitor may eat a particular food before or after an event for psychological reasons. One eats a steak the night before wrestling, another takes some honey five minutes after diving. As long as these practices remain harmless, they should be respected.

Pregame Meals The pregame meal or snack should include plenty of fluids and be light and easy to digest. It should provide between 300 and 800 kcalories, primarily from carbohydrate-rich foods that are familiar and well tolerated by the athlete. The meal should end 3 to 5 hours before competition to allow plenty of time for the stomach to empty before exertion.

Breads, potatoes, pasta, and fruit juices—that is, carbohydrate-rich foods low in fat, protein, and fiber—form the basis of the best pregame meal. Bulky, fiber-rich foods such as raw vegetables or high-bran cereals, although usually desirable, are best avoided just before competition. Fiber in the digestive tract attracts water out of the blood and can cause stomach discomfort during performance. Liquid meals are easy to digest, and many such meals are commercially available. Alternatively, athletes can mix nonfat milk or juice, frozen fruits, and flavorings in a blender.

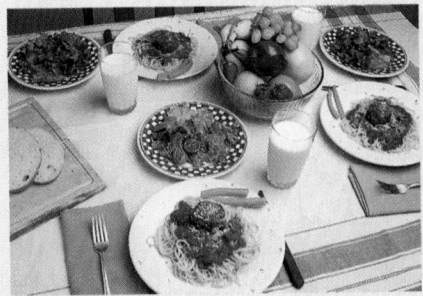

A variety of foods is the best source of nutrients for athletes.

Postgame Meals As mentioned earlier, eating high-carbohydrate foods *after* physical activity enhances glycogen storage. Since people are usually not hungry immediately following physical activity, carbohydrate-containing beverages such as a sports drink may be preferred. If an active person does feel hungry after an event, then foods high in carbohydrate and low in protein, fat, and fiber are the ones to choose—the same ones recommended prior to competition. Foods high in protein and fat should be avoided during the first few hours after activity as these foods may suppress hunger and thus limit carbohydrate intake.[13]

The person who chooses to live a physically active life can expect to enjoy the rewards of fitness and good overall health as well as the pleasures of the chosen activities themselves. Another benefit accompanies these: a person who spends more energy in activity can eat more food, which can bring added pleasure and improved nutrition status.

NOTES

1. R. S. Paffenbarger and coauthors, The association of changes in physical-activity level and other lifestyle characteristics with mortality among men, *New England Journal of Medicine* 328 (1993): 538–545; L. Sandvik and coauthors, Physical fitness as a predictor of mortality among healthy, middle-aged Norwegian men, *New England Journal of Medicine* 328 (1993): 533–537.

2. U.S. Centers for Disease Control and Prevention and American College of Sports Medicine, Summary statement: Workshop on physical activity and public health, *Sports Medicine Bulletin* 28 (1993): 7.

3. American Heart Association Position Statement on Exercise: Benefits and recommendations for physical activity programs for all Americans, *Circulation* 86 (1992): 340–344; A. M. Bovens and coauthors, Physical activity, fitness, and selected risk factors for CHD in active men and women, *Medicine and Science in Sports and Exercise* 25 (1993): 572–576; R. R. Pate and coauthors, Physical activity and public health: A recommendation from the Centers for Disease Control and Prevention and the American College for Sports Medicine, *Journal of the American Medical Association* 273 (1995): 402–407.

4. U.S. Department of Health and Human Services, *Physical Activity and Health: A Report of the Surgeon General Executive Summary* (Washington, D.C.: Government Printing Office, 1996); W. L. Haskell, Health consequences of physical activity: Understanding and challenges regarding dose-response, *Medicine and Science in Sports and Exercise* 26 (1994): 649–660.

5. U.S. Centers for Disease Control and Prevention and American College of Sports Medicine, 1993.

6. American College of Sports Medicine, The recommended quality and quantity of exercise for developing and maintaining fitness in healthy adults, *Medicine and Science in Sports and Exercise* 22 (1990): 265–274.

7. M. Hargreaves, Carbohydrates and exercise, in *Foods, Nutrition and Sports Performance: An International Scientific Consensus,* eds. C. Williams and J. T. Devlin (London: E & FN Spon, 1992), pp. 19–33.

8. P. Arnos, F. Andres, and K. Drowatzky, Fat oxidation and RPE at varied exercise intensities, *Medicine and Science in Sports and Exercise* (supplement) 25 (1993): S9; F. A. Kulling and coauthors, Identification and evaluation of the exercise intensity which maximizes fat oxidation in young women, *Medicine and Science in Sports and Exercise* (supplement) 25 (1993): S179.

9. F. Carraro and coauthors, Alanine kinetics in humans during low-intensity exercise, *Medicine and Science in Sports and Exercise* 26 (1994): 348–353.

10. Position of The American Dietetic Association and The Canadian Dietetic Association: Nutrition for physical fitness and athletic performance for adults, *Journal of the American Dietetic Association* 93 (1993): 691–695.

11. J. E. Greenleaf, Problem: Thirst, drinking behavior, and involuntary dehydration, *Medicine and Science in Sports and Exercise* 24 (1992): 645–656.

12. R. J. Maughan, Fluid and electrolyte loss and replacement in exercise, in *Foods, Nutrition, and Sports Performance: An International Scientific Consensus,* eds. C. Williams and J. T. Devlin (London: E. & FN Spon, 1992), pp. 147–178.

13. E. F. Coyle, Timing and method of increased carbohydrate intake to cope with heavy training, competition, and recovery, in *Foods, Nutrition, and Sports Performance: An International Scientific Consensus* eds. C. Williams and J. T. Devlin (London: E & FN Spon, 1992), pp. 37–61.

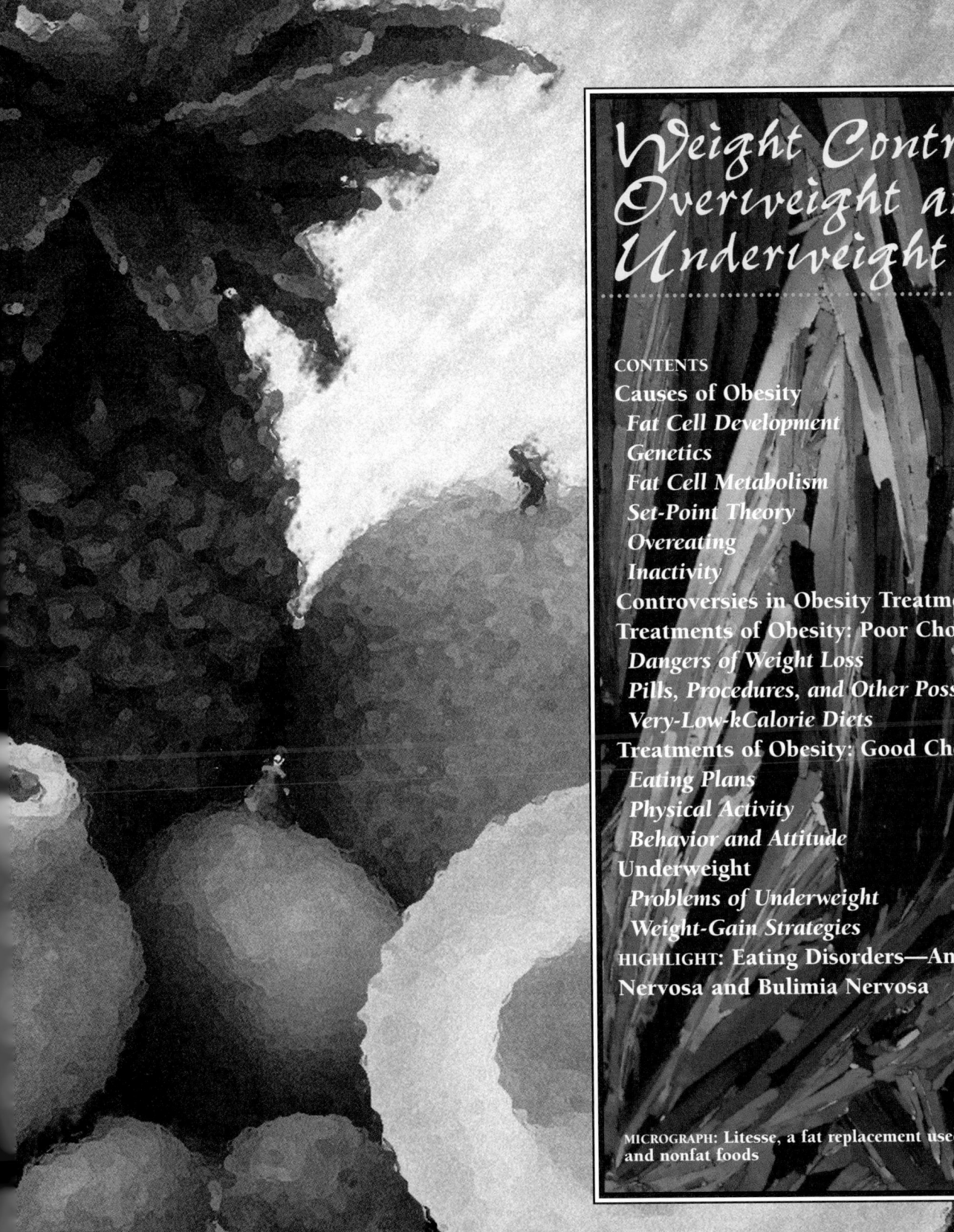

Chapter 9

Weight Control: Overweight and Underweight

CONTENTS
Causes of Obesity
Fat Cell Development
Genetics
Fat Cell Metabolism
Set-Point Theory
Overeating
Inactivity
Controversies in Obesity Treatment
Treatments of Obesity: Poor Choices
Dangers of Weight Loss
Pills, Procedures, and Other Possibilities
Very-Low-kCalorie Diets
Treatments of Obesity: Good Choices
Eating Plans
Physical Activity
Behavior and Attitude
Underweight
Problems of Underweight
Weight-Gain Strategies
HIGHLIGHT: **Eating Disorders—Anorexia Nervosa and Bulimia Nervosa**

MICROGRAPH: Litesse, a fat replacement used in low-fat and nonfat foods

Are you pleased with your body weight? If you answered yes, you are a rare individual. Nearly all people in our society think they should weigh more or less (mostly less) than they do. Usually, their primary reason is appearance, but they often perceive, correctly, that physical health is also somehow related to weight. At the extremes, both overweight and underweight present health risks.

This chapter emphasizes the problems of overweight, partly because they have been more intensively studied and partly because they are a widespread health problem in the developed countries. Information on underweight is presented wherever appropriate. The highlight that follows this chapter delves into the eating disorders anorexia nervosa and bulimia nervosa.

Despite our nation's preoccupation with body image and weight loss, the incidence of obesity continues to rise dramatically (see Figure 9–1). Approximately one out of three adults and one out of five teenagers in the United States are now overweight.[1]* The prevalance of overweight has been increasing and is especially high among women, the poor, and some ethnic groups.[2]

Figure 9–1

Prevalence of Obesity among Adults in the United States

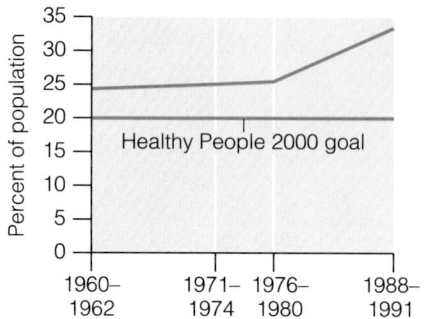

 HEALTHY PEOPLE 2000: Reduce overweight to a prevalence of no more than 20% among people aged 20 years and older and maintain prevalence at no more than 15% among adolescents aged 12 and 19 years.

Causes of Obesity

Excess body fat accumulates when people consistently take in more food energy than they spend. Why do they do this? Is it genetic? Environmental? Cultural? Behavioral? Socioeconomic? Psychological? Metabolic? All of these? Most likely, obesity has many interrelated causes; some experts in the field speak of many different *obesities*. Why an imbalance between energy intake and energy expenditure occurs is unclear; the next sections summarize possible explanations.

FAT CELL DEVELOPMENT

When more energy is consumed than is spent for whatever reason, much of the excess energy is stored in fat cells. The amount of fat on a person's body reflects both the *number* and the *size* of the fat cells. The number of fat cells increases most rapidly during the growing years of late childhood and early puberty.[3] Fat cell number increases more rapidly in obese children than in lean children, and obese children entering their teen years may already have as many fat cells as do adults of normal weight.

The fat cells can expand in size. When the cells reach their maximum size, they may also divide. Thus obesity develops when a person's fat cells increase in number, in size, or quite often both. Figure 9–2 illustrates fat cell development.

With fat loss, the fat cells shrink in size, but not in number. For this reason, people with extra fat cells may tend to regain lost weight rapidly; they may be able to shrink their cells, but not reduce the number. When they gain weight, their many fat cells readily expand. In contrast, people with a normal number of

Obesity due to an increase in the *number* of fat cells is hyperplastic obesity. Obesity due to an increase in the *size* of fat cells is hypertrophic obesity

---

*Overweight is defined as BMI ≥ 27.8 for men and ≥ 27.3 for women.

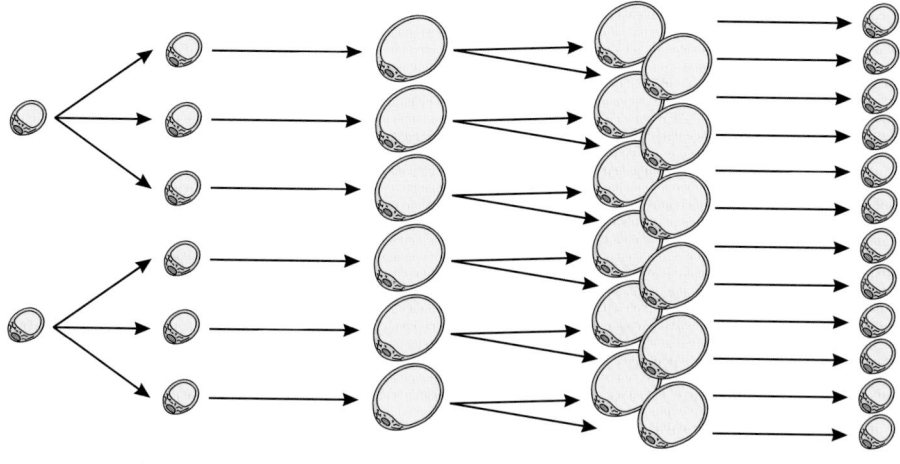

Figure 9-2

Fat Cell Development

Fat cells are capable of increasing their size by 20-fold and their number by several thousandfold.

During growth, fat cells increase in number.

When energy intake exceeds expenditure, fat cells increase in size.

When fat cells have reached their maximum size and energy intake continues to exceed energy expenditure, fat cells increase in number again.

With fat loss, the size of the fat cells shrinks, but not the number.

enlarged fat cells may be more successful in maintaining weight losses; when their cells shrink, both cell size and number are normal. Prevention of obesity is most critical, then, during the growing years when cell number is increasing.

Studies of body weight regulation have noted differences between the body's white adipose tissue and its brown adipose tissue: regular white fat primarily stores fat, whereas brown fat produces heat. When white fat is oxidized, some of the energy is released in heat and some is captured in ATP, but brown fat oxidation is uncoupled from ATP formation; it produces heat only. Radiating energy away as heat enables the body to spend, rather than store, energy. The heat is particularly important in newborns and in animals who hibernate or live in cold climates; they have plenty of brown adipose tissue. In contrast, human adults have small amounts of brown fat in strategic locations, and its role is poorly understood. Some researchers have speculated that the lack of brown fat in adults may contribute to obesity, but its role in weight regulation remains unknown.[4]

GENETICS

Genetics plays an important role in determining a person's body weight and body composition. When both parents are obese, the chances that their children will be obese are quite high (80 percent), whereas when neither parent is obese, the chances are relatively small (less than 10 percent). Adoption studies show that biological parents and their natural children tend to be similar in weight, but that adoptive parents and their adopted children do not. Studies of more than 600 pairs of twins yield similar findings: identical twins are twice as likely to weigh the same as fraternal twins—even when reared apart.[5]

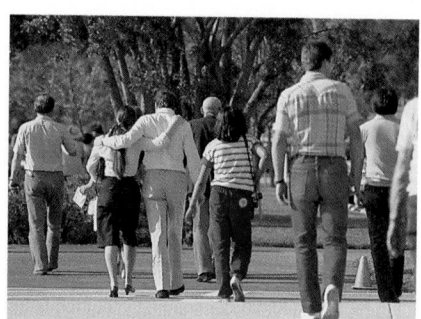

Heredity is a significant determinant of each person's weight.

Similarly, some people have the genetic tendency to *gain* more weight than others on comparable energy intakes.[6] When several sets of identical twins ate an extra 1000 kcalories a day for 100 days, some of the pairs gained 9 pounds while others gained up to 29 pounds. Within each pair, the amount of weight gained, percentage of body fat, and distribution of fat were similar.

Genetics may also influence the way energy is *spent*. Differences in basal metabolic rate (BMR) among individuals are greater than can be explained by age, sex, and body composition alone. Similarities within families suggest a genetic influence on BMR, and a low metabolic rate is a major risk factor for weight gain.[7]

Recently, researchers have discovered a gene in humans that they have named the *obese* gene.[8] Mice with a defective version of the gene weigh up to three times as much as normal mice. Scientists believe that when the gene is functioning, it is active in fat-storage cells and may signal the body to stop eating. Like all genes, the obese gene instructs cells to make a particular protein, perhaps a hormone that slows down eating as the body accumulates fat. This protein is called leptin, a Greek word meaning "thin." Scientists are currently working on determining leptin's exact role, and they are hopeful it will lead them to an understanding of how the body controls its weight.

FAT CELL METABOLISM

Reminder: The enzyme *lipoprotein lipase (LPL)* promotes fat storage.

Some of the research investigating the genetic influence on obesity focuses on the enzyme lipoprotein lipase (LPL), which promotes fat storage in both fat and muscle cells. People with high LPL activity are especially efficient at storing fat. As you might expect, obese people have much more LPL activity in their fat cells than lean people (muscle cell LPL activity is similar).[9] Consequently, even modest excesses in energy intake have a more dramatic impact on obese people than on lean people.

The activity of LPL is partially regulated by sex-specific hormones—estrogen in women and testosterone in men. In women, fat cells in the breasts, hips, and thighs produce abundant LPL, putting fat away in those body sites; in men, fat cells in the abdomen produce abundant LPL. This explains why men tend to develop central obesity whereas women more readily develop lower-body fat.

The activity of LPL may explain why lost weight is so easily regained.[10] One group of researchers measured the LPL in nine obese people before they followed a very-low-kcalorie diet and again after they had lost an average of 90 pounds. The researchers found that LPL activity *rose* after weight loss, and that it rose highest in the people who had been fattest prior to weight loss. Researchers speculate that weight loss serves as a signal to the gene that produces the LPL enzyme, saying "Make more enzyme to store fat." This response to weight loss helps explain why obese people easily regain weight after having lost it, and why their repeated efforts at weight loss are so difficult—they are battling against enzymes that want to store fat. The activity of LPL also supports the theory that some inner mechanism sets a person's weight or body composition and that if anything is done to change it, the body will adjust to restore the set point.

SET-POINT THEORY

Many internal physiological variables, such as blood glucose, blood pH, and body temperature, remain fairly stable under a variety of conditions. The hypothalamus and other regulatory centers constantly monitor and delicately adjust conditions so as to maintain homeostasis. The stability of such complex systems may depend on set-point regulators that maintain variables within specified limits.

Research on the regulation of body weight has been influenced by this set-point concept. Unlike body temperature, however, people's weight ranges vary widely. For example, a reasonable weight for an adult woman, 5 feet 4 inches tall, is about 135 pounds. Yet it is easy to find women of that height who weigh less than 100 pounds and others who weigh more than 200 pounds. These large variations within a population may seem inconsistent with a tightly regulated set-point system, but they aren't; it is the variation within an *individual* that is fairly narrow over long time spans.

Researchers speculate that the body sends out signals to *defend* the established body weight when it is challenged. Recent research confirms that the body adjusts its metabolism whenever it gains or loses weight—in the direction that returns to the initial body weight: energy expenditure increases with weight gain and decreases with weight loss.[11] These changes in energy expenditure are greater than those predicted based on body composition and help to explain why it is so difficult for an obese person to maintain weight losses.

The set-point theory remains controversial and unproven, but many researchers seem to agree that the body somehow (probably by way of genetics) stabilizes its weight. Research is focusing on whether and how a person can lower an elevated set point by manipulating environmental factors such as diet and exercise.

set point: the point at which controls are set (for example, on a thermostat). The set-point theory proposes that the body tends to maintain a certain weight by means of its own internal controls.

OVEREATING

One obvious, although not necessarily accurate, explanation for obesity is that overweight people overeat. Yet diet histories from obese people reveal energy intakes that are similar to, or even less than, those of others.[12] Diet histories may not be accurate records of actual intakes, however. Misreporting of diet and exercise patterns occurs among nonobese as well as obese people.[13]

Some obese people report that even when they follow an energy-restricted diet, they cannot lose weight. But studies have found that these people may actually be eating more and exercising less than they think they are.[14] Furthermore, they tend to believe that their obesity is caused by genetic and metabolic factors, and not by their overeating. Some clinicians dub this "denial" and say that it prevents people from recognizing and taking responsibility for their behaviors.[15]

The long-held belief that obese people do not overeat but simply have low energy needs has been challenged. Compared with others, obese people who report being unable to lose weight despite energy-restrictive dieting do not have lower measures of basal metabolic rate, thermic effect of food, or metabolic response to exercise.[16] Such findings have led some experts to conclude that obese people simply eat more and exercise less than nonobese people.[17]

INACTIVITY

People may be obese, not because they eat too much, but because they spend too little energy.[18] Some obese people are so extraordinarily inactive that even when they eat less than lean people, they still have an energy surplus. Reducing their food intake further would jeopardize health and incur nutrient deficiencies.

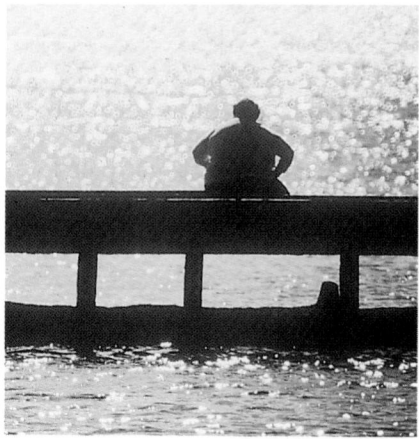

Lack of physical activity fosters obesity.

Physical activity, then, is a necessary component of nutritional health. People must be physically active if they are to eat enough food to deliver all the nutrients needed without unhealthy weight gain.

One hundred years ago, 30 percent of the energy used in farm and factory work came from muscle power; today only 1 percent does.[19] Modern technology has replaced physical activity at home, at work, and in transportation. Underactivity is probably the single most important contributor to obesity. In turn, television watching may contribute most to physical inactivity.[20]

Watching television contributes to obesity in several ways. First, television viewing requires little energy beyond the resting metabolic rate; in fact, one study reports that television viewing actually *lowers* energy expenditure.[21] Second, it replaces time spent in more vigorous activities. Third, watching television correlates with between-meal snacking, eating the high-kcalorie, high-fat foods most heavily advertised on programs, and influencing family food purchases. Nonnutritious foods and beverages appear not only in commercials, but also within the television programs themselves. People, especially children, may miss the message that eating and drinking these foods will bring about weight gain when they see television stars indulging in such behavior and remaining thin.

Children who watch the most television have the greatest prevalence of obesity: obesity increases by 2 percent for each additional hour of television viewed per day.[22] The relationship between television and obesity remains strong when control variables such as prior obesity and socioeconomic class are considered.

Like all the other "causes" of obesity, inactivity alone fails to explain it fully. Fat cell development, genetics, metabolism, set point, and overeating all offer possible, but still incomplete, explanations. Most likely, obesity has not one cause, but different causes and combinations of causes in different people. After all, no two people are alike either physically or psychologically. Some causes may be within a person's control and some may be beyond it. In recent years, the view has been gaining ground that obesity is no one's "fault"—it is not a matter of undisciplined gluttony. Philosophies of weight control and treatment have been evolving to square with this view.

Controversies in Obesity Treatment

An estimated 30 to 40 percent of all U.S. women (and 20 to 25 percent of U.S. men) are trying to lose weight at any given time, spending up to $30 to $40 billion each year to do so.[23] Many of these people do not even need to lose weight. Others need to lose weight, but are not successful. People have attached so many dreams of happiness to weight loss that they are willing to risk huge sums of money for the slightest chance of success. As a result, weight-loss schemes are one of the leading forms of fraud in the United States.

Many people assume that every overweight person can achieve slenderness and should pursue that goal. First consider that most overweight people cannot—for whatever reason—become slender: only 5 percent of all people who try to lose weight are able to maintain their losses.[24] Then consider the prejudice involved in that assumption. People come with varying weight tendencies just as they come with varying potentials for height and degrees of intelligence, yet we do not expect tall people to shrink or smart people to stop thinking in an effort to become "normal."

Our society places such enormous value on thinness that many overweight people face prejudice and discrimination: they are judged on their appearance more than on their character. Socially, overweight people are stereotyped as lazy, stupid, and lacking in self-control. They are less likely to be married than those who are not overweight.[25] Overweight people pay more for insurance and for clothing; they are also less likely to be admitted to college or hired for employment, even when they are qualified. This is especially true for women—a 250-pound man can equally easily be a lumberjack or a corporate executive, but a woman that size faces numerous obstacles. Psychologically, fat people may suffer embarrassment when others treat them with hostility and contempt, and some have even learned to view their own bodies as grotesque and loathsome.[26] Parents and friends may chide them about their weight and lack of discipline to resolve the problem. All of this hurts self-esteem. Many overweight people today are tired of our nation's obsession with weight control and simply want to be accepted as they are. Health care professionals, including dietitians, are among the chief offenders, and some of them are calling for action to stop stigmatizing obesity and to extend the Americans with Disabilities Act to include the obese.[27] To free our nation of its obsession with body weight and prejudice against obesity, we must first learn to judge others for who they are and not for what they weigh.[28]

Still, traditional medical advice urges all obese people to reduce their weight to reduce associated health risks. Obese people die younger from a host of causes, including heart attacks, strokes, certain types of cancer, and complications of diabetes (the noninsulin-dependent type).[29]* Even after the effects of diagnosed diseases are discounted, the risk of death remains twice as high for obese people, especially for those with lifelong obesity, than would otherwise be expected.

Encouraging weight loss may be justified when health benefits are clear. For example, a 30-year-old man with a body mass index (BMI) of 40 may be able to avoid the diabetes that runs in his family by losing 75 pounds. The effort required to do so may be great, but it is far less than the effort and consequences of living with diabetes. Sometimes health benefits appear with less weight loss. A 60-year-old man the same size may be able to improve the arthritis in his knees by losing 25 pounds, for example. In this case, the effort to lose more weight may not pay off.[30] Often a person's motivations for weight loss have nothing to do with health: for example, when a 20-year-old woman with a BMI of 25 wants to lose a few pounds for spring break. Sometimes a person may be healthier *not* losing weight. Such is the case in people with anorexia nervosa who want to lose weight in spite of the devastating medical consequences (see Highlight 9).

In summary, the question whether a person should lose weight depends on many factors: the extent of overweight, age, health, and genetic makeup among them. Not all obesity will cause disease or shorten life expectancy, and just as there are normal-weight people who are unhealthy, there are obese people who are

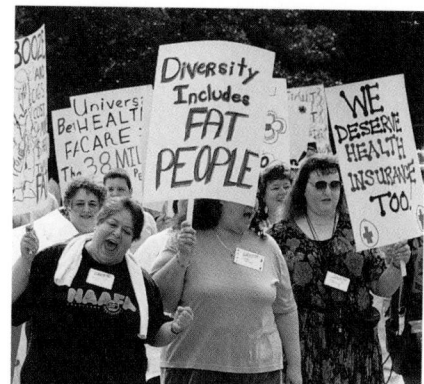

Members of the National Association to Advance Fat Acceptance protest rampant discrimination.

---

*The greater the degree of overweight, the higher the death rate, especially in the young.

healthy. The concept of "healthy obese" people is relatively new, yet it has become generally accepted; the debate focuses on how to characterize this group's health status and risks.[31] Weight-loss advice, then, does not apply equally to all overweight people. Some people may risk more in the process of losing weight than in remaining obese.

Treatments of Obesity: Poor Choices

Most obesity treatments are ineffective and possibly risky. The negative effects must be carefully considered before embarking on any weight-loss program.

DANGERS OF WEIGHT LOSS

Many states have developed a consumer bill of rights to help protect potential weight-loss clients. Such a document explains the risks associated with weight-loss programs and provides honest predictions of success (see Table 9–1). Physical problems may arise from fad diets and "yo-yo" dieting, and psychological problems may emerge from repeated "failures."[32]

Chapter 7 describes the metabolic consequences of a low-carbohydrate diet and the protein-sparing fast.

Fad Diets   Fad diets espouse exaggerated or false theories of weight loss and advise consumers to follow inadequate diets. Some fad diets are more hazardous to health than obesity itself. Adverse reactions can be as minor as headaches, nausea, and dizziness or as serious as death. Of 29,000 claims, treatments, and

Table 9–1

Weight-Loss Consumer Bill of Rights (An Example)

1. *WARNING:* Rapid weight loss may cause serious health problems. Rapid weight loss is weight loss of more than 1½ pounds to 2 pounds per week or weight loss of more than 1 percent of body weight per week after the second week of participation in a weight-loss program.
2. Consult your personal physician before starting any weight-loss program.
3. Only permanent lifestyle changes, such as making healthful food choices and increasing physical activity, promote long-term weight loss and successful maintenance.
4. Qualifications of this provider are available upon request.
5. *YOU HAVE A RIGHT TO:*
   - Ask questions about the potential health risks of this program and its nutritional content, psychological support, and educational components.
   - Receive an itemized statement of the actual or estimated price of the weight-loss program, including extra products, services, supplements, examinations, and laboratory tests.
   - Know the actual or estimated duration of the program.
   - Know the name, address, and qualifications of the dietitian or nutritionist who has reviewed and approved the weight-loss program.

theories for losing weight, fewer than 6 percent of them are effective—and 13 percent are downright dangerous. The accompanying box offers guidelines for identifying weight-loss scams. Some of the nation's largest diet programs have misled consumers with unsubstantiated claims and deceptive testimonials.[33] Furthermore, they fail to provide an assessment of the short- and long-term results of their treatment plans, even though such evaluations are possible and would permit consumers to make informed decisions.[34]

Weight Cycling   Many people who try to lose weight become trapped in weight cycling, the endless repeating rounds of weight loss and regain from "yo-yo" dieting (see Figure 9–3). When people repeatedly lose weight only to regain it, their bodies become very efficient at making and storing fat. This increased efficiency shows itself in a way familiar to dieters who have lost and gained—and lost and gained again. With each attempt, it becomes harder and takes longer to lose weight and easier and quicker to gain it back. In fact, previous weight-cycling history can predict a person's success (or lack thereof) in maintaining weight loss.[35]

Such fluctuations in body weight do not appear to produce permanent changes in body composition, but they do increase the risks of diabetes, hypertension, high blood lipids, and even death, independent of the obesity itself.[36] Some research indicates that maintaining a stable weight, even if it is overweight, may be less harmful to health than repeated bouts of weight gains and losses. Such concerns should not deter obese people who want to lose weight from trying, but rather should encourage them to commit to lifelong changes that will maintain weight losses.[37]

Psychological Problems   Some weight-loss programs are better than others in terms of cost, approach, and customer satisfaction, but none are particularly successful in helping people keep lost weight off. Most programs assume that the problem can be solved simply by applying willpower and hard work. If determination were the only factor involved, though, the success rate would be far greater than 5 percent. Overweight people may readily assume the blame for their failures to lose weight and maintain the losses when, in fact, the programs have failed to deliver on their promises.[38] Ineffective treatment and its associated sense of failure add to a person's psychological burden.[39] Figure 9–4 illustrates how the devastating psychological effects of obesity and dieting perpetuate themselves.

PILLS, PROCEDURES, AND OTHER POSSIBILITIES

A number of alternative strategies for losing weight have been set forth. Some are of limited usefulness, some are not useful at all, and some are actually harmful.

Diuretics   Temporary water retention may add several pounds on the scale, but obesity does not cause water retention.* In fact, obese people have a *smaller*

---

*Many women experience temporary water retention around the time of the menstrual period. Oral contraceptives may also cause water retention and may even promote fat gain in some women. A woman who has this problem should consult her physician about switching brands.

Figure 9–3

The Weight-Cycling Effect of Repeated Dieting

Each round of dieting is followed by a rebound of weight to a higher level than before.

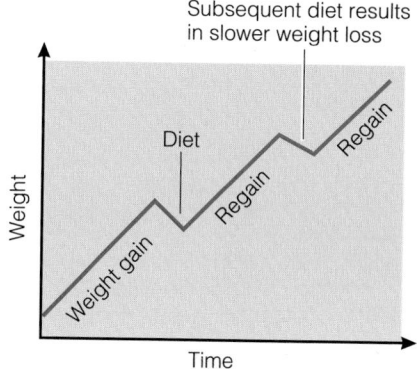

weight cycling: repeated cycles of weight loss and gain. The weight-cycling pattern is popularly called the ratchet effect or yo-yo effect of dieting.

Losing 10 pounds and keeping them off may be beneficial, but losing 100 pounds and regaining them may be quite harmful.

Figure 9–4

The Psychology of Weight Cycling

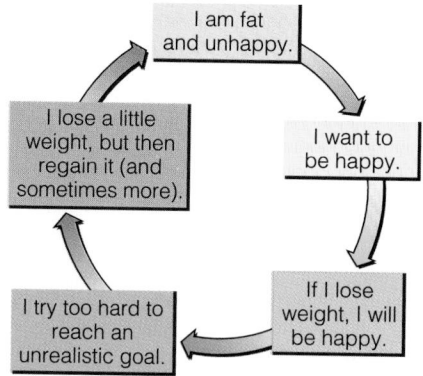

Source: Adapted with permission from J. P. Foreyt and G. K. Goodrick, *Living without Dieting* (Houston: Harrison Publishing, 1992).

How to Identify Unsound Weight-Loss Schemes and Diets

1. They promise dramatic, rapid weight loss (i.e., substantially more than 1 percent of total body weight per week).
2. They promote diets that are nutritionally unbalanced or extremely low in kcalories. Diets should provide:
   - A reasonable number of kcalories (not fewer than 1200 kcalories per day).
   - Enough, but not too much, protein (between the RDA and twice the RDA).
   - Enough, but not too much fat (between 20 and 30 percent of daily energy intake from fat).
   - Enough carbohydrate to spare protein and prevent ketosis (about 100 grams).
   - A balanced assortment of vitamins and minerals from a variety of foods from each of the food groups.
3. They use liquid formulas rather than foods and provide too little energy.
4. They attempt to make clients dependent upon special foods or devices rather than teaching them how to make good choices from the conventional food supply.
5. They fail to encourage permanent, realistic lifestyle changes, including regular exercise and behavior modification.
6. They misrepresent salespeople as "counselors" supposedly qualified to give guidance in nutrition and/or general health. Even if adequately trained, such "counselors" would still be objectionable because of the obvious conflict of interest that exists when providers profit directly from products they recommend and sell.
7. They collect large sums of money at the start or require that clients sign contracts for expensive, long-term programs. Programs should be reasonably priced and on a pay-as-you-go basis.
8. They fail to inform clients of the risks associated with weight loss in general or the specific program being promoted. They provide no information about dropout rates or long-term success of their clients.
9. They promote unproven or spurious weight-loss aids such as human chorionic gonadotrophin hormone (HCG), starch blockers, diuretics, sauna belts, body wraps, passive exercise, ear stapling, acupuncture, electric muscle-stimulating (EMS) devices, spirulina, amino acid supplements (e.g., arginine, ornithine), glucomannan, methylcellulose (a "bulking agent"), "unique" ingredients, and so forth.
10. They fail to provide for weight maintenance after the program ends.

Source: Adapted from *National Council Against Health Fraud Newsletter,* March/April 1987, National Council Against Health Fraud, Inc.

percentage of body water than people of normal weight. When people take diuretics, they lose water, not fat. The weight loss lasts only half a day or so, and the price is dehydration and mineral imbalances.

Amphetamines   Years ago physicians routinely prescribed amphetamines (pep pills) to reduce the appetite. Not only are amphetamines of little value in weight loss, but they are also highly addictive. Many dieters who used them remained overweight and were left with the additional problem of getting off the drugs. Common side effects of amphetamines include dizziness, irritability, blurred vision, nausea, vomiting, and diarrhea. Amphetamines are no longer approved by the Food and Drug Administration (FDA) for weight loss.

Other Prescription Drugs   Most prescription drugs either suppress appetite and so curb food intake or speed up energy metabolism and the use of fat for fuel.[40]* Most drugs that suppress appetite can be addictive and lose their effectiveness after a few weeks of use.[41] Drugs that accelerate energy expenditure also have serious side effects and lose their effectiveness with time.† One compound currently under investigation because of its action in reducing fat synthesis and enhancing fat utilization is DHEA—a product made in the body during the synthesis of steroid hormones.[42]‡ A hormone called leptin that regulates body fat is being studied in obese mice and has proven successful in causing them to lose a third of their weight in two weeks.

Another new drug currently under testing acts on the small intestine's fat-digesting enzymes to prevent digestion and absorption of about a third of the fat consumed. The drug, tetrahydrolipostatin, faces years of rigorous study before it can be approved by the FDA.

One nonaddicting drug that was recently approved by the FDA, dexfenfluramine, shows promise in reducing hunger and improving dietary compliance.[43] The drug works by stimulating the brain to release the neurotransmitter serotonin, which depresses appetite. Several other appetite-suppressing drugs are also under study and may one day prove their worth. Side effects vary with each obesity drug, but the overall incidence is relatively modest.

While some drugs have proved effective in promoting initial weight loss, the long-term effects of their use are unknown.[44] Government regulations restrict the use of prescription drugs for obesity to a three-month limit due to fears of potential abuse and previous indiscriminate prescription; some research indicates that long-term treatment may be beneficial.[45] In either case, drugs should be used only as one component of a comprehensive weight-loss program.

Over-the-Counter Products   The FDA has given approval to two over-the-counter medications to help with weight loss. One contains phenyl-propanolamine, which suppresses appetite and enhances weight loss when used with a low-kcalorie diet.[46] The other contains benzocaine (in a candy form), which anesthetizes the tongue, reducing taste sensations.

diuretic (dye-you-RET-ic): a drug that promotes water excretion; popularly, a "water pill."
   dia = through
   ure = urine

---

*Examples of drugs that suppress food intake include naltrexone, chlorocitric acid, cholecystokinin-octapeptide, and serotonergic agents.

†Examples of drugs that stimulate fat utilization include idazoxon, atpamezole, phenoxybenzamine, and thermogenic agents.

‡DHEA stands for dehydroepiandrosterone.

Manufacturers of many other diet products have been making weight-loss claims without having to prove their effectiveness or safety.* One company marketed guar gum, the soluble fiber commonly used as a thickener in many food products, as a weight-loss product. Guar gum forms a gel when taken with water, and in several cases (including one that led to death), people developed esophageal blockages and GI obstructions after swallowing guar tablets. Upon learning of these problems, the FDA banned the sale of guar tablets. Consumers can best protect themselves from hazards like these by remembering that weight loss does not come in tablet form.

Other Gimmicks   Other gimmicks don't help with weight loss either. Hot baths do not speed up the BMR so that pounds can be lost in hours. Steam and sauna baths do not melt the fat off the body, although they may dehydrate people so that their weights change dramatically. Machines that jiggle parts of the body while people lean passively on them provide pleasant stimulation, but no exertion and so no expenditure of energy. Brushes, sponges, and massages intended to move, burn, or break up "cellulite" do nothing of the kind, because there is no such thing as cellulite.

Surgery   Surgery, as an approach to weight loss, is justified in some specific cases of clinically severe obesity. Guidelines for client evaluation, selection, care, and follow-up have been published.[47] The person contemplating surgery for weight loss should consider all the health implications before submitting to it.

Two gastric partitioning procedures have gained wide acceptance and are illustrated in Figure 9–5.[48] Both procedures effectively limit food intake by reducing the size of the stomach's pouch. They reduce the size of the outlet as well, so they delay the passage of food from the stomach into the intestine for digestion and absorption. The long-term safety and effectiveness of gastric

---

*To obtain a list of ineffective diet aids, write to FDA, HFE-20, 5600 Fishers Lane, Rockville, MD 20857.

cellulite (SELL-you-light or SELL-you-leet): supposedly, a lumpy form of fat; actually, a fraud. The lumpy appearance in fatty areas of the body is caused by strands of connective tissue that attach the skin to underlying muscles. These points of attachment may pull tight where the fat is thick, making lumps appear between them. The fat itself is not different from fat anywhere else in the body. So, if the fat in these areas is lost, the lumpy appearance disappears.

clinically severe obesity: a BMI of 40 or greater or 100 pounds or more overweight for an average adult. A less preferred term used to describe the same condition is *morbid obesity*.

gastric partitioning: a surgical procedure used to treat clinically severe obesity. The operation limits food intake by reducing the size of the stomach and delays gastric emptying by restricting the outlet.

Figure 9–5

Surgical Procedures Used in the Treatment of Severe Obesity

The dark pink areas highlight the flow of food through the GI tract. Notice that the first procedure maintains a relatively normal flow whereas the second one bypasses most of the stomach, all of the duodenum, and some of the jejunum. The pale pink areas indicate the sections that have been bypassed.

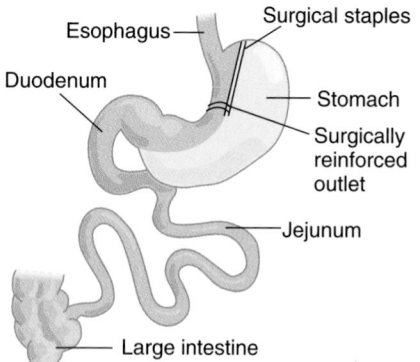

In vertical banded gastroplasty, the surgeon constructs a small gastric pouch and restricts the outlet from the stomach to the intestine.

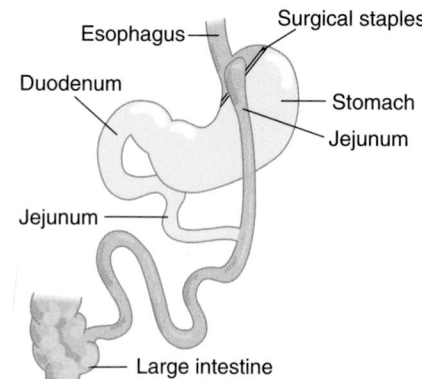

In gastric bypass, the surgeon constructs a small gastric pouch and creates an outlet directly to the jejunum.

surgery depend, in large part, on compliance with dietary instructions. Common immediate postsurgical complications include infections, nausea, vomiting, and dehydration; in the long term, vitamin and mineral deficiencies and psychiatric disorders are common.[49] Lifelong medical supervision is necessary for those who choose the surgical route, but in suitable candidates the benefits of weight loss prove worth the risks.[50]

Another surgical procedure is used, not to treat obesity, but to remove the evidence. Plastic surgeons can extract some fat deposits by suction lipectomy, or "liposuction." This cosmetic procedure has little effect on body weight, but can alter body shape slightly in specific areas.

Gastric Balloons A physician can position and inflate a balloon inside the stomach so that a person who eats too much food will feel uncomfortable. Risks of gastric ulcer, internal bruising, and intestinal blockage commonly occur during the fourth month of use, so the FDA requires removal of these balloons after three months.

Jaw Wiring Desperation leads some people to request that their jaws be wired shut so that they will be forced to consume a liquid diet. This does bring about weight loss, but when the wires are removed, most people promptly regain the lost weight because they have not learned the new eating habits that will support weight maintenance.

VERY-LOW-KCALORIE DIETS

For many obese people, compliance with a well-balanced, nutritionally adequate, energy-restricted diet offers slow results compared with the number of pounds they have to lose. Quite often, they become frustrated and lose hope before significant changes become apparent. For these people, very-low-kcalorie diets (VLCD) offered by medical centers provide rapid weight loss (sort of a "jump start" on the journey). For the duration of the VLCD, they need make no decisions about what foods to buy, how to prepare them, or how much to eat. They need only drink a formula as prescribed.

This break from food may help a person establish a new relationship with food. Unlike a recovering alcoholic, who can abstain from alcohol altogether, or a smoker, who can throw away all cigarettes, a person cannot give up food "cold turkey." A VLCD provides a break from poor eating habits and an opportunity to begin good eating habits when the VLCD ends.

VLCD plans provide 800 kcalories, at least 1 gram per kilogram of body weight of high-quality protein, little or no fat, and a little carbohydrate (not enough to spare protein); there is no advantage to providing less energy.[52] They are accompanied by an assortment of vitamins and minerals from supplements. Meals consist of a limited number of foods (primarily lean meats, fish, and poultry) each day, a powdered formula available by prescription, or a combination of the two.

VLCD formulas are designed to be nutritionally adequate, but the body responds to this severe energy restriction as if the person were starving—conserving energy and preparing to regain weight at the first opportunity. As Chapter 7 described, several changes occur in hormone concentrations, metabolic activities, fluid and electrolyte balances, and organ functions in the effort to

Recommended criteria for people on VLCD:[51]
- Motivated.
- Moderately to severely obese (BMI >30).
- No heart, kidney, gallbladder, or liver disease; cancer; or alcoholism.
- No psychiatric disorders (including eating disorders).

meet the challenge of living on a much-less-than-adequate energy intake. For these reasons, a VLCD is appropriate only for short-term use (four months) and under close medical supervision.[53] Table 9–2 lists common side effects of VLCD.

Without doubt, weight losses on VLCD are dramatic. Unfortunately, weight regains are almost certain.[54] With the weight loss comes a slower BMR and slower fat oxidation—conditions that favor weight gain.[55] Such rapid losses and steady gains are detrimental to both physical and mental health. People undertaking VLCD should be forewarned that the hard part begins at the end of the diet,

Table 9–2

Possible Physical Consequences of Very-Low-kCalorie Diets

Blood

- Blood carotene concentrations increase.
- Blood cholesterol concentrations increase.
- Blood urea concentrations increase.

Cardiovascular/Respiratory

- Blood pressure declines.
- Carbon dioxide production declines.
- Cardiac output declines.
- Heart muscle atrophies.
- Heartbeat becomes irregular.
- Low blood pressure develops.
- Oxygen consumption declines.
- Pulse rate declines.
- Respiratory rate declines.

Digestive

- Gallstones and kidney stones form.
- GI tract motility declines.
- Liver inflammation and fibrosis develop.
- Nausea, vomiting, diarrhea, abdominal discomfort, and constipation occur.

Hormonal

- Menstrual irregularity develops.
- Sex drive is lost.

Immunity

- Immune response diminishes.
- White blood cells decrease in number.

Metabolic

- Basal metabolism declines.
- Bone mineral content shifts.
- Cold intolerance occurs.
- Dehydration may occur.
- Gout may occur.
- Ketosis develops.
- Lean body tissues are lost.
- Mineral and electrolyte imbalances occur.
- Nitrogen balance becomes negative.

Other

- Body and breath odor (from ketone excretion) may become apparent.
- Cold intolerance develops.
- Hair falls out.
- Headaches occur.
- Lethargy, fatigue, and loss of stamina set in.
- Skin dries out.
- Sleeplessness may occur.
- Sudden death becomes possible.

Sources: Evidence on metabolic rate, lean body tissue, liver, gallstone, heartbeat, bones, and nitrogen balance, from various authors in *American Journal of Clinical Nutrition* (supplement) 56 (1992); immune failure reported in C. J. Field, R. Gougeon, and E. B. Marliss, Changes in circulating leukocytes and mitogen responses during very-low-energy all-protein reducing diets, *American Journal of Clinical Nutrition* 54 (1991): 123–129; reduced oxygen consumption reported in K. N. Pavlou and coauthors, Exercise as an adjunct to weight loss and maintenance in moderately obese subjects, *American Journal of Clinical Nutrition* 49 (1989): 1115–1123; low blood pressure, headache, atrophy of heart muscle, and hormonal effects from R. L. Atkinson, Low calorie diets and obesity, in *Biotechnology and Nutrition*, eds. D. D. Bills and S. D. Kung (Boston: Butterworth-Heinemann, 1992), pp. 29–45.

when they have to learn to maintain their weight loss. A weight-maintenance phase is an essential part of every VLCD program.[56]

In summary, weight-loss efforts often are misguided, and when pursued via unwise weight-loss techniques, they can be downright dangerous. This is not to say, though, that no one should attempt to lose weight. Weight loss is highly desirable for those whose health will benefit from it, who can do it, and who pursue it using safe and effective techniques.

Treatments of Obesity: Good Choices

Dietary recommendations state that for good health, a person should "achieve and maintain appropriate body weight." The goal is not weight loss, but health gains. Weight loss can improve control of diabetes and reduce the risks of heart disease by lowering blood pressure and blood cholesterol, especially for those with upper-body fat.[57] For these reasons, parameters such as blood pressure, blood cholesterol, or even self-esteem are more useful than body weight in marking success. Of course, the same eating and exercise habits that improve health often lead to an appropriate body weight and composition as well. Whether the goal is health or weight loss, expectations need to be reasonable. Unreachable targets ensure failure. It is better to aim for realistic and achievable goals. Then, if success is greater than expected, there will be rewards instead of disappointments.

In pursuing good health, keep in mind that it is a lifelong journey. Most adults are keenly aware of their body weights and shapes and realize that what they eat and what they do can make a difference to some extent. Those who are most successful at preventing weight gain or maintaining weight loss seem to have fully incorporated healthful eating and physical activity into their lives. Their approach is not "on-again-off-again," but a routine part of their daily lives. And it is a multifaceted approach, involving diet, physical activity, behavior, and attitude.

• Weight-loss pointer: Adopt reasonable expectations about health and weight goals and about how long it will take to achieve them.

HEALTHY PEOPLE 2000: Increase to at least 50% the proportion of overweight people aged 12 years and older who have adopted sound dietary practices combined with regular physical activity to attain an appropriate body weight.

EATING PLANS

No one food plan is magical, and no specific food must be included or avoided. In designing a plan, people need only consider foods that they like or can learn to like, that are available, and that are within their means.

• Weight-loss pointer: Be involved in planning.

Realistic Energy Intake   The main characteristic of a weight-loss diet is that it provides less energy than the person needs to maintain present body weight. Restricting energy intake too severely, however, may have only short-term effects and can be counterproductive.[58] Rapid weight loss means excessive loss of lean tissue. Initially, overweight people should only try to stop binge eating and start eating normally—say, three meals a day—and then examine energy intake.

Energy intake should provide nutritional adequacy without excess—that is, somewhere between kcalorie-restricted dieting and complete freedom to eat

- Weight-loss pointer: Adopt a realistic plan.

- Weight-loss pointer: Make nutritional adequacy a high priority.

- Weight-loss pointer: Emphasize nutrient-dense foods.

- Weight-loss pointer: Eat small portions of foods at each meal.
- Weight-loss pointer: Make legumes, grains, vegetables, and fruits central to your diet plan.

everything in sight. A rule of thumb is that a person needs at least 10 kcalories per pound of current weight each day to lose fat efficiently while retaining lean tissue. For example, a 140-pound woman would start by setting her energy intake at 1400 kcalories a day. Then, as she lost weight, she would adjust her energy intake downward.

Nutritional Adequacy   Nutritional adequacy is difficult to achieve on fewer than 1200 kcalories a day, and most healthy adults should not consume any less than that. Consider that 1200 kcalories a day allows a person who weighs 120 pounds to lose weight, yet hardly anyone who weighs 120 pounds is overweight. People weighing more can lose weight on higher energy intakes. A plan that provides an adequate intake supports a healthier and more successful weight loss than a restrictive plan that creates feelings of starvation and deprivation, which can lead to an irresistible urge to binge.

Take a look at Table 9–3 and notice that the 1200-kcalorie food plan represents the minimum servings suggested in the Daily Food Guide (introduced in Chapter 2) and allows a teaspoon of fat at each of three meals. Such an intake would allow most people to lose weight gradually and still meet their nutrient needs with careful, nutrient-dense food selections. (Women might need an iron supplement.) The other patterns provide for higher energy intakes.

Small Portions   Overweight people usually need to learn to eat less food at each meal—one piece of chicken for dinner instead of two, a teaspoon of butter on the vegetables instead of a tablespoon, and a cookie for dessert instead of six. The goal is to eat enough food for energy, nutrients, and pleasure, but not so much as to have an excess. This amount should leave a person feeling satisfied—not necessarily full. Keep in mind that even low-fat foods can deliver a lot of kcalories when a person eats large quantities. A low-fat cookie or two can be a sweet treat even on a weight-loss diet, but a whole box would clearly be excessive.

Table 9–3

Diet Patterns for Different Energy Intakes

Food Group	Recommended Savings for Various Energy Levels (kcal)						
	1200	1500	1800	2000	2200	2600	3000
Bread, cereal, rice, and pasta	6	7	8	9	11	13	15
Meat and meat alternates (lean)	4	5	6	6	6	7	8
Vegetables	3	4	5	5	5	6	6
Fruits	2	3	4	4	4	5	6
Milk and milk products (nonfat)	2	2	2	3	3	3	3
Fat	3	5	6	7	8	10	12

Note: These patterns follow the Daily Food Guide plan and supply less than 30 percent of kcalories as fat.

Carbohydrates, Not Fats   Center meals and snacks on complex carbohydrate foods. Fresh fruits, vegetables, legumes, and whole grains offer abundant vitamins, minerals, and fiber but little fat. They also require effort to eat—an added bonus. People who eat these foods in abundance spontaneously eat for longer times and take in fewer kcalories than when eating foods of high energy density. The satiety signal indicating fullness is sent after a 20-minute lag, so a person who slows down and savors each bite eats less before the signal reaches the brain.

Satiety plays a key role in weight-loss diets. Researchers compared a diet in which fat was restricted, but complex carbohydrates were eaten freely, with a more conventional energy-restricted diet.[59] Moderately obese women in both diet groups lost weight, but those who ate the low-fat, complex carbohydrate-rich diet rated it higher in terms of satiety and taste. They also gave higher ratings to "quality of life," perhaps because they felt less deprived when allowed to eat unrestricted quantities of low-fat, complex carbohydrate foods.

Findings from several other studies agree: restricting fat is effective in, and may even be more effective than, restricting energy for weight loss.[60] Furthermore, body composition may improve on a low-fat diet. Rats who had been on a high-fat diet were switched to a diet that provided fewer kcalories, with each group receiving either a low-, medium-, or high-fat diet.[61] Compared with rats on the low-fat diet, the rats on the high-fat diet lost less weight and kept much more of their body fat. Even worse, their LPL activity increased compared with rats that remained on the initial high-fat diet. This study suggests that body *fat* will not be lost by following a low-kcalorie diet alone, even when weight is lost—dietary fat must also be reduced.

Similarly, women who followed a low-fat diet (20 percent kcalories from fat) lost both weight and body fat.[62] In fact, the only way the women could *maintain* weight was to raise their total energy intakes. Clearly then, to lose weight and improve body composition, measure fat with extra caution. A slip of the butter knife adds more kcalories than a slip of the sugar spoon. Less fat in the diet means less fat in the body. Be careful not to take this advice to the extreme, however; too little fat in the diet or in the body carries health risks as well.

Speaking of empty kcalories, a person trying to achieve or maintain a healthy weight needs to pay attention not only to fat, but to sugar and alcohol, too. Using them for pleasure on occasion is compatible with health as long as most daily choices are of nutrient-dense foods.

Adequate Water   Learn to satisfy thirst with water. Water fills the stomach between meals and dilutes the metabolic wastes generated from the breakdown of fat. It meets the water need that was formerly met by eating extra food (remember that foods provide water).

Adopt a lifelong "eating plan for good health" rather than a "diet for weight loss." That way, you will be able to keep the lost weight off.

PHYSICAL ACTIVITY

People who combine diet and exercise are more likely to lose more fat and less likely to regain weight than those who only diet.[63] People who include physical activity in their weight-control program seem to follow their diet plan more

- Weight-loss pointer: Eat slowly.

- Weight-loss pointer: Eat complex carbohydrates in abundance.

- Weight-loss pointer: Select low-fat foods regularly.

- Weight-loss pointer: Limit concentrated sweets and alcoholic beverages.

- Weight-loss pointer: Drink plenty of water (8 glasses or more a day).

- Weight-loss pointer: Learn, practice, and follow a healthful eating plan for the rest of your life.

- Fitness pointer: Participate in some form of physical activity regularly.

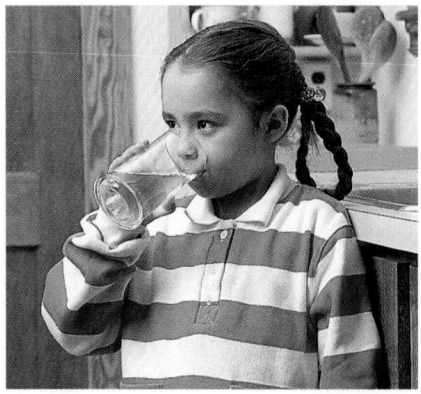

Drinking water is a healthy habit.

Benefits of physical activity in a weight-control program:
- Short-term increase in energy expenditure (from exercise and from a slight rise in BMR).
- Long-term increase (slight) in BMR.
- Appetite control.
- Stress reduction and control of stress eating.
- Physical, and therefore psychological, well-being.
- High self-esteem.

closely than those who do not exercise.[64] Consequently they benefit from both a little less energy input and the added energy output of physical activity. Table 8–2 (on p. 264) shows how much energy each of several activities uses. The table also shows that the number of kcalories spent in an activity depends more upon body weight than on how fast the exercise is done. For example, a person who weighs 150 pounds and runs a mile in 6 minutes spends about 103 kcalories. That same person walking a mile in 15 minutes uses almost the same amount—about 92 kcalories. Similarly, a 220-pound person spends about 150 kcalories on the 6-minute mile, and only a little less—about 135 kcalories—on the 15-minute walk. Whether a person chooses to run or walk the distance, the same energy will be spent; walking will just take longer. To lose fat, expend as much energy as your time allows.[65]

Activity and the BMR Activity also contributes to energy output in an indirect way—by speeding up basal metabolism. It does this both immediately and over the long term. On any given day, basal metabolism remains elevated for several hours after intense and prolonged exercise. Over the long term, daily vigorous activity for many weeks gradually changes body composition toward more lean tissue. Metabolic rate rises accordingly, and this makes a contribution toward continued weight loss or maintenance.

The raised metabolic rate continues for as long as the person keeps exercising regularly. The more energy expended in metabolic activities, the greater the energy requirement. This means that a person can eat more without gaining weight, which in turn brings both pleasure and nutrients.

Activity and Appetite Control Physical activity also helps to control appetite. People think that exercising will make them hungry, but this is not entirely true. Yes, active people do have healthy appetites, but immediately after a good workout, most people do not feel like eating. They may be thirsty and want to shower, but they are not hungry. The reason is that the body has released fuels from storage to support the exercise, so glucose and fatty acids are abundant in the blood. At the same time, the body has suppressed its digestive functions. Hard physical work and eating are not compatible. A person must calm down, put energy fuels back in storage, and relax before eating. Thus exercise helps curb appetite, especially the inappropriate appetite that accompanies boredom, anxiety, or depression and might prompt a person to eat when not hungry. Weight-control programs encourage people to use this strategy to overcome their urge to eat when not hungry: go out and exercise instead. The activity passes time, relieves anxiety, and prevents inappropriate eating.

Activity and Psychological Benefits Activity also helps reduce stress. Since stress itself is a cue to inappropriate eating for many people, activity can help here, too. Activity offers still more psychological advantages. The fit person looks and feels healthy and, as a result, gains self-esteem. High self-esteem motivates a person to persist in seeking weight control and fitness, which continues the beneficial cycle.

Choosing Activities Clearly, physical activity is a plus in a weight-control program. What kind of physical activity is best? People seeking to lose weight should choose activities that they enjoy and that they are willing to do regularly. Sustained physical activities of moderate intensity (aerobic exercises) are more effective in weight control than short bursts of vigorous exercise.[66] In addition to exercise, there are hundreds of ways to incorporate energy-spending activities into daily routines: take the stairs instead of the elevator, walk to the neighbor's apartment instead of making a phone call, and rake the grass clippings instead of using a bagger. Remember that sitting uses more kcalories than lying down, standing uses more kcalories than sitting, and moving uses more kcalories than standing. A 175-pound person who replaces a 30-minute television program with a 2-mile walk a day can spend enough energy to lose (or not gain) 18 pounds in a year. Walk a mile. Run a race. Swim a lap. Dance a jig. Ride a bike. Climb a mountain. Do whatever you enjoy doing—and do it often.

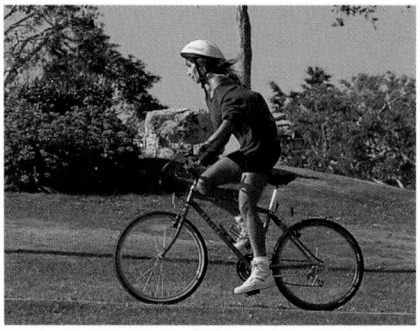

Regular physical activity, such as bicycling or walking briskly, will help to burn fat.

Spot Reducing   People sometimes ask about "spot reducing." Unfortunately, muscles do not "own" the fat that surrounds them. Fat cells all over the body release fat in response to demand, and the fat is then used by whatever muscles are active. No exercise can remove the fat from any one particular area—and, incidentally, neither can massage machines that claim to break up fat on trouble spots. Being moved passively by machines or pounded by massages neither increases energy output nor takes off fat.

Exercise can help with trouble spots in another way, though. Strengthening muscles in a trouble area can help to improve their tone; stretching to gain flexibility can help with associated posture problems. Thus aerobic, strength, and flexibility workouts can improve fitness and physical appearance.

BEHAVIOR AND ATTITUDE

Behavior and attitude are important supporting factors to achieving and maintaining appropriate body weight and composition. Behavior modification changes the hundreds of small behaviors of overeating and underexercising that lead to, and perpetuate, obesity. Making these changes requires time and effort, so you must be prepared to invest in yourself. Furthermore, it is important to adopt the right attitude. Healthy eating and activity choices are not intolerable tasks that demand herculean willpower to achieve. They are an essential part of healthy living and should simply be incorporated into the day. "They are just things one has to do"[67]—much like brushing one's teeth or wearing a seat belt.

• Behavior change pointer: A record of diet and exercise habits reveals problem areas, the first step toward improving behaviors.

Becoming Aware of Behaviors   A person who is aware of all the behaviors that created a problem has a head start toward solving it. Thus the first step in changing behaviors is to record present eating and exercise behaviors (see Figure 9–6). Keeping a diary will help the individual identify behaviors that may need changing and establish a baseline against which to measure future progress.

Making Small Changes   Behavior-modification strategies encourage making many small changes in daily behaviors. Behavior-modification experts see each behavior as the second part of a three-part sequence. Its antecedents precede it, and its consequences follow it:

$$A \text{ (antecedents)} \rightarrow B \text{ (behavior)} \leftrightarrow C \text{ (consequences)}$$

behavior modification: the changing of behavior by the manipulation of *antecedents* (cues or environmental factors that trigger behavior), the *behavior* itself, and *consequences* (the penalties or rewards attached to behavior).

Figure 9–6

Food Diary

The entries in a food diary should include the times and places of meals and snacks, the types and amounts of foods eaten, the persons present when food is eaten, and a description of the individual's feelings when eating. The diary should also record physical activities: the kind, the intensity level, the duration, and the person's feelings about them.

Time	Place	Activity or food eaten	People present	Mood
10:30–10:40	School vending machine	6 peanut butter crackers and 12 oz. cola	by myself	Starved
12:15–12:30	Restaurant	Sub sandwich and 12 oz. cola	friends	relaxed & friendly
3:00–3:45	Gym	Weight training	work out partner	tired
4:00–4:10	Snack bar	Small frozen yogurt	by myself	OK

A behavior occurs in response to antecedents (cues or stimuli); the more intense the antecedents are, the more likely the behavior will occur. The behavior in turn leads to consequences. The more intense these consequences are, positively or negatively, the more or less likely the behavior is to occur again.

Applying Behavior-Modification Strategies The box on pp. 308–309 shows how a person might apply behavior-modification strategies to a weight-control program. The strategies are designed to encourage the repeated occurrence of desired eating and exercise behaviors and to eliminate the occurrence of unwanted behaviors. A particularly attractive feature of these strategies is that they do not involve blaming oneself or putting oneself down—an important element in fostering self-esteem.

With so many possible behavior changes available, a person can choose where to begin. Start simply and don't try to master them all at once. Attempting too many changes at one time is never successful; a person must set priorities. Pick one trouble area that is manageable and start there. Practice a desired behavior until it is habitual and automatic. Then select another trouble area to work on, and so on. Another bit of advice along the same lines: don't try to tackle weight loss during a particularly stressful time of life.

Maintaining Weight Finally, be aware that it can be hard to maintain weight loss. Maintenance is only possible if the eating and activity behaviors that led to weight loss continue. If, on arriving at goal weight after months of self-discipline, the victorious weight loser "celebrates" by resuming old eating habits, then maintenance will not be successful.

Obesity is not "cured" by simply attaining a reasonable body weight; eating wisely and staying active must continue to be part of life's daily routines. Ongoing membership in a weight-control organization and regular, continued physical activity can provide indispensable support for the formerly overweight person who wants to remain trim.

• Behavior change pointer: Adopt permanent lifestyle changes to achieve and maintain a healthy weight.

Personal Attitude   Being overweight becomes a part of a person's identity. For many people, overeating and being overweight have become integral aspects of their lives, involving social, marital, and family relationships; community activities; work; health; self-concept; and emotional states. Changing diet and exercise behaviors without attention to a person's self-concept invites failure. People who fully understand their personal relationships with food are best prepared to make healthful changes in eating and exercise behaviors.

Sometimes habitual behaviors that are hazardous to health, such as smoking or drinking alcohol, contribute positively by helping people adapt to stressful situations. Similarly, many people overeat to cope with the stresses of life. To break out of that pattern, they must first identify the particular stressors that trigger the urge to overeat. Then, when faced with these situations, they must learn and practice problem-solving skills. These skills will help them to respond appropriately to difficult situations.

All this is not to imply that psychological therapy holds the magic answer to a weight problem. Still, efforts to improve one's general well-being may result in weight control even when weight loss is not the primary goal. When the problems that trigger the urge to overeat are dealt with in alternative ways, people may find they eat less and that their eating behavior begins to respond appropriately to internal cues of hunger rather than inappropriately to external signals of stress. Sound emotional health supports a person's ability to take care of health in all ways—including nutrition, weight control, and fitness.

- Behavior change pointer: Learn alternative ways to deal with emotions and stresses.

Self-esteem underlies emotional health and facilitates personal growth. Overweight people who have low self-esteem can learn to feel better about themselves even before they lose the first pound. A person can enhance self-esteem by fostering a positive view of the inner self and by developing a healthy relationship with the outer self, the body. To view the inner self positively, practice positive thinking, make affirmative statements about oneself, and visualize success. People who believe they can lose weight are more successful at losing weight than those who expect to fail; people who view themselves as "physically fit" are more successful at maintaining weight loss than those who view themselves as "fat" or even as "formerly fat."

- Behavior change pointer: Use positive self-talk—"You can do it!"

- Behavior change pointer: Believe that you can succeed in spite of past failures.

Support Groups   Group support is important when making life changes. Some people find it helpful to join a group that provides support in efforts to lose weight, such as Take Off Pounds Sensibly (TOPS), Weight Watchers (WW), Overeaters Anonymous (OA), or others. A modest expenditure for health is well worthwhile, but people need to avoid rip-offs, of course; review the box on p. 296 for help in identifying unsound weight-loss schemes. Many dieters find it helpful to form their own self-help groups.

- Behavior change pointer: Attend support groups regularly or develop supportive relationships with others.

HEALTHY PEOPLE 2000: Increase to at least 50% the proportion of worksites with 50 or more employees that offer nutrition education and/or weight management programs for employees.

A surefire remedy for obesity has yet to be found, although many people find a combination of the approaches just described to be most effective. Diet and exercise shift energy balance so that more energy is being spent than is taken in. The

How to Apply Behavior-Modification Strategies to Weight Loss

1. To eliminate inappropriate eating cues:
   - Buy foods that are low in fat.
   - Shop when you are not hungry.
   - Serve low-fat meals.
   - Let other family members buy, store, and serve their own sweets (monitor children's intakes).
   - Change channels or look away when food commercials appear on television.
   - Shop only from a list and stay away from convenience stores.
   - Carry appropriate snacks from home and avoid vending machines.

2. To suppress the cues you cannot eliminate:
   - Eat only in one place (at a table), and in one room; use plates, bowls, and eating utensils.
   - Clear plates directly into the garbage.
   - Create obstacles to the eating of problem foods (for example, make it necessary to unwrap, cook, and serve each one separately).
   - Minimize contact with excessive food (serve individual plates, don't put serving dishes on the table, and leave or clean the table when you have finished eating).
   - Make small portions of food look large by spreading food out and serving on small plates.
   - Control deprivation (eat regular meals, don't skip meals, avoid getting tired, avoid boredom by keeping cues to fun activities in sight).

3. To strengthen the cues to appropriate eating and exercise:
   - Encourage others to eat appropriate foods with you.
   - Keep your favorite appropriate foods in the front of the refrigerator.

physical activity maintains or even builds the lean body so that fat is preferentially lost and metabolic energy needs remain high. The behavior modification retrains habits so that once the weight is lost, it will not return; and the improvement in inner self helps a person to manage life without a dependency on food. This treatment package requires time, individualization, and sometimes the assistance of skilled health care professionals.

Underweight

Reminder: *Underweight* is a body weight so low as to have adverse health effects; it is generally defined as 10% or more below the standard or BMI <20.

Underweight is a far less prevalent problem than overweight, affecting no more than 10 percent of U.S. adults. Whether the underweight person needs to gain weight is a question of health and, like weight loss, a highly individual matter. People who are healthy at their present weights may stay there; those who are at risk for malnutrition and illness should try to gain. Medical advice can help make the distinction.

- Learn appropriate portion sizes and prepare one portion at a time.
- Establish specific times for meals and snacks.
- Prepare foods attractively.
- Keep your walking shoes (ski poles, tennis racket) by the door.

4. To engage in desired eating or exercise behaviors:
   - Eat only at planned times; plan not to eat after a specified time (say, 7:00 or 8:00 P.M.).
   - Slow down (pause several times during a meal, put down utensils between mouthfuls, chew thoroughly before swallowing, swallow before reloading the fork, always use utensils).
   - Leave some food on the plate.
   - Engage in no other activities while eating (such as reading or watching television).
   - Move more (shake a leg, pace, fidget, flex your muscles).
   - Join in and exercise with a group of active people.

5. To arrange or emphasize negative consequences of inappropriate eating:
   - Eat your meals with other people.
   - Ask that others respond neutrally when you deviate from your plan (make no comment). This is a negative consequence because it withholds attention.
   - If you slip, don't punish yourself.

6. To arrange or emphasize positive consequences of appropriate behaviors:
   - Update records of food intake, exercise, and weight change regularly.
   - Arrange for rewards for each unit of behavior change or weight loss.
   - Ask family and friends for reinforcement (praise and encouragement).

Some people are unalterably thin by reason of heredity or early physical influences. They may find gaining weight difficult. People who wish to gain weight for appearance's sake or to improve their athletic performance need to be aware that healthful weight gains can be achieved only by physical conditioning combined with high energy intakes. On a high-kcalorie diet alone, a person will gain weight, but it will be mostly fat. Even if the gain improves appearance, it can be as detrimental to health as being slightly underweight. For an athlete, such a weight gain might impair performance. Therefore, in weight gain, as in weight loss, physical activity and energy intake are essential components of a sound plan.

PROBLEMS OF UNDERWEIGHT

The causes of underweight may be as diverse as those of overweight—hunger, appetite, and satiety irregularities; psychological traits; metabolic factors; and hereditary tendencies. Habits learned early in childhood, especially food aversions, may perpetuate themselves.

The demand for energy to support physical activity and growth often contributes to underweight. An active, growing boy may need more than 4000 kcalories a day to maintain his weight and may be too busy to take time to eat. Underweight people find it hard to gain weight—due, in part, to their expenditure of energy in adaptive thermogenesis. So much energy may be spent adapting to a higher food intake that at first as many as 750 to 800 extra kcalories a day may be needed to gain a pound a week. Like those who want to lose weight, people who want to gain must learn new habits and learn to like new foods. They are also similarly vulnerable to potentially harmful schemes and would be wise to review the consumer bill of rights on p. 294, using the term "weight gain" instead of "weight loss" where appropriate.

WEIGHT-GAIN STRATEGIES

Weight-gain strategies center on eating foods that provide many kcalories in a small volume and exercising to build muscle. Conventional advice to the bodybuilder is to eat enough foods to provide about 700 to 1000 kcalories a day above normal energy needs and to exercise to build lean tissue.

Energy-Dense Foods   Energy-dense foods (the very ones eliminated from a successful weight-loss diet) hold the key to weight gain. Pick the highest-kcalorie items from each food group—that is, milk shakes instead of nonfat milk, salmon instead of snapper, avocados instead of cucumbers, a cup of grape juice instead of a small apple, and whole-wheat muffins instead of whole-wheat bread. Because fat contains more than twice as many kcalories per teaspoon as sugar does, fat adds kcalories without adding much bulk.

Be aware that a low-fat diet plan is recommended because the general U.S. population is overweight and at risk for heart disease. Consumption of high-fat foods is not healthy for most people, but may be essential for an underweight individual who needs to gain weight. An underweight person who is physically active and eating a nutritionally adequate diet can afford a few extra kcalories from fat. For health's sake, it would be wise to select monounsaturated and polyunsaturated fats instead of those with saturated fats: for example, sautéing vegetables in olive oil instead of butter.

Regular Meals Daily   People who are underweight need to make meals a priority and take the time to plan, prepare, and eat each meal. They should eat at least three healthy meals every day and learn to eat more food within the first 20 minutes of a meal. Another suggestion is to eat meaty appetizers or the main course first and leave the soup or salad until later.

Large Portions   It is also important to learn to eat more food at each meal. Put extra slices of ham and cheese on the sandwich for lunch, drink milk from a larger glass, and eat cereal from a larger bowl.

The person should expect to feel full. Most underweight individuals are accustomed to small quantities of food. When they begin eating significantly more, they feel uncomfortable. This is normal and passes over time.

Extra Snacks   Since a substantially higher energy intake is needed each day, in addition to eating more food at each meal, it is necessary to eat more fre-

- Weight-gain pointer: Expect weight gain to take time (1 pound per month would be reasonable).

- Weight-gain pointer: Eat energy-dense foods regularly.

- Weight-gain pointer: Eat at least three meals a day.

- Weight-gain pointer: Eat large portions of foods and expect to feel full.

quently. Between-meal snacking offers a solution. For example, a student might make three sandwiches in the morning and eat them between classes in addition to the day's three regular meals.

Juice and Milk   Beverages provide an easy way to increase energy intake. Consider that 6 cups of cranberry juice add almost 1000 kcalories to the day's intake. kCalories can be added to milk by mixing in powdered milk or packets of instant breakfast.

For people who are underweight due to illness, concentrated liquid formulas are often recommended because a weak person can swallow them easily. A physician or registered dietitian can recommend high-protein, high-kcalorie formulas to help the underweight person maintain or gain. Used in addition to regular meals, these can help considerably.

Exercising to Build Muscles   To gain weight, use strength training primarily and increase energy intake to support that exercise. Eating extra food will then support a gain of both muscle and fat.

In theory, it takes an excess of about 2000 to 2500 kcalories to support the gain of a pound of pure lean tissue.[68] The rate at which the body can build muscle tissue also depends on the person. Men and women have mixtures of both male and female hormones; people with more male hormones build muscle more easily than others, but it is not known what the limits are. (Taking anabolic steroids to stimulate muscle bulking is a dangerous and illegal practice.) About 700 to 1000 kcalories a day above normal energy needs is enough to support both the exercise and the building of muscle.

The problem of underweight is less prevalent than overweight. To gain weight, a person must train physically and increase energy intake by selecting energy-dense foods, eating regular meals, taking larger portions, and consuming extra snacks and beverages.

An extreme underweight condition known as anorexia nervosa is sometimes seen in people who employ heroic self-denial in order to control their weight. They go to such extremes that they become severely undernourished, achieving final body weights of 70 pounds or even less. The distinguishing feature of a person with anorexia nervosa, as opposed to other underweight people, is that the starvation is intentional. Anorexia nervosa is a major eating disorder seen in our society today. Another is bulimia nervosa—compulsive overeating and purging. Eating disorders are the subject of the highlight that follows this chapter.

- Weight-gain pointer: Eat snacks between meals.

- Weight-gain pointer: Drink plenty of juice and milk.

- Weight-gain pointer: Exercise and eat to build muscles.

Study Questions

1. What factors contribute to obesity?
2. List several ill-advised ways to lose weight and explain why such methods are not recommended.
3. Discuss dietary strategies suitable for achieving and maintaining a healthy body weight.
4. What are the benefits of increased physical activity in a weight-loss program?
5. Describe the behavior-modification techniques recommended for changing an individual's dietary habits. What role does personal attitude play?
6. Describe strategies for successful weight gain.

Notes

1. R. J. Kuczmarski and coauthors, Increasing prevalence of overweight among US adults: The National Health and Nutrition Examination Surveys, 1960 to 1991, *Journal of the American Medical Association* 272 (1994): 205–211; Data from the 1988–1991 National Health and Nutrition Examination Survey (NHANES III) as reported in National Heart, Lung, and Blood Institute Obesity Education Summary Report, September 1994; Prevalence of overweight among adolescents— United States, 1988–1991, *Morbidity and Mortality Weekly Report* 43 (1994): 818–821.

2. NIH Technology Assessment Conference Panel, Methods for voluntary weight loss and control, *Annals of Internal Medicine* 116 (1992): 942–949.

3. G. A. Bray, An approach to the classification and evaluation of obesity, in *Obesity*, eds. P. Björntorp and B. N. Brodoff (Philadelphia: J. B. Lippincott, 1992), pp. 294–308.

4. G. Ailhaud, P. Grimaldi, and R. Négrel, Cellular and molecular aspects of adipose tissue development, *Annual Review of Nutrition* 12 (1992): 207–233.

5. A. J. Stunkard and coauthors, The body-mass index of twins who have been reared apart, *New England Journal of Medicine* 322 (1990): 1483–1487.

6. C. Bouchard, The response to long-term overfeeding in identical twins, *New England Journal of Medicine* 322 (1990): 1477–1482.

7. E. Ravussin and C. Bogardus, A brief overview of human energy metabolism and its relationship to essential obesity, *American Journal of Clinical Nutrition* 55 (1992): 242S–245S.

8. Y. Zhang and coauthors, Positional cloning of the mouse *obese* gene and its human homologue, *Nature* 372 (1994): 425–431.

9. R. H. Eckel, Lipoprotein lipase regulation in obesity and after weight loss, an address presented at the North American Association for the Study of Obesity and Emory University School of Medicine conference on Obesity Update: Pathophysiology, Clinical Consequences, and Therapeutic Options, Atlanta, Georgia, August 31–September 2, 1992.

10. P. A. Kern and coauthors, The effects of weight loss on the activity and expression of adipose-tissue lipoprotein lipase in very obese humans, *New England Journal of Medicine* 322 (1990): 1053–1059.

11. R. L. Leibel, M. Rosenbaum, and J. Hirsch, Changes in energy expenditure resulting from altered body weight, *New England Journal of Medicine* 332 (1995): 621–628; P. Pasquet and M. Apfelbaum, Recovery of initial body weight and composition after long-term massive overfeeding in men, *American Journal of Clinical Nutrition* 60 (1994): 861–863.

12. Committee on Diet and Health, *Diet and Health: Implications for Reducing Chronic Disease Risk* (Washington, D.C.: National Academy Press, 1989), p. 144.

13. E. Danforth and E. A. H. Sims, Obesity and efforts to lose weight, *New England Journal of Medicine* 327 (1992): 1947–1948.

14. S. W. Lichtman and coauthors, Discrepancy between self-reported and actual caloric intake and exercise in obese subjects, *New England Journal of Medicine* 327 (1992): 1893–1898.

15. A. Laws, Actual versus self-reported intake and exercise in obesity (letter), *New England Journal of Medicine* 328 (1993): 1494–1495.

16. Lichtman and coauthors, 1992.

17. G. B. Forbes, Diet and exercise in obese subjects: Self-report versus controlled measurements, *Nutrition Reviews* 51 (1993): 296–300.

18. R. Rising and coauthors, Determinants of total daily energy expenditure: Variability in physical activity, *American Journal of Clinical Nutrition* 59 (1994): 800–804.

19. A. P. Simopoulos, Characteristics of obesity, in *Obesity*, eds. P. Björntorp and B. N. Brodoff (Philadelphia: J. B. Lippincott, 1992), pp. 309–319.

20. S. L. Gortmaker, W. H. Dietz, Jr., and L. W. Y. Cheung, Inactivity, diet, and the fattening of America, *Journal of the American Dietetic Association* 90 (1990): 1247–1255; E. Obarzanek and coauthors, Energy intake and physical activity in relation to indexes of body fat: The National Heart, Lung, and Blood Institute Growth and Health study, *American Journal of Clinical Nutrition* 60 (1994): 15–22.

21. R. C. Klesges, M. L. Shelton, and L. M. Klesges, Effects of television on metabolic rate: Potential implications for childhood obesity, *Pediatrics* 91 (1993): 281–286.

22. W. H. Dietz, Jr., and S. L. Gortmaker, Do we fatten our children at the television set? Obesity and television viewing in children and adolescents, *Pediatrics* 75 (1985): 807–812.

23. NIH Technology Assessment Conference Panel, 1992.

24. R. L. Atkinson and V. S. Hubbard, Report on the NIH Workshop on Pharmacologic Treatment of Obesity, *American Journal of Clinical Nutrition* 60 (1994): 153–156; F. M. Kramer and coauthors, Long-term follow-up of behavioral treatment for obesity: Patterns of weight regain among men and women, *International Journal of Obesity* 13 (1989): 123–136; T. A. Wadden and coauthors, Treatment of obesity by very low calorie diet, behavior therapy, and their combination: A five year prospective, *International Journal of Obesity* (supplement) 13 (1989): 39–46.

25. S. L. Gortmaker and coauthors, Social and economic consequences of overweight in adolescence and young adulthood, *New England Journal of Medicine* 329 (1993): 1008–1012.

26. A. J. Stunkard and T. A. Wadden, Psychological aspects of human obesity, in *Obesity*, eds. P. Björntorp and B. N. Brodoff (Philadelphia: J. B. Lippincott, 1992), pp. 352–360.

27. H. Oberrieder and coauthors, Attitude of dietetics students and registered dietitians toward obesity, *Journal of the Ameri-*

can Dietetic Association 95 (1995): 914–915; A. J. Stunkard and T. I. A. Sørensen, Obesity and socioeconomic status—A complex relation, *New England Journal of Medicine* 329 (1993): 1036–1037.

28. J. A. Cassell, Social anthropology and nutrition: A different look at obesity in America, *Journal of the American Dietetic Association* 95 (1995): 424–427.

29. L. V. Sjöström, Mortality of severely obese subjects, *American Journal of Clinical Nutrition* 55 (1992): 516S–523S.

30. J. S. Garrow, Treatment of obesity, *The Lancet* 340 (1992): 409–413.

31. R. J. Garrison, Healthy adiposity in women: The Framingham Offspring Study, *Journal of the American College of Nutrition* 12 (1993): 357–362.

32. K. A. Petersmarck, The Michigan approach: Building consensus for safe weight loss, *Journal of the American Dietetic Association* 92 (1992): 679–680.

33. FTC accuses five diet programs of deceptive advertising, *FDA Consumer*, December 1993, p. 3.

34. Committee to Develop Criteria for Evaluating the Outcomes of Approaches to Prevent and Treat Obesity, Food and Nutrition Board, Institute of Medicine, National Academy of Sciences, *Journal of the American Dietetic Association* 95 (1995): 96–105; T. A. Wadden and coauthors, A multicenter evaluation of a proprietary weight reduction program for the treatment of marked obesity, *Archives of Internal Medicine* 152 (1992): 961–966.

35. G. Haus and coauthors, Key modifiable factors in weight maintenance: Fat intake, exercise, and weight cycling, *Journal of the American Dietetic Association* 94 (1994): 409–413.

36. K. van der Kooy and coauthors, Effect of a weight cycle on visceral fat accumulation, *American Journal of Clinical Nutrition* 58 (1993): 853–857; A. M. Prentice and coauthors, Effects of weight cycling on body composition, *American Journal of Clinical Nutrition* 56 (1992): 209S–216S; L. Lissner and coauthors, Variability of body weight and health outcomes in the Framingham population, *New England Journal of Medicine* 324 (1991): 1839–1844; L. Lissner and K. D. Brownell, Weight cycling, mortality, and cardiovascular disease: A review of epidemiologic findings, in *Obesity*, eds. P. Björntorp and B. N. Brodoff (Philadelphia: J. B. Lippincott, 1992), pp. 653–661.

37. National Task Force on the Prevention and Treatment of Obesity, Weight cycling, *Journal of the American Medical Association* 272 (1994): 1196–1202; Garrow, 1992.

38. E. S. Parham, Applying a philosophy of nutrition education to weight control, *Journal of Nutrition Education* 22 (1990): 194–197.

39. S. C. Wooley and D. M. Garner, Obesity treatment: The high cost of false hope, *Journal of the American Dietetic Association* 91 (1991): 1248–1251.

40. G. A. Bray, Drug treatment of obesity, *American Journal of Clinical Nutrition* 55 (1992): 538S–544S; A. Astrup and coau-

thors, The effect of ephedrine/caffeine mixture on energy expenditure and body composition in obese women, *Metabolism: Clinical and Experimental* 41 (1992): 686–688.

41. C. D. Berdanier, Dehydroepiandrosterone (DHEA): Useful or useless as an antiobesity agent? *Nutrition Today*, November/December 1993, pp. 34–38.

42. Berdanier, 1993.

43. FDA approves obesity pill, *Journal of the American Dietetic Association* 96 (1996): 748; S. Heshka, Dexfenfluramine for the long-term management of obesity, in *Obesity: New Directions in Assessment and Management*, eds. T. B. VanItallie and A. P. Simopoulos (Philadelphia: The Charles Press, 1995), pp. 227–233; M. M. Kogon and coauthors, Psychological and metabolic effects of dietary carbohydrates and dexfenfluramine during a low-energy diet in obese women, *American Journal of Clinical Nutrition* 60 (1994): 488–493; Dexfenfluramine influences dietary compliance and eating behaviors of obese subjects, *Nutrition Reviews* 52 (1994): 65–68; L. M. H. Mathus-Vliegen and A. M. A. Res, Dexfenfluramine influences dietary compliance and eating behavior, but dietary instruction may overrule its effect on food selection in obese subjects, *Journal of the American Dietetic Association* 93 (1993): 1163–1165; N. Finer, F. Finer, and P. Naoumova, Drug therapy after very-low-calorie diets, *American Journal of Clinical Nutrition* 56 (1992): 195S–198S.

44. R. L. Atkinson, Treatment of obesity (editorial), *Nutrition Reviews* 50 (1992): 338–345.

45. D. J. Goldstein and J. H. Potvin, Long-term weight loss: The effect of pharmacologic agents, *American Journal of Clinical Nutrition* 60 (1994): 647–657.

46. D. E. Schteingart, Phenylpropanolamine in the management of moderate obesity, in *Obesity: New Directions in Assessment and Management*, eds. T. B. VanItallie and A. P. Simopoulos (Philadelphia: The Charles Press, 1995), pp. 220–226.

47. Gastrointestinal surgery for severe obesity: National Institutes of Health Consensus Development Conference Statement, *American Journal of Clinical Nutrition* 55 (1992): 615S–619S.

48. Gastrointestinal surgery for severe obesity, 1992.

49. Gastrointestinal surgery for severe obesity, 1992; W. J. Pories, Surgical approaches to the treatment of the morbidly obese, an address presented at the North American Association for the Study of Obesity and Emory University School of Medicine conference on Obesity Update: Pathophysiology, Clinical Consequences, and Therapeutic Options, Atlanta, Georgia, August 31–September 2, 1992.

50. A. M. C. Macgregor and C. S. W. Rand, Gastric surgery in morbid obesity: Outcome in patients aged 55 years and older, *Archives of Surgery* 128 (1993): 1153–1157.

51. National Task Force on the Prevention and Treatment of Obesity, *Journal of the American Medical Association* 270 (1993): 967–974.

52. G. D. Foster and coauthors, A controlled comparison of three very-low-calorie diets: Effects on weight, body composition,

and symptoms, *American Journal of Clinical Nutrition* 55 (1992): 811–817.

53. T. A. Wadden, T. B. VanItallie, and G. L. Blackburn, Responsible and irresponsible use of very-low-calorie diets in the treatment of obesity, *Journal of the American Medical Association* 263 (1990): 83–85.

54. National Task Force on the Prevention and Treatment of Obesity, 1993; A. C. Shovic and coauthors, Effectiveness and dropout rate of a very-low-calorie diet program, *Journal of the American Dietetic Association* 93 (1993): 583–584.

55. F. Froidevaux and coauthors, Energy expenditure in obese women before and during weight loss, after refeeding, and in the weight-relapse period, *American Journal of Clinical Nutrition* 57 (1993): 35–42.

56. F. X. Pi-Sunyer, The role of very-low-calorie diets in obesity, *American Journal of Clinical Nutrition* 56 (1992): 240S–243S.

57. J. A. Kanaley and coauthors, Differential health benefits of weight loss in upper-body and lower-body obese women, *American Journal of Clinical Nutrition* 57 (1993): 20–26.

58. J. P. Foreyt and G. K. Goodrick, Weight management without dieting, *Nutrition Today,* March/April 1993, pp. 4–9.

59. M. Shah and coauthors, Comparison of a low-fat ad libitum complex-carbohydrate diet with a low-energy diet in moderately obese women, *American Journal of Clinical Nutrition* 59 (1994): 980–984.

60. L. Lissner, Dietary fat and the regulation of energy intake in human subjects, *American Journal of Clinical Nutrition* 46 (1987): 886–892; A. Kendall and coauthors, Weight loss on a low-fat diet: Consequences of the imprecision of the control of food intake in humans, *American Journal of Clinical Nutrition* 53 (1991): 1124–1129; L. Sheppard, A. R. Kristal, and L. H. Kushi, Weight loss in women participating in a randomized trial of low-fat diets, *American Journal of Clinical Nutrition* 54 (1991): 821–828.

61. C. N. Boozer, A. Brasseur, and R. L. Atkinson, Dietary fat affects weight loss and adiposity during energy restriction in rats, *American Journal of Clinical Nutrition* 58 (1993): 846–852.

62. Sheppard, Kristal, and Kushi, 1991; T. E. Prewitt and coauthors, Changes in body weight, body composition, and energy intake in women fed high- and low-fat diets, *American Journal of Clinical Nutrition* 54 (1991): 304–310.

63. R. Ross, H. Pedwell, and J. Rissanen, Effects of energy restriction and exercise on skeletal muscle and adipose tissue in women as measured by magnetic resonance imaging, *American Journal of Clinical Nutrition* 61 (1995): 1179–1185; S. B. Racette and coauthors, Effects of aerobic exercise and dietary carbohydrate on energy expenditure and body composition during weight reduction in obese women, *American Journal of Clinical Nutrition* 61 (1995): 486–494; D. D. Hensrud and coauthors, A prospective study of weight maintenance in obese subjects reduced to normal body weight without weight-loss training, *American Journal of Clinical Nutrition* 60 (1994): 688–694; Haus and coauthors, 1994; S. Kayman, W. Bruvold, and J. S. Stern, Maintenance and relapse after weight loss in women: Behavioral aspects, *American Journal of Clinical Nutrition* 52 (1990): 800–807.

64. S. B. Racette and coauthors, Exercise enhances dietary compliance during moderate energy restriction in obese women, *American Journal of Clinical Nutrition* 62 (1995): 345–349.

65. M. Grediagin and coauthors, Exercise intensity does not effect body composition change in untrained, moderately overfat women, *Journal of the American Dietetic Association* 95 (1995): 661–665.

66. J. P. Flatt, Biochemistry of energy expenditure, in *Obesity,* eds. P. Björntorp and B. N. Brodoff (Philadelphia: J. B. Lippincott, 1992), pp. 100–116.

67. Garrow, 1992.

68. W. D. McArdle, F. I. Katch, and V. L. Katch, *Exercise Physiology: Energy, Nutrition, and Human Performance,* 2nd ed. (Philadelphia: Lea & Febiger, 1991), pp. 634–655.

Eating Disorders—Anorexia Nervosa and Bulimia Nervosa

For some people, dieting to lose weight progresses to a dangerous and obsessive point. An estimated 2 million people in the United States, primarily girls and young women, suffer from the eating disorders anorexia nervosa and bulimia nervosa (the glossary on p. 316 defines these and related terms). Many more do not meet the specific criteria that define these disorders but have "dieted" to the point of endangering health. Psychologists refer to these cases as "eating disorders not otherwise specified."[1]

Why do so many people in our society suffer from these disorders? Some researchers speculate that our society's excessive pressure to be thin is to blame. By making thinness the ideal, society pushes people to view normal healthy body weight as fat. Then healthy people who perceive themselves as fat adopt unhealthy eating behaviors to battle this imaginary problem. Some researchers have uncovered neurological links with depression and impulsive behaviors, and still others believe the cause to be an inability to cope. They agree that the disorders are most likely multifactorial and that treatment requires a multidisciplinary approach that addresses two sets of issues and behaviors: those relating to food and weight and those involving relationships with oneself and others.[2] The nutrition component of treatment requires both dietary intervention and education.

ANOREXIA NERVOSA

Julie is 18 years old. She is a super-achiever in school and a fine

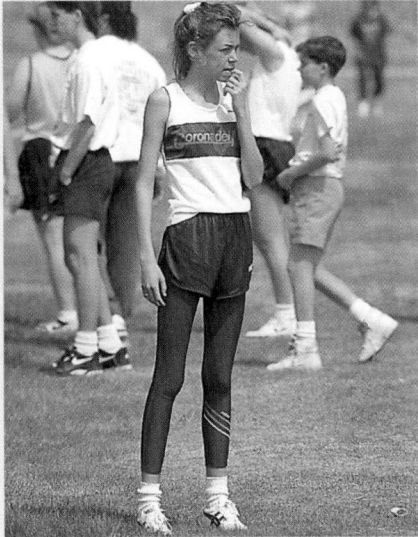

People with anorexia nervosa see themselves as fat, even when they are dangerously underweight.

dancer. She watches her diet with great care, and she exercises and practices ballet daily, maintaining a heroic schedule of self-discipline. She is thin, but she is not satisfied with her weight and is determined to lose more. She is 5 feet 6 inches tall and weighs 85 pounds. She has anorexia nervosa.

Julie is unaware that she is undernourished, and she sees no need to obtain treatment. She stopped menstruating (developed amenorrhea) several months ago and has become moody and easily depressed. She insists that she is too fat, although her eyes are sunk in deep hollows in her face. She has recently been told by her dance master that her performance is not up to her potential; she blames this on a stress fracture that is slow to heal.[3] Julie denies that she is ever tired, although she is close to physical exhaustion, and she no longer

sleeps easily. Her family is concerned, and though reluctant to push her, they have finally insisted that she see a psychiatrist. Julie's psychiatrist has diagnosed anorexia nervosa and prescribed group therapy as a start, but warns that if she does not begin to gain weight soon she will need to be hospitalized.

Characteristics of Anorexia Nervosa

Most people with anorexia nervosa are women and girls from educated, middle- or upper-class families. Men account for only about 5 to 10 percent of cases, although many more report that their most powerful fear is of gaining weight or becoming fat.[4] Among male athletes and dancers, eating disorders are much more common, possibly equaling the incidence among their female peers.[5] Athletes, in general, seem to be vulnerable to eating disorders.[6] To succeed in competition, athletes must often meet stringent weight requirements. Competitors often report being terrified of becoming fat, being obsessed with food, and using laxatives in an attempt to control weight.[7] Ballet dancers, jockeys, wrestlers, distance runners, gymnasts, and others whose body weight and appearance are frequently judged in comparison with an "ideal" are especially prone to develop problems.

Coaches, trainers, and especially parents contribute to eating disorders.[8] Such authority figures are likely to be critical and to overvalue outward appearances while undervaluing inner self-esteem. Family patterns often include parents who

Glossary

amenorrhea (ay-MEN-oh-REE-ah): the absence of or cessation of menstruation. *Primary amenorrhea* is menarche delayed beyond 16 years of age. *Secondary amenorrhea* is the absence of three to six consecutive menstrual cycles.

anorexia nervosa: an eating disorder characterized by a refusal to maintain a minimally normal body weight and a distortion in perception of body shape and weight, most commonly seen in teenage girls and young women.
  an = without
  orex = mouth
  nervos = of nervous origin

bulimia nervosa: an eating disorder characterized by repeated episodes of binge eating usually followed by self-induced vomiting, misuse of laxatives or diuretics, fasting, or excessive exercise.
  buli = ox

cathartic: a strong laxative.

eating disorder: a disturbance in eating behavior that jeopardizes a person's physical or psychological health.

emetic (em-ETT-ic): an agent that causes vomiting.

stress fractures: bone damage or breaks caused by stress on bone surfaces during exercise.

---

oppose one another's authority and vacillate between defending the anorexic child's behavior and condemning it, confusing the child and disrupting normal parental control.[9] In the extreme, parents may even be abusive. Julie is a perfectionist, and her parents expect perfection. She works hard to please her parents and identifies so strongly with their ideals and goals that she sometimes feels she has no identity of her own. She feels controlled by others, yet she earnestly desires to control her own destiny. When she does not eat, she gains control.

How can a person as thin as Julie continue to starve herself? Julie uses tremendous discipline to strictly limit her portions of low-kcalorie foods. She will deny her hunger, telling you how full she is after having eaten only a half-dozen carrot sticks. She can recite the kcalorie cost of dozens of foods and of as many exercises. If she feels that she has gained an ounce of weight, she runs or jumps rope until she is sure she has exercised it off. If she fears she has eaten too much, she takes laxatives to hasten the passage of food from her system. Her other ways of staying thin are so effective that she is unaware that laxatives have no effect on body fat. She is desperately hungry. In fact, she is starving, but she doesn't eat because her need for self-control dominates. Her obsession with dieting accelerates; the more weight she loses, the more she wants to lose.

Many people, on learning of this disorder, say they wish they had "a

People with anorexia nervosa may reluctantly eat small amounts of low-kcalorie foods.

touch" of it to get thin. They mistakenly think that people with anorexia nervosa feel no hunger. They also fail to comprehend the psychological and physical pain associated with the condition.

Central to the diagnosis of anorexia nervosa is a distorted body image that overestimates the person's own body fatness. When Julie looks at herself in the mirror, she sees her 85-pound body as fat. The more Julie overestimates her body size, the more resistant she is to treatment, and the more unwilling to examine her faulty values and misconceptions. Malnutrition itself is known to affect brain functioning and judgment in this way. Table H9–1 shows the criteria that professionals use to diagnose anorexia nervosa.

Anorexia nervosa cannot be self-diagnosed. Nearly everyone in our society is engaged in the pursuit of thinness, and denial runs high among people with anorexia nervosa. Some women have all the attitudes and behaviors associated with the condition, but without the weight loss.

Anorexia nervosa damages the body much as starvation does. In fact, after a few months, most people with anorexia nervosa have protein-energy malnutrition (PEM) that is similar to marasmus.[10] Victims are dying to be thin—quite literally. In young people, growth ceases and normal development falters. They lose so much lean tissue that basal metabolic rate slows, an effect that may remain even after treatment and regain of weight.[11]

In athletes, the loss of lean tissue affects physical performance unfavorably. Hormonal changes and nutrient deprivation compromise bone density and lead to stress fractures.[12] Losses of bone density are

Table H9–1

Criteria for Diagnosis of Anorexia Nervosa

A person with anorexia nervosa demonstrates the following:

A. Refusal to maintain body weight at or above a minimal normal weight for age and height (e.g., weight loss leading to maintenance of body weight less than 85% of that expected; or failure to make expected weight gain during period of growth, leading to body weight less than 85% of that expected).

B. Intense fear of gaining weight or becoming fat, even though underweight.

C. Disturbance in the way in which one's body weight or shape is experienced, undue influence of body weight or shape on self-evaluation, or denial of the seriousness of the current low body weight.

D. In females past puberty, amenorrhea, i.e., the absence of at least three consecutive menstrual cycles. (A woman is considered to have amenorrhea if her periods occur only following hormone, e.g., estrogen, administration.)

Two types:

Restricting type: During the episode of anorexia nervosa, the person does not regularly engage in binge eating or purging behavior (i.e., self-induced vomiting or the misuse of laxatives, diuretics, or enemas).

Binge eating/purging type: During the episode of anorexia nervosa, the person regularly engages in binge eating or purging behavior (i.e., self-induced vomiting or the misuse of laxatives, diuretics, or enemas).

Source: Reprinted with permission from the *Diagnostic and Statistical Manual of Mental Disorders,* 4th ed. (Washington, D.C.: American Psychiatric Association, 1994).

especially pronounced in female athletes who cease menstruating because of overtraining. In fact, eating disorders, premature bone loss, and irregular menstruation are a common triple threat to overtrained female athletes.[13] These three associated disorders are called "the female athlete triad" (see Figure H9–1).[14] The prevalence of amenorrhea among premenopausal women in the United States is about 2 to 5 percent overall, but among female athletes, it may be as high as 66 percent.[15] Contrary to previous notions, amenorrhea is *not* a normal adaptation to strenuous physical training: it is a symptom of something going wrong.[16] Amenorrhea is characterized by low blood estrogen, infertility, and bone mineral losses (see Highlight 12).

Starvation brings other physical consequences: the heart pumps inefficiently and irregularly, the heart muscle becomes weak and thin, the chambers diminish in size, and the blood pressure falls. Electrolytes that help to regulate heartbeat become unbalanced. Many deaths occur due to multiple organ system failure. Impaired immune response, anemia, and a loss of digestive functions worsen malnutrition. Peristalsis becomes sluggish, the stomach empties slowly, and the lining of the intestinal tract atrophies. The deteriorated GI tract fails to provide sufficient absorptive surfaces and digestive enzymes for handling any food the victim may eat. The pancreas slows its production of digestive enzymes. The person who resumes eating ample food

may have diarrhea, further worsening malnutrition.

Other effects of starvation include altered blood lipids, high blood vitamin A and vitamin E, low blood proteins, dry thin skin, abnormal nerve functioning, reduced bone density, low body temperature, low blood pressure, and the development of fine body hair (the body's attempt to keep warm). The electrical activity of the brain becomes abnormal, and insomnia is common. Both women and men lose their sex drives.

Women with anorexia nervosa develop amenorrhea (it is one of the diagnostic criteria). In one-third to one-half of all cases, that symptom precedes the weight loss.[17] Anorexia nervosa delays the onset of menstruation in young girls. Menstrual periods typically resume with recovery, although some women never restart even after they have gained weight. Should an underweight woman with anorexia nervosa become pregnant, she is likely to give birth to an underweight baby—and low-birthweight babies face many health problems (as Chapter 18 explains).[18]

Figure H9–1

The Female Athlete Triad

Eating Disorder
- Restrictive dieting (inadequate energy and nutrient intake)
- Overexercising
- Weight loss
- Lack of body fat

Osteoporosis
- Loss of calcium from bones

Amenorrhea
- Diminished hormones

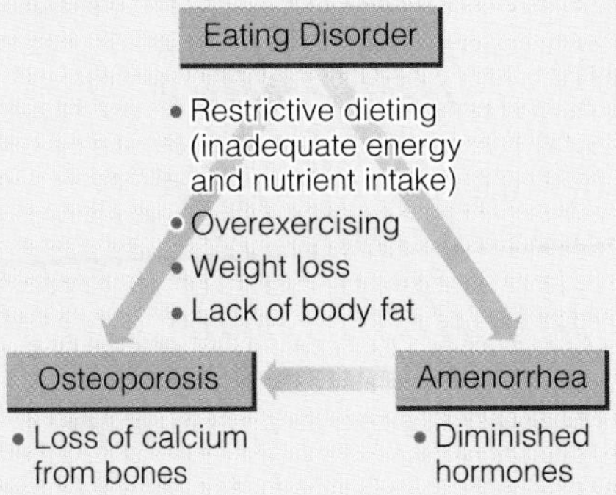

Table H9–2

Principles of Nutrition Intervention in Anorexia Nervosa

- Increase food energy intake slowly (adding 200 kcal/week).
- Prescribe well-balanced diets, with *some* individual variations according to client preferences (e.g., vegetarian).
- Give multiple vitamin-mineral supplements at RDA levels.
- Enhance elimination with dietary fiber from grain sources.
- Reduce sensations of bloating with small, frequent feedings.
- In behavioral programs, link rewards to food energy intake, not to weight gain.
- Use liquid supplements when the client cannot achieve desired intake with solid food.
- Reduce satiety sensations by offering cold or room-temperature foods and finger foods (e.g., snacks).
- Provide interactive nutrition counseling as an ongoing process.
- Reduce excessive caffeine intake.
- Provide parenteral nutritional support only in severe states of ill health, malnutrition, and wasting.

Source: Adapted from C. L. Rock and J. Yager, Nutrition and eating disorders: A primer for clinicians, *International Journal of Eating Disorders* 6 (1987): 276, as cited in *Nutrition and the M.D.*, July 1988, with permission. Reprinted with permission of John Wiley & Sons, Inc., copyright 1987.

Treatment in Anorexia Nervosa

Treatment artfully combines medical, psychosocial, and dietary facets to initiate and sustain weight gain with psychological techniques to resolve personal and family problems. Teams of physicians, nurses, psychiatrists, family therapists, and dietitians work together to treat people with anorexia nervosa.

The diet needs to be tailored individually to each client's needs; appropriate diet is crucial to recovery. Clients are seldom willing to feed themselves, but if they are, they may recover without other interventions. Table H9–2 (above) lists principles of nutrition intervention in anorexia nervosa.

Because anorexia nervosa is like starvation physically, health care professionals classify clients based on indicators of protein-energy malnutrition.* Low-risk clients need nutrition counseling. Intermediate-risk clients may need supplements such as high-kcalorie, high-protein formulas in addition to regular meals, but they may not have to be hospitalized. High-risk clients may requires hospitalization, and tube feeding may be necessary to forestall death. This step causes psychological trauma.[19] Drugs are commonly prescribed, but to date, they play a limited role in treatment.

The goals of treatment are simultaneously to facilitate weight gain

---

*Indicators of protein-energy malnutrition: a low percentage of body fat, low serum albumin, low serum transferrin, and impaired immune reactions.

and to resolve underlying personal and family problems. The first dietary objective is to stop weight loss while establishing regular eating patterns. The diet should include foods from each of the food groups, with portion sizes gradually increasing as energy intake increases. Because body weight is low and fear of weight gain is high, initial food intake may be small. At first, energy intake may be as low as whatever the person has become accustomed to, but ideally it will at least meet basal metabolic needs. As eating becomes more comfortable, energy intake should increase gradually. Vitamin and mineral supplements may be necessary to restore nutrient losses. Physicians and clients need to realize that weight gain may be difficult, especially during the first week of treatment, perhaps because the resting metabolic rate of people with anorexia nervosa is so high.[20]

Denial is so common among those with anorexia nervosa that few seek treatment on their own. Of those who are treated, about half recover fully.[21] They can maintain a healthy body weight, and many of the women begin menstruating again, although weight gain alone is not always sufficient in restoring menstruation.[22] The other half have poor or fair treatment outcomes, relapsing back into abnormal eating behaviors to some extent.[23] Over 10 percent of those treated for anorexia nervosa die—most commonly from starvation, electrolyte imbalance, or suicide.

Before drawing conclusions about someone who is extremely thin or who eats very little, remember that diagnosis and treatment require professional attention. People who are seeking help with anorexia nervosa, either for themselves or for others,

Table H9–3

Criteria for Diagnosis of Bulimia Nervosa

A person with bulimia nervosa demonstrates the following:

A. Recurrent episodes of binge eating. An episode of binge eating is characterized by both of the following:

    1. Eating, in a discrete period of time (e.g., within any two-hour period), an amount of food that is definitely larger than most people would eat during a similar period of time and under similar circumstances.

    2. A sense of lack of control over eating during the episode (e.g., a feeling that one cannot stop eating or control what or how much one is eating).

B. Recurrent inappropriate compensatory behavior in order to prevent weight gain, such as self-induced vomiting; misuse of laxatives, diuretics, enemas, or other medications; fasting; or excessive exercise.

C. Binge eating and inappropriate compensatory behaviors both occur, on average, at least twice a week for three months.

D. Self-evaluation unduly influenced by body shape and weight.

E. The disturbance does not occur exclusively during episodes of anorexia nervosa.

Two types:

    Purging type: The person regularly engages in self-induced vomiting or the misuse of laxatives, diuretics, or enemas.

    Nonpurging type: The person uses other inappropriate compensatory behaviors, such as fasting or excessive exercise, but does not regularly engage in self-induced vomiting or the misuse of laxatives, diuretics, or enemas.

Source: Reprinted with permission from *Diagnostic and Statistical Manual of Mental Disorders,* 4th ed. (Washington, D.C.: American Psychiatric Association, 1994).

can call the National Association of Anorexia Nervosa and Associated Disorders for information.*

BULIMIA NERVOSA

Kelly is a charming, intelligent, 20-year-old flight attendant of normal weight who thinks constantly about food. She alternates between starving herself and secretly binge eating; then, when she has eaten too much, she makes herself vomit. Few people would fail to recognize these symptoms as those of bulimia nervosa.

Bulimia nervosa is distinct from anorexia nervosa and is more prevalent, although the true incidence is difficult to establish because denial is equally common in this disease.[24] More men suffer from bulimia nervosa than from anorexia nervosa, but it is still more common in women.[25] The secretive nature of bulimic behaviors makes recognition of the problem difficult; once recognized, diagnosis is based on the criteria listed in Table H9–3.

Families of bulimic people often have unusually close emotional ties between members. They may be overcontrolling and intermeshed in ways that stifle individual growth and development.[26] If the member with bulimia nervosa begins taking steps toward recovery, others in the family may feel threatened. Changes in the family structure often meet with resistance, even if such changes would greatly benefit the person with bulimia nervosa. Additionally, the family may have secrets that are hidden from outsiders. Many people with bulimia nervosa report having been abused sexually or physically by family members or family friends.

Characteristics of Bulimia Nervosa

Like the typical person with bulimia nervosa, Kelly is single, female, and white. She is well educated and close to her ideal body weight, although her weight fluctuates 10 pounds or so—up and down—over a few weeks. As a flight attendant, she is required to "make weight"—that is, to weigh no more than a certain cutoff weight slightly below the weight that her body maintains naturally.

Kelly seldom lets her eating disorder interfere with work or other activities, although many bingers do. From early childhood she has been a high achiever and emotionally dependent on her parents. As a young teen, Kelly cycled on and off crash diets but could never maintain an appropriate weight. Kelly feels anxious at social events and cannot easily establish personal relationships. She is sometimes depressed and is often impulsive. Some people with bulimia nervosa abuse drugs, steal compulsively (kleptomania), or are sexually promiscuous.

Like the person with anorexia nervosa, the person with bulimia nervosa spends much time thinking about her body weight and food. Her preoccupation with food manifests itself in secretive binge-eating episodes, which usually progress

*Phone numbers and addresses are in Appendix F.

through several emotional stages: anticipation and planning, anxiety, urgency to begin, rapid and uncontrollable consumption of food, relief and relaxation, disappointment, and finally shame or disgust.

A bulimic binge is not like normal eating. It is not primarily a response to hunger; it is a compulsion to eat. Food is not consumed for its nutritional value. A typical binge occurs periodically, in secret, usually at night, and lasts an hour or more. A binge frequently follows a period of rigid dieting, so that eating is accelerated by hunger. During a binge, Kelly consumes thousands of kcalories of food. She typically chooses cookies, cakes, and ice cream—and she eats the entire bag of cookies, the whole cake, and every last spoonful of ice cream. These foods are easy-to-eat, low-fiber, smooth-textured, high-fat, and especially, high-carbohydrate foods. After the binge, Kelly pays the price with swollen hands and feet, bloating, fatigue, headache, nausea, and pain.

Binges are typically followed by self-induced vomiting, fasting, or the misuse of laxatives, diuretics, or

Figure H9–2

The Vicious Cycle of Restrictive Dieting and Binge Eating

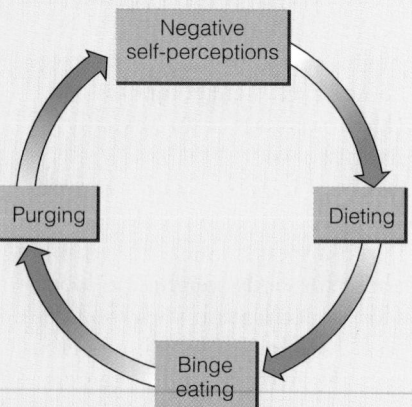

enemas. These purging behaviors are often accompanied by feelings of shame or guilt. Hence a vicious cycle develops: negative self-perceptions followed by dieting, bingeing, and purging, which in turn lead to negative self-perceptions (see Figure H9–2).[27] Bulimic behaviors often begin in late adolescence or early adulthood after a long series of various unsuccessful weight-reduction diets. People with bulimia nervosa commonly follow a pattern of restrictive dieting interspersed with binge eating and purging behaviors and experience weight fluctuations of more than 10 pounds up and down over short periods of time.

On first glance, purging seems to offer a quick and easy solution to the problems of unwanted kcalories and body weight. Many people perceive such behavior as neutral or even positive, when, in fact, binge eating and purging have serious physical consequences.[28] Signs of subclinical malnutrition are evident in a compromised immune system.[29] Fluid and electrolyte imbalance caused by vomiting or diarrhea can lead to abnormal heart rhythms and injury to the kidneys, which have to cope with the altered balance. Urinary tract infections can lead to kidney failure. Vomiting causes irritation and infection of the pharynx, esophagus, and salivary glands; ero-

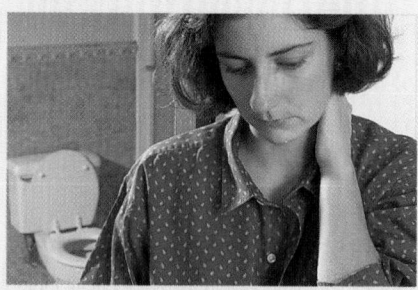

Bulimic binges are often followed by self-induced vomiting and feelings of shame or disgust.

sion of the teeth; and dental caries. The esophagus may rupture or tear, as may the stomach. Sometimes the eyes become red from pressure during vomiting. The hands may be bruised or cut by the teeth while inducing vomiting. Some people induce vomiting by using emetics—drugs that are intended as first aid for poisoning. Overuse of emetics can lead to heart failure. Others use cathartics—strong laxatives that can injure the lower intestinal tract.

Unlike Julie, Kelly is aware that her behavior is abnormal, and she is deeply ashamed of it. Feeling inadequate ("I can't even control my eating"), she tends to be passive and to look to others, primarily men, for confirmation of her sense of worth. When she is rejected either in reality or in her imagination, her bulimia nervosa becomes worse. Then Kelly's depression may deepen, and she may seek solace in drug or alcohol abuse.

Treatment in Bulimia Nervosa

The dietary goals of treatment are to help clients gain control over food, establish regular eating patterns, and restore nutritional health. Energy intake should not be severely restricted because restrictive weight-loss dieting is a strong trigger to binge. Rather than cyclic weight gains and losses, maintenance is a must for recovery. The person needs to learn to eat a quantity of nutritious food sufficient to nourish the body. Table H9–4 offers diet recommendations for the treatment of bulimia nervosa.

A mental health professional should be on the treatment team. Clinical depression is common in people with bulimia nervosa, and the rates of alcohol, marijuana, and cigarette abuse are high.[30] Some

Table H9–4
. . . .

Diet Recommendations for Bulimia Nervosa

- Avoid finger foods; eat foods that require the use of utensils.
- Enhance satiety by eating warm foods.
- Include vegetables, salad, and/or fruit at meals to prolong eating time.
- Choose whole-grain and high-fiber breads and cereals to maximize bulk.
- Eat a well-balanced diet and meals, consisting of a variety of foods.
- Use foods that are naturally divided into portions, such as potatoes (rather than rice or pasta); 4- and 8-ounce containers of yogurt or cottage cheese; precut steak or chicken parts; and frozen entreés.
- Include foods containing ample complex carbohydrates (for satiety) and some fat (to slow gastric emptying).
- Eat meals and snacks sitting down.
- Plan meals and snacks, and record plans in a food diary prior to eating.

Source: Adapted from C. L. Rock and J. Yager, Nutrition and eating disorders: A primer for clinicians, *International Journal of Eating Disorders* 6 (1987): 276, as cited in *Nutrition and the M.D.*, July 1988, with permission. Reprinted with permission of John Wiley & Sons, Inc., copyright 1987.

physicians prescribe the antidepressant drug fluoxetine in the treatment of bulimia nervosa.* Another drug that may be useful in the management of bulimia nervosa is naloxone, an opiate antagonist that suppresses the consumption of sweet and high-fat foods in binge-eaters.[31]

Anorexia nervosa and bulimia nervosa are distinct eating disorders, yet they sometimes overlap in important ways.[32] Victims of both disorders share an overconcern with body weight and the tendency to drastically undereat; many perceive foods as "forbidden" and "give in" to an eating binge. The two disorders can also appear in the same person, or one can lead to the other.

BINGE-EATING DISORDER

Cheryl is a 40-year-old schoolteacher who has been overweight

*Fluoxetine is marketed under the trade name Prozac.

all her life. Her friends and family are forever encouraging her to lose weight, and she has come to believe that if she only had more willpower, dieting would work. She periodically gives dieting her best shot—restricting energy intake for a day or two only to succumb to uncontrollable cravings, especially for high-fat foods. Like Cheryl, up to half of the obese people who try to lose weight periodically binge; unlike people with bulimia nervosa, however, they typically do not purge. Such an eating disorder does not meet the criteria for either anorexia nervosa or bulimia nervosa—yet such compulsive overeating is a problem. The 1994 American Psychiatric Association's manual includes binge eating under the category "eating disorders not otherwise specified." Table H9–5 (on p. 322) lists criteria for unspecified eating disorders, including binge eating. Obesity alone is not an eating disorder.

Clinicians note differences between people with bulimia nervosa and those with binge-eating disorder. People with binge-eating disorder consume less during a binge, rarely purge, and exert less restraint during times of dieting. Similarities also exist, including feeling out of control, disgusted, depressed, embarrassed, guilty, or distressed because of their self-perceived gluttony.[33]

There are also differences between obese binge-eaters and obese people who do not binge. Those with the binge-eating disorder report higher rates of self-loathing, disgust about body size, depression, and anxiety.[34] Their eating habits differ as well. Obese binge-eaters tend to consume more kcalories and more dessert and snack-type foods during regular meals and binges than obese people who do not binge.[35]

Binge eating is a behavioral disorder that can be resolved with treatment. Resolving such behavior may not bring weight loss, but it may make participation in weight-control programs easier. It also improves physical health, mental health, and the chances of success in breaking the cycle of rapid weight losses and gains.

EATING DISORDERS IN SOCIETY

Eating disorders have complex causes. A person's psychological problems develop within the context of society. Proof that society plays a role in eating disorders is found in their demographic distribution—they are known only in developed nations, and they become more prevalent as wealth increases and food becomes plentiful.

Some people point to the vomitoriums of ancient times and claim

Table H9–5

Unspecified Eating Disorders, including Binge Eating Disorder

Criteria for Diagnosis of Unspecified Eating Disorders, in General

Many people have eating disorders but do not meet all the criteria to be classified as having anorexia nervosa or bulimia nervosa. Some examples include those who:

A. Meet all of the criteria for anorexia nervosa, except irregular menses.

B. Meet all of the criteria for anorexia nervosa, except that their current weights fall within the normal ranges.

C. Meet all of the criteria for bulimia nervosa, except that binges occur less frequently than stated in the criteria.

D. Are of normal body weight and who compensate inappropriately for eating small amounts of food (example: self-induced vomiting after eating two cookies).

E. Repeatedly chew food, but spit it out without swallowing.

F. Have recurrent episodes of binge eating but who do not compensate as do those with bulimia nervosa.

Criteria for Diagnosis of Binge-Eating Disorder, Specifically

A person with a binge-eating disorder demonstrates the following:

A. Recurrent episodes of binge eating. An episode of binge eating is characterized by both of the following:

1. Eating, in a discrete period of time (e.g., within any two-hour period) an amount of food that is definitely larger than most people would eat in a similar period of time under similar circumstances.

2. A sense of lack of control over eating during the episode (e.g., a feeling that one cannot stop eating or control what or how much one is eating).

B. Binge-eating episodes are associated with at least three of the following:

1. Eating much more rapidly than normal.

2. Eating until feeling uncomfortably full.

3. Eating large amounts of food when not feeling physically hungry.

4. Eating alone because of being embarrassed by how much one is eating.

5. Feeling disgusted with oneself, depressed, or very guilty after overeating.

C. The binge eating causes marked distress.

D. The binge eating occurs, on average, at least twice a week for six months.

E. The binge eating is not associated with the regular use of inappropriate compensatory behaviors (e.g., purging, fasting, excessive exercise) and does not occur exclusively during the course of anorexia nervosa or bulimia nervosa.

Source: Reprinted with permission from the *Diagnostic and Statistical Manual of Mental Disorders,* fourth edition. Copyright 1994 American Psychiatric Association.

that bulimia nervosa is not new, but the two are actually distinct. Ancient people were eating for pleasure, without guilt, and in the company of others; they vomited so that they could rejoin the feast.

Bulimia nervosa is a disorder of isolation and is often accompanied by low self-esteem.

A food-centered society that favors thinness puts people in a bind. Families may encourage hearty eating and socializing around the dinner table. Party hosts take pride in the delicacies they serve, and guests are obliged to indulge. A child raised in such a setting and also encouraged to aspire to a thin ideal may see little alternative but to celebrate by indulging in food and then to vomit, crash diet, or starve to "undo" possible weight gain. Then, starving and guilty, but still reluctant to appear to be a glutton, the child may begin eating uncontrollably to relieve a desperate hunger.

There is no doubt that our society sets unrealistic ideals for body weight, especially in women, and devalues those who do not conform to them. Even professionals, including physicians and dietitians, are prone to praise people for losing weight and to suggest weight loss to people who do not need it for their health. As a result, even beautiful, normal-weight preteen girls are already worried that they are too fat. Two-thirds of adolescent girls and one-third of adolescent boys are dissatisfied with their body weight and shape.[36] Characteristics of disordered eating such as restrained eating, fasting, binge eating, purging, fear of fatness, and distortion of body image are extraordinarily common among young, white, middle- and upper-class girls.[37] Most are "on diets," and many are poorly nourished. Some eat too little food to support normal growth; thus they miss out on their adolescent growth spurts and may never catch up. Many eat so little that hunger propels them into binge-purge cycles. Magazines, newspapers, and television all convey the message that to be thin is to be beautiful and happy. Anorexia nervosa and bulimia nervosa are not a form of rebellion against these unreasonable expectations, but rather an exaggerated acceptance of them.

Perhaps a person's best defense against these disorders is to learn to appreciate his or her own uniqueness. When people discover and honor the body's real needs, they become unwilling to sacrifice health for conformity. The author Eda LeShan described her recovery from overeating this way: "Deep inside there had always been a small child begging for my attention. All I gave her was food. Now I give her love."[38] To respect and value oneself may be lifesaving.

NOTES

1. American Psychiatric Association: *DSM-IV* (Washington, D.C.: American Psychiatric Association, 1994).

2. Position of The American Dietetic Association: Nutrition intervention in the treatment of anorexia nervosa, bulimia nervosa, and binge eating, *Journal of the American Dietetic Association* 94 (1994): 902–907.

3. N. T. Frusztajer and coauthors, Nutrition and the incidence of stress fractures in ballet dancers, *American Journal of Clinical Nutrition* 51 (1990): 779–783.

4. American Psychiatric Association, 1994; A. R. Lucas and D. M. Huse, Behavioral disorders affecting food intake: Anorexia nervosa and bulimia nervosa, in *Modern Nutrition in Health and Disease*, eds. M. E. Shils, J. A. Olson, and M. Shike (Philadelphia: Lea & Febiger, 1994), pp. 977–983; M. J. Devlin and B. T. Walsh, Anorexia nervosa and bulimia, in *Obesity*, eds. P. Björntorp and B. N. Brodoff (Philadelphia: J. B. Lippincott, 1992), pp. 436–444; S. N. Collier and coauthors, Assessment of attitudes about weight and dieting among college-aged individuals, *Journal of the American Dietetic Association* 90 (1990): 276–278.

5. "Anorexia athletica," Special report on nutrition and the athlete, *Sports Medicine Digest*, 1989, p. 10; S. N. Steen and K. D. Brownell, Patterns of weight loss and regain in wrestlers: Has the tradition changed? *Medicine and Science in Sports and Exercise* 22 (1990): 762–768.

6. K. K. Yeager and coauthors, The female athlete triad: Disordered eating, amenorrhea, osteoporosis, *Medicine and Science in Sports and Exercise* 25 (1993): 775–777.

7. J. L. Walbery and C. S. Johnston, Menstrual function and eating behavior in female recreational weight lifters and competitive body builders, *Medicine and Science in Sports and Exercise* 23 (1991): 30–36.

8. M. T. Depalma and coauthors, Weight control practices of lightweight football players, *Medicine and Science in Sports and Exercise* 25 (1993): 694–701; B. J. Larson, Relationship of family communication patterns to Eating Disorder Inventory scores in adolescent girls, *Journal of the American Dietetic Association* 91 (1991): 1065–1067.

9. G. Szmukler and C. Dare, Family therapy of early-onset, short-history anorexia nervosa, in *Family Approaches in Treatment of Eating Disorders*, eds. D. B. Woodside and L. Shekter-Wolfson (Washington, D.C.: American Psychiatric Press, 1991), pp. 25–47.

10. P. Barbe and coauthors, Sex-hormone-binding globulin and protein-energy malnutrition indexes as indicators of nutritional status in women with anorexia nervosa, *American Journal of Clinical Nutrition* 57 (1993): 319–322.

11. R. C. Casper and coauthors, Total daily energy expenditure and activity level in anorexia nervosa, *American Journal of Clinical Nutrition* 53 (1991): 1143–1150; L. Scalfi and coauthors, Bioimpedance analysis and resting energy expenditure in undernourished and refed anorectic patients, *European Journal of Clinical Nutrition* 47 (1993): 61–67.

12. R. B. Mazess, H. S. Barden, and E. S. Ohlrich, Skeletal and body-composition effect of anorexia nervosa, *American Journal of Clinical Nutrition* 52 (1990): 438–441; L. K. Bachrach and coauthors, Decreased bone density in adolescent girls with anorexia nervosa, *Pediatrics* 86 (1990): 440–447.

13. R. C. Henderson, Bone health in adolescence: Anorexia and athletic amenorrhea, *Nutrition Today*, March/April 1991, pp. 25–29; F. Munning, Tackling women's health issues, *Physician and Sportsmedicine*, September 1992, p. 33.

14. A. A. Skolnick, "Female athlete triad" risk for women, *Journal of the American Medical Association* 270 (1993): 921–923.

15. Yeager and coauthors, 1993.

16. C. L. Otis, American College of Sports Medicine's Ad Hoc Task Force on Women's Issues in Sports Medicine, as quoted in Skolnick, 1993.

17. M. A. Balaa and D. A. Drossman, Anorexia nervosa and bulimia: The eating disorders, *Disease a Month* (Chicago: Year Book Medical Publishers, June 1985), pp. 1–52.

18. Committee on Nutritional Status during Pregnancy and Lactation, *Nutrition during Pregnancy* (Washington, D.C.: National Academy Press, 1990).

19. B. R. Carruth, Adolescence, in *Present Knowledge in Nutrition*, ed. M. L. Brown (Washington, D.C.: International Life Sciences Institute, 1990), pp. 325–332.

20. M. V. Solanto and coauthors, Rate of weight gain of inpatients with anorexia nervosa under two behavioral contracts, *Pediatrics* 93 (1994): 989–991; E. Obarzanek, M. D. Lesem, and D. C. Jimerson, Resting metabolic rate of anorexia nervosa patients during weight gain, *American Journal of Clinical Nutrition* 60 (1994): 666–675.

21. Devlin and Walsh, 1992.

22. E. A. Weltman and coauthors, Weight and menstrual function in patients with eating disorders and cystic fibrosis, *Pediatrics* 85 (1990): 282–287.

23. American Psychiatric Association Workgroup on Eating Disorders, Practice guidelines for eating disorders, I. Disease definition, epidemiology, and natural history, *American Journal of Psychiatry* 150 (1993): 212–228.

24. D. M. Stein, The prevalence of bulimia: A review of empirical research, *Journal of Nutrition Education* 23 (1991): 205–213.

25. American Psychiatric Association, 1994; Devlin and Walsh, 1992.

26. L. G. Roberto, Impasses in the family treatment of bulimia, in *Family Approaches in Treatment of Eating Disorders*, eds. D. B. Woodside and L. Shekter-Wolfson (Washington, D.C.: American Psychiatric Press, 1991), pp. 69–85.

27. Adapted from D. Newmark-Sztainer, R. Butler, and H. Palti, Dieting and binge eating: Which dieters are at risk? *Journal of the American Dietetic Association* 95 (1995): 586–589.

28. P. W. Meilman, F. A. von Hippel, and M. S. Gaylor, Self-induced vomiting in college women: Its relation to eating, alcohol use, and Greek life, *College Health* 40 (1991): 39–41.

29. A. Marcos, Evaluation of immunocompetence and nutritional status in patients with bulimia nervosa, *American Journal of Clinical Nutrition* 57 (1993): 65–69.

30. J. A. Bushnell and coauthors, Bulimia comorbidity in the general population and in the clinic, *Psychological Medicine* 24 (1994): 605–611; C. M. Bulik, Alcohol use and depression in women with bulimia, *American Journal of Drug and Alcohol Abuse* 13 (1987): 343–355; D. B. Herzog, Are anorexic and bulimic patients depressed? *American Journal of Psychiatry* 141 (1984): 1594–1597.

31. A. Drewnowski and coauthors, Naloxone, an opiate blocker, reduces the consumption of sweet high-fat foods in obese and lean female binge-eaters, *American Journal of Clinical Nutrition*

61 (1995): 1206–1212.

32. C. G. Fairburn and G. T. Wilson, *Binge eating: Nature, assessment, and treatment* (New York: Guilford Press, 1993).

33. J. P. Foreyt and G. K. Goodrick, Weight management without dieting, *Nutrition Today*, March/April 1993, pp. 4–9; R. L. Spitzer and coauthors, Binge eating disorder: A multisite field trial of the diagnostic criteria, *International Journal of Eating Disorders* 11 (1992): 191–203.

34. American Psychiatric Association, 1994.

35. S. Z. Yanovski and coauthors, Food selection and intake of obese women with binge-eating disorder, *American Journal of Clinical Nutrition* 56 (1992): 975–980.

36. D. C. Moore, Body image and eating behavior in adolescents, *Journal of the American College of Nutrition* 12 (1993): 505–510.

37. Moore, 1993; L. M. Mellin, C. E. Irwin, and S. Scully, Prevalence of disordered eating in girls: A survey of middle-class children, *Journal of the American Dietetic Association* 92 (1992): 851–853.

38. E. LeShan, *Winning the Losing Game: Why I Will Never Be Fat Again* (New York: Crowell, 1979).

Chapter 10

The Water-Soluble Vitamins: B Vitamins and Vitamin C

CONTENTS

The Vitamins—An Overview
The B Vitamins—As Individuals
 Thiamin
 Riboflavin
 Niacin
 Biotin
 Pantothenic Acid
 Vitamin B$_6$
 Folate
 Vitamin B$_{12}$
 Vitamin Impostors
The B Vitamins—In Concert
 B Vitamin Interactions
 B Vitamin Deficiencies
 B Vitamin Toxicities
 B Vitamin Food Sources
Vitamin C
 Vitamin C Roles
 Vitamin C Recommendations
 Vitamin C Deficiency
 Vitamin C Toxicity
 Vitamin C Food Sources
HIGHLIGHT: **Vitamin and Mineral Supplements**

MICROGRAPH: Vitamin C, the water-soluble vitamin known for its antioxidant actions

Table 10–1

The Water-Soluble Vitamins

- B vitamins
  Thiamin
  Riboflavin
  Niacin
  Biotin
  Pantothenic acid
  Vitamin B_6
  Folate
  Vitamin B_{12}
- Vitamin C

Reminder: The *vitamins* are organic, essential nutrients required in minute amounts to perform specific functions that promote growth, reproduction, or the maintenance of health and life.

vita = life
amine = containing nitrogen (the first vitamins discovered contained nitrogen)

precursors: substances that precede others; with regard to vitamins, compounds that can be converted into active vitamins; also known as provitamins.

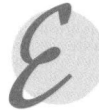arlier chapters focused on the energy-yielding nutrients, which play leading roles in the body. The vitamins and minerals are their supporting cast. This chapter begins with an overview of the vitamins and then examines each of the water-soluble vitamins (see Table 10–1); the next chapter features the fat-soluble vitamins.

The Vitamins—An Overview

The vitamins are powerful substances, as their absence attests. Vitamin A deficiency can cause blindness; a lack of niacin can cause symptoms of mental illness; and a lack of vitamin D can retard bone growth. The consequences of deficiencies are so dire, and the effects of restoring the needed vitamins so dramatic, that people spend billions of dollars every year on vitamin pills to cure a host of ailments (see Highlight 10). Vitamins certainly contribute to sound nutritional health, but they do not cure all ills. Furthermore, vitamin supplements do not offer the many benefits that come from vitamin-rich foods.

The *presence* of the vitamins also attests to their power. Vitamin C not only prevents the deficiency disease scurvy, but also seems to protect against certain types of cancer. Similarly, vitamin E seems to help protect against some facets of cardiovascular disease. The B vitamin folate helps to prevent birth defects. As you will see, the vitamins' roles in supporting optimal health extend far beyond preventing deficiency diseases. In fact, some of the credit given to low-fat diets in preventing disease actually belongs to the vitamins that such diets deliver (see Highlight 11 for more on vitamins in disease prevention). A diet that includes plenty of vegetables, fruits, and grain products is like a coin—the two sides are different but they spend the same. On the one side, such a diet is low in fat; on the other, it provides vitamins in abundance. Both attributes help to maintain health and slow the progression of disease.

The vitamins differ from the carbohydrates, fats, and proteins in the following ways:

- *Structure.* Vitamins are individual units; they are not linked in long chains.
- *Function.* Vitamins do not yield usable energy when broken down; they assist the enzymes that release energy from carbohydrates, fats, and proteins.
- *Food contents.* The amounts of vitamins people ingest daily and the amounts they require are measured in *micrograms* or *milligrams*, rather than grams.

The vitamins are similar to the energy-yielding nutrients, though, in that they are all vital to life, organic, and available in foods.

Precursors Some of the vitamins are available from foods in an inactive form known as precursors, or provitamins. Once inside the body, precursors are changed chemically to an active form of the vitamin. Thus, in measuring a person's vitamin intake, it is important to count both the amount of the active vitamin and the potential amount available from its precursors. The summary tables throughout this chapter and the next identify which vitamins have precursors.

Organic Nature   Because vitamins are organic, they can be destroyed. They can break down and become unable to perform their duties; therefore, they must be handled with care during storage and in cooking. The water-soluble vitamins thiamin, riboflavin, and vitamin C are especially vulnerable. Prolonged heating may destroy as much as 40 percent of the thiamin in food. Riboflavin can be destroyed by the ultraviolet rays of the sun or by fluorescent light; foods stored in transparent glass containers are most likely to lose riboflavin. Oxygen destroys vitamin C, so losses are closely related to the extent to which foods are cut or broken and thereby exposed to air.

The body treats vitamins with respect. It makes special provisions to absorb them, it provides most of them with special protein carriers, and it provides special enzymes to alter their forms so that they can perform different roles.

Solubility   As you may recall, carbohydrates and proteins are hydrophilic and lipids are hydrophobic. The vitamins divide along the same lines—the hydrophilic, water-soluble ones are the B vitamins and vitamin C; the hydrophobic, fat-soluble ones are vitamins A, D, E, and K.

Solubility is apparent in the food sources, and it affects the body's absorption, transport, storage, and excretion of the vitamins. The water-soluble vitamins are found in the watery compartments of foods; the fat-soluble vitamins usually occur together in the fats and oils of foods. On being absorbed, the water-soluble vitamins move directly into the blood; like fats, the fat-soluble vitamins must first enter the lymph, then the blood. Once in the blood, many of the water-soluble vitamins travel freely; many of the fat-soluble vitamins require protein carriers for transport. Upon reaching the cells, water-soluble vitamins freely circulate in the water-filled compartments of the body; fat-soluble vitamins tend to become trapped in the cells associated with fat. The kidneys, monitoring the blood that flows through them, detect and remove excess water-soluble vitamins, but do not "see" the fat-soluble vitamins. These tend to remain in fat-storage sites in the body rather than being excreted, and so are more likely to reach toxic levels when consumed in excess.

Because the body stores fat-soluble vitamins, they can be eaten in large amounts once in a while and still meet the body's needs over time. Water-soluble vitamins are retained for varying periods in the body; a single day's omission from the diet does not bring on a deficiency, but still, the water-soluble vitamins must be eaten more regularly than the fat-soluble vitamins.

In summary, the vitamins are essential nutrients that are needed in tiny amounts in the diet to both prevent deficiency diseases and support optimal health. The water-soluble vitamins are the B vitamins and vitamin C; the fat-soluble vitamins are vitamins A, D, E, and K. Table 10–2 summarizes the differences between the water-soluble and fat-soluble vitamins.

As each vitamin was discovered, it was given a name and sometimes a letter and number as well. Many of the water-soluble vitamins have multiple names, which has led to some confusion. Table 10–1 lists the standard names; summary tables throughout this chapter provide the common alternative names.[1]

The discussion of B vitamins that follows begins with a brief description of each of them, then offers a look at the ways they work together. Thus a preview of the "trees" is followed by a survey of the "forest."

Table 10–2

Water-Soluble and Fat-Soluble Vitamins Compared

Exceptions occur, but these differences between the water-soluble and fat-soluble vitamins are valid generalizations.

	Water-Soluble Vitamins: B Vitamins and Vitamin C	Fat-Soluble Vitamins: Vitamins A, D, E, and K
Absorption	Directly into the blood.	First into the lymph, then the blood.
Transport	Travel freely.	Many require protein carriers.
Storage	Freely circulate in water-filled parts of the body.	Trapped in the cells associated with fat.
Excretion	Kidneys detect and remove excess in urine.	Less readily excreted; tend to remain in fat-storage sites.
Toxicity	Unlikely to reach toxic levels when consumed in excess.	Likely to reach toxic levels when consumed in excess.
Requirements	Needed in frequent, small doses.	Needed in periodic doses.

The B Vitamins—As Individuals

Despite advertisements that claim otherwise, the vitamins are not fuels that give you energy. The energy-yielding nutrients—carbohydrate, fat, and protein—are used for fuel; the B vitamins help the body to use that fuel.

It is true, though, that without B vitamins the body would lack energy. Many of the B vitamins serve as coenzymes to the enzymes that release energy from carbohydrate, fat, and protein. Figure 10–1 illustrates coenzyme action.

Other B vitamins play other indispensable roles in metabolism. One assists enzymes that metabolize amino acids; two others help cells to multiply. Among

- The B vitamins that serve in coenzymes in energy pathways: thiamin, riboflavin, niacin, pantothenic acid, and biotin.
- The B vitamin that serves in coenzymes in amino acid metabolism: vitamin B_6.

Figure 10–1

Coenzyme Action

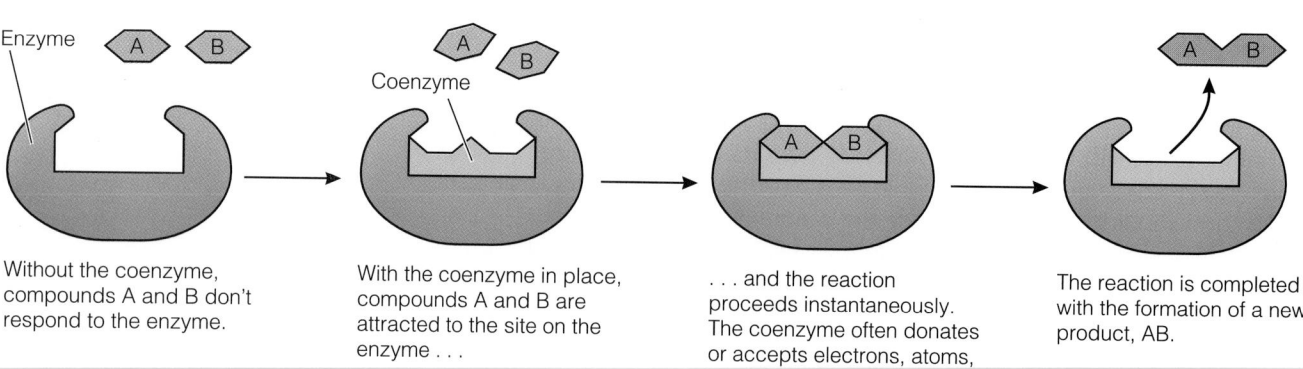

Without the coenzyme, compounds A and B don't respond to the enzyme.

With the coenzyme in place, compounds A and B are attracted to the site on the enzyme . . .

. . . and the reaction proceeds instantaneously. The coenzyme often donates or accepts electrons, atoms, or groups of atoms.

The reaction is completed with the formation of a new product, AB.

these cells are the red blood cells and the cells lining the GI tract—cells that deliver energy to all the others.

The vitamin portion of a coenzyme allows a chemical reaction to take place; the remaining portion of the coenzyme binds to the enzyme. Without its coenzyme, an enzyme cannot function. Thus symptoms of B vitamin deficiencies directly reflect the disturbances of metabolism incurred by a lack of coenzymes.

The following sections describe individual B vitamins and note many coenzymes and metabolic pathways. Keep in mind that a later section will assemble these pieces of information into a whole picture.

THIAMIN

Researchers first isolated the coenzyme form of thiamin in 1926. Since then, the world of vitamins and enzyme action has opened up, revealing its intricacies and permitting medicine and science to put vitamins and enzymes to use in a multitude of ways.

Thiamin is the vitamin part of the coenzyme TPP, which assists in energy metabolism. The TPP coenzyme promotes the conversion of pyruvate to acetyl CoA. The reaction removes one carbon from the 3-carbon pyruvate to make the 2-carbon acetyl CoA and carbon dioxide. Later TPP promotes a similar step in the TCA cycle where it helps convert a 5-carbon compound to a 4-carbon compound. Besides playing these pivotal roles in the energy metabolism of all cells, thiamin occupies a special site on the membranes of nerve cells. Processes in nerves and in their responding tissues, the muscles, depend heavily on thiamin.

Thiamin Recommendations   Because thiamin is essential in energy metabolism, the RDA is stated in milligrams per 1000 kcalories of food energy. Generally, if a person eats enough food to meet energy needs and obtains that energy from thiamin-containing foods, thiamin needs will be met. This is true even for an athlete with high energy needs because almost any nutrient-dense food supplies thiamin, and people with greater energy needs eat more food. A person who is fasting or is on a very-low-kcalorie diet still needs at least 1 milligram thiamin a day to support the body's ongoing metabolic activities.

Thiamin Deficiency   People who fail to meet energy needs risk thiamin deficiency, a condition that seems to be reappearing among the nation's malnourished and homeless people. Similarly, people who derive most of their energy from empty-kcalorie items, like alcohol, risk thiamin deficiency. Alcohol contributes energy, but provides no nutrients and often displaces food. In addition, alcohol enhances thiamin excretion in the urine, doubling the risk of deficiency.

Prolonged thiamin deficiency can result in the disease beriberi, which was first observed in East Asia when the custom of polishing rice became widespread. Rice provided 80 percent of the energy intake of the people of that area, and rice hulls were their principal source of thiamin. When the hulls were removed, beriberi spread like wildfire.

Beriberi was first believed to be caused by an infectious agent. Medical researchers wasted much time and energy seeking a microbial cause before they realized that the cause of beriberi was not something that was in the food, but something that was absent from it.

Because thiamin participates in nerve processes, paralysis sets in when it is lacking. The symptoms of beriberi include damage to the nervous system as well

• The B vitamins that help cells to divide: folate and vitamin B$_{12}$.

Reminder: A *coenzyme* is a small organic molecule that associates closely with many enzymes; many B vitamins form an integral part of coenzymes.

thiamin (THIGH-ah-min): a B vitamin; the coenzyme form is TPP (thiamin pyrophosphate).

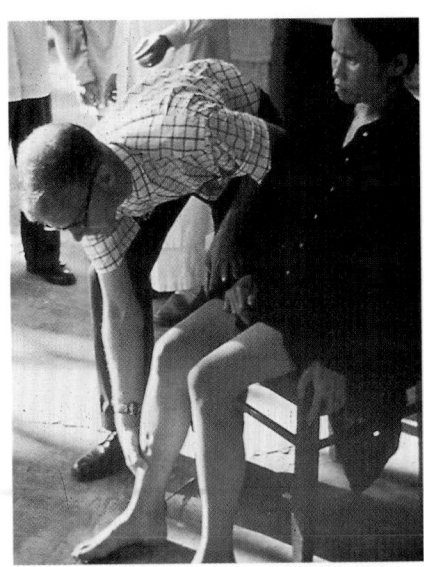

Beriberi may be characterized as "wet" (referring to edema) or "dry" (with muscle wasting, but no edema). Physical examination confirms that this woman has wet beriberi. Notice how the impression of the doctor's thumb remains on her leg.

beriberi: the thiamin-deficiency disease; it pointed the way to discovery of the first vitamin, thiamin.
    beri = weakness
    beriberi = "I can't, I can't"

The **Wernicke-Korsakoff** (VER-nee-key KORE-sah-koff) syndrome commonly seen in malnourished alcohol abusers is characterized by symptoms similar to those seen in thiamin deficiency and can be treated with thiamin supplements.

Table 10–3

Thiamin—A Summary

Other Names	Deficiency Disease Name
Vitamin B$_1$	Beriberi
Adult RDA	**Deficiency Symptoms**
	BLOOD/CIRCULATORY SYSTEM
0.5 mg/1000 kcal/day (1mg/day minimum) Men (19–50 yr): 1.5 mg/day Women (19–50 yr): 1.1 mg/day	Edema, enlarged heart, abnormal heart rhythms, heart failure
	NERVOUS/MUSCULAR SYSTEMS
Chief Functions in the Body	Degeneration, wasting, weakness, painful calf muscles, low morale, difficulty walking, loss of ankle and knee-jerk reflexes, mental confusion, paralysis
Part of the coenzyme TPP (thiamin pyrophosphate) used in energy metabolism; supports normal appetite and nerve function	
Significant Sources	
Occurs in all nutritious foods in moderate amounts; pork, ham, bacon, liver, whole-grain or enriched breads and cereals, legumes, nuts	

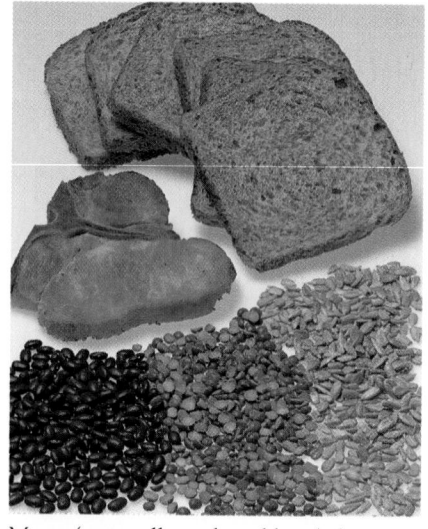

Meats (especially pork and ham), legumes such as black beans and split peas, sunflower seeds, and whole-wheat bread are thiamin-rich foods.

riboflavin (RYE-boh-flay-vin): a B vitamin; the coenzyme forms are FMN (flavin mononucleotide) and FAD (flavin adenine dinucleotide).

as to the heart and other muscles. Table 10–3 summarizes thiamin's deficiency symptoms, main functions, and food sources.

Thiamin Food Sources   Before examining Figure 10–2, you may want to read the box on p. 331 that describes the many features found in this and similar figures in this chapter and the next three chapters. When you look at Figure 10–2, notice that thiamin occurs in small quantities in many nutritious foods. The long red bars near the bottom of the graph represent meats that are exceptionally rich in thiamin—those in the pork and ham family.

As mentioned earlier, prolonged cooking can destroy thiamin. Also, like other water-soluble vitamins, thiamin leaches into water when foods are boiled or blanched. Cooking methods that require little or no water such as steaming and microwave heating conserve thiamin and other water-soluble vitamins.

RIBOFLAVIN

Like thiamin, riboflavin helps enzymes to facilitate the release of energy from nutrients in all body cells. The coenzyme forms of riboflavin are FMN and FAD; both can accept and then donate two hydrogens (see Figure 10–3 on p. 333). During energy metabolism, FAD picks up two hydrogens (with their electrons) from the TCA cycle and delivers them to the electron transport chain (see Chapter 7).

Riboflavin Recommendations   Like thiamin's RDA, riboflavin's RDA is stated in milligrams per 1000 kcalories of food energy, so recommendations vary accordingly for different age and sex groups. Growing infants and children have

How to Look to Foods for Single Nutrients

Figure 10–2 is the first of a series of figures in this and the next three chapters that present the vitamins and minerals in foods. Each figure presents the same 45 foods, which were selected to ensure a variety of choices representative of each of the food groups as suggested by the Daily Food Guide Pyramid. From the base of the pyramid, for example, a bread, a cereal, a rice, and a pasta were chosen. Other pyramid suggestions were also considered: to include dark green, leafy vegetables (spinach, broccoli); deep yellow vegetables (carrots, sweet potatoes); starchy vegetables (potatoes, corn, green peas); legumes (navy, pinto, kidney, and garbanzo beans); and other vegetables (green beans). The selection of fruits followed the pyramid suggestions to use whole fruits (apples, bananas); citrus fruits (oranges, grapefruit juice); melons (watermelon); and berries (strawberries). Items were selected from the milk and meat groups in a similar way. In addition to the 45 foods that appear in all of the figures, five different foods were selected for each of the nutrients. These five foods were chosen to add variety and often reflect excellent, and sometimes unusual, sources of the specific nutrient.

Notice that the figures list the food, the serving size, and the food energy (kcalories) on the left and graph the amount of the nutrient per serving on the right along with the RDA for adults, so you can see how many servings would be needed to meet recommendations. Serving sizes reflect those used by the Daily Food Guide plan. The colored bars show at a glance which food groups best provide a nutrient: gold for breads and cereals; green for vegetables; purple for fruits; white for milk and milk products; brown for legumes; and red for meat, fish, and poultry. (Because the pyramid mentions legumes with both the meat group and the vegetable group and because legumes are especially rich in many vitamins and minerals, they have been given their own color to highlight their nutrient contributions.) Notice how the bar graphs shift in the various figures. Careful study of all of the figures taken together will confirm that variety is the key to nutrient adequacy.

Another way to evaluate foods for their nutrient contributions is to consider their nutrient density (their calcium *per 100 kcalories*, for example). Quite often, vegetables rank higher on a nutrient-per-100 kcalories list than they do on a nutrient-per-serving list. Both listings offer valuable information, though, especially when combined with a realistic appraisal. For example, turnip greens provide more calcium per kcalorie than milk, but milk offers more calcium per serving. What matters most is which are you more likely to consume—1½ cups of turnip greens or 1 cup of milk? Both provide about 300 milligrams of calcium, but the greens save you about 50 kcalories. The left column in the figure highlights in yellow the foods that offer the best deal for your energy "dollar" (the kcalorie). Notice how many of them are vegetables.

Realistically, people cannot eat for single nutrients. Fortunately, most foods deliver more than one nutrient, allowing diet planners to combine foods into nourishing meals.

Figure 10–2 Thiamin in Selected Foods

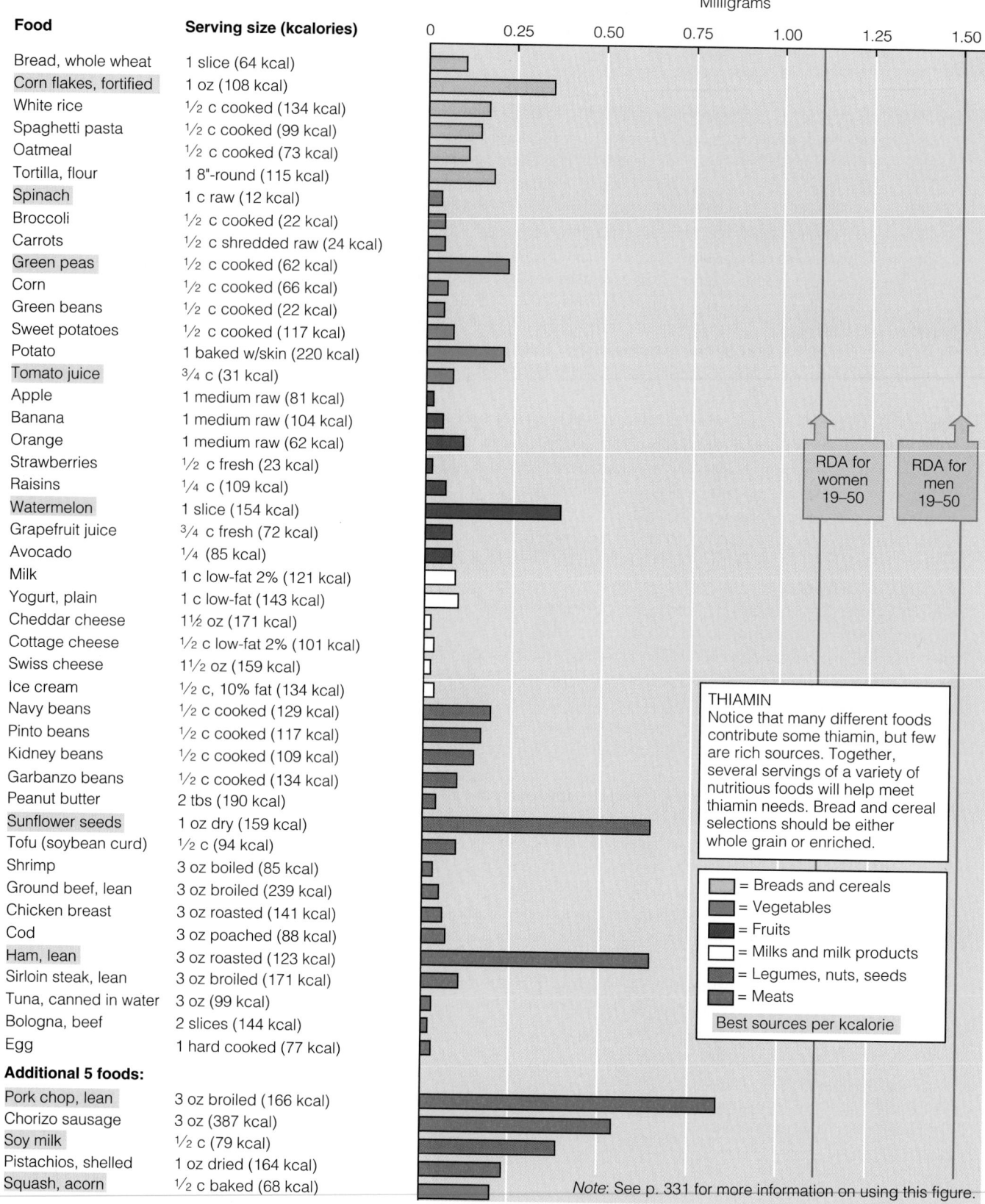

Food	Serving size (kcalories)
Bread, whole wheat	1 slice (64 kcal)
Corn flakes, fortified	1 oz (108 kcal)
White rice	½ c cooked (134 kcal)
Spaghetti pasta	½ c cooked (99 kcal)
Oatmeal	½ c cooked (73 kcal)
Tortilla, flour	1 8"-round (115 kcal)
Spinach	1 c raw (12 kcal)
Broccoli	½ c cooked (22 kcal)
Carrots	½ c shredded raw (24 kcal)
Green peas	½ c cooked (62 kcal)
Corn	½ c cooked (66 kcal)
Green beans	½ c cooked (22 kcal)
Sweet potatoes	½ c cooked (117 kcal)
Potato	1 baked w/skin (220 kcal)
Tomato juice	¾ c (31 kcal)
Apple	1 medium raw (81 kcal)
Banana	1 medium raw (104 kcal)
Orange	1 medium raw (62 kcal)
Strawberries	½ c fresh (23 kcal)
Raisins	¼ c (109 kcal)
Watermelon	1 slice (154 kcal)
Grapefruit juice	¾ c fresh (72 kcal)
Avocado	¼ (85 kcal)
Milk	1 c low-fat 2% (121 kcal)
Yogurt, plain	1 c low-fat (143 kcal)
Cheddar cheese	1½ oz (171 kcal)
Cottage cheese	½ c low-fat 2% (101 kcal)
Swiss cheese	1½ oz (159 kcal)
Ice cream	½ c, 10% fat (134 kcal)
Navy beans	½ c cooked (129 kcal)
Pinto beans	½ c cooked (117 kcal)
Kidney beans	½ c cooked (109 kcal)
Garbanzo beans	½ c cooked (134 kcal)
Peanut butter	2 tbs (190 kcal)
Sunflower seeds	1 oz dry (159 kcal)
Tofu (soybean curd)	½ c (94 kcal)
Shrimp	3 oz boiled (85 kcal)
Ground beef, lean	3 oz broiled (239 kcal)
Chicken breast	3 oz roasted (141 kcal)
Cod	3 oz poached (88 kcal)
Ham, lean	3 oz roasted (123 kcal)
Sirloin steak, lean	3 oz broiled (171 kcal)
Tuna, canned in water	3 oz (99 kcal)
Bologna, beef	2 slices (144 kcal)
Egg	1 hard cooked (77 kcal)

Additional 5 foods:

Food	Serving size (kcalories)
Pork chop, lean	3 oz broiled (166 kcal)
Chorizo sausage	3 oz (387 kcal)
Soy milk	½ c (79 kcal)
Pistachios, shelled	1 oz dried (164 kcal)
Squash, acorn	½ c baked (68 kcal)

Milligrams

0   0.25   0.50   0.75   1.00   1.25   1.50

RDA for women 19–50

RDA for men 19–50

THIAMIN
Notice that many different foods contribute some thiamin, but few are rich sources. Together, several servings of a variety of nutritious foods will help meet thiamin needs. Bread and cereal selections should be either whole grain or enriched.

= Breads and cereals
= Vegetables
= Fruits
= Milks and milk products
= Legumes, nuts, seeds
= Meats

Best sources per kcalorie

Note: See p. 331 for more information on using this figure.

Figure 10–3

Riboflavin Coenzyme, Accepting and Donating Hydrogens

This figure shows the chemical structure of the riboflavin portion of the coenzyme only; the remainder of the coenzyme structure is represented by dotted lines (see Appendix C for the complete chemical structure of FAD and FMN). The reactive sites that accept and donate hydrogens are highlighted in white.

FAD

During the TCA cycle, compounds release hydrogens, and the riboflavin coenzyme FAD picks up two of them. As it accepts two hydrogens, FAD becomes $FADH_2$.

$FADH_2$

$FADH_2$ carries the hydrogens to the electron transport chain. At the end of the electron transport chain, the hydrogens are accepted by oxygen, creating water, and $FADH_2$ becomes FAD again. For every $FADH_2$ that passes through the electron transport chain, 2 ATP are generated.

high riboflavin needs; so do pregnant women. The riboflavin RDA is generous enough to cover the needs of most physically active people and so does not differ from the RDA for sedentary people of the same age and sex.[2]

Riboflavin Deficiency   No one disease is associated with riboflavin deficiency. Lack of the vitamin affects the facial skin, eyes, and GI tract. Table 10–4 lists riboflavin's deficiency symptoms, chief roles, and food sources.

Riboflavin Food Sources   Clearly, milk, milk products such as cheese, and liver dominate the riboflavin list (see Figure 10–4 on p. 335). The need for riboflavin is a major reason for including milk and milk products in every day's meals; no other commonly eaten food can make such a substantial contribution in a single serving.

Most people easily meet their riboflavin RDA. On the average, they derive about half their riboflavin from milk and milk products, about a fourth from meats, and most of the rest from green vegetables (such as broccoli, turnip greens, asparagus, and spinach) and whole-grain or enriched bread and cereal products. A list of riboflavin sources ranked per 100 kcalories includes many dark green, leafy vegetables high on the list (notice those foods highlighted in yellow in the left column of the figure). Vegetarians who don't use milk must rely on ample servings of dark greens for riboflavin. Nutritional yeast is another rich source.

Light and irradiation destroy riboflavin. For these reasons, precautions are taken when vitamin D is added to milk by irradiation.* Also, milk is seldom sold in transparent glass or plastic containers; cardboard or opaque plastic containers are preferred. In contrast, riboflavin is stable to heat, so cooking does not destroy it.

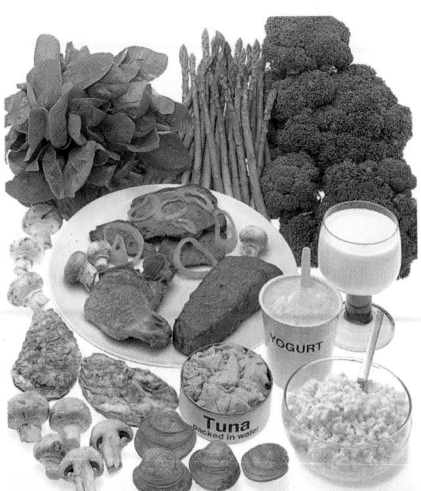

Milk and milk products provide much of the riboflavin in the diets of most people.

nutritional yeast: a preparation of yeast cells grown especially as a nutrient supplement, particularly for vegetarian diets. The type of yeast used is brewer's yeast, not baker's yeast. Different species of yeasts produce different compounds; yeast cells used in brewing produce alcohol, proteins, and B vitamins as they grow. The nutrients are removed from beer and wine in the filtering process. Yeast cells used in baking produce mostly carbon dioxide, which causes bread dough to rise.

---

*Vitamin D can be added to milk by feeding cows irradiated yeast or by irradiating the milk itself.

Table 10–4

Riboflavin—A Summary

Other Names	Deficiency Disease Name
Vitamin B$_2$	Ariboflavinosis (ay-RYE-boh-FLAY-vin-oh-sis)
Adult RDA	**Deficiency Symptoms**
0.6 mg/1000 kcal/day (1.2 mg/day minimum) Men (19–50 yr): 1.7 mg/day Women (19–50 yr): 1.3 mg/day	MOUTH, GUMS, TONGUE
	Cracks and redness at corners of mouth;[a] painful, smooth, purplish red tongue[b]
Chief Functions in the Body	NERVOUS SYSTEM AND EYES
Part of coenzymes FMN (flavin mononucleotide) and FAD (flavin adenine dinucleotide) used in energy metabolism; supports normal vision and skin health	Inflamed eyelids and sensitivity to light,[c] reddening of cornea
	OTHER
Significant Sources	Skin rash
Milk, yogurt, cottage cheese, meat, leafy green vegetables, whole-grain or enriched breads and cereals	

[a]Cracks at the corners of the mouth are termed *cheilosis* (kee-LOH-sis).
[b]Smoothness of the tongue is caused by loss of its surface structures and is termed *glossitis* (gloss-EYE-tis).
[c]Hypersensitivity to light is *photophobia*.

NIACIN

niacin (NIGH-a-sin): a B vitamin. Niacin can be eaten preformed or made in the body from its precursor, tryptophan, one of the amino acids. The active coenzyme forms are NAD (nicotinamide adenine dinucleotide) and NADP (the phosphate form of NAD).

1 NE = 1 mg niacin.
1 NE = 60 mg tryptophan.

The box on p. 337 describes how to calculate niacin equivalents in the diet.

niacin equivalents: the amount of niacin present in food, including the niacin that can theoretically be made from its precursor, tryptophan, present in the food.

pellagra (pell-AY-gra): the niacin-deficiency disease.
   pellis = skin
   agra = rough

The name niacin describes two chemical structures: nicotinic acid and nicotinamide (also known as niacinamide). The body can easily convert nicotinic acid to nicotinamide, which is the major form of niacin in the blood. The two coenzyme forms of niacin, NAD and NADP, participate in numerous metabolic activities. They are central in energy-transfer reactions, especially the metabolism of glucose, fat, and alcohol. NAD is similar to riboflavin coenzymes in that it carries hydrogens (and their electrons) during metabolic reactions, including the pathway from the TCA cycle to the electron transport chain.

Niacin Recommendations   Niacin is unique among the B vitamins in that the body can make it from the amino acid tryptophan. To make 1 milligram of niacin requires approximately 60 milligrams of dietary tryptophan. For this reason, recommended niacin intakes are stated in "equivalents." A food containing 1 milligram of niacin and 60 milligrams of tryptophan provides the equivalent of 2 milligrams of niacin, or 2 niacin equivalents (NE). Like the RDA for thiamin and riboflavin, the RDA for niacin is based on energy intake.

Niacin Deficiency   The niacin-deficiency disease, pellagra, produces the symptoms of diarrhea, dermatitis, dementia, and eventually death. In the early 1900s, pellagra caused widespread misery and some 87,000 deaths in the U.S. South, where many people subsisted on a low-protein diet centered on corn. This

Figure 10–4 Riboflavin in Selected Foods

Milligrams

0   0.2   0.4   0.6   0.8   1.0   1.2   1.4   1.6

Food	Serving size (kcalories)
Bread, whole wheat	1 slice (64 kcal)
Corn flakes, fortified	1 oz (108 kcal)
White rice	½ c cooked (134 kcal)
Spaghetti pasta	½ c cooked (99 kcal)
Oatmeal	½ c cooked (73 kcal)
Tortilla, flour	1 8"-round (115 kcal)
Spinach	1 c raw (12 kcal)
Broccoli	½ c cooked (22 kcal)
Carrots	½ c shredded raw (24 kcal)
Green peas	½ c cooked (62 kcal)
Corn	½ c cooked (66 kcal)
Green beans	½ c cooked (22 kcal)
Sweet potatoes	½ c cooked (117 kcal)
Potato	1 baked w/skin (220 kcal)
Tomato juice	¾ c (31 kcal)
Apple	1 medium raw (81 kcal)
Banana	1 medium raw (104 kcal)
Orange	1 medium raw (62 kcal)
Strawberries	½ c fresh (23 kcal)
Raisins	¼ c (109 kcal)
Watermelon	1 slice (154 kcal)
Grapefruit juice	¾ c fresh (72 kcal)
Avocado	¼ (85 kcal)
Milk	1 c low-fat 2% (121 kcal)
Yogurt, plain	1 c low-fat (143 kcal)
Cheddar cheese	1½ oz (171 kcal)
Cottage cheese	½ c low-fat 2% (101 kcal)
Swiss cheese	1½ oz (159 kcal)
Ice cream	½ c, 10% fat (134 kcal)
Navy beans	½ c cooked (129 kcal)
Pinto beans	½ c cooked (117 kcal)
Kidney beans	½ c cooked (109 kcal)
Garbanzo beans	½ c cooked (134 kcal)
Peanut butter	2 tbs (190 kcal)
Sunflower seeds	1 oz dry (159 kcal)
Tofu (soybean curd)	½ c (94 kcal)
Shrimp	3 oz boiled (85 kcal)
Ground beef, lean	3 oz broiled (239 kcal)
Chicken breast	3 oz roasted (141 kcal)
Cod	3 oz poached (88 kcal)
Ham, lean	3 oz roasted (123 kcal)
Sirloin steak, lean	3 oz broiled (171 kcal)
Tuna, canned in water	3 oz (99 kcal)
Bologna, beef	2 slices (144 kcal)
Egg	1 hard cooked (77 kcal)

Additional 5 foods:

Food	Serving size (kcalories)
Liver	3 oz fried (184 kcal)
Oysters	3 oz cooked (139 kcal)
Clams, canned	3 oz (126 kcal)
Feta cheese	1 oz (75 kcal)
Mushrooms	½ c cooked (21 kcal)

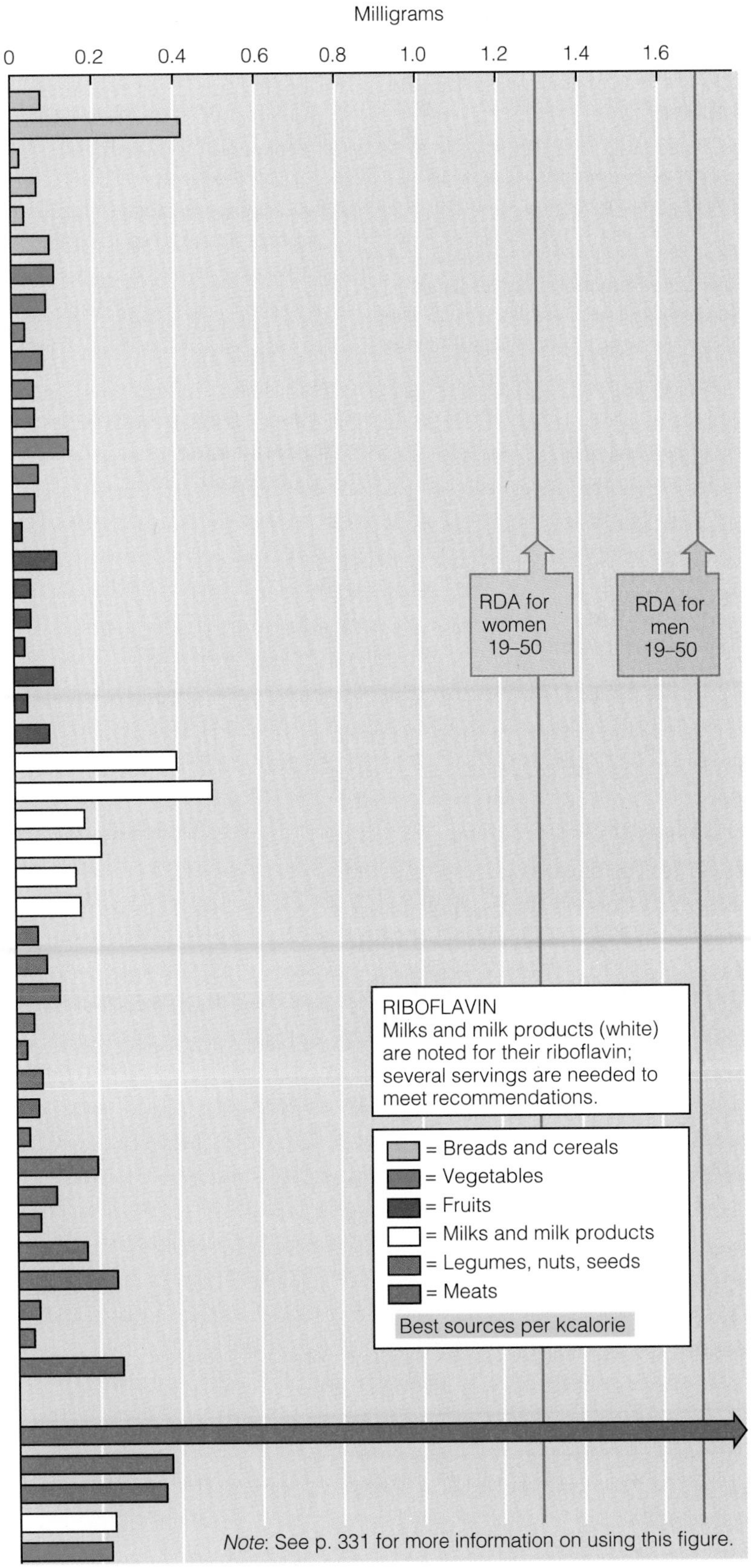

RDA for women 19–50

RDA for men 19–50

RIBOFLAVIN
Milks and milk products (white) are noted for their riboflavin; several servings are needed to meet recommendations.

= Breads and cereals
= Vegetables
= Fruits
= Milks and milk products
= Legumes, nuts, seeds
= Meats
Best sources per kcalorie

Note: See p. 331 for more information on using this figure.

See p. 337 for a photo of the dermatitis of pellagra.

When a normal dose of a nutrient (levels commonly found in foods and not exceeding 150% of the RDA) provides a normal blood concentration, the nutrient is having a physiological effect. When a large dose (two to ten times greater than the RDA) overwhelms some body system and acts like a drug, the nutrient is having a pharmacological effect.

physio = natural

pharma = drug

diet supplied neither enough niacin nor enough tryptophan. At least 70 percent of the niacin in corn is unavailable. Furthermore, corn is high in the amino acid leucine, which may contribute to the development of pellagra.[3] (See Table 10–5 for niacin's deficiency and toxicity symptoms as well as its various names, functions, and food sources.)

Niacin Toxicity   Large doses of niacin exert a druglike effect on the nervous system and on blood lipids and blood glucose. When niacin in the form of nicotinic acid is taken in doses ten times the RDA or more, it dilates the capillaries and causes a tingling sensation that can be painful, an effect known as the "niacin flush." The nicotinamide form does not produce this effect.

Physicians can effectively lower blood cholesterol with large doses of niacin, but such therapy must be closely monitored because of its adverse side effects (liver damage and peptic ulcers, among others).[4] Pharmacological doses of nicotinamide are currently being tested in a large international study to prevent diabetes (IDDM).[5]

Table 10–5

Niacin—A Summary

Other Names	Deficiency Disease Name	
Nicotinic acid, nicotinamide, niacinamide, vitamin B_3; precursor is dietary tryptophan	Pellagra	
Adult RDA	**Deficiency Symptoms**	**Toxicity Symptoms**
	DIGESTIVE SYSTEM	
6.6 mg NE/1000 kcal/day (13 NE minimum) Men (19–50 yr): 19 mg NE/day Women (19–50 yr): 15 mg NE/day	Diarrhea	Diarrhea, heartburn, nausea, ulcer irritation, vomiting
Chief Functions in the Body	MOUTH, GUMS, TONGUE	
Part of coenzymes NAD (nicotinamide adenine dinucleotide) and NADP (its phosphate form) used in energy metabolism; supports health of skin, nervous system, and digestive system	Inflamed, swollen, smooth tongue[a]	
	NERVOUS SYSTEM	
	Irritability, loss of appetite, weakness, dizziness, mental confusion progressing to psychosis or delirium	Fainting, dizziness
Significant Sources	SKIN	
Milk, eggs, meat, poultry, fish, whole-grain and enriched breads and cereals, nuts, and all protein-containing foods	Bilateral symmetrical determatitis, especially on areas exposed to sun	Painful flush and rash ("niacin flush") excessive sweating
	OTHER	
		Liver damage, low blood pressure

[a]Smoothness of the tongue is caused by loss of its surface structures and is termed *glossitis* (gloss-EYE-tis).

How to Determine Niacin Intake

To obtain a rough approximation of niacin intake:

1. Calculate total protein consumed (grams).
2. Assuming that the RDA amount of protein will be used first to make body protein, subtract the RDA to obtain "leftover" protein available to make niacin (grams). (Actually, the RDA provides a generous protein allowance, so "leftover" protein may be even greater than this.)
3. About 1 gram of every 100 grams of protein is tryptophan, so divide by 100 to obtain the tryptophan in this leftover protein (grams).
4. Multiply by 1000 to express this amount of tryptophan in milligrams.
5. Divide by 60 to get niacin equivalents (milligrams).
6. Finally, add the amount of preformed niacin obtained in the diet (milligrams).

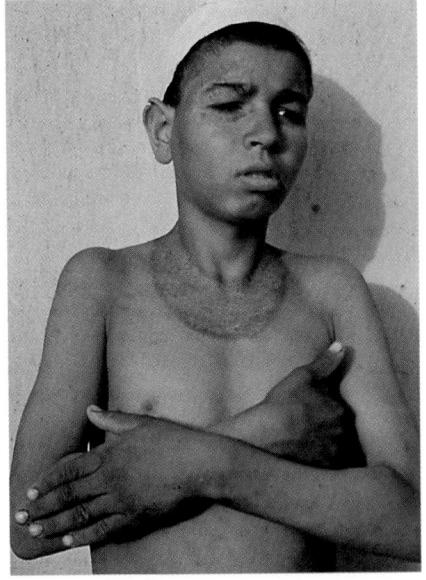

In the dermatitis of pellagra, the skin darkens and flakes away as if it were sunburned. Kwashiorkor also produces a "flaky paint" dermatitis, but the two are easily distinguished. The dermatitis of pellagra is bilateral and symmetrical and occurs only on those parts of the body exposed to the sun.

Niacin Food Sources   Tables of food composition typically list preformed niacin only, but people also obtain the vitamin from protein, which almost invariably contains the niacin precursor, tryptophan. Hence diets that are high in protein are never deficient in niacin. The accompanying box shows how to calculate the total amount of niacin available from the diet. The average diet supplies enough preformed niacin to meet daily needs, and dietary tryptophan usually meets about half the need.

The predominance of red bars in Figure 10–5 explains why meat, poultry, and fish contribute about half the niacin equivalents most people receive. About a fourth of most people's niacin comes from enriched breads and cereals. Mushrooms, asparagus, and leafy green vegetables are among the richest vegetable sources (per kcalorie) and can provide abundant niacin to the person who eats generous amounts of them.

Niacin is less vulnerable to losses during food preparation and storage than other water-soluble vitamins. Being fairly heat-resistant, niacin can withstand reasonable cooking times, but like other water-soluble vitamins, it will leach into cooking water.

BIOTIN

Biotin plays an important role in metabolism as a coenzyme that carries carbon dioxide. This role is critical to the TCA cycle: biotin delivers a carbon to 3-carbon pyruvate, thus replenishing the 4-carbon compound needed to combine with acetyl CoA to keep the TCA cycle turning. The biotin coenzyme also serves crucial roles in gluconeogenesis, fatty acid synthesis, and the breakdown of certain fatty acids and amino acids.

Biotin Recommendations   Biotin is needed in very small amounts. Recommendations for daily intakes have not been established; instead, "estimated safe and adequate daily dietary intakes" have been set.

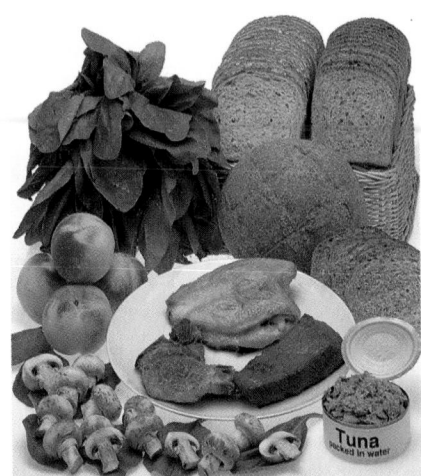

Protein-rich foods such as tuna fish and chicken contribute much of the niacin in people's diets. Enriched breads and cereals, leafy green vegetables, and a few fruits are also rich in niacin.

biotin (BY-oh-tin): a B vitamin that functions as a coenzyme in the metabolism of carbohydrates and fats.

Figure 10–5 Niacin in Selected Foods

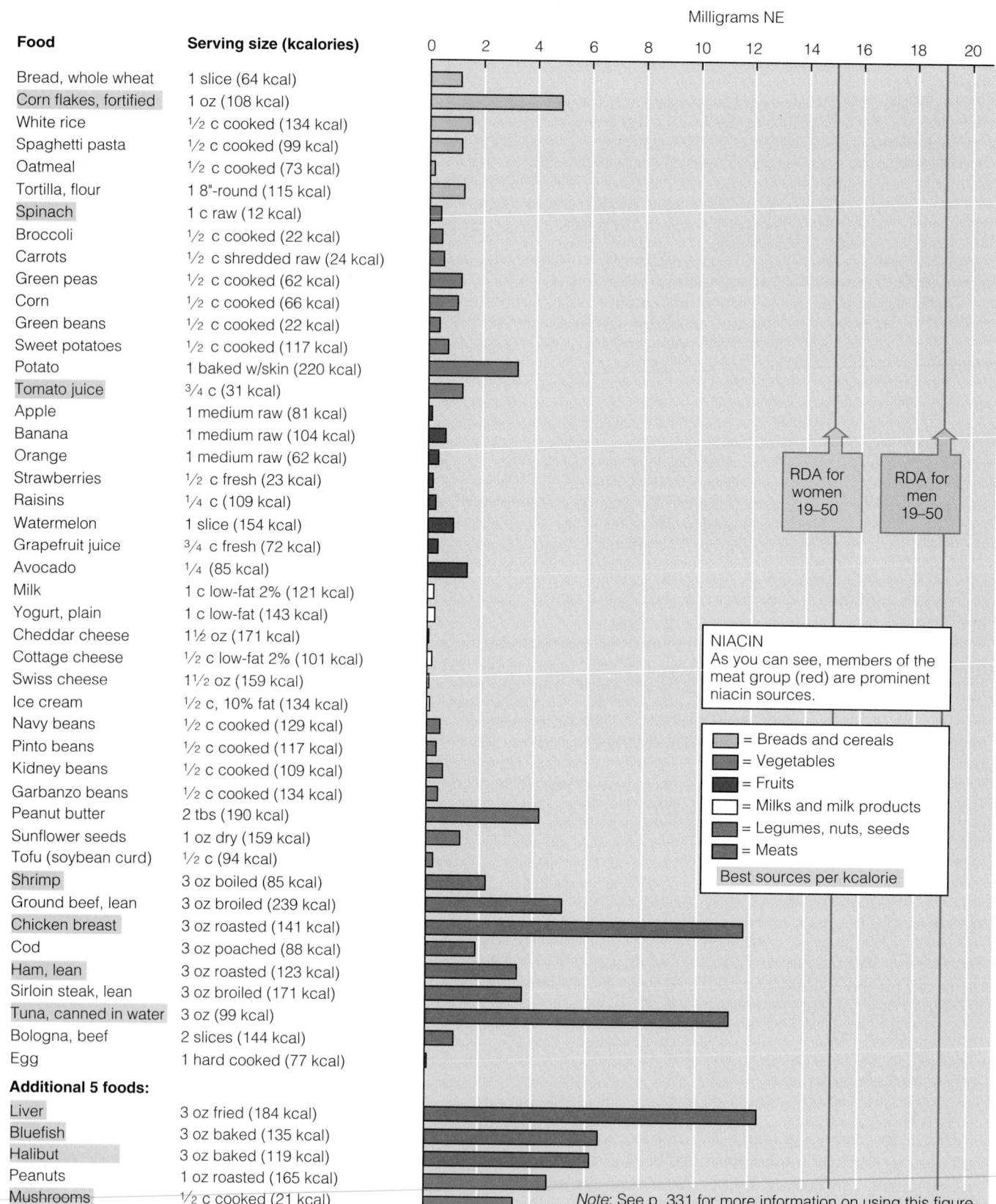

Food	Serving size (kcalories)
Bread, whole wheat	1 slice (64 kcal)
Corn flakes, fortified	1 oz (108 kcal)
White rice	½ c cooked (134 kcal)
Spaghetti pasta	½ c cooked (99 kcal)
Oatmeal	½ c cooked (73 kcal)
Tortilla, flour	1 8"-round (115 kcal)
Spinach	1 c raw (12 kcal)
Broccoli	½ c cooked (22 kcal)
Carrots	½ c shredded raw (24 kcal)
Green peas	½ c cooked (62 kcal)
Corn	½ c cooked (66 kcal)
Green beans	½ c cooked (22 kcal)
Sweet potatoes	½ c cooked (117 kcal)
Potato	1 baked w/skin (220 kcal)
Tomato juice	¾ c (31 kcal)
Apple	1 medium raw (81 kcal)
Banana	1 medium raw (104 kcal)
Orange	1 medium raw (62 kcal)
Strawberries	½ c fresh (23 kcal)
Raisins	¼ c (109 kcal)
Watermelon	1 slice (154 kcal)
Grapefruit juice	¾ c fresh (72 kcal)
Avocado	¼ (85 kcal)
Milk	1 c low-fat 2% (121 kcal)
Yogurt, plain	1 c low-fat (143 kcal)
Cheddar cheese	1½ oz (171 kcal)
Cottage cheese	½ c low-fat 2% (101 kcal)
Swiss cheese	1½ oz (159 kcal)
Ice cream	½ c, 10% fat (134 kcal)
Navy beans	½ c cooked (129 kcal)
Pinto beans	½ c cooked (117 kcal)
Kidney beans	½ c cooked (109 kcal)
Garbanzo beans	½ c cooked (134 kcal)
Peanut butter	2 tbs (190 kcal)
Sunflower seeds	1 oz dry (159 kcal)
Tofu (soybean curd)	½ c (94 kcal)
Shrimp	3 oz boiled (85 kcal)
Ground beef, lean	3 oz broiled (239 kcal)
Chicken breast	3 oz roasted (141 kcal)
Cod	3 oz poached (88 kcal)
Ham, lean	3 oz roasted (123 kcal)
Sirloin steak, lean	3 oz broiled (171 kcal)
Tuna, canned in water	3 oz (99 kcal)
Bologna, beef	2 slices (144 kcal)
Egg	1 hard cooked (77 kcal)

Additional 5 foods:

Food	Serving size (kcalories)
Liver	3 oz fried (184 kcal)
Bluefish	3 oz baked (135 kcal)
Halibut	3 oz baked (119 kcal)
Peanuts	1 oz roasted (165 kcal)
Mushrooms	½ c cooked (21 kcal)

Milligrams NE

RDA for women 19–50

RDA for men 19–50

NIACIN
As you can see, members of the meat group (red) are prominent niacin sources.

- = Breads and cereals
- = Vegetables
- = Fruits
- = Milks and milk products
- = Legumes, nuts, seeds
- = Meats

Best sources per kcalorie

Note: See p. 331 for more information on using this figure.

Table 10–6

Biotin—A Summary

Estimated Safe and Adequate Intake	Deficiency Symptoms
Adults: 30 to 100 µg/day	BLOOD/CIRCULATORY SYSTEM
Chief Functions in the Body	Abnormal heart action
	DIGESTIVE SYSTEM
Part of a coenzyme used in energy metabolism, fat synthesis, amino acid metabolism, and glycogen synthesis	Loss of appetite, nausea
	NERVOUS/MUSCULAR SYSTEMS
Significant Sources	Depression, hallucinations, muscle pain, weakness, fatigue
	SKIN
Widespread in foods	Drying, scaly dermatitis, hair loss

Biotin Deficiency   Biotin deficiencies rarely occur. Researchers can induce a biotin deficiency in animals or human beings by feeding them raw egg whites, which contain a protein that binds biotin and thus prevents its absorption. Biotin-deficiency symptoms include scaly dermatitis, hair loss, loss of appetite, nausea, hallucinations, and depression. More than two dozen egg whites must be consumed daily to produce these effects, however, and the eggs have to be raw; cooking denatures the binding protein.

Biotin Food Sources   Biotin is widespread in foods (including egg yolks), so eating a variety of foods protects against deficiencies. Biotin is also synthesized by GI tract bacteria, but how much of it is absorbed is unknown. A brief summary of biotin facts is provided in Table 10–6.

PANTOTHENIC ACID

Pantothenic acid is involved in more than 100 different steps in the synthesis of lipids, neurotransmitters, steroid hormones, and hemoglobin.[6] It serves as part of coenzyme A—the same CoA that forms acetyl CoA, the "crossroads" compound in several metabolic pathways, including the TCA cycle. Coenzyme A helps shuttle acetate (as acetyl CoA) and other small molecules along pathways in glucose, fatty acid, and energy metabolism.

Pantothenic Acid Recommendations   No RDA exists for pantothenic acid. Instead, estimated safe and adequate intakes have been set.

Pantothenic Acid Deficiency   Pantothenic acid deficiency is rare. Its symptoms involve a general failure of all the body's systems (see Table 10–7).

The protein avidin in egg whites binds biotin.
avid = greedy

pantothenic (PAN-toe-THEN-ick) acid: a B vitamin; the principal active form is part of coenzyme A, called "CoA" throughout Chapter 7.
pantos = everywhere

Table 10–7

Pantothenic Acid—A Summary

Estimated Safe and Adequate Intake	Deficiency Symptoms	Toxicity Symptoms
Adults: 4 to 7 mg/day	DIGESTIVE SYSTEM	
Chief Functions in the Body	Vomiting, intestinal distress	Occasional diarrhea
Part of coenzyme A, used in energy metabolism	NERVOUS SYSTEM	
Significant Sources	Insomnia, fatigue	
Widespread in foods	OTHER	
		Water retention (rare)

Pantothenic Acid Food Sources   Pantothenic acid is widespread in foods, and typical diets seem to provide adequate intakes. Meat, fish, poultry, whole-grain cereals, and legumes are particularly good sources. Pantothenic acid loss during food preparation can be substantial because it is readily destroyed by heat.

VITAMIN B₆

vitamin B$_6$: a family of compounds—pyridoxal, pyridoxine, and pyridoxamine; the primary active coenzyme form is PLP (pyridoxal phosphate).

Vitamin B$_6$ occurs in three forms—pyridoxal, pyridoxine, and pyridoxamine. All three can be converted to the coenzyme PLP.

The PLP coenzyme is active in amino acid metabolism because it can transfer amino groups. This feature permits the body to synthesize nonessential amino acids when amino groups are available (review Figure 7–14 on p. 234). The ability to add and remove amino groups makes PLP valuable in protein and urea metabolism as well. The conversion of the amino acid tryptophan to niacin or to the neurotransmitter serotonin also depends on PLP as does the synthesis of heme, nucleic acids, and lecithin.

serotonin (SER-oh-tone-in): a neurotransmitter important in sleep and sensory perception; it is synthesized from the amino acid tryptophan with the help of vitamin B$_6$.

A surge of vitamin B$_6$ research in the last decade has revealed that vitamin B$_6$ influences cognitive development, immune function, and steroid hormone activity.[7] Unlike other water-soluble vitamins, vitamin B$_6$ is stored extensively in muscle tissue.

Among the many drugs that interact with vitamin B$_6$, alcohol stands out. As Highlight 7 described, when the body breaks down alcohol, it first produces acetaldehyde. If allowed to accumulate, acetaldehyde has toxic effects, and so it must quickly be broken down further. Acetaldehyde dislodges PLP from its enzymes; once loose, PLP breaks down and is excreted. Thus alcohol actively promotes the destruction and loss of vitamin B$_6$ from the body.

antagonist: a competing factor that counteracts the action of another factor. When a drug displaces a vitamin from its site of action, the drug renders the vitamin ineffective and thus acts as a vitamin antagonist.

Another drug that acts as a vitamin B$_6$ antagonist is INH, a drug that inhibits the growth of the tuberculosis bacterium.* INH has saved countless lives, but as a vitamin B$_6$ antagonist, it binds and inactivates the vitamin, inducing a defi-

_____
*INH stands for *isonicotinic acid hydrazide*.

ciency. Whenever INH is used to treat tuberculosis, vitamin B_6 supplements must be given to protect the person from deficiency.

Vitamin B_6 Recommendations   Because the vitamin B_6 coenzymes play many roles in amino acid metabolism, dietary needs are roughly proportional to protein intakes. The RDA for vitamin B_6 is high enough to handle at least 100 grams of protein per day for men and 60 grams of protein per day for women. Research does not support claims that large doses of vitamin B_6 enhance physical endurance. Pills cannot compete with a nutritious diet.

Vitamin B_6 Deficiency   People given a vitamin B_6–deficient diet first experience weakness, irritability, and insomnia. Advanced symptoms include growth failure, impaired motor function, and convulsions. Immune function is also impaired in vitamin B_6 deficiency.[8]

Vitamin B_6 Toxicity   The first major report of vitamin B_6 toxicity appeared in 1983. Until that time, everyone (including researchers and dietitians) believed that, like the other water-soluble vitamins, vitamin B_6 could not reach toxic concentrations in the body. The report told of seven women who had been taking more than 2 grams of vitamin B_6 daily (the RDA for women is less than 2 *milligrams*) for two months or more.

Most of these women were attempting to treat the symptoms of premenstrual syndrome (PMS). PMS is a cluster of physical, emotional, and psychological symptoms that some women experience prior to menstruation. In about 5 percent of women with PMS, at least one physical or psychological symptom can reach such severity as to be temporarily disabling.[9]

Specific PMS symptoms vary from woman to woman, but their timing is predictable: they begin seven to ten days prior to menstruation and wane after menstruation begins. The cause of PMS remains undefined, although researchers generally agree that the hormonal changes of the menstrual cycle must be responsible. Without a full understanding of PMS causes, medical treatments flounder, and quack treatments abound. Among nutritional approaches, the taking of vitamin B_6 has received much attention, but seems to have done more harm than good.

Some people have taken vitamin B_6 supplements in an attempt to cure carpal tunnel syndrome and sleep disorders; at least one study reports that vitamin B_6 may be effective in treating carpal tunnel syndrome.[10] Self-prescribing is ill-advised, however, because large doses of vitamin B_6 taken for months or years can cause irreversible nerve damage. (Table 10–8 lists common symptoms of both deficiency and toxicity as well as chief functions and food sources of vitamin B_6.)

That vitamin B_6 is both essential and harmful may seem surprising, but the same is true of most vitamins and minerals. The effects of every substance depend on its dose, and this is one reason consumers should not self-prescribe vitamins for their own ailments. See the box, "How to Understand Dose Levels and Effects" (on p. 343), for a perspective on doses.

Vitamin B_6 Food Sources   As you can see from Figure 10–7 (on p. 344), meats, fish, and poultry (red), potatoes and a few other vegetables (green), and fruits (purple) offer vitamin B_6. As is true of most of the other vitamins, vegetables would rank considerably higher if foods were ranked by nutrient density

Common PMS symptoms:
   Headaches.
   Breast swelling and tenderness.
   Water retention.
   Weight gain.
   Irritability.
   Anxiety.
   Fatigue.
   Depression.
   Appetite changes and food cravings.
   Backaches.
   Acne.
   Constipation.

carpal tunnel syndrome: a pinched nerve at the wrist, causing pain or numbness in the hand.

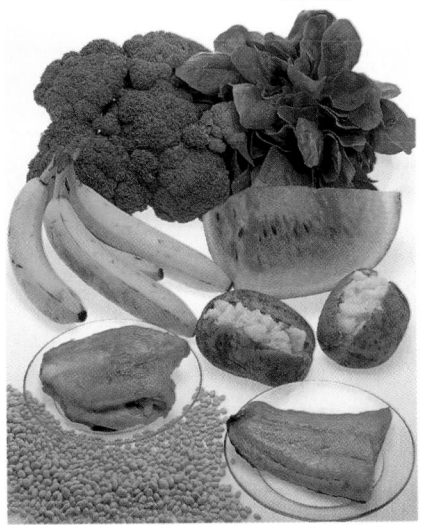

Most protein-rich foods provide ample vitamin B_6; some vegetables and fruits are good sources, too.

Table 10–8

Vitamin B$_6$—A Summary

Other Names	Deficiency Symptoms	Toxicity Symptoms
Pyridoxine, pyridoxal, pyridoxamine	**BLOOD/CIRCULATORY SYSTEM**	
	Anemia (small-cell type)[a]	Bloating
Adult RDA	**MOUTH, GUMS, TONGUE**	
0.016 mg/g protein/day	Smooth tongue,[b] cracked corners of the mouth[c]	
Men: 2.0 mg/day		
Women: 1.6 mg/day		
Chief Functions in the Body	**NERVOUS/MUSCULAR SYSTEMS**	
Part of coenzymes PLP (pyridoxal phosphate) and PMP (pyridoxamine phosphate) used in amino acid and fatty acid metabolism; helps to convert tryptophan to niacin; helps to make red blood cells	Abnormal brain wave pattern, irritability, muscle twitching, convulsions	Depression, fatigue, irritability, headaches, nerve damage leading to numbness and muscle weakness
	SKIN	
	Irritation of sweat glands, dermatitis	
Significant Sources	**OTHER**	
Green and leafy vegetables, meats, fish, poultry, shellfish, legumes, fruits, whole grains	Kidney stones	Bone pain

[a]Small-cell–type anemia is *microcytic anemia.*
[b]Smoothness of the tongue is caused by loss of its surface structures and is termed *glossitis* (gloss-EYE-tis).
[c]Cracks at the corners of the mouth are termed *cheilosis* (kee-LOH-sis).

(vitamin B$_6$ per 100 kcalories). Several servings of vitamin B$_6$–rich foods are needed to meet recommended intakes.

Foods lose vitamin B$_6$ when heated. Information is limited, but research shows that vitamin B$_6$ bioavailability from plant-derived foods is lower than from animal-derived foods; fiber does not appear to hamper absorption.

bioavailability: the rate and extent to which a nutrient is absorbed.

FOLATE

folate (FOLE-ate): a B vitamin; also known as folic acid, folacin, or pteroylglutamic (tare-o-EEL-glue-TAM-ick) acid (PGA). The coenzyme forms are DHF (dihydrofolate) and THF (tetrahydrofolate).

Folate, also known as folic acid or folacin, has a chemical name that would fit a flying dinosaur: pteroylglutamic acid (PGA for short). Its primary coenzyme form is THF. THF serves as part of an enzyme complex that handles one-carbon compounds that arise during metabolism. This action helps convert vitamin B$_{12}$ to one of its coenzyme forms and helps synthesize the DNA required for all rapidly growing cells.

Foods deliver folate mostly in the "bound" form—that is, combined with a string of amino acids (glutamate), known as polyglutamate (see Appendix C for the chemical structure). The intestine prefers to absorb the "free" folate form—folate with only one glutamate attached (the monoglutamate form). Enzymes on the intestinal cell surfaces hydrolyze the polyglutamate to monoglutamate and then attach a methyl group. Special transport systems deliver the monoglutamate form to the liver and other body cells.

How to Understand Dose Levels and Effects

A substance may have a beneficial or harmful effect, but a critical thinker would not conclude that the substance itself was beneficial or harmful without first asking what dose was used. Two corollaries to this statement might be the following:

- A substance that is poisonous at a high concentration may be an essential nutrient at a lower concentration.
- A nutrient needed at a low concentration may be toxic at a high concentration.

Figure 10–6 shows three possible relationships between dose levels and effects. The third diagram represents the situation with nutrients—more is better up to a point, but beyond that point, still more is harmful.

Figure 10–6

Dose Levels and Effects

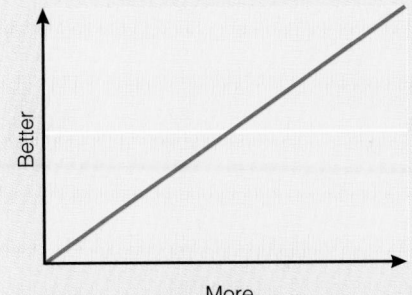

As you progress in the direction of more, the effect gets better and better, with no end in sight (real life is seldom, if ever, like this).

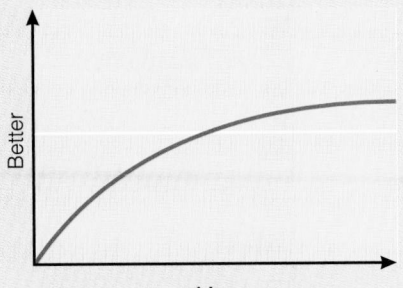

As you progress in the direction of more, the effect reaches a maximum and then a plateau, becoming no better with higher doses.

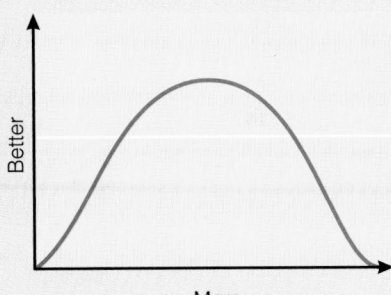

As you progress in the direction of more, the effect reaches an optimum at some intermediate dose and then declines, showing that more is better up to a point and then harmful. That too much is as harmful as too little represents the situation with nutrients.

To store folate, cells add glutamate, converting it back to the polyglutamate form. To release it, they hydrolyze it back to monoglutamate again. To dispose of excess folate, the liver secretes most of it into bile and ships it to the gallbladder, whence it returns to the intestine—an enterohepatic circulation route like that of bile itself (review Figure 5–15 on p. 157).

In order for the folate coenzyme to function, the methyl group needs to be removed from methyl-THF. The enzyme that removes the methyl group requires the help of vitamin B_{12}. Without that help, folate becomes trapped inside cells in its methyl form, unavailable to support DNA synthesis and cell growth (see Figure 10–8 on p. 345).

This complicated system for handling folate is vulnerable to GI tract injuries. Since folate is actively secreted back into the intestinal tract with bile, it has to be reabsorbed repeatedly. If the GI tract cells are harmed, then folate is rapidly lost from the body. Such is the case in alcohol abuse; folate deficiency rapidly develops and, ironically, damages the GI tract further. The folate coenzymes, remem-

Figure 10–7   Vitamin B₆ in Selected Foods

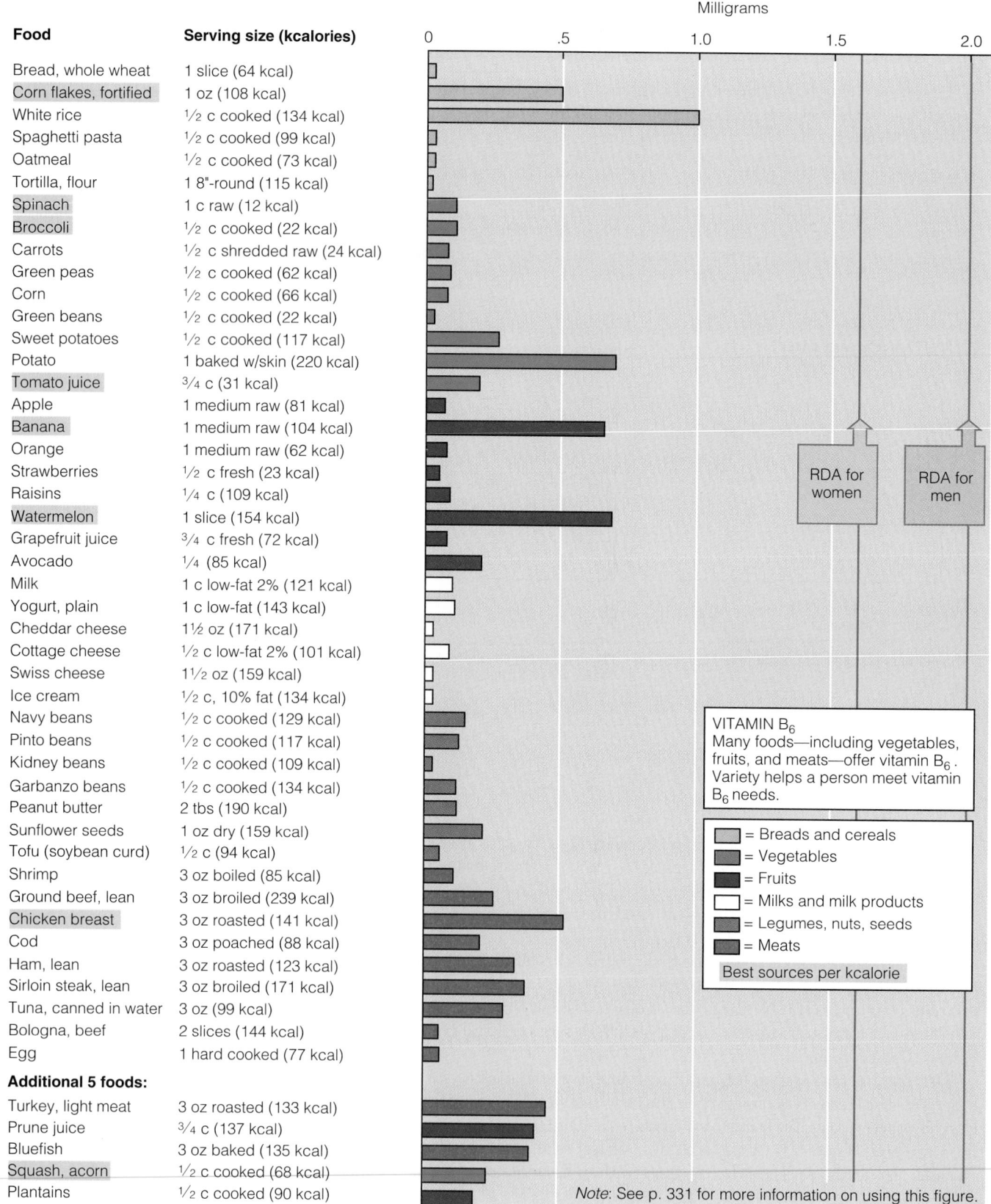

Food	Serving size (kcalories)
Bread, whole wheat	1 slice (64 kcal)
Corn flakes, fortified	1 oz (108 kcal)
White rice	½ c cooked (134 kcal)
Spaghetti pasta	½ c cooked (99 kcal)
Oatmeal	½ c cooked (73 kcal)
Tortilla, flour	1 8"-round (115 kcal)
Spinach	1 c raw (12 kcal)
Broccoli	½ c cooked (22 kcal)
Carrots	½ c shredded raw (24 kcal)
Green peas	½ c cooked (62 kcal)
Corn	½ c cooked (66 kcal)
Green beans	½ c cooked (22 kcal)
Sweet potatoes	½ c cooked (117 kcal)
Potato	1 baked w/skin (220 kcal)
Tomato juice	¾ c (31 kcal)
Apple	1 medium raw (81 kcal)
Banana	1 medium raw (104 kcal)
Orange	1 medium raw (62 kcal)
Strawberries	½ c fresh (23 kcal)
Raisins	¼ c (109 kcal)
Watermelon	1 slice (154 kcal)
Grapefruit juice	¾ c fresh (72 kcal)
Avocado	¼ (85 kcal)
Milk	1 c low-fat 2% (121 kcal)
Yogurt, plain	1 c low-fat (143 kcal)
Cheddar cheese	1½ oz (171 kcal)
Cottage cheese	½ c low-fat 2% (101 kcal)
Swiss cheese	1½ oz (159 kcal)
Ice cream	½ c, 10% fat (134 kcal)
Navy beans	½ c cooked (129 kcal)
Pinto beans	½ c cooked (117 kcal)
Kidney beans	½ c cooked (109 kcal)
Garbanzo beans	½ c cooked (134 kcal)
Peanut butter	2 tbs (190 kcal)
Sunflower seeds	1 oz dry (159 kcal)
Tofu (soybean curd)	½ c (94 kcal)
Shrimp	3 oz boiled (85 kcal)
Ground beef, lean	3 oz broiled (239 kcal)
Chicken breast	3 oz roasted (141 kcal)
Cod	3 oz poached (88 kcal)
Ham, lean	3 oz roasted (123 kcal)
Sirloin steak, lean	3 oz broiled (171 kcal)
Tuna, canned in water	3 oz (99 kcal)
Bologna, beef	2 slices (144 kcal)
Egg	1 hard cooked (77 kcal)

Additional 5 foods:

Food	Serving size (kcalories)
Turkey, light meat	3 oz roasted (133 kcal)
Prune juice	¾ c (137 kcal)
Bluefish	3 oz baked (135 kcal)
Squash, acorn	½ c cooked (68 kcal)
Plantains	½ c cooked (90 kcal)

Milligrams
0   .5   1.0   1.5   2.0

RDA for women

RDA for men

VITAMIN B₆
Many foods—including vegetables, fruits, and meats—offer vitamin B₆. Variety helps a person meet vitamin B₆ needs.

= Breads and cereals
= Vegetables
= Fruits
= Milks and milk products
= Legumes, nuts, seeds
= Meats
Best sources per kcalorie

Note: See p. 331 for more information on using this figure.

Figure 10–8

Folate's Absorption and Activation

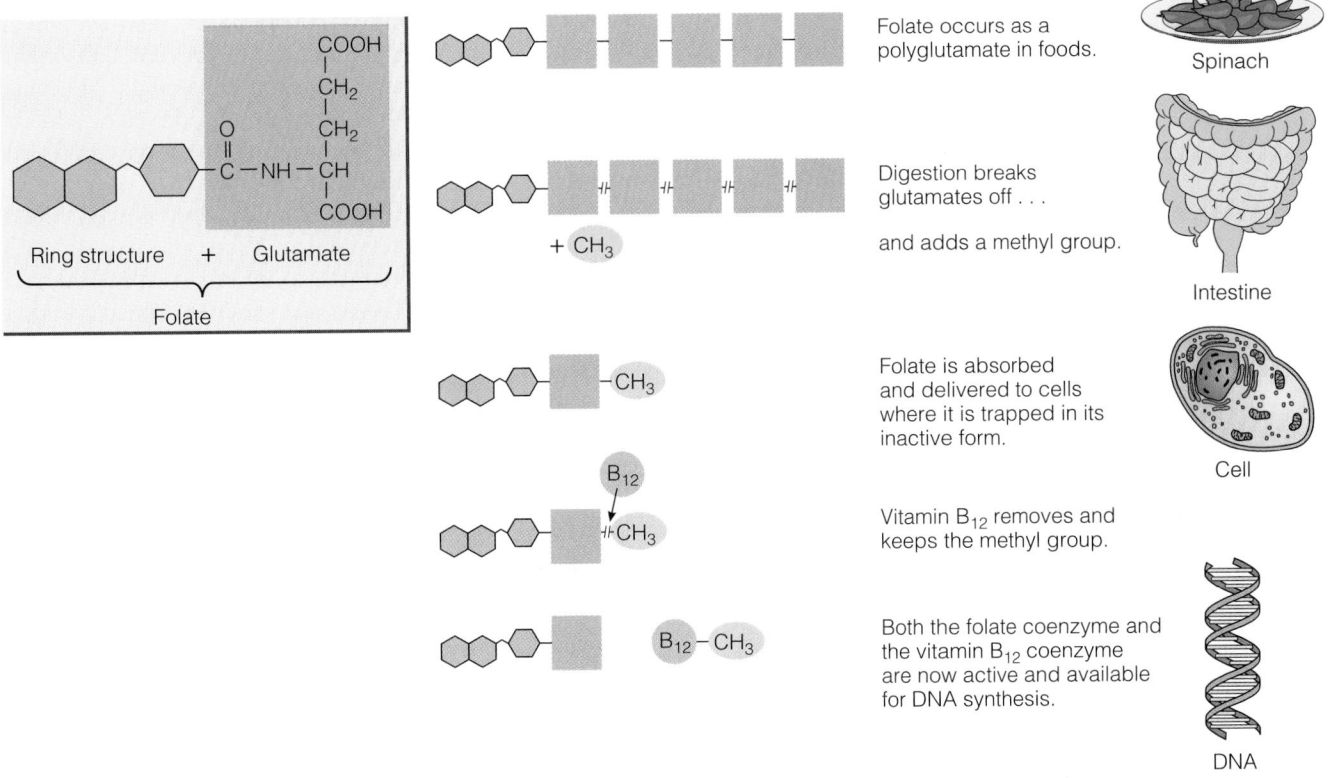

Folate occurs as a polyglutamate in foods.

Spinach

Digestion breaks glutamates off . . .

and adds a methyl group.

Intestine

Folate is absorbed and delivered to cells where it is trapped in its inactive form.

Cell

Vitamin B_{12} removes and keeps the methyl group.

Both the folate coenzyme and the vitamin B_{12} coenzyme are now active and available for DNA synthesis.

DNA

ber, are active in cell multiplication—and the cells lining the GI tract are among the most rapidly renewed cells in the body. Unable to make new cells, the GI tract deteriorates and not only loses folate, but also fails to absorb other nutrients.

Folate Recommendations   Recommendations for daily intake are set high enough to cover folate's poor bioavailability. Only about half of dietary folate is available for use in the body. The need for folate rises considerably during pregnancy and whenever cells are multiplying, so the recommendations for pregnant women are considerably higher than for other adults.

Folate and Neural Tube Defects   Several research studies have focused on the role of folate in preventing neural tube defects. The neural tube is the embryonic tissue from which the central nervous system develops. Neural tube defects cause serious disabilities and infant mortality. The defects commonly arise in the first weeks of pregnancy before a woman may realize she is pregnant.

Recent evidence suggests that folate supplements taken one month before conception and continued throughout the first trimester of pregnancy can prevent neural tube defects.[11] For this reason, the Public Health Services has recommended that all women of childbearing age who are capable of becoming pregnant should take 0.4 milligrams (400 micrograms) of folate daily.[12] This amount of folate can be met through diet rather easily—all one needs to do is eat

The brain and spinal cord develop from the neural tube, and defects in its orderly formation during early gestation may result in various central nervous system disorders. The two main types of neural tube defects are *spina bifida* (literally, "split spine,") and *anencephaly* ("no brain").

For perspective, the folate RDA for women 15 years and older is 180 μg/day.

the suggested minimum five servings of fruits and vegetables daily. But many women typically eat too few fruits and vegetables and receive only 0.2 milligrams of folate from foods daily.

For this reason, and because most pregnancies are unplanned, the Food and Drug Administration has mandated that grain products be fortified to deliver folate to the U.S. population.* Fortification is expected to prevent half of the 4000 neural tube defects each year, but it raises safety concerns as well.[13] Because high intakes of folate complicate the diagnosis of a vitamin B_{12} deficiency, folate consumption should not exceed 1 milligram daily.[14] Whether it is wise to fortify our food supply with folate is the subject of much debate.[15]

Folate's role in preventing neural tube defects is unclear. Most women whose babies develop neural tube defects are not deficient in folate and women with severe folate deficiencies typically do *not* give birth to infants with neural tube defects—so other factors must also be involved. Researchers speculate that "folate deficiency must act on an underlying nutrient-sensitive genetic defect to yield a defective newborn."[16]

Folate Deficiency Folate deficiency impairs cell division and protein synthesis—processes critical to growing tissues. In a folate deficiency, the replacement of red blood cells and GI tract cells falters. Not surprisingly, then, two of the first symptoms of a folate deficiency are anemia and GI tract deterioration.

The anemia of folate deficiency is characterized by large, immature blood cells. Without folate, DNA synthesis slows and the cells lose their ability to divide. The nucleus of the cell is not released as normally occurs during development. As a result, the immature blood cells are enlarged and oval-shaped. They cannot carry oxygen or travel through the capillaries as efficiently as normal red blood cells. (Table 10–9 provides a summary of information about folate.)

Folate deficiencies may develop from inadequate intake and have been reported in babies fed goat's milk, which is notoriously low in folate. Folate deficiency may also result from impaired absorption or an unusual metabolic need for the vitamin. Metabolic needs increase wherever cell multiplication must speed up: in pregnancies involving twins and triplets; in cancer; in skin-destroying diseases such as chicken pox and measles; and in burns, blood loss, GI tract damage, and the like.

Of all the vitamins, folate appears to be most vulnerable to interactions with drugs. Some drugs have a chemical structure similar to folate and can displace the vitamin from enzymes and interfere with normal metabolism. Many anticancer drugs are of this type. Cancer cells, like all cells, need the real vitamin to multiply; without it, they die. Unfortunately, other cells in the body also need folate, and vitamin deficiency develops.

Aspirin and antacids also interfere with the body's handling of folate. Healthy adults who use these drugs to relieve an occasional headache or upset stomach need not be concerned, but people who rely heavily on aspirin or antacids should be aware of the nutrition consequences. Oral contraceptives also impair folate status, as does smoking.[17] Abnormalities in the cervical cells of oral contraceptive users and in the lung cells of smokers seem to indicate a "localized" folate deficiency. Folate deficiency aggravates the risk of cervical cancer,[18] although it is not certain that folate supplements can normalize cervical cells.

Chapter 28 reviews recent research on the relationships between folate, homocysteine, and heart disease.

anemia: literally, "too little blood." Anemia is any condition in which too few red blood cells are present, or the red blood cells are immature (and therefore large) or too small or contain too little hemoglobin to carry the normal amount of oxygen to the tissues. It is not a disease itself but can be a symptom of many different disease conditions, including many nutrient deficiencies, bleeding, excessive red blood cell destruction, and defective red blood cell formation.

an = without
emia = blood

The large-cell anemia of a folate deficiency is known as macrocytic or megaloblastic anemia.

macro = large
cyte = cell
mega = large

---

*Beginning in 1998, grain products must be fortified with between 0.43 and 1.4 milligrams folate per pound of food.

Table 10–9

Folate—A Summary

Other Names	Deficiency Symptoms	Toxicity Symptoms
Folic acid, folacin, pteroylglutamic acid (PGA)	BLOOD/CIRCULATORY SYSTEM	
	Anemia (large-cell type)[a]	
Adult RDA	DIGESTIVE SYSTEM	
3 μg/kg body weight/day Men: 200 μg/day Women: 180 μg/day	Heartburn, diarrhea (loss of villi and their enzymes), constipation	
Chief Functions in the Body	IMMUNE SYSTEM	
	Suppression, frequent infections	
Part of coenzymes THF (tetrahydrofolate) and DHF (dihydrofolate) used in DNA synthesis and therefore important in new cell formation	MOUTH, GUMS, TONGUE	
	Smooth, red tongue[b]	
Significant Sources	NERVOUS SYSTEM	
Leafy green vegetables, legumes, seeds, liver	Depression, mental confusion, fainting, fatigue	
	OTHER	
		Masks vitamin B_{12}–deficiency symptoms

[a]Large-cell–type anemia is known as either *macrocytic* or *megaloblastic anemia*.
[b]Smoothness of the tongue is caused by loss of its surface structures and is termed *glossitis* (gloss-EYE-tis).

Folate Food Sources   Figure 10–9 shows that folate is especially abundant in legumes and vegetables. The vitamin's name suggests the word *foliage,* and indeed, leafy green vegetables are outstanding sources. The lack of red and white bars illustrates that meats, milk, and milk products are poor folate sources. Heat and oxidation during cooking and storage can destroy as much as half of the folate in foods.[19]

VITAMIN B_{12}

Vitamin B_{12} and folate are closely related: each depends on the other for activation. Recall that vitamin B_{12} removes a methyl group to activate the folate coenzyme; similarly, folate donates a methyl group to activate the vitamin B_{12} coenzyme (review Figure 10–8). The regeneration of the amino acid methionine and the synthesis of DNA and RNA depend on the folate coenzyme and therefore on both folate and vitamin B_{12}.* In addition, without any help from folate, vitamin

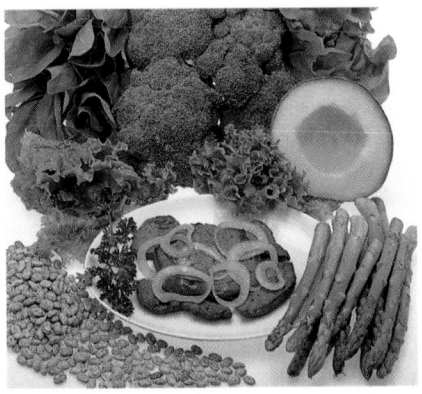

Leafy green vegetables, legumes, liver, and some fruits are rich in folate.

vitamin B_{12}: a B vitamin characterized by the presence of cobalt (see Figure 13–7 on p. 477); the active forms of coenzyme B_{12} are methylcobalamin and deoxyadenosyl-cobalamin.

---

*In the body, the essential amino acid methionine serves as a methyl (CH_3) donor. In doing so, methionine can be converted to other amino acids. While some of these amino acids can regenerate methionine, a continuous supply of methionine is still needed in the diet.

Figure 10–9   Folate in Selected Foods

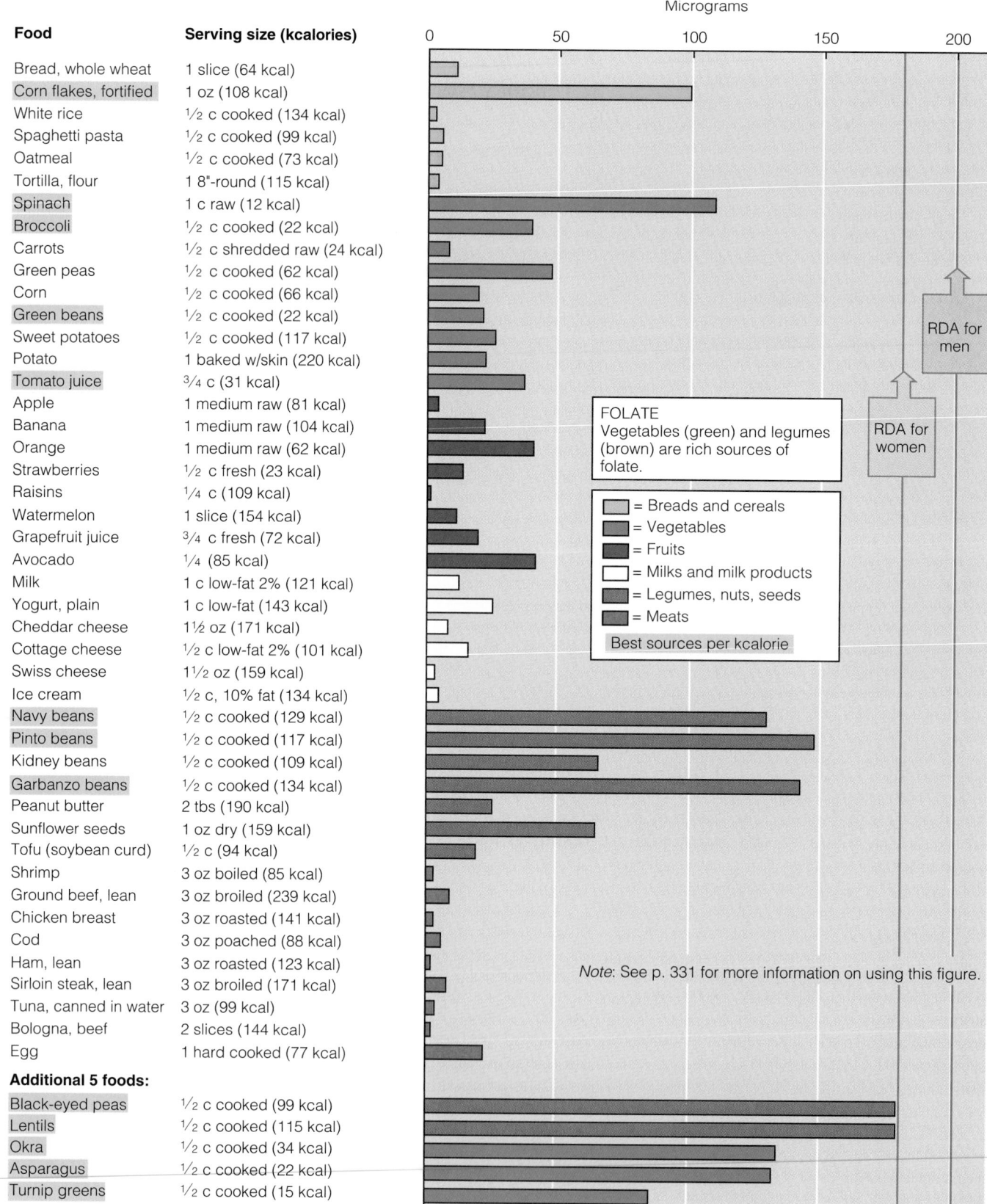

Food	Serving size (kcalories)
Bread, whole wheat	1 slice (64 kcal)
Corn flakes, fortified	1 oz (108 kcal)
White rice	½ c cooked (134 kcal)
Spaghetti pasta	½ c cooked (99 kcal)
Oatmeal	½ c cooked (73 kcal)
Tortilla, flour	1 8"-round (115 kcal)
Spinach	1 c raw (12 kcal)
Broccoli	½ c cooked (22 kcal)
Carrots	½ c shredded raw (24 kcal)
Green peas	½ c cooked (62 kcal)
Corn	½ c cooked (66 kcal)
Green beans	½ c cooked (22 kcal)
Sweet potatoes	½ c cooked (117 kcal)
Potato	1 baked w/skin (220 kcal)
Tomato juice	¾ c (31 kcal)
Apple	1 medium raw (81 kcal)
Banana	1 medium raw (104 kcal)
Orange	1 medium raw (62 kcal)
Strawberries	½ c fresh (23 kcal)
Raisins	¼ c (109 kcal)
Watermelon	1 slice (154 kcal)
Grapefruit juice	¾ c fresh (72 kcal)
Avocado	¼ (85 kcal)
Milk	1 c low-fat 2% (121 kcal)
Yogurt, plain	1 c low-fat (143 kcal)
Cheddar cheese	1½ oz (171 kcal)
Cottage cheese	½ c low-fat 2% (101 kcal)
Swiss cheese	1½ oz (159 kcal)
Ice cream	½ c, 10% fat (134 kcal)
Navy beans	½ c cooked (129 kcal)
Pinto beans	½ c cooked (117 kcal)
Kidney beans	½ c cooked (109 kcal)
Garbanzo beans	½ c cooked (134 kcal)
Peanut butter	2 tbs (190 kcal)
Sunflower seeds	1 oz dry (159 kcal)
Tofu (soybean curd)	½ c (94 kcal)
Shrimp	3 oz boiled (85 kcal)
Ground beef, lean	3 oz broiled (239 kcal)
Chicken breast	3 oz roasted (141 kcal)
Cod	3 oz poached (88 kcal)
Ham, lean	3 oz roasted (123 kcal)
Sirloin steak, lean	3 oz broiled (171 kcal)
Tuna, canned in water	3 oz (99 kcal)
Bologna, beef	2 slices (144 kcal)
Egg	1 hard cooked (77 kcal)

Additional 5 foods:

Food	Serving size (kcalories)
Black-eyed peas	½ c cooked (99 kcal)
Lentils	½ c cooked (115 kcal)
Okra	½ c cooked (34 kcal)
Asparagus	½ c cooked (22 kcal)
Turnip greens	½ c cooked (15 kcal)

Microgram axis: 0, 50, 100, 150, 200

RDA for men
RDA for women

FOLATE
Vegetables (green) and legumes (brown) are rich sources of folate.

- = Breads and cereals
- = Vegetables
- = Fruits
- = Milks and milk products
- = Legumes, nuts, seeds
- = Meats

Best sources per kcalorie

Note: See p. 331 for more information on using this figure.

B_{12} maintains the sheath that surrounds and protects nerve fibers and promotes their normal growth. Bone cell activity and metabolism also seem to depend on vitamin B_{12}.

After ingestion, vitamin B_{12} is released from the proteins to which it was attached in foods by hydrochloric acid and the enzyme pepsin in the stomach. Then the vitamin binds with an "intrinsic factor" for absorption from the intestinal tract into the bloodstream. The genes carry the code for this factor, which is synthesized in the stomach. After the intrinsic factor attaches to vitamin B_{12}, the complex passes to the small intestine, where the vitamin is gradually absorbed. Transport of vitamin B_{12} in the blood depends on specific binding proteins.

Vitamin B_{12} Recommendations   According to the RDA, adults need about 2 micrograms of vitamin B_{12} a day—only two-millionths of a gram. The ink in the period at the end of this sentence may weigh about 2 micrograms. But tiny though this amount appears to the human eye, it contains billions of molecules of vitamin B_{12}, enough to provide coenzymes for all the enzymes that need its help.

Vitamin B_{12} Deficiency   Most vitamin B_{12} deficiencies reflect inadequate absorption, not poor intake. Inadequate absorption typically occurs for one of two reasons: a lack of hydrochloric acid or a lack of intrinsic factor. Many people, especially those over 60, develop atrophic gastritis, a condition characterized by inadequate hydrochloric acid. Consequently, even with adequate intake, their vitamin B_{12} status diminishes: the vitamin is not released from the dietary proteins and so is not available for binding with the intrinsic factor.

Some people inherit a defective gene for the intrinsic factor. Without the intrinsic factor, they develop deficiency symptoms, even though they are receiving enough vitamin B_{12} from foods. In some cases, or when the stomach has been injured and cannot produce enough of the intrinsic factor, vitamin B_{12} must be injected to bypass the need for intestinal absorption. The vitamin B_{12} deficiency caused by lack of intrinsic factor is known as pernicious anemia.

Because vitamin B_{12} is required to convert folate to its active form, one of the most obvious vitamin B_{12}–deficiency symptoms is the anemia of folate deficiency. This anemia is characterized by large, immature red blood cells, which are indicative of slow DNA synthesis and an inability to divide (see Figure 10–10). When folate is trapped in its inactive (methyl folate) form due to vitamin B_{12} deficiency, or is unavailable due to folate deficiency itself, DNA synthesis slows.

First to be affected in vitamin B_{12} or folate deficiency are the rapidly growing blood cells. Either vitamin B_{12} or folate will clear up the anemia, but if folate is given when vitamin B_{12} is needed, the result is disastrous: devastating neurological symptoms. Remember that vitamin B_{12}, but not folate, maintains the sheath that surrounds and protects nerve fibers and promotes their normal growth. Folate "cures" the *blood* symptoms of a vitamin B_{12} deficiency, but allows the *nerve* symptoms to progress. By doing so, folate "masks" a vitamin B_{12} deficiency. A deficiency of vitamin B_{12} causes a creeping paralysis of the nerves and muscles, which begins at the extremities and works inward and up the spine. Early detection and correction are necessary to prevent permanent nerve damage and paralysis. With sufficient folate in the diet, the neurological symptoms of vitamin B_{12} deficiency can develop without evidence of anemia. Such interactions between folate and vitamin B_{12} highlight some of the safety issues surrounding

intrinsic: inside the system. The **intrinsic factor** is a glycoprotein (a protein with short polysaccharide chains attached) made in the stomach that aids in the absorption of vitamin B_{12}.

atrophic gastritis: chronic inflammation of the stomach accompanied by a diminished size and functioning of the mucosa and glands.
  atrophy = wasting
  gastro = stomach
  itis = inflammation

pernicious (per-NISH-us) **anemia:** a blood disorder that reflects a vitamin B_{12} deficiency caused by lack of intrinsic factor and characterized by a deficit of red blood cells, muscle weakness, and neurological disturbances.
  pernicious = destructive

Figure 10–10

Normal and Anemic Blood Cells

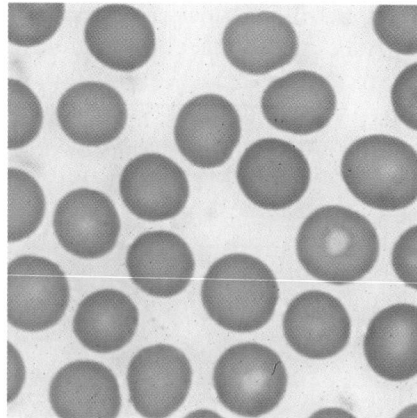

Normal blood cells. The size, shape, and color of the red blood cells show that they are normal. Mature red blood cells have lost their nuclei.

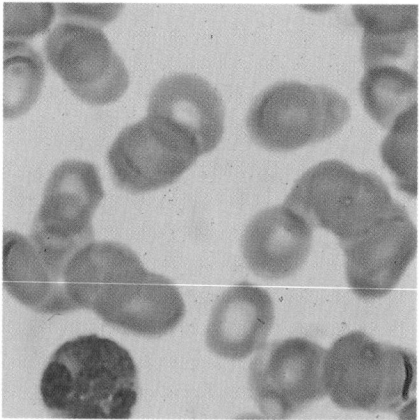

Blood cells in pernicious anemia (megaloblastic). Megaloblastic blood cells are arrested at an immature stage of development, so they still have their nuclei. For this reason, they are slightly larger than normal red blood cells, and their shapes are irregular.

the use of supplements and fortification of the food supply. Table 10–10 provides a summary of information about vitamin B_{12}.

Vitamin B_{12} Food Sources   Vitamin B_{12} is unique among the nutrients in being found almost exclusively in foods derived from animals. Anyone who eats reasonable amounts of meat is guaranteed an adequate intake, and vegetarians who use milk, cheese, and eggs are also protected from deficiency. Fermented soy products such as miso (a soybean paste) or sea algae such as spirulina do *not* provide vitamin B_{12} in its active form. Extensive research shows that the amounts listed on the labels of these plant products are inaccurate and misleading, because the vitamin B_{12} is in an inactive, unavailable form. Vegans need a reliable source, such as vitamin B_{12}–fortified soy "milk," meat replacements, or vitamin B_{12} supplements. Yeast that is grown on a vitamin B_{12}–enriched medium and mixed with that medium provides some vitamin B_{12}, but yeast itself does not contain active vitamin B_{12}.

People who stop eating foods containing vitamin B_{12} may take up to 20 years to develop deficiencies because the body recycles much of its vitamin B_{12}, reabsorbing it over and over again. Even when the body fails to absorb vitamin B_{12}, deficiency may take up to three years to develop because the body conserves its supply.

Reminder: *Meat replacements* are textured vegetable-protein products formulated to look and taste like meat, fish, or poultry and often fortified with nutrients commonly found in meats.

VITAMIN IMPOSTORS

inositol (in-OSS-ih-tall): a nonessential nutrient that can be made in the body from glucose. Inositol is used in cell membranes.

The compounds inositol, choline, and lipoic acid are sometimes called B vitamins. Researchers are exploring the possibility that these substances may be essential and one day might be considered for an RDA. Some research indicates

Table 10–10

Vitamin B$_{12}$—A Summary

Other Names	Deficiency Disease Name
Cobalamin (and related forms)	Pernicious anemia[a]
Adult RDA	**Deficiency Symptoms**
2 µg/day (0.002 mg, or two-millionths of a gram)	BLOOD/CIRCULATORY SYSTEM
	Anemia (large-cell type)[b]
Chief Functions in the Body	MOUTH, GUMS, TONGUE
Part of coenzymes methylcobalamin and deoxyadenocobalamin used in new cell synthesis; helps to maintain nerve cells; reforms folate coenzyme; helps to break down some fatty acids and amino acids	Smooth tongue[c]
	NERVOUS SYSTEM
	Fatigue, degeneration of peripheral nerves progressing to paralysis
Significant Sources	SKIN
Animal products (meat, fish, poultry, shellfish, milk, cheese, eggs)	Hypersensitivity

[a]The name *pernicious anemia* refers to the vitamin B$_{12}$ deficiency caused by lack of intrinsic factor, but not to that caused by inadequate dietary intake.
[b]Large-cell–type anemia is known as either *macrocytic* or *megaloblastic anemia*.
[c]Smoothness of the tongue is caused by loss of its surface structures and is termed *glossitis* (gloss-EYE-tis).

that they are conditionally essential under certain circumstances.[20] Even if they are essential, though, supplements are unnecessary because these compounds are abundant in foods.

Some vitamin companies include these compounds in their formulations to make their vitamin pills look more "complete" than others, but these compounds confer no advantage. For a rational way to compare different vitamin-mineral supplements, read Highlight 10.

Medical practitioners have reported overdoses of choline and its relative lecithin (which contains choline as part of its structure as Figure 5–9 on p. 151 shows). Taken in excess, these components cause short-term discomforts such as GI distress, sweating, salivation, and anorexia, as well as long-term health hazards such as injury to the nervous and cardiovascular systems.

Other substances have been mistaken for essential nutrients for human beings because they are needed for growth by bacteria or other forms of life. Among them are PABA (para-aminobenzoic acid), the bioflavonoids (vitamin P or hesperidin), and ubiquinone (coenzyme Q$_{10}$). Other names associated wrongly with vitamins are "vitamin B$_5$" (another name for pantothenic acid), "vitamin B$_{15}$" (also called "pangamic acid," a hoax), "vitamin B$_{17}$" (laetrile, an alleged "cancer cure" and not a vitamin by any stretch of the imagination), and "vitamin B$_T$" (carnitine, an important piece of cell machinery, but not a vitamin because it can be made by the body as needed).

choline (KOH-leen): a nonessential nutrient that can be made in the body from an amino acid. Choline is used to make the phospholipid lecithin and the neurotransmitter acetylcholine.

lipoic (lip-OH-ick) acid: a nonessential nutrient.

In summary, the B vitamins serve as coenzymes that facilitate the work of every cell. They are active in carbohydrate, fat, and protein metabolism and in the making of DNA and thus new cells. Historically famous B vitamin–deficiency diseases are beriberi (thiamin), pellagra (niacin), and pernicious anemia (vitamin B_{12}). Pellagra can be prevented by adquate protein because the amino acid tryptophan can be converted to niacin in the body. A high intake of folate can mask the blood symptom of a vitamin B_{12} deficiency, but it will not prevent the associated nerve damage. Vitamin B_6 participates in amino acid metabolism and can be toxic in excess. Biotin and pantothenic acid serve important roles in energy metabolism and are abundant in food. Many substances that people claim as B vitamins are not (including inositol, lipoic acid, and choline).

The B Vitamins—In Concert

Figure 10–11 (on p. 353) is intended to convey an *impression* of the ways B vitamins busily work in metabolic pathways all over the body. They are involved in every crucial step. Metabolism is the body's work, and the B vitamin coenzymes are indispensable to it. In scanning the pathways of metabolism depicted in the figure, note the abbreviations for the coenzymes that keep the processes going.

Roles of the B Vitamin Coenzymes   Look at the first step in the now-familiar pathway of glucose breakdown. To break down glucose to pyruvate, the cells must have certain enzymes. For the enzymes to work, they must have the niacin coenzyme NAD. To make NAD, the cells must be supplied with niacin (or enough of the amino acid tryptophan to make niacin). They can make the rest of the coenzyme without outside help.

The next step in glucose catabolism is the breakdown of pyruvate to acetyl CoA. The enzymes involved in this step require NAD plus the thiamin coenzyme, TPP. The cells can manufacture the TPP they need from thiamin, if thiamin is in the diet.

Another coenzyme needed for this step is CoA. Predictably, the cells can make CoA except for an essential part that must be obtained in the diet—pantothenic acid. Another coenzyme requiring biotin serves the enzyme complex involved in converting pyruvate to a compound that can combine with acetyl CoA in the TCA cycle.

These and other coenzymes are involved throughout all the metabolic pathways. When the diet provides riboflavin, the body synthesizes FAD—a needed coenzyme in the TCA cycle. Vitamin B_6 is an indispensable part of PLP—a coenzyme required for many amino acid conversions, for a crucial step in the making of the iron-containing portion of hemoglobin for red blood cells, and for many other reactions. Folate becomes THF—the coenzyme required for the synthesis of new genetic material and therefore new cells. The vitamin B_{12} coenzyme, in turn, regenerates THF to its active form; thus vitamin B_{12} is also necessary for the formation of new cells.

Thus each of the B vitamin coenzymes is involved, directly or indirectly, in energy metabolism. Some are facilitators of the energy-releasing reactions themselves; others help build new cells to deliver the oxygen and nutrients that permit the energy pathways to run.

Figure 10–11

Metabolic Pathways Involving B Vitamins

These metabolic pathways were introduced in Chapter 7 and are presented here to highlight the many coenzymes that facilitate the reactions. These coenzymes depend on the following vitamins:

- NAD and NADP: niacin.
- TPP: thiamin.
- CoA: pantothenic acid.
- B_{12}: vitamin B_{12}.
- FMN and FAD: riboflavin.
- THF: folate.
- PLP: vitamin B_6.
- Biotin.

For further details, see Appendix C.

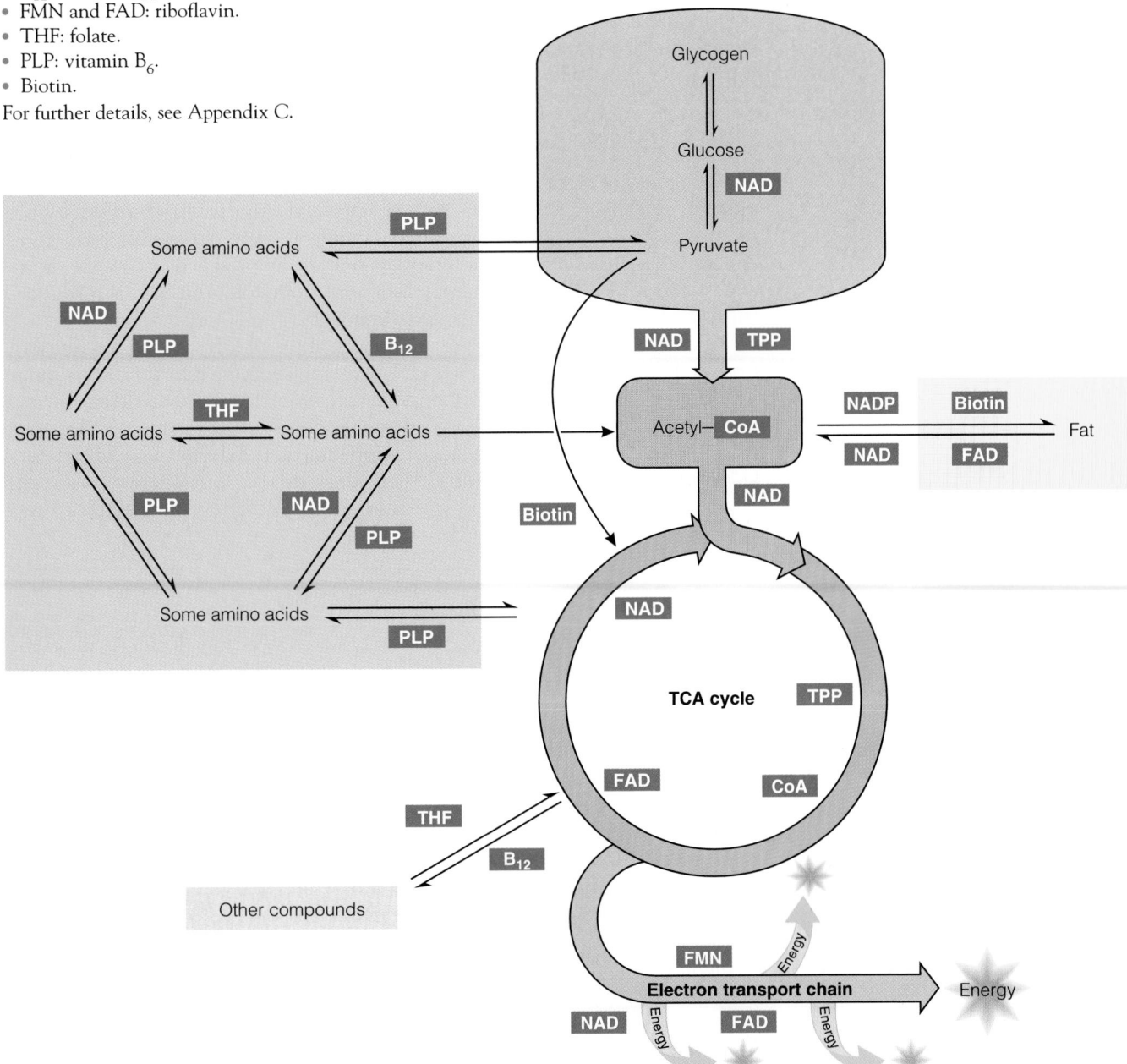

For want of a nail, a horseshoe was lost.
For want of a horseshoe, a horse was lost.
For want of a horse, a soldier was lost.
For want of a soldier, a battle was lost.
For want of a battle, the war was lost,
And all for the want of a horseshoe nail!

—Mother Goose

Effects of a Deficiency Now suppose the body's cells lack one of these B vitamins—niacin, for example. Without niacin, the cells cannot make NAD. Without NAD, the enzymes involved in every step of the glucose-to-energy pathway cannot function. Then, since all the body's activities require energy, literally everything begins to grind to a halt. This is no exaggeration. The deadly disease pellagra, caused by niacin deficiency, produces the "devastating *D*s": dermatitis, which reflects a failure of the skin; dementia, a failure of the nervous system; diarrhea, a failure of digestion and absorption; and eventually, as would be the case for any severe nutrient deficiency, death. These symptoms are the obvious ones, but a niacin deficiency affects all other organs, too, because all are dependent on the energy pathways. In short, niacin is like the horseshoe nail for want of which a war was lost. All the vitamins are like horseshoe nails.

B VITAMIN INTERACTIONS

This chapter has described some of the impressive ways that vitamins work individually, as if their many actions in the body could easily be disentangled. In fact, oftentimes it is difficult to tell which vitamin is truly responsible for a given effect because the nutrients are interdependent; the presence or absence of one affects another's absorption, metabolism, and excretion. You have already seen this interdependence with folate and vitamin B_{12}.

Riboflavin and vitamin B_6 are another example of a B vitamin relationship. One of the riboflavin coenzymes, FMN, assists the enzyme that converts vitamin B_6 to its coenzyme form PLP.[21] Consequently, a severe riboflavin deficiency can impair vitamin B_6 activity. Thus a deficiency of one nutrient may alter the action of another. Furthermore, a deficiency of one nutrient may create a deficiency of another. For example, a vitamin B_6 deficiency hinders calcium absorption and enhances magnesium excretion.[22] These interdependent relationships are evident in many of the B vitamin deficiencies.

B VITAMIN DEFICIENCIES

With any B vitamin deficiency, many body systems become deranged, and similar symptoms may appear. Removing "horseshoe nails" can have disastrous and far-reaching effects.

Deficiencies of single B vitamins seldom show up in isolation. After all, people do not eat nutrients singly; they eat foods, which contain mixtures of nutrients. Only in two cases described earlier—beriberi and pellagra—have dietary deficiencies associated with single B vitamins been observed on a large scale in human populations. Even in these cases, the deficiencies were not pure. Both diseases were attributed to deficiencies of single vitamins, but both were likely to have been deficiencies of several vitamins in which one vitamin stood out above the rest. When foods containing the vitamin known to be needed were provided, the vitamins that may have been in short supply came as part of the package.

Significantly, these deficiency diseases were eliminated by supplying foods—not pills. Vitamin pill advertisements make much of the fact that vitamins are indispensable to life, but human beings obtained their nourishment from foods for centuries before vitamin pills existed. If the diet lacks a vitamin, the solution is to adjust food intake to obtain that vitamin.

Manufacturers of so-called *natural* vitamins boast that their pills are purified from real foods rather than synthesized in a laboratory. Think back on the course of human evolution; it is not *natural* to take any kind of pill. In reality, the finest, most complete vitamin "supplements" available are meat, fish, poultry, eggs, legumes, nuts, milk and milk products, vegetables, fruits, and grain products.

The skin and the tongue appear to be especially sensitive to B vitamin deficiencies, but note that listing them in the summary tables gives them undue emphasis. Remember that these two body parts are readily visible in a physical examination. If the skin is degenerating, other tissues beneath it may be, too. Similarly, the mouth and tongue are the visible part of the digestive system; if they are abnormal, there may well be an abnormality throughout the GI tract. The impact of a vitamin deficiency is felt inside the cells of the body; what the physician sees and reports are the deficiency's outward manifestations. The accompanying box offers other insights into symptoms and their causes.

Major deficiency diseases of epidemic proportions such as pellagra and beriberi are no longer seen in the United States and Canada, but lesser deficiencies of nutrients, including the B vitamins, sometimes are observed. When they occur, it is usually in people whose food choices are poor because of poverty, ignorance, illness, or poor health habits like alcohol abuse (review Highlight 7 to fully appre-

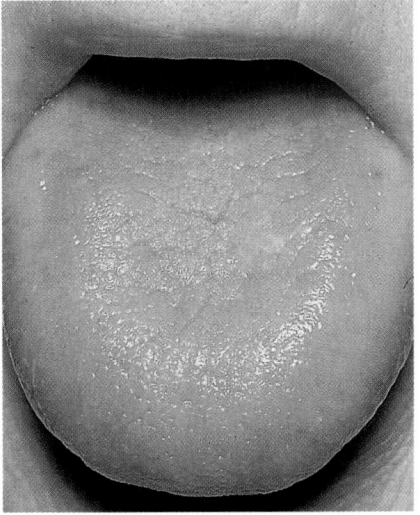

Tongue symptoms of B vitamin deficiency. The tongue is smooth due to atrophy of the tissue (glossitis).

How to Distinguish Symptoms and Causes

It is more and more apparent that no one can observe a symptom and automatically jump to a conclusion regarding its cause. The summary tables in this chapter show that deficiencies of riboflavin, niacin, and vitamin B_6 can all cause skin rashes. But so can deficiencies of protein, linoleic acid, or vitamin A. Because skin is on the outside and easy to see, it is a useful indicator of things-going-wrong-in-cells. But by itself, a skin symptom says nothing about its possible cause.

The same is true of anemia. Anemia is often caused by iron deficiency, but it can also be caused by a folate or vitamin B_{12} deficiency; by digestive tract failure to absorb any of these nutrients; or by such nonnutritional causes as infections, parasites, cancer, or loss of blood. Again, no specific nutrient will always cure a given symptom.

A person who feels chronically tired may be tempted to self-diagnose iron-deficiency anemia and self-prescribe an iron supplement. But this will relieve tiredness only if the cause is indeed iron-deficiency anemia. If the cause is a folate deficiency, taking iron will only prolong the tiredness. A person who is better informed may decide to take a vitamin supplement with iron, covering the possibility of a vitamin deficiency. But the symptom may have a nonnutritional cause. If the cause of the tiredness is actually hidden blood loss due to cancer, the postponement of a diagnosis may be equivalent to suicide. When tiredness is caused by a lack of sleep, of course, no nutrient or combination of nutrients can replace a good night's rest. A person who is chronically tired should see a physician rather than self-prescribe.

ciate how alcohol induces vitamin deficiencies and interferes with energy metabolism). Remember from Chapter 1 that deficiencies can arise not only from deficient intakes (primary causes), but also for other (secondary) reasons.

B VITAMIN TOXICITIES

Toxicities of the B vitamins are uncommon but do occur when people overuse supplements. When the cells become oversaturated with a vitamin, they must work to eliminate the excess. The cells remove water-soluble vitamins by excreting excesses in the urine, but sometimes fail to regain homeostasis. On the other hand, B vitamin toxicities from foods alone are unknown.

B VITAMIN FOOD SOURCES

The food figures presented in this chapter, taken together, sing the praises of the balanced diet. The meat group serves thiamin, niacin, vitamin B_6, and vitamin B_{12} well. The milk and milk products group stands out for riboflavin and vitamin B_{12}. The fruit and vegetable groups excel in folate. The cereal and bread group delivers thiamin, riboflavin, and niacin. A diet that offers a variety of foods from each group, prepared with reasonable care, serves up ample B vitamins.

The B vitamin coenzymes work together in energy metabolism. Some are facilitators of the energy-releasing reactions themselves; others help build cells to deliver the oxygen and nutrients that permit the energy pathways to run. These vitamins depend on each other to function optimally; a deficiency of any of them creates multiple problems. Fortunately a variety of foods from each of the five food groups will provide an adequate supply of all of the B vitamins.

Vitamin C

scurvy: the vitamin C–deficiency disease.

Two hundred and fifty years ago, any man who joined the crew of a seagoing ship knew he had only half a chance of returning alive—not because he might be slain by pirates or die in a storm, but because he might contract the dread disease scurvy. As many as two-thirds of a ship's crew might die of scurvy on a long voyage. Only men on short voyages, especially around the Mediterranean Sea, were free of scurvy. No one knew the reason: that on long ocean voyages, the ship's cook used up the fresh fruits and vegetables early and then served cereals and meats until the return to port.

The first nutrition experiment ever performed on human beings was devised in 1747 to find a cure for scurvy. James Lind, a British physician, divided 12 sailors with scurvy into six pairs. Each pair received a different supplemental ration: cider, vinegar, sulfuric acid, seawater, oranges and lemons, or a purgative mixed with spices. Those receiving the citrus fruits quickly recovered, but sadly, it was 50 years before the British navy required all vessels to provide every sailor with lime juice daily. This tradition gave British sailors the nickname "limeys."

purgative: a strong laxative.

antiscorbutic factor: the original name for vitamin C.
anti = against
scorbutic = causing scurvy

The antiscurvy "something" in limes and other foods was dubbed the antiscorbutic factor. Nearly 200 years later, the factor was isolated from lemon juice and found to be a six-carbon compound similar to glucose; it was named ascorbic acid. Shortly thereafter, it was synthesized, and today hundreds of millions of vitamin C pills are produced in pharmaceutical laboratories each year and sold for a few dollars a bottle.

VITAMIN C ROLES

Vitamin C parts company with the B vitamins in its mode of action. In some settings, vitamin C helps a specific enzyme perform its job, but in others, it acts in a more general way as an antioxidant.

As an Antioxidant   An antioxidant is any substance that prevents or inhibits the oxidation of another substance. In doing so, the antioxidant becomes oxidized itself, but this is useful because it protects the other substance from being altered or even destroyed by oxidation. Vitamin C is like a bodyguard for water-soluble substances; it stands ready to sacrifice its own life to save theirs. Figure 10–12 illustrates how vitamin C's structure can change, so that it can serve as an antioxidant.

Because of vitamin C's antioxidant property, manufacturers sometimes add it to foods as a preservative. In the cells and body fluids, vitamin C helps to prevent damage to tissues, which may be important in preventing disease. In the intestines, vitamin C protects iron from oxidation and so promotes iron absorption.

In Collagen Formation   Vitamin C helps to form the fibrous structural protein known as collagen, the single most important protein of connective tissues. Collagen serves as the matrix on which bones and teeth are formed. When a person is wounded, collagen glues the separated tissues together, forming scars. Cells are held together largely by collagen; this is especially important in the artery walls, which must expand and contract with each beat of the heart, and in the thin capillary walls, which must withstand a pulse of blood every second or so without giving way.

The body makes all proteins by stringing together chains of amino acids. In collagen, the amino acids proline and lysine appear in abundance. During the synthesis of collagen, each time a proline or lysine is added to the growing protein chain, an enzyme hydroxylates it (adds an OH group to it), making the

ascorbic acid: one of the two active forms of vitamin C (see Figure 10–12). Many people refer to vitamin C by this name.
  a = without
  scorbic = having scurvy

antioxidant: a compound that protects others from oxidation by being oxidized itself. An antioxidant donates electrons to another substance; that substance becomes reduced as the antioxidant simultaneously becomes oxidized. Chemists describe the antioxidant action of vitamin C as maintaining the "oxidation-reduction equilibrium," or "redox state."

Highlight 11 discusses the role of antioxidant nutrients in disease prevention in more detail. Chapter 13 provides more details on the relationship between vitamin C and iron.

Reminder: *Collagen* is the protein material from which connective tissues such as scars, tendons, ligaments, and the foundations of bones and teeth are made.

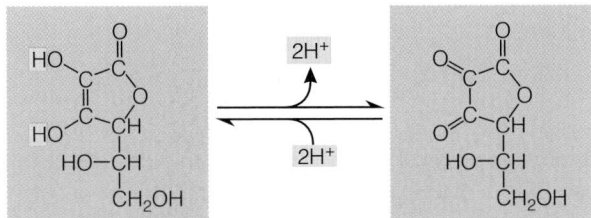

Ascorbic acid is the reduced form of vitamin C. Ascorbic acid can easily give up two hydrogens with their electrons, thereby becoming dehydroascorbic acid. Molecules with unpaired electrons (free radicals) combine with antioxidants such as vitamin C instead of causing oxidative damage to the cells.

Dehydroascorbic acid is the oxidized form of vitamin C. The reversibility of this reaction is key to vitamin C's role as an antioxidant.

Figure 10–12

Active Forms of Vitamin C

cofactor: a mineral element that, like a coenzyme, works with an enzyme to facilitate a chemical reaction. The cofactor maintains the structural integrity of the enzyme and may also facilitate the enzyme's catalytic activity.

Figure 10–13

Vitamin C's Role in Hydroxyproline Synthesis

Collagen is unique among body proteins because it contains large amounts of the amino acid hydroxyproline. The hydroxylase enzyme, which forms hydroxyproline by adding a hydroxyl group to the amino acid proline, requires vitamin C and iron.

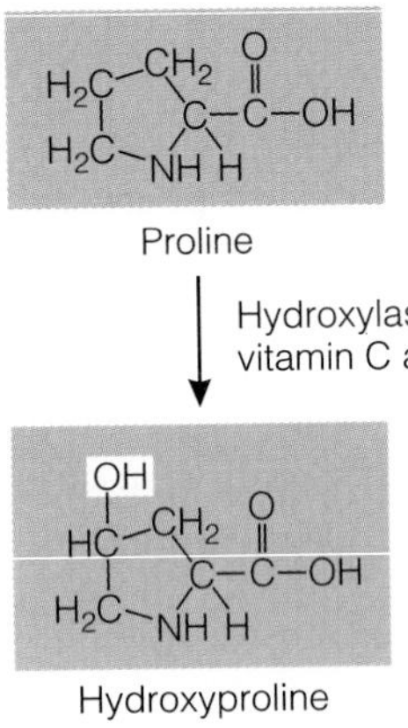

Proline

Hydroxylase + vitamin C and iron

Hydroxyproline

amino acids hydroxyproline or hydroxylysine, respectively. Figure 10–13 illustrates the conversion of proline to hydroxyproline. This hydroxylase enzyme requires both vitamin C and iron. Iron works as a cofactor in the reaction, and vitamin C maintains iron in the form that allows it to do so. Without them, the hydroxylation step does not occur. Hydroxyproline and hydroxylysine facilitate the binding together of collagen fibers to make strong, ropelike structures.

In Stress   Vitamin C assists in the metabolism of several amino acids, some of which are used to make hormones—notably, the hormones norepinephrine and thyroxin. The adrenal glands are richer in vitamin C than any other organ in the body, and during stress, these glands release the vitamin, together with hormones, into the blood.

The vitamin's exact role in the stress reaction is unclear. Psychological stress alone does not appear to raise needs above the RDA, but some physical stresses such as infections, wound healing, and exposure to cold raise vitamin C needs. When immune system cells are called into action, they use a lot of oxygen and produce oxidants that can damage the cells themselves.[23] Thus vitamin C is used as an antioxidant whenever the immune system becomes active. The hormone thyroxin (made with vitamin C's help) regulates the metabolic rate, which speeds up under extreme stress and also when the body needs to produce extra heat—for example, in fever or cold weather.

As a Cure for the Common Cold and Respiratory Infections   Newspaper headlines touting vitamin C as a cure for colds have appeared frequently over the years, but researchers have found little, if any, support for such claims. A major review of the research on vitamin C in the treatment and prevention of the common cold revealed a significant difference of one-tenth of a cold per year and an average difference in duration of one-tenth of a day per cold in favor of those taking vitamin C. The term *significant* means that *statistical* analysis suggests that the findings probably didn't arise from a chance event, but from the experimental treatment being tested. The *human* significance of the findings, however, is apparent only when considered in a real-life context: the typical cold lasts about a week, and one-tenth of a day is only 2½ hours. Is that enough savings to warrant routine supplementation? Scientists think not; supplement users seem to think so.

Interestingly, findings from one study revealed that those who received the placebo *but thought they were receiving vitamin C* had fewer colds than the group who received vitamin C *but thought they were receiving the placebo*. (Never underestimate the healing power of faith!)

Recent discoveries of the ways vitamin C works in the body provide possible links between the vitamin and the common cold. Some research suggests that vitamin C (2 grams taken daily for two weeks) reduces blood histamine.[24] Anyone who has ever had a cold knows the discomfort of a runny or stuffed-up nose. Nasal congestion develops in response to elevated blood histamine, and people commonly take antihistamines for relief. Like an antihistamine, vitamin C comes to the rescue and deactivates histamine.[25]

Vitamin C also appears to protect the lungs.[26] Researchers exploring the relationship between vitamin C and upper respiratory infections found that vitamin C supplements significantly improved symptoms of respiratory infections.[27] In a study of runners, vitamin C supplements reduced the incidence of respiratory symptoms after participation in a marathon.[28] Earlier studies had shown that marathon and ultramarathon competitors have a high incidence of upper respiratory symptoms immediately following a race.

In Disease Prevention   The role of vitamin C in the prevention of, or therapy for, cancer and other diseases is still being studied, and findings are presented in Highlight 11. An epidemiological study of over 11,000 U.S. adults reported an inverse relationship between all causes of death and vitamin C intake up to a few hundred milligrams.[29] The relationship was stronger for men than for women and remained apparent after controlling for confounding variables such as age, sex, cigarette smoking, disease history, race, and education.

VITAMIN C RECOMMENDATIONS

How much vitamin C is enough? Allowances set by different nations are based on similar research findings, but vary from 30 milligrams per day in Great Britain and Canada to 60 in the United States and 100 in Japan.[30] As Figure 10–14 illustrates, all the different recommendations fall within a broad range of possible safe intakes.

The requirement—the amount needed to prevent the overt symptoms of scurvy—is well known to be only 10 milligrams daily. However, 10 milligrams a day does not saturate all the body tissues; larger intakes increase the body's total vitamin C. At about 60 milligrams per day, the tissues in the average person stop responding to further increases in intake, and at 100 milligrams per day, 95 percent of the population probably reaches tissue saturation. After the tissues are saturated, excess vitamin C is readily excreted.

The RDA for vitamin C, like all the RDA, is intended to maintain health in healthy people, not to restore health in sick people. A variety of physical stresses deplete the body's vitamin C supply and may make higher intakes desirable. Among the stresses known to increase vitamin C needs are infections; burns; extremely high or low temperatures; intakes of toxic heavy metals such as lead, mercury, and cadmium; the chronic use of certain medications, including aspirin, barbiturates, and oral contraceptives; and cigarette smoking. Cigarette smoke contains oxidants, which greedily consume this potent antioxidant. Exposure to cigarette smoke, especially when accompanied by low intakes of vitamin C, depletes the body's pool in both active and passive smokers.[31] Whereas the RDA for nonsmokers is 60 milligrams a day, the RDA for people who smoke cigarettes regularly is 100 milligrams; the Canadian RNI provides a similar increase for those who smoke.

After oral surgery, dentists may prescribe supplemental vitamin C to hasten healing. After major operations or extensive burns, when a tremendous amount of scar tissue must form during healing, the amount needed may be as high as 1000 milligrams (1 gram) a day or even more. In individual cases, a physician may prescribe vitamin C supplements for certain conditions; self-medication is not recommended under any circumstances.

VITAMIN C DEFICIENCY

Two of the most notable signs of a vitamin C deficiency reflect its role in maintaining the integrity of blood vessels. The gums bleed easily around the teeth, and capillaries under the skin break spontaneously, producing pinpoint hemor-

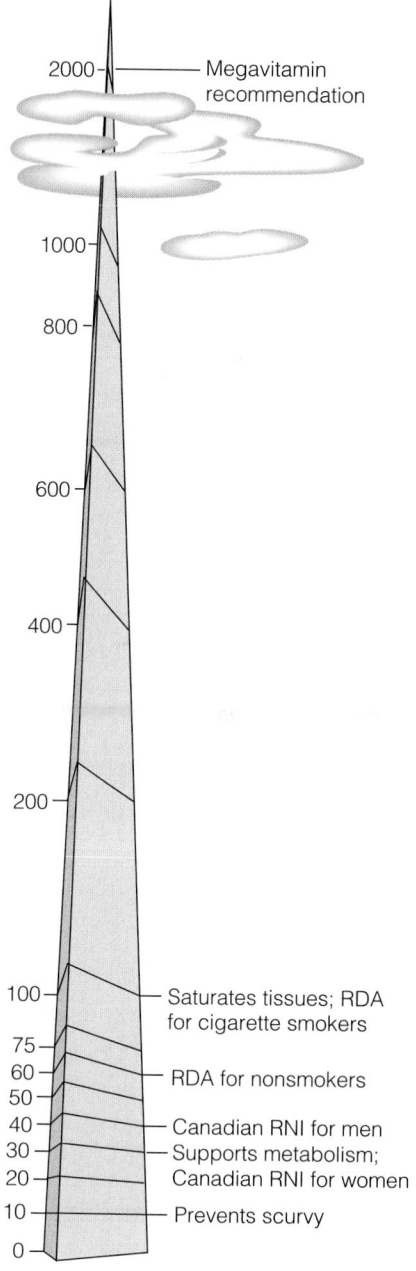

Figure 10–14

Vitamin C Intake (mg)

Recommendations differ, but all are generously above the minimum requirement and below the toxicity level. In contrast, megadoses of 2 grams a day are clearly way up in the clouds.

2000 — Megavitamin recommendation

1000

800

600

400

200

100 — Saturates tissues; RDA for cigarette smokers

75

60 — RDA for nonsmokers

50

40 — Canadian RNI for men

30 — Supports metabolism; Canadian RNI for women

20

10 — Prevents scurvy

0

rhages. Atherosclerotic plaques grow rapidly in the arteries. Table 10–11 reviews vitamin C information.

When the vitamin C pool falls to about a fifth of its optimal size (this may take several weeks on a diet lacking vitamin C), scurvy symptoms begin to appear. Failure to promote normal collagen synthesis causes further hemorrhaging. Muscles, including the heart muscle, degenerate. The skin becomes rough,

Table 10–11

Vitamin C—A Summary

Other Names	Deficiency Disease Name	
Ascorbic acid	Scurvy	
Adult RDA	**Deficiency Symptoms**	**Toxicity Symptoms**
	BLOOD/CIRCULATORY SYSTEM	
60 mg/day Smokers: 100 mg/day	Anemia (small-cell type),[a] atherosclerotic plaques, pinpoint hemorrhages	
Chief Functions in the Body	DIGESTIVE SYSTEM	
Collagen synthesis (strengthens blood vessel walls, forms scar tissue, provides matrix for bone growth), antioxidant, thyroxin synthesis, amino acid metabolism, strengthens resistance to infection, helps in absorption of iron		Nausea, abdominal cramps, diarrhea
	IMMUNE SYSTEM	
	Suppression, frequent infections	
Significant Sources	MOUTH, GUMS, TONGUE	
Citrus fruits, cabbage-type vegetables, dark green vegetables, cantaloupe, strawberries, peppers, lettuce, tomatoes, potatoes, papayas, mangoes	Bleeding gums, loosened teeth	
	NERVOUS/MUSCULAR SYSTEMS	
	Muscle degeneration and pain, hysteria, depression	Headache, fatigue, insomnia
	SKELETAL SYSTEM	
	Bone fragility, joint pain	
	SKIN	
	Rough skin, blotchy bruises	Hot flashes, rashes
	OTHER	
	Failure of wounds to heal	Interference with medical tests, aggravation of gout symptoms, urinary tract problems, kidney stones[b]

[a]Small-cell–type anemia is *microcytic anemia.*
[b]People who have a tendency toward gout and those who have a genetic abnormality that alters the breakdown of vitamin C are prone to forming kidney stones. Vitamin C is inactivated and degraded by several routes, sometimes producing oxalate, which can form stones in the kidneys.

brown, scaly, and dry. Wounds fail to heal because scar tissue will not form. Bone rebuilding falters; the ends of the long bones become softened, malformed, and painful, and fractures appear. The teeth become loose as the cartilage around them weakens. Anemia and infections are common. There are also characteristic psychological signs, including hysteria and depression. Sudden death is likely, occasioned by severe atherosclerosis or by massive bleeding into the joints and body cavities.

Once diagnosed, scurvy is readily reversed by vitamin C. Moderate doses in the neighborhood of 100 milligrams per day are sufficient, curing the scurvy within about five days. Such an intake is easily achieved by including vitamin C–rich foods in the diet.

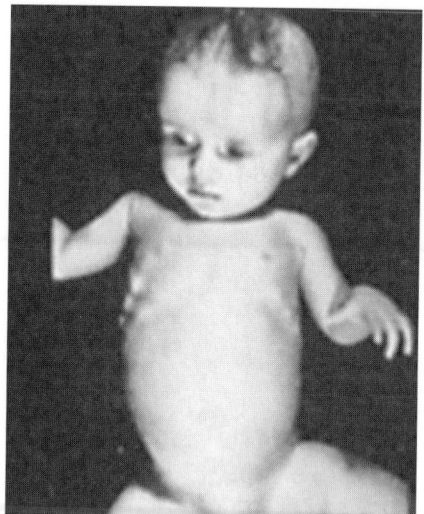

Scorbutic gums. Unlike other lesions of the mouth, scurvy presents a symmetrical appearance without infection.

VITAMIN C TOXICITY

The easy availability of vitamin C supplements and the publication of books recommending vitamin C to prevent colds and cancer have led thousands of people to take large doses of vitamin C. Not surprisingly, instances of vitamin C's causing harm have surfaced.

Toxic effects such as nausea, abdominal cramps, and diarrhea are often reported. Several instances of interference with medical regimens are also known. Large amounts of vitamin C excreted in the urine obscure the results of tests used to detect diabetes, giving a false positive result in some instances and a false negative in others. People taking anticlotting medications may unwittingly abolish the effect if they also take massive doses of vitamin C.* Those who have a tendency toward gout and those who have a genetic abnormality that alters vitamin C's breakdown to its excretion products are prone to forming kidney stones if they take large doses of vitamin C.† Vitamin C supplements are dangerous for people with iron overload; vitamin C enhances iron absorption and releases iron from body stores.[32]

A person who has taken large doses of vitamin C for a long time (say, ten times the RDA daily for several weeks) may adapt by limiting absorption and destroying and excreting more of the vitamin than usual. If the person then suddenly reduces intake to normal, the accelerated disposal system may not be able to put on its brakes fast enough to avoid destroying too much of the vitamin. It has been suggested that adults who stop taking large doses may develop scurvy on intakes that would protect most adults, but evidence is scanty on this point. If scurvy does develop, the situation is similar to the withdrawal reaction seen in drug and alcohol abusers when they discontinue drug use. When people cease taking vitamin C in excessive doses, they might be wise to do so gradually.

Few instances warrant consuming more than 100 to 300 milligrams of vitamin C a day. For adults who dose themselves with 1 to 2 grams a day, the risks may not be great; those taking more than 2 grams, and especially those taking amounts above 8 grams per day, should be aware of the distinct possibility of harm.

Infant scurvy. This is the characteristic "scorbutic pose," with legs bent and thighs rotated open. The infant's joints are painful, and she will cry if made to move.

false positive: a test result indicating that a condition is present (positive) when in fact it is not (therefore false).

false negative: a test result indicating that a condition is *not* present (negative) when in fact it is present (therefore false).

Reminder: *Gout* is a metabolic disease in which uric acid crystals precipitate in the joints.

---

*Vitamin C interferes with such anticoagulants as warfarin, dicumarol, heparin, and coumadin. It is unclear whether vitamin C inhibits the absorption or the action of these drugs.

†Vitamin C is inactivated and degraded by several routes, and sometimes oxalate, which can form kidney stones, is produced along the way. People may also develop oxalate crystals in their kidneys regardless of vitamin C status.

withdrawal reaction: a reaction to removal of a substance (usually of a drug) that reveals that the user has become dependent. One infant is reported to have been born of a mother who took massive doses of vitamin C. The infant developed rebound scurvy on an intake that would have been adequate for the average infant.

In conclusion, the range of safe vitamin C intakes seems to be broad, as is typical for water-soluble vitamins. Between the absolute minimum of 10 milligrams a day and a reasonable maximum of perhaps 300 milligrams, nearly everyone can find a suitable intake. People who venture outside these limits may be taking health risks.

VITAMIN C FOOD SOURCES

Fruits and vegetables can easily provide a generous intake of vitamin C. A cup of orange juice at breakfast, a salad for lunch, and a stalk of broccoli and a potato for dinner alone provide more than 300 milligrams. Clearly, a person making such food choices needs no vitamin C pills.

Figure 10–15 (on p. 363) shows the amounts of vitamin C in various common foods. The overwhelming abundance of purple and green bars reveals not only that the citrus fruits are justly famous for being rich in vitamin C, but that other fruits and vegetables are in the same league. A single serving of broccoli, green pepper, cauliflower, cantaloupe, and strawberries provides more than 50 milligrams of the vitamin (and an array of other nutrients) for less than 60 kcalories. Because vitamin C is vulnerable to heat, raw fruits and vegetables usually have a higher nutrient density than their cooked counterparts.

The potato is an important source of vitamin C, not because one potato by itself meets the daily need, but because potatoes are such a common staple that they make significant contributions.[33] In fact, scurvy was unknown in Ireland until the potato blight of the mid-1840s when some two million people died of malnutrition and infection.[34] Potatoes provide about 20 percent of all the vitamin C in the U.S. diet.

The lack of gold, white, brown, and red bars in Figure 10–15 confirms that grains, milk (except breast milk), legumes, and meats are notoriously poor sources of vitamin C. Organ meats (liver, kidneys, and others) and raw meats contain some vitamin C, but most people don't eat large quantities of these. Raw meats and fish contribute enough vitamin C to be significant in parts of Alaska, Canada, and Japan, but elsewhere, fruits and vegetables are necessary to supply sufficient vitamin C.

To protect the vitamin C in foods:
- Store cut produce in airtight wrappers and juices in closed containers (it's easily oxidized).
- Refrigerate produce, and avoid high temperatures and long cooking times (it's vulnerable to heat).
- Use a microwave oven or steam vegetables in a small amount of water (it's lost in the liquid).

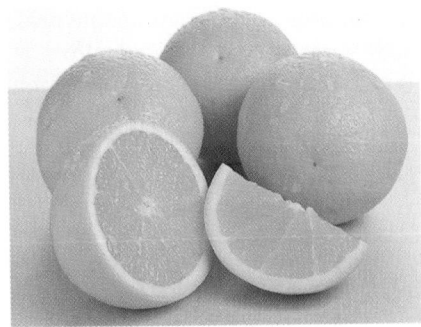

When nutritionists say "vitamin C," people think "oranges."

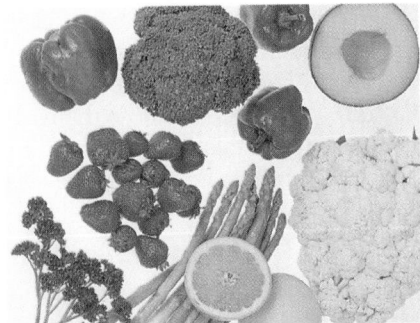

But these foods are also rich in vitamin C.

Figure 10–15 Vitamin C in Selected Foods

Milligrams

Food	Serving size (kcalories)
Bread, whole wheat	1 slice (64 kcal)
Corn flakes, fortified	1 oz (108 kcal)
White rice	½ c cooked (134 kcal)
Spaghetti pasta	½ c cooked (99 kcal)
Oatmeal	½ c cooked (73 kcal)
Tortilla, flour	1 8"-round (115 kcal)
Spinach	1 c raw (12 kcal)
Broccoli	½ c cooked (22 kcal)
Carrots	½ c shredded raw (24 kcal)
Green peas	½ c cooked (62 kcal)
Corn	½ c cooked (66 kcal)
Green beans	½ c cooked (22 kcal)
Sweet potatoes	½ c cooked (117 kcal)
Potato	1 baked w/skin (220 kcal)
Tomato juice	¾ c (31 kcal)
Apple	1 medium raw (81 kcal)
Banana	1 medium raw (104 kcal)
Orange	1 medium raw (62 kcal)
Strawberries	½ c fresh (23 kcal)
Raisins	¼ c (109 kcal)
Watermelon	1 slice (154 kcal)
Grapefruit juice	¾ c fresh (72 kcal)
Avocado	¼ (85 kcal)
Milk	1 c low-fat 2% (121 kcal)
Yogurt, plain	1 c low-fat (143 kcal)
Cheddar cheese	1½ oz (171 kcal)
Cottage cheese	½ c low-fat 2% (101 kcal)
Swiss cheese	1½ oz (159 kcal)
Ice cream	½ c, 10% fat (134 kcal)
Navy beans	½ c cooked (129 kcal)
Pinto beans	½ c cooked (117 kcal)
Kidney beans	½ c cooked (109 kcal)
Garbanzo beans	½ c cooked (134 kcal)
Peanut butter	2 tbs (190 kcal)
Sunflower seeds	1 oz dry (159 kcal)
Tofu (soybean curd)	½ c (94 kcal)
Shrimp	3 oz boiled (85 kcal)
Ground beef, lean	3 oz broiled (239 kcal)
Chicken breast	3 oz roasted (141 kcal)
Cod	3 oz poached (88 kcal)
Ham, lean [a]	3 oz roasted (123 kcal)
Sirloin steak, lean	3 oz broiled (171 kcal)
Tuna, canned in water	3 oz (99 kcal)
Bologna, beef [a]	2 slices (144 kcal)
Egg	1 hard cooked (77 kcal)

Additional 5 foods:

Food	Serving size (kcalories)
Red bell pepper	1 c raw chopped (27 kcal)
Kiwi	1 (46 kcal)
Mango	1 (134 kcal)
Brussels sprouts	½ c cooked (30 kcal)
Snow peas	½ c stir fry (35 kcal)

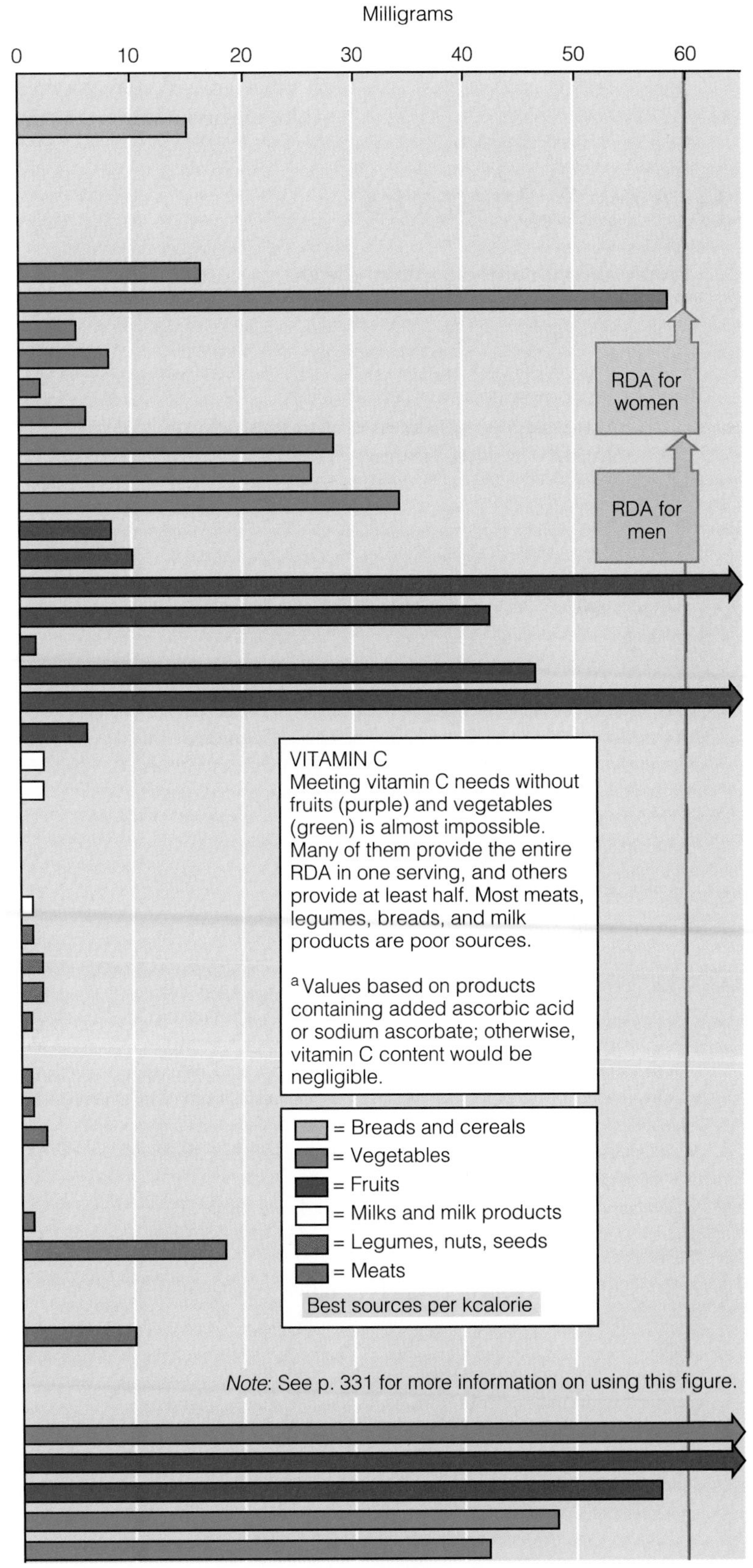

RDA for women

RDA for men

VITAMIN C
Meeting vitamin C needs without fruits (purple) and vegetables (green) is almost impossible. Many of them provide the entire RDA in one serving, and others provide at least half. Most meats, legumes, breads, and milk products are poor sources.

[a] Values based on products containing added ascorbic acid or sodium ascorbate; otherwise, vitamin C content would be negligible.

= Breads and cereals
= Vegetables
= Fruits
= Milks and milk products
= Legumes, nuts, seeds
= Meats
Best sources per kcalorie

Note: See p. 331 for more information on using this figure.

Vita means life. After this discourse on the vitamins, who could dispute that they deserve their name? Their regulation of metabolic processes makes them vital to normal growth, development, and maintenance of the body. The remarkable roles of the vitamins continue in the next chapter.

Study Questions

1. How do the vitamins differ from the energy nutrients?
2. Describe some general differences between fat-soluble and water-soluble vitamins.
3. Which B vitamins are involved in energy metabolism? Protein metabolism? Cell division?
4. For thiamin, riboflavin, niacin, biotin, pantothenic acid, vitamin B_6, folate, vitamin B_{12}, and vitamin C, state:

   - Its chief function in the body.
   - Its characteristic deficiency symptoms.
   - Its significant food sources.

5. What is the relationship of tryptophan to niacin?
6. Describe the relationship between folate and vitamin B_{12}.
7. What risks are associated with high doses of niacin? Vitamin B_6? Vitamin C?

Notes

1. The vitamin names used here are those established by the International Union of Nutritional Sciences Committee on Nomenclature, in Nomenclature policy: Generic descriptors and trivial names for vitamins and related compounds, *Journal of Nutrition* 117 (1987): 7–15.
2. Committee on Dietary Allowances, *Recommended Dietary Allowances*, 10th ed. (Washington, D.C.: National Academy Press, 1989), pp. 132–137.
3. D. A. Bender, *Nutritional Biochemistry of the Vitamins* (Cambridge: Cambridge University Press, 1992), pp. 184–222.
4. R. B. Colletti and coauthors, Niacin treatment of hypercholesterolemia in children, *Pediatrics* 92 (1993): 78–82; Y. Henkin, K. C. Johnson, and J. P. Segrest, Rechallenge with crystalline niacin after drug-induced hepatitis from sustained-release niacin, *Journal of the American Medical Association* 264 (1990): 241–243.
5. M. T. Behme, Nicotinamide and diabetes prevention, *Nutrition Reviews* 53 (1995): 137–139.
6. W. O. Song, Pantothenic acid: How much do we know about this B-complex vitamin? *Nutrition Today*, March/April 1990, pp. 19–25.
7. T. R. Guilarte, Vitamin B_6 and cognitive development: Recent research findings from human and animal studies, *Nutrition Reviews* 51 (1993): 193–198; S. N. Meydani and coauthors, Vitamin B_6 deficiency impairs interlukin 2 production and lymphocyte proliferation in elderly adults, *American Journal of Clinical Nutrition* 53 (1991): 1275–1280.
8. L. C. Rall and S. N. Meydani, Vitamin B_6 and immune competence, *Nutrition Reviews* 51 (1993): 217–225.
9. R. L. Reid, Premenstrual syndrome, *New England Journal of Medicine* 324 (1991): 1208–1210.
10. A. L. Bernstein and J. S. Dineson, Effect of pharmacologic doses of vitamin B_6 on carpal tunnel syndrome, electroencephalographic results, and pain, *Journal of the American College of Nutrition* 12 (1993): 73–76.
11. Committee on Genetics, Folic acid for the prevention of neural tube defects, *Pediatrics* 92 (1993): 493–494; M. M. Werler, S. Shapiro, and A. A. Mitchell, Periconceptional folic acid exposure and risk of occurrent neural tube defects, *Journal of the American Medical Association* 269 (1993): 1257–1261; A. E. Czeizel and I. Dudás, Prevention of the first occurrence of neural-tube defects by periconceptual vitamin supplementation, *New England Journal of Medicine* 327 (1992): 1832–1835.
12. From the Centers for Disease Control and Prevention, Recommendations for use of folic acid to reduce number of spina bifida cases and other neural tube defects, *Journal of the American Medical Association* 269 (1993): 1233–1238.
13. R. D. Williams, FDA proposes folic acid fortification, *FDA Consumer*, May 1994, pp. 11–14.
14. Folate and neural tube defects: US policy evolves, *Nutrition Reviews* 51 (1993): 358–361.
15. M. Nestle, Folate fortification and neural tube defects: Policy implications, *Journal of Nutrition Education* 26 (1994): 287–293; A. Bendich, Folic acid and prevention of neural tube birth defects: Critical assessment of FDA proposals to increase folic acid intakes, *Journal of Nutrition Education* 26 (1994): 294–299.
16. V. Herbert, Folate and neural tube defects, *Nutrition Today*, November/December 1992, pp. 30–33.

17. C. L. Krumdieck, Folic acid, in *Present Knowledge in Nutrition*, 6th ed., ed. M. L. Brown (Washington, D.C.: Nutrition Foundation, 1990), pp. 179–188.

18. C. E. Butterworth and coauthors, Folate deficiency and cervical dysplasia, *Journal of the American Medical Association* 267 (1992): 528–533.

19. Committee on Dietary Allowances, 1989, pp. 150–158.

20. Choline: A conditionally essential nutrient for humans, *Nutrition Reviews* 50 (1992): 112–114; C. D. Berdanier, Is inositol an essential nutrient? *Nutrition Today*, March/April 1992, pp. 22–26.

21. D. B. McCormick, Riboflavin, in *Present Knowledge in Nutrition*, 6th ed., ed. M. L. Brown (Washington, D.C.: Nutrition Foundation, 1990), pp. 146–154.

22. J. R. Turnlund and coauthors, Vitamin B-6 depletion followed by repletion with animal- or plant-source diets and calcium and magnesium metabolism in young women, *American Journal of Clinical Nutrition* 56 (1992): 905–910.

23. G. Wolf, Uptake of ascorbic acid by human neutrophils, *Nutrition Reviews* 11 (1993): 337–338.

24. C. S. Johnston, L. J. Martin, and X. Cai, Antihistamine effect of supplemental ascorbic acid and neutrophil chemotaxis, *Journal of the American College of Nutrition* 11 (1992): 172–176.

25. A. R. Sherman and N. A. Hallquist, Immunity, in *Present Knowledge in Nutrition*, 6th ed., ed. M. L. Brown (Washington, D.C.: Nutrition Foundation, 1990), pp. 463–476.

26. J. Schwartz and S. T. Weiss, Relationship between dietary vitamin C intake and respiratory function in the First National Health and Nutrition Examination Survey (NHANES I), *American Journal of Clinical Nutrition* 59 (1994): 110–114.

27. C. Bucca, G. Rolla, and J. C. Farina, Effect of vitamin C on transient increase of bronchial responsiveness in conditions affecting the airways, *Annals of the New York Academy of Sciences* 669 (1992): 175–186.

28. E. M. Peters and coauthors, Vitamin C supplementation reduces the incidence of postrace symptoms of upper-respiratory-tract infection in ultramarathon runners, *American Journal of Clinical Nutrition* 57 (1993): 170–174.

29. J. E. Enstrom, L. E. Kanim, and M. A. Klein, Vitamin C intake and mortality among a sample of the United States population, *Epidemiology* 3 (1992): 194–202.

30. S. N. Gershoff, Vitamin C (ascorbic acid): New roles, new requirements, *Nutrition Reviews* 11 (1993): 313–326.

31. D. L. Tribble, L. J. Giuliano, and S. P. Fortmann, Reduced plasma ascorbic acid concentrations in nonsmokers regularly exposed to environmental tobacco smoke, *American Journal of Clinical Nutrition* 58 (1993): 886–890.

32. V. Herbert, Vitamin C supplements are dangerous for iron-overloaded persons, *Journal of the American Dietetic Association* 93 (1993): 526–527.

33. G. B. Forbes, Potatoes: A reliable source of vitamin C (Scorbutus nauticus cured without citrus), *Nutrition Today*, January/February 1993, pp. 33–35.

34. A. Nikiforuk, The Irish famine: A blighted fable, in *The Fourth Horseman: A Short History of Epidemics, Plagues, Famine and Other Scourges* (New York: M. Evans & Company, 1993), pp. 110–125.

Vitamin and Mineral Supplements

Approximately 40 percent of the U.S. population takes vitamin and mineral supplements regularly, spending billions of dollars on them each year.[1] Some people take supplements as dietary insurance, "in case" they are not meeting their nutrient needs from foods alone—as kind of an all-purpose extra food. Some people take supplements as health insurance to protect against certain diseases—as kind of an all-purpose extra drug.

One out of every five people takes multinutrient pills daily.[2] Others take large doses of single nutrients, most commonly, vitamin C, iron, and calcium. In many cases, taking supplements is a costly but harmless practice; sometimes, it is both costly and harmful to health.

For the most part, people self-prescribe supplements, taking them on the advice of friends, television, or books that may or may not be reliable. Sometimes, they take supplements on the recommendation of a physician. When such advice follows a valid nutrition assessment, supplementation may be warranted, but even then the preferred course of action is to improve food choices and eating habits. Without an assessment, the advice to take supplements may be inappropriate.

When people think of supplements, they often think only of vitamins, but minerals are important, too, of course. People whose diets lack vitamins, for whatever reason, probably lack several minerals as well. Vitamin-mineral supplements may be appropriate in some circumstances.

This highlight examines several questions related to supplement tak-

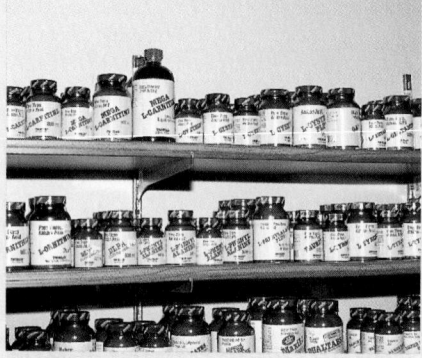

Supplements are available in a number of shapes and flavors, but none offer the full array of nutrients that a variety of foods can provide.

ing. What are the arguments for taking supplements? What are the arguments against taking them? Can athletes benefit from taking supplements? Finally, if people do take supplements, how can they choose the appropriate ones?

ARGUMENTS FOR SUPPLEMENTS

Supplements do have appropriate uses. In some cases, they can correct deficiencies; in others, they can reduce the risk of diseases.

Correct Overt Deficiencies

Vitamin deficiency diseases such as scurvy, pellagra, and beriberi are rare, but they do still occur. Correcting an overt deficiency disease may require therapeutic doses two to ten times the RDA of a nutrient. When doses exceed the amounts of nutrients commonly found in foods,

the supplements are being used more as drugs than as foods.

Improve Nutrition Status

In contrast to the classical deficiencies, which present a multitude of symptoms and are easy to recognize, subclinical deficiencies are subtle and easy to overlook—and they are also more likely to occur. People whose energy intakes are too low to deliver the needed amounts of nutrients, such as habitual dieters, strict vegetarians, and the elderly, risk developing subclinical deficiencies. If there is no way for these people to eat enough nutritious foods to meet their needs, then vitamin-mineral supplements may be appropriate to help prevent nutrient deficiencies.

While most nutrients can be obtained from a well-balanced diet, sometimes even a well-planned diet falls short of meeting the RDA for key nutrients. A person must not only follow guidelines such as the Food Guide Pyramid, but must also carefully select foods within that framework. While few people receive all of the RDA for all nutrients every day, most people receive at least their average needs for all nutrients. Supplements can help people to receive the intakes recommended by government and health authorities on a regular basis.

Consider the case of a woman who loses a lot of blood and therefore a lot of iron and other blood-building nutrients during menstruation each month. Such a woman may be able to eat well enough to make up for all nutrient deficits except that of iron: she may need an iron supplement. Chapter 13 shows ways for women to try to obtain enough iron in their diets, but also observes that it is hard to do. It also cautions that nutrition assessment is a necessary prerequisite to making the decision whether supplementation is appropriate.

Reduce Disease Risks

Many people, especially those who are intolerant to lactose or allergic to milk, may not receive enough calcium to forestall the bone degeneration of old age, osteoporosis. For them, nonmilk calcium-rich foods are especially valuable, but calcium supplements may also be appropriate (Highlight 12 provides more details).

Support Increased Nutrient Needs

Nutrient needs increase during certain stages of the life cycle, making it difficult to meet those needs without supplementation. For example, women of childbearing age may need folate supplements to reduce the risks of neural tube defects. Pregnant women and women who are breastfeeding their infants have exceptionally high nutrient needs and so usually need special supplements of iron, calcium, and folate. Newborns routinely receive a single dose of vitamin K at birth. Infants may need other supplements as well, depending on whether they are breastfed or receiving formula, and on whether their water contains fluoride.

Improve Body's Defenses

Health care professionals may provide special supplementation to people being treated for addictions to alcohol or other drugs and to people with prolonged illnesses, extensive injuries, or other severe stresses such as surgery. Nutrient

intakes are reduced in people with illnesses that interfere with appetite, eating, or nutrient absorption. Nutrient needs are increased by diseases or drugs that speed or alter nutrient metabolism. In all these cases, supplements are appropriate.

ARGUMENTS AGAINST SUPPLEMENTS

Supplement taking is risky, and the higher the dose, the greater the risk of harm. People's tolerances for high doses of nutrients vary, just as their risks of deficiencies do. Amounts that some can tolerate may be harmful for others, and no one knows who falls where along the spectrum. It is impossible to say just how much of a nutrient is enough— or too much. Assuming, however, that it is best to err on the conservative side, Table H10–1 presents suggested limits for vitamins and minerals from supplements.

Toxicity

The extent and severity of supplement toxicity remain unclear. Only a few alert health care professionals can recognize toxicity, even when it is acute. When it is chronic, with the effects developing subtly and progressing slowly, it often goes unrecognized. In one case, a woman took just 1000 RE (5000 IU) of vitamin A, an amount typically found in vitamin-mineral supplements, daily for ten years. She was diagnosed with liver disease. Only when she discontinued the supplement did the condition clear up.[3] In view of the potential hazards, some authorities believe supplements should bear warning labels, advising consumers that large doses may be toxic.

Toxic overdoses of vitamins and minerals in children are more readily recognized and, unfortunately, fairly common. Poison control centers receive more than 30,000 reports a year of children under the age of six swallowing excessively large doses of supplements. Fruit-flavored, chewable vitamins shaped like cartoon characters entice young children to eat them like candy in amounts that can cause poisoning. Iron-containing supplements are especially toxic and are the leading cause of accidental ingestion fatalities among children.[4] Even mild overdoses cause GI distress, nausea, and black diarrhea that reflects gastric bleeding. Severe overdoses result in bloody diarrhea, shock, liver damage, coma, and death.

Life-Threatening Misinformation

Another problem arises when people who are ill come to believe that high doses of vitamins or minerals can be therapeutic. These claims are exceedingly common, as this report by a watchdog consumer group illustrates:

> In 1989, volunteers of the Consumer Health Education Council (CHEC) telephoned 41 Houston-area health food stores and asked to speak with the person who provided nutritional advice. The callers explained that they had a brother sick with AIDS. . . . All 41 retailers offered products they said could strengthen the brother's immune system. . . . Thirty said they sold products that would cure AIDS.[5]

Other such inquiries led to wrong-headed advice from salespeople urging that customers use supplements to treat headaches, dizziness, fatigue, kidney stones, abnormal thirst (a diabetes warning sign), glaucoma (a progressive eye-destroying disease), and sudden weight loss (a serious

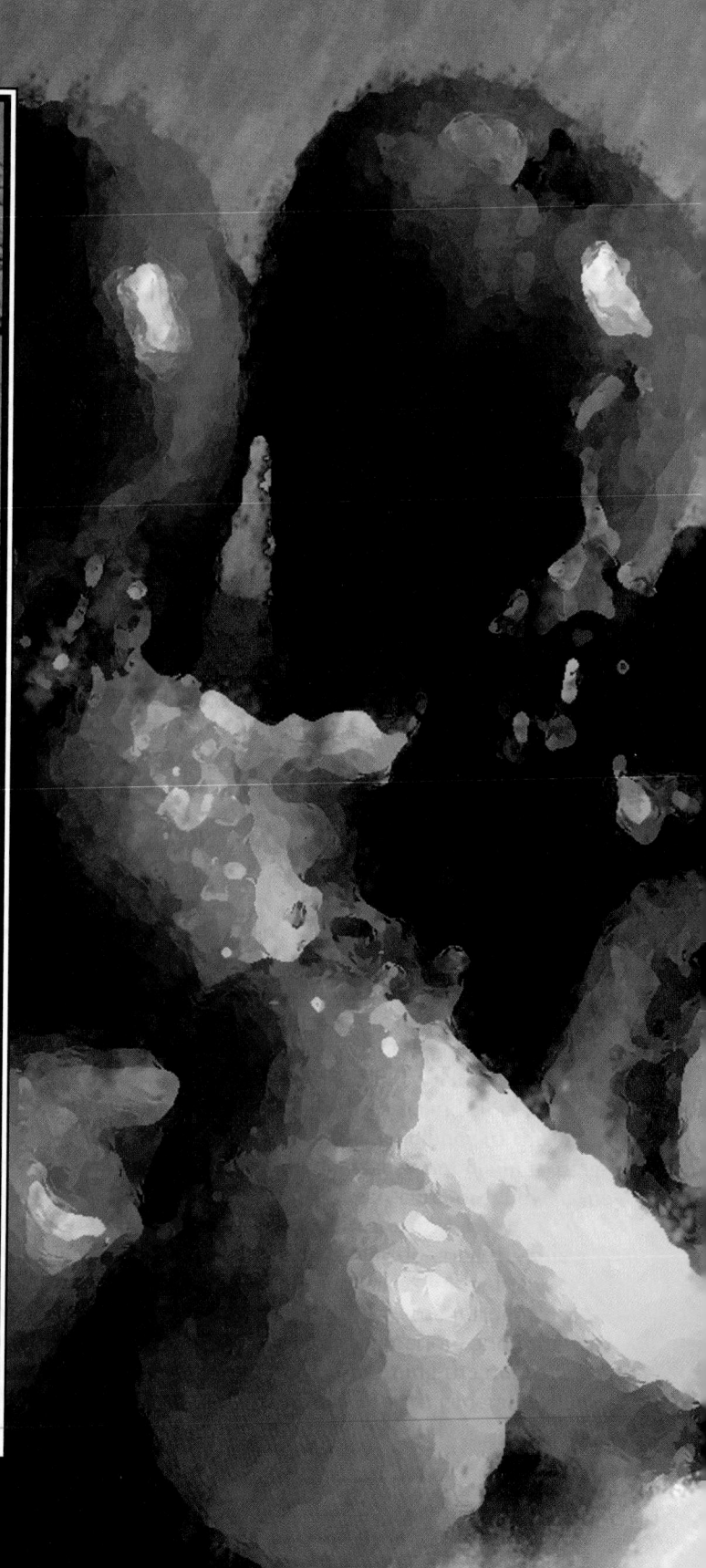

Chapter 11

The Fat-Soluble Vitamins: A, D, E, and K

CONTENTS

Vitamin A and Beta-Carotene
Roles in the Body
Vitamin A Recommendations
Vitamin A Deficiency
Vitamin A Toxicity
Vitamin A in Foods
Vitamin D
Roles in the Body
Vitamin D Deficiency
Vitamin D Toxicity
Vitamin D Recommendations and Sources
Vitamin E
Vitamin E as an Antioxidant
Vitamin E Deficiency
Vitamin E Toxicity
Vitamin E Recommendations
Vitamin E in Foods
Vitamin K
Vitamin K Deficiency
Vitamin K Toxicity
Vitamin K Recommendations and Sources
The Fat-Soluble Vitamins—In Summary
HIGHLIGHT: Antioxidant Nutrients and
Nonnutrients in Disease Prevention

MICROGRAPH: Beta carotene, the vitamin A precursor
found in fruits and vegetables

*t*he fat-soluble vitamins A, D, E, and K differ from the water-soluble vitamins in several significant ways (review Table 10–2 on p. 328). The fat-soluble vitamins are found in the fats and oils of foods. They are insoluble in water, so they require bile for digestion and chylomicrons for absorption. Upon absorption, fat-soluble vitamins enter the lymphatic system before entering the bloodstream, where many of them require protein carriers for transport. The fat-soluble vitamins are stored in the liver and adipose tissue until they are needed; they are not readily excreted, as most of the water-soluble vitamins are. Having stored these vitamins, people can eat less than their daily need for days, weeks, or even months or years without ill effects. Blood concentrations are maintained because the body retrieves the vitamins from storage as needed; thus a person need only ensure that over time *average* daily intakes approximate the RDA. By the same token, because fat-soluble vitamins are stored, the risk of toxicity is greater than it is for the water-soluble vitamins.

Vitamin A and Beta-Carotene

Vitamin A was the first fat-soluble vitamin to be recognized. More than 75 years later, vitamin A and its precursor, beta-carotene, continue to intrigue researchers with their diverse roles and profound effects on health.

Three different forms of vitamin A are active in the body: retinol, retinal, and retinoic acid. Collectively, these compounds are known as retinoids. Foods derived from animals provide preformed vitamin A as compounds (retinyl esters) that are easily hydrolyzed to retinol in the intestine. Foods derived from plants provide carotenoids, some of which have vitamin A activity. The most important of the carotenoids is beta-carotene, which can be split to form retinol in the intestine and liver. Beta-carotene's absorption and conversion are less efficient than those of preformed vitamin A. Figure 11–1 illustrates the structural similarities and differences of these vitamin A compounds.

The cells can convert retinol and retinal to the other active forms as needed. The oxidation of retinol to retinal is reversible, but the further oxidation of retinal to retinoic acid is irreversible. This irreversibility is significant because each form of vitamin A performs a function that the others cannot (see Figure 11–2).

A special transport protein, retinol-binding protein (RBP), picks up vitamin A from the liver, where it is stored, and carries it in the blood. Cells that will use vitamin A have special protein receptors for it, as if the vitamin were fragile and had to be passed carefully from hand to hand without being dropped. Each form of vitamin A has its own receptor protein (retinol has several) within the cell.

ROLES IN THE BODY

Vitamin A is a versatile vitamin. Its major roles include:

- Promoting vision.
- Promoting cell differentiation (and thereby maintaining the health of epithelial tissues and skin).
- Supporting the immune system.
- Promoting growth and bone remodeling.

Reminder: A *precursor* is a compound that can be converted into an active vitamin.

beta-carotene (BAY-tah KARE-oh-teen): an orange pigment and vitamin A precursor found in plants.

retinol (RET-ih-nol): the alcohol form of vitamin A.

retinal (RET-ih-nal): the aldehyde form of vitamin A, active in the eye.

retinoic (RET-ih-no-ick) **acid:** the acid form of vitamin A.

retinoids: chemically related compounds with biologic activity similar to retinol; metabolites of retinol.

preformed vitamin A: dietary vitamin A in its active form.

carotenoids: pigments commonly found in plants and animals, some of which have provitamin A activity. Carotenoids are among the best-known **phytochemicals**— plant chemicals that are not nutrients but have biological activity in the body (see Highlight 11 for more details).

retinol-binding protein (RBP): the specific protein responsible for transporting retinol.

Figure 11–1
. . . .

Forms of Vitamin A

In this diagram, corners represent carbon atoms, as in all previous diagrams in this book. A further simplification here is that methyl groups (CH_3) are understood to be at the ends of the lines extending from corners. (See Appendix C for complete structures.)

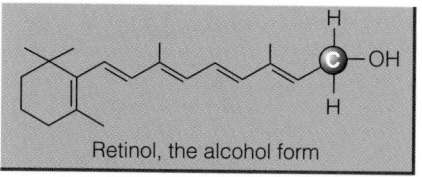

Retinol, the alcohol form

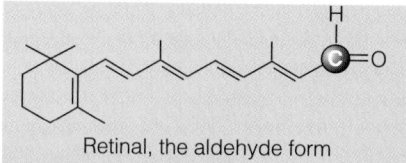

Retinal, the aldehyde form

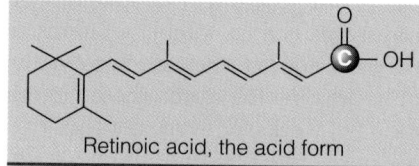

Retinoic acid, the acid form

Cleavage at this point can
yield two molecules of vitamin A*

Beta-carotene, a precursor

*Sometimes cleavage occurs at other points as well, so that one molecule of beta-carotene may yield only one molecule of vitamin A. Furthermore, not all beta-carotene is converted to vitamin A, and absorption of beta-carotene is not as efficient as vitamin A. For these reasons, 6 μg of beta-carotene are equivalent to 1 μg of vitamin A. Conversion of other carotenoids to vitamin A is even less efficient.

Each form of vitamin A performs specific tasks. Retinol supports reproduction and is the major transport and storage form of the vitamin. Retinal is active in vision and is also an intermediate in the conversion of retinol to retinoic acid. Retinoic acid acts like a hormone, regulating cell differentiation, growth, and embryonic development.[1] Animals raised on retinoic acid as their sole source of vitamin A can grow normally, but they become blind, because retinoic acid cannot be converted to retinal.[2]

Vitamin A in Vision   Vitamin A plays two indispensable roles in the eye: it helps maintain a crystal-clear outer window, the cornea, and it participates in the transportation of light energy into nerve impulses at the retina (see Figure 11–3). When light falls on the eye, it passes through the clear cornea and strikes the cells of the retina. Pigment molecules inside the cells of the retina absorb light. (The glossary on p. 378 describes these molecules—rhodopsin, iodopsin, and others.) Each pigment molecule is composed of a protein called opsin bonded to a molecule of retinal. When light energy enters the eye, the retinal portion of the pigment

Figure 11–2
. . . .

Conversion of Vitamin A Compounds

Notice that the conversion from retinol to retinal is reversible, whereas the pathway from retinal to retinoic acid is not.

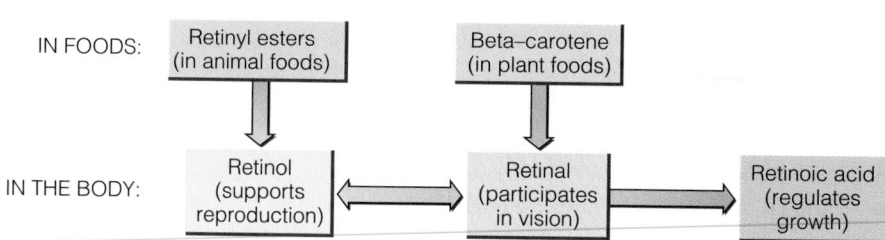

IN FOODS: Retinyl esters (in animal foods)   Beta–carotene (in plant foods)

IN THE BODY: Retinol (supports reproduction) ⟷ Retinal (participates in vision) ⟶ Retinoic acid (regulates growth)

Figure 11–3

Vitamin A's Role in Vision

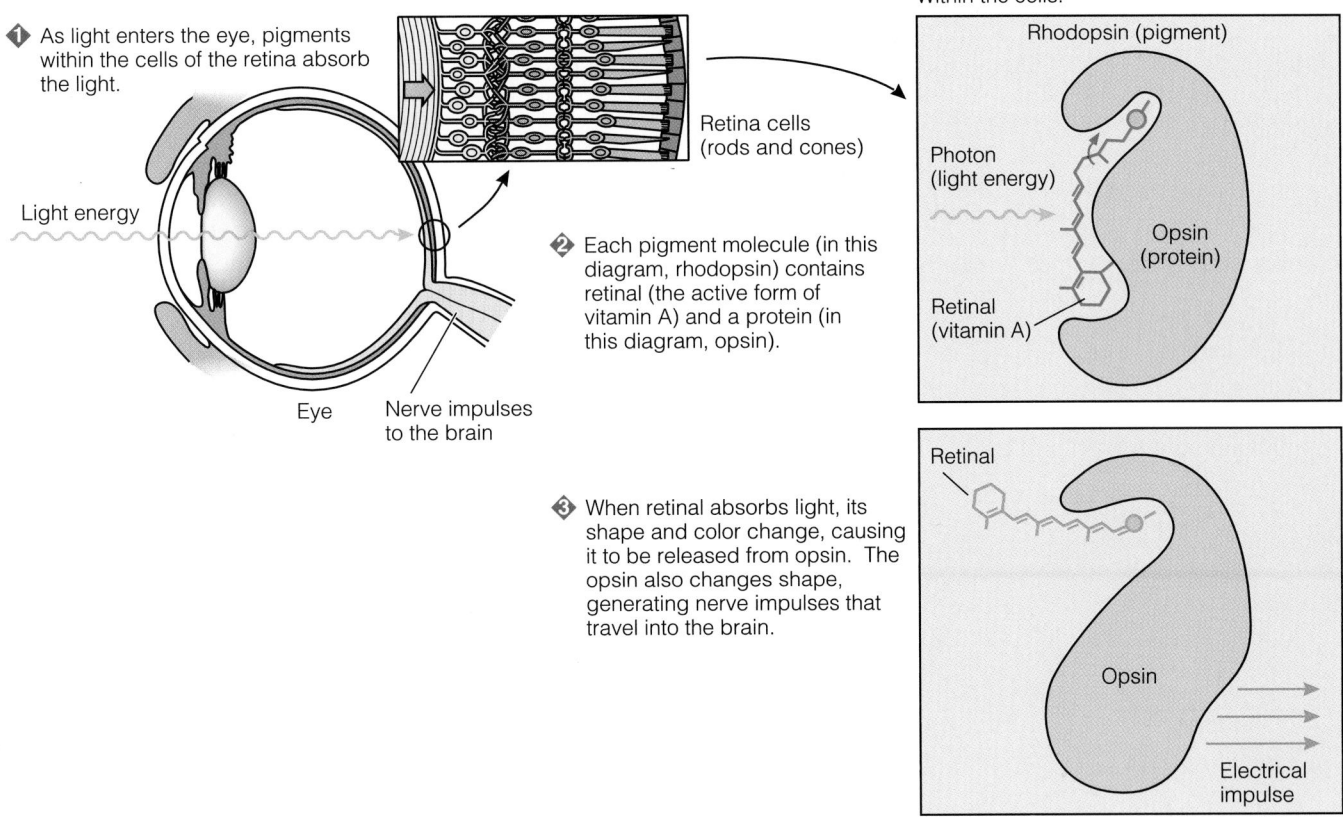

Within the cells:

1 As light enters the eye, pigments within the cells of the retina absorb the light.

Light energy

Eye

Nerve impulses to the brain

Retina cells (rods and cones)

2 Each pigment molecule (in this diagram, rhodopsin) contains retinal (the active form of vitamin A) and a protein (in this diagram, opsin).

3 When retinal absorbs light, its shape and color change, causing it to be released from opsin. The opsin also changes shape, generating nerve impulses that travel into the brain.

Rhodopsin (pigment)

Photon (light energy)

Retinal (vitamin A)

Opsin (protein)

Retinal

Opsin

Electrical impulse

molecule absorbs the photon and responds by changing shape: it shifts from a *cis* to a *trans* configuration as fatty acids do during hydrogenation (see p. 147). In the process, the retinal also changes color, becoming bleached. In its altered form, retinal cannot remain bonded to opsin and is released. This alters the shape of the opsin molecule.

The change in opsin's shape has further effects: it disturbs the membrane of the cell, generating an electrical impulse that travels along the cell's length. At the other end of the cell, the impulse is transmitted to a nerve cell, which conveys it deeper into the brain. Thus the message is sent. After sending the message, much of the retinal is converted back to its original form and rejoined to opsin to regenerate the pigment rhodopsin. Some retinal, however, may be oxidized to retinoic acid, a biochemical dead end for the visual process.

A genius could not have designed a better system. Light itself cannot be conducted through the solid material of the brain, but nerve impulses can be. To preserve the information in the different colors, or wavelengths, that light comes in, the eye uses the color-sensitive cone cells to receive them. Blue light is absorbed by one set of cells, green by another, and yellow-red by a third. By day, cones receive these colors and convey the full range of color vision to the optic center

Glossary of Vision Terms

cones: the cells of the retina that respond to bright light and are responsible for color vision.

cornea (KOR-nee-uh): the transparent membrane covering the outside of the eye.

iodopsin (eye-o-DOP-sin): the light-sensitive pigment of the cones in the retina. Both rhodopsin and iodopsin contain retinal; the protein portions of the pigments differ.

opsin (OP-sin): the protein portion of the visual pigment molecule.

photon (FOE-ton): a unit of light energy. Depending on its wavelength, a photon conveys different colors of light.

pigment: a molecule capable of absorbing certain wavelengths of light, so that it reflects only those that we perceive as a certain color.

retina (RET-in-uh): the layer of light-sensitive nerve cells lining the back of the inside of the eye; consists of rods and cones.

rhodopsin (ro-DOP-sin): the light-sensitive pigment of the rods in the retina; it contains the retinal form of vitamin A.
  rhod = rod-shaped cells
  opsin = visual protein

rods: the cells of the retina that respond to dim light and convey black-and-white vision.

---

in the brain. By night, the light entering the eye is of low intensity and can be received only by the rod cells; so by night a person can normally discern only the presence of light, not its color.

About 6 to 7 million cone cells and 100 million rod cells reside in the retina, and each contains about 30 million molecules of retinal-containing visual pigment. Visual activity leads to repeated small losses of retinal and necessitates its constant replenishment from retinol in the blood, which brings a new supply from the body stores. Ultimately, vitamin A and its relatives in foods are the source of all the retinal in the pigments of the eye.

A lot of retinal can be destroyed at night. If the body's vitamin A stores are marginal, the use of the eyes at night can lead to a vitamin A deficiency and the early, tell-tale symptom of night blindness. The eye is especially vulnerable to retinal destruction at night for three reasons. First, the pupil opens wide at night, so as to allow as much light as possible to enter the eye. Second, a shadowing pigment that protects the rods by day withdraws at night, leaving them exposed. Third, there are many more rods than cones. Hence, if a bright light suddenly shines at night through the wide-open pupil onto the unprotected rods, much of the pigment in them is bleached and momentarily inactivated. More retinal than usual is released, and more is lost. A moment passes before the pigments regenerate and sight returns. You no doubt have been temporarily "blinded" on occasion by a light shining directly into your eyes. Normally, of course, you quickly recover your ability to see.

Vitamin A in Cell Differentiation   Despite its important role in vision, only one-thousandth of the body's vitamin A is in the retina. Much more is in the cells lining the body's surfaces, where the vitamin participates in cell differentiation.[3]

All body surfaces, both inside and out, are covered by layers of cells known as epithelial cells. The epithelial tissue on the outside of the body is, of course, the

night blindness: slow recovery of vision after flashes of bright light at night or an inability to see in dim light; an early symptom of vitamin A deficiency.

differentiation: development of specific functions different from those of the original.

epithelial (ep-i-THEE-lee-ul) **cells:** cells on the surface of the skin and mucous membranes.

epithelial tissues: the layers of the body that serve as selective barriers between the body's interior and the environment (examples are the cornea, the skin, the respiratory lining, and the lining of the digestive tract).

skin. The epithelial tissues that line the inside of the body are the mucous membranes: the linings of the mouth, stomach, and intestines; the linings of the lungs and the passages leading to them; the linings of the urinary bladder and urethra; the linings of the uterus and vagina; and the linings of the eyelids and sinus passageways. Within the body, the mucous membranes of the GI tract alone line an area larger than a quarter of a football field, and vitamin A helps to maintain their integrity (see Figure 11–4).

Vitamin A promotes differentiation of both epithelial cells and goblet cells, one-celled glands that synthesize and secrete mucus. Mucus coats and protects the epithelial cells from invasive microorganisms and other harmful substances, such as gastric juices.

Vitamin A in Immunity   Vitamin A's maintenance of healthy epithelial tissues helps to fight infection by preventing the invasion of bacteria and viruses. In addition, vitamin A appears to play a direct role in immunity itself.[4] Children with even mild vitamin A deficiency develop respiratory infections and diarrhea at two and three times the rate of children with normal vitamin A status.

Vitamin A in Growth   As mentioned, vitamin A supports growth. Growth failure is common in children with vitamin A deficiency. When they are given vitamin A supplements, they gain weight and grow taller.

The growth of bones illustrates that growth is a complex phenomenon of remodeling. To convert a small bone into a large bone, the bone-remodeling cells must "undo" some parts of the bone as they go, and vitamin A participates in the undoing. The cells that break down bone contain sacs of degradative enzymes. With the help of vitamin A, these enzymes eat away at selected sites in the bone, removing the parts that are not needed. A similar process occurs when a human embryo loses its tail and becomes human-shaped; the tail "grows" shorter and shorter until it disappears. The process depends on vitamin A.

Beta-Carotene as an Antioxidant   Beta-carotene functions in the body as a vitamin A precursor, but it also has roles of its own. Not all dietary beta-carotene is converted to active vitamin A. Some beta-carotene acts as an antioxidant capable of protecting the body against disease. Highlight 11 discusses some recent findings related to this protection.

mucous membranes: the membranes, composed of mucus-secreting cells, that line the surfaces of body tissues.

urethra (you-REE-thruh): the tube through which urine from the bladder passes out of the body.

Reminder: *Goblet cells* in the epithelium of the GI tract and lungs secrete mucus.

Reminder: *Mucus* is a slippery substance secreted by the goblet cells of mucous membranes.

remodeling: the dismantling and reformation of a structure, in this case, bone.

The cells that destroy bone during growth are **osteoclasts;** those that build bone are **osteoblasts.**

> *osteo* = bone
> *clast* = break
> *blast* = build

The sacs of degradative enzymes are **lysosomes** (LYE-so-zomes).

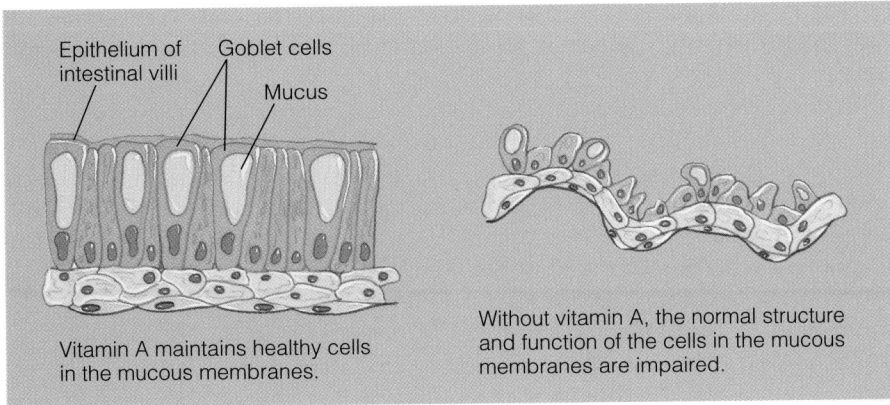

Vitamin A maintains healthy cells in the mucous membranes.

Without vitamin A, the normal structure and function of the cells in the mucous membranes are impaired.

Figure 11–4

Mucous Membrane Integrity

Figure 11–5

Vitamin A Deficiency and Toxicity
As the dose increases from zero, normalcy is reached. A wide range of intakes is safe, and then toxicity is reached.

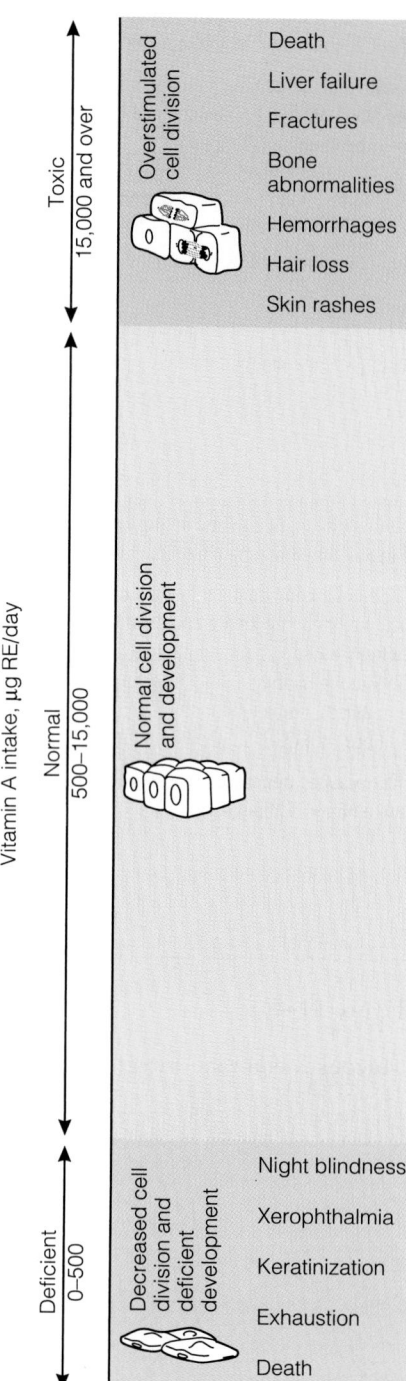

VITAMIN A RECOMMENDATIONS

Because the body can derive vitamin A either preformed or from beta-carotene, its contents in foods and its recommendations are expressed as retinol equivalents or RE. Some products still report their vitamin A contents using international units (IU), an older system of measurement that is based on some assumptions now known to be inaccurate. To evaluate vitamin A intake expressed in IU requires some computing: 1 RE is roughly equivalent to 3.33 IU of vitamin A from animal tissues or 10 IU from plant tissues.[5] Newer tables of food composition, including Appendix H in this book, report the vitamin A activity of foods in RE.

Vitamin A intakes can range widely before deficiency or toxicity symptoms appear (see Figure 11–5). Recommended intakes in both the United States and Canada are set at about double the minimum necessary to prevent deficiency. Doubtless, many people need not consume amounts this high; other countries and international agencies recommend lower values.[6] The exact upper limit of safety cannot be determined because people's tolerances to overdoses vary. Several authorities agree that the RDA are the best guidelines for safety and that higher intakes offer no benefits.[7]

VITAMIN A DEFICIENCY

Vitamin A status depends mostly on the adequacy of vitamin A stores, 90 percent of which are in the liver. Vitamin A status also depends on a person's having adequate protein, because protein provides the vitamin's carriers for inside-the-body transport. If a healthy adult were to stop eating vitamin A–rich foods, deficiency symptoms would not begin to appear until after stores were depleted, which would take one to two years; it would take less time in a growing child. Then, however, the consequences would be profound and severe. Table 11–1 (on pp. 382–383) itemizes deficiency symptoms as well as toxicity symptoms, functions in the body, and food sources.

Vitamin A deficiency is one of the developing world's major nutrition problems. More than 100 million children worldwide have some degree of vitamin A deficiency, and so are vulnerable to infectious diseases.[8]

Infectious Diseases   Since the early 1980s, several large studies conducted in Indonesia, India, Nepal, and Sudan have found that supplementing children with vitamin A can reduce death rates significantly.[9] This evidence prompted the World Health Organization (WHO) and UNICEF (the United Nations International Children's Emergency Fund) to make the control of vitamin A deficiency a major goal in their quest to improve child survival throughout the developing world.

In developing countries throughout the world, measles is a devastating infectious disease, killing as many as 2 million children each year.[10] The severity of the illness often correlates with the degree of vitamin A deficiency; deaths are usually due to related infections such as pneumonia and severe diarrhea.[11] Children with measles who receive vitamin A supplements recover faster from pneumonia and other infections than children who do not receive supplements.[12] Providing large doses of vitamin A to children hospitalized with severe measles can reduce their risk of dying by at least 50 percent.[13]

Of historical interest is a similar trial carried out in London in 1932 that showed remarkably consistent results: children hospitalized with measles who were given daily doses of cod liver oil (a rich source of vitamin A) died at a rate only half that of similar children not given the oil.[14] WHO now recommends routine vitamin A supplementation for all children with measles in areas where vitamin A deficiency is a problem or where the measles death rate is high.[15] In the United States, the American Academy of Pediatrics recommends vitamin A supplementation for certain groups of measles-infected infants and children.[16]

Night Blindness   Night blindness is one of the first detectable signs of vitamin A deficiency and permits early diagnosis of the condition. In night blindness, the blood bathing the cells of the retina does not supply sufficient retinal to rapidly regenerate visual pigments bleached by light. The person loses the ability to recover promptly from the temporary blinding that occurs following a flash of bright light at night or simply to see after the lights go out. In many parts of the world, after the sun goes down, vitamin A–deficient children become night-blind: they cannot find their shoes or toys and often cling to others or sit still, afraid that they may trip and fall or lose their way if they try to go home alone. In many developing countries, night blindness due to vitamin A deficiency is so common that the people have special words to describe it. In Indonesia, the term is *buta ayam*, which means "chicken eyes" or "chicken blindness." (Chickens do not have rods in their eyes and therefore cannot see at night.) Vitamin A–deficient children, like chickens, stumble after dark. Figure 11–6 shows the eyes' slow recovery in response to a flash of bright light in night blindness.

RE (retinol equivalent): a measure of vitamin A activity; the amount of retinol that the body will derive from a food containing preformed retinol or its precursor beta-carotene.

1 RE	=	1 μg retinol.
	=	6 μg beta-carotene.
	=	12 μg of other vitamin A precursor carotenes.

international units (IU): a measure of vitamin activity, determined by such biological methods as feeding a compound to vitamin-deprived animals and measuring growth. This system was used to measure vitamin A before direct chemical analysis was possible.

1 RE	=	3.33	IU (retinol from animal foods).
	=	10.00	IU (beta-carotene from plant foods).
	≈	5.00	IU (on average).

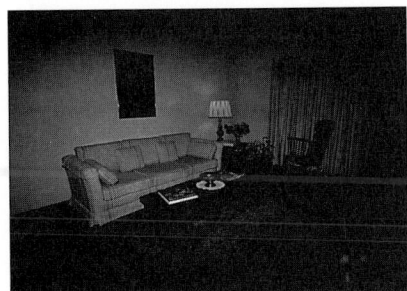

A. In dim light, you can make out the details in this room. You are using your rods for vision.

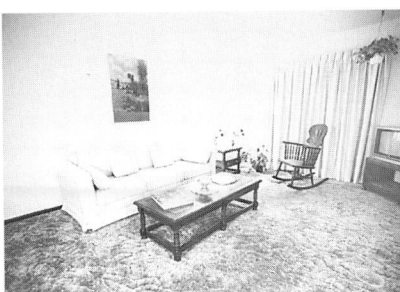

B. A flash of bright light momentarily blinds you as the pigment in the rods is bleached.

Figure 11–6

Night Blindness

These photographs illustrate the eyes' slow recovery in response to a flash of bright light at night. In animal research studies, the response rate is measured with electrodes.

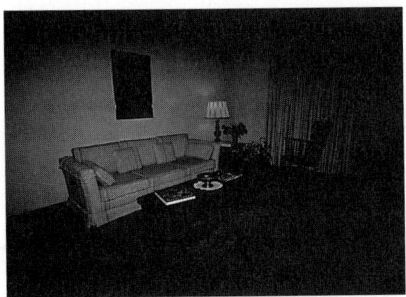

C. You quickly recover and can see the details again in a few seconds.

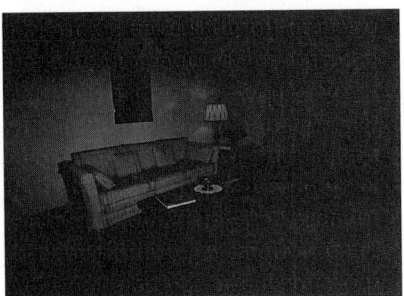

D. With inadequate vitamin A, you do not recover but remain blinded for many seconds.

Table 11–1

Vitamin A—A Summary

Other Names	Deficiency Disease Name	Toxicity Disease Name
Retinol, retinal, retinoic acid; precursor is provitamin A carotenoids such as beta-carotene	Hypovitaminosis A	Hypervitaminosis A[a]
Adult RDA	**Deficiency Symptoms**	**Toxicity Symptoms**
Men: 1000 µg RE/day Women: 800 µg RE/day	BONES/TEETH	
	Cessation of bone growth, painful joints, impaired enamel formation, cracks in teeth, tendency to decay, atrophy of dentin-forming cells	Increased activity of osteoclasts[b] causing decalcification, joint pain, fragility, stunted growth, and thickening of long bones; increase of pressure inside skull, mimicking brain tumor; headaches
Chief Functions in the Body	BLOOD	
Vision; maintenance of cornea, epithelial cells, mucous membranes, skin; bone and tooth growth; reproduction; immunity	Anemia, often masked by dehydration	Loss of hemoglobin and potassium by red blood cells, cessation of menstruation, slowed clotting time, easily induced bleeding
Significant Sources	EYES[c]	
Retinol: fortified milk, cheese, cream, butter, fortified margarine, eggs, liver	Night blindness, changes in epithelial tissue (hyperkeratinization), drying (xerosis), triangular gray spots on eye (Bitot's spots), irreversible drying (keratomalacia), and corneal degeneration (blindness)	
Beta-carotene: spinach and other dark leafy greens; broccoli, deep orange fruits (apricots, cantaloupe) and vegetables (squash, carrots, sweet potatoes, pumpkin)	SKIN	
	Plugging of hair follicles with keratin, forming white lumps (hyperkeratosis)	Dryness; itching; peeling; rashes; dry, scaling lips; cracking and bleeding of lips; nosebleeds; loss of hair; brittle nails

[a] A related condition, *hypercarotenemia*, is caused by the accumulation of too much of the vitamin A precursor beta-carotene in the blood, which turns the skin noticeably yellow. Hypercarotenemia is not, strictly speaking, a toxicity symptom.
[b] *Osteoclasts* are the cells that destroy bone during its growth. Those that build bone are *osteoblasts*.
[c] The eyes' symptoms of vitamin A deficiency are collectively known as *xerophthalmia*.

xerophthalmia (zer-off-THAL-mee-uh): progressive blindness caused by vitamin A deficiency.

xero = dry
ophthalm = eye

xerosis (zee-ROW-sis): drying of the cornea; a sign of vitamin A deficiency.

keratomalacia (KARE-ah-toe-ma-LAY-shuh): softening of the cornea seen in severe vitamin A deficiency that leads to irreversible blindness.

Blindness (Xerophthalmia)   Beyond night blindness lies total blindness—failure to see at all. Night blindness is caused by a lack of vitamin A at the back of the eye, the retina; total blindness is caused by a lack in the front of the eye, the cornea. Vitamin A deficiency is the major cause of childhood blindness in the world, causing more than half a million preschool children to lose their sight each year. Blindness due to vitamin A deficiency, known as xerophthalmia, progresses. First, the cornea becomes dry and hard, a condition known as xerosis. Corneal xerosis can quickly progress to keratomalacia, the softening of the cornea that leads to irreversible blindness. Dietary vitamin A reduces the risk of xerophthalmia significantly.[17]

Table 11–1

Vitamin A—A Summary (continued)

Deficiency Symptoms	Toxicity Symptoms
DIGESTIVE SYSTEM	
Changes in lining, diarrhea	Nausea, vomiting, abdominal pain, diarrhea, weight loss
IMMUNE SYSTEM	
Suppression of immune reactions; frequent respiratory, digestive, bladder, vaginal, and kidney infections	Overstimulation of immune reactions
NERVOUS/MUSCULAR SYSTEMS	
Brain and spinal cord growth too fast for stunted skull and spine	Loss of appetite, irritability, fatigue, insomnia, restlessness, headaches, blurred vision, nausea, vomiting, muscle weakness, interference with thyroxin
OTHER	
Kidney stones	Amenorrhea,[d] jaundice,[e] enlargement of liver[f] and spleen, massive accumulation of fat and vitamin A in liver

[d]Elevated serum carotene concentrations are associated with amenorrhea.
[e]*Jaundice* (JAWN-dice) is a symptom of liver disease, in which bile and related pigments spill into the bloodstream and the skin yellows.
[f]If liver impairment is severe, the "classic" signs seen in skin and hair may be masked.

Keratinization Elsewhere in the body, vitamin A deficiency affects other surfaces. Without vitamin A, the goblet cells in the stomach and intestines diminish in number and activity, limiting the secretion of mucus. With less mucus, the normal digestion and absorption of nutrients are hindered, and this, in turn, worsens the deficiency by impairing the absorption of whatever vitamin A the diet may deliver. Similar changes in the cells of other epithelial tissues weaken defenses, making infections of the respiratory tract, the GI tract, the urinary tract, the vagina, and possibly the inner ear likely. On the body's outer surface, the epithelial cells change shape and begin to secrete the protein keratin—the hard, inflexible protein of hair and nails. The skin becomes dry, rough, and scaly as lumps of keratin accumulate around each hair follicle (keratinization).

VITAMIN A TOXICITY

Just as a deficiency of vitamin A affects all body systems, so does a toxicity. Symptoms begin to develop when all the binding proteins are swamped, and free vitamin A damages the cells. Such effects are unlikely when a person depends on a balanced diet for nutrients, but if the person takes large amounts of the preformed vitamin from animal foods or supplements, toxicity is a real possibility.

keratin (KERR-uh-tin): a water-insoluble protein; the normal protein of hair and nails. Keratin-producing cells may replace mucus-producing cells in vitamin A deficiency.

hair follicle (FOLL-i-cul): a group of cells in the skin from which a hair grows.

keratinization: accumulation of keratin in a tissue; a sign of vitamin A deficiency.

Beta-carotene, which is found in a wide variety of plant foods, is not converted efficiently enough in the body to cause vitamin A toxicity; instead, it is stored in fat depots under the skin. Overconsumption of beta-carotene may turn the skin yellow, but this is not harmful.

Children are most vulnerable to toxicity because they need less and are more sensitive to overdoses. Serious toxicity is seen in infants and young children when they are given more than ten times the recommended amount every day for weeks at a time. A child who regards vitamin pills as candy may easily self-overdose.

Birth Defects   In animals, large doses of vitamin A during pregnancy produce malformations in all organ systems. Although a clear-cut cause-and-effect relationship between excessive vitamin A intakes during pregnancy and birth defects is not confirmed in human beings, several reports implicate excess vitamin A as a factor. Most convincing was the case of a woman who ingested a single massive dose of vitamin A (about 100 times greater than the RDA) during the second month of her pregnancy.[18] Her infant was born with numerous birth defects, including eye malformations. The lowest intake of vitamin A that causes birth defects is uncertain, but several agencies suggest limiting supplements to less than 3 times the RDA for pregnant women.[19]

acne: a chronic inflammation of the skin's follicles and oil-producing glands, which leads to an accumulation of oils inside the ducts that surround hairs; usually associated with the maturation of young adults.

Not for Acne   Adolescents need to know that massive doses of vitamin A have no corrective effect on acne, but may cause toxicity. The prescription medicine Accutane is made from vitamin A but is chemically altered. Taken orally, Accutane is effective against the deep lesions of cystic acne. It is highly toxic, however, especially during growth, and has caused birth defects in infants when women have taken it during their pregnancies. For this reason, women taking Accutane must begin using an effective form of contraception at least a month before starting to take the drug and continue using contraception a month after discontinuing its use.

Another vitamin A relative, Retin-A, fights acne, the wrinkles of aging, and other skin disorders. Applied topically, this ointment smooths and softens skin; it also lightens skin that has become darkly pigmented after inflammation.[20] During treatment, the skin becomes red and tender and peels. Although the Food and Drug Administration (FDA) has approved Retin-A, several questions remain unanswered: Does it have long-term toxic effects? How does it work? What is the minimum effective dose? How long do the benefits last?

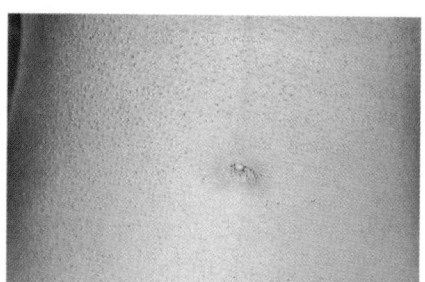

In vitamin A deficiency, the epithelial cells secrete the protein keratin in a process known as *keratinization*. (Keratinization doesn't occur in the GI tract, but mucus-producing cells dwindle, and mucus production declines.) The progression of this condition to the extreme is *hyperkeratinization* or *hyperkeratosis*. When keratin accumulates around each hair follicle, the condition is known as *follicular hyperkeratosis*.

Not for Cancer   Beta-carotene and the retinoids may help prevent cancer, but the retinoids are so toxic as to preclude their use in supplement form.[21] Still, gullible people take massive doses of vitamin A in the hope of preventing cancer. As a result, more cases of vitamin A toxicity may be reported in the years to come. Highlight 11 discusses the role of beta-carotene in cancer prevention.

VITAMIN A IN FOODS

The richest sources of preformed vitamin A are foods of animal origin—liver, fish liver oils, milk and milk products, butter, and eggs. Plants contain no preformed vitamin A, but many vegetables and some fruits contain provitamin A carotenoids, the red and yellow pigments of plants. Only a few carotenoids have vitamin A activity. The carotenoid with the greatest vitamin A activity is beta-carotene.

The Colors of Vitamin A Foods   Recommendations to eat dark green and deep orange vegetables and fruits help people to meet their vitamin A needs (see Figure 11–7). A 1-cup serving of carrots, sweet potatoes, or dark greens such as spinach provides such liberal amounts of carotenoids that even allowing for inefficient absorption and conversion, the intake of the vitamin is sufficient for many days. Alternatively, a diet including more or larger servings of medium sources also ensures an ample intake.

Most foods with vitamin A activity are brightly colored—green, yellow, orange, and red. Any plant food with significant vitamin A activity must have some color, since carotene is a rich, deep yellow, almost orange compound. The dark green, leafy vegetables contain abundant amounts of the green pigment chlorophyll, which masks the carotene in them. An attractive meal includes foods of different colors; such a meal most likely supplies vitamin A as well.

On the other hand, colorful vegetables do not invariably provide vitamin A activity. Beets and corn, for example, derive their colors from the red and yellow xanthophylls, which have no vitamin A activity. On the third hand (this chapter has three hands), white plant foods such as potatoes, cauliflower, pasta, and rice also possess little or no vitamin A activity.

Typical Intakes   In the typical United States diet, about half of the vitamin A activity comes from vegetables and fruits, and half of this comes from the dark leafy greens (like spinach—not celery or cabbage) and the rich yellow or deep orange vegetables (such as winter squash, cantaloupe, carrots, and sweet potatoes—not corn or bananas). The other half of the vitamin A activity in foods is from preformed vitamin A in milk, cheese, butter, and other dairy products; eggs; and liver. Since vitamin A is fat soluble, it is lost when milk is skimmed. To compensate, nonfat milk is often fortified so as to supply about 40 percent of the RDA per quart.* Margarine is usually fortified so as to provide the same amount of vitamin A as butter.

Vitamin A–Poor Fast Foods   Fast foods often lack vitamin A. Anyone who dines frequently on hamburgers, french fries, and colas is advised to emphasize vegetables at other meals.

Vitamin A–Rich Liver   Liver is a rich source of preformed vitamin A, because in animals, just as in humans, vitamin A is stored there.† People sometimes wonder if eating liver too frequently can cause vitamin A toxicity. Arctic explorers who have eaten large quantities of polar bear liver have become ill with symptoms suggesting vitamin A toxicity. Closer to home, vitamin A toxicity symptoms were reported in young children who regularly ate a chicken liver

vitamin A activity: a term useful for referring to both the preformed vitamin A and the carotene contents of foods without distinguishing between them.

carotene: a vitamin A precursor found in plants; an orange pigment.

chlorophyll: the green pigment of plants, which absorbs photons and transfers their energy to other molecules, thereby initiating photosynthesis.

xanthophylls (ZAN-tho-fills): pigments found in plants; responsible for the color changes seen in autumn leaves.

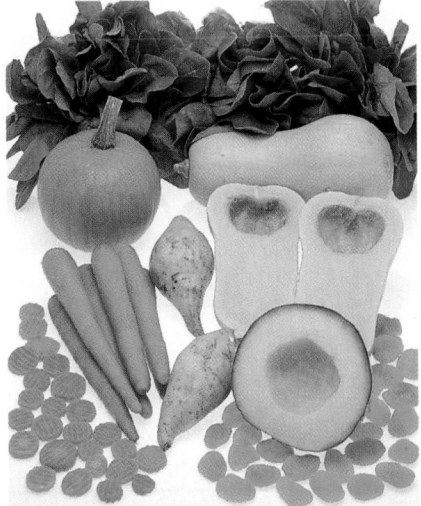

The carotenoids bring colors to meals; the retinoids allow us to see them.

---

*Vitamin A fortification of milk in Canada follows a similar standard.

†The liver is not the only organ that stores vitamin A. The kidneys, adrenals, and other organs do, too, but the liver stores the most and is the one most commonly eaten.

Figure 11–7 Vitamin A in Selected Foods

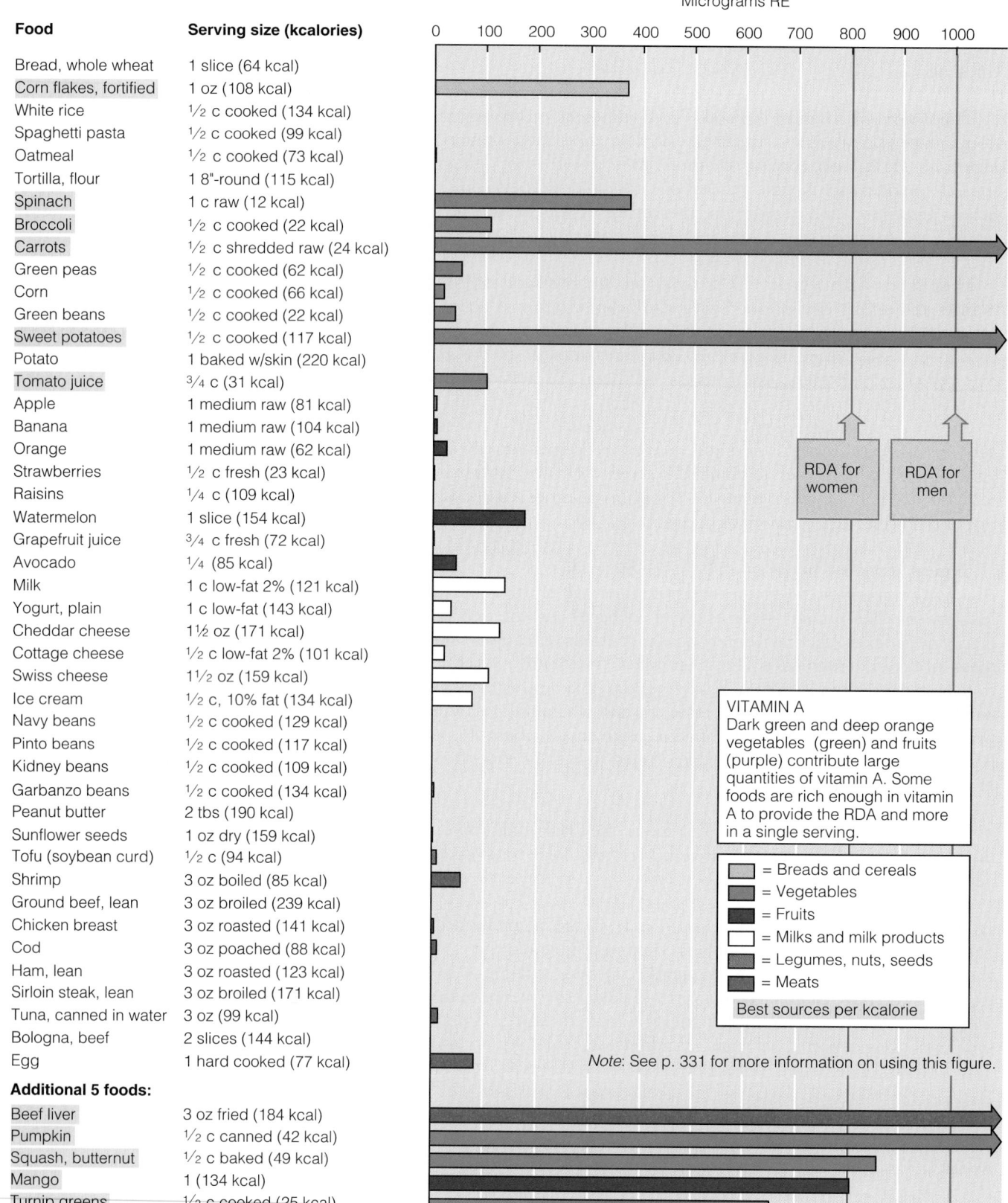

Micrograms RE

Food	Serving size (kcalories)
Bread, whole wheat	1 slice (64 kcal)
Corn flakes, fortified	1 oz (108 kcal)
White rice	½ c cooked (134 kcal)
Spaghetti pasta	½ c cooked (99 kcal)
Oatmeal	½ c cooked (73 kcal)
Tortilla, flour	1 8"-round (115 kcal)
Spinach	1 c raw (12 kcal)
Broccoli	½ c cooked (22 kcal)
Carrots	½ c shredded raw (24 kcal)
Green peas	½ c cooked (62 kcal)
Corn	½ c cooked (66 kcal)
Green beans	½ c cooked (22 kcal)
Sweet potatoes	½ c cooked (117 kcal)
Potato	1 baked w/skin (220 kcal)
Tomato juice	¾ c (31 kcal)
Apple	1 medium raw (81 kcal)
Banana	1 medium raw (104 kcal)
Orange	1 medium raw (62 kcal)
Strawberries	½ c fresh (23 kcal)
Raisins	¼ c (109 kcal)
Watermelon	1 slice (154 kcal)
Grapefruit juice	¾ c fresh (72 kcal)
Avocado	¼ (85 kcal)
Milk	1 c low-fat 2% (121 kcal)
Yogurt, plain	1 c low-fat (143 kcal)
Cheddar cheese	1½ oz (171 kcal)
Cottage cheese	½ c low-fat 2% (101 kcal)
Swiss cheese	1½ oz (159 kcal)
Ice cream	½ c, 10% fat (134 kcal)
Navy beans	½ c cooked (129 kcal)
Pinto beans	½ c cooked (117 kcal)
Kidney beans	½ c cooked (109 kcal)
Garbanzo beans	½ c cooked (134 kcal)
Peanut butter	2 tbs (190 kcal)
Sunflower seeds	1 oz dry (159 kcal)
Tofu (soybean curd)	½ c (94 kcal)
Shrimp	3 oz boiled (85 kcal)
Ground beef, lean	3 oz broiled (239 kcal)
Chicken breast	3 oz roasted (141 kcal)
Cod	3 oz poached (88 kcal)
Ham, lean	3 oz roasted (123 kcal)
Sirloin steak, lean	3 oz broiled (171 kcal)
Tuna, canned in water	3 oz (99 kcal)
Bologna, beef	2 slices (144 kcal)
Egg	1 hard cooked (77 kcal)

Additional 5 foods:

Food	Serving size (kcalories)
Beef liver	3 oz fried (184 kcal)
Pumpkin	½ c canned (42 kcal)
Squash, butternut	½ c baked (49 kcal)
Mango	1 (134 kcal)
Turnip greens	½ c cooked (25 kcal)

RDA for women

RDA for men

VITAMIN A
Dark green and deep orange vegetables (green) and fruits (purple) contribute large quantities of vitamin A. Some foods are rich enough in vitamin A to provide the RDA and more in a single serving.

= Breads and cereals
= Vegetables
= Fruits
= Milks and milk products
= Legumes, nuts, seeds
= Meats

Best sources per kcalorie

Note: See p. 331 for more information on using this figure.

spread that provided a daily average of up to three times their recommended intake.[22] Liver offers many nutrients, and eating it periodically may benefit health, but once every week or so is often enough.

In summary, vitamin A is found in the body in three forms: retinol, retinal, and retinoic acid. Together, they are essential to vision, healthy epithelial tissues, immunity, and bone growth and remodeling. Vitamin A deficiency is a major health problem worldwide, leading to infections, blindness, and keratinization of epithelial tissues. Toxicity can also cause problems and is most often associated with supplement abuse. Preformed vitamin A is found primarily in animal-derived foods such as liver and milk, whereas the precursor beta-carotene is found in brightly colored plant foods such as spinach, carrots, and pumpkins. In addition to providing vitamin A, beta-carotene acts as an antioxidant in the body.

Vitamin D

Vitamin D is different from all the other nutrients in that the body can synthesize it, with the help of sunlight, from a precursor that the body makes from cholesterol. Therefore, vitamin D is not an essential nutrient: given enough time in the sun, people need no vitamin D from foods.

Figure 11–8 diagrams the pathway by which active vitamin D is made. Ultraviolet rays from the sun hit the precursor in the skin and convert it to previtamin D_3. This compound works its way back into the interior of the body and slowly, over the next 36 hours, is converted to vitamin D_3 with the help of the body's heat. The biological activity of the active vitamin is 500- to 1000-fold higher than that of its precursor.

Regardless of whether the body manufactures vitamin D_3 or obtains it from food, two hydroxylation steps must occur before the vitamin becomes fully active. First, the liver adds an OH group, and then the kidneys add another OH group to produce the active vitamin. A review of Figure 11–8 shows how diseases affecting either the liver or the kidneys can impair the transformation of inactive vitamin D to its active form and therefore produce symptoms of deficiency.

ROLES IN THE BODY

Vitamin D acts like a hormone—a compound manufactured by one organ of the body that affects another part. Vitamin D can enter a cell, cross the nuclear membrane, attach to specific receptors on the DNA or its protein wrapping, and promote cell differentiation.[23] The best-known vitamin D target organs are the intestines, the kidneys, and the bones. All respond to vitamin D by making calcium available for bone growth. For example, in animals, vitamin D promotes the elongation of intestinal villi, which enhances calcium absorption.

Vitamin D in Bone Growth Vitamin D is a member of a large and cooperative bone-making and maintenance team composed of nutrients and other compounds, including vitamins A, C, and K; the hormones parathormone and calcitonin; the protein collagen, which underlies and supports bone; and the minerals calcium, phosphorus, magnesium, and fluoride, which compose the

Figure 11–8

Vitamin D Synthesis and Activation

The precursor of vitamin D is 7-dehydrocholesterol, which is made in the liver from cholesterol (see Figure 5–10 on p. 152 and Appendix C). This is one of the body's many "good" uses for cholesterol. The final product, active vitamin D, is 1,25-dihydroxycholecalciferol (or calcitriol). The hydroxylation of vitamin D to its active form is a closely regulated process.

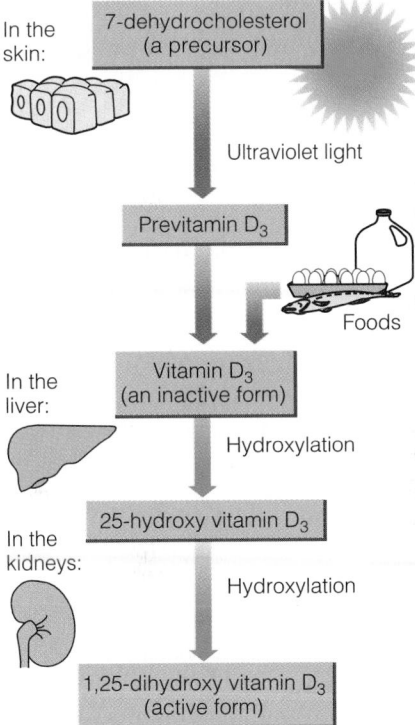

Vitamin D is also known as vitamin D_3 or cholecalciferol (KO-lee-kal-SIF-er-ol). The plant version is known as vitamin D_2 or ergocalciferol (er-go-kal-SIF-er-ol).

mineralization: the process in which calcium, phosphorus, and other minerals crystallize on the collagen matrix of a growing bone, hardening the bone.

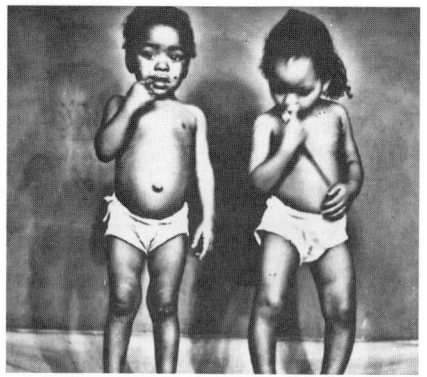

As Table 11–2 points out, rickets affects many areas of the body. The child on the left has the characteristic protruding belly resulting from lax abdominal muscles. The child on the right has the bowed legs commonly seen in rickets.

rickets: the vitamin D–deficiency disease in children characterized by inadequate mineralization of bone (manifested in bowed legs or knock-knees, outward-bowed chest, and knobs on ribs). A rare type of rickets, *not* caused by vitamin D deficiency, is known as vitamin D–refractory rickets

osteomalacia (OS-tee-o-ma-LAY-shuh): a bone disease characterized by softening of the bones; symptoms include bending of the spine and bowing of the legs. The disease occurs most often in adult women.
osteo = bone
malacia = softening

High blood calcium is known as hypercalcemia and may develop from a variety of disorders, including vitamin D toxicity. It does *not* develop from a high calcium intake.

inorganic part of bone. The special function of vitamin D is to promote normal bone mineralization. It helps to make calcium and phosphorus available in the blood that bathes the bones, to be deposited as the bones harden, or mineralize.

Vitamin D raises blood concentrations of these minerals in three ways. It stimulates their absorption from the GI tract, it stimulates their retention by the kidneys, and it helps to withdraw them from bones into the blood. The star of the show is calcium itself; vitamin D is a director. The vitamin may work alone, as it does in the GI tract, or in combination with parathormone, as it does in the bones and kidneys. Details of how calcium moves from food into the blood and into and out of bone appear in Chapter 12.

Vitamin D in Other Roles   Scientists have recently discovered many other vitamin D target tissues, including the brain and nervous system, pancreas, skin, muscles and cartilage, reproductive organs, immune cells, and some cancer cells.[24] These discoveries suggest that vitamin D has numerous functions and may be valuable in treating a number of disorders, including cancer.[25]

VITAMIN D DEFICIENCY

In vitamin D deficiency, production of the calcium-binding protein in the intestinal cells slows. Thus, even when calcium in the diet is adequate, it passes through the GI tract unabsorbed, leaving the bone undersupplied. The symptoms of a vitamin D deficiency are those of calcium deficiency, shown in Table 11–2.

Rickets   Worldwide, the vitamin D–deficiency disease rickets still affects large numbers of children. The bones fail to calcify normally, causing growth retardation and skeletal abnormalities. The bones become so weak that they bend when they have to support the body's weight. A child with rickets who is old enough to walk characteristically develops bowed legs, often the most obvious sign of the disease. Another obvious sign is the protruding belly that results from lax abdominal muscles.

Osteomalacia   Adult rickets, or osteomalacia, occurs most often in women who have low calcium intakes and little exposure to sun and who go through repeated pregnancies and periods of lactation. The bones of the legs may soften to such an extent that a young woman who is tall and straight at 20 may be condemned by repeated pregnancies to become bent, bowlegged, and stooped before she is 30.

Any failure to synthesize adequate vitamin D sets the stage for the mobilization of calcium from the bones and retardation of bone remodeling. This combination leads to a loss of bone mass, which can result in fractures. Highlight 12 describes the many factors that lead to osteoporosis, a condition of reduced bone density.

VITAMIN D TOXICITY

Whereas vitamin D deficiency depresses calcium absorption, blood calcium, and bone mineralization, an excess of the vitamin does the opposite, as shown in Table 11–2. It enhances calcium absorption, produces high blood calcium, and

Table 11–2
....

Vitamin D—A Summary

Other Names	Deficiency Disease Names	Toxicity Disease Name
Calciferol, cholecalciferol, dihydroxy vitamin D; precursor is the body's own cholesterol	Rickets, osteomalacia	Hypervitaminosis D
Adult DRI[a]	**Deficiency Symptoms**	**Toxicity Symptoms**

Other Names

Calciferol, cholecalciferol, dihydroxy vitamin D; precursor is the body's own cholesterol

Adult DRI[a]

5 μg/day (19–50 yr)

10 μg/day (51 and over)

Chief Functions in the Body

Promotes mineralization of bones (raises blood calcium and phosphorus by increasing absorption from digestive tract, withdrawing calcium from bones, stimulating retention by kidneys)

Significant Sources

Self-synthesis with sunlight; fortified milk, fortified margarine, egg yolk, liver, fatty fish

Deficiency Disease Names

Rickets, osteomalacia

Deficiency Symptoms

BONES/TEETH

Rickets in Children
Faulty calcification, resulting in misshapen bones (bowing of legs) and retarded growth; enlargement of ends of long bones (knees, wrists); deformities of ribs (bowed, with beads or knobs);[b] delayed closing of fontanel, resulting in rapid enlargement of head (see figure); slow eruption of teeth; malformed, decay-prone teeth

Osteomalacia in Adults
Softening effect: deformities of limbs, spine, thorax, and pelvis; demineralization; pain in pelvis, lower back, and legs; bone fractures

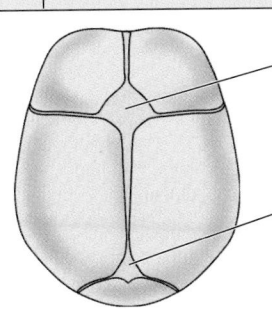

Fontanel
A fontanel is an open space in the top of a baby's skull before the bones have grown together. In rickets, closing of the fontanel is delayed.

Anterior fontanel normally closes by the end of the second year

Posterior fontanel normally closes by the end of the first year

BLOOD

Decreased calcium and/or phosphorus, increased alkaline phosphatase[c]

NERVOUS/MUSCULAR SYSTEMS

Lax muscles resulting in protrusion of abdomen; muscle spasms

Involuntary twitching, muscle spasms

EXCRETORY SYSTEM

Increased calcium in stools, decreased calcium in urine

OTHER

Abnormally high secretion of parathormone

Toxicity Disease Name

Hypervitaminosis D

Toxicity Symptoms

BONES/TEETH

Increased calcium withdrawal

BLOOD

Increased calcium and phosphorus concentration

NERVOUS/MUSCULAR SYSTEMS

Loss of appetite, headache, weakness, fatigue, excessive thirst, irritability, apathy

EXCRETORY SYSTEM

Increased excretion of calcium in urine, kidney stones, irreversible renal damage

OTHER

Calcification of soft tissues (blood vessels, kidneys, heart, lungs, tissues around joints), death

---

[a]1997 recommendations for vitamin D are called Dietary Reference Intakes (DRI).

[b]Bowing of the ribs causes the symptoms known as *pigeon breast*. The beads that form on the ribs resemble rosary beads; thus this symptom is known as *rachitic* (ra-KIT-ik) *rosary* ("the rosary of rickets").

[c]Alkaline phosphatase is an enzyme in the blood that rises during bone resorption.

promotes the return of bone calcium into the blood. Excess blood calcium tends to precipitate in the soft tissue, forming stones, especially in the kidneys where calcium is concentrated in the effort to excrete it. Calcification may also harden the blood vessels and is especially dangerous in the major arteries of the heart and lungs, where it can cause death.

The range of safe intakes of vitamin D is narrower than that of vitamin A. Half the recommended intake is too little, but more than a few times the recommended intake may be too much. In fact, vitamin D is the most likely of the vitamins to have toxic effects when consumed in amounts above recommendations on a continuous basis. The amounts of vitamin D in foods available in the United States and Canada are well within safe limits, but pills containing the vitamin in concentrated form should be kept out of the reach of children and used cautiously by adults. During the warm months of the year, when sunlight exposure may be frequent, vitamin D supplements can harm healthy children and adults who drink at least 2 glasses of vitamin D–fortified milk per day.[26] Vitamin D toxicity has also been reported in people who drank milk that was fortified with too much vitamin D by mistake.[27]

VITAMIN D RECOMMENDATIONS AND SOURCES

Neither cow's milk nor human breast milk supplies enough vitamin D to meet human needs reliably. Cow's milk is fortified, and infants are given either fortified formula or supplements.

Vitamin D in Foods Only a few foods supply significant amounts of vitamin D, notably those derived from animals: egg yolks, liver, fatty fish, butter, and fortified milk. The fortification of milk with vitamin D is the best guarantee that people will meet their needs and underscores the importance of milk in a well-balanced diet.* For those who use margarine in place of butter, fortified margarine is a significant source. A plant version of vitamin D may yield an active compound on irradiation, but its contribution is minor. Without adequate sunshine, fortification, or supplementation, a strict vegetarian diet cannot meet vitamin D needs.[28]

Most adults, especially in sunny regions, need not make special efforts to obtain vitamin D from food. People who are not outdoors much or who live in northern or predominantly cloudy or smoggy areas are advised to drink at least 2 cups of vitamin D–fortified milk a day.

Vitamin D from the Sun Most of the world's population relies on natural exposure to sunlight to maintain adequate vitamin D nutrition. The sun imposes no risk of vitamin D toxicity; prolonged exposure to sunlight degrades the vitamin D precursor in the skin, preventing its conversion to the active vitamin. Even lifeguards on southern beaches are safe from vitamin D toxicity from the sun.

Prolonged exposure to sunlight does, however, prematurely wrinkle the skin and present the risk of skin cancer. Sunscreens help reduce these risks, but unfor-

---

Tolerable Upper Intake for adults: 50 µg/day.

Vitamin D activity was previously expressed in international units (IU), but is now expressed in micrograms of cholecalciferol. To convert, use the following factor: 1 IU = 0.025 µg cholecalciferol. For example:
- 100 IU = 2.5 µg.
- 400 IU = 10 µg.

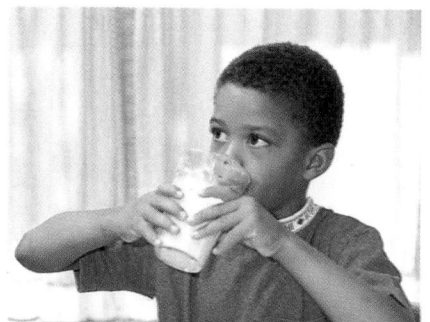

A cool glass of milk refreshes as it replenishes the bone-building nutrients.

---

*Vitamin D fortification of milk in the United States is 10 micrograms cholecalciferol (400 IU) per quart; in Canada, 360 IU per liter.

tunately, sunscreens with sun protection factors (SPF) of 8 and above also prevent vitamin D synthesis. A strategy to avoid this dilemma is to apply sunscreen after enough time has elapsed to provide sufficient vitamin D synthesis. For most people, exposing hands, face, and arms on a clear summer day for 10 to 15 minutes a few times a week should be sufficient to maintain vitamin D nutrition.

Dark-skinned people require longer sunlight exposure than light-skinned people, but by three hours, vitamin D synthesis in heavily pigmented skin arrives at the same plateau as in fair skin in 30 minutes. The ultraviolet rays of the sun that promote vitamin D synthesis are blocked by heavy clouds, smoke, or smog. Differences in skin pigmentation and smog may account for the finding that dark-skinned people in northern, smoggy cities are more prone to rickets. For these people, and for those who are unable to go outdoors frequently, dietary vitamin D is most important. Deficiency is especially likely in older adults because they typically drink little or no milk, their exposure to sunlight is limited, and the skin and kidneys lose their ability to make and activate vitamin D with advancing age.

The ultraviolet rays from tanning lamps and tanning booths may also stimulate vitamin D synthesis, but the hazards outweigh any possible benefits. The FDA warns that if the lamps are not properly filtered, people using tanning booths risk burns, damage to the eyes and blood vessels, and skin cancer.[29]

To summarize, vitamin D can be synthesized in the body with the help of sunlight or obtained from animal foods. It sends signals to three primary target sites: the GI tract to absorb more calcium, the bones to release more, and the kidneys to retain more. These actions support bone formation and maintenance. A deficiency causes rickets in childhood and osteomalacia in later life. Fortified milk is an important food source.

Smog filters out ultraviolet rays of the sun.

Vitamin E

In 1922, researchers discovered a component of vegetable oils necessary for reproduction in rats. This antisterility factor was named tocopherol, which means "to bring forth offspring."[30] A few years later, the compound was named vitamin E. When chemists isolated four different tocopherol compounds, they designated them by the first four letters of the Greek alphabet: alpha, beta, gamma, and delta. The tocopherols consist of a complex ring structure and a long saturated side chain (see Appendix C).* The numbers and positions of methyl groups on the ring distinguish one tocopherol from another. The most abundant and biologically active tocopherol in nature is alpha-tocopherol.

VITAMIN E AS AN ANTIOXIDANT

Vitamin E is a fat-soluble antioxidant and one of the body's primary defenders against oxidation, protecting the lipids and other vulnerable components of the cells and their membranes from destruction. Within the mitochondria of cells,

tocopherol (tuh-KOFF-er-ol): a general term for several chemically related compounds, most of which have vitamin E activity (see Appendix C for chemical structures).

alpha-tocopherol: the most biologically active vitamin E compound.

Reminder: An *antioxidant* is a compound that protects other compounds from oxidation by being oxidized itself.

---

*Another group of chemically related compounds, the tocotrienols (TOE-koe-try-EEN-ols), have unsaturated side chains. The tocotrienols are less abundant, less active, and less important in nutrition than the tocopherols are.

Table 11–3

Vitamin E—A Summary

Other Names	Deficiency Symptoms	Toxicity Symptoms
Alpha-tocopherol, tocopherol, tocotrienol	BLOOD/CIRCULATORY SYSTEM	
Adult RDA	Red blood cell breakage,[a] anemia	Augments effects of anticlotting medication
Men: 10 mg α-TE/day Women: 8 mg α-TE/day	DIGESTIVE SYSTEM	
		General discomfort
Chief Functions in the Body	NERVOUS/MUSCULAR SYSTEMS	
Antioxidant, stabilization of cell membranes, regulation of oxidation reactions, protection of PUFA and vitamin A	Degeneration, weakness, difficulty walking, severe pain in calf muscles	
Significant Sources		
Polyunsaturated plant oils (margarine, salad dressings, shortenings), green and leafy vegetables, wheat germ, whole-grain products, liver, egg yolks, nuts, seeds		

[a]The breaking of red blood cells is called *erythrocyte hemolysis*.

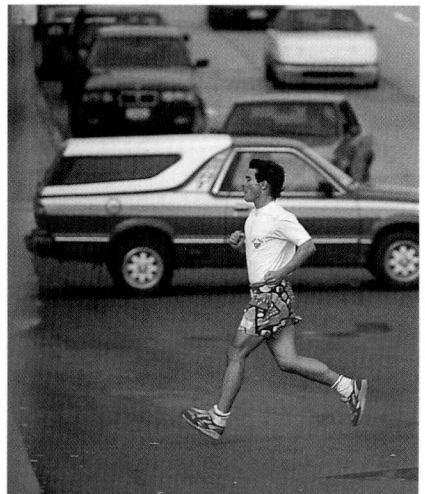

Vitamin E helps to protect the lungs against air pollutants, especially when a person is breathing hard during exercise.

vitamin E protects a part of the metabolic equipment that transforms energy fuels into ATP. Vitamin E is especially effective in preventing the oxidation of the polyunsaturated fatty acids (PUFA), but it protects all other lipids and related compounds (for example, vitamin A) as well. Table 11–3 presents a summary of vitamin E's functions, deficiency symptoms, toxicity symptoms, and food sources.

Vitamin E exerts an especially important antioxidant effect in the lungs, where the exposure of cells to oxygen is maximal. Several kinds of cells benefit from the vitamin's protection: the red and white blood cells that pass through the lungs and the cells of the lung tissue itself. Vitamin E also protects the lungs from air pollutants such as nitrogen dioxide or ozone that can initiate damaging reactions.

Vitamin E protects white as well as red blood cells and thus participates in the body's immune defenses. Recent studies have found that vitamin E supplementation significantly above the RDA improves the immune response of healthy, older adults.[31] The researchers speculate that vitamin E's support of immunity may be due to its protection of cell lipids. Highlight 11 provides more on vitamin E's role in protecting against chronic disease.

While research continues to reveal possible roles for vitamin E, it also has clearly discredited claims that vitamin E improves physical performance, enhances sexual performance, or cures sexual dysfunction in males. Vitamin E does not slow or prevent the processes of aging such as hair turning gray or skin wrinkling. Nor does it slow the progression of Parkinson's disease.[32]

VITAMIN E DEFICIENCY

In human beings, dietary vitamin E deficiency is rare; deficiency is usually associated with diseases of fat malabsorption such as cystic fibrosis. When the blood concentration of vitamin E falls below a certain critical level, the red blood cells tend to break open and spill their contents, probably due to oxidation of the PUFA in their membranes. This classic sign of vitamin E deficiency, known as erythrocyte hemolysis, is seen in premature infants, born before the transfer of vitamin E from the mother to the infant that takes place in the last weeks of pregnancy. Vitamin E treatment corrects erythrocyte hemolysis.

Prolonged vitamin E deficiency also causes neuromuscular dysfunction involving the spinal cord and retina. Common symptoms include loss of muscle coordination and reflexes and impaired vision and speech. Vitamin E treatment corrects these neurological symptoms of vitamin E deficiency.

The neuromuscular weakness and atrophy that accompany a vitamin E deficiency can be cured by reintroducing the vitamin into the diet, but vitamin E does *not* prevent or cure the herditary muscular dystrophy that afflicts children. Children with hereditary muscular dystrophy do not benefit from vitamin E treatment and usually die at an early age when their respiratory muscles deteriorate.

Two other conditions seem to respond to vitamin E therapy, although results are inconsistent. One is a nonmalignant breast disease (fibrocystic breast disease), and the other is an abnormality of blood flow that causes cramping in the legs (intermittent claudication).

VITAMIN E TOXICITY

Even though many claims have been discredited, many people continue to take vitamin E supplements for all kinds of reasons. In fact, vitamin E supplement use has risen recently as its antioxidant action against disease has been recognized. Still, toxicity is not as common, and its effects are not as detrimental, as with vitamins A and D. Extremely high doses of vitamin E may interfere with the blood-clotting action of vitamin K and enhance effects of drugs used to oppose blood clotting, causing hemorrhage.

VITAMIN E RECOMMENDATIONS

Tocopherols occur in two forms, D and L, of which the D form is more active. The most active vitamin E compound is D-alpha-tocopherol. Different tocopherols vary in their vitamin E activity; to reconcile them, recommended intakes are expressed in tocopherol equivalents (TE). One TE equals the amount of vitamin E activity in 1 milligram of D-alpha-tocopherol.*

A person who consumes a large amount of PUFA needs more vitamin E. Fortunately, vitamin E and PUFA tend to occur together in the same foods.

erythrocyte hemolysis: the breaking open of red blood cells; a symptom of vitamin E–deficiency disease in human beings.

erythrocyte (eh-REETH-ro-cite): red blood cell.

> *erythro* = red
> *cyte* = cell

hemolysis (he-MOLL-uh-sis): bursting of red blood cells.

> *hemo* = blood
> *lysis* = breaking

muscular dystrophy (DIS-tro-fee): a hereditary disease in which the muscles gradually weaken; its most debilitating effects arise in the lungs.

fibrocystic breast disease: a harmless condition in which the breasts develop lumps, sometimes associated with caffeine consumption. In some, it responds to treatment by abstinence from caffeine; in others, it can be treated with vitamin E.

> *fibro* = fibrous tissue
> *cyst* = closed sac

intermittent claudication: severe calf pain caused by inadequate blood supply; it occurs when walking and subsides during rest.

> *intermittent* = at intervals
> *claudicare* = to limp

D, L: *D* stands for *dextro*, or "right-handed," and *L*, for *levo*, or "left-handed," referring to the shapes of the molecules, which are mirror images of each other.

tocopherol equivalents (TE): the units in which vitamin E activity is measured. One TE equals the amount of vitamin E activity in 1 mg of D-alpha-tocopherol.

---

*The activities of beta- and gamma-tocopherol and alpha-tocotrienol are one-half, one-tenth, and one-third the activity of D-alpha-tocopherol, respectively.

VITAMIN E IN FOODS

Vitamin E is widespread in foods (see Figure 11–9 on facing page). About 20 percent of the vitamin E in the diet comes from vegetable oils and products made from them, such as margarine, salad dressings, and shortenings. Another 20 percent comes from fruits and vegetables. Fortified cereals and other grain products contribute about 15 percent of the vitamin E in the diet, and smaller percentages come from meats, poultry, fish, eggs, nuts, and seeds.[33] Wheat germ oil is especially rich in vitamin E; corn and soybean oils rank second, with a tablespoon of either of these supplying more than 10 milligrams (more than the RDA) of the vitamin. Other oils contain less (for example, peanut oil supplies about a third as much per tablespoon). Animal fats such as meat and milk fat contain little or no vitamin E.

Vitamin E is readily destroyed by heat processing (such as deep-fat frying) and oxidation, so fresh or lightly processed foods are preferable sources. Most processed and convenience foods do not contribute enough vitamin E to ensure an adequate intake.

To review, vitamin E acts as an antioxidant, defending lipids and other components of the cells against oxidative damage. Deficiencies are rare, but do occur in premature infants, the primary symptom being erythrocyte hemolysis. Vitamin E is found predominantly in vegetable oils and appears to be one of the least toxic of the fat-soluble vitamins.

Vitamin K

K stands for the Danish word koagulation *("coagulation" or "clotting").*

Chapter 15 describes the interaction between vitamin K and anticoagulant medicines.

hemorrhagic (hem-o-RAJ-ik) disease: a disease characterized by excessive bleeding.

hemophilia: a hereditary disease that has no relation to vitamin K, but is caused by a genetic defect; the blood is unable to clot because it lacks the ability to synthesize certain clotting factors.

Blood has a remarkable ability to remain a liquid even though it carries many large molecules and cells through the circulatory system. But blood can also turn solid within seconds when the integrity of that system is disturbed. (If blood did not clot, a single pinprick could drain the entire body of all its blood, just as a tiny hole in a bucket makes the bucket forever useless for holding water.) Vitamin K acts primarily in blood clotting, where its presence can make the difference between life and death. At least 13 different proteins and the mineral calcium are involved in making a blood clot. Vitamin K is essential for the synthesis of at least four of these proteins, among them prothrombin, made by the liver as a precursor of the protein thrombin (see Figure 11–10 on p. 396). When any of the blood-clotting factors is lacking, hemorrhagic disease results. If an artery or vein is cut or broken, bleeding goes unchecked. (Of course, this is not to say that hemorrhaging is always caused by vitamin K deficiency. Another cause is hemophilia, which is not curable by vitamin K.)

Vitamin K also participates in the synthesis of a bone protein. The rate of synthesis of this protein is regulated by the more famous bone vitamin—vitamin D. Without vitamin K, the bones produce an abnormal protein that cannot bind to the minerals that normally form bones.

Like vitamin D, vitamin K can be obtained from a nonfood source. Bacteria in the GI tract synthesize vitamin K that the body can absorb, but bacterial synthesis alone is insufficient to meet all of a person's needs.

Figure 11–9   Vitamin E in Selected Foods

Milligrams α-TE

Food	Serving size (kcalories)
Bread, whole wheat	1 slice (64 kcal)
Corn flakes, fortified	1 oz (108 kcal)
White rice	½ c cooked (134 kcal)
Spaghetti pasta	½ c cooked (99 kcal)
Oatmeal	½ c cooked (73 kcal)
Tortilla, flour	1 8"-round (115 kcal)
Spinach	1 c raw (12 kcal)
Broccoli	½ c cooked (22 kcal)
Carrots	½ c shredded raw (24 kcal)
Green peas	½ c cooked (62 kcal)
Corn	½ c cooked (66 kcal)
Green beans	½ c cooked (22 kcal)
Sweet potatoes	½ c cooked (117 kcal)
Potato	1 baked w/skin (220 kcal)
Tomato juice	¾ c (31 kcal)
Apple	1 medium raw (81 kcal)
Banana	1 medium raw (104 kcal)
Orange	1 medium raw (62 kcal)
Strawberries	½ c fresh (23 kcal)
Raisins	¼ c (109 kcal)
Watermelon	1 slice (154 kcal)
Grapefruit juice	¾ c fresh (72 kcal)
Avocado	¼ (85 kcal)
Milk	1 c low-fat 2% (121 kcal)
Yogurt, plain[a]	1 c low-fat (143 kcal)
Cheddar cheese	1½ oz (171 kcal)
Cottage cheese	½ c low-fat 2% (101 kcal)
Swiss cheese	1½ oz (159 kcal)
Ice cream	½ c, 10% fat (134 kcal)
Navy beans	½ c cooked (129 kcal)
Pinto beans	½ c cooked (117 kcal)
Kidney beans	½ c cooked (109 kcal)
Garbanzo beans	½ c cooked (134 kcal)
Peanut butter	2 tbs (190 kcal)
Sunflower seeds	1 oz dry (159 kcal)
Tofu (soybean curd)	½ c (94 kcal)
Shrimp	3 oz boiled (85 kcal)
Ground beef, lean	3 oz broiled (239 kcal)
Chicken breast	3 oz roasted (141 kcal)
Cod	3 oz poached (88 kcal)
Ham, lean	3 oz roasted (123 kcal)
Sirloin steak, lean	3 oz broiled (171 kcal)
Tuna, canned in water	3 oz (99 kcal)
Bologna, beef	2 slices (144 kcal)
Egg	1 hard cooked (77 kcal)

Additional 5 foods:

Food	Serving size (kcalories)
Wheat germ oil	1 tbs (120 kcal)
Soybean oil	1 tbs (120 kcal)
Corn oil	1 tbs (120 kcal)
Canola oil	1 tbs (120 kcal)
Cashews	1 oz (163 kcal)

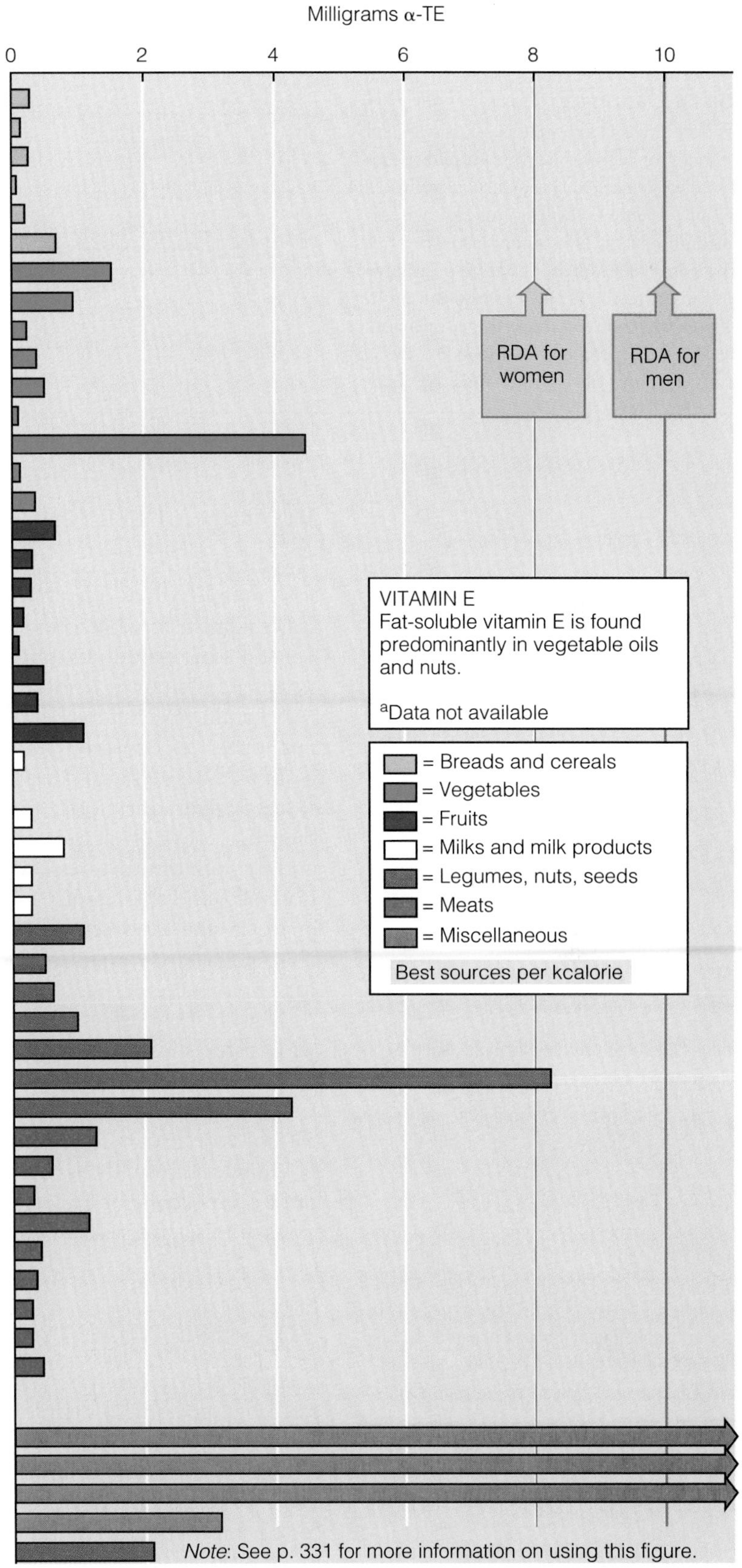

RDA for women

RDA for men

VITAMIN E
Fat-soluble vitamin E is found predominantly in vegetable oils and nuts.

[a]Data not available

= Breads and cereals
= Vegetables
= Fruits
= Milks and milk products
= Legumes, nuts, seeds
= Meats
= Miscellaneous

Best sources per kcalorie

Note: See p. 331 for more information on using this figure.

Figure 11–10

Blood-Clotting Process

When blood is exposed to air, foreign substances, or secretions from injured tissues, platelets (small, cell-like structures in the blood) release a phospholipid known as thromboplastin. Thromboplastin catalyzes the conversion of the inactive protein prothrombin to the active enzyme thrombin. Thrombin then catalyzes the conversion of the precursor protein fibrinogen to the active protein fibrin that forms the clot.

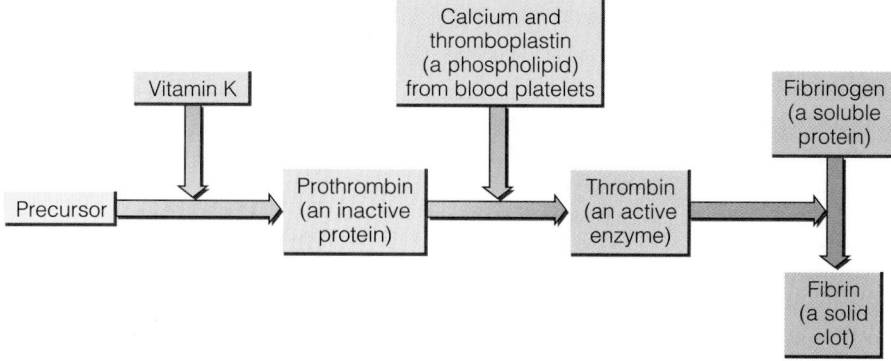

sterile: free of microorganisms, such as bacteria.

A synthetic form of vitamin K is menadione (men-uh-DYE-own); see Appendix C.

jaundice: yellowing of the skin, due to spillover of the bile pigments bilirubin (bill-ee-ROO-bin) from the liver into the general circulation; also known as hyperbilirubinemia (HIGH-per-BILL-eh-roo-bin-EE-me-ah). When these pigments invade the brain, the condition is kernicterus (ker-NICK-ter-us). Jaundice may be caused by obstruction of bile passageways, hemolysis, or dysfunctional liver cells.

VITAMIN K DEFICIENCY

A deficiency of vitamin K may occur whenever absorption of fat is impaired—for example, when bile production is faulty or in diarrhea. The vitamin is sometimes administered before operations to reduce bleeding in surgery, but is only of value at this time if a vitamin K deficiency exists. Table 11–4 (on facing page) summarizes vitamin K information.

Vitamin K deficiency is seldom seen except when an unusual combination of circumstances conspires to bring it about. When it does occur, however, it can be fatal. The scenario goes like this. A hospital client with marginal vitamin K stores is given antibiotics to prevent or overcome infection and is fed a formula diet that does not include vitamin K. The antibiotics kill the intestinal bacteria, and the vitamin K stores become depleted. During surgery, the blood fails to clot normally, and the client bleeds to death. The combination of antibiotics, inadequate intake, and surgery raises a warning flag that clotting time should be checked before surgery is performed. People taking sulfa drugs, which destroy intestinal bacteria, may also become deficient in vitamin K.

Newborn babies present a unique case of vitamin K nutrition. A baby is born with a sterile digestive tract, and the vitamin K–producing bacteria take weeks to establish themselves in the baby's intestines. At the same time, plasma prothrombin concentrations are low (this makes fatal blood clotting unlikely during the stress of birth). To prevent hemorrhagic disease in the newborn, a single dose of vitamin K (usually as the naturally occurring form, phylloquinone) is given at birth either orally or by intramuscular injection. Concerns that vitamin K given at birth raises the risks of childhood cancer are unproven and unlikely.[34]

VITAMIN K TOXICITY

Toxicity is not common but can result when vitamin K supplements are prescribed, especially to infants or to pregnant women. High doses of vitamin K can reduce the effectiveness of anticoagulant drugs used to prevent blood clotting. People taking these drugs should eat vitamin K–rich foods in moderation and keep their intakes consistent from day to day. Toxicity symptoms include red blood cell hemolysis, jaundice, and brain damage.

Table 11–4

Vitamin K—A Summary

Other Names	Deficiency Symptoms	Toxicity Symptoms
	BLOOD/CIRCULATORY SYSTEM	
Menadione, menaquinone, phylloquinone, naphthoquinone	Hemorrhaging	Interference with anticlotting medication; vitamin K analogues may cause jaundice, red blood cell hemolysis, and brain damage
Adult RDA	**Chief Functions in the Body**	

1 μg/kg body weight/day
Men: 70 μg/day (19–24 yr)
     80 μg/day (25 and over)
Women: 60 μg/day (19–24 yr)
        65 μg/day (25 and over)
	Participates in the synthesis of blood-clotting proteins and a bone protein that regulates blood calcium	

	Significant Sources	
	Bacterial synthesis in the digestive tract; liver; leafy green vegetables, cabbage-type vegetables; milk	

VITAMIN K RECOMMENDATIONS AND SOURCES

As mentioned earlier, vitamin K is made in the GI tract by the billions of bacteria that normally reside there. Once synthesized, vitamin K is absorbed and stored in the liver. The total need for vitamin K cannot be met by bacterial synthesis alone. People eating vitamin K–rich foods such as liver, leafy green vegetables, and members of the cabbage family can easily meet their needs. Milk, meats, eggs, cereals, fruits, and vegetables provide smaller, but still significant, amounts.

To sum up, vitamin K helps with blood clotting, and its deficiency causes uncontrolled bleeding. Bacteria in the GI tract can make the vitamin; people typically receive about half of their requirements from bacterial synthesis and half from foods such as liver, leafy green vegetables, and members of the cabbage family. Because people depend on bacterial synthesis for vitamin K, deficiency is most likely in newborn infants and in people taking antibiotics.

The Fat-Soluble Vitamins—In Summary

The four fat-soluble vitamins play many specific roles in the growth and maintenance of the body. Their presence affects the health and function of the eyes, skin, GI tract, lungs, bones, teeth, nervous system, and blood; their deficiencies become apparent in these same areas. Toxicities of the fat-soluble vitamins are possible, especially when people use supplements because the body stores excesses.

As with the water-soluble vitamins, the function of one fat-soluble vitamin often depends on the presence of another. Recall that vitamin E protects vitamin

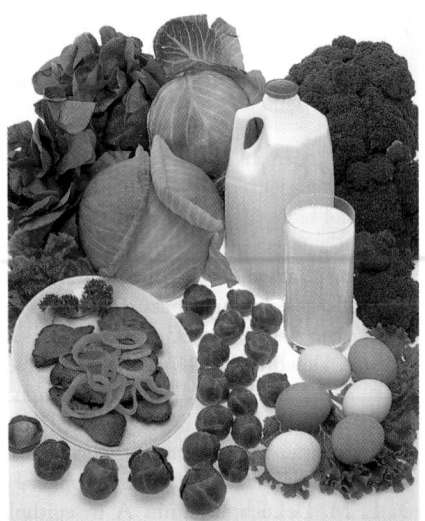

Notable food sources of vitamin K include milk, eggs, brussels sprouts, liver, cabbage, spinach, and broccoli.

Antioxidant Nutrients and Nonnutrients in Disease Prevention

*C*ount on supplement manufacturers to proclaim the day's hot topics in nutrition. The moment bits of research news surface, new supplements appear—and terms like "antioxidants" become household words. Friendly faces in TV commercials begin to persuade us that these antioxidants are new magic bullets in the fight against aging, disease, and death. Then the antioxidants hit the market and cash registers ring. Vitamin C, long the leading single nutrient supplement, gains new popularity, and sales of beta-carotene and vitamin E supplements soar as well.

In the meantime, scientists and medical experts around the world continue their work to clarify and confirm the roles of these antioxidant nutrients in preventing chronic diseases.[1] This highlight summarizes some of the accumulating evidence on nutrients, *nonnutrients*, and their antioxidant actions.

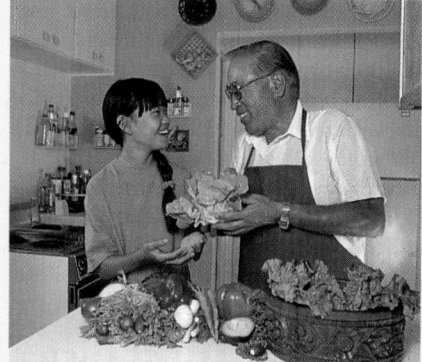

People who eat generous amounts of fruits and vegetables daily are helping their bodies to fight disease.

It also revisits the advantages of foods over supplements.

FREE-RADICAL FORMATION AND THE BODY'S DEFENSES

All of the body's cells use oxygen to produce energy for their work. During these normal metabolic processes, oxygen sometimes reacts with body compounds to produce highly unstable molecules known as free radicals—molecules with unpaired electrons (the glossary on p. 402 defines free radicals and related terms).* An electron without a partner is unstable and highly reactive; it needs to pair up with another electron in order to return to a stable state. Free radicals quickly react with other compounds in an attempt to capture that needed electron (see Figure H11–1).

When two free radicals react with each other, their unpaired electrons form a bond. In some cases, this is fine, but in others, the product is toxic. Generally, though, free radicals simply attack the nearest stable molecule in the body,

---

*Many free radicals exist, but the oxygen-derived ones are most common in the human body. Examples of oxygen-derived free radicals include superoxide radical ($O_2^{\cdot-}$), hydroxyl radical ($OH^{\cdot}$), and nitric oxide ($NO^{\cdot}$). (The dots in the symbols represent the unpaired electrons.) Technically, hydrogen peroxide (H_2O_2) and singlet oxygen are not free radicals because they contain paired electrons, but their unstable conformation of electrons makes radical-producing reactions likely. Scientists sometimes use the term *reactive oxygen species* to describe all of these compounds.

"stealing" an electron. With the loss of an electron, the stable molecule becomes a free radical itself, and a chain reaction is under way. Antioxidants neutralize free radicals by donating one of their own electrons, thus ending the electron-snatching reactions. (Review Figure 10–12 on p. 357 to see how ascorbic acid can give up two hydrogens with their electrons and become dehydroascorbic acid; antioxidants do not become free radicals when they lose electrons because they are stable in either form.)

Free radicals not only arise spontaneously during metabolism, but also are made on purpose by cells of the immune system to help them inactivate viruses and bacteria. In addition to these normal body processes, environmental factors such as radiation, pollution, and herbicides can generate free radicals. Free radicals are also involved in the oxidative damage caused by cigarette smoking.[2]

The body's natural defense and repair systems try to handle all free radicals, but these systems are not 100 percent effective. If antioxidants are unavailable, or if free-radical production becomes excessive, problems develop.[3] Unrepaired damage accumulates with age.

Free radicals are like tornadoes, causing damage wherever they go. They commonly attack lipoproteins and unsaturated fatty acids in cell membranes, starting chain reactions called lipid peroxidation.[4] Left uncontrolled, lipid peroxidation

Figure H11–1
. . . .

The Actions of Free Radicals and Antioxidants

❶ FREE-RADICAL FORMATION

During normal energy metabolism, hydrogens and electrons are added to oxygen in a series of reactions known as the electron transport chain (introduced in Chapter 7). This sequence eventually produces water, but some of the intermediate compounds inevitably created during the process are free radicals. Reminder: the dot in the symbols represents the unpaired electrons.

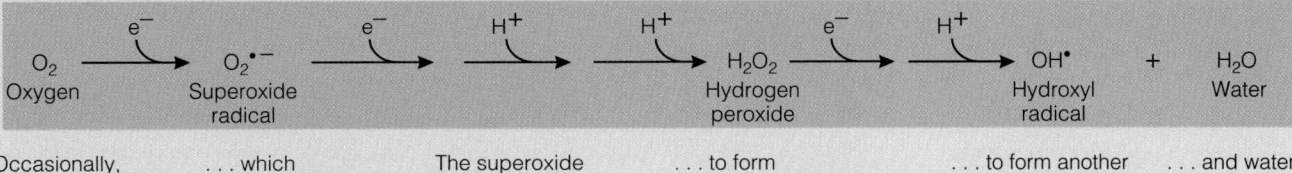

| Occasionally, oxygen gains an extra electron from the electron transport chain . . . | . . . which generates the free radical called superoxide radical (a molecule of oxygen with an extra, unpaired electron). | The superoxide radical can gain another electron (again, from the electron transport chain) and react with two hydrogen ions . . . | . . . to form hydrogen peroxide. Hydrogen peroxide can react with an electron and hydrogen . . . | . . . to form another free radical called a hydroxyl radical . . . | . . . and water. |

❷ FREE-RADICAL CHAIN REACTION AND DAMAGE

Hydroxyl radicals are highly reactive, wanting to match their unpaired electrons. For example, they might take electrons from the lipids in a cell membrane, which causes damage that gives rise to degenerative diseases.

$$Lipid \ + \ OH^• \longrightarrow Lipid^• \ + \ H_2O$$

| When a hydroxyl radical takes a hydrogen atom from a lipid (such as a polyunsaturated fatty acid) . . . | . . . it generates a lipid radical . . . | . . . and water. | The lipid radical can, in turn, react with oxygen to form another lipid radical, which can, in turn, remove hydrogen atoms from other lipids, producing new radicals, thereby initiating a chain reaction. |

❸ ANTIOXIDANT PROTECTION

Antioxidants interact with free radicals and break the destructive chain reaction that damages tissues.

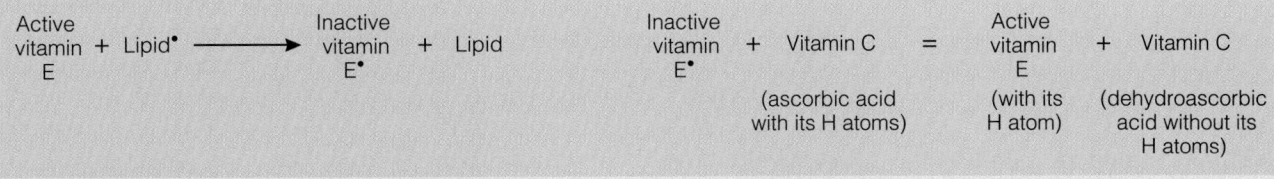

| Vitamin E gives up one of its hydrogens to a lipid radical.* | The result is that vitamin E is no longer active, but it has successfully stopped the radicals from causing more damage and generating more radicals. | Vitamin E can be reactivated by accepting a hydrogen atom from fellow antioxidant vitamin C. Vitamin C's two structures are presented in Figure 10–12 on p. 357. |

*The compound is actually a lipid peroxyl radical.

Glossary

free radical: an atom or molecule that has one or more unpaired electron(s) in the outer orbital (see Appendix B for a review of basic chemistry concepts). This electron imbalance makes free radicals unstable and highly reactive. Radicals typically arise during oxidation reactions and readily attack other molecules with which they come in contact.

oxidant: a compound (such as oxygen itself) that oxidizes other compounds. Compounds that prevent oxidation are called *antioxidants*, whereas those that encourage it are called *prooxidants*.
  anti = against
  pro = for

oxidative stress: damage to biological systems caused by free-radical formation.

peroxidation: the production of unstable molecules containing more than the usual amount of oxygen. Hydrogen peroxide, H_2O_2, for example, may be produced from water, H_2O.

phytochemicals: nonnutrient compounds in plant-derived foods that have biological activity in the body.
  phyto = plant

Reminder: *Nonnutrients* are compounds in foods with no known nutritional value.

---

damages cell structures and impairs their functions. Free radicals also damage proteins and DNA.

Rampant free-radical formation and the resulting damage together are called oxidative stress. This stress has been implicated in the aging process and in the development of diseases such as cancer, arthritis, cataracts, and heart disease.[5] Not unreasonably, researchers have predicted, and to some extent confirmed, that dietary antioxidants help the body fight oxidative stress. Vitamin E, for example, has been credited with reducing the oxidative stresses that accompany diabetes.[6] Daily supplements of vitamin E enhance the action of insulin, perhaps by stabilizing the membranes of responding cells. The result is to improve glucose control in diabetes.[7]

THE ANTIOXIDANT NUTRIENTS

Much research has focused on the theory that antioxidant nutrients

act as scavengers of oxygen-derived free radicals, thereby helping to prevent cell and tissue damage that otherwise would give rise to degenerative diseases. The beneficial effects of fruits, vegetables, and grains in fighting degenerative diseases have been attributed, in part, to the antioxidants they provide. The antioxidant roles of several vitamins that these plant foods are famous for—beta-carotene, vitamin C, and vitamin E—are under especially extensive study.

Beta-Carotene

For many years scientists believed beta-carotene's sole function was to serve as a vitamin A precursor. Now they recognize that beta-carotene also serves as an antioxidant, important in human health.

Vitamin C

Vitamin C is the most abundant water-soluble antioxidant in the body and is active primarily in

extracellular fluid. Its actions are most notable in combating the free radicals of polluted air and cigarette smoke. Not only does vitamin C scavenge many free radicals, but it helps return vitamin E to its active form.

Vitamin E

Vitamin E is the most abundant fat-soluble antioxidant and one of the body's primary defenders against oxidation. It protects the polyunsaturated fatty acids, all other lipids, and related fat-soluble compounds such as vitamin A.

Vitamin E serves as the body's first line of defense against lipid peroxidation by effectively breaking the chain reaction. In fact, vitamin E is one of the most efficient chain-breaking antioxidants available, reacting 200 times faster than the antioxidant BHT (butylated hydroxytoluene) commonly used in commercial bakery products. For this reason, a small amount of vitamin E can protect a large amount of lipid. Of course, in protecting other substances, vitamin E is used up and so needs to be replenished from dietary sources.

Other vitamins may serve not as antioxidants, but in supporting roles. For example, riboflavin forms part of the coenzymes that are required by several enzymes active in oxidative metabolism.[8]

ANTIOXIDANT NUTRIENTS AND CANCER

Cancers arise when cellular DNA is damaged—perhaps by free-radical attacks.[9] Antioxidant nutrients may reduce cancer risks by protecting DNA from this damage. Epidemiological reports indicate a correlation between low intakes of foods rich in antioxidant nutrients and high cancer rates. Laboratory studies with animals and cells in tissue culture seem to support such findings.

Many studies using animals as subjects have shown that beta-carotene protects against cancer.[10] The protective effects vary, depending on the experimental conditions, the types of animals tested, and the cancer types and sites.[11]

Research on human beings also produces diverse results. Researchers have compared groups of people with high cancer rates with groups that have low cancer rates, but are similar in other characteristics—for example, smoking history and age. They report a consistent relationship between low intakes of vegetables and fruits (specifically of those containing beta-carotene and its relatives) and high rates of lung cancer.[12] Such findings suggest that beta-carotene is protective, but researchers are quick to add that other constituents of fruits and vegetables may be responsible for the effect. When researchers collect blood samples, though, they find that low concentrations of beta-carotene consistently correlate with the development of both lung and breast cancers.[13]

Research has not always made it clear whether preformed vitamin A, beta-carotene, or both are protective against cancer.[14] Some research indicates that dietary vitamin A—from whatever source—seems to play a role in inhibiting the development of breast cancer.[15] Evidence of protection against cancers of the colon or prostate is less convincing.

Large-scale studies of populations suggest that vitamin C also helps protect against certain types of cancers, especially those of the mouth, larynx, and esophagus.[16] A dozen or so different studies have correlated high vitamin C intakes with low rates of cancer. Such a correlation may reflect the benefits of a diet rich in fruits and vegetables and low in fat and does not necessarily support the taking of vitamin C supplements to treat or prevent cancer.

Some research suggests that vitamin C protects against stomach cancer specifically, by preventing the formation of carcinogenic nitrite compounds in the stomach.[17] More research is needed, but the results so far are promising.

Evidence that vitamin E helps guard against cancer is less consistent than for beta-carotene and vitamin C. One large population study showed the highest risks of certain cancers in the people with lowest blood vitamin E.[18] The association was strongest for some gastrointestinal cancers and for cancers not related to smoking.

ANTIOXIDANTS AND HEART DISEASE

Much of the research on antioxidant nutrients has focused on cancer prevention, but antioxidants, especially vitamin E, may protect against cardiovascular disease as well.[19] Research confirms that high blood cholesterol carried in low-density lipoproteins (LDL) correlates directly with cardiovascular disease. Researchers are now asking how high LDL exert their damage. Some of the most promising research suggests that LDL first undergo oxidation by free radicals inside the artery wall and then promote the formation of artery-clogging plaques.[20] Evidence thus far is persuasive but not conclusive.

If oxidized LDL are a factor in heart disease, might antioxidant nutrients offer some protection? Some research suggests that they do. Findings from an epidemiological study suggest a negative correlation between vitamin E status and death rates from heart disease.[21] Researchers selected groups of men in 16 European regions where rates of death from heart disease varied six-fold. The researchers measured plasma vitamin E, cholesterol, and blood pressure in men from each region. When the groups were compared, high death rates from heart disease correlated more strongly with low vitamin E concentrations than with either cholesterol or blood pressure. The authors cautioned that the evidence for the "antioxidant hypothesis" of heart disease was suggestive, but indirect.

Two other large epidemiological studies found that large doses of vitamin E supplements were associated with a significantly reduced risk of heart disease.[22] This correlation remained strong after the researchers analyzed for coronary risk factors and other dietary antioxidants.

Vitamin C may also affect the susceptibility of LDL to oxidation. Some epidemiological studies have found an association between vitamin C and cardiovascular disease; others have not.[23] Research suggests a synergism between vitamin C and vitamin E in defending LDL against oxidation; vitamin C defends against free radicals in the water compartments of cells, and vitamin E acts in lipid environments. Together, they effectively protect LDL against oxidation. In addition, vitamin C may regenerate vitamin E from its oxidized form, making it available to act as an antioxidant once again.[24] Some studies also suggest that vitamin C may raise HDL, lower total cholesterol, and improve blood pressure.[25]

SUPPLEMENTS VERSUS FOODS

Of course, researchers are genuinely excited to learn that the antioxidant nutrients might help prevent such life-threatening diseases as cancer and cardiovascular disease, but their findings have sparked new controversies.[26] Some research suggests a protective effect from as little as a daily glass of orange juice and carrot juice (rich sources of vitamin C and beta-carotene, respectively).[27] Other current intervention studies, however, are using levels of nutrients that far exceed the RDA and can only be achieved by taking supplements. What if research finds a true benefit in taking vitamin pills as opposed to eating a healthy diet alone? Members of the Food and Nutrition Board of the National Research Council are reconsidering their long-held bias against vitamin supplements. They realize that it may be necessary to broaden the concept of the RDA to include both a recommended daily intake to prevent classic deficiency diseases and another substantially higher intake to help protect against chronic diseases.[28]

While awaiting final answers, should people anticipate the go-ahead and start taking vitamin E or other antioxidant supplements now?[29] Most scientists agree that it is too early to make such a recommendation. While fruits and vegetables that contain many antioxidant nutrients have been associated with a diminished risk of many cancers, supplements of beta-carotene and vitamins C and E have not always

proven beneficial.[30] Clinical studies will take several years to complete, and until they prove a clear benefit from taking antioxidant supplements, it would be irresponsible for health care professionals to make such recommendations. We do not know the consequences of taking large doses of antioxidants, even naturally occurring ones, over the long term, much less over a lifetime. Without data to confirm the benefits, we cannot accept the potential risks. And the risks are real.

Consider the findings from a study to determine whether daily supplements of vitamin E, beta-carotene, or both would reduce the incidence of lung cancer among smokers.[31] After five to eight years of supplementation, there was no reduction in the incidence of lung cancer; in fact, there was a higher incidence of lung cancer among those receiving the beta-carotene. Such findings were surprising, to say the least, especially given the association between high beta-carotene intakes and low rates of lung cancer reported in earlier epidemiological studies. These discrepancies highlight the importance of considering research findings from a variety of studies and the need for replication, already emphasized in Chapter 1. The findings also suggest that remedies to life-threatening diseases such as lung cancer may not be as simple as taking daily pills. Smokers are much wiser to stop smoking than to rely on vitamin supplements to protect them from lung cancer. Much more research is needed to define optimal and dangerous levels of intake. The Food and Drug Administration (FDA) is now in the process of establishing guidelines for the safe use of nutrient supplements in quantities greater than those

needed to meet basic nutrient requirements.

This much we know: antioxidant nutrients behave differently at various levels of intake. At physiological levels typical of a healthy diet, they act as antioxidants, but at pharmacological doses typical of supplements, they may act as *prooxidants*, *stimulating* the production of free radicals, especially when metal ions such as iron are present.[32] As long as the risks of supplement use remain unclear, the best way to supplement antioxidant nutrients is to eat generous servings of fruits and vegetables, especially citrus fruits and green and yellow vegetables.

FOODS MAKING HEALTH CLAIMS

Results of clinical studies may one day support the use of selected supplements to prevent disease, but until then, people will want to select foods rich in all of the vitamins and minerals—particularly the antioxidants. Which foods to select?

The FDA examined the available scientific evidence concerning antioxidant vitamins and cancer to determine whether a health claim on food labels was appropriate. The agency concluded that *diets* high in fruits and vegetables, which are good sources of two antioxidant vitamins (vitamin A as beta-carotene and vitamin C), are strongly associated with reduced risks of several types of cancer. Still, the FDA rejected the antioxidant health claim, stating that the reduction in risk could not be attributed directly and solely to the antioxidant effect of the vitamins. Therefore labels may not claim an association between antioxidant vitamins and cancer; the health claim must be stated in terms of "fruits and vegetables and cancer."

NONNUTRIENTS IN DISEASE PREVENTION

What do fruits and vegetables have in them besides nutrients? They must have something, for as research has shown, the nutrients alone are not fully responsible for the beneficial effects fruits and vegetables have on disease prevention. Other, nonnutrient compounds must also be involved.

The nonnutrient compounds found in plants are called phytochemicals, and they have been the topic of much recent research. In foods, these compounds may impart flavors and colors, but in the body, they can have profound physiological effects, including suppression of the development of cancer.[33] Table H11–1 summarizes the common food sources and actions of selected phytochemicals.

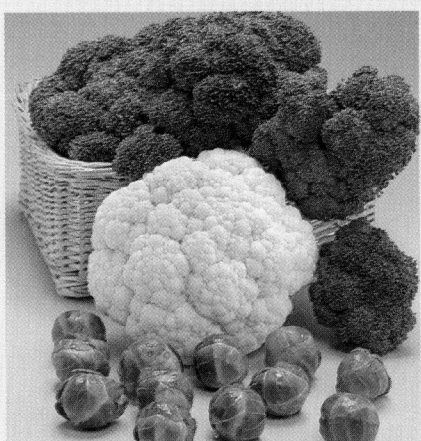

Cruciferous vegetables, such as cauliflower, broccoli, and brussels sprouts contain nutrients and nonnutrients that may inhibit cancer development.

This book has focused primarily on the nutrients, but foods deliver thousands of other chemicals. For this reason, researchers must be careful in giving credit for particular health benefits to any one nutrient. Diets rich in whole grains, legumes, vegetables, and fruits seem to be protective against cancer, but identifying *the* specific foods or components of foods that are responsible is difficult. Green leafy vegetables such as spinach and kale, for example, contain lutein, an antioxidant more active than beta-carotene. The anticancer benefits of green leafy vegetables may be due to beta-carotene, but they may be due to lutein—or to another as yet unnamed character. Perhaps credit even belongs to the unique *combination* of chemicals found in leafy greens. Similarly, soybeans contain several compounds that appear to have anticancer activity.[34] We simply do not have all the answers.

Other nonnutrients with antioxidant activity are the flavonoids commonly found in vegetables, fruits, beverages such as tea and wine, and spices such as oregano. These compounds may offer important health benefits and explain, in part, why people who drink wine and others who have high intakes of flavonoids have reduced risks of heart diseases.[35]

Everyone eats a variety of phytochemicals in small quantities every day. This approach may be more beneficial than taking large doses of any one phytochemical.[36] In large doses, some phytochemicals can be toxic. The regulation of phytochemicals depends on how they are used.[37] Consider garlic, for example. A clove of garlic is a food. The FDA classifies dehydrated garlic and garlic extracts as generally recog-

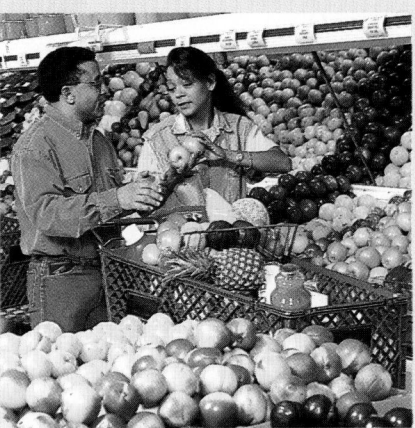

Many cancer-fighting products are available now at your local produce counter.

nized as safe (GRAS) substances. A product derived from garlic that makes a special health claim, on the other hand, is classified as a drug.

Of course, as soon as science discovers a role for phytochemicals in disease prevention, manufacturers will begin marketing supplements. (Highlight 10 explained how some manufacturers have already tried to sell antioxidant supplements marketed as "nutraceuticals.") It should be clear by now, though, that we cannot know the identity and action of every chemical in every food. Even if we did, why create a supplement to replicate a food? Why not eat foods and enjoy the pleasure, nourishment, and health benefits they provide? The beneficial constituents in foods are widespread among plants.[38] Don't try to single out one particular food for its magic phytochemical. Instead, eat a wide variety of fruits and vegetables in generous quantities every day— and get *all* the magic compounds these foods have to offer.

Table H11–1

. . . .

Phytochemicals—Their Food Sources and Actions

Food Source	Name	Action in the Body
Deeply pigmented fruits and vegetables (carrots, sweet potatoes, tomatoes, spinach, broccoli, cantaloupe, pumpkin, apricots)	Carotenoids[a] (including beta-carotene)	Act as antioxidants, reducing the risk of cancer.
Citrus fruits	Limonene	Triggers enzyme production to facilitate carcinogen excretion.
	Phenols	Inhibit lipid oxidation; block formation of carcinogenic nitrosamines in the body.
Garlic/onions	Allyl sulfides	Trigger enzyme production to facilitate carcinogen excretion.
Broccoli and other cruciferous vegetables (cauliflower and brussels sprouts)	Sulforaphane	Protects against cancer.
	Dithiolthiones	Trigger enzyme production to block carcinogen damage to cells' DNA.
	Indoles	Trigger enzymes to inhibit estrogen action, reducing the risk of breast cancer.
	Isothiocyanates	Trigger enzyme production to block carcinogen damage of cells' DNA.
Grapes	Ellagic acid	Scavenges carcinogens.
Soy/legumes	Protease inhibitors	Suppress enzyme production in cancer cells, slowing tumor growth.
	Phytosterols	Inhibit cell reproduction in GI tract, preventing colon cancer.
	Isoflavones[b]	Block estrogen activity in cells, reducing the risk of breast and ovarian cancer.
	Saponins	Interfere with DNA reproduction, preventing cancer cell multiplication.
Flaxseed	Lignans[b]	Block estrogen activity in cells, reducing the risk of breast and ovarian cancer.
Fruits (blueberries, prunes, grapes), oats, soybeans	Caffeic acid	Triggers enzyme production to make carcinogens water soluble, facilitating excretion.
	Ferulic acid	Binds to nitrates in stomach, preventing the conversion to nitrosamines.
Grains	Phytic acid	Binds to minerals, preventing cancer-causing free-radical formation.
Fruits, vegetables, tea, wine, oregano	Flavonoids	Act as antioxidants, reducing the risk of cancer.

[a]In addition to beta-carotene, other carotenoids include alpha-carotene, beta-cryptoxanthin, lectein, zeaxanthin, and lycopene.

[b]Isoflavones and lignans are types of phytoestrogens—compounds that bind to estrogen receptors and reduce estrogen activity.

NOTES

1. Health promotion and disease prevention: The role of antioxidant vitamins, *American Journal of Medicine* 97 (supplement 3A) (1994): 1S–28S; B. Halliwell, J. M. C. Gutteridge, and C. E. Cross, Free radicals, antioxidants, and human disease: Where are we now? *Journal of Laboratory and Clinical Medicine* 119 (1992): 598–620; A. T. Diplock, Antioxidant nutrients and disease prevention: An overview, *American Journal of Clinical Nutrition* 53 (1991): 189S–193S.

2. J. D. Morrow and coauthors, Increase in circulating products of lipid peroxidation (F_2-

isoprostanes) in smokers—Smoking as a cause of oxidative damage, *New England Journal of Medicine* 332 (1995): 1198–1203.

3. B. Halliwell, Free radicals and antioxidants: A personal view, *Nutrition Reviews* 52 (1994): 253–265.

4. G. W. Burton and M. G. Traber, Vitamin E: Antioxidant activity, biokinetics, and bioavailability, *Annual Review of Nutrition* 10 (1990): 357–382.

5. Diplock, 1991; L. Packer, Protective role of vitamin E in biological systems, *American Journal of Clinical Nutrition* 53 (1991): 1050S–1055S.

6. B. Caballero, Vitamin E improves the action of insulin, *Nutrition Reviews* 51 (1993): 339–340.

7. G. Paolisso and coauthors, Pharmacologic doses of vitamin E improve insulin action in healthy subjects and non-insulin-dependent diabetic subjects, *American Journal of Clinical Nutrition* 57 (1993): 650–656.

8. R. S. Rivlin and P. Dutta, Vitamin B2 (riboflavin)—Relevance to malaria and antioxidant activity, *Nutrition Today* 30 (1995): 62–67.

9. I. T. Johnson, G. Williamson, and S. R. R. Musk, Anticarcinogenic factors in plant foods: A new class of nutrients? *Nutrition Research Reviews* 7 (1994): 175–204; B. N. Ames, M. K. Shigenaga, and T. M. Hagen, Oxidants, antioxidants, and the degenerative diseases of aging, *Proceedings of the National Academy of Sciences* 90 (1993): 7915–7922.

10. N. I. Krinsky, Effects of carotenoids in cellular and animal systems, *American Journal of Clinical Nutrition* 52 (1991): 238S–246S.

11. T. Byers and G. Perry, Dietary carotenes, vitamin C, and vitamin E as protective antioxidants in human cancers, *Annual Review of Nutrition* 12 (1992): 139–159.

12. R. G. Ziegler, Vegetables, fruits, and carotenoids and the risk of cancer, *American Journal of Clinical Nutrition* 53 (1991): 251S–259S.

13. H. B. Stahalein and coauthors, Beta-carotene and cancer prevention: The Basel Study, *American Journal of Clinical Nutrition* 53 (1991): 265S–269S; N. Potischman and coauthors, Breast cancer and dietary and plasma concentrations of carotenoids and vitamin A, *American Journal of Clinical Nutrition* 52 (1990): 909–915.

14. W. C. Willett and D. J. Hunter, Vitamin A and cancers of the breast, large bowel, and prostate: Epidemiologic evidence, *Nutrition Reviews* (supplement) 52 (1994): S53–S59.

15. D. J. Hunter and coauthors, A prospective study of the intake of vitamins C, E, and A and the risk of breast cancer, *New England Journal of Medicine* 329 (1993): 234–240.

16. G. Block, Vitamin C and cancer prevention: The epidemiologic evidence, *American Journal of Clinical Nutrition* 53 (1991): 270S–282S.

17. S. R. Tannenbaum, J. S. Wishnok, and C. D. Leaf, Inhibition of nitrosamine formation by ascorbic acid, *American Journal of Clinical Nutrition* 53 (1991): 247S–250S.

18. P. Knekt and coauthors, Vitamin E and cancer prevention, *American Journal of Clinical Nutrition* 53 (1991): 283S–286S.

19. T. Byers, Vitamin E supplements and coronary heart disease, *Nutrition Reviews* 51 (1993): 333–336; K. F. Gey and coauthors, Increased risk of cardiovascular disease at suboptimal plasma concentrations of essential antioxidants: An epidemiological update with special attention to carotene and vitamin C, *American Journal of Clinical Nutrition* 57 (1993): 787S–797S.

20. B. Halliwell, Oxidation of low-density lipoproteins: Questions of initiation, propagation, and the effect of antioxidants, *American Journal of Clinical Nutrition* 61 (1995): 670S–677S.

21. K. F. Gey and coauthors, Inverse correlation between plasma vitamin E and mortality from ischemic heart disease in cross-cultural epidemiology, *American Journal of Clinical Nutrition* 53 (1991): 326S–334S; Gey and coauthors, 1993.

22. M. J. Stampfer and coauthors, Vitamin E consumption and the risk of coronary disease in women, *New England Journal of Medicine* 328 (1993): 1444–1449; E. B. Rimm and coauthors, Vitamin E consumption and the risk of coronary disease in men, *New England Journal of Medicine* 328 (1993): 1450–1456.

23. Gey and coauthors, 1993; D. L. Trout, Vitamin C and cardiovascular risk factors, *American Journal of Clinical Nutrition* 53 (1991): 322S–325S; Stampfer and coauthors, 1993; Rimm and coauthors, 1993.

24. D. Kritchevsky, Antioxidant vitamins in the prevention of cardiovascular disease, *Nutrition Today*, January/February 1992, pp. 30–33.

25. Trout, 1991; J. P. Moran and coauthors, Plasma ascorbic acid concentrations relate inversely to blood pressure in human subjects, *American Journal of Clinical Nutrition* 57 (1993): 213–217.

26. J. Blumberg, Are antioxidants at an awkward age? *Journal of the American College of Nutrition* 13 (1994): 218–219.

27. M. Abbey, M. Noakes, and P. J. Nestel, Dietary supplementation with orange and carrot juice in cigarette smokers lowers oxidation products in copper-oxidized low-density lipoproteins, *Journal of the American Dietetic Association* 95 (1995): 671–675.

28. W. A. Pryor, The antioxidant nutrients and disease prevention—What do we know and what do we need to find out? *American Journal of Clinical Nutrition* 53 (1991): 391S–393S.

29. D. Steinberg, Antioxidant vitamins and coronary heart disease, *New England Journal of Medicine* 328 (1993): 1487–1489.

30. E. R. Greenberg and coauthors, A clinical trial of antioxidant vitamins to prevent colorectal adenoma, *New England Journal of Medicine* 331 (1994): 141–147.

31. O. P. Heinonen, J. K. Huttunen, and D. Albanes (and other participants in the alpha-tocopherol, beta carotene cancer prevention study group), The effect of vitamin E and beta carotene on the incidence of lung cancer and other cancers in male smokers, *New England Journal of Medicine* 330 (1994): 1029–1035.

32. T. Repka and R. P. Hebbel, Hydroxyl radical formation by sickle erythrocyte membranes: Role of pathological iron deposits and cytoplasmic reducing agents, *Blood* 78 (1991): 2753–2758; V. Herbert, The antioxidant supplement myth, *American Journal of Clinical Nutrition* 60 (1994): 157–158; B. Halliwell, Antioxidants: Sense or speculation? *Nutrition Today*, November/December 1994, pp. 15–19.

33. L. W. Wattenberg, Inhibition of carcinogenesis by minor dietary constituents, *Cancer Research* 52 (1992): 2085s–2091s.

34. M. Messina and S. Barnes, The role of soy products in reducing risk of cancer, *Journal of the National Cancer Institute* 83 (1991): 541–546.

35. Dietary flavonoids and risk of coronary heart disease, *Nutrition Reviews* 52 (1994): 59–61.

36. L. U. Thompson, Antioxidants and hormone-mediated health benefits of whole grains, *Critical Reviews in Food Science and Nutrition* 34 (1994): 473–497.

37. J. N. Hathcock, Safety and regulatory issues for phytochemical sources: "Designer foods," *Nutrition Today*, November/December 1993, pp. 23–25.

38. Position of The American Dietetic Association: Phytochemicals and functional foods, *Journal of the American Dietetic Association* 95 (1995): 493–496; E. A. Decker, The role of phenolics, conjugated linoleic acid, carnosine, and pyrroloquinoline quinone as nonessential dietary antioxidants, *Nutrition Reviews* 53 (1995): 19–58.

Chapter 12

Water and the Major Minerals

CONTENTS

Water and the Body Fluids
Water Balance and Recommended Intakes
Blood Volume and Blood Pressure
Fluid and Electrolyte Balance
Fluid and Electrolyte Imbalance
Acid-Base Balance
The Minerals—An Overview
Sodium
Chloride
Potassium
Calcium
Calcium Roles in the Body
Calcium Recommendations and Intakes
Calcium Deficiency
Phosphorus
Magnesium
Sulfur
HIGHLIGHT: Osteoporosis and Calcium

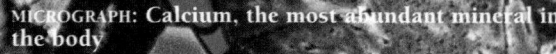

MICROGRAPH: Calcium, the most abundant mineral in the body

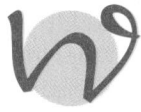

ater is an essential nutrient, as important to life as any of the others. In fact, you can survive only a few days without water, whereas a deficiency of the other nutrients may take weeks, months, or even years to develop.

This chapter begins with a look at water and the body's fluids. The body maintains an appropriate balance and distribution of water with the help of another class of nutrients—the minerals. In addition to introducing the minerals that help regulate body fluids, the chapter describes many of the other important functions minerals perform in the body.

Water and the Body Fluids

In the body, water becomes the fluid in which all life processes occur. Every cell contains intracellular fluid of the exact composition that is best for that cell and is bathed externally in another such fluid (interstitial fluids.) (Figure 6–9 on p. 191 illustrates a cell and its associated fluids.) The interstitial fluid provides each cell with the ingredients it requires and receives the end products of the chemical reactions that take place within the cells' boundaries. The water molecules of the intracellular fluid nestle around the cell's giant proteins, glycogen, and other large molecules, helping to maintain their structures and participating in many chemical reactions.

These fluids are constantly losing and replacing their constituent parts, yet the composition in each compartment remains remarkably constant at all times. The entire system of cells and fluids remains in a delicate but firmly maintained state of homeostasis. The water in the body fluids:

- Carries nutrients and waste products throughout the body.
- Helps to form the structure of large molecules.
- Actively participates in many chemical reactions.
- Serves as the solvent for minerals, vitamins, amino acids, glucose, and a multitude of other small molecules.
- Acts as a lubricant and cushion around joints.
- Serves as a shock absorber inside the eyes, spinal cord, and, in pregnancy, the amniotic sac surrounding the fetus in the womb.
- Aids in the body's temperature regulation.
- Maintains blood volume.

Because water is so vital to these and other functions, the body directs many of its activities toward maintaining an appropriate balance.

WATER BALANCE AND RECOMMENDED INTAKES

Water constitutes about 60 percent of an adult's body weight and a higher percentage of a child's. The proportion of water is generally lower in females, obese people, and the elderly. The amount of fluid in the body is tightly controlled because imbalances can be devastating. The body attempts to restore homeostasis as promptly as possible, adjusting both water intake and excretion as needed.

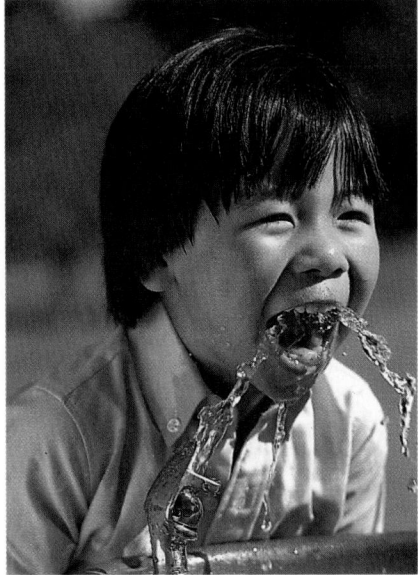

Water is the most indispensable nutrient.

intracellular fluid: fluid within the cells, usually high in potassium and phosphate. Intracellular fluid accounts for approximately two-thirds of the body's water.

intra = within

interstitial fluid (IN-ter-STISH-al): fluid between the cells, usually high in sodium and chloride. Interstitial fluid is a large component of **extracellular fluid** (fluid outside the cells), which also includes plasma and the water of structures such as the skin and bones. Extracellular fluid accounts for approximately one-third of the body's water.

inter = in the midst, between
extra = outside

Reminder: *Homeostasis* is the maintenance of relatively constant conditions within the body's systems.

water balance: the balance between water intake and output (losses).
Water balance = intake − output.

thirst: a conscious desire to drink.

hypothalamus (high-po-THAL-ah-mus): a brain center that controls activities such as maintenance of water balance and regulation of body temperature.

dehydration: the condition in which body water output exceeds water input.

water intoxication: the condition in which body water contents are too high.

Water Intake   Thirst and satiety influence water intake, apparently in response to changes sensed by the mouth, hypothalamus, and nerves. When the blood is too concentrated (having lost water, but not the dissolved substances within it), the mouth becomes dry, and the person responds by drinking. When the hypothalamus detects that the blood is too concentrated, it also initiates drinking behavior. The nerves also play a role: thirsty animals drink until stretch receptors in the stomach turn off the drinking. Similarly, receptors in the heart monitor blood volume and suppress thirst when the volume is elevated.

Thirst drives a person to seek water, but it lags behind the body's need. A water deficiency that develops slowly can switch on drinking behavior in time to prevent serious dehydration, but a deficiency that develops quickly may not. Also, thirst itself does not remedy a water deficiency; a person must notice the thirst signal, pay attention, and take the time to get a drink. The long-distance runner, the gardener in hot weather, the child busy playing, and the elderly person whose thirst sensation may be blunted can experience serious dehydration if they fail to drink promptly in response to their need for water.

Dehydration may easily develop with either water deprivation or excessive water losses. The symptoms progress rapidly from thirst, to weakness, to exhaustion and delirium and end in death if not corrected. Water intoxication, on the other hand, is rare but can occur with excessive water ingestion and kidney disorders that reduce urine output. The symptoms may include confusion, convulsion, and even death in extreme cases.

Water Sources   The obvious dietary sources of water are water itself and other beverages, but nearly all foods also contain water. Most fruits and vegetables contain up to 95 percent water; many meats and cheeses contain at least 50 percent (see Appendix H). Water is also generated during metabolism. Recall that when the energy-yielding nutrients break down, their carbons and hydrogens combine with oxygen to yield carbon dioxide (CO_2)—and water (H_2O). The water derived daily from these three sources totals, on the average, about 2½ liters (about 2½ quarts), as Table 12–1 shows.

Table 12–1

Water Balance

Water Sources	Amount (ml)	Water Excretion	Amount (ml)
Liquids	550 to 1500	Kidneys	500 to 1400
Foods	700 to 1000	Skin	450 to 900
Metabolic water	200 to 300	Lungs	350
		Feces	150
	1450 to 2800		1450 to 2800

Note: These values reflect data from several sources and are compatible with those cited in many other references. For further information, see L. Sherwood, *Fundamentals of Physiology: A Human Perspective* (St. Paul, Minn.: West Publishing, 1995), pp. 396–417; Committee on Dietary Allowances, *Recommended Dietary Allowances*, 10th ed. (Washington, D.C.: National Academy Press, 1989), pp. 247–261; J. L. Groff, S. S. Gropper, and S. M. Hunt, *Advanced Nutrition and Human Metabolism* (St. Paul, Minn.: West Publishing, 1995), pp. 423–438.

Water Losses   The body must excrete a minimum of about 500 milliliters of water each day as urine—enough to carry away the waste products generated by a day's metabolic activities. Above this amount, excretion adjusts to balance intake. If a person drinks more water, the urine becomes more dilute. In addition, water is lost from the lungs as vapor and from the skin as sweat; some is also lost in feces.* The losses from all of these sources total about 2½ liters a day on the average. Table 12–1 shows how water excretion balances intake.

The amount of water the body has to excrete each day to dispose of its wastes is the **obligatory** (ah-BLIG-ah-TORE-ee) **water excretion**—about 500 ml, or a pint.

Water Recommendations   Water needs vary, depending primarily on diet, activity, environmental temperature, and humidity. Accordingly, a general water requirement is difficult to establish. Recommendations for adults are expressed in proportion to the amount of energy expended under average environmental conditions.[1] A person who expends 2000 kcalories a day needs about 2 to 3 liters of water (about 7 to 11 cups).

Fluid needs are best met by water, but milk and juices can account for part of the day's recommended intake.[2] In addition to their high water content, these beverages deliver valuable nutrients. Alcoholic beverages and those containing caffeine, such as coffee, tea, and sodas, however, are not good substitutes for water. Both alcohol and caffeine act as diuretics, causing the body to lose fluids.

Fluid needs before, during, and after exercise are addressed in Highlight 8.

Water recommendation for adults:
- 1.0 to 1.5 ml/kcal expended.
- 4.2 to 6.3 ml/kJ expended.

Water recommendation for infants:
- 1.5 ml/kcal expended.

Note: 1 ml = 0.03 fluid oz.
125 ml ≈ ½ c.

Easy estimation: ½ c per 100 kcal expended.

BLOOD VOLUME AND BLOOD PRESSURE

Water balance is critical to maintaining the blood volume, which in turn influences blood pressure. If too much water is lost from the body, blood volume and blood pressure fall.

ADH and Water Retention   The hypothalamus stimulates the pituitary gland to release the antidiuretic hormone (ADH) whenever the blood becomes too concentrated, or whenever blood volume or blood pressure falls too low. ADH stimulates the kidneys to reabsorb water, so they recirculate it, rather than excrete it. Consequently, the more water you need, the less you excrete.

ADH (antidiuretic hormone): a hormone released by the pituitary gland in response to highly concentrated blood. The kidneys respond by reabsorbing water, thus preventing water loss. In addition to its antidiuretic effect, ADH also elevates blood pressure and is called **vasopressin.**

anti = against
di = through
ure = urine
vaso = vessel
press = pressure

Recall from Highlight 7 how alcohol depresses ADH activity, thus promoting fluid losses and dehydration.

Angiotensin and Blood Vessel Constriction   Cells in the kidneys respond to low blood pressure by releasing an enzyme called renin. Through a complex series of events, renin causes the kidneys to reabsorb sodium. Sodium reabsorption, in turn, is always accompanied by water retention, which helps to restore blood volume and blood pressure. Renin activates a protein in the blood called angiotensinogen to its active form, angiotensin. Angiotensin is a powerful vasoconstrictor: it narrows blood vessel diameters, thereby raising the blood pressure.

renin: an enzyme from the kidneys that works by activating angiotensin.

angiotensin: a blood protein that helps to raise blood pressure. Its precursor protein is called **angiotensinogen.**

vasoconstrictor: a substance that constricts or narrows the blood vessels.

Aldosterone and Sodium Retention   Angiotensin also mediates the release of the hormone aldosterone from the adrenal glands. Aldosterone causes the kidneys to retain more sodium (and thus more water). Again, the effect is that when more water is needed, less is excreted.

In summary, in response to low blood volume or highly concentrated blood, these three actions effectively restore homeostasis (see Figure 12–1):

aldosterone (al-DOS-ter-own): a hormone secreted by the adrenal glands that stimulates the reabsorption of sodium by the kidneys; aldosterone also regulates chloride and potassium concentrations.

adrenal glands: glands adjacent to, and just above, each kidney.

---

*Water lost from the lungs and skin accounts for almost one-half of the daily losses even when a person is not visibly perspiring; these losses are commonly referred to as *insensible water losses*.

Figure 12–1

How the Body Regulates Water Excretion

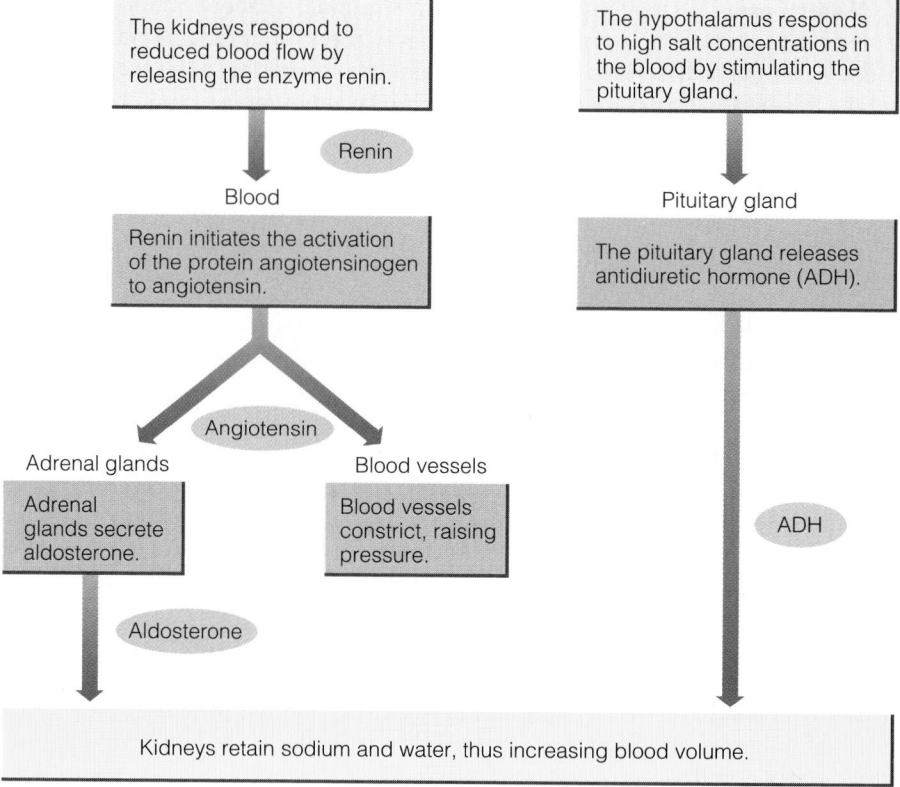

Reminder: *Fluid and electrolyte balance* is the maintenance of the proper amounts and kinds of fluid and minerals in each compartment of the body fluids.

The cell membrane is selectively permeable; that is, it permits some, but not all, substances to pass freely.

salts: compounds composed of a positive ion other than H⁺ and a negative ion other than OH⁻. An example is sodium chloride (Na⁺Cl⁻).
  Na = sodium.
  Cl = chloride.

dissociation: the physical separation of a compound into ions.

ions (EYE-uns): atoms or molecules that have gained or lost electrons and therefore have electrical charges. Examples include the positively charged sodium ion (Na⁺) and the negatively charged chloride ion (Cl⁻). For a closer look at ions, see Appendix B.

- ADH causes water retention.
- Angiotensin constricts blood vessels.
- Aldosterone causes sodium retention.

These mechanisms cannot maintain water balance by themselves, however; they work only if a person drinks enough water.

FLUID AND ELECTROLYTE BALANCE

The body cells, with only a few exceptions, cannot move water from place to place; they need to use minerals and other constituents to regulate the distribution of body fluids. About two-thirds of the body fluids reside inside the cells and one-third outside. This balance is vital to the life of the cells. If too much water entered the cells, it might rupture them; if too much water were to leave, they would collapse. To control the movement of water, the body uses its major minerals, which form salts that dissolve in the body fluids. The cells direct the movement of these salts, and this determines where the fluids flow because *water follows salt.* (This simple statement sums up how osmotic pressure works; a later section describes osmosis in more detail.)

Dissociation of Salt in Water   When a mineral salt such as sodium chloride (NaCl) dissolves in water, it separates (dissociates) into ions—positively and negatively charged particles (Na^+ and Cl^-). The positive ions are cations; the negative ones are anions. Unlike pure water, which conducts electricity poorly, ions dissolved in water carry electrical current. For this reason, ions are called electrolytes, and the fluids of the body, which contain water and dissociated salts, are electrolyte solutions.

In all electrolyte solutions, anion and cation concentrations balance. If a fluid contains 1000 "−" charges, it must contain 1000 "+" charges, too. If an anion enters the fluid, a cation must accompany it or another anion must leave so that electroneutrality will be maintained.

It is not necessary, though, to have the same number of Na^+ and Cl^- ions in a body fluid. Na^+ ions can leave a cell, provided that some other + ions enter: potassium (K^+) ions, for example. Table 12–2 shows that, indeed, the numbers of each kind of ion inside and outside cells differ over a wide range, but the + and − charges are perfectly balanced.

Inside the cells, in each liter of fluid, there are 150 K^+, 2 Ca^{++}, and 40 Mg^{++} charges for each 10 Na^+. (Chemists count these charges in milliequivalents, mEq.) The + charges total 202. The − charges inside the cells balance these perfectly. Outside the cells, the amounts of ions and their proportions differ from those inside, but again the + and − charges balance.

Electrolytes Attract Water   Because electrolytes are charged, they attract water molecules, which are polar. Although each water molecule bears a net

cations (CAT-eye-uns): positively charged ions.

anions (AN-eye-uns): negatively charged ions.

electrolytes: salts that dissolve in water and dissociate.

electrolyte solutions: solutions that can conduct electricity due to the presence of ions.

milliequivalents (mEq): the concentration of electrolytes in a volume of solution. The number of milliequivalents is a useful measure when considering ions, because the number of charges reveals characteristics about the solution that are not evident when expressed in terms of weight.

polar: describes a neutral molecule that has opposite charges spatially separated within the molecule; see Appendix B for more details.

Table 12–2

Important Body Electrolytes

Electrolyte	Extracellular Concentration (mEq/L)	Intracellular Concentration (mEq/L)
Cations		
Sodium (Na^+)	142	10
Potassium (K^+)	5	150
Calcium (Ca^{++})	5	2
Magnesium (Mg^{++})	3	40
	155	202
Anions		
Chloride (Cl^-)	103	2
Bicarbonate (HCO_3^-)	27	10
Phosphate ($HPO_4^=$)	2	103
Sulfate ($SO_4^=$)	1	20
Organic acids (lactate, pyruvate)	6	10
Proteins	16	57
	155	202

Note: The number of positive and negative charges in a given fluid is the same. For example, in extracellular fluid, the cations and anions both equal 155 milliequivalents per liter (mEq/L). Of the cations, sodium ions make up 142 mEq/L; and potassium, calcium, and magnesium ions make up the remainder. Of the anions, chloride ions number 103 mEq/L; bicarbonate ions number 27; and the rest are provided by phosphate ions, sulfate ions, organic acids, and protein.

Figure 12–2

Water Dissolves Salts and Follows Electrolytes

The structural arrangement of the two hydrogen atoms and one oxygen atom enables water to dissolve solutes. Water's role as a solvent is one of its most valuable characteristics.

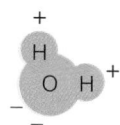

Water is polar, because the negatively charged electrons that bond the hydrogens to the oxygen spend most of their time near the oxygen atom. As a result, the oxygen is slightly negative, and the hydrogen is slightly positive (see Appendix B).

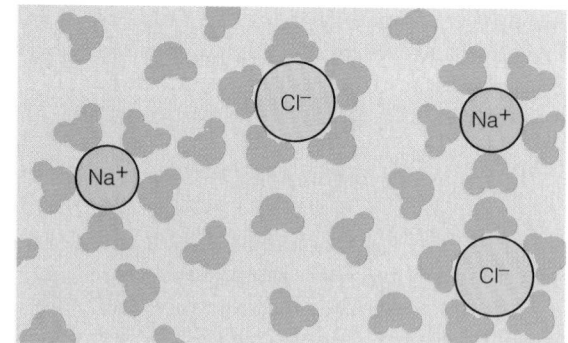

In an electrolyte solution, therefore, water molecules are attracted to both anions and cations. Notice that the negative oxygen atoms of the water molecules are drawn to the sodium cation (Na^+) here, while the positive sides of the water molecules are drawn to the chloride ions (Cl^-).

The word ending -ate denotes a salt of the mineral.

solutes (SOLL-yutes): the substances that are dissolved in a solution.

osmotic pressure: the pressure that develops when two solutions of different concentrations are separated by a membrane that permits water, but not the solutes, to cross. Water flows *toward* the side of the membrane on which the solutes are more concentrated.

The pump activity exchanges sodium for potassium across the cell membrane, maintaining a strong *concentration gradient* of each. Known as the sodium-potassium pump, it uses ATP (Chapter 7) as an energy source and the enzyme sodium-potassium ATPase (A-T-P-ace) to release that energy from ATP.

charge of zero, the oxygen side of the molecule is slightly negatively charged, and the hydrogens are slightly positively charged. Figure 12–2 shows the result in an electrolyte solution: both positive and negative ions attract clusters of water molecules around them. It is this attraction that dissolves salts in water and enables the body to move fluids into appropriate compartments.

Water Follows Electrolytes   Some electrolytes reside primarily outside the cells (notably, sodium and chloride), while others are predominantly inside the cells (notably, potassium, magnesium, phosphate, and sulfate). Cells can move the electrolytes in and out, and water will follow them.

The statement that water follows salt means that a force moves water toward concentrated solutes. This force, known as osmotic pressure, moves water across a membrane whenever the solute concentrations on the two sides are not equal—the solutes themselves cannot cross the membrane. Figure 12–3 (on facing page) shows this principle in operation.

Proteins Regulate Flow of Fluids and Ions   Transport proteins in the cell membranes also regulate the passage of positive ions and other substances from one side of the membrane to the other. Negative ions follow positive ions, and water flows toward the more concentrated solution.

A well-understood member of this class of proteins is the sodium pump, an enzyme that pumps sodium out of cells faster than it can diffuse back in. Simultaneously, the enzyme pumps potassium ions the other way, into the cell. Figure 6–10 on p. 192 illustrates this action.

Maintenance of Fluid and Electrolyte Balance   The amounts of various salts in the body must remain nearly constant. If salts are lost, they must be replaced from external sources—meaning foods and beverages. The body has discrete regulatory mechanisms to help ensure that the concentrations of all minerals stay within bounds. Regulation occurs chiefly at two sites: the GI tract and the kidneys.

Figure 12–3

Osmotic Pressure
Water flows in the direction of the higher concentration of solute.

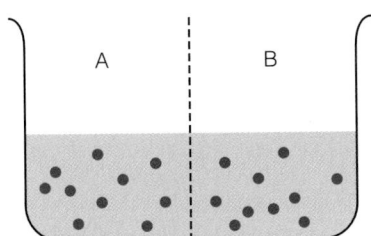

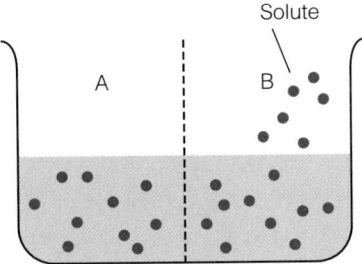

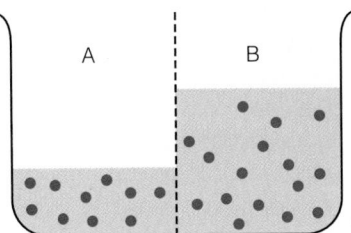

❶ With equal numbers of solute particles on both sides, the concentrations are equal, and the tendency of water to move in either direction is about the same.

❷ Now additional solute is added to side B. Solute cannot flow across the divider (in the case of a cell, its membrane).

❸ Water can flow both ways across the divider, but has a greater tendency to move from side A to side B, where there is a greater concentration of solute. The volume of water becomes greater on side B, and the concentrations on sides A and B become equal.

Regulation by the GI Tract   The GI tract continuously pours minerals out into its upper portions (stomach and small intestine) in the digestive juices and bile it secretes. It then reabsorbs these minerals and those from foods in its lower segment (the colon) as needed. In a day, 8 liters of fluids and associated minerals are recycled this way, providing ample opportunity for the regulation of electrolyte balance.

Regulation by the Kidneys   The kidneys' control of the body's *water* content has already been described; the hormone ADH determines how much water the kidneys will release in urine and how much they will reabsorb into the bloodstream. To regulate the *electrolyte* contents, the kidneys depend on the adrenal glands, which send out the hormone aldosterone to convey messages. If the body's sodium is low, aldosterone promotes sodium reabsorption from the kidney tubules. As sodium is reabsorbed, potassium is excreted, obeying the rule that total positive charges must remain the same. (A review of kidney function may be helpful: see Figure 3–8 on p. 88.)

FLUID AND ELECTROLYTE IMBALANCE

Normally, the body defends itself successfully against fluid and electrolyte imbalances. However, a person may encounter situations of imbalance for which the cell membranes, kidneys, and thirst instinct cannot compensate. Vomiting, diarrhea, heavy sweating, burns, wounds, and the like may incur great fluid and electrolyte losses, precipitating a medical emergency.

The details of electrolyte balances are among the most important concepts that health care professionals must learn. They are emphasized in physiology courses and in medical and nursing curricula. Everyone, however, should appre-

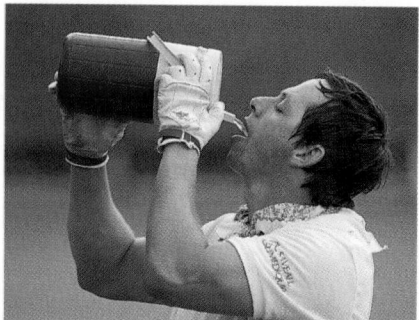

Physically active people must remember to replace their body fluids.

The administration of a simple solution of sugar, salt, and water, taken by mouth, to treat dehydration caused by diarrhea is called oral rehydration therapy (ORT). A simple ORT recipe: 1 c boiling water.
  2 tsp sugar.
  A pinch of salt.

pH: a measure of the concentration of H^+ ions (see Appendix B). The lower the pH, the stronger the acid. Thus, at pH 2, a solution is a strong acid, and at pH 6, a solution is a weak acid (pH 7 is neutral). A pH above 7 is alkaline, or base (a solution in which OH^- ions predominate).

Reminder: *Buffers* are compounds that help keep a solution's acidity or alkalinity constant. The buffering action of proteins is described in Chapter 6.

carbonic acid: a compound with the formula H_2CO_3 that results from the combination of carbon dioxide (CO_2) and water (H_2O), of particular importance in the body's buffer system.

ciate the importance of the balance and the principles by which it is maintained. Knowledge of the situations that threaten fluid and electrolyte balance enables a person to take the appropriate action and seek medical help. People usually take water and salts for granted and ignore them, but the rapid loss of fluid and electrolytes can threaten life.

Sodium and Chloride Most Easily Lost Because sodium and chloride are the body's principal extracellular cation and anion, they are first to be lost when fluid is lost by sweating, bleeding, or renal or fecal excretion. It is no accident that after sweating excessively or losing fluid in other ways, a person craves salty foods and refreshing drinks.

Different Solutes Lost by Different Routes If fluid is lost by vomiting or diarrhea, sodium is lost indiscriminately. If the adrenal glands oversecrete aldosterone, as occurs when a tumor develops, the kidneys may excrete too much potassium. And the person with uncontrolled diabetes may lose a solute not normally excreted: glucose, and with it, large amounts of water. All three situations bring on dehydration, but just drinking water cannot restore balance. In each case, medical intervention is required.

Replacing Lost Fluids and Electrolytes In many cases, people can replace the fluids and minerals lost in sweat or in a temporary bout of diarrhea by drinking plain cool water and eating regular foods. Some cases, however, demand rapid replacement of fluids and electrolytes—for example, when diarrhea threatens the life of a malnourished child.

Caretakers around the world have learned to use simple formulas to treat mild-to-moderate cases of diarrhea. These lifesaving formulas do not require hospitalization and can be prepared from ingredients available locally. Caretakers must only learn to measure ingredients carefully and use sanitary water. Once rehydrated, children can begin eating foods.

ACID-BASE BALANCE

The body uses its ions not only to help maintain water balance, but also to help regulate the acidity (pH) of its fluids. The pH scale of Chapter 3 is repeated here, in Figure 12–4, with the normal and abnormal pH ranges of body fluids added.

Regulation by Buffers Some of the electrolyte mixtures in the body fluids, as well as some of the proteins, protect the body against changes in acidity by acting as buffers—substances that can neutralize acids or bases. The body's buffer systems serve as a first line of defense against changes in the fluids' acid-base balance.

Regulation by Excretion The lungs, skin, GI tract, and kidneys provide other defenses. Carbon dioxide, which is formed all the time by cellular respiration, forms carbonic acid in the blood, pushing the balance toward acid. If too much acid builds up, the respiration rate speeds up, and more carbon dioxide is exhaled. If base builds up, the respiration rate slows; more carbon dioxide is retained and forms more carbonic acid. The skin can excrete acid in sweat, and

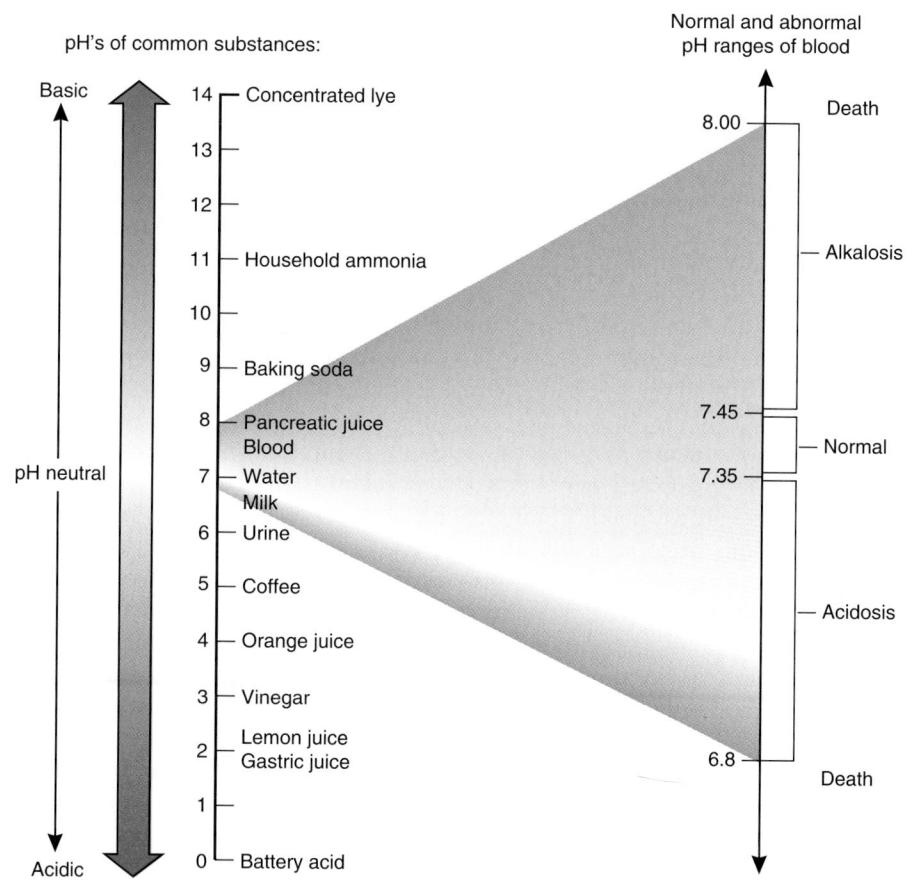

Figure 12–4

The pH Scale

Note: Each step is ten times as concentrated in base ($\frac{1}{10}$ as much acid, or H^+) as the one below it.

the specialized tear ducts can alter the composition of tears. These are of minor, although not negligible, importance; the kidneys play the primary role in maintaining acid-base balance.

   Regulation by the Kidneys   The kidneys adjust the acid-base balance by selecting which ions to retain and which to excrete. Their work is complex, but their net effect is easy to sum up. The *body's* total acid burden remains nearly constant; to a great extent, what a person ingests affects the acidity, not of the body, but of the *urine*.

In summary, water makes up about 60 percent of the body's weight. It assists with transportation of nutrients and waste products throughout the body, participates in chemical reactions, acts as a solvent, serves as a shock absorber, and regulates body temperature. To maintain water balance, intake from liquids, foods, and metabolism must equal losses from kidneys, skin, lungs, and feces. The antidiuretic hormone (ADH) signals the kidneys to retain water, and the hormone aldosterone causes the kidneys to retain sodium; together, they increase blood volume and restore normal blood pressure. Because water follows salt, electrolytes (charged minerals) in the fluids help distribute the fluids inside and outside of cells, thus ensuring the appropriate balance to support all life processes.

The Minerals—An Overview

Reminder: *Minerals* are inorganic elements; some minerals are required in small amounts and are therefore essential nutrients.

major minerals: essential mineral nutrients found in the human body in amounts larger than 5 g.

trace minerals: essential mineral nutrients found in the human body in amounts less than 5 g.

Figure 12–5 shows the amounts of the major minerals and, for comparison, some of the trace minerals found in the body. The distinction between the major and trace minerals does not mean that one group is more important than the other—all are vital. The major minerals are so named because they are the minerals present, and needed, in the largest amounts in the body. The major minerals, sometimes referred to as macrominerals, are shown at the top of the figure and are discussed in this chapter. The trace minerals (shown at the bottom), sometimes referred to as microminerals, are discussed in Chapter 13.

A few generalizations pertain to all of the minerals and distinguish them from the vitamins. Especially notable is their chemical nature.

Inorganic Elements Unlike the vitamins, which are organic compounds, minerals are inorganic elements that always retain their chemical identity. For example, iron may reversibly combine with other charged elements in salts, but it is always iron. Once minerals enter the body proper, they remain there until excreted; they cannot be changed into anything else. Neither can minerals be destroyed by heat, air, acid, or mixing; only a little care is needed to preserve minerals during food preparation. In fact, the ash that remains when a food is burned contains all the minerals that were in the food originally. Minerals can be lost from food only when they leach into water that is then thrown away.

The Body's Handling of Minerals The minerals also differ from the vitamins in the amounts the body can absorb and in the extent to which they must be specially handled. Some minerals are easily absorbed into the blood, transported freely, and readily excreted by the kidneys, much like the water-soluble vitamins. Some minerals are more like fat-soluble vitamins in that they must have carriers to be absorbed and transported. And, like the fat-soluble vitamins, minerals taken in excess can be toxic.

Figure 12–5

The Amounts of Minerals in a 60-kilogram (132-pound) Human Body

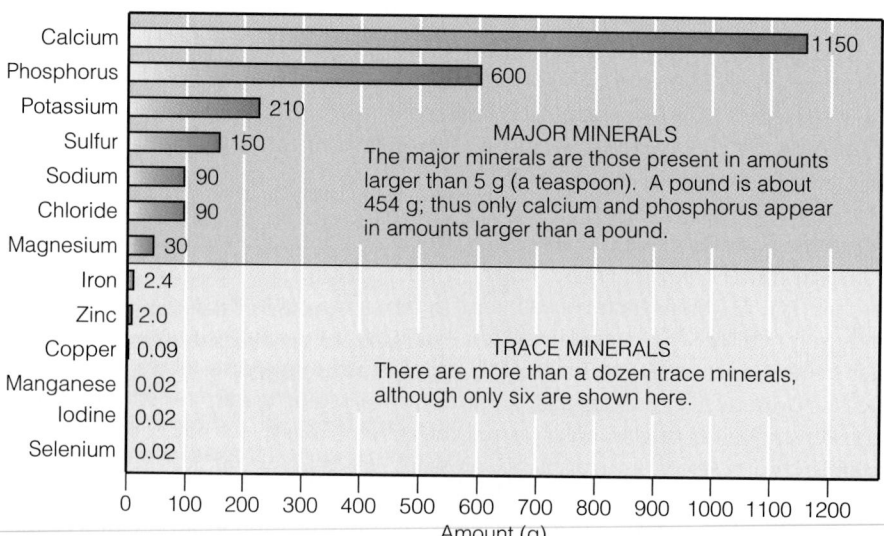

Variable Bioavailability   Some foods contain binders that combine chemically with minerals, preventing their absorption and carrying them out of the body with other wastes. For example, phytic acid makes the calcium (as well as iron and zinc) in certain foods less available than it might be otherwise; oxalic acid also binds calcium and iron. Phytic acid is found primarily in legumes and grains; oxalic acid is present in rhubarb and spinach, among other foods.

To quickly review, the major minerals are found in larger quantities in the body, whereas the trace minerals occur in smaller amounts. Minerals are inorganic elements that retain their chemical identities; they usually receive special handling and regulation in the body; and they may bind with other substances, thus limiting their absorption.

While all the major minerals help to maintain the body's fluid balance described earlier, sodium, chloride, and potassium are most noted for that role. For this reason, these three minerals are discussed first here. Later sections describe the minerals most noted for their roles in bone growth and maintenance—calcium, phosphorus, and magnesium.

Sodium

People have held salt (sodium chloride) in high regard throughout recorded history. We say "you are the salt of the earth" to someone we admire and "you are not worth your salt" to someone we consider worthless. Even the word *salary* comes from the Latin word for salt.

Sodium Roles in the Body   Sodium is the principal cation of the extracellular fluid and the primary regulator of its volume. Sodium also helps maintain acid-base balance and is essential to nerve transmission and muscle contraction.* Table 12–3 summarizes information about sodium.

Foods usually provide more sodium than the body needs. The intestinal tract absorbs sodium readily, and it travels freely in the blood, but the kidneys filter all the sodium out of the blood; then, with great precision, they return to the bloodstream the exact amount the body needs. Normally, the amount excreted is approximately equal to the amount ingested on a given day. When blood sodium rises, as when a person eats salted foods, thirst signals the person to drink until the appropriate sodium-to-water ratio is restored. Then the kidneys secrete the extra water and the extra sodium together.

Sodium Recommendations   Diets rarely lack sodium. For this reason, no RDA is set; instead, the Committee on Dietary Allowances estimated the *minimum* sodium requirement for adults to be 500 milligrams (0.5 grams). Similarly, Canada has not established an RNI for sodium, but has estimated the minimum requirement for adults to be 115 milligrams. Such differences between countries' recommendations are not unusual and typically reflect differences in judgment more than differences in research data. The minimum average requirement for adults without active sweating has been estimated to be 115 milligrams, but the

Reminder: *Bioavailability* refers to the rate and extent to which a nutrient is absorbed. Some nutrients are not readily released from foods during digestion or are not efficiently absorbed, which reduces their bioavailability.

binders: chemical compounds occurring in foods that can combine with nutrients (especially minerals) to form complexes the body cannot absorb. Examples of such binders include phytic (FIGHT-ic) acid and oxalic (ox-AL-ic) acid.

sodium: the principal cation in the extracellular fluids of the body, critical to the maintenance of fluid balance, nerve transmissions, and muscle contractions.

---

*One of the ways the kidneys regulate acid-base balance is by excreting hydrogen ions in exchange for sodium ions.

Table 12–3

Sodium—A Summary

Adult Estimated Minimum Requirement	Chief Functions in the Body	Deficiency Symptoms	Toxicity Symptoms	Significant Sources
500 mg/day	An electrolyte that maintains normal fluid and electrolyte balance; assists in nerve impulse transmission and muscle contraction	Muscle cramps, mental apathy, loss of appetite	Edema, acute hypertension	Table salt, soy sauce; moderate amounts in meats, milks, breads, and vegetables; large amounts in processed foods

Salt (sodium chloride) is about 40% sodium.
1 g salt contributes 400 mg sodium.
5 g salt = 1 tsp.
1 tsp salt contributes 2000 mg sodium.

U.S. Committee on Dietary Allowances set its recommendation slightly higher to accommodate a wide variety of physical activities and climates.

The *Diet and Health* recommendations, which emphasize moderation, not adequacy, advise limiting daily *salt* intake to less than 6 grams (the equivalent of 2.4 grams or 2400 milligrams *sodium*). Similarly, the American Heart Association recommends limiting sodium intake to 3 grams daily; people with mild-to-moderate hypertension may benefit from restriction to 2 grams of sodium daily.[3]

HEALTHY PEOPLE 2000: Decrease salt and sodium intake so at least 65% of home meal preparers prepare foods without adding salt, at least 80% of people avoid using salt at the table, and at least 40% of adults regularly purchase foods modified or lower in sodium.

Sodium and Hypertension   For years, a high *sodium* intake was considered *the* primary factor responsible for high blood pressure. Then research pointed to *salt* (sodium chloride) as the dietary culprit. Salt has a greater effect on blood pressure than either sodium or chloride alone or in combination with other ions.[4]

Some individuals are genetically sensitive and experience high blood pressure from excesses in salt intake. People with chronic renal disease, those who have one or two parents with hypertension, blacks, and people over 50 years of age are most likely to be salt sensitive.* Salt avoidance promises to help prevent hypertension in salt-sensitive individuals, but for the majority of people with hypertension, salt restriction does not lower blood pressure. The most effective dietary treatment for hypertension is weight loss.

Sodium Intakes   Cultures vary in their use of salt. The most recent food intake survey in the United States estimates that men consume an average of 3300 milligrams of sodium (equivalent to 8 grams of salt) a day, which is slightly more than the American Heart Association recommends.[5] Asian people, whose staple sauces and flavorings are based on soy sauce and monosodium glutamate (MSG), consume the equivalent of about 30 to 40 grams of salt per day. The

---

*Salt-sensitive individuals have elevated concentrations of renin in their blood, compared with others.

prevalence of high blood pressure in China, Japan, and Korea is equal to or greater than that in the United States.[6]

Sodium in Foods   In general, processed foods have the most sodium, while unprocessed foods such as fresh fruits and vegetables have the least. In fact, as much as 75 percent of the sodium in people's diets comes from salt added to foods by manufacturers; about 15 percent comes from salt added during cooking and at the table; and only 10 percent comes from the natural salt in foods.[7]

Because processed foods may contain sodium without chloride, as in additives such as sodium bicarbonate or sodium saccharin, they do not always taste salty. Most people are surprised to learn that 1 ounce of cornflakes (a 1¼-cup serving) contains more sodium than 1 ounce of salted peanuts—and that ½ cup of instant chocolate pudding contains still more. (A reason the peanuts taste saltier is that the salt is all on the surface, where the tongue's sensors immediately pick it up.)

Figure 12–6 shows that processed foods contain not only more sodium but also less potassium than their less-processed counterparts. Low potassium may be as significant as excess sodium when it comes to blood pressure regulation, so these foods have two strikes against them. The accompanying box offers strategies for

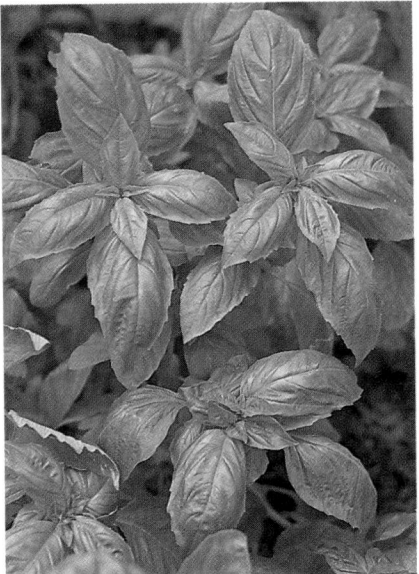

Fresh herbs add flavor to a recipe without adding salt.

How to Cut Salt Intake

Most people eat more salt and sodium than they need, and some people can lower their blood pressure by avoiding highly salted foods and removing the saltshaker from the table. Foods eaten without salt may seem less tasty at first, but with repetition, people can learn to enjoy the natural flavors of many unsalted foods. Strategies to cut salt intake include:

- Cook with only small amounts of added salt.
- Prepare foods with sodium-free spices such as basil, bay leaves, curry, garlic, ginger, lemon, mint, oregano, pepper, rosemary, and thyme.
- Add little or no salt at the table.
- Read labels with an eye open for salt. (See Table 2–8 on p. 60 for terms used to describe the sodium contents of foods on labels.)
- Eat high-salt foods in moderation and use low-salt or salt-free products regularly.

Use these foods sparingly:

- Foods prepared in brine, such as pickles, olives, and sauerkraut.
- Salty or smoked meats, such as bologna, corned or chipped beef, frankfurters, ham, lunch meats, salt pork, sausage, and smoked tongue.
- Salty or smoked fish, such as anchovies, caviar, salted and dried cod, herring, sardines, and smoked salmon.
- Snack items such as potato chips, pretzels, salted popcorn, salted nuts, and crackers.
- Bouillon cubes; seasoned salts; soy, Worcestershire, and barbeque sauces.
- Cheeses, especially processed types.
- Canned and instant soups.
- Prepared horseradish, catsup, and mustard.

cutting sodium/salt intake. Chapter 28 reviews the research on sodium, potassium, and hypertension in relation to heart disease.

Sodium Deficiency   Overly strict use of low-sodium diets in the treatment of hypertension, kidney disease, or heart disease can deplete the body of needed

Figure 12–6

What Processing Does to the Sodium and Potassium Contents of Foods

People who eat foods high in salt often happen to be eating fewer potassium-containing foods at the same time. Note how the *same* food loses potassium and gains sodium as it goes through processing, so that its potassium-to-sodium ratio falls dramatically. Limiting sodium intake may help in two ways, then—by lowering blood pressure in salt-sensitive individuals and by indirectly raising potassium intakes in all individuals.

Note how potassium is lost and sodium is gained as foods become more processed.

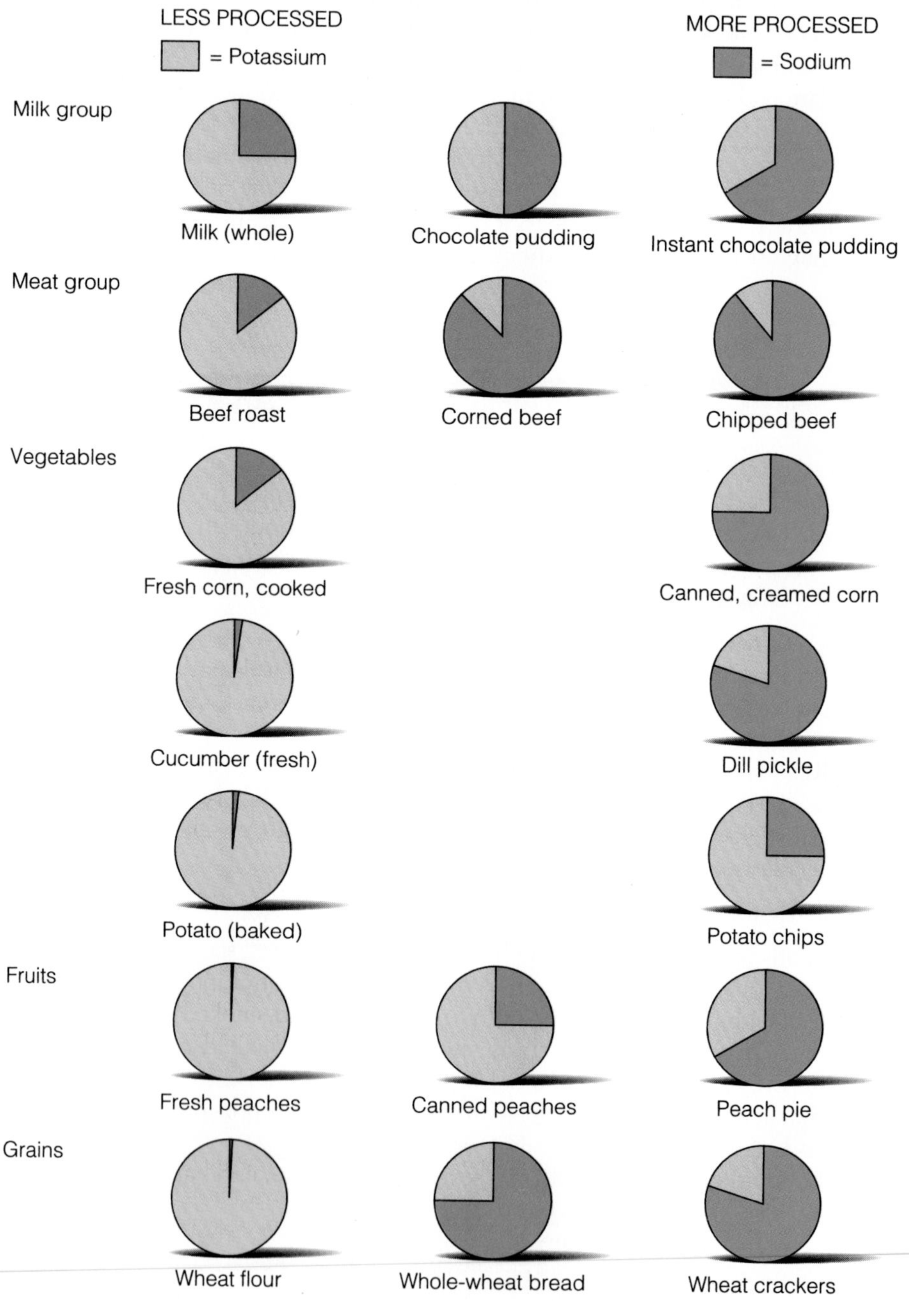

LESS PROCESSED   MORE PROCESSED

☐ = Potassium   ☐ = Sodium

Milk group — Milk (whole) — Chocolate pudding — Instant chocolate pudding

Meat group — Beef roast — Corned beef — Chipped beef

Vegetables — Fresh corn, cooked — Canned, creamed corn

Cucumber (fresh) — Dill pickle

Potato (baked) — Potato chips

Fruits — Fresh peaches — Canned peaches — Peach pie

Grains — Wheat flour — Whole-wheat bread — Wheat crackers

sodium. Vomiting, diarrhea, or heavy sweating can, too. If blood sodium drops, both sodium and water must be replenished. Under normal conditions of sweating due to exercise, salt losses can easily be replaced later in the day with ordinary foods. Salt tablets are not recommended because too much salt, especially if taken with too little water, can induce dehydration.

Sodium Toxicity   The immediate symptoms of acute sodium toxicity are edema and hypertension, but such toxicity is not a problem as long as water needs are met. Prolonged excessive sodium intake, especially when the sodium is derived from salt, may be related to the development of hypertension in sensitive people, as explained earlier.

Chloride

The element *chlorine* (Cl_2), is a poisonous gas. When chlorine reacts with sodium or hydrogen, however, it forms the negative chloride ion (Cl^-). *Chloride* is required in the diet.

Chloride Roles in the Body   Chloride is the major anion of the extracellular fluids, where it occurs mostly in association with sodium (Table 12–4 summarizes information on chloride). Chloride can move freely across membranes and so also associates with potassium inside cells. Like sodium, chloride is critical to maintaining fluid and electrolyte balance.

In the stomach, the chloride ion is part of hydrochloric acid, which maintains the strong acidity of the gastric juice. One of the most serious consequences of vomiting is the loss of this acid from the stomach, which upsets the acid-base balance.*

Chloride Recommendations and Intakes   Chloride is abundant in foods (especially processed foods) as part of sodium chloride and other salts. The Committee on Dietary Allowances has not set an RDA for chloride, but has estimated a minimum requirement for adults.

Chloride Deficiency and Toxicity   Diets rarely lack chloride. A case is on record in which chloride was omitted from an infant formula and the deficiency caused illness and death before it was discovered. Chloride losses may occur in sodium-depleting conditions such as heavy sweating or chronic diarrhea and vomiting. The only known cause of high blood chloride concentrations is dehydration due to water deficiency.[8] In both cases, consuming ordinary foods and beverages can restore chloride balance.

chloride: the major anion in the extracellular fluids of the body. Chloride is the ionic form of chlorine, Cl^-; see Appendix B for a description of the chlorine-to-chloride conversion.

Reminder: The loss of acid can lead to *alkalosis*, an above-normal alkalinity in the blood and body fluids.

---

*Hydrochloric acid secretion into the stomach involves the addition of bicarbonate ions to the plasma. These bicarbonate ions are neutralized by hydrogen ions from the gastric secretions that are reabsorbed into the plasma. When hydrochloric acid is lost during vomiting, these hydrogen ions are no longer available for reabsorption, which in effect increases the concentration of bicarbonate ions in the plasma. In this way, excessive vomiting of acidic gastric juices leads to *metabolic alkalosis*.

Table 12–4

Chloride—A Summary

Adult Estimated Minimum Requirement	Chief Functions in the Body	Deficiency Symptoms	Toxicity Symptoms	Significant Sources
750 mg/day	An electrolyte that maintains normal fluid and electrolyte balance; part of hydrochloric acid found in the stomach, necessary for proper digestion	Do not occur under normal circumstances	Vomiting	Table salt, soy sauce; moderate amounts in meats, milks, eggs; large amounts in processed foods

Potassium

potassium: the principal cation within the body's cells, critical to the maintenance of fluid balance, nerve transmissions, and muscle contractions.

Like sodium, potassium is a positively charged ion. In contrast to sodium, potassium is the body's principal cation *inside* the body cells.

Potassium Roles in the Body Potassium plays a major role in maintaining fluid and electrolyte balance and cell integrity. During nerve transmission and muscle contraction, potassium and sodium briefly trade places across the cell membrane. The cell then quickly pumps them back into place. The control of potassium distribution is a high priority for the body because it affects many aspects of homeostasis, including a steady heartbeat.

Potassium Recommendations and Intakes As for sodium and chloride, the Committee on Dietary Allowances has estimated a minimum potassium requirement for adults. Potassium is abundant inside all living cells, both plant and animal. Because cells remain intact unless foods are processed, the richest sources of potassium are *fresh* foods of all kinds, as Figure 12–7 shows. People who emphasize fresh fruits and vegetables in their diets have intakes as high as 11 grams per day, but toxicity is normally not a concern when the source is foods.[9]

Fresh foods, especially fruits, contain much more potassium than sodium. In contrast, most processed foods such as canned vegetables, ready-to-eat cereals, and luncheon meats contain more sodium and less potassium (recall Figure 12–6).

Potassium and Hypertension Some authorities believe that potassium might both prevent and help to correct hypertension. Low-potassium diets raise blood pressure in men with normal blood pressure and in those who are hypertensive, whereas a high potassium intake seems to protect against stroke.

Potassium Deficiency A dietary deficiency of potassium is unlikely, but with a regular diet low in fresh fruits and vegetables, it is possible. Potassium deficiency occurs more often due to excessive losses than to deficient intakes. Conditions such as diabetic acidosis, dehydration, or prolonged vomiting or diarrhea can create a potassium deficiency, as can the regular use of certain drugs, includ-

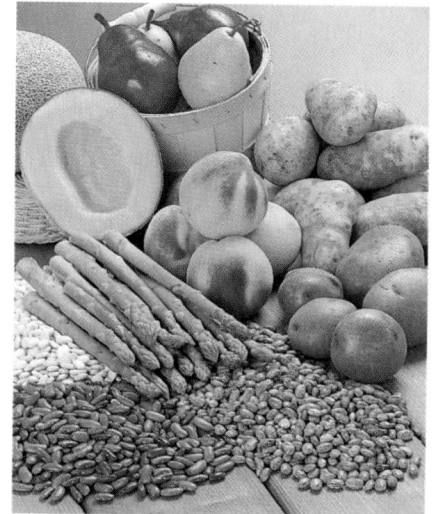

Fresh fruits and vegetables provide potassium in abundance.

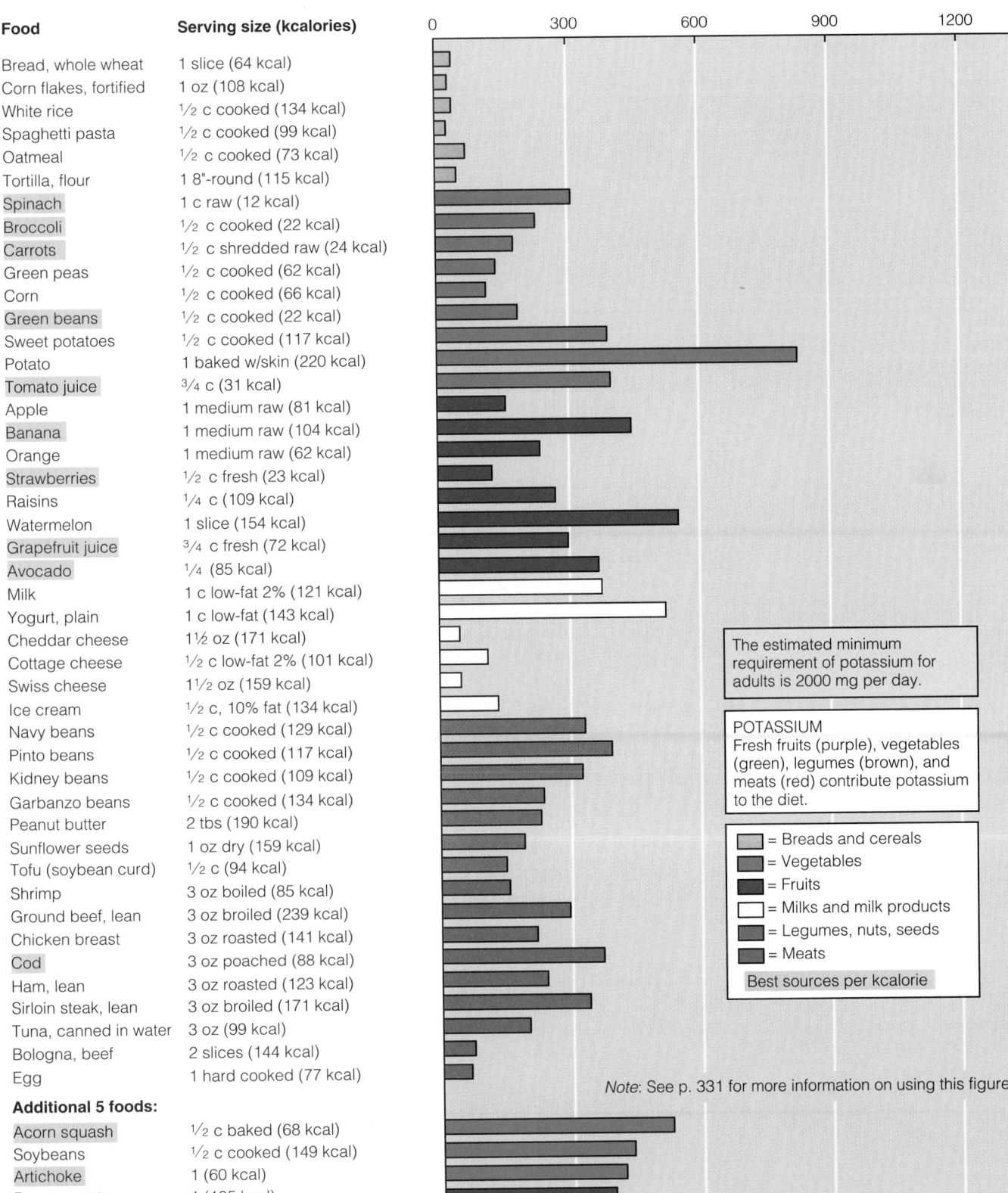

Milligrams

Food	Serving size (kcalories)
Bread, whole wheat	1 slice (64 kcal)
Corn flakes, fortified	1 oz (108 kcal)
White rice	½ c cooked (134 kcal)
Spaghetti pasta	½ c cooked (99 kcal)
Oatmeal	½ c cooked (73 kcal)
Tortilla, flour	1 8"-round (115 kcal)
Spinach	1 c raw (12 kcal)
Broccoli	½ c cooked (22 kcal)
Carrots	½ c shredded raw (24 kcal)
Green peas	½ c cooked (62 kcal)
Corn	½ c cooked (66 kcal)
Green beans	½ c cooked (22 kcal)
Sweet potatoes	½ c cooked (117 kcal)
Potato	1 baked w/skin (220 kcal)
Tomato juice	¾ c (31 kcal)
Apple	1 medium raw (81 kcal)
Banana	1 medium raw (104 kcal)
Orange	1 medium raw (62 kcal)
Strawberries	½ c fresh (23 kcal)
Raisins	¼ c (109 kcal)
Watermelon	1 slice (154 kcal)
Grapefruit juice	¾ c fresh (72 kcal)
Avocado	¼ (85 kcal)
Milk	1 c low-fat 2% (121 kcal)
Yogurt, plain	1 c low-fat (143 kcal)
Cheddar cheese	1½ oz (171 kcal)
Cottage cheese	½ c low-fat 2% (101 kcal)
Swiss cheese	1½ oz (159 kcal)
Ice cream	½ c, 10% fat (134 kcal)
Navy beans	½ c cooked (129 kcal)
Pinto beans	½ c cooked (117 kcal)
Kidney beans	½ c cooked (109 kcal)
Garbanzo beans	½ c cooked (134 kcal)
Peanut butter	2 tbs (190 kcal)
Sunflower seeds	1 oz dry (159 kcal)
Tofu (soybean curd)	½ c (94 kcal)
Shrimp	3 oz boiled (85 kcal)
Ground beef, lean	3 oz broiled (239 kcal)
Chicken breast	3 oz roasted (141 kcal)
Cod	3 oz poached (88 kcal)
Ham, lean	3 oz roasted (123 kcal)
Sirloin steak, lean	3 oz broiled (171 kcal)
Tuna, canned in water	3 oz (99 kcal)
Bologna, beef	2 slices (144 kcal)
Egg	1 hard cooked (77 kcal)
Additional 5 foods:	
Acorn squash	½ c baked (68 kcal)
Soybeans	½ c cooked (149 kcal)
Artichoke	1 (60 kcal)
Pomegranate	1 (105 kcal)
Buttermilk, nonfat	1 c (99 kcal)

The estimated minimum requirement of potassium for adults is 2000 mg per day.

POTASSIUM
Fresh fruits (purple), vegetables (green), legumes (brown), and meats (red) contribute potassium to the diet.

☐ = Breads and cereals
☐ = Vegetables
☐ = Fruits
☐ = Milks and milk products
☐ = Legumes, nuts, seeds
☐ = Meats
Best sources per kcalorie

Note: See p. 331 for more information on using this figure.

Table 12–5

Potassium—A Summary

Adult Estimated Minimum Requirement	Chief Functions in the Body	Deficiency Symptoms[a]	Toxicity Symptoms	Significant Sources
2000 mg/day	An electrolyte that maintains normal fluid and electrolyte balance; facilitates many reactions; supports cell integrity; assists in nerve impulse transmission and muscle contractions	Muscular weakness, paralysis, confusion	Muscular weakness; vomiting; if given into a vein, can stop the heart	All whole foods: meats, milks, fruits, vegetables, grains, legumes

[a]Deficiency accompanies dehydration.

ing diuretics, steroids, and strong laxatives.* For this reason, many physicians prescribe potassium supplements along with drugs. One of the earliest symptoms of deficiency is muscle weakness. Table 12–5 summarizes facts about potassium.

Potassium Toxicity   Potassium toxicity can result from the overuse of potassium salt, especially in an infant or a person with heart disease; it does not result from overeating foods high in potassium. Given more potassium than the body needs, the kidneys accelerate excretion. If the GI tract is bypassed, however, and potassium is injected rapidly into a vein, it can stop the heart.

To summarize, the electrolytes primarily responsible for maintaining fluid balance are sodium, chloride, and potassium. Sodium is the main cation outside cells; dietary deficiency is rare, and excesses may aggravate hypertension in some people. The kidneys regulate blood sodium in response to hormonal signals from ADH and aldosterone. Chloride is the major anion outside cells, and it associates closely with sodium. In addition to its role in fluid balance, chloride is part of the stomach's hydrochloric acid, which facilitates protein digestion and iron absorption. Potassium is the primary cation inside cells; fresh fruits and vegetables are its best sources.

Calcium

calcium: the most abundant mineral in the body, found primarily in the body's bones and teeth.

Calcium is the most abundant mineral in the body. It receives much emphasis in this chapter and in the highlight that follows because an adequate intake early in life helps grow a healthy skeleton and minimize bone loss in later life. Calcium's roles, deficiency symptoms, and food sources appear in Table 12–6.

*People using diuretics to control hypertension should know that some cause potassium excretion and can induce a deficiency. Those using these drugs must be particularly careful to include rich sources of potassium in their daily diets. (Some diuretics are designed to spare potassium.)

Table 12–6

Calcium—A Summary

Adult DRI[a]	Chief Functions in the Body	Deficiency Symptoms	Toxicity Symptoms	Significant Sources
1000 mg/day (19–50 yr) 1200 mg/day (51 and older)	The principal mineral of bones and teeth; also involved in muscle contraction and relaxation, nerve functioning, blood clotting, blood pressure, and immune defenses	Stunted growth in children; bone loss (osteoporosis) in adults	Constipation; increased risk of urinary stone formation and kidney dysfunction; interference with absorption of other minerals	Milk and milk products, small fish (with bones), tofu (bean curd), greens (broccoli, chard), legumes

[a]1997 recommendations for calcium are called Dietary Reference Intakes (DRI).

CALCIUM ROLES IN THE BODY

Ninety-nine percent of the body's calcium is in the bones, where it plays two roles. First, it is an integral part of bone structure, providing a rigid frame that holds the body upright and serves as attachment points for muscles, making motion possible. Second, it serves as a calcium bank, offering a readily available source of the mineral to the body fluids should a drop in blood calcium occur.

Calcium in Bones   Many people have the idea that once a bone is built, it is inert like a rock. Actually, the bones are in a state of constant flux, with formation and dissolution simultaneously taking place. As bones begin to form, calcium salts form crystals on a matrix of the protein collagen. These crystals, called hydroxyapatite, invade the collagen and gradually lend more and more strength and rigidity to the maturing bones until they are able to support the weight they will have to carry. Thus the long leg bones of children can support their weight by the time they have learned to walk.

The formation of teeth follows a pattern similar to that of bones. Hydroxyapatite crystals form on a collagen matrix to create the dentin that gives strength to the teeth (see Figure 12–8). The turnover of minerals in teeth is not as rapid as in bone, but some withdrawal and redepositing do take place throughout life. Fluoride hardens and stabilizes the crystals of teeth, opposing the withdrawal of minerals from them.

Calcium in Body Fluids   The 1 percent of the body's calcium that circulates in the fluids as ionized calcium is vital to life. The calcium ion participates in the regulation of muscle contraction, the clotting of blood, the transmission of nerve impulses, the secretion of hormones, and the activation of some enzyme reactions.

Calcium also serves as a cofactor in a protein that helps convey signals, received at the cell surface, to the inside of the cell. The protein that relays these messages is calmodulin. Several of the messages it delivers help to maintain normal blood pressure.

Calcium and Disease Prevention   Calcium may be useful in both preventing and treating hypertension. Epidemiological studies show that low dietary calcium correlates with a high prevalence of hypertension.[10] Reports that an

Figure 12–8

A Tooth

The inner layer of dentin is a bonelike material that forms on a protein (collagen) matrix, which requires a variety of substances, including vitamin C, for proper formation. The outer layer of enamel is harder than bone and forms on a protein (keratin) matrix, which depends in part on vitamin A for its synthesis. Both dentin and enamel contain hydroxyapatite (highdrox-ee-APP-ah-tite), crystals made of calcium and phosphorus. The crystals of enamel may become even harder when exposed to the trace mineral fluoride.

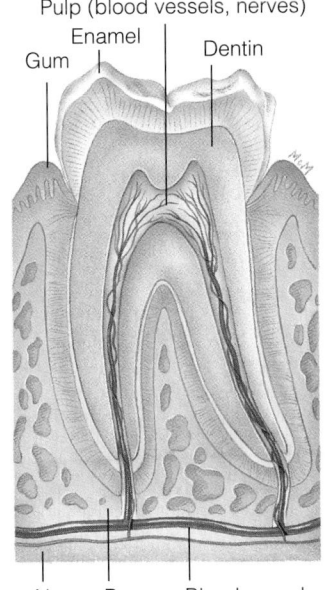

Pulp (blood vessels, nerves)
Enamel
Gum   Dentin
Nerve Bone   Blood vessel

calmodulin (cal-MOD-you-lin): an inactive protein that becomes active when bound to calcium; then it becomes a messenger that tells other proteins what to do. The system serves as interpreter for hormone- and nerve-mediated messages arriving at cells.

The hormones parathormone (PAIR-ah-THOR-moan) from the parathyroid and calcitonin (KAL-see-TOE-nin) from the thyroid glands, as well as vitamin D, regulate calcium balance. Parathormone raises blood calcium, while calcitonin lowers it by inhibiting release of calcium from bone. Vitamin D raises blood calcium by acting at the three sites listed.

increase in calcium intake can lower blood pressure in people with and without hypertension further support this hypothesis. Some evidence also suggests relationships between dietary calcium and blood cholesterol, diabetes, and cancer.[11]

Calcium Balance   Calcium homeostasis is one of the body's highest priorities and involves a system of hormones and vitamin D that promotes calcium deposits into bone whenever blood calcium rises too high. Whenever blood calcium falls too low, three organ systems may raise it:

- Intestines: absorb more calcium.
- Bones: release more calcium.
- Kidneys: excrete less calcium.

Thus blood calcium can return to normal. Figure 12–9 illustrates how hormones regulate blood calcium.

The calcium in bone provides a nearly inexhaustible bank of calcium for the blood. The blood borrows and returns calcium as needed, so that even with a dietary deficiency, blood calcium remains normal—even as bone calcium diminishes. Blood calcium changes only in response to abnormal regulatory control, not to diet. This makes a developing calcium deficiency completely silent. A per-

Figure 12–9

Calcium Balance in Bone

Blood calcium is regulated in part by vitamin D and two hormones—calcitonin and parathormone. Bone serves as a source of calcium when blood calcium is low and as a reservoir when blood calcium is high. Osteoclasts break down bone and release calcium into the blood; osteoblasts build new bone using calcium from the blood.

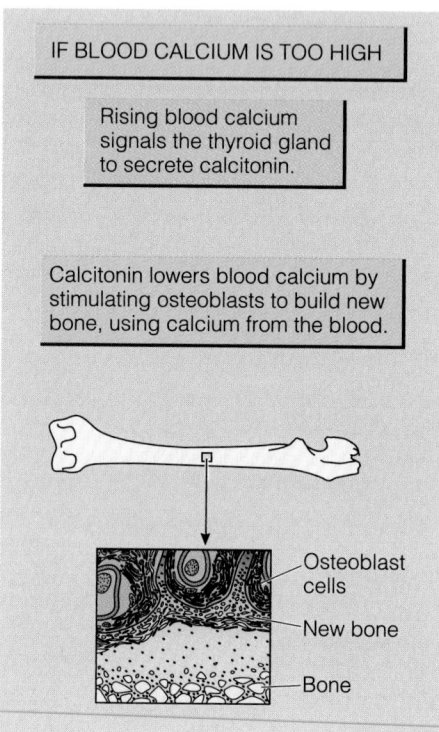

IF BLOOD CALCIUM IS TOO HIGH

Rising blood calcium signals the thyroid gland to secrete calcitonin.

Calcitonin lowers blood calcium by stimulating osteoblasts to build new bone, using calcium from the blood.

Osteoblast cells
New bone
Bone

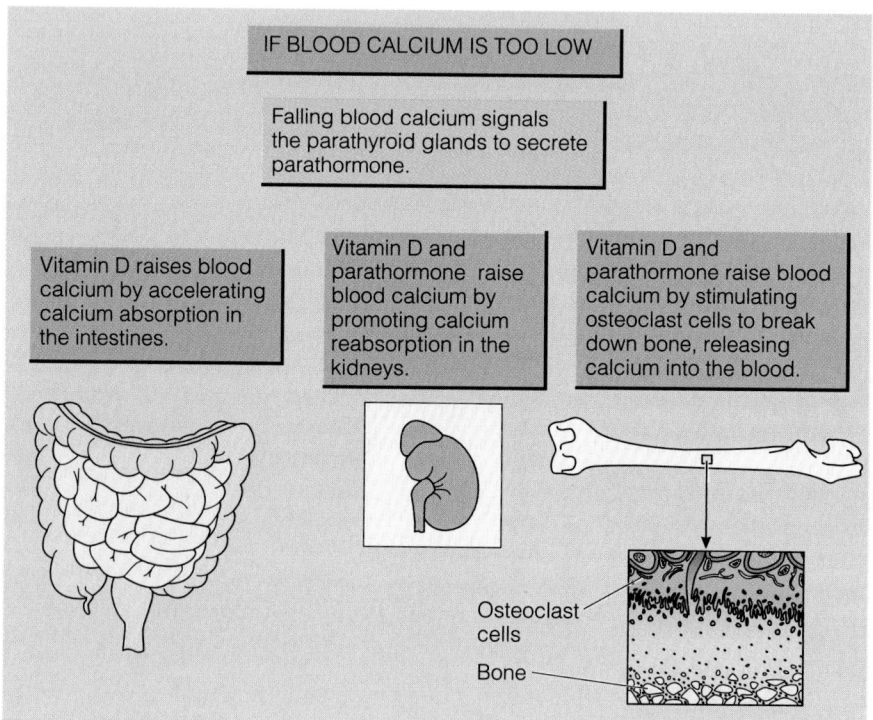

IF BLOOD CALCIUM IS TOO LOW

Falling blood calcium signals the parathyroid glands to secrete parathormone.

Vitamin D raises blood calcium by accelerating calcium absorption in the intestines.

Vitamin D and parathormone raise blood calcium by promoting calcium reabsorption in the kidneys.

Vitamin D and parathormone raise blood calcium by stimulating osteoclast cells to break down bone, releasing calcium into the blood.

Osteoclast cells
Bone

son can have an inadequate calcium intake for years and suffer no noticeable symptoms. Only late in life does it become apparent that the integrity of the bones has been compromised.

Blood calcium above normal results in calcium rigor; the muscles contract and cannot relax. Similarly, blood calcium below normal causes calcium tetany—also characterized by uncontrolled muscle contraction. These conditions do *not* reflect a *dietary* excess or lack of calcium; they are caused by a lack of vitamin D or by abnormal secretion of the regulatory hormones. A chronic *dietary* deficiency of calcium, or a chronic deficiency due to poor absorption over the years, depletes the savings account in the bones. Again: it is the *bones*, not the blood, that are robbed by calcium deficiency.

Calcium Absorption Many factors affect calcium absorption, but on the average, adults absorb about 30 percent of the calcium they ingest. The stomach's acidity helps to keep calcium soluble, and absorption is enhanced when calcium is consumed with a meal. Vitamin D helps the absorptive cells of the GI tract to make the necessary calcium-binding protein. It is no accident that calcium-rich milk is the chosen vehicle for fortification with vitamin D. The lactose in milk also enhances calcium absorption. Also, calcium seems to be better absorbed if accompanied by an approximately equal amount of phosphorus.

The body regulates calcium absorption by altering its production of the calcium-binding protein, making more if more calcium is needed. The result is obvious in the case of a pregnant woman, who absorbs 50 percent of the calcium from the milk she drinks. Similarly, growing children absorb 50 to 60 percent of ingested calcium. Then, when their bones' growth slows or stops, their absorption falls to the adult level of about 30 percent. In addition, calcium absorption is more efficient at low intakes than at high intakes.

Many of the conditions that enhance calcium absorption hinder its absorption when they are absent. For example, sufficient vitamin D supports absorption, while a deficiency impairs it. In addition, fiber, in general, and phytate and oxalate, in particular, interfere with calcium absorption, but their effects are relatively minor at intakes typical of U.S. diets. Vegetables with oxalates and whole grains with phytates are nutritious foods, of course, but they are not useful calcium sources. Table 12–7 summarizes the factors influencing calcium absorption.

calcium rigor: hardness or stiffness of the muscles caused by high blood calcium concentrations.

calcium tetany (TET-ah-nee): intermittent spasm of the extremities due to nervous and muscular excitability caused by low blood calcium concentrations.

calcium-binding protein: a protein in the intestinal cells, made with the help of vitamin D, that facilitates calcium absorption.

Reminder: Phytate and oxalate are *binders* that combine with minerals to form complexes that the body cannot absorb. Phytates are common in cereal grain husks; oxalates occur in beets, rhubarb, spinach, and peanuts.

CALCIUM RECOMMENDATIONS AND INTAKES

The ideal calcium intake for people is difficult to determine. Calcium is unlike most other nutrients, in that its blood concentration does not reflect the body's calcium status. Calcium recommendations are therefore arrived at by way of balance studies. These studies, which measure daily absorption and excretion, determine how much calcium must be ingested daily to maintain calcium balance.

Calcium Recommendations Because obtaining enough calcium during early life helps to ensure that the skeleton will be strong and dense, recommendations have been set high at 1300 milligrams daily for adolescents up to the age of 18 years. Such an intake can be difficult to achieve, since the best source, milk, has only 300 milligrams per cup. Between the ages of 19 and 50, recommendations are lowered to 1000 milligrams a day: for later life, recommendations are raised again to 1200 milligrams a day to minimize the bone loss that tends to

Table 12–7

Factors Influencing Calcium Absorption

Calcium absorption is a complex process that is influenced to various degrees by several dietary and physiological factors.

Factors That Promote Calcium Absorption	Factors That Interfere with Calcium Absorption
• Hormones that promote growth.	• Diminished absorption with aging.
• Ingestion with a meal; stomach acid.	• Lack of stomach acid.
• Vitamin D.	• Vitamin D deficiency.
• Lactose.	• High phosphorus intake.
• Phosphorus in an optimal ratio.	• High-fiber diet.
	• Phytates and oxalates.
	• High protein intake.

occur late in life. Some authorities advocate as much as 1500 milligrams a day for women over 50. Many people in the United States and Canada, particularly women, have calcium intakes below current recommendations.

Unfortunately, many people perceive milk as fattening and omit it from their diets in their attempts to lose weight. Whole milk and many cheeses are high in fat, but low-fat options are available and many people have switched from whole milk to nonfat or low-fat milk and milk products.[12] Such choices help a person both meet calcium needs and stay within a reasonable energy and fat allowance.

Internationally, calcium recommendations vary widely. Calcium intakes are low in most of the world, but given long times to adjust, adults can adapt to very low intakes. The World Health Organization recommends only 400 to 500 milligrams per day for adults. Protein intakes are also low in most of the world. As Chapter 6 mentioned, high protein intakes seem to accelerate calcium excretion, and so perhaps the higher intakes of protein by North Americans warrant the setting of higher calcium allowances.

Recommended daily milk servings:
- Children: 2 c
- Teenagers: 3 c
- Adults: 2 c
- Pregnant or lactating women: 3 c
- Pregnant or lactating teens: 4 c

 HEALTHY PEOPLE 2000: Increase calcium intake so that at least 50% of people aged 25 years and older consume two or more servings of calcium-rich foods daily.

Calcium Sources Figure 12–10 shows that calcium is found most abundantly in a single class of foods—milk and milk products. For this reason, dietary recommendations advise daily consumption of low- or nonfat milk products. Milk offers about 300 milligrams of calcium per cup, so an adult who drinks 2 to 3 cups of milk a day should have no problem meeting calcium needs, given the additional contributions from other foods; teenagers and young adults need 3 to 4 cups of milk daily. The word *daily* should be stressed because the body has a limited ability to absorb calcium, and so needs frequent opportunities to take in small amounts. The consumption of *milk* products, not just *dairy* products, should also be stressed. Dairy products such as butter and cream are milk fats that contain negligible calcium because calcium is not soluble in fat.

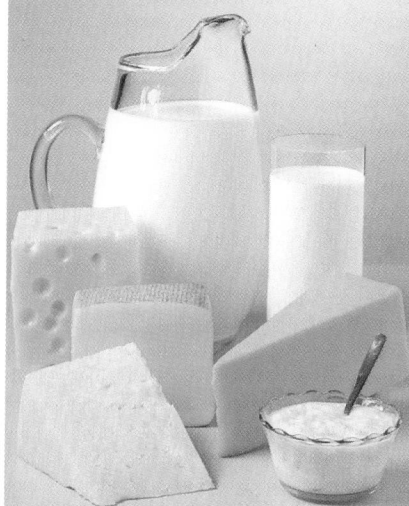

Milk and milk products are rightly famous for their calcium contents.

Figure 12–10 Calcium in Selected Foods

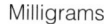

Food	Serving size (kcalories)
Bread, whole wheat	1 slice (64 kcal)
Corn flakes, fortified	1 oz (108 kcal)
White rice	1/2 c cooked (134 kcal)
Spaghetti pasta	1/2 c cooked (99 kcal)
Oatmeal	1/2 c cooked (73 kcal)
Tortilla, flour	1 8"-round (115 kcal)
Spinach[a]	1 c raw (12 kcal)
Broccoli	1/2 c cooked (22 kcal)
Carrots	1/2 c shredded raw (24 kcal)
Green peas	1/2 c cooked (62 kcal)
Corn	1/2 c cooked (66 kcal)
Green beans	1/2 c cooked (22 kcal)
Sweet potatoes	1/2 c cooked (117 kcal)
Potato	1 baked w/skin (220 kcal)
Tomato juice	3/4 c (31 kcal)
Apple	1 medium raw (81 kcal)
Banana	1 medium raw (104 kcal)
Orange	1 medium raw (62 kcal)
Strawberries	1/2 c fresh (23 kcal)
Raisins	1/4 c (109 kcal)
Watermelon	1 slice (154 kcal)
Grapefruit juice	3/4 c fresh (72 kcal)
Avocado	1/4 (85 kcal)
Milk	1 c low-fat 2% (121 kcal)
Yogurt, plain	1 c low-fat (143 kcal)
Cheddar cheese	1 1/2 oz (171 kcal)
Cottage cheese	1/2 c low-fat 2% (101 kcal)
Swiss cheese	1 1/2 oz (159 kcal)
Ice cream	1/2 c, 10% fat (134 kcal)
Navy beans	1/2 c cooked (129 kcal)
Pinto beans	1/2 c cooked (117 kcal)
Kidney beans	1/2 c cooked (109 kcal)
Garbanzo beans	1/2 c cooked (134 kcal)
Peanut butter	2 tbs (190 kcal)
Sunflower seeds	1 oz dry (159 kcal)
Tofu (soybean curd)[b]	1/2 c (94 kcal)
Shrimp	3 oz boiled (85 kcal)
Ground beef, lean	3 oz broiled (239 kcal)
Chicken breast	3 oz roasted (141 kcal)
Cod	3 oz poached (88 kcal)
Ham, lean	3 oz roasted (123 kcal)
Sirloin steak, lean	3 oz broiled (171 kcal)
Tuna, canned in water	3 oz (99 kcal)
Bologna, beef	2 slices (144 kcal)
Egg	1 hard cooked (77 kcal)

Additional 5 foods:

Sardines, with bones[c]	3 oz canned (117 kcal)
Molasses, blackstrap[d]	1 tbs (47 kcal)
Pudding	1/2 c (148 kcal)
Bok choy (Chinese cabbage)	1/2 c cooked (10 kcal)
Almonds	1 oz (167 kcal)

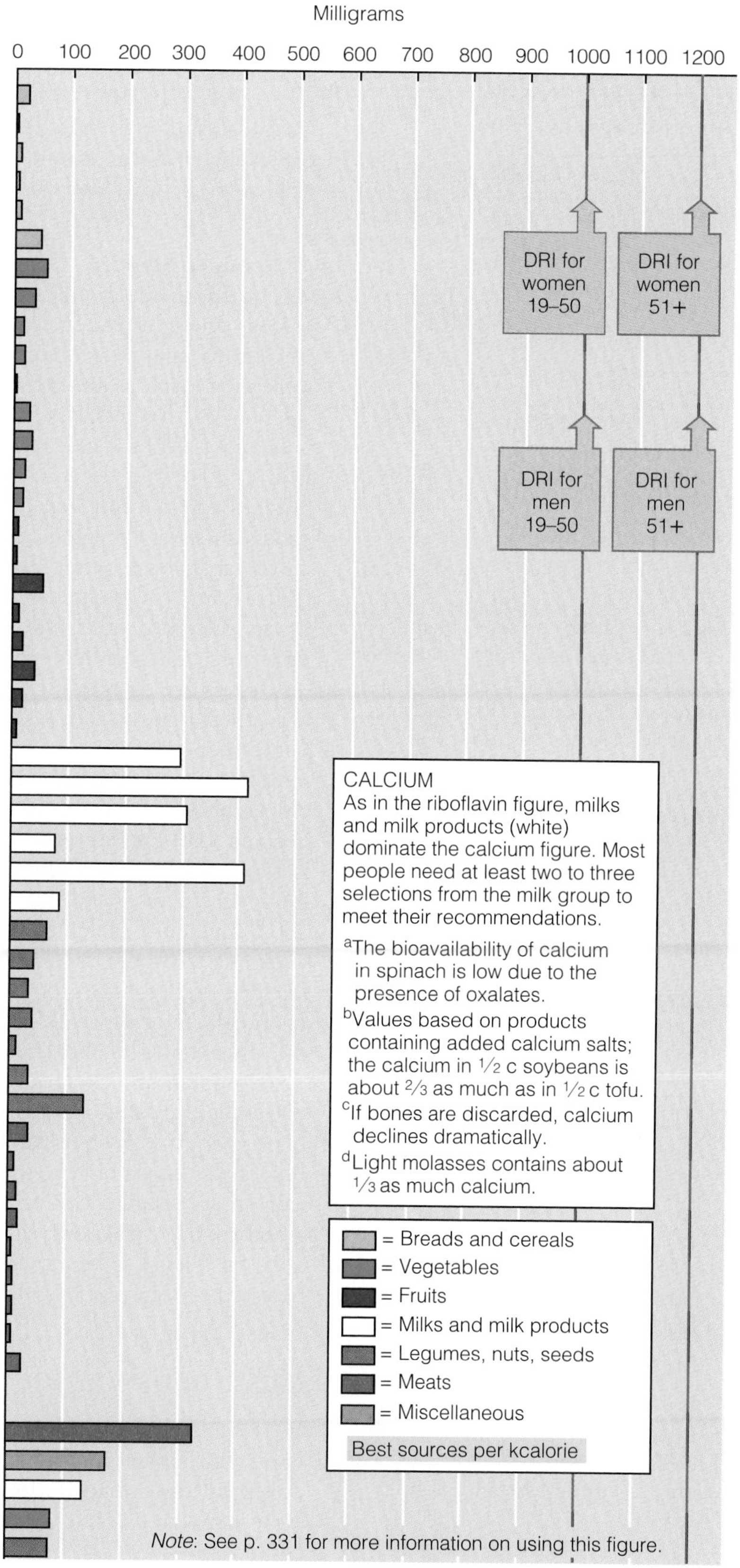

Milligrams — scale: 0 100 200 300 400 500 600 700 800 900 1000 1100 1200

DRI for women 19–50
DRI for women 51+
DRI for men 19–50
DRI for men 51+

CALCIUM
As in the riboflavin figure, milks and milk products (white) dominate the calcium figure. Most people need at least two to three selections from the milk group to meet their recommendations.

[a]The bioavailability of calcium in spinach is low due to the presence of oxalates.

[b]Values based on products containing added calcium salts; the calcium in 1/2 c soybeans is about 2/3 as much as in 1/2 c tofu.

[c]If bones are discarded, calcium declines dramatically.

[d]Light molasses contains about 1/3 as much calcium.

■ = Breads and cereals
■ = Vegetables
■ = Fruits
□ = Milks and milk products
■ = Legumes, nuts, seeds
■ = Meats
■ = Miscellaneous

Best sources per kcalorie

Note: See p. 331 for more information on using this figure.

Figure 12–11

Foods Ranked According to Absorbability of Calcium

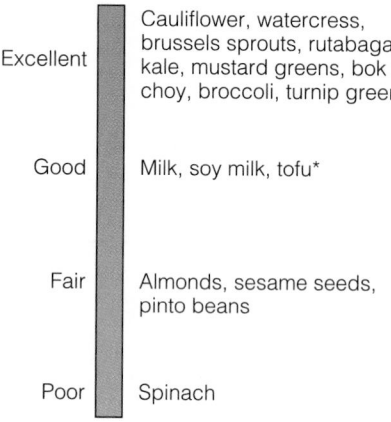

Excellent	Cauliflower, watercress, brussels sprouts, rutabaga, kale, mustard greens, bok choy, broccoli, turnip greens
Good	Milk, soy milk, tofu*
Fair	Almonds, sesame seeds, pinto beans
Poor	Spinach

*Calcium–set tofu

Note: For reference, calcium absorption for foods categorized as excellent was greater than 50%; for those considered good, it was about 30%; for those listed as fair, it was about 20%; and for poor, it was 5%.

Source: Figure created based on data from C. M. Weaver and K. L. Plawecki, Dietary calcium: Adequacy of a vegetarian diet, *American Journal of Clinical Nutrition* 59 (1994): 1238S–1241S.

Calcium supplements are discussed in Highlight 12.

peak bone mass: the highest attainable bone density for an individual, developed during the first three decades of life.

For the person who doesn't like to drink milk, milk and milk products can be concealed in foods. Powdered nonfat milk, which is an excellent and inexpensive source of protein, calcium, and other nutrients, can be added to casseroles, meat loaf, and other mixed dishes in preparation; 5 heaping tablespoons offer the equivalent of a cup of milk. This simple step is probably the best way for older women to obtain added calcium beyond what they can get from liquid milk.

Nonmilk Sources   Some cultures do not use milk in their cuisines; some vegetarians exclude milk as well as meat; and some people are allergic to milk protein or are lactose intolerant. These people need to find nonmilk sources of calcium to help meet their calcium needs. Some brands of tofu, corn tortillas, some nuts (such as almonds), and some seeds (such as sesame seeds) can supply calcium for the person who doesn't use milk products. Wheat bread contains only about 1/10 of the calcium found in milk, but can be a major source for people who eat a lot of it because the calcium is well absorbed. Among the vegetables, mustard and turnip greens, bok choy, kale, parsley, watercress, and broccoli are good sources of available calcium. So are some seaweeds such as the nori popular in Japanese cooking. Some dark green, leafy vegetables—notably spinach, rhubarb, and Swiss chard—appear to be calcium-rich but actually provide little, if any, calcium to the body because of the binders they contain. Figure 12–11 ranks selected foods according to the absorbability of their calcium.

Oysters are also a rich source of calcium, as are small canned fish prepared with their bones, such as canned sardines. Many Asians prepare a stock from bones that helps account for their adequate calcium intake without the use of milk. To make a high-calcium extract, they soak the cracked bones from chicken, turkey, pork, or fish in vinegar and then slowly boil the bones until they become soft. The bones release calcium into the acid medium, and most of the vinegar taste boils off. Then the cooks use the stock in place of water to prepare soup, vegetables, rice, or stew. One tablespoon of such stock may contain over 100 milligrams of calcium.

Some foods offer large amounts of calcium because they are fortified. Calcium-fortified orange juice, for example, provides as much calcium as regular milk. High-calcium milk (milk with extra calcium added) and calcium-fortified bread are other examples of calcium-fortified foods.

A generalization that has been gaining strength throughout this book is supported by the information given here about calcium. A balanced diet that supplies a variety of foods is the best assurance of adequacy for all essential nutrients. All food groups should be included, and none should be overused. In our culture, calcium is usually lacking wherever milk is underemphasized in the diet—whether through ignorance, poverty, simple dislike, fad dieting, lactose intolerance, or allergy. By contrast, iron is usually lacking whenever milk is overemphasized, as Chapter 13 will show.

CALCIUM DEFICIENCY

Bone mass peaks at the time of skeletal maturity (about age 30), and a dense bone mass is the best protection against later age-related bone loss and fracture. A low calcium intake during the growing years impairs acquisition of an optimal bone mass and density.[13] All adults lose bone as they grow older, beginning before they are 40. When bone loss reaches the point at which bones fracture under common, everyday stresses, the condition is known as osteoporosis. Osteoporosis afflicts over 25 million people in the United States, mostly older women.

The urgency of protecting oneself against osteoporosis has to be learned through education because the body sends no signals saying bone loss is occurring. Many diseases make themselves known by symptoms that can be felt or seen, such as pain, shortness of breath, skin lesions, tiredness, and the like, but bone loss is silent. No evidence can be found in a blood sample because blood calcium remains normal no matter what the bone content may be. Measures of bone density are not often taken. Highlight 12 suggests strategies to protect against bone loss, of which obtaining enough calcium is only one.

osteoporosis (OSS-tee-oh-pore-OH-sis): a condition of older persons in which the bones become porous and fragile due to a loss of minerals; also called adult bone loss.
  osteo = bone
  porosis = porous

Phosphorus

Phosphorus is the second most abundant mineral in the body. About 85 percent of it is found combined with calcium in the hydroxapatite crystals of bones and teeth.

phosphorus: a major mineral found mostly in the body's bones and teeth.

Phosphorus Roles in the Body The concentration of phosphorus salts (phosphates) in blood plasma is less than half that of calcium. Phosphates are in all body cells as part of a major buffer system (phosphoric acid and its salts). Phosphorus is also part of DNA and RNA, the genetic code material present in every cell, and therefore is necessary for all growth.

Phosphorus assists in energy transfers during cellular metabolism. Many enzymes and the B vitamins become active only when a phosphate group is attached. (Recall that the B vitamins play major roles in energy metabolism.) ATP itself, the energy carrier of the cells, uses three phosphate groups to do its work.

Lipids containing phosphorus as part of their structures (phospholipids) help to transport other lipids in the blood. Phospholipids are also the major structural components of cell membranes, where they affect transport of nutrients into and out of the cells. Some proteins, such as the casein in milk, contain phosphorus as part of their structures (phosphoproteins). Table 12–8 lists functions and food sources of phosphorus.

Table 12–8

Phosphorus—A Summary

Adult DRI[a]	Chief Functions in the Body	Deficiency Symptoms	Toxicity Symptoms	Significant Sources
700 mg/day	A principal mineral of bones and teeth; part of every cell; important in genetic material, part of phospholipids, used in energy transfer and in buffer systems that maintain acid-base balance	Weakness, bone pain[b]	Low blood calcium levels	All animal tissues (meat, fish, poultry, eggs, milk)

[a]1997 recommendations for phosphorus are called Dietary Reference Intakes (DRI).
[b]Dietary deficiency rarely occurs, but some drugs can bind with phosphorus making it unavailable and resulting in bone loss that is characterized by weakness and pain.

Phosphorus Recommendations   Recommended intakes of phosphorus were recently revised and now differ from those for calcium. Diets that provide adequate energy and protein also supply adequate phosphorus.

Phosphorus Intakes   Dietary deficiencies of phosphorus are unknown. Animal protein is the best source of phosphorus, because the mineral is so abundant in cells. In addition to foods from the milk and meat groups, processed foods (including soft drinks) are usually high in phosphorus. Phosphorus from additives in processed foods can add significantly to people's intakes.

Magnesium

magnesium: a cation within the body's cells, active in many enzyme systems.

Magnesium barely qualifies as a major mineral: only about 1 ounce of magnesium is present in the body of a 130-pound person. Over half of the body's magnesium is in the bones. Most of the rest is in the muscles and soft tissues, with only 1 percent in the extracellular fluid. Bone magnesium seems to be a reservoir to ensure that some will be on hand for vital reactions, regardless of recent dietary intake.

Magnesium Roles in the Body   Magnesium is important to more than 300 of the body's enzyme systems. Magnesium acts in all the cells of the soft tissues, where it forms part of the protein-making machinery and is necessary for energy metabolism. A major role seems to be as a catalyst in the reaction that adds the last phosphate to the high-energy compound ATP. As a required component for ATP metabolism, magnesium is essential to the body's use of glucose; the synthesis of protein, fat, and nucleic acids; and the cells' membrane transport systems. Together with calcium, magnesium is involved in muscle contraction and blood clotting: calcium promotes the processes, whereas magnesium inhibits them. This dynamic interaction between the two minerals helps regulate the functioning of the lungs.[14] Magnesium also helps prevent dental caries by holding calcium in tooth enamel. Like many other nutrients, magnesium supports the normal functioning of the immune system.[15] Table 12–9 offers a summary.

Table 12–9

Magnesium—A Summary

Adult DRI[a]	Chief Functions in the Body	Deficiency Symptoms	Toxicity Symptoms	Significant Sources
420 mg/day (men, 31 + yr) 320 mg/day (women, 31 + yr)	Involved in bone mineralization, the building of protein, enzyme action, normal muscular contraction, nerve impulse transmission, maintenance of teeth, and functioning of immune system	Weakness; confusion; if extreme, convulsions, bizarre muscle movements (especially of eye and face muscles), hallucinations, and difficulty in swallowing; in children, growth failure[b]	Not known; large doses have been taken in the form of the laxative Epsom salts without ill effects except diarrhea	Nuts, legumes, whole grains, dark green vegetables, seafood, chocolate, cocoa

[a]1997 recommendations for magnesium are called Dietary Reference Intakes (DRI).
[b]A still more severe deficiency causes tetany, an extreme, prolonged contraction of the muscles similar to that caused by low blood calcium.

Magnesium Intakes   Dietary magnesium intakes average about three-quarters of the recommended intake for U.S. adults.[16] Dietary intake data, however, do not include the contribution made by water. In some parts of the country, the water contains both calcium and magnesium ("hard" water) and contributes significantly to intakes.

The brown bars in Figure 12–12 indicate that legumes, seeds, and nuts make significant magnesium contributions. Magnesium is part of the chlorophyll molecule, so leafy green vegetables are magnesium-rich.

Magnesium Deficiency   Even when average magnesium intakes are below recommendations, deficiency symptoms are not apparent except with disease.[17] Magnesium deficiency develops in alcohol abuse, protein malnutrition, renal or endocrine disorders, or diseases that cause prolonged vomiting or diarrhea. People using diuretics may also show symptoms. A severe magnesium deficiency causes a tetany similar to the calcium tetany described earlier. Magnesium deficiencies also impair central nervous system activity and are thought to cause the hallucinations experienced by people withdrawing from alcohol intoxication.

Magnesium and Hypertension   The magnesium ion appears critical to heart function and seems to protect against hypertension and heart disease. With magnesium deficiency, the walls of arteries and capillaries undergo visible changes and tend to constrict, a possible mechanism for the hypertensive effect. Studies have reported that magnesium intakes are lower in men who have heart attacks and that injections of magnesium can be used successfully in the treatment of heart attack victims.[18]

To sum up, most of the body's calcium is in the bones where it provides a rigid structure and reservoir of calcium for the blood. Blood calcium participates in muscle contraction, blood clotting, and nerve impulses and is closely regulated by a system of hormones and vitamin D. Phosphorus accompanies calcium both in the crystals of bone and in many foods such as milk. Magnesium also supports bone mineralization and is involved in numerous enzyme systems.

Sulfur

The body does not use sulfur by itself as a nutrient (see Table 12–10). The reason sulfur is mentioned here is that it occurs in essential nutrients that the body does use, such as thiamin and the amino acids methionine and cysteine. Sulfur plays a well-known role in determining the contour of protein molecules. The sulfur-containing side chains in cysteine molecules can link to each other, forming disulfide bridges, which stabilize the protein structure. Skin, hair, and nails contain some of the body's more rigid proteins, which have a high sulfur content.

There is no recommended intake for sulfur, and no deficiencies are known. Only when people lack protein to the point of severe deficiency will they lack the sulfur-containing amino acids.

Like the other nutrients, the minerals' actions are coordinated to get the body's work done. The major minerals, especially sodium, chloride, and potassium, influence the body's fluid balance; whenever an anion moves, a cation moves—always maintaining homeostasis. Sodium, chloride, potassium, calcium, and magnesium

sulfur: a mineral present in the body as part of some amino acids.

Cysteine in one part of a protein chain can bind to cysteine in another part of the chain by way of a disulfide bridge (see the drawing of insulin with its disulfide bridge on p. 182). Two cysteine molecules linked this way are called cystine.

Figure 12–12 Magnesium in Selected Foods

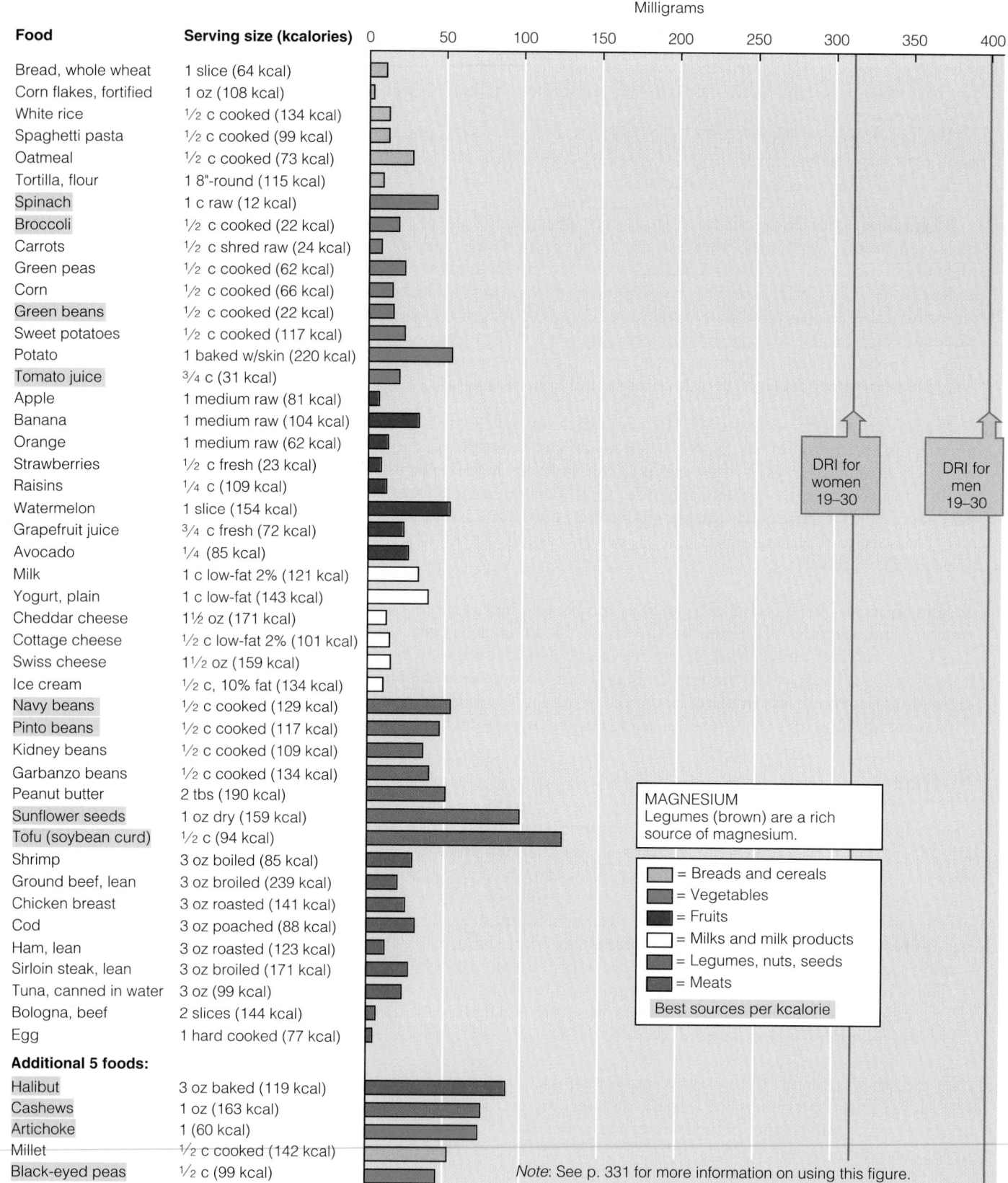

Food	Serving size (kcalories)
Bread, whole wheat	1 slice (64 kcal)
Corn flakes, fortified	1 oz (108 kcal)
White rice	½ c cooked (134 kcal)
Spaghetti pasta	½ c cooked (99 kcal)
Oatmeal	½ c cooked (73 kcal)
Tortilla, flour	1 8"-round (115 kcal)
Spinach	1 c raw (12 kcal)
Broccoli	½ c cooked (22 kcal)
Carrots	½ c shred raw (24 kcal)
Green peas	½ c cooked (62 kcal)
Corn	½ c cooked (66 kcal)
Green beans	½ c cooked (22 kcal)
Sweet potatoes	½ c cooked (117 kcal)
Potato	1 baked w/skin (220 kcal)
Tomato juice	¾ c (31 kcal)
Apple	1 medium raw (81 kcal)
Banana	1 medium raw (104 kcal)
Orange	1 medium raw (62 kcal)
Strawberries	½ c fresh (23 kcal)
Raisins	¼ c (109 kcal)
Watermelon	1 slice (154 kcal)
Grapefruit juice	¾ c fresh (72 kcal)
Avocado	¼ (85 kcal)
Milk	1 c low-fat 2% (121 kcal)
Yogurt, plain	1 c low-fat (143 kcal)
Cheddar cheese	1½ oz (171 kcal)
Cottage cheese	½ c low-fat 2% (101 kcal)
Swiss cheese	1½ oz (159 kcal)
Ice cream	½ c, 10% fat (134 kcal)
Navy beans	½ c cooked (129 kcal)
Pinto beans	½ c cooked (117 kcal)
Kidney beans	½ c cooked (109 kcal)
Garbanzo beans	½ c cooked (134 kcal)
Peanut butter	2 tbs (190 kcal)
Sunflower seeds	1 oz dry (159 kcal)
Tofu (soybean curd)	½ c (94 kcal)
Shrimp	3 oz boiled (85 kcal)
Ground beef, lean	3 oz broiled (239 kcal)
Chicken breast	3 oz roasted (141 kcal)
Cod	3 oz poached (88 kcal)
Ham, lean	3 oz roasted (123 kcal)
Sirloin steak, lean	3 oz broiled (171 kcal)
Tuna, canned in water	3 oz (99 kcal)
Bologna, beef	2 slices (144 kcal)
Egg	1 hard cooked (77 kcal)
Additional 5 foods:	
Halibut	3 oz baked (119 kcal)
Cashews	1 oz (163 kcal)
Artichoke	1 (60 kcal)
Millet	½ c cooked (142 kcal)
Black-eyed peas	½ c (99 kcal)

Milligrams: 0, 50, 100, 150, 200, 250, 300, 350, 400

DRI for women 19–30

DRI for men 19–30

MAGNESIUM
Legumes (brown) are a rich source of magnesium.

- = Breads and cereals
- = Vegetables
- = Fruits
- = Milks and milk products
- = Legumes, nuts, seeds
- = Meats

Best sources per kcalorie

Note: See p. 331 for more information on using this figure.

Table 12–10

Sulfur—A Summary

Chief Functions in the Body	Deficiency Symptoms	Toxicity Symptoms	Significant Sources
As part of proteins, stabilizes their shape by forming disulfide bridges; part of the vitamins biotin and thiamin and the hormone insulin	None known; protein deficiency would occur first	Toxicity would occur only if sulfur-containing amino acids were eaten in excess; this (in animals) depresses growth	All protein-containing foods (meats, fish, poultry, eggs, milk, legumes, nuts)

are key members of the team of nutrients that direct nerve transmission and muscle contraction; they are also the primary nutrients involved in regulating blood pressure.[19] Phosphorus and magnesium participate in many reactions involving glucose, fatty acids, amino acids, and the vitamins. Calcium, phosphorus, and magnesium combine to form the structure of the bones and teeth. Each major mineral also plays other specific roles in the body. With all of the tasks these minerals perform, they are of great importance to life. Consuming enough of each of them every day is not difficult, given a variety of food choices from each of the food groups. Whole-grain breads supply magnesium; fruits, vegetables, and legumes also provide magnesium and potassium, too; milks offer calcium and phosphorus; meats also offer phosphorus and sulfur as well; all foods provide sodium and chloride, excesses being more problematic than inadequacies. The message is quite simple and has been repeated throughout this text: for an adequate intake of all the nutrients, including the major minerals, choose different foods from each of the five food groups. And drink plenty of water.

Study Questions

1. List the roles of water in the body.
2. List the sources of water intake and routes of water excretion.
3. What is ADH? Where does it exert its action? What is aldosterone? How does it work?
4. How does the body use electrolytes to regulate fluid balance?
5. What do the terms *major* and *trace* mean when describing the minerals in the body?
6. Describe some characteristics of minerals that distinguish them from vitamins.
7. What is the major function of sodium in the body? Describe how the kidneys regulate blood sodium. Is a dietary deficiency of sodium unlikely? Why?
8. List calcium's roles in the body. How does the body keep blood calcium constant regardless of intake?
9. Name significant food sources of calcium. What are the consequences of inadequate intakes?
10. List the roles of phosphorus in the body. Discuss the relationships between calcium and phosphorus. Is a dietary deficiency of phosphorus likely? Why?
11. State the major functions of chloride, potassium, magnesium, and sulfur in the body. Are deficiencies of these nutrients likely to occur in your own diet? Why?

Notes

1. Committee on Dietary Allowances, *Recommended Dietary Allowances,* 10th ed. (Washington, D.C.: National Academy Press, 1989), pp. 247–261.

2. Pamphlet from The American Dietetic Association, Water: The beverage of life, 1994.

3. Nutrition Committee, American Heart Association, *Dietary Guidelines for Healthy American Adults: A Statement for Physicians and Health Professionals* (Dallas, Tex.: American Heart Association, 1988).

4. T. A. Kotchen and J. M. Kotchen, Nutrition, diet, and hypertension, in *Modern Nutrition in Health and Disease,* 8th ed., eds. M. E. Shils, J. A. Olson, and M. Shike (Philadelphia; Lea & Febiger, 1994), pp. 1287–1297.

5. H. S. Wright and coauthors, The 1978–88 Nationwide Food Consumption Survey: An update on the nutrient intake of respondents, *Nutrition Today,* May/June 1991, pp. 21–27.

6. Committee on Diet and Health, *Diet and Health: Implications for Reducing Chronic Disease Risk* (Washington, D.C.: National Academy Press, 1989), pp. 99–135.

7. R. D. Mattess, Discretionary salt use, *American Journal of Clinical Nutrition* (1990 ASCN Annual Meeting) 51 (1990): 519.

8. Committee on Dietary Allowances, 1989, pp. 247–261.

9. Committee on Dietary Allowances, 1989, pp. 247–261.

10. D. A. McCarron and coauthors, Dietary calcium and blood pressure: Modifying factors in specific populations, *American Journal of Clinical Nutrition* (supplement) 54 (1991): 215–219.

11. J. Sharlin and coauthors, Nutrition and behavioral characteristics and determinants of plasma cholesterol levels in men and women, *Journal of the American Dietetic Association* 92 (1992): 434–440; G. A. Golditz and coauthors, Diet and risk of clinical diabetes in women, *American Journal of Clinical Nutrition* 55 (1992): 1018–1023; C. F. Garland, F. C. Garland, and E. D. Gorham, Can colon cancer incidence and death rates be reduced with calcium and vitamin D? *American Journal of Clinical Nutrition* 54 (1991): 193S–201S; K. K. Carroll and coauthors, Calcium and carcinogenesis of the mammary gland, *American Journal of Clinical Nutrition* 54 (1991): 206S–208S.

12. *Nutrition Monitoring in the United States: Selected Findings from the National Nutrition Monitoring and Related Research Program* (Hyattsville, Md.: Public Health Service, 1993), pp. 29, 31.

13. V. Matkovic, Calcium metabolism and calcium requirements during skeletal modeling and consolidation of bone mass, *American Journal of Clinical Nutrition* 54 (1991): 245–260.

14. R. A. Landon and E. A. Young, Role of magnesium in regulation of lung function, *Journal of the American Dietetic Association* 93 (1993): 674–677.

15. H. McCoy and M. A. Kenney, Magnesium and immune function: Recent findings, *Magnesium Research* 5 (1992): 281–293.

16. Wright and coauthors, 1991.

17. Committee on Dietary Allowances, 1989, pp. 190–191.

18. P. C. Elwood and coauthors, Dietary magnesium and prediction of heart disease, *The Lancet* 340 (1992): 483; K. L. Woods and coauthors, Intravenous magnesium sulphate in suspected acute myocardial infarction: Results of the second Leicester Intravenous Magnesium Intervention Trial (LIMIT-2), *The Lancet* 339 (1992): 1553–1558.

19. M. E. Reusser and D. A. McCarron, Micronutrient effects on blood pressure regulation, *Nutrition Reviews* 52 (1994): 367–375.

Osteoporosis and Calcium

Osteoporosis is one of the most prevalent diseases of aging, affecting more than 25 million people in the United States—most of them women. Each year more than 1.5 million people suffer bone breaks in their hips, backs, and wrists due to osteoporosis.

Osteoporosis develops without warning. People cannot tell that they are losing bone tissue until late in life: Then dramatic symptoms suddenly emerge. The causes are tangled, and it is not yet clear whether abundant dietary calcium can prevent or forestall osteoporosis. This highlight addresses several questions: What is osteoporosis? What factors contribute to it? What, if anything, can people do to reduce their risks? And where does calcium fit into the picture?

THE PROBLEM OF OSTEOPOROSIS

Osteoporosis often first becomes apparent when someone's hip suddenly gives way. People say, "She fell and broke her hip," but in fact the hip may have been so fragile that it broke *before* she fell. Even stepping down off a curb may be enough to shatter a porous bone into fragments so numerous and scattered that they cannot be reassembled. Removing them and replacing them with an artificial joint requires major surgery. About a fifth of the patients die of complications within a year. Half of those who survive will never walk independently again.

Bone has two compartments: the outer, hard shell of cortical bone, and the inner, lacy structural matrix

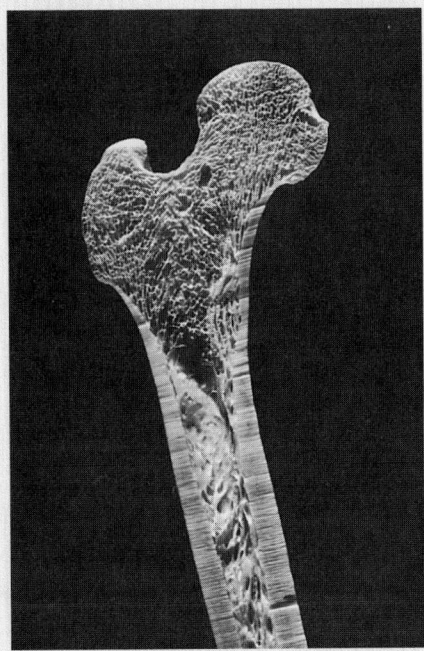

Trabecular bone is the lacy network of calcium-containing crystals that fills the interior. Cortical bone is the dense, ivorylike bone that forms the exterior shell.

of trabecular bone. Both can lose minerals, but in different ways and at different rates. (The accompanying glossary defines relevant terms.) The opening photograph shows a human

leg bone sliced lengthwise, exposing the lacy, calcium-containing crystals inside the bone. These crystals give up calcium to the blood when the day's supply from the diet runs short, and they take up calcium again when the dietary supply is plentiful. For people who have invested in their body's calcium bank during the bone-forming years of their childhood and young adulthood, these deposits provide a nearly inexhaustible fund of calcium.

In contrast to trabecular bone, cortical bone forms the dense, ivorylike exterior shell that surrounds and protects each bone. Cortical bone composes the shafts of the long bones, and a thin cortical shell caps the end of the bone, too. Both compartments confer strength on bone: cortical bone provides the sturdy outer wall, while trabecular bone provides support along the lines of stress.

The two types of bone play different roles in calcium balance and osteoporosis. Trabecular bone is generally supplied with blood vessels and is metabolically active. It is sensitive to hormones that govern day-to-day

Glossary

bone density: a measure of bone strength. When minerals fill the bone matrix, they give it strength.

cortical bone: the ivorylike outer bone layer that forms a shell surrounding trabecular bone and comprises the shaft of a long bone.

trabecular (tra-BECK-you-lar) **bone:** the lacy inner structure of calcium crystals

that supports the bone's structure and provides a calcium storage bank.

type I osteoporosis: osteoporosis characterized by rapid bone losses, primarily of trabecular bone.

type II osteoporosis: osteoporosis characterized by gradual losses of both trabecular and cortical bone.

deposits and withdrawals of calcium, and it readily gives up minerals whenever blood calcium needs replenishing. Losses of trabecular bone start becoming significant for men and women in their 30s, although losses can occur whenever calcium withdrawals exceed deposits.

Cortical bone also gives up calcium, but slowly and at a steady pace. Cortical bone losses typically begin at about 40 years of age and continue slowly but surely thereafter.

Researchers have associated losses of trabecular and cortical bone with two types of osteoporosis, which cause two types of bone breaks. Type I osteoporosis involves losses of trabecular bone (see Figure H12–1). These losses sometimes exceed three times the expected rate, and bone breaks may occur suddenly. Trabecular bones become so fragile that even the body's own weight can overburden the spine—vertebrae may suddenly disintegrate and crush down, painfully pinching major nerves. Wrists may break as bone ends weaken, and teeth may loosen or fall out as the trabecular bone of the jaw recedes. Women are most often the victims of this type of osteoporosis, outnumbering men six to one. Taking estrogen for at least seven years after menopause is the most effective preventive measure against this type of osteoporosis.[1]

In type II osteoporosis, the calcium of both cortical and trabecular bone is drawn out of storage, but slowly over the years. As old age approaches, the vertebrae may compress into wedge shapes, forming what is often called "dowager's hump," the posture many older people assume as they "grow shorter." Figure H12–2 (on facing page) shows

Figure H12–1

Healthy and Osteoporotic Trabecular Bones

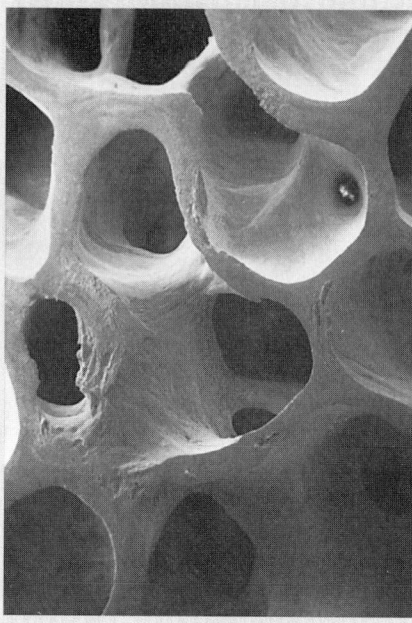

Electron micrograph of healthy trabecular bone.

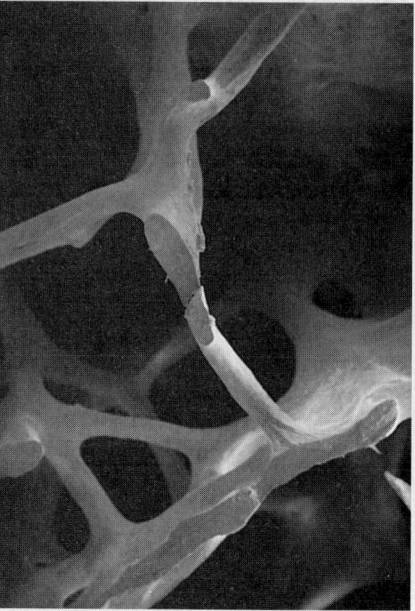

Electron micrograph of trabecular bone affected by osteoporosis.

the effect of compressed spinal bone on a woman's height and posture. Because both the cortical shell and the trabecular interior weaken, breaks most often occur in the hip, as in the opening example. A woman is twice as likely as a man to suffer type II osteoporosis. Table H12–1 summa-

Table H12–1

Types of Osteoporosis Compared

	Type I	Type II
Other name	Postmenopausal osteoporosis	Senile osteoporosis
Age of onset	50 to 70 years old	70 years and older
Bone loss	Trabecular bone	Both trabecular and cortical bone
Fracture sites	Wrist and spine	Hip
Gender incidence	6 women to 1 man	2 women to 1 man
Primary causes	Rapid loss of estrogen in women following menopause; loss of testosterone in men with advancing age	Reduced calcium absorption, increased bone mineral loss, increased propensity to fall

Source: Adapted from C. Niewoehner, Calcium and osteoporosis, *Cereal Foods World* 33 (1988): 784–787.

Figure H12–2
. . . .

Loss of Height in a Woman Caused by Osteoporosis

The woman on the left is about 50 years old. On the right, she is 80 years old. Her legs have not grown shorter: only her back has lost length, due to collapse of her spinal bones (vertebrae). Collapsed vertebrae cannot protect the spinal nerves from pressure that causes excruciating pain.

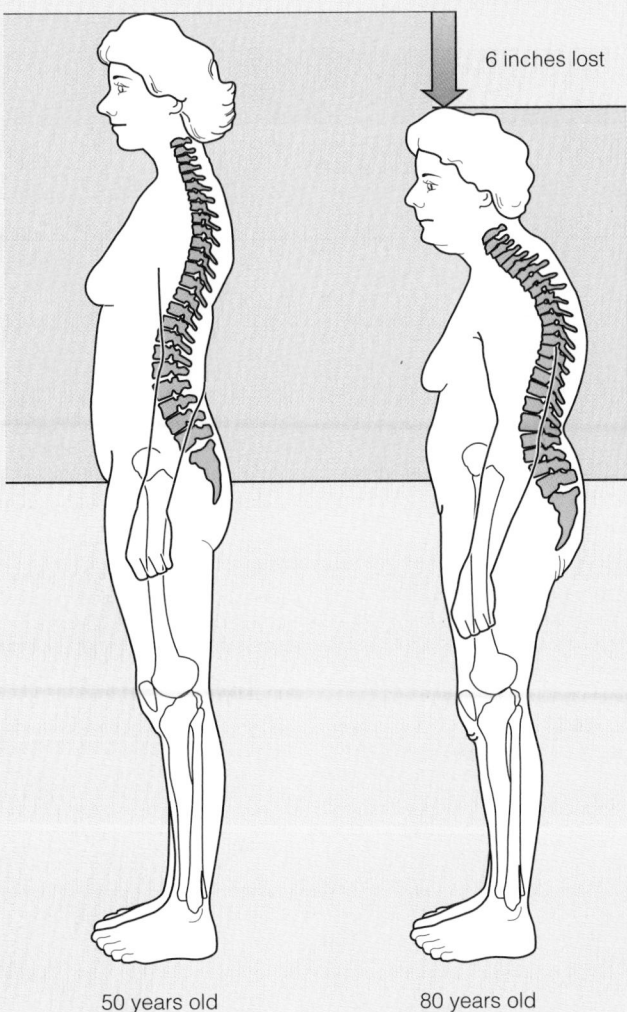

6 inches lost

50 years old   80 years old

rizes the differences between the two types of osteoporosis.

Whether a person develops osteoporosis seems to depend partly on heredity and partly on other factors, including nutrition. The strongest predictor of bone density is age, followed by sex. Other predictors, whose order of importance is not known, are hormonal status, racial inheritance, physical activity, body weight, smoking, alcohol, drugs, and nutrition.

AGE AND BONE CALCIUM

During the first two decades of life, the skeleton grows stronger and denser as it accumulates minerals. Then, in the late 20s to early 30s, the bones stop growing. As the years pass, the cells that build bone gradually become less active, while those that dismantle bone continue working. Thus, with advancing age, bones lose strength and density (see Figure H12–3).

Calcium intakes of older adults are typically low, and calcium absorption declines after about the age of 65 years. The kidneys do not activate vitamin D as well as they did earlier (recall that active vitamin D promotes calcium absorption). Also, sunlight is needed to form vitamin D, and many older people spend little or no time outdoors in the sunshine. For these reasons, and because intakes of vitamin D are typically low anyway, blood vitamin D decreases. A recent study found the rate of fractures was significantly reduced in women with osteoporosis who received a regular vitamin D supplement (0.25 μg twice daily for three years).[2]

Some of the hormones that regulate bone and calcium metabolism also change with age and accelerate bone mineral withdrawal.* Together, these age-related factors probably contribute to bone loss: inefficient bone remodeling, reduced calcium intakes, impaired calcium absorption, poor vitamin D status, physical inactivity, and hormonal changes that favor bone mineral withdrawal.

---

*Among the hormones suggested as influential are parathormone, calcitonin, and estrogen.

SEX AND HORMONES

After age, sex is the next strongest predictor of loss of bone density with aging: women have much more substantial losses than men in later life. Menopause imposes special perils on women's bones. Bone dwindles rapidly when the hormone estrogen diminishes and menstruation ceases. Accelerated losses continue for 6 to 8 years following menopause, then taper off, so that women again lose bone at the same rate as men their age (see Figure H12–4). Losses of bone minerals continue throughout the remainder of a woman's lifetime, but not at the free-fall pace of the menopause years.

When *young* women experience reduced estrogen secretion and cease menstruating, they, too, lose bone rapidly. Highlight 9 described how women who overexercise and unreasonably restrict their body weights develop athletic amenorrhea and become susceptible to bone fractures. The combination of irregular or absent menstrual periods and low body weights explains much of the bone loss seen in young athletes.[3] Estrogen taken as a prescription drug can help nonmenstruating women prevent further bone loss and reduce the incidence of fractures.[4]

If estrogen deficiency is a major cause of osteoporosis in women, what is the cause of bone loss in men? Men produce only a little estrogen, yet they resist osteoporosis better than women. Male hormones must also play a role because men suffer more fractures after removal of the testes (in cases of disease) or when their testes lose functional ability with aging. Men who have delayed puberty also appear to have

Figure H12–3

Phases of Bone Development throughout Life

The active growth phase occurs from birth to approximately age 20. The next phase of peak bone mass development occurs between the ages of 12 and 40. The final phase, when bone resorption exceeds formation, begins between age 30 and 40 and continues throughout the remainder of life.

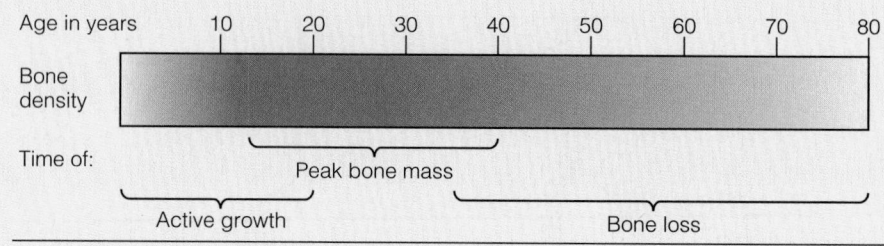

Figure H12–4

High Peak Bone Mass Early in Life Postpones Osteoporosis

Over a lifetime, women lose 30 to 40 percent of their bone mass and men, 20 to 30 percent. Can you see why it is so important for young people to consume enough calcium to attain a maximum bone mass?

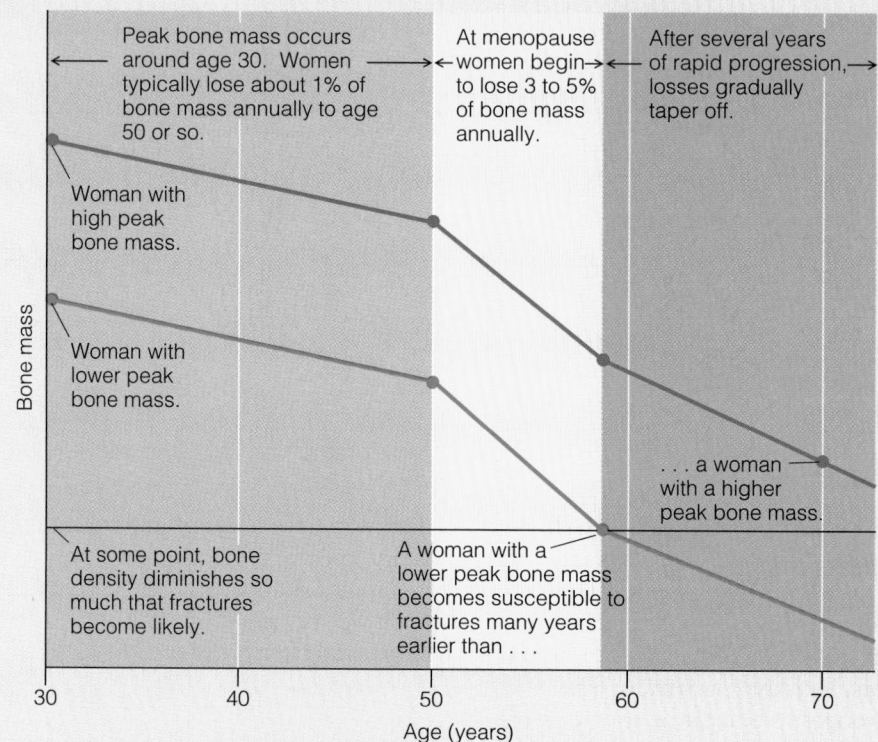

more fractures, suggesting that timing of puberty influences peak bone density.[5] Thus both male and female sex hormones appear to play roles in the development of osteoporosis.

One more complication of the estrogen theory is that some women lose bone tissue in middle age before they reach menopause, as though they were predisposed to do so. Clearly, hormones are only one of several factors affecting bones. Still, being female and experiencing menopause remain prime risk factors for the development of osteoporosis.

GENETIC INHERITANCE AND RACE

Studies of mothers and daughters confirm that heredity plays an influential role in bone density.[6] Most likely, inheritance influences both peak bone mass achieved during growth and the extent of bone loss during menopause. The extent to which a given genetic potential is realized, however, depends on many outside factors. Nutrition and physical activity, for example, can maximize peak bone density during growth, whereas alcohol and tobacco abuse can accelerate bone losses later in life.

Risks of osteoporosis appear to run along racial lines. Significant differences in bone metabolism divide elderly African Americans from Caucasians.[7] Black people have denser bones than do white people, and these differences are evident even before birth.[8] Greater bone density expresses itself in a lower rate of osteoporosis among blacks. Hip fractures, for example, are about three times more likely at 80 years of age in white women than in African-American women.

Other ethnic groups have *less* dense bones than do many people of European heritage. Asians from China and Japan, Mexican Americans, Hispanic people from Central and South America, and Inuit people from St. Lawrence Island all have lower bone density than do people with a northern European background. One might predict that these groups would suffer more bone fractures, but this is not always the case. Chinese people living in Singapore have low bone density, but their hip fracture rates are among the lowest in the world. In the countries of the Balkan peninsula (former Yugoslavia), bone fracture rates correlate with calcium nutrition—lower rates in areas of high calcium intake, higher rates in areas of low calcium intake—despite racial similarities. These findings demonstrate that although a person's genes may lay the groundwork for a likely outcome, environmental factors influence the genes' ultimate expression. From the findings reported in the Balkans, calcium nutrition appears to be one of those environmental factors. Others include physical activity, body weight, smoking, alcohol, and protein intake—all factors within a person's control.

PHYSICAL ACTIVITY AND BODY WEIGHT

When people are idle—for example, when they are confined to bed—their bones lose strength just as their muscles do. Astronauts who live with reduced gravity for days or weeks at a time also lose bone and muscle strength.

Muscle strength and bone strength tend to go together. When muscles work, they pull on the bones, stimulating them to lay down more trabeculae and grow stronger. Also, when muscles work, the hormones that promote new muscle growth also favor the building of bone. As a result, active bones are denser than sedentary bones.[9] Even modest increases in physical activity and calcium intake help to maximize bone gains in young adulthood and minimize further losses that occur with inactivity.[10]

To keep the bones healthy, weight-bearing physical activity, such as walking, dancing, or jogging, are especially effective. Even swimming may be beneficial, perhaps because it increases muscle strength. Dr. Robert Heaney of Omaha's Creighton University stated the case for taking an active (quite literally) stand against osteoporosis: "Osteoporosis is a total life-style problem. You can't cure a bad life-style with a pill, and it's a terrible strategic mistake to encourage people to think you can. If I'm sitting all day, don't walk to work, don't carry loads or work in the garden on the weekend, I'm going to lose bone. You can give me all the calcium in the world, and it's not going to stop it."[11] Cells do not helplessly accept what is given to them; instead they respond, with the help of the necessary regulators, to the demands put upon them. Then they select the nutrients they need from what is offered. The way to increase bone density is to put a demand on the bones, make them work, and then provide the raw materials from which they can grow strong: calcium, other minerals, all the nutrients in the right balance.

Heavier body weights also place stress on the bones and promote their maintenance. In fact, body weight (and to some extent, body fatness) is a significant and consistent predictor of bone density and risk of fractures.[12] As mentioned earlier, the combination of a too-slender body, severely restricted energy intake, extreme daily exercise, and the absence of menstruation reliably predict bone loss.[13]

SMOKING, ALCOHOL, AND CAFFEINE

Smokers experience more fractures from slight injury than do nonsmokers. A study of twins reports that women who smoke a pack of cigarettes a day throughout adulthood lose an extra 5 to 10 percent of their bone density by menopause.[14] Although the mechanism of action remains undefined, both the lower body weights of smokers and the earlier menopause of female smokers may be factors.[15]

People who abuse alcohol often suffer from osteoporosis and experience more bone breaks than others. Several factors appear to be involved: alcohol promotes fluid excretion that leads to excessive calcium losses in the urine; alcohol may upset the hormonal balance required for healthy bones; alcohol may slow bone formation, leading to lower bone density; and alcohol abuse increases the risk of falling.

Caffeine has been considered a possible risk factor for the development of osteoporosis, but evidence is inconclusive.[16] Some studies indicate that caffeine accelerates calcium excretion; other studies have found no significant effects.[17] The effects of caffeine on calcium balance may be deleterious only when calcium intake is low.

Table H12–2 summarizes the risk factors and protective factors covered so far and includes some others, among them nutrition factors, discussed next. The more risk factors that apply to a person, the greater the chances of bone loss. Notice that several factors are more influential than diet in the development of osteoporosis.

PROTEIN NUTRITION

Extra dietary protein seems to promote calcium excretion in the urine. A lifetime of consuming excess dietary protein may well accelerate bone loss.[18] Many women in the United States may have protein intakes high enough and calcium intakes low enough to compromise bone integrity.[19]

The converse is also true: diets low in protein help to conserve bone density. This is seen both in laboratory animals and in strict vegetarians, who consume a lower-than-average amount of protein. Vegetarians who center meals on

Table H12–2

Risk and Protective Factors That Correlate with Osteoporosis

Risk Factors	Protective Factors
HIGH CORRELATION	
Advanced age	African American
Alcohol abuse	Estrogens, long-term use
Anorexia nervosa	
Caucasian	
Chronic steroid use	
Female sex	
Rheumatoid arthritis	
Surgical removal of ovaries	
Thinness	
MODERATE CORRELATION	
Chronic thyroid hormone use	Having given birth
Cigarette smoking	High body weight
Diabetes (insulin-dependent type)	
Early menopause	
Excessive antacid use	
Low-calcium diet	
Sedentary lifestyle	
Vitamin D deficiency	
PROBABLY IMPORTANT BUT NOT YET PROVED	
Alcohol taken in moderation	High-calcium diet
Caffeine use	Regular physical activity
Family history of osteoporosis	
High-fiber diet	
High-protein diet	

Source: Adapted from C. D. Arnaud and S. D. Sanchez, The role of calcium in osteoporosis, *Annual Review of Nutrition* 10 (1990): 397–414.

eggs and dairy products, however, can consume as much protein and lose bone just as rapidly as do meat eaters.[20] A tentative link has been suggested between the hormone insulin, released in response to dietary protein, and calcium losses in the urine.[21] Diabetes (IDDM) also seems to alter the body's handling of calcium and magnesium with possible harmful effects on the health of the bones.[22]

Too little protein can be as harmful as too much, of course. Protein deprivation also stimulates calcium losses.[23] These facts seem to conflict at first glance, but they really just demonstrate a sound nutrition principle—that moderation is best.

CALCIUM NUTRITION

As stated earlier, a low calcium uptake into bones during the growing years makes a person susceptible to osteoporosis later. Nutritional causes of poor calcium status early in life include deficiencies of vitamin D and calcium and possibly of fluoride. Fluoride taken during the bone-building years seems to increase bone density, but supplementation has not been effective in treating osteoporosis. When women with osteoporosis were given fluoride supplements for four years, their spinal bone mass increased, but their other bones fractured more, as compared with the control group.[24] Fluoride-treated women also experienced side effects such as stomach irritation and pain in the lower extremities.

As important as calcium may be to bone health, osteoporosis is not a calcium-deficiency disease comparable to iron-deficiency anemia. In iron-deficiency anemia, high iron intakes reliably reverse the condi-

tion; in osteoporosis, though, high calcium intakes alone during adulthood may do little or nothing to reverse bone loss.

Most experts agree that there must be a lower limit for calcium intakes, below which bone loss accelerates. Recommendations for adults in the United States and Canada are set well above this minimum, although exactly how much calcium is minimal is a point of disagreement. Defining an exact minimum is complicated because people who consume less calcium absorb more, and vice versa.

Some people question how certain ethnic groups can use no dairy products and have low calcium intakes, yet still maintain calcium balance. Part of the answer is the body's adaptation to low calcium intakes. Another part of the answer is that bone loss is not always apparent. Women in regions of China who have high calcium intakes have greater bone densities than women in other areas.[25]

CALCIUM RECOMMENDATIONS

Throughout life, many factors can either hasten or slow the bone loss that occurs in everyone. Scientists agree that bone strength later in life depends on how well the bones are developed and maintained during youth, and that adequate calcium nutrition during the growing years is essential to achieving optimal peak bone mass.[26] On the basis of this agreement, the Committee on Dietary Reference Intakes recommends 1300 milligrams of calcium per day for everyone 9 through 18 years of age. Once a person reaches the bone-losing years of middle age, those who formed dense bones dur-

ing youth have the advantage: they can afford to lose more bone tissue before beginning to suffer ill effects. After bone loss has begun, a person can still do a few things to maintain the bones, as discussed earlier.

Unfortunately, few girls meet the recommended intake for calcium during their bone-forming years. (Boys generally obtain intakes close to those recommended because they eat more food.) Even if girls do meet the recommended intake, it may not be high enough to achieve the maximum bone mass.[27] This may mean that most girls start their adult lives with less than optimal bone density. As for adults, women rarely meet the recommended intake of 1000 to 1200 milligrams from food within their energy allowances. Furthermore, evidence is accumulating that calcium recommendations should be higher still, especially for postmenopausal women.[28] Some authorities suggest 1500 milligrams of calcium for postmenopausal women who are not receiving estrogen.

A PERSPECTIVE ON SUPPLEMENTS

People who do not consume milk products or other calcium-rich foods in amounts that provide even half the recommended calcium may benefit from calcium supplements.[29] During the menopausal years, calcium supplements of 1 gram may slow, but cannot fully prevent, the inevitable bone loss.[30] Supplements are commonly used as a part of therapy for osteoporosis, along with gentle exercise and, for women, estrogen replacement, but supplements should not be used as a substitute for estrogen.[31] As a rule, women taking estrogen need no more calcium than other women their age.

Regular vitamin-mineral pills contain little or no calcium. The label may list a few milligrams of calcium, but remember that the recommended intake is a gram or more for adults.

Anyone contemplating the use of calcium supplements should do so only on a physician's advice. Taking calcium supplements may present risks, as described in Table H12–3. If these risks are deemed acceptable, the consumer still has several decisions to make when selecting a calcium supplement.[32] Supplements are available in three forms. Simplest are the purified calcium compounds, such as calcium carbonate, citrate, gluconate, lactate, malate, or phosphate, and compounds of calcium with amino acids (called amino acid chelates). Then there are mixtures of calcium with other compounds, such as calcium carbonate with magnesium carbonate, with aluminum salts (as in some antacids), or with vitamin D. Then there are powdered, calcium-rich materials such as bone meal, powdered bone, oyster shell, or dolomite (limestone). (See Table H12–4's description of supplement terms.)

The first question to ask is how well the body absorbs and uses the calcium from various supplements. Based on limited research to date, it seems that most healthy people absorb calcium equally well—and as well as from milk—from any of these supplements: amino acids chelated with calcium; calcium phosphate dibasic; or calcium acetate, carbonate, citrate, gluconate, or lactate. People absorb calcium less well from a mixture of calcium and magnesium carbonates, from oyster shell calcium fortified with inorganic magnesium, from a chelated calcium-magnesium combination, or from calcium carbonate fortified with vitamins and iron.

A way to circumvent adverse nutrient interactions may be to take calcium supplements between, not with, meals. But for anyone with reduced stomach acid secretion, this is not a satisfactory solution because only a meal stimulates sufficient acid secretion to permit the absorption of the calcium. (Score a point here for food sources of calcium.)

Consider another point for food. Some people absorb calcium better from milk and milk products than from even the most absorbable supplements named above.

The next question to ask is how much calcium the supplement provides. Healthy people have consumed up to 2500 milligrams of calcium per day without problems.[33] To be safe, though, supplements should provide less than this, since foods also provide calcium. Read the label to find out how much a dose supplies. Calcium carbonate is 40 percent calcium, whereas calcium gluconate is only 9 percent. The user should select a low-dose supplement and take it several times a day rather than taking a large-dose supplement all at once. Divided doses can improve a day's total absorption by up to 20 percent.

Table H12–3

Problems Arising from Calcium Supplementation

People who take calcium supplements risk:

- Impaired iron status. (This is due to the change in stomach pH caused by calcium, which interferes with iron absorption. Calcium citrate, calcium phosphate, calcium carbonate, and calcium chloride taken with meals interfere with iron absorption. Taking calcium supplements between meals limits calcium absorption.)
- Accelerated calcium loss. (Calcium-containing antacids that also contain aluminum and magnesium hydroxide cause a net calcium loss.)
- Urinary tract stones or kidney damage in susceptible individuals. (People who have a history of kidney stones need to be monitored by a physician and to use calcium citrate supplements, which are most soluble.)
- Exposure to contaminants. (Some preparations of bone meal and dolomites are contaminated with hazardous amounts of arsenic, cadmium, mercury, and lead.)
- Vitamin D toxicity. (Vitamin D is needed to enhance calcium absorption, but continued high intakes of vitamin D, which is present in many calcium supplements, can be toxic. Users must eliminate other concentrated vitamin D sources and take enough, but not too much, vitamin D to normalize calcium absorption.)
- Excess blood calcium. (This complication is seen only with doses of calcium fourfold or more greater than customarily prescribed.)
- Milk alkali syndrome. (This alkalosis is also only seen with doses of calcium of 4 to 10 grams/day. This condition disappears when supplementation is discontinued.)
- Other nutrient interactions. (Calcium phosphate dibasic inhibits magnesium absorption.)
- Drug interactions. (Calcium and tetracycline form an insoluble complex that impairs both mineral and drug absorption.)
- Constipation, intestinal bloating, and excess gas; confusion. (Older people are especially prone to these conditions.)

Table H12–4
....

Calcium Supplements

- **Amino acid chelates** (KEY-lates) are compounds of minerals (such as calcium) combined with amino acids in a form that favors their absorption. A *chelating agent* is a molecule that surrounds another molecule and can then either promote or prevent its movement from place to place; *chele* means claw.

- **Antacids** are acid-buffering agents used to counter excess acidity in the stomach. Calcium-containing preparations (such as Tums) contain available calcium. Antacids with aluminum or magnesium hydroxides (such as Rolaids) can accelerate calcium losses.

- **Bone meal** or **powdered bones** are crushed or ground bone preparations intended to supply calcium to the diet. Calcium from bone is not well absorbed and is often contaminated with toxic materials such as arsenic, mercury, lead, and cadmium.

- **Dolomite** is a compound of minerals (calcium magnesium carbonate) found in limestone and marble. Dolomite is powdered and is sold as a calcium-magnesium supplement, but may be contaminated with toxic minerals, is not well absorbed, and interacts adversely with absorption of other essential minerals.

- **Oyster shell** is a product made from the powdered shells of oysters that is sold as a calcium supplement, but is not well absorbed by the digestive system.

Then consider that when manufacturers compress large quantities of calcium into small pills, the stomach acid has difficulty penetrating the pill. To test a supplement's absorbability, drop it into a 6-ounce cup of vinegar, and stir occasionally. A high-quality formulation will dissolve within half an hour.

Finally, having chosen a supplement, a person must take it regularly. Clearly, taking supplements for calcium can be a burdensome choice.

Experts agree that it remains highly desirable to adjust food and beverage intakes to provide calcium. The Consensus Conference on Osteoporosis recommends milk. The American Society for Bone and Mineral Research recommends foods as a source of calcium in preference to supplements. The *Diet and Health* report urges people to eat low- or nonfat dairy products and dark green vegetables to meet their calcium needs and concludes that current research does not justify the use of calcium supplements.[34] Seldom is such a consensus seen among nutritionists.

SOME CLOSING THOUGHTS

Unfortunately, many of the strongest risk factors for osteoporosis are beyond people's control: age, sex, genetics, and race. But several factors within people's control can help to reduce the risk: a calcium-rich diet, a moderate protein intake, daily physical activity, abstinence from cigarette smoking, and moderation in, or abstinence from, alcohol use. Women should be evaluated for possible estrogen replacement therapy at menopause. The reward for taking these steps is the best possible chance of preserving bone health throughout life.

NOTES

1. D. T. Felson and coauthors, The effect of postmenopausal estrogen therapy on bone density in elderly women, *New England Journal of Medicine* 329 (1993): 1141–1146; L. G. Tolstoi and R. M. Levin, Osteoporosis—The treatment controversy, *Nutrition Today,* July/August 1992, pp. 6–12.

2. M. W. Tilyard and coauthors, Treatment of postmenopausal osteoporosis with calcitriol or calcium, *New England Journal of Medicine* 326 (1992): 357–362.

3. B. L. Drinkwater, B. Bruemner, and C. H. Chestnut III, Menstrual history as a determinant of current bone density in young athletes, *Journal of the American Medical Association* 263 (1990): 545–548.

4. B. L. Riggs and L. J. Melton, The prevention and treatment of osteoporosis, *New England Journal of Medicine* (1992): 620–627; C. D. Arnaud and S. D. Sanchez, The role of calcium in osteoporosis, *Annual Review of Nutrition* 10 (1990): 397–414.

5. J. S. Finkelstein and coauthors, Osteopenia in men with a history of delayed puberty, *New England Journal of Medicine* 326 (1992): 600–604.

6. S. R. Cummings and coauthors, Risk factors for hip fractures in white women, *New England Journal of Medicine* 332 (1995): 767–773; J. Lutz and R. Tesar, Mother-daughter pairs: Spinal and femoral bone densities and dietary intakes, *American Journal of Clinical Nutrition* 52 (1990): 878–888.

7. H. M. Perry and coauthors, A preliminary report of vitamin D and calcium metabolism in older African Americans, *Journal of the American Geriatric Society* 41 (1993): 612–616.

8. A history of racial and ethnic differences in regard to bone health is found in W. S. Pollitzer and J. J. B. Anderson, Ethnic and genetic differences in bone mass: A review with a hereditary vs environmental perspective, *American Journal of Clinical Nutrition* 50 (1989): 1244–1259.

9. J. A. Metz, J. J. B. Anderson, and P. N. Gallagher, Jr., Intakes of calcium, phosphorus, and protein, and physical activity are related to radial bone mass in young adult women, *American Journal of Clinical Nutrition* 58 (1993): 537–542; C. N. Meridith, Exercise in the prevention of osteoporosis, in *Nutrition of the Elderly,* eds. H. Munro and G. Schlierf (New York: Raven Press, 1992), pp. 169–175.

10. ACSM Position stand on osteoporosis and exercise, *Medicine and Science in Sports and Exercise* 27 (1995): i–vii; R. R. Recker and coauthors, Bone gain in young adult women, *Journal of the American Medical Association* 268 (1992): 2403–2408.

11. Health & Fitness: Going crazy over calcium—It sells a rainbow of products, but does it work? *Time*, February 23, 1987.

12. J. F. Aloia and coauthors, To what extent is bone mass determined by fat-free or fat mass? *American Journal of Clinical Nutrition* 61 (1995): 1110–1114; Cummings and coauthors, 1995; S. L. Edelstein and E. Barrett-Connor, Relation between body size and bone mineral density in elderly men and women, *American Journal of Epidemiology* 138 (1993): 160–169; I. R. Reid and coauthors, Determinants of total body and regional bone mineral density in normal post-menopausal women—A key role for fat mass, *Journal of Clinical Endocrinology and Metabolism* 75 (1992): 45–51.

13. Drinkwater, Bruemner, and Chestnut III, 1990; J. H. Wilson, Nutrition, physical activity and bone health in women, *Nutrition Research Reviews* 7 (1994): 67–91.

14. J. L. Hopper and E. Seeman, The bone density of female twins discordant for tobacco use, *New England Journal of Medicine* 330 (1994): 387–392.

15. C. W. Slemenda, Cigarettes and the skeleton, *New England Journal of Medicine* 330 (1994): 430–431.

16. Arnaud and Sanchez, 1990; Cummings and coauthors, 1995.

17. M. J. Barger-Lux, R. P. Heaney, and M. R. Stegman, Effects of moderate caffeine intake on the calcium economy of premenopausal women, *American Journal of Clinical Nutrition* 52 (1990): 722–725.

18. Committee on Dietary Allowances, *Recommended Dietary Allowances*, 10th ed. (Washington, D.C.: National Academy Press, 1989); Arnaud and Sanchez, 1990; R. P. Heaney, Pro-tein intake and the calcium economy, *Journal of the American Dietetic Association* 93 (1993): 1259–1260; J. C. Howe, Postprandial response of calcium metabolism in post menopausal women to meals varying in protein level/source, *Metabolism Clinical and Experimental* 39 (1990): 1246–1252.

19. Heaney, 1993.

20. R. Tesar and coauthors, Axial peripheral bone density and nutrient intakes of post menopausal vegetarian and omnivorous women, *American Journal of Clinical Nutrition* 56 (1992): 699–704.

21. Howe, 1990.

22. G. Saggese and coauthors, Hypomagnesemia and the parathyroid hormone–vitamin D endocrine system in children with insulin-dependent diabetes mellitus, *Journal of Pediatrics* 118 (1991): 220–225.

23. J. Bonjour and coauthors, Hip fracture, femoral bone mineral density, and protein supply in elderly patients, in *Nutrition of the Elderly*, eds. H. Munro and G. Schlierf (New York: Raven Press, 1992), pp. 151–159.

24. B. L. Riggs and coauthors, Effect of fluoride treatment on the fracture rate in post-menopausal women with osteoporosis, *New England Journal of Medicine* 322 (1990): 802–809.

25. J. F. Hu and coauthors, Dietary calcium and bone density among middle-aged and elderly women in China, *American Journal of Clinical Nutrition* 58 (1993): 219–227.

26. R. P. Heaney, Nutritional factors in osteoporosis, *Annual Review of Nutrition* 13 (1993): 287–316; F. Bronner, Calcium and osteoporosis, *American Journal of Clinical Nutrition* 60 (1994): 831–836.

27. V. Matkovic and J. Z. Ilich, Calcium requirements for growth: Are current recommendations adequate? *Nutrition Reviews* 51 (1993): 171–180.

28. D. V. Porter, Washington update: NIH consensus Development Conference Statement Optimal Calcium Intake, *Nutrition Today*, September/October 1994, pp. 37–40; R. P. Heaney, Thinking straight about calcium, *New England Journal of Medicine* 328 (1993): 503–505.

29. B. Dawson-Hughes and coauthors, A controlled trial of the effect of calcium supplementation on bone density in postmenopausal women, *New England Journal of Medicine* 323 (1990): 878–883.

30. B. Dawson-Hughes, Calcium supplementation and bone loss: A review of controlled clinical trials, *American Journal of Clinical Nutrition* 54 (1991): 274S–280S; I. R. Reid and coauthors, Effect of calcium supplementation on bone loss in postmenopausal women, *New England Journal of Medicine* 328 (1993): 460–464.

31. Arnaud and Sanchez, 1990: B. Ettinger, H. K. Genant, and C. E. Cann, Long-term estrogen replacement therapy prevents bone loss and fractures, *Annals of Internal Medicine* 102 (1985): 319–324.

32. D. I. Levenson and R. S. Bockman, A review of calcium preparations, *Nutrition Reviews* 52 (1994): 221–232.

33. Committee on Dietary Allowances, 1989, pp. 174–184.

34. Committee on Diet and Health, *Diet and Health: Implications for Reducing Chronic Disease Risk* (Washington, D.C.: National Academy Press, 1989), p. 17.

Chapter 13

The Trace Minerals

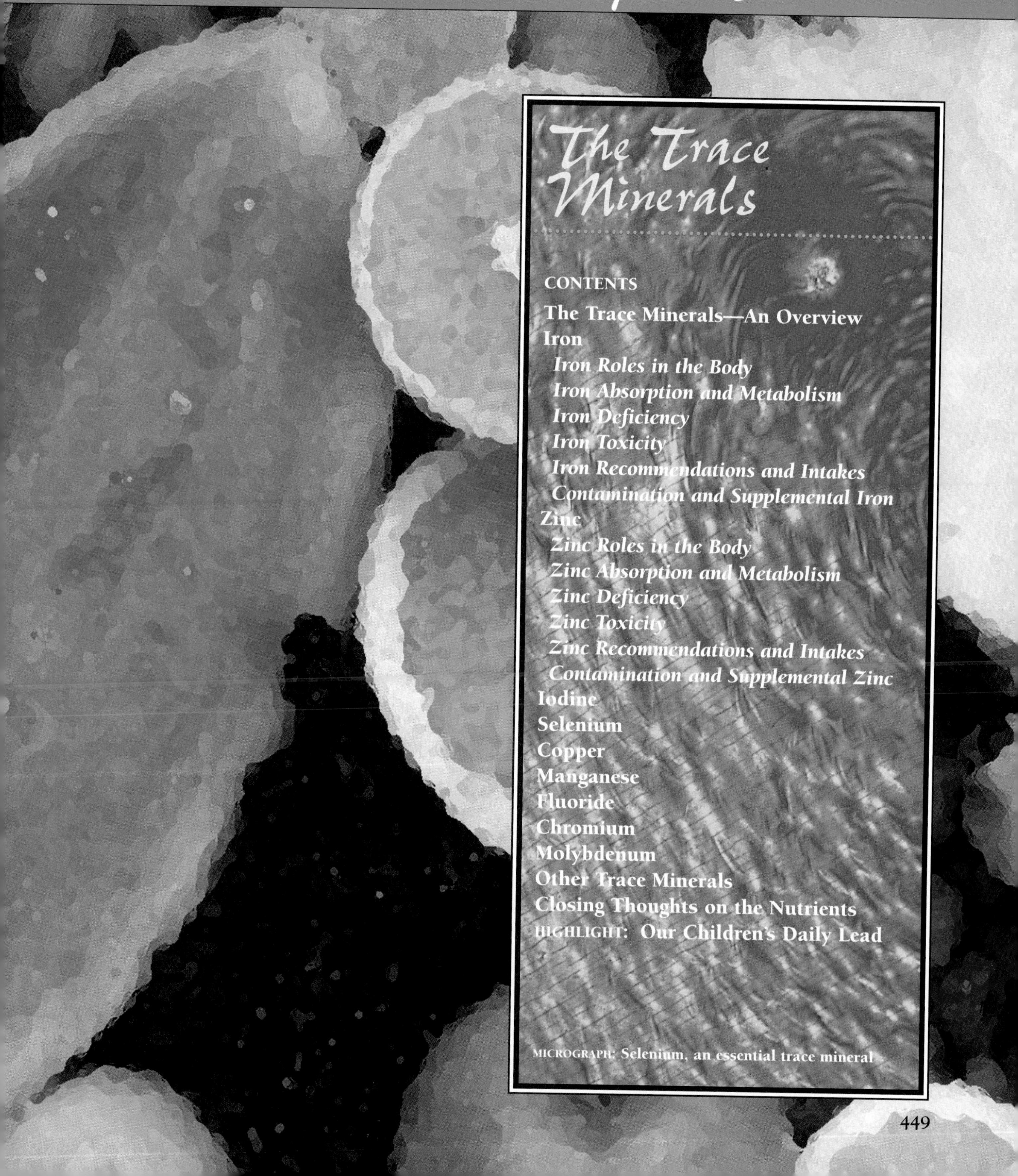

CONTENTS

The Trace Minerals—An Overview
Iron
Iron Roles in the Body
Iron Absorption and Metabolism
Iron Deficiency
Iron Toxicity
Iron Recommendations and Intakes
Contamination and Supplemental Iron
Zinc
Zinc Roles in the Body
Zinc Absorption and Metabolism
Zinc Deficiency
Zinc Toxicity
Zinc Recommendations and Intakes
Contamination and Supplemental Zinc
Iodine
Selenium
Copper
Manganese
Fluoride
Chromium
Molybdenum
Other Trace Minerals
Closing Thoughts on the Nutrients
HIGHLIGHT: **Our Children's Daily Lead**

MICROGRAPH: Selenium, an essential trace mineral

449

The trace elements (minerals):
- Iron
- Zinc   ⎤
- Iodine   ⎦— RDA nutrients
- Selenium

- Copper
- Manganese ⎤
- Fluoride   ⎦— Safe and adequate daily dietary intakes established
- Chromium
- Molybdenum

- Arsenic
- Nickel   ⎤— Known essential for animals; human requirements under study
- Silicon
- Boron

igure 12–5 in the last chapter (p. 418) showed how tiny the quantities of trace minerals in the human body are. Taken all together, they are only a bit of dust, hardly enough to fill a teaspoon. Yet each of the trace minerals performs some vital role. A deficiency of any of them may be fatal, and an excess of many is equally deadly. Remarkably, people's diets normally supply just enough of these minerals to maintain health.

The best-known trace elements—iron, zinc, iodine, and selenium—have been extensively studied, and the Committee on Dietary Allowances has established RDA for them. For five others, the committee has published tentative ranges for safe and adequate daily intakes. Still others are recognized as essential for some animals, but data from which to estimate human requirements are lacking.[1] Many other trace elements are currently under study as possible nutrients.

The Trace Minerals—An Overview

A few statements apply to the trace minerals as a group. The body requires them in minuscule quantities, and they function in some similar ways, assisting enzymes in diverse tasks all over the body. In addition, each one has special duties that only it can perform.

Food Sources   The trace mineral contents of foods are unpredictable, because they depend on soil and water quality and on how foods are processed. Furthermore, many factors in the diet and within the body affect bioavailability and absorption. Still, it is probably safe to say that a list of outstanding food sources for each of the trace minerals, just like the lists of outstanding foods for the other nutrients, would include a wide variety of foods, especially whole foods.

Deficiencies   Severe deficiencies of the better-known minerals are easy to recognize. Deficiencies of less well-known minerals are harder to diagnose, and for all minerals, mild deficiencies are easy to overlook. In general, the most common result of a deficiency is failure of children to grow and thrive, for the minerals are active in all the body systems—the GI tract, cardiovascular system, blood, muscles, bones, and central nervous system.

Toxicities   The trace elements are toxic at an intake not far above the estimated requirements. Thus it is important not to overdose. The Committee on Dietary Allowances places a special warning on its trace mineral table not to habitually exceed the upper end of the range of recommended intakes.

Supplements   Many vitamin-mineral pills contain trace minerals, making it easy for pill takers to have excessive intakes. The Food and Drug Administration (FDA) is not permitted to limit the amounts of trace minerals in supplements; consumers have demanded the freedom to choose their own doses of nutrients. Individuals who take vitamin-mineral pills must therefore be aware of the possible dangers and avoid supplements that contain more than the RDA. They would be wiser to select foods from a variety of sources than to try to put together a combination of pills to meet all their needs without causing toxicity.

Interactions   As research on the trace minerals unfolds, many interactions among them have come to light. An excess of one may cause a deficiency of another. (A slight manganese overload, for example, may aggravate an iron deficiency.) A deficiency of one may open the way for another to cause a toxic reaction. (Iron deficiency, for example, makes the body much more susceptible than normal to lead poisoning.) A deficiency of one may exacerbate the problems associated with the deficiency of another. (A combined iodine and selenium deficiency, for example, reduces thyroid hormone production more than an iodine deficiency alone.)[2] These examples point out the need to balance intakes and to steer clear of supplement use. A good food source of one nutrient may be a poor food source of another; and factors that cooperate with some trace elements may oppose others. (Vitamin C, for example, enhances the absorption of iron but depresses that of copper.) The continuous outpouring of new information about the trace minerals is a sign that we have much more to learn about them.

Iron

Iron is an essential nutrient that is vital to the processes by which cells generate energy. Iron can also be damaging when it accumulates in the body. In fact, iron is a problem nutrient for millions of people: some people simply don't eat enough iron-containing foods to support their health optimally, while others have so much iron that it threatens their well-being. The principle that too little or too much of a nutrient is harmful seems particularly apropos for iron.

IRON ROLES IN THE BODY

Iron has a knack of switching back and forth between two ionic states. In the reduced state, iron has lost two electrons and therefore has a net positive charge of two. Iron in the reduced state is known as ferrous iron. In the oxidized state, iron has lost a third electron, has a net positive charge of three, and is known as ferric iron. Because it can exist in different ionic states, iron can serve as a cofactor to enzymes involved in oxidation-reduction reactions. In every cell, iron works with several of the electron-transport-chain proteins that perform the final steps of the energy-yielding metabolic pathways.* These proteins transfer hydrogens and electrons from energy-yielding nutrients to oxygen, forming water, and in the process make ATP for the cell's use.

Most of the body's iron is found in two proteins: hemoglobin in the red blood cells and myoglobin in the muscle cells. In both, iron helps accept, carry, and then release oxygen. Iron is also found in many enzymes that oxidize compounds—reactions so widespread in metabolism that they occur in all cells. Iron is required by enzymes involved in the making of amino acids, hormones, and neurotransmitters.

Iron's two ionic states:
- Ferrous iron (reduced): Fe^{++}.
- Ferric iron (oxidized): Fe^{+++}.

For details about these ions, oxidation, and reduction, see Appendix B.

Reminder: A *cofactor* is a mineral element that works with an enzyme to facilitate a chemical reaction.

Reminder: *Hemoglobin* is the oxygen-carrying protein of the red blood cells that transports oxygen from the lungs to tissues throughout the body; hemoglobin accounts for 80% of the body's iron.

myoglobin: the oxygen-holding protein of the muscle cells.
   myo = muscle

---

*The iron-containing proteins at the end of the metabolic pathway include several TCA cycle enzymes and the electron carriers of the electron transport chain—known as *cytochromes*. See Appendix C for these pathways.

IRON ABSORPTION AND METABOLISM

The body conserves iron zealously and has devised many special provisions for its handling, depicted in Figure 13–1. Because iron losses are usually limited, balance is maintained primarily through absorption.

Iron Absorption   Two special proteins in the intestinal mucosal cells help the body absorb iron from food. One protein, called *mucosal ferritin*, receives iron from the GI tract and stores it in the mucosal cell. When the body needs iron, mucosal ferritin releases some iron to another protein, called *mucosal transferrin*. Mucosal transferrin transfers the iron to a carrier in the blood called *blood transferrin*, which transports iron to the rest of the body. Intestinal mucosal cells are replaced about every three days; when the cells are shed from the intestinal

Mucosal ferritin (FERR-ih-tin), holds iron in the cell, and mucosal transferrin (trans-FERR-in) passes the iron on to blood transferrin.

Figure 13–1

Iron Routes in the Body

Most iron is recycled. Some is lost with body tissues and must be replaced by eating iron-containing food.

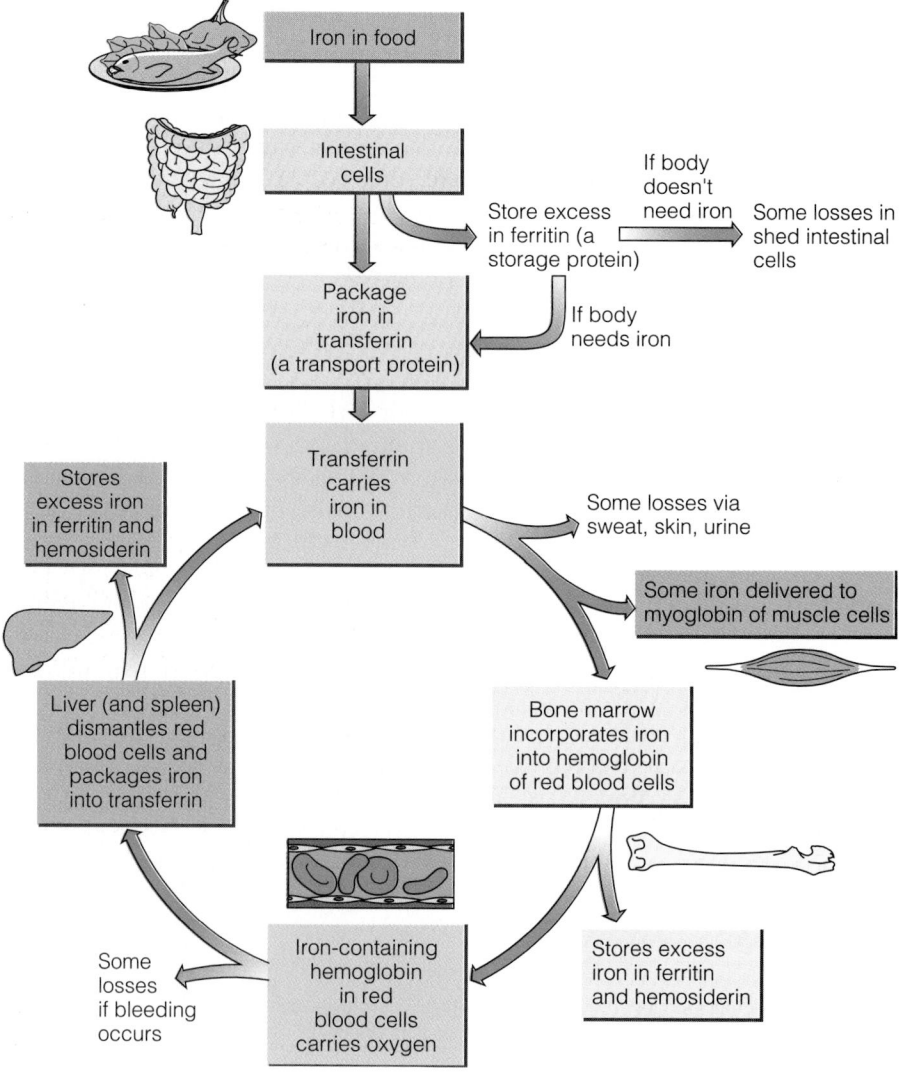

Figure 13–2

Heme and Nonheme Iron in Foods

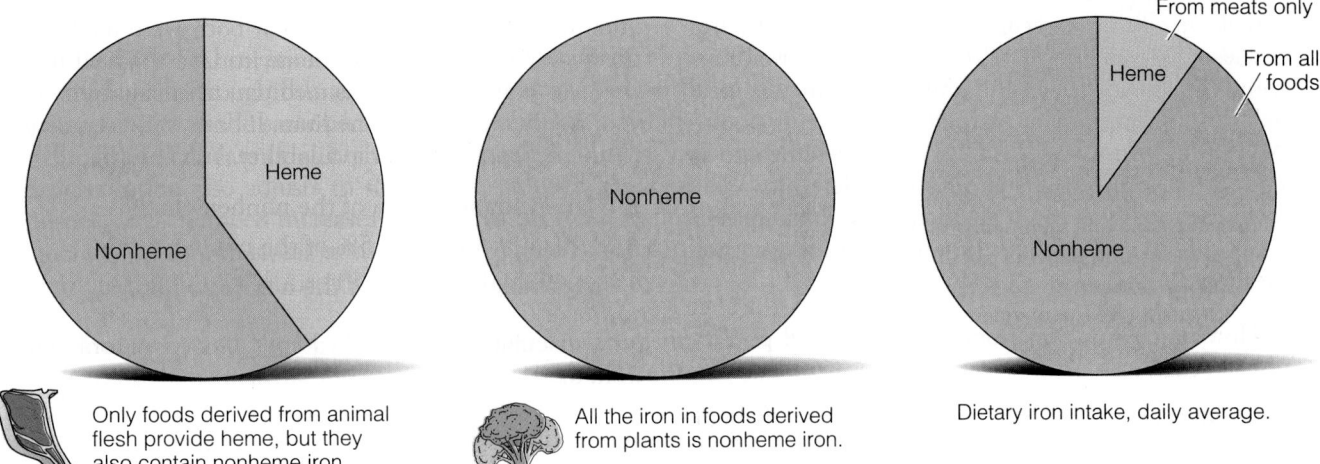

Only foods derived from animal flesh provide heme, but they also contain nonheme iron.

All the iron in foods derived from plants is nonheme iron.

Dietary iron intake, daily average.

mucosa and excreted in the feces, they carry some iron out with them. The iron-holding capacity of these cells provides a buffer against short-term changes in iron need or supply.

Heme and Nonheme Iron   How much iron is absorbed depends in part on its source. Iron occurs in two forms in foods: as heme iron, which is found only in foods derived from the flesh of animals, such as meats, poultry, and fish; and as nonheme iron, which is found in both plant-derived and animal-derived foods (see Figure 13–2). Heme iron contributes only about 10 percent of the iron the average person consumes in a day; most of the rest is nonheme iron from vegetables, fruits, grains, eggs, meat, fish, and poultry. Even though heme iron accounts for a small proportion of the intake, it is so well absorbed that it contributes significant iron: heme iron is absorbed at a relatively constant rate of about 23 percent. The rates of absorption of nonheme iron are lower, ranging from 2 to 20 percent, and are strongly influenced by dietary factors and body iron stores. People with severe iron deficiencies absorb both heme and nonheme iron more efficiently and are more sensitive to dietary enhancing factors than people with better iron status.

Absorption-Enhancing Factors: MFP and Vitamin C   Meat, fish, and poultry contain not only the highly bioavailable heme iron, but also a factor (MFP factor) that promotes the absorption of nonheme iron from other foods eaten with them.[3] Vitamin C, which also enhances nonheme iron absorption from foods eaten in the same meal, is the most potent promoter of nonheme iron absorption.[4] Vitamin C captures iron and keeps it in the ferrous form, ready for absorption. A system of calculating the iron absorbed from a meal has been developed and reveals some factors worthy of attention (see the box on p. 454).[5]

Absorption Inhibitors   Some dietary factors bind with nonheme iron, inhibiting absorption. These include the phytates and fibers in whole-grain cere-

heme (HEEM): the iron-holding part of the hemoglobin and myoglobin proteins. About 40% of the iron in meat, fish, and poultry is bound into heme; the other 60% is nonheme iron.

MFP factor: a factor associated with the digestion of meat, fish, and poultry that enhances iron absorption.

Factors that enhance nonheme iron absorption:
- Vitamin C (ascorbic acid).
- MFP factor.
- Citric acid and lactic acid from foods and HCl acid from the stomach.
- Sugars (including the sugars in wine).

Factors that reduce iron absorption:
- Phytates and fibers.
- EDTA (in food additives).
- Calcium and phosphorus (milk).
- Tannic acid (and other polyphenols).

Figure 13–3

Normal and Anemic Blood Cells

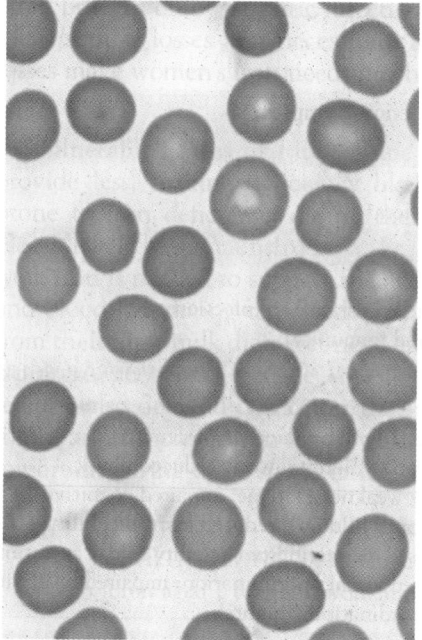 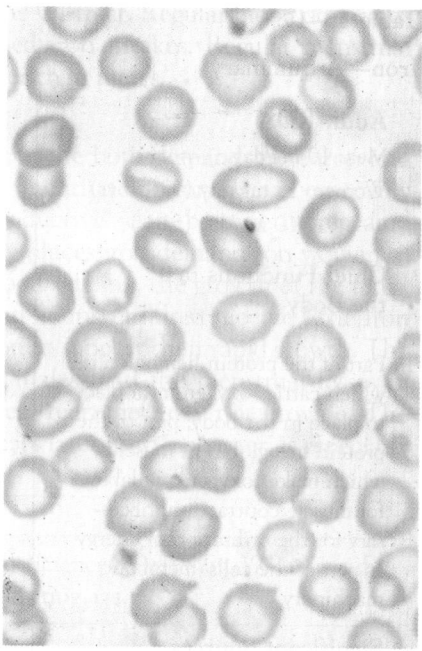

Normal blood cells. Both size and color are normal.

Blood cells in iron-deficiency anemia. These cells are small (microcytic) and pale (hypochromic) because they contain less hemoglobin.

gram for Women, Infants, and Children (WIC), which provides foods high in iron to low-income families, appears also to have helped.

The effects of iron deficiency on children's behavior are discussed in Chapter 19.

Iron Deficiency and Behavior   Long before the red blood cells are affected and anemia is diagnosed, a developing iron deficiency affects behavior. Even at slightly lowered iron levels, the complete oxidation of pyruvate is impaired, reducing physical work capacity and productivity. With reduced energy available to work, plan, think, play, sing, or learn, people simply do these things less. They have no obvious deficiency symptoms; they just appear unmotivated, apathetic, and less physically fit.

Many of the symptoms associated with iron deficiency are easily mistaken for behavioral or motivational problems. A restless child who fails to pay attention in class might be thought contrary. An apathetic homemaker who has let housework pile up might be thought lazy. No responsible nutritionist would ever claim that all behavioral problems are caused by nutrient deficiencies, but poor nutrition is always a possible contributor to problems like these. When investigating a behavioral problem, it makes sense to check the adequacy of the diet and to seek a routine physical examination before undertaking more expensive, and possibly harmful, treatment options.

pica (PIE-ka): a craving for nonfood substances. Also known as geophagia (gee-oh-FAY-gee-uh) when referring to clay eating and pagophagia (pag-oh-FAY-gee-uh) when referring to ice craving.

  picus = woodpecker or magpie
  geo = earth
  phagein = to eat
  pago = frost

Iron Deficiency and Pica   A curious behavior seen in some iron-deficient people, especially in women and children of low-income groups, is pica—an appetite for ice, clay, paste, and other nonfood substances. It is not clear whether iron deficiency precedes or follows pica. These substances contain no iron and cannot remedy a deficiency; in fact, clay actually inhibits iron absorption, which may explain the iron deficiency that accompanies such behavior.

IRON TOXICITY

The body normally absorbs less iron if its stores are full, but some individuals are poorly defended against iron toxicity. Once considered rare, iron overload has emerged as an important disorder of iron metabolism.

Iron Overload   Iron overload is known as hemochromatosis and is usually caused by a gene that enhances iron absorption. Other causes of iron overload include repeated blood transfusions, massive doses of dietary iron, and rare metabolic disorders. Long-term overconsumption of iron may cause hemosiderosis, a condition characterized by large deposits of the iron storage protein hemosiderin in the liver and other tissues.

Some of the signs and symptoms of iron overload are similar to those of iron deficiency: fatigue, headache, irritability, lowered work performance, and anemia. Therefore, taking iron supplements before measuring iron status is clearly unwise; hemoglobin tests alone would fail to make the distinction.[15]

Iron overload is most often diagnosed when tissue damage occurs, especially in iron-storing organs such as the liver. Infections are likely to develop because bacteria thrive on iron-rich blood. Other common symptoms include enlarged liver, skin pigmentation, lethargy, joint diseases, loss of body hair, amenorrhea, and impotence. These effects are most severe in people who drink large quantities of alcohol because alcohol damages the intestine, further impairing its defenses against absorbing excess iron. Untreated hemochromatosis aggravates the risks of diabetes, liver cancer, heart disease, and arthritis.

In the United States, an estimated 10 percent of the population is in positive iron balance, with 1 percent having iron overload. Iron overload is more common in men than in women and is twice as prevalent among men as is iron deficiency. Some people have expressed concerns about the widespread iron fortification of foods.[16] Widespread fortification does make it hard for people with hemochromatosis to follow a low-iron diet, but greater dangers lie in the indiscriminate use of iron and vitamin C supplements.

Iron and Heart Disease   Recent research has found that the risk of heart disease is markedly higher for the small proportion of people who have both high blood iron and high LDL cholesterol.[17] For every 1 percent rise in blood iron, there was a 4 percent rise in the risk; only smoking predicted heart attacks better than iron status. High LDL alone was not a major risk factor in this study; it only became a risk factor when accompanied by high iron. Free iron oxidizes LDL, and oxidized LDL is most damaging to the cardiovascular system. This is an important finding in light of this nation's extensive use of vitamin C supplements: vitamin C not only enhances iron absorption, but releases iron from ferritin, allowing free iron to wreak the damage typical of free radicals.[18] This is an example of how vitamin C acts as a *prooxidant* when taken in high doses (see Highlight 11).

Prior to these findings, scientists had speculated that premenopausal women were protected against heart disease by their estrogen (women's rate of heart dis-

iron overload: toxicity from excess iron.

hemochromatosis (heem-oh-crome-a-TOCE-iss): a hereditary defect in iron metabolism characterized by deposits of iron-containing pigment in many tissues, with tissue damage.

hemosiderosis (heem-oh-sid-er-OH-sis): a condition characterized by the deposition of hemosiderin in the liver and other tissues.

ease is lower and begins to approach that of men only after menopause). Now scientists are asking whether low iron stores from repeated menstrual losses might be the protective factor. (Women's iron stores tend to catch up with men's after menopause.)

Iron and Cancer   There also appears to be a positive association between iron and cancer.[19] Explanations for how iron might be involved in causing cancer focus on its involvement in lipid peroxidation (see Highlight 11). These reactions generate free radicals that can damage DNA, possibly causing cancer. One of the beneficial effects of a high-fiber diet may be that its phytate binds iron, making it less available for such reactions.

Iron Poisoning   The most common cause of accidental poisoning in small children is ingestion of iron supplements or multivitamin supplements with iron. Symptoms of intoxication include nausea, vomiting, diarrhea, a rapid heartbeat, a weak pulse, dizziness, shock, and confusion. As few as 6 to 12 iron tablets have caused death in a child within four hours. A child suspected of iron poisoning should be rushed to the hospital to have the stomach pumped; 30 minutes may make a crucial difference.

IRON RECOMMENDATIONS AND INTAKES

To obtain enough iron, people must first select iron-rich foods and then eat so as to maximize iron absorption. This discussion begins by identifying iron-rich foods, then reviews factors affecting absorption.

Recommended Iron Intakes   The usual Western mixed diet provides only about 6 to 7 milligrams of iron in every 1000 kcalories. The RDA for an adult man is 10 milligrams and most men eat more than 2000 kcalories a day, so men can meet their iron needs without special effort. The RDA for a woman during her childbearing years, however, is 15 milligrams.[20] (The box on p. 461 explains how the recommended intake is calculated.) Because women have higher iron needs and typically need fewer than 2000 kcalories per day, they have trouble obtaining sufficient iron. On the average, women receive only 10 to 11 milligrams iron per day, not enough until after menopause. To meet their iron needs from foods, premenopausal women must emphasize the most iron-rich foods in every food group at every meal.

Iron in Foods   Figure 13–4 (on p. 462) shows the amounts of iron in selected foods. Meats, fish, and poultry contribute the most iron; other protein-rich foods such as legumes and eggs provide less. Foods in the milk group are as poor in iron as they are rich in calcium. Although an indispensable part of the diet, milk products should not be overemphasized. Grain foods vary; whole-grain and enriched breads and cereals are the richest in iron. Finally, among other plant foods, legumes, dark greens, and some fruits (especially when dried) contribute iron.

Iron-Enriched Foods   Iron is one of the enrichment nutrients for breads and cereals. One serving of enriched bread or cereal provides only a little iron, but because people eat many servings of these foods, the contribution can be significant. Iron added to foods is not absorbed as well as iron occurring naturally in

How to Estimate the Recommended Daily Intake for Iron

To calculate the recommended daily iron intake, a number of factors need to be considered. For example, for an adult woman:

- Losses from shed skin: 1.0 milligram.
- Losses through menstruation (about 15 milligrams total averaged over 30 days): 0.5 milligram.
- Average daily need (total): 1.5 milligrams.
- Average iron intake: 10 to 11 milligrams per day (provides adequate stores for most women).
- Added margin of safety to cover the needs of essentially all adult women.

Assuming that an average of 10 to 15 percent of ingested iron is absorbed, the RDA is set at 15 milligrams.

foods, but eaten with absorption-enhancing foods, enrichment iron can make a difference. In some cases, enrichment may even contribute to iron overload, at least in men. At present, 25 percent of all the iron consumed in the United States derives from enriched breads, fortified breakfast cereals, and the like.

Maximizing Iron Absorption In general, the bioavailability of iron in meats, fish, and poultry is high; in grains and legumes, intermediate; and in most vegetables, especially those high in oxalate such as spinach, low. The amount of iron ultimately absorbed from a meal depends on the interplay between enhancing and inhibiting factors. For maximum absorption of nonheme iron, eat meat for MFP and fruits or vegetables for vitamin C. The iron of baked beans, for example, will be enhanced by the MFP in a piece of ham served with them; the iron of bread will be enhanced by vitamin C in a slice of tomato on a sandwich.

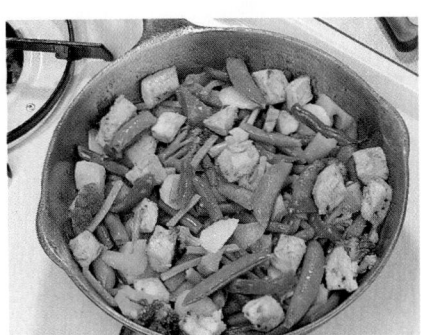

An old-fashioned iron skillet adds iron to foods.

CONTAMINATION AND SUPPLEMENTAL IRON

In addition to the iron from foods, contamination iron from nonfood sources of inorganic iron salts can contribute to the day's intakes. People can also ingest iron in supplement form.

Contamination Iron Foods cooked in iron cookware take up iron salts. A half cup of spaghetti sauce simmered in a glass dish provides 3 milligrams of iron, but the iron increases to 87 milligrams when the sauce is simmered for three hours in an iron skillet. The more acidic the food, and the longer it is cooked in iron cookware, the higher the iron content. Even in the short time it takes to scramble eggs, the cook can triple their iron content by cooking them in an iron pan. Similarly, dried peaches or raisins contain more iron than the fresh fruits do, because they are dried in iron pans. Admittedly, the absorption of this iron may be poor (perhaps only 1 to 2 percent, depending on what else is eaten with the meal), but every little bit counts.

contamination iron: iron found in foods as the result of contamination by inorganic iron salts from iron cookware, iron-containing soils, and the like.

Figure 13–4 Iron in Selected Foods

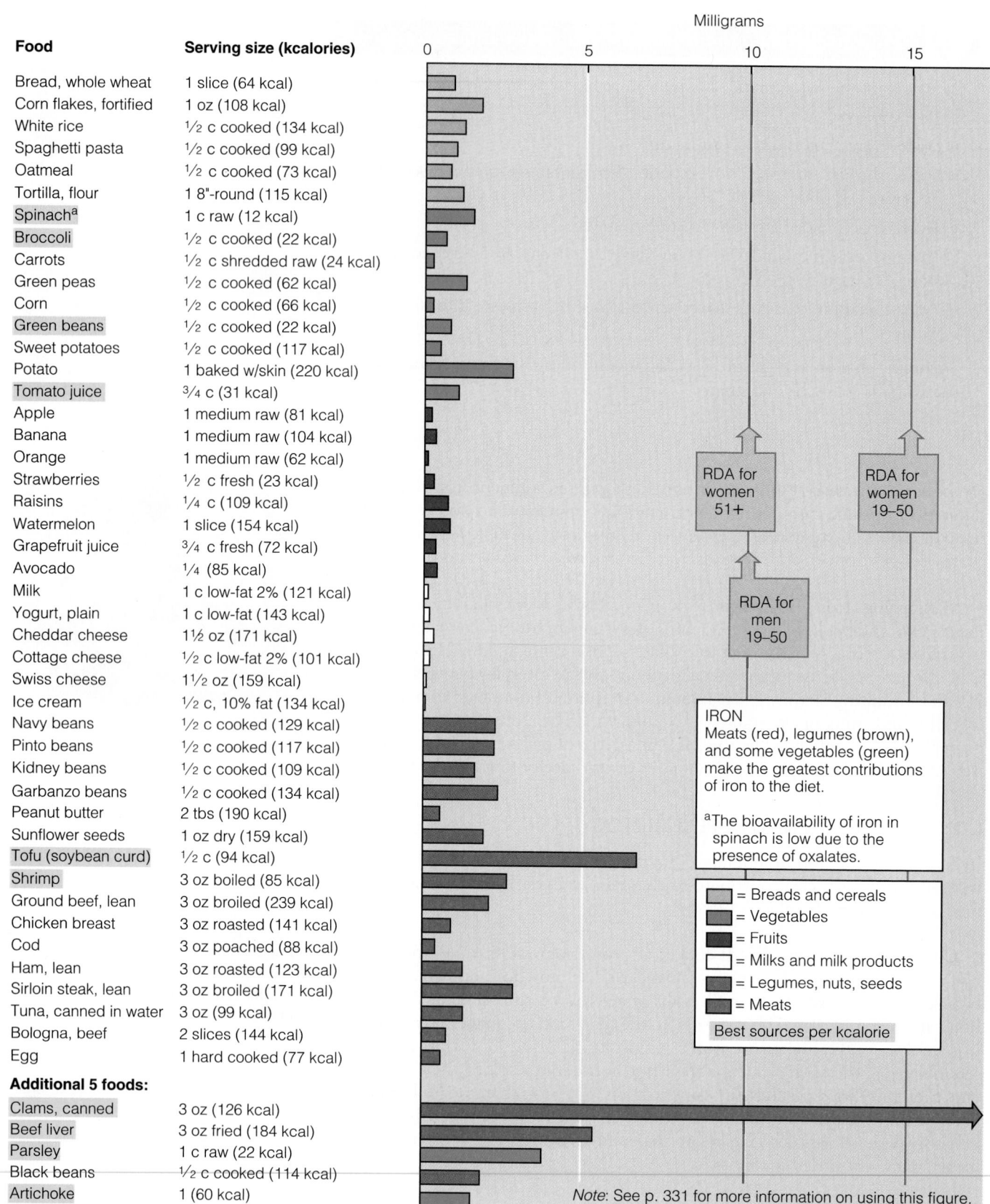

Food	Serving size (kcalories)
Bread, whole wheat	1 slice (64 kcal)
Corn flakes, fortified	1 oz (108 kcal)
White rice	½ c cooked (134 kcal)
Spaghetti pasta	½ c cooked (99 kcal)
Oatmeal	½ c cooked (73 kcal)
Tortilla, flour	1 8"-round (115 kcal)
Spinach[a]	1 c raw (12 kcal)
Broccoli	½ c cooked (22 kcal)
Carrots	½ c shredded raw (24 kcal)
Green peas	½ c cooked (62 kcal)
Corn	½ c cooked (66 kcal)
Green beans	½ c cooked (22 kcal)
Sweet potatoes	½ c cooked (117 kcal)
Potato	1 baked w/skin (220 kcal)
Tomato juice	¾ c (31 kcal)
Apple	1 medium raw (81 kcal)
Banana	1 medium raw (104 kcal)
Orange	1 medium raw (62 kcal)
Strawberries	½ c fresh (23 kcal)
Raisins	¼ c (109 kcal)
Watermelon	1 slice (154 kcal)
Grapefruit juice	¾ c fresh (72 kcal)
Avocado	¼ (85 kcal)
Milk	1 c low-fat 2% (121 kcal)
Yogurt, plain	1 c low-fat (143 kcal)
Cheddar cheese	1½ oz (171 kcal)
Cottage cheese	½ c low-fat 2% (101 kcal)
Swiss cheese	1½ oz (159 kcal)
Ice cream	½ c, 10% fat (134 kcal)
Navy beans	½ c cooked (129 kcal)
Pinto beans	½ c cooked (117 kcal)
Kidney beans	½ c cooked (109 kcal)
Garbanzo beans	½ c cooked (134 kcal)
Peanut butter	2 tbs (190 kcal)
Sunflower seeds	1 oz dry (159 kcal)
Tofu (soybean curd)	½ c (94 kcal)
Shrimp	3 oz boiled (85 kcal)
Ground beef, lean	3 oz broiled (239 kcal)
Chicken breast	3 oz roasted (141 kcal)
Cod	3 oz poached (88 kcal)
Ham, lean	3 oz roasted (123 kcal)
Sirloin steak, lean	3 oz broiled (171 kcal)
Tuna, canned in water	3 oz (99 kcal)
Bologna, beef	2 slices (144 kcal)
Egg	1 hard cooked (77 kcal)

Additional 5 foods:

Clams, canned	3 oz (126 kcal)
Beef liver	3 oz fried (184 kcal)
Parsley	1 c raw (22 kcal)
Black beans	½ c cooked (114 kcal)
Artichoke	1 (60 kcal)

Milligrams: 0   5   10   15

RDA for women 51+

RDA for women 19–50

RDA for men 19–50

IRON
Meats (red), legumes (brown), and some vegetables (green) make the greatest contributions of iron to the diet.

[a]The bioavailability of iron in spinach is low due to the presence of oxalates.

- = Breads and cereals
- = Vegetables
- = Fruits
- = Milks and milk products
- = Legumes, nuts, seeds
- = Meats

Best sources per kcalorie

Note: See p. 331 for more information on using this figure.

Iron Supplements   People who are iron deficient may need supplements as well as an iron-rich, absorption-enhancing diet. In addition, many physicians routinely recommend iron supplements to pregnant women, infants, and young children. Iron from supplements is less well absorbed than that from food, so the doses have to be high. The absorption of iron taken as ferrous sulfate or as an iron chelate is better than that from other iron supplements. Absorption also improves when supplements are taken between meals or at bedtime on an empty stomach, and with liquids other than milk, tea, or coffee, which inhibit absorption. There is no benefit to taking iron supplements with orange juice because vitamin C does not enhance absorption from supplements as it does for dietary iron. (Vitamin C helps iron absorption by converting insoluble ferric iron in foods to the more soluble ferrous iron, and supplemental iron is already in the ferrous form.) Constipation is a common side effect of iron supplementation; a plentiful fluid intake may help to relieve this problem.

A **chelate** (KEY-late) is a substance that can grasp the positive ions of a metal.
chele = claw

In summary, most of the body's iron is in hemoglobin and myoglobin where it carries oxygen for use in energy metabolism; some iron is also a cofactor for enzymes involved in a variety of reactions. Special proteins assist with iron absorption, transport, and storage—all helping to maintain an appropriate balance, because both too little and too much iron can be damaging. Iron deficiency is most common among infants and young children, teenagers, women of childbearing age, and pregnant women; symptoms include fatigue and anemia. Iron overload is most common in men and has been linked with heart disease. Heme iron, which is found only in meat, fish, and poultry, is better absorbed than nonheme iron, which occurs in most foods. Nonheme iron absorption is improved by eating iron-containing foods with foods containing the MFP factor and vitamin C.

Zinc

Zinc is a versatile trace element required as a cofactor by more than 100 enzymes in every organ in the body. Wherever protein is, zinc is. Virtually all cells contain zinc, but the highest concentrations are in bone, the prostate gland, and the eyes.[21] Muscle contains the highest proportion of total body zinc (60 percent), however, because it accounts for most of the body's mass. Tissues do not readily give up their zinc when blood levels fall, so frequent dietary intakes are necessary.[22]

Reminder: A *cofactor* is a mineral element that works with an enzyme to facilitate a chemical reaction.

metalloenzyme (MEH-tal-oh-EN-zime): an enzyme that contains one or more minerals as part of its structure.

ZINC ROLES IN THE BODY

Zinc supports the work of numerous proteins in the body—among them are the metalloenzymes, which are involved in a variety of metabolic processes.* Zinc also assists in immune function and in growth and development. Zinc associates with the hormone insulin in the pancreas, although it does not appear to play a direct role in insulin's action.[23] Zinc interacts with platelets in blood clotting, affects thyroid hormone function, and influences behavior and learning

A sampling of enzymes that zinc assists:
- Enzymes that help make parts of the genetic materials DNA and RNA.
- An enzyme that manufactures heme for hemoglobin.
- An enzyme involved in essential fatty acid metabolism.
- An enzyme that releases vitamin A from liver stores.
- Enzymes that metabolize carbohydrates.
- Enzymes that synthesize proteins.
- An enzyme that metabolizes alcohol in the liver.
- An eyzyme that disposes of damaging free radicals.

---

*Among the metalloenzymes requiring zinc are carbonic anhydrase, deoxythymidine kinase, DNA and RNA polymerase, and alkaline phosphatase.

performance. It is necessary to produce the active form of vitamin A (retinal) in visual pigments and the retinol-binding protein that transports vitamin A. It is essential to normal taste perception, wound healing, the making of sperm, and fetal development. A zinc deficiency impairs all these and other functions, underlining the vast importance of proteins as the body's working machines.

Zinc, like iron, helps protect the body from heavy metal poisoning—for example, poisoning by lead. This is especially important during fetal development and early childhood. Highlight 13 reveals the damage heavy metals can do and shows how iron and zinc help ward it off.

ZINC ABSORPTION AND METABOLISM

The body's handling of zinc resembles that of iron in some ways and differs in others. A key difference is that the mucosal cells in the intestine provide a two-way passage for zinc from the intestine to the blood and back again.

Zinc Absorption   Upon absorption into an intestinal cell, zinc has several options. It may become involved in the metabolic functions of the cell itself. Alternatively, it may be retained within the cell by metallothionein, a special binding protein that is similar to the iron storage protein ferritin.

metallothionein (meh-TAL-oh-THIGH-oh-neen): a sulfur-rich protein that avidly binds with metals such as zinc.
  metallo = containing a metal
  thio = containing sulfur
  ein = a protein

Metallothionein, the Zinc-Binding Protein   The synthesis of metallothionein in the intestinal cells helps to regulate zinc absorption. When zinc intakes are high, more metallothionein is made; it holds zinc in reserve, thus inhibiting absorption.[24] (Similarly, metallothionein in the liver binds zinc until other body tissues signal a need for it.) When the body needs zinc, intestinal metallothionein releases it into the blood where it can be transported around the body. Some zinc eventually reaches the pancreas.

Enteropancreatic Circulation of Zinc   Many of the digestive enzymes released from the pancreas into the intestine at mealtimes contain zinc. The intestine thus receives two doses of zinc with each meal—one from ingested foods and the other from the zinc-rich pancreatic secretions. The circulation of zinc in the body from the pancreas to the intestine and back to the pancreas is referred to as the enteropancreatic circulation of zinc. Thus even zinc that has already entered the body is rescreened periodically by the intestine and can be refused entry or tied up in intestinal cells on any of its times around (see Figure 13–5).

enteropancreatic (EN-ter-oh-PAN-kree-AT-ik) **circulation**: the circulatory route from the pancreas to the intestine and back to the pancreas.

Factors Affecting Absorption   The rate of zinc absorption varies from about 15 to 40 percent, depending on a person's zinc status: if more is needed, more is absorbed. Also, dietary constituents influence zinc absorption. Zinc bioavailability from beef is about four times greater than from high-fiber cereals.[25] Fiber and phytates bind zinc, thus limiting its bioavailability. Cow's milk protein (casein) also binds zinc avidly and seems to hinder absorption somewhat; infants absorb zinc better from breast milk. Milk does not inhibit adults' zinc absorption, however, so long as they ingest adequate animal protein.

Zinc Transport by Albumin   Zinc's main transport vehicle in the blood is the protein albumin, which is a major determinant of zinc absorption. This may

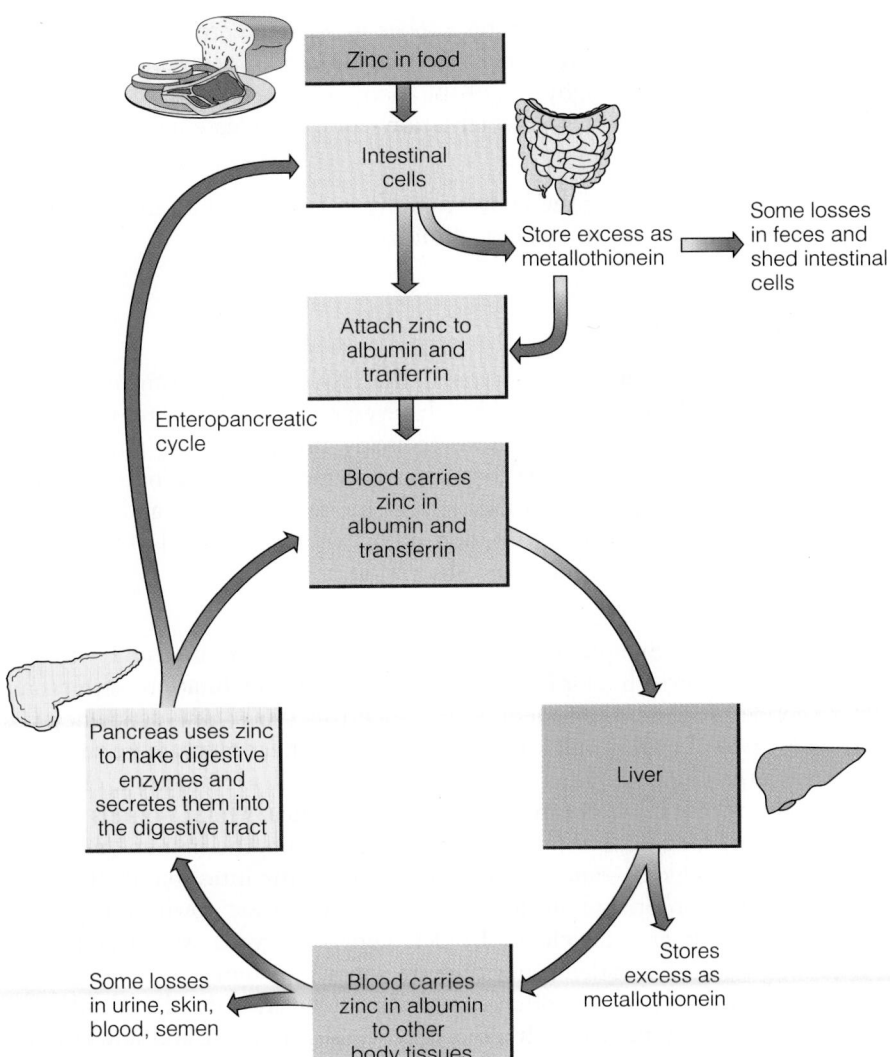

Figure 13–5
. . . .

Zinc's Routes in the Body
Notice the enteropancreatic circulation of zinc from the intestine to the pancreas and back to the intestines.

Zinc in food

Intestinal cells

Store excess as metallothionein

Some losses in feces and shed intestinal cells

Attach zinc to albumin and tranferrin

Enteropancreatic cycle

Blood carries zinc in albumin and transferrin

Pancreas uses zinc to make digestive enzymes and secretes them into the digestive tract

Liver

Stores excess as metallothionein

Some losses in urine, skin, blood, semen

Blood carries zinc in albumin to other body tissues

account for observations that zinc absorption declines in conditions that lower albumin concentrations—for example, pregnancy and malnutrition.

Zinc Interactions with Iron and Copper   Some plasma zinc also binds to transferrin—the same transferrin that carries iron in the blood. In healthy individuals, transferrin is usually less than 50 percent saturated with iron, but in iron overload, it is more saturated. Dietary iron-to-zinc ratios of greater than 2 to 1 leave too few transferrin-binding sites available for zinc and thereby impair zinc absorption. The converse is also true: large doses of zinc inhibit iron absorption.

Large doses of zinc create a similar problem with another essential mineral, copper. Recall that when zinc intakes are high, the intestinal cells synthesize large amounts of the binding protein metallothionein. This protein binds copper

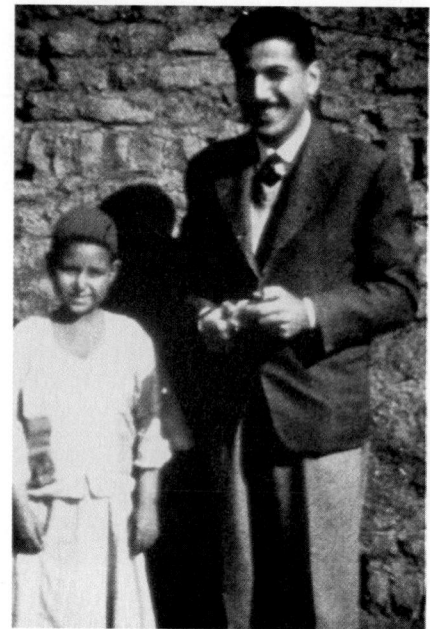

The Egyptian man on the right is an adult of average height. The Egyptian boy on the left is 17 years old but is only 4 feet tall, like a 7-year-old in the United States. His genitalia are like those of a 6-year-old. The retardation, known as *dwarfism*, is rightly ascribed to zinc deficiency because it is partially reversible when zinc is restored to the diet.

more strongly than zinc and captures copper in a nonabsorbable form.[26] This binding impairs copper absorption and may result in a copper deficiency. These nutrient interactions highlight one of the many reasons why people should use supplements conservatively: supplementation can easily create imbalances.

Zinc Losses Zinc exits the body primarily in feces. Smaller losses occur in urine, shed skin, hair, sweat, menstrual fluids, and semen.

ZINC DEFICIENCY

Human zinc deficiency was first reported in the 1960s in children and adolescent boys in Egypt, Iran, and Turkey. Children have especially high zinc needs because they are growing rapidly and synthesizing many zinc-containing proteins; the native diets among those populations were not meeting these needs. Middle Eastern diets are typically low in the richest zinc source, meats, and the staple foods are beans, unleavened breads, and other whole-grain foods—all high in fiber and phytates, which inhibit zinc absorption.*

Zinc-Deficiency Symptoms The zinc deficiency seen in the 1960s was marked by severe growth retardation and arrested sexual maturation—symptoms that responded to zinc supplementation. Since the 1960s, zinc deficiency has been recognized elsewhere, and it is now known to affect much more than just growth. It alters digestive function by impairing pancreatic function, chylomicron formation, and GI tract function. It causes diarrhea, which worsens malnutrition not only for zinc, but for all nutrients. It impairs the immune response, making infections likely—among them, infections of the intestinal tract, which worsen malnutrition, including zinc malnutrition (a classic downward spiral of events).[27] Chronic zinc deficiency hinders central nervous system and brain functioning. Because zinc deficiency directly impairs vitamin A metabolism, vitamin A–deficiency symptoms often appear. Zinc deficiency also disturbs thyroid function and the metabolic rate. It alters taste, causes anorexia, and slows wound healing—in fact, its symptoms are so all-pervasive that generalized malnutrition and sickness are more likely to be the diagnosis than simple zinc deficiency. Table 13–2 (on facing page) includes a list of zinc-deficiency symptoms.

Vulnerable Stages of Life Severe zinc deficiencies are not widespread in developed countries, but they do occur in vulnerable groups—pregnant women, young children, the elderly, and the poor. Research shows that even a mild zinc deficiency can result in poor growth, poor appetite, impaired immune response, abnormal taste, and abnormal vision in darkness.[28]

ZINC TOXICITY

Accidental high doses (2 grams or more) of zinc may cause vomiting, diarrhea, fever, exhaustion, and other symptoms (see Table 13–2). A dose of just a few milligrams above the RDA, especially when taken regularly over time, lowers the

---

*Unleavened bread contains no yeast, which normally breaks down phytates during fermentation.

Table 13–2

Zinc—A Summary

Adult RDA	Deficiency Symptoms[a]	Toxicity Symptoms
Men: 15 mg/day	**BLOOD**	
Women: 12 mg/day	High ammonia, low alkaline phosphatase, low insulin	Anemia: reduced hemoglobin production
Chief Functions in the Body	**BONES**	
	Growth retardation, abnormal collagen synthesis	Growth in length, but without normal zinc content
Part of many enzymes; associated with the hormone insulin; involved in making genetic material and proteins, immune reactions, transport of vitamin A, taste perception, wound healing, the making of sperm, and the normal development of the fetus	**CELLS/METABOLISM**	
	Slow DNA synthesis, impaired cell division and protein synthesis	Raised LDL, lowered HDL
	DIGESTIVE SYSTEM	
	Weak sense of smell, poor sensitivity to the taste of salt, weight loss, delayed glucose absorption, diarrhea, nausea, impaired folate absorption	Diarrhea, vomiting, decreased calcium and copper absorption
Significant Sources	**EYES**	
	Night blindness	
Protein-containing foods: meats, fish, poultry, whole grains, vegetables	**GLANDULAR SYSTEM**	
	Delayed onset of puberty, small gonads in males, decreased synthesis and release of testosterone, abnormal glucose tolerance, reduced synthesis of adrenocortical hormones, altered thyroid function	
	IMMUNE SYSTEM	
	Altered skin test responses, low white blood cell count, few antibody-forming cells, thymus atrophy, susceptibility to infection	Fever, elevated white blood cell count
	KIDNEY	
		Renal failure
	LIVER/SPLEEN	
	Enlargement	
	NERVOUS/MUSCULAR SYSTEMS	
	Anorexia (poor appetite), mental lethargy, irritability	Muscular pain and incoordination, heart muscle degeneration, exhaustion, dizziness, drowsiness
	REPRODUCTIVE SYSTEM	
	Impaired reproductive function (rats), low sperm counts	Reproductive failure
	SKIN	
	Generalized hair loss; lesions; rough, dry appearance; slow healing of wounds and burns	

[a]A rare inherited disease, *acrodermatitis enteropathica*, causes additional and more severe symptoms.

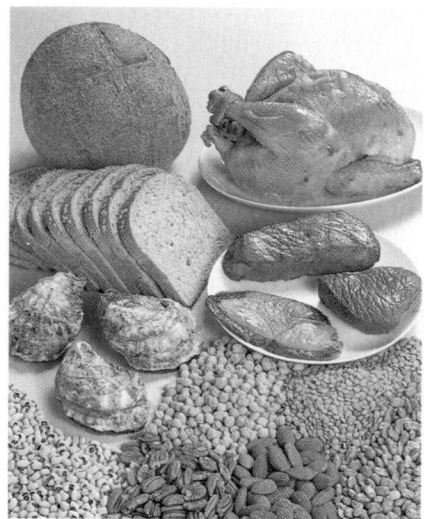

Zinc-rich foods include oysters, meat, and poultry; whole-grain breads; and legumes and nuts.

galvanized: a term referring to metals that have been treated with a zinc-containing coating to prevent rust.

body's copper content—an effect that, in animals, leads to degeneration of the heart muscle. High doses also affect cholesterol metabolism, alter lipoprotein levels, and appear to accelerate the development of atherosclerosis.

ZINC RECOMMENDATIONS AND INTAKES

In setting the zinc RDA, the Committee on Dietary Allowances assumed that 20 percent of dietary zinc is available to the body.[29] Average intakes in the United States are about 10 milligrams per day, so most people are probably not meeting the RDA. Requirements for infants and children are relatively higher than for adults due to zinc's role in normal growth and development.

Figure 13–6 (on facing page) shows zinc amounts in foods per serving. Zinc is highest in protein-rich foods such as shellfish (especially oysters), meats, poultry, and liver. Legumes and whole-grain products are good sources of zinc if large quantities are eaten; in typical U.S. diets, phytate intake from grains is not high enough to impair zinc absorption. Vegetables vary in zinc content depending on the soil in which they are grown.

CONTAMINATION AND SUPPLEMENTAL ZINC

In earlier times, galvanized cooking pots and storage vessels, contributed zinc to foods, especially to acid foods. Galvanized pipes, used in plumbing in earlier times, may also have contributed zinc to people's intakes. With today's use of stainless steel and plastic, these sources of zinc have been largely eliminated.

Zinc supplements are seldom appropriate. A decade ago, much excitement surrounded the publication of a research study that showed that zinc lozenges shortened the duration of the common cold.[30] However, results from many other studies attempting to confirm this finding have contradicted it.[31]

Zinc supplements are known to be useful in two instances: to remedy an accurately diagnosed zinc deficiency and to displace other ions in unusual medical circumstances. Otherwise, it should be possible to obtain enough zinc from the diet without resorting to supplements.

To summarize, zinc assists enzymes in a multitude of reactions affecting growth, vitamin A activity, and pancreatic digestive enzyme synthesis, among others. Both dietary zinc and zinc-rich pancreatic secretions (via enteropancreatic circulation) are available for absorption. Absorption is monitored by a special binding protein (metallothionein) in the intestine. High-protein foods derived from animals are the best sources of zinc of high bioavailability. Fiber and phytates in cereals bind zinc, limiting absorption. Growth retardation and sexual immaturity are hallmark symptoms of zinc deficiency.

Iodine

Like chlorine gas, iodine gas is poisonous; however, the iodine ion that occurs in foods is far less toxic, and traces of it are indispensable to life. Any iodine ingested in foods is converted to the iodide ion in the GI tract; this chapter uses *iodine* when referring to the nutrient in foods and *iodide* when referring to it in

Figure 13–6   Zinc in Selected Foods

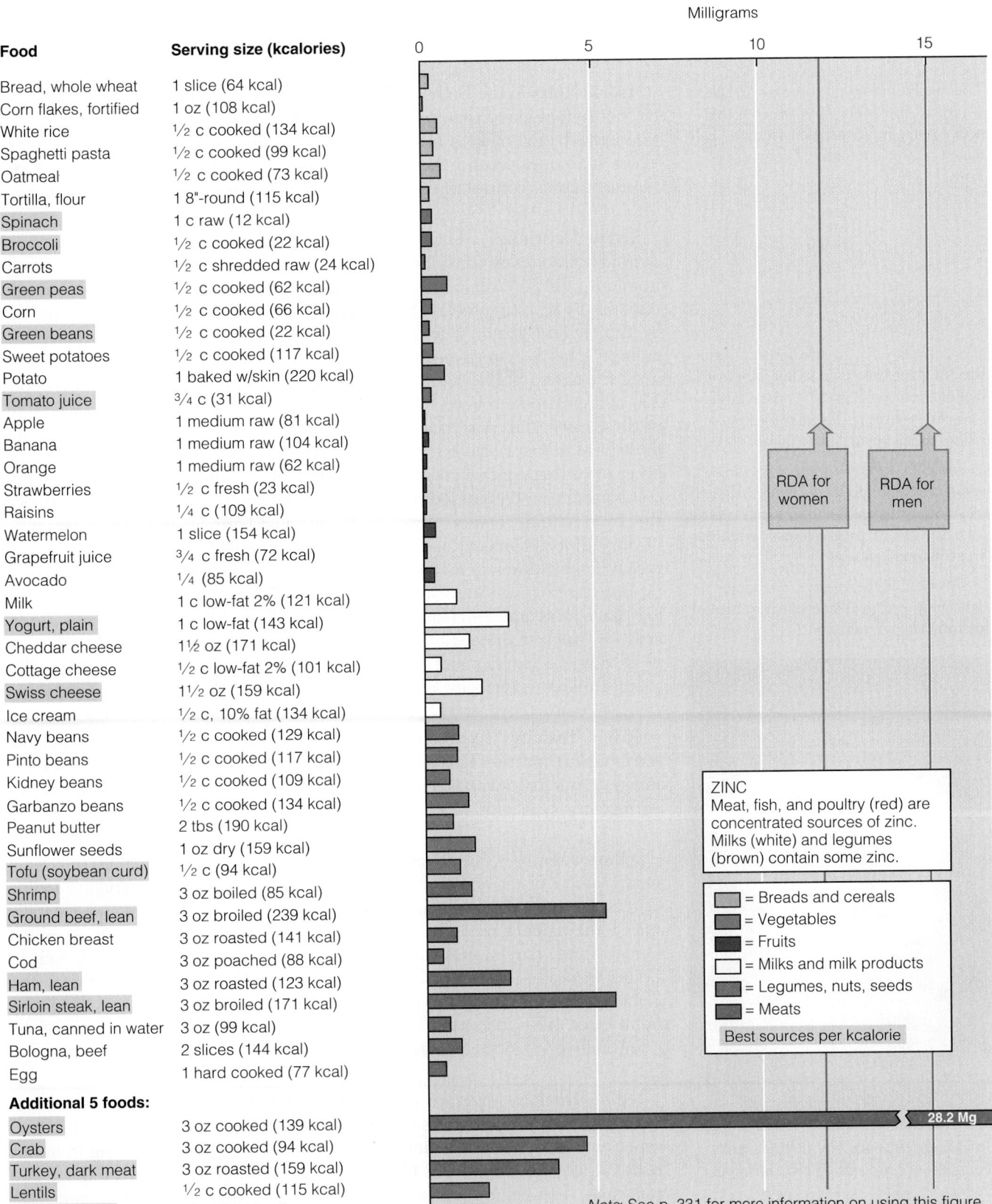

Food	Serving size (kcalories)
Bread, whole wheat	1 slice (64 kcal)
Corn flakes, fortified	1 oz (108 kcal)
White rice	½ c cooked (134 kcal)
Spaghetti pasta	½ c cooked (99 kcal)
Oatmeal	½ c cooked (73 kcal)
Tortilla, flour	1 8"-round (115 kcal)
Spinach	1 c raw (12 kcal)
Broccoli	½ c cooked (22 kcal)
Carrots	½ c shredded raw (24 kcal)
Green peas	½ c cooked (62 kcal)
Corn	½ c cooked (66 kcal)
Green beans	½ c cooked (22 kcal)
Sweet potatoes	½ c cooked (117 kcal)
Potato	1 baked w/skin (220 kcal)
Tomato juice	¾ c (31 kcal)
Apple	1 medium raw (81 kcal)
Banana	1 medium raw (104 kcal)
Orange	1 medium raw (62 kcal)
Strawberries	½ c fresh (23 kcal)
Raisins	¼ c (109 kcal)
Watermelon	1 slice (154 kcal)
Grapefruit juice	¾ c fresh (72 kcal)
Avocado	¼ (85 kcal)
Milk	1 c low-fat 2% (121 kcal)
Yogurt, plain	1 c low-fat (143 kcal)
Cheddar cheese	1½ oz (171 kcal)
Cottage cheese	½ c low-fat 2% (101 kcal)
Swiss cheese	1½ oz (159 kcal)
Ice cream	½ c, 10% fat (134 kcal)
Navy beans	½ c cooked (129 kcal)
Pinto beans	½ c cooked (117 kcal)
Kidney beans	½ c cooked (109 kcal)
Garbanzo beans	½ c cooked (134 kcal)
Peanut butter	2 tbs (190 kcal)
Sunflower seeds	1 oz dry (159 kcal)
Tofu (soybean curd)	½ c (94 kcal)
Shrimp	3 oz boiled (85 kcal)
Ground beef, lean	3 oz broiled (239 kcal)
Chicken breast	3 oz roasted (141 kcal)
Cod	3 oz poached (88 kcal)
Ham, lean	3 oz roasted (123 kcal)
Sirloin steak, lean	3 oz broiled (171 kcal)
Tuna, canned in water	3 oz (99 kcal)
Bologna, beef	2 slices (144 kcal)
Egg	1 hard cooked (77 kcal)

Additional 5 foods:

Food	Serving size (kcalories)
Oysters	3 oz cooked (139 kcal)
Crab	3 oz cooked (94 kcal)
Turkey, dark meat	3 oz roasted (159 kcal)
Lentils	½ c cooked (115 kcal)
Ricotta cheese	½ c (170 kcal)

Milligrams

RDA for women

RDA for men

ZINC
Meat, fish, and poultry (red) are concentrated sources of zinc. Milks (white) and legumes (brown) contain some zinc.

= Breads and cereals
= Vegetables
= Fruits
= Milks and milk products
= Legumes, nuts, seeds
= Meats

Best sources per kcalorie

28.2 Mg

Note: See p. 331 for more information on using this figure.

The two hormones from the thyroid gland are triiodothyronine (T$_3$), which is the active form, and tetraiodothyronine (T$_4$), which is more commonly known as *thyroxin*.

goiter (GOY-ter): an enlargement of the thyroid gland due to an iodine deficiency, malfunction of the gland, or overconsumption of a goitrogen. Goiter caused by iodine deficiency is simple goiter.

goitrogen (GOY-troh-jen): a thyroid antagonist found in food; causes toxic goiter. Goitrogens are found in such foods as cabbage, kale, brussels sprouts, cauliflower, broccoli, and kohlrabi.

cretinism (CREE-tin-ism): an iodine-deficiency disease characterized by mental and physical retardation.

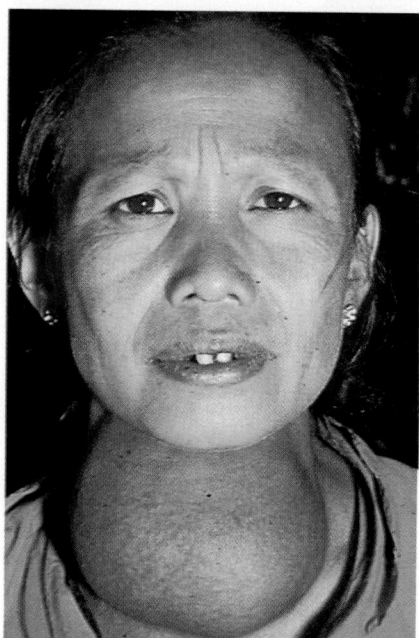

In iodine deficiency, the thyroid gland enlarges—a condition known as simple goiter.

the body. Iodide occurs in the body in a tiny quantity, but its principal role in human nutrition is well known, and the amount needed is well established.

Iodide Roles in the Body   Iodide is an integral part of two hormones released by the thyroid gland that regulate body temperature, metabolic rate, reproduction, growth, the making of blood cells, nerve and muscle function, and more. These hormones control the rate at which the cells use oxygen; that is to say, these hormones control the rate at which energy is released during metabolism.

Iodine Deficiency   The hypothalamus regulates the plasma concentrations of thyroid hormones by controlling the release of the pituitary's thyroid-stimulating hormone (TSH). With iodine deficiency, thyroid hormone declines, and the body responds by secreting more TSH in a futile attempt to accelerate iodide uptake by the thyroid gland. If a deficiency persists, the cells of the thyroid gland enlarge, so as to trap as much iodide as possible. Sometimes the gland enlarges until it makes a visible lump in the neck, a simple goiter. Goiter afflicts about 200 million people the world over, many of them in Africa. In all but 4 percent of these cases, the cause is iodine deficiency. As for the 4 percent (8 million), most have goiter because they overconsume plants of the cabbage family and other foods that contain an antithyroid substance (goitrogen) whose effect is not counteracted by dietary iodine. The goitrogens present in plants serve notice that even natural components of foods can cause harm when eaten in excess.

An iodine deficiency causes sluggishness and weight gain. During pregnancy, it may impair development of the fetus, causing the extreme and irreversible mental and physical retardation known as cretinism. An infant with cretinism may have a mental deficiency and a face and body with many physical abnormalities. Much of the mental retardation of cretinism can be averted by diagnosis of iodine deficiency and treatment early in pregnancy. Iodine deficiency in young children is typically associated with goiter and poor school performance.

Iodine Toxicity   Excessive intakes of iodine can enlarge the thyroid gland, just as deficiency can. This goiterlike condition can be so severe as to block the airways in infants and cause suffocation. The toxic dose is thought to be over 2000 micrograms per day for an adult—several times higher than average intakes.

Iodine Sources   The ocean is the world's major source of iodine. In coastal areas, seafood, water, and even iodine-containing sea mist are dependable iodine sources. Further inland, the amount of iodine in foods is variable and generally reflects the amount present in the soil in which plants are grown or on which animals graze. Landmasses that were once under the ocean have soils rich in iodine; those that were not have iodine-poor soils. In the United States and Canada, the soil around the Great Lakes and the inland valleys of Oregon is iodine-poor. The iodization of salt eliminated widespread misery caused by iodine deficiency in the people of these regions during the 1930s.

Iodine Intakes   Average consumption of iodine in the United States is about 200 to 500 micrograms—more than the RDA, but below toxic levels as well. Some of the excess iodine in the U.S. diet seems to be coming from fast foods, which use iodized salt liberally. Some comes from bakery products and from milk. The baking industry uses iodates as dough conditioners, and most

Table 13–3

Iodine—A Summary

Adult RDA	Deficiency Disease Name	
150 μg/day	Simple goiter, cretinism	
Chief Functions in the Body	**Deficiency Symptoms**	**Toxicity Symptoms**
A component of two thyroid hormones that help to regulate growth, development, and metabolic rate	Enlargement of the thyroid gland, weight gain, mental and physical retardation of an infant	Enlargement of the thyroid gland, depressed thyroid activity
Significant Sources		
Iodized salt, seafood, bread, dairy products, plants grown in iodine-rich soil and animals fed those plants		

dairies feed cows iodine-containing medications and use iodine to disinfect milking equipment. Now that these sources have been identified, food industries have reduced their use of these compounds, but the sudden emergence of this problem points to a need for continued surveillance of the food supply. Table 13–3 provides a summary of iodine.

Iodine Recommendation   The recommended intake of iodine for adults is a minuscule amount. The need for iodine is easily met by consuming seafood, vegetables grown in iodine-rich soil, and iodized salt. In the United States, labels state whether salt is iodized; in Canada, all table salt is iodized.

2 g iodized salt (less than ½ tsp) contains the RDA for iodine.

Selenium

The essential mineral selenium is one of the body's antioxidants, working closely with the enzyme glutathione peroxidase. Glutathione peroxidase prevents free-radical formation, thus blocking the chain reaction before it begins. (Highlight 11 describes free-radical formation, chain reactions, and antioxidant action in detail.) Glutathione peroxidase and vitamin E work in concert: if free radicals do form and a chain reaction starts, vitamin E halts it. Selenium also works closely with the enzyme that converts thyroid hormone to its active form.

selenium (se-LEEN-ee-um): a trace element.

Selenium Deficiency   At first, selenium's antioxidant function was the only evidence that it was essential for human beings. Then, in the 1970s, the discovery that selenium deficiency was associated with a heart disease in hundreds of thousands of children in China intensified research efforts to learn more about this mineral. The heart disease is prevalent in regions of China where the soil and foods are selenium-poor. The primary cause of this heart disease is probably a virus, but selenium deficiency appears to predispose people to it, and adequate selenium seems to prevent it.

The heart disease associated with selenium deficiency is named Keshan disease for one of the provinces of China where it was studied. Keshan disease is characterized by heart enlargement and insufficiency; the middle layer of the walls of the heart, which are normally composed of muscle tissue, are replaced with fibrous tissue.

Selenium and Cancer   In other parts of the world, selenium-poor soil correlates with a high incidence of certain kinds of cancer. This finding has stimulated research with both animal and human subjects seeking to find out whether

Table 13–4

Selenium—A Summary

Adult RDA	Chief Functions in the Body	Deficiency Symptoms	Toxicity Symptoms	Significant Sources
Men: 70 μg/day Women: 55 μg/day	Part of an enzyme system that works with vitamin E to protect body compounds from oxidation	Predisposition to heart disease characterized by cardiac tissue becoming fibrous	Digestive system disorders, loss of hair and nails, skin lesions, nervous system disorders, tooth damage	Seafood, meat, grains

dietary selenium adequacy is one of the many factors that may protect against cancer. So far, research results are inconclusive.

Selenium Intakes   Some regions in the United States and Canada produce crops on selenium-poor soil, but the people are protected from deficiency, partly because they eat supermarket foods transported from other regions, and partly because of their high intakes of selenium-rich meats. Meats and other animal products are reliable sources of selenium because selenium is associated with the protein parts of foods.

Selenium Toxicity   High doses (a milligram or more daily) of selenium are toxic. Selenium toxicity causes vomiting, diarrhea, loss of hair and nails, and lesions of the skin and nervous system. The inappropriate use of selenium supplements as an anticancer agent poses the possibility of selenium overdose.[32] See Table 13–4 for a summary of selenium.

Copper

The body contains about 100 milligrams of copper.[33] About one-third is in the muscles, one-third is in the liver and brain, and the rest is in the bones, kidneys, blood, and other tissues.

Copper Roles in the Body   Copper serves as a constituent of enzymes. The copper-containing enzymes have diverse metabolic roles with one common characteristic: all involve reactions that consume oxygen or oxygen radicals. For example, copper-containing enzymes catalyze the oxidation of ferrous iron to ferric iron.* Copper's role in iron metabolism makes it a key factor in hemoglobin synthesis. Another copper- and zinc-containing enzyme functions as an antioxidant.† Still another copper enzyme helps to manufacture collagen and heal wounds.‡ Copper, like iron, is needed in many of the reactions related to respiration and the release of energy.**

---

*The copper-requiring enzymes ceruloplasmin and ferroxidase II participate in the oxidation of ferrous iron to ferric iron.

†The copper-requiring enzyme superoxide dismutase protects cell membranes against free-radical damage.

‡The copper-requiring enzyme lysyl oxidase helps synthesize connective tissues.

**The copper-requiring enzyme cytochrome C oxidase is part of the electron transport chain.

Table 13–5

Copper—A Summary

Estimated Safe and Adequate Intake	Chief Functions in the Body	Deficiency Symptoms	Toxicity Symptoms	Significant Sources
Adults: 1.5–3.0 mg/day	Necessary for the absorption and use of iron in the formation of hemoglobin; part of several enzymes	Anemia, bone abnormalities (rare in human beings)	Vomiting, diarrhea	Meat, drinking water

Copper Deficiency and Toxicity   Copper deficiency is rare, but not unknown. It has been seen in malnourished children, and it can severely disturb growth and metabolism. Excess zinc, as mentioned, interferes with copper absorption and can cause deficiency. Copper deficiency in animals raises blood cholesterol and damages blood vessels, leading researchers to explore whether low dietary copper might contribute to cardiovascular disease.[34] Copper toxicity from foods is unlikely, but supplements can cause it.

Copper Recommendations and Intakes   The richest food sources of copper are legumes, grains, nuts, organ meats, and seeds. About a third of the copper taken in food is absorbed, and the rest is eliminated in the feces. Water also provides copper; its content varies with the type of plumbing pipe and hardness of the water. See Table 13–5 for a summary of copper facts.

Manganese

The human body contains a tiny 20 milligrams of manganese, mostly in the bones and metabolically active organs such as the liver, kidneys, and pancreas. Manganese acts as cofactor for many enzymes that facilitate dozens of different metabolic processes. For example, manganese metalloenzymes assist in urea synthesis, the conversion of pyruvate to a TCA cycle compound, and the prevention of lipid peroxidation by free radicals.

Manganese Deficiency   Deficiencies of manganese have not been seen in human beings. In animals, manganese deficiency alters fat metabolism and deranges many systems, including the skeletal, reproductive, and nervous systems. Manganese requirements are low, and many plant foods contain significant amounts of this trace mineral, so deficiencies are unlikely. As is true of other trace minerals, however, dietary factors influence manganese absorption: both iron and calcium inhibit manganese absorption. This interaction may depress the manganese status of people who use iron and calcium supplements regularly.

Manganese Toxicity   Toxicity is more likely to occur when the environment is contaminated with manganese than from dietary intake. Miners who inhale large quantities of manganese dust on the job over prolonged periods show symptoms of a brain disease, along with abnormalities of appearance and behavior. A summary of manganese appears in Table 13–6.

Table 13–6

Manganese—A Summary

Estimated Safe and Adequate Intake	Chief Functions in the Body	Deficiency Symptoms	Toxicity Symptoms	Significant Sources
Adults: 2–5 mg/day	Facilitator, with enzymes, of many cell processes	(In experimental animals): poor growth, nervous system disorders, reproductive abnormalities	Nervous system disorders	Widely distributed in foods

Fluoride

Fluoride is present in virtually all soils, water supplies, plants, and animals. Only a trace of fluoride occurs in the human body, but with this amount, the crystalline deposits in bones and teeth are larger and more perfectly formed. Table 13–7 summarizes fluoride information.

Reminder: *Hydroxyapatite* is the major calcium-containing crystal of bones and teeth.

fluorapatite (floor-APP-uh-tite): the stabilized form of bone and tooth crystal, in which fluoride has replaced the hydroxyl groups of hydroxyapatite.

Fluoride Roles in the Body   When bones and teeth become mineralized, a crystal called hydroxyapatite forms from calcium and phosphorus. Then fluoride replaces the hydroxyl (OH) portions of the hydroxyapatite crystal, forming fluorapatite, which makes the bones stronger and the teeth more resistant to decay.

Fluoridation and Dental Caries   Dental caries ranks as the nation's most widespread health problem: an estimated 95 percent of the population have decayed, missing, or filled teeth. Dental problems interfere with a person's ability to chew and eat a wide variety of foods, and this can lead to a multitude of nutrition problems. Where fluoride is lacking, dental decay is common. By fluoridating the drinking water, a community offers its residents, particularly the children, a safe, economical, practical, and effective way to defend against dental caries.[35]

All normal diets contain some fluoride, but drinking water is usually the most significant source. The National Research Council of the National Academy of Sciences recommends fluoridation of drinking water to raise the concentration

Table 13–7

Fluoride—A Summary

Adult DRI[a]	Chief Functions in the Body	Deficiency Symptoms	Toxicity Symptoms	Significant Sources
3.8 mg/day (men) 3.1 mg/day (women)	An element involved in the formation of bones and teeth; helps to make teeth resistant to decay	Susceptibility to tooth decay	Fluorosis (discoloration of teeth), nausea, diarrhea, chest pain, itching, vomiting	Drinking water (if fluoride containing or fluoridated), tea, seafood

[a]1997 recommendations for fluoride are called Dietary Reference Intakes (DRI).

to about 1 part fluoride per 1 million parts water. Water with 1 part per million (1 ppm) fluoride offers the greatest protection against dental caries at virtually no risk of toxicity.

Fluoride and Osteoporosis The role of fluoride in protecting against adult bone loss (osteoporosis) is less clear than its role in protecting against tooth decay. Early studies reported that osteoporosis was more common in areas where the water was low in fluoride than in high-fluoride areas. Subsequent research shows that fluoride (administered as sodium fluoride) clearly affects bone, but the effects may be detrimental.[36] Highlight 12 mentions research findings on the use of fluoride in osteoporosis treatment.

Fluorosis and Other Toxic Effects In communities where the water naturally contains elevated levels of fluoride (2 to 8 parts per million), fluorosis, or discoloration of the teeth, may occur. More serious cases of fluoride poisoning have been reported in communities where the public water system failed and allowed fluoride concentrations to reach 150 parts per million.[37] Symptoms of fluoride poisoning include nausea, vomiting, diarrhea, abdominal pain, and numbness or tingling of the face and extremities.

Fluoride Intakes About half of the U.S. population has access to water with an optimal fluoride concentration, which typically delivers about 1 milligram per person per day. Fish and most teas contain appreciable amounts of natural fluoride.

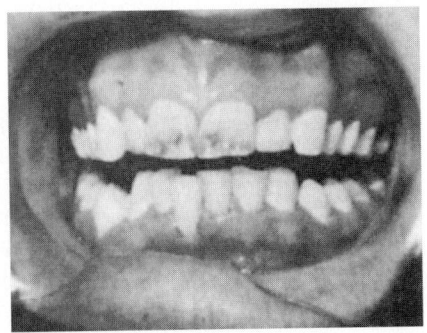

Fluorosis.

1 ppm = 1 mg per liter.

fluorosis: discoloration of tooth enamel caused by excess fluoride.

Chromium

Chromium is an essential mineral that participates in carbohydrate and lipid metabolism. Like iron, chromium can have different charges. In the case of chromium, the Cr^{+++} ion seems to be the best absorbed and most effective in living systems. The percentage of chromium absorbed rises with low dietary intake and falls with high dietary intake.

Chromium Roles in the Body Chromium helps maintain glucose homeostasis. Experiments on animals have shown that chromium works closely with the hormone insulin to facilitate glucose uptake into cells and energy release. When chromium is lacking, a diabeteslike condition of high blood glucose results. Research on human beings suggests that diets low in chromium may impair glucose tolerance, insulin response, and glucagon response.[38]

Early research identified chromium as a part of a small organic compound called the glucose tolerance factor (GTF) that enhances insulin's action. Recent studies have identified other glucose tolerance factors that do not contain chromium. Because nonchromium factors may also enhance insulin's action, "biologically active chromium" may better describe the chromium-containing compounds. Although the details remain somewhat unclear, most researchers agree that chromium participates in insulin's action.

glucose tolerance factor (GTF): a small organic compound that enhances insulin's action.

Chromium Recommendations and Intakes Chromium is present in a variety of foods.[39] Still, an estimated 90 percent of U.S. adults consume less than the suggested minimum intake of 50 micrograms a day.[40] Unrefined foods are the

Table 13–8

Chromium—A Summary

Estimated Safe and Adequate Intake	Chief Functions in the Body	Deficiency Symptoms	Toxicity Symptoms	Significant Sources
Adults: 50–200 μg/day	Associated with insulin and required for the release of energy from glucose	Diabeteslike condition marked by an inability to use glucose normally	Unknown as a nutrition disorder; occupational exposures damage skin and kidneys	Meat, unrefined foods, fats, vegetable oils

best sources, particularly liver, brewer's yeast, whole grains, nuts, and cheeses. The more refined foods people eat, the less chromium they ingest. Older people are most susceptible to marginal intakes because many lack appetite or the desire to prepare and eat meals. Table 13–8 provides a summary of chromium.

Molybdenum

molybdenum (mo-LIB-duh-num): a trace element.

Molybdenum is an important mineral in human and animal physiology. It acts as a working part of several metalloenzymes. Deficiencies of molybdenum are unknown in animals and human beings because the amounts needed are minuscule—as little as 0.1 part per million parts of body tissue. Legumes, breads and other grains, leafy green vegetables, milk, and liver are molybdenum-rich foods.[41] Average daily intakes fall within the suggested range of intakes.

Molybdenum toxicity is rare, but has been reported in workers exposed to its dust. Characteristics include goutlike symptoms in human beings. For a summary of molybdenum facts, see Table 13–9.

Other Trace Minerals

Several trace minerals have been known for decades, and understanding their roles in the body has become a rapidly growing research area. Research to determine whether other trace minerals are essential is difficult, both because their

Table 13–9

Molybdenum—A Summary

Estimated Safe and Adequate Intake	Chief Functions in the Body	Deficiency Symptoms	Toxicity Symptoms	Significant Sources
Adults: 75–250 μg/day	Facilitator, with enzymes, of many cell processes	Unknown	Enzyme inhibition, goutlike symptoms	Legumes, cereals, organ meats

quantities in the body are so small and because human deficiencies are unknown. Much of the available knowledge comes from research using animals.

Nickel is now recognized as important for the health of many body tissues; deficiencies harm the liver and other organs. Silicon is needed for healthy bones, brains, and blood vessels in animals; some researchers believe it may be essential for human beings as well.[42] Tin is necessary for growth in animals. Vanadium, too, is necessary for growth and bone development and also for normal reproduction; human intakes of vanadium may barely exceed the minimum needed for health. Cobalt is a key mineral in the large vitamin B_{12} molecule (see Figure 13–7), but it is not an essential nutrient and no RDA has been established. Boron may play a key role in bone development and oppose demineralization in osteoporosis.[43] In the future many other trace minerals may turn out to play key nutritional roles: silver, mercury, lead, barium, and cadmium. Even arsenic—famous as a poison used by murderers and known to be a carcinogen—may turn out to be essential for human beings in tiny quantities.

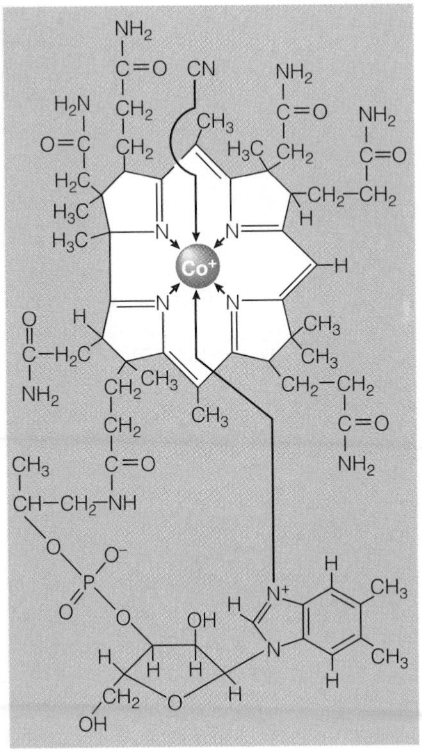

Closing Thoughts on the Nutrients

This chapter completes the introductory lessons on the nutrients. Each nutrient from the amino acids to zinc has been described rather thoroughly—its chemistry, roles in the body, sources in the diet, symptoms of deficiency and toxicity, and influences on health and disease. Such a detailed examination is informative, but it can also be misleading. It is important to step back from the myopic study of the individual nutrients to look at them as a whole. After all, people eat foods, not nutrients, and most foods deliver several nutrients. Furthermore, nutrients work cooperatively with each other in the body; their actions are most often *interactions*. This chapter alone mentioned how iron needs vitamin C to keep it in its active form and copper to incorporate it into hemoglobin; how zinc is needed to activate and transport vitamin A; and how both iodine and selenium are needed in the synthesis of thyroid hormones.

Estimates of how much of each particular nutrient the body needs are based on principles that are changing.[44] Nutrient needs fall into the broad area between intakes that are inadequate and cause illness and intakes that are excessive and cause illness. Between deficiency and toxicity lies a wide range of intakes that support health—to varying degrees. In the past, nutrient needs were determined by how much was needed to cure deficiency symptoms. If lack of a nutrient caused illness, it was defined as essential.

Today's research is rethinking nutrient needs based on how much is needed to support optimal health. The amount of vitamin C needed to prevent scurvy is much less than the amount correlated with reducing the risk of cancer, for example. Furthermore, nutrients are being examined within the context of the whole diet. Health benefits are not credited to vitamin C alone, but to the vitamin C–rich fruits and vegetables that also provide many other nutrients—and nonnutrients—important to health.

Yet foods can also pose hazards to health. The next chapter looks at consumer concerns about foods and the possible hazards they may present.

Figure 13–7

Cobalt with Vitamin B_{12}

The intricate vitamin B_{12} molecule contains one atom of cobalt. The alternative name for vitamin B_{12}, cobalamin, reflects the presence of cobalt in its structure.

Study Questions

1. Distinguish between heme and nonheme iron. Discuss the factors that enhance iron absorption.
2. Distinguish between iron deficiency and iron-deficiency anemia. What are the symptoms of iron-deficiency anemia?
3. What causes iron overload? What are its symptoms?
4. Discuss possible reasons for a low intake of zinc. What factors affect the bioavailability of zinc?
5. Describe the similarities and differences in the absorption and regulation of iron and zinc.
6. Describe the principal functions of iodide, selenium, copper, fluoride, and chromium in the body.
7. What public health measure has been used in preventing simple goiter? What measure has been recommended for protection against tooth decay?
8. Discuss the importance of balanced and varied diets in obtaining the essential minerals and avoiding toxicities.
9. Describe some of the ways trace minerals interact with each other and with other nutrients.

Notes

1. Committee on Dietary Allowances, *Recommended Dietary Allowances*, 10th ed. (Washington, D.C.: National Academy Press, 1989), pp. 262–271.
2. G. J. Beckett and coauthors, Effects of combined iodine and selenium deficiency on thyroid hormone metabolism in rats, *American Journal of Clinical Nutrition* 57 (1993): 240S–243S.
3. R. D. Baynes and T. H. Bothwell, Iron deficiency, *Annual Review of Nutrition* 10 (1990): 133–148.
4. Baynes and Bothwell, 1990.
5. E. R. Monsen and coauthors, Estimation of available dietary iron, *American Journal of Clinical Nutrition* 31 (1978): 134–141.
6. M. Tuntawiroon and coauthors, Dose-dependent inhibitory effect of phenolic compounds in foods on nonheme iron absorption in men, *American Journal of Clinical Nutrition* 53 (1991): 554–557.
7. E. R. Monsen, Iron nutrition and absorption: Dietary factors which impact iron bioavailability, *Journal of the American Dietetic Association* 88 (1988): 786–790.
8. H. Munro, The ferritin genes: Their response to iron status, *Nutrition Reviews* 51 (1993): 65–73.
9. D. C. Rockey and J. P. Cello, Evaluation of the gastrointestinal tract in patients with iron-deficiency anemia, *New England Journal of Medicine* 329 (1993): 1691–1695.
10. V. Herbert, Everyone should be tested for iron disorders, *Journal of the American Dietetic Association* 92 (1992): 1502–1509.
11. P. R. Dallman, Iron, in *Present Knowledge in Nutrition*, 6th ed., ed. M. L. Brown (Washington, D.C.: International Life Sciences Institute—Nutrition Foundation, 1990), pp. 241–250.
12. Baynes and Bothwell, 1990.
13. Baynes and Bothwell, 1990.
14. F. A. Oski, Iron deficiency in infancy and childhood, *New England Journal of Medicine* 329 (1993): 190–193.
15. Herbert, 1992.
16. C. B. Gable, Hemochromatosis and dietary iron supplementation: Implications from U.S. mortality, morbidity, and health survey data, *Journal of the American Dietetic Association* 92 (1992): 208–212.
17. J. T. Salonen and coauthors, High stored iron levels are associated with excess risk of myocardial infarction in Eastern Finnish men, *Circulation* 86 (1992): 803–811.
18. V. Herbert, S. Shaw, and E. Jayatilleke, Vitamin C supplements are harmful to lethal for the over 10% of Americans with high iron stores, *FASEB Journal* 8 (1994): A678.
19. R. L. Nelson and coauthors, Body iron stores and risk of colonic neoplasia, *Journal of the National Cancer Institute* 86 (1994): 455–460.
20. Committee on Dietary Allowances, 1989.
21. R. J. Cousins and J. M. Hempe, Zinc, in *Present Knowledge in Nutrition*, 6th ed., ed. M. L. Brown (Washington, D.C.: International Life Sciences Institute—Nutrition Foundation, 1990), pp. 251–260.
22. C. L. Keen, Zinc deficiency and immune function, *Annual Review of Nutrition* 10 (1990): 415–431.
23. M. C. Linder, Nutrition and the metabolism of trace elements, in *Nutritional Biochemistry and Metabolism with Clinical Implications*, ed. M. C. Linder (New York: Elsevier, 1991), pp. 215–276.
24. Cousins and Hempe, 1990.
25. J. Zheng and coauthors, Measurement of zinc bioavailability from beef and a ready-to-eat high-fiber breakfast cereal in humans: Application of a whole-gut lavage technique, *American Journal of Clinical Nutrition* 58 (1993): 902–907.
26. Cousins and Hempe, 1990; B. L. O'Dell, Copper, in *Present Knowledge in Nutrition*, 6th ed., ed. M. L. Brown (Washington, D.C.: International Life Sciences Institute—Nutrition Foundation, 1990), pp. 261–267.
27. Keen, 1990.

28. A. S. Prasad, Discovery of human zinc deficiency and studies in an experimental human model, *American Journal of Clinical Nutrition* 53 (1991): 403–412.

29. Committee on Dietary Allowances, 1989, pp. 205–213.

30. G. A. Eby, D. R. David, and W. W. Halcomb, Reduction in duration of common colds by zinc gluconate lozenges in a double-blind study, *Antimicrobial Agents and Chemotherapy* 25 (1984): 20–24.

31. J. C. Godfrey, Zinc for the common cold: Antimicrobial prophylaxis and treatment of rhinovirus colds with zinc gluconate lozenges, *Journal of Antimicrobial Chemotherapy* 20 (1987): 893–901; B. M. Farr and coauthors, Two randomized controlled trials of zinc gluconate lozenge therapy of experimentally induced rhinovirus colds, *Antimicrobial Agents and Chemotherapy* 31 (1987): 1183–1187.

32. A. M. Fan and K. W. Kizer, Selenium—Nutritional, toxicologic, and clinical aspects, *The Western Journal of Medicine* 153 (1990): 160–167.

33. M. A. Johnson and S. E. Kays, Copper: Its role in human nutrition, *Nutrition Today*, January/February 1990, pp. 6–14.

34. G. E. Bunce, Hypercholesterolemia of copper deficiency is linked to glutathione metabolism and regulation of hepatic HMG-CoA reductase, *Nutrition Reviews* 51 (1993): 305–307; Decreased dietary copper impairs vascular function, *Nutrition Reviews* 51 (1993): 188–189; Low-copper diets increase aortic lipid peroxides in rats, *Nutrition Reviews* 51 (1993): 88–89.

35. Position of The American Dietetic Association: The impact of fluoride on dental health, *Journal of the American Dietetic Association* 94 (1994): 1428–1431.

36. M. Kleerekoper and R. Balena, Fluorides and osteoporosis, *Annual Review of Nutrition* 11 (1991): 309–324.

37. B. D. Gessner and coauthors, Acute fluoride poisoning from a public water system, *New England Journal of Medicine* 330 (1994): 95–99; D. E. Leland, K. E. Powell, and R. S. Anderson, Jr., A fluoride overfeed incident at Harbor Springs, Mich., *Journal of the American Water Works Association* 72 (1980): 238–243; L. R. Petersen and coauthors, Community health effects of a municipal water supply hyperfluoridation accident, *American Journal of Public Health* 78 (1988): 711–713; Acute fluoride poisoning—North Carolina, *Morbidity and Mortality Weekly Report* 23 (1974): 199.

38. R. A. Anderson and coauthors, Supplemental-chromium effects on glucose, insulin, glucagon, and urinary chromium losses in subjects consuming controlled low-chromium diets, *American Journal of Clinical Nutrition* 54 (1991): 909–916.

39. E. G. Offenbacher and F. X. Pi-Sunyer, Chromium in human nutrition, *Annual Review of Nutrition* 8 (1988): 543–563.

40. J. McBride, Chromium supplementation helps keep blood glucose levels in check (Of Interest to You), *Journal of the American Dietetic Association* 91 (1991): 178.

41. K. V. Rajagopalan, Molybdenum: An essential trace element in human nutrition, *Annual Review of Nutrition* 8 (1988): 401–427.

42. C. D. Seaborn and F. H. Nielsen, Silicon: A nutritional beneficence for bones, brains, and blood vessels? *Nutrition Today*, July/August 1993, pp. 13–18.

43. H. McCoy and coauthors, Relation of boron to the composition and mechanical properties of bone, *Environmental Health Perspectives* (supplement) 102 (1994): 49–53.

44. W. Mertz, Essential trace metals: New definitions based on new paradigms, *Nutrition Reviews* 51 (1993): 287–295.

Our Children's Daily Lead*

At nine months, Joey crawled about exploring the world around him—touching and tasting everything, as all babies do. He chewed on table legs, toys, and spindles of flaky paint railings—whatever was in his reach. He eagerly drank his morning bottle of formula, which his mother prepared with the first water drawn from the tap. Not until he was two did he begin to toddle about while his parents watched proudly. At four, he amused his parents when he'd chase after balls tossed his way, but he couldn't catch them. By age five, he was a cautious, quiet preschooler who clung tightly to stair railings with both hands as he slowly climbed up or down.

Joey was late in walking, small for his age, seldom played as vigorously as other children, and was prone to small health disturbances such as diarrhea, irritability, and lethargy. His kindergarten teacher reported that Joey had some difficulty hearing and that his progress was slower than expected. While his health quietly deteriorated, his parents thought these subtle symptoms were within the range of normal variations seen in children. Finally, a pediatrician detected lead toxicity and started treating Joey with lead-scavenging drugs.[1] Joey is now growing normally and playing vigorously, although he still has minor learning disabilities. His physician expects the deficits in brain function to persist into adulthood.[2]

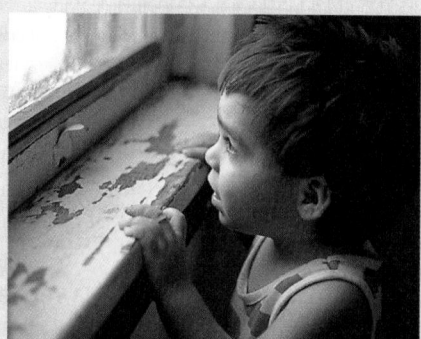

Old, lead-based paint threatens the health of an exploring child.

For children like Joey, the diagnosis often comes too late. Even one year of lead exposure can permanently injure the brain, nervous system, and psychological functioning. Furthermore, the effects occur with even low exposure.[3] The lead poisoning threshold—the amount of lead in the blood recognized to cause harm —is now known to be 10 micrograms per 100 milliliters of blood; earlier it was thought to be 25.[4] Health agencies point to lead poisoning as the most serious environmental threat to young children.[5] The Food and Drug Administration (FDA) has proposed reducing the acceptable level of lead in foods tenfold—from its 1958 limit of 10 parts per million to 0.5 to 1.0 parts per million.[6]

This highlight describes how lead disrupts the body processes and impairs nutrition status then points out sources of lead in the environment. Perhaps, with awareness, we can make changes that will safeguard the health of our children.

LEAD IN THE BODY

Chapters 12 and 13 told of the many ways minerals serve the body—maintaining fluid and electrolyte balance, providing structural support to the bones, transporting oxygen, and assisting enzymes. In contrast to those minerals that the body requires, the mineral lead impairs the body's growth, work, and general heath.

Like other minerals, lead is indestructible; the body cannot change its chemistry. Chemically similar to nutrient minerals like iron, calcium, and zinc, lead displaces them from some of the slots they normally occupy, but is then unable to perform their roles. For example, lead interferes with the enzymes that facilitate heme formation (see Figure H13–1). Lead damages many body systems, particularly the vulnerable nervous system, kidneys, and bone marrow. It impairs such normal activities as growth by interfering with hormone activity.[7] Table H13–1 lists symptoms of lead toxicity. The greater the exposure, the more damaging the effects.

LEAD AND GROWING CHILDREN

The body absorbs lead greedily, especially during times of rapid growth. Thereafter, it hoards lead possessively. During pregnancy, lead readily moves across the placenta, inflicting severe damage on the developing fetal nervous system. Infants and young children absorb five to ten times as much lead as adults do. One out of every six children from six months to five years old and one out of every nine fetuses are exposed to harmful doses of lead. Lead toxicity is most prevalent among children under six—as many

---

*Title borrowed form M. A. Wessel and A. Dominski, Our children's daily lead, *American Scientist* 65 (1977): 294–298.

Figure H13–1

Lead Displaces Iron

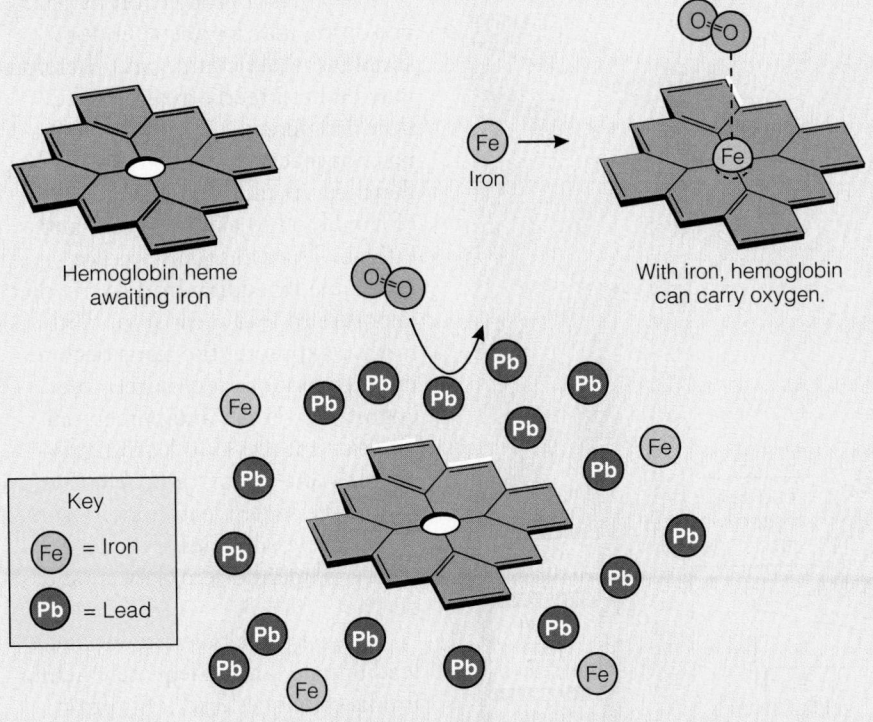

Hemoglobin heme awaiting iron

Iron

With iron, hemoglobin can carry oxygen.

Key

Fe = Iron

Pb = Lead

With high levels of lead, the placement of iron in the heme structure is blocked, and so hemoglobin cannot carry oxygen.

Excess lead in the blood also deranges the structure of red blood cell membranes, making them leaky and fragile. Lead interacts with white blood cells, too, impairing their ability to fight infection, and it binds to antibodies, thereby impairing the body's resistance to disease.

THE MALNUTRITION-LEAD CONNECTION

Among children, those who are malnourished are most vulnerable to lead poisoning. Children absorb more lead if their stomachs are empty, if they have low calcium or zinc intakes, and, of greatest concern because it is so common, if they have iron deficiencies.

As Chapter 13 mentioned, lead poisoning can cause iron deficiency, and iron deficiency weakens the body's defenses against lead absorption. In fact, the interactions

as 3 to 4 million children (10 to 15 percent of all preschoolers) may have blood lead concentrations high enough to cause mental, behavioral, and other health problems.[8]

Lead poisoning in infants most often comes from infant formula made with contaminated water.[9] The water, in turn, receives its lead burden from lead-soldered plumbing. The first water drawn from the tap each day is highest in lead—therefore, a person living in a house with old, lead-soldered plumbing should let the water run a few minutes before drinking or using it to prepare formula or food.

Lead intoxication in young children comes from their own behav-iors and activities—putting their hands in their mouths, playing in dirt, and eating nonfood items (see Figure H13–2 on p. 482). The toddler years see a marked rise in blood lead. Tragically, a child's neuromuscular system is maturing at precisely the same time. No wonder children with high blood lead experience impairment of balance, motor development, and the relaying of nerve messages to and from the brain. Children two and three years old with the highest blood lead suffer the greatest developmental delays at age four. Researchers studying young children's development must now consider the possible effects of lead poisoning.

Table H13–1

Symptoms of Lead Toxicity

In children:
- Learning disabilities
- Low IQ
- Behavior problems
- Slow growth
- Iron-deficiency anemia
- Nervous system disorders
- Impaired concentration
- Reduced short-term memory
- Slow reaction time
- Seizures
- Impaired hearing
- Poor coordination

In adults:
- Hypertension
- Reproductive complications

Figure H13–2
. . . .

Sources of Lead Exposure
Lead finds its way into the bodies of children when they ingest lead-containing foods, water, dust, or paint chips, or when they breathe lead-laden air.

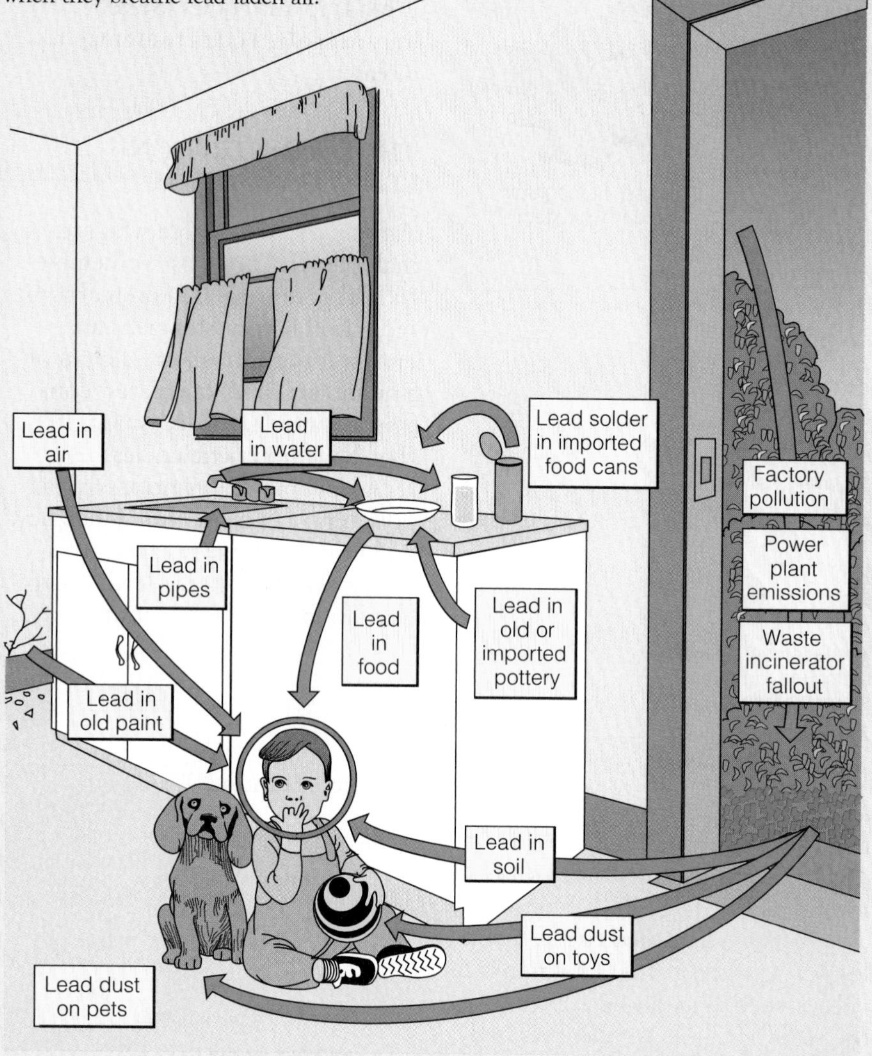

Lead in air

Lead in water

Lead solder in imported food cans

Factory pollution

Power plant emissions

Waste incinerator fallout

Lead in pipes

Lead in food

Lead in old or imported pottery

Lead in old paint

Lead in soil

Lead dust on toys

Lead dust on pets

for nonfood items. Many children with lead poisoning eat dirt or newspapers, two common sources of lead.

The anemia brought on by lead poisoning may be mistaken for a simple iron deficiency, and therefore may be incorrectly treated. Like iron deficiency, mild lead toxicity has nonspecific symptoms, including diarrhea, irritability, reduced ability of the blood to carry oxygen, and fatigue. The symptoms are not reversible by adding iron to the diet; exposure to lead must stop. With further exposure, the signs become more pronounced: children lose cognitive, verbal, and perceptual abilities and develop learning disabilities and behavior problems. Still more severe lead toxicity can cause irreversible nerve damage, paralysis, mental retardation, and death.

Just as iron deficiency enhances lead uptake, an inadequate calcium intake enhances lead absorption and retention. Zinc deficiency also enhances both tissue accumulation of lead and sensitivity to its effects; serum zinc is frequently low in children with high blood lead. Prevention of lead toxicity rests primarily on reduced exposure, but parents can protect their children, at least to some degree, by making sure that they eat adequate foods rich in iron, calcium, zinc, and other nutrients.

between lead poisoning and iron deficiency are so strong that lead poisoning is considered an adverse consequence of iron deficiency. A child with adequate iron stores is not immune, but a child with iron-deficiency anemia is three times as likely to have high blood lead. Common to both iron deficiency and lead poisoning is a low socio-economic background. Another common factor is pica—a craving

LEAD IN THE ENVIRONMENT

All foods contain some lead. Most, perhaps all, of it derives from industrial pollution. People are exposed to lead in some types of gasoline, paint, newspaper ink, batteries, shotgun ammunition, and pesticides as well as in the air and water that carry lead from industrial processes and landfills. Lead works its way through rainfall and soil into plants and animals that people use for food. Lead also enters food from containers such as tin cans sealed with lead solder. (Manufacturers in the United States no longer use lead solder in canning, but many in foreign countries still do.) Old, handmade, or imported pottery decorated with lead glazes can also leach lead into foods.

Pipelines soldered with lead or coupled with brass fixtures also release lead into drinking water, making lead the nation's most significant water contaminant. A recent sampling by the Environmental Protection Agency (EPA) found unsafe levels of lead in the public water systems that serve 30 million people. Exposures are highest in older communities along the nation's east coast; in urban and industrial areas; near highways; and in slums where old leaded paint peels from the buildings. People suffering the effects of lead exposure are most often black, male, and from low-income families, but it is also seen in upper-middle-class families as they move into inner-city areas and renovate older homes.

Federal law has mandated reductions in the use of leaded gasolines, lead-based solder, and other products in recent years. These efforts have helped to reduce the amounts of lead in the environment—and in children's blood. The decline in blood lead in children during the late 1970s paralleled exactly the decline in the nation's use of leaded gasolines, leaded house paints, and lead-soldered food cans. Even so, lead still contaminates the blood of some 4 percent of our nation's children. Paint remains the primary source;[10] 70 percent of homes built before 1960 are covered with lead paint and are likely to cause lead

poisoning, especially during times of renovation. A routine question asked when screening children for lead poisoning is whether they have ever lived in a house built before 1960.[11] If leaded surfaces in these homes are peeling and deteriorating, the children are either already poisoned or at immediate risk of lead poisoning.

STRATEGIES FOR PROTECTION

Three major discoveries about lead toxicity occurred simultaneously: lead poisoning has *subtle* effects; the effects are *permanent*; and they occur at *low levels of exposure*. Consumers would be wise to take ultraconservative measures to protect themselves, and especially their infants and young children, from lead poisoning.

Defensive strategies include:

- Test children for lead poisoning; lead screening is essential to preventing its devastating effects.[12]
- In contaminated environments, keep small children from putting dirty or old painted objects in their mouths, and make sure children wash their hands before eating.
- Be aware that other countries do not have the same regulations protecting consumers against lead. Children have been poisoned by eating crayons made in China and drinking fruit juice canned in Mexico.
- Make baby formula from lead-free ingredients. Do not use milk from lead-soldered cans and do not use lead-contaminated water.
- Once you have opened canned food, immediately move it to a lead-free storage container to prevent lead migration into the food.

- Do not store acidic foods or beverages (such as orange juice) in ceramic dishware.
- Many manufacturers are now making lead-safe products.* Old, handmade, or imported ceramic cups and bowls may contain lead and should not be used to heat coffee or tea, or acidic foods such as tomato soup.
- Do not store alcoholic beverages in pewter or crystal decanters.
- Some wineries still use lead in their foil seals; to be safe, wipe the foil-sealed rim of the wine bottle with water or lemon juice before removing the cork.
- Feed children nutritious meals regularly (see Chapter 19 for more details).
- Confirm with the publisher that your newspaper uses no lead in its ink before using the paper to wrap food, mulch garden plants, or add to your compost.

The EPA also publishes a booklet, *Lead and Your Drinking Water*, in which the following cautions appear:

- Have the water in your home tested by a competent laboratory.
- Use only cold water for drinking, cooking, and making formula (cold water absorbs less lead).
- When water has been standing in pipes for more than two hours, flush the cold-water pipes by running water through them for at least a minute before using it for drinking, cooking, or mixing formulas.

---

*Shopper's Guide to Low-Lead China is available from the Environmental Defense Fund, 257 Park Avenue South, New York, NY 10010; telephone (212) 505–2100.

- If lead contamination of your water supply seems probable, obtain additional information and advice from the EPA and your local public health agency.[13]

By taking these steps, parents can protect themselves and their children from this preventable danger.*

This highlight may appear to have been just about lead, but its actions typify the ways all heavy metals behave in the body: they interfere with nutrients that are trying to do their jobs. The "good guy" nutrients are shoved aside by the "bad guy" contaminants. Then the contaminants—whether lead, mercury, cadmium, or some other—cannot perform the roles of the nutrients, and health declines. To safeguard our health, we must defend ourselves against contamination by eating

---

*The National Lead Information Center provides two hotlines; call (800) LEAD–FYI (532–3394) for general information or (800) 424–LEAD (424–5323) with specific questions.

nutrient-rich foods and preserving a clean environment.

NOTES

1. The majority of children with high blood lead levels (45 µg/dL) are treated using a process called chelation—using drugs (most often succimer or calcium-disodium EDTA) that bind to lead in the blood and carry it out in the urine. American Adademy of Pediatrics Committee on Drugs, Treatment guidelines for lead exposure in children, *Pediatrics* 96 (1995): 155–160.

2. P. A. Baghurst and coauthors, Environmental exposure to lead and children's intelligence at the age of seven years, *New England Journal of Medicine* 327 (1992): 1279–1284; D. C. Bellinger, K. M. Stiles, and H. L. Needleman, Low-level lead exposure, intelligence and academic achievement: A long-term follow-up study, *Pediatrics* 90 (1992): 855–961; H. L. Needleman and coauthors, The long-term effects of exposure to low doses of lead in childhood: An 11-year follow-up report, *New England Journal of Medicine* 322 (1990): 83–88.

3. K. N. Dietrich, O. G. Berger, and P. A. Succop, Lead exposure and the motor developmental status of urban six-year-old children in the Cincinnati Prospective Study, *Pediatrics* 91 (1993): 301–307.

4. J. Murphy, Federal agencies gearing up for new efforts against lead, *Nation's Health*, May/June 1991, pp. 1, 23.

5. A. Greeley, Getting the lead out of just about everything, *FDA Consumer*, July/August 1991, pp. 27–36.

6. FDA seeks lower lead levels in food additives and GRAS ingredients, *Journal of the American Dietetic Association* 94 (1994): 495.

7. C. A. Huseman, M. M. Varma, and C. R. Angle, Neuroendocrine effects of toxic and low blood lead levels in children, *Pediatrics* 90 (1992): 186–189.

8. Murphy, 1991.

9. M. W. Shannon and J. W. Graef, Lead intoxication in infancy, *Pediatrics* 89 (1992): 87–90.

10. Childhood lead poisoning: A disease for the history texts (editorial), *American Journal of Public Health* 81 (1991): 685.

11. H. J. Binns, Is there lead in the suburbs? Risk assessment in Chicago suburban pediatric practices, *Pediatrics* 93 (1994): 164–171.

12. Committee on Environmental Health, Lead poisoning: From screening to primary prevention, *Pediatrics* 92 (1993): 176–183; S. J. Schaffer, P. G. Szilagyi, and M. Weitzman, Lead poisoning risk determination in an urban population through the use of a standardized questionnaire, *Pediatrics* 93 (1994): 159–163.

13. U.S. Environmental Protection Agency, Office of Water, *Lead and Your Drinking Water*, publication no. OPA 87–006 (Washington, D.C.: Government Printing Office, April 1987).

Chapter 14

Consumer Concerns about Foods

CONTENTS

Food-Borne Illnesses
*Food-Borne Infections and Food
    Intoxications*
Food Hazards in the Marketplace
Food Safety in the Kitchen
Food Safety while Traveling
Nutritional Adequacy of Foods and Diets
Environmental Contaminants
*Harmfulness of Environmental
    Contaminants*
Examples of Environmental Contaminants
Natural Toxicants in Foods
Pesticides
Food Additives
Regulations Governing Additives
Intentional Food Additives
Indirect Food Additives
Hormones
Radiation
Food Biotechnology
HIGHLIGHT: **Consumer Concerns about
Public Water**

MICROGRAPH: Capsaicin, the nonnutrient that makes
hot peppers hot

*M*uch of this book has focused on the nutrients in foods and in the body, but no chapter has focused on what is in foods besides nutrients. What causes food poisoning? Are the amounts of contaminants and pesticides found in foods harmful? Are food additives safe? What does public water contain, and is it safe to drink?

This chapter takes up these concerns in the order listed in the margin. This is the order in which the Food and Drug Administration (FDA) has ranked them according to the risks they pose. The rank order of these food hazards is remarkably similar for nations around the world.[1] The highlight features a look at public drinking water.

By way of introduction, take a moment to consider the vastness of the task at hand—supplying food to over 250 million people in the United States. To feed this nation requires farmers to grow and harvest crops; dairy producers to supply milk products; ranchers to raise livestock; shippers to deliver foods to manufacturers by land, sea, and air; manufacturers to prepare, process, preserve, and package products for refrigerated food cases and grocery-store shelves; and grocers to store the food and supply it to consumers. After much time, much labor, and extensive transport, an abundant supply of a large variety of safe foods finally reaches consumers at reasonable market prices.

Government and international agencies monitor this huge system using a nationwide network of people and sophisticated equipment. The accompanying glossary identifies the various food regulatory agencies by their acronyms. These agencies focus on the potential hazard of foods, which differs from the toxicity of a substance—a distinction worth understanding. Anything can be toxic. Toxicity simply means that a substance *can* cause harm *if* enough is consumed. We eat lots of things that are toxic, without risk, because the amounts consumed are so

FDA's food safety concerns:

1. Food-borne illnesses.
2. Nutritional adequacy of foods.
3. Environmental contaminants.
4. Naturally occurring toxicants.
5. Pesticide residues.
6. Food additives.

risk: a measure of the probability and severity of harm.

hazard: source of danger; used to refer to circumstances in which toxicity is possible under normal conditions of use.

toxicity: the ability of a substance to harm living organisms. All substances are toxic if high enough concentrations are used.

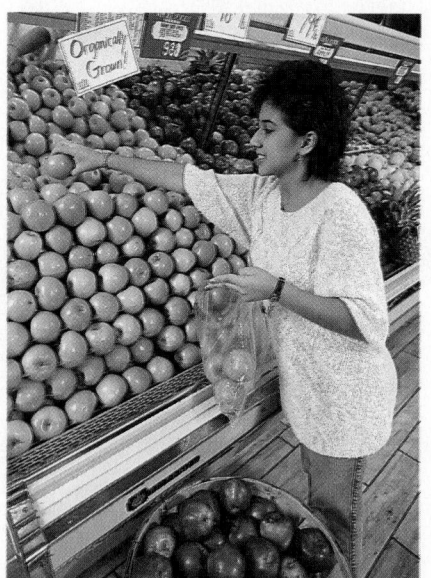

With the benefits of a safe and abundant food supply comes the responsibility to select, prepare, and store foods safely.

Glossary of Agencies That Monitor the Food Supply

CDC (Centers for Disease Control): a branch of the Department of Health and Human Services that is responsible for, among other things, monitoring food-borne diseases.

EPA (Environmental Protection Agency): a federal agency that is responsible for, among other things, regulating pesticides and establishing water quality standards.

FAO (Food and Agriculture Organization): an international agency (part of the United Nations) that has adopted standards to regulate pesticide use among other responsibilities.

FDA (Food and Drug Administration): a part of the Department of Health and Human Services' Public Health Service that is responsible for ensuring the safety and wholesomeness of all foods sold in interstate commerce except meat, poultry, and eggs (which are under the jurisdiction of the USDA); inspecting food plants and imported foods; and setting standards for food composition.

USDA (U.S. Department of Agriculture): the federal agency responsible for enforcing standards for the wholesomeness and quality of meat, poultry, and eggs produced in the United States; conducting nutrition research; and educating the public about nutrition.

WHO (World Health Organization): an international agency that has adopted standards to regulate pesticide use among other responsibilities.

small. The term *hazard*, on the other hand, is more relevant to our daily lives because it refers to the harm that is *likely* under real-life conditions. Consumers rely on these monitoring agencies to set sound standards and can learn to protect themselves from food hazards by taking a few preventive steps.

Food-Borne Illnesses

The FDA lists food-borne illness as the leading food safety concern because episodes of food poisoning far outnumber episodes of any other kind of food contamination. Just about everyone experiences a food-borne illness (whether they realize it or not) at least once a year. Some 6.5 million cases of food-borne illness are reported in the United States each year; millions more go unreported. For some 9000 people each year, the symptoms can be so severe as to cause death.[2] Most vulnerable are the very young, the very old, the sick, and the malnourished. By taking the proper precautions, however, people can minimize their chances of contracting food-borne illnesses.

FOOD-BORNE INFECTIONS AND FOOD INTOXICATIONS

The term *food-borne illness* refers to both infections and intoxications. Table 14–1 summarizes some of the more common food-borne illnesses, their most frequent food sources, general symptoms, and prevention methods.

Food-Borne Infections   Food-borne infections are caused by eating foods contaminated by infectious microbes. Two of the most common infectious microbes are *Campylobacter jejuni* and *Salmonella*, which enter the GI tract in contaminated foods such as undercooked poultry and unpasteurized milk. Symptoms generally include abdominal cramps, fever, and diarrhea. If a person experiences these symptoms as the major or only symptoms of a bout of "flu," chances are excellent that what the person really has is a food-borne illness.*

Food Intoxications   Food intoxications are caused by eating foods containing natural toxins or, more likely, microbes that produce toxins. The most infamous, but not common, example is *Clostridium botulinum*, the organism that produces a deadly toxin in improperly canned foods. Botulism requires immediate medical attention, and even then, survivors may suffer the effects for months or years. An amount of toxin as tiny as a single crystal of salt can kill several people within an hour.

FOOD HAZARDS IN THE MARKETPLACE

Commercially prepared food is usually safe, but infected food from one major supplier can make thousands of people sick. Milk producers, for example, rely on pasteurization to make milk safe for consumption. When a major dairy in Chicago experienced a flaw in its pasteurization system, over 16,000 confirmed, and as many as 200,000 suspected, cases of food-borne illness resulted. Similarly,

food-borne illnesses: illnesses transmitted to human beings through food, caused by either an infectious agent (*food-borne infection*) or a poisonous substance (*food intoxication*); commonly known as food poisoning.

Reminder: *Botulism* is an often-fatal food-borne illness caused by the ingestion of foods containing a toxin produced by bacteria that grow without oxygen in improperly canned nonacidic foods. The botulinum (BOT-chew-line-um) toxin responsible for botulism is called botulin (BOT-chew-lin).

Botulism danger signs:
- Double vision.
- Slurred speech.
- Weakening muscles.
- Difficulty swallowing.
- Difficulty breathing.

pasteurization: a process of heating milk sufficiently to kill many disease-causing microbes commonly transmitted through milk; not a sterilization process. Pasteurized milk retains bacteria that cause milk spoilage. Unpasteurized ("certified" raw) milk transmits many food-borne diseases to people each year and should be avoided.

---

*Some viruses do cause intestinal distress, and those that do are usually transmitted via food; true influenza viruses cause symptoms primarily in the upper respiratory tract.

Table 14–1

Food-Borne Illnesses

Disease and Organism That Causes It	Most Frequent Food Source	Onset and General Symptoms	Prevention Methods[a]
FOOD-BORNE INFECTIONS			
Campylobacteriosis *Campylobacter jejuni* bacterium	Raw poultry, beef, lamb, unpasteurized milk (foods of animal origin eaten raw or undercooked or recontaminated after cooking).	Onset: 2 to 5 days. Diarrhea, nausea, vomiting, abdominal cramps, fever; sometimes bloody stools; lasts 7 to 10 days.	Cook foods thoroughly; use pasteurized milk; use sanitary food-handling methods.
Giardiasis *Giardia lamblia* protozoa	Contaminated water; uncooked foods.	Onset: 5 to 25 days. Diarrhea (but occasionally constipation), abdominal pain, gas, abdominal distention, digestive disturbances, anorexia, nausea, and vomiting.	Use sanitary food-handling methods; avoid raw fruits and vegetables where protozoa are endemic; dispose of sewage properly.
Hepatitis Hepatitis A virus	Undercooked or raw shellfish.	Onset: 15 to 50 days (28 to 30 days average). Inflammation of the liver with tiredness; nausea, vomiting, or indigestion; jaundice (yellowed skin and eyes from buildup of wastes); muscle pain.	Cook foods thoroughly.
Listeriosis *Listeria monocytogenes* bacterium	Raw meat and seafood, raw milk, and soft cheeses.	Onset: 7 to 30 days. Mimics flu; blood poisoning, complications in pregnancy, and meningitis (stiff neck, severe headache, and fever).	Use sanitary food-handling methods; cook foods thoroughly; use pasteurized milk.
Perfringens food poisoning *Clostridium perfringens* bacterium	Meats and meat products stored at between 120 and 130°F.	Onset: 8 to 12 hr (usually 12). Abdominal pain, diarrhea, nausea, and vomiting; symptoms last a day or less and are usually mild; can be serious in old or weak people.	Use sanitary food-handling methods; cook foods thoroughly; refrigerate foods promptly and properly.
Salmonellosis *Salmonella* bacterium	Raw or undercooked eggs, meats, poultry, milk and other dairy products, shrimp, frog legs, yeast, coconut, pasta, and chocolate.	Onset: 6 to 48 hr. Nausea, fever, chills, vomiting, abdominal cramps, diarrhea, and headache; can be fatal.	Use sanitary food-handling methods; use pasteurized milk; cook foods thoroughly; refrigerate foods promptly and properly.

some 1000 residents of St. Paul became sick after eating *Samonella*-contaminated ice cream made by a local manufacturer. In another episode, over 100 people in California got sick and 50 of them died of listeriosis from eating contaminated cheese. In still another, a fast-food restaurant in Seattle served burgers tainted with the infectious organism *Escherichia coli*, causing illness in some 500 patrons and at least one child's death. The meat had been improperly handled at the slaughterhouse and undercooked at the restaurant.

Fortunately, such large-scale incidents, though dramatic, make up only a small fraction of total food poisoning cases each year. Most arise from one person's error in a small setting and affect just a few victims. Some people have come to accept a yearly bout or two of intestinal illness as inevitable, but in truth, most of these illnesses can be prevented.

Disease and Organism That Causes It	Most Frequent Food Source	Onset and General Symptoms	Prevention Methods[a]
FOOD-BORNE INFECTIONS *(continued)*			
Traveler's diarrhea *Escherichia coli* (usually)	Contaminated water, undercooked ground beef, raw foods, imported soft cheeses.	Onset: 12 to 18 hr. Loose and watery stools, nausea, bloating, and abdominal cramps.	Cook foods thoroughly; use safe, treated water and pasteurized milk; wash fruits and vegetables.
Trichinosis *Trichinella spiralis* parasite	Raw or undercooked pork or wild game (bear). Worms burrow through the body tissues to reach muscle tissue where they remain alive.	Onset: 24 hr. Abdominal pain, nausea, vomiting, diarrhea, and fever. One to two weeks later, muscle pain, low-grade fever, pain on breathing, edema (swelling), skin eruptions, loss of appetite, and weight loss. Drug therapy kills the worms and deaths are rare.	Cook foods thoroughly.
FOOD INTOXICATIONS			
Botulism Botulinum toxin (produced by *Clostridium botulinum* bacterium)	Anaerobic environment of low acidity (canned corn, peppers, green beans, soups, beets, asparagus, mushrooms, ripe olives, spinach, tuna, chicken, chicken liver, liver pâté, luncheon meats, ham, sausage, stuffed eggplant, lobster, and smoked and salted fish).	Onset: 4 to 36 hr. Nervous system symptoms, including double vision, inability to swallow, speech difficulty, and progressive paralysis of the respiratory system; often fatal; leaves prolonged symptoms in survivors.	Use proper canning methods for low-acid foods; avoid commercially prepared foods with leaky seals or with bent, bulging, or broken cans.
Staphylococcal food poisoning Staphylococcal toxin (produced by *Staphylococcus aureus* bacterium)	Toxin produced in meats, poultry, egg products, tuna, potato and macaroni salads, and cream-filled pastries.	Onset: ½ to 8 hr. Diarrhea, nausea, vomiting, abdominal cramps, and fatigue; mimics flu; lasts 24 to 48 hr; rarely fatal.	Use sanitary food-handling methods; cook food thoroughly; refrigerate foods promptly and properly.

[a]The box on pp. 490–491 provides more details on the proper handling, cooking, and refrigeration of foods.

Canned and packaged foods sold in grocery stores are controlled more easily than raw foods, but still, rare accidents do happen. Batch numbering makes it possible for suppliers to recall contaminated foods through public announcements via newspapers, television, and radio. In the grocery store, consumers can carefully inspect the seals, safety "buttons," and wrappers of packages. A broken seal or mangled package fails to protect the product against microbes, insects, spoilage, or even vandalism.

Raw foods from the grocery store, especially meats and poultry, contain microbes. Whether microbes multiply and cause illness depends, in part, on what consumers do or fail to do in their kitchens.

Figure 14–1

Safe Internal Temperatures for Cooking Meats and Poultry (Fahrenheit)

Source: USDA, 1993.

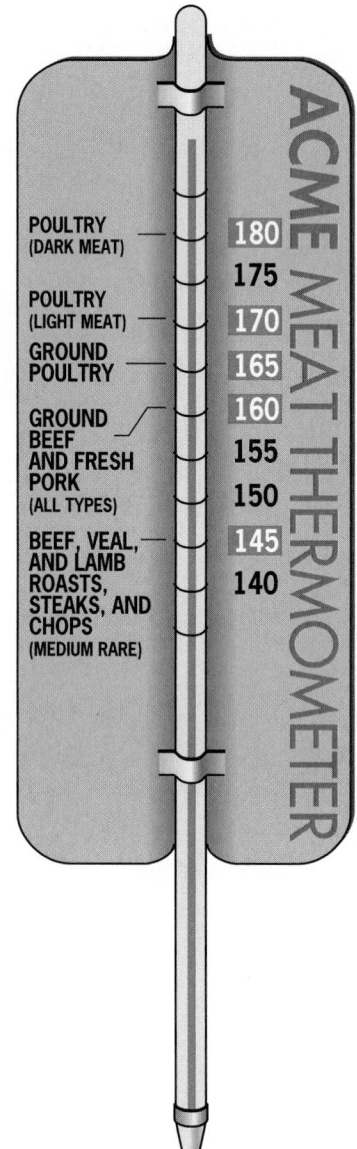

POULTRY
(DARK MEAT) — 180

175

POULTRY
(LIGHT MEAT) — 170

GROUND
POULTRY — 165

GROUND
BEEF — 160
AND FRESH
PORK — 155
(ALL TYPES) — 150

BEEF, VEAL,
AND LAMB — 145
ROASTS,
STEAKS, AND — 140
CHOPS
(MEDIUM RARE)

ACME MEAT THERMOMETER

How to Prevent Food-Borne Illnesses

Most food-borne illnesses can be prevented by following three simple rules: keep hot foods hot, keep cold foods cold, and keep a clean kitchen.

Keep Hot Foods Hot

- When cooking meats or poultry, use a thermometer to test the internal temperature. Insert the thermometer between the thigh and the body of a turkey or into the thickest part of other meats, making sure the tip of the thermometer is not in contact with bone or the pan. Cook to the temperature indicated for that particular meat; cook hamburgers to at least medium well-done. If you have safety questions, call the USDA Meat and Poultry Hotline: (800) 535–4555.
- Cook stuffing separately, or stuff poultry just prior to cooking.
- Do not cook large cuts of meats or turkeys in a microwave oven; it leaves some parts undercooked while overcooking others.
- Marinate meats in the refrigerator, not on the counter. Don't use marinade that was in contact with raw meat for basting or sauces.
- Cook eggs before eating them (soft-boiled for at least 3½ minutes; scrambled until set, not runny; fried for at least 3 minutes on one side and 1 minute on the other).
- Cook seafood thoroughly. If you have safety questions call the FDA Seafood Hotline: (800) FDA–4010.
- When serving foods, maintain temperatures at 140°F or higher.
- Heat leftovers thoroughly to at least 165°F.

Keep Cold Foods Cold

- When running errands, stop at the grocery store last. When you get home, refrigerate the perishable groceries (such as meats and dairy products) immediately. Do not leave perishables in the car any longer than it takes for ice cream to melt.
- Buy only those foods that are solidly frozen and stored below the frost line in store freezers.
- Keep cold foods at 40°F or less; keep frozen foods at 0°F or less (keep a thermometer in the refrigerator).
- Refrigerate leftovers promptly; use shallow containers to cool foods faster.
- Thaw meats or poultry in the refrigerator, not at room temperature. If you must hasten thawing, use cool running water or a microwave oven.

Keep a Clean and Safe Kitchen

- Wash fruits and vegetables with a scrub brush.
- Use hot, soapy water to wash hands, utensils, dishes, nonporous cutting boards, and countertops. Use a bleach solution on wooden cutting boards.
- Cover cuts with clean bandages before food preparation; dirty bandages carry harmful microorganisms.
- Avoid cross-contamination by washing all surfaces that have been in contact with raw meats, poultry, or eggs before reusing.

- Mix foods with utensils, not hands; keep hands and utensils away from mouth, nose, and hair.
- Anyone may be a carrier of bacteria and should avoid coughing or sneezing over food. A person with a skin infection or infectious disease should not prepare food.
- Wash or replace sponges and towels regularly.
- Clean up food spills and crumb-filled crevices.

In General

- Do not taste food that is suspect. "If in doubt, throw it out."
- Throw out foods with danger-signaling odors. Be aware, though, that most food poisoning bacteria are odorless, colorless, and tasteless.
- Do not buy or use items that appear to have been opened; check safety seals, buttons, and expiration dates.
- Follow label instructions for storing and preparing packaged and frozen foods.
- Discard foods that have decayed or been contaminated by insects or rodents.

For Specific Food Items

- *Canned goods*. Carefully discard food from cans that leak or bulge so that other people and animals will not accidentally ingest it; before canning, seek professional advice from the USDA Extension Service (check your phone book under U.S. government listings, or ask directory assistance).
- *Milk and cheeses*. Use only pasteurized milk and milk products. Aged cheeses, such as cheddar and swiss, do well for an hour or two without refrigeration, but should be refrigerated or stored in an ice chest for longer periods.
- *Eggs*. Use clean eggs with intact shells. Do not eat eggs raw.
- *Honey*. Honey may contain dormant bacterial spores, which can awaken in the human body to produce botulism. In adults, this poses little hazard, but infants under one year of age should never be fed honey. Honey can accumulate enough toxin to kill an infant; it has been implicated in several cases of sudden infant death. (Honey can also be contaminated with environmental pollutants picked up by the bees.)
- *Mayonnaise*. Commercial mayonnaise may actually help a food to resist spoilage because of the acid content. Still, keep it cold after opening.
- *Mixed salads*. Mixed salads of chopped ingredients spoil easily because they have extensive surface area for bacteria to invade, and they have been in contact with cutting boards, hands, and kitchen utensils that easily transmit bacteria to food (regardless of their mayonnaise content). Chill them well before, during, and after serving.
- *Picnic foods*. Choose foods that last without refrigeration such as fresh fruits and vegetables, breads and crackers, and canned spreads and cheeses that can be opened and used immediately. Pack foods cold, layer ice between foods, and keep foods out of water.

FOOD SAFETY IN THE KITCHEN

Almost one-third of all food-borne illnesses arise from mistakes made in home kitchens.[3] For the most part, these illnesses can be prevented by doing three simple things: keeping hot foods hot; keeping cold foods cold; and keeping hands, utensils, and the kitchen clean.

Keeping hot foods hot includes cooking foods long enough to reach internal temperatures that will kill microbes, keeping them hot enough to prevent bacterial growth until served, and refrigerating them immediately after serving a meal. Keeping cold foods cold entails going directly home upon leaving the grocery store and immediately unpacking foods into the refrigerator or freezer upon arrival. Keeping a clean, safe kitchen requires that cooks wash the countertops, their hands, and utensils in hot, soapy water before and after each step of food preparation. See the box on pp. 490–491 for specific food safety tips.

The "2–40–140" rule will help you to remember the time and temperature danger zone for foods—allow them to stay for no more than 2 hr between 40°F and 140°F.

Meat   Meat requires special handling. It contains bacteria, and its moist, nutrient-rich environment favors microbial growth. Ground meat is especially susceptible because it receives more handling than other kinds of meat and has more surface exposed to bacterial contamination. Consumers have no way to detect the harmful bacteria in or on meat. A USDA seal indicates that the product has been inspected for quality. It does not guarantee that the meat is free of potentially harmful bacteria, although the USDA has recently strengthened its inspection system to include microbial testing and prohibit fecal contamination.

When buying meat, consumers take on the responsibility of handling it in such a way that the bacteria present won't cause a food-borne illness (see Figure 14–2). Wash any utensils and surfaces (such as cutting boards or platters) that have been in contact with raw meat with hot, soapy water before using them again for the cooked meat or raw produce. Bacteria inevitably left on the surfaces from the raw meat can recontaminate the cooked meat or start to grow in the other foods—a problem known as *cross-contamination*. Cook meat thoroughly, using a thermometer to test the internal temperature (see Figure 14–1).

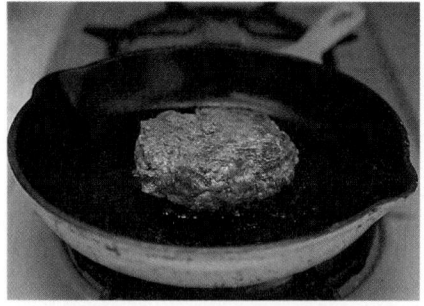

Cook hamburgers until they are brown (not pink) throughout, the juices run clear, and the inside is steaming hot.

Figure 14–2

Safe Handling Instructions for Meat and Poultry

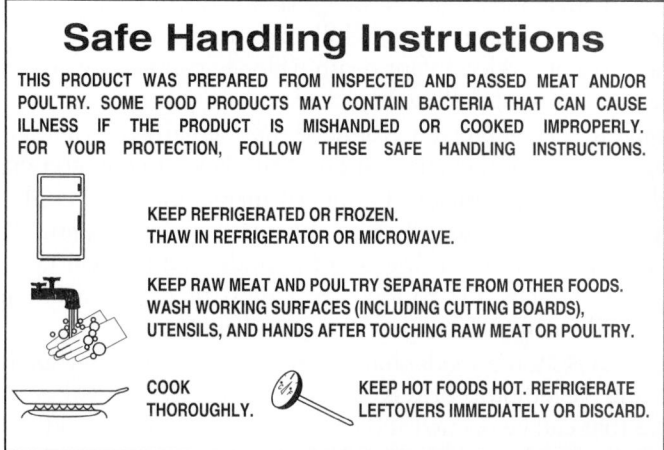

Safe Handling Instructions

THIS PRODUCT WAS PREPARED FROM INSPECTED AND PASSED MEAT AND/OR POULTRY. SOME FOOD PRODUCTS MAY CONTAIN BACTERIA THAT CAN CAUSE ILLNESS IF THE PRODUCT IS MISHANDLED OR COOKED IMPROPERLY. FOR YOUR PROTECTION, FOLLOW THESE SAFE HANDLING INSTRUCTIONS.

KEEP REFRIGERATED OR FROZEN.
THAW IN REFRIGERATOR OR MICROWAVE.

KEEP RAW MEAT AND POULTRY SEPARATE FROM OTHER FOODS.
WASH WORKING SURFACES (INCLUDING CUTTING BOARDS), UTENSILS, AND HANDS AFTER TOUCHING RAW MEAT OR POULTRY.

COOK THOROUGHLY.

KEEP HOT FOODS HOT. REFRIGERATE LEFTOVERS IMMEDIATELY OR DISCARD.

Seafood   Most seafoods available in the United States and Canada are safe, but eating undercooked seafood or raw seafood can cause severe illnesses—hepatitis, worms, parasites, viral intestinal disorders, and other diseases. The microorganisms in raw seafood are undetectable, even to an expert. Rumor has it that freezing fish will make it safe to eat raw, but this is only partly true. Freezing fish will kill mature parasitic worms, but only cooking can kill all worm eggs and other microorganisms that can cause illness. For safety's sake, all seafood should be cooked. Even sushi can be enjoyed this way: many sushi chefs combine cooked seafood, vegetables, avocado, and other ingredients into delicacies that are perfectly safe to enjoy.

At least 10 species of bacteria found in raw oysters cause illness in people. Raw oysters may also carry the hepatitis A virus, which can cause liver disease. Some hot sauces can kill many of these bacteria, but not the virus; alcohol may also protect against oyster-borne illnesses, but not completely. One study reported that among people who had eaten contaminated oysters, those who consumed an alcoholic beverage were less likely to have gotten sick, or their symptoms were less severe, than those who had not consumed alcoholic beverages.[4] Of course, this is not sufficient evidence to guarantee protection or to recommend drinking alcohol.

As population density increases along the shores of seafood-harvesting waters, pollution inevitably invades the seafood living there. Watchdog agencies monitor commercial fishing waters to keep harvesters out of contaminated areas, but some unwholesome foods taken illegally from closed harvesting areas do reach the market.[5] Preventing seafood-borne illness is in large part a task of controlling water pollution.

Chemical pollution and microbial contamination lurk not only in the water, but in the boats and warehouses where seafood is cleaned, prepared, and refrigerated. Seafood is one of the most perishable foods: time and temperature are critical to its freshness and flavor. To keep seafood as fresh as possible, people in the industry "keep it cold, keep it clean, and keep it moving."[6] Wise consumers eat it cooked.

Precautions and Procedures   Fresh food generally smells fresh. Not all types of food poisoning are detectable by odor, but some bacterial wastes produce "off" odors. If an abnormal odor exists, the food is spoiled. Throw it out or, if it was recently purchased, return it to the grocery store. Do not taste it. Table 14–2 lists safe storage times for selected foods.

Local health departments and the USDA Extension Service can provide further information about food safety. Should precautions fail and mild food-borne illness develop, drink clear liquids to replace fluids lost through vomiting and diarrhea. If serious food-borne illness is suspected, first call a physician. Then wrap the remainder of the suspected food and label its container so that it cannot be mistakenly eaten, place it in the refrigerator, and hold it for possible inspection by health authorities.

New advances in biotechnology offer promise for the future purity of foods, and especially of seafoods. Geneticists can couple a strand of synthetic DNA with one from bacteria to create a combined version that possesses a new talent—the hybrid is a biosensor that can detect chemicals that disease-causing microorganisms produce in foods.[7] These biosensors surpass today's methods in their sensitivity, simplicity, and reliability in detecting harmful organisms.[8]

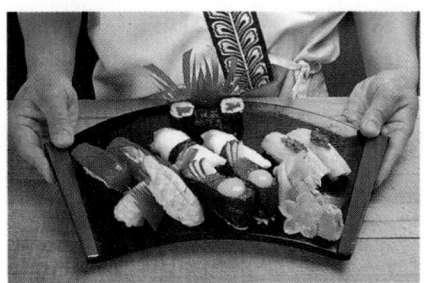

Eating raw seafood is a risky proposition even if it is prepared in sushi by a master chef.

sushi: vinegar-flavored rice and seafood, typically wrapped in seaweed and stuffed with colorful vegetables. Some sushi is stuffed with raw fish; other varieties contain only cooked ingredients.

Frequently unsafe:
- Raw milk.
- Raw or undercooked seafood, meat, or eggs.

Occasionally unsafe:
- Soft cheeses (Mexican style, feta, brie, camembert, blue-veined).
- Salad bar items.
- Unwashed berries and grapes.
- Sandwiches.
- Hamburgers.
- Airline food.

Rarely unsafe:
- Peeled fruit.
- High-sugar foods.
- Steaming-hot foods.

Call a doctor if you develop these potentially dangerous conditions:
- Bloody diarrhea.
- A stiff neck, severe headache, and fever (signs of meningitis).
- Excessive diarrhea or vomiting.
- Any food poisoning symptoms that last longer than 3 days.

biosensor: a genetically altered microbe that provides a rapid, low-cost, and accurate test for the products of spoilage in foods.

Table 14–2

Safe Refrigerator Storage Times (40°F)

1 to 2 Days

Raw ground meats, breakfast or other raw sausages, raw fish or poultry; gravies

3 to 5 Days

Raw steaks, roasts, or chops; cooked meats, vegetables, and mixed dishes; ham slices; mayonnaise salads (chicken, egg, pasta, tuna)

1 Week

Hard-cooked eggs, bacon or hot dogs (opened packages); smoked sausages

2 to 4 Weeks

Raw eggs (in shells); bacon or hot dogs (packages unopened); dry sausages (pepperoni, hard salami); most aged and processed cheeses (swiss, brick)

2 Months

Mayonnaise (opened jar); most dry cheeses (parmesan, romano)

Sources: A. Hecht, Preventing food-borne illnesses, *FDA Consumer*, January/February 1991, p. 21; Refrigerator storage times for selected foods, *Consumer Reports on Health*, December 1991, p. 93.

pathogens (PATH-oh-jens): microorganisms or substances capable of producing disease.

How to Achieve Food Safety while Traveling

Food-borne illnesses contracted while traveling are colloquially known as traveler's diarrhea. A bout of this ailment can ruin the most enthusiastic tourist's trip. To avoid food-borne illness while traveling:

- Wash your hands often with soap and water, especially before handling food or eating.
- Eat only cooked or canned foods. Eat raw fruits or vegetables only if you have washed them in boiled water and peeled them yourself. Skip salads and raw fish and shellfish.
- Be aware that water, and ice made from it, may be unsafe. Take along disinfecting tablets or a device to boil water. Do not use the local water supply, even to brush your teeth, unless you boil or disinfect it first. Do not use ice.
- Drink no beverages made with tap water. Drink only treated, boiled, canned, or bottled beverages, and drink them without ice, even if they are not chilled to your liking. Refuse dairy products unless they have been properly pasteurized and refrigerated.
- Before you leave on the trip, ask your physician to recommend medicines to take with you in case your efforts to avoid illness fail.

One journalist succinctly sums up these recommendations, "Boil it, cook it, peel it, or forget it."[a] Chances are excellent that if you follow these rules, you will remain well.

---

[a]R. D. Williams, Boil it, cook it, peel it or forget it, *FDA Consumer*, September 1991, p. 17.

Someday their use may dramatically improve the safety of fish and other foods for sale on the market.

FOOD SAFETY WHILE TRAVELING

People who travel to other countries have a 50–50 chance of contracting traveler's diarrhea. Like many other food-borne illnesses, traveler's diarrhea is a sometimes serious, always annoying bacterial infection of the digestive tract. The risk is high because, for one thing, some countries' cleanliness standards for food and water may be lower than those in the United States and Canada. For another, every region's microbes are different, and while people are immune to those in their own neighborhoods, they have had no chance to develop immunity to the pathogens in places they are visiting for the first time. The accompanying box offers tips to travelers on avoiding food-borne infections.

In summary, millions of people suffer from mild to life-threatening symptoms caused by food-borne illnesses. As the box on pp. 490–491 describes, most of these illnesses can be prevented by storing and cooking foods at their proper temperatures and by preparing them in sanitary conditions.

Nutritional Adequacy of Foods and Diets

Among the FDA's priority concerns, the nutritional adequacy of foods and diets ranks second only to food-borne illness. In years past, when most foods were whole and farm fresh, the task of meeting nutrient needs primarily involved balancing servings from the various food groups. Today, however, foods have changed. Many "new" foods are available to appeal to people's tastes and health needs, but not necessarily to deliver a balanced assortment of needed nutrients.

To assist consumers in finding their way among these foods, the FDA has developed extensive nutrition labeling regulations intended to help consumers combine foods into healthful diets, as Chapter 2 described. In addition, the USDA's dietary guidelines help consumers "eat to stay healthy," and the Food Guide Pyramid helps them to put those recommendations into practice (see Chapter 2).

Environmental Contaminants

The third concern, environmental contamination of foods, is growing in importance as the world becomes more populated and more industrialized. A food contaminant is anything that does not belong there.

contaminant: a substance that does not normally occur in a food.

HARMFULNESS OF ENVIRONMENTAL CONTAMINANTS

The potential harmfulness of a contaminant depends in part on its persistence—the extent to which it lingers in the environment or in the body. Some contaminants in the environment are short-lived because microorganisms or agents such as sunlight or oxygen can break them down. Some contaminants in the body may linger for only a short time because the body rapidly excretes them or metabolizes them to harmless compounds. These contaminants present little cause for concern. Some contaminants, however, resist breakdown and can accumulate. Each level of the food chain, then, has a greater concentration than the one below (bioaccumulation). Figure 14–3 shows how bioaccumulation leads to high concentrations of toxins in people at the top of the food chain, and Figure 14–4 (on p. 497) shows how contaminants find their way into food.

How much of a threat do environmental contaminants pose to the food supply? For the most part, the hazards appear to be small because the FDA regulates the presence of contaminants in foods and requires foods with unsafe amounts to be removed from the market. In the event of an accidental spill, however, the hazards can suddenly become great.

persistence: stubborn or enduring continuance; with respect to food contaminants, the quality of persisting, rather than breaking down, in the bodies of animals and human beings.

food chain: the sequence in which living things depend on other living things for food.

bioaccumulation: the accumulation of contaminants in the flesh of animals high on the food chain.

EXAMPLES OF ENVIRONMENTAL CONTAMINANTS

The following paragraphs describe how two different types of contaminants have found their way into the food supply in the past. One is a heavy metal that was released into waterways by industry and ingested by fish that people ate. The other is an organic halogen that was accidentally spilled into livestock feed and ingested by animals that people ate.

heavy metal: any of a number of mineral ions such as mercury and lead, so called because they are of relatively high atomic weight. Many heavy metals are poisonous.

organic halogen: an organic compound containing one or more atoms of a halogen—fluorine, chlorine, iodine, or bromine.

Figure 14–3

Bioaccumulation of Toxins in the Food Chain

If none of the chemicals are lost along the way, one person ultimately receives all of the toxic chemicals that were present in the original several tons of producer organisms.

❹ A person whose principal animal-protein source is fish may consume about 100 pounds of fish in a year.

❸ These fish consume a few tons of plankton-eating fish in the course of their lifetimes—and the toxic chemicals become more concentrated.

❷ The toxic chemicals become more concentrated in the plankton-eating fish that consume several tons of producer organisms in their lifetimes.

❶ Producer organisms may become contaminated with toxic chemicals.

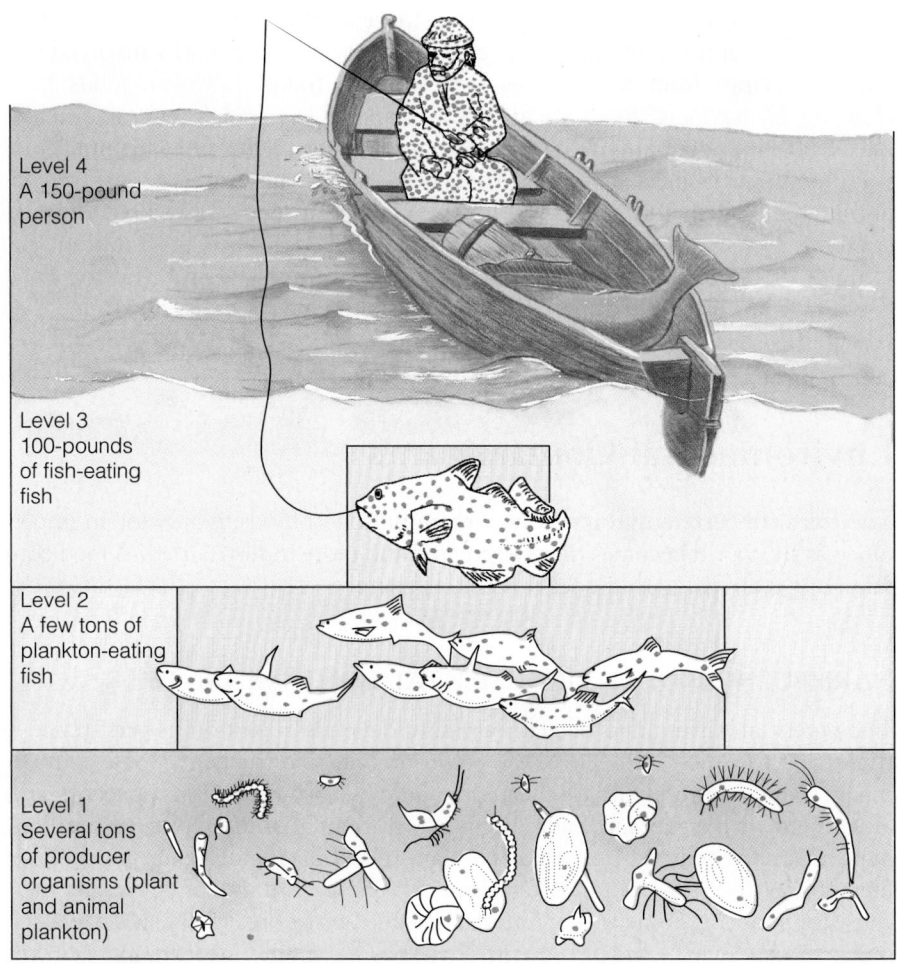

Level 4
A 150-pound person

Level 3
100-pounds of fish-eating fish

Level 2
A few tons of plankton-eating fish

Level 1
Several tons of producer organisms (plant and animal plankton)

Toxic chemicals ⋮

Methylmercury A classic example of acute contamination occurred in 1953 when a number of people in Minamata, Japan, became ill with a disease no one had seen before. By 1960, 121 cases had been reported, including 23 in infants. Mortality was high; 46 died, and the survivors suffered blindness, deafness, incoordination, and intellectual deterioration. The cause was ultimately revealed to be methylmercury contamination of fish from the bay where these people lived. The infants who contracted the disease had not eaten any fish, but their mothers had, and even though the mothers exhibited no symptoms during their pregnancies, the poison had been affecting their unborn babies. Manufacturing plants in the region were discharging mercury into the waters of the bay, the mercury was turning to methylmercury on leaving the factories, and the fish in the

Figure 14–4

Contaminants Find Their Way into Foods

Heavy metals and other contaminants entering the air in smokestack emissions return to the soil in rainfall. Contaminants in the soil are absorbed by plants. People either eat the plants (fruits and vegetables) or the meat from livestock that have eaten the plants. Sewage sludge and pesticides leave residues in the soil; runoff pollutes ground and surface water and contaminates the seafood that people eat.

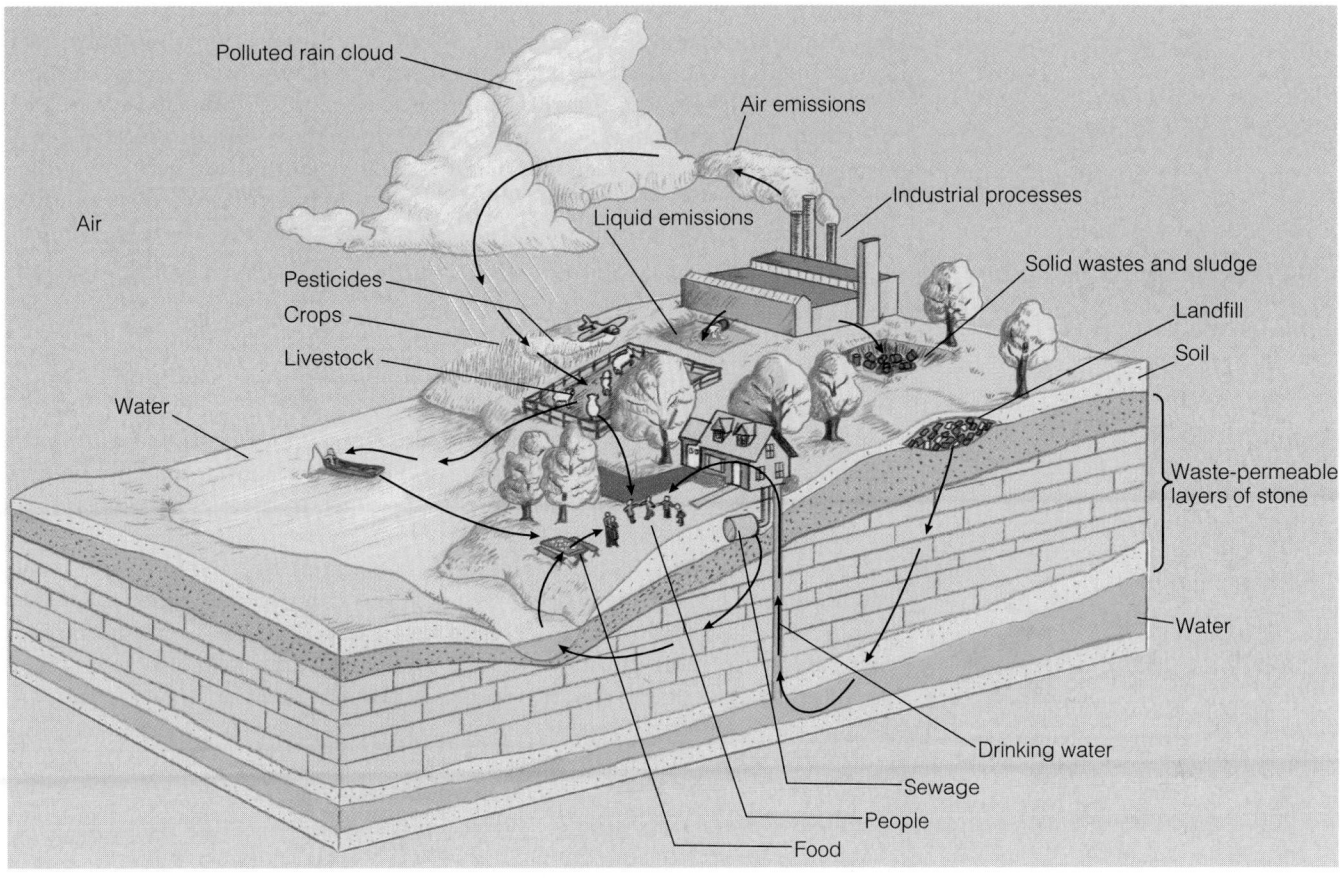

bay were accumulating this poison in their bodies. Some of the affected families had been eating fish from the bay every day.

PBB   In 1973, in Michigan, half a ton of polybrominated biphenyl (PBB), a toxic organic compound, was accidentally mixed into some livestock feed that was distributed throughout the state. The chemical found its way into millions of animals and then into people who ate the meat. The seriousness of the accident began to come to light when dairy farmers reported their cows were going dry, aborting their calves, and developing abnormal growths on their hooves. Although more than 30,000 cattle, sheep, and swine and more than a million chickens were destroyed, an estimated 97 percent of Michigan's residents had been exposed to PBB. Some of the exposed farm residents suffered nervous system aberrations and liver disorders.

Methylmercury and PCB (polychlorinated biphenyl, a compound similar to PBB) are still found in our food supply today. Fish harvested from contaminated waters have relatively high amounts of these two pollutants. Thousands of other contaminants exist as well; Highlight 13 focused on the heavy metal lead and its toxic effects.

To briefly sum up, environmental contamination of foods is a growing concern, but so far, the hazards appear small. In all cases, two principles apply: First, remain alert to the possibility of contamination of foods, and keep an ear open for public health announcements and advice. Second, do not eat any one food too often; vary your choices. Switching from food to food is an effective defensive strategy against the accumulation of toxins in your body. This is the principle of dilution: each food eaten dilutes contaminants that may be present in other components of the diet.

Natural Toxicants in Foods

Consumers concerned about food contamination may naively think that they can eliminate all poisons from their diets by eating only "natural" foods. On the contrary, nature has provided plants with an abundant array of toxicants. A few examples will show how even "natural" foods may contain potentially harmful substances. They also show that while the *potential* for harm exists, actual harm rarely occurs.

Poisonous mushrooms are a familiar example of plants that everyone knows can be harmful when eaten. Few people know, though, that other foods they commonly eat contain substances that can cause illnesses. Cabbage, turnips, mustard greens, and radishes contain small quantities of goitrogens—compounds that can enlarge the thyroid gland. Eating exceptionally large amounts of goitrogen-containing vegetables can aggravate a preexisting thyroid problem, but usually does not initiate one.

Lima beans and fruit seeds such as apricot pits contain cyanogens—inactive compounds that produce the deadly poison cyanide upon activation by a specific plant enzyme. For this reason, many countries restrict commercially grown lima beans to those varieties with the lowest cyanogen contents. As for fruit seeds, they are seldom deliberately eaten. An occasional swallowed seed or two presents no danger, but a couple of dozen seeds can be fatal to a small child. Perhaps the most infamous cyanogen in seeds is laetrile—a compound erroneously represented as a cancer cure. True, laetrile kills cancer, but only at doses that kill the person, too. Research over the past hundred years has never proven laetrile to be an effective cancer treatment. In fact, laetrile is more dangerous than no treatment at all. The combination of cyanide poisoning and lack of medical attention is life-threatening.

Potatoes contain many natural poisons including solanine—a powerful narcotic-like substance. The small amounts of solanine normally found in potatoes are harmless, but solanine is toxic and presents a hazard when consumed in large quantities. Solanine production increases when potatoes are improperly stored in the light and in either very cold or fairly warm places. Cooking does not destroy solanine, but because most of a potato's solanine is in the green layer that develops just beneath the skin, it can be peeled off, making the potato safe to eat.

Reminder: *Goitrogens* are thyroid antagonists found in such foods as cabbage, kale, brussels sprouts, cauliflower, broccoli, and kohlrabi.

solanine (SO-lah-neen): a poisonous narcotic-like substance present in potato peels and sprouts. Physical symptoms of solanine poisoning include headache, vomiting, abdominal pain, diarrhea, and fever; neurological symptoms include apathy, restlessness, drowsiness, confusion, stupor, hallucinations, and visual disturbances.

To review, natural toxicants include the goitrogens in cabbage, cyanogens in lima beans, and solanine in potatoes. These examples of naturally occurring toxicants illustrate two familiar principles. First, any substance can be toxic when consumed in excess. Second, poisons are poisons, whether made by people or by nature. Remember: it is not the source of a chemical that makes it hazardous, but its chemical structure and the quantity consumed.

Pesticides

The use of pesticides is controversial. They do help to ensure the survival of some crops, but they leave residues in the environment and on some of the foods we eat.

Ideally, a pesticide would destroy the pest, not accumulate in the food chain, and quickly degenerate to nontoxic products. Then, by the time consumers ate the food, no harmful residues would remain. Unfortunately, no such perfect pesticide exists. Developing new pesticides and monitoring their use are ongoing activities that require continued vigilance on the part of government agencies.

Hazards of Pesticides   Many pesticides are broad-spectrum poisons that damage all living cells, not just those of pests. Their use, therefore, is hazardous to those who work with them: manufacturers, field workers, truck drivers, and anyone else who is exposed to them. The danger of misuses or accidental spills is ever present, despite safety regulations and precautions.

Consumers have reason to be concerned, too, because pesticides may linger in the foods to which they were applied in the field.[9] Health risks from pesticide exposure are probably small for healthy adults, but children may be vulnerable to some types of pesticide poisoning.[10] The FDA, EPA, and USDA are considering proposals to revise food safety and pesticide laws to protect infants and children from pesticide risks.[11] When setting tolerance levels, the agencies will first identify foods that children commonly eat in large amounts and then consider the effects of pesticide exposure during developmental stages.[12]

Whether consumers are ingesting pesticide residues depends on a number of factors. How much of a given food is the consumer eating? What pesticide was used on it? How much was used? How long ago was the food last sprayed? Did environmental conditions promote pest growth or pesticide breakdown? How well was the produce washed? Was it peeled or cooked? With so many factors, consumers cannot know for sure whether any pesticide residues remain on foods.

Regulation of Pesticides   Consumers depend on the EPA and the FDA to keep pesticide use within safe limits. These two agencies have joint responsibility for registering pesticides and regulating their use. To register a pesticide, the manufacturer submits results of studies on its biological effects, persistence in crops, and environmental fate to the EPA. The EPA then evaluates the risks and benefits of the pesticide's use by asking such questions as, How dangerous is it? How much residue is left in the crop? How much harm does the pesticide do to the environment? How necessary is it? What are the alternatives to its use?

If the pesticide is approved, the EPA registers the chemical and establishes a tolerance level for its presence in foods, well below that at which it could cause

pesticides: chemicals used to control insects, diseases, weeds, fungi, and other pests on plants, vegetables, fruits, and animals. Used broadly, the term includes herbicides (to kill weeds), insecticides (to kill insects), and fungicides (to kill fungi).

residues: whatever remains. In the case of pesticides, those amounts that remain on or in foods when people buy and use them.

tolerance level: the maximum amount of a residue permitted in a food when a pesticide is used according to label directions.

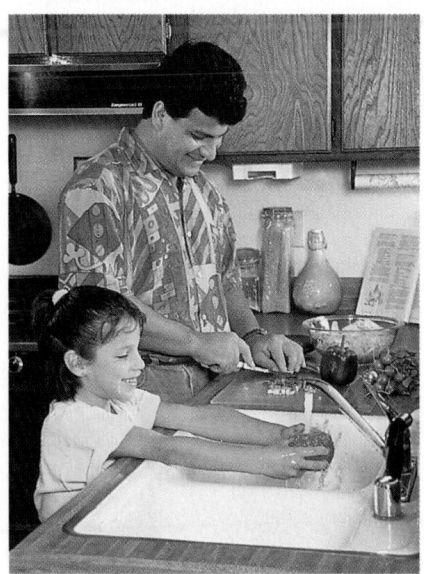

Washing fresh fruits and vegetables removes most, if not all, of the pesticide residues that might have been present.

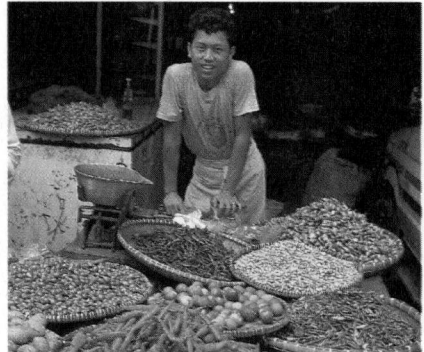

Foods imported from other countries may contain residues of pesticides that are banned from use here.

certification: the process in which a private laboratory inspects shipments of a product for selected chemicals and then, if the product is free of violative levels of those chemicals, issues a guarantee to that effect.

any conceivable harm. Tolerance levels are generally 1/100 to 1/1000 the amount that caused "no effect" in laboratory animals; actual residues may be much lower than that. Tolerance regulations also state the specific crops for which each pesticide can be used. If a pesticide is misused, growers risk fines, lawsuits, and destruction of their crops.

Once tolerances are set, the FDA enforces them by monitoring foods and livestock feeds for the presence of pesticides. In 25 years of testing, the FDA has seldom found residues above tolerance levels, so it appears that pesticides are generally used according to regulations. Minimal pesticide use means lower costs for growers. In addition to costs, many farmers are concerned about the environment, the quality of their farmland, and a safe food supply. Where violations are found, they are usually due to unusual weather conditions, use of unapproved pesticides, or misuse—for example, use of a particular pesticide on a crop for which it has not been approved.

Pesticides from Other Countries   Regulations in foreign countries differ from those in the United States. Imported foods may contain both pesticides that have been banned in this country and permitted pesticides at concentrations higher than are allowed in domestic foods. A loophole in federal regulations allows U.S. companies to manufacture and sell, to other countries, pesticides that are banned in this country. The banned pesticides then return to the United States on imported foods—a circuitous route that concerned consumers have called the "circle of poison." Federal inspectors do monitor imported foods and refuse entry if they are found to contain illegal residues.

Monitoring Pesticides: Food in the Fields   The FDA collects and analyzes samples of both domestic and imported foods. If the agency finds samples in violation of regulations, it can seize the products or order them destroyed. The FDA may also invoke a certification requirement that forces manufacturers, at their own expense, to have their foods periodically inspected and certified safe by an independent testing agency. Individual states can also scan for pesticides (as well as for industrial chemicals) and share information with the FDA.

In addition to its ongoing surveillance, the FDA also conducts selective surveys to determine the presence of particular pesticides in specific crops. For example, selective surveys for one year included a search for aldicarb in potatoes, captan in cherries, and diaminozide (the chemical name for Alar) in apples, among others. Actions taken that year required several certifications. Thus one shipper in Australia had to certify apples; one in Canada, peppers; one in Costa Rica, chayotes; eight in the Dominican Republic, eggplant; 11 in Spain, lemons; and there were other similar actions. All grapes from Mexico had to be certified and so did all mangoes from anywhere. This shows, incidentally, how many foods come from abroad—not only those already named, but also bitter melons, long beans, okra, snow peas, squash, broccoli, coriander, cucumbers, grapes, strawberries, and currants—and that the FDA monitors them as carefully as it does the domestic food supply.

Monitoring Pesticides: Food on the Plate   In addition to monitoring foods in the field for pesticides, the FDA also monitors people's actual intakes. The agency conducts the Total Diet Study (sometimes called the "Market Basket Survey") to estimate the dietary intakes of pesticide residues by eight age and sex groups from infants to senior citizens. Four times a year, FDA surveyors buy over

200 foods from U.S. grocery stores, each time in several cities, prepare the foods table ready, and then analyze them not only for pesticides, but for essential minerals, industrial chemicals, heavy metals, and radioactive materials. In all, the survey reports on over 10,000 samples a year, and recently more than half have been imported foods. Most heavily sampled are fresh vegetables, then fruits, and then dairy foods.

The Total Diet Study provides a direct estimate of the amounts of pesticide residues that remain in foods as they are usually eaten—after they have been washed, peeled, and cooked. The FDA finds the intake of almost all pesticides to be less than 1 percent of the amount considered acceptable. The amount considered acceptable is "the daily intake of a chemical which, if ingested over a lifetime, appears to be without appreciable risk"; it is established by the United Nations Food and Agriculture Organization and the World Health Organization. All in all, these findings corroborate "the continuing safety of the U.S. food supply relative to pesticide residues."[13]

safety: a judgment that considers the risks acceptable.

Consumer Concerns Despite these reassuring reports, consumers still worry that the monitoring of foods may not be adequate. For one thing, new pesticides keep appearing before the EPA can evaluate and register them. For another, as described, other countries use pesticides that are illegal for use here. For still another, although the regulations described here may protect U.S. foods adequately, they do not necessarily protect the environment or the people who work with them nearly as well. Concerns over poisoning of soil, waterways, wildlife, and workers may well be valid.

The FDA does not sample *all* food shipments and test for *all* pesticides in each sample. Budget constraints limit the FDA to fewer than 700 inspectors and scientists nationwide to test food samples from a multitude of farms, groves, docks, airports, warehouses, and processing plants. The FDA is a *monitoring* agency, and as such, it cannot, nor can it be expected to, guarantee 100 percent safety in the food supply. Instead, it sets conditions so that substances do not become a hazard, checks enough samples to adequately assess average food safety, and acts promptly when problems or suspicions arise.

Minimizing Risks Consumers must assume some responsibility for their own health and safety with respect to pesticides. They can learn about the potential benefits and possible dangers of pesticide use, discuss regulations and alternatives with others, advise their government representatives of their findings, and apply pressure wherever it will help change procedures. Meanwhile, people can minimize their risks by following the guidelines offered on the next page.

In addition to the suggestions in the box, consumers can buy fresh foods grown locally, especially when they can confirm that produce has been grown using responsible methods. Consumers who want pesticide-free produce shouldn't look for "perfect" fruits and vegetables; pesticide-free produce may have a few blemishes, but minor blemishes are not a hazard. It is also important to buy a variety of foods and not to rely too heavily on any one. The food supply is protected well enough that consumers who take these precautions can feel secure that the foods they eat are safe.

Alternatives to Pesticides To feed a nation while employing fewer pesticides requires creative farming methods. Such methods have been recommended

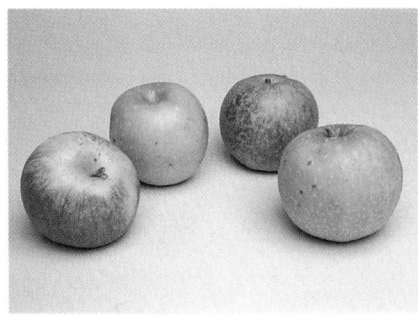

Pesticide-free produce may not be perfectly free of blemishes, but may be a healthy choice.

How to Prepare Foods to Minimize Pesticide Residues

To remove or reduce any pesticide residues from foods:

- Trim the fat from meat, and remove the skin from poultry and fish; discard fats and oils in broths and pan drippings. (Pesticide residues concentrate in the animal's fat.)
- Wash fresh produce in water. Use a scrub brush, and rinse thoroughly.
- Use a knife to peel an orange or grapefruit; do not bite into the peel.
- Discard the outer leaves of leafy vegetables such as cabbage and lettuce.
- Peel waxed fruits and vegetables; waxes don't wash off and can seal in pesticide residues.
- Peel vegetables such as carrots and fruits such as apples when appropriate. (Peeling removes pesticides that remain in or on the peel, but also removes fibers, vitamins, and minerals.)

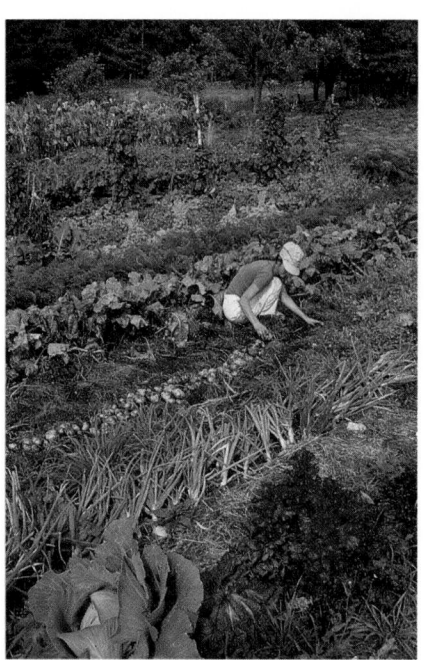

People can avoid the use of pesticides and fertilizers when their gardens or farms are relatively small.

by the National Academy of Sciences as part of a system known as alternative, or sustainable, agriculture. This system depends on crop rotation and the use of plants that produce natural pesticides rather than on synthetic, toxic pesticides. Among natural pesticides are the nicotine in tobacco and psoralens in celery. Natural pesticides are less damaging to other living things and less persistent in the environment than most human-made ones.

Other alternatives to heavy pesticide use include releasing organisms into fields to destroy pests and planting nonfood crops nearby to kill pests or attract them away from the food crops. For example, sterile male fruit flies have been released into orchards, thus helping to curb the population growth of these pests; some flowers, such as marigolds, release natural insecticides and are often planted near crops such as tomatoes. In addition, farmers can plow compost into the soil, which enriches the nutrient content of the soil, increases moisture retention, and reduces erosion. Such alternative farming methods are more labor-intensive and may produce smaller yields than conventional methods, at least initially. Given a fair chance to compete with present methods, however, these alternatives may actually cut costs more than they cut yields, by eliminating expensive pesticides, fertilizers, and fuels.

Consumers with questions about pesticides can call the pesticide hotline.* Meanwhile, the most important thing consumers can do to protect their *food* supply is to defend the *environment*.

In short, pesticides can safely improve crop yields when used according to regulations, but can also be hazardous when used inappropriately. The FDA tests both domestic and imported foods for pesticide residues in the fields and in market basket surveys of foods prepared table ready. Consumers can minimize their ingestion of pesticide residues on foods by following the suggestions in the box above.

*The National Pesticide Hotline, funded by the EPA, is 1–800–858–PEST. Call anytime day or night, 365 days a year. The Canadian Pesticide Information Line is 1–800–267–6315.

Food Additives

Additives confer many benefits on foods. Some reduce the risk of food-borne illness (for example, nitrites used in curing meat prevent poisoning from the botulinum toxin). Others enhance nutrient quality (as in vitamin D–fortified milk). Most additives help prevent spoilage during the time it takes to deliver foods long distances to grocery stores and then to kitchens. Some additives simply make foods look and taste good.

Intentional additives are put into foods on purpose, while indirect additives may get in unintentionally before or during processing. This discussion begins with the regulations that govern additives, then presents intentional additives class by class, and finally goes on to say a word about the indirect additives.

REGULATIONS GOVERNING ADDITIVES

The FDA's concern with additives hinges primarily on their safety. To receive permission to use a new additive in food products, a manufacturer must satisfy the FDA that the additive is:

- Effective (it does what it is supposed to do).
- Detectable and measurable in the final food product.
- Safe (when fed in large doses to animals under strictly controlled conditions, it causes no cancer, birth defects, or other injury).

On approving an additive's use, the FDA writes a regulation stating in what amounts and in what foods the additive may be used. No additive receives permanent approval; all must undergo periodic review.

The GRAS List   Many familiar substances are exempted from complying with this procedure because they are generally recognized as safe (GRAS), based either on their extensive, long-term use in foods or on current scientific evidence. Several hundred substances are on the GRAS list, including such items as salt, sugar, caffeine, and herbs. Whenever substantial scientific evidence or public outcry has questioned the safety of any substance on the GRAS list, it has been reevaluated. All substances about which any legitimate question has been raised have been removed or reclassified. Meanwhile, the entire GRAS list is subjected to ongoing review.

The Delaney Clause   One risk that the U.S. law on additives refuses to tolerate at any level is the risk of cancer. To remain on the GRAS list, an additive must not have been found to be a carcinogen in any test on animals or human beings. The Delaney Clause (the part of the law that states this criterion) is uncompromising in addressing carcinogens in foods and drugs; in fact, it has been under fire for many years for being too strict and inflexible.

The Delaney Clause states that "no additive shall be deemed to be safe if it is found to induce cancer when ingested [at any level] by man or animal." That sounds clear enough, yet some products that fail to meet that standard still remain on the market. The artificial sweetener saccharin was the first exception to the rule. In the 1970s, when the FDA tried to ban saccharin because tests had revealed that it caused cancer in animals, consumers raised an outcry asking that it still be allowed in foods. In response, Congress created a special exception that

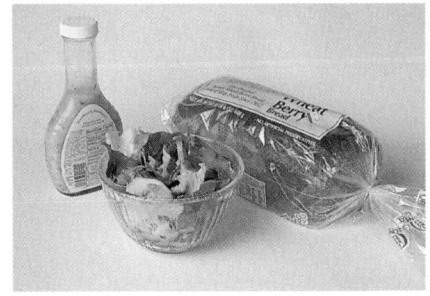

Without additives, bread would quickly get moldy and salad dressing would go rancid.

additives: substances not normally consumed as foods but added to food either intentionally or by accident.

intentional additives: additives intentionally added to foods, such as nutrients, colors, and preservatives.

indirect additives: substances that can get into food as a result of contact with foods during growing, processing, packaging, storing, cooking, or some other stage before the foods are consumed; also called **incidental** or **accidental additives**.

GRAS (generally recognized as safe) list: a list, established by the FDA in 1958, of food additives that had long been in use and were believed safe. The list is subject to revision as new facts become known.

Delaney Clause: a clause in the Food Additive Amendment to the Food, Drug, and Cosmetic Act that states that no substance that is known to cause cancer in animals or human beings at any dose level shall be added to foods.

Reminder: A *carcinogen* is a substance that initiates cancer development.

For perspective, one part per trillion is equivalent to about one grain of sugar in an Olympic-sized swimming pool; or 1 second in 32,000 years; or one hair on 10 million heads, assuming none are bald.

The *de minimis* rule defines risk as a cancer rate of less than one cancer per million people exposed to a contaminant over a 70-year lifetime.

margin of safety: when speaking of food additives, a zone between the concentration normally used and that at which a hazard exists. For common table salt, for example, the margin of safety is 1/5 (five times the amount normally used would be hazardous).

allowed saccharin to remain on the market as long as products containing it carried a warning. This was an attempt to balance the Delaney Clause with current food safety and cancer knowledge.

The Delaney Clause is best understood as a product of a different historical era. It was adopted more than 35 years ago at a time when scientists knew little about carcinogens and cancer development and most substances were detectable in foods only in relatively large amounts, such as parts per thousand. Today, scientific understanding of cancer has progressed, and technology has advanced so that carcinogens in foods can be detected even when they are present only in parts per billion or even per trillion. Earlier, "zero risk" may have seemed attainable, but today we know it is not: all substances, no matter how pure, can be shown to be contaminated at some level with one carcinogen or another. For these reasons, the FDA prefers to deem additives (and pesticides and other contaminants) safe if lifetime use presents no more than a one-in-a-million risk of cancer to human beings. Thus, instead of the "zero-risk" policy of the Delaney Clause, the FDA used a "negligible-risk" standard, sometimes referred to as a *de minimis* rule. This policy was challenged and overruled in court, rekindling the debate on the controversial Delaney Clause.[14] A congressional report called the Delaney Clause "scientifically unmanageable" and noted that it does not allow food safety to keep up with science.[15] New legislation was enacted to exempt pesticide residues from the Delaney Clause and require a "reasonable certainty of no harm" instead.

Margin of Safety Whatever risk level is permitted, actual risks must be determined by experiments. Experiments to determine risks posed by an additive involve feeding test animals the additive at several concentrations throughout their lives. The additive is then permitted in foods 100 times below the lowest level that is found to cause any harmful effect, that is, at a 1/100 margin of safety. In many foods, *naturally* occurring substances occur with narrower margins of safety, such as 1/10. Even nutrients pose risks at dose levels above those normally consumed: the margin of safety for vitamins A and D is 1/25 to 1/40 for adults and may be less than 1/10 for infants. For some trace elements, the margin of safety is about 1/5. People consume common table salt daily in amounts only three to five times less than those that pose a hazard.

Risks versus Benefits Of course, additives would not be added to foods if they only presented risks. Additives are in foods because they offer benefits that outweigh the risks they present, or make the risks worth taking. In the case of color additives that only enhance the appearance of foods but do not improve their health value or safety, no amount of risk may be deemed worth taking. In contrast, the FDA finds that it is worth taking the small risks associated with the use of nitrites on meat products, for example, because nitrites inhibit the formation of the deadly botulinum toxin. The choice involves a compromise between the risks of using additives and the risks of doing without them.

It is the manufacturers' responsibility to use only the amounts of additives that are necessary to get the needed effect, and no more. The FDA also requires that additives *not* be used:

- To disguise faulty or inferior products.
- To deceive the consumer.

- Where they significantly destroy nutrients.
- Where their effects can be achieved by economical, sound manufacturing processes.

INTENTIONAL FOOD ADDITIVES

Intentional food additives are added to foods to give them some desirable characteristic: resistance to spoilage, color, flavor, texture, stability, or nutritional value. The accompanying glossary defines the categories of additives, and the next sections describe additives people most often ask about.

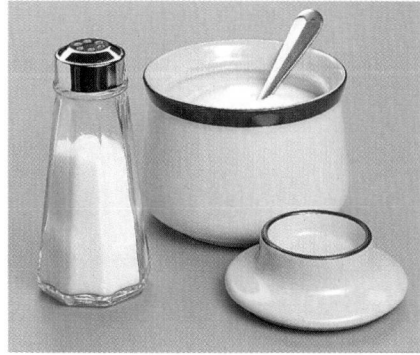

Both salt and sugar act as preservatives by withdrawing water from food; microbes cannot grow without water.

Antimicrobial Agents   Foods can go bad in two ways. One way is relatively harmless: by losing their flavor and attractiveness. (Additives to prevent this kind of spoilage include antioxidants, discussed later.) The other way is by becoming contaminated with microbes that cause food-borne illnesses, a hazard that justifies the use of antimicrobial agents.

The most widely used antimicrobial agents are ordinary salt and sugar. Salt has been used throughout history to preserve meat and fish; sugar serves the same purpose in canned and frozen fruits and in jams and jellies. Both exert their protective effect primarily by capturing water and making it unavailable to microbes. Other additives, such as potassium sorbate and sodium propionate, are used to extend the shelf life of baked goods, cheeses, beverages, mayonnaise, margarine, and other products.

Other antimicrobial agents, the nitrites and nitrates, are added to foods for three main purposes: to preserve color, especially the pink color of hot dogs and other cured meats; to enhance flavor by inhibiting rancidity, especially in cured meats; and to protect against bacterial growth. In amounts smaller than those needed to confer color, nitrites prevent the growth of the bacteria that produce the deadly botulinum toxin.

Nitrites clearly serve a useful purpose, but their use has been controversial. In the human body, nitrites can be converted to nitrosamines. At nitrite levels higher than those used in food products, nitrosamine formation causes cancer in

Common examples of antimicrobial additives:
- Salt.
- Sugar.
- Nitrites and nitrates (such as sodium nitrate).

nitrites: salts added to food to prevent botulism; one example is sodium nitrite, which is used to preserve meats.

nitrates: salts that are converted to nitrites by bacteria.

nitrosamines (nigh-TROHS-uh-meens): derivatives of nitrites that may be formed in the stomach when nitrites combine with amines; nitrosamines are carcinogenic in animals.

Glossary of Intentional Food Additives

antimicrobial agents: preservatives that prevent microorganisms from growing.

artificial colors: certified food colors added to enhance appearance. (*Certified* means approved by the FDA.)

artificial flavors, flavor enhancers: chemicals that mimic natural flavors and those that enhance flavor.

nutrient additives: vitamins and minerals added to improve nutritive value.

preservatives: antimicrobial agents, antioxidants, and other additives that retard spoilage or maintain desired qualities, such as softness in baked goods.

radiation: ionizing rays used to sterilize and protect food.

Reminder: An *antioxidant* is a compound that protects others from oxidation; with respect to food additives, chemicals that prevent rancidity of fats and other damage to food caused by oxygen.

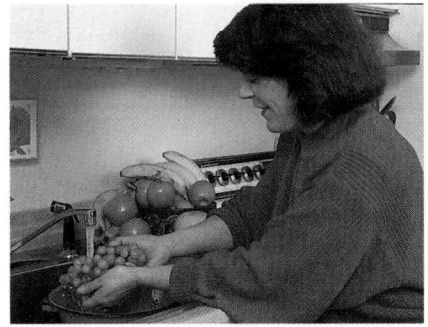

Raw grapes may legally be treated with sulfites, so wash them thoroughly before eating them.

Common examples of antioxidant additives:
- Vitamin C (ascorbate).
- Vitamin E (tocopherol).
- Sulfites.
- BHA and BHT.

sulfites: salts containing sulfur that are added to foods to prevent spoilage.

Sulfites appear on food labels as:
- Sulfur dioxide.
- Sodium sulfite.
- Sodium bisulfite.
- Potassium bisulfite.
- Sodium metabisulfite.
- Potassium metabisulfite.

BHA and **BHT:** preservatives commonly used to slow the development of off-flavors, odors, and color changes caused by oxidation.

Common examples of color additives:
- Carotenoids.
- Blue (brilliant blue and indigotine).
- Green (fast green).
- Red (allura red and erythrosine).
- Yellow (tartrazine and sunset yellow).

animals. The food industry uses the minimal amount of nitrites necessary to achieve results, and nitrosamine formation has not been shown to cause cancer in human beings.

Detectable amounts of nitrosamine-related compounds are found in malt beverages (beer) and cured meats (primarily, bacon). Yet even the quantities found in beer and bacon hardly make a difference in a person's overall exposure to nitrosamine-related compounds. An average cigarette smoker inhales 100 times the nitrosamines that the average bacon eater ingests. A beer drinker ingests twice as much as the bacon eater, but even so, exposure from new car interiors and cosmetics is higher than this.

Antioxidants Another way food can go bad is by undergoing changes in color and flavor caused by exposure to oxygen (oxidation). Oftentimes, these changes involve no hazard to health, but they damage the food's appearance, flavor, and nutritional quality. Oxidation is easy to see when sliced apples or potatoes turn brown or when oil goes rancid. Antioxidants prevent these reactions. Among the antioxidants approved for use in foods are vitamin C (ascorbate) and vitamin E (tocopherol).

Another group of antioxidants, the sulfites, cost less than the vitamins. Sulfites prevent oxidation in many processed foods, alcoholic beverages (especially wine), and drugs. Restaurant owners used to use sulfites to keep raw fruits and vegetables on salad bars looking fresh, but this practice was banned after some people experienced adverse reactions. The FDA now prohibits sulfite use on foods intended to be consumed raw, with the exception of grapes, and requires foods and drugs that contain sulfite additives to declare it on their labels. For most people, sulfites pose no hazard in the amounts used in products, but there is one more consideration: sulfites destroy thiamin. For this reason, the FDA prohibits their use on foods that are important sources of the vitamin, such as enriched grain products.

Two other antioxidants in wide use are BHA and BHT, which prevent rancidity in baked goods and snack foods.* Several tests have shown that animals fed large amounts of BHT developed *less* cancer when exposed to carcinogens and lived *longer* than controls. BHT apparently protects against cancer through its antioxidant effect, which is similar to that of the antioxidant vitamins. The amount of BHT ingested daily from the U.S. diet, however, contributes little to the body's antioxidant defense system. A caution: at intake levels higher than those that protect against cancer, the substance has experimentally *produced* cancer. Vitamin E and vitamin C remain the most important dietary antioxidants to strengthen defenses against cancer.

Artificial Colors Only a few artificial colors remain on the FDA's list of color additives approved for use in foods—a highly select group that has survived considerable testing. Artificial colors are among the most intensively investigated of all additives. In fact, coloring agents are much better known than the natural pigments of plants, and the safety of their use can be stated with greater certainty. Examples of natural pigments commonly used by the food industry are the caramel that tints cola beverages and the carotenoids that color margarine, cheeses, and pastas.

---

*BHA is butylated hydroxyanisole; BHT is butylated hydroxytoluene.

Artificial Flavors and Flavor Enhancers   Flavoring agents are the largest single group of food additives. One of the best-known members of this group is monosodium glutamate, or MSG—a sodium salt of the amino acid glutamic acid. MSG is used widely in a number of foods, and especially in Asian foods, as a flavor enhancer. Besides enhancing the well-known sweet, salty, bitter, and sour tastes, MSG may, itself, possess a pleasant flavor.

MSG has received publicity because it may produce an adverse reaction in some individuals—the so-called Chinese restaurant syndrome—involving burning sensations, chest and facial flushing or pain, and throbbing headaches. MSG has been investigated extensively enough to be deemed safe for all adults except the 1 to 2 percent of the population who are sensitive to it. Food labels require ingredient lists to itemize all additives, including MSG.

Nutrient Additives   As mentioned earlier, manufacturers sometimes add nutrients to improve or maintain the nutritional quality of foods. Included among nutrient additives are the four nutrients added to refined grains to enrich them; the iodine added to salt; the vitamins A and D added to milk products; and the nutrients added to fortified breakfast cereals. A nutrient-poor food with nutrients added may appear to be nutrient-rich, but it is rich only in those nutrients chosen for addition, and the absorption of these nutrients may be poor. Appropriate uses of nutrient additives are to:

- Correct dietary deficiencies known to result in deficiency diseases.
- Restore nutrients to levels found in the food before storage, handling, and processing.
- Balance the vitamin, mineral, and protein contents of a food in proportion to the energy content.
- Correct nutritional inferiority in a food that replaces a more nutritious traditional food.

Nutrients are sometimes also added for other purposes. Vitamins C and E were already mentioned for their antioxidant properties; beta-carotene (a vitamin A precursor) is sometimes used for its color.

On the whole, the benefits of food additives seem to justify the risks associated with their use. The FDA closely regulates and monitors all intentional additives.

INDIRECT FOOD ADDITIVES

Indirect or incidental additives are substances that find their way into foods during harvesting, production, processing, storage, or packaging. For example, incidental additives include tiny bits of plastic, glass, paper, tin, and other substances from packages as well as chemicals from processing, such as the solvent used to decaffeinate some types of coffee. The following paragraphs discuss three different types of indirect additives that sometimes make headline news.

Microwave Packaging   When the FDA regulations were established in the 1950s, the writers did not foresee the use of microwave ovens. Consequently,

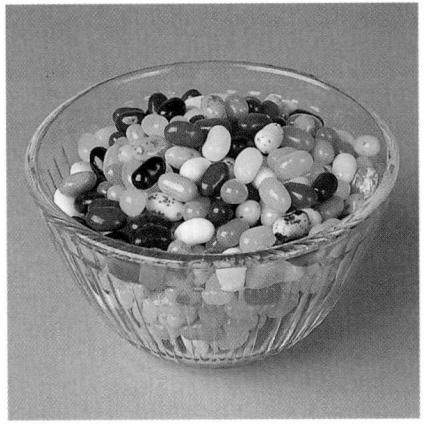

Color additives not only make foods attractive, but identify flavors as well. Everyone agrees that yellow jellybeans should taste lemony and black ones like licorice.

Chinese restaurant syndrome: an intolerance reaction that may occur in 1 to 2% of the population 20 min after the ingestion of the additive MSG (monosodium glutamate). Symptoms include burning sensations, chest and facial flushing and pain, and throbbing headaches.

Common examples of nutrient additives:
- Thiamin, niacin, riboflavin, and iron in grain products (beginning in 1998, grain products will also be fortified with folate).
- Iodine in salt.
- Vitamins A and D in milk.
- Vitamin C in fruit drinks.

they did not specify temperatures at which packages should be tested to determine if incidental additives migrated to foods at high temperatures. Some microwave products are sold in "active packaging" that helps to cook the food; for example, pizzas are often heated on a metalized film laminated to paperboard. This film absorbs the microwave energy in the oven and reaches temperatures as high as 500°F. In testing such products, the FDA found that packaging components migrate into the food.[16]

Most microwave products are sold in "passive packaging" that is transparent to microwaves and simply holds the food as it cooks. These containers don't get much hotter than the foods, but materials still migrate at high temperatures. Migration from packages may turn out to be harmless, but until more is known, consumers are advised to use only glass or ceramic containers designed for use in microwave ovens and to avoid reusing disposable containers such as margarine tubs.

Dioxins Coffee filters, milk cartons, paper plates, and frozen food packages, if made from bleached paper, can contaminate foods with minute quantities of dioxins—compounds formed during chlorine treatment of wood pulp during paper manufacture. Dioxin contamination of foods from such products appears only in trace quantities—in the parts per trillion range (recall, for perspective, that one part per trillion is equal to 1 second in 32,000 years). Such levels appear to present no health risks to people, but scientists recognize that dioxins are extremely toxic, and they are known to cause cancer in animals. Accordingly, the paper industry has reduced its use of chlorine to cut dioxin exposure; in the meantime, the FDA has concluded that drinking milk from bleached-paper cartons presents no health hazard.[17]

Decaffeinated Coffee Many consumers have tried to eliminate caffeine from their diets by selecting decaffeinated coffee. Is decaffeinated coffee a safe alternative? To answer that question, one first has to learn the facts about the decaffeination process.[18] What substances do manufacturers use? How much remains in the final cup of coffee? And are those residues harmful to health?

To remove caffeine from coffee beans, manufacturers often use methylene chloride in a process that leaves traces of the chemical in the final product. The FDA estimates that the average cup of coffee treated this way contains about 0.1 part per million of methylene chloride, which seems to pose no significant threat. A person drinking 2½ cups of decaffeinated coffee containing 100 times as much methylene chloride every day for a lifetime has a one in a million chance of developing cancer from it. People are exposed to much more methylene chloride from other sources such as hair sprays and paint stripping solutions. Still, some consumers prefer either to return to caffeine or to select coffee decaffeinated in another way. Unfortunately, manufacturers are not required to state on their labels the type of decaffeination process used in their products. Many labels provide consumer-information telephone numbers for those who have such questions.

Incidental additives sometimes find their way into foods, but adverse effects are rare. All food packagers are required to perform specific tests to discover whether materials are migrating into foods; if they are, their safety must be confirmed by strict procedures similar to those governing intentional additives.

Quick test for using glass containers in a microwave:
Microwave the empty container for 1 min.
- If it's warm, it's unsafe for the microwave.
- If it's lukewarm, it's safe for short-term reheating in the microwave.
- If it's cool, it's safe for long-term cooking in the microwave.

dioxins: any of 75 structurally related compounds that contain both nitrogen and chlorine.

HORMONES

Hormones are a unique type of incidental additive in that their use is intentional, but their presence in the final food product is not. The FDA has approved about a dozen hormones for use in food-producing animals, and the USDA has established limits for residues allowed in meat products.

BGH   Some ranchers in the United States treat young calves with bovine growth hormone (BGH). Hormone-treated meat animals produce leaner meats, and dairy cows produce more milk.[19] All cows make BGH naturally: the pituitary gland produces it and releases it into the bloodstream. Now scientists can stimulate bacteria to produce BGH, which allows laboratories to harvest huge quantities of the hormone and sell it to farmers as a drug.[20] This practice has some consumers concerned that an "artificial" drug is being given to cows that will be used for meat and milk.

Indeed, traces of BGH do remain in the meat and milk of both hormone-treated and untreated cows. BGH residues have not been tested for safety in human beings because residues of the natural hormone have always been present in milk and meat and the amount found in treated cows is within the range that can occur naturally.[21] Furthermore, BGH, being a peptide hormone, is denatured by the heat used in processing milk and cooking meat and is also digested by enzymes in the GI tract. If any BGH were to enter the bloodstream, it would have no effect because the chemical structures of animal growth hormones differ from those in human beings; BGH does not stimulate receptors for *human* growth hormone. In a report from its Technology Assessment Conference, the National Institutes of Health concludes, "As currently used in the United States, meat and milk from [hormone] treated cows are as safe as those from untreated cows."[22]

Opponents of BGH   Whether treating animals with hormones is wise is debated. Opponents say that a vast surplus of milk will flood the market, driving milk prices down. Huge farms that can weather price fluctuations will not be affected, but small farms may be forced to close, further reducing an already dwindling agricultural landscape across the United States.

Another concern is that BGH-treated cows suffer more udder infections (mastitis) and so are given more antibiotics—then, these drugs show up in the cows' milk and meat.[23] Furthermore, increased agricultural use of antibiotics helps to spread antibiotic-resistant microorganisms. These microorganisms can cause life-threatening food-borne illnesses that do not respond to antibiotic therapy.

Proponents of BGH   Supporters of BGH say that we need and use all the milk that can be produced. A greater output of milk per cow will simply mean fewer cows to feed, smaller feed bills, and larger profits for farmers. Similarly, beef cattle will reach their market weights earlier and require less food and care. The environment will suffer less damage. Smaller herds can live on smaller plots of cleared land and eat less food, which means less production, transportation, and overall environmental degradation.

Despite reassurances, some U.S. consumers still have concerns. The outcry against BGH has prompted farmers and grocers in several milk-producing states

bovine growth hormone (BGH): a hormone produced naturally in the pituitary gland of a cow that promotes growth and milk production; now produced for agricultural use by transgenic bacteria (described in the text).

bovine = of cattle

to pledge not to produce or sell milk from hormone-treated cows. The beef industry has responded by providing beef "certified as untreated." Several European countries refuse to import meat from animals treated with hormones. Consumers will have the final word on BGH by deciding whether to accept milk and meat from hormone-treated animals.

RADIATION

The FDA has approved the use of ionizing radiation on certain foods and treats irradiation as an additive. Radiation kills microorganisms and insects in postharvest wheat, spices, and teas (postharvest pesticide fumigation); kills *Trichinella*, the parasitic worms that sometimes contaminate pork; kills *Salmonella*, the bacteria that contaminate poultry; inhibits the growth of sprouts on potatoes and onions; and delays ripening in some fruits such as strawberries and mangoes.[24] Milk products change flavor when irradiated and so are not candidates for the treatment. (Incidentally, the milk in those boxes kept at room temperature on grocery-store shelves is not irradiated, but processed with an ultrahigh temperature treatment for just long enough to sterilize it.)

In many cases, the flavor, texture, and color of foods treated with radiation do not change. Vitamin loss is minimal and comparable to amounts lost from foods processed by other commercial processing methods.

Consumer Concerns   Irradiation does not make foods radioactive and therefore does not expose people to radiation. Radiation sterilizes foods and, as a side effect, slightly alters their chemistry. When radiation strikes the atoms in the molecules of the food, they lose electrons and form ions or free radicals. How these particles react with one another and with other food constituents is the focus of much research.

Compounds produced as a result of the irradiation process are called radiolytic products. A few radiolytic products are unique to irradiated foods. The higher the radiation dose, the more unique radiolytic products are formed. Most radiolytic products (approximately 90 percent), however, are also found in foods that have not been irradiated, leading to the conclusion that radiolytic products are probably not hazardous.[25] Research on irradiation safety continues.

Many customers, associating radiation with cancer, birth defects, and mutations, have strong negative emotions about the use of radiation on foods. Some confuse it with food contamination by radioactive particles, such as occurs in the aftermath of a nuclear accident. Many food producers are eager to use irradiation, but hesitate to do so until consumers are ready to accept it. Proponents believe that once consumers understand the benefits of irradiation and are no longer afraid of it, they will demand to have foods sterilized by this process. Some proponents suggest renaming irradiation *pico wave,* because consumers readily accepted microwaves.

Speaking of microwaves, like irradiation, microwaves can sterilize foods under certain conditions of time and temperature.* Unlike irradiation, though, microwaves cook food, and they do not create unique radiolytic products.

ultrahigh temperature (UHT) treatment: sterilizing a food by short-time exposure to temperatures above those normally used.

radiolytic (RAY-dee-oh-LIT-ic) products: chemicals formed during the irradiation of food.

---

*Gamma waves (pico waves) used in the irradiation of foods have a wavelength of 10^{-12} meters; microwaves have a wavelength of 10^{-2} meters. As a point of reference, lightbulbs emit wavelengths in the range of 10^{-7} meters.

Irradiation cuts down on food wastage and can replace some costly pesticides, thus reducing those residues in food. Alternatively, the same goals could be achieved by less expensive methods—such as higher cleanliness standards for food-animal facilities to prevent microbial contamination and selective breeding of produce to achieve longer storage times. These methods pose none of the hazards associated with transport and handling of radioactive materials, and they are proven safe for the human food supply. Whether irradiation will become widely used for food processing may depend on the ability of its backers to prove its safety beyond doubt.

Where irradiation technology is available, its use must be carefully scrutinized. There is no possibility of a meltdown or nuclear disaster because food irradiation plants are not nuclear reactors. However, strict controls on the transport of radioactive materials, adequate safety operations at facilities, and proper disposal of the wastes generated are indispensable to prevent hazards to workers and the environment.

This international symbol identifies retail foods that have been irradiated. The words "Treated by irradiation" or "Treated with irradiation" must accompany the symbol. The irradiation label is not required on commercially prepared foods that contain irradiated ingredients, such as spices.

Regulation of Radiation   The FDA has established regulations governing the specific uses of irradiation and allowed doses. Each food that has been treated with radiation must say so on its label. Labels can be misleading however, if consumers interpret the *absence* of the irradiation symbol to mean that the food was produced without any kind of treatment. This is not true; it is just that the FDA does not require label statements for other treatments used for the same purpose, such as postharvest fumigation with pesticides. If all treatment methods were declared, consumers could make fully informed choices.

FOOD BIOTECHNOLOGY

For centuries farmers have manipulated the genetics of plants and animals to shape the characteristics of their crops and livestock. Consider corn, for example. Wild, native corn bears only two or three kernels on a cob, but many years of patient selective breeding have produced the large, full, sweet ears people enjoy today, and many types of wild corn are now all but extinct. Half of the increases in U.S. crop yields in this century are due to such genetic improvements; the use of irrigation, fertilizers, and pesticides have also contributed.[26] Farmers are still using selective breeding to provide consumers with low-fat meats, high-yield grains, and a seemingly endless variety of fruits and vegetables.

Recently, scientists have discovered a way of speeding up the process of genetic change through biotechnology. Farmers need no longer wait patiently for breeding to yield improved crops and animals, nor must they even respect natural lines of reproduction among species. Laboratory scientists can now select desirable traits from any of a number of species and insert those traits into the genetic material of crops and animals.

biotechnology: the use of biological systems or organisms to create or modify products; also called **biogenetic engineering.**

So far, most of the traits that have been selected for transfer help to produce foods more efficiently. For example, the enzyme rennin, which is essential for making cheese, was previously harvested from the stomachs of calves, a costly process. Now scientists can convey into bacteria the genetic material to mass-produce rennin.

Among the new products of biotechnology are tomatoes that stay fresh much longer than others and so promise less waste and higher profits. Soybeans may soon be implanted with a gene that will upgrade soy protein to a quality approaching that of milk. Corn may be modified to contain lysine and trypto-

rennin: an enzyme that coagulates milk; found in the gastric juice of cows, but not human beings.

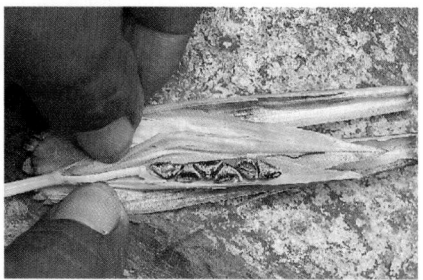

Today's large, full, sweet ears bear little resemblance to the original wild, native corn with its sparse two or three kernels to a cob.

recombinant DNA technology: methods of joining (recombining) pieces of the genetic material DNA in order to change the proteins produced by the altered DNA.

transgenic organism: an organism that grows from an embryonic, stem, or germ cell into which a gene is inserted; the organism then carries the new gene in all of its cells.

antisense gene: the chemical opposite of a native gene that adheres to the native working gene and blocks its production of proteins.

phan, its two limiting amino acids.[27] Fats and oils with a predetermined fatty acid composition may be possible within the decade.[28] Crops that produce their own insecticides upon receiving genes from bacteria may render pesticides unnecessary. Shrimp may soon fight diseases with genetic ammunition borrowed from sea urchins. Livestock may receive growth-promoting hormones from bacteria as mentioned earlier. Overall, biotechnology offers opportunities to enhance the quality, nutritional value, and variety of foods.[29] The possibilities seem unlimited, and though they sound fantastic, many are waiting on laboratory shelves for the time when they will be fully employed in agriculture.

While food industrialists hail biotechnology as a miracle, some other people fear that tampering with genetics may change organisms in ways not yet fully understood, even by the scientists who developed the techniques. They wonder what unknown changes take place when the genes of living things are manipulated, and what the long-term consequences might be.

DNA Technology   To understand the issues, it is necessary to understand the basic process of recombinant DNA technology.[30] To transfer genes, scientists first employ enzymes to snip from an organism's genetic material the bit of DNA responsible for a desirable trait. Then, they "recombine" the snipped bit with the DNA from viruses, yeasts, bacteria, or other sources to yield a complete DNA molecule. They then insert this "recombinant DNA" into the target plant, animal, or bacterial cell where it produces the proteins responsible for the desired trait. When the receiving cell happens to be an embryonic, stem, or germ cell, it gives rise to a whole new transgenic organism.

The transgenic organism carries the desired DNA code in every one of its cells. For example, when scientists implant a piece of DNA from a virus that attacks potato plants into a stem cell, that cell develops into a new potato plant that replicates a piece of the viral protein coat in each of its cells. That transgenic potato plant can then effectively repel the virus when it attacks.

The technique just described allows an organism to make proteins native to another living thing. Another way that biotechnology can change the internal chemistry of an organism is by blocking, or suppressing, production of a protein the organism normally makes. One example is the long-lasting tomato, mentioned earlier. Normally, tomatoes produce a protein that softens them after they have been picked. Scientists introduce into a tomato plant an antisense gene, that is, a gene that is a mirror image of the one that codes for the "softening" enzyme. The antisense gene fastens itself to the RNA of the native gene and blocks its action. A vine-ripe tomato with the antisense gene rots much more slowly than a normal tomato. This means growers can harvest tomatoes at their most flavorful and nutritious red stage, and the tomatoes will still last much longer during shipping and marketing than regular, green-harvested tomatoes.

Safety and Regulation   The case for regulating technology's products is strong.[31] New substances, additives in a sense, are present in genetically engineered foods. The source of the new materials may be unique—never before seen in foods in exactly the same way. If a disease-producing microorganism donates genetic material to make recombinant DNA, scientists must prove that no dangerous characteristic from the microorganism exists in the food. If the new genetic material creates proteins never before encountered by the human body, their effects should be understood and their presence regulated to ensure their safety for human consumption.[32]

So far, FDA safety and labeling regulations apply only if the technology creates new ingredients in the food. The FDA has taken the position that foods produced through biotechnology that are not substantially different from others require no special safety testing or labeling.[33] A product with an antisense gene, such as the tomato described earlier, need not be tested since antisense genes *prevent* synthesis of a protein and add nothing but a tiny fragment of genetic material. On the other hand, any substances introduced into a food by way of bioengineering must meet the same safety standards applied to all additives.[34] A tomato plant with a gene that, for example, produces an insecticide cannot be marketed until it proves safe for consumption. Foods produced via biotechnology are not required to be labeled as such unless they pose known problems, such as allergy, to some people.

Some people object to genetic tampering and want labels to help them identify "old-fashioned" tomatoes. They may not realize that most foods available today have already been altered genetically by selective breeding. The new vegetable broccoflower, a product of sophisticated cross-breeding of broccoli with cauliflower, met no testing or approval barriers on its way to the dinner plate. Only after the vegetables became popular with consumers did scientists study its nutrient contents (see Appendix H for their findings).

Scientists are continuing to study the effects not only of biotechnology but of all sorts of new food-processing techniques. Their efforts to enhance food production will help meet the challenge of feeding an ever-increasing world population.[35]

To summarize food additives, the FDA regulates the use of the following intentional additives: antimicrobial agents (such as nitrites) to prevent microbial spoilage; antioxidants (such as vitamins C and E, sulfites, and BHA and BHT) to prevent oxidative changes; colors (such as tartrazine) and flavor enhancers (such as MSG) to appeal to senses; and nutrients (such as iodine in salt) to enrich or fortify foods. Incidental additives sometimes get into foods during processing, but rarely present a hazard. Other processes such as treating livestock with hormones, irradiating fruits and vegetables, and using biotechnology enhance crop yields and make some foods safer to eat, but raise consumer concerns.

As this chapter said at the start, supplying food safely to over 250 million people is an incredible challenge—one that gets met, for the most part, with remarkable efficiency. The following highlight describes a similar situation—that of delivering clean water safely to the people.

Study Questions

1. To what extent does food poisoning present a real hazard to U.S. consumers eating U.S. foods? How often does it occur?
2. Distinguish between the two types of food-borne illnesses and provide an example of each. Describe measures that help prevent food-borne illnesses at home and while traveling.
3. What special precautions apply to meats? To seafood?
4. What is meant by a "persistent" contaminant of foods? Describe how contaminants get into foods and build up in the food chain.
5. What dangers do natural toxicants present?
6. How do pesticides become a hazard to the food supply, and how are they monitored? In what ways can people reduce the concentrations of pesticides in and on foods that they prepare?
7. What is the difference between a GRAS substance and a regulated food additive? Give examples of each. Name and describe the different classes of additives.

Notes

1. R. L. Hall, Food safety and biotechnology, *Nutrition Today*, May/June 1991, pp. 15–20.

2. M. P. Doyle, Reducing foodborne diseases—What are the priorities? *Nutrition Reviews* 51 (1993): 346–347.

3. A. Hecht, The unwelcome dinner guest: Preventing food-borne illness, *FDA Consumer*, January/February 1991, pp. 19–25.

4. J. A. Desenclos and coauthors, The protective effect of alcohol on the occurrence of epidemic oyster-borne hepatitis A, *Epidemiology* 3 (1992): 371–374.

5. M. Segal, Operation pearl, *FDA Consumer*, January/February 1991, pp. 35–36.

6. P. M. Schantz, The dangers of eating raw fish, *New England Journal of Medicine* 320 (1989): 1143–1145.

7. J. H. T. Luong, C. A. Groom, and K. B. Male, The potential role of biosensors in the food and drink industries, *Biosensors and Bioelectronics* 6 (1991): 547–554.

8. P. I. Peterkin, E. S. Idziak, and A. N. Sharpe, Detection of *Listeria monocytogenes* by direct colony hybridization on hydrophobic grid-membrane filters by using a chromogen-labeled DNA probe, *Applied and Environmental Microbiology* 57 (1991): 586–591; M. Hoshi, Y. Sasamoto, and M. Nonaka, Microbial sensor system for nondestructive evaluation of fish meat quality, *Biosensors and Bioelectronics* 6 (1991): 15–20.

9. C. F. Chaisson, B. Petersen, and J. S. Douglass, *Pesticides in Foods: A Guide for Professionals* (Chicago: American Dietetic Association, 1991), pp. 2–3.

10. National Academy of Sciences Committee, as quoted by J. Raloff and D. Pendick, Pesticides in produce may threaten kids, *Science News* 144 (1993): 4–5.

11. Three agencies propose pesticide reforms, *FDA Consumer*, January/February 1994, p. 3.

12. C. Marwick, Pesticides pose concern about children's diet, *Journal of the American Medical Association* 270 (1993): 802, 805.

13. Food and Drug Administration Pesticide Program, 1991.

14. C. K. Winter, Pesticide residues and the Delaney Clause, *Food Technology* 47 (1993): 81–86; Government regulation of food safety: Interaction of scientific and societal forces, *Food Technology* 46 (1992): 73–80.

15. Federal update: Delaney Clause called "scientifically unmanageable," *Journal of the American Dietetic Association* 93 (1993): 268.

16. D. Farley, Keeping up with the microwave revolution, *FDA Consumer*, March 1990, pp. 17–21.

17. D. Blumenthal, Deciding about dioxins, *FDA Consumer*, February 1990, pp. 11–13.

18. Much of the discussion on decaffeinated coffee came from P. L. Cerrato, Is decaffeinated coffee dangerous to your health? *Issues in Nutrition*, ed. A Heinz (New York: American Council on Science and Health, 1991), pp. 107–108.

19. T. D. Etherton and coauthors, Mechanisms by which somatotropin decreases adipose tissue growth, *American Journal of Clinical Nutrition* (supplement) 58 (1993): 287S–295S; Bovine somatotropin and the safety of cow's milk: National Institutes of Health Technology Assessment Conference Statement, *Nutrition Reviews* 49 (1991): 227–232.

20. T. D. Etherton, P. M. Kris-Etherton, and E. W. Mills, Recombinant bovine and porcine somatotropin: Safety and benefits of these biotechnologies, *Journal of the American Dietetic Association* 93 (1993): 177–180.

21. J. C. Juskevich and C. G. Guyer, Bovine growth hormone: Human food safety evaluation, *Science* 249 (1990): 875–884; R. W. Rhein, BST = A Safe, More Plentiful Milk Supply (1990), a booklet available from the American Council on Science and Health at 1995 Broadway, 16th floor, New York, NY 10023–5860.

22. Bovine somatotropin and the safety of cow's milk, 1991.

23. Bovine somatotropin and the safety of cow's milk, 1991.

24. D. Blumenthal, Food irradiation: Toxic to bacteria, safe for humans, *FDA Consumer*, November 1990, pp. 11–15.

25. Blumenthal, 1990.

26. R. L. Phillips, Plant genetics: Out with the old, in with the new? *American Journal of Clinical Nutrition* (supplement) 58 (1993): 259S–263S.

27. B. A. Larkins, C. R. Lending, and J. C. Wallace, Modification of maize-seed-protein quality, *American Journal of Clinical Nutrition* (supplement) 58 (1993): 264S–269S.

28. C. R. Somerville, Future prospects for genetic modification of the composition of edible oils from higher plants, *American Journal of Clinical Nutrition* (supplement) 58 (1993): 270S–275S.

29. Position of The American Dietetic Association: Biotechnology and the future of food, *Journal of the American Dietetic Association* 93 (1993): 189–192.

30. W. L. Carroll, Introduction to recombinant-DNA technology, *American Journal of Clinical Nutrition* (supplement) 58 (1993): 249S–258S.

31. R. J. Goldburg, Why the U.S. should regulate gene-altered foods, 1991; American Medical Association Council on Scientific Affairs, Biotechnology and the American agricultural industry, *Journal of the American Medical Association* 265 (1991): 1429–1436.

32. Goldburg, 1991.

33. Statement of policy: Foods derived from new plant varieties, *Federal Register*, May 29, 1992, pp. 22983–23005.

34. Biotechnology of food: Background information from the FDA, *Nutrition Today*, July/August 1994, pp. 19–20.

35. T. D. Etherton, The impact of biotechnology on animal agriculture and the consumer, *Nutrition Today*, July/August 1994, pp. 12–18.

Consumer Concerns about Public Water

ater may contain the same impurities that foods do: microorganisms, environmental contaminants, pesticides, and additives such as chlorine used to kill pathogenic microorganisms and fluoride used to protect against dental caries. A glass of "water" is more than just H_2O. This highlight describes various sources of drinking water and some of the regulations that help to ensure its safety.

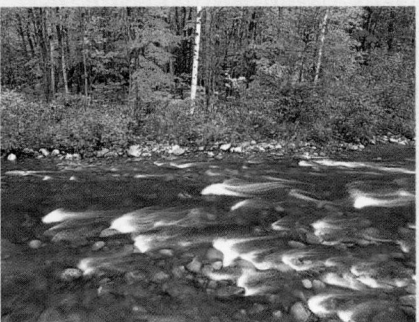

Clean rivers represent irreplaceable water resources.

SOURCES OF DRINKING WATER

Drinking water comes from two sources—surface water and groundwater. Each source supplies water for about half of the population.

Surface Water

Surface water comes from lakes, rivers, and reservoirs and supplies drinking water for most major cities. Surface water is readily contaminated because it is directly exposed to acid rain, runoff from highways and urban areas, pesticide runoff from agricultural areas, and industrial wastes that are dumped directly into it. Surface water contamination is reversible, however, because the water is constantly replaced by fresh rain. It is also cleansed to some degree by aeration, sunlight, and the plants and microorganisms that live in it.

Groundwater

Groundwater comes from underground aquifers—rock formations that are saturated with and yield

usable water. People who live in rural areas rely mostly on groundwater pumped up from private wells.

Groundwater is contaminated more slowly than surface water, but also more permanently. Contaminants deposited on the ground migrate slowly through the soil before reaching groundwater. Slow replacement combined with lack of aeration, sunlight, and aerobic microorganisms means that contaminants break down more slowly in groundwater than in surface water. Groundwater is especially susceptible to contamination from hazardous waste sites, dumps and landfills, underground tanks storing gasoline and other chemicals, and improperly discarded household chemicals and solvents.

Contaminants via Plumbing

Contamination can also occur as water travels from the main water supply to homes. Lead or asbestos from corroded pipes can contaminate drinking water, as can bacteria and dirt from leaking pipes. People who suspect contamination of their

water should have it tested where it flows out, at the tap.

The Cleansing Process

In the wilderness, water is purified each time it cycles through living systems. The soil filters out animal waste excreted onto the earth, preventing it from reaching the groundwater; plants use the waste as fertilizer instead. Soil holds pollutants, too—not beneficial to the soil, of course, but protective of the water. Surface waters also leave behind their pollutants as rivers flow along. But neither the soil nor the rivers can completely purify the heavily polluted water expelled as city sewage or industrial waste. Water leaving a factory may contain higher and higher concentrations of toxic metals as time passes, especially if the same water cycles repeatedly through the factory. Human technology is responsible for purifying water contaminated by human technology.

Public water systems treat water to remove contaminants that have been detected above acceptable levels. During treatment, a disinfectant (usually, chlorine) is added to kill bacteria. The addition of chlorine to public water is an important public health measure that appears to offer both great benefits and small risks.[1] On the one hand, chlorinated water has eliminated such water-borne diseases as typhoid fever, which once ravaged vast areas, killing thousands of people. On the other hand, it has been associated with a slight increase in bladder and rectal cancers and with contamination of the environment with the toxic by-product dioxin. Private well water is usually not chlorinated or cleansed, so the 40 million Americans who consume water from private wells are most at risk of drinking contaminated water.

DRINKING WATER CONTAMINANTS

Hundreds of contaminants, including heavy metals, pathogenic microorganisms, and organic compounds, have been detected in public drinking water. The health implications of these contaminants are just becoming known.

Heavy Metals

The metals of greatest concern are mercury, cadmium, and lead. These metals may be absorbed into the body, where they damage cell structures and impair enzyme or coenzyme functions. When combined with organic compounds, these metals may be absorbed especially rapidly and may damage body tissues even more. Heavy metals can alter the genetic material DNA, causing mutations that can produce cancer or birth defects. If the mutations occur in the DNA of the germ cells (eggs or sperm), the changes are hereditary.

Pathogenic Microorganisms

While the water supply naturally contains few, if any, heavy metals, it does naturally contain bacteria from the soil and from contamination with sewage. Before a sewage treatment plant releases water into the public supply, it must cut the bacterial count.

High standards for sewage treatment in the developed countries

Glossary

artesian water: water that is drawn from a well that taps a confined aquifer in which the water level stands above the natural water table.

distilled water: water that has been vaporized and recondensed, leaving it free of dissolved minerals.

fluoridated water: water that has been treated so as to contain at least 0.8 mg fluoride per liter.

hard water: water with a high calcium and magnesium concentration.

mineral water: water from a spring or well that typically contains 250 to 500 ppm of minerals. Minerals give water a distinctive flavor. Many mineral waters are high in sodium.

natural water: water obtained from a spring or well that is certified to be safe and sanitary. The mineral content may not be changed, but the water may be treated in other ways such as by filtration or ozonization.

potable (POTE-ah-bul) water: water that is suitable for drinking.

public water: water from a municipal or county water system that has been treated and disinfected.

purified water: water that has been processed through distillation, deionization, or reverse osmosis and meets U.S. Pharmacopoeia standards for medical and research purposes.

soft water: water with a high sodium concentration.

spring water: water originating from an underground spring or well. It may be carbonated or not ("flat" or "still"). Brand names such as "Spring Pure" do not necessarily mean that the water comes from a spring.

well water: water drawn from groundwater by tapping into an aquifer.

ensure that most people have safe drinking water. For the rest of the world, however, microbial contamination remains the primary cause of human diseases and epidemics. Two of the most basic public health needs of the world's people are safe drinking water and an acceptable standard of waste disposal.

Organic Compounds

Organic compounds from sewage, pesticides, petroleum-based industries, highway runoff, and other sources may also appear in water. Researchers have found that some of these compounds cause birth defects, some cause cancer, and some cause genetic mutations.

Many of these organic compounds contain chlorine, and some may be formed during the chlorination of water. The risks they present remain unknown; standards are being established, and if public water exceeds them, new treatment systems may be needed.

WATER SYSTEMS AND REGULATIONS

The EPA is responsible for ensuring that public water systems meet minimum standards for protecting the public health. The agency's tasks include developing maximum permitted levels for all regulated contaminants, monitoring for contaminants in drinking water, identifying the appropriate technology for removing excess contaminants, and providing protection for ground-water sources. Critics have charged that existing laws are inadequate to protect drinking water supplies and are not enforced. Some consumers have adopted alternatives to the public water system.

Home Water Treatments

To ease concerns about drinking water quality, some people purchase home water-treatment systems. Manufacturers offer a variety of units for removing contaminants from drinking water. None of them removes all contaminants, and each has its own advantages and disadvantages. Choosing the right treatment unit depends on the kinds of contaminants in the water. Therefore, before purchasing a home water-treatment unit, a consumer must first determine the quality of the water. In some cases, a state or county health department will test water samples or can refer the consumer to a certified laboratory.

Rather than purchasing a home treatment unit, some people boil their water. This kills microorganisms and removes some organic chemicals, but may concentrate inorganic chemicals such as lead.

Bottled Water

Many people turn to bottled water as an alternative to tap water. Bottled water is classified as a food, so it is regulated nationwide by the FDA and locally by state health and environmental agencies. The FDA has established quality and safety standards for bottled drinking waters compatible with those set by the EPA for public water systems. In addition, all bottled waters must be processed, packaged, and labeled in accordance with FDA regulations.

Approximately 75 percent of bottled waters derive from protected ground-water (from springs or wells) that has been disinfected with ozone rather than chlorine. Ozone kills microorganisms, then disintegrates spontaneously into water and oxygen, leaving behind no toxic by-products. Other bottled waters derive from municipal tap water that has been treated by carbon filtration to remove chlorine and inorganic compounds. Bottled waters may also be treated by reverse osmosis or ion exchange to remove inorganic compounds. Alternatively, the water may be distilled or deionized to remove dissolved solids. Some bottled waters may also have minerals or carbonation added. "Carbonated," "seltzer," "soda," and "tonic" waters are not considered waters, however, but soft drinks.

The FDA has proposed regulations for labels to disclose the sources of bottled waters and to use legally defined descriptive terms.[2] Some of the terms used to describe water are listed in the glossary.

Despite government regulations, some contamination has been detected in some bottled waters.[3] While the amounts of most contaminants found in bottled waters are probably insignificant, consumers should be aware that bottled water is not always purer than the water from their taps.

Protection of drinking water is, and will continue to be, the subject of an ongoing battle between environmentalists and industry. Many consumers and industries are unwilling to pay the financial costs of a clean, safe environment. Long-term solutions are most likely to emerge when consumers demand safe environmental practices and stringent environmental legislation and, especially, enforcement. Better handling of industrial wastes in some areas is an obvious need. Alternative farming techniques are also needed to reduce large-scale use of pesticides. Consumer education for proper disposal of solvents and household wastes is also important. A lack of attention to the problem of water contamination will only ensure that it gets worse. To learn about the water supply in your area, call the local public health agency.

NOTES

1. K. Napier, Chlorinated water: Risks and benefits, *Priorities*, Fall 1992, p. 23.
2. V. Lambert, Bottled water: New trends, new rules, *FDA Consumer*, June 1993, pp. 8–11.
3. D. Farley and coauthors, Contaminated bottled water dumped, *FDA Consumer*, January/February 1991, pp. 39–40.

Chapter 15

The Nutrition Care Process: Assessing Historical and Physical Data

CONTENTS

The Nutrition Care Process

Assessing Nutrition Status

Historical Information

  Health History

  Drug History

  Socioeconomic History

  Diet History

Physical Examinations

HIGHLIGHT: Diet and Health

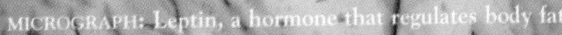

MICROGRAPH: Leptin, a hormone that regulates body fat.

*t*he earlier chapters of this book have shown how a physically fit body and an alert mind depend on good nutrition. Turning now to clinical nutrition, the remaining chapters show how poor nutrition can accelerate the development of certain degenerative diseases and how nutrition therapy can improve the quality of life for people who have become ill.

Health care professionals who recognize the indispensable roles nutrition plays in supporting health make a conscientious effort to think "nutrition." They bridge the gap between knowledge and action by carefully identifying nutrition needs and developing realistic plans of action. This chapter defines the nutrition care process, emphasizing the use of histories and physical examinations in assessing nutrition status. The next chapter shows how anthropometric and biochemical findings complete the assessment process and explains how assessment data then provide the foundation upon which to build nutrition care plans.

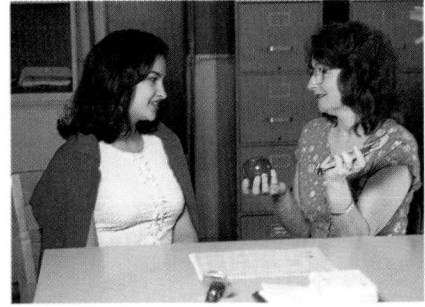

Health care professionals develop nutrition care plans to meet clients' nutrition and nutrition education needs.

The Nutrition Care Process

The nutrition care process is a systematic and logical approach used to identify and meet each person's nutrient and nutrition education needs. Appropriate medical nutrition therapy and skillful communication are two complementary parts of effective nutrition care.

The nutrition care process consists of five steps:

1. Assess nutrition status.
2. Analyze assessment data to determine nutrient requirements.
3. Develop a plan of action for meeting nutrition needs, including client education.
4. Implement the nutrition care plan.
5. Evaluate the effectiveness of the nutrition care plan through ongoing assessment and make changes as needed.

The dietitian has the primary responsibility for assessing nutrition status and developing and implementing nutrition care plans. The physician, nurse, dietetic technician, social worker, pharmacist, physical therapist, and occupational therapist also make valuable contributions (see Highlight 17). To the extent that all of these people apply their nutrition knowledge, technical skills, and interpersonal skills, the care plan will be realistic and attainable.

To ensure the success of the nutrition care process, health care professionals should make sure that, whenever possible, the client is an active participant in the process. In cases where active participation is not possible, such as for infants and young children, people who are very ill or unconscious, people with mental disabilities, or people who are uncooperative, health care professionals can enlist the involvement of family members or other support people.

Health care professionals use the nutrition care process to systematically assess, analyze, plan, implement. and evaluate their clients' nutrition and nutrition education needs. The contributions of all members of the health care team enhance the accuracy and effectiveness of the nutrition care plan.

nutrition care process: an organized approach to nutrition intervention that consists of five steps (assessing, analyzing, planning, implementing, and evaluating). The nutrition care process parallels the *nursing care process* except that it focuses on nutrition concerns.

medical nutrition therapy: a term introduced by the American Dietetic Association in 1994 to emphasize the role of nutrition in medical care. In this book, the terms *medical nutrition therapy* and *diet therapy* are used interchangeably.

nutrition care plan: a plan that translates nutrition assessment data into a strategy for meeting a client's nutrient and nutrition education needs.

health care team: a group of professionals representing several disciplines who work together to resolve their clients' medical problems; see Highlight 17.

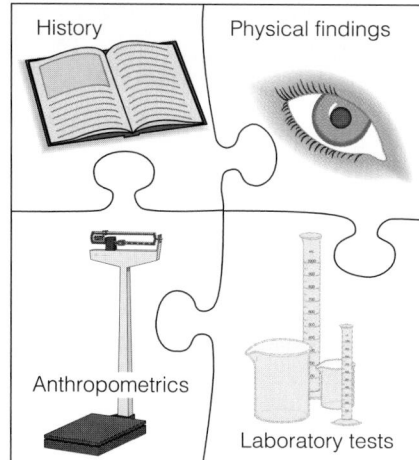

History

Physical findings

Anthropometrics

Laboratory tests

Taken as a whole, the information gathered during a nutrition assessment helps define a person's nutrition status.

nutrition assessment: the evaluation of many factors that influence or reflect nutritional health; the tools used for nutrition assessment include historical information, physical examinations, anthropometric findings, and biochemical analyses.

Nurses and registered dietetic technicians are the professionals who most often assist dietitians in completing nutrition assessments.

Assessing Nutrition Status

Nutrition assessment provides the information needed to determine how well a client's nutrient needs are being met. From the information, the assessor can develop a plan of action to prevent or correct any imbalances. The assessor, usually a registered dietitian assisted by other qualified health care professionals, relies on many sources of data including:

- Historical information.
- Physical examinations.
- Anthropometric data.
- Biochemical analyses (laboratory tests).

By accurately gathering this information and carefully interpreting each finding in relation to the others, the assessor obtains the basis for a meaningful evaluation. Assessors frequently use computer programs to perform many of the mathematical calculations required and to check the results against standards.

The following sections describe many techniques for assessing nutrition status. Using every technique for each assessment is not practical or necessary. Instead, health care professionals determine which techniques to use for different clients and different situations. Chapter 16 provides more information about screening clients for risk factors that suggest the need for a complete nutrition assessment.

A thorough nutrition assessment provides the basis for a nutrition care plan. This chapter and the next emphasize the four components of nutrition assessments: histories, physical examinations, anthropometric data, and biochemical analyses.

Historical Information

Table 15–1 sums up the types of historical data that may provide clues to nutrition status. Form 15–1 shows the data typically collected in recording a client's history. A thorough history alerts the assessor to potential problems that can be further investigated using other assessment techniques.

Table 15–1

Historical Data Used in Nutrition Assessments

Type of History	What It Identifies
Health history	Health factors that affect nutrition status
Drug history	Medications and nutrient supplements that affect nutrition status
Socioeconomic history	Personal, financial, and environmental influences on food intake, nutrient needs, and diet therapy options
Diet history	Nutrient intake excesses or deficiencies and the reasons for imbalances

Name_____   Date _____
Address_____   Date of last medical checkup _____
_____   Age _____   Sex _____
_____   Height _____   Weight _____
Phone_____   Usual weight _____
Reason for admission_____   Desirable weight range _____
_____

Health History

1. Have you been told that you have (check any that apply):
   - ☐ Diabetes   ☐ Heart disease   ☐ Ulcers
   - ☐ GI disorders   ☐ Lung disease   ☐ Cancer
   - ☐ High blood pressure   ☐ Kidney disease   ☐ Other _____
   - ☐ Hardening of arteries   ☐ Liver disease

2. Do you have complaints about any of the following:
   - ☐ Lack of appetite   ☐ Diarrhea   ☐ Nausea
   - ☐ Difficulty chewing or swallowing   ☐ Indigestion   ☐ Vomiting
   - ☐ Constipation   ☐ Fever   ☐ Other

3. Do you use tobacco in any way?____ How much?_____

4. For females:
   Are you pregnant?_____ How many months?_____
   How many pregnancies have you carried to term? _____
   When was your last child born? _____
   Are your menstrual periods normal? _____If not, please explain: _____

Drug History

1. Do you take medication, either prescribed by a doctor or over-the-counter?

Name of drug	Reason for taking	Dose	Frequency	Duration of intake
_____	_____	_____	_____	_____
_____	_____	_____	_____	_____
_____	_____	_____	_____	_____

2. Have you noticed any side effects from taking these medications?_____ If so, please explain: _____
3. Do you take vitamins or any kind of supplements?_____ Which ones? _____
   How often? _____ For what reason? _____

Socioeconomic History

1. Last grade of school completed _____ Still in school?_____
2. Are you employed? _____Occupation _____
3. Does someone else live with you?_____ Who? _____
4. Do you regularly eat alone or with others?_____
5. Do you have a refrigerator?_____Stove?_____
6. How often do you shop for food?_____ Where? _____

Diet History

1. Have you recently lost or gained more than 10 lb? _____ If yes, explain the surrounding circumstances (including associated illness, dietary changes, and time frame): _____
2. Do you eat at regular times each day? _____ How many times per day? _____
3. Where do you eat most of your meals? _____
4. Do you usually eat snacks? _____When? _____
5. What foods do you particularly like? _____
6. Are there foods you don't eat for other reasons? _____
7. Do you have difficulty eating? _____
8. How would you describe your feelings about food? _____
9. Do your eating habits change when you are emotionally upset? _____ How? _____
10. Are you, or any member of your family, on a special diet? _____If yes, who and what kind? _____
11. Do you drink alcohol? _____ How much? _____ How often? _____
12. How would you describe your exercise habits?_____ Type of exercise _____
    Intensity_____ Duration _____ Frequency _____
13. Are there any other facts about your lifestyle that you think might be related to your nutritional health? _____
    Explain _____

Note: Use the appropriate form to record food intake data (Forms 15–2 and 15–3).

How to Conduct Successful Interviews

To solicit accurate and reliable information from clients, the successful interviewer respects, and shows genuine concern for, the individual. Techniques to help clients feel comfortable and communicate openly and freely include:

- Each time you visit a client, introduce yourself, verify the client's name, and explain the purpose of your visit. In so doing, you confirm that you are talking with the right person, you set the tone for the discussion, and you let the person know who you are and what to expect.
- Arrange for privacy and reassure the client that all the information provided will be treated confidentially.
- Be sure that the client is comfortable and that the physical environment is conducive to an interview. If the client is in pain or is tired, it may be best to arrange another time for the interview. To facilitate communication, you might modify the physical environment by, for example, adjusting the lighting, turning off the television, changing the temperature in the room, providing a glass of water, or repositioning the client.
- Position yourself so that you are comfortable and can maintain eye contact. To do so, you may have to sit down. If you are uncomfortable or if you stand while the client sits or lies in bed, you may nonverbally communicate an unfriendly, overpowering, or hurried feeling.
- Allow adequate time for the interview. Hurrying through an interview conveys to the client that your discussion is not very important and that you really do not care enough to get all the facts.
- Allow others to be themselves. In other words, accept and value people for who and what they are. If an interviewer reacts with advice, criti-

An adept history taker uses the interview not only to gather facts, but also to establish rapport with the client and to assess motivation, education, and ability level. Interviewers who establish a caring and trusting relationship while they gather information are best equipped to deliver effective care. The interviewer must obtain personal facts and information about lifelong habits that are influenced by complex medical, social, cultural, psychological, religious, and economic factors. No one would share this much without trusting that the interviewer truly cared and would accept the information, whatever it might be. The accompanying box provides pointers for conducting successful interviews.

HEALTH HISTORY

Physical and mental health both affect and reflect nutrition status; the history taker makes note of all conditions that increase the risk of malnutrition (see Table 15–2). Figure 15–1 on p. 525 illustrates some of the relationships between illness and nutrition.

An assessor is wise to review the client's health, or medical, history before visiting the client. During the interview, the assessor can then keep in mind the factors that may affect the person's nutrition status. Conversations with the client

health history: an account of the client's current and past health status and risk factors for disease. Traditionally, the health history has been called the *medical history*. The term *health history* now seems more appropriate, however, since the contents describe the client's health status, and current trends in the medical profession now emphasize health promotion and disease prevention.

cism, or judgment, the client may withhold important information, not wanting to risk belittlement. To avoid such pitfalls, use open-ended questions, which allow a wide choice of answers. In contrast, closed-ended questions narrowly limit a client's responses. For example, if you ask a client if she prefers orange juice or tomato juice, you aren't giving her an opportunity to say she'd really rather have grapefruit juice or a slice of melon.

- Be an active listener. Let the client do most of the talking and control the direction of the conversation. Don't interrupt the person's thoughts. Try not to follow a set guide for asking important questions; rather, use forms as guides, and ask questions based on the client's responses.

- Avoid giving diet advice when seeking information. If a person tells you he eats a candy bar for breakfast, and you react with advice about better choices for breakfast, the client may be hesitant to tell you he eats two more candy bars before going to bed. Reserve nutrition education sessions for a later time.

- Regularly provide the client with feedback to make sure you understand each other correctly. Repeat key phrases and ask for further information when clarity is needed.

- Prior to ending an interview, let the client know what to expect next. For example, "I'll come back tomorrow to talk with you about your eating plan."

While interviews serve as a tool for gathering information, they also provide an opportunity for establishing a relationship with the client. That relationship will influence all future communications with the client.

Open-versus closed-ended questions:
- *Open-ended:* What is the first time you usually eat during the day?
- *Closed-ended:* What do you usually eat for breakfast?
- *Open-ended:* What foods do you usually eat at that time?
- *Closed-ended:* Do you usually have cereal or eggs for breakfast?

can also uncover valuable health-related information that might otherwise be overlooked because no one thought to ask.

Appetite and Food Intake   Loss of appetite commonly accompanies illness. A child with a fever frequently is unable to eat; so is an adult with cancer. Nausea, mouth dryness, problems with chewing or swallowing, and obstructions in the digestive tract can all lead to malnutrition.

The secondary effects of illness can also affect nutrient intake. Pain and anxiety associated with illness can make it difficult or impossible to eat; pain in the mouth or throat is especially problematic. Anxiety stimulates stress hormone activity and suppresses digestive activity, making clients lose their appetites. Medical treatments and procedures may require that a person not eat at the very time when nutrient needs are especially high due to illness.

Digestion and Absorption   Illnesses that interfere with digestion or absorption usually affect several nutrients and can cause nutrition status to deteriorate rapidly. Examples include cystic fibrosis, pancreatitis, and inflammatory bowel diseases. (Chapter 22 describes these disorders in more detail.)

Table 15–2

Health Factors That Can Affect or Reflect Nutrition Status

- Acquired immune deficiency syndrome (AIDS)
- Alcoholism
- Alzheimer's disease
- Anorexia (lack of appetite)
- Anorexia nervosa
- Bulimia
- Cancer
- Chewing or swallowing difficulties (including poorly fitted dentures, dental caries, missing teeth, and mouth ulcers)
- Chronic obstructive pulmonary disease
- Circulatory problems
- Constipation
- Crohn's disease
- Decubitus ulcers
- Dementia
- Depleted blood proteins

- Diabetes mellitus
- Diarrhea
- Diseases of the GI tract
- Drug addiction
- Dysphagia
- Failure to thrive
- Fever
- Heart disease
- HIV infection
- Hormonal imbalance
- Hyperlipidemia
- Hypertension
- Infection
- Kidney disease
- Liver disease
- Lung disease
- Malabsorption
- Mental illness
- Mental retardation
- Multiple pregnancies

- Nausea
- Neurologic disorders
- Organ failure
- Overweight
- Pancreatic insufficiency
- Paralysis
- Physical disability
- Pneumonia
- Pregnancy
- Radiation therapy
- Recent major illness
- Recent major surgery
- Recent weight loss or gain
- Surgery of the GI tract
- Tobacco use
- Trauma
- Ulcerative colitis
- Ulcers
- Underweight
- Vomiting

Metabolism　Illnesses can directly alter metabolism (Chapters 25 and 30) and change nutrient needs. They can also alter organ function and thereby alter metabolism indirectly; examples are liver disease (Chapter 26), diabetes (Chapter 27), renal failure (Chapter 29), cancer (Chapter 30), and AIDS (also in Chapter 30).

Excretion　Illnesses can also interfere with the excretion of nutrients. The result can be either excessive retention of nutrients, as in renal failure (Chapter 29), or excessive loss of nutrients, as in diarrhea (Chapter 22) or nephrotic syndrome (Chapter 29).

Highlight 7 describes nutrition concerns associated with alcohol abuse (one type of substance abuse), and Highlight 9 explores eating disorders and their nutrition consequences.

Emotional and Mental Health　Emotional and nutritional health go together. Emotionally healthy people have the capacity to feed themselves well. Well-nourished people experience none of the nutrient deficiencies that might impair mental health. Malnourished people, on the other hand, may suffer the mental symptoms of nutrient deficiencies. People with B vitamin deficiencies, for example, often exhibit "mental" symptoms ranging from confusion, apathy, fatigue, and irritability to delirium and psychoses.

The effects of mental illnesses on nutrition status may be less readily apparent than those of physiological illnesses, but are no less important. Mental illnesses frequently alter emotional health and may lead to anxiety, depression, and severe mood swings, which, in turn, impair nutritional health. People with mental illnesses characterized by illogical thinking or dementia may have little interest in food or may be unable to make appropriate food choices. Those who are paranoid may believe that foods are being used to poison them. People suffering from

Figure 15–1

Relationships between Illness and Nutrition
(Nutrition for people with cancer is discussed in Chapter 30.)

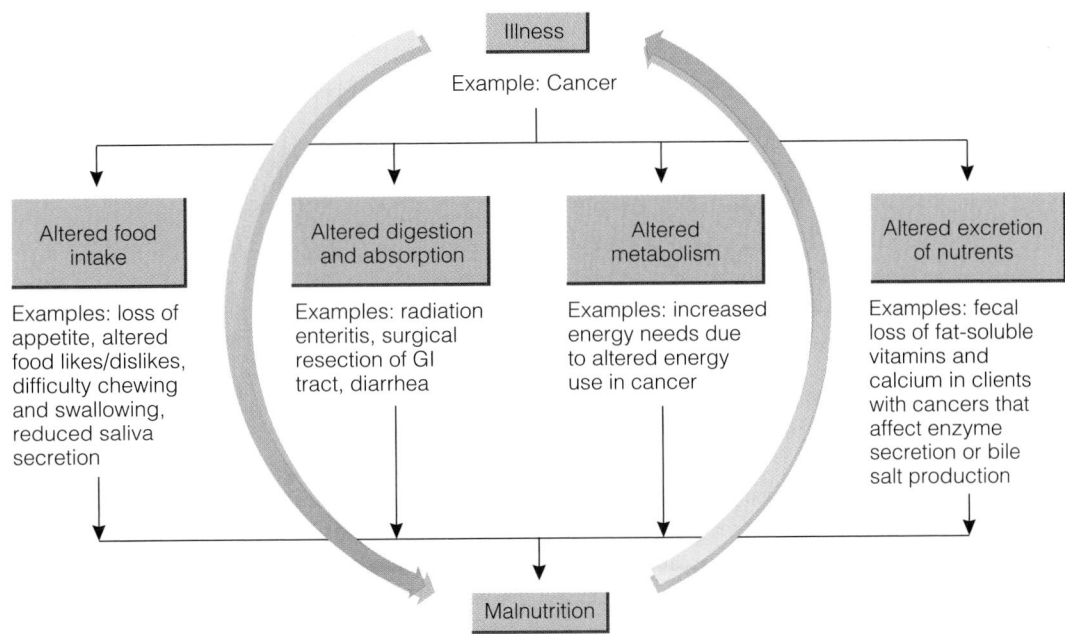

delusions may attribute magical powers to certain foods and insist on eating only those foods. Drugs used to treat mental illnesses can also affect nutrition status. (Drug interactions are described later in this chapter.)

To reflect on the interrelationships between mental, emotional, and nutritional health, consider a typical scenario of an elderly woman who lives alone. Over the years she may have become increasingly isolated from family and friends. As her loneliness progresses, she may become depressed and begin to eat less. Her malnutrition worsens the apathy she feels from the loneliness. Consequently, she has even less energy with which to feed herself. Watch for such a downward spiral in all people who are lonely, especially the elderly or those who have recently lost a loved one.

DRUG HISTORY

Medical drugs are often involved in the treatment of illness, and nearly every drug affects nutrition status to some degree. Therefore, obtaining a drug history is an important part of the assessment process. All medications are of interest: prescription drugs, nonprescription or over-the-counter (OTC) drugs, illicit drugs, and even nutrient supplements. If a person is taking any medication routinely, the assessor records the name of the medication or supplement with the dose, frequency, and duration of intake; the reason for taking the medication; and signs of any adverse or positive effects (see Form 15–1).

Hundreds of medications and nutrients interact, which can lead to imbalances or interfere with drug effectiveness.[1] This discussion focuses on medical drugs. Adverse drug-nutrient interactions are most likely to occur if medications

drug history: a record of all the medications, over-the-counter and prescribed, that a person takes routinely.

The trend toward making formerly prescription drugs available over-the-counter underscores the need to ask clients about all nonprescription medications they may be taking.

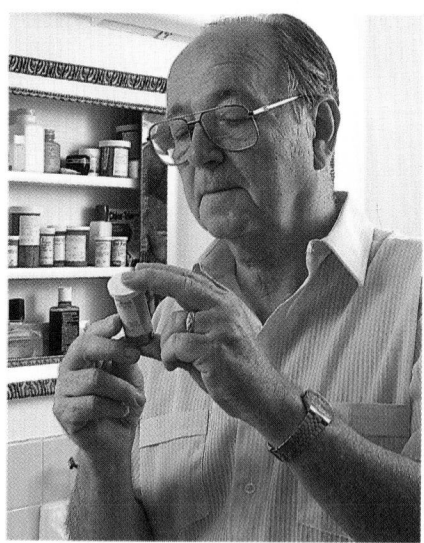

Taking several medications over long periods intensifies the risk of drug-nutrient interactions.

are taken over long periods, if several medications are taken, or if nutrition status is poor or deteriorating. Understandably, then, elderly people with chronic diseases and people with illnesses that dramatically raise nutrient needs are most at risk. Studies of institutionalized elderly people suggest that multiple medication use may significantly affect nutrition status in this population.[2]

Nutrients and medications may interact in many ways:

- Medications can alter food intake and the absorption, metabolism, and excretion of nutrients.
- Foods and nutrients can alter the absorption, metabolism, and excretion of medications.

Table 15–3 lists the general classes of medications notable for their interactions with nutrients. The following sections describe these interactions, and Table 15–4 summarizes this information and provides specific examples. Table E–1 in Appendix E provides details on specific interactions, drug by drug.

Medications and Food Intake Many medications can lead to malnutrition by interfering with food intake. Amphetamines used to treat hyperactivity in children provide an example: they may effectively improve behavior, but they also suppress appetite, alter taste perceptions, dry the mouth, and cause nausea. Conversely, some medications stimulate the appetite and lead to undesirable weight gain. An example is astemizole (Hismanal), an antihistamine used by some people to relieve allergy symptoms.

Absorption and Medications Laxatives provide an example of how medications can interfere with nutrient absorption. Laxatives cause foods to move so rapidly through the intestine that many vitamins do not have enough time to be absorbed. The use of mineral oil as a laxative robs the person of the fat-soluble vitamins, notably vitamin D. The vitamins from foods dissolve in the indigestible oil and are excreted; calcium, too, is excreted. A person who uses laxatives daily for a long time may find that the intestines can no longer function without them. This dependence can lead to malnutrition.

Table 15–3

Classes of Medications That Can Affect Nutrition Status

- Amphetamines and other stimulants
- Analgesics
- Antacids
- Antibiotics
- Anticonvulsants
- Antidepressants
- Antidiabetic agents
- Antidiarrheals
- Antihyperlipemics
- Antihypertensives
- Antineoplastics
- Antiulcer agents
- Catabolic steroids
- Diuretics
- Hormonal agents
- Immunosuppressive agents
- Laxatives
- Oral contraceptives
- Vitamin and other nutrient preparations

Note: Specific examples, drug by drug, appear in Appendix E, Table E–1.

Table 15–4

Mechanisms and Examples of Food-Medication Interactions

Drugs Can Alter Food Intake by:

- Altering the appetite (amphetamines suppress the appetite).
- Interfering with taste or smell (methotrexate changes taste perceptions).
- Inducing nausea or vomiting (digitalis can do both).
- Changing the oral environment (phenobarbital can cause dry mouth).
- Irritating the GI tract (cyclophosphamide induces mucosal ulcers).
- Causing sores or inflammation of the mouth (methotrexate can cause painful mouth ulcers).

Drugs Can Alter Nutrient Absorption by:

- Changing the acidity of the digestive tract (antacids can interfere with iron absorption).
- Altering digestive juices (cimetidine can improve fat absorption).
- Altering motility of the digestive tract (laxatives speed motility, causing the malabsorption of many nutrients).
- Inactivating enzyme systems (neomycin may reduce lipase activity).
- Damaging mucosal cells (chemotherapy can damage mucosal cells).
- Binding to nutrients (some antacids bind phosphorus).

Foods Can Alter Drug Absorption by:

- Changing the acidity of the digestive tract (candy can change the acidity, thereby causing slow-acting asthma medication to dissolve too quickly).
- Stimulating secretion of digestive juices (griseofulvin is absorbed better when taken with foods that stimulate the release of digestive enzymes).
- Altering rate of absorption (aspirin is absorbed more slowly when taken with food).
- Binding to drugs (calcium binds to tetracycline, limiting drug absorption).
- Competing for absorption sites in the intestines (dietary amino acids interfere with levodopa absorption this way).

Drugs and Nutrients Can Interact and Alter Metabolism by:

- Acting as structural analogs (as anticoagulants and vitamin K do).
- Competing with each other for metabolic enzyme systems (as phenobarbitol and folate do).
- Altering enzyme activity and contributing pharmacologically active substances (as monoamine oxidase inhibitors and tyramine do).

Drugs Can Alter Nutrient Excretion by:

- Altering reabsorption in the kidneys (some diuretics increase the excretion of sodium and potassium).
- Displacing nutrients from their plasma protein carriers (aspirin displaces folate).

Foods Can Alter Drug Excretion by:

- Changing the acidity of the urine (vitamin C can alter urinary pH and limit the excretion of aspirin).

A classic example of how foods can interfere with medication absorption is the interaction between the antibiotic tetracycline and the minerals calcium and iron. When calcium and tetracycline, or iron and tetracycline, are taken at the same time, they bind to each other, thus reducing the absorption of both. Clients are therefore instructed not to take tetracycline with milk, milk products, or calcium-containing antacids (such as Tums). Similarly, clients must take their iron supplements two hours apart from their tetracycline doses.

Another example is the interaction between acidic foods and the nicotine gum that is used to help people quit smoking cigarettes. Certain acid-containing foods and beverages interfere with the absorption of nicotine through the lining of the mouth into the blood. For maximum effectiveness, people should refrain from ingesting foods and beverages for 15 minutes before, and while, chewing the gum. When a food or beverage blocks nicotine's absorption from the mouth, the person swallows the nicotine, and this may cause nausea and hiccups as well as interfere with the drug's effectiveness.

Some medications are absorbed better with foods than without them. For this reason, the antifungal drug griseofulvin is always given with meals. In many cases, though, foods delay the rate at which medications are absorbed. In some instances this, too, can be helpful. An aspirin taken on an empty stomach works faster than when it is given with food, but because aspirin can irritate the GI tract, taking it with food can reduce nausea.

Metabolism and Medications　To appreciate how drug-nutrient interactions can affect metabolism, consider medications that resemble vitamins in structure. Vitamin K and the anticlotting medication warfarin (Coumadin) provide an example. Warfarin opposes clotting by interfering with vitamin K. To be clinically effective, the warfarin dose must be large enough to counteract whatever vitamin K is in the person's diet. If a person's vitamin K intake increases, as it may in summer when lettuces and greens are in season, then the physician has to increase the medication dose. Another example is methotrexate, which is used to treat certain cancers and rheumatoid arthritis; methotrexate is structurally similar to folate and can cause severe folate deficiencies (see Figure 15–2).

Aspirin can also alter folate metabolism but in a different way. Aspirin competes with folate for its protein carrier, thus hindering the body's use of the vitamin. When aspirin is used over long periods of time, health care professionals should ensure that either the diet or supplements supply sufficient folate to meet the added demands.

The effects of tyramine provide another example of a substance in foods that alters a medication's action. Tyramine is a substance found in some foods, and it interacts with monoamine oxidase inhibitors (MAO inhibitors), which are prescribed to treat certain forms of severe depression. Normally, a certain enzyme in the brain inactivates tyramine, but the MAO inhibitors block the action of that enzyme. When people take the medication, the enzyme fails to act. Thus tyramine remains active and stimulates the release of the neurotransmitter norepi-

Figure 15–2

Folate and Methotrexate

Methotrexate (an antineoplastic drug) is structurally similar to the vitamin folate. When this medication is used, it competes for the enzyme that normally activates folate, creating a secondary deficiency of folate.

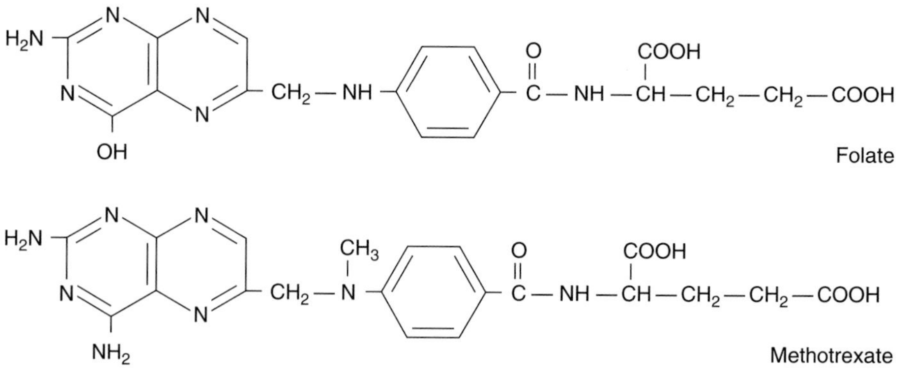

nephrine. This action can lead to severe hypertension and headaches. If blood pressure rises high enough, it can be fatal. For this reason, people taking MAO inhibitors must restrict their intakes of foods rich in tyramine (see Table 15–5).

Excretion and Medications   Urinary acidity affects drug reabsorption from the kidneys back into the blood. An acidic urine limits the excretion of acidic drugs like aspirin. Large doses of vitamin C given with aspirin increase the urine's acidity, and aspirin remains in the blood longer.

Medications can also alter urinary excretion of nutrients. For example, some diuretics accelerate the excretion of the minerals calcium, potassium, magnesium, and zinc.

Other Ingredients in Medications   Besides the active ingredients, medications may contain other substances such as sugar, sorbitol, sodium, alcohol, and caffeine. For most people who use medications on occasion and in small amounts, such ingredients pose no problem. When medications are taken regularly or in large doses, however, people on special diets may need to be aware of these additional ingredients and their effects.

Many liquid preparations contain sugar or sorbitol to make them taste better. For people who must regulate their intakes of simple sugars, such as people with diabetes, the amount of sugar in medications must be considered. Large doses of liquids containing sorbitol may result in diarrhea.

Antibiotics and antacids often contain sodium. People who take Alka Seltzer may not realize that a single 2-tablet dose may exceed their safe sodium intakes for a whole day. Another antacid (Tums) contains a considerable amount of cal-

Table 15–5

Foods Restricted in a Tyramine-Controlled Diet

Beverages:	Red wines including chianti, sherry[a]
Cheeses:	Aged cheeses, American, camembert, cheddar, gouda, gruyère, mozzarella, parmesan, provolone, romano, roquefort, stilton[b]
Meats:	Liver; dried, salted, smoked, or pickled fish; sausage; pepperoni; salami; dried meats
Vegetables:	Fava beans; Italian broad beans; sauerkraut; snow peas; fermented pickles and olives
Other:	Brewer's yeast;[c] all aged and fermented products; soy sauce in large amounts; cheese-filled breads, crackers, and desserts; salad dressings containing cheese

Note: The tyramine contents of foods vary from product to product depending on the methods used to prepare, process, and store the food. In some cases, as little as 1 ounce of cheese can cause a severe hypertensive reaction in people taking monoamine oxidase inhibitors. In general, the following foods contain small enough amounts of tyramine that they can be consumed in small quantities: ripe avocado, banana, yogurt, sour cream, acidophilus milk, buttermilk, raspberries, and peanuts.
[a]Most wine and domestic beer can be consumed in small quantities.
[b]Unfermented cheeses, such as ricotta, cottage cheese, and cream cheese, are allowed.
[c]Products made with baker's yeast are allowed.

cium. Although Tums are sometimes recommended as a calcium supplement, they are less than ideal for this purpose. For one, the form of calcium in Tums is poorly absorbed. For another, antacids neutralize stomach acid, on which the absorption of many nutrients (possibly including calcium itself) depends. Taking any antacid regularly will reduce the absorption of many nutrients.

Medications given by vein provide water and frequently provide sodium, potassium, and other electrolytes, or dextrose (a form of sugar). Assessors must consider these contributions when clients' diets must be modified in any of these nutrients. Administering medications through a feeding tube requires additional precautions (see Chapter 23).

A Note to Assessors   Hundreds of drug-nutrient interactions have been identified, and information continues to accumulate. It would be difficult, if not impossible, to remember all the potential effects of drug-nutrient interactions on nutrition status. Instead, assessors serve their clients best if they:

- Keep in mind that drug-nutrient interactions can and do occur, especially when the medication use is long term.
- Record the complete drug and diet histories of clients; review these histories with potential interactions in mind. Keep a reference handy, such as Table E–1 in Appendix E, and check it frequently.
- Be aware of groups of people who are likely to develop drug-related nutrient deficiencies, and be prepared to look up the nutrition effects of medications these clients are taking.
- Reassess nutrition status frequently for high-risk clients.
- Become familiar with the nutrient interactions of the medications commonly used to treat the disorders of their clients. For example, nurses working with people who have heart disease should become familiar with the nutrition effects of medications used to treat that condition.

SOCIOECONOMIC HISTORY

Socioeconomic factors can profoundly affect nutrition status and food choices (see Table 15–6 and Form 15–1). Age affects both nutrient requirements and food choices (see Chapters 18–20). Infants and children depend on caregivers to provide nutritious and acceptable foods; so do adults who are unable to care for themselves. Therefore, assessors must sometimes evaluate caregivers as well as clients.

A person's occupation provides clues to the person's education and income. It can also reveal certain eating habits and physical activity levels. One job, for example, may entail desk work and eating out; another may require vigorous physical activity and only a short lunch break.

The ethnic background, religious affiliation, and educational level of both the client and the other members of the household often influence food availability and food choices. These factors also suggest how the interviewer should word questions, interpret answers, and plan for nutrition education. The community environment may also influence the client's nutrition status. The interviewer should be familiar with the food habits of the major ethnic and religious groups within the locale, regional food preferences, local crops, and nutrition resources

socioeconomic history: a record of a person's social and economic background, including such factors as education, income, and ethnic identity.

Table 15–6

Socioeconomic Factors That Can Affect Food Choices

- Access to grocery stores
- Activities
- Age
- Education
- Ethnic identity
- Income
- Geographical area
- Kitchen facilities
- Number of people in household
- Occupation
- Religious affiliation

and programs available in the community. Local health departments and social agencies can often provide such information.

Income level also influences the diet. In general, diet quality declines as income falls; an inadequate income puts an adequate diet out of reach. Agencies use poverty indexes to identify people at risk for poor nutrition and to qualify people for government food assistance programs. Highlight 18 addresses additional issues regarding poverty and hunger.

Low income affects not only the power to purchase foods but also the ability to shop for, store, and cook them. A skilled assessor will note whether the person has transportation to a grocery store that sells a sufficient variety of low-cost foods and whether the person has access to a refrigerator and stove.

DIET HISTORY

A diet history provides a record of eating habits and food intake and can help identify possible nutrient imbalances (see Table 15–7) and factors that affect food intake. Information about the person's eating habits also provides the background for developing realistic and attainable nutrition goals.

Constructing an accurate diet history requires skill. Eating habits are an important part of lifestyle and often reflect a person's philosophy. The assessor who makes nonjudgmental responses and asks open-ended questions about eating habits and food intake encourages trust and enhances the likelihood of obtaining accurate information.

Form 15–1 (on p. 521) shows questions about eating habits and lifestyle that can clue assessors to possible nutrient imbalances and factors that affect food intake. In addition to determining food habits, assessors can evaluate food intake using various tools such as the 24-hour recall, the usual intake record, the food frequency checklist, the food record, and direct observation of food intake. The assessor relies on clinical judgment to select the best tool or tools to obtain the needed information about nutrient intake or food habits. Each tool depends on an accurate account of portion sizes and food composition.[3] Food models or photos and measuring devices can help clients identify the types of foods and quantities consumed. The assessor also needs to know how the foods are prepared and when they are eaten. In addition to asking about foods, assessors ask about beverage consumption, including beverages containing alcohol or caffeine.

24-Hour Recall The 24-hour recall provides data for one day only and is commonly used in nutrition surveys to obtain estimates of the typical food intakes for a population. For individuals, the assessor uses the 24-hour recall to get an idea of general eating habits and meal times. The assessor asks the client to recount everything eaten or drunk in the past 24 hours or for the previous day. Form 15–2 shows a typical 24-hour recall form.

An advantage of the 24-hour recall is that it is easy to obtain. It is also more likely to provide accurate data, at least about the past 24 hours, than estimates of average intakes over long periods. It does not, however, provide enough information to allow accurate generalizations about an individual's usual food intake. Only when 24-hour recalls are collected on several nonconsecutive days, including both weekdays and weekend days, is this limitation overcome.

Table 15–7

Dietary Factors That Can Affect Nutrition Status

- Deficient or excessive food intake
- Frequently eating out
- Intravenous fluids (other than total parenteral nutrition) for 7 or more days
- No intake for 7 or more days
- Omission from diet of any food group (for example, vegetables)
- Poor appetite
- Restrictive or fad diets
- Monotonous diet (lack of variety)

diet history: a record of eating behaviors and the foods a person eats.

Judgmental versus nonjudgmental responses:
- *Helper:* Do you take any type of vitamin or mineral supplements?
- *Client:* I take a vitamin E capsule and 2 grams of vitamin C every day.
- *Judgmental helper response:* You know, of course, that there is no reason for taking these vitamin supplements.
- *Nonjudgmental helper response:* For what reasons do you take these vitamin supplements?

24-hour recall: a record of foods eaten by a person for one 24-hour period.

Form 15–2   Food Intake for a 24-Hour Recall or Usual Intake Pattern

Name and address _____   Date _____

_____

_____

Did or do you take vitamin-mineral supplements? _____

If yes, what kind?_____   Dose _____

Please record the type and amount of foods and beverages consumed today. [Or: Please record the types and amounts of foods and beverages you typically consume each day.]

Time of Day	Food	Amount (c, tbs, or piece)	Description (how cooked, how served)

Usual Intake   To obtain data about a person's usual intake, an inquiry might begin with "What is the first thing you usually eat or drink during the day?" Similar questions follow until a typical daily intake pattern emerges. This method uses the same form as the 24-hour recall (Form 15–2), and can be useful, especially in verifying food intake when the past 24 hours have been atypical. It also helps the assessor verify ususal eating habits. For example, one person may always eat an afternoon snack; another may never eat breakfast. A person whose intake varies widely from day to day, however, may find it difficult to answer such general questions, and in such a case, another food intake tool should be used to estimate nutrient intake.

food frequency checklist: a checklist of foods on which a person can record the frequency with which he or she eats different types of foods.

Food Frequency Checklist   A less common approach is to use a food frequency checklist to ascertain how often an individual eats a specific type of food. This information helps pinpoint food groups, and therefore nutrients, that may be excessive or deficient in the diet. That a person ate no vegetables yesterday may not seem particularly significant, but never eating vegetables is a warning sign of possible nutrient deficiencies. When used with the usual intake or 24-hour recall approach, the food frequency record enables the assessor to double-check the accuracy of the information obtained. Form 15–3 (on pp. 534–535) is a food frequency checklist.

Food Records   A food record maintained over several days can be a valuable tool for gathering food intake data. The assessor instructs the person keeping the record to write down all foods and beverages consumed, the time of day, the amounts consumed, and methods of preparation. Often the person must record other information as well, depending on the purpose of the food record. When the purpose of the record is to help a person change eating behaviors and lose weight, the record might also include information about the person's mood, the occasion (party, holiday, family meal), behaviors associated with eating food (watching TV, driving in the car on the way to work, sitting at the table with the family), and physical activity. When the purpose of the food record is to establish blood glucose control (see Chapter 27), records include details of drug administration, physical activity, and the results of blood glucose monitoring. When the purpose of the record is to establish food tolerances (such as the amount of lactose a person can handle), food records also include symptoms associated with eating (for example, cramps, diarrhea, nausea, or hives).

Food records, when carefully kept, provide an accurate account of food intake, food behaviors, and food tolerances. The assessor can use the record to identify problem food behaviors and find solutions. The record keeper assumes an active role and may learn to take responsibility for personal food choices and eating habits.

Observing Food Intake   Direct observation of clients' food intakes is possible in health care facilities such as hospitals or nursing homes. Dietitians, dietetic technicians, and nurses frequently work together to keep records of the kinds and quantities of foods a client both receives and leaves on the plate. From these records, the dietitian deduces what has been eaten and estimates nutrient intakes as described in the next section. Often, direct observations are used to estimate a client's current energy and protein intake, and the procedure is simply called a *kcalorie count*.

Analysis of Food Intake Data   After collecting food intake data, the assessor estimates nutrient intakes, either informally by using food guides or formally by using food composition tables. Food intakes are then compared with standards, usually nutrient recommendations or dietary guidelines to determine how closely a diet meets the standards. Are the types and amounts of proteins, carbohydrates (including fiber), and fats (including cholesterol) appropriate? Are all food groups included in appropriate amounts? Is caffeine or alcohol consumption excessive? Are intakes of any vitamins or minerals (such as sodium or iron) excessive or deficient? An informal evaluation is possible only if the assessor has enough prior experience with formal calculations to "see" nutrient amounts in reported food intakes without calculations. Assessors often use the exchange system, described in Chapter 17, to estimate nutrient intake. Even then, such an informal analysis is best followed by actual calculations to spot-check for key nutrients.

Formal calculations can be performed either manually (by looking up each food in a table of food composition, recording its nutrients, and adding them up) or by using a computer diet analysis program. The assessor then compares the intakes with standards such as the RDA.

food record: an extensive, accurate log of all foods eaten over a period of several days or weeks.

Form 15–3   Food Frequency Checklist

The assessor helps the client estimate portion sizes and frequency of use.

	Number of Servings	Frequency[a]
1. How often do you eat the following foods?		
Bread, toast, rolls, muffins	_____	_____
Cereal (type?) _____ . . .	_____	_____
Rice or other cooked grains	_____	_____
Noodles (macaroni, spaghetti)	_____	_____
Pancakes or waffles	_____	_____
Crackers or pretzels	_____	_____
Fruits or fruit juices	_____	_____
Vegetables other than potatoes	_____	_____
Vegetable juice	_____	_____
Potatoes	_____	_____
Dried beans and peas	_____	_____
Beef	_____	_____
Pork or ham	_____	_____
Veal	_____	_____
Poultry	_____	_____
Fish	_____	_____
Organ meats (such as liver)	_____	_____
Bacon	_____	_____
Sausage	_____	_____
Lunch meat	_____	_____
Hot dogs	_____	_____
Other meats (type?) _____ . . .	_____	_____
Eggs	_____	_____
Peanut butter or nuts	_____	_____
Milk (including on cereal)	_____	_____
Cheese or cheese dishes	_____	_____
Yogurt or tofu	_____	_____
Other milk products (type?)_____ . . .	_____	_____
Butter or margarine (type?) _____ . . .	_____	_____
Salt pork	_____	_____
Mayonnaise or salad dressing (type?)_____ . . .	_____	_____
Oil (type?) _____ . . .	_____	_____
Cream	_____	_____
Sugar, jam, jelly, syrup, honey	_____	_____
Bakery goods (type?)_____ . . .	_____	_____
Candy	_____	_____
Soft drinks (types?) _____ . . .	_____	_____
Potato or snack chips (type?) _____ . . .	_____	_____
Coffee or tea (type?) _____ . . .	_____	_____
Alcoholic beverages (type?) _____ . . .	_____	_____
Fast foods eaten out (type?) _____ . . .	_____	_____
TV dinners, pot pies, other prepared meals (type?) _____ . . .	_____	_____
Instant meals such as breakfast bars or diet meal beverages (type?)_____ . . .	_____	_____

Form 15–3	(continued)

2. What specific kinds of the following foods do you eat? Include the name of the food; whether it is fresh, canned, or frozen; and how it is prepared.

Fruits and fruit juices _____

Vegetables _____

Milk and milk products _____

Meats and meat alternates _____

Breads and cereals _____

Desserts _____

Snack foods _____

3. Please list the names of any liquid, powder, or pill forms of vitamin or mineral products you take, and state how often you take them. Please also list any diet supplement you use (such as protein milk shakes or brewer's yeast), how much you use, and how often you use it. _____

_____

4. Is there anything else you can relate about your food/nutrient intake?

_____

ªNumber of servings per day, week, month, or year.

Limitations of Food Intake Analysis   Food intake data can be informative, but the skillful assessor also keeps their limitations in mind. For example, a computer diet analysis tends to imply greater accuracy than is possible to obtain from data as uncertain as the starting information. Nutrient contents of foods listed in tables of food composition or stored in computer databases are averages and, for some nutrients, are incomplete. In addition, the available data on nutrient contents of foods do not reflect the amounts of nutrients a person actually absorbs. Iron is a case in point: its availability from a given meal may vary from as high as 50 percent to below 2 percent, depending on the person's iron status; the relative amounts of heme iron, nonheme iron, vitamin C, meat, fish, and poultry eaten at the meal; and the presence of inhibitors of iron absorption such as tea, coffee, and nuts. (Chapter 13 explains how to calculate iron absorption from a meal.)

Furthermore, reported portion sizes may not be correct. The person who reports eating "a serving" of greens may not distinguish between ¼ cup and 2 whole cups. Children tend to remember the serving sizes of foods they like as being larger than serving sizes of foods they dislike.

Interpretation of Food Intake Data   The assessor must remember that adequate nutrient *intakes* do not guarantee adequate nutrient *status* for an individual. Likewise, insufficient intakes do not always indicate deficiencies, but instead alert the assessor to possible problems. Each person digests, absorbs, metabolizes, and excretes nutrients in a unique way; individual needs vary. Intakes of nutrients identified by diet histories are only pieces of a puzzle that must be put together with other indicators of nutrition status in order to extract meaning.

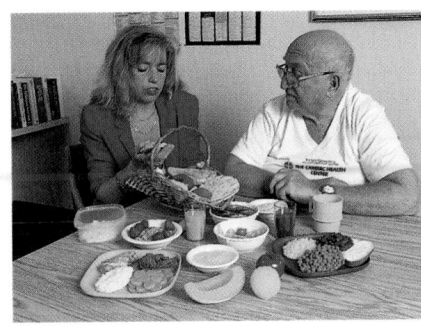

Help clients estimate food sizes by using food models and measuring utensils. When these items are not available, provide comparisons. For example, a small chicken leg is about 2 oz; a slice of luncheon meat is about 1 oz.

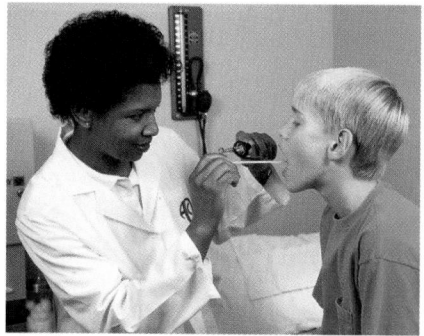

A physical examination provides valuable clues about a person's nutrition status.

Table 15–8

Physical Signs of Dehydration and Fluid Retention

Dehydration
- Sunken eyes
- Hollow cheekbones
- Dry mucous membranes
- Loss of skin turgor (elasticity)[a]
- Weak cry[b]
- Depression of the anterior fontanel[b]
- Deep, gasping respirations
- Weak, rapid pulse
- Thirst
- Reduced urinary output
- Weight loss

Fluid retention
- Edema
- Ascites (abdominal fluid retention)
- Elevated blood pressure
- Increased urinary output
- Weight gain

[a]May not be a useful parameter in the elderly.
[b]Findings specific to infants.

Histories alert health care professionals to potential nutrition problems. Diet and socioeconomic histories pinpoint food intake, eating behaviors, and factors that influence food choices and food habits. Medical and drug histories identify health factors and drugs that can alter nutrient requirements. To substantiate findings, other assessment tools including physical examinations (described next) and anthropometric and biochemical measurements (described in the next chapter) are useful.

Physical Examinations

One clinician astutely summarized the role of the physical examination in nutrition assessment this way: "To me, physical examination proves the saying 'A picture is worth a thousand words.' "[4] Indeed, health care professionals can simply look at people to see if they are overweight, underweight, lethargic, confused, or unable to feed themselves, to give a few examples.

With closer examination, a skilled assessor can use a physical examination to search for signs of nutrient deficiency or toxicity. Many tissues and organs can reflect signs of malnutrition. Malnutrition appears most rapidly in parts of the body where cell replacement occurs at a high rate, such as the hair, skin, and digestive tract (including the mouth and tongue). The summary tables in Chapters 10 through 13 list physical signs of vitamin and mineral malnutrition.

Fluid Balance   Among the most useful physical signs of nutrition status are those that reflect dehydration and fluid retention. As Chapter 16 describes, to interpret laboratory tests and anthropometric measurements accurately, the assessor must consider the state of hydration. In addition, many conditions significantly upset fluid balances, and attention to physical signs and laboratory tests that reflect fluid balance help guide therapy. Table 15–8 lists physical signs that may occur in dehydration and fluid retention. Considering the causes of fluid imbalances vary, however, the clinical manifestations vary as well.

Limitations of Physical Findings   Like the other assessment methods, such an examination requires knowledge, skill, and clinical judgment. Many physical signs are nonspecific; they can reflect any of several nutrient deficiencies as well as conditions not related to nutrition (see Table 15–9). For example, cracked lips may be caused by sunburn, windburn, dehydration, or any of several B vitamin deficiencies. For this reason, physical findings are most valuable for revealing problems for other assessment techniques to confirm or for confirming other assessment measures. A diet history can provide further support for a suspected vitamin deficiency, for example. Weight and height meaurements (anthropometric measurements) can confirm that a person is underweight and quantify the degree of underweight. Laboratory data can help verify a person's state of hydration or vitamin-mineral status.

Together with historical information, physical examinations provide important clues to a person's nutrition status. The next chapter describes anthropometric and biochemical measurements that further define nutrition status.

Table 15–9

Physical Findings Used in Nutrition Assessments

Body System	Acceptable Findings	Malnutrition Findings	What the Findings Reflect
Hair	Shiny, firm in the scalp	Dull, brittle, dry, loose; falls out	PEM
Eyes	Bright, clear pink membranes; adjust easily to light	Pale membranes; spots; redness; adjust slowly to darkness	Vitamin A, the B vitamins, zinc and iron status
Teeth and gums	No pain or caries, gums firm, teeth bright	Missing, discolored, decayed teeth; gums bleed easily and are swollen and spongy	Mineral and vitamin C status
Face	Clear complexion without dryness or scaliness	Off-color, scaly, flaky, cracked skin	PEM, vitamin A, and iron status
Glands	No lumps	Swollen at front of neck	PEM and iodine status
Tongue	Red, bumpy, rough	Sore, smooth, purplish, swollen	B vitamin status
Skin	Smooth, firm, good color	Dry, rough, spotty; "sandpaper" feel or sores; lack of fat under skin	PEM, essential fatty acid deficiency, vitamin A, the B vitamins, and vitamin C status
Nails	Firm, pink	Spoon-shaped, brittle, ridged, pale	Iron status
Internal systems	Regular heart rhythm, heart rate, and blood pressure; no impairment of digestive function, reflexes, or mental status	Abnormal heart rate, heart rhythm, or blood pressure; enlarged liver, spleen; abnormal digestion; burning, tingling of hands, feet; loss of balance, coordination; mental confusion, irritability, fatigue	PEM and mineral status
Muscles and bones	Muscle tone; posture, long bone development appropriate for age	"Wasted" appearance of muscles; swollen bumps on skull or ends of bones; small bumps on ribs; bowed legs or knock-knees	PEM, mineral, and vitamin D status

Study Questions

1. What are the steps in the nutrition care process?
2. What two services should the nutrition care plan deliver to the client?
3. Identify the four components of nutrition assessment.
4. How can a client's health history affect nutrition status?
5. What factors in a client's drug history suggest a likelihood of drug-nutrient interactions? Describe the mechanisms by which medications and nutrients can interact.

6. In what ways do socioeconomic factors affect nutrition status and food choices?
7. List two important uses for diet histories.
8. Describe ways of gathering food intake data and suggest uses for each method.
9. Itemize the major limitations of two methods of analyzing food intake data.
10. What is the primary use of the physical examination in nutrition assessment?

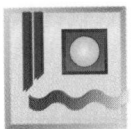

Clinical Applications

1. Considering the many factors that can affect nutrient intake addressed in this chapter, explain why it is important to follow a systematic approach to nutrition care. Describe some ways in which a physician, nurse, dietetic technician, pharmacist, and social worker might assist the dietitian in the assessment process.

2. Describe the possible nutrition implications of these findings from a client's history and physical examination: age 73, lives alone, recently lost spouse, uses a walker, no teeth, pale skin, lack of energy, history of hypertension and diabetes, several medications prescribed.

3. Nurses and nurse's aides often shoulder much of the responsibility for collecting food intake data for kcalorie counts because they often deliver food trays and snacks and later retrieve them. Why is it important for a nurse or aide to verify and record both what the client receives (both the foods and the amounts) and the foods that remain uneaten? When might clients be enlisted to aid in the collection of food intake data, and when might such a course be unwise?

4. During an initial nutrition assessment of a hospitalized client, the dietitian noted that the client appeared to be pale, thin, weak, and apathetic. Upon follow-up two weeks later, the dietitian noted that although the client was still quite thin, her color looked better and she appeared more energetic and talkative. The nurses noted that the client had been eating better and her weight had increased by two pounds. Does the dietary and weight information confirm or contradict the dietitian's observations?

Notes

1. J. A. Thomas, Drug-nutrient interactions, *Nutrition Reviews* 53 (1995): 271–282.

2. C. W. Lewis, E. A. Frongillo, and D. A. Roe, Drug-nutrient interactions in long-term care facilities, *Journal of the American Dietetic Association* 95 (1995): 309–315; R. N. Varma, Risk for drug-induced malnutrition is unchecked in elderly patients in nursing homes, *Journal of the American Dietetic Association* 94 (1994): 192–194.

3. L. R. Young and M. Nestle, Portion sizes in dietary assessment: Issues and policy implications, *Nutrition Reviews* 53 (1995): 149–158.

4. K. Hammond, Nutrition focused physical assessment, *Support Line*, August 1996, pp. 1–4.

Diet and Health

A century ago, our ancestors feared infectious and communicable diseases such as smallpox—diseases that claimed many children's lives and limited the average life expectancy of adults. Today far fewer infectious diseases threaten us, thanks to medial science's ability to identify disease-causing microorganisms and develop vaccines and effective treatments. In developed nations, immunizations protect individuals from some infections, purification of water prevents the spread of infection, and antimicrobial drugs successfully treat infections.

Although some infectious diseases remain serious threats in developed countries, most of today's life-threatening diseases develop and become chronic as a result of physiological deterioration of the body induced by such factors as genetics, age, gender, lifestyle, and environment. Diet is one of many lifestyle factors that influence the risks of developing chronic diseases, and dietary factors that advance or prevent the progression of chronic disease are the focus of this highlight.

MAJOR CHRONIC DISEASES AND THEIR RISK FACTORS

Table H15–1 lists the ten leading causes of death in the United States.[1] Four of these causes, including the top three, have some relationship with diet. Taken together, these four conditions account for two-thirds of the nation's 2 million deaths each year. Earlier chapters described individual nutrients' connections with diseases and may

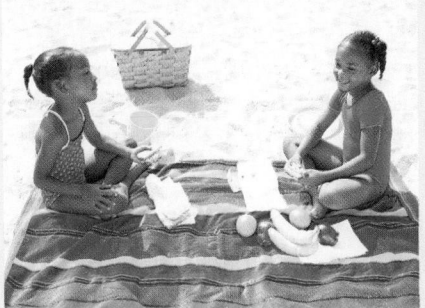

Establishing healthful habits in childhood lowers the risk of developing chronic diseases in adulthood.

have left the mistaken impression that these relationships can be described in terms of "one disease–one nutrient."[2] Indeed, valid links do exist between fat and heart disease, calcium and osteoporosis, and antioxidant vitamins and cancer, but to focus just on these links oversimplifies the story. In reality, each nutrient may have connections with several diseases because its role in the body is not

Table H15–1

Ten Leading Causes of Death in the United States

1. **Heart disease.**
2. **Cancers.**
3. **Strokes.**
4. Chronic obstructive lung disease.
5. Unintentional injuries.
6. Pneumonia and influenza.
7. **Diabetes mellitus.**
8. HIV infection.
9. Suicide.
10. Homicide.

Note: The diseases in bold type have documented relationships with diet.

specific to a disease, but to a body function. For example, vitamin C—because it acts as an antioxidant—helps prevent both cancer and heart disease. Furthermore, each of the chronic diseases develops in response to multiple factors, including many nondietary factors such as genetics, physical activity, and smoking. An integrated and balanced approach to disease prevention therefore includes attention to all factors involved. Figure H15–1 on p. 540 illustrates some of the relationships between risk factors and degenerative diseases.

RECOMMENDATIONS FOR POPULATIONS VERSUS INDIVIDUALS

Most chronic diseases that are influenced by diet are also influenced by genetics. Hypertension, obesity, high blood lipids, atherosclerosis, diabetes, and some types of cancer are common in families primarily for genetic reasons. Just as people's hereditary susceptibility to diseases varies, so do their responses to dietary measures. Logically, therefore, preventive efforts may be most beneficial for persons with strong family histories of disease, and health care professionals should single those people out for treatment. In reality, though, such a person-to-person approach is not feasible.

To determine whether dietary recommendations may be important to you personally, examine your family history to see which diseases are common to your parents and grandparents (see Figure H15–2 on p. 542 for a hypothetical "medical family tree"). In addition to family history,

Figure H15–1

Diet/Lifestyle Risk Factors and Degenerative Diseases

The chart at the top shows that the same risk factor can affect many chronic diseases. Notice, for example, how many diseases have been linked to a high-fat diet. The chart also shows that a particular disease, such as atherosclerosis, may have several risk factors.

The flow chart at the bottom shows that many of these conditions are themselves risk factors for other chronic diseases. For example, a person with diabetes is likely to develop atherosclerosis and hypertension. These two conditions, in turn, worsen each other. Notice how all of these diseases are linked to obesity.

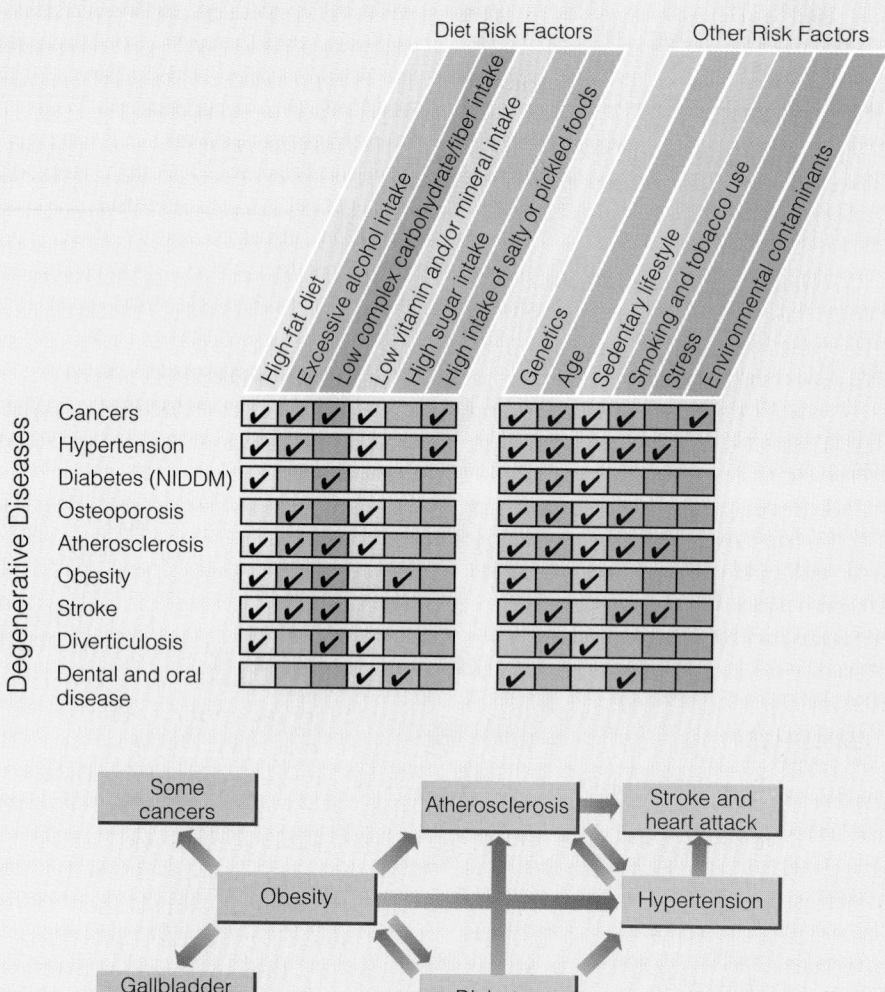

PUTTING IT ALL TOGETHER

Dietary excesses, particularly excess food energy and fat intakes, increase the likelihood of all of today's major diseases. Several of the recommendations are aimed at weight control: cut fat, add complex carbohydrates, and balance food intake with activity. The problems of overweight people multiply when medical problems develop. Overweight people with diabetes usually have hypertension and high blood lipids as well. Such a combination of problems may require only one treatment: lose the excess weight by adopting a healthful diet combined with regular physical activity.

Dietary deficiencies, particularly deficiencies in fiber, vitamin, and mineral intakes, also increase the likelihood of the major diseases. Following the recommendation to eat a variety of foods and to include plenty of grains, fruits, and vegetables in the diet addresses this concern.

Not all recommendations apply equally to all of the diseases or to all people with the disease (salt has a special relationship with hypertension in some cases, for example), but fortunately for the consumer, the dietary recommendations to help prevent these diseases do not contradict one another. Thanks to the fruits of recent research, healthy adults have a great opportunity: they can employ the benefits of a nutritious diet to help preserve their health into their later years.

NOTES

1. Centers for Disease Control, Mortality patterns—United States, 1989, *Morbidity and Mortality Weekly Report* 41 (1992): 121–125.
2. W. Mertz, A balanced approach to nutrition for health: The need for biologically essential minerals and vitamins, *Journal of the American Dietetic Association* 94 (1994): 1259–1262.

personal history is also important: take note of your own medical problems, weight, blood pressure, blood test results, and lifestyle habits such as smoking and physical activity.

Table H15–2 applies information from the *Dietary Guidelines for Americans* (see p. 541) and shows the medical risk factors that alert people to the personally relevant ones.

Table H15–2
. . . .

Nutrition Recommendations and Health Risks

Nutrition Changes Recommended for Most People	This Is Especially Important if Your Family Health History Indicates:	And/or if Your Personal Health History Indicates:
Energy, energy nutrients, and weight control: • Achieve and maintain a healthy body weight.[a] • Reduce consumption of total fat, saturated fat, and cholesterol.[b] • Increase consumption of complex carbohydrates and fibers.[c]	Obesity, diabetes, cancer, or any form of cardiovascular disease	Unhealthy weight, glucose intolerance, elevated blood cholesterol or triglycerides, hypertension, other cardiovascular disease
Salt/sodium: Reduce intake of salt/sodium.[d]	Hypertension, diabetes, or any form of cardiovascular disease	Hypertension, glucose intolerance
Alcohol: • Take alcohol only in moderation, if at all.[e]	Alcohol abuse or osteoporosis	Unhealthy weight, glucose intolerance, elevated blood cholesterol and triglycerides, any sign of adult bone loss
• Abstain from alcohol.		Pregnancy, alcohol abuse, liver disease, pancreatitis

[a]To achieve and maintain desirable body weight, choose a dietary pattern in which food energy intake matches energy expenditure. To reduce energy intake, limit foods relatively high in kcalories, fats, and sugars and minimize alcohol consumption. Increase energy expenditure through regular and sustained physical activity.

[b]Choose foods relatively low in fats and cholesterol, such as vegetables, fruits, whole-grain foods, fish, poultry, lean meats, and low-fat dairy products. Use food preparation methods that add little or no fat.

[c]To increase consumption of complex carbohydrates and fiber, eat more whole-grain foods and cereal products, vegetables, dried beans and peas, and fruits.

[d]To reduce intake of salt/sodium, choose foods relatively low in sodium, and limit the amount of salt added in food preparation and at the table.

[e]To exercise moderation in the use of alcohol, research suggests that men take no more than two to six drinks per week and that women take no more than one to three drinks per week (see Highlight 28). Avoid drinking any alcohol before or while driving, operating machinery, taking medications, or engaging in any other activity requiring judgment.

Figure H15–2

Hypothetical Medical Family Tree

A "medical family tree" notes the types of diseases family members have had, their ages at the times of major medical events or death, and their pesonal medical histories.

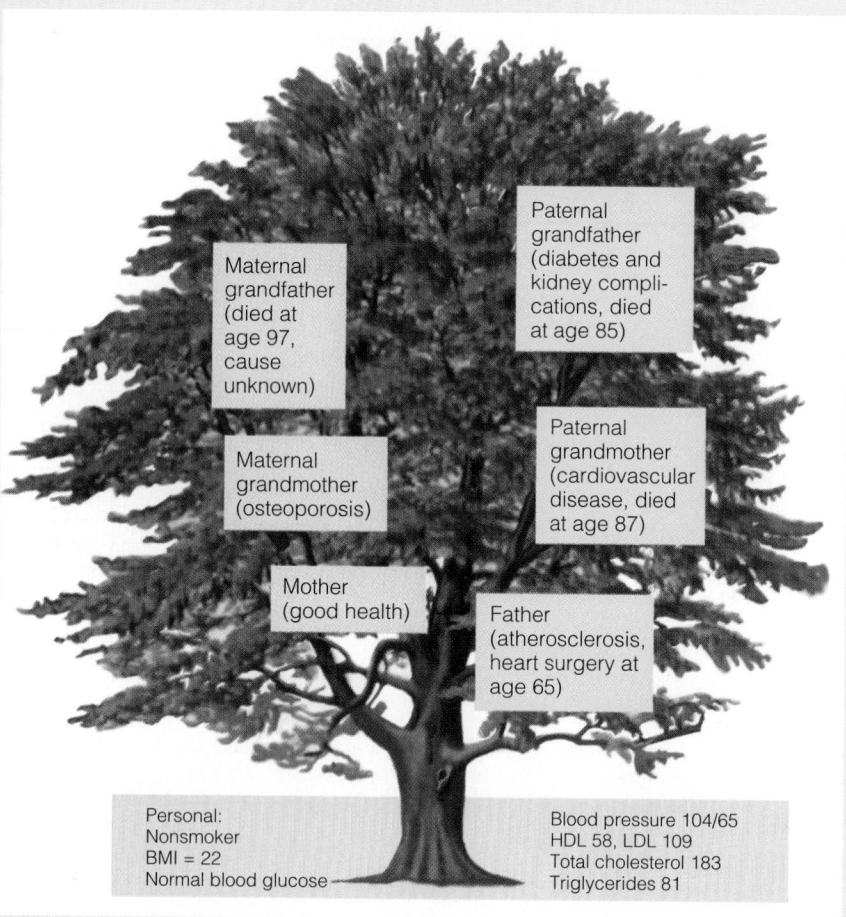

Maternal grandfather (died at age 97, cause unknown)

Paternal grandfather (diabetes and kidney complications, died at age 85)

Maternal grandmother (osteoporosis)

Paternal grandmother (cardiovascular disease, died at age 87)

Mother (good health)

Father (atherosclerosis, heart surgery at age 65)

Personal:
Nonsmoker
BMI = 22
Normal blood glucose

Blood pressure 104/65
HDL 58, LDL 109
Total cholesterol 183
Triglycerides 81

Chapter 16

The Nutrition Care Process: Assessing Anthropometric and Biochemical Data

CONTENTS

Anthropometric Measurements
  Measures of Growth and Development
  Measures of Body Fat and Lean Tissue
  Functional Measures of Nutrition Status
Biochemical Analyses
  Limitations of Biochemical Tests
  Biochemical Tests of Protein Status
Nutrition Screening
HIGHLIGHT: Nutrition and Diagnostic Tests

MICROGRAPH: Vitamin A, the most common vitamin deficiency among the hungry people of the world.

C hapter 15 introduced the nutrition care process and nutrition assessments and showed how the assessor can use historical information and physical examinations to look for signs of nutrient imbalances. This chapter shows how physical and biochemical measurements complete the assessment process.

Anthropometric Measurements

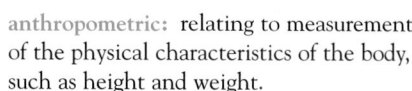

anthropometric: relating to measurement of the physical characteristics of the body, such as height and weight.

 anthropos = human

 metric = measure

Anthropometrics are physical measurements that provide an indirect assessment of body composition and development (see Table 16–1 on p. 546). They serve three main purposes: first, to evaluate the progress of growth in pregnant women, infants, children, and adolescents; second, to detect undernutrition and overnutrition in all age groups; and third, to measure changes in body composition over time.

Assessors compare anthropometric measurements taken on an individual with population standards specific for gender and age to see how body composition compares to norms. Assessors may also take measurements periodically and compare them with previous measurements to reveal changes in an individual's status.

Height and weight are well-recognized anthropometrics; others include fatfold measurements and various measures of lean tissue. Still other measures are useful in specific situations. For example, a head circumference measurement may help to assess brain development in an infant, and an abdominal girth measurement supplies information about abdominal fluid retention or enlargement of abdominal organs.

Mastering the techniques for taking anthropometric measurements requires proper instruction and practice to ensure reliability. Once the correct techniques are learned, taking the measurements is easy and generally requires minimal equipment.

MEASURES OF GROWTH AND DEVELOPMENT

Height and weight are among the most common and useful anthropometric measurements. Length measurements for infants and children up to age three and height measurements for children over three are particularly valuable in assessing growth, which depends on adequate nutrition. Poor growth in children is an important indicator of malnutrition. For adults, height measurements alone do not reflect current nutrition status but help to estimate desirable weight, to interpret other assessment data, and to estimate energy needs. Once adult height has been reached, changes in body weight may reveal either overnutrition or undernutrition.

Height For infants and children younger than three, health care professionals may use special equipment to measure length. The assessor lays the barefoot infant on a measuring board that has a fixed headboard and movable footboard attached at right angles to the surface. Often two people are needed to obtain an accurate measurement: one to hold the infant's head against the headboard and keep the legs straight, and the other to do the measuring. This method provides the most accurate measure possible, but many health care professionals

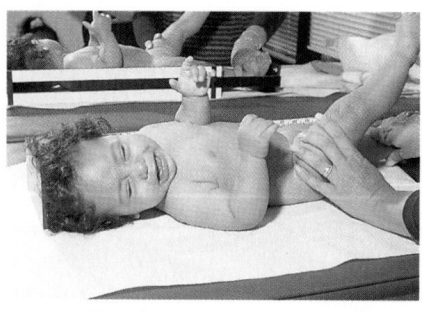

Lying still with legs straight for a length measurement can be a trying experience.

use a less exacting method. They may simply hold the infant straight with its head against the headboard or other vertical support, mark the blanket with a chalk or pen at the infant's heel, and then measure the distance from the head-board to the mark. Even more informally and less accurately, they may lay the infant on a flat surface and extend a nonstretchable measuring tape along the infant's side from the top of the head to the heel of the foot.

The procedure for measuring a child who can stand erect and cooperate is the same as for an adult. The best way to measure standing height is with the person's back against a flat wall to which a nonstretchable measuring tape or stick has been fixed. The person stands erect, without shoes, with heels together. The person's line of sight should be horizontal, with the heels, buttocks, shoulders, and head touching the wall. The assessor places a ruler, book, or other stiff object on top of the head at a right angle to the wall, carefully checks the height measurement, and records it immediately in either inches or centimeters. Immediate recording prevents the assessor from forgetting the correct measurement.

The measuring rod of a scale is commonly used to measure height, but is less accurate because of its movability. The assessor follows the same general procedure, asking the person to face away from the scale and to stand erect.

Many health care professionals merely ask clients how tall they are rather than measuring their height. Self-reported height is often inaccurate and should be used only as a last resort when measurement is impractical, as in the case of an uncooperative client or an emergency admission.

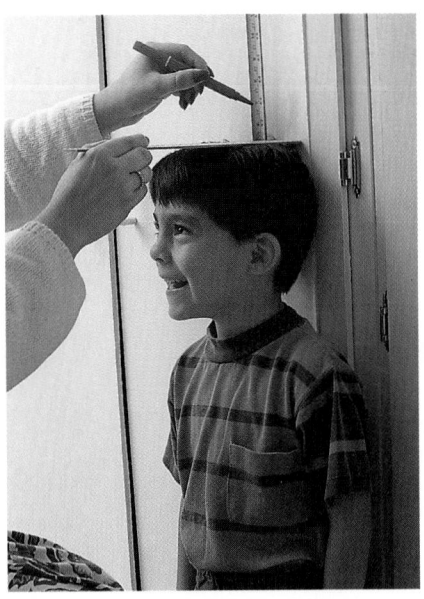

Standing "at attention" allows for an accurate height measurement.

Weight   Valid weight measurements require functional scales that have been carefully maintained, calibrated, and checked for accuracy at regular intervals. Beam balance and electronic scales are the most accurate types of scales. Special scales and hospital beds with built-in scales are available for weighing people who are bedridden. Bathroom scales are inaccurate and inappropriate for use in professional settings.

To measure an infant's weight, assessors use special scales that allow infants to lie or sit. Weighing infants naked, without diapers, is standard procedure. Children who can stand are weighed in the same way as adults. Standardized conditions are necessary if repeated measures are to be useful. Each weighing should take place at the same time of day (preferably before breakfast), in the same amount of clothing (without shoes), after the person has voided, and on the same scale. As with all measurements, the assessor records observed weight immediately in either pounds or kilograms.

Head Circumference   Assessors may also measure head circumference to confirm that infant growth is proceeding normally or to help detect protein-energy malnutrition (PEM) and evaluate the extent of its impact on brain size. To measure head circumference, the assessor places a nonstretchable tape so that it encircles the largest part of the infant's head: just above the eyebrow ridges, just above the point where the ears attach, and around the occipital prominence at the back of the head. To ensure accurate recording, the assessor immediately notes the measure in either inches or centimeters.

Analysis of Measures in Infants and Children   Health professionals evaluate physical development by monitoring the growth rate of a child and comparing this rate with standard charts (see Appendix E for more information).

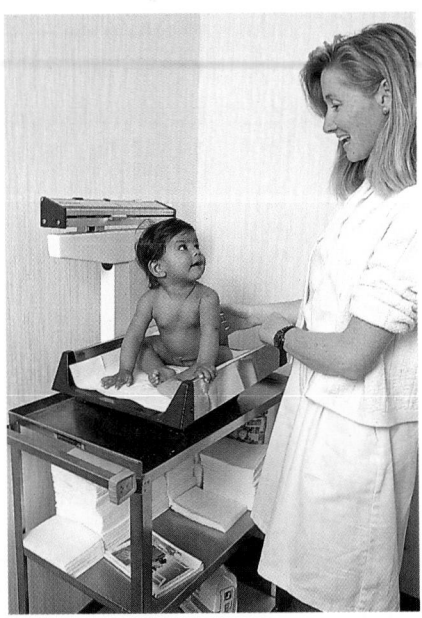

Special scales allow infants to sit and watch while they are being weighed.

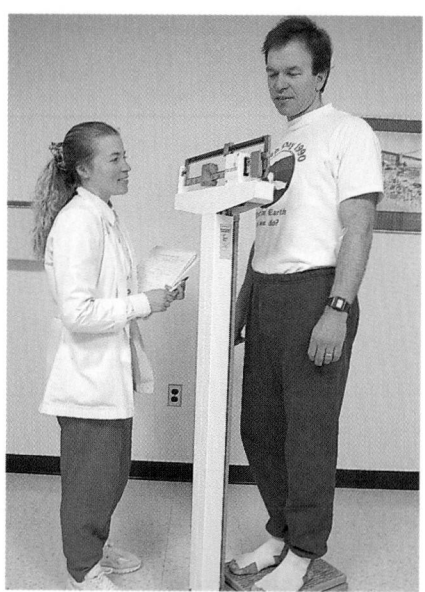

Beam balance scales provide accurate weight measurements for adults.

Table 16–1
•••••••••••

Anthropometric Measurements Used in Nutrition Assessments

Type of Measurement	What It Reflects
Abdominal girth measurement	Abdominal fluid retention
Height-weight	Overnutrition and undernutrition; growth in children
Head circumference	Brain growth and development in infants and children under two
Fatfold	Subcutaneous and total body fat
Midarm muscle circumference	Muscle mass (i.e., protein status)

Standard growth charts compare weight to age, height to age, and weight to height; ideally, height and weight are in roughly the same percentile. Although individual growth patterns may vary, a child's growth curve will generally stay at about the same percentile throughout childhood. Measurements below standard for height, weight, or head circumference in infants and young children indicate growth retardation, which is an important sign of malnutrition. (Chapter 19 describes the expected growth patterns and consequences of malnutrition for infants and children.)

In children whose growth has been retarded, nutrition rehabilitation will ideally induce height and weight to increase to higher percentiles. Obesity is also an important sign requiring intervention. In overweight children, the goal is for weight to remain stable as height increases, until weight becomes appropriate for height.

Head circumference is a useful indicator of brain growth in children under two years of age. Since the brain grows rapidly before birth and during early infancy, extreme and chronic malnutrition during these times can impair brain development, curtailing the number of brain cells and the head circumference. Head circumference percentiles should be similar to the child's weight and height percentiles. Nonnutritional factors, such as certain disorders and genetic variation, can also influence head circumference.

Analysis of Measures for Adults   Chapter 8 (pp. 268–271) discussed healthy body weight and described the controversies regarding weight standards for adults. Health care professionals typically compare weights with weight-for-height standards. Each facility or practitioner decides which standard to use based on review of the literature and clinical judgment. The commonly used standards for nutrition assessment include:

1. The body mass index (BMI) and tables based on the BMI observed to be consistent with health (see pp. 270–271 and inside back cover).
2. The Metropolitan Life Insurance weight-for-height tables (see Appendix E).
3. A quick method of estimating desirable body weight described in the accompanying box.

Reminder: The *body mass index (BMI)* is an index of a person's weight in relation to height, determined by dividing the weight in kilograms by the square of the height in meters:

$$\text{BMI} = \frac{\text{weight (kg)}}{\text{height (m)}^2}$$

How to Quickly Estimate Ideal Body Weight

In the health care setting, professionals may bypass standard height and weight tables and simply use a rule of thumb to estimate an "ideal" weight based on height and gender. The assessor considers 106 pounds a reasonable weight for a man who is 5 feet tall and then adds 6 pounds for each inch over 5 feet (or subtracts 6 pounds for each inch under 5 feet). For example, the calculation for a man who is 5 feet 8 inches tall would be:

$$5 \text{ ft} = 106 \text{ lb.}$$
$$8 \text{ in} = 48 \text{ lb } (8 \text{ in} \times 6 \text{ lb}).$$
$$5 \text{ ft } 8 \text{ in} = 154 \text{ lb.}$$

A reasonable estimate, then, for this man is 154 pounds. Large-framed individuals may need to add 10 percent, whereas small-framed individuals may need to subtract 10 percent. Thus the range for men of this height is 139 to 169. Compared with the range of 125 to 164 pounds listed in the standard "suggested weights" table found on p. 269, this estimated range is close enough for most purposes.

Similarly, the assessor considers 100 pounds a reasonable weight for a woman who is 5 feet tall and than adds 5 pounds for each inch over 5 feet (or subtracts 5 pounds for each inch under 5 feet). The calculation for a woman who is 5 feet 5 inches tall would be:

$$5 \text{ ft} = 100 \text{ lb.}$$
$$5 \text{ in} = 25 \text{ lb } (5 \text{ in} \times 5 \text{ lb}).$$
$$5 \text{ ft } 5 \text{ in} = 125 \text{ lb.}$$

A reasonable estimate for this woman is 125 pounds. Because large-framed individuals may need to add 10 percent, and small-framed individuals may need to subtract 10 percent, the estimated range for women of this height is 112 to 138. Again this range is similar to the suggested range of 114 to 150 (p. 269).

Reminder: Height and weight tables suggest a weight range, rather than pinpointing one ideal weight—a helpful reminder that no weight is perfect for everyone.

The assessor can compare the standard chosen with the person's actual weight to generate a figure known as the percent ideal body weight (%IBW). Current weight can also be compared to usual body weight to generate the percent usual body weight (%UBW), which considers what is normal for a particular individual. The client, family, friends, and older medical records can provide information about usual body weight. The %UBW is particularly useful for evaluating weight changes in cases where an individual has weighed considerably more or less than average throughout life. Additionally, in cases where an overweight individual becomes acutely ill and is rapidly losing weight, the health care professional relying on the %IBW may inadvertently overlook malnutrition. The rate of any recent weight change is important—a 5 percent weight loss within a month might be significant, yet the same loss over five months might not be. The box on p. 549 and Table 16–2 show how to calculate and evaluate the %IBW and the %UBW.

Table 16–2

Weight as an Indicator of Nutrition Status

%IBW	%UBW	Nutrition Status
>120	—	Obese
110–120	—	Overweight
90–109	—	Adequate
80–89	85–95	Mildly underweight
70–79	75–84	Moderately underweight
<70	<75	Severely underweight

Weight Change during Pregnancy One of the anthropometric measures most predictive of an infant's birthweight is the mother's amount and pattern of weight gain or loss during pregnancy. Chapter 18 describes normal weight gains related to pregnancy, and Appendix E provides an example of a chart used to monitor weight gain during pregnancy. Patterns of weight gain that deviate from these require further investigation.

MEASURES OF BODY FAT AND LEAN TISSUE

Significant weight changes in both children and adults can reflect overnutrition or undernutrition with respect to energy and protein. To estimate the degree to which fat stores or lean tissues are affected by weight changes, several anthropometric measurements are useful.

Body Fat As Chapter 8 explained, both the amount and the distribution of body fat are important. Body fat measurements include fatfold measures, waist-to-hip ratios, hydrodensitometry, and bioelectrical impedance, all described in Chapter 8. Another anthropometric measurement—the midarm muscle circumference—provides information about skeletal muscle mass.

Isotope studies, ultrasonography, and computerized axial topography (CAT scan) are other methods that have been used to determine body composition. The expense of these tests limits their clinical use, although they are useful in specific situations and in research.

Appendix E shows the proper techniques for measuring triceps fatfold and provides standards for comparison.

Midarm Muscle Circumferences Just as subcutaneous fat provides an indirect estimate of total body fat, measurable muscles provide an indirect measure of the protein status of muscular organs such as the heart. To determine whether a person has a depleted muscle mass, an indirect measure of arm muscle size is useful: the *midarm muscle* circumference. This measure is estimated by subtracting the amount of fat on the arm from the total area (derived from the arm's circumference). Appendix E shows how this is done and presents standards for comparison.

Cautious Interpretation of Measures The reliability of anthropometric measurements is limited by the skills of the measurer and the accuracy of the equipment used for measuring. Sometimes taking measurements is difficult for physical reasons, such as when a person cannot be moved to be weighed or measured for height. Triceps fatfolds and arm circumferences are sometimes difficult to measure in people with wounds or loose, hanging skin on their arms. In the elderly, the distribution of fat and the compressibility of the skin change, complicating the measurement and interpretation of fatfolds.

How to Estimate %IBW and %UBW

To estimate %IBW, compare the individual's current weight with the ideal body weight from standard height and weight tables:

$$\%IBW = \frac{\text{actual weight}}{\text{ideal weight}} \times 100.$$

For example, to calculate %IBW in a man who is 5 feet 8 inches tall and weighs 115 pounds, follow these steps. For ideal weight, use the midpoint of the weight range in Table 8–5 on p. 269. In this example, the ideal weight is 144 pounds.

$$\%IBW = \frac{115 \text{ lb}}{144 \text{ lb}} \times 100 = 80\%.$$

The man in this example is at 80 percent of his ideal body weight. Look to Table 16–2 to find that 80 percent IBW indicates that he is mildly underweight.

This man has lost 15 pounds in the last month. To calculate %UBW for this man, follow these steps:

$$\%UBW = \frac{\text{actual weight}}{\text{usual weight}} \times 100.$$

Calculate the usual weight (130 pounds) by adding the weight loss (15 pounds) to the current body weight (115 pounds).

$$\%UBW = \frac{115 \text{ lb}}{130 \text{ lb}} \times 100 = 88\%.$$

The man is at 88 percent of his usual body weight. A look at Table 16–2 reveals that a person at 88 percent UBW is mildly underweight. Based on %UBW, the degree of underweight is less severe than the %IBW implied, because the person has consistently weighed less than standard weight. Nevertheless, his recent rate of weight change is significant: he lost almost 4 pounds per week.

Even when measurements are taken accurately, interpreting them can present problems. A person's state of hydration, for example, significantly influences anthropometric measurements, because body composition reflects total body water as well as lean body mass and body fat. Diseases or medications that cause fluid retention can mask significant weight loss. Dehydration affects measurements of weight, fatfolds, and midarm muscle circumference. Besides the state of hydration, exercise alters anthropometric measurements. Exercise enhances muscle size, and lack of exercise may diminish muscle mass, independently of nutrition factors.[1]

Accurate interpretations of anthropometric measurements are also confounded by problems with the standards used for comparison. The controversies surrounding weight standards have already been described in Chapter 8. Another difficulty is that fatfold and muscle circumference standards were devel-

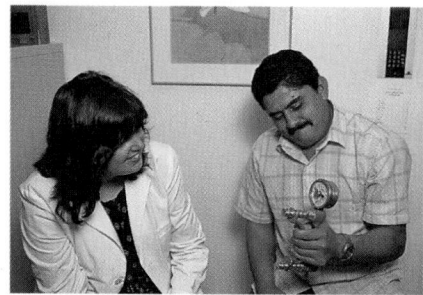

An instrument called a dynamometer measures hand grip strength.

oped for specific populations, often of healthy people in their middle years of life. The application of such standards to people who are sick or who are not within the age groups studied requires cautious clinical judgment.

Another limitation of anthropometrics is their inability to describe small changes in body composition that occur over short periods of time. Thus anthropometrics are of limited value in quantifying the effects of acute illnesses on nutrition status. Furthermore, research is needed to determine if internal fat stores change at the same rate as subcutaneous fat during illnesses that markedly raise the metabolic rate (see Chapter 25).

FUNCTIONAL MEASURES OF NUTRITION STATUS

Two tests of nutrition status, hand grip strength and skin tests, measure the function of organ systems, rather than a specific body compartment. Technically, these tests are not anthropometric measurements, but they both require physical measurements and so are described here.

Hand Grip Strength   The measurement of hand grip strength is a practical and inexpensive tool for assessing nutrition status that relates changes in body composition to organ function. The assessor asks the person to grip an instrument (called a dynamometer) as tightly as possible. Low grip strength (weak muscle function) indicates risk for poor nutrition status, which must be confirmed by other tests. People with severe arthritis or muscular disorders may have low grip strengths unrelated to nutrition status.

induration: a raised, hardened area of skin.

durus = hard

Conditions other than PEM that can affect skin tests include metabolic stress, liver disease, kidney disease, and the use of many drugs including corticosteroids and general anesthesia.

Skin Tests   Just as hand grip strength measures muscle function, antigen skin tests measure immune function. Organisms (usually three or four kinds) that produce an immune reaction in most people are injected just under the skin.* Raised, hardened areas (induration) appear after 24 to 48 hours in well-nourished people, but are minimal or absent in people with PEM. Many factors other than nutrition interfere with immune responses, however, and skin testing alone cannot identify PEM.

Anthropometric measurements, including height, weight, fatfolds, muscle circumference, and others, provide valuable information regarding body weight and composition. Hand grip strength reflects muscle function and skin tests reflect immune function; poor nutrition may be responsible for test results, but these tests alone may not be conclusive. Anthropometric measurements require properly working equipment and trained assessors to render accurate results that can then be compared to standards for interpretation. Biochemical tests, described next, help define nutrition status, organ function, body composition, and response to medical nutrition therapy.

Biochemical Analyses

All of the approaches to nutrition assessment discussed so far are external approaches. Biochemical analyses or laboratory tests help to determine what is

---

*Typical antigens include *Candida*, mumps, purified protein derivative (PPD), streptokinase-streptodornase (SK-SD), and *Monilla*.

happening to the body internally. Common tests are based on analysis of blood and urine samples, which contain nutrients, enzymes, and metabolites. Some directly reflect nutrition status. Other tests, such as serum glucose or tests that define fluid and electrolyte balance, acid-base balance, and organ function, help pinpoint disorders or problems with nutrition implications. Table 16–3 identifies some biochemical tests with nutrition implications and shows what these tests reflect. Tests important in specific disorders will be discussed in the appropriate chapters.

LIMITATIONS OF BIOCHEMICAL TESTS

The interpretation of biochemical data requires skill. The person's state of hydration greatly influences laboratory values, and indeed, laboratory tests are often used to detect dehydration and fluid retention. With dehydration, lab results may be deceptively high; with overhydration, lab results may be deceptively low.

No single test is sufficient to diagnose nutrient deficiencies because many factors influence test results. The low blood concentration of a nutrient may reflect a primary deficiency of that nutrient, but it may also be secondary to the deficiency of one or several other nutrients or to a factor unrelated to nutrition. Nutrient concentrations in the blood and urine sometimes reflect recent intakes rather than long-term intakes. Thus blood concentrations of a nutrient may be normal, even when tissue levels are deficient. Assessors who keep these limitations in mind and use lab tests along with other assessment data, however, can create a total picture that becomes clear with careful interpretation.

It is beyond the scope of this text to describe all lab tests used to assess nutrition status, define organ function, and develop nutrition care plans. Instead, the emphasis is on lab tests used to evaluate protein status. Appendix E provides tables of lab tests useful in detecting various vitamin and mineral deficiencies, including nutrition–related anemias.

BIOCHEMICAL TESTS OF PROTEIN STATUS

Protein is found in skeletal muscles, serum, and internal organs. Muscle proteins perform the physical work of the body, and serum and organ proteins maintain fluid balances, synthesize enzymes and hormones, mount immune responses, heal wounds, and much more. When the body is deprived of adequate energy to use as fuel, protein is sacrificed to make glucose. If energy deprivation continues long enough, the function of muscular organs such as the heart and organs that depend on muscles such as the lungs is compromised. Eventually, protein is unavailable to maintain these vital body functions.

While anthropometric measurements and hand grip strength evaluate skeletal muscle mass, lab tests of serum proteins and skin tests help evaluate internal proteins. Serum proteins are synthesized in the liver, and serum levels can reflect liver function, the availability of amino acids (protein intake), the distribution of proteins (proteins may shift from the blood to the intravascular or intracellular compartments, for example), and the rate of protein use by the body. Therefore, when evaluating serum proteins, assessors must consider disorders of metabolism and organ function, the body's rate of use of each protein, and protein status. Table 16–4 provides standards for evaluating the serum proteins most widely used in nutrition assessments. Other biochemical tests useful in assessing protein status include the total lymphocyte count, a measure of immune

The taking of several measurements during a single blood test is referred to as SMA (simultaneous multiple analysis). SMA is followed by a number (for example, SMA-12) that indicates how many tests will be run.

The serum is the watery portion of the blood that remains after removal of the cells and clot-forming material; plasma is the fluid that remains when unclotted blood is centrifuged. In most cases, serum and plasma concentrations are similar. Lab technicians usually prefer serum samples because plasma samples occasionally clog mechanical blood analyzers.

Recall that lab tests that confirm dehydration or fluid retention, including sodium, BUN (blood urea nitrogen), hemoglobin, and hematocrit, alert the assessor to interpret anthropometric measurements cautiously.

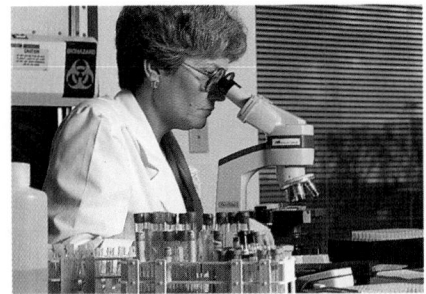

Blood and urine samples offer valuable clues for assessing nutrition status.

Table 16–3

Routine Hospital Laboratory Tests

Test	Uses
HEMATOLOGY	
Hemoglobin (Hg)	To detect anemia and determine state of hydration.
Hematocrit (Hct)	To detect anemia and determine state of hydration.
White blood cells (WBC)	To detect infection and determine total lymphocyte count.
Mean corpuscular volume (MCV)	To detect anemia and determine its causes.
Mean corpuscular hemoglobin (MCH)	To detect anemia and determine its causes.
Mean corpuscular hemoglobin concentration (MCHC)	To detect anemia and determine its causes.
BLOOD CHEMISTRY	
Proteins	
Total protein[a]	To detect PEM and various nutrient imbalances.
Albumin	To detect PEM and determine state of hydration.
Transferrin	To detect PEM and monitor response to feeding.
Prealbumin	To detect PEM and monitor response to feeding.
Electrolytes	
Sodium	To check state of hydration.
Potassium	To monitor acid-base balance and renal function and detect imbalances.
Chloride	To monitor acid-base balance and detect GI losses of chloride (from vomiting or nasogastric suctioning).
Carbon dioxide	To monitor acid-base balance.
Other	
Glucose	To detect diabetes mellitus, pancreatic tumors, and hypoglycemia and monitor glucose intolerance.
Blood urea nitrogen	To monitor renal function and determine state of hydration.
Calcium	To detect hormonal imbalances, certain malignancies, and steatorrhea (malabsorption).
Phosphorus	To detect hormonal imbalances and PEM and monitor renal function and response to feeding.
Magnesium	To monitor renal function and response to feeding and detect PEM.
Cholesterol	To assess risk of heart disease and possibility of obstructive jaundice.
Uric acid	To detect gout and determine state of hydration.
Serum creatinine	To monitor renal function and determine state of hydration.
Serum enzymes	
Creatinine phosphokinase (CPK)	To monitor heart function and muscle damage.
Lactic dehydrogenase (LDH)	To monitor heart and renal function.
Alanine transaminase (ALT, formerly SGPT)	To monitor heart and liver function.
Aspartate transaminase (AST, formerly SGOT)	To monitor heart and liver function.
Alkaline phosphatase	To monitor liver function.
Serum amylase	To monitor pancreatic function.
Serum lipase	To monitor pancreatic function.

Note: This table presents a partial listing of the major uses of certain commonly performed lab tests that have implications for nutrition.
[a]More than half of the total protein is albumin.

Table 16–4

Relationship between Degree of Undernutrition and Serum Proteins

Indicator	Degree of Depletion			
	NORMAL	MILD	MODERATE	SEVERE
Albumin (g/100 ml)	≥3.5	2.8–3.4	2.1–2.7	<2.1
Transferrin (mg/100 ml)	>200	150–200	100–149	<100
Prealbumin (mg/100 ml)	16–30	10–15	5–9	<5
Retinol-binding protein[a] (mg/100 ml)	2.6–7.6	—	—	—

Note: To convert albumin (g/100 ml) to standard international units (g/L), multiply by 100. To convert transferrin (mg/100 ml) to standard international units (g/L), multiply by 0.01.
[a]Levels less than normal suggest compromised protein status. The actual degree of depletion (mild, moderate, and severe) has not been defined.

function; urinary nitrogen, used to evaluate nitrogen balance; and urinary creatinine, a measure of skeletal muscle mass.

Serum Albumin   Albumin accounts for over 50 percent of the total serum proteins. Serum albumin is slow to reflect changes in nutrition status because it is plentiful in the body and breaks down slowly.[*] Therefore, low serum albumin reflects prolonged protein depletion. Likewise, albumin concentrations increase slowly with appropriate nutrition support, so measuring albumin as an indicator of response to nutrition therapy is of limited value. Serum albumin levels appear to correlate well with survival among people in the hospital.[2]

Note that albumin concentrations can be depressed by many conditions besides malnutrition, including liver disease, kidney disease (nephrotic syndrome), eclampsia, and disorders that can markedly raise the metabolic rate (metabolic stress) including infection, cancer, and burns.

Serum Transferrin   Transferrin is a protein that transports iron; consequently, its concentrations reflect both protein and iron status. Interpreting transferrin levels as an indicator of protein status is difficult when an *iron* deficiency is present. Transferrin rises as iron deficiency grows worse and falls as iron status improves. Markedly reduced transferrin levels indicate severe PEM; in mild-to-moderate PEM, transferrin levels may vary, limiting their usefulness.[3] Although transferrin breaks down in the body more quickly than albumin, it is still relatively slow to respond to changes in protein intake. Thus it is not a sensitive indicator of response to medical nutrition therapy.[†]

Conditions other than protein status that lower transferrin concentrations include liver disease, kidney disease (nephrotic syndrome), and metabolic stress. Pregnancy, iron-deficiency anemia, hepatitis, blood loss, and the use of oral contraceptive agents can elevate transferrin levels.

Prealbumin is also known as *thyroxin-binding prealbumin* or *transthyretin*.

Prealbumin and Retinol-Binding Protein   Prealbumin and retinol-binding protein[††] respond quickly to changes in protein intake, and both measure response to nutrition therapy.[4] Lab tests of prealbumin and retinol-binding protein are more expensive than the relatively inexpensive test of serum albumin,

Conditions other than protein status that can lower prealbumin levels include metabolic stress, hemodialysis, and hypothyroidism; levels may be elevated in kidney disease and with the use of corticosteroids.

---

[*]The half-life of albumin is about 20 days, an indication of a slow degradation rate.
[†]Transferrin has a half-life of 4 to 8 days.
[††]The half-lives of prealbumin and retinol-binding protein are 2 days and 12 hours, respectively.

Conditions other than protein status that can lower retinol-binding protein levels include vitamin A deficiency, metabolic stress, hyperthyroidism, liver disease, and cystic fibrosis; levels may be elevated in kidney disease.

Somatomedin-C is also known as *insulin-like growth factor (IGF-1)*.

Conditions other than protein status that affect the total lymphocyte count include metabolic stress (including infection) and the use of chemotherapy, immunosuppressives, and corticosteroids.

Appendix E shows the equations used for calculating nitrogen balance and the creatinine height index.

which is routinely available. Therefore, tests of prealbumin and retinol-binding protein are often reserved for clients with disorders that markedly change metabolic rates and can rapidly and profoundly affect nutrition status.

Other Serum Proteins   Other serum proteins that may be useful in protein assessment include serum somatomedin-C and fibronectin. These indicators of protein status are less practical and more expensive to measure than the other serum proteins used in nutrition support and are not in common use.

Total Lymphocyte Count   PEM compromises the immune system, reducing the number of white blood cells (lymphocytes), which are important in resisting and fighting infections. The total lymphocyte count, derived from the number of white blood cells and the percentage of lymphocytes (see the box below), is inexpensive and easy to obtain, but the many variables that affect the levels of the total lymphocyte count limit its value in nutrition assessment.[5]

Urinary Tests of Protein Status   Two biochemical tests of protein status—urinary urea nitrogen (UUN) and urinary creatinine excretion—require the collection of urine over a 24-hour period. Both tests require normal kidney function for accurate results. Assessors use the 24-hour UUN measurement, along with an accurate record of the client's energy and protein intake during the same period, to calculate nitrogen balance (see p. 194). Results of nitrogen balance studies determine whether protein intake is adequate to meet needs.

Urinary creatine excretion provides an indirect measure of skeletal muscle mass. By comparing urinary creatinine excretion to standards for sex and height (creatinine height index), assessors determine if muscle mass is adequate or depleted.

Twenty-four-hour urine collections are invalid if even one urine specimen is discarded or if samples are not stored properly. Nitrogen balance studies further

How to Calculate the Total Lymphocyte Count

To calculate the total lymphocyte count (TLC), look at the laboratory report and find the complete blood count (CBC). Two figures from this report, the number of white blood cells (WBC) in cubic millimeters (mm^3) and the percentage of lymphocytes are used to determine the total lymphocyte count:

$$TLC (mm^3) = WBC (mm^3) \times \% \text{ lymphocytes.}$$

A person with a WBC count of 7500 mm^3 with 15 percent lymphocytes would have a total lymphocyte count of:

$$TLC (mm^3) = 7500 \ mm^3 \times 0.15 = 1125 \ mm.^3$$

The standard lymphocyte count is 2500 mm^3. Values below 1500 mm^3 suggest mild depletion; below 1200 mm^3, moderate depletion; and below 800 mm^3, severe depletion. In the example, then, a TLC of 1125 mm^3 suggests moderate depletion.

require careful measurement of the food portions presented to and eaten by the client. Such difficulties explain why these tests are not routinely performed in most facilities. Nevertheless, nitrogen balance studies are very useful for evaluating protein needs for clients with severe metabolic stresses.

Laboratory tests help to define protein status, vitamin-mineral status, and alterations of metabolism or organ function with nutrition implications. The most common laboratory tests of protein status include serum levels of albumin, transferrin, prealbumin, and retinol-binding protein; the total lymphocyte count; and urinary urea nitrogen and creatinine. Compared to the serum proteins albumin and transferrin, which reflect long-term protein status, serum prealbumin and retinol-binding protein and urinary urea nitrogen respond more quickly to changes in diet. Urinary creatinine indirectly reflects skeletal muscle mass. The many variables that affect each laboratory test, however, remind assessors to ascertain findings using other assessment techniques.

Nutrition Screening

The numerous markers of nutrition status described in this chapter and the last provide clinicians with a variety of tools for evaluating malnutrition, the risk of malnutrition, and the response to diet therapy. Cost considerations, staffing, and individual preferences determine which tests are routinely available in different facilities and which will be used under specific circumstances. For a person with an elevated cholesterol detected during a routine physical, the assessor might measure height and weight, take a diet history to determine current eating habits, and repeat laboratory tests periodically to evaluate the nutrition care plan. A client admitted to the hospital who is suffering a hypermetabolic stress needs a more detailed assessment. Some hospitals may routinely measure serum albumin; others may not. One approach, the Subjective Global Assessment (SGA), relies on historical, anthropometric, and physical findings to assess nutrition status.[6] Often facilities use readily available information from histories and routine laboratory tests to identify high-risk clients and reserve in-depth assessments for individuals as needed.

Nutrition-screening policies vary from facility to facility but typically include the following:[7]

- *Assessment of health history.* Does the person's health history reveal risk factors for poor nutrition status (review Table 15–2)? Do the current medical problems include metabolic stress, malabsorption, depressed appetite, swallowing problems (dysphagia), or altered organ function?

- *Assessment of diet history.* Do the person's intake data reveal the exclusion of food groups or poor eating habits? Are certain food groups routinely excluded? Has the person been following an extremely restrictive diet?

- *Assessment of height and weight data.* Is the person's weight for height adequate, but not excessive? Has the person lost or gained weight? How much? How fast?

- *Physical assessment.* Does the individual appear to have obvious muscle wasting? Excessive weight? Fluid retention?

- *Assessment of available lab reports.* Do serum albumin and total lymphocyte count suggest malnutrition?

nutrition screening: the use of routine nutrition assessment procedures to identify people who are malnourished or are at risk for malnutrition.

In addition to these screening procedures, health care professionals can use other techniques to screen clients including:

- Check the client's tray to see if food is being eaten.
- If the client is to receive no food or is unable to eat, how long has it been since the client has eaten? Ask if the client is expected to be able to eat soon.
- If the client is unable to eat, determine whether adequate nutrients are being delivered by tube or by vein. (Chapter 24 shows how to calculate the nutrient content of intravenous solutions.)

Regardless of the health care setting in which the client is seen, communicate any problems that you discover and follow up to make sure the problem is being addressed. Always record problems in the medical record to ensure that whoever cares for a particular client will be alert to the problem. A dietitian will perform a more in-depth nutrition assessment if a problem is detected. Be persistent if you suspect that a problem is being ignored.

Nutrition screening provides a cost-effective method for identifying clients who need in-depth nutrition assessments using selected tools described in this chapter and the last. The case study that follows shows how the assessor uses assessment data.

Case Study   Nutrition Assessment of a Computer Scientist Following a Car Accident

Ms. Green, a 38-year-old computer scientist, was admitted to the hospital for surgery to repair a broken hip following a car accident. Other injuries included a wound over her left eye and bruises on her arm. After screening her health record, the physician referred Ms. Green to a dietitian for further nutrition assessment. Before visiting the client, the dietitian reviewed the medical record and noted the following:

- Ms. Green has been in good health over the past ten years, although she has experienced a gradual weight gain (height, 5 feet 7 inches; current weight, 150 pounds). She is in stable condition following surgery.
- Prior to hospitalization, Ms. Green was taking one multivitamin-mineral supplement daily and no medications. Morphine sulfate is now being administered for pain.
- Available information from the lab report shows a mildly depleted serum albumin (3 g/100 ml) and a moderately depleted total lymphocyte count (1000 mm^3).

From this information the dietitian keeps these points in mind before visiting the client:

- Even though Ms. Green is overweight, her nutrient requirements are temporarily increased.
- Pain mediation may make it difficult for Ms. Green to provide a detailed diet history.

Once in the client's room, the dietitian confirms Ms. Green's identity, introduces himself, and states the purpose of his visit. He takes time to establish rapport and get a sense of the client's ability to answer questions. Ms. Green appears to be alert, and the dietitian learns that she lives alone. Her busy schedule seldom leaves time for her to prepare meals. Using a usual food intake, the dietitian finds that Ms. Green usually skips breakfast and often eats out. She enjoys foods from all food groups, although she seldom eats the recommended amounts from the fruits and vegetable groups. For the past three weeks, she has been trying to lose weight, and her intake has been less than usual. She has lost 10 pounds during this time. Money for food and facilities for food preparation are not a problem. She appears to be overweight and pale.

Reviewing the elements of typical nutrition-screening procedures described on p. 555, what factors might have alerted the health care team to the need for a complete nutrition assessment? What factors in Ms. Green's health, drug, socioeconomic, and diet histories or physical findings suggest malnutrition?

Determine Ms. Green's ideal body weight and calculate her percent ideal body weight and percent usual body weight. Consider Ms. Green's recent weight change. What is a safe rate of weight loss (see p. 547)? How does Ms. Green's weight loss compare with the safe rate? Does her recent weight change increase her risk of poor nutrition status? What do Ms. Green's lab values indicate with respect to her protein status? What factors besides malnutrition need to be considered when interpreting Ms. Green's lab test results?

Study Questions

1. How do anthropometric measurements help define nutrition status? What anthropometric measurements are frequently used in nutrition assessments? Describe the limitations of anthropometric measurements.

2. How do lab tests help define nutrition status? What factors influence lab test results?
3. Describe the lab tests used to uncover PEM.
4. What is the purpose of nutrition screening? List various screening techniques.

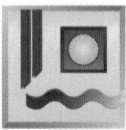

Clinical Applications

1. Calculate percent ideal body weight and percent usual body weight for a man who is 5 feet 11 inches tall with a current weight of 160 pounds and a usual body weight of 180 pounds. Select a weight standard for comparison and briefly defend your choice. What additional information will be important for you to find out about this man's weight loss?

2. Recall that serum proteins are influenced by metabolic stresses. With this in mind, what possible explanations can you suggest for these findings from a nutrition screening: client suffering a metabolic stress, 15-pound weight loss over the last four months (unintentional), depleted serum albumin, elevated serum transferrin, elevated total lymphocyte count. How might one sort through the possible explanations?

Notes

1. K. N. Jeejeebhoy, A. S. Detsky, and J. P. Baker, Assessment of nutrition status, *Journal of Parenteral and Enteral Nutrition* (supplement) 14 (1990): 193–196.

2. J. P. Doweiko and D. J. Nompleggi, The role of albumin in human physiology and pathophysiology, Part III: Albumin and disease states, *Journal of Parenteral and Enteral Nutrition* 15 (1991): 476–483.

3. A. Spiekerman, Proteins used in nutritional assessment, *Clinical Laboratory Medicine* 13 (1993): 353–369.

4. P. Charney, Nutrition assessment in the 1990s: Where are we now? *Nutrition in Clinical Practice* 10 (1995): 131–195; M. Russell, Serum proteins and nitrogen balance: Evaluating response to nutrition support, *Support Line*, February 1995, pp. 3–7.

5. Charney, 1995.

6. A. S. Detsky and coauthors, What is Subjective Global Assessment of nutrition status? *Journal of Parenteral and Enteral Nutrition* 11 (1987): 8–13.

7. Charney, 1995.

Nutrition and Diagnostic Tests

Chapter 16 introduced the laboratory tests that help diagnose malnutrition. Laboratory tests also play a pivotal role in the identification and treatment of many other disorders. Diagnostic tests include laboratory analysis of the blood, stool, urine, and breath and other procedures such as X rays, endoscopy, and other imaging techniques. Nutrition may influence the results of these tests and their interpretations. As you read through the examples presented in this highlight, keep in mind that the concepts introduced may apply to other tests as well.

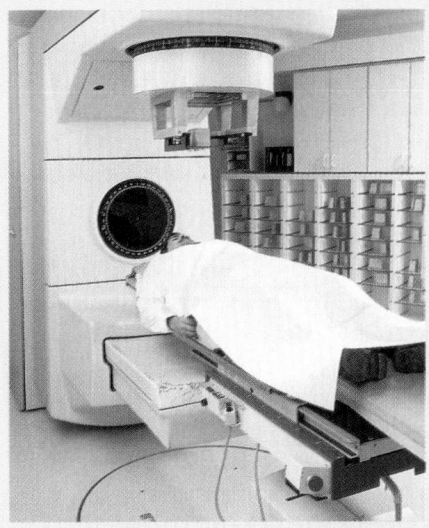

Clients must often adjust their diets in preparation for diagnostic tests.

EFFECTS OF FOODS ON LABORATORY VALUES

After a meal, the concentration of nutrients in the blood rises—a reflection of recent nutrient absorption. These levels may affect the test results for some blood constituents directly; for example, vitamin and mineral tests often reflect recent intake.

In some cases, the expected effect of a food on a lab value is known, and it may even be desirable to study that effect. Such is the case with a glucose tolerance test—a test of glucose metabolism. A person is given a dose of dietary glucose, and blood glucose is checked at regular intervals. By looking at the person's response to the glucose load, the clinician can tell if the person is metabolizing glucose normally. To improve the validity of the test, the person needs to receive a diet adequate in kcalories and protein, and at least 150 grams of carbohydrate, for at least 3 days before the test.[1]

Another test requiring that a set amount of a nutrient be consumed is that for fat malabsorption. To diagnose fat malabsorption, clinicians aim to provide about 100 grams (900 kcalories) of fat per day for 2 to 3 days; during the same period, the person's stools are collected.[2] Some people, however, simply cannot eat that much fat, particularly when they are ill. In those cases, diets can be planned to include from 60 to 80 grams of fat, and different standards are used to determine malabsorption.

Alternatively, some blood tests require that people fast for 8 to 12 hours before blood is drawn. After a meal, triglyceride levels rise and cause the blood sample to become cloudy. The cloudiness interferes with many chemical reactions that affect test results.[3] Fasting blood samples are often recommended when multiple tests will be performed on one blood sample.

Sometimes, tests require specific dietary restrictions to obtain valid results. One example is a stool test used to detect GI bleeding, an aid to the detection of cancer of the colon. The person often takes this test at home as part of a routine physical examination. For 48 to 72 hours before the test, and during the times stools are collected, the person should follow a high-fiber diet and eat no red meats, poultry, fish, turnips, and horseradish. The high-fiber foods speed up intestinal transit time and maximize the likelihood of detecting significant blood loss if it is present. Omitting the red meats and other foods listed above helps prevent false positive results—that is, results that suggest significant GI blood loss, when in fact there was none.

Vitamin C and iron supplements are also restricted during this GI test. Vitamin C supplements (more than 500 milligrams per day) can cause falsely normal test results, even when the person is experiencing significant GI bleeding. In contrast, iron supplements may produce GI bleeding in some people, even though there is no lesion.

A urinary test that requires a restrictive diet is used to detect certain tumors by looking for a compound called 5-hydroxyindoleacetic acid (5-HIAA) in the urine. If present, 5-HIAA signifies abnormal production of the brain neurotransmitter serotonin. Some foods contain significant amounts of serotonin and can interfere with test results. For the 24 hours preceding the test, clients are instructed not to eat avocado, bananas, kiwi, pineapple, plantain, plums, eggplant, tomatoes, butternuts, pecans, and walnuts. Clients must also abstain from alcohol because it suppresses 5-HIAA levels.

Even breath tests can be affected by diet. An analysis of hydrogen in the breath is used to detect lactose intolerance. Breads and pastas made from wheat flour and legumes can contribute significant quantities of hydrogen in the breath, so the person is cautioned not to eat these foods the day before the test. The person must fast from at least midnight until the next morning when breath hydrogen is collected to obtain a baseline hydrogen level; then the person is given an oral dose of lactose. Breath hydrogen is measured thereafter at intervals.

So far, all of the diagnostic tests described have been laboratory tests. X rays, endoscopy, and other imaging techniques may also require special dietary restriction. X rays of the intestinal tract, for example, may require that the person fast from midnight the day before the test. Likewise, endoscopy procedures frequently require fasting.

ASSURING DIET COMPLIANCE

To assure that clients receive appropriate diets for diagnostic tests depends on cooperation and communication between various health care professionals. First, the physician ordering the test must specify the test diet. The diet order may read simply, "diet for breath hydrogen test." In the hospital, the dietary department is then responsible for sending the appropriate diet, which is specified in the diet manual. The nurse working with the client can check the diet manual to see what the diet entails and instruct the client, explaining how long the special diet (or fast) will last. The laboratory analyzing the test may also provide information about testing procedures. To make sure the test is valid, clients are advised to eat only those foods provided by the health care facility.

For tests that require ingestion of a certain amount of a nutrient, such as the fat malabsorption tests, nurses and dietitians frequently share responsibility for monitoring and recording the client's intake. The dietitian is often responsible for calculating expected fecal fat excretion when intakes fall below desirable levels. Nurses are responsible for stool and urine collections; laboratory technicians draw blood for blood tests.

Extra care must be taken when clients are being tested in an outpatient setting. Clients who are at home during the test period have free access to a wide variety of foods, nutrient supplements, and drugs. Like foods and nutrients, drugs can interfere with some test results. The dietitian or nurse is wise to provide oral and clearly written instructions about foods, nutrients, and drugs that may affect test results. Clients may be instructed to keep food and drug records, so that their test results can be assessed.

Finally, it is important to note that diagnostic procedures change from time to time. When new tests are developed, precautions needed earlier may not apply. Regular communication between the department performing the test and the physician, nursing service, and dietary departments can help keep everyone up to date.

NOTES

1. A. Ateshkadi and coauthors, *Basic Skills in Interpreting Laboratory Data* (Bethesda, Md.: American Society of Health-System Pharmacists, 1996), p. 259.
2. J. K. Nelson and coauthors, *Mayo Clinic Diet Manual* (St. Louis: Mosby, 1994), p. 413.
3. *Diagnostic Tests Handbook* (Springhouse, Pa.: Springhouse Corporation, 1993), p. XVI.

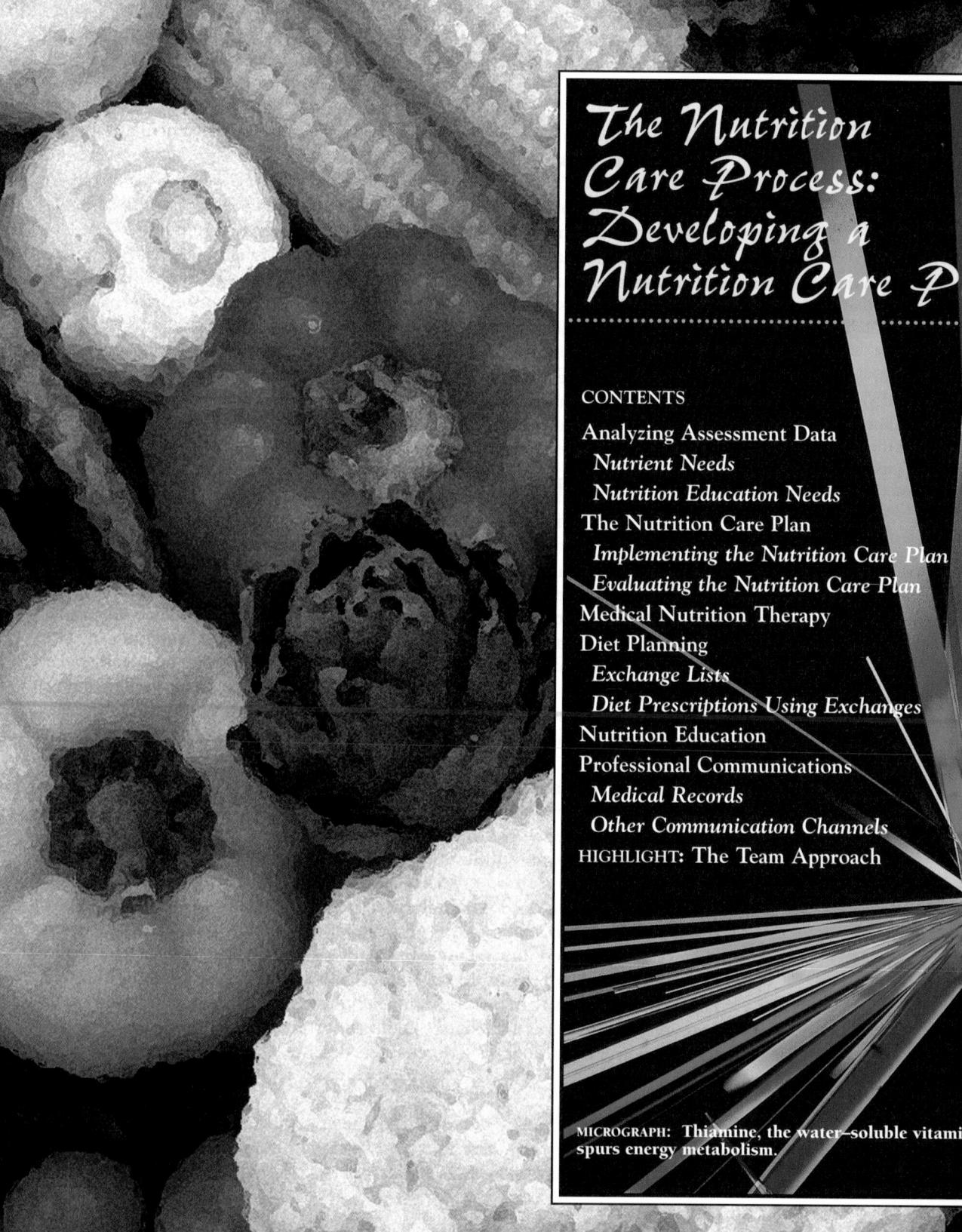

Chapter 17

The Nutrition Care Process: Developing a Nutrition Care Plan

CONTENTS

Analyzing Assessment Data
  Nutrient Needs
  Nutrition Education Needs
The Nutrition Care Plan
  Implementing the Nutrition Care Plan
  Evaluating the Nutrition Care Plan
Medical Nutrition Therapy
Diet Planning
  Exchange Lists
  Diet Prescriptions Using Exchanges
Nutrition Education
Professional Communications
  Medical Records
  Other Communication Channels
HIGHLIGHT: The Team Approach

MICROGRAPH: Thiamine, the water–soluble vitamin that spurs energy metabolism.

Figure 17–1   The Exchange System: Examples of Foods, Portion Sizes, and Energy-Nutrient Contributions

THE CARBOHYDRATE GROUP

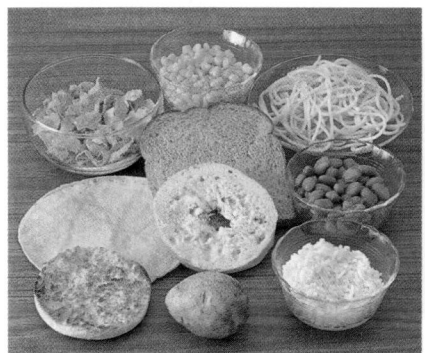

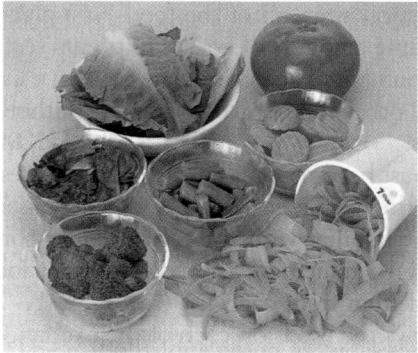

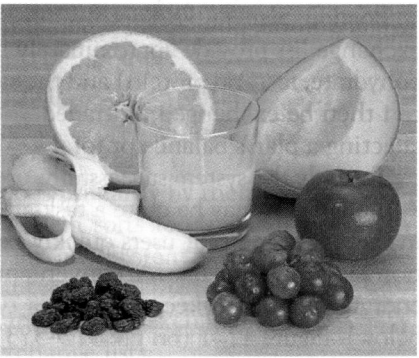

Starch
1 starch exchange is like:
1 slice bread.
¼ c ready-to-eat cereal.
½ c cooked pasta.
⅓ c cooked rice.
½ c cooked beans.ᵃ
½ c corn, peas, or yams.
1 small (3 oz) potato.
½ bagel, English muffin, or bun.
1 tortilla, waffle, or roll.
(1 starch = 15 g carbohydrate, 3 g protein,
0–1 g fat, and 80 kcal.)
ᵃ½ c cooked beans = 1 very lean meat
exchange *plus* 1 starch exchange.

Vegetables
1 vegetable exchange is like:
½ c cooked carrots, greens, green beans,
brussels sprouts, beets, broccoli, cauliflower, or spinach.
1 c raw carrots, radishes, or salad greens.
1 lg tomato.
(1 vegetable = 5 g carbohydrate, 2 g protein, and 25 kcal.)

Fruits
1 fruit exchange is like:
1 small banana, nectarine, apple, or
orange.
½ large grapefruit or pear.
½ c orange, apple, or grapefruit juice.
17 small grapes.
⅓ cantaloupe (or 1 c cubes).
2 tbs raisins.
(1 fruit = 15 g carbohydrate and 60 kcal.)

THE MEAT AND MEAT SUBSTITUTES GROUP (PROTEIN)

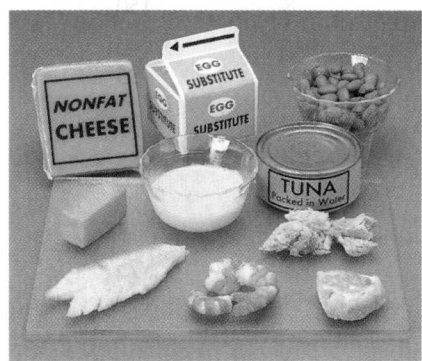

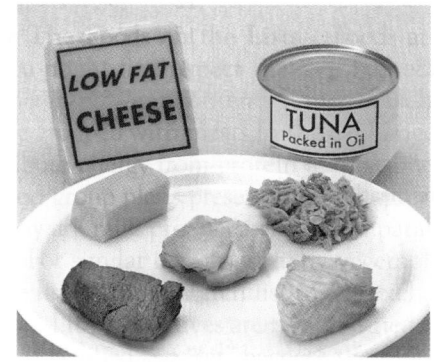

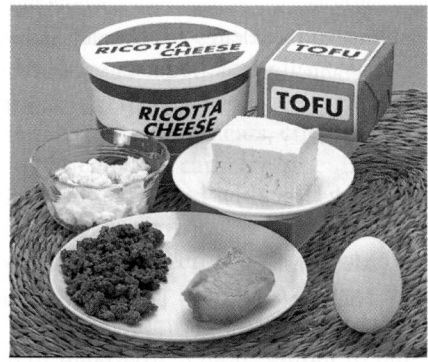

Meat and substitutes (very lean)
1 very lean meat exchange is like:
1 oz chicken (white meat, no skin).
1 oz cod, flounder, or trout.
1 oz tuna (canned in water).
1 oz clams, crab, lobster, scallops, shrimp,
or imitation seafood.
1 oz fat-free cheese.
½ c cooked beans, peas, or lentils.
¼ c nonfat or low-fat cream cheese.
2 egg whites (or ¼ c egg substitute).
(1 very lean meat = 7 g protein, 0–1 g fat,
and 35 kcal).

Meats and substitutes (lean)
1 lean meat exchange is like:
1 oz beef or pork tenderloin.
1 oz chicken (dark meat, no skin).
1 oz herring or salmon.
1 oz tuna (canned in oil, drained).
1 oz low-fat cheese or luncheon meats.
(1 lean meat = 7 g protein, 3 g fat, and
55 kcal.)

Meats and substitutes (medium-fat)
1 medium-fat meat exchange is like:
1 oz ground beef.
1 oz pork chop.
1 egg.
¼ c ricotta cheese.
4 oz tofu.
(1 medium-fat meat = 7 g protein, 5 g fat,
and 75 kcal.)

Figure 17–1   *(continued)*

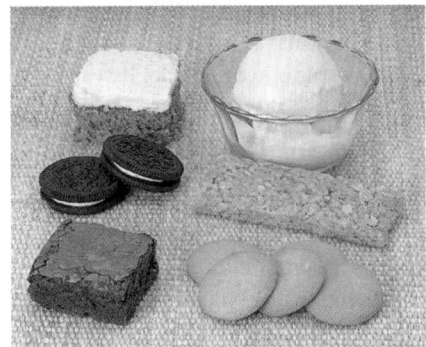

Other carbohydrates
1 other carbohydrates exchange is like:
2 small cookies.
1 small brownie or cake.
5 vanilla wafers.
1 granola bar.
½ c ice cream.
(1 other carbohydrate = 15 g carbohydrate and may be exchanged for 1 starch, 1 fruit, or 1 milk. Because many items on this list contain added sugar and fat, their fat and kcalorie values vary and their portion sizes are small.)

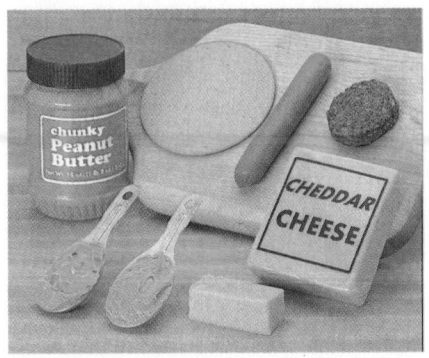

Meats and substitutes (high-fat)
1 high-fat meat exchange is like:
1 oz pork sausage.
1 oz luncheon meat (such as bologna).
1 oz regular cheese (such as cheddar or swiss).
1 small hot dog (turkey or chicken).[b]
2 tbs peanut butter.[c]
(1 high-fat meat = 7 g protein, 8 g fat, and 100 kcal.)

[b]A beef or pork hot dog counts as 1 high-fat meat exchange *plus* 1 fat exchange.

[c]Peanut butter counts as 1 high-fat meat exchange *plus* 1 fat exchange.

Milks (nonfat and very-low fat)
1 nonfat milk exchange is like:
1 c nonfat milk.
¾ c nonfat yogurt, plain.
1 c nonfat or lowfat buttermilk.
½ c evaporated nonfat milk.
⅓ c dry nonfat milk.
(1 nonfat milk = 12 g carbohydrate, 8 g protein, 0–3 g fat, and 90 kcal.)

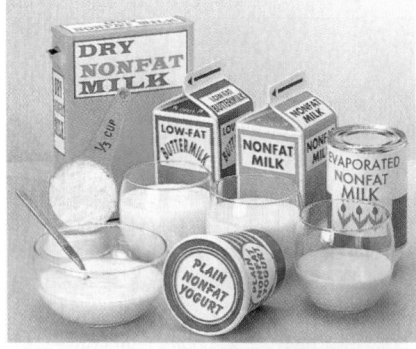

Milks (low-fat)
1 low-fat milk exchange is like:
1 c 2% milk.
¾ c low-fat yogurt, plain.
(1 low-fat milk = 12 g carbohydrate, 8 g protein, 5 g fat, and 120 kcal.)

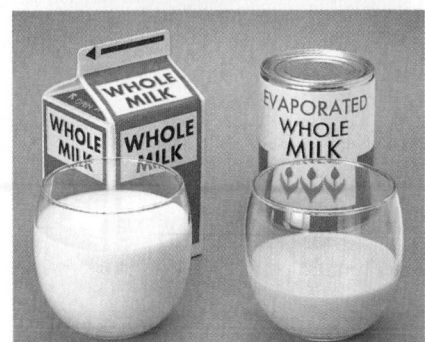

Milks (whole)
1 whole milk exchange is like:
1 c whole milk.
½ c evaporated whole milk.
(1 whole milk = 12 g carbohydrate, 8 g protein, 8 g fat, and 150 kcal.)

THE FAT GROUP
Fats
1 fat exchange is like:
1 tsp butter.
1 tsp margarine or mayonnaise (1 tbs reduced fat).
1 tsp any oil.
1 tbs salad dressing (2 tbs reduced fat).
8 large black olives.
10 large peanuts.
⅛ medium avocado.
1 slice bacon.
2 tbs shredded coconut.
1 tbs cream cheese (2 tbs reduced fat).
(1 fat = 5 g fat and 45 kcal.)

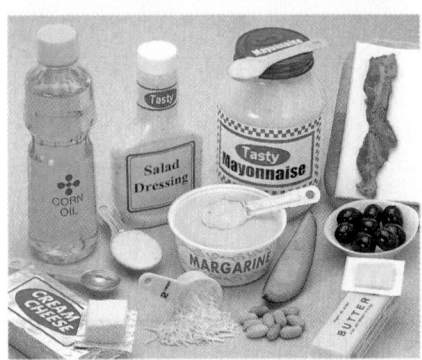

Note: Health recommendations urge people to limit their intakes of saturated fats; butter, bacon, coconut, and cream cheese contain saturated fat.

Figure 17–2

Using Labels to Calculate Exchanges

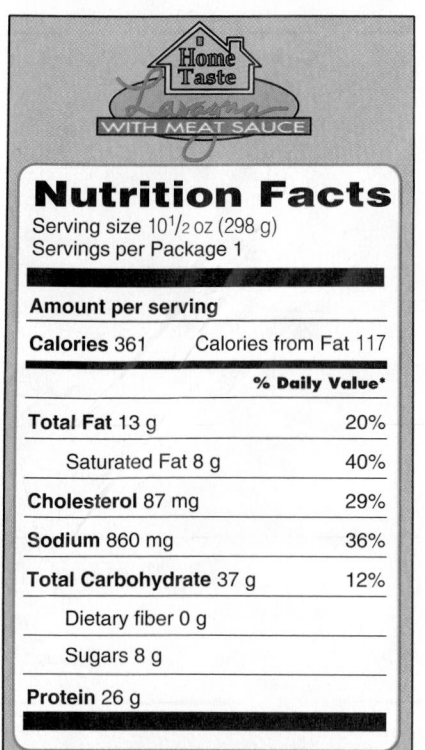

Nutrition Facts

Serving size 10½ oz (298 g)
Servings per Package 1

Amount per serving

Calories 361	Calories from Fat 117

% Daily Value*

Total Fat 13 g	20%
Saturated Fat 8 g	40%
Cholesterol 87 mg	29%
Sodium 860 mg	36%
Total Carbohydrate 37 g	12%
Dietary fiber 0 g	
Sugars 8 g	
Protein 26 g	

Can you "see" these exchanges
in the label above?

Exchange	Carbohydrate	Protein	Fat
2 starches	**30 g**	**6 g**	—
1 vegetable	**5 g**	**2 g**	—
3 medium-fat meats	—	**21 g**	**15 g**
Total	**35 g**	**29 g**	**15 g**

Note that a *portion* in the exchange system is not the same as a *serving* in the Daily Food Guide, especially when it comes to meats. The exchange system lists meats and most cheeses in single ounces; that is, 1 *portion* (or *exchange*) of meat is 1 ounce, whereas one *serving* is 2 to 3 ounces. Thus, if a person's diet plan allows for 3 ounces of meat at dinner, the diet plan would specify 3 meat exchanges. Taking actual portion sizes into account is pivotal to the successful use of the diet.

Food Mixtures   Users of the exchange lists learn to view mixtures of foods, such as casseroles and soups, as combinations of foods from different exchange lists. They also learn to interpret food labels with the exchange system in mind (see Figure 17–2). Knowing that foods on the starch list provide 15 grams of carbohydrate and those on the vegetable list provide 5, you can count a lasagna dinner that provides 37 grams of carbohydrate as "2 starches and 1 vegetable"; knowing that foods on the meat list provide 7 grams of protein, you might count it as "3 meats"; the grams of fat suggest that the meat (and cheese) is probably medium-fat.

DIET PRESCRIPTIONS USING EXCHANGES

Once the dietitian has determined the total energy and the percentage of kcalories from carbohydrate, protein, and fat to be included in a client's diet, the next step is to translate the prescription into exchange lists. Table 17–3 provides examples of sample diets at different kcalorie levels. (The box in Chapter 27 shows the steps a dietitian uses to derive such a pattern of exchanges for a client with diabetes.)

Combining Food Group Plans and Exchange Lists   Although exchange systems make excellent diet-planning tools, they do not guarantee adequate intakes of vitamins and minerals. Food group plans work better from that standpoint because the food groupings are based on similarities in vitamin-mineral content. To take advantage of the strengths of both exchange patterns and food group plans, diet planners check the exchange pattern to ensure that the diet contains adequate servings from each food group.

Table 17–3

Diet Patterns for Different Energy Intakes

Exchange	Energy Level (kcal)						
	1200	1500	1800	2000	2200	2600	3000
Starch/bread	6	7	8	9	11	13	15
Meat (lean)	4	5	6	6	6	7	8
Vegetable	3	4	5	5	5	6	6
Fruit	2	3	4	4	4	5	6
Milk (nonfat)	2	2	2	3	3	3	3
Fat	3	5	6	7	8	10	12

Note: These patterns follow the Daily Food Guide plan and supply less than 30 percent of kcalories as fat.

Translating Exchanges into Meals   The next step in diet planning is to assign the exchanges to meals and snacks. The final plan for a 2000-kcalorie diet might look like the one in Table 17–4. The person uses the plan by filling in real foods to create a menu (use Figure 17–1 and Appendix G). For example, the breakfast plan calls for 2 starches, 1 fruit, 1 nonfat milk and 2 fats. A person might select a bowl of shredded wheat with banana slices and milk (1 cup shredded wheat = 2 starches, 1 small banana = 1 fruit, and 1 cup nonfat milk = 1 milk) and save the fat for another meal; or a bagel with two teaspoons of margarine and a bowl of cantaloupe pieces topped with yogurt (1 bagel = 2 starches, ⅓ cantaloupe melon = 1 fruit, and ¾ cup nonfat plain yogurt = 1 milk, 2 teaspoons margarine = 2 fat). Alternatively, the person could have pancakes with strawberries and milk (4 small pancakes = 2 starches plus 2 fats, 1 ¼ cup strawberries = 1 fruit, and a cup of nonfat milk = 1 milk). Then the person could move on to complete the menu for lunch, dinner, and snacks.

Exchange list systems provide a practical tool for diet planning and estimating nutrient intakes. Unlike food group plans, foods on exchange lists are divided by their energy, protein, carbohydrate, and lipid contents. Once the dietitian designs a diet and meal plan for a client, the next step is to explain the diet plan to the client and caregivers.

Nutrition Education

Nutrition education is a continuous process that requires active participation between the dietitian and client. For temporary dietary adjustments (such as a diet for a diagnostic test), the dietitian, dietetic technician, or nurse describes the foods allowed and not allowed on the diet, the length of time the diet will be necessary, and the reasons for the diet. For long-term dietary adjustments, more extensive counseling is required. In such cases, nutrition education is best accomplished in stages, allowing time for the client to assimilate information, ask questions, and recognize potential obstacles in following the diet.

Table 17–4

A Sample 2000-kCalorie Diet Plan

Exchange	Breakfast	Lunch	Snack	Dinner	Evening Snack
9 starch	2	2	1	3	1
6 vegetable		3		3	
5 fruit	1	1	1	1	1
5 lean meat		2		3	
3 nonfat milk	1	1			1
6 fat	2	2		2	

Note: This diet plan is one of many possibilities. It follows the number of servings suggested by the Daily Food Guide and meets dietary recommendations to provide 55 to 60 percent of its kcalories from carbohydrate, 15 to 20 percent from protein, and less than 30 percent from fat.

Responsibility for Nutrition Education   In health care facilities that employ dietitians, the primary responsibility for nutrition education lies with the dietitian, but physicians, nurses, and dietetic technicians can help to reinforce and clarify nutrition information. For example, while helping a client prepare for breakfast, a nurse listens as the client comments that breakfast just isn't the same without milk for his cereal now that he is on a low-fat diet. The nurse acknowledges that things will be a bit different, thus reinforcing the importance of making the necessary changes in accordance with the low-fat diet. The nurse adds, however, that the client need not do without milk altogether, but instead can include nonfat and some low-fat milks. Because the nurse sees that the client is confused about his diet, she asks the dietitian to talk with the client again.

In some outpatient clinics, nursing homes, and other facilities, dietitians are not available to provide nutrition education. In these facilities, the nurse or physician most often assumes the responsibility.

Application of Nutrition Education   Our abundant knowledge of the relationships between diet and health is purely academic until people can apply that knowledge to their lives. Successful counselors gather thorough client histories and use the information wisely to plan diets and provide diet and health information in a way that helps clients integrate the needed changes into their lifestyles. Just as important, if not more so, successful counselors motivate clients to make the needed changes. Although it is beyond the scope of this text to provide all the details of nutrition counseling, the following paragraphs highlight some key points. The checklist in Table 17–5 shows measures that can facilitate successful counseling.

Establish a caring relationship.

Establishing a Caring Relationship   Counselors who show they care about their clients are more likely to gain their clients' trust. A trusting client will provide honest feedback, which is essential to successful nutrition education. To promote trust, work on establishing rapport and empathy. To establish rapport, spend a little time expressing your interest in and concern for your client. To establish empathy, put yourself in your client's shoes: this will lay the foundation for developing understanding between the two of you.

Positive feelings foster learning.

A caring counselor realizes that the client is a whole person and that nutrition is only a part of that person's life. Major life stresses, pain, anger, and resentment may interfere with a client's motivation to change and may block messages from getting through. In some cases, the counselor may fare better by rescheduling a session than by forcing information on an unwilling learner.

Encouraging Behavior Changes   Changing behaviors is difficult to say the least. Consider that for most of their lives, clients select foods based on taste, socioeconomic factors, convenience, and persuasive messages from friends and advertisers. Then one day, a nutrition counselor advises a client to make most food selections based on health. To accomplish this goal every time the choice arises—and it arises every time the person eats—requires an incredibly strong commitment.

Changing long-term behaviors takes time, and a person's level of motivation often progresses in stages. A small change that produces a positive result may motivate the person to make further changes. Thus successful counselors plan for several counseling sessions. They present information in a way their client can

Table 17–5

Nutrition Counseling Checklist

PREPARATION

Successful communication begins with adequate preparation. Before beginning a counseling session, be sure to:

- *Assess your client's needs*—nutritional, educational, and motivational. This information allows you to make the information relevant to, and appropriate for, each individual client.
- *Assess your own knowledge* of the diet, medical condition, and treatment plans of your client. Gather the information you might need and be prepared, but don't worry that a client might ask a question or two that you can't answer.
- *Develop objectives* for meeting your client's needs. Define specific, realistic objectives in terms of behaviors that can be observed and measured.
- *Determine the content* of (the type and amount of information to present), as well as the methods used for the counseling session (for example, a filmstrip, a diet booklet, food models, practice menus, or a food record). Let the client's level of interest, motivation, and education guide you in these decisions. For example, an illiterate adult or a child might appreciate diet instructions in picture form. One person may find the in-depth details about the body's response to diet fascinating, whereas another person wants just the diet without the background.
- *Establish a time frame* for accomplishing objectives. The time frame can be tentative and somewhat flexible to reflect the client's needs.
- *Arrange for appropriate others* to be present at the session.

IMPLEMENTATION

When counseling, remember to establish a caring environment, allow others to be themselves, be a good listener, use familiar language and appropriate nonverbal gestures, and maintain eye contact. You will also want to use open-ended questions, center the session around the client, provide positive feedback, and summarize your discussion. In addition, be sure to:

- *Establish rapport* by spending a little time creating a trusting and caring atmosphere before beginning diet instructions.
- *Identify and communicate the objectives* of counseling clearly. If clients know, for example, that they will be told how dietary changes will improve their health, they may listen more closely to the explanation of the diet. Furthermore, this gives the client an opportunity to modify your expectations.
- *Discuss the rationale for diet changes* and show your clients how nutrition supports recovery. Clients who do not understand the benefits will not be motivated to change.
- *Answer all questions accurately,* even if you must explain that you will check on the information and convey it at a later time. This action clearly surpasses giving incorrect advice or ignoring a question.
- *Stress to clients that they carry the responsibility* for their health and for making the necessary diet changes.
- *Encourage client participation* in the counseling session. You will often hear statements such as "You need to talk to my wife; she does the cooking." It does help if the family member who prepares the food participates in the counseling session and understands the diet. However, clients must accept that they—not their spouses and not the counselor—need to accept the responsibility for their diets.
- *Be realistic* when applying principles of diet to lifestyle. Be sure that the person can actually apply the changes. The busy executive who frequently eats restaurant meals must know how to make appropriate food choices in restaurants. A person with a low income may need help with incorporating lower-cost food items into the diet, as well as tips on shopping economically. A person who follows a strictly kosher diet must know how to plan meals around the Jewish dietary laws (see Highlight 2).
- *Make diet instructions relevant* to clients by using many examples consistent with their own eating habits. Do this by becoming familiar with diet histories, having clients plan personal menus, asking them to tell you what they would select in a restaurant, or observing them make selections from the hospital cafeteria line.
- *Encourage active participation* in the sessions and allow clients to arrive at conclusions on their own.
- *Reinforce all positive responses* and acknowledge your client's cooperation during the session.
- *Arrange for follow-up* if needed.

EVALUATION

When a counseling session is complete, consider whether:

- The objectives have been met.
- The content and methods of instruction were appropriate. Ask yourself which methods worked well and which were less effective.
- The time was adequate and whether additional counseling is needed.
- The client's needs have changed.
- Your counseling skills were effective. Ask yourself how you can improve your instructional techniques for future counseling sessions.

A little information remembered and applied is better than a lot of information forgotten and disregarded.

understand, and they limit the amount of information they present at any one session. At each session, the nutrition counselor assesses the client's level of motivation and understanding, sets goals that realistically reflect the client's commitment and knowledge, and modifies the goals as the client's progress indicates.[1]

Counseling Limitations   As described, nutrition education to promote long-term behavior changes is most likely to succeed when clients can proceed at their own pace. Unfortunately, many clients receive nutrition education under less than ideal circumstances. In the hospital, for example, dietitians must often begin counseling clients when they are still ill and overwhelmed with a diagnosis and its implications. Even if clients learn to make proper food selections from the hospital menu, they may feel lost when it comes to planning a menu at home. Furthermore, after the immediate danger of illness has passed, the person may lose the motivation to keep following nutrition advice. For these reasons, it is advisable for the dietitian to provide follow-up in any way possible—personally through a phone call, home visit, or scheduled visit by the client to the counselor or through the client's physician.

Whether nutrition counseling is effective depends on the extent to which clients change their eating habits in response to it. Clearly, nutrition counselors face a challenge; they need to use both their nutrition knowledge and their counseling skills. Counseling skills improve with practice, but even the best counselor experiences some failures. In the end, the client, not the counselor, must accept responsibility for making the necessary diet changes.

Professional Communications

Maintaining strong professional communication networks benefits both health care professionals and their clients. Conversely, miscommunication between professionals can result in inappropriate therapy with serious consequences for clients' health. Professionals communicate through the medical record and other written records. In addition, many opportunities exist for professionals to discuss clients' medical conditions, concerns, and progress.

MEDICAL RECORDS

medical record: a continuous written account of a client's health history, diagnosis, therapy, and prognosis.

diagnosis: the disease a person has or is thought to have.
   dia = through
   gnosis = knowing

prognosis: the predicted course and outcome of a disease.
   pro = ahead of time, before

Medical records are legal documents that record a client's history, the assessment and diagnosis of medical problems, the measures being taken to treat those problems, and the results of tests and therapy. Reading the medical record at regular intervals allows health care professionals to continuously assess the client's condition and response to therapy. Writing in the medical records allows health care professionals to document the actions taken to comply with physicians' orders, the client's responses to those actions, and recommendations.

   Medical records can be organized in many ways. Most commonly, health care professionals use the problem-oriented medical record (POMR) approach. In this approach, health care team members list each of the client's problems to generate a problem list. Subsequently, each entry in the record addresses the actions being taken to deal with a problem. As new problems arise, they are added to the list.

The Medical Record and Nutrition Care   Learn how to effectively use the record in the facility where you work. Regardless of the type of medical record approach used, be sure the client's medical record includes important nutrition-related information. Examples of important information include:

- Evaluation of the client's current diet.
- Nutrition assessment data.
- Recommended medical nutrition therapy.
- The client's acceptance and tolerance of the diet.
- Problems with the client's food intake.
- Documentation of diet counseling.
- Any planned follow-up or referral to another person or agency.
- The client's response to nutrition care.
- The client's response to diet counseling.

Other Records   In addition to the formal medical record, various health care professionals keep records of their own. For example, nurses keep nursing care plans, just as dietitians keep the nutrition care plans described earlier. These records contain some of the same information that is in the formal medical record, but they also include more detailed plans and notes specifically pertinent to the individual health team member. For example, a nutrition care plan may have details about a client's reaction to a diet, which the dietitian will later use in preparation for diet counseling. Nursing care plans often contain information that relates to nutrition care. A nurse caring for a client may note that a client isn't eating, is having problems chewing foods, or needs assistance while eating. In the course of a busy day, these problems may not be communicated to the physician or dietitian. The dietitian who reads these notes, however, can initiate actions to correct the problems.

OTHER COMMUNICATION CHANNELS

Opportunities for communication other than by way of written records also exist among health team members. Health team members in a hospital often phone or page each other when they identify problems or when questions arise. Outside the hospital, health team members may be reached in their offices or through their answering services.

Bedside rounds provide an ideal opportunity for professional communication (see Highlight 17). Use these discussions to call attention to nutrition-related problems, recommend changes, or exchange information about clients' concerns and attitudes.

Nurses also report to one another at the end of each shift. Use this time to pass along information about clients' special nutrition and diet needs and requests.

Effective nutrition care addresses the unique needs of the individual, framing nutrient needs in the context of the person's educational, socioeconomic, and medical needs. This chapter has described techniques for building effective nutrition care plans. Later chapters describe how nutrient needs change due to illness and how therapeutic diets can meet them.

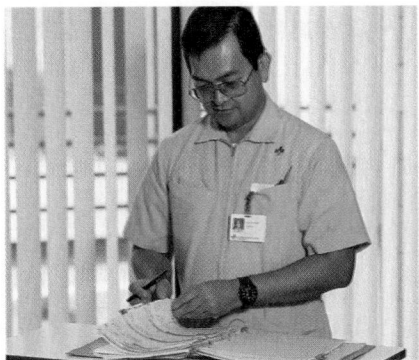

Take time to record important nutrition information in the client's medical record.

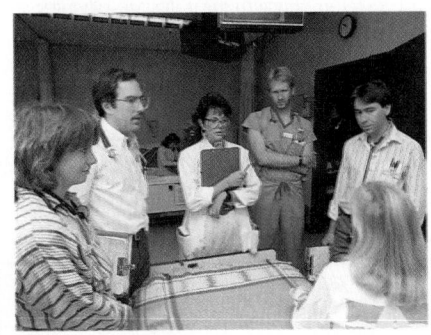

Bedside rounds provide an excellent opportunity to discuss your concerns regarding a person's nutrition status.

Study Questions

1. How does the analysis of assessment data contribute to the nutrition care plan?
2. What are the parts of a nutrition care plan? What two services should the plan deliver to a client? Why must the plan be evaluated from time to time?
3. What is medical nutrition therapy? In what ways can diets be modified to meet individual needs?
4. Describe the exchange lists used for diet planning. How do exchange lists differ from food group plans? What are the strengths of each system? How can the strengths of the two systems be combined?
5. Why is it important to present nutrition information in stages when a client must be on a special diet for a long time? Who is responsible for nutrition education? Describe some of the ways in which counselors can motivate clients to make diet changes.
6. How can you use the medical record to communicate a client's nutrition needs to other health care professionals? What kinds of information about nutrition should you record? Where else can you find written information about a client's nutrient or nutrition education needs?
7. Discuss some other ways that health care professionals can share concerns about a client's nutrition needs.

Clinical Applications

1. Refer to the case study about Ms. Green on p. 566. The physician prescribes a weight-loss diet for Ms. Green, and the dietitian plans a 1200-kcalorie, weight-reduction diet. Using Table 17–3 and the exchange lists in Appendix G, plan menus for one day's meals.
2. You are nurse visiting a client who recently suffered a heart attack and is now on a special diet. The client tells you that the dietitian has talked to him about his diet and he is totally confused. He confides in you that the diet is the last thing on his mind right now. What actions should you take?
3. A client has been losing weight while in the hospital, and the physician orders a kcalorie count. The physician's written order is recorded in the medical record, as is a note from the dietitian verifying the details of the procedure. Considering the communications channels described in this chapter, what steps might the dietitian take to ensure that the client's intake will be recorded through all shifts?

Note

1. American Diabetes Association and American Dietetic Association, *Facilitating Lifestyle Change: A Resource Manual* (The American Diabetes Association, Inc., and The American Dietetic Association, 1996), pp. 2–3.

The Team Approach

Human beings depend on one another to accomplish many tasks in everyday life. When several people work together, ideas flow and tasks become manageable. Consider a group of citizens planning a relief effort to deliver food and clothes to victims of a devastating tornado. After discussing the many tasks to be completed, the members of the committee decide how each of them can best contribute to accomplishing their goal. One person volunteers to make flyers to pass out—she has access to a copying machine. Another offers storage space for collecting goods—his business recently expanded and he has some extra space. Still another will call the local radio stations to ask them to make public service announcements. Another knows the owner of a trucking company who can lend a truck for transporting the food and clothes to the areas where they are needed. Working together, the committee members complete a large project efficiently. In much the same way, health care professionals can work together, sharing their unique expertise and skills to benefit their clients' health. Fortunately, the value of the health care team is increasingly being recognized. This highlight illustrates the principles of the team approach and describes some of the responsibilities of health care team members.

HEALTH CARE TEAMS

The number and types of health care teams vary from institution to institution. A health care team consists of a group of professionals specializing in a particular medical specialty. For example, the cardiac

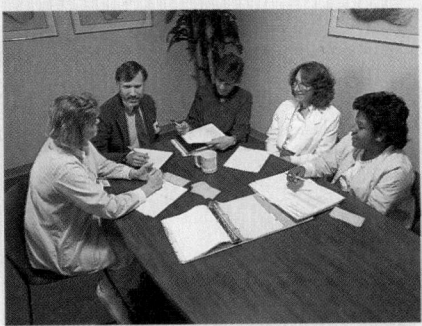

The team approach helps to ensure safe and effective nutrition support.

rehabilitation team works with clients recovering from heart attacks or cardiac surgery. Many health care teams include physicians, nurses, dietitians, pharmacists, and mental health workers among their core members. Other members vary according to the team specialty. A respiratory therapist would be a primary member of a pulmonary rehabilitation team, for example. Physical therapists and occupational therapists frequently participate on rehabilitation or burn teams. Social workers provide solutions to financial problems and coordinate home care programs.

Dietitians participate on health care teams that recognize medical nutrition therapy as essential to client care. Some examples include teams that specialize in disorders of the heart, blood vessels, lungs, endocrine system (such as diabetes mellitus), gastrointestinal tract, liver, and kidneys. Dietitians also serve on teams in cases where multiple organ systems may be involved such as severe trauma, burns, acquired immune deficiency syndrome (AIDS), cancer, and metabolic disorders.

Additionally, many institutions have nutrition support teams that develop protocols for nutrition screening and nutrition assessment, identify people who have nutrition problems, and oversee the care of people who must be fed by tube or by vein (Chapters 23 and 24) either in the hospital or at home.[1] Figure H17–1 shows the core members of the nutrition support team and illustrates how team members interact. Members of the nutrition support team share many of the responsibilities for client care, but each one also provides unique services. By working together, team members integrate their knowledge and provide the client with the benefits of their combined expertise. Team members also benefit—by learning how the others contribute to the care process, they learn to delegate responsibilities to the person who can do each job most effectively.

RESPONSIBILITIES OF TEAM MEMBERS

Team members maintain records and, both individually and as a team, review the progress of each client in their care. They often serve as consultants to the rest of the hospital staff, providing information, answering questions, and solving problems that arise in client care. Team members also carry responsibility for keeping abreast of new developments in their respective fields. They analyze new products, review current research, and communicate their findings to other team members.

The team physician assumes primary responsibility for client care:

Figure H17–1

. . . .

The Nutrition Support Team

The physician
- Diagnoses medical problems
- Performs medical procedures
- Coordinates and prescribes therapy
- Directs and supervises team
- Approves guidelines and protocols
- Consults with other physicians

The nurse
- Assesses nursing needs
- Performs direct client care
- Explains medical procedures and treatment plans
- Instructs clients regarding medical care
- Acts as a liaison between team and nursing staff
- Coordinates discharge plans

All team members
- Review current research
- Analyze new products
- Develop guidelines
- Provide in-service training
- Monitor clients
- Correct problems
- Educate clients
- Evaluate the outcome of the care provided

The dietitian
- Assesses nutrition status
- Determines clients' nutrient needs
- Recommends appropriate diet therapy
- Reevaluates clients regularly
- Instructs clients about their diets
- Acts as a liaison between the team and the dietary department

The pharmacist
- Recommends appropriate drug therapy
- Identifies drug-drug and drug-nutrient interactions
- Identifies drug-related complications
- Educates clients about their medications
- Acts as a liaison between the team and the pharmacy

diagnosing the client's medical problems, performing medical procedures, and coordinating and prescribing appropriate therapy. The physician frequently supervises the activities of other team members, monitors any complications that may arise, and makes the final decision on what steps to take to correct problems.

Team physicians also direct the development and approval of guidelines and protocols pertinent to the team's area of specialization. They oversee in-hospital educational and training programs for the profes-sional staff and act as consultants to other physicians who require their professional expertise.

The team nurse plays a central role in client care management and communications with the client, caregivers, and nursing staff. The nurse often explains medical procedures and treatment plans to clients and their care-givers. In addition, the team nurse supervises other nurses who care for each client to assure that they are delivering optimal care. The team nurse teaches staff nurses, as a group and individually, the ratio-nales for various procedures and the appropriate administration techniques. The nurse also assists in training physicians and other health care professionals.

The team nurse often coordinates the client's discharge from the hos-pital. Discharge responsibilities include discussing with clients any steps they will need to follow at home, making sure they have writ-ten instructions, providing appropri-ate supplies and equipment, and arranging for follow-up care.

The dietitian, as the team's nutri-tion expert, assesses the client's nutrition status, determines nutrient requirements, recommends appro-priate diet therapy, and translates diet orders into foods or formulas. Dietitians calculate nutrient intake data and nitrogen balance. The dietitian also instructs clients about their diets and prepares them to fol-low special diets at home.

Team dietitians provide in-service training on nutrition-related topics in their specialty areas for other dietitians, nurses, or other health care professionals. If particu-lar nutrition problems arise, dieti-tians actively investigate the cause, devise solutions, and see that they are carried out. The team dietitian also acts as a liaison between the team and the dietary department.

The pharmacist assists the health care team in managing the client's drug therapy; alerts team members to interactions of drugs with other drugs, nutrients, or nutrient solu-tions; and identifies complications that may be drug related. The phar-macist may recommend an optimal drug administration schedule and educates clients about the proper use of their medications. The phar-macist also serves as a liaison between the pharmacy and the health care team.

HOW THE TEAM APPROACH WORKS

Team members communicate with each other both informally and formally. They may share office space and see each other throughout the day, but their primary avenue for managing team responsibilities is during rounds, when the entire team discusses each client in the team's care. During rounds, the physician oversees the discussions and takes recommendations for changes. For example, the dietitian may express concern for a client who is unable to eat dinners because painful treatments have been scheduled just prior to dinner. The pharmacist recommends pain medication that will be effective through dinner to help alleviate this problem. The physician and pharmacist see no problem with adding this drug to the client's therapy, and the physician writes the medication order. The nurse makes sure that staff nurses working with the client

understand the rationale for the new drug therapy and the importance of its timing. Working together, the team has efficiently identified and solved a problem that might otherwise go unresolved.

Team rounds also serve as an avenue of communication for general problems that affect more than one client's care. For example, while discussing a client who has undergone a nitrogen balance study, the physician mentions that problems have occurred repeatedly with this procedure in the last month. The nurse recalls that many of the new nurses are having difficulty with the procedure and suggests an in-service training session on the proper techniques for nitrogen balance studies. The nurse and dietitian agree to jointly conduct the in-service training.

During rounds, team members may bring up current research that may affect the care they give clients, or they may share informa-

tion about new products they wish to evaluate for use with their clients. The team then decides if further action is warranted.

In these ways, health care teams contribute to optimal client care by combining and coordinating the expertise of various health care professionals. In addition, health care teams can effectively reduce hospital costs by providing the most efficient use of personnel and supplies.

To appreciate the team approach, remember the old adage, "Two heads are better than one." In this case, several heads are better still. Clients benefit when they have many eyes noting problems and many brains searching for solutions. In short, teamwork works.

NOTE

1. J. R. Wesley, Nutrition support teams: Past, present, and future, *Nutrition in Clinical Practice* 10 (1995): 219–228.

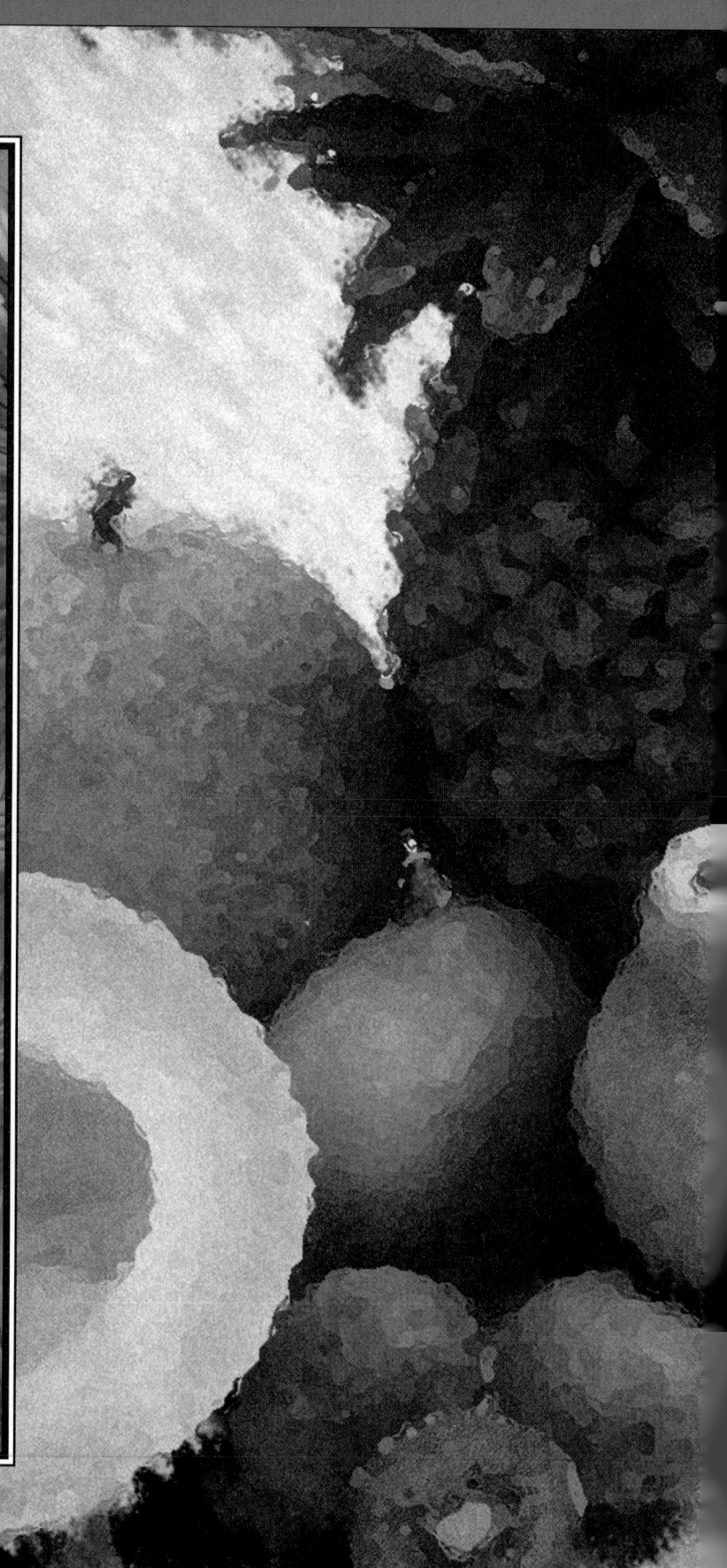

Chapter 18

Life Cycle Nutrition: Pregnancy and Lactation

CONTENTS

Growth and Development during Pregnancy
Placental Development
Fetal Growth and Development
Critical Periods
Maternal Weight
Weight for Height prior to Conception
Weight Gain and Exercise during Pregnancy
Nutrition during Pregnancy
Energy and Nutrient Needs during Pregnancy
Common Nutrition-Related Concerns of
Pregnancy
High-Risk and Low-Risk Pregnancies
Malnutrition and Pregnancy
The Infant's Birthweight
The Mother's Health Status
Adolescent Pregnancy
Fetal Alcohol Syndrome
Other Practices Incompatible with Pregnancy
Nutrition during Lactation
Breastfeeding: A Learned Behavior
The Mother's Nutrient Needs
Concerns of Breastfeeding Mothers
HIGHLIGHT: **Hunger and Global**
Environmental Problems

MICROGRAPH: **Folate, a B vitamin critical in preventing birth defects**

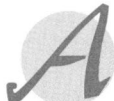ll people need the same nutrients, but the amounts needed vary depending on the stage of life. This chapter focuses on nutrition in preparation for, and support of, pregnancy and lactation.

Growth and Development during Pregnancy

A whole new life begins at conception. Organ systems develop rapidly, and nutrition plays many supportive roles. This section describes placenta and fetal development, paying close attention to times of intense activity.

PLACENTAL DEVELOPMENT

In the early days of pregnancy, a new organ develops within the uterus—the placenta, shown in Figure 18–1. Two associated structures also form. One is the amniotic sac, a fluid-filled balloonlike structure that houses the developing fetus. The other is the umbilical cord, a ropelike structure containing fetal blood vessels that extends through the fetus's "belly button" (the umbilicus) to the placenta. These three structures serve crucial roles during the pregnancy and then are expelled from the uterus following childbirth.

The placenta is composed of spongy tissue in which fetal blood and maternal blood flow side by side, each in its own vessels. The maternal blood transfers oxygen and nutrients to the fetus's blood and picks up fetal waste products. By exchanging oxygen, nutrients, and waste products, the placenta performs the respiratory, absorptive, and excretory functions that the fetus's lungs, digestive system, and kidneys will provide after birth.

The placenta is a versatile, metabolically active organ. Like all body tissues, the placenta uses energy and nutrients to support its work. Like a gland, it produces an array of hormones that maintain pregnancy and prepare the mother's breasts for lactation (making milk). A healthy placenta is essential for normal fetal development.

FETAL GROWTH AND DEVELOPMENT

Fetal development begins with the fertilization of an ovum by a sperm. Three stages follow: the zygote, the embryo, and the fetus.

The Zygote The newly fertilized ovum, or zygote, begins as a single cell and divides to become many cells during the days after fertilization. Within two weeks, the zygote embeds itself in the uterine wall—a process known as implantation. Cell division continues—each set of cells divides into many other cells. Later in gestation, as development proceeds, the zygote becomes an embryo.

The Embryo The embryo accomplishes amazing developmental feats. The number of cells at first doubles approximately every 24 hours; later the rate slows, and only one doubling occurs during the final ten weeks of pregnancy. The embryo's size changes very little, but at eight weeks, the 1¼-inch embryo has a complete central nervous system, a beating heart, a digestive system, well-defined fingers and toes, and the beginnings of facial features.

uterus (YOU-ter-us): the muscular organ within which the infant develops before birth; the womb.

placenta (plah-SEN-tuh): the organ that develops inside the uterus early in pregnancy, in which maternal and fetal blood circulate in close proximity so that materials can be exchanged between them. The fetus receives nutrients and oxygen across the placenta; the mother's blood picks up carbon dioxide and other waste products to be excreted.

amniotic (am-nee-OTT-ic) **sac:** the "bag of waters" in the uterus, in which the fetus floats.

umbilical (um-BILL-ih-cul) **cord:** the ropelike structure through which the fetus's veins and arteries reach the placenta; the route of nourishment and oxygen into the fetus and the route of waste disposal from the fetus. The scar in the middle of the abdomen that marks the former attachment of the umbilical cord is the **umbilicus** (um-BILL-ih-cus), commonly known as the "belly button."

ovum: the female reproductive cell, capable of developing into a new organism upon fertilization; commonly referred to as an egg.

sperm: the male reproductive cell, capable of fertilizing an ovum.

zygote (ZY-goat): the product of the union of ovum and sperm; so-called for the first two weeks after fertilization.

implantation: the stage of development in which the zygote embeds itself in the wall of the uterus and begins to develop; occurs during the first two weeks after conception.

gestation (jes-TAY-shun): the period from conception to birth; for human beings gestation lasts from 38 to 42 weeks. Pregnancy is often divided into thirds, called **trimesters**

embryo (EM-bree-oh): the developing infant from two to eight weeks after conception.

Figure 18–1

The Placenta and Associated Structures

To understand how placental villi absorb nutrients without maternal and fetal blood interacting directly, think of how the intestinal villi work. The GI side of the intestinal villi is bathed in a nutrient-rich fluid (chyme). The intestinal villi absorb the nutrient molecules and release them into the body via capillaries. Similarly, the maternal side of the placental villi is bathed in nutrient-rich maternal blood. The placental villi absorb the nutrient molecules and release them to the fetus via fetal capillaries.

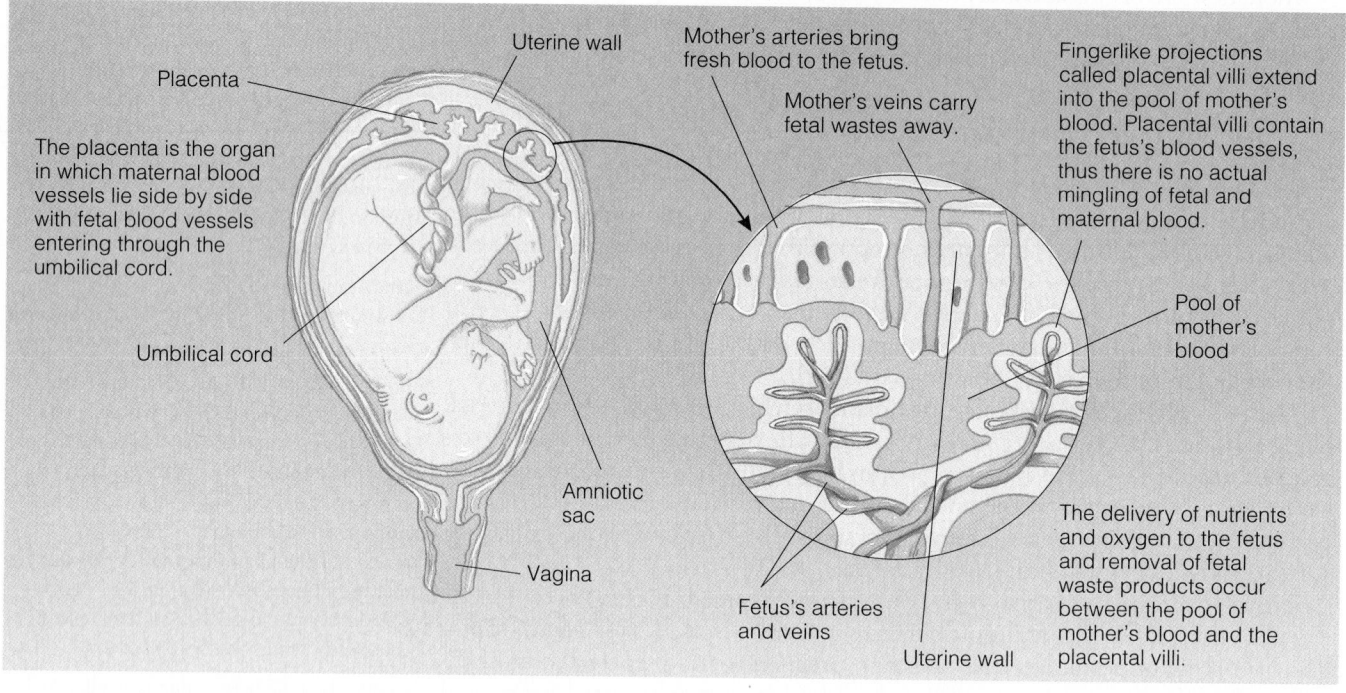

Uterine wall

Placenta

The placenta is the organ in which maternal blood vessels lie side by side with fetal blood vessels entering through the umbilical cord.

Umbilical cord

Amniotic sac

Vagina

Mother's arteries bring fresh blood to the fetus.

Mother's veins carry fetal wastes away.

Fingerlike projections called placental villi extend into the pool of mother's blood. Placental villi contain the fetus's blood vessels, thus there is no actual mingling of fetal and maternal blood.

Pool of mother's blood

Fetus's arteries and veins

Uterine wall

The delivery of nutrients and oxygen to the fetus and removal of fetal waste products occur between the pool of mother's blood and the placental villi.

---

fetus (FEET-us): the developing infant from eight weeks after conception until term.

critical periods: finite periods during development in which certain events may occur that will have irreversible effects on later developmental stages. In a body organ, a critical period is usually a period of rapid cell division.

The neural tube forms the beginnings of the brain and spinal cord, key structures in the central nervous system.

The Fetus   During the next seven months, each organ grows to maturity on its own schedule. As Figure 18–2 shows, fetal growth is phenomenal: weight increases from less than a gram to about 3500 grams (7½ pounds).

CRITICAL PERIODS

Times of intense development and rapid cell division are called critical periods—critical in the sense that the events scheduled for those times can occur only then, not later. If cell division and the final cell number achieved in an organ are limited during a critical period, full recovery will not occur (see Figure 18–3 on p. 588).

Each organ and tissue is most vulnerable to adverse influences during its own critical period. The critical period for neural tube development, for example, is from 17 to 30 days gestation.[1] Consequently, neural tube development is most vulnerable to nutrient deficiencies or toxins during this time—a time most women do not even realize that they are pregnant. Any abnormal development of the neural tube or its failure to close completely can produce major defects in the central nervous system, causing serious disabilities and infant death.

Figure 18–2

Stages of Embryonic and Fetal Development

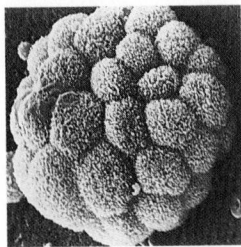

1. A newly fertilized ovum is about the size of the period at the end of this sentence. This zygote at less than one week after fertilization is not much bigger and is ready for implantation.

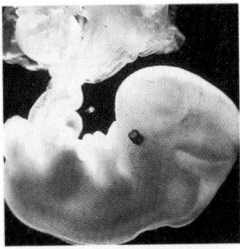

3. A fetus after 11 weeks of development is just over an inch long. Notice the umbilical cord and blood vessels connecting the fetus with the placenta.

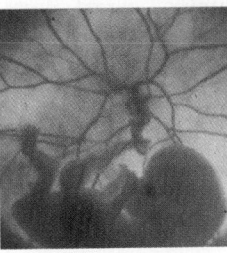

2. After implantation, the placenta develops and begins to provide nourishment to the developing embryo. An embryo five weeks after fertilization is about ½ inch long.

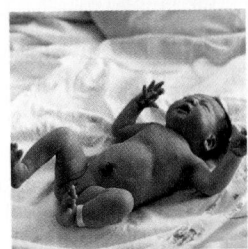

4. A newborn infant after nine months of development measures close to 20 inches in length. From eight weeks to term, this infant grew 20 times longer and 50 times heavier.

Spina Bifida   One of the most common types of neural tube defects is spina bifida, a disorder characterized by incomplete closure of the spinal cord and its bony encasement. The membranes covering the spinal cord often protrude as a sac, which may rupture and lead to meningitis, a life-threatening inflammation of the membranes. Spina bifida is accompanied by varying degrees of paralysis, depending on the extent of spinal cord damage. Mild cases may not even be noticed, but severe cases lead to death. Common problems include clubfoot, dislocated hip, kidney disorders, curvature of the spine, muscle weakness, mental handicaps, and motor and sensory losses.

In the United States, approximately 1 of every 1000 newborns has a neural tube defect; some 2500 to 3000 infants are affected each year.* Many other pregnancies with neural tube defects end in abortion or stillbirths.

Folate Supplementation   Chapter 10 described how folate supplements taken one month before conception and continued throughout the first trimester can prevent neural tube defects.[2] For this reason, the Public Health Service recommends that all women of childbearing age who are capable of becoming pregnant take 0.4 milligrams of folate daily. This amount of folate is easy to obtain from a diet that includes plenty of fruits and vegetables, but supplements offer women a convenient way to ingest sufficient folate regularly and continuously enough to benefit pregnancy. Most over-the-counter multivitamin supplements contain 0.4 milligrams of folate; prenatal supplements usually contain at least 0.8 milligrams. A woman who has previously had an infant with a neural tube defect may be advised by her physician to take folate supplements in doses

Folate RDA:
- For women: 180 μg (0.18 mg)/day.
- During pregnancy: 400 μg (0.4 mg)/day.

---

*Worldwide, some 300,000 to 400,000 infants are born with neural tube defects each year.

Figure 18–3

The Concept of Critical Periods

Critical periods occur early in development. An adverse influence felt early can have a much more severe and prolonged impact than one felt later on.

Normal development

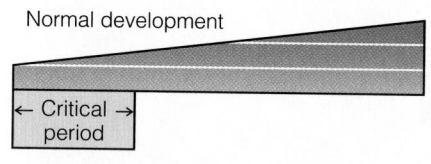

An adverse influence felt late temporarily impairs development, but a full recovery is possible.

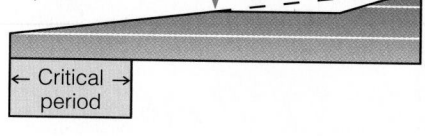

An adverse influence felt early permanently impairs development, and a full recovery never occurs.

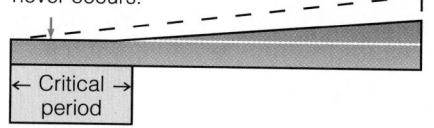

Underweight is defined as BMI <19.8.

preterm (infant)**:** an infant born prior to the 38th week of pregnancy; also called a **premature** infant. A **term** infant is born between the 38th and 42nd week of pregnancy.

ten times larger—4 milligrams daily. The risks associated with high doses of folate are not all known, but they can mask the pernicious anemia of a vitamin B_{12} deficiency. For this reason, quantities of 1 milligram or more require a prescription.

To deliver folate to the U.S. population, the Food and Drug Administration (FDA) has mandated fortification of grain products. In making this decision, the agency carefully weighed the benefits of fortification against the risks of overconsumption. On the one hand, an adequate folate intake is expected to reduce the incidence of neural tube defects by 50 percent. On the other hand, if vitamin B_{12} deficiency is masked by folate and left untreated, irreversible nerve damage may occur. The FDA regulation requires manufacturers to fortify foods to provide 140 micrograms of folate per 100 grams of foods, which should increase average daily intakes by 100 micrograms. Fortified foods include cereal, pasta, flour, rolls, buns, farina, grits, cornmeal, and rice.

Maternal nutrition before and during pregnancy affects both the mother's health and the infant's growth. As the infant develops through its three stages—the zygote, embryo, and fetus—its organs and tissues grow, each on its own schedule. Times of intense development are critical periods that depend on nutrients to proceed smoothly. Without folate, for example, the neural tube fails to develop completely during the first month of pregnancy, prompting recommendations for all women of childbearing age to take folate daily.

Because critical periods occur throughout pregnancy, a woman should continuously take good care of her health. That care should include, first, achieving and maintaining a healthy body weight and, then, gaining sufficient weight to support a healthy pregnancy.

Maternal Weight

Birthweight is the most reliable indicator of an infant's health. In general, higher birthweights present lower risks for infants. Two characteristics of the mother's weight influence an infant's birthweight: her weight for height prior to conception and her weight gain during pregnancy.

WEIGHT FOR HEIGHT PRIOR TO CONCEPTION

A woman's weight for height prior to conception influences fetal growth. Even with the same weight gain during pregnancy, underweight women tend to have smaller babies than heavier women.

Underweight An underweight woman has a high risk of having a low-birthweight infant, especially if she is unable to gain sufficient weight during pregnancy. In addition, the rates of preterm births and infant mortality are higher for underweight women. An underweight woman improves her chances of having a healthy infant by gaining sufficient weight prior to conception or by gaining extra pounds during pregnancy. To increase food energy intake, an underweight woman can follow the dietary recommendations for pregnant women (described in Table 18–3 on p. 593).

Overweight   Like underweight women, overweight women face problems related to pregnancy and childbirth. Overweight women face an especially high risk of medical complications such as hypertension, gestational diabetes, and postpartum infections. Compared with other women, overweight women are also more likely to require induced labor and cesarean section.

Infants of overweight women are likely to be born post term and to weigh more than 9 pounds. Overweight women are unlikely to have premature infants, but if they do, the infants may be large for their gestational age. Weight-loss dieting during pregnancy is never advisable, however. An overweight woman should try to achieve a healthy body weight before becoming pregnant, avoid excessive weight gain during pregnancy, and postpone weight loss until after childbirth. Weight loss is best achieved by eating moderate amounts of nutritious foods and exercising to lose body fat.

Overweight is defined as BMI >26.0 to 29.0, which corresponds with 20% over the reference weight in standard weight-for-height tables. Obese is defined as BMI >29.0.

cesarean section: a surgically assisted birth involving removal of the fetus by an incision into the uterus, usually by way of the abdominal wall.

post term (infant): an infant born after the 42nd week of pregnancy.

WEIGHT GAIN AND EXERCISE DURING PREGNANCY

All women must gain weight during pregnancy—fetal growth and maternal health depend on it. Maternal weight gain during pregnancy correlates closely with infant birthweight, and as mentioned earlier, infant birthweight is a strong predictor of the health and subsequent development of the infant.

Recommended Weight Gains   The recommended gain for a woman who begins pregnancy at a healthy weight and is carrying a single fetus is 25 to 35 pounds.[3] An underweight woman needs to gain between 28 and 40 pounds; and an overweight woman, between 15 and 25 pounds. Some women should strive for gains at the upper end of the target range, notably, adolescents who are still growing themselves. Short women (5 feet 2 inches and under) should strive for gains at the lower end of the target range. Women who are carrying twins should aim for a weight gain of 35 to 45 pounds. For the normal-weight woman, weight gain ideally follows a pattern of about 5 pounds during the first trimester, and about 1 pound per week thereafter. Health care professionals monitor weight gain using charts; Appendix E presents a prenatal weight gain grid.

If a woman gains more than is recommended early in pregnancy, she should not restrict her energy intake later in order to lose weight. To be a little overweight is healthier than to be underweight. A sudden large weight gain, however, may be the first sign of preeclampsia, a serious medical complication discussed later.

Weight-gain recommendations:
- Underweight women: 28 to 40 lb (12.5 to 18 kg).
- Normal-weight women: 25 to 35 lb (11.5 to 16 kg).
- Overweight women: 15 to 25 lb (7 to 11.5 kg).
- Obese women: 13 lb minimum (6 kg minimum).

Components of Weight Gain   Women often express concern about the weight gain that accompanies a healthy pregnancy. They may find comfort in a reminder that most of the gain supports the growth and development of the placenta, uterus, blood, and breasts, as well as an optimally healthy 7½-pound infant. A small amount goes into maternal fat stores, and even that fat is there for a special purpose: to provide energy for labor and lactation. Table 18–1 shows the components of a typical 30-pound weight gain.

Weight Loss after Pregnancy   The pregnant woman loses some of the weight at delivery. In the following weeks, she loses more as her blood volume returns to normal and she sheds accumulated fluids. The typical woman does not, however, return to her prepregnancy weight. In general, the more weight a woman gains beyond what she needs for pregnancy, the more she will retain.

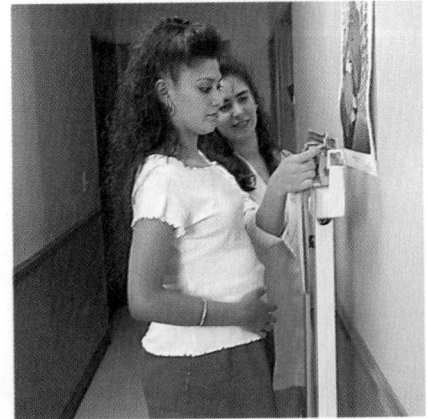

Fetal growth and maternal health depend on a sufficient weight gain during pregnancy.

Table 18–1

Components of Weight Gain during Pregnancy

Development	Weight Gain (lb)
Infant at birth	7½
Placenta	1½
Increase in mother's blood volume to supply placenta	4
Increase in mother's fluid volume	4
Increase in size of uterus and supporting muscles	2
Increase in size of mother's breasts	2
Fluid to surround infant in amniotic sac	2
Mother's fat stores	7
Total	30

Source: ACOG Guide to Planning for Pregnancy, Birth, and Beyond (Washington, D.C.: The American College of Obstetricians and Gynecologists, 1990), p. 109.

Even with an average weight gain, though, most women tend to retain a couple of pounds with each pregnancy.[4]

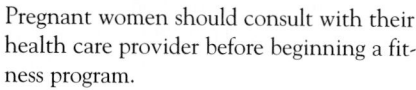
Pregnant women should consult with their health care provider before beginning a fitness program.

Exercise   The active, physically fit woman experiencing a normal pregnancy can continue to exercise throughout pregnancy, adjusting the duration and intensity as the pregnancy progresses. Staying active can improve fitness, prevent gestational diabetes, facilitate labor, and reduce stress.[5] It also maintains the habits that help a woman lose excess weight and get back into shape after the birth. A pregnant woman should avoid sports in which she might fall or be hit by other people or objects. For example, playing tennis with one person on each side of the net is safer than a fast-moving game of racquetball in which the two competitors can collide. Swimming is ideal because it allows the body to remain cool and move freely with the water's support. Table 18–2 provides some guidelines for exercise during pregnancy.[6] Several of the guidelines listed are aimed at

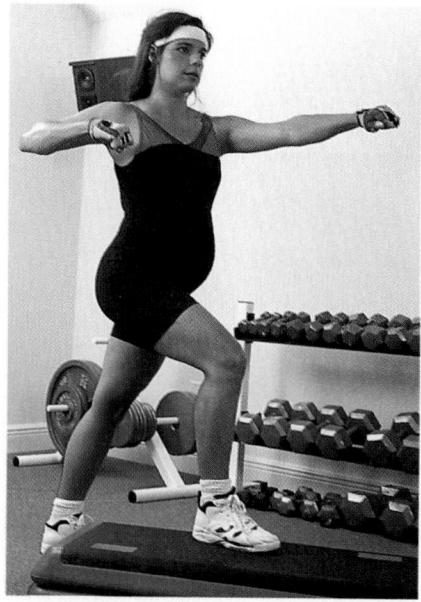
Pregnant women can enjoy the benefits of exercise.

Table 18–2

Exercise Guidelines for Pregnancy

- Exercise regularly (at least three times a week), not intermittently.
- Avoid standing motionless for long periods or lying on the back after the first trimester (the enlarged uterus can obstruct the vena cava and cut off the blood flow to the fetus).
- Lower the intensity of activity or stop exercising when tired or uncomfortable; do not work to exhaustion. Heart rate should not exceed 140 beats per minute.
- Avoid activities that involve the potential for even mild abdominal trauma.
- Eat enough to support the additional needs of both pregnancy and physical activity.
- Drink plenty of fluids before and after exercise; wear appropriate clothing; and avoid physical activity in hot, humid weather.
- After the birth, resume prepregnancy levels of intensity and duration gradually.

preventing excessively high internal body temperature and dehydration, both of which can harm fetal development. To this end, pregnant women should also stay out of saunas, steam rooms, and hot whirlpools.

A healthy pregnancy depends on a sufficient weight gain. Women who begin their pregnancies at a healthy weight need to gain about 30 pounds, which covers the growth and development of the placenta, uterus, blood, breasts, and infant.

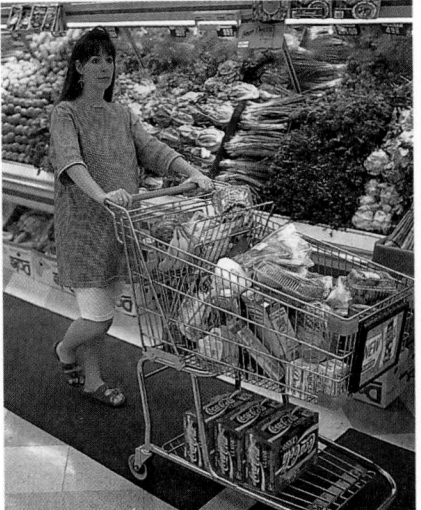

A pregnant woman's nutrition choices support both her health and her infant's growth and development.

Nutrition during Pregnancy

A woman's body changes dramatically during pregnancy. Her blood volume expands; her uterus and its supporting muscles increase in size and strength; her joints become more flexible in preparation for childbirth; her feet swell in response to high concentrations of the hormone estrogen, which promotes water retention and helps to ready the uterus for delivery; and her breasts grow in preparation for lactation. The hormones that mediate all these changes may influence her mood. She can best prepare to handle these changes given a nutritious diet, regular physical activity, plenty of rest, and caring companions. This section highlights the role of nutrition.

ENERGY AND NUTRIENT NEEDS DURING PREGNANCY

From conception to birth, all parts of the infant—bones, muscles, organs, blood cells, skin, and other tissues—are made of nutrients from maternal stores and diet. For most women, nutrients needs during pregnancy and lactation are higher than at any other time (see Figure 18–4).

The RDA table (inside front cover, left) provides separate listings for women during pregnancy and lactation, reflecting their heightened nutritional needs.

Energy Nutrients   A pregnant woman needs extra food energy, but only a little extra—300 kcalories above the allowance for nonpregnant women—and only during the second and third trimesters. A woman can easily get 300 kcalories by taking just one extra serving from each of the five food groups—a slice of bread, a serving of vegetables, an ounce of lean meat, a piece of fruit, and a cup of nonfat milk (see Table 18–3 and the sample menu on p. 593). Pregnant teenagers, underweight women, and exceptionally active women may require more.

Energy RDA during pregnancy (2nd and 3rd trimesters):
    +300 kcal/day.
Canadian RNI during pregnancy:
    +100 to 300 kcal/day.*

For women of average size and moderate physical activity, 300 kcalories represent only 15 percent more food energy than before pregnancy. Nutrient needs expand more than this, however, so nutrient-dense foods should supply the 300 kcalories: foods such as nonfat milk; lean meats, fish, and poultry; eggs; legumes; dark green vegetables; citrus fruits; and whole-grain breads and cereals. Ample carbohydrate is needed to spare the protein for growth.

Protein   The RDA for pregnancy is 10 grams per day higher than for non-pregnant women. Because people in the United States typically exceed the

Protein RDA during pregnancy:
    +10 g/day.
Canadian RNI during pregnancy:
    +5 to 24/g day.†

---

*For all Canadian RNI values during pregnancy, the lower value indicates recommendations for the first trimester, and the higher value indicates those for the second and third trimesters.

†For the first trimester, the RNI is an additional 5 grams/day; for the second trimester, it is an additional 20 grams/day; and for the third trimester, it is 24 grams/day.

Figure 18–4

Comparison of Nutrient RDA of Nonpregnant, Pregnant, and Lactating Women

For actual values, turn to the table on the inside front cover, left.

ªReflect DRI values.

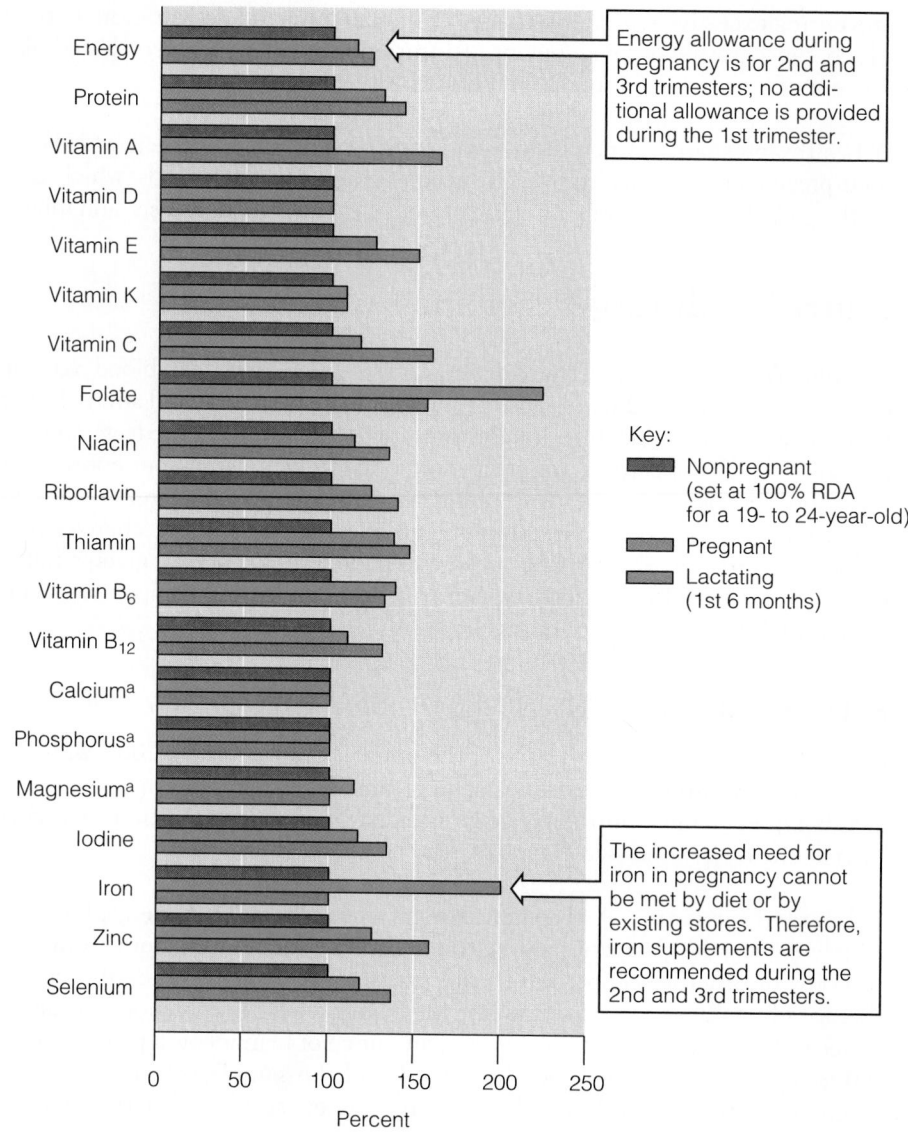

Energy allowance during pregnancy is for 2nd and 3rd trimesters; no additional allowance is provided during the 1st trimester.

Key:
- Nonpregnant (set at 100% RDA for a 19- to 24-year-old)
- Pregnant
- Lactating (1st 6 months)

The increased need for iron in pregnancy cannot be met by diet or by existing stores. Therefore, iron supplements are recommended during the 2nd and 3rd trimesters.

Thiamin RDA during pregnancy:
  1.5 mg/day.
Canadian RNI during pregnancy:
  +0.1 mg/day.

Riboflavin RDA during pregnancy:
  1.6 mg/day.
Canadian RNI during pregnancy:
  +0.1 to 0.3 mg/day

Niacin RDA during pregnancy:
  17 mg NE/day.
Canadian RNI during pregnancy:
  +1 to 2 NE/day.

RDA, most women need not add the full 10 grams to their diets. In fact, pregnant women in the United States—even those with low incomes who are not participating in food assistance programs—generally receive between 75 and 110 grams of protein a day.[7] Pregnant vegetarian women who meet their energy needs by eating ample servings of protein-containing plant foods such as legumes, whole grains, nuts, and seeds meet their protein needs as well. Use of high-protein supplements during pregnancy can be harmful and is discouraged.

B Vitamins Associated with Energy Intake   Extra B vitamins are needed in proportion to the increase in energy requirements. The Committee on Dietary Allowances recommends a slight increase above the nonpregnant woman's RDA for thiamin, riboflavin, and niacin. The usual intake of these nutrients is adequate for most pregnant women in the United States.

Table 18–3

Daily Food Choices for Pregnant and Lactating Women

Food Group	Number of Servings	
	ADULT	PREGNANT OR LACTATING WOMEN
Breads/cereals	6 to 11	7 to 11
Vegetables	3 to 5	4 to 5
Fruits	2 to 4	3 to 4
Meat/meat alternatives	2 to 3	3
Milk/milk products	2	3 to 4

Note: Figure 2–1 in Chapter 2 provides a detailed summary of the Daily Food Guide.

Vitamin B_6 Associated with Protein Intake   Vitamin B_6 recommendations rise in parallel with protein recommendations. The RDA provides enough additional vitamin B_6 to cover the protein recommendation.

Folate and Vitamin B_{12} for Blood Production and Cell Growth   New cells are laid down at a tremendous pace as the fetus grows and develops. At the same time, the mother's red blood cell mass expands, so the RDA for folate more than doubles during pregnancy. It is possible to obtain sufficient folate, without supplements, from a diet that includes fruits, juices, green vegetables, and whole-grain or fortified cereals. When dietary folate is inadequate, daily supplementation is recommended.

Vitamin B_6 RDA during pregnancy: 2.2 mg/day.
Canadian RNI during pregnancy: 0.015 mg/g dietary protein.

Folate RDA during pregnancy: 400 µg/day.
Canadian RNI during pregnancy: +200 µg/day.

Menu

Breakfast
2 medium bran muffins
2 tsp butter/margarine
1 c vanilla yogurt
½ c fresh strawberries
1 c orange juice
Midmorning snack
1 medium apple

Lunch
Sandwich (2 oz ham,
   1 oz swiss cheese, 2
   slices rye bread, 2 tsp
   mayonnaise, lettuce)
1 ¼ c salad (lettuce,
   tomatoes, carrots)
1 tbs salad dressing
1 c low-fat milk
Afternoon snack
1 c low-fat milk
3 oatmeal cookies

Dinner
Chicken cacciatore
   4 oz chicken
   ¾ c stewed tomatoes
1 c rice
¾ c summer squash
1 ½ c salad (spinach,
   mushrooms, onions)
1 tbs salad dressing
2 slices Italian bread
2 tsp butter/margarine
1 c low-fat milk

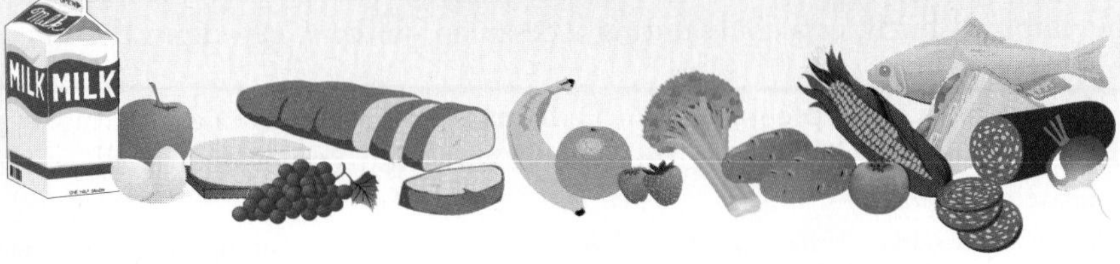

Sample Menu for Pregnant and Lactating Women

This sample meal plan follows the Daily Food Guide for pregnant and lactating women and provides about 2500 kcalories (50 percent from carbohydrate, 20 percent from protein, and 30 percent from fat).

Vitamin B$_{12}$ RDA during pregnancy:
    2.2 μg/day.
Canadian RNI during pregnancy:
    +0.2 μg/day.

Reminder: *Osteomalacia* is the vitamin D–deficiency disease characterized by softening of the bones.

Vitamin D DRI during pregnancy:
    5 μg/day.

Calcium DRI during pregnancy:
    1300 mg/day (14 to 18 yr).
    1000 mg/day (19 to 50 yr).

Iron RDA during pregnancy:
    30 mg/day.
Canadian RNI during pregnancy:
    +0 to 10 mg/day.

The pregnant woman also has a slightly greater need for the B vitamin that activates folate—vitamin B$_{12}$. Generally, even modest amounts of meat, fish, eggs, or milk products together with body stores easily meet the need for vitamin B$_{12}$. Strict vegetarians who exclude all foods of animal origin, however, may need daily supplements to prevent deficiency.

Vitamin D and Calcium for Bone Development   Vitamin D and the bone-building minerals calcium, phosphorus, and magnesium are in great demand during pregnancy. Insufficient intakes may produce abnormal fetal bones and teeth.

Vitamin D plays a vital role in calcium absorption and utilization. Consequently, maternal vitamin D deficiency is associated with underdeveloped tooth enamel in the fetus and osteomalacia in the mother. Exposure to sunlight and vitamin D–fortified milk is usually sufficient to provide the recommended amount of vitamin D during pregnancy. Routine supplementation is not recommended because of the toxicity risk. Vegetarians who avoid milk, eggs, and fish may receive enough vitamin D from daily exposure to sunlight or from fortified soy milk.

Calcium absorption more than doubles early in pregnancy, and the mother's bones store the mineral. Whether calcium added to the mother's bones early in pregnancy is withdrawn to provide sufficient calcium to the fetus later in gestation is unclear.[8] During the last trimester, as the fetal bones begin to calcify, a dramatic shift of calcium across the placenta occurs. In the final weeks of pregnancy, over 300 milligrams are transferred to the fetus every day. An adequate calcium intake during pregnancy helps conserve maternal bone while meeting fetal needs.

Most pregnant women drink more milk than other women, but still their calcium intakes typically fall below recommendations. Because a woman under 25 may still be actively depositing minerals in her own bones, adequate calcium is especially important for young women. Pregnant women under age 25 who receive less than 600 milligrams of dietary calcium daily need to increase their consumption of milk, cheese, yogurt, and other calcium-rich foods. Alternatively, and less preferably, they may need a daily supplement of 600 milligrams of calcium.

 HEALTHY PEOPLE 2000: Increase calcium intake so at least 50% of pregnant and lactating women consume three or more servings daily of foods rich in calcium.

Iron   The body makes several adaptations to help meet iron needs during pregnancy. Menstruation, the major route of iron loss in women, ceases, and iron absorption nearly triples due to a rise in blood transferrin, the body's iron-absorbing and iron-carrying protein. Still, iron stores dwindle during pregnancy.

A pregnant woman needs iron to support her enlarged blood volume and to provide for placental and fetal needs. The developing fetus draws on maternal iron stores to create stores of its own to last through the first four to six months after birth when iron-poor milk will be its sole food. Also, the blood losses inevitable at birth, especially during a cesarean delivery, can drain the mother's supply.*

Few women enter pregnancy with adequate iron stores, so a daily iron supplement is recommended during the second and third trimesters for all pregnant

---

*The average blood loss during a cesarean delivery is almost twice that occurring during the average vaginal delivery of a single fetus.

women.[9] To enhance absorption, the supplement should be taken between meals or at bedtime on an empty stomach and with liquids other than milk, coffee, or tea, which inhibit iron absorption.[10] Vitamin C does not enhance iron absorption from supplements as it does from foods; supplemental iron is already in the ferrous form.

Zinc   Zinc is required for DNA and RNA synthesis and thus for protein synthesis and cell development. Low blood zinc is a significant predictor of low birthweight.[11] Typical zinc intakes are lower than recommendations, but routine supplementation is not advised.[12] Large doses of iron interfere with the body's absorption and use of zinc, so women taking iron supplements (more than 30 milligrams per day) may need zinc supplementation.

Nutrient Supplements   A balanced diet can meet most of a pregnant woman's nutrient needs, except for iron. As mentioned, iron supplements (30 milligrams per day) are recommended during the second and third trimesters of pregnancy. Daily multivitamin-mineral supplements are recommended for women who do not eat adequately and for those in high-risk groups: women carrying multiple fetuses, cigarette smokers, and alcohol and drug abusers. Table 18–4 lists recommended amounts for supplements.

The nutrients mentioned earlier are those most intensely involved in blood production, cell growth, and bone growth. Of course, other nutrients are also needed during pregnancy. Without adequate nutrient and energy intakes, the growth and health of both fetus and mother may be compromised. Even with adequate nutrition, repeated pregnancies less than a year apart deplete nutrient reserves: fetal growth may be protected, but maternal health may decline.[13]

COMMON NUTRITION-RELATED CONCERNS OF PREGNANCY

Nausea, constipation, heartburn, and food sensitivities are common nutrition-related concerns during pregnancy. A few simple strategies can help avert them.

Nausea   Many women have uneasy stomachs in the early months of pregnancy. The nausea of "morning" (actually, anytime) sickness ranges from mild queasiness to debilitating nausea and vomiting. Severe and continued vomiting, known as hyperemesis, may require hospitalization if it results in acidosis, dehydration, or excessive weight loss. The hormonal changes of early pregnancy seem to be responsible for a woman's sensitivities to a food's appearance, texture, or smell. Traditional strategies for quelling nausea are listed in the margin, but some women benefit most from simply eating the foods they want when they feel like eating.[14]

Constipation and Hemorrhoids   As the hormones of pregnancy alter muscle tone and the growing infant crowds intestinal organs, an expectant mother may experience constipation. She may also develop hemorrhoids (swollen veins of the anus and rectum). These can be painful, and straining during bowel movements makes them worse. The strategies listed in the margin may provide relief.

Heartburn   Heartburn is another common complaint during pregnancy. As the growing fetus puts increasing pressure on a woman's stomach, acid may back

---

Zinc RDA during pregnancy: 15 mg/day.
Canadian RNI during pregnancy: +6 mg/day.

Table 18–4

Nutrient Supplements during Pregnancy[a]

Nutrient	Amount
Folate	300 µg
Vitamin B$_6$	2 mg
Vitamin C	50 mg
Vitamin D	5 µg
Calcium	250 mg
Copper	2 mg
Iron	30 mg
Zinc	15 mg

[a]For pregnant women at nutritional risk (see Table 18–5).

Source: Reprinted with permission from *Nutrition during Pregnancy* © by the National Academy of Sciences. Published by the National Academy Press, Washington, D.C., 1990.

To alleviate the nausea of pregnancy:
- On waking, arise slowly.
- Eat dry toast or crackers.
- Chew gum or suck hard candies.
- Eat small, frequent meals.
- Avoid foods with offensive odors.
- When nauseated, do not drink citrus juice, water, milk, coffee, or tea.

To prevent or alleviate constipation:
- Eat foods high in fiber.
- Exercise daily.
- Drink at least 8 glasses of liquids a day.
- Respond promptly to the urge to defecate.
- Use laxatives only as prescribed by a physician; do not use mineral oil because it impairs fat-soluble vitamin absorption.

To prevent or relieve heartburn:
- Eat small, frequent meals.
- Drink liquids between meals.
- Avoid spicy or greasy foods.
- Sit up while eating.
- Wait an hour after eating before lying down.
- Wait 2 hours after eating before exercising.

If this small infant is a female, she may develop poorly and in turn will have an elevated risk of having a poor pregnancy outcome. Thus a woman's malnutrition during or even before her pregnancy can adversely affect not only her children but her *grandchildren*.

Malnutrition and Fetal Development   Without adequate nutrition during pregnancy, fetal growth and infant health are compromised. In general, consequences of malnutrition during pregnancy include:

- Fetal growth retardation.
- Congenital malformations (birth defects).
- Spontaneous abortion and stillbirth.
- Premature birth.
- Low infant birthweight.

Of these, birthweight is most frequently used as a predictor of an infant's survival and health. Malnutrition coupled with low birthweight contributes to more than half of all deaths of children under five worldwide.

THE INFANT'S BIRTHWEIGHT

low birthweight (LBW): a birthweight of 5½ lb (2500 g) or less; indicates probable poor health in the newborn and poor nutrition status in the mother during pregnancy, before pregnancy, or both. Normal birthweight for a full-term baby is 6½ to 8¾ lb (about 3000 to 4000 g).

Some preterm infants are of a weight appropriate for gestational age (AGA); others are small for gestational age (SGA), often reflecting malnutrition. The latter type are also called small-for-date babies.

The most common outcome of a high-risk pregnancy is low birthweight. Low-birthweight infants, defined as infants who weigh 5½ pounds or less, are classified according to gestational age. Preterm, or premature, infants are born before they are fully developed; they are often underweight and have trouble breathing because their lungs are immature. Preterm infants may be small, but if their size and weight are appropriate for their age, they can catch up in growth given adequate nutrition support. In contrast, small-for-gestational-age infants have suffered growth failure in the uterus and do not catch up as well. For the most part, survival improves with increased gestational age and birthweight.[16]

Low-birthweight infants are more likely to experience complications during delivery than normal-weight babies. They also have a statistically greater chance of having physical and mental birth defects, contracting diseases, and dying early in life. Of infants who die before their first birthdays, about two-thirds are low-birthweight babies.

A strong relationship has been established between socioeconomic disadvantage and low birthweight. Low socioeconomic status impairs fetal development by causing stress and by limiting access to medical care and to nutritious foods. Low socioeconomic status often accompanies teen pregnancies, smoking, and alcohol and drug abuse—all predicators of low birthweight.

THE MOTHER'S HEALTH STATUS

Normal weight gain and adequate nutrition support the health of the mother and growth of the infant. Conversely, maternal diseases detract from growth and health. If discovered early, many diseases can be controlled—another reason early prenatal care is recommended.

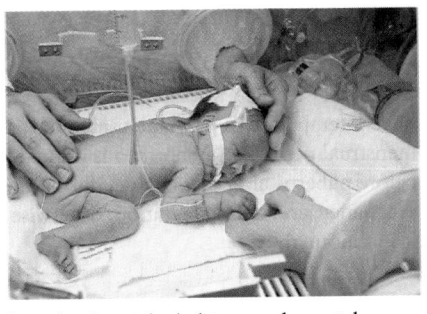
Low-birthweight babies need special care and nourishment.

Preexisting Diabetes   The extent to which diabetes presents risks depends on how well it is controlled before and during pregnancy. Without proper management, women with diabetes face an exceptionally high infertility rate, and those who do conceive may experience episodes of severe hypoglycemia or hyperglycemia, spontaneous abortions, and pregnancy-related hypertension. Ideally, a woman with diabetes will have it under control before becoming pregnant and will be able to maintain glucose control throughout pregnancy.

Gestational Diabetes   Placental hormones elevate blood insulin and alter insulin resistance during pregnancy. In some women, this can precipitate a condition known as gestational diabetes. Gestational diabetes usually develops during the second half of pregnancy, with subsequent return to normal glucose tolerance after childbirth. In about one-third of such cases, however, women develop diabetes (NIDDM) within five years. To ensure that the problems of gestational diabetes are dealt with promptly, health care professionals look for the risk factors listed in the margin.[17] Gestational diabetes requires dietary management just as other forms of diabetes do. Diet alone may control gestational diabetes, but insulin therapy may be required if blood glucose fails to normalize.

gestational diabetes: the appearance of abnormal glucose tolerance during pregnancy, with subsequent return to normal postpartum.

Risk factors for gestational diabetes:
- Previous gestational diabetes.
- History of large infants (9 lb or more).
- Age 30 or older.
- Obesity or excessive weight gain.
- Complications in previous pregnancies.
- Symptoms of diabetes.
- Family history of diabetes.

Preexisting Hypertension   Hypertension complicates pregnancy. In addition to the threats hypertension always carries (such as heart attack and stroke), high blood pressure raises the risks of having a low-birthweight baby or of having the placenta detach from the wall of the uterus before the birth, resulting in stillbirth. Ideally, before a woman with hypertension becomes pregnant, her blood pressure will be normalized by diet, weight loss, and possibly medication.

Transient Hypertension of Pregnancy   Some women first develop hypertension during the second half of pregnancy.* Most often, the rise in blood pressure is mild and does not affect the pregnancy adversely.[18] Blood pressure usually returns to normal during the first few weeks after childbirth. This transient hypertension of pregnancy differs from the pregnancy-induced hypertension that accompanies preeclampsia.†

pregnancy-induced hypertension (PIH): high blood pressure that develops in the second half of pregnancy.

Preeclampsia   Hypertension may signal the onset of preeclampsia, a condition characterized not only by high blood pressure but by protein in the urine and fluid retention (edema). Preeclampsia usually occurs with first pregnancies after 20 weeks gestation, most often near term. Symptoms typically regress within two days of delivery. The edema of preeclampsia is a whole-body edema, distinct from the localized fluid retention women normally experience late in pregnancy. Preeclampsia affects almost all of the mother's organs—the circulatory system, liver, kidneys, and brain.

Blood flow through the vessels that supply oxygen and nutrients to the placenta diminishes. For this reason, preeclampsia often retards fetal growth. In some cases, the placenta separates from the uterus, resulting in stillbirth.

preeclampsia: a condition characterized by hypertension, fluid retention, and protein in the urine.

The normal edema of pregnancy responds to gravity; fluid pools in the ankles. The edema of preeclampsia is a generalized edema. The differences between these two types of edema help with the diagnosis of preeclampsia.

---

*Blood pressure of 140/90 millimeters mercury during the second half of pregnancy in a woman who has not previously exhibited hypertension indicates high blood pressure. So does a rise in systolic blood pressure of 30 millimeters or in diastolic blood pressure of 15 millimeters on at least two occasions more than six hours apart. By this rule, an apparently "normal" blood pressure of 120/85 would be high for a woman whose normal value was 90/70.

†The Working Group on High Blood Pressure in Pregnancy, convened by the National High Blood Pressure Education Program of the National Heart, Lung, and Blood Institute, has suggested abandoning the term "pregnancy-induced hypertension" because it fails to differentiate between the mild, transient hypertension of pregnancy and the life-threatening hypertension of preeclampsia.

eclampsia: a condition characterized by convulsions and coma that develops in some women with untreated preeclampsia.

Warning signs of preeclampsia:
• Hypertension.
• Protein in the urine.
• Upper abdominal pain.
• Severe and constant headaches.
• Swelling, especially of the face.
• Dizziness.
• Blurred vision.
• Sudden weight gain (1 lb/day).

Preeclampsia can progress rapidly to eclampsia—a condition characterized by convulsions and coma. Maternal mortality during pregnancy and childbirth is extremely rare in developed countries, but eclampsia is a common cause.

Preeclampsia demands prompt medical attention. Treatment focuses on regulating blood pressure and preventing convulsions. If preeclampsia develops early and is severe, induced labor or cesarean birth may be necessary. The infant will be preterm, with all of the associated problems, including poor lung development, and will need special care.

Several approaches have been proposed to prevent preeclampsia, including salt restriction, calcium supplementation, and low-dose aspirin therapy. Salt restriction does not improve the incidence or severity of preeclampsia and is not a part of treatment until and unless the kidneys prove unable to handle sodium.

Several studies have reported an inverse relationship between calcium intake and preeclampsia.[19] Furthermore, research has determined that calcium supplementation during pregnancy can lower high blood pressure.[20] In a group of over 1000 pregnant women given either a calcium supplement or a placebo during the second half of pregnancy, the women who received calcium supplements (2000 milligrams per day) had a reduced risk of hypertensive disorders.[21] Such findings are promising, but at this time evidence is insufficient to recommend routine supplementation; furthermore, calcium supplementation may create risks of its own, including the development of kidney stones.[22]

Another promising option is the use of low doses of aspirin (60 to 100 milligrams a day). Low-dose aspirin appears to reduce the incidence of preeclampsia, and some clinicians recommend its use in high-risk pregnancies (women with a history of preeclampsia, fetal death, or placental insufficiency).[23]

PREGNANCY IN ADOLESCENCE

Most adolescents become sexually active before age 19, and one million adolescent girls face pregnancies each year in the United States. About half of them continue their pregnancies. Put another way, about one out of every five babies is born to a teenager, and more than a tenth of these mothers are age 15 or younger. Clearly, teenage pregnancy is a major public health problem. Even when not pregnant, a teenage girl has difficulty meeting her nutrient needs. Nourishing a growing fetus adds to her burden. The competition between maternal and fetal needs places both mother and infant at risk. Simply being young increases these risks independently of important socioeconomic factors.[24]

To support the needs of both mother and fetus, young teenagers (13 to 16 years old) are encouraged to strive for the highest weight gains recommended for pregnancy. For a teen who enters pregnancy at a healthy body weight, a weight gain of approximately 35 pounds is recommended; this minimizes the risk of delivering a low-birthweight infant.[25] Gaining less may limit fetal growth.[26] Pregnant and lactating teenagers can use the Daily Food Guide presented in Table 18–3 (on p. 593), making sure to select at least 4 servings of milk or milk products daily.

Pregnant adolescents have unique economic, psychosocial, and physical vulnerabilities that jeopardize a healthy pregnancy.[27] To improve their chances for a successful pregnancy and healthy infant, they must seek prenatal care. WIC helps pregnant teenagers obtain adequate food to support a reasonable weight gain.

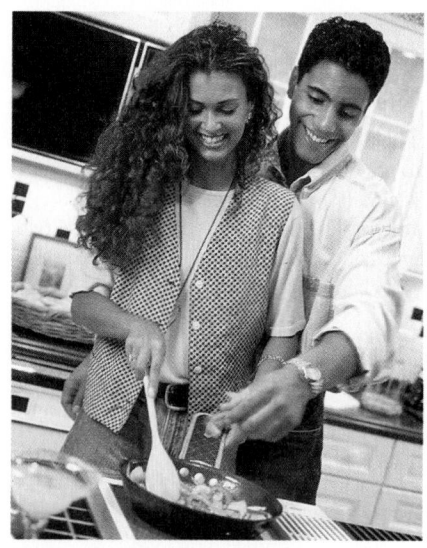

Young adults can prepare themselves for a healthy pregnancy by taking care of themselves today.

PREGNANCY IN OLDER WOMEN

In the last three decades, as many women have pursued their education and careers, they have delayed childbearing. As a result, the number of first births to women 35 and older has increased dramatically.

Each year, 994 out of 1000 pregnant women over the age of 35 have healthy pregnancies.[28] Most of the complications associated with later childbearing reflect chronic conditions such as hypertension and diabetes. These complications often result in a cesarean delivery, which is twice as common in women over 35 as among younger women. For all these reasons, maternal mortality rates are higher in women over 35 than in younger women.

The babies of older mothers face problems of their own. Because 1 out of 50 pregnancies in older women produces an infant with genetic abnormalities, obstetricians routinely screen women older than 35. Birth defects, preterm births, growth retardation, and death are common among infants born to women over 35. For a 40-year-old mother, the risk of having a child with Down syndrome, for example, is about 1 in 100 compared with 1 in 300 for a 35-year-old and 1 in 10,000 for a 20-year-old. Fetal mortality is twice as high for women 35 years and older than for younger women.[29] Why this is so remains a bit of a mystery. One possibility is that the uterine blood vessels of older women cannot fully adapt to the increased demands of pregnancy.

Down syndrome: a genetic abnormality that causes mental retardation, short stature, and flattened facial features.

FETAL ALCOHOL SYNDROME

Drinking alcohol during pregnancy endangers the fetus. Alcohol crosses the placenta freely and deprives the developing fetal brain of both nutrients and oxygen. The result may be fetal alcohol syndrome (FAS), a cluster of symptoms that includes:[30]

See Highlight 7 for additional alcohol-related information.

fetal alcohol syndrome (FAS): the cluster of symptoms seen in an infant or child whose mother consumed excess alcohol during pregnancy, including retarded growth, impaired development of the central nervous system, and facial malformations.

- Prenatal and postnatal growth retardation.
- Impairment of the brain and nerves, with consequent mental retardation, poor coordination, and hyperactivity.
- Abnormalities of the face and skull (see Figure 18–5).
- Increased frequency of major birth defects: cleft palate, heart defects, and defects in ears, genitals, and urinary system.

Tragically, the damage evident at birth persists: children with FAS never fully recover.[31]

Of every 10,000 children born in the United States some 6 or 7 suffer health problems because their mothers drank alcohol during pregnancy—a sixfold increase over the past 15 years.[32] In addition, many infants are born with the less serious, yet still significant, damage some clinicians describe as fetal alcohol effects (FAE).[33] Some children with FAE have no outward signs; others may be short or have only minor facial abnormalities. Often children with FAE go undiagnosed even when problems develop in the early school years: learning disabilities, behavioral abnormalities, motor impairments, and more.

fetal alcohol effects (FAE): a subclinical version of FAS, with hidden defects including learning disabilities, behavioral abnormalities, and motor impairments; also called **alcohol-related birth defects (ARBD).**

The surgeon general states that pregnant women should drink absolutely no alcohol. Abstinence from alcohol is the best policy for pregnant women both because alcohol consumption during pregnancy has such severe consequences, and because FAS can only be prevented—it cannot be treated.[34] And because

Figure 18–5

Typical Facial Characteristics of FAS

The severe facial abnormalities shown here are just outward signs of the severe mental impairments within. The internal organs also suffer irreversible damage that, while hidden, may create major problems for a child's health.

Source: Adapted from J. O. Beattie, Alcohol exposure and the fetus, *European Journal of Clinical Nutrition* 46 (1992): S7–S17.

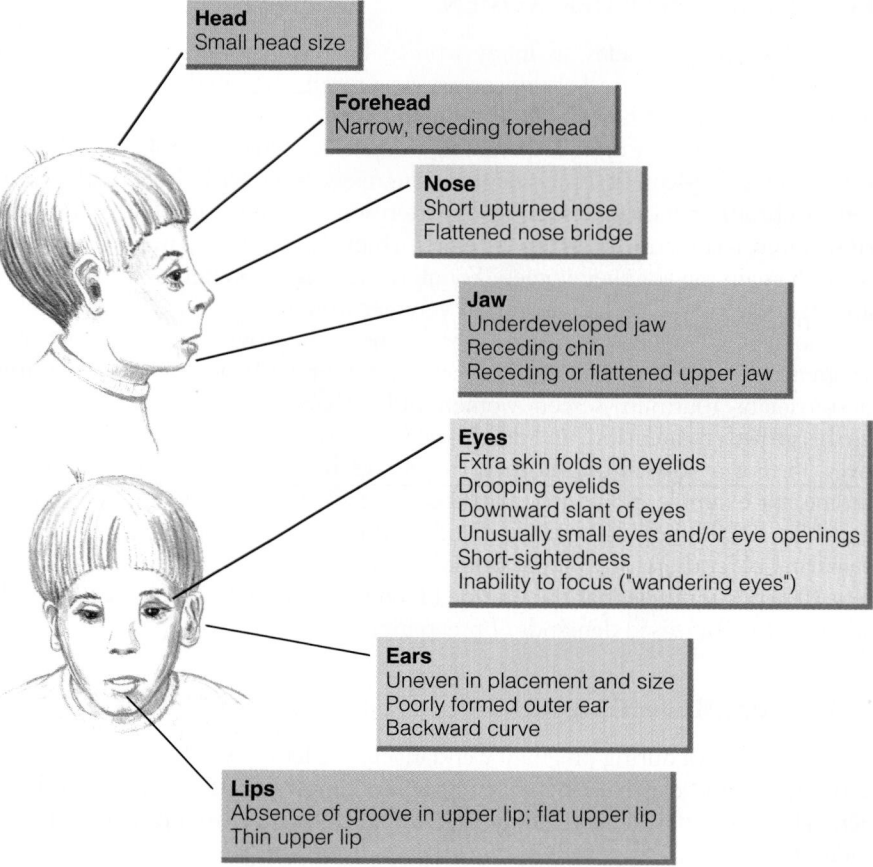

Head
Small head size

Forehead
Narrow, receding forehead

Nose
Short upturned nose
Flattened nose bridge

Jaw
Underdeveloped jaw
Receding chin
Receding or flattened upper jaw

Eyes
Extra skin folds on eyelids
Drooping eyelids
Downward slant of eyes
Unusually small eyes and/or eye openings
Short-sightedness
Inability to focus ("wandering eyes")

Ears
Uneven in placement and size
Poorly formed outer ear
Backward curve

Lips
Absence of groove in upper lip; flat upper lip
Thin upper lip

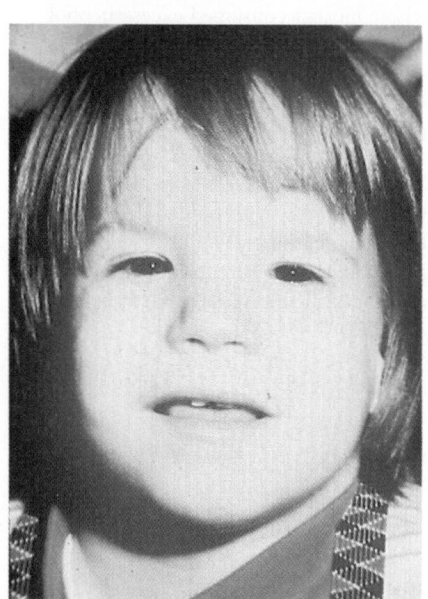

The most obvious symptoms of FAS are the abnormal facial features, but the most tragic ones are the mental disabilities.

the most severe damage occurs around the time of conception—*before a woman may even realize that she is pregnant*—even a woman planning to conceive should abstain.

Drinking during Pregnancy When a woman drinks during pregnancy, she causes damage in two ways: directly, by intoxication, and indirectly, by malnutrition. Prior to the complete formation of the placenta (approximately 12 weeks), alcohol diffuses directly into the tissues of the developing embryo, causing incredible damages. When alcohol crosses the placenta, fetal blood alcohol rises until it reaches an equilibrium with maternal blood alcohol. The mother may not even appear drunk, but the fetus may be poisoned. The fetus's body is small, its detoxification system is immature, and alcohol remains in fetal blood long after it has disappeared from maternal blood. Alcohol interferes with many developmental events, reducing the number of cells produced and damaging those that are produced.

Alcohol also impairs maternal nutrition status. People who abuse alcohol often are malnourished, and as described earlier, maternal malnutrition impedes fetal development. Even if the mother eats well and maintains adequate nutrient stores, alcohol damages the placenta, and so interferes with the transport of nutrients to the fetus, causing fetal malnutrition.

How Much Alcohol Is Too Much?   Alcohol damages the fetus to an extent that correlates directly with the quantity the mother consumes: the number of defects rises with increasing amounts of alcohol. A pregnant woman need not have an alcohol-abuse problem to give birth to a baby with FAS. She need only drink in excess of her liver's capacity to detoxify alcohol. About four drinks a day dramatically worsens the risk of having physical malformations. Even one to two drinks a day threatens to retard growth.

Does this mean that drinking, say, one drink every day or so might be safe? Probably not, for researchers have not yet defined the relationship between alcohol consumption and damage that precisely, nor do they agree on the criteria used to define safety. Although some of alcohol's effects are obvious (such as the physical malformations), others are more subtle (the neurological defects) and often become evident only after several years. Even with those ambiguities resolved, researchers could not specify an amount that would be safe for every woman because individuals respond differently to varying levels of alcohol intake.

In addition to total alcohol intake, drinking patterns play an important role. Most FAS studies report their findings in terms of average intake per day, but people usually drink more heavily on some days than on others. For example, a woman who drinks an *average* of 1 ounce of alcohol (2 drinks) a day may not drink at all during the week but then have 14 drinks on Saturday night, exposing the fetus to highly toxic quantities of alcohol. Whether drinking a certain number of drinks during binges or spreading them out over several days causes more damage depends on the frequency of the binges, the quantity consumed, and the stage of fetal development at the time of each drinking episode.

An occasional drink may be innocuous, but researchers are unable to say how much alcohol is safe to consume during pregnancy. For this reason, health care professionals urge women to stop drinking alcohol as soon as they realize they are pregnant, or better, as soon as they *plan* to become pregnant.[35] Why take any risk? Only the woman who abstains is sure of protecting her infant from FAS.

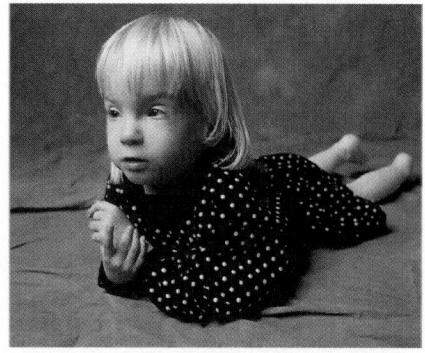

Characteristic facial features may diminish with time, but children with FAS typically continue to be short and underweight for their age.

When Is the Damage Done?   The type of abnormality observed in an FAS infant depends on the developmental events occurring at the times of alcohol exposure. During the first trimester, developing organs such as the brain, heart, and kidneys may be malformed. During the second trimester, the risk of spontaneous abortion increases. During the third trimester, body and brain growth may be retarded.

In experiments on laboratory animals, the effects of alcohol on fetal development are most marked when the female takes alcohol during the earliest period—that of organ formation. Effects also appear when the female takes alcohol just *prior* to conception. Studies on human beings also find that alcohol is most potent in causing birth defects within the first eight weeks of gestation.

Male alcohol ingestion may also affect fertility and fetal development. Animal studies have found smaller litter sizes, lower birthweights, reduced survival rates, and impaired learning ability in the offspring of males consuming alcohol prior to conception.[36] One human study found an association between paternal alcohol intake one month prior to conception and low infant birthweight.[37] (Paternal alcohol intake was defined as an average of two or more drinks daily or at least five drinks on one occasion.) This relationship was independent of either parent's smoking and of the mother's use of alcohol, caffeine, or other drugs.

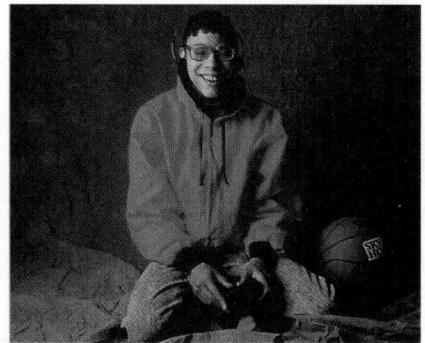

Children born with FAS must live with the long-term consequences of prenatal brain damage.

In view of these findings, it is important to advise women not to drink during pregnancy. Everyone should know of the potential dangers. Heavy drinkers who are sexually active urgently need effective contraception to prevent pregnancy.

All containers of beer, wine, and liquor carry the warning: "Drinking during pregnancy may cause mental retardation and other birth defects. Avoid alcohol during pregnancy." Everyone should hear the message loud and clear: Don't drink alcohol prior to conception or during pregnancy. Once present, FAS has no cure.

OTHER PRACTICES INCOMPATIBLE WITH PREGNANCY

Besides malnutrition and alcohol consumption, which present many hazards to pregnancy, a variety of other lifestyle factors can have adverse impacts; and some may be teratogenic. People who are planning to have children need to know what practices to avoid.

teratogenic (ter-AT-oh-jen-ik): causing abnormal fetal development and birth defects.

> *terato* = monster
> *genic* = to produce

Medicinal Drugs Drugs other than alcohol can also cause complications during pregnancy, problems in labor, and serious birth defects. For these reasons, pregnant women should not take any medicines without consulting their physicians. Drug labels warn: As with any drug, if you are pregnant or nursing a baby, seek the advice of a health professional before using this product. For aspirin and ibuprofen, an additional warning immediately follows: It is especially important not to use aspirin (or ibuprofen) during the last three months of pregnancy unless specifically directed to do so by a doctor because it may cause problems in the unborn child or (excessive bleeding) during delivery.

Illicit Drugs The recommendation to avoid drugs during pregnancy includes illicit drugs, of course. Unfortunately, use of illicit drugs, such as cocaine and marijuana, is common among pregnant women. One study of over 700 pregnant women found that 15 percent of them tested positive for illicit drugs—regardless of race or socioeconomic status.[38]

Drugs of abuse, such as cocaine, pass easily through the placenta and impair fetal development.[39] Furthermore, they are responsible for preterm births, low-birthweight infants, and sudden infant deaths.[40] If these newborns survive, their cries and behaviors at birth are abnormal, and their cognitive development later in life is impaired.[41] They may be hypersensitive or underaroused; those who test positive for drugs suffer the greatest effects of toxicity and withdrawal.[42]

Fetal effects of abused drugs:
- Amphetamines: Suspected nervous system damage; behavioral abnormalities.
- Barbiturates: Drug withdrawal symptoms in the newborn, lasting up to six months.
- Cocaine (including "crack"): Uncontrolled jerking motions; paralysis; permanent mental and physical damage.
- Marijuana: Short-term irritability at birth.
- Opiates (including heroin): Drug withdrawal symptoms in the newborn; permanent learning disability (attention deficit disorder).

Smoking during pregnancy increases the risk of:
- Fetal growth retardation.
- Low birthweight.
- Complications at birth.
- Mislocation of the placenta.
- Premature separation of the placenta.
- Vaginal bleeding.
- Spontaneous abortion.
- Fetal death.
- SIDS.

Smoking and Chewing Tobacco Smoking and chewing tobacco at any time exerts harmful effects, and pregnancy dramatically magnifies the hazards of these practices. Smoking restricts the blood supply to the growing fetus and so limits oxygen and nutrient delivery and waste removal. Also, smokers tend to eat less nutritious foods during their pregnancies than do nonsmokers, which in turn impairs fetal nutrition.[43]

Of all preventable causes of low birthweight in the United States, smoking has the greatest impact. The more a mother smokes, the smaller her baby will be. Furthermore, smoking causes death in otherwise healthy fetuses and newborns. There is a positive relationship between sudden infant death syndrome (SIDS) and both cigarette smoking during pregnancy and postnatal exposure to passive smoke.[44] Smoking during pregnancy may even harm the intellectual and behavioral development of the child later in life.[45] Infants of mothers who chew tobacco also have lower birthweights and higher rates of fetal deaths than infants born to women who do not use tobacco.

The prevalence of smoking in pregnancy is an estimated 20 percent, with higher rates for unmarried women, teenagers, and those who lack education. A woman who smokes and is considering pregnancy or who is already pregnant should try to quit or at least cut back on the number of cigarettes smoked.

Environmental Contaminants Evidence of exposure to environmental contaminants such as lead and mercury has been detected in the amniotic fluid of pregnant women.[46] Infants and young children of these mothers show signs of impaired cognitive development.[47] For this reason, it is particularly important that pregnant women receive foods and beverages grown and prepared in environments free of contamination.

Vitamin-Mineral Megadoses The pregnant woman who is trying to eat well may mistakenly assume that more is better when it comes to vitamin-mineral supplements. This is simply not true; many vitamins are toxic when taken in excess, and the minerals are even more so, some at levels not far above recommendations. A pregnant woman can obtain most of the vitamins and minerals she needs by eating whole foods and should take supplements only on the advice of a registered dietitian or physician.

Caffeine Pregnant women may wonder whether they should give up coffee, tea, and colas because of their caffeine contents. Research studies have not proven that caffeine (even in high doses) causes birth defects in human babies (as it does in animal studies), but limited evidence suggests that moderate-to-heavy use may lower infant birthweight.[48] All things considered, it might be most sensible to limit caffeine consumption to the equivalent of a cup of coffee or two 12-ounce cola beverages a day.

Weight-Loss Dieting Weight-loss dieting, even for short periods, is hazardous during pregnancy. Low-carbohydrate diets or fasts that cause ketosis deprive the fetal brain of needed glucose and may impair its development. Such diets are also likely to lack other nutrients vital to fetal growth. Regardless of prepregnancy weight, pregnant women should never intentionally lose weight.

Sugar Substitutes Artificial sweeteners have been extensively investigated and found to be safe for use during pregnancy.[49] (Women with phenylketonuria should not use aspartame, as Highlight 4 explains.) It would be prudent for pregnant women to use sweeteners in moderation and within an otherwise nutritious and well-balanced diet.

To recap, high-risk pregnancies, especially for teenagers, threaten the life and health of both mother and infant. Proper nutrition and abstinence from smoking, alcohol, and other drugs improve the outcome. In addition, prenatal care includes monitoring pregnant women for gestational diabetes and preeclampsia.

sudden infant death syndrome (SIDS): the unexpected and unexplained death of an apparently well infant; the most common cause of death of infants between the second week and the end of the first year of life; also called *crib death*.

Highlight 13 describes how lead toxicity impairs a child's development.

The caffeine contents of selected beverages, foods, and drugs are listed on p. H–3 of Appendix H.

For infants, breastfeeding:
- Prevents a variety of infections.
- Protects against some chronic diseases, such as NIDDM.
- Makes food allergies less likely.

For mothers, breastfeeding:
- Contracts the uterus.
- Lengthens birth intervals.
- Conserves iron stores (amenorrhea).
- Reduces risk of breast cancer.
- Protects bone density.
- Saves money and offers convenience.

To learn about breastfeeding, a pregnant woman can read at least one of the many books available. Appendix F provides a list of other nutrition resources, including La Leche League International.

Some hospitals employ *certified lactation consultants* who specialize in helping new mothers to establish a healthy breastfeeding relationship with their newborns. These consultants are often registered nurses with specialized training in breast and infant anatomy and physiology.

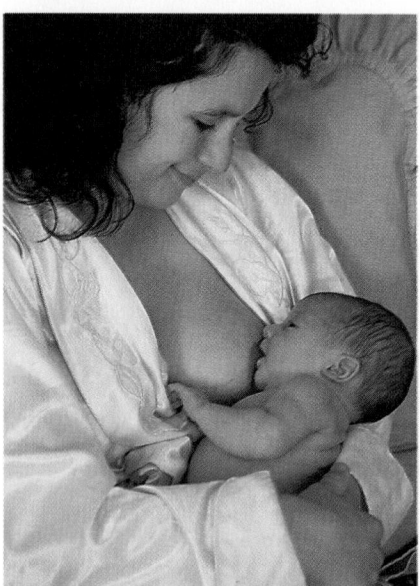

Breastfeeding is a natural extension of pregnancy—of the mother's body nourishing the infant.

Nutrition during Lactation

Before the end of her pregnancy, a woman will need to consider whether to feed her infant breast milk, infant formula, or both. These options are the only recommended foods for an infant during the first four to six months of life.

HEALTHY PEOPLE 2000: Increase to at least 75% the proportion of mothers who breastfeed their babies in the early weeks and to at least 50% the proportion who continue breastfeeding until their babies are five to six months old.

Breastfeeding offers many benefits to both mother and infant, and every pregnant woman should seriously consider it. Still, there are valid reasons for not breastfeeding, and formula-fed infants grow and develop into healthy children. After all, the primary goal is to provide the infant with optimal nourishment in a relaxed and loving environment.

BREASTFEEDING: A LEARNED BEHAVIOR

In many countries around the world, a woman breastfeeds her newborn without considering the alternatives or consciously making a decision. In other parts of the world, a woman feeds her newborn formula simply because she knows so little about breastfeeding. She may have misconceptions or feel uncomfortable about a process she has never seen or experienced.

Although lactation is an automatic physiological process, breastfeeding is a learned behavior that is most successful in a supportive environment. Health care professionals play an important role in providing encouragement and accurate information on breastfeeding. Of women who do breastfeed, 25 to 50 percent stop within the first month, and 50 to 70 percent stop by four months; those who receive early and repeated information and support breastfeed their infants longer than other breastfeeding women.

Fathers also play an important role in encouraging breastfeeding.[50] One study reported that most of those fathers whose partners planned to breastfeed supported that decision and respected breastfeeding women. By comparison, those whose partners planned to bottle feed believed that breastfeeding would make the breasts ugly and interfere with sex. Clearly, educating fathers could change attitudes and promote breastfeeding.

In societies where few women breastfeed, appropriate breastfeeding etiquette remains undefined. A woman faces conflict, confusion, and frustration. Must she retreat to a private place to nurse? What if she cannot find such a place in a public setting? A hungry infant is impatient, and a mother must act quickly. As role models become more numerous, a consensus will develop as to what behaviors are accepted and will provide nursing mothers with more guidance and confidence. Many public buildings now provide "baby rooms" with tables for changing diapers and comfortable chairs for nursing.

Parents in today's society also have to coordinate work and family. All mothers are working women—many of them with jobs outside the home. A social system that provides extended, paid maternity leaves, breaks on the job to nurse infants or pump breasts, and job-site child care promotes breastfeeding as a feasible option.

Most healthy women who want to breastfeed can do so with a little preparation; physical obstacles to breastfeeding are rare. Successful breastfeeding requires adequate nutrition and rest. This, plus the support of all who care, will help to enhance the well-being of mother and infant.

THE MOTHER'S NUTRIENT NEEDS

By continuing to eat nutrient-dense foods throughout lactation, the mother who chooses to breastfeed her infant will be nutritionally prepared to do so. An adequate diet is needed to support the stamina, patience, and self-confidence that nursing an infant demands.

lactation: production and secretion of breast milk for the purpose of nourishing an infant.

Energy Intake and Exercise   A nursing mother produces about 25 ounces of milk a day, with considerable variation from woman to woman and in the same woman from time to time, depending primarily on the infant's demand for milk.[51] To produce milk, a woman needs extra food energy—almost 650 kcalories a day above her regular need during the first six months of lactation. To meet this energy need, the woman is advised to eat an extra 500 kcalories of food each day and let the fat reserves she accumulated during pregnancy provide the rest. Some research suggests that many women need less energy for milk production; other research findings confirm current recommendations.[52] Severe energy restriction, however, hinders milk production.

Energy RDA during lactation:
+500 kcal/day (1800 kcal/day minimum).
Canadian RNI during lactation:
+450 kcal/day.

After the birth of the infant, many women are in a hurry to lose the extra body fat they accumulated during pregnancy. One study reports that the amount of weight lost does not depend on whether a woman breastfeeds her infant.[53] Another study suggests that breastfeeding enhances weight loss initially, especially fat loss from the lower body, but not thereafter.[54] Still another study indicates that weight loss is significant only if breastfeeding continues for at least six months.[55] A woman who breastfeeds her infant will gradually lose weight if she chooses nutrient-dense foods, even though her energy intake may be greater than normal. Most women lose 1 to 2 pounds a month during the first four to six months of lactation; some may lose more, and others may maintain or even gain weight.[56] Regardless of a woman's prepregnancy weight, the more weight she gains during pregnancy, the more weight she loses following delivery (when measured at six weeks and one year).[57]

Women often exercise to reduce body fat and improve fitness, and this is compatible with breastfeeding.[58] Studies have found that lactating women who exercise compensate for their high energy expenditures by increasing their energy intakes.[59] Intense exercise can raise the lactic acid concentration of breast milk, which influences the milk's taste. Infants appear to prefer milk produced prior to exercise (which has a lower lactic acid content).[60] For this reason, mothers may want to breastfeed their infants before exercise or express their milk before exercise for use afterward.

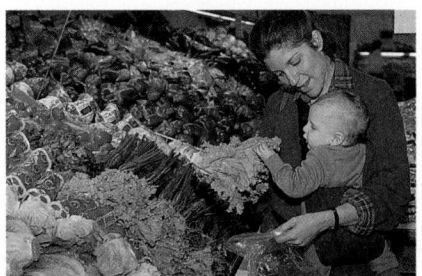

Nutritious foods support successful lactation.

Vitamins and Minerals   In addition to providing energy, the foods consumed by the nursing mother should offer abundant nutrients and plenty of fluid. Review Figure 18–4 (on p. 592) to compare a lactating woman's nutrient needs with those of pregnant and nonpregnant women.

A question often raised is whether a mother's milk may lack a nutrient if she fails to get enough in her diet. The answer differs from one nutrient to the next,

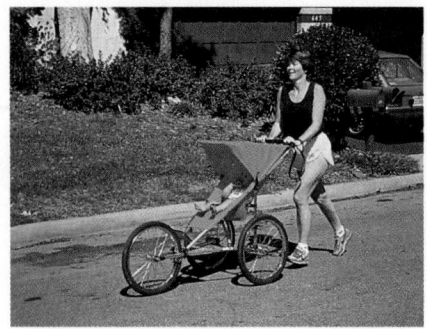

A brisk walk through the neighborhood offers a refreshing opportunity for physical activity and fresh air.

but in general, nutritional inadequacies reduce the *quantity,* not the *quality,* of breast milk. Women can produce milk with adequate protein, carbohydrate, fat, and most minerals, even when their own supplies are limited.[61] For these nutrients and for folate as well, milk quality is maintained at the expense of maternal stores. Nutrients in breast milk are most likely to decline in response to prolonged inadequate intakes of the vitamins—especially vitamins B_6, B_{12}, A, and D.[62]

Water   A lactating woman needs to drink plenty of fluids to protect herself from dehydration. A sensible rule of thumb is to drink a glass of milk, juice, or water at each meal and each time the baby nurses. Despite previous misconceptions, a mother who drinks more fluid does not produce more breast milk.[63]

Supplements   Most lactating women can obtain all the nutrients they need from a well-balanced diet without taking vitamin-mineral supplements; some, however, may need iron supplements. Maternal iron stores dwindle during pregnancy, when the fetus takes iron to meet its own needs during the first four to six months after birth. In addition, childbirth may have incurred blood losses. A woman may therefore need iron supplements during lactation, not to augment the iron in her breast milk, but to refill her depleted iron stores.

Particular Foods   Foods with strong or spicy flavors (such as garlic) may alter the flavor of breast milk.[64] A sudden change in the taste of the milk may annoy some infants. Infants who are sensitive to particular foods such as cow's milk protein may become uncomfortable when the mother's diet includes these foods. Only a few infants exhibit this sensitivity, so only a few nursing mothers need avoid cow's milk. Generally, nutrients from milk products support both the infant's and the mother's health.

In general, a nursing mother can eat whatever nutritious foods she chooses. If she suspects a particular food is causing the infant discomfort, her physician may recommend a dietary challenge: eliminate the food from the diet to see if the infant's reactions subside; then return the food to the diet, and again monitor the infant's reactions. If a food must be eliminated for an extended time, appropriate substitutions must be made to ensure nutrient adequacy.

CONCERNS OF BREASTFEEDING MOTHERS

Some substances impair milk production or enter breast milk and interfere with infant development. Some medical conditions prohibit breastfeeding. This section describes these effects.

Alcohol   Alcohol easily enters breast milk. One study showed that the alcohol concentration of breast milk peaks within one hour after ingestion.[65] In this study, even small amounts of alcohol (equivalent to a can of beer) consumed by lactating women significantly reduced their infants' intakes of breast milk. The researchers suggest three possible reasons, acting separately or together. For one, the alcohol may have altered the flavor of the breast milk and thereby the infants' acceptance of it. For another, because infants metabolize alcohol inefficiently, even low doses may be potent enough to suppress their feeding behavior. Third, the alcohol may have reduced the women's milk production.

In the past, alcohol has been recommended to mothers to facilitate lactation despite a lack of scientific evidence that it does so. The research summarized here suggests that alcohol actually hinders breastfeeding. An occasional glass of wine or beer is considered within safe limits, but in general, lactating women should consume little or no alcohol.

Caffeine Caffeine taken during lactation may make a breastfed infant irritable and wakeful. As during pregnancy, caffeine consumption should be moderate—say, one to two cups of coffee a day. Larger doses of coffee may interfere with the availability of iron from the milk and impair the infant's iron status.

Smoking Cigarette smoking reduces milk volume, so smokers may produce too little milk to meet their infants' energy needs. One study of lactating women found that infants of smoking mothers gained less weight than infants of nonsmoking mothers.[66] Furthermore, infant exposure to passive smoke negates the protective effect breastfeeding offers against SIDS and increases the risks dramatically.[67]

Medical Considerations If a woman has an ordinary cold, she can go on nursing without worry. If susceptible, the infant will catch it from her anyway. (Thanks to immunological protection, a breastfed baby may be less susceptible than a formula-fed baby would be.) If a woman has a communicable disease such as tuberculosis or hepatitis that could threaten the infant's health, then mother and baby have to be separated; mothers can pump their breasts several times a day and feed breast milk by bottle.

For mothers with HIV infections, advice differs depending on the context.[68] Where safe alternatives are available, the Centers for Disease Control and the American Academy of Pediatrics recommend that HIV-positive women not breastfeed their infants. In developing countries, however, the feeding of inappropriate or contaminated formulas is the cause of 1.5 million infant deaths each year, so WHO and UNICEF urge mothers to breastfeed irrespective of HIV infection.

Women with chronic diseases such as diabetes (IDDM) may need careful monitoring and counseling to ensure successful lactation.[69] Women with IDDM need to adjust their energy intakes and insulin doses to meet the heightened needs of lactation. Maintaining good glucose control helps to initiate lactation and support milk production.[70]

Many drugs are compatible with breastfeeding, but some medicines are contraindicated, either because they suppress lactation or because they are secreted into breast milk and can harm the infant.[71] As a precaution, a nursing mother should consult with her physician prior to taking any drug. Illicit drugs, of course, are harmful to the physical and emotional health of both the mother and the nursing infant. Breast milk can deliver such high doses of illicit drugs as to cause irritability, tremors, and hallucinations in infants.

Women who breastfeed experience prolonged postpartum amenorrhea. Absent menstrual periods, however, do not protect a woman from pregnancy. To prevent pregnancy, a couple must use some form of contraception—but not oral contraceptive agents. Standard oral contraceptives contain estrogen, which reduces milk volume and the protein content of breast milk.[72]

postpartum amenorrhea: the normal temporary absence of menstrual periods immediately following childbirth.

Some women fear that breastfeeding will cause their breasts to sag. The breasts do swell and become heavy and large immediately after the birth, but even when they are producing enough milk to nourish a thriving infant, they eventually shrink back to their prepregnant size. Given proper support, diet, and exercise, breasts often return to their former shape and size after weaning. Breasts change their shape as the body ages, but breastfeeding does not accelerate this process.

Environmental Contaminants Environmental contaminants, such as DDT, PCBs, and methylmercury can find their way into breast milk. Inuit mothers living in Arctic Québec who eat seal and beluga whale blubber have concentrations of DDT and PCBs in their breast milk two to ten times greater than those found in breast milk from women in southern Québec.[73] The impact of contaminated breast milk on infant development is unclear, however. Preliminary studies indicate the children of these Inuit mothers are developing normally. Researchers speculate that the abundant omega-3 fatty acids of the Inuit diet may protect against damage to the central nervous system.

In summary, the lactating woman needs extra fluid and enough energy and nutrients to produce about 25 ounces of milk a day. Alcohol, other drugs, smoking, and contaminants may impair milk production or enter breast milk and impair infant development.

This chapter has focused on the nutrition needs of the mother during pregnancy and lactation. The next chapter explores the dietary needs of infants, children, and adolescents.

Study Questions

1. Describe the placenta and its function.
2. Describe the normal events of fetal development. How does malnutrition impair fetal development?
3. Define the term *critical period*. How do adverse influences during critical periods affect later health?
4. Explain why women of childbearing age need folate in their diets. How much is recommended, and how can women ensure that these needs are met?
5. How does nutrition *prior* to conception influence a pregnancy?
6. What is the recommended pattern of weight gain during pregnancy for a woman at a healthy weight? For an underweight woman? For an overweight woman?
7. What does a pregnant woman need to know about exercise?
8. Which nutrients are needed in the greatest amounts during pregnancy? Why are they so important? Describe wise food choices for the pregnant woman.
9. Define low-risk and high-risk pregnancies. What is the significance of infant birthweight in terms of the child's future health?
10. Describe some of the special problems of the pregnant adolescent. Which nutrients are needed in increased amounts?
11. What practices should be avoided during pregnancy? Why?
12. How do nutrient needs during lactation differ from nutrient needs during pregnancy?

Notes

1. Committee on Nutritional Status during Pregnancy and Lactation, *Nutrition during Pregnancy* (Washington, D.C.: National Academy Press, 1990), pp. 412–419.

2. American Academy of Pediatrics, Committee on Genetics, Folic acid for the prevention of neural tube defects, *Pediatrics* 92 (1993): 493–494.

3. Committee on Nutritional Status during Pregnancy and Lactation, 1990, p. 10.

4. Committee on Nutritional Status during Pregnancy and Lactation, 1990, p. 229.

5. K. G. Dewey and M. A. McCrory, Effects of dieting and physical activity on pregnancy and lactation, *American Journal of Clinical Nutrition* (supplement) 59 (1994): 446S–453S.

6. *ACOG Technical Bulletin 189: Exercise during Pregnancy and the Postpartum Period* (Washington, D.C.: The American College of Obstetricians and Gynocologists, 1994).

7. Committee on Nutritional Status during Pregnancy and Lactation, 1990, p. 384.

8. Committee on Dietary Reference Intakes, *Dietary Reference Intakes for Calcium, Phosphorus, Magnesium, Vitamin D, and Fluoride* (Washington, D.C.: National Academy Press, 1997), 4–38.

9. Committee on Nutritional Status during Pregnancy and Lactation, 1990, pp. 272–298.

10. Committee on Nutritional Status during Pregnancy and Lactation, 1990 pp. 285–293.

11. Y. H. Neggers and coauthors, A positive association between maternal serum zinc concentration and birth weight, *American Journal of Clinical Nutrition* 51 (1990): 678–684.

12. Committee on Nutritional Status during Pregnancy and Lactation, 1990, pp. 299–317.

13. K. Merchant, R. Martorell, and J. D. Haas, Consequences for maternal nutrition of reproductive stress across consecutive pregnancies, *American Journal of Clinical Nutrition* 52 (1990): 616–620.

14. M. Erick, Battling morning (noon and night) sickness: New approaches for treating an age-old problem, *Journal of the American Dietetic Association* 94 (1994): 147–148.

15. Transplacental nutrient transfer and intrauterine growth retardation, *Nutrition Reviews* 50 (1992): 56–57.

16. D. L. Phelps and coauthors, 28-day survival rates of 6676 neonates with birth weights of 1250 grams or less, *Pediatrics* 87 (1991): 7–17.

17. *ACOG Guide to Planning for Pregnancy, Birth, and Beyond* (Washington, D.C.: The American College of Obstetricians and Gynecologists, 1990), pp. 128–140.

18. F. G. Cunningham and M. D. Lindheimer, Hypertension in pregnancy, *New England Journal of Medicine* 326 (1992): 927–932.

19. Calcium supplementation prevents hypertensive disorders of pregnancy, *Nutrition Reviews* 50 (1992): 233–236.

20. K. B. Knight and R. E. Keith, Calcium supplementation on normotensive and hypertensive pregnant women, *American Journal of Clinical Nutrition* 55 (1992): 891–895; J. R. Repke and J. Villar, Pregnancy-induced hypertension and low birth weight: The role of calcium, *American Journal of Clinical Nutrition* 54 (1991): 237S–241S.

21. J. M. Belizan and coauthors, Calcium supplementation to prevent hypertensive disorders of pregnancy, *New England Journal of Medicine* 325 (1991): 1399–1405.

22. T. F. Ferris, Pregnancy, preeclampsia, and the endothelial cell, *New England Journal of Medicine* 325 (1991): 1439–1440.

23. F. G. Cummingham and N. F. Gant, Prevention of preeclampsia—A reality? *New England Journal of Medicine* 321 (1989): 606–607.

24. A. M. Fraser, J. E. Brockert, and R. H. Ward, Association of young maternal age with adverse reproductive outcomes, *New England Journal of Medicine* 332 (1995): 1113–1117.

25. M. L. Hediger and coauthors, Rate and amount of weight gain during adolescent pregnancy: Associations with maternal weight-for-height and birth weight, *American Journal of Clinical Nutrition* 52 (1990): 793–799.

26. Committee on Nutritional Status during Pregnancy and Lactation, 1990, pp. 1–23; J. M. Rees and coauthors, Weight gain in adolescents during pregnancy: Rate related to birth-weight outcome, *American Journal of Clinical Nutrition* 56 (1992): 868–873.

27. Position of The American Dietetic Association: Nutrition care for pregnant adolescents, *Journal of the American Dietetic Association* 94 (1994): 449–450.

28. F. G. Cunningham and K. J. Leveno, Childbearing among older women—The message is cautiously optimistic, *New England Journal of Medicine* 333 (1995): 1002–1004.

29. R. C. Fretts and coauthors, Increased maternal age and the risk of fetal death, *New England Journal of Medicine* 333 (1995): 953–957.

30. Committee on Substance Abuse and Committee on Children with Disabilities, American Academy of Pediatrics, Fetal alcohol syndrome and fetal alcohol effects, *Pediatrics* 91 (1993): 1004–1006; J. O. Beattie, Alcohol exposure and the fetus, *European Journal of Clinical Nutrition* 46 (1992): S7–S17.

31. H. L. Spohr, J. Willms, and H. C. Steinhausen, Prenatal alcohol exposure and long-term developmental consequences, *Lancet* 341 (1993): 907–910.

32. Update: Trends in fetal alcohol syndrome—United States, 1979–1993, *Morbidity and Mortality Weekly Report* 44 (1995): 249–251.

33. J. M. Aase, K. L. Jones, and S. K. Clarren, Do we need the term "FAE"? *Pediatrics* 95 (1995): 428–430.

34. Committee on Nutritional Status during Pregnancy and Lactation, *Nutrition during Pregnancy* (Washington, D.C.: National Academy Press, 1990), pp. 390–411.

35. Committee on Substance Abuse and Committee on Children with Disabilities, 1993; *The Surgeon General's Report on Nutrition and Health* (Washington, D.C.: Government Printing Office, 1988), p. 72.

36. When dad drinks: Can his liquor intake impair his future offspring? *Scientific American*, February 1990, p. 23; L. F. Soyka and J. M. Joffe, Male mediated drug effects on offspring, *Progress in Clinical and Biological Research* 36 (1980): 49–66.

37. R. E. Little and C. F. Sing, Father's drinking and infant birth weight: Report of an association, *Teratology* 36 (1987): 59–65.

38. I. J. Chasnoff and coauthors, The prevalence of illicit-drug or alcohol use during pregnancy and discrepancies in mandatory

reporting in Pinellas County, Florida, *New England Journal of Medicine* 322 (1990): 1202–1206.

39. D. B. Petitti and C. Coleman, Cocaine and the risk of low birth weight, *American Journal of Public Health* 80 (1990): 25–28; S. Parker and coauthors, Jitteriness in full-term neonates: Prevalence and correlates, *Pediatrics* 85 (1990): 17–23; M. van de Bor, F. J. Walther, and M. Ebrahimi, Decreased cardiac output in infants of mothers who abused cocaine, *Pediatrics* 85 (1990): 30–32; B. Zuckerman and coauthors, Effects of maternal marijuana and cocaine use on fetal growth, *New England Journal of Medicine* 320 (1989): 762–768.

40. W. T. Weathers and coauthors, Cocaine use in women from a defined population: Prevalence at delivery and effects on growth in infants, *Pediatrics* 91 (1993): 350–354.

41. S. D. Azuma and I. J. Chasnoff, Outcome of children prenatally exposed to cocaine and other drugs: A path analysis of three-year data, *Pediatrics* 92 (1993): 396–402; M. J. Corwin and coauthors, Effects of in utero cocaine exposure on newborn acoustical cry characteristics, *Pediatrics* 89 (1992): 1199–1203; L. N. Eisen and coauthors, Perinatal cocaine effects on neonatal stress behavior and performance on the Brazelton Scale, *Pediatrics* 88 (1991): 477–480; M. Mirochnick and coauthors, Circulating catecholamine concentrations in cocaine-exposed neonates: A pilot study, *Pediatrics* 88 (1991): 481–485.

42. Corwin and coauthors, 1992; L. C. Mayes and coauthors, Neurobehavioral profiles of neonates exposed to cocaine prenatally, *Pediatrics* 91 (1993): 778–783.

43. F. M. Haste and coauthors, Nutrient intakes during pregnancy: Observations on the influence of smoking and social class, *American Journal of Clinical Nutrition* 51 (1990): 29–36.

44. H. S. Klonoff-Cohen and coauthors, The effect of passive smoking and tobacco exposure through breast milk on sudden infant death syndrome, *Journal of the American Medical Association* 273 (1995): 795–798; E. A. Mitchell and coauthors, Smoking and the sudden infant death syndrome, *Pediatrics* 91 (1993): 893–896; K. C. Schoendorf and J. L. Kiely, Relationship of sudden infant death syndrome to maternal smoking during and after pregnancy, *Pediatrics* 90 (1992): 905–908; M. G. Bulterys, S. Greenland, and J. F. Kraus, Chronic fetal hypoxia and sudden infant death syndrome: Interaction between maternal smoking and low hematocrit during pregnancy, *Pediatrics* 86 (1990): 535–540; B. Haglund and S. Cnattingius, Cigarette smoking as a risk factor for sudden infant death syndrome: A population-based study, *American Journal of Public Health* 80 (1990): 29–32.

45. D. L. Olds, C. R. Henderson, Jr., and R. Tatelbaum, Intellectual impairment in children of women who smoke cigarettes during pregnancy, *Pediatrics* 93 (1994): 221–227; D. M. Fergusson, L. J. Horwood, and M. T. Lynskey, Maternal smoking before and after pregnancy: Effects on behavioral outcomes in middle childhood, *Pediatrics* 92 (1993): 815–822.

46. M. Lewis and coauthors, Prenatal exposure to heavy metals: Effect on childhood cognitive skills and health status, *Pediatrics* 89 (1992): 1010–1015.

47. Lewis and coauthors, 1992; M. W. Shannon and J. W. Graef, Lead intoxication in infancy, *Pediatrics* 89 (1992): 87–90.

48. Committee on Nutritional Status during Pregnancy and Lactation, 1990, pp. 397–399.

49. Position of The American Dietetic Association: Use of nutritive and nonnutritive sweeteners, *Journal of the American Dietetic Association* 93 (1993): 816–821.

50. G. L. Freed, J. K. Fraley, and R. J. Schanler, Attitudes of expectant fathers regarding breast-feeding, *Pediatrics* 90 (1992): 224–227.

51. K. G. Dewey and coauthors, Maternal versus infant factors related to breast milk intake and residual milk volume: The DARLING Study, *Pediatrics* 87 (1991): 829–837; Committee on Nutrition Status during Pregnancy and Lactation, *Nutrition during Lactation* (Washington, D.C.: National Academy Press, 1991), pp. 1–19.

52. M. A. Guillermo-Tuazon and coauthors, Energy intake, energy expenditure, and body composition of poor rural Philippine women throughout the first 6 mo of lactation, *American Journal of Clinical Nutrition* 56 (1992): 874–880; C. Frigerio and coauthors, A new procedure to assess the energy requirements of lactation in Gambian women, *American Journal of Clinical Nutrition* 54 (1991): 526–533; J. M. A. van Raaij and coauthors, Energy cost of lactation, and energy balances of well-nourished Dutch lactating women: Reappraisal of the extra energy requirements of lactation, *American Journal of Clinical Nutrition* 53 (1991): 612–619.

53. S. Potter and coauthors, Does infant feeding method influence maternal postpartum weight loss? *Journal of the American Dietetic Association* 91 (1991): 441–446.

54. F. M. Kramer and coauthors, Breast-feeding reduces maternal lower-body fat, *Journal of the American Dietetic Association* 93 (1993): 429–433.

55. K. G. Dewey, M. J. Heinig, and L. A. Nommsen, Maternal weight-loss patterns during prolonged lactation, *American Journal of Clinical Nutrition* 58 (1993): 162–166.

56. Committee on Nutritional Status during Pregnancy and Lactation, 1991, pp. 1–19.

57. Potter and coauthors, 1991.

58. Dewey and McCrory, 1994; K. G. Dewey and coauthors, A randomized study of the effects of aerobic exercise by lactating women on breast-milk volume and composition, *New England Journal of Medicine* 330 (1994): 449–453.

59. Dewey and coauthors, 1994; C. A. Lovelady, B. Lonnerdal, and K. G. Dewey, Lactation performance of exercising women, *American Journal of Clinical Nutrition* 52 (1990): 103–109.

60. J. P. Wallace, G. Inbar, and K. Ernsthausen, Infant acceptance of postexercise breast milk, *Pediatrics* 89 (1992): 1245–1247.

61. Committee on Nutritional Status during Pregnancy and Lactation, 1991, p. 140.

62. Committee on Nutritional Status during Pregnancy and Lactation, 1991, p. 140.

63. L. B. Dusdieker and coauthors, Prolonged maternal fluid supplementation in breast-feeding, *Pediatrics* 86 (1990): 737–740.

64. J. A. Mennella and G. K. Beauchamp, Maternal diet alters the sensory qualities of human milk and the behavior of the nursing infant, *Pediatrics* 88 (1991): 737–747.

65. J. A. Mennella and G. K. Beauchamp, The transfer of alcohol to human milk: Effects on flavor and the infant's behavior, *New England Journal of Medicine* 325 (1991): 981–985.

66. F. Vio, G. Salazar, and C. Infante, Smoking during pregnancy and lactation and its effects on breast-milk volume, *American Journal of Clinical Nutrition* 54 (1991): 1011–1016.

67. Klonoff-Cohen and coauthors, 1995.

68. R. F. Black, Transmission of HIV-1 in the breast-feeding process, *Journal of the American Dietetic Association* 96 (1996): 267–274.

69. A. M. Ferris and E. A. Reece, Nutritional consequences of chronic maternal conditions during pregnancy and lactation: Lupus and diabetes, *American Journal of Clinical Nutrition* (supplement) 59 (1994): 465S–473S; A. M. Ferris and coauthors, Perinatal lactation protocol and outcome in mothers with and without insulin-dependent diabetes mellitus, *American Journal of Clinical Nutrition* 58 (1993): 43–48.

70. C. M. van Beusekom and coauthors, Milk of patients with tightly controlled insulin-dependent diabetes mellitus has normal macronutrient and fatty acid composition, *American Journal of Clinical Nutrition* 57 (1993): 938–943.

71. American Academy of Pediatrics, Committee on Drugs, The transfer of drugs and other chemicals into human milk, *Pediatrics* 93 (1994): 137–150.

72. American Academy of Pediatrics, Committee on Drugs, Transfer of drugs and other chemicals into human milk, *Pediatrics* 84 (1989): 924–936.

73. E. Dewailly and coauthors, Inuit exposure to organochlorines through the aquatic food chain in Arctic Québec, *Environmental Health Perspectives* 101 (1993): 618–620.

Hunger and Global Environmental Problems

*I*n the early 1990s, one person in every ten worldwide was experiencing hunger—not the healthy hunger we all feel, which leads us to sit down and eat a hearty meal, but the chronic, painful hunger people feel when no food is available. Today, hundreds of millions of people are suffering from chronic hunger, both in the developing world and at home in the United States. Many are dying of starvation: tens of thousands each day, one every two seconds.[1] Many are children. Tragic scenes of people starving in drought- and flood-stricken areas are a familiar sight on television. Some of the causes (such as war) are obvious, but the environmental factors that often underlie these situations are less apparent.

This highlight examines hunger in the United States and around the world and discusses how environmental problems contribute to world hunger. Aside from the constant struggle to overcome the devastation wrought by civil unrest and wars, the ultimate solutions to the problem of world hunger involve both large- and small-scale choices made with an awareness of environmental consequences. The objective is to identify sustainable ways of doing things (the glossary below defines sustainable and other terms). Sustainable development permits economic growth without environmental destruction. Sustainable use consumes resources at a rate that nature, forestry, or agriculture can replace. Numerous examples of environmentally conscious choices related to food consumption are presented at the end of this highlight.

HUNGER IN THE UNITED STATES

Much as it should surprise us, even in the United States, hunger is a problem. It is estimated that 30 million Americans, including 12 million children, cannot afford to buy enough food to maintain good health.[2] Soup kitchens are numerous and are needed as badly in some regions of the country as were the bread lines of the Great Depression in the 1930s. The prevalence of malnutrition and other health problems associated with chronic hunger—stunted growth, failure to thrive, low-birthweight babies, infant mortality, and anemia—is declining more slowly than in earlier decades; some problems are growing worse. Some studies show that one of every five children in the United States is chronically hungry; these children live in families that do not know where their next meal is coming from or when it will come.[3] Their hunger stems, not from the lack of available food, but from the lack of money with which to buy it.[4]

Who Are the Hungry in the United States?

Hunger is not always easy to recognize. The accompanying box shows

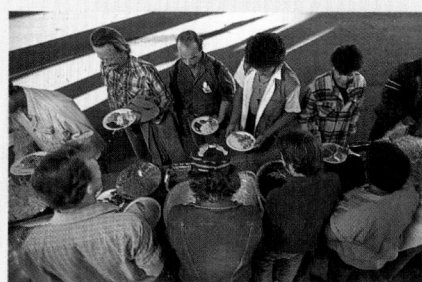

Feeding the hungry—in the United States.

Glossary

cash crops: crops grown for cash, as opposed to crops grown for food; examples include cotton and tobacco.

food insecurity: intermittent hunger caused by lack of money or lack of control over other resources needed to assure a reliable food supply; the predominant form of hunger in the United States today.

Food Stamp Program: a federal food assistance program. The USDA issues food stamp coupons through state social services or welfare agencies to households—people who buy and prepare food together. The number of stamps a household receives depends on the household's size and income. Recipients may use the coupons like cash to purchase food and seeds, but not to buy tobacco, cleaning items, alcohol or other nonfood items.

fossil fuel: coal, oil, and natural gas; these are nonrenewable fuels that pollute. (Renewable or alternative fuels, such as solar and wind energy, pollute less or not at all.)

sustainable: able to continue indefinitely. Here, the term means the use of resources at such a rate that the earth can keep on replacing them—for example, cutting trees no faster than new ones grow and producing pollutants at a rate with which the environment and human cleanup efforts can keep pace, so that no net accumulation of pollution occurs.

How to Identify Food Insecurity in a U.S. Household

Questions like these are asked on surveys to determine the extent of food insecurity in a household. The more questions that receive a "Yes" answer, the more intense the hunger the household is experiencing.

- Do you usually have enough food to eat? If you don't have enough food to eat, is it because:
  a. you sometimes run out of money to buy food?
  b. you do not have transportation?
  c. you do not have working appliances (stove, refrigerator)?

- Do you ever rely on nutritionally inferior foods to feed yourself or your children because you lack any of these resources?

- Do you ever eat less than you feel you should because you lack any of these resources?

- Do you ever skip meals or cut the size of meals because you lack any of these resources?

- Do you ever rely on neighbors, friends, relatives, or schools to feed any of your children because there is not enough food in the house?

- Do your children ever say they are hungry because there is not enough food in the house?

- Do you or any of your children ever go to bed hungry because there is not enough food in the house?

Sources: Adapted from C. A. Wehler, R. I. Scott, and J. J. Anderson, The Community Childhood Hunger Identification Project: A model of domestic hunger—demonstration project in Seattle, Washington, *Journal of Nutrition Education* (1 supplement) 24 (1992): 29S–35S; R. R. Briefel and C. E. Woteki, Development of food sufficiency questions for the Third National Health and Nutrition Examination Survey, *Journal of Nutrition Education* (1 supplement) 24 (1992): 24S–28S.

how national surveys identify "food insecurity" and hunger in the United States. Questions like these provide crude, but necessary, data to estimate the degree of hunger in this country.

Hunger has many causes, but a major one is poverty. Other causes that contribute to hunger are abuse of alcohol and other drugs; physical and mental illness; lack of awareness of available food assistance programs; and the reluctance of people, particularly the elderly, to accept what they perceive as "welfare" or "charity."[5] Still, poverty remains the major cause of hunger, and solving the poverty problem would do a lot to solve the hunger problem.

In the United States, poverty and hunger reach into all segments of society, affecting not only the chronic poor (migrant workers, the unskilled and unemployed, the homeless, and some elderly) but also the so-called new poor. Some are displaced farm families. Some are former blue-collar and white-collar workers forced out of their trades and professions into minimum-wage jobs. These people outnumber the chronic poor, and they are not on welfare; they have jobs, but the pay is low. Families with incomes below a certain level are simply unable to buy sufficient amounts of nourishing foods, even if they are wise food shoppers.

Assistance Programs Aimed at Hunger and Malnutrition

At present, many programs aimed at preventing or remediating domestic malnutrition and hunger are in effect in the United States. To what extent these federal programs will continue to feed those who are hungry is unknown, given the current political climate; many federal programs are being targeted in cost saving measures.

Several food assistance programs are described in other chapters: the school lunch, breakfast, and child care food programs for children; the WIC program for low-income pregnant women, mothers, and their young children; and food assistance

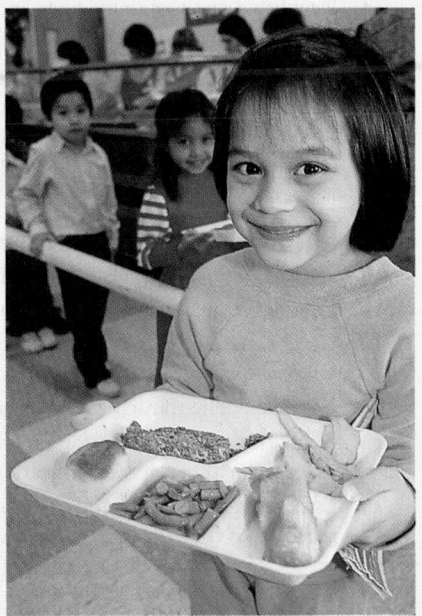

School lunches provide children with nourishment at little or no charge.

ENVIRONMENTAL DEGRADATION AND HUNGER

Today, environmental degradation is beginning to threaten the world's ability to produce enough food to feed its people. Not only are we losing our resources, but we are losing our ability to compensate for the losses.

Environmental Problems and Food Production

One element of environmental degradation is soil erosion, which is occurring in every nation and is resulting in crop losses estimated at 6 percent per year.[17] Other environmental problems slowing food outputs are deforestation, air pollution, climate change, water scarcity, deterioration of rangelands, and declining fisheries.

Deforestation   Deforestation along the watersheds of the Blue Nile led to erosion and during just nine years laid down so much silt behind the Roseires Reservoir dam in Sudan, which supplies irrigation water for the dry season, that one-third of its capacity was lost.[18] In Sierra Leone, where 60 percent of the land was primarily rainforest in 1961, only 6 percent is now.[19] For the world as a whole, if present rates continue, by 2010 per capita forested area will have dropped 30 percent.[20]

Air Pollution   Damage to crops from air pollution is now measurable in the car-centered societies of Western Europe, the United States, and Canada and in societies that burn coal to generate electricity—notably, Eastern Europe and China. In the United States, according to a seven-year study by two government

agencies, the most damaging air pollutants are ozone, sulfur dioxide, and nitrous oxide, which come from the burning of fossil fuels. Crops are especially sensitive to ground-level ozone concentrations, which increasingly are detected and measured in rural as well as urban areas in ranges that reduce crop yields. An estimate puts the increase in annual crop losses ascribable to ozone pollution at 1 percent per year.

Not only is ground-level ozone pollution reducing agricultural outputs, but outer-atmosphere ozone depletion is doing so, too—especially to radiation-sensitive crops such as soybeans. For each 1 percent loss of outer-atmosphere ozone, the amount of damaging ultraviolet radiation reaching the earth increases by 2 percent. Based on studies of experimental plots, soybean yields fall 1 percent for each 1 percent rise in radiation. Soybeans are the world's leading protein crop, and at last report, no one was monitoring radiation-induced losses.

Climate Change   Crop yields may also be affected by climate change caused by increased atmospheric concentrations of heat-trapping, carbon dioxide, produced by fossil fuels. At whatever rate climate change is occurring, it is potentially disruptive. If summers become hotter, droughts during the growing season may become more common. An unusually hot and dry summer in 1988 pushed the U.S. grain harvest below consumption for the first time in history. In 1994, new heat records were set throughout the western United States, northern Europe, the Baltic, and Japan.[21] A rise of only a degree or so in average global temperature may reduce soil moisture, impair pollination of major food crops such as rice and

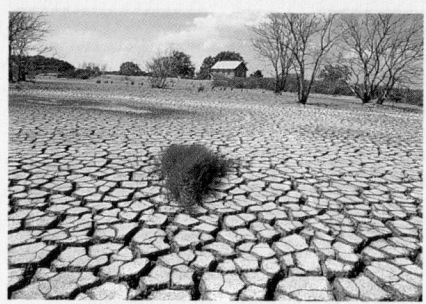

As groundwater is used up, deserts spread.

corn, slow growth, weaken disease resistance, and disrupt many other factors affecting crop yields.

Water Scarcity   Water supplies, too, are becoming limited. Decreases in available water result in reduced crop yields, most obviously on irrigated cropland. Two-thirds of all water taken from rivers and underground aquifers is used for irrigation.[22] Agricultural lands that require irrigation water play a disproportionate role in meeting the world's food needs. Although they account for only one-sixth of total cropland, irrigated croplands yield more than one-third of the total global harvest. The amount of irrigated land per capita, however, peaked in 1978 and has fallen almost 6 percent since then.[23]

Deteriorating Rangelands   Grazing land is decreasing along with agricultural cropland. Grasslands for raising beef are already being fully used or misused on every continent. One-fifth of the world's land area is rangeland, twice as much area as is farmed. This land supports most of the world's 3.2 billion cattle, sheep, and goats.[24] Although world beef and mutton production per capita increased 37 percent between 1950 and 1972, more recent yields have dropped.[25] These decreases reflect deterioration in the condition of the rangelands due to environmental problems and extensive overgrazing. The feed needs of livestock in nearly all developing countries now exceed the capacity of their rangelands. In Africa, where this problem is most visible, the annual loss of rangeland productivity is estimated at $7 billion, more than the gross national product of Ethiopia and Uganda combined.[26]

Diminishing Fisheries The yield of fish from the oceans is also declining, for the first time in history, due to overfishing and pollution. Big fish, such as tuna, swordfish, and shark, are becoming threatened because they are being overfished. Atlantic stocks of the heavily fished bluefin tuna have dropped by 94 percent.[27] Cod are rapidly disappearing off the New England coast and are almost gone farther north.

Inland fisheries have also suffered tremendous drops in yield as a result of environmental damage. The Aral Sea, located between Kazakhstan and Uzbekistan, yielded 40,000 tons of fish per year in 1960 and today is biologically dead. As water was diverted for irrigation over the last 30 years, the sea became increasingly salty until finally fish could no longer live in it.[28] Acidification has also taken a toll on inland fisheries. In Canada, 14,000 lakes are considered biologically dead as a result of acid rain.[29]

Limitations in Food Production

All in all, then, environmental problems are reducing the world's ability to feed its people. With fish yields and rangelands decreasing, can advances in agriculture compensate for the losses caused by environmental degradation? Historically, agricul-

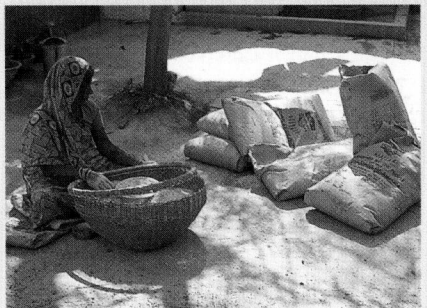
International efforts help to relieve hunger and poverty around the world.

ture has improved yields by making greater investments in irrigation, fertilizer, and improved genetic strains. Today, however, the contributions these measures can make are reaching limits for the first time in history: the improvements are leveling off. Irrigation can no longer compensate by improving crop yields because almost all the land that can benefit from irrigation is already receiving it. In fact, rising concentrations of salt in the soil—a by-product of irrigation—are *lowering* yields on close to a quarter of the world's irrigated cropland. Nor can fertilizer use enhance agricultural production much. Much of the fertilizing that can be done is being done—and with great effect; fertilizer use supports some 40 percent of the world's total crop yields. Adding more fertilizer, however, brings no further rise in yield. As for the development of high-yielding strains of crops, some advances have been dramatic, but they show little potential to change the overall trends described here. Furthermore, the raw materials necessary for developing new crops are becoming less and less available as genetic variety is lost due to the extinction of many plant species. Of the 5000 food plants used through-

out the world a few centuries ago, only 150 are grown in modern agriculture today. Most of the world's population relies on only five cereals, three legumes, and three root crops to meet their energy needs. Even among these, valuable strains are vanishing.[30]

Estimates are that the world grain harvest can be increased by no more than 1 percent a year. The increase might be higher, but for the many forms of environmental degradation described earlier. Meanwhile, the world's population is rising at the rate of at least 2 percent per year.[31] Many authorities in many fields—and more every year—are calling for a reduction in the growth rate of the world's population as the only way to enable the world's food output to keep pace with people's growing numbers.

The world still produces enough food to feed all its people, and the problem of hunger today remains a problem of unequal distribution of resources. If present trends continue, however, the time is approaching when there will be an absolute deficit of food. This conclusion seems inescapable. The world's increasing population threatens the world's capacity to produce adequate food. Population control has become one of the most pressing needs of this time in history. Until the nations of the world resolve the population problem, they can neither support the lives of people already born nor remedy global trends toward environmental deterioration. And to resolve the population problem, a necessary first step is to remedy the poverty problems, for reasons discussed next. Of the 90 million people being added to the population each year, the vast majority are in the most poverty-stricken areas of the world.

POVERTY AND OVERPOPULATION

Population growth is one of many factors contributing to poverty and hunger. The reverse is also true: poverty and hunger contribute to population growth.

Population Growth Leads to Hunger and Poverty The first of these cause-effect relationships is easy to understand. Population growth contributes to poverty and hunger, for the more mouths there are to feed, the worse poverty and hunger become. The sheer magnitude of our annual population increase of 90 million people is difficult to comprehend. Each month the world adds the equivalent of another New York City.[32] During six months of the terrible 1992 famine in Somalia, an estimated 300,000 people starved to death. Yet it took the world only 29 *hours* to replace their numbers! Ninety million people a year, spread over 365 days, comes to a quarter-million people a day—or just over 10,000 people born every hour.[33]

Population growth also contributes to hunger indirectly by preempting good agricultural land for growing cities and industry and forcing people onto marginal land, where they cannot produce sufficient food for themselves. The

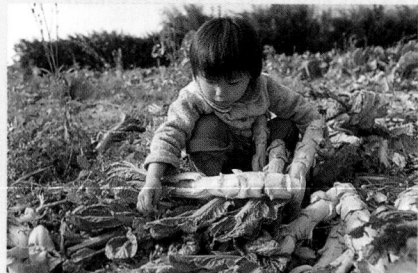

Families in developing countries depend on their children to help provide for daily needs.

world's poorest people live in the world's most damaged and inhospitable environments. There they experience, daily, tens of thousands of early deaths from malnutrition and disease.

Hunger and Poverty Lead to Population Growth Overpopulation, then, together with the environmental degradation that it causes, worsens poverty. How, though, does poverty lead to overpopulation? Poverty and hunger are believed to exert an ironic effect on people, making them bear more children. Poverty and hunger typically go hand in hand with ignorance, including ignorance of how to control family size. Also, a family depends on its children to farm the land, haul water, and care for adults in their old age. If a family faces ongoing poverty with its associated high rates of childhood disease and mortality, the parents will choose to have many children to ensure that some will survive to adulthood. People are willing to risk having fewer children only if they are sure that their children will live.

Relieving poverty and hunger, then, may be a necessary first step in curbing population growth. When people attain better access to health care, education, and family planning, the death rate falls. At first there is a "bulge" in the population, because births outnumber deaths, but as the standard of living continues to improve, families become willing to risk having fewer children. Then the birth rate falls. Thus, after a short but necessary lag time, improvements in economic status help stabilize the population.

The link between improved economic status and slowed population growth has been demonstrated in country after country.[34] Sustainable

development is central to this success and must include not only economic growth, but a sharing of resources among all groups. In parts of Sri Lanka, Taiwan, Malaysia, and Costa Rica, where this has happened, population growth has slowed the most. Where economic growth has occurred but only the rich have grown richer, population growth has remained high. Examples include Brazil, Mexico, the Philippines, and Thailand, where large families continue to be a major economic asset for the poor.

SOLUTIONS

Both the poor and the rich nations must contribute to solving the world's hunger, environmental, and poverty problems, but in different ways. The poor nations need to gain control of their rampaging population growth and to slow and reverse the destruction of their environmental resources: forests, waterways, and soil. To do this, they must, among other things, find ways to relieve their people's poverty. The rich nations need to stem their wasteful and polluting uses of resources and energy, which are contributing to global environmental degradation. They also must become willing to help relieve the debtor nations of their poverty in ways that effectively reach the poor.

Sustainable Development Worldwide

Many nations now recognize that improving all nations' economies is a prerequisite to meeting the world's other urgent needs: relief of hunger, population stabilization, arrest of environmental degradation, and sustainable treatment of resources. An important step was taken when a

United Nations convention on the Rights of the Child was ratified by over 100 nations. Significantly, for the first time in world history, the convention cited *nutrition* as an internationally recognized human right.[35]

Another important step was taken in 1992, when more than 100 nations met for the Earth Summit in Rio de Janeiro, Brazil, and discussed the relationship of the environment to poverty and hunger.* At this meeting, many nations agreed for the first time to 27 principles of sustainable development, which the conferees defined as development that would equitably meet both the economic and the environmental needs of present and future generations.

Participants discussed climate change and the possibility of setting legally binding targets and timetables for every nation to cut its emissions of global-warming gases. They began to approach agreement on this issue. They also signed agreements to protect the earth's remaining species of plants and animals and to preserve the world's forests.

The Earth Summit's discussions opened vistas of hope. Much remains to be done, and all nations have major parts to play. For our part, in the United States, the challenges are many. Can we reduce our consumption of fossil fuel and thereby our disproportionate contribution to global environmental degradation? The willingness of U.S. consumers to take responsibility for their individual shares in solving global problems could make a substantial contribution to the

*The formal name of the summit was the United Nations Conference on Environment and Development: UNCED, for short.

quality of life for future generations. Our decision to use fewer goods, devour fewer resources, create less pollution, and consume less energy would go a long way toward remedying global environmental problems and conditions that contribute to world hunger. In addition, the United States can help directly by supporting international moves to relieve poverty and environmental degradation worldwide. The following steps have been recommended:

- First, the developing countries need to be relieved of the gigantic interest payments they have been making to U.S. and international banks.
- Second, the debt relief needs to reach those within the countries who need it, and not just the wealthy.
- Third, rather than emphasizing *technology*-intensive methods of *harvesting* their resources, developing countries might shift toward *labor*-intensive means of *maintaining* their resources.
- Fourth, to account for the great value of environmental resources, soil, water, and trees should be counted in economic balance sheets.

The United States can exert international leadership by adopting these strategies and encouraging other developed nations to support similar measures. The idea behind all these measures is that relieving poverty will help relieve environmental degradation and hunger. To rephrase a well-known adage: If you give a man a fish, he will eat for a day. If you teach him to fish and enable him to buy and maintain his own gear and bait, he will eat for a lifetime and help to feed others. Unlike food giveaways and money doles, which are only stop-gap mea-

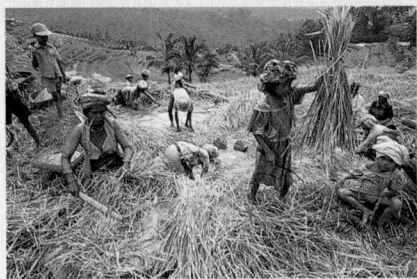

Labor-intensive technology is most often the appropriate technology in developing countries.

sures, social programs that will permanently better the lot of the poor can permanently solve the hunger problem.

Activism and Simpler Lifestyles at Home

Every segment of our society can have a place in the fight against hunger, poverty, and environmental degradation. The federal government, the states, local communities, big business and small companies, educators, and all individuals, including dietitians and foodservice managers, have many opportunities to forward the effort.

Government Action   Government policies can change to promote sustainability. For example, the government can stop using tax money to pay for the wasteful use of fossil fuels and of fertilizers and pesticides made from them. Instead, it can pay for energy conservation services and crop protection. Tax laws could be revised to reward energy conservation efforts, which would have a major impact on the research and development of conservation industries and sustainable agriculture. All of these actions are possible, but they depend on the support of elected officials. Keep in mind that you can affect the direction of such government actions by voting and writing letters that express your views on hunger, poverty, and environmental degradation.

Business Involvement   Businesses can take initiative to help; some already have. Several large corporations are currently major supporters of antihunger programs. Many grocery stores and restaurants give their out-of-date and leftover food to hunger organizations such as Third Harvest, which then distribute the food where needed in the community.

Education   Educators, including nutrition educators, can teach others about the underlying social and political causes of poverty, the root cause of hunger. At the college level, they can teach the relationship between hunger and population, hunger and environmental degradation, hunger and the status of women, and hunger and the global debt crisis. They can advocate legislation to address these problems. They can teach the poor to develop and run nutrition programs in their own communities and to fight on their own behalf for antipoverty, antihunger legislation.

Foodservice Efforts   Dietitians and foodservice managers have a special role to play. Their professional organization, the American Dietetic Association (ADA), is urging them to promote the saving of resources by reuse, recycling (including composting), energy conservation, and water conservation, in both their professional and their personal lives. In addition, the ADA urges its members to work for policy changes in private and gov-

ernment food assistance programs, to intensify education about hunger, and to be advocates on the local, state, and national levels to help end hunger in the United States.[36]

Other Opportunities   Individuals can support organizations that lobby for the needed economic policy changes toward developing countries. They can join and work for international hunger relief organizations. Appendix F includes some of the major ones.

Most importantly, at every level, individuals can try to make lifestyle choices that consider the environmental consequences. Several possible choices relating to typical U.S. foodways are presented in Table H18–2. These suggested lifestyles changes can easily be extended from food to other areas. All aspects of our lifestyles relate to global problems. Recommendations include personal actions: reduce, reuse, recycle, and cut energy use. Admittedly, these approaches to solving today's global problems seem simplistic, but because we number 5 billion plus, individual actions can add up to exert an immense impact. The problems are complex, they are not fully understood, and high-level scientific research is needed to solve them. But even as that research is being done and the world's best minds are translating the results into recommended actions, individuals can be doing what they already know how to do. As Margaret Mead said, "Never doubt that a small group of thoughtful, committed people can change the world. Indeed, it is the only thing that ever has."

Emphasis on personal lifestyle choices is important because it raises awareness and paves the way for larger actions. Individual choices

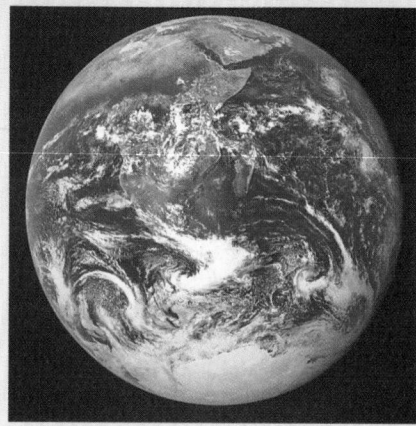

Good planets are hard to find.

are, however, only part of the solution to today's problems. Institutional changes are the other part—changes in the way agriculture, industry, and governments do their business domestically and internationally. Students can become involved in promoting both kinds of change: make personal lifestyle changes and then vote for government changes.

"Be part of the solution, not part of the problem," an adage says. In other words, don't waste time or energy moaning and groaning about how tough things are; do something to improve them. This adage is as applicable to today's global environmental problems as it is to an unwashed dish in the kitchen sink. They are our problems: human beings created them, and human beings must solve them.

NOTES

1. L. N. Burby, *World Hunger* (San Diego, Calif.: Lucent Books, 1995), pp. 13–16; P. L. Kutzner, *World Hunger: A Reference Handbook* (Santa Barbara, Calif.: ABC–CL10, 1991) pp. 158–159.

2. *Tallahassee Democrat*, October 14, 1994; P. Univ, The state of world hunger, *Nutrition Reviews* 52 (1994): 151–161.

Table H18–2
• • • • • • • • • • • • • •

Environmentally Conscious Foodways

Food production taxes environmental resources and causes pollution. Consumers can make environmentally conscious choices at every step from food shopping to cooking and use of kitchen appliances to serving, cleanup, and waste disposal.

Food Shopping

Transportation:
- Whenever possible, walk or ride a bicycle; use car pools and mass transit.
- Shop only once a week, share trips, or take turns shopping for each other.
- When buying a car, choose an energy-efficient one.

Food choices:
- Eat low on the food chain; that is, eat plants, rather than animals that eat plants (this suggestion complements the Food Guide Pyramid recommendations for eating for good health).
- Avoid buying canned beef products (many of these foods come at the expense of cleared rainforest land).
- Eat small portions of meat; select range-fed beef, buffalo, poultry, and fish.
- Select local foods (they are transported shorter distances and less fuel is required to pack them, label them, and keep them cold if they are fresh).

Food packages:
- Whenever possible, select foods with no packages; next best are minimal, reusable, or recyclable ones.
- Buy juices and sodas in large glass or recyclable plastic bottles (not small individual cans or cartons); grains in bulk (not separate little packages); and eggs in pressed fiber cartons (not foam, unless it is recycled locally).
- Carry reusable shopping bags; alternatively, ask for plastic bags if they are recyclable.

Cooking Food

- Cook foods quickly in a pressure cooker or microwave oven.
- When using the oven, bake a lot of food at one time and keep the door closed tightly.
- Refuse throwaway utensils.
- Avoid spray products.

Kitchen Appliances

- Do without small electrical appliances such as can openers, mixers, knife sharpeners, and food processors.
- When buying a refrigerator, choose an energy-efficient one.
- Consider the possibility of using solar energy to meet home electrical needs.
- Set the water heater at 130°F (54°C), no hotter; put it on a timer; wrap it and the hot-water pipes in insulation; install water-saving faucets.

Food Serving, Dish Washing, and Waste Disposal

- Use "real" plates, cups, and glasses instead of disposable ones.
- Use cloth towels and napkins, reusable storage containers with lids, and dishcloths instead of paper towels, plastic wrap, plastic storage bags, and sponges.
- Run the dishwasher only when it is full.
- Recycle all glass, plastic, and aluminum.
- Compost all vegetable scraps, fruit peelings, and leftover plant foods.

3. *Fact Sheet on Childhood Hunger and Poverty*, (c. 1992), available from Bread for the World, 802 Rhode Island Avenue NE, Washington, DC 20018.
4. S. Lewis, Food security, environment, poverty, and the world's children, *Journal of Nutrition Education* (1 supplement) 24 (1992): 3S–5S.
5. L. D. McBean, ed., with D. Derelian, R. J. Fersh, and L. Parker, Hunger and undernutrition in America, *Dairy Council Digest*, March/April 1992.
6. U.S. Department of Commerce, *Statistical Abstract of the United States, 1994* (Washington, D.C.: Bureau of the Census, 1994), p. 386.
7. Food Research and Action Center, *Community Childhood Hunger Identification Project: A Survey of Childhood Hunger in the United States*, Executive Summary (Washington, D.C.: Food Research and Action Center, March 1991), as cited in McBean, 1992.
8. *Fact Sheet on Childhood Hunger and Poverty*, c. 1992.
9. J. C. Wolgemuth and coauthors, Wasting malnutrition and inadequate nutrient intakes identified in a multiethnic homeless population, *Journal of the American Dietetic Association* 92 (1992): 834–839; M. A. Drake, The nutritional status and dietary adequacy of single homeless women and their children in shelters, *Public Health Reports* 107 (1992): 312–319; B. E. Cohen, N. Chapman, and M. R. Burt, Food sources and intake of homeless persons, *Journal of Nutrition Education* (1 supplement) 24 (1992): 45S–51S.
10. World Bank, *World Development Report 1991* (New York: Oxford University Press, 1991); S. Postel, Denial in the decisive decade, in L. R. Brown and coauthors, *State of the World 1992* (New York: W. W. Norton, 1992), pp. 3–8.
11. L. Timberlake, *Only One Earth*, cited in Food for thought, *Seeds*, Sprouts edition, 1988.
12. R. W. Kates, Ending deaths from famine: The opportunity in Somalia, *New England Journal of Medicine* 328 (1993): 1055–1057.
13. *Tallahassee Democrat*, October 14, 1994.
14. Kates, 1993.
15. U.S. Department of Commerce, 1994, pp. 854–855.
16. L. R. Brown and coauthors, *State of the World 1995* (New York: W. W. Norton, 1995), p. 11; *Tallahassee Democrat*, June 10, 1995.
17. L. R. Brown and J. E. Young, Feeding the world in the nineties, in L. R. Brown, *State of the World 1990* (New York: W. W. Norton, 1990).
18. J. W. Clay and coauthors, *The Spoils of Famine: Ethiopian Famine Policy and Peasant*

Agriculture (Cambridge, Mass.: Cultural Survival, 1988), as cited in L. R. Brown and H. Kane, *Full House* (New York: W. W. Norton, 1994), pp. 146–157.

19. R. D. Kaplan, The coming anarchy, *Atlantic Monthly*, February 1994, pp. 44–76.

20. L. R. Brown and coauthors, *State of the World, 1994* (New York: W. W. Norton, 1994), p. 202.

21. Brown and coauthors, 1995, p. 191.

22. Brown and coauthors, 1995, p. 192.

23. Brown and coauthors, 1994, p. 201.

24. FAO, *FAO Production Yearbook 1992* (Rome: 1993); FAO, *FAO Production Yearbook 1991* (Rome: 1992); FAO, *1948–1985 World Crop and Livestock Statistics* (Rome: 1987), as cited in L. R. Brown and H. Kane, *Full House* (New York: W. W. Norton, 1994), pp. 89–95.

25. U.S. Department of Agriculture (USDA), *Dairy, Livestock, and Poultry: World Livestock Situation* (Washington, D.C.: October 1993), as cited in L. R. Brown and H. Kane, *Full House* (New York: W. W. Norton, 1994), pp. 89–95.

26. H. Dregne and coauthors, A new assessment of the world status of desertification, *Desertification Control Bulletin 20* (1991), as cited in L. R. Brown and H. Kane, *Full House* (New York: W. W. Norton, 1994), pp. 89–95.

27. FAO, cited in World Resources Institute (WRI), *World Resources 1992–93* (New York: Oxford University Press, 1992); bluefin tuna figure from D. Meadows and coauthors, *Beyond the Limits* (Post Mills, Vt.: Chelsea Green Publishing Company, 1992), as cited in L. R. Brown and H. Kane, *Full House* (New York: W. W. Norton, 1994), pp. 75–88.

28. L. Brown, The Aral Sea: going, going . . ., *World Watch*, January/February 1991.

29. Government of Canada, *The State of Canada's Environment* (Ottawa: 1991).

30. K. Dixit, The shrinking pool, *New Internationalist*, March 1991, p. 20.

31. Brown and Young, 1990, pp. 64–65.

32. Population Reference Bureau (PRB), *1993 World Population Data Sheet* (Washington, D.C.: 1993), as cited in L. R. Brown and H. Kane, *Full House* (New York: W. W. Norton, 1994), pp. 49–61.

33. Centers for Disease Control, Population based mortality assessment: Baidoa and Afgoi, Somalia, 1992, *Journal of the American Medical Association* (1993), as cited in L. R. Brown and H. Kane, *Full House* (New York: W. W. Norton, 1994), pp. 49–61.

34. P. S. Dasgupta, Population, poverty and the local environment, *Scientific American*, February 1995, pp. 40–45.

35. Lewis, 1992.

36. Position of The American Dietetic Association: Environmental issues, *Journal of the American Dietetic Association* 93 (1993): 589–591; Position of The American Dietetic Association: Domestic hunger and inadequate access to food, *Journal of the American Dietetic Association* 90 (1990): 1437–1441.

Chapter 19

Life Cycle Nutrition: Infancy, Childhood, and Adolescence

CONTENTS

Nutrition during Infancy
  Energy and Nutrient Needs
  Breast Milk versus Infant Formula
  Breast Milk
  Infant Formula
  Special Needs of Preterm Infants
  Introducing First Foods
  Mealtimes with Infants
Nutrition during Childhood
  Energy and Nutrient Needs
  Hunger and Malnutrition in Children
  Nutrition, Hyperactivity, and "Hyper"
      Behavior
  Television and Children's Nutrition
  Adverse Reactions to Foods
  Mealtimes at Home
  Nutrition at School
Nutrition during Adolescence
  Growth and Development
  Energy and Nutrient Needs
  Food Choices and Health Habits
  Problems Adolescents Face
HIGHLIGHT: Childhood Obesity and the
Early Development of Chronic Diseases

MICROGRAPH: Growth hormone, a chemical messenger active during infancy, childhood, and adolescence

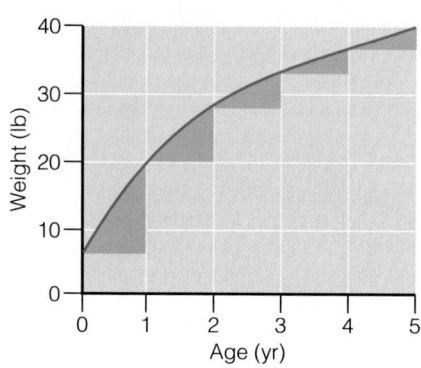

Figure 19–1

Weight Gain of Human Infants in Their First Five Years of Life

In the first year, an infant's birthweight may triple, but over the following several years, the rate of weight gain gradually diminishes.

A newborn baby requires about 650 kcalories per day, whereas most adults require about 2000 kcalories per day. In comparison to body weight, the difference is remarkable.

Recommended water intake for infants:
1.5 mL/kcal energy expenditure.
For example, a six-month-old infant who expends 850 kcal a day needs:

1.5 mL/kcal × 850 kcal = 1275 mL, or about 5 c of water/day.

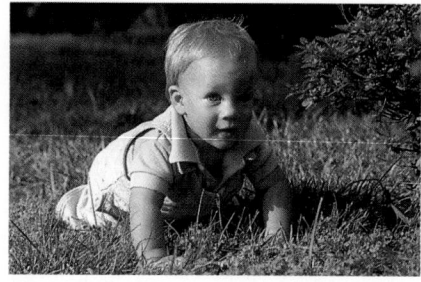

After six months, energy saved by slower growth is spent in increased activity.

*t*he first year of life is a time of phenomenal growth and development. After the first year, a child continues to grow and change, but more slowly. Still, the cumulative effects over the next decade are remarkable. Then, as the child enters the teen years, the pace toward adulthood accelerates dramatically. This chapter examines the special nutrient needs of infants, children, and teenagers.

Nutrition during Infancy

For a while, the infant drinks only breast milk or formula, but later begins to eat some foods, as appropriate. Trends change and experts argue about the fine points, but properly nourishing a baby is relatively simple overall. Common sense in the selection of infant foods and a nurturing, relaxed environment go far to promote an infant's health and well-being.

ENERGY AND NUTRIENT NEEDS

An infant grows faster during the first year than ever again, as Figure 19–1 shows. Growth directly reflects nutrient intake and is an important parameter in assessing the nutrition status of infants and children. Health care professionals measure the heights and weights of infants and children at intervals and compare measures both with standard growth curves for sex and age and with previous measures of each child (see Figure 19–2).

Energy Intake and Activity A healthy infant's birthweight doubles by about four months of age and triples by the age of one year, typically reaching 20 to 25 pounds. (If an adult were to do this, a person weighing 150 pounds would increase to 450 pounds in a single year.) By the end of the first year, infant growth slows considerably; an infant gains less than 10 pounds during the second year.

Not only do infants grow rapidly, but their basal metabolic rate is remarkably high—about twice that of an adult, based on body weight.[1] Infants require about 100 kcalories per kilogram of body weight per day, whereas most adults need fewer than 40. (A 170-pound adult who tried to eat like an infant would have to ingest over 7000 kcalories a day.) After six months, metabolic needs decline as the growth rate slows down, but some of the energy saved by slower growth is spent in increased activity.

Vitamins and Minerals Vitamin and mineral recommendations are based on the contents of human milk, which seems appropriate considering that neither deficiencies nor toxicities develop when infants receive these amounts.[2] Figure 19–3 (on p. 628) compares a five-month-old infant's needs per unit of body weight with those of a man and shows that some of the differences are extraordinary.

Water An important nutrient for infants, as for everyone, is the one easiest to forget: water. The younger the infant, the greater the percentage of body weight that is present as fluids between the cells and in the vascular space—fluids *outside* the cells that are easy to lose. Breast milk or infant formula normally provides enough water to replace a healthy infant's fluid losses, but an infant who is exposed to hot weather, has diarrhea, or vomits repeatedly needs supplemen-

Figure 19–2

Examples of Growth Charts

These two charts are used for girls from birth to 36 months. The first chart gives percentiles for length and weight for age; the other, percentiles for head circumference for age and weight for length. Appendix E describes how to monitor growth and provides these and six other growth charts for both boys and girls of various ages.

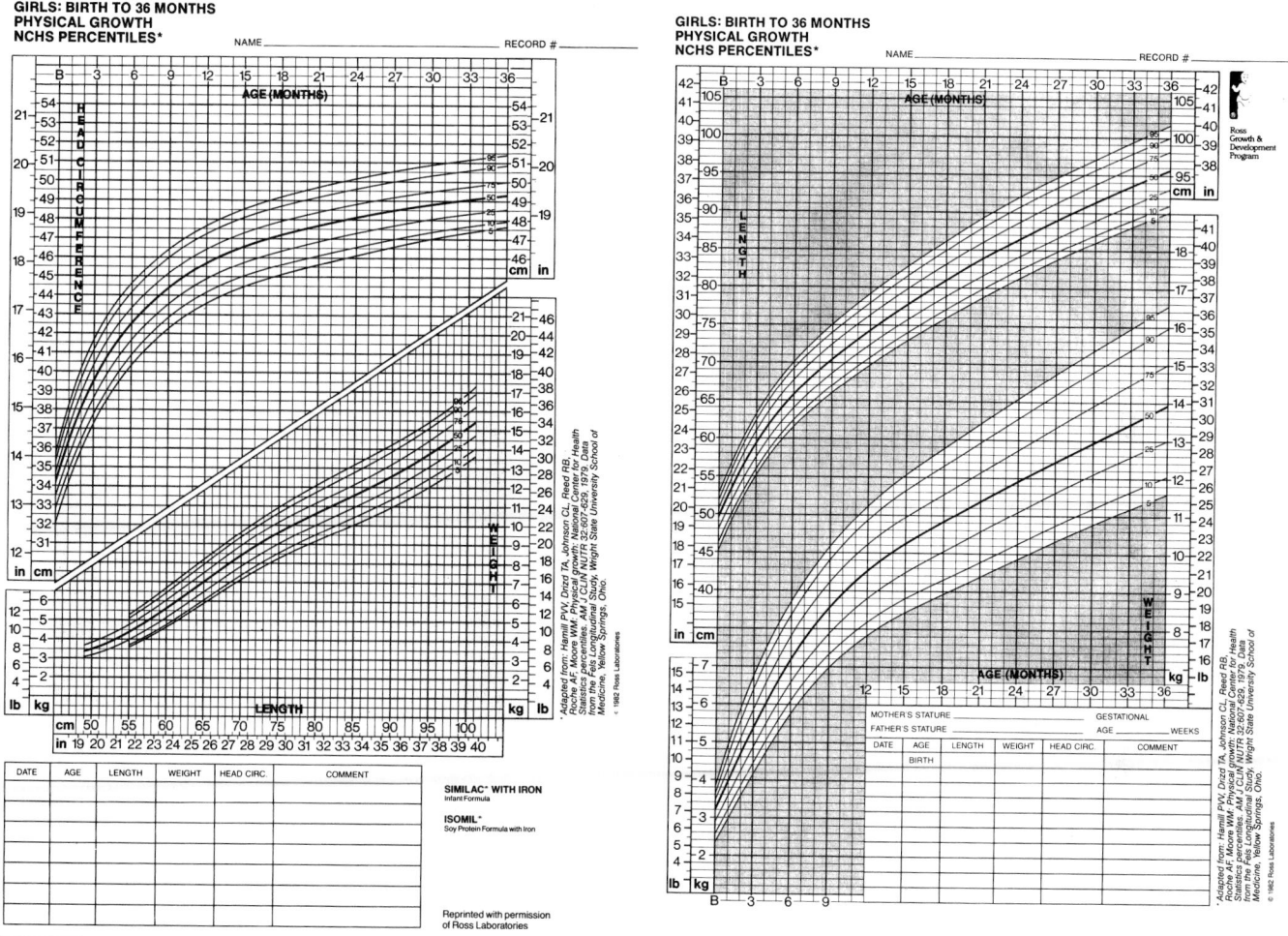

tal water to prevent life-threatening dehydration.[3] Infants cannot explain why they are crying; adults must remember that an infant may need water, and then provide as much as the infant will drink.

BREAST MILK VERSUS INFANT FORMULA

The American Academy of Pediatrics recommends that infants receive breast milk for the first 6 to 12 months.[4] The American Dietetic Association also advocates breastfeeding because of its many benefits to both infant and mother.[5] Breast milk's unique nutrient composition and protective factors promote optimal infant health and development. Experts add, though, that iron-fortified for-

Figure 19–3

Nutrient RDA of a Five-Month-Old Infant and an Adult Male Compared on the Basis of Body Weight

Because infants are small, they need smaller total amounts of the nutrients than adults do, but when comparisons are based on body weight, infants need over twice as much of many nutrients. Infants use large amounts of energy and nutrients, in proportion to their body size, to keep all their metabolic processes going.

Infant's metabolism:
- Heart rate: 120 to 140 beats per minute.
- Respiration rate: 20 per minute.
- Energy needs: 45 kcalories per pound (100 kcalories per kilogram) body weight.

Adult's metabolism:
- Heart rate: 70 to 80 beats per minute.
- Respiration rate: 12 to 14 per minute.
- Energy needs: <18 kcalories per pound (<40 kcalories per kilogram) body weight.

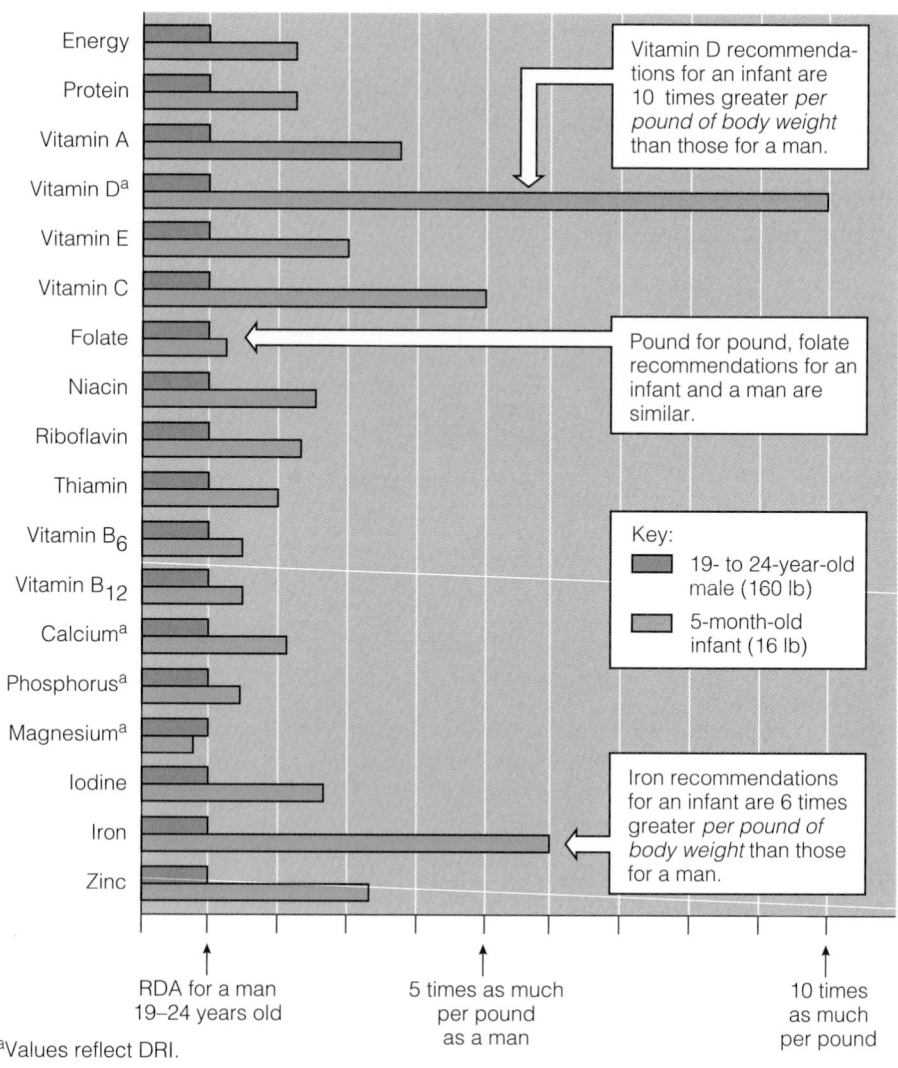

aValues reflect DRI.

mula is an acceptable alternative to breast milk, for it imitates the composition of breast milk as closely as possible.

Even two or three months of breastfeeding give the infant immunological protection and other special advantages during the most critical period after birth—protection that persists beyond the breastfeeding period itself.[6] The mother can then shift to formula, if necessary, knowing she has given her infant those benefits.

In the United States and Canada, the two dietary practices that have the most effect on an infant's nutrition status are, first, the milk the infant receives, and second, the age at which solid foods are introduced. The next sections are devoted to feeding the infant and identifying common nutrient deficiencies.

BREAST MILK

Breast milk excels as a source of nutrients for the young infant.[7] The American Academy of Pediatrics and the Canadian Pediatric Society have issued this joint statement: "Breastfeeding is strongly recommended for full-term infants, except in the few instances where specific contraindications exist."

Breastfed infants generally gain weight at about the same rate as formula-fed infants during the first two or three months, even though they usually drink less milk and therefore have lower energy intakes.[8] For the next six months, breastfed infants tend to gain slightly less weight than formula-fed infants, but then resume gaining at a similar rate again.[9]

With the possible exception of vitamin D, breast milk provides all the nutrients a healthy infant needs for the first four to six months of life. Breast milk also confers immunological protection, described later.

Energy Nutrients   The energy-nutrient composition of breast milk differs dramatically from the dietary recommendations for adults (see Figure 19–4). Yet for infants, breast milk is the most nearly perfect food, proving that people at different stages of life really do have different nutrient needs.

Breast milk's carbohydrate is lactose, which enhances calcium absorption. Breast milk's fat offers a generous proportion of the essential fatty acid linoleic acid. The total protein in breast milk is less than in cow's milk, which is good because it places less stress on the infant's immature kidneys to excrete the major end product of protein metabolism, urea. The main protein in breast milk is alpha-lactalbumin, which is easy for infants to digest.

Vitamins   With the possible exception of vitamin D, the vitamins in breast milk are ample to support infant growth. Even vitamin C, for which cow's milk is a poor source, is abundant in the breast milk of a well-nourished mother. The vitamin D in breast milk is low, however, and vitamin D deficiency impairs bone mineralization in infants and children.[10] Manufacturers fortify cow's milk and infant formulas with vitamin D, and physicians may prescribe vitamin D supplements for breastfed infants who do not receive sufficient exposure to sunlight.

Infants who are exposed to sunlight regularly can make enough vitamin D to meet their needs. The amount formed depends on skin color, exposure time, atmospheric pollution, time of year, and latitude. Vitamin D deficiency is a risk for infants who are not exposed to sunlight daily, who receive breast milk without supplementation, and who have darkly pigmented skin.

Figure 19–4

Percentages of Energy-Yielding Nutrients in Human Milk and in Recommended Adult Diets

The proportions of energy-yielding nutrients in human breast milk differ from those recommended for adults.

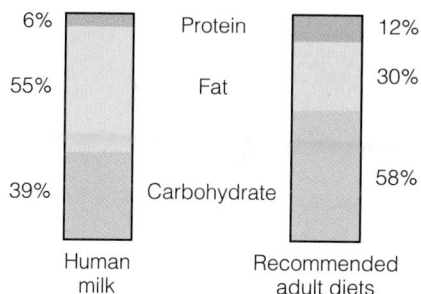

alpha-lactalbumin (lact-AL-byoo-min): the chief protein in human breast milk, as opposed to casein (CAY-seen), the chief protein in cow's milk.

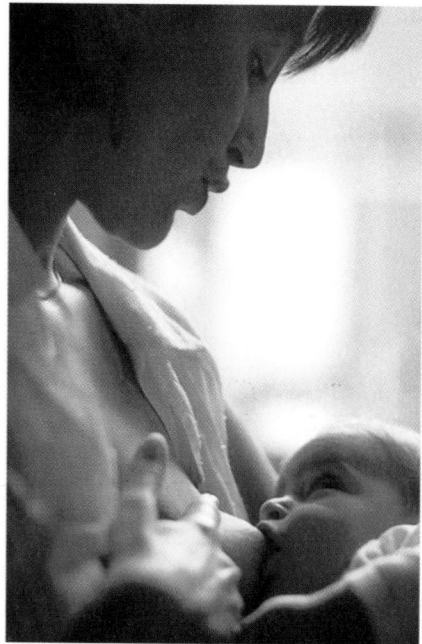

Women are encouraged to breastfeed whenever possible because breast milk offers infants many nutrients and health advantages.

colostrum (co-LAHS-trum): a milklike secretion from the breast, present during the first day or so after delivery before milk appears; rich in protective factors.

All newborns receive a single dose of vitamin K at birth.

Minerals   The calcium-to-phosphorus ratio of breast milk is ideal for calcium absorption. The iron in breast milk is highly absorbable, as is the zinc, thanks to the presence of a zinc-binding protein. Breast milk is low in sodium, another benefit for immature kidneys.

Fluoride is not an essential nutrient, but it does help to prevent dental caries. Breast milk provides little fluoride, regardless of the mother's intake.

Supplements   Breastfed newborns usually require no supplements, with the possible exception of vitamin D. At six months, depending on food and water intake, infants may require iron and fluoride supplements (see Table 19–1).

Immunological Protection   Breast milk offers unsurpassed protection against infection during a time when an infant's immune system is not fully functional. It contains antiviral agents such as immunoglobulins, antibacterial agents such as lactoferrin, and other infection inhibitors.

During the first two or three days of lactation, the breasts produce colostrum, a premilk substance containing antibodies and white cells from the mother's blood. Because it contains maternal immune factors, colostrum helps protect the newborn from infections the mother has developed immunity against. These diseases are the ones in her environment and are precisely those against which the infant needs protection. The maternal antibodies swallowed with the milk inactivate disease-causing bacteria within the digestive tract before they can start infections. This explains, in part, why breastfed infants have fewer intestinal infections than formula-fed infants. Later, breast milk also delivers antibodies, although not as many as colostrum.

Table 19–1

Supplements for Full-Term Infants

	Vitamin D[a]	Iron[b]	Fluoride[c]
Breastfed infants:			
Birth to six months of age	✓		
Six months to one year	✓	✓	✓
Formula-fed infants:			
Birth to six months of age			
Six months to one year		✓	✓

[a]Vitamin D supplements are recommended only for as long as breast milk is the infant's major milk.

[b]Infants four to six months of age need additional iron, preferably in the form of iron-fortified cereal for both breastfed and formula-fed infants and iron-fortified infant formula for formula-fed infants.

[c]The Committee on Nutrition of the American Academy of Pediatrics recommends initiating fluoride supplements at six months of age for breastfed infants, formula-fed infants who receive ready-to-use formulas (these are prepared with water low in fluoride), and those who receive formula mixed with water that contains little or no fluoride (less than 0.3 ppm).

Sources: Adapted from Committee on Nutrition, American Academy of Pediatrics, Vitamin and mineral supplement needs of normal children in the United States, in *Pediatric Nutrition Handbook*, 3rd ed., ed. L. A. Barness (Elk Grove Village, Ill.: American Academy of Pediatrics, 1993), pp. 34–42; American Academy of Pediatrics, Committee on Nutrition, Fluoride supplementation for children: Interim policy recommendations, *Pediatrics* 95 (1995): 777.

In addition to antibodies, colostrum and breast milk provide other powerful agents that help to fight against bacterial infection. Among them are bifidus factors, which favor the growth of the "friendly" bacterium *Lactobacillus bifidus* in the infant's digestive tract, so that other, harmful bacteria cannot gain a foothold there. An iron-grabbing protein in breast milk, lactoferrin, keeps bacteria from getting the iron they need to grow, helps absorb iron into the infant's bloodstream, and kills some bacteria directly. Also present is a growth factor that stimulates the development and maintenance of the infant's digestive tract and its protective factors. Several breast milk enzymes, hormones, and lipids also help protect the infant against infection. Much remains to be learned about the composition and characteristics of human milk, but clearly it is a very special substance.

bifidus (BIFF-id-us, by-FEED-us) **factors:** factors in colostrum and breast milk that favor the growth of the "friendly" bacterium *Lactobacillus* (lack-toh-ba-SILL-us) *bifidus* in the infant's intestinal tract, so that other, less desirable intestinal inhabitants will not flourish.

lactoferrin (lack-toh-FERR-in): a factor in breast milk that binds iron and keeps it from supporting the growth of the infant's intestinal bacteria.

INFANT FORMULA

Breastfeeding offers many benefits to both mother and infant, and every woman should seriously consider it. Still, there are valid reasons for not breastfeeding, and formula-fed infants grow and develop into healthy children. The mother who chooses to feed formula to her infant can offer the same closeness, warmth, and stimulation during feedings as the breastfeeding mother can. Other family members can help with feedings, thus allowing the mother additional time to rest.

Formula preparation:
- Liquid concentrate (inexpensive, relatively easy)—mix with equal part water.
- Powdered formula (cheapest, lightest for travel)—read label directions.
- Ready-to-feed (easiest, most expensive)—pour directly into clean bottles.
- Whole milk—do not use during first year.

Appropriate Uses of Formula A woman who breastfeeds for a year can wean her infant to cow's milk, bypassing the need for infant formula. Many breastfeeding women use some infant formula, however. Some substitute formula for breastfeeding on occasion. Some wean from breast milk to formulas within the first year. And some women, of course, feed formula to their infants from birth. Whatever the case, a woman who uses formula must select an appropriate formula and learn to prepare it.

wean: to gradually replace breast milk with infant formula or other foods appropriate to an infant's diet.

Infant Formula Composition Formulas made from cow's milk closely resemble human milk in nutrient content. Figure 19–5 illustrates the energy-nutrient balance of both, and Table 19–2 compares breast milk, cow's milk, and a standard infant formula.

The American Academy of Pediatrics recommends iron-fortified infant formula for all formula-fed infants. The increasing use of iron-fortified formulas during the past few decades is a major reason for the decline in iron-deficiency anemia among U.S. infants.

Infant formulas contain no protective antibodies for infants, but in general, vaccinations, clean water, and clean environments in the developed countries make this deficit less important than in the past. Formulas can be prepared safely by following the rules of proper food handling and using water that is sanitary and free of contamination. Lead-contaminated water is a major source of lead poisoning in infants (see Highlight 13).[11]

Risks of Formula Feeding In developing countries and in poor areas of this country, formula may be unavailable or may be prepared with contaminated water or overdiluted in an attempt to save money. More than 1.2 billion people in developing countries have no safe drinking water. Contaminated formulas often cause infections, leading to diarrhea, dehydration, and failure to absorb

Figure 19–5

Percentages of Energy-Yielding Nutrients in Human Milk and in Infant Formula

The proportions of energy-yielding nutrients in human breast milk and formula differ slightly.

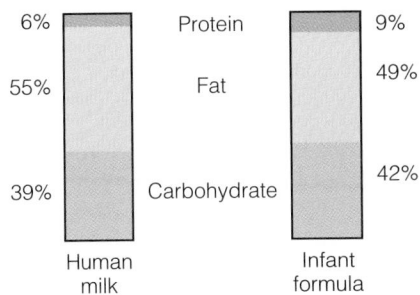

Table 19–2

Comparison of Human Milk, Cow's Milk, and Infant Formula

Nutrient (per 100 mL)	Human Milk	Cow's Milk	Infant Formula[a]
ENERGY-YIELDING NUTRIENTS			
Energy (kcal)	64	66	67
Protein (g)	0.9	3.4	1.5
Fat (g)	3.4	3.7	3.7
Carbohydrate (g)	6.6	4.9	7.1
MINERALS			
Sodium (mg)	17	58	20
Potassium (mg)	55	138	68
Chloride (mg)	43	103	43
Calcium (mg)	26	125	47
Phosphorus (mg)	14	96	35
Magnesium (mg)	4	12	5
Iron (mg)	0.5	0.5	1.2[b]
Zinc (mg)	0.2	0.4	0.5
Copper (mg)	0.04	0.01	0.06
VITAMINS			
Vitamin A (IU)	190	103	255
Thiamin (μg)	16	44	63
Riboflavin (μg)	36	175	110
Vitamin B_6 (μg)	10	64	41
Niacin (μg)	159	93	700
Pantothenic acid (μg)	198	352	277
Biotin (μg)	1	4	1.4
Folate (μg)	5	5	9
Vitamin B_{12} (μg)	0.04	0.04	0.14
Vitamin C (mg)	4.6	1.2	5.6
Vitamin D (IU)	2.2	3.4	41
Vitamin E (IU)	0.2	0.04	1.7
Vitamin K (μg)	1.5	6.0	5.7
Inositol (μg)	37	17	3
Choline (μg)	6	20	10

[a] Values represent the average for three major commercial products: (1) Similac, Ross Laboratories; (2) Enfamil, Mead-Johnson Laboratories; and (3) SMA, Wyeth Laboratories.
[b] The value represents formulas with iron fortification. The value for unfortified formula is 0.1 milligram.

Source: Adapted with permission from K. J. Motil, Breast-feeding: Public health and clinical overview, in *Pediatric Nutrition,* eds. R. J. Grand, J. L. Sutphen, and W. H. Dietz, Jr. (Boston: Butterworths, 1987), pp. 251–263.

nutrients. Without sterilization and refrigeration, bottles of formula are an ideal breeding ground for bacteria. Whenever such risks are present, breastfeeding can be a life-saving option. Wherever sanitation is poor, breastfeeding is preferred: breast milk is sterile, and its antibodies enhance an infant's resistance to disease. An infant who lives in a house without indoor plumbing and is not breastfed is twice as likely to die early in life as a breastfed infant who lives in a house with good sanitation.

Infant Formula Standards   National and international standards have been set for the nutrient contents of infant formulas. U.S. standards are based on American Academy of Pediatrics recommendations, and the Food and Drug Administration (FDA) mandates quality control procedures to ensure that they are met. All formulas that meet the standards are nutritionally similar; small differences are sometimes confusing, but usually not important unless infants have special needs.

Special Formulas   Standard formulas are inappropriate for some infants. For example, infants with inherited diseases may need special formulas. Special formulas based on soy protein are available for infants allergic to milk protein. Soy formulas are usually lactose-free, and so can be used for infants with lactose intolerance as well. Other variations have been formulated for infants with other special needs.

Inappropriate Formulas   Caretakers must use only products designed for infants; soy *beverages*, for example, are nutritionally incomplete and inappropriate for infants.[12] Goat's milk is also inappropriate for infants because of its low folate content. An infant receiving goat's milk is likely to develop "goat's milk anemia," an anemia characteristic of folate deficiency.

Nursing Bottle Tooth Decay   Dentists advise against putting a baby to bed with a bottle. Salivary flow, which normally cleanses the mouth, diminishes as the baby falls asleep. Sucking for long times pushes the jawline out of shape and causes a bucktoothed profile, with protruding upper and receding lower teeth. Furthermore, prolonged sucking on a bottle of formula, milk, or juice bathes the upper teeth in a carbohydrate-rich fluid that nourishes decay-producing bacteria. (The tongue covers and protects most of the lower teeth, but they, too, may be affected.) The result is extensive and rapid tooth decay. To prevent it, no child should be put to bed with a bottle of nourishing fluid. If a bottle is given, it should contain water. In fact, caregivers are wise to offer infants water after each feeding to rinse the mouth.

 HEALTHY PEOPLE 2000: Increase to at least 75% the proportion of parents and caregivers who use feeding practices that prevent nursing bottle tooth decay.

SPECIAL NEEDS OF PRETERM INFANTS

The terms *preterm* and *premature* imply incomplete fetal development, or immaturity, of many body systems. The preterm infant faces physical independence

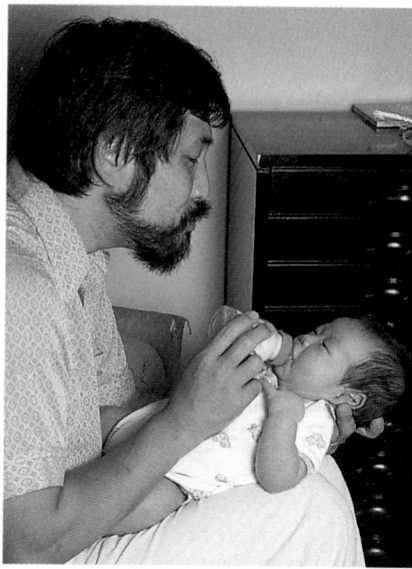

The infant thrives on infant formula offered with affection.

nursing bottle tooth decay: extensive tooth decay due to prolonged tooth contact with formula, milk, fruit juice, or other carbohydrate-rich liquid offered to an infant in a bottle.

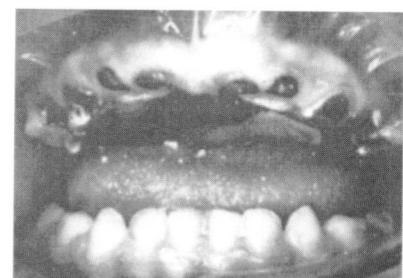

An extreme example of nursing bottle tooth decay. This child was frequently put to bed sucking on a bottle filled with apple juice, so that the teeth were bathed in carbohydrate for long periods of time— a perfect medium for bacterial growth. The upper teeth have decayed all the way to the gum line.

before some of the organs and tissues are ready. The fastest fetal weight gain occurs during the last trimester of gestation, so a preterm infant is most often a low-birthweight infant. With a premature birth, the infant is forced to endure the time of maximal growth without the continued nutritional support of the placenta.

The last trimester of gestation is also a time when nutrients are stored for later use. Having limited nutrient stores intensifies the precarious situation for premature infants, and their metabolic immaturity further compromises their nutrition status. Their absorption of nutrients, especially of fat and calcium, is also limited. Preterm, low-birthweight infants are likely candidates for nutrient deficiencies.

Infants who are born eight to ten weeks prior to term have acquired only about 30 percent as much calcium as full-term infants, so their calcium requirements are high. They miss out on the normal mineralization of bone that takes place during the last trimester of gestation. As a result, they often develop the metabolic bone disease osteopenia, the rickets of prematurity. Susceptibility to osteopenia varies directly with the infant's weight: the smaller the infant, the greater the risk.

osteopenia: a metabolic bone disease common in preterm infants; also called rickets of prematurity

Preterm infants often receive both breast milk and formula. Breast milk provides protection against infection, and its composition is excellent for the immature intestine, kidneys, and liver. Breast milk cannot, however, fully meet the calcium and phosphorus needs of the preterm infant. Formulas for preterm infants contain more highly concentrated calcium and phosphorus than standard formulas, and breastfed preterm infants receive human milk supplemented with these minerals.[13] Special formulas designed for preterm infants offer the advantages of known composition and precise measurement of intake.

INTRODUCING FIRST FOODS

Changes in body organs during the first year affect the baby's readiness to accept solid foods. For example, the stomach and intestines can easily digest the milk sugar lactose at birth, but they cannot digest starch for several months. One reason why breast milk or formula is the ideal first food is that its easily digested carbohydrate can best supply energy for the baby's intense growth and activity. Breast milk or infant formula should therefore be the baby's major food, at first. Cow's milk is inappropriate during the first year because it provides insufficient vitamin C and iron and excessive sodium and protein. If introduced too soon, cow's milk displaces iron-fortified formula or breast milk and causes GI blood loss in many infants.

Supplemental, or weaning, foods are sometimes called beikost (BYE-cost).

When to Introduce Solid Food In addition to formula or breast milk, an infant needs to begin eating other foods around four to six months. Infants who do not receive solid foods before the end of the first year may suffer delayed growth.

Physical readiness for solid foods develops in small steps. Teeth begin to erupt, and the infant develops the ability to swallow solid foods at around four to six months. Offering food by spoon and liquids by cup helps an infant learn to swallow. At nine months to a year, a baby can sit up and handle objects; at that time, hard crackers and other finger foods can help the infant develop manual dexterity and control of the jaw muscles.

Table 19–3

First Foods for the Infant

Breast milk or iron-fortified formula is the only source of nourishment for the first 4 to 6 months. Throughout the first year, the infant's intake of breast milk or iron-fortified formula will gradually decline as solid food intake increases.

Age (mo)	Addition
4 to 6	Iron-fortified rice cereal, followed by other single-grain cereals, mixed with breast milk, formula, or water
	Pureed vegetables and fruits, one by one (perhaps vegetables before fruits, so the baby will learn to like their less sweet flavors)
6 to 8	Infant breads and crackers
	Mashed vegetables and fruits, and their juices[a]
8 to 10	Breads and cereals from the table
	Soft, cooked vegetables and fruit from the table
	Finely cut meats, fish, chicken, casseroles, cheeses, yogurts, tofu, eggs, and legumes
10 to 12	Continue to introduce a variety of nutritious foods

[a]All baby juices are fortified with vitamin C. Orange juice may cause allergies; apple juice may be a better juice to feed first. Dilute juices with water and offer in a cup to prevent nursing bottle tooth decay.

Source: Adapted in part from Committee on Nutrition, American Academy of Pediatrics, *Pediatric Nutrition Handbook*, 3rd ed., ed. L. A. Barness (Elk Grove Village, Ill.: American Academy of Pediatrics, 1993), pp. 23–33.

Infants differ, and each program of adding foods should depend on the infant, not on a rigid schedule. Indications of readiness for solid foods include:

- The infant's birthweight has doubled.
- The infant can sit with support and can control head movements.
- The infant is four to six months old.

Table 19–3 presents a suggested sequence for adding foods to the infant's diet.

Some parents want to feed solids at an earlier age on the mistaken belief that "stuffing the baby" at bedtime promotes sleeping through the night. On the average, babies start to sleep through the night at about three to four months, regardless of when solid foods are introduced.

The Need for Water   An infant's kidneys are unable to concentrate waste efficiently, so the infant must excrete relatively more water than an adult to carry off a comparable amount of waste. When solid foods are introduced, the risk of dehydration becomes greater, and infants may require supplemental water.

Allergy-Causing Foods   New foods should be introduced singly and at intervals spaced to permit detection of allergies. For example, when cereals are introduced, rice cereal is offered first for several days because it is least likely to cause an allergy. When it is clear that rice cereal is not causing an allergy, another grain is introduced. Wheat cereal is offered last because it is the most common

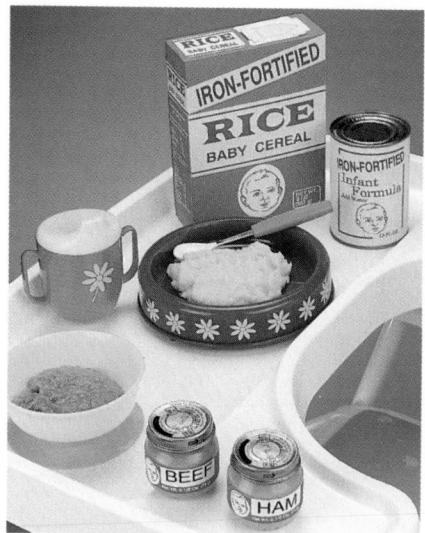

Foods such as iron-fortified cereals and formulas, mashed legumes, and strained meats provide iron.

offender. If a cereal causes an allergic reaction such as skin rash, digestive upset, or respiratory discomfort, its use should be discontinued before introducing the next food. A later section in this chapter offers more on food allergies.

Choice of Infant Foods   Commercial baby foods in the United States and Canada are generally safe, nutritious, and of high quality. They contain little or no salt, less sugar than in the past, and few or no additives. Except for mixed dinners and heavily sweetened desserts, commercial baby foods typically have high nutrient density. Alternatively, parents who want to feed the baby family foods can follow safe food handling practices, cook foods without salt, and "blenderize" small portions at each meal. The foods offered should include good sources of iron and vitamin C.

Foods to Provide Iron   Iron deficiency is common in children throughout the world, especially between six months and three years when they are growing fast and milk, which is a poor source of iron, has a large place in their diets. The iron an infant stored during gestation typically runs out after the birthweight doubles, long before the end of the first year.

In addition to breast milk or formula with iron, infants can receive iron from iron-fortified cereals and, later, from meat or meat alternates such as legumes. Iron-fortified cereals contribute a significant amount of iron to an infant's diet, but the iron's bioavailability is poor. Consequently, cereal alone, or in combination with cow's milk, is insufficient to meet iron needs.[14] During the first year, cereals should be mixed with iron-fortified formula, breast milk, or water rather than cow's milk. Parents or caretakers can enhance iron absorption from iron-fortified cereals by selecting vitamin C–rich foods to go with meals.

Foods to Provide Vitamin C   The best sources of vitamin C are fruits and vegetables. Some authorities suggest that an infant who is introduced to fruits before vegetables may develop a preference for sweets and find the vegetables less palatable. To prevent this, introduce vegetables first, fruits later.

Fruit juices should be diluted and served in a cup, not a bottle. They should also be served in reasonable quantities as part of a balanced selection of foods. Cases have been reported of children failing to grow and thrive because they were drinking such large amounts of juice daily that other more energy- and nutrient-dense foods were displaced from their diets.[15] Such findings prove that any one food—even a healthful and nutritious one—can create nutrient imbalances and impair growth when consumed in excess.

Foods to Omit   Sweets of any other kind, including baby food "desserts," have no place in an infant's diet. They convey no nutrients to support growth, and the extra food energy can promote obesity. Canned vegetables are also inappropriate for infants, as they often contain too much sodium. Honey and corn syrup should never be fed to infants because of the risk of botulism.* Babies and even young children cannot safely chew and swallow popcorn, whole grapes,

botulism (BOT-chew-lism): an often fatal food-borne illness caused by the ingestion of foods containing a toxin produced by bacteria that grow in improperly canned acidic foods (see Chapter 14 for details).

---

*In infants, but not in older individuals, ingestion of *Clostridium botulinum* spores can cause illness when the spores germinate in the intestine and produce toxin, which is absorbed. Symptoms include poor feeding, constipation, loss of tension in the arteries and muscles, weakness, and respiratory compromise. Infant botulism has been implicated in 5 percent of cases of sudden infant death syndrome (SIDS).

Menu

Breakfast
½ c whole milk
3 tbs cereal
1 to 2 tbs fruit
Teething crackers
Morning snack
½ c whole milk
1 to 2 tbs fruit
Teething crackers

Lunch
1 c whole milk
2 to 3 tbs vegetables
2 tbs chopped meat or
    well-cooked, mashed
    legumes
Afternoon snack
½ c whole milk
Teething crackers
1 tbs peanut butter

Dinner
1 c whole milk
1 egg
2 tbs cereal or potato
2 to 3 tbs vegetables
2 to 3 tbs fruit

Sample Menu for a One-Year-Old

Note: Fruit choices need to include citrus fruits, melons, and berries and vegetable choices need to include dark green, leafy and deep yellow vegetables.

whole beans, hot dog slices, hard candies, and nuts; they can easily choke on these foods, a risk not worth taking.

Foods at One Year   At one year of age, whole cow's milk becomes the primary source of most of the nutrients an infant needs; 2 to 3½ cups a day meets those needs sufficiently. More milk than this displaces foods necessary to provide iron and can lead to milk anemia. Children one to two years old should drink whole milk, not low-fat or nonfat milk. If they use powdered milk, it should be one of the fat-containing varieties. Other foods—meats, iron-fortified cereals, enriched or whole-grain breads, fruits, and vegetables—should be supplied in variety and in amounts sufficient to round out total energy needs. Ideally, a one-year-old will sit at the table, eat many of the same foods everyone else eats, and drink liquids from a cup, not a bottle. The accompanying menu shows a sample meal plan that meets a one-year-old's requirements.

milk anemia: iron-deficiency anemia that develops when an excessive milk intake displaces iron-rich foods from the diet.

MEALTIMES WITH INFANTS

The wise parent of a one-year-old offers nutrition and love together. "Feeding with love" produces better growth and brain development than feeding the same food without love.

The person feeding a one-year-old has to be aware that exploring and experimenting are normal and desirable behaviors at this time in a child's life. The child is developing a sense of autonomy that, if fostered, will provide the foundation for later confidence and effectiveness as an individual. The child's impulses, if consistently denied, can turn to shame and self-doubt. In light of the developmental needs of one-year-olds and their often willful behavior, a few

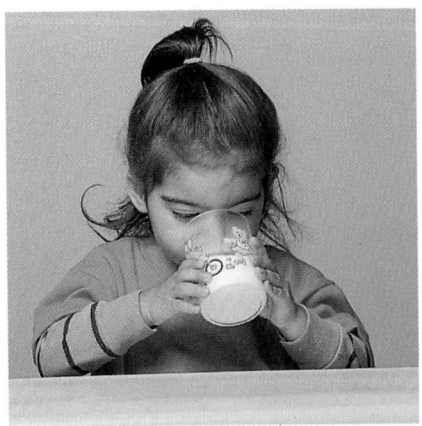

Toddlers need vitamin A– and vitamin D–fortified whole milk.

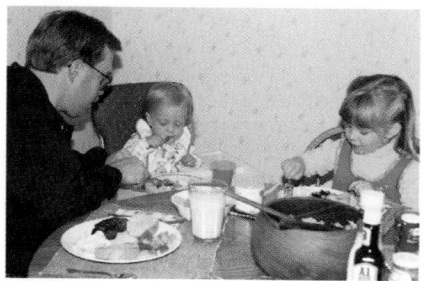

Ideally, a one-year-old eats many of the same foods as the rest of the family.

feeding guidelines may be helpful:

- Discourage unacceptable behavior, such as standing at the table or throwing food, by removing the child from the table to wait until later to eat. Be consistent and firm, not punitive. The child will soon learn to sit and eat.
- Let the child explore and enjoy food, even if this means eating with fingers for a while. Use of the spoon will come in time.
- Don't force food on children. Rejecting new foods is normal; acceptance is more likely as infants and children become familiar with new foods through repeated opportunities to taste them.[16]
- Provide children with nutritious foods, and let them choose which ones and how much they will eat. Gradually, they will acquire a taste for different foods.
- Limit sweets. Infants have little room in their daily energy allowance for empty-kcalorie foods. Do not use sweets as a reward for eating meals.
- Don't turn the dining table into a battleground. Make mealtimes enjoyable. Teach children healthy food choices and eating habits in a pleasant environment.

These recommendations reflect the spirit of tolerance that best serves the emotional and physical interests of the young child.

To recap, the primary food for infants during the first 6 to 12 months is either breast milk or iron-fortified formulas. In addition to nutrients, breast milk also offers immunological protection. At about 4 to 6 months, infants should gradually begin eating solid foods so that by 1 year, they are drinking from a cup and eating many of the same foods as the rest of the family.

Nutrition during Childhood

Each year from age one to adolescence, a child typically grows taller by 2 to 3 inches and heavier by 5 or so pounds. Growth charts provide valuable clues to a child's health. Weight gains out of proportion to height gains may reflect overeating and inactivity, whereas measures significantly below the standard suggest malnutrition.

Increases in height and weight are only two of the many developmental changes occurring during childhood. At age one, children can stand alone and are learning to toddle; by two, they can walk and are learning to run; by three, they can jump and are climbing with confidence. Bones and muscles increase in mass and density to make these accomplishments possible. Thereafter, further lengthening of the long bones and increases in musculature proceed, unevenly and more slowly, until adolescence.

ENERGY AND NUTRIENT NEEDS

Children's appetites begin to diminish around one year, consistent with the slowing of growth. Thereafter, children spontaneously vary their food intakes to coincide with their growth patterns; they demand more food during periods of rapid growth than during slow periods. At times they seem to be insatiable, and at other times they seem to live on air and water.

Although children's energy intakes may vary widely from meal to meal, their total daily intakes are remarkably constant.[17] If children eat less at one meal, they typically eat more at the next, and vice versa. Overweight children are an exception: they do not always adjust their energy intakes appropriately and may eat in response to external cues, disregarding appetite-regulation signals.

Energy Intake and Activity A one-year-old child needs perhaps 1000 kcalories a day; a three-year-old needs only 300 kcalories more. By age ten, a child needs about 2000 kcalories a day. Total energy needs increase slightly with age, but energy needs per kilogram body weight actually decline gradually.

Individual children's energy needs vary widely, depending on their physical activity. Inactive children can become obese even when they eat less food than the average. They would do well to learn to enjoy physical play and exercise.

Vitamins and Minerals Steady growth during childhood implies gradually increasing needs of all nutrients. Before adolescence, children accumulate stores of nutrients. Then, when they take off on the adolescent growth spurt and their nutrient intakes cannot meet the demands of rapid growth, they draw on those stores. This is especially true of calcium; the denser the bones grow in childhood, the better they can support teen growth and still withstand the inevitable bone losses of later life. The way preteen children eat, then, influences their nutritional health during childhood, during their teen years—and in their old age.

Planning Children's Meals To provide all the needed nutrients, children's meals should include a variety of foods from each food group—in amounts suited to their appetites and needs. Serving sizes increase with age. A portion of meat, grains, fruits, or vegetables for children is loosely defined as 1 tablespoon per year. Thus, at four years of age, a portion is about 4 tablespoons, or ¼ cup. This rule of thumb applies until they reach the teen years. Table 19–4 offers a daily food pattern for children.

To ensure that children have healthy appetites and plenty of room for nutritious foods when they are hungry, parents and teachers must limit access to candy, cola, and other concentrated sweets. If such foods are permitted in large quantities, the only possible outcomes are nutrient deficiencies, obesity, or both. The preference for sweets is innate; most children do not naturally select nutritious foods on the basis of taste. In one study, when children were allowed to create meals freely from a variety of foods, they selected foods that provided 25 percent of the kcalories from sugar.[18] When their parents were watching, or even when they thought their parents were watching, the children improved their selections. Overweight children, especially, need help in sticking to nutrient-dense foods that will meet their nutrient needs within their energy allowances.

Sweets need not be banned altogether. Children who are exceptionally active can enjoy high-kcalorie foods such as ice cream or pudding from the milk group or pancakes or cookies from the bread group. These foods carry valuable nutrients and bring pleasure. As for sedentary children, they need to become more active, and then they, too, can enjoy some of these foods without unhealthy weight gain.

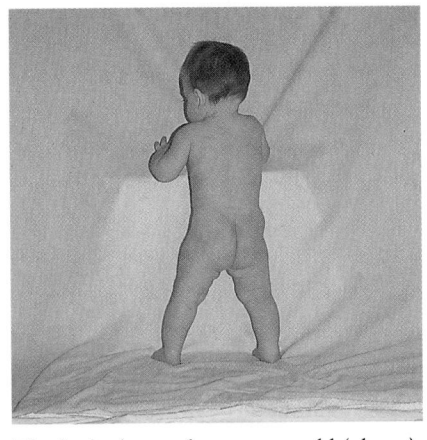

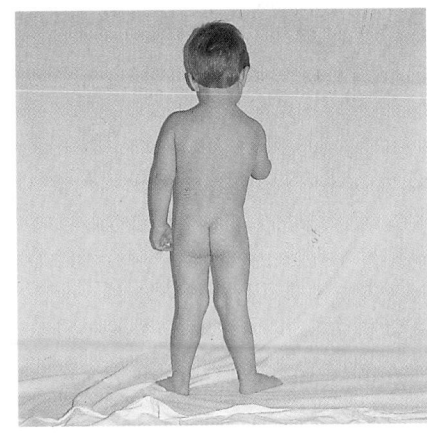

The body shape of a one-year-old (above) changes dramatically by age two (below). The two-year-old has lost much of the baby fat; the muscles (especially in the back, buttocks, and legs) have firmed and strengthened; and the leg bones have lengthened.

Table 19–4
....
Children's Daily Food Patterns for Good Nutrition

Food Group	Servings per Day	Average Size of Serving		
		1 TO 3 YEARS	4 TO 6 YEARS	7 TO 12 YEARS
Bread and cereals (whole grain or enriched)[a]	6 or more	½ slice	1 slice	1 to 2 slices
Vegetables[b]	3 or more	2–4 tbs or ½ c juice	¼–½ c or ½ c juice	½–¾ c or ½ c juice
Fruits[b]	2 or more	2–4 tbs or ½ c juice	¼–½ c or ½ c juice	½–¾ c or ½ c juice
Meat and meat alternates[c]	2 or more	1–2 oz	1–2 oz	2–3 oz
Milk and milk products[d]	3 to 4	½–¾ c	¾ c	¾–1 c

[a]1 slice bread = ¾ c dry cereal, ½ c cooked cereal, ½ c potato, rice, or noodles.
[b]Vitamin C source (citrus fruits, berries, tomatoes, broccoli, cabbage, cantaloupe) daily; vitamin A source (spinach, carrots, squash, tomato, cantaloupe) 3 to 4 times weekly.
[c]1 oz meat, fish, poultry = 1 egg, 1 frankfurter, 2 tbs peanut butter, ½ c cooked legumes.
[d]½ c milk = ½ c cottage cheese, pudding, yogurt; ¾ oz cheese; 2 tbs dried milk.
Source: Adapted from P. M. Queen and R. R. Henry, Growth and nutrient requirements of children, in *Pediatric Nutrition*, eds. R. J. Grand, J. L. Sutphen, and W. H. Dietz, Jr. (Boston: Butterworths, 1987), p. 347.

HUNGER AND MALNUTRITION IN CHILDREN

Most U.S. and Canadian children are well nourished. Their average energy intakes are sufficient to support normal growth, and their average nutrient intakes, except for iron, meet or exceed recommendations. Some low-income children, however, are malnourished and have suffered growth retardation. An estimated 11 million U.S. children under age 12 are hungry and living in poverty.

Highlight 18 examines the causes and consequences of hunger in the United States and around the world.

HEALTHY PEOPLE 2000: Reduce growth retardation among low-income children aged five years and younger to less than 10%.

Malnutrition and Health   When hunger is chronic, children become malnourished. Worldwide, malnutrition takes a devastating toll on children, contributing to nearly half of the deaths of children under four years old. Vitamin A deficiency afflicts more than 5 million children worldwide, inducing blindness, stunted growth, and infections. Zinc deficiency also retards growth and typically accompanies protein-energy malnutrition and vitamin A deficiency.

Hunger and Behavior   Even when hunger is temporary, as when a child misses one meal, behavior and academic performance are affected. Children who eat nutritious breakfasts function better than their peers who do not. Young children who participate in the federally funded School Breakfast Program improve their scores on achievement tests and are tardy or absent significantly less often than children who qualify for the program, but do not participate. Without breakfast, children perform poorly in tasks requiring concentration, their attention spans are shorter, and they even show lower IQs on testing than their well-fed peers; malnourished children are particularly vulnerable. Common sense dictates that it is unreasonable to expect anyone to learn and perform work when no fuel has been provided. By late morning, discomfort from hunger may become distracting even if a child has eaten breakfast.

The problem children face when attempting morning schoolwork on an empty stomach appears to be at least partly due to low blood glucose. The average child up to age ten or so needs to eat every four to six hours to maintain a blood glucose concentration high enough to support the activity of the brain and nervous system. A child's brain is as big as an adult's, and the brain is the body's chief glucose consumer. A child's liver is much smaller than an adult's, however, and the liver is the organ responsible for storing glucose as glycogen and releasing it into the blood as needed. A child's liver can store only about four hours' worth of glycogen—hence the need to eat fairly often. Teachers aware of the late-morning slump in their classrooms wisely request that midmorning snacks be provided; snacks improve classroom performance all the way to lunchtime. For the child who hasn't had breakfast, the morning's lessons may be lost altogether.

Eating breakfast also helps children to meet their nutrient needs each day. Children who skip breakfast typically do not make up the deficits at later meals—they simply have lower intakes of energy, vitamins, and minerals than those who eat breakfast.[19]

Iron Deficiency   Iron-deficiency anemia is a major problem worldwide, as well as being the most prevalent nutrient deficiency among U.S. and Canadian children. The high iron needs of growth combined with typically low iron intakes leave many children with marginal iron status. Reducing iron deficiency among young children is one of the foremost health priorities in the United States.[20] Internationally, the World Health Organization is collaborating with a United Nations subcommittee on nutrition to develop a ten-year plan to eliminate iron deficiency.[21]

 HEALTHY PEOPLE 2000: Reduce iron deficiency to less than 3% among children aged one through four years.

To prevent iron deficiency, children's foods must deliver approximately 10 milligrams of iron per day. To achieve this goal, snacks and meals should include the iron-rich foods listed in Table 19–5, and milk should be limited to 3 or 4 cups a day, so that it will not displace lean meats, fish, poultry, eggs, legumes, and whole-grain or enriched products.

Iron Deficiency and Behavior   Iron deficiency has well-known and widespread effects on children's behavior. In addition to carrying oxygen in the blood, iron transports oxygen within cells, which use it to help produce energy. Iron is also used to make neurotransmitters—most notably, those that regulate the ability to pay attention, which is crucial to learning. An iron deficiency not only causes an energy crisis but also directly affects mood, attention span, and learning ability.

Iron deficiency is usually diagnosed by a deficit of iron in the *blood*, after the deficiency has progressed all the way to anemia. A child's *brain*, however, is sensitive to low iron concentrations long before the blood effects appear. Research has shown that iron deficiency lowers the "motivation to persist in intellectually

The brain uses about three times as much glucose per day as the rest of the body.

Table 19–5

Iron-Rich Foods Children Like[a]

Breads, cereals, and grains
Canned macaroni (½ c)
Canned spaghetti (½ c)
Cream of wheat (¼ c)
Fortified dry cereals (1 oz)[b]
Noodles, rice, or barley (½ c)
Tortillas (1 flour, 2 corn)
Whole-wheat, enriched, or fortified bread (1 slice)
Bran muffins
Vegetables
Baked flavored potato skins (½ skin)
Cooked mushrooms (½ c)
Cooked mung bean sprouts or snow peas (½ c)
Green peas (½ c)
Mixed vegetable juice (1 c)
Fruits
Apple juice (1 c)
Canned plums (3 plums)
Cooked dried apricots (½ c)
Dried peaches (4 halves)
Raisins (1 tbs)
Meats and legumes
Bean dip (¼ c)
Canned pork and beans (⅓ c)
Mild chili or other bean/meat dishes (¼ c) such as burritos
Liverwurst (½ oz)
Meat casseroles (½ c)
Peanut butter and jelly sandwich (½ sandwich)
Lean roast beef or cooked ground beef (1 oz)
Sloppy joes (½ sandwich)

[a]Each serving provides at least 1 milligram iron, or one-tenth of a child's RDA for iron. Vitamin C–rich foods included with these snacks increase iron absorption.

[b]Some fortified breakfast cereals contain more than 10 milligrams iron per half-cup serving (read the labels).

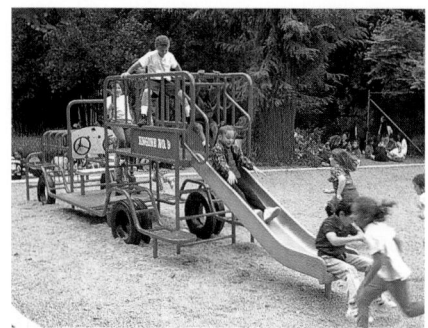

Healthy, well-nourished children are alert in the classroom and energetic at play.

challenging tasks," shortens the attention span, and impairs overall intellectual performance. Anemic children perform less well on tests and are more disruptive than their nonanemic classmates. At least one study found that children who had had iron-deficiency anemia *as infants* still continued to perform poorly at age five compared with their peers, even though they had regained excellent iron status.[22] The long-term damaging effects on mental development make prevention of iron deficiency during infancy and early childhood a high priority.[23]

Other Nutrient Deficiencies and Behavior   Iron is not the only nutrient that can be displaced from a diet by nutrient-poor foods. Several dozen other nutrients may be lacking as well, causing both physical and behavioral symptoms.

A child with nutrient deficiencies may be irritable, aggressive, disagreeable, or sad and withdrawn. Such a child may be labeled "hyperactive," "depressed," or "unlikable," when in fact these traits may arise from simple, even marginal, malnutrition. In any such case, inspection of the child's diet by a qualified health care professional is clearly in order. Should suspicion of dietary inadequacies be raised, no matter what causes may be implicated, the people responsible for feeding the child should take steps to correct those inadequacies promptly.

Lead Toxicity and Malnutrition   Malnutrition is quite often a complex condition involving multiple nutrients and other environmental factors. An example of a possible complicating factor is lead poisoning. Lead toxicity can cause iron deficiency, and iron deficiency can impair the body's defenses against lead absorption. Highlight 13 describes the mental, behavioral, and other health problems associated with lead toxicity. Such problems are important to investigate, but even before they have been identified, the child should be fed properly.

Parents and medical practitioners often overlook the possibility that malnutrition may account for abnormalities of appearances and behavior. Any departure from normal healthy appearance and behavior is a sign of possible poor nutrition (see Table 19–6).

NUTRITION, HYPERACTIVITY, AND "HYPER" BEHAVIOR

Because malnutrition can impair children's functioning in many ways, people tend to look to food habits for explanations of hyperactivity. Hyperactivity is not caused by a poor diet, but a poor diet may be part of a cluster of factors seen in a hyperactive child's life.

Tension-Fatigue Syndrome   Children can become excitable, rambunctious, and unruly out of a desire for attention, lack of sleep, overstimulation, too much television, or a lack of physical activity. Together, these factors produce the tension-fatigue syndrome, which suggests that more consistent care, and not just better food, is needed. It helps most to insist on regular hours of sleep, regular mealtimes, and regular outdoor activity.

Hyperactivity   Hyperactivity is a condition that may affect behavior and learning in about 5 percent of young school-age children. Left untreated, hyperactivity can interfere with a child's social development and ability to learn. Treatment focuses on relieving the symptoms and controlling the associated problems; there is no cure.

tension-fatigue syndrome: apparent hyperactivity produced in a child by the combination of lack of sleep, overstimulation, and anxiety.

hyperactivity: a condition of excessive activity. When hyperactivity is accompanied by an inability to pay attention and poor impulse control, professionals call this syndrome **attention deficit hyperactivity disorder (ADHD)**

Table 19–6

Physical Signs of Health and Malnutrition in Children

	Healthy	Malnourished
Hair:	Shiny, firm in the scalp	Dull, brittle, dry, loose; falls out
Eyes:	Bright, clear pink membranes; adjust easily to darkness	Pale membranes; spots; redness; adjust slowly to darkness
Teeth and gums:	No pain or cavities, gums firm, teeth bright	Missing, discolored, decayed teeth; gums bleed easily and are swollen and spongy
Face:	Good complexion	Off-color, scaly, flaky, cracked skin
Glands:	No lumps	Swollen at front of neck and cheeks
Tongue:	Red, bumpy, rough	Sore, smooth, purplish, swollen
Skin:	Smooth, firm, good color	Dry, rough, spotty; "sandpaper" feel or sores; lack of fat under skin
Nails:	Firm, pink	Spoon-shaped brittle, ridged
Behavior:	Alert, attentive, cheerful	Irritable, apathetic, inattentive, hyperactive
Internal systems:	Heart rate, heart rhythm, and blood pressure normal; normal digestive function; reflexes and psychological development normal	Heart rate, heart rhythm, or blood pressure abnormal; liver and spleen enlarged; abnormal digestion; mental irritability, confusion; burning, tingling of hands and feet; loss of balance and coordination
Muscles and bones:	Good muscle tone and posture; long bones straight	"Wasted" appearance of muscles; swollen bumps on skull or ends of bones; small bumps on ribs; bowed legs or knock-knees

Note: The physical signs shown here are consistent with malnutrition but not diagnostic of it.

Physicians often manage hyperactivity through behavior modification, special educational techniques, psychological counseling, and drug therapy. The drugs most commonly prescribed are stimulants. Normally, stimulants speed up people's activity, but they have a paradoxical effect on hyperactivity: they normalize it by stimulating control centers in the brain. If a child calms down when given stimulant drugs, the response indicates that the drugs may be correcting a biochemical imbalance in the nervous system and can help control the behavior.

Many parents mistakenly believe a solution may lie in manipulating the diet—most commonly, by eliminating sugar or food additives. Diet is one area of a child's life in which parents feel they can exert some control. If problems can be solved by adding carrots or eliminating candy, then parents are eager to give diet advice a try. While nutrition should be considered whenever a person's health is less than optimal, it is unwise to jump at appealing solutions that are unfounded. Several studies have found no convincing evidence that sugar causes hyperactivity or worsens behavior.[24] Recommendations to restrict sugar in children's diets to prevent or treat behavior problems are groundless. Sugar can influence children's behavior only by displacing nutritious foods and contributing to nutrient deficiencies.

Caffeine and Behavior   Caffeine is often overlooked as a source of "hyper" behavior in children, but it is a matter of some concern to pediatricians. A 12-

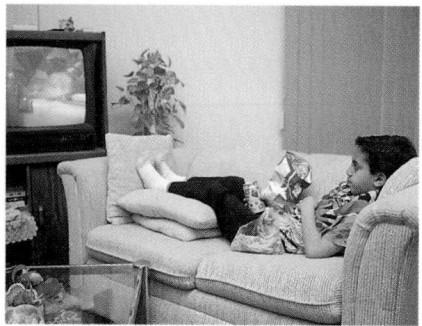

Television watching influences children's eating habits and activity patterns.

TV fosters obesity because it:
- Requires no energy beyond basal metabolism.
- Replaces vigorous activities.
- Encourages snacking.
- Promotes a sedentary lifestyle.

Playing computer games influences activity patterns similarly.

adverse reactions: unusual responses to food (including intolerances and allergies).

food intolerances: adverse reactions to foods that do not involve the immune system.

food allergies: adverse reactions to foods that involve an immune response; also called *food-hypersensitivity reactions.*

ounce cola beverage may contain as much as 50 milligrams caffeine; in the body of a 60-pound child, two or more such beverages are equivalent to the caffeine in 8 cups of coffee for a 175-pound adult. Children who are troubled by sleeplessness, restlessness, and irregular heartbeats may need to limit their caffeine consumption. Children not accustomed to caffeine who are given doses equivalent to about two cola beverages a day become noticeably inattentive and restless. As long as children are surrounded by attractive temptations such as cola beverages, adults must prevent abuse until the children learn to control consumption themselves. (Appendix H presents a table that lists the caffeine contents of foods, beverages, and medicines.)

TELEVISION AND CHILDREN'S NUTRITION

The average child watches 5000 hours of television before the end of preschool and has seen 19,000 hours by the end of high school.[25] Watching programs or videos on television is second only to sleeping among children's uses of time.

Besides contributing to tension-fatigue syndrome, watching television adversely affects children's nutritional health in several ways. As Chapter 9 reported, studies have found that the prevalence of obesity increases with each hour of television viewed; even daydreaming appears to use more energy than watching television.[26] Children who watch more than two hours of television per day also have higher serum cholesterol than do more active children.

The average child sees an estimated 10,000 commercials a year—almost all luring viewers to purchase sugar-coated breakfast cereals, candy bars, chips, fast foods, and carbonated beverages. These foods add sugar, fat, and salt to the diet and displace foods that provide needed nutrients. Many parents and pediatricians believe that food ads aimed at children should be banned because they support corporate profits rather than children's health. Alternatively, parents can teach their children how to evaluate food ads and make healthful choices.

ADVERSE REACTIONS TO FOODS

Adverse reactions to foods can threaten nutritional health to varying extents, depending on the severity and duration of the reactions and the foods they involve. Temporary reactions may lead to permanent avoidance of foods; permanent reactions, if not detected and treated, can cause chronic illness.

Food Intolerances Not all adverse reactions to foods are food allergies, although even physicians may describe them as such. Signs of adverse reactions to foods include stomachaches, headaches, pain, rapid pulse rate, nausea, wheezing, hives, bronchial irritation, coughs, and other such discomforts. Among the causes may be reactions to chemicals in foods, such as the flavor enhancer monosodium glutamate (MSG), the natural laxative in prunes, or the mineral sulfur; digestive diseases, such as obstructions or injuries; enzyme deficiencies, such as lactose intolerance; and even psychological aversions. These reactions involve symptoms but no antibody production. Therefore, they are food intolerances, not allergies.[27]

Food Allergies A true food allergy occurs when a whole food protein or other large molecule enters the body and elicits an immunologic response. (Recall that large molecules of food are normally dismantled in the digestive tract to smaller ones that are absorbed without such a reaction.) The body's immune system reacts to a large food molecule as it does to other antigens—by producing antibodies, histamines, or other defensive agents.

Allergies may have one or two components. They always involve antibodies; they may or may not involve symptoms. This means that allergies can be diagnosed only by testing for antibodies. Even symptoms exactly like those of an allergy may not be caused by one.

Allergic reactions to food may be immediate or delayed. In both cases, the antigen interacts immediately with the immune system, but the timing of symptoms varies from minutes to 24 hours. Identifying the food that causes an immediate allergic reaction is easy because the symptoms correlate closely with the time of eating the food. Identifying the food that causes a delayed reaction is more difficult because the symptoms may not appear until a day later. By this time, many other foods have been eaten, complicating the picture.

Almost 75 percent of adverse reactions are caused by three major foods—eggs, peanuts, or milk.[28] Allergic reactions to single foods are common. Reactions to multiple foods are the exception, not the rule.

Identifying a true food allergy requires a thorough health history, physical examination, and diagnostic tests to eliminate other diseases.[29] Skin pricks with food extracts are one of the most common tests for food allergies, even though the high incidence of false positive results can complicate diagnosis. Physicians also conduct dietary trials that first eliminate the offending food and then reintroduce it in small quantities to substantiate that reactions occur only when that particular food is eaten.[30] Once a food allergy has been diagnosed, therapy requires strict elimination of the offending food.

Food allergies are most common during the first few years of life, but then children typically outgrow (become tolerant to) their hypersensitivity. Between 2 and 8 percent of young children are allergic to certain foods, whereas only 2 percent of adults have food allergies.[31] Tolerance is most likely if the offending food can be identified and eliminated from the diet for at least a year or two.[32]

When parents stop serving a suspected food to their child, they risk the child's suffering nutrient deficiencies. They should be sure to include other foods that offer the same nutrients as the omitted food. Children with allergies, like all children, need all their nutrients.

Healthful food choices and regular physical activity both promote growth and help prevent the degenerative diseases of later life—cardiovascular disease, cancer, diabetes, and osteoporosis. In contrast, poor food choices and lack of exercise can lead to obesity, elevated cholesterol levels, and hypertension—major risk factors for degenerative diseases. The highlight that follows this chapter describes how behaviors during the childhood and teen years influence disease in adulthood. The next two sections examine how children's eating behaviors are shaped both at home and at school.

MEALTIMES AT HOME

The childhood years represent a parent's best, and maybe last, chance to influence food choices. Parents are gatekeepers; they determine what foods and activities will be available in their children's environments. Then the children make their own selections. One survey reports that 65 percent of fourth through eighth graders choose their own breakfasts, 46 percent select their lunches, and 74 per-

For help with food allergies, call the Food Allergy network at (800) 929-4040.

histamine (HISS-tah-mean, or HISS-tah-men): a substance produced by cells of the immune system as part of a local immune reaction to an antigen; participates in causing inflammation.

A person who produces antibodies *without* having any symptoms has an **asymptomatic allergy**; a person who produces antibodies *and* has symptoms has a **symptomatic allergy**.

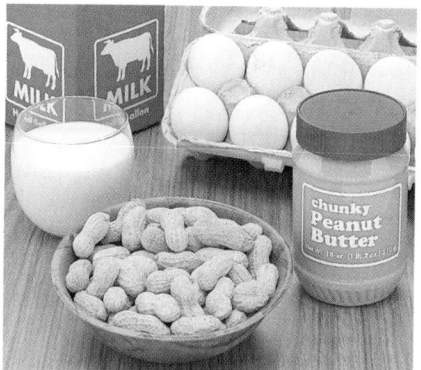

Eggs, peanuts, and milk are most likely to induce symptoms in people with food allergy.

gatekeepers: with respect to nutrition, key people who control other people's access to foods and thereby exert profound impacts on their nutrition. Examples are the spouse who buys and cooks the food, the parent who feeds the children, and the caretaker in a day-care center.

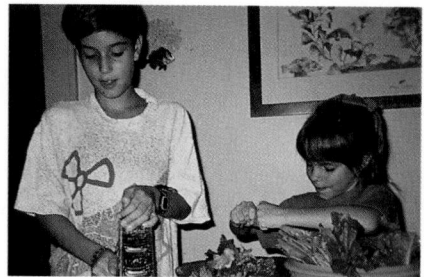

Children enjoy eating the foods they help to prepare.

- Child feeding pointer: Provide child-sized portions and utensils.

- Child feeding pointer: Serve vegetables raw or slightly undercooked and crunchy.

- Child feeding pointer: Encourage children to help plan and prepare meals.

- Child feeding pointer: Offer children nutritious foods, but don't insist that they eat.

cent select their snacks.[33] Gatekeepers who want to promote nutritious choices and healthful habits provide access to nutrient-dense, delicious foods and opportunities for active play at home.

Honoring Children's Preferences   Little children like to eat at little tables and to be served little portions of food. They also like to eat with other children, and they tend to eat more in the company of their peers. Children also more easily overcome their prejudices against foods when they see their peers eating them.

Children usually like raw vegetables better than cooked ones, so it is wise to offer vegetables that are raw or slightly undercooked and crunchy, served separately, and easy to eat. Foods should be warm, not hot, because a child's mouth is much more sensitive than an adult's. The flavor should be mild because a child has more taste buds, and smooth foods such as mashed potatoes or pea soup should contain no lumps (a child wonders, with some disgust, what the lumps might be). Children prefer foods that are familiar, so offer various foods regularly.

Learning through Participation   Helping to plan and prepare family meals can be an enjoyable learning experience. Children are also more likely to eat the foods they have prepared. Vegetables are pretty, especially when fresh, and provide opportunities for children to learn about color, about growing things and their seeds, and about shapes and textures—all of which are fascinating to young children. Measuring, stirring, washing, and arranging vegetables are skills that even a young child can practice with enjoyment and pride.

Avoiding Power Struggles   When introducing new foods at the table, parents are advised to offer them one at a time and only in small amounts at first. The more often a food is presented to a young child, the more likely the child will like that food. Whenever possible, offer the new food at the beginning of the meal, when the child is hungry, and allow the child to make the decision to accept or reject it. Never make an issue of food acceptance, not even to reward acceptance. Children who are pushed to try new foods are less likely to try those foods again than children who are left to decide for themselves. The parent is responsible for *what* the child is offered to eat, but the child is responsible for *how much* and even *whether* to eat.

A bright, unhurried atmosphere free of conflict is conducive to good appetite. Parents who serve meals in a relaxed and casual manner, without anxiety, provide a climate that minimizes a child's negative emotions. Unaware parents can promote conflicts, despite their good intentions. Parents who beg, cajole, and demand that their children eat deny opportunities to develop self-control. Instead, the children engage in battles that take on more importance than their own hunger. A power struggle almost invariably results in a confirmed pattern of resistance and a permanently closed mind on the child's part.

- Child feeding pointer: To prevent choking, watch children eat and enforce a "sit-down" rule.

Young children can easily choke on:
- Popcorn.
- Hot dog slices.
- Whole grapes.
- Hard candies.
- Whole beans.
- Nuts.

- Child feeding pointer: Play first, then eat.

Choking Prevention   Parents must always be alert to the dangers of choking. A choking child is a silent child, and an adult should be present whenever a child is eating. Serve foods cut into small bite-size pieces and encourage children to sit when eating; choking is more likely when a child is running or falling. (Highlight 3 describes the Heimlich maneuver for children.)

Play First   Ideally, each meal is preceded, not followed, by fun activities. A number of schools have discovered that children eat a much better lunch if recess occurs before, rather than after, the meal—otherwise children "hurry up and eat" so that they can go play.

Snacks　　Parents may find that their children snack so much that they aren't hungry at mealtimes. Instead of teaching children *not* to snack, parents might be wise to teach them *how* to snack. Provide snacks that are as nutritious as the foods served at mealtime. Snacks can even be mealtime foods served individually over time, instead of all at once on one plate. When providing snacks to children, a smart parent thinks of the food groups and offers such snacks as pieces of cheese, tangerine slices, carrot sticks, and peanut butter on whole-wheat crackers. Snacks need to be easy to prepare, especially for children who arrive home from school before parents.

- Child feeding pointer: Provide healthful snacks.

Preventing Dental Caries　　Children frequently snack on sticky, sugary foods that stay on the teeth and provide an ideal environment for the growth of bacteria that cause dental caries. Teach children to eat sweets at mealtimes, to brush and floss after meals, to brush or rinse after eating snacks, to avoid sticky foods, and to select crisp or fibrous foods instead. Table 19–7 lists food suggestions for controlling dental caries.

Serving as Role Models　　In an effort to practice these many tips, parents may overlook perhaps the single most important influence on their children's food habits—themselves. Parents who don't eat carrots shouldn't be surprised when their children refuse to eat carrots. Likewise, parents who dislike the smell

- Child feeding pointer: Set a good example—enjoy nutritious foods.

Table 19–7

Food Suggestions for Controlling Dental Caries

Food Group	Frequent Use Recommended	Infrequent Use Suggested[a]
Milk/milk products	Milk, cheese, plain yogurt	Chocolate milk, ice cream, ice milk, milk shakes, fruited yogurt
Meat/meat alternates	Lean meat, fish, poultry; eggs; legumes	Peanut butter with added sugar, lunch meats with added sugar, meats with sugared glazes
Fruits	Fresh or packed in water	Dried, packed in syrup or juice, jams, jellies, preserves, fruit juices or drinks
Vegetables	Salad greens, cauliflower, cucumbers, radishes, carrots, celery	Candied sweet potatoes, glazed carrots
Bread/cereal	Popcorn, soda crackers, toast, hard rolls, pretzels, corn chips, pizza	Cookies, sweet rolls, pies, cakes, potato chips, ready-to-eat sweetened cereals as between-meal snacks
Other	Sugarless gum	Sugared soft drinks, candy, fudge, caramels, honey, sugars, syrups

[a]It is particularly important to brush, floss, and rinse after eating these foods.

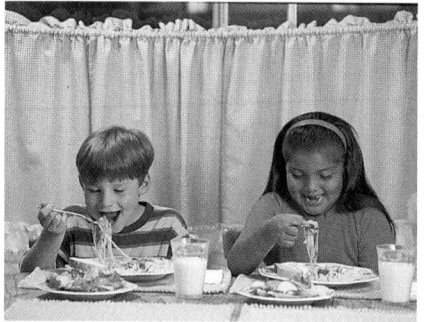

Eating is more fun when your friends are there.

of brussels sprouts may not be able to persuade children to try them. Children learn much through imitation. Parents and older siblings set an irresistible example by enjoying nutritious foods.

While serving and enjoying food, caretakers can promote both physical and emotional growth at every stage of a child's life. They can help their children to develop both a positive self-concept and a positive attitude toward food. If the beginnings are right, children will grow without the conflicts and confusions over food that can lead to nutrition and health problems.

NUTRITION AT SCHOOL

While parents are doing what they can to establish good eating habits in their children at home, child-care centers and schools are introducing foods prepared and served by others. In addition, children begin to learn about food and nutrition in the classroom. Meeting the nutrition and education needs of children is critical to supporting their healthy growth and development.[34]

School Meals   The U.S. government funds several programs to provide nutritious meals for children at school. Both the School Breakfast Program and the National School Lunch Program provide meals at a reasonable cost to children from families with the financial means to pay. Meals are available free or at reduced cost to children from low-income families. (School lunches in Canada are administered locally and therefore vary from area to area.) Several studies have reported that children who participate in school food programs show improvements in learning. The accompanying box describes food programs for children, and Table 19–8 shows school lunch patterns for children of different ages.

 HEALTHY PEOPLE 2000: Increase to at least 90% the proportion of school lunch and breakfast services and increase to at least 50% the proportion of child-care foodservices with menus that are consistent with the nutrition principles in the *Dietary Guidelines for Americans*.

Table 19–8

School Lunch Patterns for Different Ages

Food Group	Preschool (Age)		Grade School through High School (Grade)		
	1 TO 2	3 TO 4	K TO 3	4 TO 6	7 TO 12
Meat or meat alternate 1 serving:					
Lean meat, poultry, or fish	1 oz	1½ oz	1½ oz	2 oz	3 oz
Cheese	1 oz	1½ oz	1½ oz	2 oz	3 oz
Large egg(s)	1	1½	1½	2	3
Cooked dry beans or peas	½ c	¾ c	¾ c	1 c	1½ c
Peanut butter	2 tbs	3 tbs	3 tbs	4 tbs	6 tbs
Vegetable and/or fruit					
2 or more servings, both to total	½ c	½ c	½ c	¾ c	¾ c
Bread or bread alternate					
Servings	5 per week	8 per week	8 per week	8 per week	10 per week
Milk					
1 serving of fluid milk	¾ c	¾ c	1 c	1 c	1 c

Food Assistance Programs for Children

The federal School Lunch and School Breakfast Programs assist schools financially so that every student can receive a nutritious lunch, breakfast, or both. These programs enable schools to provide low-income students with meals at no cost while charging other students somewhat less than the full costs of their meals. In addition, schools that participate in the programs can obtain food commodities. Nationally, the U.S. Department of Agriculture (USDA) administers the programs; on the state level, state departments of education operate them (although Congress may change this arrangement in its efforts to cut federal spending). The programs usually cost school districts little.

Nearly 25 million children receive lunches through the National School Lunch Program—half of them at a free or reduced price. School lunches are designed to provide at least a third of the RDA for each of many nutrients and must include specified numbers of servings of milk, protein-rich foods (meat, poultry, fish, cheese, eggs, legumes, or peanut butter), vegetables, fruits, and breads or other grain foods.

The School Breakfast Program is available in slightly more than half of the nation's schools, and about 5 million children participate in it. The school breakfast must provide at least a fourth of the RDA for each of many nutrients and contain at least one serving of milk; one serving of fruit, juice, or vegetable; and either two servings of bread (or bread alternates), two servings of meat (or meat alternates), or one serving of each.

Another federal program, the Child Care Food Program, operates similarly and provides funds to organized child-care programs. All eligible children, centers, and family day-care homes have the right to participate. Meal reimbursements cover most of the meal and administration costs. Sponsors may also receive USDA commodity foods.

School lunches offer a variety of food choices and are available to most children. To their credit, these lunches help our nation's children meet at least one-third of their daily RDA. These lunches are supposed to meet the *Dietary Guidelines*, but unfortunately, almost all of the participating schools exceed recommendations for fat, saturated fat, and sodium and fall short on recommendations for carbohydrate.[35] Yet given the choice, many children will select low-fat meals.[36] Schools that have made special efforts to lower fat in school lunches typically have trouble providing enough energy and nutrients, especially iron, to meet the RDA specifications. The American Dietetic Association (ADA) advocates the development of dietary guidelines specifically for children to ensure that school lunches will both provide adequate energy and nutrients and support health.[37] According to the ADA, the guidelines currently used may be appropriate for adults, but may not be adequate to meet children's unique needs.

Nutrition Education at School   Coincident with the school breakfast and lunch programs is a program of nutrition education and training (NET) in all the public schools. This program is minimally funded, but program administrators are ingenious and creative in accomplishing its highest-priority objectives. Children need to be fed well *and* learn enough about nutrition to make healthful food choices when the choices become theirs to make.

 HEALTHY PEOPLE 2000: Increase to at least 75% the proportion of the nation's schools that provide nutrition education from preschool through grade 12, preferably as part of quality school health education.

In summary, children's appetites and nutrient needs reflect their stage of growth. Those who are chronically hungry and malnourished suffer growth retardation; when hunger is temporary and nutrient deficiencies are mild, the problems are usually more subtle—such as poor academic performance. Iron deficiency is widespread and has many physical and behavioral consquences. "Hyper" behavior is not caused by poor nutrition, but may reflect too much caffeine and inconsistent care, including too much television watching, which can contribute to obesity by promoting inactivity and an overconsumption of snack foods. Adults at home and at school need to provide children with nutrient-dense foods and teach them how to make healthful choices.

Nutrition during Adolescence

adolescence: the period from the beginning of puberty until maturity.

Nutrient needs are greater during adolescence than at any other time of life, except for pregnancy and lactation. In general, nutrient needs rise throughout childhood and then level off or even diminish slightly as the adolescent passes into adulthood.

Teenagers make many more choices for themselves than they did as children. They are not fed, they eat; they are not sent out to play, they choose to go. At the same time, social pressures thrust choices at them: whether to drink alcoholic beverages and whether to develop their bodies to meet extreme ideals of slimness or athletic prowess.

Adolescents learn about nutrition—both valid information and misinformation—from personal, immediate experiences. They are concerned with how diet can improve their lives now—they engage in crash dieting in order to buy a new bathing suit, avoid greasy foods in an effort to clear acne, or eat a pile of spaghetti to prepare for a big sporting event. The person concerned with the nutrition and health of adolescents, then, must learn about these subjects of interest and show the relationships with nutrition.

GROWTH AND DEVELOPMENT

The steady growth of childhood speeds up abruptly and dramatically with the onset of adolescence, and female and male growth patterns become distinct. A female's adolescent growth spurt begins at age 10 or 11 and reaches its peak at 12. A male's growth spurt begins at 12 or 13 and peaks at 14.

Gender differences become apparent in the skeletal system, lean body mass, and fat stores. In females, fat becomes a larger percentage of the total body weight, and in males, the lean body mass—muscle and bone—becomes much greater. On the average, males grow 8 inches taller during the growth spurt;

females, 6 inches. Males add approximately 45 pounds to their weight; females, about 35 pounds. Hormonal changes profoundly affect every organ of the body, including the brain, and within two or three years, physically mature adults emerge.

Teenagers' rates and patterns of growth exhibit such wide variations that growth charts used for children must be abandoned when the signs of puberty begin to appear. Age in years indicates little about development; one way to be sure a teenager is growing normally is to compare his or her height and weight with previous measures. To record developmental changes during puberty, health care professionals use standard rating scales based on stages of adolescent development.[38]

puberty: the period in life in which a person becomes physically capable of reproduction.

ENERGY AND NUTRIENT NEEDS

As children become adults, they change in many ways. Their physical changes make their nutrient needs high, and their emotional, intellectual, and social changes make meeting those needs a challenge.

Energy Intake and Activity   The energy needs of adolescents vary to a great extent, depending on the current rate of growth, body size, and physical activity. Boys' energy needs may be especially high; they grow faster and, as mentioned, develop more lean body mass. An active boy of 15 may need 4000 kcalories or more a day just to maintain his weight. Girls start growing earlier than boys and attain lower body weights, so their energy needs peak sooner and decline more quickly than those of their male peers. An inactive girl of 15 whose growth is nearly at a standstill may need fewer than 2000 kcalories a day if she is to avoid excessive weight gain. Thus adolescent girls need to pay special attention to being physically active and selecting foods of high nutrient density in order to meet their nutrient needs without exceeding their energy needs.

The insidious problem of obesity becomes apparent in adolescence and often continues into adulthood; it occurs mostly in females, especially in African-American females.[39] Young women who become interested in nutrition may make choices that will benefit their fitness, or they may become unhealthily obsessed with weight control (see Highlight 9).

Iron   Iron remains a nutrient of special concern. Iron needs increase in females as they start to menstruate and in males as their lean body mass develops. Adolescent iron intakes often fail to keep pace with increasing needs, especially for females, who typically consume less iron-rich meat and fewer total kcalories than males.[40]

Iron RDA during adolescence:
12 mg/day (males).
15 mg/day (females).

Calcium   Adolescence is a crucial time for bone development, and the requirement for calcium reaches its peak during these years.[41] Unfortunately, many adolescents have calcium intakes below current recommendations.[42] Low calcium intakes during the adolescent growth spurt, especially if paired with physical inactivity, may compromise the development of peak bone mass. As emphasized earlier, the attainment of maximal bone mass is considered the best protection against age-related bone loss and fractures.[43] Once again, teenage girls are at greatest risk, for their milk—and therefore calcium—intakes begin to decline at the time when their calcium needs are greatest.

Calcium DRI during adolescence:
1300 mg/day.

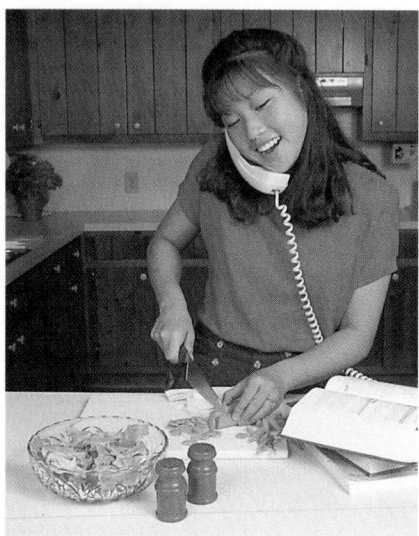

Nutritious snacks play an important role in an active teen's diet.

The nutritive values of selected fast foods are presented in Appendix H.

Table 19–10

Selected Nutrients in a Hamburger, Chocolate Shake, and Small Serving of French Fries

Nutrient	Male[a] % RDA	Female[a] % RDA
Energy	30	35
Protein	47	64
Fat[b]	26	31
Calcium[c]	35	35
Iron	30	24
Zinc	16	20
Vitamin A	9	11
Thiamin	41	48
Riboflavin	42	49
Niacin	35	41
Folate	18	20
Vitamin C	7	7
Sodium[b]	34	34

[a]RDA for a 15- to 18-year-old, moderately active person of average height and weight.
[b]Daily Values used for fat and sodium.
[c]Reflects DRI value.

HEALTHY PEOPLE 2000: Increase calcium intake, so that at least 50% of youth aged 12 through 24 years consume three or more servings of calcium-rich foods daily.

FOOD CHOICES AND HEALTH HABITS

Teenagers come and go as they choose and eat what they want when they have time. With a multitude of after-school, social, and job activities, they almost inevitably fall into irregular eating habits. The teenage snacker who finds only nutritious foods around the house is well provided for.

Snacks   Snacks typically provide at least a fourth of the average teenager's daily food energy intake. Snacks often fail to provide enough calcium, iron, vitamin A, and folate. Many adolescents need to eat a greater variety of foods to obtain these nutrients. Table 19–9 shows how to combine foods from different food groups to create healthy snacks. Most vending machines offer few nutrient-dense options, and nutrition information alone does not convince people to make healthy choices.[44]

Eating Away from Home   Inevitably, adolescents do a lot of eating away from home, and their nutritional welfare is enhanced or hindered by the choices they make. A lunch of a hamburger, a chocolate shake, and french fries supplies substantial quantities of many nutrients, as shown in Table 19–10, at a kcalorie cost of 800, an energy cost many adolescents can afford. When they eat this sort of lunch, teens can balance their diets by adjusting their breakfast and dinner choices. They need to select fruits and vegetables for vitamins A, C, folate, and fiber, and lean meats for iron and zinc at their other meals.

Peer Influence   Many of the food and health choices adolescents make reflect the opinions and actions of their peers. When others perceive milk as "babyish," a teen will choose soft drinks instead; when others skip lunch and hang out in the parking lot, a teen may join in for the camaraderie, regardless of hunger. Adults need to remember that teenagers have the right to make their own decisions—even if they are contrary to the adults' views. Gatekeepers can set up the environment so that nutritious foods are available and can stand by with reliable nutrition information and advice, but the rest is up to the adolescents. Ultimately, they make the choices. Highlight 9 examines the influence of social pressures on the development of eating disorders.

PROBLEMS ADOLESCENTS FACE

Physical maturity and growing independence present adolescents with new choices to make. The consequences of those choices will influence their nutritional health both today and throughout life. Some teenagers begin using drugs, alcohol, and tobacco; others wisely refrain. Information about the use of these substances is presented here because most people are first exposed to them during adolescence, but it actually applies to people of all ages.

Marijuana   Three of every five high school seniors report that they have at least tried an illicit drug, most commonly marijuana. The body processes all sub-

Table 19–9

Healthful Snack Ideas—Think Food Groups, Alone and in Combination

Selecting two or more foods from different food groups adds variety and nutrient balance to snacks. The combinations are endless, so be creative.

Grain Products

Grain products are filling snacks, especially when combined with other foods:
- Cereal with fruit and milk.
- Crackers and cheese.
- Wheat toast with peanut butter.
- Popcorn with grated cheese.
- Oatmeal raisin cookies with milk.

Vegetables

Cut-up fresh, raw vegetables make great snacks alone or in combination with foods from other food groups:
- Celery with peanut butter.
- Broccoli, cauliflower, and carrot sticks with a flavored cottage cheese dip.

Fruits

Fruits are delicious snacks and can be eaten alone—fresh, dried, or juiced—or combined with other foods:
- Apples and cheese.
- Bananas and peanut butter.
- Peaches with yogurt.
- Raisins mixed with sunflower seeds or nuts.

Meats and Meat Alternates

Meat and meat alternates add protein to snacks:
- Refried beans with nachos and cheese.
- Tuna on crackers.
- Luncheon meat on wheat bread.

Milk and Milk Products

Milk can be used as a beverage with any snack, and many other milk products, such as yogurt and cheese, can be eaten alone or with other foods as listed above.

stances, and marijuana is no exception. The active ingredients are rapidly and almost completely absorbed from the lungs.* Then, being fat soluble, these substances are packaged in lipoproteins before traveling in the blood to the various body tissues. The liver and other tissues metabolize these substances, and their remnants linger in the body for several days, being gradually excreted for a week or more after the smoking of a single marijuana cigarette. With repeated exposure, these substances accumulate in body fat, the lungs, the liver, the reproductive organs, and the brain.

---

*The active ingredient of marijuana, which is primarily responsible for its intoxicating effects, is delta-9-tetrahydrocannabinol, or THC.

Smoking a marijuana cigarette seems to enhance the enjoyment of eating, especially of sweets, a phenomenon commonly known as "the munchies." Why or how this effect occurs is not known; it may be a social effect induced by suggestibility, or it may be that the drug stimulates appetite. Prolonged use of the drug does not seem to bring about a weight gain.

Marijuana users may think that because they usually smoke fewer marijuana cigarettes in a day than they would tobacco cigarettes, their lungs will incur fewer harmful, long-term effects. This is a myth. One marijuana cigarette is as bad for the body as four or five tobacco cigarettes, because people who smoke marijuana inhale more smoke and hold it in their lungs longer. People who regularly smoke several marijuana cigarettes a day face the same risk of lung cancer as people who smoke a pack of tobacco cigarettes a day.[45]

Cocaine One in 20 high school seniors reports having used cocaine at least once.[46] Cocaine elicits diverse effects: intense euphoria, restlessness, heightened self-confidence, irritability, insomnia, and loss of appetite. Weight loss is common, and cocaine abusers often develop eating disorders. Notably, the craving for cocaine replaces hunger; rats given unlimited cocaine will choose it over food until they starve to death. Thus, unlike marijuana use, cocaine use has major nutritional consequences.

Cocaine can cause rapid and irregular heartbeats, heart attacks, and even death. Its use continues to escalate as cheaper and more addictive forms become available. In its smokable form, crack cocaine is more addicting than any other drug. One former crack addict tells of holding a gun to his brother's head to steal money for his next drug purchase.

Drug Abuse, in General The effects of other addictive drugs vary in degree but are similar in kind to those caused by cocaine. Drug abusers face the multiple nutrition problems listed in the margin. During withdrawal from drugs, an important part of treatment is to identify and correct these nutrition problems.

Alcohol Abuse Sooner or later all teenagers face the decision whether to drink alcohol. The law forbids the sale of alcohol to people under a specific age, but most adolescents who seek alcohol find it easy to obtain.

Many adolescents find that alcohol and marijuana serve similar purposes, and the pattern of substance use indicates parallel consumption, not a displacement of one by the other. Some adolescents use alcohol as an escape or for support—an ineffective way to cope with problems that leads to greater problems. Dependency on any drug severely impairs development and deserves attention, but is beyond the scope of this text.

Highlight 7 describes how alcohol affects nutrition status. To sum it up, alcohol is an empty-kcalorie beverage that can displace nutritious foods from the diet. It alters nutrient absorption and metabolism, so that imbalances develop. People who cannot keep their alcohol use moderate must abstain to maintain their health.

Tobacco Cigarette smoking is a pervasive health problem causing thousands of people to suffer from cancer and diseases of the cardiovascular, digestive, and respiratory systems. These effects are beyond the scope of nutrition, but smoking cigarettes does influence hunger, body weight, and nutrient status. Links between nutrients and lung cancer are also known.

Reminder: *Euphoria* is an inflated sense of well-being and pleasure brought on by some drugs; popularly called a *high*.

Nutrition problems of drug abusers:
- They buy drugs with money that could be spent on food.
- They lose interest in food during "highs."
- Some drugs depress appetite.
- Their lifestyle fails to promote good eating habits.
- If they use intravenous (IV) drugs, they may contract AIDS, hepatitis, or other infectious diseases, which increase their nutrient needs. Hepatitis also causes taste changes and loss of appetite.
- Medicines used to treat drug abusers may alter their nutrition status.

Smoking a cigarette eases feelings of hunger. When smokers receive a hunger signal, they can quiet it with cigarettes instead of food. Such behavior ignores body signals and postpones energy and nutrient intake. Studies on rats confirm that nicotine reduces food intake, causing weight loss.[47]

Indeed, smokers tend to weigh less than nonsmokers and to gain weight when they stop smoking.[48] Weight gain is often a concern for people contemplating giving up cigarettes. They should know that the average person who quits smoking gains less than 10 pounds. Smokers wanting to quit need to prepare for this possibility and adjust their diet and activity habits so as to maintain weight during and after quitting. Smoking cessation programs need to include strategies for weight management.

Nutrient intakes of smokers and nonsmokers differ. Smokers tend to have lower intakes of dietary fiber, vitamin A, beta-carotene, folate, and vitamin C.[49] The association between smoking and low vitamin intake may be noteworthy, considering the altered metabolism of vitamin C in smokers and the protective effect of vitamin A and beta-carotene against lung cancer.

Research shows that compared to nonsmokers, smokers require almost twice as much vitamin C to maintain steady body pools. Oxidants in cigarette smoke accelerate vitamin C metabolism and deplete smokers' body stores of this antioxidant; this depletion is even evident to some degree in nonsmokers who are exposed to passive smoke.[50]

Beta-carotene enhances the immune response and protects against some cancer activity.[51] Specifically, the risk of lung cancer is greatest for smokers who have the lowest intakes of carotene. Of course, such evidence should not be misinterpreted. It does not mean that as long as people eat their carrots, they can safely use tobacco. Smokers are ten times more likely to get lung cancer than nonsmokers. Both smokers and nonsmokers can, however, reduce their cancer risks by eating fruits and vegetables rich in carotene (see Highlight 11 for details on antioxidant nutrients and disease prevention).

To review, nutrient needs rise dramatically as children enter the rapid growth phase of the teen years. The busy lifestyles of teenagers add to the challenge of meeting their nutrient needs—especially for iron and calcium. In addition to making wise foods choices, teenagers need to refrain from using substances that will impair their health—including illicit drugs, tobacco, and alcohol.

The nutrition and lifestyle choices people make as children and teenagers have long-term, as well as immediate, effects on their health. Highlight 19 describes how sound choices and good habits during childhood can help prevent disease later in life.

The vitamin C RDA for people who regularly smoke cigarettes is 100 mg/day. The Canadian RNI suggests smokers should add 50% to the vitamin C recommendation.

Study Questions

1. Describe some of the nutrient and immunological attributes of breast milk.
2. What are the appropriate uses of formula feeding? What criteria would you use in selecting an infant formula?
3. Why are solid foods not recommended for an infant during the first few months of life? When is an infant ready to start eating solid food?
4. Name foods that are inappropriate for infants and explain why they are inappropriate.

(continued on the next page)

5. What nutrition problems are most common in children? What strategies can help prevent them?

6. Describe the relationships between nutrition and behavior. How does television influence nutrition?

7. Describe a true food allergy. Which foods most often cause allergic reactions? How do food allergies influence nutrition status?

8. List strategies for introducing nutritious foods to children.

9. What impact do school meal programs have on the nutrition status of children?

10. Describe the changes in nutrient needs from childhood to adolescence. Why is a teenaged girl more likely to develop an iron deficiency than is a boy?

11. How do teen eating habits influence their nutrient intakes?

12. How does the use of illicit drugs influence nutrition status?

13. How do the nutrient intakes of smokers differ from those of nonsmokers? What impacts can those differences exert on health?

Notes

1. P. S. W. Davies, Energy requirements and energy expenditure in infancy, *European Journal of Clinical Nutrition* (supplement 4) 46 (1992): S29–S35.

2. H. L. Greene and coauthors, Vitamins for newborn infant formulas: A review of recommendations with emphasis on data from low birth-weight infants, *European Journal of Clinical Nutrition* 46 (1992): S1–S8.

3. Committee on Nutrition, American Academy of Pediatrics, *Pediatric Nutrition Handbook*, 3rd ed., ed. L. A. Barness (Elk Grove Village, Ill.: American Academy of Pediatrics, 1993), pp. 23–33.

4. American Academy of Pediatrics, Committee on Nutrition, The use of whole cow's milk in infancy, *Pediatrics* 89 (1992): 1105–1109.

5. Position of The American Dietetic Association: Promotion and support of breast feeding, *Journal of the American Dietetic Association* 93 (1993): 467–469.

6. J. S. Forsyth, Is it worthwhile breast-feeding? *European Journal of Clinical Nutrition* (supplement 1) 46 (1993): 519–525.

7. A. C. Goedhart and J. G. Bindels, The composition of human milk as a model for the design of infant formulas: Recent findings and possible applications, *Nutrition Research Reviews* 7 (1994): 1–23.

8. N. F. Butte, E. O. Smith, and C. Garza, Energy utilization of breast-fed and formula-fed infants, *American Journal of Clinical Nutrition* 51 (1990): 350–358.

9. M. J. Heinig and coauthors, Energy and protein intakes of breast-fed and formula-fed infants during the first year of life and their association with growth velocity: The DARLING Study, *American Journal of Clinical Nutrition* 58 (1993): 152–161.

10. Committee on Nutritional Status during Pregnancy and Lactation, *Nutrition during Lactation* (Washington, D.C.: National Academy Press, 1991), pp. 155–156.

11. M. W. Shannon and J. W. Graef, Lead intoxication in infancy, *Pediatrics* 89 (1992): 87–90.

12. D. Stehlin, Soy beverages not complete formulas, *FDA Consumer,* September 1990, p. 29.

13. S. Ryan, Bone mineralization and growth, *European Journal of Clinical Nutrition* 46 (1992): S41–S44.

14. T. Walter and coauthors, Effectiveness of iron-fortified infant cereal in prevention of iron deficiency anemia, *Pediatrics* 91 (1993): 976–982; G. J. Fuchs and coauthors, Iron status and intake of older infants fed formula vs cow milk with cereal, *American Journal of Clinical Nutrition* 58 (1993): 343–348.

15. M. M. Smith and F. Lifshitz, Excess fruit juice consumption as a contributing factor in nonorganic failure to thrive, *Pediatrics* 93 (1994): 438–443.

16. S. A. Sullivan and L. L. Birch, Infant dietary experience and acceptance of solid foods, *Pediatrics* 93 (1994): 271–277.

17. L. L. Birch and coauthors, Effects of a nonenergy fat substitute on children's energy and macronutrient intake, *American Journal of Clinical Nutrition* 58 (1993): 326–333; S. Shea and coauthors, Variability and self-regulation of energy intake in young children in their everyday environment, *Pediatrics* 90 (1992): 542–546; L. L. Birch and coauthors, The variability of young children's energy intake, *New England Journal of Medicine* 324 (1991): 232–235.

18. R. E. Klesges and coauthors, Parental influence on food selection in young children and its relationships to childhood obesity, *American Journal of Clinical Nutrition* 53 (1991): 859–864.

19. T. A. Nicklas and coauthors, Breakfast consumption affects adequacy of total daily intake in children, *Journal of the American Dietetic Association* 93 (1993): 886–891.

20. P. L. Splett and M. Story, Child nutrition: Objectives for the decade, *Journal of the American Dietetic Association* 91 (1991): 665–668.

21. N. S. Scrimshaw, Iron deficiency, *Scientific American*, October 1991, pp. 46–52.

22. B. Lozoff, E. Jimenez, and A. W. Wolf, Long-term developmental outcome of infants with iron deficiency, *New England Journal of Medicine* 325 (1991): 687–694.

23. F. A. Oski, Iron deficiency in infancy and childhood, *New England Journal of Medicine* 329 (1993): 190–193; S. J. Fairweather-Tait, Iron deficiency in infancy: Easy to prevent—or is it? *European Journal of Clinical Nutrition* (supplement 4) 46 (1992): S9–S14.

24. D. A. Gans, Sucrose and unusual childhood behavior, *Nutrition Today*, May/June 1991, pp. 8–14; E. H. Wender and M. V. Solanto, Effects of sugar on aggressive and inattentive behavior in children with attention deficit disorder with hyperactivity and normal children, *Pediatrics* 88 (1991): 960–966; J. A. Bachorowshi and coauthors, Sucrose and delinquency: Behavioral assessment, *Pediatrics* 86 (1990): 244–253.

25. R. Zoglin, Is TV ruining our children? *Time*, October 15, 1990, p. 75.

26. R. C. Klesges, M. L. Shelton, and L. M. Klesges, Effects of television on metabolic rate: Potential implications for childhood obesity, *Pediatrics* 91 (1993): 281–286.

27. H. A. Sampson and D. D. Metcalfe, Food allergies, *Journal of the American Medical Association* 268 (1992): 2840–2844.

28. S. A. Bock and F. M. Atkins, Patterns of food hypersensitivity during sixteen years of double-blind, placebo-controlled food challenges, *Journal of Pediatrics* 117 (1990): 561–567.

29. Sampson and Metcalfe, 1992.

30. V. L. Olejer, Food hypersensitivities, *Handbook of Pediatric Nutrition* (Gaithersburg, Md.: Aspen Publishers, 1993), pp. 206–231.

31. A. T. Hingley, Food allergies: When eating is risky, *FDA Consumer*, December 1993, pp. 27–31.

32. Sampson and Metcalfe, 1992.

33. National Center for Nutrition and Dietetics, International Food Information Council, Kids at the table: Who's placing the orders? (Chicago: American Dietetic Association, 1991).

34. Position of The American Dietetic Association: Nutrition standards for child care programs, *Journal of the American Dietetic Association* 94 (1994): 323.

35. K. Schuster, Feds put schools on a lowfat diet, *Food Management* 29 (1994): 78–84; J. Burghardt and B. Devaney, The School Nutrition Dietary Assessment Study: Summary of findings, Food and Nutrition Service, U.S. Department of Agriculture, October 1993.

36. R. C. Whitaker and coauthors, An environmental intervention to reduce dietary fat in school lunches, *Pediatrics* 91 (1993): 1107–1111.

37. Timely statement of The American Dietetic Association: Dietary guidance for healthy children, *Journal of the American Dietetic Association* 95 (1995): 370.

38. L. E. Underwood, Normal adolescent growth and development, *Nutrition Today*, March/April 1991, pp. 11–16.

39. T. A. Wadden and coauthors, Obesity in black adolescent girls: A controlled clinical trial of treatment by diet, behavior modification, and parental support, *Pediatrics* 85 (1990): 345–352.

40. J. B. Anderson, The status of adolescent nutrition, *Nutrition Today*, March/April 1991, pp. 7–10.

41. S. M. Ott, Bone density in adolescents, *New England Journal of Medicine* 325 (1991): 1646–1647.

42. S. I. Barr, Associations of social and demographic variables with calcium intakes of high school students, *Journal of the American Dietetic Association* 94 (1994): 260–266, 269.

43. V. Matkovic, Diet, genetics, and peak bone mass of adolescent girls, *Nutrition Today*, March/April 1991, pp. 21–24.

44. S. M. Hoerr and V. A. Louden, Can nutrition information increase sales of healthful vended snacks? *Journal of School Health* 63 (1993): 386–390.

45. T. C. Wu and coauthors, Pulmonary hazards of smoking marijuana as compared with tobacco, *New England Journal of Medicine* 318 (1988): 347–351.

46. American Council on Science and Health, *Cocaine: Facts and Dangers* (New York: American Council on Science and Health, 1990).

47. S. R. Schwid, M. D. Hirvonen, and R. E. Keesey, Nicotine effects on body weight: A regulatory perspective, *American Journal of Clinical Nutrition* 55 (1992): 878–884.

48. D. F. Williamson and coauthors, Smoking cessation and severity of weight gain in a national cohort, *New England Journal of Medicine* 324 (1991): 739–745.

49. T. A. B. Sanders and coauthors, Essential fatty acids, plasma cholesterol and fat-soluble vitamins in subjects with age-related maculopathy and matched control subjects, *American Journal of Clinical Nutrition* 57 (1993): 428–433; A. F. Subar, L. C. Harlan, and M. E. Mattson, Food and nutrient intake differences between smokers and non-smokers in the US, *American Journal of Public Health* 80 (1990): 1323–1329.

50. D. L. Tribble, L. J. Giuliano, and S. P. Fortmann, Reduced plasma ascorbic acid concentrations in nonsmokers regularly exposed to environmental tobacco smoke, *American Journal of Clinical Nutrition* 58 (1993): 886–890.

51. G. van Poppel, S. Spanhaak, and T. Ockhuizen, Effect of β-carotene on immunological indexes in healthy male smokers, *American Journal of Clinical Nutrition* 57 (1993): 402–407; T. V. Ringer and coauthors, Beta-carotene's effects on serum lipoproteins and immunologic indices in humans, *American Journal of Clinical Nutrition* 53 (1991): 688–694.

Childhood Obesity and the Early Development of Chronic Diseases

When people think of the health problems of children and adolescents, they typically think of measles and acne, not cardiovascular disease (CVD). They think of CVD as the number one killer of adults in the United States and Canada, but CVD begins in childhood.[1]

Much of our knowledge about the early development of CVD comes from the Bogalusa Heart Study, a long-term epidemiological study of some 14,000 young people. For nearly three decades, researchers have been observing how changes in body weight, blood lipids, blood pressure, and individual behaviors correlate with the development of CVD over time—from infancy to childhood through adolescence and into young adulthood. Some major findings have emerged from the research:

- Changes inside the arteries—changes predictive of CVD—are evident in childhood.
- Obesity in children affects these changes.
- Behaviors that influence the development of obesity and of CVD are learned and begin early in life. These behaviors include overeating, eating high-fat foods, physical inactivity, and cigarette smoking.

This highlight focuses on efforts to prevent childhood obesity and CVD, but the benefits extend to cancer, diabetes, and other chronic diseases as well. The years of childhood are emphasized here, for the earlier in life health-promoting

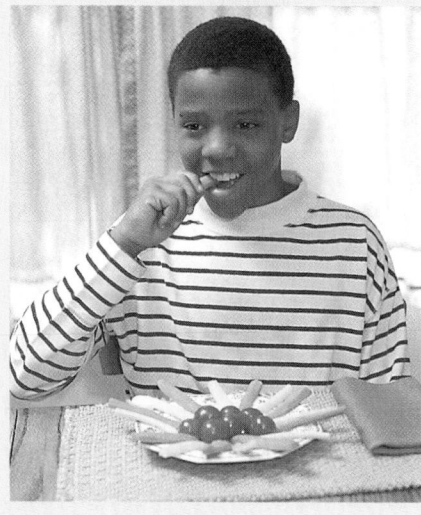

Take care of your body and your body will take care of you.

habits become established, the better they will stick.

Invariably, questions arise as to what extent genetics is involved in CVD development. Children who are obese and who have high blood lipids and high blood pressure are often from families with a history of CVD. Genetics does not appear to play a *determining* role in CVD; that is, a person is not simply destined at birth to develop CVD.[2] Instead, genetics appears to play a *permissive* role—the potential is inherited and then will develop, if given a push by poor health choices such as excessive weight gain, poor diet, sedentary lifestyle, and cigarette smoking.

EARLY DEVELOPMENT OF CVD

Most people consider CVD to be an adult disease: its incidence rises with advancing age, and symptoms

rarely appear before age 30. The disease process begins much earlier, though.

Atherosclerosis

Most CVD involves atherosclerosis—the accumulation of cholesterol and other blood lipids along the walls of the arteries. Atherosclerosis eventually blocks the flow of blood to the heart and causes a heart attack, or cuts off blood flow to the brain and causes a stroke. Infants are born with healthy, smooth, clear arteries, but within the first decade of life, fatty streaks may begin to appear (see Figure H19–1). During adolescence, these fatty streaks may begin to turn to fibrous plaques. By early adulthood, the fibrous plaques may begin to calcify and become raised lesions, especially in boys and young men.[3] As the lesions grow more numerous and enlarge, the heart disease rate begins to rise, and the rise becomes dramatic at about age 45 in men and 55 in women.[4] From this point on, arterial damage and blockage progress rapidly, and heart attacks and strokes threaten life. In short, the consequences of atherosclerosis, which become apparent only in adulthood, have their beginnings in the first decades of life.[5]

Atherosclerosis is not inevitable; people can grow old with relatively clear arteries. Early lesions may either progress or regress, depending on several factors, many of which reflect lifestyle behaviors. Smoking, for example, is strongly associated

Figure H19–1

The Formation of Plaques in Atherosclerosis

When plaques have covered 60 percent of the coronary artery walls, the critical phase of heart disease begins.

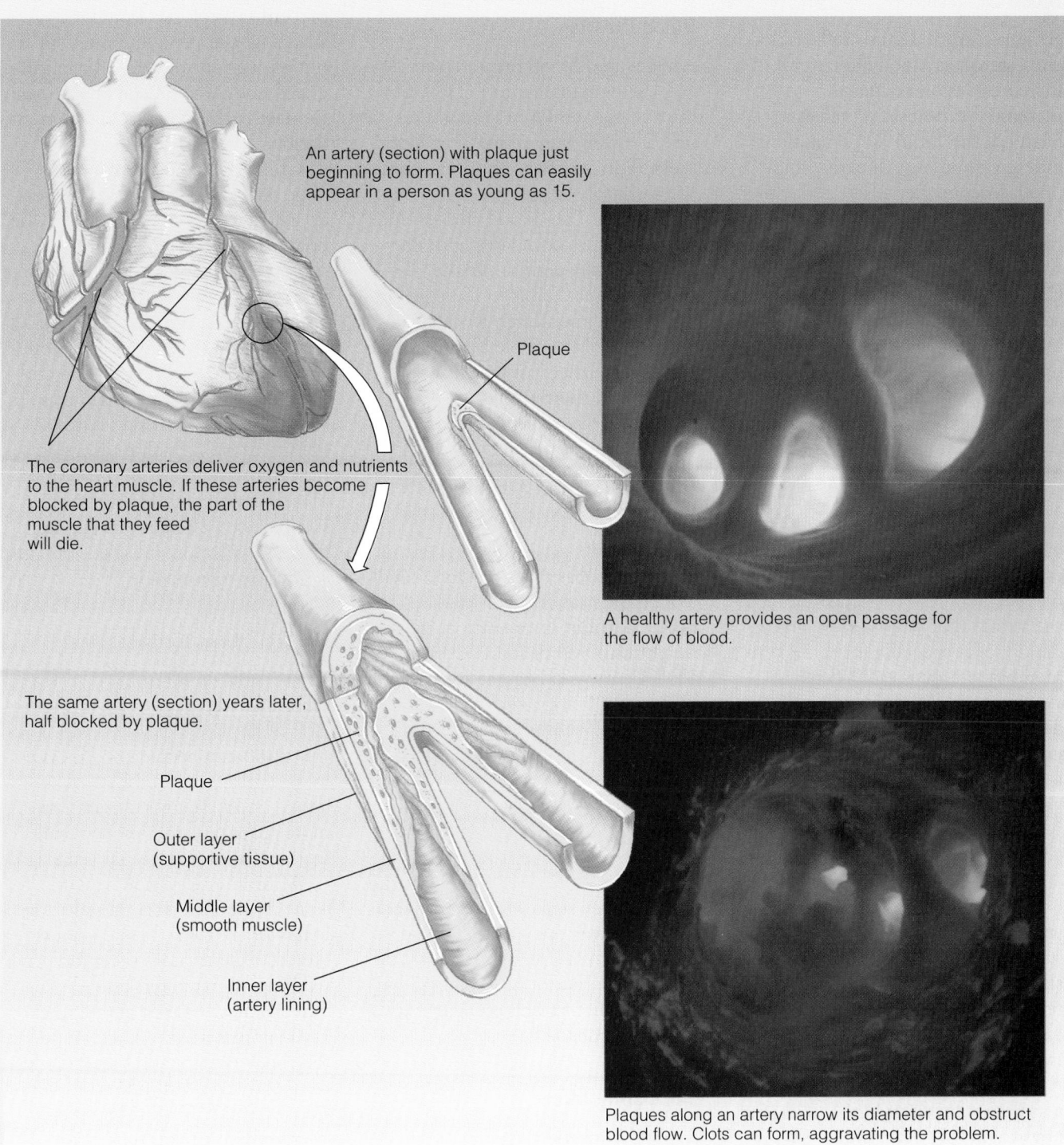

An artery (section) with plaque just beginning to form. Plaques can easily appear in a person as young as 15.

Plaque

The coronary arteries deliver oxygen and nutrients to the heart muscle. If these arteries become blocked by plaque, the part of the muscle that they feed will die.

A healthy artery provides an open passage for the flow of blood.

The same artery (section) years later, half blocked by plaque.

Plaque

Outer layer (supportive tissue)

Middle layer (smooth muscle)

Inner layer (artery lining)

Plaques along an artery narrow its diameter and obstruct blood flow. Clots can form, aggravating the problem.

with the prevalence of raised lesions, even in young adults.[6]

Blood Cholesterol

Atherosclerotic lesions reflect blood cholesterol: as blood cholesterol increases, lesion coverage increases.[7] Cholesterol values at birth are similar in all populations; differences emerge in early childhood. In countries where the adults have high blood cholesterol and high rates of CVD, the children also tend to have high blood cholesterol. Conversely, in countries where the adults have low blood cholesterol and low rates of CVD, the children tend to have low blood cholesterol, suggesting that adult heart disease tracks early trends and that early preventive efforts might reduce the incidence of later CVD.[8]

The studies just described examined population trends; but individual cholesterol status also becomes established in early childhood. At one year, cholesterol values predict the values that will be seen later in childhood, especially for those with high blood cholesterol.[9] Studies examining children for more than a decade have found that the best predictor of their blood cholesterol is earlier baseline values: childhood values correlate with values in young adulthood.[10] Quite simply, if you want to know a child's future cholesterol, measure it now.

Blood cholesterol also correlates with obesity, especially central obesity. LDL cholesterol correlates positively, and HDL negatively.[11] These relationships are apparent throughout childhood, and their magnitude increases with age.

Research has also confirmed an association between blood lipids and physical activity in children similar to that seen in adults.[12] Inactive children have higher total cholesterol and LDL and lower HDL than physically active children.

Blood Pressure

An elevated blood pressure accelerates the development of CVD. On the average, children's blood pressure is lower than adults', but blood pressure increases as children grow, rising sharply at puberty and then leveling off. Like blood cholesterol, blood pressure correlates with obesity, especially central obesity.[13] Blood pressure tends to increase at a slower rate in children who participate in regular aerobic activity or who have either lost weight or maintained their weight as they grew taller.[14]

DEVELOPMENT OF OBESITY IN CHILDREN

Many experts agree that preventing or treating obesity in childhood will reduce the rate of CVD in adulthood. Without intervention, overweight children become overweight adolescents who become overweight adults, and being overweight exacerbates every chronic disease that adults face.[15]

Growing Fatter

Children are heavier today than they were 10 to 20 years ago. On the average, they have gained more than 5 pounds over the past two decades. This pattern is a secular trend—that is, one that cannot be explained by genetics. Diet and physical activity must be responsible.

Not Eating More

Reports from the Bogalusa Heart Study indicate that children's energy intakes have remained relatively stable over the past 15 years. There has even been a slight decline in fat intake, from 38 to 36 percent of kcalories from fat daily.[16] This slight decline in dietary fat is not enough, however, to have influenced body weight, nor is it enough to meet current dietary recommendations.

Children's dietary fat intakes vary, of course, and some children do eat high-fat diets. Children who prefer high-fat foods tend to consume a relatively large percentage of their energy intake from fat.[17] They also tend to be more overweight than their peers. Particularly noteworthy is the finding that the children's fat preferences and consumption correlate with their parents' obesity as well. Such findings confirm the significant roles parents play—teaching children about healthy food choices, providing children with low-fat selections, and serving as role models.

Growing Less Active

Most likely, children have grown more overweight because of their lack of physical activity.[18] An inactive child can become obese even while eating less food than an active child. Today's children are more sedentary and less physically fit than children were 20 years ago.

Watching television accounts for some 24 hours a week of sedentary behavior. Beyond these 24 hours, children spend more sedentary time working at computers and playing video games. As mentioned in earlier chapters, studies have found that both obesity and blood cholesterol correlate with hours of television viewed.[19] TV uses no more energy than it takes to rest, displaces participation in more vigorous activities, and fosters snacking on high-fat foods.

Just as blood cholesterol and obesity track over the years, so does a person's level of physical activity. A study of almost 1000 teenagers reported that over half of those who were initially described as inactive remained inactive six years later.[20] Similarly, almost half of those who were physically active remained so. Compared with inactive teens, those who were physically active weighed less, smoked less, ate a diet lower in saturated fats, and had a better blood lipid profile. The message is clear: physical activity offers numerous health benefits and children who are active today are most likely to be active for years to come.

PREVENTING CHILDHOOD OBESITY

In light of all these findings, parents and teachers of children are encouraged to make major efforts to prevent child obesity. Among directives are the following: encourage children to eat slowly, to pause and enjoy their table companions, and to stop eating when they are full. Teach them how to select low-fat snacks and to serve themselves appropriate portions. Never force children to clean their plates. Encourage physical activity daily to promote strong skeletal, muscular, and cardiovascular development and to instill in children the desire to be physically active throughout life. Physical activity is a natural and lifelong behavior of healthy living.[21] It can be as simple as riding a bike, playing tag, jumping rope, or doing chores. It need not be an organized sport; it just needs to be some activity on a regular basis.

It is important to use sensitivity in teaching children nutrition prin-

ciples that can help to prevent obesity. Children can easily get the idea that their worth is tied to their body weight. Some parents fail to realize that society's ideal of slimness can be perilously close to starvation, and that a child encouraged to "diet" cannot obtain the energy and nutrients required for normal growth and development. Even healthy children without diagnosable eating disorders have been observed to limit their growth through "dieting."[22] Weight gain in truly overweight children can be controlled safely without compromising growth, but should be overseen by a health care professional.

DEALING WITH CHILDHOOD OBESITY

The child who is already obese needs careful management. Weight loss is not ordinarily recommended because restrictive diets can easily impair growth in children. Instead, aim to maintain a constant weight while the child grows taller. The object is to support normal lean body development, while letting children "grow out" of their obesity.

CHOLESTEROL SCREENING FOR CHILDREN

Many children in the United States are not only overweight but also have high blood cholesterol.[23] The question of whether to screen children for high blood cholesterol is controversial.[24] Currently, selective screening for children and adolescents whose parents or grandparents have CVD is recommended.[25] Since blood cholesterol in children is a good predictor of adult values, however, some experts recommend universal screening to identify all children with high blood choles-

terol.[26] They note that many children who have high blood cholesterol do not have family histories of CVD and would be missed under current screening criteria.[27] Opponents argue that some children with high blood cholesterol may reach adulthood with normal blood cholesterol and that treating adults who have high blood cholesterol should be sufficient. They believe screening will create unnecessary anxiety and lead to an overuse of drug therapy and overly restrictive dieting during childhood and adolescence.[28] Furthermore, studies have found that few children follow up with additional testing or dietary changes anyway.[29] Standard values for cholesterol screening in children and adolescents are listed in Table H19–1.

In some cases, parents are too young to have a CVD history. In many other cases, children, or their parents, may not know their family histories. For these reasons, it may be most effective for physicians of adult heart patients to refer the children and grandchildren of these patients for cholesterol screening.[30]

Some research shows that overweight children should also be con-

Table H19–1

Cholesterol Values for Children and Adolescents

Disease Risk	Total Cholesterol (mg/dL)	LDL Cholesterol (mg/dL)
Acceptable	<170	<110
Borderline	170–199	110–129
High	≥200	≥130

Note: Adult values appear in Chapter 28.

sidered for cholesterol screening, even if they do not satisfy the current criteria.[31] The incidence of high blood cholesterol in obese children with no other criteria is similar to that of nonobese children with family histories of CVD.

Considering the many lifestyle factors that accompany the development of CVD, questions regarding a child's health behaviors might also be informative. Health care professionals should determine whether children smoke, and how physically active they are, especially when family history is unknown.[32]

Early—but not advanced—atherosclerotic lesions are reversible, making screening and education a high priority. Both those with family histories of CVD and those with multiple risk factors need intervention. Children with the highest risks of developing CVD are sedentary and obese, with high blood pressure and high blood cholesterol. In contrast, children with the lowest risks of heart disease are physically active and of normal weight, with low blood pressure and favorable lipid profiles. Routine pediatric care should identify these known risk factors and provide education when needed (see Table H19–2).

DIETARY RECOMMENDATIONS FOR CHILDREN

An expert panel on blood cholesterol in children and adolescents recommends that, regardless of family history, all children over age two should eat a variety of foods and maintain desirable weight.[33] Children should receive less than 30 percent of total energy from fat, less than 10 percent from saturated fat, and less than 300 milligrams of cholesterol per day. The American

Table H19–2
· · · · · · · · · · · · · ·
Health Professional's Schedule of Cardiovascular Disease Assessment in Children

Birth	• Family history for early heart disease, high blood lipids (if positive, discuss risk factors and refer parents to health care).
	• Start growth chart.
	• Parental smoking history (if positive, refer to smoking cessation program).
0–2 years	• Update family history, growth chart.
	• With introduction of solids, begin teaching about healthy diet (nutritionally adequate, low in salt, low in saturated fats).
	• Recommend healthy snacks as finger foods.
	• Change to whole milk from formula or breastfeeding at approximately 1 year of age.
2–6 years	• Update family history, growth chart (review growth chart[a] with family and discuss concept of weight for height).
	• Introduce moderately low-fat diet.
	• Change to low-fat milk.
	• Start blood pressure chart at approximately 3 years of age;[b] review for concept of lower salt intake.
	• Encourage active parent-child play.
	• Lipid determination in children with positive family history or with parental cholesterol >240 mg/dl (if abnormal, initiate nutrition counseling).
6–10 years	• Update family history, blood pressure, and growth charts.
	• Complete cardiovascular health profile with child; determine family history, smoking history, blood pressure percentile, weight for height, fingerstick cholesterol, and level of activity and fitness.
	• Reinforce low-fat diet.
	• Begin active antismoking counseling.
	• Introduce fitness for health and encourage lifelong sport activities for child and family.
	• Discuss role of watching television in sedentary lifestyle and obesity.
>10 years	• Update family history, blood pressure, and growth charts annually.
	• Review low-fat diet, risks of smoking, fitness benefits whenever possible.
	• Consider lipid profile in all patients.
	• Final review of personal cardiovascular health status.

[a]If weight is >120% of normal for height, diagnosis of obesity should be considered and the subject addressed with the child and family.
[b]If three consecutive interval blood pressure measurements exceed the 90th percentile and blood pressure is not explained by height or weight, diagnosis of hypertension should be made and appropriate evaluation considered.

Source: Adapted with permission from W. B. Strong and coauthors, Integrated cardiovascular health promotion in childhood: A statement for health professionals from the Subcommittee on Atherosclerosis and Hypertension in Childhood of the Council on Cardiovascular Disease in the Young, American Heart Association, *Circulation* 85 (1992): 1638–1650. Copyright 1992 American Heart Association.

Academy of Pediatrics agrees, but cautions against fat intakes of less than 30 percent of total kcalories for growing children.

Not before Two

Recommendations limiting fat and cholesterol are not intended for infants or children under two years old. Infants and toddlers need a higher percentage of fat to support their rapid growth.

Moderation, Not Deprivation

Healthy children over age two can begin the transition to eating according to recommendations. Even then, meals can include moderate amounts of a child's favorite foods, even if they are high-fat selections such as french fries and ice cream.[34] Without such additions, diets might be too low in fat, not to mention unappetizing and boring.

Balanced meals need to provide lean meat, poultry, fish, and vegetable sources of protein; fruits and vegetables; whole grains; and low-fat milk products. Such meals can provide enough food energy and nutrients to support growth and maintain blood cholesterol within a healthy range.[35] Pediatricians warn parents to avoid extremes; they caution that while intentions may be good, excessive food restriction may create nutrient deficiencies and impair growth. Furthermore, parental control over eating may instigate battles and foster attitudes about foods that can lead to inappropriate eating behaviors.

Diet First, Drugs Later

Experts agree that children at high risk should first be treated with diet.

If, in children ten years and older, blood cholesterol remains high after 6 to 12 months of dietary intervention, then drugs may be used to lower blood cholesterol.[36] Pharmacological doses of niacin effectively lower LDL cholesterol in children, but adverse effects are common; such treatment should be reserved only for severe cases.[37]

SMOKING

Another risk factor for CVD that starts in childhood and carries over into adulthood is cigarette smoking. Each day 3000 children begin to use tobacco, 40 percent of them in grade school. Among high school students, two out of three have tried smoking, and one in eight smokes regularly. Over half of all adult smokers began smoking before the age of 18.

Efforts to teach children about the dangers of smoking need to be aggressive to compete with the tobacco industry's promotional campaigns. The tobacco industry spends millions of dollars on advertising aimed at young people and makes over $200 million a year on sales to children under 18. Cigarette companies use cartoon characters, advertise in youth-oriented publications,

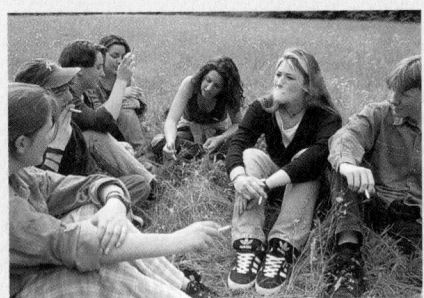

Cigarette smoking is the number-one cause of premature deaths.

and sponsor sporting events. Children and teenagers are not likely to consider the long-term health consequences of tobacco use. They are more likely to be struck by the immediate health consequences, such as shortness of breath when playing sports, or social consequences, such as having bad breath. Whatever the context, the message to all children and teens should be clear: don't start smoking. If you've already started, quit.

In conclusion, *adult* CVD is a major *pediatric* problem. Without intervention, some 60 million children are destined to suffer its consequences within the next 30 years. Optimal prevention efforts focus on children, especially on those who are overweight.

Just as young children receive vaccinations against infectious diseases, they need screening for, and education about, CVD. Many health education programs have been implemented in schools around the country.[38] These programs are most effective when they include education in the classroom, heart-healthy meals in the lunchroom, fitness activities on the playground, and parental involvement at home.

NOTES

1. G. S. Berenson and coauthors, Review: Atherosclerosis and its evolution in childhood, *American Journal of the Medical Sciences* 30 (1987): 429–440; W. B. Strong and coauthors, Integrated cardiovascular health promotion in childhood: A statement for health professionals from the Subcommittee on Atherosclerosis and Hypertension in Childhood of the Council on Cardiovascular Disease in the Young, American Heart Association, *Circulation* 85 (1992): 1638–1650.

2. W. B. Kannel, R. B. D'Agostino, and A. Belanger, Concept of bridging the gap from

youth to adulthood—The Framingham Study, an address presented at the Recognition and Prevention of Heart Disease: State of the Art conference, New Orleans, Louisiana, April 27 and 28, 1994.

3. G. S. Berenson and coauthors, Atherosclerosis of the aorta and coronary arteries and cardiovascular risk factors in persons aged 6 to 30 years and studied at necropsy (the Bogalusa Heart Study), *American Journal of Cardiology* 70 (1992): 851–858.

4. Kannel, D'Agostino, and Belanger, 1994.

5. Committee on Nutrition, Statement on cholesterol, *Pediatrics* 90 (1992): 469–473; National Cholesterol Education Program, Report of the Expert Panel on Blood Cholesterol Levels in Children and Adolescents, Overview and summary, *Pediatrics* (supplement) 89 (1992): 525–527.

6. Pathobiological Determinants of Atherosclerosis in Youth (PDAY) Research Group, Relationship of atherosclerosis in young men to serum lipoprotein cholesterol concentrations and smoking: A preliminary report from the Pathobiological Determinants of Atherosclerosis in Youth (PDAY) Research Group, *Journal of the American Medical Association* 264 (1990): 3018–3024.

7. Pathobiological Determinants of Atherosclerosis in Youth (PDAY) Research Group, 1990.

8. L. Snetselaar and R. M. Lauer, Childhood, diet and the atherosclerotic process, *Nutrition Today*, January/February 1992, pp. 22–28.

9. M. J. T. Kallio and coauthors, Tracking of serum cholesterol and lipoprotein levels from the first year of life, *Pediatrics* 91 (1993): 949–954.

10. S. Guo and coauthors, Serial analysis of plasma lipids and lipoproteins from individuals 9–21 years of age, *American Journal of Clinical Nutrition* 58 (1993): 61–67.

11. W. A. Wattigney and coauthors, Increasing impact of obesity on serum lipids and lipoproteins in young adults: The Bogalusa Heart Study, *Archives of Internal Medicine* 151 (1991): 2017–2022.

12. E. Suter and M. R. Hawes, Relationship of physical activity, body fat, diet, and blood lipid profile in youths 10–15 yr, *Medicine and Science in Sports and Exercise* 25 (1993): 748–754.

13. C. L. Shear and coauthors, Body fat patterning and blood pressure in children and young adults: The Bogalusa Heart Study, *Hypertension* 9 (1987): 236–244.

14. S. Shea and coauthors, The rate of increase in blood pressure in children 5 years of age is related to changes in aerobic fitness and body mass index, *Pediatrics* 94 (1994): 465–470.

15. S. S. Guo and coauthors, The predictive value of childhood body mass index values for overweight at age 35 y, *American Journal of Clinical Nutrition* 57 (1994): 810–819.

16. T. A. Nicklas and coauthors, Secular trends in dietary intakes and cardiovascular risk factors of 10-year-old children: The Bogalusa Heart Study (1973–1988), *American Journal of Clinical Nutrition* 57 (1993): 930–937.

17. J. O. Fisher and L. L. Birch, Fat preferences and fat consumption of 3- to 5-year-old children are related to parental obesity, *Journal of the American Dietetic Association* 95 (1995): 759–764.

18. S. A. Schlicker, S. T. Borra, and C. Regan, The weight and fitness status of United States children, *Nutrition Reviews* 52 (1994): 11–17.

19. E. Obarzanek and coauthors, Energy intake and physical activity in relation to indexes of body fat: The National Heart, Lung, and Blood Institute Growth and Health Study, *American Journal of Clinical Nutrition* 60 (1994): 15–22.

20. O. T. Raitakari and coauthors, Effects of persistent physical activity on coronary risk factors in children and young adults: The Cardiovascular Risk in Young Finns Study, *American Journal of Epidemiology* 140 (1994): 195–205.

21. Committee on Sports Medicine and Fitness, Fitness, activity, and sports participation in the preschool child, *Pediatrics* 90 (1992): 1002–1004.

22. F. Lifshitz and N. Moses, Nutritional dwarfing: Growth, dieting, and fear of obesity, *Journal of the American College of Nutrition* 7 (1988): 367–376.

23. G. S. Berenson, S. R. Srinivasan, and L. S. Webber, Cardiovascular risk prevention in children: A challenge or a poor idea? *Nutrition, Metabolism and Cardiovascular Diseases* 4 (1994): 46–52.

24. S. S. Gidding, The rationale for lowering serum cholesterol levels in American children, *American Journal of Diseases of Children* 147 (1993): 386–392; P. T. Einhorn and B. M. Rifkind, Cholesterol measurement in children, *American Journal of Diseases of Children* 147 (1993): 373–375; G. S. Berenson, Cholesterol: Myth vs reality in pediatric practice, *American Journal of Diseases of Children* 147 (1993): 371–373.

25. Report of the Expert Panel on Blood Cholesterol Levels in Children and Adolescents, *Pediatrics* 89 (1992): entire supplement.

26. Berenson, Srinivasan, and Webber, 1994.

27. S. J. Wadowski and coauthors, Family history of coronary artery disease and cholesterol: Screening children in disadvantaged inner-city population, *Pediatrics* 93 (1994): 109–113; K. Resnicow and D. Cross, Are parents' self-reported total cholesterol levels useful in identifying children with hyperlipidemia? An examination of current guidelines, *Pediatrics* 92 (1993): 347–354.

28. National Cholesterol Education Program, Overview and summary, 1992.

29. C. M. Lannon and J. Earp, Parents' behavior and attitudes toward screening children for high serum cholesterol levels, *Pediatrics* 89 (1992): 1159–1163.

30. L. E. Muhonen and coauthors, Coronary risk factors in adolescents related to their knowledge of familial coronary heart disease and hypercholesterolemia: The Muscatine Study, *Pediatrics* 93 (1994): 444–451.

31. M. S. Glassman and S. M. Schwarz, Cholesterol screening in children: Should obesity be a risk factor? *Journal of the American College of Nutrition* 12 (1993): 270–273.

32. Committee on Nutrition, 1992.

33. NCEP Expert Panel on Blood Cholesterol Levels in Children and Adolescents, National Cholesterol Education Program (NCEP): Highlight of the report of the Expert Panel on Blood Cholesterol Levels in Children and Adolescents, *Pediatrics* 89 (1992): 495–501.

34. N. Sigman-Grant, S. Zimmerman, and P. M. Kris-Etherton, Dietary approaches for reducing fat intake of preschool-age children, *Pediatrics* 91 (1993): 955–960.

35. Timely statement on NCEP report on children and adolescents, *Journal of the American Dietetic Association* 91 (1991): 983; Is there a relationship between dietary fat and stature or growth in children three to five years of age? *Pediatrics* 92 (1993): 579–586.

36. Committee on Nutrition, 1992.

37. R. B. Colletti and coauthors, Niacin treatment of hypercholesterolemia in children, *Pediatrics* 92 (1993): 78–82.

38. A. M. Downey, J. L. Cresanta, and G. S. Berenson, Cardiovascular health promotion in children: "Heart Smart" and the changing role of physicians, *American Journal of Preventive Medicine* 5 (1989): 279–295.

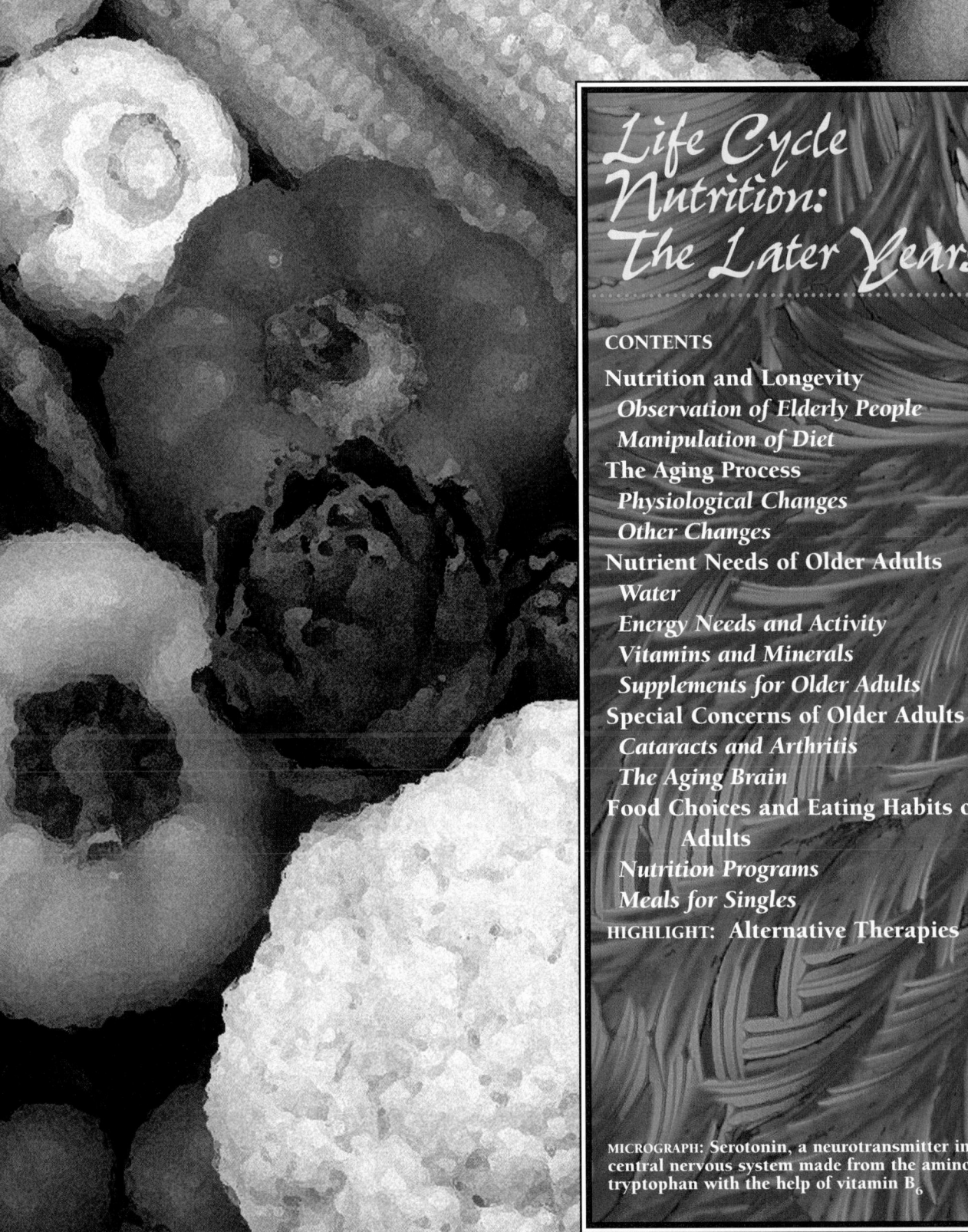

Chapter 20

Life Cycle Nutrition: The Later Years

CONTENTS

Nutrition and Longevity
  Observation of Elderly People
  Manipulation of Diet
The Aging Process
  Physiological Changes
  Other Changes
Nutrient Needs of Older Adults
  Water
  Energy Needs and Activity
  Vitamins and Minerals
  Supplements for Older Adults
Special Concerns of Older Adults
  Cataracts and Arthritis
  The Aging Brain
Food Choices and Eating Habits of Older Adults
  Nutrition Programs
  Meals for Singles
HIGHLIGHT: **Alternative Therapies**

MICROGRAPH: Serotonin, a neurotransmitter in the central nervous system made from the amino acid tryptophan with the help of vitamin B_6

life expectancy: the average number of years lived by people in a given society.

longevity: long duration of life.

life span: the maximum number of years of life attainable by a member of a species.

Figure 20–1

The Aging of the U.S. Population (![person icon] = 65 years or older)

In 1940, 6.8 percent of the population was 65 or older. In 1990, 12.7 percent of us had reached age 65, with 1.2 percent of the population 85 years or older; by 2040, 21.7 percent will have reached age 65; and a century from now, nearly one of four Americans will be 65 and older. An estimated 25,000 Americans now living are 100 years old or older.

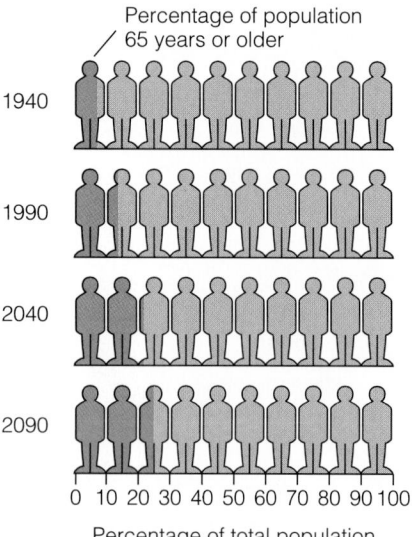

Percentage of population
/ 65 years or older

1940

1990

2040

2090

0 10 20 30 40 50 60 70 80 90 100
Percentage of total population

ise food choices, made throughout adulthood, can support a person's ability to meet physical, emotional, and mental challenges and to achieve freedom from disease. Three goals inspire adults to take responsibility for their nutritional health: promotion of overall wellness, prevention of disease, and slowing of aging. Much of this text has focused on nutrition to support wellness during adulthood; this chapter presents information on aging and the nutrition needs of older adults.

The U.S. population is "graying." The majority is now middle-aged, and the ratio of old people to young is becoming greater, as Figure 20–1 shows. Our society uses the arbitrary age of 65 years to define the transition point between middle age and old age, but growing "old" happens day by day, with change occurring gradually over time. Since 1950 the population of those over 65 has more than doubled. Remarkably, the fastest-growing age group is people over 85 years (see Figure 20–2).[1]

The life expectancy for U.S. women is 79 years and for men, 72 years—up from about 47 years in 1900. Advances in medical science—antibiotics and other treatments—are largely responsible for almost doubling the life expectancy in this century. Improved nutrition and an abundant supply of food have also contributed to lengthening life expectancy.[2] Still, there appears to be an upper limit on human longevity that even nutrition cannot extend. The human life span is about 115 years and has not changed much over the years.

Nutrition and Longevity

Only in this century have human beings achieved a life expectancy that permits science to study aging. Research in the field now is active—and difficult. Researchers are challenged by the diversity of older adults. When older adults experience health problems, it is hard to know whether to attribute them to normal, age-related processes or to other reasons and relationships. If some of the health problems of later life are preventable, then research that focuses on how nutrition and other factors affect aging and disease processes is of great value. The findings will be vital to ensuring that more and more people can look forward to long, healthy lives.

The idea that nutrition can influence the aging process is particularly appealing, because people can control and change their eating habits. Among the questions researchers are asking are:

- To what extent is aging inevitable, and can it be slowed through changes in lifestyle and environment?
- What role does nutrition play in the aging process, and what role can it play in retarding aging?

With respect to the first question, it seems that aging is an inevitable, natural process, programmed into the genes at conception. People can, however, slow the process within the natural limits set by heredity. They need to adopt healthy lifestyle habits such as engaging in physical activity.

With respect to the second question, good nutrition helps to maintain a healthy body and can therefore ease the aging process in many significant ways. Clearly, nutrition can improve the quality of the life in later years.

OBSERVATION OF ELDERLY PEOPLE

One approach researchers use to search out the secret of long life has been to study older people. No doubt, you have noticed that some people are young for their ages, others old for their ages. What makes the difference?

Healthy Habits   Six healthy habits seem to have a profound influence on physiological age:[3]

- Abstinence from, or moderation in, alcohol use.
- Regularity of meals.
- Weight control.
- Regular, adequate sleep.
- Abstinence from smoking.
- Regular physical activity.

The effects of all these factors are cumulative—that is, those who follow all of the practices are in better health, even if older in chronological age, than people who fail to do so. In fact, the physical health of people who report all positive health practices is comparable to that of people *30 years younger* who follow few or none. Other studies have confirmed that these health habits both extend longevity and support independence in later life.[4] The findings suggest that even though people cannot alter the years of their births, they can alter the probable lengths and quality of their lives.

Especially Physical Activity   Vigorous physical activity and long life seem to go together.[5] Even a moderate amount of physical activity—for example, a brisk 30-minute walk each day—is protective against early mortality. An extensive study of more than 16,000 men demonstrates this clearly.[6] The men were between 35 and 74 years of age and were studied for 12 to 16 years. The group whose members expended 2000 or more kcalories in exercise per week (equal to walking or running about 20 miles per week) had a death rate 25 to 33 percent lower than the less active group's rate. Exercise seemed to affect the risk of death even more than did heredity, smoking, hypertension, or extremes in body weight. Physical activity slows cardiovascular aging and reduces heart disease risks. The numerous benefits derived from regular physical activity emphasize the importance of making it a priority in everyone's life.

MANIPULATION OF DIET

Another approach researchers use to learn about longevity has been to manipulate animals' diets. This research has given rise to some interesting and suggestive findings.

physiological age: a person's age as estimated from her or his body's health and probable life expectancy.

chronological age: a person's age in years from his or her date of birth.

Figure 20–2

U.S. Population Growth, 1960 to 1990

The "oldest old"—those 85 years and older—are the fastest-growing age group in the United States. Between 1960 and 1990, the U.S. population grew 39 percent, but the population of those over 85 more than doubled.

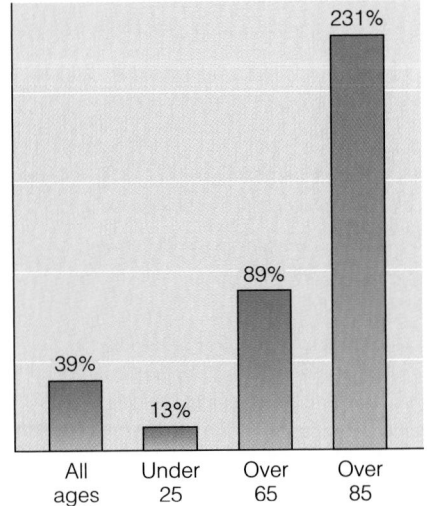

To extend the life span, rats were restricted to 60 percent of their regular intake.

Energy Restriction in Rats Rats live longer when their food intakes are restricted in the early weeks of their lives or even after they are mature. Extensive research shows that it is the restriction of food energy rather than restriction of a specific nutrient that exerts the antiaging effect.[7]

Several mechanisms to explain how energy restriction prolongs life in rats have been proposed but not proven. Food restriction may extend the life span by delaying age-related diseases, retarding growth and development, reducing body fat, slowing the metabolic rate, controlling blood glucose, and preventing lipid oxidation.[8]

While restricting energy intake is the most effective way to lengthen rats' lives, no evidence suggests that these findings apply to human beings. To apply the results of animal studies to human beings is often unrealistic and, in this case, would even be dangerous. The animals given restricted feedings suffered distinct disadvantages: half of them died *very* early (before 300 days); the surviving animals were retarded and malformed in a number of ways. Extreme starvation to extend life, like any extreme, is probably never worth the price.

Energy Restriction in Human Beings One group of researchers studied the relationship between *moderate* energy restriction and the retardation of aging in human beings.[9] Sixteen middle-aged, nonobese men were studied during 10 weeks of energy restriction (80 percent of their usual weight-maintaining intake). They lost weight, mostly due to loss of fat. Their blood pressures dropped significantly, and their HDL cholesterol concentrations rose significantly. Energy restriction had no adverse effects on their mental and physical performances. For these men, moderate energy restriction favorably changed disease risk factors such as obesity, blood pressure, and blood cholesterol.

In summary, life expectancy in the United States has increased dramatically in the last century. Factors that enhance longevity include limited or no alcohol use, regular balanced meals, weight control, adequate sleep, abstinence from smoking, and regular physical activity. Nutrition alone, even if ideal, cannot guarantee a long and robust life. At the very least, however, nutrition can influence aging and longevity in human beings by helping to prevent disease. Later chapters present the relationships between diet and disease prevention; the focus here is on changes that commonly accompany the aging process.

The Aging Process

stress: any threat to a person's well-being; a demand placed on the body to adapt.

stressor: an environmental element, physical or psychological, that causes stress.

stress response: the body's response to stress, mediated initially by both nerves and hormones; begins with an *alarm reaction*, proceeds through a stage of *resistance*, and then leads to *recovery* or, if prolonged, to *exhaustion*. This three-stage response has also been termed the general adaptation syndrome.

As people get older, each person becomes less and less like anyone else. Everyday stresses and habits have had more time to affect the body's health. Both physical stressors, such as alcohol abuse, other drug abuse, smoking, pain, heat, and illness, and psychological stressors, such as exams, divorce, moving, and death of a loved one, elicit the body's stress response. The body responds to such stressors with an elaborate series of physiological steps, using the nervous and hormonal systems to bring about defensive readiness in every body part. The effects all favor physical action—the classic fight-or-flight response. Stress that is prolonged or severe can drain the body of its reserves and leave it weakened, aged, and vulnerable to illness, especially if physical action is not taken. As people age, they lose their ability to adapt to both external and internal disturbances. When disease strikes, the reduced ability to adapt makes the aging individual more vulnerable to death than a younger person.

PHYSIOLOGICAL CHANGES

As aging progresses, inevitable changes in each of the body's organs contribute to the body's declining function. These physiological changes influence nutrition status, just as growth and development do in the earlier stages of the life cycle.

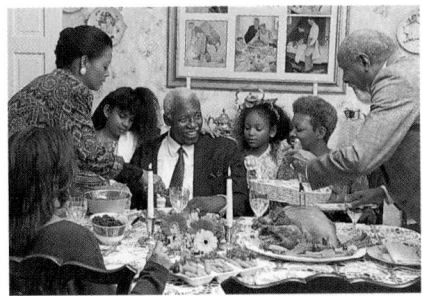

Growing old is enjoyable for people who take care of their health and live each day fully.

Body Composition   Optimal nutrition and physical activity can minimize the body composition changes associated with aging. In general, though, older people tend to lose bone and lean body mass and gain body fat.[10] Many of these changes in body composition occur because some hormones that regulate metabolism become less active with age while others become more active. The action of insulin, for example, diminishes with age as the pancreas begins to secrete less of the hormone and the cells lose their ability to respond efficiently.*

Immune System   Changes in the immune system also bring declining function with age.[11] The immune system is also compromised by nutrient deficiencies, and so the combination of age and malnutrition makes older people vulnerable to infectious diseases.[12] Adding insult to injury, antibiotics often are not effective against infections in people with compromised immune systems.[13] Consequently, infectious diseases are a major cause of death in older adults.

GI Tract   In the GI tract, the intestinal wall loses strength and elasticity with age, and this slows motility. Constipation is four to eight times more common in the elderly than in the young.[14] Atrophic gastritis, a condition that affects almost one-third of those over 60, is characterized by an inflamed stomach, abundant bacteria, and a lack of hydrochloric acid—all of which can impair the digestion and absorption of nutrients, most notably, vitamin B_{12}, biotin, calcium, and iron.

Reminder: *Atrophic gastritis* is a condition characterized by chronic inflammation of the stomach accompanied by a diminished size and functioning of the mucosa and glands.

Tooth Loss   Tooth loss and gum disease are common in old age, making chewing difficult or painful. Dentures, even when they fit properly, are less effective than natural teeth, and inefficient chewing can cause choking. People with tooth loss, gum disease, and ill-fitting dentures tend to limit their selections to soft foods. If foods such as corn on the cob, apples, and hard rolls are replaced by creamed corn, applesauce, and rice, then nutrition status may not be greatly affected, but when food groups are eliminated and variety is limited, inadequate intakes of vitamins, minerals, and fiber follow.

Sensory Losses   A multitude of sensory losses can also interfere with an older person's ability to obtain adequate nourishment. Failing eyesight, for example, can make driving to the grocery store impossible and shopping for food a frustrating experience. It may become so difficult to read food labels and count

---

*Other examples of hormones that change with age include the growth hormone and androgens, which decline with advancing age, thus contributing to the decrease in lean body mass, and the hormone prolactin, which increases with age, helping to maintain body fat.

money that the person doesn't buy the needed foods. Carrying bags of groceries may be an unmanageable task. Similarly, a person with limited mobility may find cooking and cleaning up too hard to do.

Sensory losses can interfere with a person's ability or willingness to eat. Taste and smell sensitivities tend to diminish with age and may make eating less enjoyable.[15] Loss of vision and hearing may contribute to social isolation.[16]

OTHER CHANGES

In addition to the physiological changes that accompany aging, adults are changing in many other ways that influence their nutrition status. Psychological, economic, and social factors play big roles in a person's ability and willingness to eat.

Psychological Changes Though not an inevitable component of aging, depression is common among older adults. It is frequently accompanied by loss of appetite and of the motivation to cook. These feelings are especially apparent when a person has recently lost a loved one. When a person is suffering the heartache and loneliness of bereavement, cooking meals may not seem worthwhile. The support and companionship of family and friends, especially at mealtimes, can help overcome depression and enhance appetite. In addition to depression, older adults are often troubled by insomnia, worry, anxiety, apathy, and forgetfulness.

Economic Changes Overall, the older population today has a higher income than their cohorts of previous generations. Still, poverty is a major problem for about 20 percent of the people over age 65. Factors such as living arrangements and income make significant differences in the food choices, eating habits, and nutrition status of older adults, especially those over age 80.[17] People of low socioeconomic status are likely to have inadequate food and nutrient intakes. For example, studies report a consistent relationship between low income and low intakes of vitamin B_6.[18]

Social Changes Malnutrition among older adults is most likely to occur among those with the least education, those living alone in federally funded housing (an indicator of low income), and those who have recently experienced a change in lifestyle. The risk of nutrient deficiencies is high among people living alone, especially men.[19] One study of home-delivered meals confirmed that men living alone eat less than men living with others; interestingly, women living alone eat more than women living with others.[20] Adults who live alone do not necessarily make poor food choices, but they often consume too little food: loneliness is directly related to nutritional inadequacies, especially of energy intake.[21]

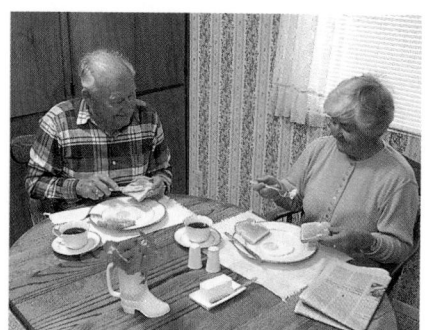

Shared meals can brighten the day and enhance the appetite.

To quickly review, many changes that accompany aging can impair nutrition status. Among physiological changes, hormone activity alters body composition, immune system changes raise the risk of infections, atrophic gastritis interferes with nutrient digestion and absorption, and tooth loss limits food choices. Psychological changes such as depression, economic changes such as loss of income, and social changes such as loneliness contribute to poor food intake.

Nutrient Needs of Older Adults

Knowledge about the nutrient needs and nutrition status of older adults has grown considerably in the last decade or so. The 1989 RDA, however, combine all people over 50 into one group. The 1997 revision split this group into two age categories—one group of 51 to 70 years old and one of 71 and over.[22]* After all, the needs of people 50 to 60 years old may be very different from those of people over 80. The need for more age-specific recommendations is becoming more and more urgent as the population ages.

Setting standards for older people is difficult, though, because individual differences become more pronounced as people grow older. One person may tend to omit vegetables from his diet, and by the time he is old, he will have an associated set of nutrition problems. Another may have omitted milk and milk products all her life—her nutrition problems will be different. Also, as people age, they suffer different chronic diseases and take different drugs—both having impacts on nutrient needs. Even before all this, people start out with different genetic predispositions and ways of handling nutrients, and the effects of these became magnified with the years. Researchers have difficulty even defining "healthy aging," a prerequisite to developing recommendations that are designed to meet the "needs of practically all healthy persons."[23] Still some generalizations are valid, and although new recommendations are needed, the present RDA for adults are of some use. The next sections give special attention to a few nutrients of concern.

WATER

Dehydration is a risk for older adults, who may not notice or pay attention to their thirst, or who find it difficult and bothersome to get a drink or to get to a bathroom. Older adults who have lost bladder control may be afraid to drink too much water. Despite real fluid needs, older people do not seem to feel thirsty or notice mouth dryness.[24] Many nursing home employees say it is hard to persuade their elderly clients to drink enough water and fruit juices.

Total body water also decreases as people age, so that even mild stresses such as fever or hot weather can precipitate rapid dehydration in older adults. Chapter 12 described the importance of water and recommended an intake of 6 to 8 glasses of water a day. Milk and juices may replace some of this water, but beverages containing alcohol or caffeine should be limited because of their diuretic effect.[25]

Water recommendation for adults: 1 to 1½ oz/kg actual body weight.

- Older adult feeding pointer: Drink plenty of water.

ENERGY NEEDS AND ACTIVITY

Energy needs decline with advancing age. As a rule of thumb, adult energy needs decline an estimated 5 percent per decade. For one thing, as people age, they usually reduce their physical activity, although they need not do so. For another, lean body mass diminishes, slowing the basal metabolic rate. The lower energy expenditures require that older adults eat less food energy to maintain their weights. Accordingly, the energy RDA for adults decreases slightly, beginning at

---

*The Canadian RNI divide older people into two age groups—50 to 74, and 75 and older.

age 51. Energy intakes typically decline in parallel with needs. Still, many older adults are overweight, indicating that their food intakes do not decline enough to compensate for their reduced energy expenditure.[26]

- Older adult feeding pointer: Select nutrient-dense foods low in fats, sugars, and alcohol.

On limited energy allowances, people must select mostly nutrient-dense foods. There is little leeway for sugars, fats, oils, or alcohol. Because overweight creates many health problems and shortens the life span, these seem to be life-sustaining recommendations. The Daily Food Guide (on pp. 42–43) offers a dietary framework for adults of all ages. Those who need additional food energy should choose extra servings from each of the groups listed.[27]

Regular Physical Activity   The many and remarkable benefits of regular physical activity are not limited to the young: older adults who are active weigh less and have greater flexibility, more endurance, and better balance than those who are inactive.[28] They reap additional benefits as well; for example, evening exercise helps to eliminate late night trips to the bathroom, and strength training significantly improves mobility and resistance to injury.[29]* In fact, regular physical activity is the most powerful predictor of a person's mobility in the later years.[30]

- Older adult pointer: Exercise to maintain muscle and bone mass.

Activities of all kinds are recommended to maintain and promote health: strength training can build muscles, and aerobic exercise can improve cardiorespiratory endurance and lower blood lipid concentrations.[31] Although aging affects both speed and endurance to some degree, older adults can still train and achieve exceptional performances.

Ideally, physical activity should be part of each day's schedule and should be intense enough to prevent muscle atrophy and to speed up the heartbeat and respiration rate. Healthy older adults who have not been active can ease into a suitable routine. They can start by walking short distances until they can walk at least a mile three times a week; then they can gradually increase their pace to achieve a 20- to 25-minute mile.[32]

Muscle mass and muscle strength tend to decline with aging, making older people vulnerable to falls and immobility. Falls are a major cause of fear, injury, disability, dependence, and even death among older adults. Regular exercise tones, firms, and strengthens muscles, helping to improve confidence, reduce the risk of falling, and minimize the risk of injury should a fall occur. Strength training, even in frail, elderly people over 85 years of age, has been shown to not only improve muscle strength and mobility but to increase energy expenditure and energy intake, thereby enhancing nutrient intakes.[33] This finding highlights another reason to exercise: a person spending energy on physical activity can afford to eat more food and with it, more nutrients. People who are committed to an ongoing fitness program can maintain their body weights and have higher energy and nutrient intakes than more sedentary people.[34]

One expert suggests the following physical activity program to maintain good health and function in older adults:[35]

- *Every day.* 60 minutes of some physical activity: gardening, walking, climbing

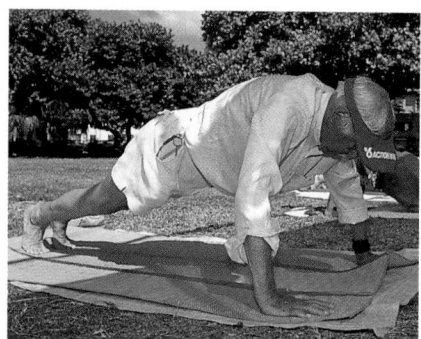

Strength training promotes strong muscles and bones and healthy appetites.

---

*Exercising keeps body fluids circulating; when sedentary people lie down, the excess fluid that has pooled in their lower extremities begins to circulate again, creating the need to urinate. Interview with W. E. Wooldridge, MD, professor emeritus of clinical medicine at the University of Missouri in Columbia as reported in *The Physician and Sportsmedicine* 19 (1991): 49.

stairs, or simply moving about. This can be for 5 minutes at a time, 12 times a day; 12 minutes at a time, 5 times a day; or any combination of activity to total 60 minutes.

- *Three days a week.* 30 to 45 minutes of vigorous and continuous physical activity, such as swimming, dancing, rowing, or brisk walking.

With persistence, people can achieve great improvements at any age. Training not only tones, firms, and strengthens muscles but also increases the blood flow to the brain, thereby improving mental ability.

Protein The protein needs of older adults appear to be about the same as, or even greater than, those of younger people. Since energy needs decrease, however, the protein has to be obtained from low-kcalorie sources of high-quality protein, such as lean meats, poultry, fish, and eggs; nonfat and low-fat milk products; and legumes and grains.

Carbohydrate Abundant carbohydrate is needed to protect protein from being used as an energy source. Complex carbohydrate foods such as vegetables, whole grains, and fruits are also rich in fiber and essential vitamins and minerals.

The combination of ample water and high-fiber foods can alleviate constipation—a condition common among older adults, and especially among nursing home residents. Physical inactivity and medications probably contribute to the high incidence of constipation, but lack of water and fiber does, too, in many cases. In fact, average fiber intakes are lower than current recommendations.

Fat As is true for people of all ages, fat needs to be limited in the diet of most older adults. Cutting fat may help retard the development of cancer, atherosclerosis, and other degenerative diseases. Restricting fat intakes to less than 30 percent of total energy presents a challenge for many older adults, given their limited energy allowances and food intakes. For some older adults, limiting fat intake too severely may lead to nutrient deficiencies and weight loss—two problems that carry greater health risks in the elderly than overweight.[36]

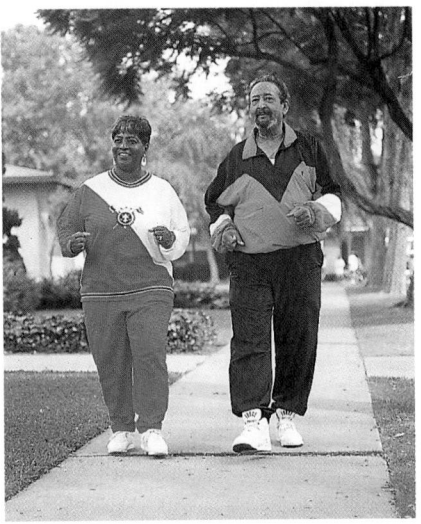

A walk in the neighborhood provides many physical benefits and a time to visit with others.

VITAMINS AND MINERALS

Most people can achieve adequate vitamin and mineral intakes simply by including foods from all food groups in their diets, but studies show that older adults often omit fruits and vegetables.[37] About 18 percent of people 60 years and older are reported to eat no vegetables at all, and up to one of every three older adults reports never eating fruit. When almost 500 participants in a meal program were asked about their food likes and dislikes, nine of the ten most-disliked foods were vegetables. Similarly, few older adults consume the recommended amounts of milk products.[38]

Vitamin A Vitamin A stands alone in that it is absorbed and stored more efficiently by the aging GI tract and liver, although its processing within the body slows slightly.[39] Several studies have reported that healthy older adults have normal levels of plasma vitamin A even when their dietary intakes fall below the RDA, suggesting that the current RDA may be too high.[40] The Committee on Dietary Allowances has hesitated in lowering the RDA, recognizing both the need to prevent vitamin A deficiency and the possibility that the vitamin A precursor beta-carotene might delay the onset of some age-related diseases.

Vitamin D   Older adults face a greater risk of vitamin D deficiency than younger people do. Only vitamin D–fortified milk provides significant vitamin D, and many older adults drink little or no milk. Consequently, many older adults have vitamin D intakes of less than half of the recommended intake. Further compromising the vitamin D status of many older people, especially those in nursing homes, is their limited exposure to sunlight. Finally, aging reduces the skin's capacity to make vitamin D and the kidneys' ability to convert it to its active form. Not only are older adults not getting enough vitamin D, but they may actually need more than the RDA to maintain bone health.[41] The recommended intake for vitamin D was recently raised from 5 to 10 micrograms daily to prevent bone loss and to maintain vitamin D status in older people, especially in those who engage in minimal outdoor activity.[42]

Vitamin B$_6$ Studies of vitamin B$_6$ reveal that its metabolism is altered with age, resulting in a higher requirement. The current RDA for people over 50 may need to be raised.[43]

Vitamin B$_{12}$ People with atrophic gastritis are particularly vulnerable to vitamin B$_{12}$ deficiency for two reasons. First, digestion in the inflamed stomach is inefficient. Second, the abundant bacteria that accompany this condition use the vitamin. Given the devastating effects of a vitamin B$_{12}$ deficiency, an RDA higher than the current one may be appropriate.[44]

Iron   Among the minerals, iron deserves first mention. Iron-deficiency anemia is less common in older adults than in younger people, but it still occurs in some, especially in those with low food energy intakes. Aside from diet, other factors in many older people's lives make iron deficiency likely: chronic blood loss from disease conditions and medicines, and poor iron absorption due to reduced stomach acid secretion and antacid use. Anyone concerned with older people's nutrition should keep these possibilities in mind.

Zinc   Zinc intake is commonly low in older people. As many as 95 percent of older adults may not get the zinc they need, and many receive less than half of the recommended amount.[45] In addition, older adults may absorb zinc less efficiently than younger people do. A number of different factors, including medications that older adults commonly use, can impair zinc absorption or enhance its excretion and thus lead to deficiency.[46] Older adults who do not make special efforts to eat zinc-rich foods such as meats, fish, and poultry will no doubt fail to meet the zinc RDA. Some of the symptoms of zinc deficiency resemble symptoms associated with aging—for example, decline in taste acuity and dermatitis. Whether these symptoms are attributable to zinc deficiency remains unclear.

Calcium DRI for older adults: 1200 mg/day.

Calcium   The appropriate calcium intake for older adults remains controversial. A National Institutes of Health panel has concluded that women over 50 who are not on estrogen replacement therapy and all adults over 65 should receive 1500 milligrams of calcium daily.[47] Recommended intakes for older adults were recently raised from 800 to 1200 milligrams of calcium daily.[48]

While researchers attempt to reach agreement about the calcium requirements of older adults, especially those of women, one thing is clear: the calcium intakes of many people, especially women, in the United States are well below recommendations. If fresh milk causes stomach discomfort, as some older people report, then special efforts should be made to eat other calcium-rich foods. One simple solution is to incorporate dry nonfat milk into recipes; Chapter 12 offers many other strategies.

The importance of abundant dietary calcium throughout life, and especially for women after menopause, to protect against osteoporosis was discussed in Chapter and Highlight 12.

HEALTHY PEOPLE 2000: Increase calcium intake so that at least 50% of people aged 25 years and older consume two or more servings of calcium-rich foods daily.

Malnutrition   It has been estimated that as many as 50 percent of nursing home residents may be malnourished and underweight.[49] For these people, a diet that emphasizes fiber-rich foods such as whole grains, fruits, and vegetables may be too low in concentrated protein and energy. Protein- and energy-dense snacks such as hard-boiled eggs, tuna fish and crackers, peanut butter on graham crackers, and homemade soups are valuable additions to the diets of underweight or malnourished older adults. Table 20–1 lists risk factors for malnutrition in elderly people.

SUPPLEMENTS FOR OLDER ADULTS

Advertisers target older people with appeals to take supplements and eat "health" foods, claiming that these products prevent disease and promote longevity. About half of all women over 65 years of age take some type of nutrient supplement, while about one-fifth of older men do. Quite often those who take supplements are not deficient in the nutrients being supplemented.[50] Certain diseases or health problems may necessitate the taking of supplements, but quite often, supplements have not been prescribed by health care professionals and are inappropriate.

When recommended by a physician, vitamin D and calcium supplements for osteoporosis or iron for iron-deficiency anemia may be beneficial. In most cases, though, the money spent on supplements would be better spent on nutritious foods. Older adults with food energy intakes less than about 1500 kcalories should probably take supplements—not megavitamins, but just the once-daily type of vitamin-mineral supplements.

People with small energy allowances would do well to become more active and earn the right to eat more food. Food is the best source of nutrients for everybody. Supplements are just that—supplements to foods, not substitutes for them. For anyone who is motivated to obtain the best possible health, it is never too late to learn to eat well, drink water, exercise regularly, and adopt other lifestyle changes such as quitting smoking, moderating alcohol use, and the like.

Table 20–1

Risk Factors for Malnutrition in Older Adults

Difficulties in chewing or swallowing
Difficulties in procuring or preparing food
Recent loss of spouse
Oral health problems
Poverty
Multiple drug use
Confusion or depression
Neurologic disorders
Chronic lung disease
Eating fewer than three meals per day
Anorexia
Institutionalization
Inability to self-feed
Alcoholism
Altered taste or smell
Recent surgery
Diabetes
Loneliness

Source: Adapted from R. Chernoff, Meeting the nutritional needs of the elderly in the institutional setting, *Nutrition Reviews* 52 (1994): 132–136.

Table 20–2

Summary of Nutrient Concerns in Aging

Nutrient	Effect of Aging	Comments
Energy	Need decreases.	Physical activity moderates the decline.
Fiber	Likelihood of constipation increases with low intakes and changes in the GI tract.	Inadequate water intakes and lack of physical activity, along with some medications, compound the problem.
Protein	Needs stay the same.	Low-fat, high-fiber legumes and grains meet both protein and other nutrient needs.
Vitamin A	Absorption increases.	RDA may be high.
Vitamin D	Increased likelihood of inadequate intake; skin synthesis declines.	Daily limited sunlight exposure may be of benefit.
Water	Lack of thirst and decreased total body water make dehydration likely.	Mild dehydration is a common cause of confusion. Difficulty obtaining water or getting to the bathroom may compound the problem.
Iron	In women, status improves after menopause; deficiencies are linked to chronic blood losses and low stomach acid output.	Adequate stomach acid is required for absorption; antacid or other medicine use may aggravate iron deficiency; vitamin C and meat increase absorption.
Zinc	Often inadequate intakes and reduced absorption; but needs may also decrease.	Medications interfere with absorption; deficiency may depress appetite and sense of taste.
Calcium	Intakes may be low; osteoporosis common.	Stomach discomfort commonly limits milk intake; calcium substitutes are needed.

Table 20–2 summarizes the nutrient concerns of aging. While some nutrients need special attention in the diet, supplements are not routinely recommended. The ever-growing number of older people in the world presents an urgent need to know more about how their nutrient requirements differ from those of younger people and how such knowledge can enhance their health.

Special Concerns of Older Adults

Nutrition through the prime years may play a greater role than has been realized in preventing many changes once thought to be inevitable consquences of growing older. The following discussions of cataracts, arthritis, and the aging brain show that nutrition may provide at least some protection against some of the conditions associated with aging.

CATARACTS AND ARTHRITIS

Two common causes of distress among older people are cataracts and arthritis. Both of these conditions have nutrition links.

Cataracts Cataracts are age-related thickenings in the lenses of the eye that impair vision. If not surgically removed, they ultimately lead to blindness. Cataracts occur even in well-nourished individuals due to ultraviolet light expo-

cataracts: thickenings of the eye lenses that impair vision and can lead to blindness.

sure, free-radical damage, injury, viral infections, toxic substances, and genetic disorders. Many cataracts, however, are vaguely called senile cataracts—meaning "caused by aging." In the United States, some 46 percent of people between the ages of 75 and 85 have cataracts, compared to only 5 percent of those between the ages of 52 and 64.[51]

Oxidative stress appears to play a significant role in the development of cataracts, and the antioxidant nutrients may help minimize the damage.[52] Studies have reported an inverse relationship between cataracts and dietary intakes of vitamin C, vitamin E, and carotenoids.[53] One study found that people who had no cataracts took significantly more supplements of vitamins C and E than those who had cataracts.[54]

Arthritis Another condition that disables older people is arthritis, a painful swelling of the joints. During movement, the ends of bones are normally protected from wear by cartilage and by small sacs of fluid that act as a lubricant; but with age, bones sometimes disintegrate, and the joints become malformed and painful to move. Arthritis afflicts millions of people around the world, especially the elderly. Nutrition quackery to treat arthritis is abundant, but no known diet prevents, relieves, or cures.

One possibly valid link between arthritis and diet is through the immune system. Researchers believe that in rheumatoid arthritis, the immune system mistakenly attacks the bone coverings as if they were made of foreign tissue.[55] The integrity of the immune system depends on adequate nutrition, and a poor diet may worsen arthritis. It is also possible that in some individuals, certain foods may stimulate the immune system to attack. For example, milk and milk products seem to aggravate arthritis in some people.[56]

Another nutrient linked to arthritis is the omega-3 fatty acid found in fish oil, EPA. Research shows that the same diet recommended for heart health—one low in saturated fat from meats and milk products and high in oils from fish—helps prevent or reduce the inflammation in the joints that makes arthritis so painful.[57] Researchers theorize that EPA probably interferes with the action of prostaglandins, chemicals involved in inflammation.

Another possible link between nutrition and arthritis involves the lipid peroxidation reaction described in Highlight 11—which vitamin E helps to prevent. Lipid peroxidation of the membranes within joints causes inflammation and swelling.[58] Vitamin E has not improved active cases of arthritis, but this is not surprising since the vitamin's role in lipid peroxidation is preventive, not restorative.

A known connection between arthritis and nutrition is overweight. Weight loss is important for overweight persons with arthritis, partly because the joints affected are often weight-bearing joints that are stressed and irritated by having to carry excess poundage. Interestingly, though, weight loss often relieves the worst of the pain of arthritis in the hands as well, even though they are not weight-bearing joints. Jogging and other weight-bearing exercises do not worsen arthritis, even in marathon runners.

Drugs used to relieve arthritis can impose nutrition risks.[59] Many drugs affect appetite and alter the body's use of nutrients, as Chapter 15 explains.
These brief discussions of cataracts and arthritis show that nutrition may provide

Reminder: *Free radicals* are highly reactive molecules that arise during oxidative reactions and readily attack other molecules; see Highlight 11 for more details.

arthritis: a usually painful inflammation of a joint caused by many conditions, including infections, metabolic disturbances, or injury; joint structure is usually altered, with loss of function.

Not effective against arthritis:
- Alfalfa tea.
- Amino acid supplements.
- Blackstrap molasses.
- Burdock root.
- Calcium.
- Celery juice.
- Cod liver oil.
- Copper supplements.
- Dimethyl sulfoxide (DMSO).
- Fasting.
- Fresh fruit.
- Garlic.
- Honey.
- Inositol.
- Kelp.
- Lecithin.
- Para-amino benzoic acid (PABA).
- Raw liver.
- *Aloe vera* liquid.
- Superoxide dismutase (SOD).
- Vitamin D.
- Vitamin megadoses.
- Watercress.
- Yeast.
- 100 other substances.

at least some protection against certain conditions associated with aging. In fact, it is beginning to look as though nutrition through the prime years may play a greater role than has been realized in preventing many changes once thought to be inevitable consequences of growing older.

THE AGING BRAIN

The brain, like all of the body's organs, responds to both inherited and environmental factors that can enhance or diminish its amazing capacities. One of the challenges researchers face when studying aging of the brain in human beings is to distinguish among normal age-related physiological changes, changes caused by diseases, and changes that result from cumulative, extrinsic factors such as diet.

The brain normally changes in some characteristic ways as it ages. For one thing, its blood supply decreases. For another, the number of neurons, the brain cells that specialize in transmitting information, diminishes as people age. When the number of nerve cells in one part of the cerebral cortex diminishes, hearing and speech are affected. Losses of neurons in other parts of the cortex can impair memory and cognitive function. When the number of neurons in the hindbrain diminishes, balance and posture are affected. Losses of neurons in other parts of the brain affect still other functions.

Clinicians now recognize that much of the cognitive loss and forgetfulness generally attributed to aging is due in part to extrinsic, and therefore controllable, factors such as nutrient deficiencies. In some instances, the degree of cognitive loss is extensive and attributable to a specific disorder such as a brain tumor. In cases such as Alzheimer's disease, deterioration may be genetically determined and will not yet yield to external approaches.

Alzheimer's Disease   Much attention has focused on the *abnormal* deterioration of the brain called senile dementia of the Alzheimer's type (SDAT), which affects 5 percent of U.S. adults by age 65 and 20 percent of those over 80.[60] Diagnosis of SDAT depends on its characteristic symptoms: the victim gradually loses memory and reasoning, the ability to communicate, physical capabilities, and eventually life itself. Nerve cells in the brain die and communication between the cells breaks down.

To date, the causes of SDAT continue to elude researchers, although genetic factors are apparently involved. Consequently, researchers have yet to find a cure for this devastating degenerative disease. Treatment involves providing care to clients and support to their families. One drug (trade-named Tacrine) seems to slow the advance of the disease in about 20 percent of those who use it, but it does not reverse the damage already done. Meanwhile, some drugs seem to favorably influence the ability to remember and so hold promise for improving the lives of those with Alzheimer's disease. Other drugs may be used to control depression or behavior problems.

Nutrition may be somehow linked to SDAT. For example, as blood flow to the brain diminishes with age, the brain normally compensates by absorbing more glucose and oxygen. In SDAT, no such compensation occurs, so the glucose and oxygen uptake declines. Whether the brain's diminished capacity to take up glucose and oxygen causes or results from SDAT remains unclear.

Another abnormality of interest involves the extremely low concentrations of the enzyme that makes the neurotransmitter acetylcholine from choline and acetyl CoA. Acetylcholine is essential to memory. To date, supplements of

---

neuron: a nerve cell; the structural and functional unit of the nervous system. Neurons initiate and conduct nerve transmissions.

cerebral cortex: the outer surface of the cerebrum.

senile dementia: the loss of brain function beyond the normal loss of physical adeptness and memory that occurs with aging.

senile dementia of the Alzheimer's type (SDAT): a degenerative disease of the brain involving memory loss and major structural changes in neuron networks; also known as **primary degenerative dementia of senile onset** or **chronic brain syndrome**, but often simply called Alzheimer's disease.

Reminder: A *neurotransmitter* is a chemical that is released by one nerve cell and acts upon a second nerve cell, altering its electrical state or activity.

choline (or of lecithin, which contains choline) have had no effect on memory or on the progression of the disease. Trials of lecithin in combination with drugs show some improvement in limited areas of cognitive deficiencies.

Most people have heard of an association between aluminum and the development of SDAT, although a causal connection seems unlikely. Brain concentrations of aluminum in SDAT people exceed normal brain concentrations by some 10 to 30 times, but blood and hair aluminum remains normal, indicating that the accumulation is caused by something in the brain itself, not by an overload of aluminum in the body. Thus the high brain aluminum must be at least partly a result, rather than a cause, of SDAT. Researchers are still investigating the relationship between dietary aluminum and SDAT in individuals, and the question is still open whether aluminum cookware, which slightly increases the aluminum content of foods, significantly affects the progress of SDAT.

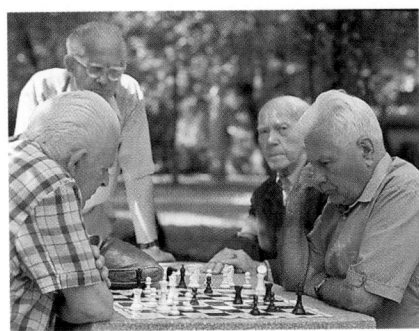

The brain is nourished by both foods and mental challenges.

Maintaining appropriate body weight may be the most important nutrition concern for the person with SDAT. Depression and forgetfulness can lead to poor food intake, and restlessness may increase energy needs. Perhaps the best that a caretaker can do nutritionally for an SDAT client is to supervise food planning and mealtimes. Providing well-liked and well-balanced meals and snacks in a cheerful atmosphere encourages food consumption. To minimize confusion, offer a few ready-to-eat foods, in bite-size pieces, with seasonings and sauces. To avoid mealtime disruptions, control distractions such as television, children, and the telephone.

SDAT is an identifiable disease, the course of which is probably not influenced by nutrition. But poor nutrition in general does affect the brain in other ways.

Nutrient Deficiencies and Brain Function Moderate, long-term nutrient deficiencies may contribute to the loss of memory and cognition that some older adults experience. For example, the ability of neurons to synthesize specific neurotransmitters depends in part on the availability of precursor nutrients that are obtained from the diet. The neurotransmitter serotonin derives from the amino acid tryptophan. To function properly, the enzymes involved in neurotransmitter synthesis require vitamins and minerals. Severe dietary deficiencies of thiamin, vitamin B_6, vitamin B_{12}, folate, and vitamin C impair mental ability, including memory. Trace elements such as iron and zinc also support normal brain function. Table 20–3 summarizes some of the better known connections between impaired brain function and severe nutrient deficiencies. If long-term,

Table 20–3

Summary of Nutrient-Brain Relationships

Brain Function	Inadequate Intake or Deficiency of:
Short-term memory loss	Vitamin B_{12}, vitamin C
Poor performance in problem-solving tests	Riboflavin, folate, vitamin B_{12}, vitamin C
Dementia	Thiamin, zinc
Cognition	Folate, vitamin B_6, vitamin B_{12}, iron
Degeneration of brain tissue	Vitamin B_6

moderate nutrient deficiencies influence the loss of cognitive function that accompanies aging, then the loss may be preventable or at least diminished or delayed through diet.

Senile dementia and other losses of brain function afflict millions of older adults. As the number of people over age 65 continues to grow, the need for solutions to the problems that this major portion of the population faces is becoming urgent. Some problems may be inevitable, but others are preventable.

We can now state with certainty that a person's nutrition status affects the health and functioning of the whole body. Eating a nutritious, balanced diet throughout life seems a small effort in light of the rewards of continued health and enjoyment in later life.

In addition, there is much people can do, besides obtaining adequate nutrition, to support a high quality of life into old age. By practicing stress-management skills, maintaining physical fitness, participating in activities of interest, and cultivating spiritual health, a person can grow old gracefully (see Table 20–4 for some strategies).

Table 20–4

Strategies for Growing Old Gracefully

- Choose nutrient-dense foods.
- Maintain appropriate body weight.
- Reduce stress.
- For women, see a physician about estrogen replacement.
- For people who smoke, quit.
- Expect to enjoy sex, and learn new ways of enhancing it.
- Use alcohol only moderately, if at all; use drugs only as prescribed.
- Take care to prevent accidents.
- Expect good vision and hearing throughout life; obtain glasses and hearing aids if necessary.
- Be alert to confusion as a disease symptom, and seek diagnosis.
- Control depression through activities and friendships.
- Drink 8 glasses of water every day.
- Practice mental skills. Keep on solving math problems and crossword puzzles, playing cards or other games, reading, writing, imagining, and creating.
- Make financial plans early to ensure security.
- Accept change. Work at recovering from losses; make new friends.
- Cultivate spiritual health. Cherish personal values. Make life meaningful.
- Go outside for sunshine and fresh air as often as possible.
- Be physically active. Walk, run, dance, swim, bike, row, or climb for aerobic activity. Lift weights, do calisthenics, or pursue some other activity to tone, firm, and strengthen muscles. Change activities to suit changing abilities and tastes.
- Be socially active—play bridge, join an exercise group, take a class, teach a class, eat with friends, volunteer time to help others.
- Stay interested in life—pursue a hobby, spend time with grandchildren, take a trip, read, grow a garden, or go to the movies.
- Enjoy life.

Food Choices and Eating Habits of Older Adults

Older people are an incredibly diverse group, and for the most part they are independent, socially sophisticated, mentally lucid, fully participating members of society who report themselves to be happy and healthy. Most people over 65 live in their own or relatives' homes; only 5 percent of those 65 to 85, and 20 percent of those over 85, live in facilities such as nursing homes.

Older people spend more money per person on foods to eat at home than other age groups and less money on foods away from home. Manufacturers would be wise to cater to the preferences of older adults by providing good-tasting, nutritious foods in easy-to-open, single-serving packages with labels that are easy to read. Such services enable older adults to maintain their independence; most of them want to take care of themselves and need to feel a sense of control and involvement in their own lives.

Familiarity, taste, and health beliefs are most influential on older people's food choices. Eating foods that are familiar, especially those that recall family meals and pleasant times, can be comforting. The importance of diet and health beliefs in food selection is evidenced by surveys indicating that older adults are choosing low-fat poultry and fish, low-fat milk and milk products, and high-fiber breads and grains.[61] People 65 and over are less likely to diet to lose weight than younger people are, but are more likely to diet in pursuit of medical goals such as controlling blood glucose, cholesterol, and sodium.

- Older adult feeding pointer: Try to maintain independence.

- Older adult feeding pointer: Select familiar foods, especially ethnic favorites.

NUTRITION PROGRAMS

Nutrition services are an integral part of health care, and different subgroups of the aging population need different programs designed to meet their specific needs.[62] People living alone can benefit from congregate meal programs; people confined to their homes need meals delivered. The Nutrition Screening Initiative is part of a national effort to identify and treat nutrition problems in older persons; it uses a screening checklist (see Table 20–5 on p. 682). To *determine* the risk of malnutrition in older clients, health care providers can keep in mind the characteristics listed in the margin.[63]

Risk factors for malnutrition in older adults:
- **D**isease.
- **E**ating poorly.
- **T**ooth loss or oral pain.
- **E**conomic hardship.
- **R**educed social contact.
- **M**ultiple medications.
- **I**nvoluntary weight loss or gain.
- **N**eeds assistance with self-care.
- **E**lderly person older than 80 years.

 HEALTHY PEOPLE 2000: Increase to at least 80% the receipt of home food-services by people aged 65 and older who have difficulty in preparing their own meals or are otherwise in need of home-delivered meals.

The U.S. government funds programs to provide nutritious meals to older adults at congregate meal sites. These meals are a valuable source of nutrients for many older adults. Like the school lunches, though, congregate meals do not typically meet current dietary recommendations to limit sodium, fat, and cholesterol.[64] The box on p. 683 describes food assistance programs for older adults.

MEALS FOR SINGLES

Singles of all ages face difficulties in purchasing, storing, and preparing food. Large packages of meat and vegetables are often intended for families of four or more, and even a head of lettuce can spoil before one person can use it all. Many

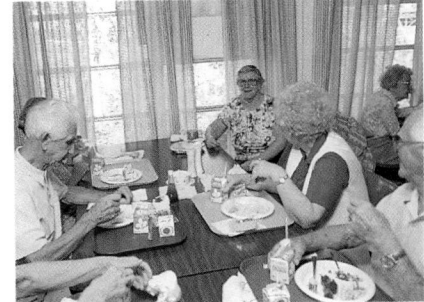
Social interactions at a congregate meal site can be as nourishing as the foods served.

Table 20–5

Nutrition Screening Initiative Checklist

Circle the number to the right if the statement applies to you. Statement	Yes
I have an illness or condition that made me change the kind and/or amount of food I eat.	2
I eat fewer than 2 meals per day.	3
I eat few fruits or vegetables or milk products.	2
I have 3 or more drinks of beer, liquor, or wine almost every day.	2
I have tooth or mouth problems that make it hard for me to eat.	2
I don't always have enough money to buy the food I need.	4
I eat alone most of the time.	1
I take 3 or more different prescribed or over-the-counter drugs a day.	1
Without wanting to, I have lost or gained 10 pounds in the last 6 months.	2
I am not always physically able to shop, cook, and/or feed myself.	2
Total	

SCORE:

0–2: Good. Recheck your score in 6 months.

3–5: Moderate nutritional risk. Visit your local office on aging, senior nutrition program, senior citizens center, or health department for tips on improving eating habits.

6 or more: High nutritional risk. See your doctor, dietitian, or other health care professional for help in improving your nutrition status.

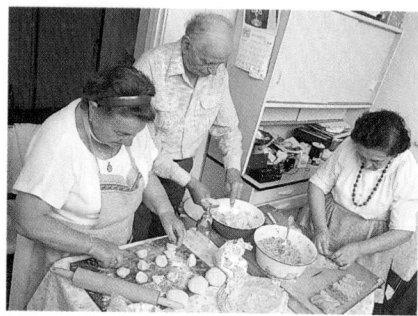

Taking time to nourish your body well is a gift you give yourself.

singles live in small dwellings and have little storage space for foods. A limited income presents additional obstacles. This section presents ideas that can help to solve some of these problems.

Spend Wisely   People who have the means to shop and cook for themselves can cut their food bills just by being wise shoppers. The first decision a person with a tight grocery budget must make is where to shop. Large supermarkets are usually less expensive than convenience stores, but the cost of transportation to the market is a consideration. A grocery list helps reduce impulse buying, and specials and coupons can save money when the items featured are those that the shopper needs and uses.

Buy Bulk   Many foods that offer a variety of nutrients for practically pennies have a long shelf life and can be purchased in bulk. Staples such as rice, pastas, nonfat dry powdered milk, and dried beans and peas can be stored on a shelf for months at room temperature. Other foods that are usually a good buy include whole pieces of cheese rather than sliced or shredded cheese; fresh produce in season; variety meats such as chicken livers; and cereals that require cooking instead of ready-to-serve cereals.

A person who has ample freezing space can buy large packages of meat, such as pork chops, ground beef, or chicken, when they are on sale. Then, the package

Food Assistance Programs for Older Adults

The federal Nutrition Program for Older Americans (Title III) is intended to improve older people's nutrition status and enable them to avoid medical problems, continue living in communities of their own choice, and stay out of institutions. Its specific goals are to provide low-cost, nutritious meals; opportunities for social interaction; homemaker education and shopping assistance; counseling and referral to social services; and transportation.

Title III provides for congregate meal programs. Administrators try to select sites for congregate meals so as to feed as many eligible people as possible. Volunteers may also deliver meals to those who are homebound either permanently or temporarily; these efforts are known as Meals on Wheels. The home-delivery program ensures nutrition, but its recipients miss out on the social benefit of the congregate meal sites; every effort is made to persuade older people to come to the shared meals, if they can. All persons aged 60 years and older are eligible to receive meals from these programs, regardless of their income. Priority is given to those who are economically and socially needy. These programs provide at least one meal a day that meets a third of the RDA for this age group; they must operate five or more days a week. Many programs voluntarily offer additional services: provisions for therapeutic diets, food pantries, ethnic meals, and delivery of meals to the homeless.

Older adults can learn about the available programs in their communities by looking in the yellow pages of the telephone book under "Social Services" or "Senior Citizens' Organizations." In addition, the local senior center and hospital can usually direct people to programs providing nutrition and other health-related services.

congregate meal sites: nutrition programs that provide food for the elderly in a conveniently located setting such as a community center.

---

can be immediately divided into individual servings and wrapped in aluminum foil, not freezer paper: the foil can become the liner for the pan in which to bake or broil the meat, thus saving work. All the individual servings can be put in a bag marked appropriately with the contents and the date. The bag will be easy to locate in the freezer, and a person can see when the supply is running low.

Frozen vegetables are more economical in large bags than in small boxes. The amount needed can be taken out, and the bag closed tightly with a rubber band. If the package is returned quickly to the freezer each time, the vegetables will stay fresh for a long time.

Finally, breads and cereals usually must be purchased in larger quantities. Again the amount needed for a few days can be taken out and the rest stored in the freezer.

Buy Small Buying the right amount in order not to waste any food is a challenge for people eating alone. They can buy fresh milk in the size best suited for personal needs. Pint-size and even cup-size boxes of milk are also available and can be stored unopened on a shelf for up to three months without refrigeration.

Boxes of milk kept at room temperature on the shelves of grocery stores have been treated with a process called **ultrahigh temperature (UHT)**; the milk is exposed to temperatures above those of pasteurization just long enough to sterilize it.

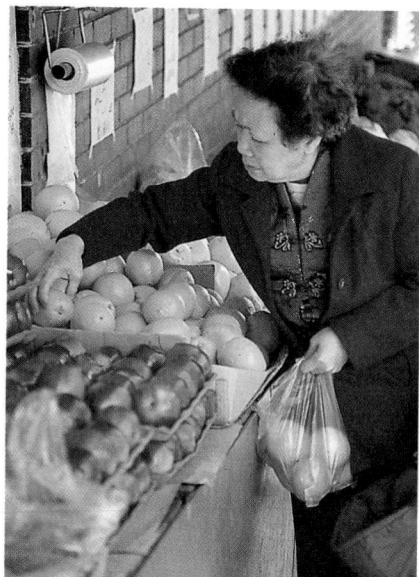

Buy only what you will use.

Grocers will break open a package of wrapped meat and rewrap the portion needed. Similarly, eggs can be purchased by the half-dozen. Eggs do keep for long periods, though, if stored properly in the refrigerator.

Fresh fruits and vegetables can be purchased individually. A person can buy three pieces of each kind of fresh fruit: a ripe one to eat right away, a semiripe one to eat soon after, and a green one to ripen on the windowsill. If vegetables are packaged in large quantities, the grocer can break open the package so that a smaller amount can be purchased. Small cans of fruits and vegetables, even though they are more expensive per unit, are a reasonable alternative, considering that it is expensive to buy a regular-size can and let the unused portion spoil.

Be Creative   For times when a person has to buy more food than one person can use, here are a few hints. Mixtures of leftovers can be prepared and served again. A thick stew made from leftover green beans, carrots, cauliflower, broccoli, and any meat with added onion, pepper, celery, and potatoes makes a complete and balanced meal—except for milk, but then powdered milk can be added to the stew.

Glass jars are ideal for storing shelf staple items—rice, tapioca, lentils or other dry beans, flour, cornmeal, nonfat dry milk, macaroni, cereal, and the like. Freezing each filled jar for one night first kills any insect eggs that might be present. The jars will then keep bugs out of the food indefinitely. They make an attractive display and serve to remind the cook of different choices to vary menus. The directions-for-use labels from the packages can be stored in the jars.

Creative chefs think of various ways to use a vegetable when only large amounts are available. For example, a head of cauliflower can be divided into thirds. Then one-third is cooked and eaten hot. Another third is put into a vinegar and oil marinade for use in a salad. And the last third can be used in a casserole or stew.

Also, single people shouldn't hesitate to invite someone to share meals with them whenever there is a lot of food. It's likely that that person will return the invitation, and both parties will get to enjoy companionship and a meal prepared by others.

An occasional frozen TV dinner can also be useful—although expensive—if it makes the difference between a person's eating and not eating. Many such dinners that are now available are low in fat and nutritious. Adding a fresh salad, a whole-wheat roll, and a glass of milk can make a nice meal. Another option for those who can afford it is to eat meals from restaurants. Most restaurants offer take-out meals and many provide delivery services.

One more suggestion for those who are alone at mealtime is this: make it a special occasion. One way to do this is to set the table with a tablecloth, a napkin, a full set of utensils, and fresh flowers. Set a pot of stew or homemade soup with vegetables and fresh herbs on low heat to cook, and make a salad. Get comfortable in a stuffed chair, and enjoy a book or some soothing music until the rich aroma of a simmering dinner beckons. After serving your plate, light a candle, dim the lights, savor the food, and relish some of the best company you will have—your own.

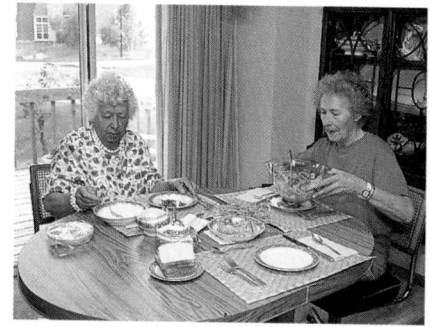

Invite guests to share a meal.

Study Questions

1. What roles does nutrition play in aging, and what roles can it play in retarding aging?
2. What are some of the physiological changes that occur in the body's systems with aging? To what extent can aging be prevented?
3. Why does the risk of dehydration increase as people age?
4. Why do energy needs usually decline with advancing age?
5. Which vitamins and minerals need special consideration for the elderly? Explain why. Name some factors that complicate the task of setting nutrient standards for older adults.
6. Discuss the relationships between nutrition and cataracts and between nutrition and arthritis.
7. What characteristics contribute to malnutrition in older people?

Notes

1. R. Chernoff, Demographics of aging, in *Geriatric Nutrition: The Health Professional's Handbook*, ed. R. Chernoff (Gaithersburg, Md.: Aspen Publishers, 1991), pp. 1–9.
2. K. G. Kinsella, Changes in life expectancy 1900–1990, *American Journal of Clinical Nutrition* 55 (1992): 1196S–1202S; S. Kobayashi, A scientific basis for the longevity of Japanese in relation to diet and nutrition, *Nutrition Reviews* 50 (1992): 353–359.
3. L. Breslow and N. Breslow, Health practices and disability: Some evidence from Alameda County, *Preventive Medicine* 22 (1993): 86–95.
4. A. Z. LaCroix and coauthors, Maintaining mobility in late life: Smoking, alcohol consumption, physical activity, and body mass index, *American Journal of Epidemiology* 137 (1993): 858–869.
5. R. S. Paffenbarger and coauthors, The association of changes in physical-activity level and other lifestyle characteristics with mortality among men, *New England Journal of Medicine* 328 (1993): 538–545; S. N. Blair and coauthors, Physical fitness and all-cause mortality, *Journal of the American Medical Association* 262 (1989): 2395–2401.
6. R. S. Paffenbarger and coauthors, Physical activity, all-cause mortality, and longevity of college alumni, *New England Journal of Medicine* 314 (1986): 605–611.
7. E. J. Masoro, Retardation of aging processes by food restriction: An experimental tool, *American Journal of Clinical Nutrition* (supplement) 55 (1992): 1250–1252.
8. E. J. Masoro, Assessment of nutritional components in prolongation of life and health by diet, *Proceedings of the Society for Experimental Biology and Medicine* 193 (1990): 31–34; Energy intake restriction and oxidant defense, *Nutrition Reviews* 49 (1991): 278–280.
9. E. J. M. Velthuis-te Wierik and coauthors, Energy restriction, a useful intervention to retard human ageing? Results of a feasibility study, *European Journal of Clinical Nutrition* 48 (1994): 138–148.
10. R. Roubenoff and L. C. Rall, Humoral mediation of changing body composition during aging and chronic inflammation, *Nutrition Reviews* 51 (1993): 1–11.
11. T. Tada, Nutrition and the immune system in aging: An overview, *Nutrition Reviews* 50 (1992): 360.
12. R. K. Chandra, Nutrition and immunity in the elderly, *Nutrition Reviews* 50 (1992): 367–371.
13. K. Hirokawa, Understanding the mechanism of the age-related decline in immune function, *Nutrition Reviews* 50 (1992): 361–366.
14. S. Hosoda and coauthors, Age-related changes in the gastrointestinal tract, *Nutrition Reviews* 50 (1992): 374–377.
15. C. Murphy, Age-associated changes in taste and odor sensation, perception, and preference, in *Nutrition of the Elderly*, eds. H. Munro and G. Schlierf (New York: Raven Press, 1992), pp. 79–87.
16. C. O. Mitchell and R. Chernoff, Nutritional assessment of the elderly, in *Geriatric Nutrition: The Health Professional's Handbook*, ed. R. Chernoff (Gaithersburg, Md.: Aspen Publishers, 1991), pp. 363–395.
17. J. V. White and coauthors, Consensus of the Nutrition Screening Initiative: Risk factors and indicators of poor nutritional status in older Americans, *Journal of the American Dietetic Association* 91 (1991): 783–787.
18. A. K. Kant and G. Block, Dietary vitamin B-6 intake and food sources in the US population: NHANES II, 1976–1980, *American Journal of Clinical Nutrition* 52 (1990): 707–716.
19. M. A. Davis and coauthors, Living arrangements and dietary quality of older U.S. adults, *Journal of the American Dietetic Association* 90 (1990): 1667–1672; I. Darnton-Hill, Psychosocial aspects of nutrition and aging, *Nutrition Reviews* 50 (1992): 476–479.
20. E. Fogler-Levitt and coauthors, Utilization of home-delivered meals by recipients 75 years of age or older, *Journal of the American Dietetic Association* 95 (1995): 552–557.
21. D. Walker and R. E. Beauchene, The relationship of loneliness, social isolation, and physical health to dietary adequacy of independently living elderly, *Journal of the American Dietetic*

Association 91 (1991): 300–304.

22. Committee on Reference Intakes, *Dietary Reference Intakes for Calcium, Phosphorus, Magnesium, Vitamin D, and Fluoride* (Washington, D.C.: National Academy Press, 1997).

23. A. Bendich, Criteria for determining recommended dietary allowances for healthy older adults, *Nutrition Reviews* 53 (1995): S105–S110.

24. B. J. Rolls and P. A. Phillips, Aging and disturbances of thirst and fluid balance, *Nutrition Reviews* 48 (1990): 137–144.

25. Water: The beverage of life (Chicago, Ill.: The American Dietetic Association, 1994).

26. E. T. Poehlman and E. S. Horton, Regulation of energy expenditure in aging humans, *Annual Review of Nutrition* 10 (1990): 255–275.

27. A. Greeley, Nutrition and the elderly, *FDA Consumer*, October 1990, pp. 25–28.

28. L. E. Voorrips and coauthors, The physical condition of elderly women differing in habitual physical activity, *Medicine and Science in Sports and Exercise* 25 (1993): 1152–1157.

29. M. A. Fiatarone and coauthors, High-intensity strength training in nonagenarians: Effects on skeletal muscle, *Journal of the American Medical Association* 263 (1990): 3029–3034; W. E. Wooldridge as cited by *The Physician and Sportsmedicine* 19 (1991): 49.

30. A. Z. LaCroix and coauthors, Maintaining mobility in late life: Smoking, alcohol consumption, physical activity, and body mass index, *American Journal of Epidemiology* 137 (1993): 858–869; Breslow and Breslow, 1993.

31. Fiatarone and coauthors, 1990; D. E. Danforth and coauthors, Report on the fourth conference for federally supported human nutrition research units and centers, *American Journal of Clinical Nutrition* 54 (1991): 164–168; M. Whitehurst and E. Menendez, Endurance training in older women, *The Physician and Sportsmedicine* 19 (1991): 95–102.

32. J. Posner, M. D., professor of medicine and chief of the divisions of Geriatric Medicine at the Medical College of Pennsylvania in Philadelphia, as cited in C. L. Pollock, Breaking the risk of falls, *The Physician and Sports Medicine* 20 (1992): 146–156.

33. M. A. Fiatarone and coauthors, Exercise training and nutritional supplementation for physical fraility in very elderly people, *New England Journal of Medicine* 330 (1994): 1769–1775; W. W. Campbell and coauthors, Increased energy requirements and changes in body composition with resistance training in older adults, *American Journal of Clinical Nutrition* 60 (1994): 167–175.

34. D. E. Butterworth and coauthors, Exercise training and nutrient intake in elderly women, *Journal of the American Dietetic Association* 93 (1993): 653–657.

35. P. Astrand, Physical activity and fitness, *American Journal of Clinical Nutrition* (supplement) 55 (1992): 1231–1236.

36. P. J. Nestel, Dietary fat for the elderly: What are the issues? in *Nutrition of the Elderly*, eds. H. Munro and G. Schlierf (New York: Raven Press, 1992), pp. 119–127.

37. V. Holt, J. Nordstrom, and M. B. Kohrs, Food preferences of older adults, *Journal of Nutrition for the Elderly* 6 (1987): 47.

38. J. G. Fischer and coauthors, Dairy product intake of the oldest old, *Journal of the American Dietetic Association* 95 (1995): 918–921.

39. Processing of dietary retinoids is slowed in the elderly, *Nutrition Reviews* 49 (1991): 116–119.

40. Russell and Suter, 1993.

41. Russell and Suter, 1993.

42. A. R. Webb and coauthors, An evaluation of the relative contributions of exposure to sunlight and of diet to the circulating concentrations of 25-hydroxyvitamin D in an elderly nursing home population in Boston, *American Journal of Clinical Nutrition* 51 (1990): 1075–1081; Committe on Dietary Reference Intakes, 1997.

43. Russell and Suter, 1993.

44. Russell and Suter, 1993.

45. C. A. Swanson and coauthors, Zinc status of elderly adults: Response to supplement, *American Journal of Clinical Nutrition* 48 (1988): 343–349.

46. G. J. Fosmire, Trace mineral requirements, in *Geriatric Nutrition: The Health Professional's Handbook*, ed. R. Chernoff (Gaithersburg, Md.: Aspen Publishers, 1991), pp. 77–105.

47. D. V. Porter, Washington update: NIH consensus development conference statement optimal calcium intake, *Nutrition Today*, September/October 1994, pp. 37–40.

48. Committee on Dietary Reference Intakes, 1997.

49. A. A. Abbase and D. Rudman, Undernutrition in the nursing home: Prevalence, consequences, causes and prevention, *Nutrition Reviews* 52 (1994): 113–122.

50. W. A. McIntosh and coauthors, The relationship between beliefs about nutrition and dietary practices of the elderly, *Journal of the American Dietetic Association* 90 (1990): 671–675; H. Payette and K. Gray-Donald, Do vitamin and mineral supplements improve the dietary intake of elderly Canadians? *Canadian Journal of Public Health* 82 (1993): 58–60.

51. G. E. Bunce, J. Kinoshita, and J. Horwitz, Nutritional factors in cataract, *Annual Review of Nutrition* 10 (1990): 233–254.

52. Bunce, Kinoshita, and Horwitz, 1990; S. D. Varma, Scientific basis for medical therapy of cataracts by antioxidants, *American Journal of Clinical Nutrition* 53 (1991): 335S–345S.

53. P. F. Jacques and L. T. Chylack, Epidemiologic evidence of a role for the antioxidant vitamins and carotenoids in cataract prevention, *American Journal of Clinical Nutrition* 53 (1991): 352S–355S; G. E. Bunce, Antioxidant nutrition and cataract in women: A prospective study, *Nutrition Reviews* 51 (1993): 84–86.

54. J. M. Robertson, A. P. Donner, and J. R. Trevithick, A possible role for vitamins C and E in cataract prevention, *American Journal of Clinical Nutrition* 53 (1991): 346S–351S.

55. E. D. Harris, Rheumatoid arthritis: Pathophysiology and implications for therapy, *New England Journal of Medicine* 322 (1990): 1277–1289.

56. R. S. Panush, Nutritional therapy for rheumatic diseases, *Annals of Internal Medicine* 106 (1987): 619–621.

57. J. M. Kremer and coauthors, Fish-oil fatty acid supplementation in active rheumatoid arthritis: A double-blind, controlled crossover study, *Annals of Internal Medicine* 106 (1987): 497–503.

58. P. Merry and coauthors, Oxidative damage to lipids within the inflamed human joint provides evidence of radical-mediated hypoxic-reperfusion injury, *American Journal of Clinical Nutrition* 53 (1991): 362S–369S.

59. R. Roubenoff and coauthors, Catabolic effects of high-dose corticosteroids persist despite therapeutic benefit in rheumatoid arthritis, *American Journal of Clinical Nutrition* 52 (1990): 1113–1117.

60. R. N. Butler, Senile dementia of the Alzheimer type (SDAT), in *The Merck Manual of Geriatrics* (Rahway, N.J.: Merck & Co., Inc., 1990), pp. 933–938.

61. Are older Americans making better food choices to meet diet and health recommendations? *Nutrition Reviews* 51 (1993): 20–22.

62. Position of The American Dietetic Association: Nutrition, aging, and the continuum of health care, *Journal of the American Dietetic Association* 93 (1993): 80–82.

63. J. Dwyer and coauthors, Screening older Americans' nutritional health: Future possibilities, *Nutrition Today*, September/October 1991, pp. 21–24.

64. M. B. Moran and E. Reed, Are congregate meals meeting clients' needs for "heart healthy" menus? *Journal of Nutrition for the Elderly* 13 (1993): 3–10.

Alternative Therapies

*I*f you suffered from migraine headaches or severe joint pain, where would you turn for relief? Would you visit a physician? Or are you more likely to go to an herbalist or an acupuncturist? Most physicians diagnose and treat medical conditions in ways that are accepted by the established medical community; by comparison, herbalists and acupuncturists, among others, use unconventional methods that offer alternatives to standard medical practice. Instead of taking two aspirin, for example, you might be advised to chew two fresh leaves of the herb feverfew or to swallow a tincture of white willow bark. Or you might receive a massage and several acupuncture needles.

Alternative therapies have become increasingly popular in recent years. Many consumers have become distrustful of, and feel overwhelmed by, the high-tech diagnostic tests and costly treatments that conventional medicine offers. They want to take more responsibility for maintaining their own health and finding cures for their own diseases, especially when traditional medical therapies prove ineffective. This highlight explores alternative therapies in search of their possible benefits and with an awareness of their potential harms.

DEFINING ALTERNATIVE MEDICINE

By definition, alternative therapies lie outside the realm of conventional medicine. An alternative therapy is any intervention that:

- Is not taught by most medical schools in the United States.

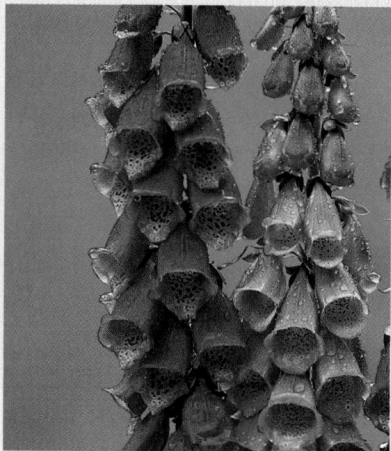

Digoxin, a drug commonly prescribed for abnormal heart rhythms, derives from the foxglove plant.

- Is not reimbursable by most health insurance providers in the United States.

- Is not well supported by scientific tests establishing its safety and effectiveness.

If it is proven safe and effective, an alternative therapy may gradually become part of mainstream conventional medicine. Cancer radiation therapy, for example, was once considered an unconventional therapy, but now is commonly accepted as standard medical practice. In some cases, a therapy that is accepted by traditional medicine for a specific ailment is used for a different purpose in an alternative therapy. For example, chelation therapy, the preferred biomedical treatment for lead poisoning, is a common alternative therapy for cardiovascular disease.

Table H20–1 lists selected fields of alternative medicine, and the accompanying glossary defines terms. Notice that most alternative medicines fall outside the field of

nutrition, but that nutrition itself can be an alternative therapy. Furthermore, many alternative therapies prescribe specific dietary regi-

Table H20–1

Fields of Alternative Medicine and Selected Examples

Mind-body interventions
  Biofeedback
  Faith healing
  Hypnotherapy
  Imagery
  Meditation
Bioelectromagnetic applications in medicine
  Electroacupuncture
  Microwave resonance therapy
Alternative systems of medical practice
  Acupuncture
  Ayurveda
  Homeopathic medicine
  Naturopathic medicine
Manual healing methods
  Biofield therapeutics
  Chiropractic
  Massage therapy
Pharmacological and biological treatments
  Cartilage therapy
  Chelation therapy
  Ozone therapy
Herbal medicine
Diet and nutrition in the prevention and treatment of chronic disease
  Macrobiotic diets
  Orthomolecular medicine

Source: Alternative Medicine: Expanding Medical Horizons, A report to the National Institutes of Health and Alternative Medical Systems and Practices in the United States (Washington, D.C.: Government Printing Office, 1992).

Glossary

acupuncture (AK-you-PUNK-cher): a technique that involves piercing the skin with long thin needles at specific anatomical points to relieve pain or illness. Acupuncture sometimes uses heat, pressure, friction, suction, or electromagnetic energy to stimulate the points.

alternative therapies: approaches to medical diagnosis and treatment that are not fully accepted by the established medical community; as such, they are not widely taught at U.S. medical schools or practiced in U.S. hospitals; also called *adjunctive*, *unconventional*, or *unorthodox* therapies.

aroma therapy: a technique that uses oil extracts from plants and flowers (usually applied by massage or baths) to enhance physical, psychological, and spiritual health.

ayurveda (EYE-your-VAY-dah): a traditional Hindu system of improving health by using herbs, diet, meditation, massage, and yoga to stimulate the body to make its own natural drugs.

bioelectromagnetic medical applications: the use of electrical energy, magnetic energy, or both to stimulate bone repair, wound healing, and tissue regeneration.

biofeedback: the use of special devices to convey information about heart rate, blood pressure, skin temperature, muscle relaxation, and the like to enable a person to learn how to consciously control these medically important functions.

biofield therapeutics: a manual healing method that directs a healing force from an outside source (commonly God or another supernatural being) through the practitioner and into the client's body; commonly known as "laying on of hands."

cartilage therapy: the use of cleaned and powdered connective tissue, such as collagen, to improve health.

chelation therapy: the use of ethylene diamine tetraacetic acid (EDTA) to bind with metallic ions, thus healing the body by removing toxic metals.

chiropractic (KYE-roe-PRAK-tik): a manual healing method of manipulating vertebrae to relieve musculoskeletal pain suspected of causing problems with internal organs.

DHEA (dehydroepiandrosterone): a hormone secreted by the adrenal glands. DHEA is available without prescription and is sold as an anti-aging remedy to improve energy, strength, and immunity. Proof of safety or effectiveness is lacking.

faith healing: healing by invoking divine intervention without the use of medical, surgical, or other traditional therapy.

garlic oil: extract of garlic; proof of effectiveness is lacking.

hemlock: a poisonous herb having finely divided leaves and small white flowers.

herbal medicine: the use of plants to treat disease or improve health; also known as *botanical medicine* or *phytotherapy*.

homeopathic (home-ee-OP-ah-thick) **medicine:** a practice based on the theory that "like cures like," that is, that substances that cause symptoms in healthy people can cure those symptoms when given in very dilute amounts.
  homeo = like
  pathos = suffering

hypnotherapy: a technique that uses hypnosis and the power of suggestion to improve health behaviors, relieve pain, and heal.

imagery: a technique that guides clients to achieve a desired physical, emotional, or spiritual state by visualizing themselves in that state.

iridology: the study of changes in the iris of the eye and their relationships to disease.

macrobiotic diet: a diet consisting of brown rice, miso soup, sea vegetables, and other traditional Japanese foods.

massage therapy: a healing method in which the therapist manually kneads muscles to reduce tension, increase blood circulation, improve joint mobility, and promote healing of injuries.

meditation: a self-directed technique of relaxing the body and calming the mind.

melatonin: a hormone secreted by the pineal gland believed to help regulate the body's daily rhythms and promote sleep. Proof of safety or effectiveness is lacking.

naturopathic medicine: a system that integrates traditional medicine with botanical medicine, clinical nutrition, homeopathy, acupuncture, East Asian medicine, hydrotherapy, and manipulative therapy.

orthomolecular medicine: the use of large doses of vitamins to treat chronic disease.

ozone therapy: the use of ozone gas to enhance the body's immune system.

---

mens. The many dietary recommendations presented throughout this text are based on scientific evidence and do *not* fall into the alternative category; strategies that are still experimental, however, do. For example, alternative therapists may recommend megadoses of antioxidant supplements or macrobiotic

689

diets to help prevent chronic diseases, whereas most registered dietitians would advise people to eat at least five servings of vegetables and fruits daily instead.

SOUND RESEARCH, LOUD CONTROVERSY

Most information on alternative therapies comes from folklore, tradition, and testimonial accounts. The clinical trials that have been conducted generally suffer from such poor methodology as to invalidate their findings.[1] In short, scientific evidence proving the safety and effectiveness of alternative therapies is lacking. Some say that alternative therapies simply do not work; others argue that the established medical community has not given these therapies a fair trial.

Sound research would answer two important questions. First, does the treatment offer better results than either doing nothing or giving a placebo? Second, do the benefits clearly outweigh the risks? Each of these points is worthy of elaboration.

Placebo Effect

As Chapter 1 explained, a placebo is an inert, harmless medication used in research studies to control for the beneficial effect that a treatment—even an inactive one—has on recovery. Placebos are inert, but they can also be effective, accounting for an apparent benefit about as often as not.[2] Traditional medicine tends to neglect this most powerful remedy, whereas many alternative therapies embrace it. While health professionals cannot conceal serious illnesses or intentionally deceive a client, they might be wise to provide a caring confidence in the appropriate treatment and likelihood of recovery.

Risks versus Benefits

Ideally, a therapy provides benefits with little or no risk. The use of ginseng as an adjunct in the management of diabetes (NIDDM), for example, correlates with an improved fasting blood glucose and glycated hemoglobin without adverse side effects.[3] Though still in the experimental stage, such findings, if replicated, hold promise that this alternative therapy may one day become accepted medical practice.

Some alternative therapies are innocuous, providing little or no benefit for little or no risk. Sipping a cup of warm tea with a pleasant aroma, for example, won't cure heart disease, but it may improve the person's mood and help release tension. Given no physical hazard and little financial risk, such therapies are acceptable.

In contrast, other products and procedures are downright dangerous, posing great risks while providing no benefits. One example is the folk practice of geophagia (eating earth or clay), which can cause GI impaction and impair iron absorption. Clearly, such therapies are too harmful to be used.

Perhaps most controversial are alternative therapies that may provide benefits, but also carry significant, unknown, or debatable risks. These therapies tend to appeal most to those who are most vulnerable—people with very serious illnesses. Smoking marijuana is a current example of such an alternative therapy: it seems to provide relief from symptoms such as nausea, vomiting, and pain that commonly accompany cancer, AIDS, and other diseases, but also poses risks that some people, including many physicians, consider acceptable and others, mainly politicians, deem intolerable.[4] Physicians have focused on individuals and recognize that marijuana stimulates the appetite in their nauseated clients; politicians and others have focused on society and realize that marijuana is one of many drugs that can be abused. Figure H20–1 summarizes the relationships between risks and benefits.

Funds and Findings

The public's growing interest in unorthodox remedies, coupled with the soaring costs of traditional medical approaches, opened the way for alternative medicine to prove itself. In 1992, Congress passed legislation requiring the National Institutes of Health (NIH) to create an Office of Alternative Medicine. Its task is "to more adequately explore unconventional medical practices."[5]

The use of tax dollars to fund research in alternative therapies has many medical professionals concerned.[6] They claim that establishing a special office lends credibility to these unproven methods of health care. Others demand that these methods be given a fair chance to prove themselves through scientifically valid research. Alternative therapies currently under study include:[7]

- Acupuncture to treat depression, attention deficit hyperactivity disorder, osteoarthritis, and postoperative dental pain.

- Hypnosis to treat chronic low back pain and to speed fracture healing.

- Ayurvedic herbals to treat Parkinson's disease.

Figure H20–1

Risk-Benefit Relationships

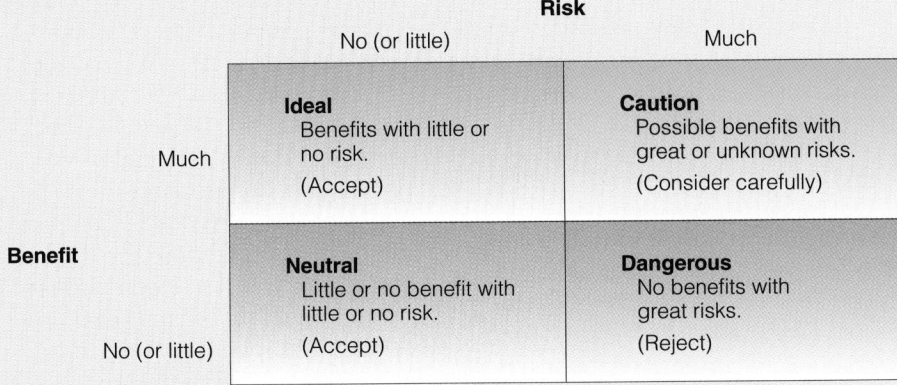

	Risk	
	No (or little)	Much
Much	**Ideal** Benefits with little or no risk. (Accept)	**Caution** Possible benefits with great or unknown risks. (Consider carefully)
No (or little)	**Neutral** Little or no benefit with little or no risk. (Accept)	**Dangerous** No benefits with great risks. (Reject)

Benefit (row label, left side)

- Biofeedback to treat diabetes, low back pain, and face and mouth pain caused by jaw disorders.

- Electric currents to treat tumors.

- Imagery to treat asthma and breast cancer.

NUTRITION AND HERBAL MEDICINES

Of greatest interest to students of nutrition is the use of foods and herbs to prevent and treat illnesses. With the proliferation of research on antioxidants and disease prevention (see Highlight 11), medical science has begun to accept the health-promoting powers of vitamin-rich vegetables. It is even beginning to consider the possibility that supplementation might someday be an appropriate preventive therapy. Herbs, on the other hand, continue to meet with resistance.[8]

Herbal Traditions

From earliest times, people have used a myriad of herbs and other plants to cure aches and ills with varying degrees of success. Upon scientific study, dozens of these folk remedies reveal their secrets. For example, myrrh, a plant resin used as a painkiller in ancient times, does indeed have an analgesic effect.[9] The herb valerian, which has long been used as a tranquilizer, contains oils that have a sedative effect. Senna leaves, brewed as a laxative tea, produce compounds that act as a potent cathartic drug. The compounds that plants make are so beneficial that today they contribute to more than half of our modern medicines. Once analyzed, the chemicals in plants can be synthesized in pharmaceutical labs, thus cutting costs and conserving endangered species. Without laboratory production, valued plants could quickly disappear; consider that it took all of the bark from one 40-foot-tall, 100-year-old Pacific yew tree to obtain one 300-milligram dose of the anticancer drug paclitaxel (Taxol), until scientists learned how to synthesize it.[10]

Herbal Precautions

Simply because plants are "natural" does not mean that they are beneficial or even safe. Nothing could be more natural—and deadly—than hemlock. Several herbal remedies have toxic effects. The popular Chinese herbal potion Jin Bu Huan, which is used as a pain and insomnia remedy, has been linked with several cases of acute hepatitis. Germanium, an ingredient in many herbal products, has been associated with chronic renal failure. Paraguay tea produces symptoms of agitation, confusion, flushed skin, and fever. Kombucha tea, commonly used in the hopes of preventing cancer, relieving arthritis, curing insomnia, and stimulating hair regrowth, can cause severe metabolic acidosis.[11]

When used to diagnose, treat, or prevent disease, herbs are drugs. Yet few herbalists have the understanding of botany, chemistry, or pharmacology necessary to prescribe plant drugs.[12] Instead, they rely on hearsay and folklore. The herbs they prescribe are not regulated by the Food and Drug Administration (FDA). Under the Dietary Supplement Health and Education Act, rather than the herb manufacturers having to prove the safety of their products, the FDA has the burden of proving that a product is not safe.[13] Because information on the safety and effectiveness of herbs derives largely from users' reports, consumers may lack information about or find discrepancies regarding:

- True identification of herbs. Most mint teas are safe, for instance, but some varieties contain the highly toxic pennyroyal oil. Mistakenly used to treat colic, mint tea laden with pennyroyal has been blamed for the liver and neurological injuries of at least two infants, one of whom died.[14]

- Purity of herbal preparations. Potentially toxic quantities of arsenic and mercury have been detected in traditional Chinese herbal balls used to treat fever, rheumatism, and cataracts.[15] Analysis of one tea prescribed by a Chinese herbalist contained lead at 20,000 times the Environmental Protection Agency's allowable level; arsenic was over 1000 times the allowable level.[16]

- Appropriate uses and contraindications of herbs. Herbal remedies may be appropriate for minor ailments—a cup of chamomile tea to ease gastric discomfort or the gel of an aloe vera plant to soothe a sunburn, for example—but not for major health problems such as cancer.

- Safe dosages of herbs. Herbs that are effective contain active ingredients that need to be administered in proper doses. Each of these active ingredients has a different potency, time of onset, duration of activity, and consequent effects, making the plant itself too unpredictable to be useful. Foxglove leaves, for example, contain dozens of compounds that have an effect on the heart; digoxin, a drug derived from foxglove, offers a standard dosage that allows for a more predictable cardiac response.

- Interactions of herbs with medicines and other herbs. Like drugs, herbs may interfere with, or potentiate, the effects of other herbs and drugs. Chewing foxglove leaves when taking the drug digoxin, for example, could be catastrophic.

- Adverse reactions and toxicity levels of herbs. As is true of all drugs,

herbs may produce undesirable reactions. The herb ephedra, commonly known as ma huang and used to promote weight loss, acts as a strong central nervous system stimulant, causing rapid heart rate, nervousness, headaches, insomnia, and even death.

Not only are herbal preparations not regulated, but their labels may carry unsubstantiated health claims as long as the following disclaimer also appears: "has not been evaluated by the Food and Drug Administration." Consumers who decide to use herbs do so at their own risk.

THE CLIENT'S PERSPECTIVE

Health care professionals may quickly dismiss alternative therapies as ineffective and perhaps even dangerous, but their clients think otherwise. In a survey of more than 1500 people, one out of every three had used at least one alternative therapy in the past year for a variety of medical complaints from anxiety and headaches to cancer and tumors.[17] Visits to alternative therapists outnumbered visits to primary care physicians.

Most often, people use alternative therapies in addition to, rather than in place of, conventional therapies. Only a few of the people surveyed saw an alternative therapist without also seeing a physician; all of those with life-threatening conditions such as cancer, diabetes, or lung problems who used alternative therapies saw a medical doctor as well. In fact, most people seem to seek alternative therapies for nonserious medical conditions or health promotion. They simply want to feel better and access is easy. Sometimes their symptoms are chronic and subjective, such as pain and

fatigue, and difficult to treat. In these cases, the chances of finding relief are often as good with an alternative therapy as they are with a placebo, standard medical intervention, or even nonintervention.

Consumers spend an estimated $13.7 billion on alternative health services a year.[18] This figure does not include expenditures on products such as herbs, crystals, and aromas, which would raise the total considerably. When revenues soar to this extent, consumers need to beware. (To review how a person can identify health fraud and quackery, turn to pp. 33–34. For a list of credible sources of nutrition information see p. 35.)

THE HEALTH CARE PROFESSIONAL'S PERSPECTIVE

How should health care professionals react to clients who use alternative therapies? Those who condemn alternative therapies risk driving clients away, especially if alternative therapists appear more understanding and less judgmental.[19] When listening to clients, health care professionals will want to:

- Be culturally sensitive; acknowledge and respect the beliefs, attitudes, and lifestyles of their clients.[20]

- Keep an open mind; standard medical treatments simply don't work for some people in some situations.

- Accept and integrate alternative therapies into the care plan if they bring comfort without harm.

- Provide accurate information, not unsubstantiated opinions; an accurate diagnosis and information on all treatment options will help clients make their health care decisions.

- Discourage practices only if they are harmful.

Some health care professionals have begun to embrace some of the alternative therapies and incorporate them into their medical practice. In much of Europe, biomedicine and alternative therapies have been combined into a system of "complementary medicine," which takes advantage of the best of both approaches. Many practitioners in the United States would like to see such an integrated approach used here as well.[21]

In closing, remember that alternative therapies come in a variety of shapes and sizes. Both their benefits and their risks may be either small, none, or great. Accept the beneficial, or even neutral, practices with an open mind and reject only those practices known to cause harm. Making healthful choices requires knowing what all the choices are.

NOTES

1. J. Kleijnen, P. Knipschild, and G. terRiet, Clinical trials of homeopathy, *British Medical Journal* 302 (1991): 316–323.

2. M. M. Lipman, The power of placebos, *Consumer Reports on Health*, February 1996, p. 23.

3. E. A. Sotaniemi, E. Haapakoski, and A. Rautio, Ginseng therapy in non-insulin-dependent diabetic patients: Effects on psychophysical performance, glucose homeostasis, serum lipids, serum aminoterminalpropeptide concentration, and body weight, *Diabetes Care* 10 (1995): 1373–1375.

4. J. P. Kassirer, Federal foolishness and marijuana, *New England Journal of Medicine* 336 (1997): 366–367.

5. Alternative Medicine: Expanding Medical Horizons, A report to the National Institutes of Health and Alternative Medical Systems and Practices in the United States (Washington, D.C.: Government Printing Office, 1992).

6. M. Larkin, NIH's office of alternative medicine: A wise use of tax dollars? *Priorities*, vol. 6, no. 4, 1994, pp. 32–36.

7. I. B. Stehlin, An FDA guide to choosing medical treatments, *FDA Consumer*, June 1995, pp. 10–14.

8. K. McNutt, Medicinals in food—Part I: Is science coming full circle? *Nutrition Today* 30 (1995): 218–222.

9. P. Lipkin, An ancient salve dampens pain, *Science News* 149 (1996): 20.

10. A photo finish for total taxol synthesis, *Science News* 145 (1994): 223.

11. Unexplained severe illness possibly associated with consumption of kombucha tea—Iowa, 1995, *Journal of the American Medical Association* 275 (1996): 96–98.

12. V. E. Tyler, *The Honest Herbal: A Sensible Guide to the Use of Herbs and Related Remedies* (New York: Pharmaceutical Products Press, 1993).

13. K. McNutt, Medicinals in food: What's new and what's not? *Nutrition Today* 30 (1995): 261–262.

14. J. A. Bakerink and coauthors, Multiple organ failure after ingestion of pennyroyal oil from herbal tea in two infants, *Pediatrics* 98 (1996): 944–947.

15. E. O. Espinoza, M. J. Mann, and B. Bleasdell, Arsenic and mercury in traditional Chinese herbal balls, *New England Journal of Medicine* 333 (1995): 803–804.

16. S. B. Markowitz and coauthors, Lead poisoning due to *Hai Ge Fen*: The prophyrin content of individual erythrocytes, *Journal of the American Medical Association* 271 (1994): 932–934.

17. D. M. Eisenberg and coauthors, Unconventional medicine in the United States: Prevalence, costs, and patterns of use, *New England Journal of Medicine* 328 (1993): 246–252.

18. J. Langone, Challenging the mainstream, *Time*, Fall 1996, pp. 40–43.

19. E. W. Campion, Why unconventional medicine? *New England Journal of Medicine* 328 (1993): 282–283.

20. L. M. Pachter, Culture and clinical care: Folk illness beliefs and behaviors and their implications for health care delivery, *Journal of the American Medical Association* 271 (1994): 690–694.

21. C. Marwick, Complementary medicine congress draws a crowd, *Journal of the American Medical Association* 274 (1995): 106–107.

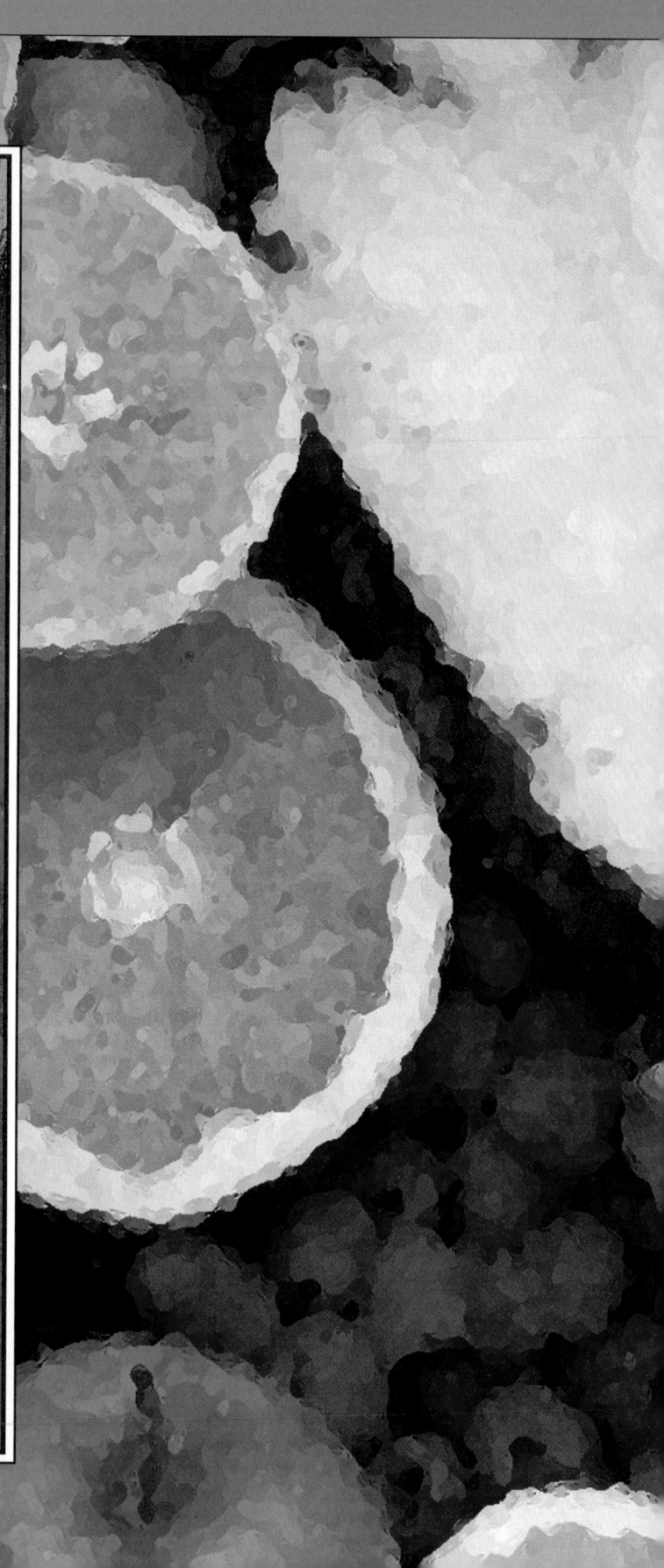

Nutrition and Disorders of the Upper GI Tract

CONTENTS

Disorders of the Mouth and Esophagus
Difficulties Chewing
Dysphagia
Disorders of the Stomach
Indigestion and Reflux Esophagitis
Nausea and Vomiting
Gastritis
Ulcers
Gastric Surgery
HIGHLIGHT: Living with Feeding Disabilities

MICROGRAPH: Vitamin B_{12}.

*T*he remarkable GI tract serves as a conduit from the external world to the internal body environment. It wisely distinguishes nutrients from substances for which the body has no use. Over the course of the life cycle, the GI tract undergoes changes that affect the absorption of nutrients and modify nutrient needs. As the healthy newborn's GI tract matures, it progressively allows the body to ingest, digest, and absorb nutrients in many forms—functions essential to life. With aging, the muscular functions of the GI tract gradually decline, and the stomach frequently changes in ways that affect the absorption of several nutrients. By adjusting diets to accommodate these normal physiologic changes, optimal nourishment can be provided. Similarly, dietary adjustments can ease symptoms, prevent malnutrition, and treat disorders that affect the functions of the GI tract. With this chapter, you begin your study of medical nutrition therapy, specifically how diet can aid the treatment of some upper GI tract symptoms and disorders. The next chapter presents disorders of the lower GI tract and their relationships to diet and nutrition status.

Disorders of the Mouth and Esophagus

Figure 21–1 on p. 696 illustrates the upper GI tract and reviews the functions of its various organs and sphincters. In the mouth, the teeth and jaw muscles work together to break down food to a consistency that can be easily swallowed and digested. The upper esophagus assists in the swallowing process, and the remaining esophagus transports food from the mouth to the stomach. The muscles controlling the esophagus push foods down and prevent them from moving back toward the throat.

A variety of dental, medical, and surgical conditions that affect the mouth and esophagus can temporarily or permanently interfere with chewing (see Table 21–1). Without appropriate adjustments in diet, people with these conditions may find eating a difficult or painful experience. They may eat too little, lose too much weight, and suffer the consequences of a deteriorating nutrition status.

The process of chewing is sometimes called mastication.

Table 21–1

Conditions That May Interfere with Chewing and Swallowing

Achalasia	Ill-fitting dentures
Acquired immune deficiency syndrome (AIDS)	Missing teeth
	Multiple sclerosis
Alzheimer's disease	Myasthenia gravis
Broken jaw	No teeth
Cancer	Oral Surgery
Chemotherapy	Parkinson's disease
Congenital defects of upper GI tract	Periodontal disease
Dental caries	Radiation therapy of the head and neck
Dryness of mouth	Sensitivity of mouth to hot or cold
Dysphagia	Strokes
Guillain-Barré syndrome	Surgery of the head and neck
Head injury	Ulceration of mouth, gums, or esophagus

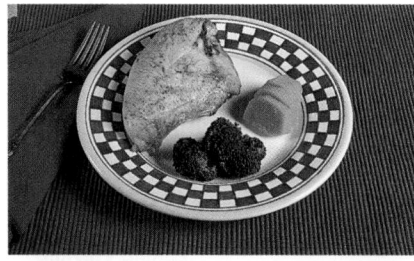

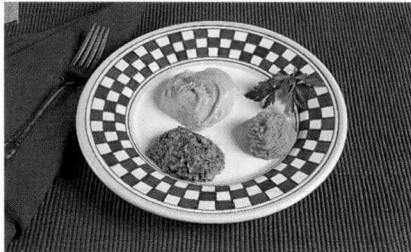

Pureed foods make an appetizing meal when chosen with an eye for color and served attractively.

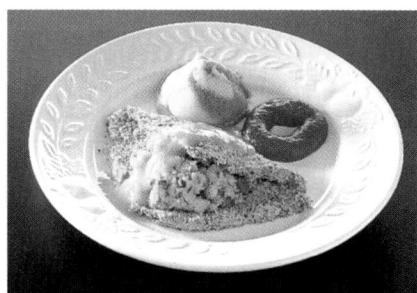

Adding commercial thickeners to pureed foods greatly enhances their appeal.

Reminder: When food becomes lodged in the trachea, *choking* occurs (see pp. 94–96).

How to Improve Acceptance of Pureed Diets

Take a moment to think about a pureed diet. A typical dinner of baked chicken, boiled potatoes, and green beans is pureed to white mush, more white mush, and a green blob. The foods may taste great, but on seeing the plate, the person may have a hard time taking the first bite. To stimulate the appetite, use creative techniques for preparing and serving food such as these:

- Encourage clients and their caregivers to prepare a variety of favorite foods and blenderize them to a tolerable consistency. The smells of favorite foods cooking and the thought of consuming a favorite food often stimulate the appetite.

- Consider color when planning meals. The meal of baked chicken, mashed potatoes, and green beans, described above, can be made more appealing by substituting mashed sweet potatoes for the white potatoes. Arranging the foods attractively on a plate with appropriate garnishes also adds color and eye appeal.

- Serve foods at the right temperature and puree them so that they are smooth and thick—not watery and thin. Commercially available thickeners add shape, texture, and even nutrients to food.

- Experiment with seasonings and spices to enliven food flavors, excluding only those that the person cannot tolerate or are not allowed for medical reasons. When clients and their caregivers choose to use baby foods for convenience, seasoning the food to accommodate adult tastes adds flavor and improves the appetite.

- Supplement the diet with nutritious liquids such as milk, instant breakfast drinks, or liquid formulas (described in Chapter 23).

Efforts to improve the acceptance of pureed diets can go a long way toward helping people to eat and maintain or improve their weights.[a] When efforts to improve clients' intakes of pureed foods are unsuccessful, feeding the person by tube becomes an option (see Chapter 23).

[a]D. Cassens, E. Johnson, and S. Keelan, Enhancing taste, texture, appearance, and presentation of pureed food improved resident quality of life and weight status, *Nutrition Reviews* (supplement) 11 (1996): 51–54.

and causing pneumonia. In healthy people, the presence of food in the trachea elicits a coughing response, which prevents food from entering the lungs. Some people with dysphagia, however, fail to cough when food slips into the trachea. Such "silent" aspiration, which has been observed in people following strokes, carries the risk of serious pneumonia and death.[1]

Signs of Dysphagia Health care professionals should be alert to subtle symptoms of dysphagia including an unexplained decline in food intake or repeated bouts of pneumonia.[2] Other symptoms include pain upon swallowing, weight loss, a fear of eating certain foods or any food at all, a feeling that food is sticking in the throat, a tendency to hold food in the mouth rather than swallowing it, coughing or choking during meals, frequent throat clearing, drooling, or a change in voice quality. Depending on the cause of dysphagia, the voice may be hoarse, nasal, or have a "wet" sound. Diagnosis is based on extensive testing that may include cranial nerve assessment, X rays, fluoroscopy, and measurements of esophageal sphincter pressure and esophageal peristalsis.

Dietary Interventions for Dysphagia   The mechanical soft diet for dysphagia leaves little room for error or experimentation. A person may appear to be tolerating a particular food when, in fact, the food is being aspirated.[3] Speech pathologists, dietitians, physicians, and nurses work together to assess a person's swallowing abilities and design an individualized diet. Often, the person can handle only semisolid foods or thickened liquids, which flow slowly enough to allow time to coordinate swallowing movements. Smooth solids such as puddings, custards, and smooth yogurts are frequently good choices; commercial thickeners, tapioca pudding, or baby cereal can be used to thicken liquids. Many of the suggestions offered in the box on p. 698 apply to diets for dysphagia.

With time, swallowing function may improve. The health care team continuously monitors the person and expands the diet to include additional foods as tolerated. Ideally, the diet is progressed to a solid diet, although this is not always possible.

Tube Feedings   Feedings by tube (described in Chapter 23) are necessary only if attempts to feed the person orally are unsuccessful. Tube feedings may be particularly beneficial for severely malnourished individuals who are unable to take adequate nourishment orally and for those whose swallowing function continues to deteriorate. Tube feedings delivered into the stomach, however, may be contraindicated due to the high risk of aspiration pneumonia in people with dysphagia. Intestinal tube feedings often provide a safer alternative.

Many disorders that affect the mouth and esophagus can interfere with chewing and swallowing and may require a modification in food consistency. Dysphagia, a serious swallowing disorder that frequently goes undiagnosed, can lead to repeated bouts of pneumonia and even death. Management includes a highly individualized mechanical soft diet. The nutrition assessment checklist on p. 700 highlights important considerations in maintaining nutrition status for people with chewing and swallowing problems.

Disorders of the Stomach

Once swallowed, food travels down the esophagus into the stomach. The stomach retains the bolus for a while, adding acids, fluids, and enzymes to the mixture before slowly releasing its contents into the intestine. Disorders of the stomach range from occasional bouts of indigestion to serious conditions that require surgical resections.

INDIGESTION AND REFLUX ESOPHAGITIS

Indigestion, or dyspepsia, is a vague term used to describe epigastric pain and fullness, early satiety, and belching. Highlight 3 (pp. 98–99) describes the causes and

The fear of eating is called sitophobia (SIGH-toe-FOE-bee-ah).

sitos = food

phobos = fear

Conditions that may lead to dysphagia:
- Acquired immune deficiency syndrome (AIDS).
- Aging.
- Alzheimer's disease.
- Brain tumors.
- Cancers of the head and neck.
- Developmental feeding disorders.
- Guilain-Barré syndrome.
- Head injuries.
- Lou Gehrig's disease (amyotrophic lateral sclerosis).
- Multiple sclerosis.
- Myasthenia gravis.
- Parkinson's disease.
- Polio.
- Reflux esophagitis.
- Strokes.

dyspepsia: vague abdominal pain; a symptom, not a disease.

dys = bad

peptein = to digest

epigastric: the region of the body just above the stomach.

epi = above

gastric = stomach

Nutrition Assessment Checklist
For People with Chewing and Swallowing Disorders

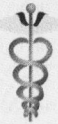

Medical Determine if the client's primary medical condition requires further dietary alterations; treatment of the primary medical condition may ease problems with chewing and swallowing. Healthy people who require short-term modifications (following wisdom tooth extraction, for example) can make up nutrient deficits when they resume their normal diets.

Drug Review the client's drug therapy for possible drug-nutrient interactions.

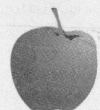

Food Intake Regularly assess the client's intake to pinpoint tolerable food consistencies and quickly address problems with failing appetite and possible nutrient deficiencies.

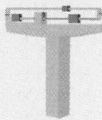

Anthropometric   Take accurate baseline height and weight measurements. For people with long-term swallowing disorders, monitor changes in height and weight in children and weight in adults as frequently as possible. Adjust diet to support growth in children and desirable weight in adults.

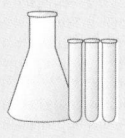

Laboratory   Monitor changes in serum albumin. Serum electrolytes and blood urea nitrogen can help detect dehydration, a common problem in people with swallowing disorders. Hemoglobin and hematocrit levels help in detecting dehydration and anemia.

Physical   Check for physical signs of nutrient deficiencies and dehydration; assess the client's energy level and emotional state.

reflux esophagitis (eh-sof-ah-JYE-tis): the backflow or regurgitation of gastric contents from the stomach into the esophagus, causing inflammation of the esophagus; also called gastroesophageal reflux, gastric reflux, or acid indigestion.

re = back

fluxus = flow

The continuous reflux of gastric juices may cause scarring of the esophageal mucosa. As scar tissue forms, the diameter of the esophagus narrows, a condition referred to as an esophageal stricture.

esophageal ulcers: lesions or sores in the lining of the esophagus.

consequences of occasional bouts of indigestion including belching, hiccups, heartburn, and regurgitation of the stomach's acid fluids into the mouth. Acid indigestion can become a chronic problem. When the reflux of highly acidic gastric fluids occurs frequently, the esophagus becomes irritated, causing a painful inflammation called reflux esophagitis. Severe inflammation and scarring may narrow the inner diameter of the esophagus. Dysphagia and its potential complications (see p. 697), esophageal ulcers, and bleeding are possible consequences.

Certain drugs, aging, and the use of feeding tubes that pass from the nose through the stomach are associated with an increased risk of reflux esophagitis. Most often, however, reflux esophagitis develops as a consequence of a hiatal hernia.

Hiatal Hernia   The esophagus joins the stomach at the cardiac sphincter. Normally, this sphincter sits right in the hiatus of the diaphragm and is reinforced by it. The esophagus lies completely above, and the stomach completely below, the diaphragm. Sometimes, however, the diaphragm weakens, and a portion of the stomach protrudes up through it, an abnormality called a hiatal hernia. Once a hiatal hernia forms, the cardiac sphincter is no longer reinforced by the surrounding diaphragm, and it becomes easy for gastric juices to reflux into the esophagus. Because reflux occurs more readily in people with hiatal hernias, they frequently suffer from heartburn, acid regurgitation into the mouth, and esophagitis; treatment aims to prevent these consequences. Figure 21–2 shows the normal relationship of the upper GI tract to the diaphragm and the changes that occur with reflux and with a hernia.

Dietary Prevention and Treatment   The tips for preventing acid indigestion described in Highlight 3 also apply to people who suffer from reflux esophagitis; the box on p. 702 reviews these suggestions and their rationale. Treatment for active reflux esophagitis aims to alleviate reflux and irritation of the inflamed esophagus by reducing gastric acidity and eliminating foods, substances, and activities that weaken the cardiac sphincter (see Table 21–2).

The **cardiac sphincter** is also called the **lower esophageal sphincter** (LES) or the **gastroesophageal sphincter.**

hiatus (high-AY-tus): the opening in the diaphragm through which the esophagus passes.

  hiatus = to yawn

hiatal hernia: a protrusion of a portion of the stomach through the esophageal hiatus of the diaphragm. There are several types of hiatal hernias, but the *sliding hiatal hernia* is the most common (see Figure 21–2).

Figure 21–2

Relationship of the Upper GI Tract to the Diaphragm

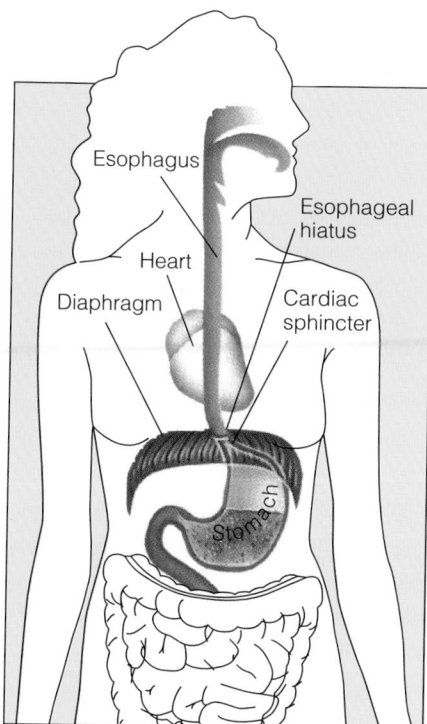

NORMAL
The stomach lies below the diaphragm, and the esophagus passes through the esophageal hiatus. The cardiac sphincter prevents reflux of stomach contents.

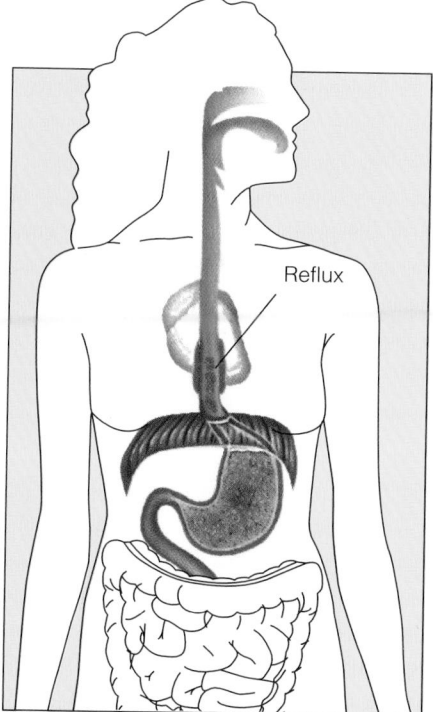

REFLUX
Overeating and overdrinking can increase pressure in the stomach. Whenever the pressure in the stomach exceeds the pressure in the esophagus, there is a greater chance of reflux. The resulting "heartburn" is so-named because it is felt in the area of the heart.

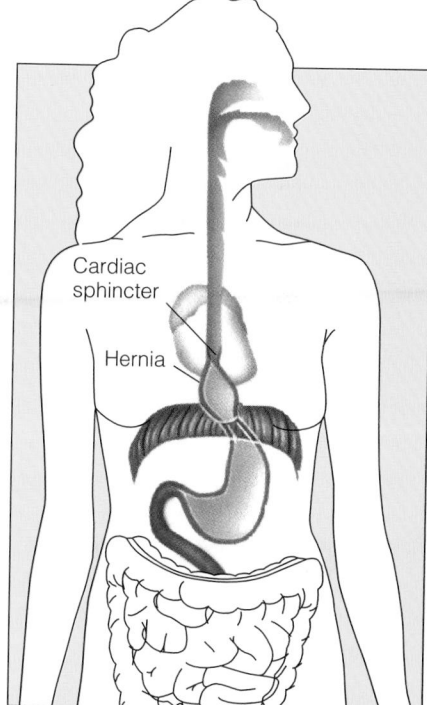

SLIDING HIATAL HERNIA
A sliding hiatal hernia results when part of the stomach, with the cardiac sphincter, slips through the diaphragm. This type of hiatal hernia is the most common.

Table 21–2

Substances That Relax the Cardiac Sphincter

Alcohol

Anticholinergic agents

Calcium channel blockers

Chocolate

Cigarette smoking

Diazepam

Garlic

High-fat foods

Meperidine

Onions

Peppermint and spearmint oils

Theophylline

antacids: acid-buffering agents used to counter excess acidity in the stomach.

Most antiulcer agents suppress or inhibit gastric acid secretion. Those that do are also classed as antisecretory agents or anti-GERD (GastroEsophageal Reflux Disease).

 PRESCRIPTION PAD

Drugs used in the treatment of reflux esophagitis may include:

● Antacids
● Antiulcer agents
● Cholinergics (metoclopramide and bethanecol, see *antinauseants*)

See Appendix E for timing with meals and nutrition-related side effects.

 How to Prevent and Treat Reflux Esophagitis

To prevent and treat reflux esophagitis and its associated discomfort, instruct clients to:

● Eat small meals and drink liquids one hour before or one hour after meals to avoid distending the stomach.
● Relax during mealtimes, eat foods slowly, and chew foods thoroughly to avoid swallowing air and distending the stomach.
● Limit foods that weaken cardiac sphincter pressure or increase gastric acid secretion, including fat, alcohol, caffeine, decaffeinated coffee and tea, chocolate, spearmint, and peppermint.
● Avoid foods and beverages that irritate the esophagus, such as citrus fruits and juices, tomatoes and tomato-based products, pepper, spices, and very hot or very cold foods according to individual tolerances.
● Lose weight, if overweight.
● Refrain from lying down or bending over and from wearing tight-fitting clothing or belts, particularly after eating, to avoid increasing stomach pressure.
● Elevate the head of the bed by 4 to 6 inches. Keeping the chest higher than the stomach helps to prevent reflux.
● Refrain from smoking cigarettes.

Individual tolerances to types and amounts of foods and spices vary markedly. Health care professionals can help clients pinpoint individual intolerances by advising them to record the types and amounts of foods and beverages consumed, the time of consumption, GI symptoms, and time of occurrence. Assessment of the record by a dietitian provides the basis for determining the types and amounts of food or food components that the client can handle without discomfort.

Drug Therapy   Turn on the television set and quite likely you will see several advertisements touting a new generation of over-the-counter medications that are highly effective in both preventing and relieving indigestion. Physicians frequently prescribe such drugs to ease the discomfort of reflux esophagitis. Antacids neutralize gastric acidity, and antiulcer agents suppress or inhibit gastric acid secretion. Medications that strengthen cardiac sphincter pressure (cholinergics) are used when other measures prove unsuccessful in controlling symptoms. If drug therapy fails, however, surgery may be indicated. The case study provides questions that review the nutrition needs of a client with a hiatal hernia and reflux esophagitis.

NAUSEA AND VOMITING

Nausea, another vague term, is used to describe the feeling that one is about to vomit. The discussion here focuses on prolonged nausea and vomiting, unrelated

Case Study   Accountant with Reflux Esophagitis

Mrs. Scarlatti, a 49-year-old accountant, recently underwent a complete physical examination. She told her physician that she had been feeling fairly well, except for heartburn, which had been occurring with increasing frequency. The attacks usually occurred after she had eaten a large meal, particularly when she lays down after eating. She told the doctor that her life was pretty hectic because it is the middle of the tax season.

Mrs. Scarlatti's past medical history shows no signs of significant health problems. During her last physical, the physician did advise her to stop smoking cigarettes and to lose 20 pounds, which she has yet to do. A diet history taken by the nurse shows that Mrs. Scarlatti usually skips breakfast, eats lunch hurriedly while she continues to work, and eats a large dinner around 8:00 P.M. She generally enjoys one or two alcoholic beverages in the evening before going to sleep. She drinks 6 to 8 cups of coffee during the day. Her current height and weight are 5 feet 6 inches and 170 pounds. After inspecting the interior of her esophagus, stomach, and duodenum with a long tube equipped with a special optical device called a gastroscope, the physician diagnosed a sliding hiatal hernia.

Can you explain to Mrs. Scarlatti what a sliding hiatal hernia is and how its leads to heartburn? Describe the care plan you would develop for Mrs. Scarlatti. What suggestions can you make to help her relieve the symptoms associated with the hernia? What other therapy might her physician prescribe?

---

to eating habits, which can lead to weight loss and malnutrition. As later chapters show, nausea is a symptom of many medical conditions that arise either within or outside of the GI tract. Nausea is also a common side effect of many drugs and medical treatments. Emotional tension or even the sight or smell of certain foods can precipitate or worsen nausea.

As Highlight 3 describes, simple vomiting is certainly unpleasant and wearying for the nauseated person but is not cause for alarm. Prolonged vomiting, however, can be serious and dangerous enough to require professional medical care. When nausea leads to vomiting, foods and medications fail to reach the intestine and are unavailable to the body. Large amounts of fluids and electrolytes from the body's cells are expelled along with the foods, further increasing the likelihood of dehydration and nutrient deficiencies.

Treatment of Nausea   Treatment of nausea depends on its severity and cause. The longer the person suffers from nausea and the greater its severity, the greater the risk of significant dehydration, weight loss, and malnutrition. Treatment of the related medical condition or a change in drug therapy, if possible, often alleviates the problem. Emotional stresses may require counseling to resolve underlying emotional conflicts. The next box (see p. 704) suggests other measures to ease nausea.

Dietary Interventions for Vomiting   Controlling nausea is often successful in preventing vomiting. During episodes of vomiting, foods are withheld. If possible, fluids and electrolytes are replaced orally using clear liquids. If oral liquids cannot be tolerated, intravenous (IV) fluids may be given to provide fluids, glucose, and electrolytes until the vomiting resolves. When vomiting continues for long periods of time, IV fluids that meet all nutrient needs (described in Chapter 24) may be indicated.

nausea (NAW-see-ah): the feeling that one is about to vomit.

Conditions that can lead to indigestion and nausea include pregnancy, reflux esophagitis, peptic ulcers, gallbladder disorders, pancreatic disorders, kidney disorders, cancer, and delayed gastric emptying.

intravenous (IV): through a vein.
intra = within
vena = vein

Notice that the suggestions in Chapter 18 for alleviating the indigestion and nausea associated with pregnancy parallel the suggestions provided here.

How to Minimize Nausea

The following suggestions can help alleviate nausea:

- Encourage clients to relax before they eat and to avoid overeating. Eating small meals and saving liquids for between meals prevent distention of the stomach.

- Remind clients to drink liquids between meals, especially when vomiting is a problem. Although individual tolerances vary, many clients tolerate cold or carbonated liquids and juices best.

- Help clients identify individual food intolerances and aromas that precipitate nausea; clients should avoid these foods and aromas, if possible. High-fat foods and highly spiced foods are often poorly tolerated. Cold or room-temperature foods may be better tolerated than hot foods, especially if food aromas trigger nausea. Recommend that others prepare foods for the client, if possible.

- Advise clients who experience nausea to eat carbohydrate-rich, low-fat foods before they get out of bed. Crackers or bread can be kept at bedside.

- Recommend a meal and snack schedule for clients who experience nausea at specific times of the day. Clients should avoid eating or drinking immediately before or during those times.

- Suggest that clients relax after eating, but not lie down. Getting fresh air after meals and wearing nonconstrictive clothing can also help.

Physicians may also prescribe antinauseants or antiemetic drugs to help control nausea and vomiting. Counsel clients to take these drugs at least 30 minutes before eating to ensure effectiveness during mealtimes.

GASTRITIS

gastritis: inflammation of the stomach lining.

Bacterial infection with *Helicobacter pylori* can cause acute or chronic gastritis.

Gastritis is a common disorder in which the mucosal lining of the stomach becomes inflamed and painful. The person with gastritis may complain of anorexia, indigestion, nausea, vomiting, and epigastric pain. Although gastritis generally resolves with treatment, unresolved gastritis can lead to hemorrhage, shock, obstruction, perforation, and gastric cancer.

Acute Gastritis Acute gastritis most often follows the repeated use of aspirin or other drugs that irritate the gastric mucosa. Alcohol abuse, food irritants, food allergies, food poisoning, radiation therapy, metabolic stress, and bacterial infection can also cause gastritis.

For the person with gastritis who cannot eat because of nausea or vomiting, foods are generally withheld for a day or two. Then, the diet progresses from liquids to a bland diet as tolerated. Bland diets (see Table 21–3) are highly individualized diets that eliminate foods that stimulate gastric acid secretion or irritate the gastric mucosa. Antacids, antiulcer drugs, and antibiotics may also be prescribed.

Chronic Gastritis Chronic gastritis presents the same symptoms as acute gastritis, but persists over time. Chronic gastritis may be associated with gastric

℞ PRESCRIPTION PAD

Drugs used in the treatment of gastritis may include:

- Antacids
- Antibiotics
- Antiulcer agents

See Appendix E for timing with meals and nutrition-related side effects.

Table 21–3

The Bland Diet

A bland diet provides three meals a day and includes all foods except those that irritate the gastric mucosa. Substances generally contraindicated on a bland diet include:

- Any foods an individual identifies as irritating to the GI tract.
- Alcohol.
- Caffeine and caffeine-containing beverages (including cola beverages, cocoa, coffee, and tea).
- Decaffeinated coffee and tea.
- Pepper and spicy foods except as tolerated.

Note: The liberal bland diet shown here has replaced the earlier "traditional bland diet," which was invalidated by research.

surgery, chronic diseases of the stomach or liver, bacterial infection, or may have no known cause. It is common in the elderly. As gastritis progresses, the gastric cells atrophy, gastric secretions decline, and the production of intrinsic factor is reduced.

Chronic gastritis requires diagnosis and treatment before damage progresses too far. Interventions need to begin early enough to prevent complications such as dehydration, malnutrition, or damage to the esophagus. An individualized bland diet may help relieve GI symptoms in some cases.

The reduced production of intrinsic factor can result in vitamin B_{12} malabsorption, which can lead to pernicious anemia. When necessary, vitamin B_{12} is given by injection to bypass the need for absorption.

Reminder: *Intrinsic factor* is a glycoprotein made in the stomach that is necessary for the absorption of vitamin B_{12}.

In atrophic gastritis all of the layers of the stomach's mucosal cells are inflamed.

ULCERS

The term *ulcers* brings to mind the image of a frantic businessman rushing through the day with coffee cup in hand, gulping down high-fat, spicy foods, and working until midnight while suppressing the pain of bleeding sores caused by excessive acid in his stomach. But like other aspects of ulcer prevention and treatment, this stereotype has fallen by the wayside. Neither a stressful lifestyle nor male gender typifies the person with ulcers; ulcers occur in stressed and unstressed men and women alike.

Ulcers can develop both inside and outside the body, but the term *ulcer* generally refers to a *peptic ulcer*—an erosion of the top layer of cells from the GI tract lining. This erosion leaves the underlying layers of cells exposed to gastric juices. When the gastric juices reach the capillaries, the ulcer bleeds, and when they reach the nerves, they cause pain.

peptic ulcer: an erosion of the top layer of cells from the mucosa of the stomach (gastric ulcer) or duodenum (duodenal ulcer). Ulcers may also develop in the mouth, esophagus, and intestines and on the skin.

Causes of Ulcers Highlight 3 introduced the three major causes of ulcers: bacterial infection, the use of certain anti-inflammatory drugs, and disorders that cause excessive gastric acid secretion. One such disorder, the Zollinger-Ellison syndrome, results from a tumor of the pancreas that produces gastrin, which, in turn, stimulates the production of gastric acid. Severe peptic ulcer disease follows.

The bacterial infection frequently associated with ulcers is caused by *Helicobacter pylori*, the same bacterium that can cause gastritis. The drugs associated with ulcers are nonsteroidal anti-inflammatory agents such as ibuprofen and naproxen.

Zollinger-Ellison syndrome: marked hypersecretion of gastric acid and consequent peptic ulcers caused by a tumor of the pancreas, which releases gastrin.

Rx **PRESCRIPTION PAD**

Drugs used in the treatment of ulcers may include:

- Antacids
- Antibiotics
- Antiulcer agents

See Appendix E for timing with meals and nutrition-related side effects.

In a subtotal or partial gastrectomy, a portion of the stomach is removed; in a total gastrectomy, the entire stomach is removed.

vagotomy: surgery that severs the nerves to the stomach that stimulate gastric acid secretion.

The surgical procedures used in the treatment of obesity are discussed on pp. 298–299.

Therapy for Ulcers   As mentioned in Highlight 3, treatment aims at relieving pain, healing the ulcer, and minimizing the likelihood of recurrence. Drug therapy plays the primary role in the treatment; the specific type of drug depends on the cause of the ulcer. Antibiotics are used to treat bacterial infections. Antiulcer drugs may be used to suppress or inhibit gastric acid secretion or otherwise protect the stomach and duodenal wall from acid erosion. As for diet, the client need only eliminate foods that cause pain or discomfort. In rare cases, surgical intervention is necessary.

For clients with Zollinger-Ellison syndrome, surgical removal of the tumor, when possible, reduces gastric acid production. Often surgery is necessary to sever the nerves that stimulate gastric acid production, and in some cases, surgery that removes all or part of the stomach, described next, may be indicated.

GASTRIC SURGERY

Several surgical procedures affect the functions of the stomach. During a gastrectomy, the surgeon removes either a portion or all of the stomach. Figure 21–3 illustrates three common gastrectomy procedures. Another type of gastric surgery, pyloroplasty, enlarges the pyloric sphincter (the sphincter that joins the stomach and small intestine) so that the basic intestinal fluids reflux into the stomach and neutralize gastric acidity. During a vagotomy, the surgeon severs the nerves that stimulate gastric acid production. A vagotomy may accompany either a gastrectomy or a pyloroplasty in some cases. In gastric partitioning, a treatment for severe obesity, the stomach remains intact, but all or a portion of the stomach is bypassed. Figure 9–5 on p. 298 shows two gastric partitioning procedures.

Chapter 25 describes nutrition care for surgical clients in general, and those considerations apply to gastric surgery as well. This section addresses nutrition concerns that arise specifically in clients undergoing gastric surgery.

Dumping Syndrome   One problem that may occur when the portion of the stomach containing the pyloric sphincter has been removed, bypassed, or disrupted is dumping syndrome (see Figure 21–4). A typical scenario goes something

Figure 21–3

Typical Gastric Surgery Resections
In a gastric resection, part, or all, of the stomach is surgically removed. The dashed lines show the removed section.

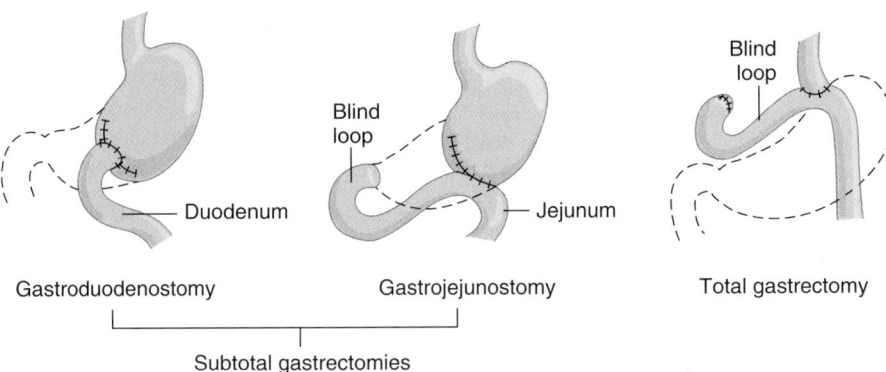

Gastroduodenostomy — Duodenum

Gastrojejunostomy — Jejunum   Blind loop

Total gastrectomy   Blind loop

Subtotal gastrectomies

like this: Mr. Clark had a fairly extensive gastric resection about a week ago and has just begun to eat solid foods. He swallows the food and about 15 minutes later begins to feel weak and dizzy. He looks pale, his heart beats rapidly, and he breaks out in a sweat. Shortly thereafter, he develops diarrhea. What causes this sequence of events?

Mr. Clark has lost an important function of his stomach: its control of the rate at which food empties into the intestine. Now, food gets "dumped" rapidly into the jejunum. (The duodenum is short, and even if it had not been bypassed during surgery, food would still pass quickly through it into the jejunum.) As the mass of food is digested, the intestinal contents rapidly become concentrated

dumping syndrome: the symptoms that result from the rapid emptying of undigested food into the jejunum: sweating, weakness, and diarrhea shortly after eating and hypoglycemia later. Dumping syndrome is common following pyloroplasties, vagotomies, total gastrectomies, and gastric bypass surgery (see Figure 21–3).

Figure 21–4
. . . .

Dumping Syndrome
When partially digested food rapidly enters the jejunum, it is quickly digested and creates a hyperosmolar load. Fluid from the intestinal capillaries enters the jejunum, diminishing blood volume and stimulating peristalsis. The result: low blood pressure and diarrhea.

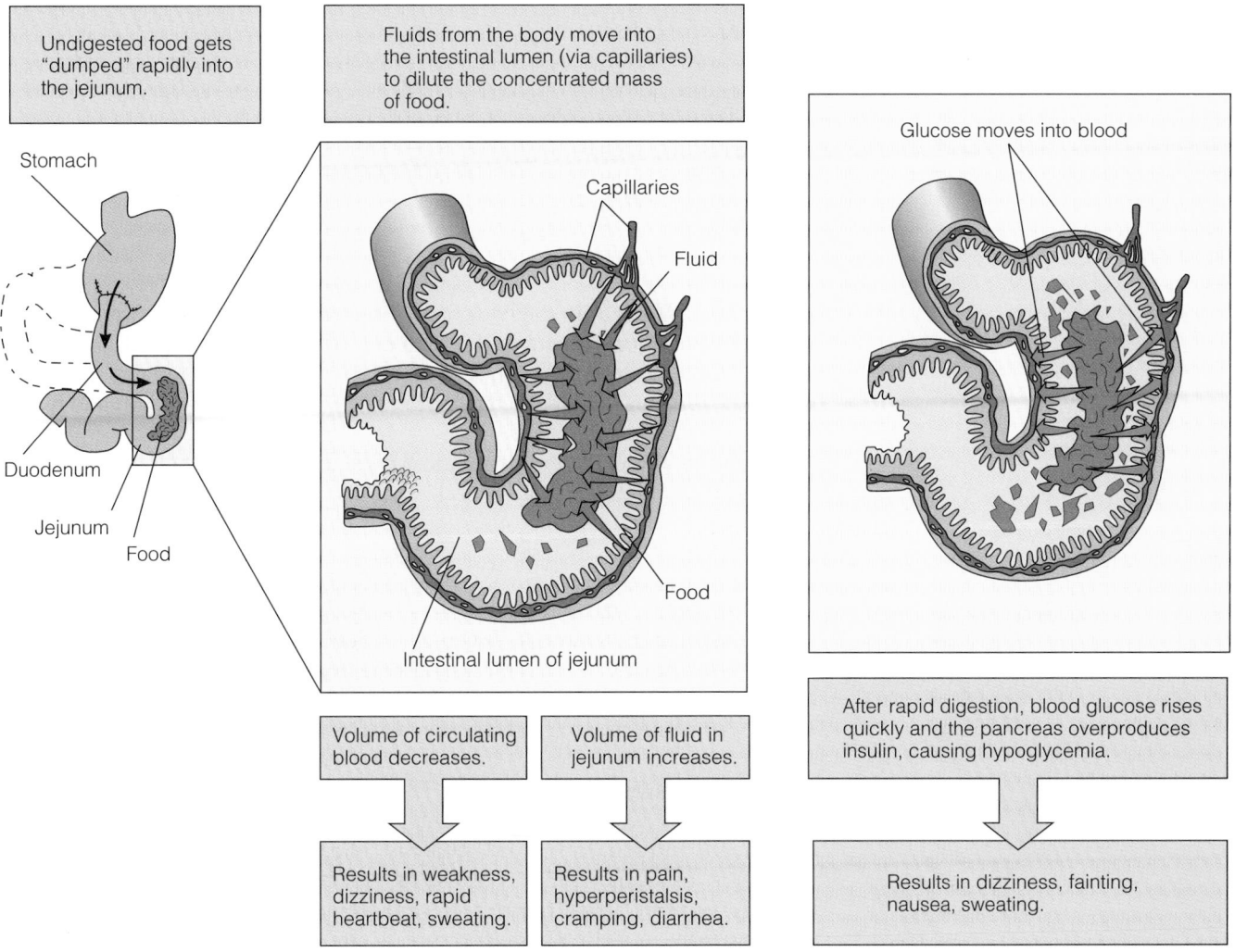

How to Adjust Meals to Prevent Dumping Syndrome

Advice for the person who has had gastric surgery includes the following suggestions:

- Eat no concentrated sweets (sugar, cookies, cakes, pies, or soft drinks) because the body digests these carbohydrates rapidly and breaks them down into many particles that attract fluids into the intestines.
- Eat frequent small meals to fit the reduced storage capacity of the stomach.
- Drink liquids in small amounts about 45 minutes before or after meals, not with them. This precaution prevents overloading the stomach's reduced storage capacity and slows the rate at which food passes from the stomach to the intestine.
- Lie down immediately after eating to help slow the transit of food to the intestine. Clients who experience gastric reflux, however, should not lie down after eating.
- Be aware that lactose intolerance (see Chapter 4) may develop and produce discomfort in response to milk and milk products. Enzyme-treated milk and milk products should also be avoided because the enzymes break down lactose to glucose and galactose, simple sugars that may promote dumping. Discontinue use of these products until recovery is under way. Then reintroduce them gradually in small amounts.

(hypertonic). Water from the body moves into the intestinal lumen to dilute the concentration. Consequently, the volume of circulating blood diminishes rapidly, causing weakness, dizziness, and a rapid heartbeat. The large volume of hypertonic fluid and unabsorbed material in the jejunum causes pain and hyperperistalsis, and diarrhea results.

Two to three hours later, Mr. Clark experiences many of the same symptoms again: dizziness, fainting, nausea, and sweating. This time the cause is different. The intestines efficiently absorbed so much glucose from the meal that blood glucose rose quickly. The pancreas responded by overproducing insulin, which made the blood glucose *fall* quickly. Now, hypoglycemia is causing the symptoms.

Not all people who have had gastric surgery or vagotomies experience the diarrhea of dumping syndrome. Even fewer develop hypoglycemia. Most people who initially experience dumping syndrome gradually adapt to a fairly regular diet. However, dietary modifications benefit clients during the immediate post-surgical period and in prolonged or severe cases.

The Postgastrectomy Diet In the immediate postsurgical period, the client receives no foods or fluids by mouth. After several days, liquids and solids are gradually introduced in small amounts. The postgastrectomy diet limits carbohydrates, especially simple sugars, in order to alleviate the symptoms of dumping syndrome. Health care professionals monitor fluid and electrolyte balances carefully, and the physician corrects any imbalances promptly. The diet emphasizes foods containing protein and fat, which are digested more slowly

The type of hypoglycemia that occurs following gastric surgery is called alimentary (AL-ee-MEN-tah-ree) or postgastrectomy hypoglycemia. Chapter 27 provides more information about hypoglycemia.

postgastrectomy diet: a carbohydrate-controlled diet given to prevent the symptoms of dumping syndrome and hypoglycemia that sometimes follow gastric surgery.

and produce fewer particles than carbohydrates and therefore do not attract fluid as rapidly as carbohydrates do. Table 21–4 on p. 710 lists foods included on, and excluded from, the postgastrectomy diet. Diet advice to offer with the postgastrectomy diet is provided in the box on p. 708 and the sample menu (below) shows a day's meals.

Dietitians carefully tailor the postgastrectomy diet to meet individual needs. Initially, visits to the client after each meal reveal food intolerances. With time, the symptoms of dumping syndrome resolve or improve in most people. Gradually, most people begin to tolerate limited amounts of concentrated sweets, larger quantities of food, and some liquids with meals. Sometimes adding pectin and guar gum (types of dietary fiber) to the diet can help prevent dumping syndrome. If dietary and medical management of dumping syndrome fail to resolve the problem, additional surgery may be necessary.

Unintentional Weight Loss and Malabsorption After gastric surgery, many people experience weight loss and develop nutrient deficiencies. Early satiety, postsurgical pain, and the desire to prevent the symptoms of dumping syndrome often limit food intake. Epigastric pain from reflux esophagitis, and sometimes dysphagia, can further interfere with nutrient intake. Weight loss is the goal for people undergoing gastric partitioning, but people with severe peptic ulcer disease or cancer often suffer significant weight loss before surgery and risk serious malnutrition.

Be aware that protein and fat malabsorption can be a problem for any client who has had a total gastrectomy or who has had the stomach surgically connected directly to the jejunum. Normally, food entering the duodenum triggers the release of the hormones secretin and cholecystokinin. These hormones, in

℞ PRESCRIPTION PAD

Drugs used in the treatment of dumping syndrome may include:

- Anticholinergics (atropine, see *antidiarrheals*)
- Antihistamines (cyprohepatine, see *miscellaneous*)
- Hormones (octreotide, see *miscellaneous*)

See Appendix E for timing with meals and nutrition-related side effects.

Sample Postgastrectomy Diet Menu

Menu

Breakfast	Lunch	Supper
1 scrambled egg	2 oz hamburger patty	2 oz boiled ham
1 slice toast	½ c mashed potatoes	⅓ c rice
1 tsp butter	1 tsp margarine	½ c carrots
Coffee (take 30–60 minutes after meal)	½ small banana	2 tsp butter
	Iced tea (take 30–60 minutes after meal)	¼ c unsweetened peach slices
		Tea (take 30–60 minutes after meal)
Midmorning Snack	**Midafternoon Snack**	**Evening Snack**
¼ c cottage cheese	2 tbs peanut butter	¼ c tuna
3 saltine crackers	3 butter crackers	1 tsp mayonnaise
		1 slice bread

Table 21–4
. . . .
Postgastrectomy Diet[a]

Meat and Meat Alternatives
Any type allowed.

Milk and Milk Products
Withheld initially and then gradually introduced as tolerated.

Grains and Starchy Vegetables
Allowed (up to 5 servings per day): Plain breads, crackers, rolls, unsweetened cereal, rice, pasta, corn, lima beans, parsnips, peas, white potatoes, sweet potatoes, pumpkin, yams, winter squash.

Excluded: Sweetened cereal; cereal containing dates, raisins, or brown sugar.

Nonstarchy Vegetables
Allowed (unlimited): Cabbage, Chinese cabbage, celery, cucumbers, lettuce, parsley, radishes, watercress.

Allowed (up to two ½ c servings per day as individual tolerances permit): Asparagus, bean sprouts, beets, broccoli, brussels sprouts, carrots, cauliflower, eggplant, green pepper, greens, mushrooms, okra, onions, rhubarb, sauerkraut, string beans, summer squash, tomatoes, turnips, zucchini.

Excluded: Vegetables prepared with sugar or creamed.

Fruits
Allowed (up to 3 servings per day): Unsweetened fruits and fruit juices.

Excluded: Sweetened fruits and fruit juices, dates, raisins.

Fats
Any type allowed.

Beverages
Allowed: Coffee, tea, artificially sweetened drinks.

Excluded: Alcohol; sweetened milk, beverages, and fruit drinks; cocoa.

Other
Excluded: Cakes, cookies, ice cream, sherbet, honey, jam, jelly, syrup, and sugar.

[a]Clients with dumping syndrome who are unable to tolerate a sufficient variety or volume of foods over long periods of time often require nutrient supplements.

turn, mediate the secretion of digestive enzymes and bile into the duodenum. When the duodenum is bypassed, these processes are also bypassed and cannot aid fat digestion and absorption as usual. In addition, malabsorption results whenever food passes rapidly through the GI tract.

Reduced gastric acid secretion can also lead to bacterial overgrowth in the stomach or upper small intestine, which results in the malabsorption of fat, fat-soluble vitamins (especially vitamin D), folate, vitamin B_{12}, and calcium. Chapter 22 describes the problems of malabsorption related to bacterial overgrowth, called the *blind loop syndrome,* in greater detail.

Case Study   Commercial Artist Requiring Gastric Surgery

Mr. Miyamoto, a 58-year-old commercial artist, was admitted to the hospital for gastric surgery after numerous attempts to medically manage his severe peptic ulcer disease had failed. A gastrojejunostomy and vagotomy were performed, and Mr. Miyamoto is recovering as expected. The health care team members anticipate nutrition-related problems and are taking measures to prevent them.

Review Figure 21–3 to understand the surgical procedure that Mr. Miyamoto underwent. Consider the possibilities that he might experience early satiety, nausea, vomiting, weight loss, dumping syndrome, malabsorption, anemia, and bone disease. Describe how these conditions might occur.

What type of diet will the physician prescribe for Mr. Miyamoto after he begins eating orally? Describe the diet and how it progresses. What advice can you give Mr. Miyamoto to prevent dumping syndrome?

Discuss the nutrition-related concerns associated with fat malabsorption and anemia. How can these concerns be handled?

Anemia   Iron-deficiency anemia is another common problem following gastrectomies and gastric partitioning procedures, although it may take several years to develop. When iron's exposure to gastric acid is limited, less iron is converted to its absorbable form. Furthermore, 50 percent of iron absorption normally takes place in the duodenum. Following gastric surgery, the transit time through the duodenum may be rapid, or the duodenum may be bypassed altogether. Inadequate intake of iron and gastrointestinal blood loss can also contribute to the problem. An iron supplement helps to correct the deficiency.

Inadequate intake and malabsorption can also lead to anemia caused by folate and, less often, vitamin B_{12} deficiencies. To correct deficiencies, clients receive supplements. Use the case study above to review the needs of a client following a gastrectomy.

Bone Disease   People who experience fat malabsorption following gastric surgery also malabsorb vitamin D and calcium. After many years, a significant number of people who have undergone gastrectomies develop a bone disease similar to osteomalacia.[4] Although the bone disease usually does not respond well to treatment, vitamin D and calcium supplements are often provided.

Gastric Partitioning   Unlike other gastric surgeries, weight loss is a goal following gastric partitioning. In addition, diet therapy aims to prevent nutrient deficiencies related to reduced food intake and malabsorption and promote eating and lifestyle habits that will help the client maintain a desirable weight.

The long-term safety and effectiveness of gastric partitioning depend, in large part, on compliance with dietary instructions. Poor dietary habits may prevent weight loss, rupture staples, or obstruct the small passage into the lower stomach. Other postsurgical complications include infections, nausea, vomiting, dehydration, dumping syndrome, esophageal reflux, and, as a result of all this and more, depression. Although the reasons are unclear, clients undergoing gastric bypass surgery frequently say that foods taste sweeter to them than before surgery; others develop an aversion to red meats.[5]

Diet following Gastric Partitioning   After surgery, clients initially follow a liquid diet. Liquids reduce the risk of disrupting the line of surgical staples and

Although one might expect vitamin B_{12} deficiencies to be common after gastric surgery because intrinsic factor production might be affected, surgeons often avert this problem by leaving intact a small part of the stomach that produces intrinsic factor. This step generally prevents the malabsorption of vitamin B_{12} due to a lack of intrinsic factor.

Reminder: *Osteomalacia* is a bone disease characterized by softening of the bones.

flow easily through the opening to the lower stomach (or jejunum). Clients gradually begin to eat pureed foods, then soft foods, and then regular foods. Regardless of food consistency, clients can tolerate only small amounts at one time because of the reduced size of the stomach; overeating or overdrinking can cause nausea, reflux, and vomiting. Although individual tolerances vary, most clients can eat regular foods by 12 weeks after surgery, provided they chew foods thoroughly.[6] Foods must be chewed thoroughly to prevent large pieces of food from obstructing the gastric outlet.

Food Selections   Clients must understand that their selections of foods and beverages influence the extent of their weight loss. If they drink high-kcalorie liquids or eat high-kcalorie foods all the time, even if only in small quantities, they will not lose weight. Their selections also affect the nutritional quality of the diet. Nutrient deficiencies, particularly of vitamin B_{12}, folate, and iron, are common after gastric bypass surgery. Careful planning, diligent compliance with the prescribed diet, and vitamin-mineral supplements are needed to ensure the adequacy of an energy-restricted diet that strictly limits intake.[7]

Indigestion, reflux esophagitis, nausea, and vomiting are frequent GI problems that can lead to weight loss and malnutrition. When treatment for a medical condition requires gastric surgery, the impact on nutrition status can be severe. The accompanying nutrition assessment checklist reminds health care professionals of factors to assess and monitor for clients with disorders of the upper GI tract.

This chapter has described how problems of the upper GI tract can affect dietary intake and how dietary intake, in turn, can affect these problems. The next chapter examines problems of the lower GI tract.

Nutrition Assessment Checklist
For People with Upper GI Tract Disorders

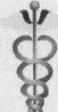 **Medical**   Assess the client's medical history for conditions and treatments that produce symptoms of indigestion, nausea, and vomiting. Medical conditions that are likely to produce severe symptoms for long periods of time alert the assessor to anticipate serious nutrition problems and to work diligently to prevent or correct them.

 Drug   Review the client's drug therapy for possible drug-nutrient interactions. Antacids and antiulcer agents are often used in the treatment of indigestion, reflux esophagitis, gastritis, and ulcers. Aluminum-containing antacids may lead to phosphorus deficiencies. Magnesium-containing antacids may cause diarrhea. Calcium- and sodium-containing antacids contribute calcium and sodium, respectively, to the diet. Some antiulcer agents (cimetidine and omeprazole) may interfere with iron absorption; iron supplements should be given 2 hours before or after taking these medications. Antiemetics may cause mouth dryness.

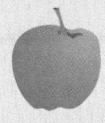 **Food Intake**   Assess food intake to determine individual food tolerances for people with indigestion, nausea, vomiting, or dumping syndrome. Instruct clients to keep records of food intake and GI symptoms to help identify food intolerances. Reassess clients to make sure they are eating sufficiently to maintain nutrition status.

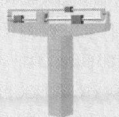 **Anthropometric**   Be alert to unintentional weight loss in people with severe indigestion, early satiety, nausea, vomiting, and dumping syndrome. Clients with reflux esophagitis should lose weight if overweight. Safe weight loss is also the goal for people undergoing gastric partitioning.

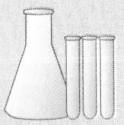 **Laboratory**   Monitor changes in serum albumin. Serum electrolytes, blood urea nitrogen, and hemoglobin and hematocrit can help detect electrolyte imbalances and dehydration, especially important for people with persistent vomiting or dumping syndrome. Anemia is a frequent problem for people with chronic gastritis or following gastric surgery. Hemoglobin and hematocrit help uncover anemia; mean corpuscular volume, serum ferritin, total iron-binding capacity, serum iron, serum folate, serum vitamin B_{12}, and tests of vitamin B_{12} absorption can help differentiate between anemias caused by iron, folate, and vitamin B_{12} deficiencies (see Appendix E).

 Physical   Check for physical signs of dehydration for people experiencing vomiting or dumping syndrome; vitamin B_{12} deficiencies for people with reflux esophagitis, gastritis, and ulcers; and protein-energy malnutrition and vitamin D, folate, iron, and calcium deficiencies for people undergoing gastric surgery.

Study Questions

1. List conditions of the mouth that can affect the ability to chew foods. What diet would you advise in each case?
2. Discuss ways to stimulate the appetite for people on pureed diets.
3. What is dysphagia, and how is the diet managed to ease its symptoms? Why does dysphagia often go unrecognized? What are its potential consequences?
4. What is reflux esophagitis, and what are its primary symptoms? Why is reflux more likely to occur in people with hiatal hernias?
5. What advice can you give the person with reflux to prevent and treat its symptoms? What long-term complications can result from chronic reflux esophagitis?
6. Under what circumstances can indigestion, nausea, and vomiting present a risk to nutrition status?
7. What is gastritis? Describe the role of diet therapy in acute and chronic gastritis.
8. Discuss the therapy for peptic ulcers.
9. What are the possible nutrition consequences of gastric surgery? Describe the relationship of gastric surgery to these consequences. What dietary interventions might help to prevent these consequences?
10. Discuss the dietary recommendations, and the rationale behind them, for a person who undergoes gastric partitioning for clinically severe obesity.

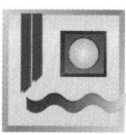

Clinical Applications

1. People on mechanical soft diets differ in the kinds of foods they can handle, in the amounts of time they remain on the diets, and in the help they need from health care professionals. Think about the difference between working with a person who has been edentulous for years and a person who recently had mouth surgery and is just beginning to eat again. Describe some nutrition-related concerns you might have for the person who has been following a mechanical soft diet for years. How would these concerns differ for a person who needs the mechanical soft diet only temporarily? Contrast the amounts of time the nurse or dietitian might spend working with the two clients.
2. Many of the diets described in this chapter are highly individualized. A particular food may give one person indigestion and have no effect on another. One person with a gastrectomy may experience lactose intolerance, while another may not. Describe practical ways to identify food tolerances.
3. Many symptoms and disorders of the upper GI tract are interrelated. Consider, for example, a person with clinically severe obesity who undergoes gastric partitioning. Explain why nausea, vomiting, indigestion, and reflux esophagitis might develop in this person. Consider further how chronic reflux might lead to dysphagia.
4. Review the chapter to find disorders that often occur as a consequence of aging. Referring to Chapter 20, describe the effects of aging on the upper GI tract and relate these changes to the disorders you find.

Notes

1. J. Horner and E. W. Massey, Silent aspiration following stroke, *Neurology* 38 (1988): 317–319.
2. E. M. Pardoe, Development of a multistage diet for dysphagia, *Journal of the American Dietetic Association* 93 (1993): 568–571.
3. Pardoe, 1993.
4. J. Grant, G. Chapman, and M. K. Russell, Malabsorption associated with surgical procedures and its treatment, *Nutrition in Clinical Practice* 11 (1996): 43–52.
5. J. C. Burge and coauthors, Changes in patients' taste acuity after Roux-en-Y gastric bypass for clinically severe obesity, *Journal of the American Dietetic Association* 95 (1995): 666–670.
6. J. K. Nelson and coauthors, *Mayo Clinic Diet Manual*, 7th ed. (St. Louis: Mosby, 1994), p. 198.
7. T. Andersen and U. Larsen, Dietary outcome in obese patients treated with gastroplasty program, *American Journal of Clinical Nutrition* 50 (1989): 1328–1340.

Living with Feeding Disabilities

Thousands of people face obstacles in the ordinary task of eating. These obstacles can arise at any time in a person's life and from any number of conditions. An infant may be born with a physical impairment such as cleft palate, an adolescent may suffer injuries in a car accident, a middle-aged adult may lose motor control following a stroke, or an older adult may struggle with the pain of arthritis. Table H21–1 lists some of the conditions that might lead to feeding problems.

This highlight deals primarily with the kinds of disabilities that make it difficult for people to eat, although disabilities do have other nutrition-related aspects. As one example, a disability may make it difficult for a person to engage in enough physical activity to support a healthy appetite. As another example, a person who has lost a limb to amputation has altered energy needs. Energy needs are reduced in proportion to the weight and metabolism represented by the missing limb, but may be increased if extra effort is necessary to do ordinary things—such as walking on crutches. As still another example, people with involuntary motor activity may have exceedingly high energy needs.

The dietitian, nurse, and occupational therapist most often become involved with feeding disabilities. They can help people achieve as much independence in eating as possible and can teach caregivers to help.

WAYS DISABILITIES CAN IMPAIR EATING

When you consider the number of individual coordinated motions that are required to get food from the table to the stomach, you may be amazed. Think about what an infant experiences when learning to feed himself. At first, the infant cannot sit upright and finds it impossible even to hold a spoon. Every single little action—from picking up the utensils, to biting and chewing, to swallowing—requires coordinated movements. Any injury or disability that interferes with these movements can lead to feeding problems. Some of the feeding skills that might be affected include:

- Sitting and balancing oneself.
- Moving the head and neck in a coordinated way.
- Moving the jaw, lips, and tongue.
- Sucking, swallowing, chewing, and drinking.
- Employing protective reflexes that prevent choking, cutting oneself, biting one's tongue, and others.
- Moving the eyes and hands.
- Making grasping motions.

Other disabilities do not involve oral-motor skills. For example, a person who has problems with sight, or who cannot drive or walk or carry groceries, or who cannot plan meals and think through what to buy has a disability that affects eating. Disabilities of any type can cause people to have trouble maintaining adequate nutrition status.[1] As you might expect, their number one problem is inadequate food intake, which leads to malnutrition, underweight, and, in children, poor growth.[2] Many conditions that lead to feeding problems also alter metabolism and require medications, which further affect nutrition status.

On top of nutrition-related problems, people who have difficulty eating often encounter emotional and social problems. For example,

Table H21–1

Conditions Leading to Feeding Problems

The following conditions may lead to feeding problems by interfering with a person's ability to suck, bite, chew, swallow, or coordinate hand-to-mouth movements.

• Accidents	• Language, visual, or hearing impairment
• Amputations	• Microcephalia
• Arthritis	• Multiple sclerosis
• Birth defects	• Muscle weakness
• Cerebral palsy	• Muscular dystrophy
• Cleft palate	• Neuromotor dysfunction
• Down's syndrome	• Parkinson's disease
• Head injuries	• Polio
• Huntington's chorea	• Spinal cord injuries
• Hydrocephalia	• Stroke

children fail to receive the social training that mealtimes provide, and older people miss the social stimulation that goes with eating in the company of others.

INDEPENDENT EATING FOR PEOPLE WITH DISABILITIES

The evaluation and treatment of a feeding problem require the joint efforts of several health care professionals, possibly including a dietitian, psychologist, occupational therapist, physical therapist, speech pathologist, dentist, and one or several nurses.[3] Table H21–2 provides a checklist of observations health care professionals use to assess feeding skills and nutrition needs. Because each case is different, it makes sense for everyone on the health care team to be familiar with all of these variables.

The dietitian assesses the client's nutrition status, plans a diet, and provides nutrition counseling. The most valuable assessment tool is observation of the client during mealtimes. While observing the client's feeding skills, the assessor can conduct a complete nutrition assessment and provide appropriate nutrition counseling. The dietitian must also ensure that the diet provides foods appropriate for the client's oral-motor capabilities. For example, people with swallowing problems prefer thickened liquids and pureed foods, which flow slowly enough to allow time to coordinate oral movements (see Chapter 21). If the client's abilities to eat improve, the diet can gradually progress through all stages from pureed foods to a regular diet.[4] The planner faces many challenges in designing a diet that coordinates the client's energy and nutrient needs, stage of development, and personal preferences.[5]

Nutrition Assessment Checklist
For People with Feeding Disabilities

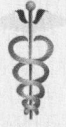

Medical Determine if the client's primary medical problem imposes further dietary changes.

Drug Be aware that anticonvulsant drugs used to treat some disorders may induce folate deficiency, impair vitamin D status, and raise blood cholesterol; drugs prescribed for attention deficit hyperactivity disorder may suppress appetite and slow growth. Remember that some drugs may slow GI tract motility, contributing to constipation; other drugs may cause gastric irritability, drowsiness, nausea, and altered taste sensations—factors that diminish appetite and food intake. Remember that clients on long-term drug therapy and those taking multiple drugs are particularly vulnerable to nutrient imbalances.

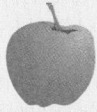

Food Intake When taking a diet history, interview all parents and caregivers responsible for feeding the client. Take into account the differences between food offered and food eaten; spills can contribute to substantial food losses.

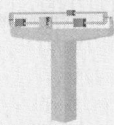

Anthropometric Obtain anthropometric measures as accurately as possible. In cases where standing height cannot be measured, use arm span length instead (measured from the tip of the middle finger on one hand to the tip of the middle finger on the other hand with arms stretched out as far as possible). Use standards specific to the medical disorder if available.

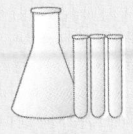

Laboratory Monitor serum albumin to ensure adequate protein status, serum ferritin to detect iron deficiency, and vitamin and mineral status as needed.

Physical Use Table H21–2 to assess the client's feeding disabilities. Note any dental problems that may interfere with food intake.

But seeing a client's ability to swallow improve due to a change in the diet's texture and consistency can be very rewarding.[6] The accompanying nutrition assessment checklist focuses on topics of notable concern for people with feeding disabilities.

The occupational therapist evaluates oral-motor abilities and feeding skills and then develops a care plan, educates the client, and shows the caregiver, if there is one, ways to implement feeding techniques at home. For example, it may be necessary to teach the client (or caregiver) the proper sitting position for ease of eating. The therapist may instruct the client to sit in a chair with the head and trunk in midline, the back straight and supported, the

717

Table H21–2

Feeding Evaluation

Oral ability

Sucking
Oral prehension
Swallowing
Breathing and swallowing coordinated
Drooling
Lips
Tongue size, thrust, mobility
Biting
Munching
Chewing
Drinking
Response to input

Dental health

Structural malformation
Impaired oral-motor ability
Delayed weaning
Use of cariogenic foods or drugs
Occlusion
Teeth
Caries
Gingiva
Oral hygiene
Palate
Pain on exam
Hypersensitivity
Teething stage

Body position

General tone and movement
Reflex activity
Head control
Sitting balance
Placement of feet
Usual feeding position

Hand use

Palmar grasp
Pincer grasp
Opposition finger/thumb
Hand-to-mouth control

Developmental feeding

Breast ___ bottle ___ weaned ___
Baby food ___ junior food ___ mashed table food ___ minced foods ___

Cut table foods ___ regular table foods ___
Closes hands in on bottle
Hand to mouth/sucks on fingers
Teething biscuit, holds and brings to mouth
Finger feeds
Opposes lips to rim of cup
Attempts to grasp spoon
Grasps spoon
Dips spoon in dish
Brings spoon to mouth
Holds bottle and drinks independently
Grasps cup
Raises cup to mouth
Lifts cup, drinks, and replaces
Scoops well with spoon
Feeds independently with spoon
Drinks with straw
Spears with fork
Spreads with knife

Feeding environment

Time of feedings (note number and length of feedings)
Atmosphere of feedings (tense, pleasant, unpleasant)
Person responsible for feeding
Parental and/or caregivers' attitude toward feeding
Past successful and unsuccessful methods
Identify positive and negative reinforcing behavior
Behavioral problems

Diet history, including:

Total fluid intake
Types of foods consumed
Method of feeding
Texture modifications
Food aversions, intolerances, or allergies
Use of food as rewards

Medications

Type
Dosage
Time given

Bowel concerns

Regular
Constipation
Diarrhea

Sources: Adapted from J. J. Cafferky, Nutrition assessment of children with developmental disabilities: Special considerations, *Support Line* (a newsletter of Dietitians in Nutrition Support) June 1993; R. B. Howard, Nutritional support of the developmentally disabled child, *Textbook of Pediatric Nutrition*, ed. R. M. Suskind (New York: Raven Press, 1981), pp. 577–582.

Figure H21–1

Examples of Special Feeding Devices

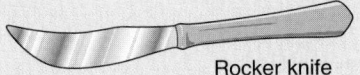

Rocker knife

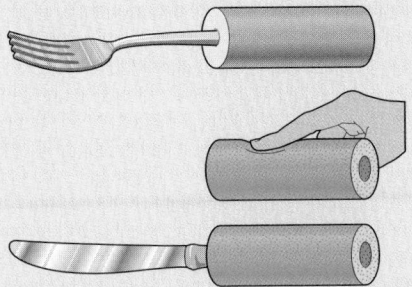

Roller knife

People with only one arm or hand may have difficulty cutting foods and may appreciate using a *rocker knife* or a *roller knife.*

People with a limited range of motion can feed themselves better when they use *flatware with built-up handles.*

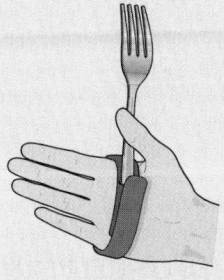

People with extreme muscle weakness may be able to eat with a *utensil holder.*

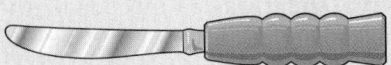

For people with tremors, spasticity, and uneven jerky movements, *weighted utensils* can aid the feeding process.

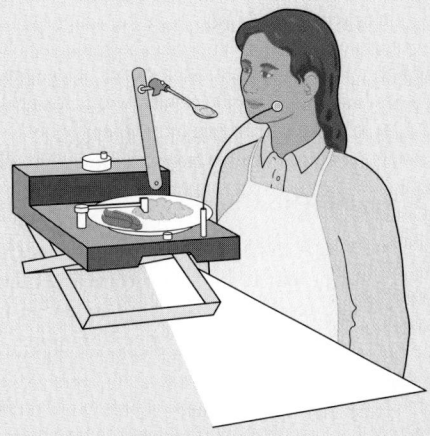

Battery-powered feeding machines enable people with severe limitations to eat with less assistance from others.

Plates

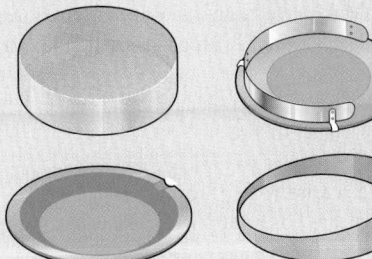

People who have limited dexterity and difficulty maneuvering food find *scoop dishes* or *food guards* useful.

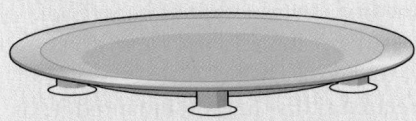

People with uncontrolled or excessive movements might move dishes around while eating and may benefit from using *unbreakable dishes with suction cups.*

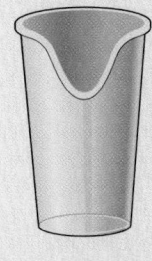

People with limited neck motion can use a *cutout plastic cup.*

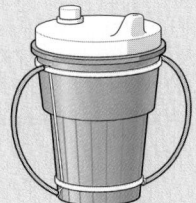

Two-handed cups enable people with moderate muscle weakness to lift a cup with two hands.

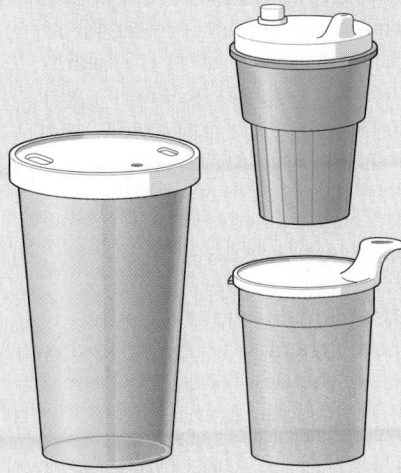

People with uncontrolled or excessive movements might prefer to drink liquids from a *covered cup* or glass with a *slotted opening* or *spout.*

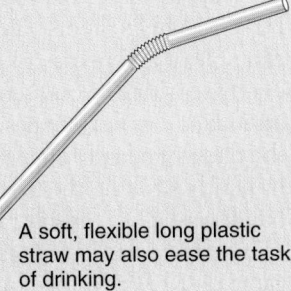

A soft, flexible long plastic straw may also ease the task of drinking.

hips and knees at right angles, and the feet flat and supported on a surface.

Special feeding devices can make a remarkable difference in a person's ability to eat independently. For a person who cannot grasp an ordinary fork, for example, a usable fork may be the key to future health. Becoming independent often improves nutrition status; people who can feed themselves seem to have better appetites and eat more food than those who require assistance.

The occupational therapist selects the appropriate feeding devices and trains the client and caregivers in their use (see Figure H21-1). Everyone on the health care team should be familiar with these devices, however, and should keep track of improved utensils that regularly become available.

Clients may need help in developing eating skills—for example, in learning to swallow. Commonly, a care plan allocates this task to a speech therapist, who trains clients to use the lips, tongue, and throat in both speaking and eating. A dentist may also be needed to evaluate the client's dental health and provide instructions on oral hygiene.

Developing feeding skills requires practice. Helpers can employ strategies such as those listed in Table H21-3 to help clients gain skills. For example, if a hyperreactive child is overly sensitive to oral sensations, an attendant can help by desensitizing the client gradually over time. Start by gently stroking the face with a hand, washcloth, or soft pliable toy. (This can be done playfully, making a game of it.) When the child can tolerate touch on less sensitive areas of the face such as the forehead, cheeks, and lips, then slowly and firmly rub the gums, palate, and tongue.

Table H21–3

Areas of Concern and Suggested Strategies for Developing Feeding Skills

Inability to Suck

- Use cold substances around lips to stimulate sucking.
- Use a cloth soaked with water for child to suck.
- Try different types of nipples.
- As child's ability begins to improve, change to nipple with a smaller hole.

Inability to Chew

- Place a small amount of food between back teeth and move jaw up and down. A mirror may help demonstrate and point out various body parts.
- Place foods such as peanut butter on lips and encourage client to wash lips with tongue. Gradually change from pureed foods to solid foods (sprinkle crackers in soup, etc.).

Inability to Swallow

- Close jaw and lips of client together (swallowing is easiest when the mouth is closed).
- Stroke throat upward under chin.
- Offer next bite of food only after client swallows.
- Demonstrate—let client feel *you* swallow.

Inability to Grasp

- Allow client to finger feed.
- Guide client in exploring mouth.
- Cut food into small pieces.
- Place your hand over client's hand and help client grasp spoon.
- Use adaptive equipment (plastic spoon, etc.).
- Make sure bowl is stabilized (suction, tape).
- Use plates with high straight sides, or build higher edge using aluminum foil.

Poor Hand-Mouth Coordination

- Pour sand, etc.
- Exercise with ball.
- Exercise with push-pull objects.
- Study body parts with client, if appropriate.

This discussion of ways to help clients achieve independence in feeding themselves has been brief, but the principles are clear. Accurate identification of the eating-related skills that are impaired leads to appropriate treatment. The treatment can be considered a success if the client becomes independent—that is, able to prepare, serve, and eat nutritionally adequate food daily without help.

THE ROLES OF HELPERS

In the best-case scenario, a person with a disability learns to plan, serve, and eat meals independently. In some cases, however, the person cannot function without help. To ensure that long-term care is successful, the health care team addresses the caregiver's personal needs and develops the caregiver's knowledge and skills.

Impaired Vision

- Place meats and vegetables consistently in same areas of plate.

Overweight

- Cut down snacks and high-kcalorie foods.,
- Refrain from rewarding with food.
- Increase exercise and leisure-time activities.

Underweight

- Increase number of meals per day.
- Include high-kcalorie foods, especially liquid supplements.
- Encourage proper exercise.

Lack of Nutrition Education

- Work with families.
- Stress the importance of proper nutrition for *all* family members.
- Teach proper feeding environment (good eating habits, eating positions).
- Provide nutrition-instruction materials.

Source: Adapted with permission from S. Calvert and F. Davies, Nutrition of children with handicapping conditions, *Dietetic Currents* 4 (1977): 13–17.

The health care team offers support and encouragement and recognizes that the caregiver's role demands a great deal of responsibility and many personal sacrifices. To learn how to effectively feed another, a caregiver needs training.[7] Training may cover how to prepare and serve foods, as well as what to expect at each level of development in terms of food acceptance, readiness for different textures, correct feeding techniques, messiness, and self-feeding abilities.

The caregiver also needs to learn how to cope with inappropriate feeding behaviors. Otherwise the emotional distress of a difficult situation can escalate during feedings and cause both the person being fed and the caregiver to dislike mealtimes. Negative feelings during mealtimes can hinder efforts to learn appropriate eating behaviors and independent self-feeding.

Consider an example. Children with cerebral palsy can take ten times longer to eat than other children. Some mothers have reported spending up to seven hours a day feeding these children.[8] The caregiver must not only put in this extra time, but ideally also try to establish an emotionally pleasant atmosphere at mealtimes. This means dealing with any feelings of hostility or resentment at other times and places. Psychologists can offer counseling for caregivers; all members of the health care team need to be alert to a caregiver's emotional frustrations.[9]

The basic human drive to eat without assistance supports nutrition adequacy. Fortunately, some people with disabilities can attain this independence with training. In other cases, caregivers can obtain the necessary education and training to provide appropriate support.

The combined efforts of the health care team support both clients and caregivers in achieving feeding independence on every level—physically, mentally, and emotionally. To whatever degree independence can be achieved, it enhances the quality of life.

NOTES

1. Position of The American Dietetic Association: Nutrition in comprehensive program planning for persons with developmental disabilities, *Journal of the American Dietetic Association* 92 (1992): 613–615.

2. M. Thommessen and coauthors, Energy and nutrient intakes of disabled children: Do feeding problems make a difference? *Journal of the American Dietetic Association* 91 (1991): 1522–1525; R. K. Johnson and M. Maeda, Establishing outpatient nutrition services for children with cerebral palsy, *Journal of the American Dietetic Association* 89 (1989): 1504–1507; L. M. Thommessen and coauthors, Nutrition and growth retardation in 10 children with congenital deaf-blindness, *Journal of the American Dietetic Association* 89 (1989): 69–73.

3. L. A. Wodarski, An interdisciplinary nutrition assessment and intervention protocol for children with disabilities, *Journal of the American Dietetic Association* 90 (1990): 1563–1568.

4. E. M. Pardoe, Development of a multistage diet for dysphagia, *Journal of the American Dietetic Association* 93 (1993): 568–571.

5. M. Williams, Dysphagia—the new frontier, *Nutrition Today*, May/June 1992, pp. 26–31.

6. Pardoe, 1993; B. C. Sonies and M. C. Dalakas, Dysphagia in patients with the postpolio syndrome, *New England Journal of Medicine* 324 (1991): 1162–1167.

7. H. N. Sanders, S. B. Hoffman, and C. A. Lund, Feeding strategy for dependent eaters, *Journal of the American Dietetic Association* 92 (1992): 1389–1390.

8. Johnson and Maeda, 1989.

9. Thommessen and coauthors, 1991.

Chapter 22

Nutrition and Disorders of the Lower GI Tract

CONTENTS

Severe Diarrhea and Irritable Bowel Syndrome
  Diarrhea
  Irritable Bowel Syndrome
Nutrition Consequences of Malabsorption
  Fat Malabsorption
  Treatments for Fat Malabsorption
Malabsorption Syndromes
  Pancreatitis
  Cystic Fibrosis
  Crohn's Disease
  Malabsorption Caused by Bacterial Overgrowth
  Short-Bowel Syndrome
  Celiac Disease
Disorders of the Large Intestine
  Diverticular Disease of the Colon
  Ulcerative Colitis
  Resections of the Large Intestine
HIGHLIGHT: Promoting Intestinal Adaptation

MICROGRAPH: Vitamin D.

s Chapter 3 noted, the intestine is "the" organ of digestion and absorption. The intestine also provides a physical barrier against invading organisms and contains many immune cells that help protect against disease. (Figure 22–1 shows the intestinal tract and related organs for your review.) Any disorder of the intestine, particularly if it results in malabsorption, can seriously impair nutrition status. This chapter describes disorders of the lower GI tract that either influence nutrition status or are affected by diet. It begins with common disorders, then takes up disorders that cause malabsorption, and finally examines disorders of the large intestine. (Some common digestive problems that do not seriously affect nutrition status, such as gas and short bouts of diarrhea and constipation, were already discussed in Highlight 3.)

Figure 22–1

The Lower GI Tract and Related Organs

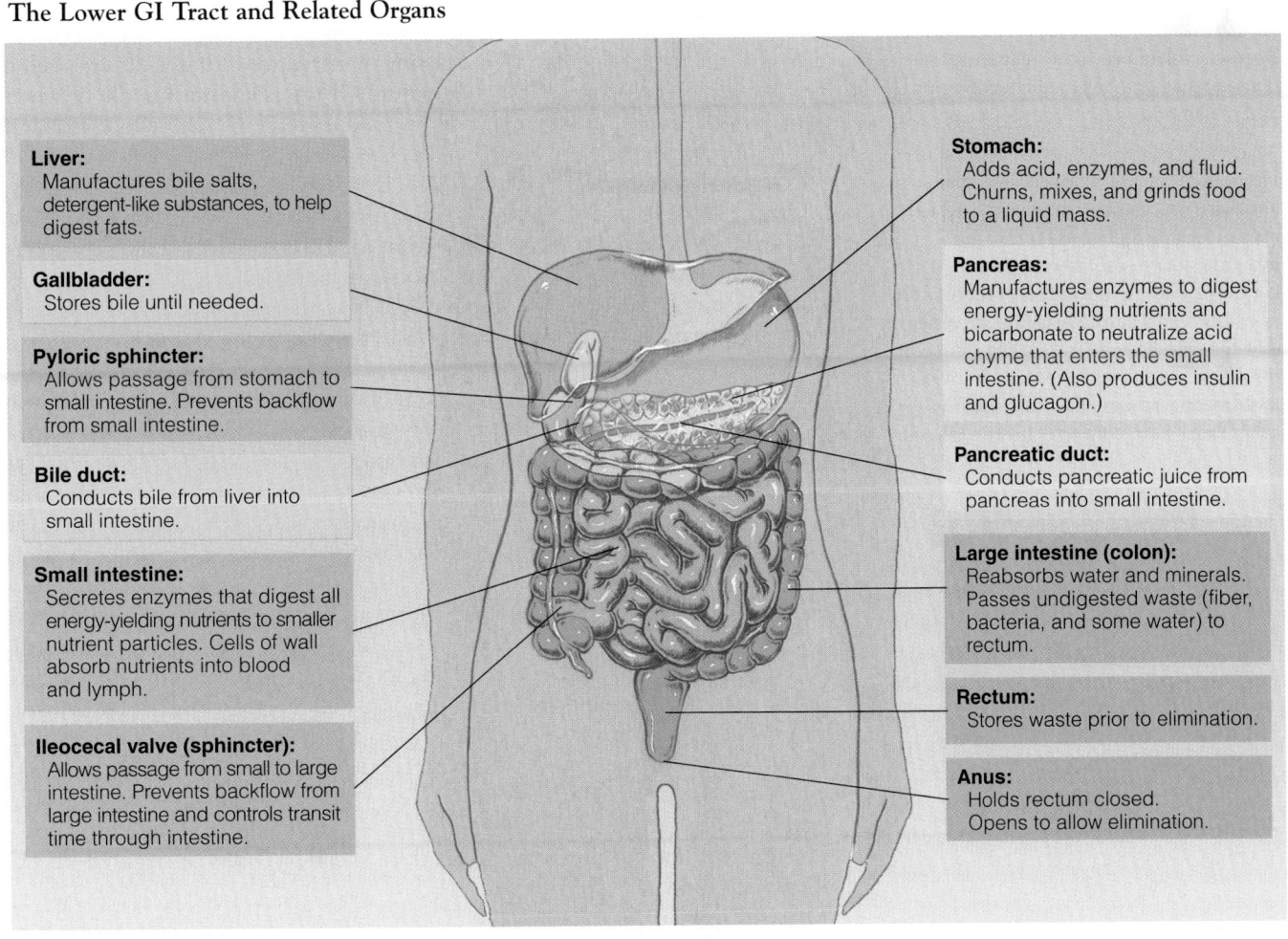

Liver:
Manufactures bile salts, detergent-like substances, to help digest fats.

Gallbladder:
Stores bile until needed.

Pyloric sphincter:
Allows passage from stomach to small intestine. Prevents backflow from small intestine.

Bile duct:
Conducts bile from liver into small intestine.

Small intestine:
Secretes enzymes that digest all energy-yielding nutrients to smaller nutrient particles. Cells of wall absorb nutrients into blood and lymph.

Ileocecal valve (sphincter):
Allows passage from small to large intestine. Prevents backflow from large intestine and controls transit time through intestine.

Stomach:
Adds acid, enzymes, and fluid. Churns, mixes, and grinds food to a liquid mass.

Pancreas:
Manufactures enzymes to digest energy-yielding nutrients and bicarbonate to neutralize acid chyme that enters the small intestine. (Also produces insulin and glucagon.)

Pancreatic duct:
Conducts pancreatic juice from pancreas into small intestine.

Large intestine (colon):
Reabsorbs water and minerals. Passes undigested waste (fiber, bacteria, and some water) to rectum.

Rectum:
Stores waste prior to elimination.

Anus:
Holds rectum closed. Opens to allow elimination.

Severe Diarrhea and Irritable Bowel Syndrome

Two common disorders of the GI tract are diarrhea and irritable bowel syndrome. Their causes may not always be known, but nutrition support may help alleviate their symptoms until a diagnosis is made.

DIARRHEA

Diarrhea refers to an increased frequency or volume of stools. Like other GI complaints, diarrhea is not a disease but a symptom of many medical conditions and treatments. It can be acute, lasting less than 2 weeks, or chronic, lasting longer. Mild diarrhea that remits in 24 to 48 hours is seldom a cause for concern unless the person is already dehydrated. A person with severe, persistent diarrhea may rapidly become dehydrated, lose weight, and develop multiple nutrient deficiencies. A child or infant can lose proportionately more fluid and weight and can develop dehydration and malnutrition in a short time.

Causes of Diarrhea   Acute diarrhea that occurs abruptly in a healthy person frequently results from viral, bacterial, or protozoal infections or as a side effect of medications. It can also occur in the person who begins to eat foods or begins a tube feeding after a period of fasting or starvation. Infants often develop diarrhea when given formulas their immature GI tracts cannot handle or when they are ill. When used in large quantities, food ingredients such as sorbitol and olestra may cause diarrhea in some people.

Chronic diarrhea can occur as a result of disorders that alter GI tract motility, such as the irritable bowel syndrome (described next); from any disorder that causes malabsorption (described later); from food intolerances (lactose intolerance, for example); and from some infections, including some parasitic infections and human immunodeficiency virus (HIV). The diarrhea associated with the dumping syndrome was described in the last chapter.

Treatment of Diarrhea   The treatment of diarrhea requires treatment of the primary medical condition. If a food is responsible for diarrhea, then that food must be omitted from the diet. If a drug is responsible, a different drug, when possible, or different drug form (injectable versus oral, for example) may alleviate the problem. Infections are treated with appropriate drugs. Drugs that slow GI motility are often recommended along with other therapies to treat diarrhea.

Oral Diets   Often people with diarrhea can tolerate regular diets. They may benefit from temporarily avoiding highly seasoned foods, fatty foods, gas-forming foods (see Table 22–1), lactose-containing foods, caffeinated beverages, and any food that aggravates the diarrhea. In other cases, clients may be advised to drink only clear liquids (see Table 22–2 on p. 726) to avoid irritating the GI tract while replacing fluids and electrolytes. For these clients, homemade or commercial oral rehydration formulas—simple solutions of water, salts, and sugar—provide needed fluids and electrolytes. For mild cases of diarrhea, fluids and electrolytes can be replaced using fruit juices, sport drinks, caffeine-free carbonated beverages, tea, and broth with crackers.

Once the diarrhea remits, the client may gradually advance to a regular diet by adding moderately seasoned, low-fiber, low-fat foods as tolerated. Frequent small meals are easiest to tolerate at first. The diet temporarily excludes lactose

Diarrhea that results from an accelerated movement of fluids and electrolytes from the intestinal capillaries into the lumen of the intestine is called secretory diarrhea.

Diarrhea that results from an increase in the osmolarity of the intestinal contents due to unabsorbed water and electrolytes is called osmotic diarrhea.

Severe, chronic diarrhea that does not respond to treatment is often called intractable diarrhea.

Permanent and temporary problems with lactose intolerance occur frequently as a consequence of many medical conditions and malabsorption syndromes (see pp. 115–116).

Drugs used to treat diarrhea are called antidiarrheal agents. Some antidiarrheal agents include diphenoxylate with atropine sulfate, kaolin- and pectin-containing drugs, loperamide, and tincture of opium. Antidiarrheal agents are generally contraindicated for diarrhea caused by infectious agents, because they slow GI motility and prolong the time that the toxin remains in contact with the GI cells.

℞ PRESCRIPTION PAD

Drugs used in the treatment of diarrhea may include:

- Antidiarrheals
- Anti-Infective Agents

See Appendix E for timing with meals and nutrition-related side effects.

Table 22–1
....

Foods That May Produce Gas

Apples	Garlic
Artichokes, Chinese	Gravy
Asparagus	High-fat meats
Barley	Honey
Beer	Kohlrabi
Bran	Legumes (dried beans and peas)
Broccoli	Mannitol
Brussels sprouts	Milk
Cabbage	Molasses
Carbonated beverages	Nuts
Cauliflower	Onions
Celery	Pastries
Coconut	Prunes
Cream sauces	Radishes
Cucumbers	Raisins
Eggplant	Sorbitol
Eggs	Soybeans
Figs	Wheat
Fish	Yeast
Fried foods	

and any foods believed to have irritated the GI tract. Permanent dietary changes may be necessary for diarrhea caused by food sensitivities or allergies.

Bowel Rest　In severe cases of diarrhea, it may become necessary to stop placing demands on the GI tract by withholding all foods and beverages until the diarrhea remits, usually in about 24 to 48 hours. During bowel rest, intravenously administered fluids and electrolytes replace losses. After a day or so of bowel rest, the person tries a clear-liquid diet and then, as tolerance permits, advances to a regular diet as described in the previous paragraph.

Alternative Feedings　Clients who are still unable to tolerate adequate amounts of foods after a few days on an oral diet may benefit from nutritionally complete, lactose-free liquid formulas (see Chapter 23) provided orally, if the client can drink them, or by tube, if oral intake remains inadequate. For people with severe diarrhea who are unable to tolerate any type of oral or tube feeding, intravenous nutrition (see Chapter 24) is indicated, and nothing is given by mouth (NPO).

The World Health Organization recipe for rehydration in diarrheal disease is: Dissolve 3.5 g sodium chloride (table salt), 2.5 g sodium bicarbonate (baking soda), 1.5 g potassium chloride, and 20 g glucose in enough water to make 1 liter.

Formulas given by mouth or by tube are called enteral formulas; formulas given by vein are parenteral formulas.

IRRITABLE BOWEL SYNDROME

Irritable bowel syndrome is another common disorder characterized by a disturbance in the motility of the GI tract. The person with irritable bowel syndrome may experience a variety of symptoms including indigestion, nausea, abdominal

Table 22–2

Foods Included on Liquid Diets

Clear-Liquid Diets	Full-Liquid Diets
Bouillon	All clear liquids
Broth, clear	Butter
Carbonated beverages	Cheese, cottage[a]
Coffee, regular and decaffeinated	Commercially prepared liquid formulas (all)
Commercially prepared clear liquid formulas	Cooked cereals, strained
Fruit drinks	Cream
Fruit ices	Custard
Fruit juices, strained	Egg, soft cooked or scrambled[a]
Gelatin	Flavorings
Hard candy	Ice cream, plain
Honey	Instant breakfast drinks
Lemonade	Margarine
Popsicles	Milk, all types
Salt	Potatoes, mashed and diluted in cream soups
Salt substitutes	Pudding
Sugar substitutes	Sherbet
Tea, regular and decaffeinated	Soups, strained vegetables, meat, or cream
	Sugar
	Sour cream
	Vegetable juices, strained
	Vegetable purees, diluted in cream soups
	Yogurt

[a]As tolerated.

 PRESCRIPTION PAD

Drugs used in the treatment of irritable bowel syndrome may include:

- Anticholinergics (to relax GI tract muscles)
- Antidiarrheals
- Antiflatulents (to relieve symptoms due to excess gas)
- Laxatives

See Appendix E for timing with meals and nutrition-related side effects.

pain, bloating, flatulence, diarrhea, constipation, or alternating diarrhea and constipation. Emotional stress may worsen the symptoms, which frequently occur shortly after a person eats and often resolve temporarily following a bowel movement. The next box provides dietary and other suggestions that may help to reduce the symptoms of irritable bowel syndrome.

Dietary adjustments can help ease the symptoms of diarrhea and irritable bowel syndrome. The dietary treatment of diarrhea depends on its medical cause and its severity. Mild diarrhea may remit without treatment, whereas severe diarrhea can lead to dehydration, electrolyte imbalances, and malnutrition. During treatment, diet therapy may range from complete bowel rest to individualized regular diets. Diarrhea is often a symptom of irritable bowel syndrome, a motility disorder that also causes other uncomfortable GI symptoms. Dietary treatment of irritable bowel syndrome hinges on identifying and avoiding individual foods that cause intolerance. For most people, a low-fat diet provided in small meals, with a gradual increase in fiber, is helpful. The next section of this chapter describes malabsorption syndromes, disorders that frequently result in chronic diarrhea and malnutrition.

How to Lessen the Symptoms of Irritable Bowel Syndrome

To reduce the discomforts associated with irritable bowel syndrome, recommend that clients:

- Identify individual food intolerances by keeping a food record that includes symptoms and the time they occur in relation to meals.

- Avoid offending foods or substances. Common intolerances include milk and milk products (lactose), fatty foods, gas-forming foods and beverages (review Table 22–1), caffeine, alcohol, and foods containing large amounts of fructose or sorbitol.

- Eat frequent small meals at a relaxed pace and at regular times.

- Gradually add dietary fiber to the diet by including more whole-grain breads and cereals, fruits and vegetables, dried beans and peas, and nuts. (Table 4–4 on p. 129 shows the fiber content of selected foods.) Because high-fiber foods are often gas producing, add fiber gradually to allow the GI tract time to adapt.

- Drink plenty of fluids. Fiber attracts water as it moves through the GI tract, so more water is needed.

- Get regular physical activity to reduce stress.

Physicians may also recommend bran or hydrophilic colloids to help relieve constipation. Bran is likely to produce gas, so hydrophilic colloids may be a better choice for some people.

hydrophilic colloid: a type of laxative that attracts water in the intestine to form a bulky stool, which then stimulates peristalsis. (Metamucil and Fiberall are examples of hydrophilic colloids.)

Nutrition Consequences of Malabsorption

Many disorders lead to malabsorption, and any nutrient can be involved. Chapter 21 described vitamin B_{12} malabsorption resulting from chronic gastritis and general malabsorption resulting from the dumping syndrome. The lower GI disorders that affect nutrition most profoundly are those that cause fat malabsorption, which consequently affects the absorption and metabolism of many other nutrients. Unabsorbed fat is excreted from the body in the stools, causing the type of diarrhea known as steatorrhea. Protein may also be malabsorbed, although usually to a lesser degree, further contributing to malnutrition.

steatorrhea (stee-ah-toe-REE-ah): fatty diarrhea characteristic of fat malabsorption; stools are loose, foamy, and foul smelling.

FAT MALABSORPTION

The body's process for absorbing fat (see pp. 154–160) depends on lipase from the pancreas and bile from the liver and is more complex than the process for absorbing protein and carbohydrate. Thus malabsorption syndromes affect fat absorption more profoundly than protein and carbohydrate absorption. The loss of fat in the stools means that valuable food energy, fat-soluble vitamins, and some minerals are lost as well (see Figure 22–2). The loss of food energy affects protein metabolism as well; protein will be sacrificed for energy, limiting its availability to maintain its vital functions.

Figure 22–2

The Effects of Fat Malabsorption

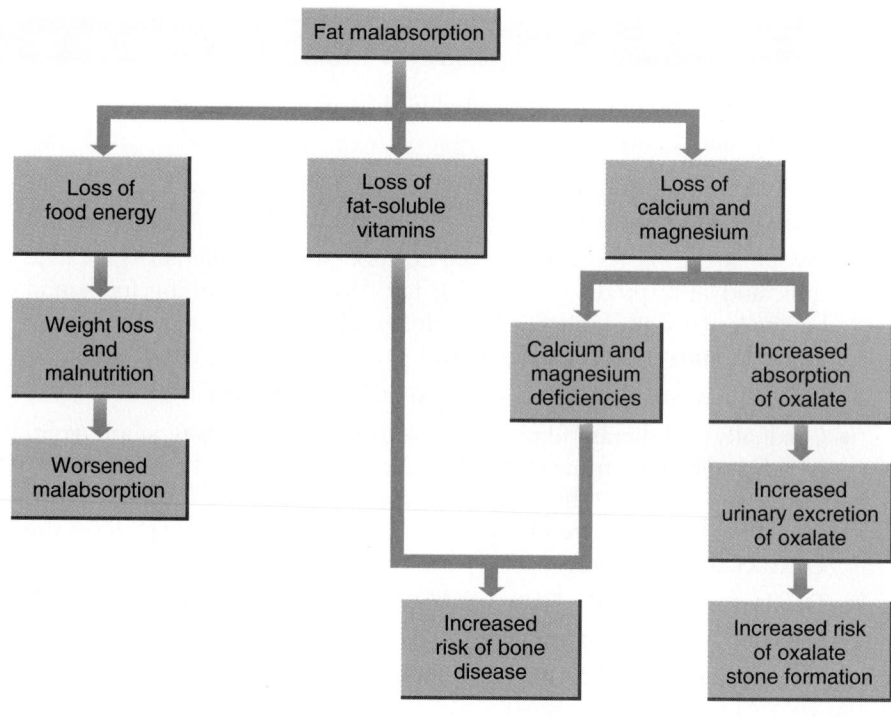

Vitamin and Mineral Malabsorption Fat-soluble vitamins normally travel through the intestine with fat, so they are lost when fat is excreted in steatorrhea. Minerals normally are absorbed in the colon, but when fat malabsorption occurs, unabsorbed fatty acids form soaps with calcium and magnesium and carry these minerals out of the body. Vitamin D losses further aggravate calcium malabsorption.

Oxalate Stones The binding of calcium to fatty acids can cause another problem, enteric hyperoxaluria. Oxalate, which is present in some foods, normally binds with some of the calcium in the gut and is excreted with it. But when fatty acids bind the calcium, the oxalate remains unbound. The intestine absorbs the unbound oxalate, but the body cannot metabolize it and so excretes it in the urine. High urinary oxalate favors the formation of kidney stones (see Highlight 29).

TREATMENTS FOR FAT MALABSORPTION

To treat steatorrhea successfully, the underlying disorder must be diagnosed and treated. Drug therapy, and sometimes surgery, may be necessary. Dietary fat is often restricted; otherwise, enzyme replacements (described later) are provided to aid absorption.

Fat-Restricted Diets Individual tolerances determine the specific amount of fat prescribed, but usually it ranges from 20 to 40 percent of total energy. Typically, the person with malabsorption begins with a diet containing 35 to 45 grams of fat. The person may gradually increase fat intake to provide additional energy as needed. Tolerance improves if fat is consumed in frequent small meals.

enteric hyperoxaluria (en-TER-ick HIGH-per-oxa-LOO-ree-ah): a condition of excess oxalate absorption that comes about because calcium is unable to bind oxalate in the gut; may lead to kidney stone formation.

enteric = intestinal

As you read through these sections on diets for fat malabsorption syndromes, keep in mind the following diet-planning principles:

• Fat is best tolerated when taken in frequent small meals.
• Part of the fat allowance may be supplied by medium-chain triglycerides (MCT).
• Fat-soluble vitamins may be given in a water-miscible form when malabsorption is severe.

Table 22–3

Fat-Restricted Diet (35 grams)

Use:

1. Nonfat milk, cheeses and yogurt made from nonfat milk, sherbet, and fruit ices.
2. Low-fat egg substitutes and up to three regular eggs per week.
3. Up to 6 oz of lean meats and poultry without skin daily.
4. Up to 3 servings of fat daily. One serving is any one of the following:
   1 tsp butter, margarine, shortening, oil, or mayonnaise
   1 strip crisp bacon
   1 tbs salad dressing
   ⅛ avocado
   2 tbs cream (half and half)
   10 small nuts
   8 large olives
   If fat is used to cook or season food, it must be taken from this allowance.
5. All vegetables prepared without fat.
6. All fruits prepared without fat.
7. Plain white or whole-grain bread; nonfat cereals, pasta, rice, noodles, and macaroni.
8. Clear soups.
9. Angel food cake and fruit whips made with gelatin, sugar, and egg-white meringues.
10. Jelly, jam, honey, gumdrops, jelly beans, and marshmallows.

Do Not Use:

1. Whole milk, chocolate milk, whole-milk cheeses, and ice cream.
2. Pastries, cakes, pies, sweet rolls, breads, or vegetables made with fat.
3. More than one egg a day, fried or fatty meats (sausage, luncheon meats, spareribs, frankfurters), duck, goose, or tuna packed in oil (unless well drained).
4. More than 3 servings of fat.
5. Desserts, candy, or anything made with chocolate, nuts, or foods not allowed.
6. Creamed soups made with whole milk.

Suggestions:

1. To make the diet still lower in fat, reduce the fat and meat (and egg) servings.
2. To raise the fat content, give additional fat or meat servings.
3. To improve acceptance of the diet, check the fat content of a well-liked food and allow that food if possible. Use the exchange system fat list for alternate suggestions for fat servings (see Appendix G).

Note: The box on p. 168 provides additional tips for lowering fat in the diet.

Table 22–3 provides instructions for a fat-restricted diet, and a sample fat-restricted diet menu is shown on p. 730.

Medium-Chain Triglycerides Note that the diet is not severely restricted in fat for any longer than is necessary; the person needs food energy. Instead, the diet may provide some fat from medium-chain triglycerides (MCT) rather than long-chain triglycerides (LCT). Products made from MCT oil and formulas con-

Sample Fat-Restricted Diet Menu
All foods are prepared without added fat.

Menu

Breakfast
1 soft-cooked egg
½ c dry cereal
4 oz orange juice
1 slice whole-wheat toast
½ tsp margarine
Nonfat milk
Coffee, sugar

Lunch
3 oz broiled chicken
½ c rice
½ c green beans
1 tsp margarine
Tossed salad
1 tbs low-fat French
   dressing
Fresh apple
Iced tea, sugar

Supper
3 oz lean roast beef
½ c mashed potatoes
½ c peas
1 slice bread
1 tsp margarine
Peaches
Nonfat milk

Snack
Fruit ice

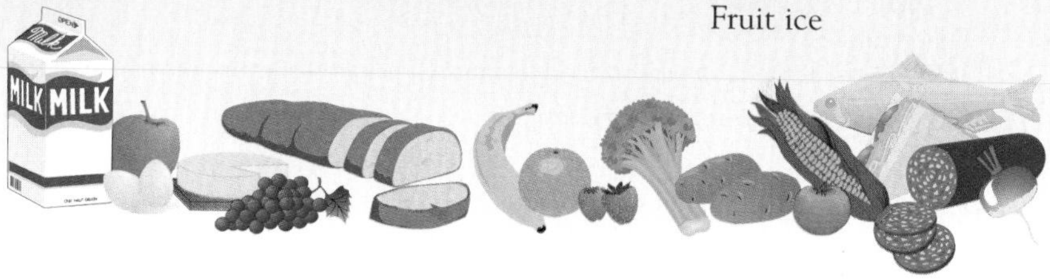

Most naturally occurring fats are LCT; LCT contain fatty acid side chains with at least 14 carbon atoms, and they require lipase and bile for absorption. MCT contain fatty acid side chains with 8 to 12 carbon atoms, and they can be absorbed with minimal lipase and bile.

taining MCT supply about as many kcalories as regular fats, but people who cannot digest and absorb LCT can digest and absorb MCT. MCT oil does not contain essential fatty acids, however, so the diet must include some LCT. The accompanying box offers suggestions for improving acceptance of fat-restricted diets and includes tips for using MCT oil.

water-miscible (MISS-ih-bul) **vitamins:** fat-soluble vitamins that readily mix with water and can be absorbed without fat.

Water-Miscible Fat-Soluble Vitamins   Most often, the person with malabsorption absorbs enough fat-soluble vitamins so that a standard supplement can be given. For people who fail to maintain adequate vitamin pools, however, fat-soluble vitamins can be supplemented in a water-miscible form that facilitates absorption.

Oxalate-Restricted Diets   To reduce the risk of oxalate stones, clients with fat malabsorption may be advised to limit foods high in oxalate. Foods notable for their high oxalate contents include spinach, rhubarb, beets, nuts, chocolate, tea, wheat bran, and strawberries.

enzyme replacements: extracts of pork or beef pancreatic enzymes that are taken as supplements to help with digestion.

Enzyme Replacement Therapy   Enzyme replacements are used when the person suffers malabsorption related to chronic and severe damage to the pancreas or whenever steatorrhea is severe. They improve digestion and absorption, thereby helping to control steatorrhea. Enzyme replacements taken with meals may lessen the malabsorption of protein and fat, but may not fully correct it.

Of the energy nutrients, fat undergoes the most complex process of digestion and absorption and, therefore, is the most likely to be affected by disorders that cause malabsorption. The loss of fat in the stools leads to the loss of food energy; the malabsorption of fat-soluble vitamins, calcium, and magnesium; and the

How to Improve Acceptance of Fat-Restricted Diets

Fat-restricted diets can be difficult for people to follow. Fats give flavors to foods—flavors that people may miss. Unlike some diets that can be introduced gradually, a fat-restricted diet must be implemented right away without giving the person time to adapt to the changes. These suggestions may help:

- Provide clients with tips for making foods palatable while lowering the fat intake, such as those found in the box on p. 168.
- Suggest that clients use cookbooks that feature low-kcalorie and low-fat recipes.
- Remind clients that new fat-free and low-fat products appear on market shelves daily, and most people find these products very acceptable.

People who use MCT oil need additional advice:

- Advise clients to add MCT to the diet gradually. Nausea, vomiting, abdominal pain, and distention can result from using too much MCT at once.
- Recommend that clients improve the palatability of MCT oil by substituting it for regular oil in salad dressing and for baking and cooking and by adding it to beverages, desserts, and other dishes.
- Warn clients that MCT products are expensive, and explain that these products can be purchased at pharmacies and may be covered by insurance.

increased absorption of oxalate. Dietary therapy for fat malabsorption may include fat- and oxalate-restricted diets and the use of MCT, water-miscible fat-soluble vitamins, and enzyme replacements. Disorders that result in malabsorption are described next.

Malabsorption Syndromes

Malabsorption syndromes and their treatments profoundly threaten nutrition status and may lead to wasting by reducing nutrient intakes, accelerating nutrient losses, and raising nutrient needs (see Table 22–4). Malabsorption can occur when the flow of enzymes from the pancreas or bile from the liver is disrupted, when the surface area of the bowel is reduced, or when normal mechanisms for absorbing nutrients are impaired. Many drugs and disorders can cause malabsorption; several are discussed throughout the remainder of this chapter, but whatever the cause, malnutrition always threatens.

Because the pancreas is an accessory organ in digestion and absorption, some pancreatic disorders result in malabsorption and cause nutrition consequences similar to those of intestinal disorders and so are described here. Malabsorption caused by other disorders such as liver disease, cancer, and HIV infection, which have additional nutrition consequences, are described in later chapters.

PANCREATITIS

Pancreatic secretions contain many enzymes necessary for the digestion of protein, fat, and carbohydrate, together with bicarbonate-rich juices that provide

Table 22–4
....
Possible Causes of Wasting in Malabsorption Syndromes

Reduced Nutrient Intake	Excessive Nutrient Losses	Raised Nutrient Needs
Abdominal pain	Blood loss	High basal energy expenditure
Anorexia	Diarrhea	Infection
Bowel rest	Fistulas	Medications
Emotional stress	General malabsorption	Surgery
Food intolerance	Intestinal losses of serum proteins	
Indigestion	Medications	
Medications	Steatorrhea	
Nausea	Vomiting	
Obstructions		

the optimal pH necessary to activate these enzymes. Consequently, pancreatic disorders can impair digestion and result in malabsorption and poor nutrition status.

pancreatitis: inflammation of the pancreas.

Acute Pancreatitis   Normally, the pancreas stores digestive enzymes in an inactive form to protect itself from digestion. In pancreatitis, however, digestive enzymes are activated within the pancreas and begin to damage the organ itself. The blood picks up some of these enzymes; thus elevated serum amylase and lipase serve as indicators of pancreatitis. Typical symptoms of pancreatitis include severe abdominal pain, nausea, and vomiting. In some cases, pancreatitis leads to serious complications including reduced blood volume, acute renal failure (see Chapter 29), respiratory failure, pancreatic hemorrhages, fistulas, and abscesses.[1] Pancreatitis most often develops as a consequence of gallstones or alcoholism; sometimes, though, the reasons are unclear because a variety of medical conditions and some drugs can also precipitate pancreatitis.[2]

fistula (FIS-too-lah): an abnormal opening between two organs or from an organ to the skin.

fistula = pipe

abscess: an accumulation of pus, caused by a local infection, that builds up and may eventually burst.

Treatment of Pancreatitis   The treatment of acute pancreatitis depends on its severity, although initial therapy in all cases aims to suppress pancreatic secretions. Food is withheld, because food stimulates pancreatic secretions. In some cases, a nasogastric tube is inserted to suction out the stomach's secretions and further reduce stimulation of the pancreas. Edema within the pancreas, losses through nasogastric suction, and lack of oral intake can disrupt fluid and electrolyte balance, making intravenous fluids necessary.

Mild-to-Moderate Pancreatitis   In most cases, pancreatitis resolves in less than a week; the person can begin oral intake when abdominal pain subsides and serum amylase levels return to normal or near normal. The diet progresses from a clear-liquid diet to a low-fat diet and, finally, to a regular diet as tolerated. If eating aggravates the pain, or if serum amylase rises, food is withheld; when these signs and symptoms subside, food can again be reintroduced. Clients may tolerate frequent small meals better at first.

If pancreatitis is severe or if complications arise, and if food intake fails to meet nutrient needs for more than a week, tube feeding is indicated.[3] The presence of nutrients in the stomach stimulates pancreatic secretions, but studies suggest that feedings delivered by tube directly into the jejunum do not significantly stimulate pancreatic secretions.[4] Thus people with pancreatitis may benefit from tube feedings of easy-to-absorb formulas delivered into the jejunum. If enteral feedings worsen abdominal pain, edema, or drainage from fistulas, or if vomiting is a problem, intravenous feedings may be necessary.

Chronic Pancreatitis   If an acute episode of pancreatitis doesn't subside or if episodes recur at frequent intervals, the pancreatic cells can be permanently destroyed, leading to chronic pancreatitis. Chronic alcohol abuse is the most frequent cause of chronic pancreatitis.

The pancreas normally excretes enzymes far in excess of needs, so even after considerable damage has occurred, digestion may proceed normally. With extensive degeneration of the pancreas and chronic pancreatitis, however, digestion, especially of fat, becomes permanently impaired. Abdominal pain is often severe and unrelenting, vomiting is frequent, and severe weight loss is common.

Nutrition Support   The goals of diet therapy in chronic pancreatitis are to maintain optimal nutrition status, reduce steatorrhea (if present), minimize pain, and avoid subsequent attacks of active pancreatitis. Health care professionals recommend a moderate fat-restricted diet; restricting fat too severely makes it difficult for the person to gain or maintain weight. Small meals may be easiest to digest. Absolutely no alcohol is permitted.

Enzyme replacements taken with meals aid in the digestion and absorption of protein and fat. Enzyme replacements, like naturally occurring enzymes, work best in a basic pH. To improve the effectiveness of enzyme replacements, people with pancreatic insufficiency often need to take drugs to limit gastric acid production, because the basic secretions from the pancreas may be reduced.

Complicating Conditions   During active attacks of pancreatitis, diet therapy reverts to that described earlier for acute pancreatitis. Sometimes pancreatitis damages the cells that produce the hormones insulin and glucagon. In these cases, clients become glucose intolerant, as in diabetes (see Chapter 27), and must follow a diet for diabetes. Deficiencies of glucagon, which lead to hypoglycemia, complicate the task of regulating blood glucose. The case study on p. 734 provides a review of pancreatitis and its treatment.

CYSTIC FIBROSIS

People with cystic fibrosis, the most common fatal genetic disorder in North America, produce thick, sticky mucus secretions that may seriously impair the function of many organs, most notably the lungs and pancreas.[5] Just a few decades ago, an infant born with cystic fibrosis seldom survived to adulthood. Today, thanks to advances in medical therapy and nutrition care, the outlook is much brighter, with some surviving into their forties and even fifties.

Cystic fibrosis has three major consequences: chronic lung disease, pancreatic insufficiency, and abnormally high electrolyte concentrations in the sweat. Chronic lung disease develops because the airways in the lungs become

---

℞ PRESCRIPTION PAD

Drugs used in the treatment of pancreatitis may include:

- Analgesics (to relieve pain)
- H2-blockers (to improve efficiency of enzyme replacements)
- Insulin (to control blood glucose levels)
- Pancreatic enzyme replacements

See Appendix E for timing with meals and nutrition-related side effects.

---

cystic fibrosis: a hereditary disorder characterized by the production of thick mucus that affects many organs, including the lungs, pancreas, liver, heart, gallbladder, and small intestine.

fibrous: composed of fibers. The development of excess fibrous tissue is **fibrosis**.

Case Study   Homemaker with Pancreatitis

Mrs. Corey is a 52-year-old homemaker who was admitted to the hospital with severe abdominal pain, nausea, and vomiting. Laboratory tests reveal very high serum amylase, low serum albumin, and red blood cell indices consistent with folate-deficiency anemia. Mrs. Corey is diagnosed as having pancreatitis. She is 5 feet 3 inches tall and weighs 100 pounds. Mrs. Corey's family has told her physician that she may have a problem with alcohol abuse. The health care team is concerned not only with the diagnosis of pancreatitis, but also with Mrs. Corey's nutrition status and possible alcohol abuse.

How would you describe pancreatitis to Mrs. Corey? Why is her serum amylase elevated? How can

pancreatitis lead to poor nutrition status? Discuss factors in Mrs. Corey's medical history that put her at risk for poor nutrition status. (Assume alcohol abuse for the purposes of this question, and review Highlight 7's description of how alcohol impairs nutrition status.)

Describe when and how Mrs. Corey should be fed. What factors would determine the need for tube feedings or parenteral nutrition?

If Mrs. Corey develops chronic pancreatitis, how should her diet be modified? What other measures should be taken to ensure adequate digestion and absorption?

congested with mucus, causing breathing to be labored. As the thick mucus stagnates in the bronchial tubes, bacteria multiply there. Lung infections are the usual cause of death in people with cystic fibrosis.

Cystic fibrosis probably causes some degree of pancreatic insufficiency in all cases, with about 90 percent of cases serious enough to require enzyme replacement therapy. With aging, damage to the pancreas worsens. The thick mucus obstructs the small pancreatic ducts and interferes with the secretion of digestive enzymes, pancreatic juices, and pancreatic hormones. Eventually, the pancreatic cells are surrounded by mucus and are gradually replaced by fibrous tissues. Malabsorption of many nutrients including fat, protein, vitamins, and minerals often leads to malnutrition. Additionally, the secretion of insulin may be affected resulting in glucose intolerance and diabetes.

Treatment of Cystic Fibrosis   Therapy for cystic fibrosis aims to promote appropriate growth and development and prevent respiratory failure and complications. Treatment includes respiratory, diet, and drug therapy.

Energy and Nutrient Needs   Nutrient losses through malabsorption, frequent infections, rapid turnover of protein and essential fatty acids, high protein catabolism, and high basal energy expenditures raise energy needs for people with cystic fibrosis to between 120 and 150 percent of the RDA for sex and age. Extra energy is needed simply to breathe. Dietitians estimate individual energy requirements based on basal metabolic rate, activity level, pulmonary function, and degree of malabsorption.

Obtaining enough energy can be complicated, however, because people with cystic fibrosis frequently experience a loss of appetite that is aggravated by repeated infections, emotional stress, and drug therapy. Coughing to clear the lungs may trigger vomiting or reflux of foods from the stomach. Thus the person with cystic fibrosis finds it difficult to take in enough food energy, protein, and other nutrients to meet needs.

R̲x̲ PRESCRIPTION PAD

Drugs used in the treatment of cystic fibrosis may include:

- Antibiotics
- Bronchodilators (to ease breathing)
- H2-blockers
- Insulin (to control blood glucose)
- Mucolytics (to thin mucous secretions)
- Pancreatic enzyme replacements

See Appendix E for timing with meals and nutrition-related side effects.

With the widespread use of supplemental vitamins for people with cystic fibrosis, overt vitamin deficiencies are uncommon. Abnormal electrolyte losses through the sweat or from vomiting require replacement.

Diet and Enzyme Replacement Therapy   With such high energy needs, fat restrictions are inappropriate; instead, pancreatic enzyme replacements are used to control steatorrhea, relieve abdominal pain, and reduce the mass and frequency of stools passed. To improve the effectiveness of the enzyme replacements, H2-blockers are often provided as well. Even with enzyme replacements, from 10 to 20 percent of food energy is lost in the stools.[6]

Feeding Infants   How can the enhanced energy and nutrient needs of infants with cystic fibrosis be met? For some infants with cystic fibrosis, breastfeeding can sustain normal growth, if enzyme replacements are given.[7] These infants must be closely monitored, however, to ensure that they meet their high energy and nutrient needs. Additionally, the breastfed infant with cystic fibrosis needs about ⅛ to ¼ teaspoon of table salt daily, given with water to replace sweat-induced electrolyte losses.[8]

Infants who are not breastfed can usually tolerate regular infant formulas. Infants who cannot tolerate regular formulas often receive special formulas that are easy to digest and absorb. Regardless of the type of feeding—human milk, regular infant formula, or hydrolyzed formula—enzyme replacements are always given as well. As for solid foods, the recommendations for feeding infants and for introducing solid foods during the first year, shown on p. 635, apply to infants with cystic fibrosis.

Formulas that are easy to digest and absorb are called hydrolyzed formulas (see Chapter 23).

Feeding Children and Adults   A child with cystic fibrosis is weaned from breast milk or infant formula to a high-kcalorie, nutritionally balanced diet carefully tailored to the child's tolerances. Indirect calorimetry may provide a more accurate assessment of energy needs than formula estimates, especially in preadolescent children.[9]

Nutrient Supplementation   Carbohydrate supplements, MCT oil and protein powders can be added to foods to boost energy and protein intakes (see Appendix K). Liquid formulas taken orally to improve energy and nutrient intake can also be used.[10]

Multivitamin supplements are prescribed to help meet the high vitamin requirements that a high-energy, high-protein intake demands. As the disorder progresses, fat-soluble vitamins may be given in addition to a multivitamin supplement. For people with severe steatorrhea, the water-miscible vitamin form is appropriate.

As for minerals, as mentioned earlier, abnormally high concentrations of electrolytes (sodium and chloride) in sweat are characteristic of cystic fibrosis. Fever, high environmental temperatures, vomiting, and malabsorption can further deplete electrolytes and lead to dehydration in people with cystic fibrosis. The liberal use of table salt and fluids is encouraged.

Fluids help liquefy thick secretions and prevent dehydration.

Alternate Feedings   People with cystic fibrosis need regular nutrition assessments to ensure that their diets are supporting their growth and well-being. Height and weight measurements are particularly relevant. For adults, the goal is

Case Study   Child with Cystic Fibrosis

Ryan is a seven-year-old boy diagnosed with cystic fibrosis. Symptoms of steatorrhea and failure to gain weight during infancy prompted tests that led to the diagnosis. Ryan is currently in the hospital to treat a respiratory infection. He has a temperature of 102°F. He is 43½ inches tall and weighs 38 pounds.

Describe the medical consequences of cystic fibrosis. Why are growth failure and repeated respiratory infections hallmarks of the disorder? Look at the growth chart appropriate for Ryan's age and sex in Appendix E. Plot Ryan's height and weight. What does the chart tell you about his growth?

What type of diet should Ryan follow? How can enzyme replacements be used effectively? What important measure should be taken to ensure that Ryan's diet is adequate?

How can the people caring for Ryan and his family offer emotional support?

to maintain a healthy weight for height. For children, every effort should be made to maintain weight at greater than 90 percent of that appropriate for height, gender, and age.[11] If weight falls below 85 percent of standard weight, feeding by tube is indicated.[12] Weight below 75 percent indicates advanced malnutrition that necessitates feeding by tube or by vein. Clients may benefit from home nutrition programs that include oral diets during waking hours and tube feedings or intravenous nutrition during sleep.

Emotional Support   People with cystic fibrosis face repeated hospitalizations and often an early death. They, and their caregivers, must deal with many aspects of care important to survival, of which nutrition is only one. They must manage daily respiratory therapy treatments, enzyme replacements, and, often, antibiotics. Caregivers must also help people with cystic fibrosis to adjust to their disease, maintain their social life, keep up with work or schoolwork, and assume as much responsibility for their health as possible. The accompanying case study discusses the needs of a child with cystic fibrosis.

CROHN'S DISEASE

Crohn's disease: inflammation and ulceration along the length of the GI tract, often with granulomas; also called regional ileitis (ILL-ee-EYE-tis).

granulomas (gran-you-LOH-mahs): granular tumors or growths.
  granulum = little grain
  oma = tumor

The two most prevalent disorders that inflame the bowel are Crohn's disease and ulcerative colitis (described later). Inflammatory bowel diseases (IBD) share some clinical features but are distinct conditions. Their causes remain unknown, although heredity, environment, and immune functions are thought to be contributing factors.[13]

In Crohn's disease, cracklike ulcers and many granulomas accompany inflammation of the bowel. Crohn's disease most often affects the ileum and colon, but can affect the entire GI tract and even the liver, kidneys, joints, eyes, and skin. The incidence of Crohn's disease is highest in people from 20 to 40 years of age and in Jews. There is no medical cure for Crohn's disease, and even after acute symptoms resolve, recurrences are likely.

Complications   As the disease progresses, fibrous tissue forms in the intestine, reducing its absorptive ability, narrowing the intestinal lumen, and sometimes causing an obstruction. The intestine may also rupture and cause a severe, and sometimes fatal, infection (peritonitis).

Reminder: A fistula is an abnormal opening between two organs or from an organ to the skin.

Fistulas may develop if an inflamed loop of intestine sticks to another loop of intestine, to another organ, or to the skin and gradually erodes. If a fistula forms between the stomach or the upper portion of the small intestine and the colon, ingested food is shunted directly into the colon, and further malabsorption results. Bacteria from the colon can then invade the stomach or upper small intestine, contributing to further malabsorption (described next), increasing the risk of serious infections, and causing severe inflammation, nausea, and vomiting. If a fistula forms between the small intestine and the skin, significant malabsorption can occur if large volumes of fluid are lost. Surgery to remove a diseased or obstructed portion of the intestine or to repair a fistula further taxes nutrition status.

Fistulas through which 100 ml or more of fluid per day are lost are called *high-output fistulas*.

Nutrition Status   Nutrition status is severely threatened in Crohn's disease. The person with Crohn's disease often experiences emotional stress, anorexia, weight loss, fever, diarrhea, malabsorption, and cramping abdominal pain—all of which can lead to nutrient deficiencies. Oral intake may be withheld so that the bowel can rest, particularly when an obstruction develops or a fistula forms. In addition, bleeding from lesions can lead to anemia, and inflammation can cause the secretion and loss of serum proteins, with resulting hypoalbuminemia.[14] The accompanying drug therapy can further impair nutrition status. If the person requires surgery or develops an infection, nutrient needs become even greater. Because surgery removes a portion of the bowel, the procedure itself may contribute to malabsorption (see "Short-Bowel Syndrome" later in this chapter).

The intestinal loss of serum proteins is called protein-losing enteropathy.

Because children with Crohn's disease need additional nutrients to support growth and maturation, nutrition problems are compounded. Growth failure is common and may be the manifestation of the disease that leads to its diagnosis.

Restoring and maintaining nutrition status for the person with Crohn's disease can be a challenging task. Protein-energy malnutrition (PEM) and deficiencies of calcium, magnesium, zinc, iron, vitamin B_{12}, folate, vitamin C, and fat-soluble vitamins are commonly reported. Low serum albumin and multiple nutrient deficiencies threaten immune function and may reduce the effectiveness of drug therapy.

℞ PRESCRIPTION PAD

Drugs used in the treatment of Crohn's disease may include:

- Antibiotics (metronidazole, sulfasalazine)
- Anti-inflammatory agents (prednisone)

See Appendix E for timing with meals and nutrition-related side effects.

Nutrition Support   People with active Crohn's disease benefit from formulas provided by mouth or by tube or total nutrition by vein (see Chapters 23 and 24).[15] Enteral nutrition is the preferred feeding route, and easy-to-absorb (hydrolyzed) formulas may offer some advantages over standard formulas or table foods.[16] Hydrolyzed formulas may be unpalatable to some people, however, and if the formula cannot be taken orally, it may be given by tube. In some cases, feeding tubes can be placed so as to bypass fistulas or partial obstructions, allowing feeding by tube without adding to the risk of complications. Feedings by vein are used to deliver needed nutrients when oral or tube feedings significantly aggravate pain and diarrhea; when the bowel is obstructed or the client is at risk for obstruction; when complete bowel rest might help a fistula to close; or when oral or tube feedings cannot meet nutrient requirements.

Oral Diets   As the acute stage of Crohn's disease resolves, the person gradually progresses, as tolerance permits, to an oral diet, often a high-kcalorie, high-protein diet. A fat-restricted diet is necessary for people with fat malabsorption. Low-fiber diets are sometimes recommended for those with partial obstructions of the intestine. Clients may be intolerant to certain foods or food components, including lactose, and these should be identified and eliminated from the diet.

Case Study College Student with Crohn's Disease

Lilinoe, a 19-year-old college student, was first diagnosed with Crohn's disease when she was 18 years old. At that time, she weighed 120 pounds and was 5 feet 7 inches tall. Her normal weight had been 130 pounds until the disease symptoms began to appear. Since then, she has been hospitalized several times for recurrent attacks of Crohn's disease. As anticipated from her weight-loss history, Lilinoe's nutrition assessment shows that she is suffering from severe PEM. In talking with Lilinoe, you discover that she is very particular about the foods she eats and often simply does not eat. Her physician has ordered an easy-to-absorb formula diet to be fed to Lilinoe by tube.

Review Lilinoe's weight history. What is her desirable body weight? What measures could have been taken to avoid weight loss?

What possible benefits might an easy-to-absorb formula offer Lilinoe? Why might the physician prefer a tube feeding rather than oral feedings?

Consider Lilinoe's long-term dietary management. What type of diet should she eventually follow? What goals should be set for weight gain? Why is it important to reassess her nutrition status regularly?

Given Lilinoe's age and stage of development, what emotional concerns might she be experiencing? What interventions might be planned to enhance her sense of hope, self-esteem, and well-being?

Supplemental vitamin-mineral preparations are frequently prescribed. Encourage clients to eat a nutrient-rich, well-balanced diet, and reassess nutrition status frequently to ensure that nutrient needs are being met. Later sections of this chapter describe additional nutrition concerns for clients who have undergone ileostomies, colostomies, or intestinal resections. A case study describing a person with Crohn's disease is presented in the accompanying box.

MALABSORPTION CAUSED BY BACTERIAL OVERGROWTH

Although the colon normally houses a bacterial population, the small intestine is protected from bacterial overgrowth by gastric acid, which kills bacteria, and peristalsis, which flushes microorganisms through the small intestine before they can flourish. Sometimes, however, these protective mechanisms fail, allowing bacteria to thrive in the small intestine. Gastric surgeries, for instance, can interfere with gastric acid secretions and alter peristalsis. In some types of gastric surgery, a portion of the small intestine is bypassed, causing stasis in the intestine and allowing bacteria to flourish. The bypassed portion is called a blind loop, and the symptoms associated with bacterial overgrowth are called the blind loop syndrome. Figure 22–3 on p. 739 shows blind loops created by gastric surgeries.

Bacterial overgrowth can also occur for other reasons besides gastric surgery. Chronic gastritis (see p. 704), drug therapy (antiulcer agents), and HIV infections, for instance, can significantly reduce gastric acid secretions and lead to bacterial overgrowth in the stomach and upper small intestine. Small bowel obstructions and nerve dysfunction associated with diabetes can also lead to bacterial overgrowth by altering peristalsis.

Consequences of Bacterial Overgrowth Bacteria in the small intestine partly dismantle the bile salts, which are essential for fat digestion and absorp-

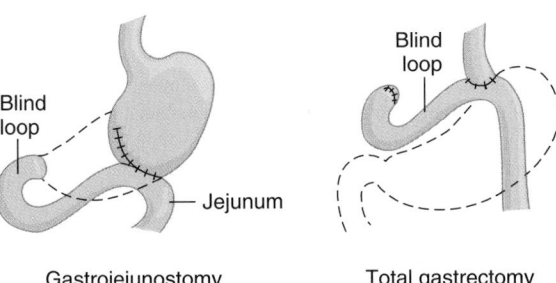

Figure 22–3

**Blind Loops Created
by Gastric Surgery**

In some gastric resections or bypass surgeries, a portion of the intestine is
bypassed (the blind loop), peristalsis
through the segment is disrupted, and bacteria flourish.

tion. Fat malabsorption and its related consequences occur as a result. Figure
22–4 repeats the figure from Chapter 5 (p. 156) that shows how bile prepares fat
for digestion, this time illustrating how bacteria interfere with that process. The
bacteria also compete with the body for vitamin B_{12} and folate, limiting the
available supply and leading to deficiencies.

   Treatment of Bacterial Overgrowth   To control bacterial overgrowth,
physicians prescribe antibiotics. Along with drug therapy, clients receive fat-
restricted diets, parenterally administered vitamin B_{12}, and oral folate supplements. If medical treatment fails, people with surgically created blind loops may
need additional surgery to remove the blind loop.

SHORT-BOWEL SYNDROME

Short-bowel, or short-gut, syndrome is characterized by diarrhea, weight loss,
muscle wasting, bone disease, protein and fat malabsorption, hypocalcemia,

short-bowel or **short-gut syndrome:**
severe malabsorption that may occur when
the absorptive surface of the small bowel is
reduced, resulting in diarrhea, weight loss,
bone disease, hypocalcemia, hypomagnesemia, and anemia.

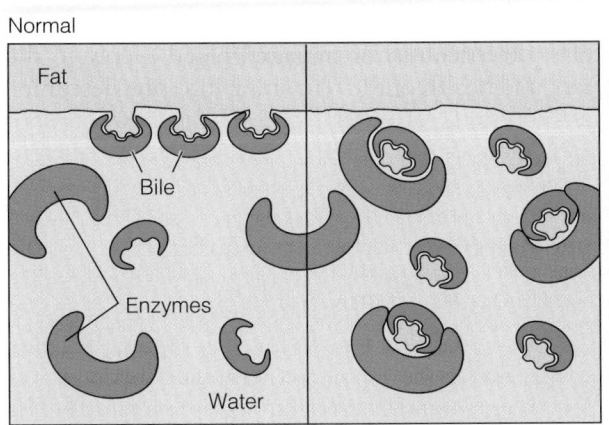 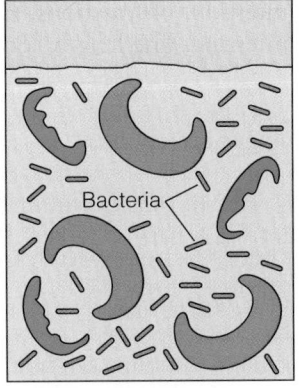

Figure 22–4

**Bacterial Overgrowth
and Steatorrhea**

When fat enters the small
intestine, bile arrives.
Bile has an affinity for both
fat and water, so it can
bring the fat into solution
in the water.

After emulsification, the fat
is mixed in the water solution,
so the enzymes have access
to it.

In blind loop syndrome,
bacteria damage the bile,
so that it is ineffective in fat
digestion and absorption.
The result is fat malabsorption
and steatorrhea.

Figure 22–5

Nutrient Absorption and Consequences of Intestinal Surgeries

About 90 to 95 percent of nutrient absorption takes place in the first half of the small intestine. After a resection, nutrient absorption is reduced.

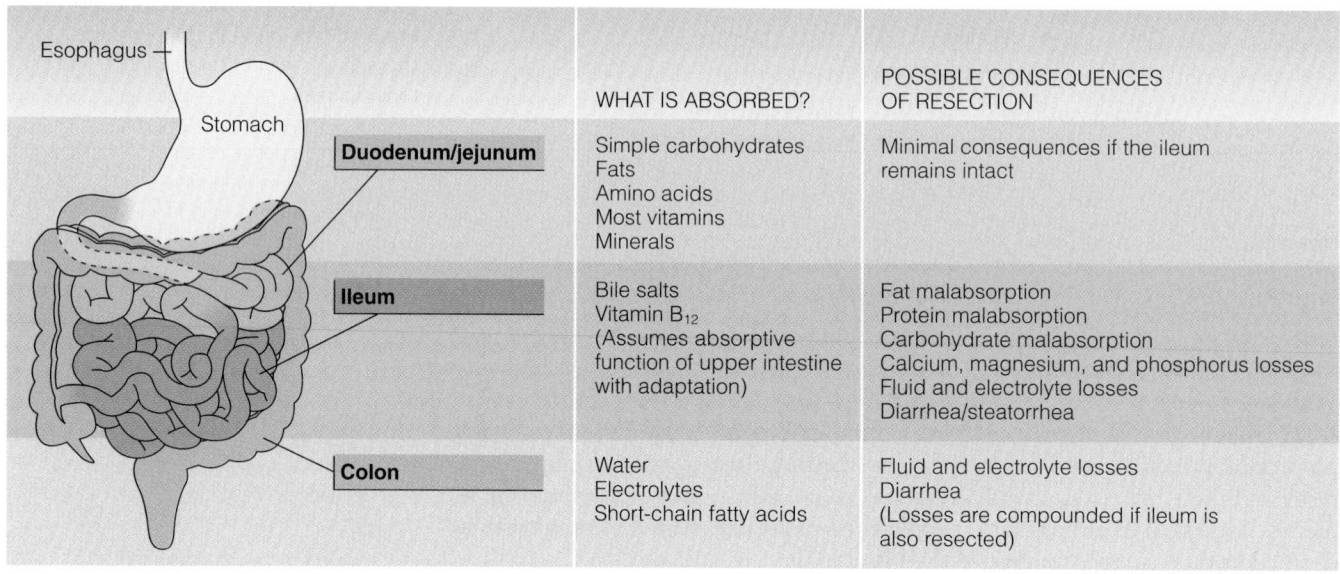

	WHAT IS ABSORBED?	POSSIBLE CONSEQUENCES OF RESECTION
Duodenum/jejunum	Simple carbohydrates Fats Amino acids Most vitamins Minerals	Minimal consequences if the ileum remains intact
Ileum	Bile salts Vitamin B_{12} (Assumes absorptive function of upper intestine with adaptation)	Fat malabsorption Protein malabsorption Carbohydrate malabsorption Calcium, magnesium, and phosphorus losses Fluid and electrolyte losses Diarrhea/steatorrhea
Colon	Water Electrolytes Short-chain fatty acids	Fluid and electrolyte losses Diarrhea (Losses are compounded if ileum is also resected)

hypomagnesemia, and anemia. It can occur whenever the absorptive surface of the small intestine is significantly reduced. Short-bowel syndrome frequently results from surgery to remove a significant portion of the small intestine, which may be necessary for people with inflammatory bowel diseases, cancer of the intestine, obstructions, fistulas, diverticulitis, or impaired blood supply to the intestine. The length, location, and health of the remaining intestine determine the degree to which nutrient absorption is affected. Figure 22–5 reviews nutrient absorption in the GI tract and describes how absorption is affected by different surgical resections.

Extent and Location of the Resection   Generally, up to 50 percent of the intestine can be resected without serious nutrition consequences. Remarkably, even resections of up to 80 percent may be well tolerated, provided that the terminal ileum, the ileocecal valve, and the colon remain intact.[17] When the ileum has been resected, however, the absorption of fat, protein, carbohydrate, fat-soluble vitamins, vitamin B_{12}, calcium, and magnesium can be impaired. The ileum is also where bile salts are normally reabsorbed. Without bile salt reabsorption, the body's pool of bile salts diminishes, and fat malabsorption worsens.

The Ileocecal Valve   The ileocecal valve controls the rate at which the intestinal contents move from the small to the large bowel. Without the valve, transit time through the small intestine is rapid, and the time available for nutrient absorption is limited. Consequently, the colon receives large volumes of unabsorbed nutrients, fluids, electrolytes, and bile salts. Nutrient absorption is impaired and diarrhea results. If the colon is resected as well, severe fluid and electrolyte imbalances threaten health.

The Colon Recent studies suggest that an intact colon plays a significant role in reducing carbohydrate and, to a lesser extent, protein malabsorption following intestinal resections.[18] Bacteria in the colon salvage energy from some of the unabsorbed carbohydrate by metabolizing it to short-chain fatty acids, which can then be absorbed and utilized for energy. This salvage function appears to be enhanced in people with intestinal resections—a form of adaptation.

Adaptation After an intestinal resection, a remarkable adaptive response occurs in the portion of the intestine that remains: it gets longer, thicker, and wider, and it either absorbs nutrients more efficiently or begins to absorb nutrients it did not absorb before. Maximum bowel adaptation may take as long as one to two years following a resection.[19] The presence of nutrients in the remaining gut appears to stimulate this adaptation—a good reason to begin enteral nutrition as early as possible. Specific dietary constituents, such as the amino acid glutamine, short-chain fatty acids, and fiber, and growth hormone may also aid in this adaptation (see Highlight 22). With an extensive bowel resection, however, even adaptation will fail to compensate for the reduced surface area.

Nutrition Support following Small Bowel Resections Immediately after surgery, the primary nutrition concern is to maintain fluid and electrolyte balance. For resections of less than 50 percent of the intestine, oral nutrition begins a few days after surgery. A moderate fat-restricted diet with supplemental vitamin B_{12} is recommended.[20] For more extensive resections, parenteral nutrition is often provided initially to ensure that nutrient needs are met until adaptation has occurred. Enteral nutrition (usually by tube feeding) is initiated as early as possible to stimulate adaptation. Drugs are also used to treat the disorder.

Once oral intake begins, people whose colons remain intact following surgery benefit from diets that are high in complex carbohydrates (60 percent of kcalories), restricted in fat (20 percent of kcalories), and low in oxalate.[21] With time, fat intake can be liberalized if additional energy is needed and if the fat does not precipitate steatorrhea or diarrhea. People with short-bowel syndrome who do not have intact colons have greater difficulty absorbing energy from either fat or carbohydrates than those with intact colons. These people are more likely to need parenteral nutrition to supply part or all of their nutrient needs.

CELIAC DISEASE

Celiac disease provides an example of how food sensitivities can cause malabsorption. Celiac disease is a hereditary disorder with an incidence of about 1 in every 2000 to 3000 births. It alters the intestinal mucosal cells, so that they become sensitive to gliadin, a fraction of the protein gluten, which is found in wheat, oats, rye, and barley. Gliadin acts as a toxic substance, causing the

PRESCRIPTION PAD

Drugs used in the treatment of short-bowel syndrome may include:

- Antidiarrheals
- Calcium carbonate antacids (to bind oxalate)
- H2-blockers

See Appendix E for timing with meals and nutrition-related side effects.

celiac (SEE-lee-ack) **disease:** a sensitivity to gliadin that causes flattening of the intestinal villi and generalized malabsorption; also called **gluten-sensitive enteropathy** (EN-ter-OP-ah-thee) or **celiac sprue.**

gliadin (GLIGH-ah-din): a fraction of the gluten protein.

gluten (GLUE-ten): a protein found in wheat, oats, rye, and barley. (Remember the acronym "WORB" to recall these grains.)

intestinal villi to atrophy and seriously reducing the absorptive surface of the intestinal tract. The disaccharidases (including lactase) and the carrier molecules normally found on the villi disappear. The result is malabsorption of many nutrients, including fat, protein, carbohydrate, fat-soluble vitamins, iron, calcium, magnesium, zinc, and some water-soluble vitamins.

Nutrition Status   The person with celiac disease often experiences steatorrhea, diarrhea, weight loss, and malnutrition. Anemia may occur as a result of iron, folate, or vitamin B_{12} deficiency. Because protein is malabsorbed, serum protein levels can fall dramatically, inducing edema. A vitamin K deficiency may precipitate clotting abnormalities, and the person may bleed easily. Furthermore, calcium deficiency can cause tetany and bone pain.

Treatment of Celiac Disease   Unlike most malabsorption syndromes, which often benefit from fat-restricted diets, the malabsorption caused by celiac disease responds to gluten restriction. Once gluten is removed from the diet, the intestinal changes reverse almost completely. Generally, improvement occurs within a few weeks of strict adherence to the diet. Lactase deficiency and lactose intolerance may be permanent. If the person fails to follow the gluten-restricted diet, the symptoms will return.

Gluten-Restricted Diets   The treatment of celiac disease sounds deceptively simple: eliminate gluten. Such a diet is easier to prescribe than follow, however, for wheat, oats, rye, and barley are common in many foods, as Table 22–5 shows. In particular, processed foods such as ice cream, salad dressings, and canned foods often use wheat flour as an extender. People with celiac disease and their caregivers need help understanding what foods they can eat and what foods they must avoid. Be sure they understand how to read food labels.

Suggestions   Dietitians often suggest the use of corn, potato, rice, and soybean flours as substitutes for wheat flour in recipes. A low-gluten wheat starch flour is also available. People who are lactose intolerant will also need to exclude milk and milk products as discussed on pp. 115–116. A family with a member who has celiac disease needs a lot of support from the health care team. Dietitians can offer tips about support groups, books, recipes, and special food products that can help clients manage their diet restrictions.

Disorders of the Large Intestine

Diverticular disease, ulcerative colitis, and resections of the large intestine are conditions that affect the colon and have nutrition implications. In diverticular disease, described next, diet plays a role in both prevention and treatment.

DIVERTICULAR DISEASE OF THE COLON

Reminder: The outpocketings of the intestinal wall that balloon through the weakened muscles of the intestine are known as *diverticula* (the singular is *diverticulum*).

Sometimes pouches of the intestinal wall (called diverticula) bulge out through the muscles surrounding the large intestine, often at points where blood vessels enter the muscles (see Figure 4–14 on p. 128). Evidence suggests that the pouches result from high pressure in the intestinal lumen combined with weak-

Table 22–5

Gluten-Restricted Diet

Meat and Meat Alternates

Any allowed except those that are breaded, prepared with bread crumbs, or creamed.

Milk and Milk Products

Any allowed if client is not intolerant to lactose except milk mixed with Ovaltine, commercial chocolate milk with a cereal additive, pudding thickened with wheat flour, or ice cream or sherbet containing gluten stabilizers.

Fruits and Vegetables

Any allowed except those that are breaded, prepared with bread crumbs, or creamed.

Starches and Grains

Allowed: Bread, cereal, or dessert products made from cornmeal, soybean flour, rice flour, potato flour, and gluten-free starch; gluten-free macaroni and porridge; tapioca; cornmeal, cornflakes, popcorn, and hominy; rice, cream of rice, puffed rice, and rice flakes; potato chips.

Not allowed: Bread, cereal, or dessert products made from wheat, rye, oats, or barley; commercially prepared mixes for biscuits, cornbread, muffins, pancakes, buckwheat pancakes, cakes, cookies, or waffles; bran; pasta, macaroni, and noodles; malt; pretzels; wheat germ; doughnuts; ice cream cones; matzo.

Other

Not allowed: Beer; ale; certain whiskeys (Canadian rye); cereal beverages (Postum); root beer; commercial salad dressings that contain gluten stabilizers; soups containing any ingredients not allowed (such as barley or noodles).

ness of the supporting muscles in the intestinal wall. Strong intestinal contractions pinch off segments of the intestine; pressure then builds in these segments and forces parts of the intestinal membrane to balloon outward through the muscle layer. Aging and low-fiber diets (see p. 127) may increase the risk of diverticular disease.

Diverticulosis and Diverticulitis   People with diverticulosis are frequently symptom-free and unaware of the disorder. In some people, however, fecal material and bacteria get trapped in the diverticula. A localized area of inflammation and infection develops, a condition called diverticulitis. People with diverticulitis may suffer from abdominal pain, alternating periods of diarrhea and constipation, dyspepsia, flatus, abdominal distention, and fever. Occasionally, a diverticulum ruptures, causing localized or sometimes life-threatening infection (peritonitis). If the diverticula become inflamed repeatedly, the intestinal wall can thicken (fibrosis), narrowing the intestinal lumen and creating an obstruction. An inflamed bowel segment can also stick to other pelvic organs, forming a fistula.

Reminder: The term *diverticulosis* describes the condition of having diverticula. The term *diverticulitis* describes the condition when the diverticula become inflamed.

Nutrition Support   Both drugs and diet play a role in the treatment of diverticular disease. For many years, health care professionals advised low-fiber diets for people with diverticulosis in the belief that fiber tended to become trapped in the diverticula and cause irritation. This advice has changed dramatically. Now, health care professionals believe a high-fiber diet may actually reduce the incidence of diverticulosis by stimulating normal GI action and maintenance. Many people with established diverticular disease have been observed to remain symptom-free while following a high-fiber diet. They may need to avoid foods with seeds such as okra and strawberries, however; the seeds may get trapped in the diverticula and cause irritation.

A high-fiber diet includes generous servings of plant foods: grains, fruits, and vegetables, especially legumes (see Table 4–4 on p. 129). Tips for adapting to a high-fiber diet are provided on p. 128, and a sample high-fiber diet menu is shown below. The accompanying case study presents an example of diverticular disease.

People with diverticular disease benefit from high-fiber diets to help them maintain GI tract function. Although diverticular diseases do not affect the intestine's absorptive functions, ulcerative colitis and intestinal resections can have a serious impact on these functions.

ULCERATIVE COLITIS

ulcerative colitis (ko-LYE-tis): inflammation and ulceration of the colon. See also *Crohn's disease* on p. 736.

Ulcerative colitis is an inflammatory bowel disease that develops in the large intestine. It causes severe diarrhea, rectal bleeding, cramping, abdominal pain, anorexia, and weight loss. Diarrhea can be almost continuous, resulting in malabsorption and major losses of fluids and electrolytes. Anemia may develop due to bleeding and nutrient losses. For people with active ulcerative colitis who fail to respond to medical therapy, surgery to remove the colon and rectum

Sample High-Fiber Diet Menu

Menu

Breakfast	Lunch	Supper
1 c multigrain cereal	1 c black bean soup	3 oz baked fish
½ banana	3 oz broiled chicken	1 baked potato with skin
1 c nonfat milk	½ c steamed broccoli	½ c peas
½ grapefruit	½ c baked sweet potatoes	1 whole-wheat dinner roll
2 slices whole-wheat toast	1 fresh pear	2 tsp margarine
2 tbs peanut butter	1 whole-wheat dinner roll	1 piece carrot cake
1 c coffee	1 tsp margarine	1 c nonfat milk
	Iced tea	
		Snack
		3 c popcorn
		1 c tomato juice

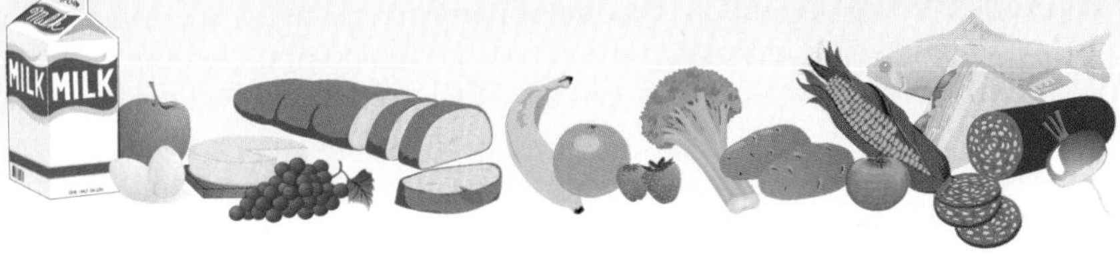

Case Study   Retired Schoolteacher with Diverticular Disease

Mr. Stavros is a 69-year-old retired school teacher. He recently told his doctor that he had been experiencing abdominal pain and fever. He also described a change in bowel function: he is frequently constipated, although he occasionally experiences diarrhea. He further complained of indigestion and a bloated feeling. Mr. Stavros was admitted to the hospital. After an examination that included X rays of the intestine, the physician made a diagnosis of diverticulitis, for which Mr. Stavros was treated. No food or drink was allowed by mouth, and a tube was inserted to suction gastric contents. An intravenous (IV) solution of fluid and electrolytes was started to prevent dehydration and maintain electrolyte balance. Antibiotics were given to treat the infection, and analgesics were given for pain and to lower Mr.

Stavros's fever. After several days, suction was discontinued, and oral intake was initiated. Once Mr. Stavros was tolerating adequate liquids orally, the IV was discontinued. He is now symptom-free and ready for discharge from the hospital.

Describe diverticular disease to Mr. Stavros. Be sure to distinguish between diverticulosis and diverticulitis. How do diverticula form, and what consequences may follow?

Are Mr. Stavros's symptoms typical of people with diverticulitis? Do all people with diverticular disease have such symptoms?

What diet would you recommend for Mr. Stavros to treat the diverticular disease? What advice can you give him about adjusting to such a diet?

(described in the next section) is often recommended. Unlike intestinal surgery for Crohn's disease, which fails to cure the disorder, removal of the colon and rectum does cure ulcerative colitis.

Nutrition Support   For people with active ulcerative colitis, no dietary interventions seem to lessen disease activity. People with severe abdominal pain and diarrhea need complete bowel rest with no enteral stimulation. Parenteral nutrition can help maintain nutrition status, especially when surgery is anticipated.[22] Meanwhile, medications can help to control disease symptoms.

Oral Diets   Many of the dietary principles outlined for Crohn's disease apply to ulcerative colitis. A primary concern is to ensure adequate intakes of fluids and electrolytes. The diet often emphasizes high-kcalorie, high-protein foods and restricts fat if the client has symptoms of fat malabsorption. Individual tolerances determine if other foods should be restricted. A low-residue or low-fiber diet is necessary for some clients: others may tolerate a regular diet. Milk and milk products may need to be eliminated if lactose intolerance is present. Supplemental vitamins and minerals may be necessary.

RESECTIONS OF THE LARGE INTESTINE

People with ulcerative colitis or cancer of the colon sometimes need surgery to remove the affected portion of the colon. Resections of the large intestine are less likely to create nutrient deficiencies than resections of the small intestine, because most nutrients are absorbed before the intestinal contents reach the colon. Fluids and electrolytes are normally reabsorbed in the colon, however, so their losses can be a problem.

 PRESCRIPTION PAD

Drugs used in the treatment of ulcerative colitis may include:

- Analgesics
- Antidiarrheals
- Anti-Infective agents
- Anti-Inflammatory agents

See Appendix E for timing with meals and nutrition-related side effects.

stoma (STOH-ma): a surgically formed opening. After an ileostomy or colostomy, a stoma is formed from the cutoff end of the intestine and brought out through the abdominal wall, rerouting the excretion of wastes.

stoma = window

In a colostomy, a segment of the colon, rectum, or both is removed. The remaining portion is then brought out through the abdominal wall via a stoma to allow for defecation (see Figure 22–6). In an ileostomy, both the entire colon and the rectum are removed, and the ileum becomes the terminal GI segment. In an alternative to an ileostomy, called the ileal pouch/anal anastomosis, the surgeon removes the diseased colon and rectal tissue and connects the ileum to the anus. Thus defecation can occur through the anus, rather than through a stoma, and a more normal bowel movement results. A temporary ileostomy is made at the time of surgery to give the intestine time to heal. After about two to three months, the ileostomy is closed.

The consistency of the stools following colostomies and ileostomies varies depending on both the length and the portion of the resected bowel. In general, ileostomies result in watery stools and colostomies in more formed stools.

Nutrition Support following Ostomies Once oral intake is permitted following surgery, people who have undergone colostomies or ileostomies often receive low-fiber, bland diets to prevent obstructions, help promote healing of

Figure 22–6

Colostomy and Ileostomy

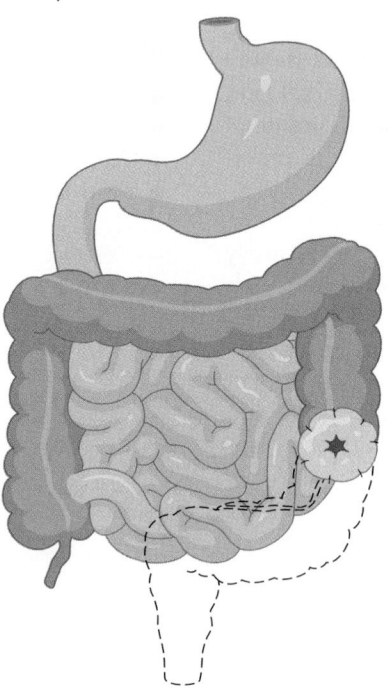

In a colostomy, the rectum and anus are removed, and the stoma is formed from the remaining colon.

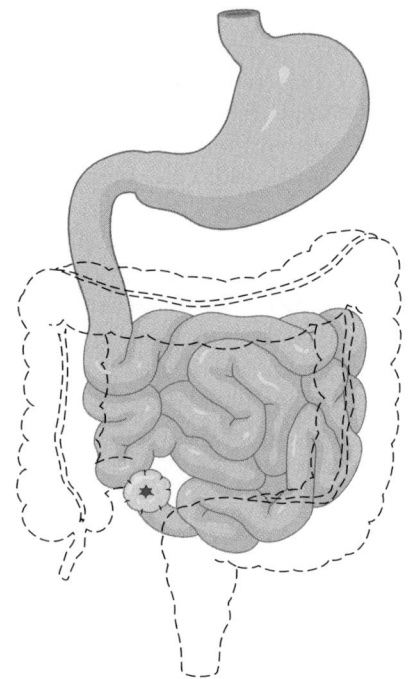

In an ileostomy, the entire colon, rectum, and anus are removed, and the stoma is formed from the ileum.

Case Study   Accountant with an Ileostomy

Tim is a 24-year-old accountant who recently developed a severe small bowel obstruction secondary to recurrent bouts of Crohn's disease. Medical and dietary management failed, and Tim underwent an ileostomy in which the ileocecal valve remained intact. Tim was malnourished on admission, and he began receiving parenteral nutrition in the immediate postoperative period. After several days, he was placed on an oral diet.

Describe the nutrients most likely to be affected by Tim's surgery.

Tim will be coping with many fears and concerns associated with his ileostomy. How can you help him make the necessary adjustments? Remember that diet is only a small part of that adjustment.

What diet will be appropriate for Tim once he has advanced to a solid diet? What advice can you give him for trying new foods, preventing obstructions, getting enough fluids, controlling diarrhea, and reducing gas and odors? How can he keep track of foods that give him problems?

the stoma, and prevent GI upsets. Encourage people to try other foods as soon as possible, however. They should add foods one at a time and in small amounts so that their effects can be assessed. If a new food presents problems, the person can try it again in a few weeks or months.

Preventing Obstructions   Some foods are more likely than others to be incompletely digested and cause obstructions for ostomates. These include stringy foods such as celery, spinach, and bean sprouts; foods with tough skins such as dried fruits, raw apples, and corn; foods with seeds; mushrooms; and nuts. Practitioners report that some of these foods can be used if the client cuts the food into small pieces and chews them thoroughly. An undigested mushroom, for example, may act as a plug and obstruct an ostomy, but it will not be a problem if it arrives in the intestine in very small pieces.

ostomate (OSS-toe-mate): a person who has a surgically formed opening from the bowel to the outside of the body, bypassing the anus. An **ileostomate** (ILL-ee-OSS-toe-mate) has an ileostomy; a **colostomate** (ko-LOSS-toe-mate) has a colostomy.

Encouraging Fluids   Ostomates need extra fluids because they are absorbing less fluid from the large intestine. They may tend to restrict their fluid intakes, however, for fear of aggravating diarrhea. Explain to ostomates that drinking fluids helps prevent constipation and dehydration, and reassure them that excess fluid taken above and beyond the amount lost through the ostomy will be absorbed by the kidneys and excreted in the urine; it will not aggravate diarrhea.

Controlling Diarrhea   Ostomates may benefit from foods that thicken the stool and help control diarrhea. These foods include applesauce, bananas, cheese, creamy peanut butter, and starchy foods such as breads, rice, and potatoes. Foods that may aggravate diarrhea include apple, grape, and prune juices; highly seasoned foods; and caffeine. The foods mentioned here are suggestions only; what works for the individual is determined by trial and error.

Reducing Gas and Odors   Ostomates are often concerned about gas and odors associated with eating certain foods. Table 22–1 provides a general list of gas-forming foods, and some ostomates identify the following as particularly bothersome: asparagus, beans, beer, broccoli, brussels sprouts, cabbage, carbon-

Nutrition Assessment Checklist
For People with Disorders of the Lower GI Tract

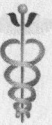

Medical   Review the client's medical record daily for test results that pinpoint the cause of diarrhea or malabsorption, improvements in the medical condition, or the development of complications (such as obstructions or fistulas) that might call for dietary adjustments. Review Table 22–4 and make note of any conditions that might affect nutrition status.

Drug   Review the client's drug therapy for possible drug-nutrient interactions. Many anti-infective agents have potential interactions. Anti-inflammatory agents may cause nausea, esophagitis, abdominal pain, fluid retention (may mask weight loss), and glucose intolerance. Laxatives may cause nausea and interfere with the absorption of fat-soluble vitamins. People taking mucolytics need adequate fluids to help liquefy thick mucous secretions.

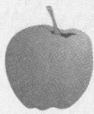

Food Intake   Determine if energy and protein intake is adequate to support a desirable weight and maintain protein status. Assess food intake to determine individual tolerances for people with diarrhea, irritable bowel syndrome, Crohn's disease, or ulcerative colitis and for people who have undergone intestinal resections. For people with steatorrhea, fat-restricted diets aim to reduce the frequency and volume of steatorrhea. Individual nutrient deficiencies accompany many of the lower GI tract disorders—assess diet and supplement intake to be sure that these needs are met.

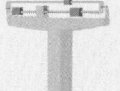

Anthropometric   Adjust diet to support growth in children and desirable weight in adults.

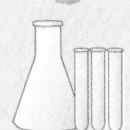

Laboratory   Monitor lab values for signs of protein malnutrition (serum albumin), dehydration (electrolytes, blood urea nitrogen, hemoglobin, and hematocrit), anemia (hemoglobin and hematocrit), and serum nutrient levels (as appropriate to the disorder). Table 22–6 shows the laboratory tests useful in detecting fat malabsorption and its severity.

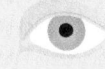

Physical   Check for physical signs of nutrient deficiencies, dehydration, and anemia; assess the client's energy level and emotional state.

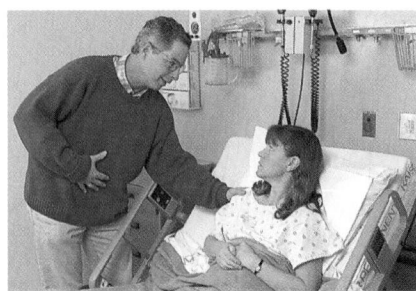

A person who has adjusted to an ostomy can greatly encourage a new ostomy client.

ated beverages, cauliflower, eggs, fish, garlic, and onions. Foods thought to reduce odors include buttermilk, cranberry juice, parsley, and yogurt.

Providing Emotional Support   Ostomates will have many adjustments to make after surgery, so emotional support is best begun before surgery occurs. Often ostomates feel they have lost control over a basic and private function.

Table 22–6

Laboratory Tests Useful in Assessing Malabsorption Syndromes

- Direct stool examinations: Stool checked for weight (greater than normal weight suggests malabsorption) and oily materials (excess fat in stool suggests steatorrhea).
- Chemical analysis of fecal fat: Fecal fat of greater than 7 g/day when the diet includes 100 g of fat/day indicates fat malabsorption.
- Serum carotene: Low serum levels accompany steatorrhea.
- Serum calcium: Low levels seen in calcium or vitamin D malabsorption. (Recall that steatorrhea can lead to calcium and vitamin D malabsorption.)
- D-xylose test: Test of carbohydrate absorption.
- Chemical analysis of fecal nitrogen: Normal fecal nitrogen is less than 2 g/day.
- Schilling test: Identifies vitamin B_{12} malabsorption.

The training required to care for the ostomy and maintain bowel function may be difficult. Ostomates may also worry that loved ones, particularly spouses, will find them unattractive. The health care team must work closely with each person and the family to help everyone make the necessary adjustments and resume normal activities.

This chapter has shown how diseases of the intestine and their treatments can seriously impair nutrition status. The nutrition assessment checklist provides guidelines for the nutrition care of people with lower GI tract disorders. Careful attention to diet and medical intervention can help people maintain their quality of life and, in some cases, recover from their diseases.

An enterostomal (en-ter-oh-STOME-al) therapist (ET) is a health care professional specially educated to assist ostomates in learning the proper methods of caring for ostomy sites and adjusting to the ostomy.

Study Questions

1. Describe the dietary treatment of diarrhea. When is diarrhea a cause for alarm?
2. What is irritable bowel syndrome, and how is diet used to control its symptoms?
3. Discuss various conditions that can lead to malabsorption. Why does fat most frequently cause problems for people with malabsorption? What roles do fat-restricted diets, low-oxalate diets, enzyme replacements, and water-miscible fat-soluble vitamins play in the treatment of fat malabsorption?
4. Recommend ways to improve acceptance of a fat-restricted diet. How should MCT be introduced into the diet?
5. How can pancreatitis lead to the malabsorption of nutrients? Contrast the dietary treatment of the person with acute pancreatitis with the dietary treatment of a person with chronic pancreatitis.
6. What are the nutrition needs of people with cystic fibrosis? How can an infant with cystic fibrosis be fed? What is the optimal diet for a child or adult with cystic fibrosis? How and why are enzyme replacements used in the treatment of cystic fibrosis?
7. What is Crohn's disease? Describe the diet therapy for a person with Crohn's disease. What special concerns arise in children with the disorder?
8. How can bacteria in the stomach or upper intestine lead to fat malabsorption? What are the other nutrition consequences of bacterial overgrowth?
9. Describe short-bowel syndrome and its effect on nutrition status. What factors affect absorption after small bowel surgery?
10. Describe the adaptive process that occurs in the remaining intestine after a portion of the intestine

is resected. What diet is most useful following intestinal resections?

11. What dietary protein and protein fraction are of particular concern in the person with celiac disease? What diet is useful in treatment? Discuss the difficulties involved in following the diet.

12. What theory explains the development of diverticula in the intestine? What dangers are associated with diverticular disease? What diet is useful for treating diverticular disease?

13. What is the recommended diet for a person with ulcerative colitis? What is the primary nutrition concern in this disorder?

14. What is an ileostomy? What is a colostomy? What diet, if any, can benefit the person who has undergone one of these procedures?

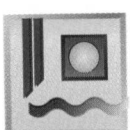 *Clinical Applications*

1. Using Table 22–3 as a guide, plan a day's menu for a diet containing 35 grams of fat. Take care to make the menu both palatable and nutritious. How can this menu be improved using the suggestions on p. 168?

2. Treatments for a disease often aim to alleviate disease symptoms rather than the disease itself. With this in mind, describe the similarities in the treatments of chronic pancreatitis and cystic fibrosis. In what ways do the treatments differ and why?

3. As stated in this chapter, treatment of celiac disease is deceptively simple—eliminate gluten. Take a trip to the grocery store and randomly select 20 to 25 of your favorite snack and convenience foods. Check the labels of these products and see if they are allowed on gluten-restricted diets. Find acceptable substitutes for the products that are not allowed. No doubt, this will be a tough assignment.

Notes

1. J. Hurst and A. L. Gallagher, Pathophysiology and nutrition management in acute pancreatitis, *Support Line*, December 1994, pp. 6–11.

2. S. Marulendra and D. F. Kirby, Nutrition support in pancreatitis, *Nutrition in Clinical Practice* 10 (1995): 45–53.

3. A.S.P.E.N. Board of Directors, Practice guidelines: Pancreatitis, *Journal of Parenteral and Enteral Nutrition* (supplement) 17 (1993): 16.

4. S. A. McClave and coauthors, Comparison of the safety of early enteral *vs* parenteral nutrition in mild acute pancreatitis, *Journal of the American Society for Parenteral and Enteral Nutrition* 21 (1997): 14–20.

5. M. R. Dambro, *Griffith's 5 Minute Clinical Consult* (Baltimore: Williams & Wilkins, 1995), pp. 278–279.

6. J. Dowsett, Nutrition in the management of cystic fibrosis, *Nutrition Reviews* 54 (1996): 31–33.

7. B. W. Ramsey and coauthors, Nutritional assessment and management in cystic fibrosis: A consensus report, *American Journal of Clinical Nutrition* 55 (1992): 108–116.

8. Ramsey and coauthors, 1992.

9. M. D. Murphy and coauthors, Resting energy expenditures measured by indirect calorimetry are higher in preadolescent children with cystic fibrosis than expenditures calculated from prediction equations, *Journal of the American Dietetic Association* 95 (1995): 30–33.

10. A. L. Rettammel and coauthors, Oral supplementation with a high-fat, high-energy product improves nutritional status and alters serum lipids in patients with cystic fibrosis, *Journal of the American Dietetic Association* 95 (1995): 454–459.

11. Ramsey and coauthors, 1992.

12. A.S.P.E.N. Board of Directors, Practice guidelines: Cystic fibrosis—pediatric, *Journal of Parenteral and Enteral Nutrition* (supplement) 17 (1993): 44.

13. Y. Kim, Can fish oil maintain Crohn's disease in remission? *Nutrition Reviews* 54 (1996): 248–257.

14. M. D. Sitrin, Nutrition support in inflammatory bowel disease, *Nutrition in Clinical Practice* 7 (1992): 53–60.

15. A.S.P.E.N. Board of Directors, Practice guidelines: Inflammatory bowel disease, *Journal of Parenteral and Enteral Nutrition* (supplement) 17 (1993): 18–19.

16. M. H. Giaffer, G. North, and C. D. Holdsworth, Controlled trial of polymeric versus elemental diet in treatment of active Crohn's disease, *Lancet* 335 (1990): 816–819; S. Klein, Elemental versus polymeric feeding in patients with Crohn's disease—Is there really a winner? *Gastroenterology* 99 (1990): 893–894; A.S.P.E.N. Board of Directors, Inflammatory bowel disease, 1993, pp. 18–19.

17. Presented by W. D. Heizer, Short bowel syndrome: Treatment strategies, *Fourth Annual Advances and Controversies in Clinical Nutrition,* sponsored by the Mayo Clinic, Jacksonville, Fla., April 18, 1994.

18. I. Nordgaard, B. S. Hansen, and P. B. Mortensen, Importance of colonic support for energy absorption as small-bowel failure proceeds, *American Journal of Clinical Nutrition* 64 (1996): 222–231.

19. T. A. Byrne and coauthors, A new treatment option for patients with short bowel syndrome: Bowel rehabilitation with growth hormone, glutamine, and a modified diet, *Support Line,* February 1996, pp. 1–7.

20. J. P. Grant, G. Chapman, and M. K. Russell, Malabsorption associated with surgical procedures and its treatment, *Nutrition in Clinical Practice* 11 (1996): 43–52.

21. Byrne and coauthors, 1996.

22. A.S.P.E.N. Board of Directors, Inflammatory bowel disease, 1993, pp. 18–19.

Promoting Intestinal Adaptation

The ability to survive a massive intestinal resection is a relatively recent medical advance spurred largely by the development of techniques for providing all needed nutrients by vein (total parenteral nutrition or TPN) and the adaptation of these techniques for use at home. Early studies report that prior to the availability of TPN, only 20 percent of people who survived the surgery itself lived for more than one year.[1] Currently, estimates suggest that most people who survive the surgery are still living after a year.[2] Without TPN, the medical team could only provide simple intravenous solutions of fluids, electrolytes, and minimal energy and hope that the person would be able to eat before malnutrition was irreversible.

As experience with TPN grew, clinicians began to recognize that although long-term TPN was a lifesaving strategy, it was accompanied by serious complications and extremely high costs. (Chapter 24 discusses these issues in more detail.) While recognizing the limitations to adaptation imposed by the extent and location of the resection, the person's age, and the health of the remaining intestine, clinicians sought ways to foster adaptation to the fullest extent possible.[3] What strategies might improve the likelihood of maintaining nutrition status with an oral diet or minimal TPN? This highlight focuses on research aimed at promoting optimal adaptation in the remaining small bowel, or bowel rehabilitation. Controversies remain, of course, partly because much of the research has been conducted on animals and partly because studies in human beings

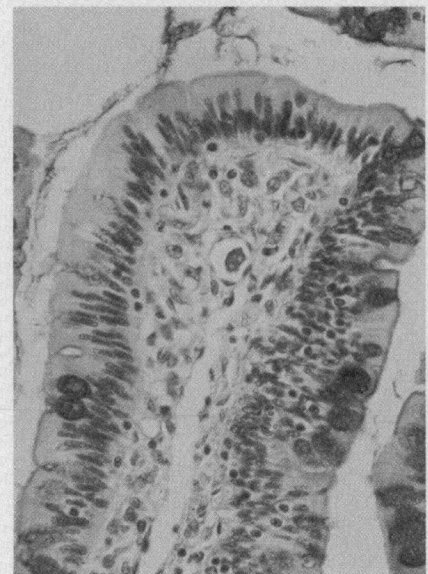

The need for intravenous feedings after extensive intestinal resections may be eliminated or reduced by taking full advantage of the remaining intestinal cells' ability to adapt.

require further elucidation and confirmation.

DIETARY FACTORS AND ADAPTATION

For some time, clinicians have accepted that intestinal adaptation can occur only when the GI tract is stimulated by enteral nutrients.[4] Animal studies further suggest that providing enteral nutrients as early as possible after an intestinal resection improves the chances that the person will be able to tolerate enteral nutrition and not be dependent on TPN.[5] Spurred by such findings, researchers and clinicians have begun to identify specific factors, including dietary components, that might optimally stimulate adaptation.

Glutamine

The amino acid glutamine is common in food and is the most abundant amino acid in the blood. Glutamine provides fuel for rapidly dividing cells and is the major fuel for the intestinal cells. After the intestinal cells have metabolized glutamine, the liver uses the end products, alanine and ammonia, to make glucose and urea, respectively. Glutamine is also important for the replication of all body cells, which use it to synthesize purines, pyrimidines, and nucleotides, as well as other amino acids.

In healthy individuals, glutamine is a nonessential amino acid. If food sources fail to meet the body's needs, the body can synthesize more glutamine from the branched-chain amino acids of skeletal muscle. Following an intestinal resection, however, the body may need more glutamine than it receives from typical nutrient sources or than it can synthesize. Under such conditions, glutamine becomes a conditionally essential amino acid.

Various animal studies show that adding glutamine to intravenous feeding solutions helps to promote adaptation following intestinal resections.[6] Animal studies further suggest that enteral, but not parenteral, glutamine facilitates glucose absorption.[7] Human studies suggest that oral glutamine raises growth hormone levels, which may further promote adaptation, as described in a later section.

Short-Chain Fatty Acids

As Chapter 22 noted, bacteria in the colon degrade dietary fibers to short-chain fatty acids. Short-chain fatty acids possess two characteristics that enhance their importance following intestinal resections. First, they stimulate intestinal cell growth, enhance intestinal blood flow, bolster secretion of pancreatic enzymes, and promote sodium and water absorption in the colon.[8] Animal studies show that short-chain fatty acids stimulate intestinal cell growth following resections, even when they are provided intravenously.[9]

Second, short-chain fatty acids provide the body with usable energy. The remarkable capacity of colonic bacteria to salvage energy following extensive small bowel resections has only recently been realized.[10]

In healthy people with full-length intestinal tracts, short-chain fatty acids normally provide about 5 to 10 percent of the total daily energy needs (about 100 to 200 kcalories per day). Following extensive small bowel resections in which the colon remains intact, however, adaptation occurs in the colon so that it assumes a greater role in providing energy. When the bacteria in the colon are confronted with more substrates in the form of dietary fiber, unabsorbed carbohydrate, and, to a lesser extent, unabsorbed protein, they step up production of short-chain fatty acids and can provide about 1000 kcalories per day of usable energy.[11] This contribution represents a substantial source of energy sorely needed by people with malabsorption.

Thus, for people whose colons remain intact following intestinal resections, providing a diet high in complex carbohydrates supports adaptation and improves energy conservation. Because the colonic bacteria cannot convert fat to short-chain fatty acids, unabsorbed fat

reaching the colon provides no additional energy and can contribute further to malabsorption as described in Chapter 22.

Researchers have also found that factors unrelated to diet can foster adaptation. Growth hormone and insulin-like growth factor-1 (IGF-1), described next, are two such factors.

HORMONES AND ADAPTATION

Research suggests that both growth hormone and IGF-1 play significant roles in promoting intestinal adaptation.[12] As its name implies, growth hormone stimulates the growth of tissues. It mediates its effects on intestinal cells through the regulation of IGF-1, which appears to directly stimulate intestinal cell growth.[13] Some studies show that IGF-1 stimulates the growth of intestinal cells to a greater degree than diet alone.[14] (Recall that oral glutamine may mediate some of its positive effects on intestinal adaptation by raising growth hormone levels.)

PRACTICAL APPLICATIONS

Following extensive small bowel resections, clinicians strive to promote maximum absorptive capacity in the remaining bowel. The most desirable outcome is for the person to be able to meet all nutrient needs orally. When that is not possible, the goal is to minimize the need for TPN, thus reducing the complications and costs associated with it.

Very impressive results have been obtained from clinical studies designed to assess the effectiveness of a combination therapy in promoting bowel rehabilitation.[15] The therapy consisted of growth hormone admin-

istration, glutamine supplementation, and a diet high in complex carbohydrates, low in fat, and supplemented with fiber. Eight clients with severe short-bowel syndrome comprised the first study group; all were believed to be dependent on TPN for life and past the period of intestinal adaptation. They were able to consume oral foods as tolerated but were unable to maintain nutrition status or adequate fluid balance without parenteral nutrition. After only three weeks of treatment, clients showed significant improvements in their energy intake and abilities to absorb protein, carbohydrates, water, and sodium.

The positive study results prompted a subsequent study of 47 clients to determine if the combination therapy could eliminate or reduce TPN requirements.[16] Again, all clients were considered to be dependent on TPN for life and past the period of intestinal adaptation. All clients received the combination therapy for a minimum of 26 days, after which time growth hormone was discontinued. Clients were discharged from the research facility and instructed to continue oral glutamine supplements and the modified diet. After about a year, 40 percent of the clients were able to maintain nutrition status with an oral diet, and another 40 percent were able to reduce their TPN requirements.

The promising results of these studies offer hope of improved treatments and outcomes for people with severe short-bowel syndrome. They also raise questions requiring further research. Would even better results occur if combination therapy was provided soon after surgery, before adaptation has occurred? Might an individual component of the combination therapy prove just as effective as all three in minimizing or reducing the need for TPN?

Medical research is a continuously evolving quest to lengthen life and improve its quality. Often research in one area overlaps with research in another. For example, severe stresses cause atrophy of the intestinal cells and significantly reduce their absorptive capacity. Factors that stimulate intestinal cell growth and adaptation for short-bowel syndrome might also help correct the intestinal atrophy that accompanies stress. Indeed, current research is examining how glutamine and growth hormone might benefit people suffering from severe stresses (Chapter 25).

NOTES

1. H. E. Haymond, Massive resection of the small intestine, *Surgery, Gynecology, and Obstetrics*, 61 (1935): 693–705.

2. G. J. Blatchford, J. S. Thompson, and L. F. Rikkers, Intestinal resection in adults: Causes and consequences, *Digestive Surgery* 6 (1989): 57–61.

3. F. Carbonnel and coauthors, The role of anatomic factors in nutritional autonomy after extensive small bowel resection, *Journal of Parenteral and Enteral Nutrition* 20 (1996): 275–280.

4. T. A. Byrne and coauthors, A new treatment option for patients with short bowel syndrome: Bowel rehabilitation with growth hormone, glutamine, and a modified diet, *Support Line*, February 1996, pp. 1–7.

5. W. D. A. Ford and coauthors, Total parenteral nutrition inhibits intestinal adaptation in young rats: Reversal by feeding, *Surgery* 96 (1983): 527–534.

6. M. C. Gouttebel and coauthors, Influence of N-acetylglutamine or glutamine infusion on plasma amino acid concentrations during the early phase of small-bowel adaptation in the dog, *Journal of Parenteral and Enteral Nutrition* 16 (1992): 117–121; H. Tamada and coauthors, Alanyl glutamine-enriched total parenteral nutrition restores intestinal adaptation after either proximal or distal massive resection in rats, *Journal of Parenteral and Enteral Nutrition* 17 (1993): 236–242.

7. A. Gardemann and coauthors, Increases in intestinal glucose absorption and hepatic glucose uptake elicited by luminal but not vascular glutamine in the jointly perfused small intestine and liver of the rat, *Biochemistry Journal* 283 (1992): 759–765.

8. M. M. Gottschlich, Selection of optimal lipid sources in enteral and parenteral nutrition, *Nutrition in Clinical Practice* 7 (1992): 152–165.

9. S. A. Kripke and coauthors, Stimulation of intestinal mucosal cell growth with intracolonic infusion of short-chain fatty acids, *Journal of Parenteral and Enteral Nutrition* 13 (1989): 109–116; M. J. Koruda and coauthors, Effect of parenteral nutrition supplemented with short-chain fatty acids on adaptation to massive small bowel resection, *Gastroenterology* 95 (1988): 715–720.

10. I. Kelberman and coauthors, Effect of fiber and its fermentation on colonic adaptation after cecal resection in the rat, *Journal of Parenteral and Enteral Nutrition* 19 (1995): 100–106; I. Nordgaard, B. S. Hansen, and P. B. Mortensen, Importance of colonic support for energy absorption as small-bowel failure proceeds, *American Journal of Clinical Nutrition* 64 (1996): 222–231.

11. Nordgaard, Hansen, and Mortensen, 1996.

12. J. A. Vanderhoof, Results of IGF-1 studies show promise in the treatment of intestinal disorders, *Journal of Parenteral and Enteral Nutrition* 20 (1996): 315–316; D. I. Shulman and coauthors, Effects of short-term growth hormone therapy in rats undergoing 75% small intestinal resection, *Journal of Pediatric Gastroenterology and Nutrition* 14 (1992): 3–11; A. B. Lemmey, IGF-1 and the truncated analogue des-(1-3) IGF-1 enhance growth in rats after gut resection, *American Journal of Physiology* 260 (1991): E213–E219.

13. T. Inaba and coauthors, Effects of growth hormone and insulin-like growth factor 1(IGF-1) treatments on nitrogen metabolism and hepatic IGF-1 messenger RNA expression in postoperative parenterally fed rats, *Journal of Parenteral and Enteral Nutrition* 20 (1996): 325–331; K. Chen and coauthors, Insulin-like growth factor-1 prevents gut atrophy and maintains intestinal integrity in septic rats, *Journal of Parenteral and Enteral Nutrition* 19 (1995): 119–124.

14. J. A. Vanderhoof and coauthors, Truncated and native insulin-like growth factors (IGF-1) treatments on the nitrogen metabolism and hepatic IGF-1–messenger RNA expression in postoperative parenterally-fed rats, *Gastroenterology* 102 (1992): 1949–1956.

15. T. A. Byrne and coauthors, Growth hormone, glutamine, and a modified diet enhance nutrient absorption in patients with short bowel syndrome, *Journal of Parenteral and Enteral Nutrition* 19 (1995): 296–302.

16. T. A. Byrne and coauthors, A new treatment for patients with short bowel syndrome: Growth hormone, glutamine and a modified diet, *Annals of Surgery* 222 (1995): 243–255.

Chapter 23

Enteral Nutrition

CONTENTS

Enteral Formulas
 Types of Formulas
 Distinguishing Characteristics
 Formula Selection
 Enteral Formulas Provided Orally
Tube Feedings
 Feeding Tube Placement
 Formula Preparation
 Formula Administration
 Drug Administration through Feeding Tubes
Addressing Tube-Feeding Complications
 *Failure to Achieve or Maintain Adequate
    Nutrition Status*
 Diarrhea
 What to Chart
From Tube Feedings to Table Foods
HIGHLIGHT: **Enteral Formulas: Who's
Minding the Market?**

MICROGRAPH: Glutamine, the amino acid that supports the health of the intestinal tract.

*t*o meet nutrient needs, a person must be able to eat, digest, and absorb nutrients in the amounts necessary to satisfy metabolic demands. Most people, whether healthy or ill, can meet these needs with conventional foods. Some illnesses, however, interfere with eating, digestion, and absorption, as Chapters 21 and 22 described. Other illnesses raise the metabolic rate to such a degree that conventional foods fail to deliver necessary nutrients. If poor appetite is the primary nutrition problem, health care professionals diligently encourage clients to eat. The accompanying box provides suggestions for helping clients to eat enough foods to meet their needs. Alternatively, liquid formulas, given orally in sufficient amounts, may help meet nutrient needs.

For clients who cannot eat or drink, it may be necessary to deliver nutrients by tube or by vein. Feedings provided either orally or by tube are *enteral* feedings, the subject of this chapter. Enteral feedings can be used whenever a client can digest and absorb nutrients via the GI tract. Otherwise, feedings are given by vein as *parenteral* feedings, the subject of the next chapter. Figure 23–1 summarizes some of the factors involved in deciding the most appropriate way to feed a client.

Enteral Formulas

enteral formulas: liquid diets intended for oral use or for tube feedings.
enteron = intestine

The number of enteral formulas on the market is staggering (several are listed in Appendix K). Most formulas are available in ready-to-use or powered form. They are designed to meet a variety of medical and nutrition needs and can be used

Figure 23–1

Selecting a Feeding Method

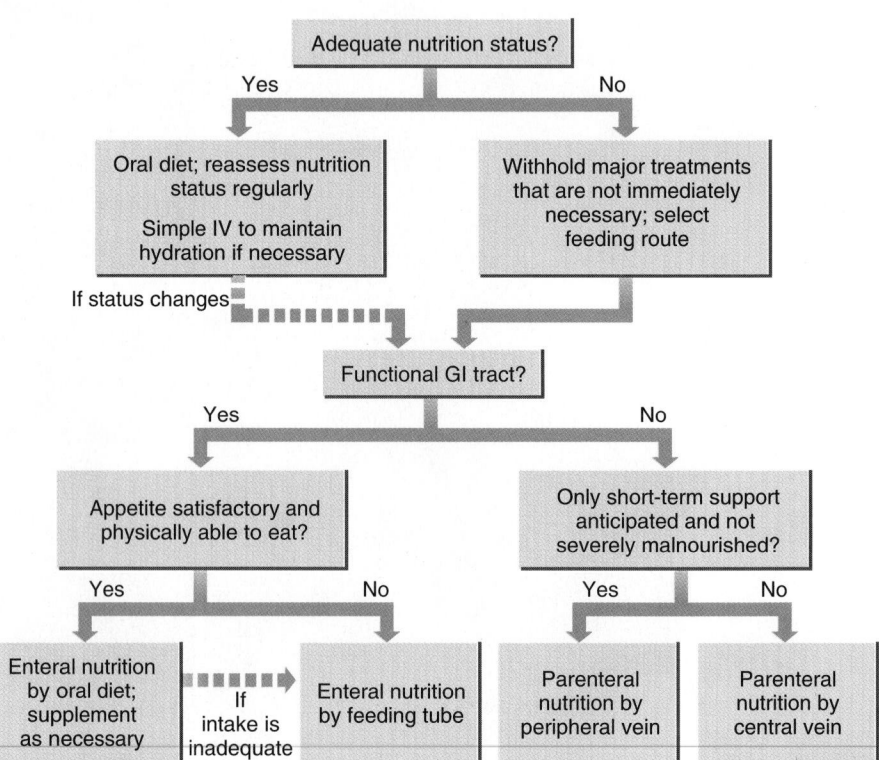

How to Help Clients Meet Nutrient Needs with Ordinary Foods

1. **Empathize.** If the person is frightened, angry, or confused, show that you care and are there to help. Imagine feeling too sick to move or too tired to sit up. Show that you understand how difficult it is to eat.

2. **Motivate.** Be sure the client understands how important nutrition is to recovery.

3. **Help clients select foods they like and mark menus appropriately.** Call the dietitian, if the client needs extra help. When appropriate and permissible, let a friend or family member bring in favorite foods from outside the hospital. This may be especially helpful for clients with strong ethnic, religious, or personal food preferences.

4. **Solve eating problems.** Encourage clients who feel full after a short time to eat the most nutritious foods first and save liquids until after meals. For clients who are weak or tired, suggest foods that require little effort to eat. Eating a roast beef sandwich, for example, requires less effort than cutting and eating a steak; drinking soup is easier than eating it with a spoon. For clients who either fill up quickly when eating or are weak or tired, smaller meals combined with snacks, such as a sandwich at bedtime and milk shakes or instant breakfast drinks between meals, can improve intake considerably.

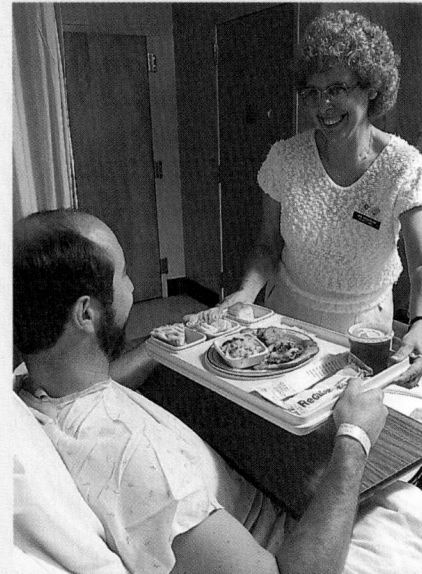

People enjoy eating when they feel comfortable and cared for.

5. **Suggest that clients add extra energy to the foods they eat** by using extra sugar or fats. Dry milk powder added to milk-based drinks, soups, and casseroles boosts nutrient intake.

6. **Help clients prepare for meals.** Encourage clients to wash their hands and faces and to brush their teeth or rinse their mouths before eating. Help them get comfortable, either in bed or in a chair. Adjust the extension table to a comfortable distance and height, and make sure it is clean. A clean, odor-free room also helps. Take these steps before the tray arrives, so the meal can be served promptly and at the right temperature.

7. **Check for accuracy and appearance.** When the food cart arrives, check the client's tray. Confirm that the client is receiving the right diet, that the foods on the tray are the ones the client marked on the menu, and that the foods look appealing. Order a new tray if foods are not appropriate.

8. **Help with eating.** Help clients who need assistance in opening containers or cutting meats and those who are unable to feed themselves.

9. **Take a positive attitude toward the hospital's food.** Never say something like "I couldn't eat this stuff either." Instead, say, "The dietary department really tries to make foods appetizing. Let me call the dietitian. I'm sure we can find a solution."

either alone or given along with foods. The client's specific nutrition needs, identified through a careful medical and nutrition assessment, guides selection of the most appropriate formula. Highlight 23 describes some of the concerns regarding appropriate marketing and use of formulas.

Whenever formula is the primary source of nutrients, complete formulas are necessary. Such is the case when a client is on a tube-feeding or an oral liquid diet for more than a few days. Complete formulas, when provided in appropriate amounts, supply all the nutrients a client needs. Complete formulas can also be (and often are) used in smaller quantities to supplement regular diets.

complete formulas: enteral formulas designed to supply all needed nutrients when given in sufficient volume.

TYPES OF FORMULAS

Formulas are classified in many ways, but for purposes of this book, it is reasonable to think of two major kinds categorized by the type of protein they supply. Standard, or intact, formulas contain complete proteins, whereas hydrolyzed formulas contain small fragments of protein, which may include free amino acids, dipeptides, and tripeptides.

standard formula: a liquid diet that contains complete molecules of proteins; also called intact or polymeric formulas.

protein isolate: a protein that has been separated from a food. Examples include casein from milk and albumin from egg.

Standard, or Intact, Formulas   Standard, or intact, formulas are appropriate for people who are able to digest and absorb nutrients without difficulty; they come as either protein isolate formulas or blenderized formulas. A protein isolate formula contains a purified protein. Blenderized formulas may contain pureed meat, vegetables, fruits, milk, and starches with vitamins and minerals added as necessary; they can be made in a blender or purchased commercially.

hydrolyzed formula: a liquid diet that contains broken-down molecules of protein, such as amino acids and short peptide chains; also called a monomeric formula.

Hydrolyzed Formulas   To simplify the body's work, a complete protein can be hydrolyzed—that is, partially broken down to yield small peptides. Alternatively, a formula can be made from free amino acids. In this text we call both types *hydrolyzed* for simplicity. Hydrolyzed formulas are often also low in fat because fat is difficult to digest and absorb. People who cannot digest or adequately absorb standard formulas may benefit from hydrolyzed formulas.

modules: formulas or foods that provide a single nutrient and are designed to be added to other formulas or foods to alter nutrient composition; they can also be combined together to create a highly individualized formula.

CAUTION: Although formulas designed to be delivered intravenously can also be delivered enterally, the reverse is not true. Enteral formulas cannot be delivered by vein without serious consequences.

Modular Formulas   Unlike complete formulas, a few formulas, called modules, provide essentially a single nutrient (protein, carbohydrate, or fat). In addition to commercial modular formulas, intravenous nutrients can serve as modules; enteral or intravenous modules can be added to enteral formula to alter its nutrient composition (for example, to add kcalories or protein). Modules can also be combined with other modules to construct individualized formulas for clients with unique nutrient needs. Designing, preparing, and delivering such a formula is a challenge that requires an in-depth knowledge of enteral nutrition and the skills of a committed nutrition support team.[1]

DISTINGUISHING CHARACTERISTICS

Formulas vary not only in the form of protein they contain but in other characteristics as well. The physician or dietitian considers these characteristics when selecting a formula for an individual client.

Nutrient Composition   The formulas available offer a wide variety of nutrient compositions. These variations allow clinicians to select formulas with particular types or proportions of nutrients to meet the needs of clients with a variety of medical conditions.

For practical purposes, 1 ml (milliliter) is equivalent to 1 cc (cubic centimeter).

Standard formulas provide about 1 kcalorie per milliliter. Formulas containing 1.5 to 2.0 kcalories per milliliter meet energy and nutrient needs in a smaller volume. One formula may provide a higher percentage of energy from fat, another from carbohydrate, and still another from protein. A person with fat malabsorption may need a formula low in fat; a person with constipation may benefit from a formula with part of the carbohydrate derived from fiber. Percentage of vitamins with minerals also vary from one formula to the next.

Formulas also derive their nutrients from different sources. One formula may derive its protein from beef. another from milk, and still another from free amino acids. Some formulas provide all of their fat from long-chain triglycerides (LCT); others provide varying amounts of medium-chain triglycerides (MCT) in addition to LCT. Sources of carbohydrate also vary; one client may benefit from a formula containing fiber, another may prefer the taste of a formula sweetened with simple sugars.[2]

Although formulas differ, many fit into general categories, and some can be used interchangeably. For example, several intact formulas provide similar amounts of kcalories, protein, carbohydrate, fat, and other nutrients. They may derive their protein from different sources, but both sources are high-quality proteins. One may provide more vitamins in a smaller volume, but that may be of little consequence to the person who is receiving a large volume of formula. In some cases, however, such differences can be significant. One client may be allergic to milk protein, for example, and another might be on a fluid-restricted diet and benefit from a formula with a high nutrient density.

Residue and Fiber   Residue and fiber contribute to fecal bulk. Low-residue formulas are well tolerated and are useful in the treatment of some GI tract disorders, following surgeries of the GI tract, and as early feedings after GI tract disuse. Since hydrolyzed formulas are almost completely absorbed, they leave little residue in the gut. Most standard formulas have a low-to-moderate residue content.

Adding fiber to a formula adds residue because dietary fibers cannot be digested by enzymes in the human digestive tract. Blenderized formulas contain fiber; other formulas may have fiber added. High-fiber formulas can cause gas and GI upsets in some clients, but help to maintain GI tract integrity in those who can tolerate them. Because formula diets are usually used for relatively short periods, determining which people might benefit from them is difficult.[3] Research suggests that fiber might most benefit people with diarrhea or constipation and those who must have tube feedings for long periods.[4] Fiber is also beneficial when it is degraded to short-chain fatty acids by bacteria in the colon (see Highlight 22). These fatty acids provide fuel to support the growth, maintenance, and repair of the intestinal lining, enabling it to adapt more readily after large portions of the small bowel have been resected.

Osmolality   Osmolality is a measure of the concentration of molecular and ionic particles in a solution. A formula that approximates the osmolality of blood serum (about 300 milliosmoles per kilogram) is referred to as an isotonic formula. A hypertonic formula has a higher osmolality than serum.

Most formulas are isotonic or only moderately hypertonic and are well tolerated by most people. When delivered directly into the intestine, however, hypertonic formulas are initially provided at a slow, even rate to improve tolerance.[5]

Cost   Costs of individual products vary greatly in different parts of the country and for different hospitals. As a general rule, however, hydrolyzed formulas and products formulated for specific disorders (renal or respiratory failure, for example) are more expensive than standard formulas.

residue: the total amount of material in the colon; it includes dietary fiber and also undigested food, intestinal secretions, bacterial cell bodies, and cells shed from the intestinal mucosa.

fiber: see pp. 108–111; the portion of the intestinal contents that remains in the colon because people don't have the enzymes to digest it—mostly plant fibers such as cellulose, lignin, and pectin.

osmolality: (OZ-mow-LAL-eh-tee): the concentration of particles in a solution, expressed as the number of milliosmoles (mOsm) per kilogram.

isotonic formula: a formula with an osmolality similar to that of blood serum (300 mOsm/kg).
  iso = the same
  ton = tension

hypertonic formula: a formula with an osmolality higher than that of blood serum.
  hyper = greater, more

FORMULA SELECTION

Choosing a formula can be a complicated process. Dietitians and physicians can use a logical approach to simplify the process (see Figure 23–2). In a nutshell, the formula that meets the client's medical and nutrient needs with the lowest risk of complications and at the lowest cost is the best choice. If no formula can be found that meets all of the client's nutrient needs, then modules can be used to construct an appropriate formula.

Digestive and Absorptive Function   Most people on tube feedings tolerate standard formulas. Hydrolyzed formulas should be reserved for people with minimal digestive and absorptive capacity. A person whose GI tract is not functioning is not a candidate for an enteral formula.

Nutrient Requirements   Nutrient requirements are estimated based on careful nutrition assessment. The client's age, medical condition, nutrition status, and metabolic rate are all important considerations in estimating nutrient requirements. If a nutrient must be restricted, a formula must be selected that delivers no more than the prescribed amount of that nutrient per day. The choice of formulas is narrowed when a person needs a low-residue or high-fiber diet.

Individual Tolerances   Food allergies or intolerances sometimes limit formula selection. Lactose-free formulas are frequently selected because temporary and permanent lactose intolerances are common problems following surgery, stress, or long periods of GI tract disuse.

For more information about lactose intolerance, see Chapter 4.

Figure 23–2

Selecting a Formula

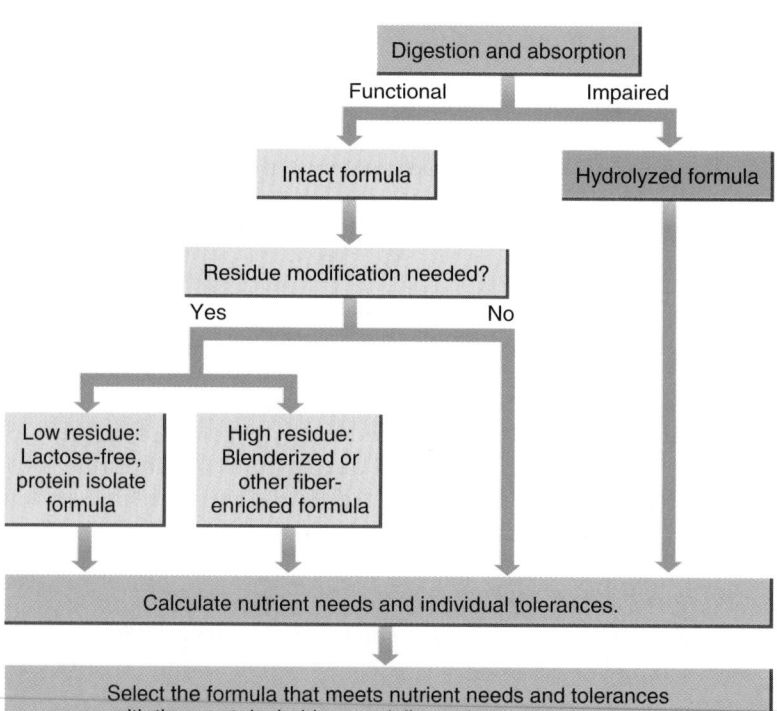

Availability   A health care facility cannot stock all of the vast number of formulas available. Instead, the nutrition support team or other qualified professionals review their client's needs and evaluate products to find the most appropriate choices. Then those formulas are kept on hand.

In the final analysis, health care professionals can only make an educated guess about the best formula for an individual. They monitor each person's nutrition status and tolerance to the formula and are prepared to make or recommend changes to help ensure that individual needs are being met.

ENTERAL FORMULAS PROVIDED ORALLY

Sometimes a formula meets nutrient needs in ways foods cannot. For people who can tolerate only liquids for long periods and for those who need hydrolyzed formulas, formulas are the major source of nutrients. If people can drink the formula, and drink enough of it, they can avoid being fed by tube.

More often, formulas are used orally to supplement a conventional diet. Some people can eat table foods, but not in sufficient quantities to meet their nutrient needs. Enteral formulas provide a reliable source of nutrients and work particularly well for adding energy and protein to the diet. Psychologically, liquids seem less filling than foods, and they are easier for debilitated, weak, or tired people to handle.

When used as an oral diet, the formula's taste must be acceptable to the individual. As a general guide, the more hydrolyzed the formula and the lower its fat content, the less tasty it will be. Remember, however, that people's likes and dislikes vary greatly, and what is unpalatable to one person might be acceptable to another. Limited evidence suggests that hydrolyzed formulas may become more acceptable over time.[6] Allowing clients to sample different flavors of formula and select the ones they like best is helpful in promoting acceptance. The box on p. 762 offers suggestions for helping clients accept oral formulas.

TUBE FEEDINGS

Tube feedings are simply complete formulas delivered by tube into the stomach or intestine. A thorough nutrition assessment provides the data needed to plan a successful tube feeding. Based on the assessment, the health care team can evaluate the client's need for a tube feeding, select the formula that will best meet the client's nutrient needs, and choose the tube and method that will deliver nutrients most effectively.

Candidates for Tube Feedings   An individual who has a functioning GI tract but is unable to ingest enough nutrients (or the appropriate type of nutrients) by mouth is a candidate for a tube feeding. Such a person may have physical problems that make chewing and swallowing difficult; have no appetite for an extended period of time; have an obstruction, fistula, or altered motility in the upper GI tract; be in a coma; have very high nutrient requirements; or be unable to ingest a hydrolyzed formula orally. Table 23–1 on p. 762 lists indications and contraindications for feeding people by tube.

Advantages of Tube Feedings   Tube feedings are always preferred to parenteral nutrition because enteral nutrition helps maintain normal gut function, causes fewer complications, and costs less than feeding by vein (see Highlight

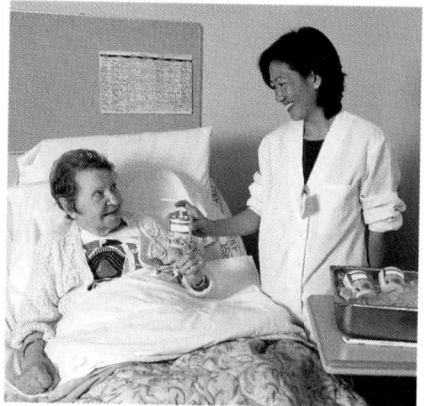

With help from caring professionals, a client can meet nutrient needs with enteral formula supplements.

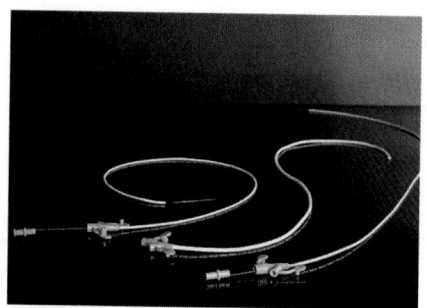

Feeding tubes provide access to the stomach and intestine for clients who cannot eat oral diets.

How to Help Clients Accept Oral Formulas

People on enteral formulas are often quite ill and frequently have poor appetites. Even when a person enjoys a formula, palatability can become a problem after a while. Hydrolyzed formulas are often less palatable than standard formulas, and clients may find them difficult to accept. Caring professionals can help by using these suggestions:

- Ask the dietitian to let the client try both different flavors and different formulas appropriate for the client's needs; use those the client likes best.

- Serve formulas attractively and remind clients to drink them. Formulas offered in a glass are more appealing than those served from a can with an unfamiliar name. Some people find the smell of formulas unappealing. Covering the top of the glass with plastic wrap or a lid, leaving just enough room for a straw, can help.

- Provide easy access. Keep the formula close to the client's bed where little effort is required to reach it, and within sight to remind the client to drink it. Clients who are very ill may lack the motivation even to reach for formula, let alone drink it. In such cases, offer the formula ready-to-drink and in small amounts frequently through the day.

- Keep formula in an ice bath, so that it will be cool and refreshing when the client drinks it.

- Ask the dietitian for help if the client stops drinking the formula after a while. The dietitian may be able to recommend different flavors or another formula to help relieve boredom.

30).[7] Enteral feedings can also stimulate intestinal adaptation following intestinal resections or following long periods of GI tract disuse. Evidence also suggests that early enteral feedings during critical illness may speed wound healing, reduce bacterial infections, and reduce the need for intensive care.[8]

FEEDING TUBE PLACEMENT

Feeding tubes are inserted into different locations along the GI tract depending on the client's medical problems and the estimated length of time that the feedings will be required. Figure 23–3 shows various tube feeding placement sites and the glossary describes various feeding tube placement sites (see p. 764).

Insertion Methods   When clients are not expected to be on tube feedings for more than about four weeks, feeding tubes are frequently inserted through the nose and passed into the stomach or intestine.[9] The client often remains fully alert during the procedure and helps pass the tube by swallowing. Health care professionals can insert a feeding tube transnasally with minimal discomfort to the client when a tube of the correct size and type is used and the client has been

For infants, feeding tubes are frequently passed from the mouth to the stomach before each feeding and removed after each feeding to allow the infant to breathe easily and reduce the risk of regurgitation.

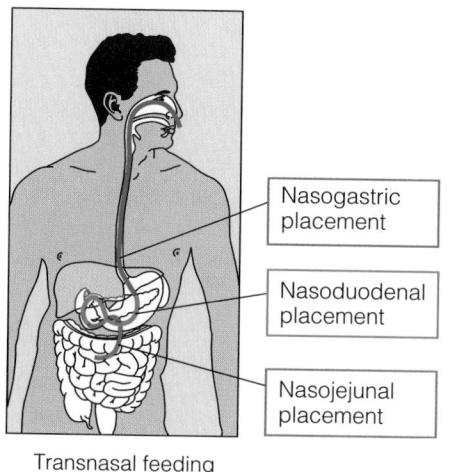

Nasogastric placement

Nasoduodenal placement

Nasojejunal placement

Transnasal feeding tube placements

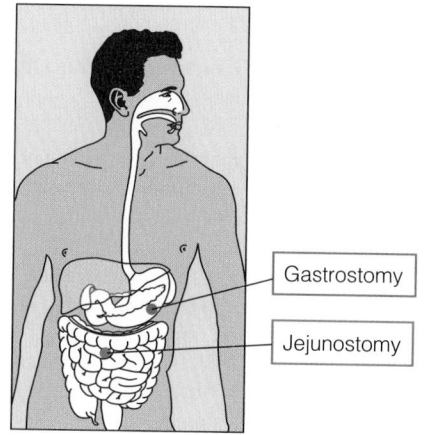

Gastrostomy

Jejunostomy

Enterostomies

Figure 23–3

Feeding Tube Placement Sites

Glossary of Feeding Tube Placement Sites

These terms are listed in order from the nose to lower organs of the digestive system.

transnasal: through the nose. A *transnasal feeding tube* is one that is inserted through the nose.

    naso = nose

nasogastric (NG): from the nose to the stomach.

nasoenteric: from the nose to the stomach or intestine. *Nasoenteric feedings* include nasogastric, nasoduodenal, and nasojejunal feedings. Most clinicians use *nasoenteric* to refer to nasoduodenal and nasojejunal feedings only.

nasoduodenal (ND): from the nose to the duodenum.

nasojejunal (NJ): from the nose to the jejunum.

orogastric: from the mouth to the stomach. This method is often used to feed infants because they breathe through their noses, and tubes inserted through the nose can hinder the infant's breathing. The tube is inserted before, and removed after, each feeding.

enterostomy (EN-ter-OSS-toe-mee): a gastric or jejunal opening made surgically or under local anesthesia through which a feeding tube can be passed.

gastrostomy (gas-TROSS-toe-mee): an opening in the stomach made surgically or under local anesthesia through which a feeding tube can be passed. The technique for creating a gastrostomy under local anesthesia is called percutaneous endoscopic gastrostomy, or PEG for short. When the feeding tube is guided from such an opening into the jejunum, the procedure is called percutaneous. endoscopic jejunostomy (PEJ), a misnomer because the enterostomy site is in the stomach.

jejunostomy (JEE-ju-NOSS-toe-mee): an opening in the jejunum made surgically or under local anesthesia through which a feeding tube can be passed. A duodenostomy (DEW-odd-eh-NOSS-toe-mee) is not used as a feeding site because the duodenum swings toward the back of the body and is not easily accessible. The technique for creating a jejunostomy under local anesthesia is called a direct endoscopic jejunostomy (DEJ). Note: Some clinicians also refer to this procedure as a PEJ, which is a more accurate use of the term than the more common use described above.

Table 23–1

Indications and Contraindications for the Use of Tube Feedings

Indications

Protein-energy malnutrition with inadequate oral nutrient intake for 5 or more days
Less than 50% of required nutrient intake orally for 7–10 days
Severe dysphasia (difficulty swallowing)
Metabolic stress
Major bowel resections (see Chapter 22) when used along with parenteral nutrition
Low-output fistulas (between the GI tract and the skin)

Contraindications

Intestinal obstruction that prohibits use of the intestine
Paralytic ileus (paralysis of the intestine)
Intractable vomiting
Peritonitis
Severe diarrhea
High-output fistulas between the GI tract and the skin
Severe acute pancreatitis

Note: In all cases, tube feedings are recommended only when the GI tract is functional.

emotionally prepared. Careful procedures must be followed to ensure that the tube is placed in the GI tract rather than in the respiratory tract. A major disadvantage of transnasal tube placement is that a client who is disoriented or uncooperative can easily pull the tube out. Furthermore, if an inappropriate tube is selected, or if feedings continue for long periods, the nasal passages and esophagus can become irritated.

When a client will be on tube feedings for a longer period, or when a feeding tube cannot be passed through the nose, esophagus, or stomach due to an obstruction or for other medical reasons, a feeding tube can be passed through an opening made into the stomach or jejunum. Enterostomies can be made either surgically or nonsurgically using local anesthesia. Surgeons who anticipate the need for a tube feeding during an earlier surgery (intestinal resections, for example) may create a gastrostomy or jejunostomy during the procedure. Gastrostomy and jejunostomy feedings offer advantages for clients receiving long-term tube feedings, because the feeding site is invisible under clothing and feeding tube irritation is eliminated. Friction from the tube and leakage of GI secretions can cause skin irritation, however. Close attention to skin care is usually effective in minimizing skin irritation.

Clinicians may use fluoroscopy, endoscopy, or laparoscopy to guide feeding tubes to their intended location or to make sure tubes have remained in their appropriate location. To help feeding tubes pass into the intestine, some clinicians also use drugs that promote gastrointestinal motility, such as metoclopramide or erythromycin. Table 23–2 on p. 765 compares some of the features of various feeding tube placement sites. The box on p. 766 suggests ways to reduce anxiety for clients beginning a tube feeding.

Table 23–2

Features of Feeding Tube Sites

Site	Insertion	Potential Irritations	Risk of Regurgitation[a]	Long-Term Tolerance	Chance of Removal by Uncooperative Client
Nasogastric	Nonsurgical	Nasal passages, esophagus	High	Fair[b]	Likely
Nasoduodenal	Nonsurgical	Nasal passages, esophagus	Moderate	Fair[b]	Likely
Nasojejunal	Nonsurgical	Nasal passages, esophagus	Low	Fair[b]	Likely
Gastrostomy	Surgery may be required	Skin	Moderate	Good	Unlikely
Jejunostomy	Surgery may be required	Skin	Low	Good	Unlikely

[a]Relative to the other feeding sites. The absolute risk of regurgitation depends on the person's medical condition.
[b]When the appropriate tube and placement site are selected.

Gastric Feedings   Using the nasogastric or gastrostomy routes allows the digestive process to begin in the stomach, just as an oral diet does. The stomach empties it contents at a controlled rate and delivers small volumes of nutrients into the intestine. Gastric feedings are not possible for people with gastric obstructions or conditions that significantly interfere with the stomach's ability to empty. A major disadvantage of gastric feedings is that some clients tend to regurgitate them. If regurgitated fluids are inhaled into the lungs, a fatal infection (aspiration pneumonia) may develop. To minimize the risk of aspiration, clinicians may prefer a nasoenteric feeding for clients with a compromised cardiac sphincter or delayed gastric emptying. Alternatively, for clients with a very high risk of aspiration, some clinicians prefer gastrostomies or jejunostomies, which allow the cardiac sphincter to remain tightly closed.

Gastric feedings are contraindicated in clients with gastric outlet obstructions.

aspiration pneumonia: an infection of the lungs caused by inhaling fluids regurgitated from the stomach. Aspiration pneumonia can be a fatal complication of a tube feeding.

Intestinal Feedings   Following severe stress (see Chapter 25), GI motility may be temporarily disrupted, but activity resumes more quickly in the small intestine than in the stomach. Thus, after severe stress, the delivery of formulas into the small intestine can be initiated earlier than gastric feedings. Intestinal feedings are also less likely to cause regurgitation of fluids. The fluids are delivered farther down the tract, and both the pyloric and cardiac sphincters are working to keep them there. The major disadvantage of intestinal feedings is loss of the controlled emptying action of the stomach. Assuring passage of the feeding tube into the appropriate location is also more difficult, and placement of the tube must be confirmed before the feeding begins. Formulas must be carefully administered to avoid diarrhea and dehydration.

The final location of the feeding tube determines the type of feeding. If a feeding tube is passed through a gastrostomy into the duodenum or jejunum, the feeding is intestinal rather than gastric.

Transnasal Feeding Tubes   Transnasal feeding tubes are soft and flexible and come in a variety of diameters and lengths. Many have characteristics that make them desirable for specific purposes. Some tubes are weighted at one end, for example, to facilitate placement and retention in the intestine, although controversies over the value of such tubes abound.

How to Help Clients Cope with Tube Feedings

The thought of being "force-fed" is frightening to many people. One person may envision a large feeding tube and fear that the procedure will be extremely painful. Another may have heard about tube feedings only from the popular press and associate them with irreversible comas. All clients benefit when they understand the insertion procedure, the expected duration of the tube feeding, and the strategic role that nutrition plays in recovery from disease. These pointers can help health care professionals prepare clients for transnasal tube feedings:

- Allow clients to see and touch the feeding tube. Seeing first hand that the tube is soft and narrow (only about half the diameter of a pencil) often alleviates anxiety. Show clients how the feeding apparatus is attached to the feeding tube and explain how the feeding will work. Use dolls or stuffed toys to demonstrate tube insertion and feeding procedures to a young child.

- Explain that the client remains fully alert during the procedure and helps pass the tube by swallowing. A numbing solution sprayed on the back of the throat minimizes discomfort and prevents gagging during the procedure.

- Tell the client that once the tube has been inserted, most people become accustomed to its presence within a few hours. In most cases, the client can easily swallow foods and liquids with the tube in place. If permitted, favorite foods or beverages can still be enjoyed.

- Assure the client that the tube feeding will be temporary, if such assurance is appropriate.

Although tube feeding may be frightening for some, for others, it is a relief. People who understand that they should eat, but can't, may be relieved to receive sound nutrition without any effort. As they feel better and begin to eat again, the tube feeding can often be reduced or discontinued.

Some people feel a loss of control over their lives; others feel self-conscious about how the feeding tube looks or awkward about moving around with the equipment. A few simple measures can help:

- Involve older children, teens, and adults in the decision-making and care process whenever possible. Clients can help arrange daily feeding schedules, and some can also perform many of the feeding procedures themselves.

- Show clients how to manipulate the feeding equipment so that they can get out of bed and move around.

- Recommend that clients walk around and socialize with other clients, if permissible.

- Recommend that clients maintain contact with friends and keep busy with hobbies and activities they enjoy. This measure is especially important for children, teens, and for those on long-term feedings.

- For infants and children, keep the developmental age of the child in mind and work with parents to ensure that appropriate feeding skills are mastered (see Highlight 21). For infants, providing a pacifier during feedings helps maintain the associations between sucking, swallowing, eating, and fullness. When possible, some of the tube-feeding formula may be provided by bottle or by spoon to further develop skills.

The more complex the procedure that a health care professional is responsible for, the easier it becomes to focus on the procedure and forget about the client's emotions. No matter how many technicalities you have to keep in mind, remember to stay focused on the person receiving your care.

The inner open space of a tube or hollow organ (such as the intestine) is called the lumen.

Which feeding tube is appropriate depends on the client's age, how the tube will be placed (for example, nasogastric or gastrostomy), where it will be placed (stomach or intestine), and its inner diameter. Once the appropriate length is selected, the smallest tube through which the formula will flow without clogging is best. Unclogging a tube is a difficult procedure that interrupts the feeding schedule and is frequently unsuccessful.[10] Insertion of a new tube can cause undue stress and anxiety.

Following selection of a feeding site, formula, and tube for a feeding, attention turns to preparing and administering the formula. Thereafter, faithful and frequent monitoring helps ensure success.

FORMULA PREPARATION

Most individuals beginning a tube feeding are seriously ill or malnourished. Many risk developing infections; people with suppressed immune systems are particularly vulnerable to infection from food-borne illness.[11] Unfortunately, bacterial contamination of formulas is commonly reported, opening the way for more serious illness. To prevent contamination, all personnel involved in preparing or delivering formulas should handle them only in clean environments, using clean equipment and clean hands.

At the Preparation Site   Formulas that must be mixed or diluted are most often prepared and packaged in the dietary department or pharmacy. Once a formula has been mixed or diluted, the container is labeled with the client's name, room, date, and time of preparation and sent to the nursing station. Ready-to-use cans of formulas are often sent unopened to the nursing station; they, too, should be labeled with the client's name and room number.

At the Nursing Station   Once a formula reaches the nursing station, the nursing staff assumes responsibility for its safe handling. The following steps reduce the likelihood of formula contamination:

- Before opening a can of formula, carefully clean the lid. If you do not use the entire can at one feeding, label the can with the time it was opened.
- Cover opened cans. Store mixed or diluted formulas in clean, closed containers. Refrigerate the unused portion of formula promptly.
- Discard unlabeled or improperly labeled containers and all opened containers of formula not used within 24 hours.

At Bedside   Prevent the risk of bacterial contamination by following these procedures:

- Before adding formula to the feeding bag or bottle, rinse the feeding container and the attached tubing with water and allow them to air dry. Never add fresh formula to formula still in the container.
- Flush the feeding tube with water before and after each use.
- Change the feeding bag or bottle and the attached tubing (except the feeding tube itself) every 12 to 24 hours.

Tube feedings sometimes come prepackaged in closed containers that can be connected directly to the feeding tube without having to be transferred to another feeding container. Such systems save nursing time and significantly reduce the risk of bacterial contamination.

FORMULA ADMINISTRATION

Recommended formula administration schedules vary between institutions, and many protocols are based on clinical judgment rather than research. Most people can receive undiluted formula (either isotonic or hypertonic) at the start of a

As an example of volume progression for a tube feeding, start the feeding at 50 ml/hour at full strength and then progress as follows:

- After 6 hours: 75 ml/hour.
- After 12 hours: 100 ml/hour.
- After 18 hours: 125 ml/hour.

A can of ready-to-feed formula typically contains 240 ml of formula, and feedings are often divided so that one can of formula can be given at each feeding.

Delivery of no more than 250 ml of formula over 30 minutes is sometimes called an intermittent feeding.

Delivery of about 300 to 400 ml of formula over 10 minutes or less is called a bolus feeding.

gastric residual: the volume of formula that remains in the stomach from a previous feeding. It is measured by gently withdrawing the gastric contents through the feeding tube using a syringe. If the measured gastric residual is acceptable, the residual is returned to the client through the feeding tube.

feeding.[12] People under severe stress, those who have not eaten for several weeks, or those receiving intestinal feedings, however, may not be able to tolerate large volumes of hypertonic formulas initially. In such cases, formulas may need to be given slowly at first, at about 25 to 50 milliliters per hour. If the person tolerates the formula, the rate can be increased by about 25 milliliters per hour every 4 to 12 hours (see the margin note), depending on the location of the feeding tube (gastric, duodenal, or jejunal) as well as the person's medical condition. If the new rate is not tolerated, back up and proceed more slowly, giving the person more time to adapt. In a few cases, formulas may need to be diluted at first, the strength increased gradually, and then the rate advanced.

For infants, the formula's concentration, infusion rate, and volume must be changed one by one and in small increments. Infants' stomachs are very small, their rate of gastric emptying is slow, and their immature GI tracts are highly sensitive to even minor changes in formula composition.

Delivery Techniques   When people are receiving formula, they should not be lying flat; the risk of aspiration is too great. Instead, elevate the client's upper body to at least a 30-degree angle during, and for at least 30 minutes after, a feeding, whenever possible.

A day's volume of formula can be given either intermittently or continuously over a period of 8 to 24 hours. Each method has its specific uses, advantages, and disadvantages.

Intermittent Feedings   Intermittent feedings are best tolerated when they are delivered into the stomach and no more than 250 to 400 milliliters is given in 20 to 30 minutes using the gravity drip method or an infusion pump. The larger the volume of formula required to meet nutrient needs, the more frequently feedings are delivered. (People who have very high nutrient needs benefit from either high–nutrient density formulas or large volumes of formula delivered continuously.) Rapid delivery (in 10 minutes or less) of a large volume of formula (300 to 400 milliliters)—called a bolus feeding—often leads to complaints of abdominal discomfort, nausea, fullness, and cramping. This makes sense. After all, people do not gobble down a meal in just a few minutes, especially when they are not feeling well.

Nurses measure gastric residuals to ensure that the stomach is emptying properly and to prevent nausea, vomiting, and possible aspiration of formula into the lungs. For intermittent feedings, the gastric residual is measured before each feeding and should not exceed 100 milliliters. If the residual is excessive, the feeding is withheld for about an hour, and then the residual is rechecked. If excessive residuals persist, the physician may withhold the feeding, reduce the rate of administration, or begin drug therapy to stimulate gastric emptying.

Intermittent feedings work well for clients able to tolerate them. Often clients gradually adapt to larger volumes of formula given over shorter periods of time. Such feedings mimic the usual pattern of eating and allow clients freedom of movement between meals. They also require less time, making them less costly and easier for people to use at home.

Continuous Feedings   Continuous feedings are delivered slowly and in constant amounts over a period of 8 to 24 hours. Such feedings benefit people who

How to Plan a Tube-Feeding Schedule

After selecting a formula that meets the client's medical and nutrient needs, the planner, usually a dietitian, determines the volume of formula per day that meets those needs. Consider a client who needs 2000 milliliters of formula per day. If the client is to receive the formula intermittently six times a day, he needs about 330 milliliters of formula at each feeding (2000 ml ÷ 6 feedings = 333 ml/feeding). Alternatively, if he is to receive the same volume of formula eight times a day, then he needs 250 milliliters (or about one can of ready-to-feed formula) at each feeding (2000 ml ÷ 8 feedings = 250 ml/feeding). He will probably tolerate this volume of formula best if it is given to him over 20 to 30 minutes at each feeding. If the client is to receive the formula continuously over 24 hours, he needs 85 milliliters of formula each hour (2000 ml ÷ 24 hr = 83 ml/hr).

have received no food through the GI tract for a long time, those who are hypermetabolic, and those receiving intestinal feedings. Infusion pumps help ensure accurate and constant flow rates. Gastric residuals for people receiving continuous feedings are measured every 4 to 6 hours and should not exceed the volume of formula infused during the preceding 2 hours. The accompanying box explains several ways to schedule tube feedings.

Supplemental Water   In addition to the formula itself, water can also be provided through the feeding tube. Using water to flush the feeding tube before and after a feeding or when the feeding apparatus is being changed helps prevent clogged feeding tubes and keeps the client hydrated. (Water can also be given orally if the person can drink it.) Supplemental water is often needed to meet the client's daily fluid requirements. As a guideline, adults require about 2000 milliliters (approximately 2 quarts) of water daily. Fever, excessive sweating, severe vomiting, diarrhea, blood loss, and burns raise water requirements. In kidney, liver, and heart diseases, water may need to be restricted.

Attention to indicators of body water balance can help determine how much additional water an individual needs. In alert adults, thirst is a good indicator of water needs; a person complaining of thirst generally needs water. In the elderly, however, thirst may be slow to develop in response to dehydration. Other clues to dehydration include unexplained weight loss, high serum electrolytes or hematocrit, and low blood pressure.

CAUTION: Young children may be attracted to the bright lights, interesting sounds, and many controls of an infusion pump. Keep infusion pumps at a safe distance to prevent children from changing the flow rate or toppling the infusion pump or intravenous pole and possibly injuring themselves or damaging the pump.

Formulas themselves contain considerable amounts of water. A standard formula (1.0 kcal/ml) contains about 850 ml of water per liter of formula. Higher-kcalorie formulas contain less water: formulas that contain 1.5 kcal/ml or 2.0 kcal/ml provide about 775 ml and 600 ml of water per liter of formula, respectively.

CAUTION: Fluid needs must be carefully monitored in infants, the elderly, and people who are unconscious.

DRUG ADMINISTRATION THROUGH FEEDING TUBES

Clients receiving tube feedings are usually quite ill and are also likely to be receiving numerous medications. Often these medications are delivered through feeding tubes, and in some cases, complications can occur.

Keep in mind that enteral formulas can interact with drugs in the same ways that foods can. The health care team must consider the effects of drug therapy on nutrient requirements, the effects of the formula on drug absorption, the effects of drugs on formulas, and the prevention of tube-feeding complications.

Drug Forms   A drug may come in any of several forms including tablet, liquid, injectable, and intravenous. People on tube feedings have functioning GI tracts, and oral drugs are less costly and easier to deliver than injectable or intravenous forms. Thus clinicians often prefer to use oral drugs for clients on tube feedings. The following guidelines may be helpful in preventing drug-drug interactions, drug-formula interactions, or clogged feeding tubes when drugs are delivered through feeding tubes:

- Give the medication orally whenever possible.
- Do not mix medications together or mix medications with the formula. Instead, stop the feeding temporarily and give each drug individually. Flush the feeding tube with warm water before and after administering each drug.
- Deliver liquid drugs through the tube using a syringe, if possible. If liquid medications are thick or sticky, dilute them with water first.
- Consider using the injectable or intravenous form if the drug is not available in liquid form. Ideally, tablets should not be crushed and administered through feeding tubes. If using tablets is unavoidable, crush the tablets to a *fine* powder and mix them with water before administering them. Do not crush tablets or capsules intended to release their contents slowly; in these cases, another drug form must be given.
- Avoid drugs known to be incompatible with formulas, such as those listed in Table 23–3.

Additional Considerations   The location of the feeding tube (whether gastric or intestinal) is also relevant to drug administration. Some drugs are designed to dissolve in the stomach's acidic environment. Such drugs may not be readily

Table 23–3

Selected Drugs That Are Incompatible with Some Formulas

Aluminum hydroxide	MCT oil
Chlorpromazine concentrate	Mellaril concentrate
Cibalith-S syrup	Mellaril oral solution
Cimetidine	Paregoric elixir
Dimetane elixir	Potassium chloride
Dimetapp elixir	Reglan syrup
Feosol elixir	Riopan
Fleet's phosphosoda	Robitussin expectorant
Gevrabon liquid	Sudafed syrup
Klorvess syrup	Throazine concentrate
Mandelamine Forte suspension	Zinc sulfate capsules

Note: These substances may be compatible with some formulas and not others.

Sources: P. E. Burns, L. McCall, and R. Wirsching. Physical compatibility of enteral formulas with various common medications, *Journal of the American Dietetic Association* 88 (1988): 1094–1096; A. J. Cutle, E. Altman, and L. Lenkel, Compatibility of enteral products with commonly employed drug additives, *Journal of Parenteral and Enteral Nutrition* 7 (1983): 186–191; Z. M. Pronsky, *Food-Medication Interactions*, 9th ed. (Pottstown, Pa.: Food-Medication Interactions, 1995).

absorbed if delivered directly to the duodenum or jejunum. Similarly, a drug that is optimally absorbed in the duodenum may be poorly absorbed in the jejunum. In such cases, oral, intravenous, or injectable forms of the drug should be used.

In some cases, formulas alter drug absorption. One example is phenytoin, a drug used to control seizures. Absorption of phenytoin may be markedly reduced for a person who is on continuous tube feedings. Although opinions of the best way to handle this problem differ, clinicians often suggest that for most clients on either intermittent or continuous feedings, the feeding should be stopped for 2 hours before and 2 hours after giving phenytoin.[13] For clients requiring continuous feedings, the rate of delivery is increased during the times the feeding is given to ensure that nutrient needs are met.

Some clients have a specific type of feeding jejunostomy called a *needle catheter jejunostomy* through which phenytoin cannot be delivered. In such cases, phenytoin is given intravenously.

To sum up, enteral formulas may be used whenever a client can digest and absorb nutrients via the GI tract, but cannot eat enough food to meet nutrient needs. Among the choices are standard formulas, which contain complete proteins, and hydrolyzed formulas, which contain free amino acids, dipeptides, and tripeptides. Complete formulas may be used to supply all the nutrients a person needs; alternatively, modular formulas, which supply individual nutrients, may be used to construct or supplement formulas as needed. Each type of formula has distinguishing characteristics that influence the formula selection (see Figure 23–2). When giving formulas by mouth, clinicians can improve palatability by adding flavors and serving them cold and attractively. When giving formulas by tube, attention must be given to the appropriate preparation of the formula, selection of the tube, delivery schedule, and administration of medications.

Addressing Tube-Feeding Complications

When formulas are correctly selected, prepared, and administered, and problems are promptly identified and corrected, chances are good that the formulas will successfully support nutritional health. Table 23–4 on p. 772 provides a monitoring schedule that helps detect problems before they become serious.

Mechanical problems, such as a clogged feeding tube, a malfunctioning feeding pump, or a tube that has become dislodged from its appropriate location, can interrupt the feeding schedule and prevent the delivery of nutrients. Complications related to the formula or its administration can result in such GI complaints as nausea, vomiting, diarrhea, cramps, constipation, delayed gastric emptying, and abdominal distention. Metabolic complications such as dehydration, electrolyte imbalance, and elevated blood glucose can also occur. Table 23–5 on p. 773 summarizes problems associated with tube feedings, their causes, and ways to prevent them. These complications have been discussed in appropriate sections throughout this chapter, but two of them deserve further attention here: failure to achieve or maintain adequate nutrition status and diarrhea.

FAILURE TO ACHIEVE OR MAINTAIN ADEQUATE NUTRITION STATUS

Sometimes a client does not respond to a tube feeding as expected. If the client continues to lose weight, for example, health care professionals must find out why. Perhaps they have underestimated energy and nutrient requirements.

Table 23–4

Checklist for Monitoring Clients Recently Placed on Tube Feedings

Before starting a new feeding:	Complete a nutrition assessment.
	Check tube placement.
Before each intermittent feeding:	Check gastric residual.
Every half hour:	Check gravity drip rate, when applicable.
Every hour:	Check pump drip rate, when applicable.
Every 4 hours:	Check vital signs, including blood pressure, temperature, pulse, and respiration.
Every 6 hours:	Check blood glucose; monitoring blood glucose can be discontinued after 48 hours if test results are consistently negative in a nondiabetic client.
Every 4 to 6 hours of continuous feeding:	Check gastric residual.
Every 8 hours:	Check intake and output.
	Check specific gravity of urine.
	Check tube placement.
	Chart client's total intake of, acceptance of, and tolerance to tube feeding.
Every day:	Weigh client.
	Check electrolytes and blood urea nitrogen until stabilized.
	Clean feeding equipment.
Every 7 to 10 days	Check all laboratory findings.
	Reassess nutrition status.
As needed:	Observe client for any undesirable responses to tube feeding; for example, delayed gastric emptying, nausea, vomiting, or diarrhea
	Check nitrogen balance.
	Check laboratory data.
	Chart significant details.

Remember that even the best calculations for determining energy and protein needs are only estimates. One study of people in a nursing home who were being tube fed found that those who developed pressure sores were malnourished, even though they were receiving formulas that were high in energy and protein.[14]

Inappropriate formula selection may explain failure to reach nutrition goals. If a formula is prescribed without calculating its nutrient composition, the formula may not be meeting all of the client's nutrient needs. The selected formula may need to be changed; a client with fat malabsorption, for example, may need a lower-fat formula, additional calcium, or extra fat-soluble vitamins.

Table 23–5

Causes and Prevention or Correction of Tube-Feeding Complications

Complications	Possible Causes	Preventive/Corrective Measures
Aspiration pneumonia	Compromised gastroesophageal sphincter, delayed gastric emptying, gastric obstruction	Use nasoenteric, gastrostomy, or jejunostomy feedings in high-risk clients; use small-diameter transnasal tube; elevate head of bed during and 30 minutes after feeding; use continuous drip method of delivery; check gastric residual.
Clogged feeding tube	Formula too thick for tube	Select appropriate tube size; dilute formula with water; flush tubing with water before and after giving formula.
	Medications	Use oral, liquid, or injectable drugs whenever possible; dilute thick or sticky liquid drugs with water before administering; crush tablets to a fine powder and mix with water; flush tubing with water before and after drugs are given; give drugs individually; do not mix drugs with formula.
Constipation	Low-fiber formula	Provide additional fluids; use high-fiber formula.
	Lack of exercise	Encourage walking and other activities, if appropriate.
	Drug therapy	Change drug therapy if possible; give laxatives or enemas if indicated.
Dehydration and electrolyte imbalance[a]	Excessive diarrhea	See items under *Diarrhea.*
	Inadequate fluid intake	Provide additional fluid.
	Carbohydrate intolerance	Use continuous drip administration of formula; monitor blood glucose; consider administering insulin; change amount or type of carbohydrate.
	Excessive protein intake	Monitor blood electrolyte levels; reduce protein intake.
Diarrhea, cramps, distention	Bacterial contamination	Use fresh formula every 24 hours; store opened or mixed formula in a refrigerator; rinse feeding bag and tubing before adding fresh formula; change feeding bag every 24 hours; prepare formula with clean hands using clean equipment in a clean environment.
	Lactose intolerance	Use lactose-free formula in lactose-intolerant and high-risk clients.
	Hypertonic formula	Use a small volume of formula and increase volume gradually; dilute formula; use isotonic formula.
	Rapid formula administration	Slow administration rate or use continuous drip feedings.
	Malnutrition/low serum albumin	Use a small volume of dilute formula and increase volume and concentration gradually.
	Drug therapy	Use antidiarrheal agents; change drug, drug form, or dosage; if possible.
Hyperglycemia	Primary medical condition	Treat disorder.
	Diabetes, hypermetabolism, drug therapy	Check blood glucose; slow administration rate; provide adequate fluids; limit type or amount of carbohydrate; consider administering insulin.
Nausea and vomiting	Obstruction	Discontinue tube feeding.
	Delayed gastric emptying	Check gastric residual; slow administration rate, use continuous drip feedings, or discontinue tube feeding.
	Intolerance to concentration or volume of formula	Use small volume of dilute formula and increase volume and concentration gradually; use continuous drip feedings.
	Drug therapy	Change drug, drug form, or dosage if possible; use antinausea and antiemetic drugs.
	Psychological reaction to tube feeding	Address client's concerns.
Skin irritation at enterostomy site	Leakage of GI secretions and friction caused by the tube	Keep site clean; inspect area for redness, tenderness, and drainage; use protective skin cream.

Note: Many of the complications presented here can be caused by the client's primary disorder rather than the tube feeding itself. In such a case, the corrective measure would include treatment of the disorder. Additionally, many of the corrective measures require a physician's order.
[a]This cluster of symptoms is sometimes called the tube-feeding syndrome. Imbalances of any electrolytes are possible, and corrective measures would vary.

It is also possible that the formula is not being delivered as intended. Sometimes feedings are withheld to perform medical procedures or to deal with complications; gastric retention of formula, inadvertent removal of the feeding tube, GI intolerances, or difficulty in positioning or retaining the tube in the appropriate feeding site (duodenum, jejunum) can all necessitate stopping the feeding. Whenever a client fails to achieve or maintain adequate nutrition status while on a tube feeding, the health care team should investigate the causes. Some questions to answer include:

- Is the client receiving the prescribed formula?
- Is the client receiving the amount of formula that has been ordered? If not, why not? When changing the feeding bag or adding fresh formula to a bag that has been rinsed with water, check and record the amount of formula left from the previous feeding.
- Is the formula being delivered at the correct flow rate? If a pump is being used, is it working correctly?
- If the formula is being delivered as prescribed, has the nutrient content of the formula been calculated to ensure that it meets the client's needs?
- Have the client's nutrient needs changed, or have they been incorrectly estimated?

Be alert to signs that the tube feeding is not being delivered as ordered so that problems can be corrected early and nutrient needs met.

DIARRHEA

Diarrhea is a commonly cited and troublesome complication associated with tube feedings. Its actual incidence and significance are difficult to determine, because diarrhea in tube-fed clients has not been clearly defined.[15] Traditionally, the enteral formula was blamed for diarrhea. It now seems clear, however, that diarrhea may often be related to the client's illness or its treatments.[16] Drug therapy is frequently the culprit. Liquid drugs (frequently used to deliver medications through feeding tubes) often contain sorbitol, a sugar alcohol that causes diarrhea when given in large doses. This scenario is particularly likely when an adult receives a liquid pediatric preparation in high doses. When drugs cause diarrhea, the client's medications must be carefully reviewed, and corrective steps taken, if possible. In some cases, a substitute drug with similar pharmaceutical action, but without the side effects, can be used to reduce GI problems. In other cases, giving the drug more frequently in smaller doses may be effective. Oftentimes, antidiarrheal agents are prescribed.

For more information about lactose intolerance, see Chapter 4.

Other reasons for diarrhea include bacterial contamination of the formula, lactose intolerance, rapid delivery of the formula, use of nutrient- or kcalorie-dense formulas, or use of high-fat formulas. Following the suggestions provided earlier (see p. 767) can reduce the risk of formula contamination. Carefully selecting formula suitable to the client's needs and delivering it appropriately can minimize diarrhea as well.

WHAT TO CHART

Chapter 17 emphasized the importance of the medical record as a communication tool. The health care team should document tube-feeding information in each client's medical record, including:

- Education of the client regarding the tube-feeding procedures.
- Type of feeding tube.
- Tube placement.
- Client's response to tube insertion.
- Administration schedule (concentration and rate).
- Method of delivery (intermittent or continuous, gravity drip or infusion pump).
- Client's tolerance to tube feeding (note any complications and any corrective actions taken).
- Client's emotional and physical responses to tube feeding.
- Reasons that a tube feeding was interrupted or could not be delivered as ordered, if necessary.
- Drugs, drug form, and problems noted when drugs are delivered through feeding tubes.

The dietitian records the client's estimated nutrient needs, the selected formula's name, and its nutrient composition. If a person on a tube feeding does not seem to be responding adequately, investigate to see if the feeding has been delivered as intended. Be sure to correct any problems early.

To review, problems with tube feedings can usually be detected and alleviated by monitoring clients regularly and taking corrective measures promptly (see Tables 23–4 and 23–5). Careful charting also helps to identify and correct problems early. The checklist on p. 776 reviews key points for assessing nutrition status in people receiving tube feedings.

From Tube Feedings to Table Foods

Once the problem causing the need for a tube feeding resolves, the client can gradually shift to an oral diet as the volume of formula is tapered off. The client should be eating adequate amounts of foods by mouth before the tube feeding is discontinued. In many cases, the person can drink the same formula that was earlier given by tube. Some people cannot make the transition to oral intake for medical reasons and go home on tube feedings. Chapter 24 discusses specialized nutrition support at home. The case study on p. 777 reviews the many factors involved in tube feedings.

Tube feeding is a practical solution to feeding the person who is unable to consume adequate nutrients by mouth. A person without a functional GI tract cannot benefit from a tube feeding, however. In such a case, intravenous nutrition (the subject of the next chapter) can be a life-saving treatment option.

Nutrition Assessment Checklist
For People Receiving Tube Feedings

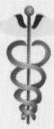

Medical   Review the client's medical record for the information necessary to select the appropriate feeding site (gastric versus intestinal), insertion procedure (transnasal or enterostomy), and formula. The development of undesirable symptoms associated with the client's medical condition, therapy (especially drug), or formula selection requires prompt intervention.

Drug   Review the client's drug therapy for possible drug-nutrient interactions and GI side effects that may affect the client's tolerance for the tube feeding. If the feeding tube is used to deliver drugs, follow the precautions on pp. 769–771.

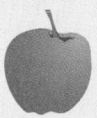

Nutrient Intake   Ensure that formula is being delivered as prescribed, and take corrective actions as needed (see p. 774). For clients beginning to eat, determine the degree to which nutrient needs are being met by table foods or formula taken orally, and reduce the volume of the tube feeding accordingly.

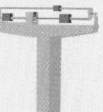

Anthropometric   Assess the client's weight daily to make sure that the client is meeting nutrition goals.

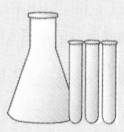

Laboratory   Monitor serum and urine lab values for signs of fluid and electrolyte imbalances and glucose intolerance. Check serum protein levels to ensure that they are improving or being maintained. When available, assess nitrogen balance to determine if the tube feeding is meeting the client's protein needs.

Physical   Check gastric residual for signs of delayed gastric emptying to prevent GI complications and reduce the risk of aspiration. Check tube placement and gravity drip rate or infusion pump drip rate as needed (see Table 23–4). Assess blood pressure, temperature, pulse, and respiration every 4 hours. Look for physical signs of malnutrition or dehydration.

Case Study   Graphics Designer Requiring Enteral Nutrition

Mrs. Innis is a 24-year-old graphics designer who suffered multiple fractures when she fell from a cliff while hiking. She has been in the hospital for seven days and has no appetite. Mrs. Innis has lost 8 pounds over the course of her hospitalization. Due to the nature of her injuries, Mrs. Innis is in traction and is immobile, although the head of her bed can be elevated to 30 degrees. From the history, the dietitian determined that Mrs. Innis's nutrition status was adequate prior to hospitalization. The health care team agrees that a nasoduodenal tube feeding should be instituted before nutrition status deteriorates further. The standard formula selected for the feeding is lactose-free, and Mrs. Innis's nutrient requirements can be met with 2200 milliliters of the formula per day.

What steps can the health care team take to prepare Mrs. Innis for tube feeding? Why might nasoduodenal placement of the feeding tube be preferred to nasogastric placement for Mrs. Innis? Based on the limited information available, is the choice of formula appropriate?

The physician's orders specified that the feeding should be given continuously over 18 hours. Develop a tube-feeding schedule for Mrs. Innis.

What parameters should be monitored to ensure that Mrs. Innis's fluid needs are being met? How can additional fluids be given? Describe precautions that should be taken if Mrs. Innis is to receive medications through the feeding tube.

After three days of feeding, Mrs. Innis develops diarrhea. Look at Table 23–5 on p. 773 to determine the possible causes. What measures can be taken to correct the various causes of diarrhea?

What tube-feeding information should be charted in Mrs. Innis's medical record? When Mrs. Innis is ready to eat table foods again, what steps will the health care team take?

Study Questions

1. Describe standard formulas, hydrolyzed formulas, complete formulas, and modular formulas, explaining the characteristics of each and how they differ.

2. What factors are considered in selecting an appropriate formula for an oral or tube feeding? Explain how each of the following narrows the formula choice: medical and nutrient needs; digestive and absorptive function; feeding route; and individual tolerances.

3. Suggest ways for improving acceptance of enteral formulas by mouth.

4. What are tube feedings? In what ways and in what locations can feeding tubes be placed?

5. Discuss the ways in which tube feedings can be administered to clients. Why are feeding tubes usually removed after each feeding when an infant is tube fed?

6. Describe the problems that can occur when drugs are delivered through feeding tubes. What guidelines can be used to help prevent these problems?

7. What complications are associated with tube feedings? What steps help to identify and prevent complications before they become serious?

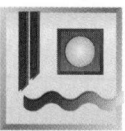

Clinical Applications

1. Complex procedures, such as those necessary to deliver enteral nutrition, require attention to many technical details, making it easy to focus on the procedure and forget about the client. Imagine that you need a transnasal tube feeding. How might you react to news that you need the feeding and to the insertion procedure? What would you miss most about eating table foods? Think of ways health care professionals might help you deal with these feelings.

2. Take a look at the checklist for monitoring clients on tube feedings (Table 23–4). You can see that the person on a tube feeding requires a great deal of care. Discuss the advantages of a nutrition support team in monitoring clients on tube feedings. What contributions might various members of the health care team make in working with tube-fed clients (see Highlight 17)?

3. Review Chapters 21 and 22 and note the symptoms and disorders that may require the use of tube feedings. For each symptom or disorder, consider when and why a tube feeding might be appropriate and which conditions might require a hydrolyzed formula. Also note those conditions associated with a risk for gastric reflux that might preclude the use of a nasogastric feeding. What alternatives are possible in these cases?

Notes

1. D. K. Bernard, J. Mandt, and E. P. Shronts, Creation of a unique modular enteral feeding system, *Support Line,* April 1993, pp. 10–14.

2. H. M. Storm and P. Lin, Forms of carbohydrate in enteral formulas, *Support Line,* June 1996, pp. 7–9.

3. D. C. Frankenfield and P. L. Beyer, Dietary fiber and bowel function in tube-fed patients, *Journal of the American Dietetic Association* 91 (1991): 590–596; J. Slavin, Commercially available enteral formulas with fiber and bowel function measures, *Nutrition in Clinical Practice* 5 (1990): 247–250.

4. J. C. Palacios and J. L. Rombeau, Dietary fiber: A brief review and potential application to enteral nutrition, *Nutrition in Clinical Practice* 5 (1990): 99–106; K. Shankardass and coauthors, Bowel function of long-term tube-fed patients consuming formulae with or without dietary fiber, *Journal of Parenteral and Enteral Nutrition* 14 (1990): 508–512.

5. D. F. Bowers, The logistics of enteral nutrition support: Current practices for the initiation and progression of tube feeding, A summary, in *Enteral Nutrition Support for the 1990s: Innovations in Nutrition, Technology, and Techniques,* Report of the Twelfth Ross Roundtable on Medical Issues, Ross Laboratories, 1992.

6. K. Teahon and coauthors, Practical aspects of enteral nutrition in the management of Crohn's disease, *Journal of Parenteral and Enteral Nutrition* 19 (1995): 365–368.

7. W. W. Souba, Nutritional support, *New England Journal of Medicine,* 336 (1997): 41–48: E. P. Shronts, Enteral vs. parenteral nutrition: A clinical review, *Support Line,* June 1996, pp. 10–13.

8. Shronts, 1996.

9. F. W. Clevenger and D. J. Rodriguez, Decision-making for enteral feeding administration: The why behind where and how, *Nutrition in Clinical Practice* 10 (1995): 104–113; Q. Duh, Decision tree for route of enteral nutrition support: Placement techniques, A summary, in *Enteral Nutrition Support,* Report of the First Ross Conference on Enteral Devices, Ross Laboratories, 1996.

10. S. P. Marcuard, K. L. Stegall, and S. Trogdon, Clearing obstructed feeding tubes, *Journal of Parenteral and Enteral Nutrition* 13 (1989): 81–83.

11. G. Moe, Enteral feeding and infection in the immunocompromised patient, *Nutrition in Clinical Practice* 6 (1991): 55–64.

12. G. P. Zaloga, Enteral nutrition in hospitalized patients: A summary, in *Enteral Nutrition Support for the 1990s: Innovations in Nutrition, Technology, and Techniques,* Report of the Twelfth Ross Roundtable on Medical Issues, Ross Laboratories, 1992.

13. J. Hatton and B. Magnuson, How to minimize interaction between phenytoin and enteral nutrition: Two approaches, *Nutrition in Clinical Practice* 11 (1996): 28–31.

14. R. A. Breslow, J. Hallfrisch, and A. P. Goldberg, Malnutrition in tubefed nursing home patients with pressure sores, *Journal of Parenteral and Enteral Nutrition* 15 (1991): 663–668.

15. S. Mobarhan and M. DeMeo, Diarrhea induced by enteral feeding, *Nutrition Reviews* 53 (1995): 67–70.

16. P. G. Eisenberg, Causes of diarrhea in tube-fed patients: A comprehensive approach to diagnosis and management, *Nutrition in Clinical Practice* 8 (1993): 119–123.

Enteral Formulas: Who's Minding the Market?

The medical marketplace offers an astounding array of enteral formulas. New products appear regularly, paralleling the trend that favors the use of enteral over parenteral nutrition to feed people who cannot meet their nutrient needs with conventional foods. Enteral formulas were originally manufactured simply to provide the nutrients of table foods in a liquid form. Gradually, formulas with specific nutrition profiles were developed for specific uses; lactose was eliminated from some formulas to improve GI tolerance, for example, and free amino acids replaced whole proteins in other formulas to improve absorption. Even more recently, formulas have been designed not only to meet nutrient needs, but also to directly affect the disease process.[1] Some of these formulas contain nutrients or other dietary constituents in types or amounts that differ considerably from those found in standard diets. Are such formulas foods or drugs? This highlight addresses the concerns of health care professionals about the expanding enteral formula market and its regulation.

CURRENT PRACTICE

In the United States, enteral formulas are exempt from the testing for safety and effectiveness that drugs must go through before they can be marketed. Enteral formulas are currently regulated as medical foods.[2] The Food and Drug Administration (FDA) notes that to qualify as medical foods, products must meet the following criteria:

- They must be specifically formulated and processed, as opposed to

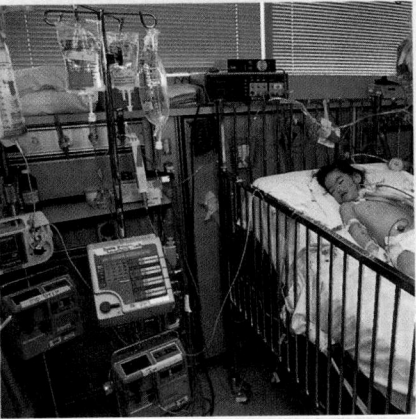

Enteral formulas, which serve as the primary source of nutrients for some people who are ill, are exempted from regulations that govern labeling, nutrient content claims, and health claims.

a naturally occurring food used in a natural state.
- They must be designed for oral or tube feeding.
- They must be labeled for the dietary management of a disorder that has distinctive nutritional requirements.
- They must be intended for use with medical supervision.[3]

Products that do not qualify as medical foods include parenteral nutrients, single-nutrient preparations, weight-loss products, and foods recommended by a physician or other health care professional as part of an overall diet to reduce the risk of a medical disease.

As medical foods, enteral formulas must conform to the manufacturing standards applied to all foods. These standards ensure that products are prepared in a sanitary environment and are free of contamination. Manufacturers, motivated to protect their reputations and limit their legal liabilities,

generally conduct clinical trials before marketing their products and maintain high quality control standards.[4]

Potential Problems

Medical foods are exempt from regulations that govern nutrition labeling, nutrient content claims, and health claims.[5] A medical food can technically be sold without any nutrition information on its label. The product may reach the market before the formulation's suitability for its intended purpose has been evaluated. Furthermore, a label on a medical food may make unsubstantiated health claims.

These exemptions would probably not be a cause for concern if enteral formula use was always supervised by a physician (as the definition of medical foods asserts), but such is not always the case. Many formulas are marketed directly to the public on television and in print and are widely available without a prescription in pharmacies and grocery stores.

In effect, medical foods, which are intended for use with people who are ill, receive less scrutiny than table foods, which are intended for the general population. Thus the public is currently not protected from potential safety hazards or inappropriate treatment claims for these products.

Standard and Special Formulas

Standard enteral formulas mimic regular diets in their sources of nutrients and proportions of protein, carbohydrate, and fat. Thus these formulas are nutritionally similar to traditional foods, and they are generally considered safe.

Other formulas, designed for use in specific medical situations, differ from standard formulas in either the types or the amounts of nutrients they supply. Hydrolyzed formulas, for example, are special because they supply free amino acids rather than intact proteins; they are also much lower in fat than standard formulas. Other special formulas may go a step further—for example, they may provide high levels of certain amino acids and low levels of others. Still other formulas may contain added amounts of dietary constituents that are not known to be essential. Formulas designed to stimulate immune function, for example, have added nucleotides, omega-3 fatty acids, and the nonessential amino acid arginine.

Special formulas pose a greater potential risk to client health than standard formulas, primarily because far less is known about nutrient requirements in specific medical conditions and because such products are often the sole source of nutrients. Manufacturers can develop formulas for a specific medical condition and market them before their safety and effectiveness have been fully documented. For example, preliminary studies suggest that glutamine, a nonessential amino acid, may help protect the integrity of the GI tract during severe stress (see Chapter 25). Because the body may not be able to make enough glutamine to meet its needs, researchers are examining whether supplemental glutamine might be a safe and effective therapy. Spurred by these potentially important studies, formulas with added glutamine have been quickly developed and marketed. The potential benefits and risks of these products, however, have not been satisfactorily documented. Consider some of these unanswered questions:

- Is glutamine a conditionally essential amino acid during stress?
- How are glutamine needs during stress affected by the degree of stress or by the person's age, gender, or other medical conditions?
- At what level should glutamine be supplemented?
- Is there a measurable benefit from using a glutamine-enriched formula over a standard formula provided in appropriate amounts?
- Are any risks associated with providing too much glutamine?

These questions remain to be answered. An example of a potential risk associated with glutamine-enriched formulas involves their use in people with compromised liver and kidney function. End products of glutamine metabolism include ammonia and urea, substances that can be toxic to people with inadequate liver and kidney function, respectively.

As mentioned, an enteral formula often represents the sole source of nutrients for the person who needs it. In addition, the person may be quite ill, and there may be little leeway for errors that could hinder recovery. Clinical trials could help to refine the art of selecting and administering enteral formulas, but conducting truly adequate clinical trials in human beings is extremely difficult, particularly in people with metabolic stresses. The type and degree of stress, individual responses to stress, prior nutrition status, age, preexisting medical conditions, and varying techniques for providing care are but a few of many factors that complicate clinical studies and limit their application to other clinical situations.

Finally, highly modified formulas are often considerably more expensive than standard formulas. In today's cost-conscious health care environment, it is important to know whether such a formula provides benefits that justify its cost.

PROPOSED REGULATIONS

Since the 1970s, the FDA has considered proposals for medical food regulations, although none have been approved to date. The FDA's most recent notice of proposed rulemaking for medical foods appeared late in 1996.[6] With the formula market expanding and new manufacturers entering the field, the FDA is aware of the increased potential for injury to consumers and fraudulent claims. For these reasons, the FDA is seeking comments from medical professionals, industry, and consumers to help it determine the most effective ways to regulate the medical food industry.

The FDA's proposed rules note that labeling regulations for medical foods might include:

- Labeling of nutrient content and inclusion of adequate directions for use.
- Assurances of product composition and quality.
- Substantiation of suitability for intended purpose and for health claims.

As of this writing, the enteral formulas are still governed as medical foods, and no further action has been taken.

PROFESSIONAL RESPONSIBILITY

In the meantime, how can health care professionals ensure the safe and effective use of enteral formulas? First of all, most clients on tube feedings are on standard formulas that have been used safely for many years. The benefits of these formulas outweigh the risks of starving or subsisting on nutrient-deficient intakes.

Special formulas should be thoroughly investigated by the nutrition support team or by a skilled dietitian or physician. The investigation should include evaluating clinical studies, reviewing product literature, and determining the values of different formulas for their intended uses. Sound medical judgment that weighs the expected benefits against the potential risks of different formulas will factor heavily in the final selection of new products.

Both individuals and organizations with extensive experiences with enteral formulas should submit their recommendations to the FDA to ensure that the final regulations will be adequate and feasible. The comments of the American Society for Parenteral and Enteral Nutrition (A.S.P.E.N.) have recently been published.[7]

Conscientious professionals know that availability of an enteral formula does not ensure safety and effectiveness. These professionals will keep abreast of new regulations and consider how these regulations will affect formula development and selection.

NOTES

1. S. B. Heymsfield, Enteral solutions: Is there a solution? *Nutrition in Clinical Practice* 10 (1995): 4–7.
2. C. Mueller and M. Nestle, Regulation of medical foods: Toward a rational policy, *Nutrition in Clinical Practice* 10 (1995): 8–15.
3. Regulation of Medical Foods, *Federal Register*, November 29, 1996, pp. 60661–60671.
4. I. S. Bass, A legal overview of the status of medical foods in the United States, *Food Drug Cosmetic Law Journal* 44 (1989): 467–477.
5. Regulation of Medical Foods, 1996.
6. Regulation of Medical Foods, 1996.
7. A.S.P.E.N. Medical Foods Task Force, A.S.P.E.N.'s response to FDA notice of proposed rulemaking, *Nutrition in Clinical Practice* 12 (1997): 131–136.

Chapter 24

Parenteral Nutrition

CONTENTS

Intravenous Nutrition
Intravenous Solutions
Types of Intravenous Feedings
Intravenous Nutrition Techniques
Insertion and Care of the Catheter
Administration of the TPN Solution
From Parenteral to Enteral Feedings
Specialized Nutrition Support at Home
The Basics of Home Programs
Home Enteral Nutrition
Home Total Parenteral Nutrition
HIGHLIGHT: Ethical Issues in Nutrition Care

MICROGRAPH: Arginine, the amino acid that assists the body's immune responses.

*t*he science of medical nutrition as we know it today was shaped tremendously by the demonstration in 1968 that all nutrient needs could be met by vein.[1] Practitioners now had a way to feed people who otherwise might have died from malnutrition before their primary medical disorders could be corrected. With time, clinicians learned which solutions and which delivery methods served their clients best. They also discovered that while intravenous nutrition is a life-saving treatment, it is very costly and is associated with serious complications including liver dysfunction, progressive kidney problems, bone disorders, and many nutrient deficiencies. These findings prompted a renewed appreciation for the GI tract and for the value of using it to deliver nutrients whenever possible. Health care professionals first make every effort to feed clients an oral diet of conventional foods, supplements (including enteral formulas), or a combination of foods and supplements. When a person with a functional GI tract cannot, will not, or should not eat an oral diet, tube feedings provide an alternative. Only when people cannot meet their nutrient requirements using the enteral route should they receive parenteral or intravenous (IV) nutrition.

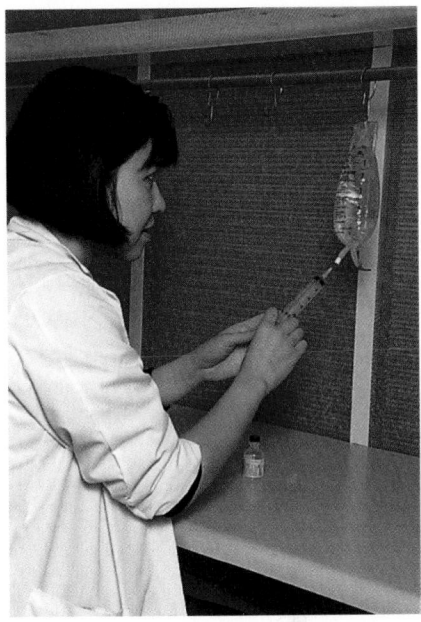

Skilled pharmacists carefully compound IV solutions under sterile conditions to ensure safety and stability.

Intravenous Nutrition

As is true of all medical nutrition therapy, the decision to use intravenous solutions, the method of delivery, and the type and amount of nutrients to provide are based on a thorough assessment of the client's medical condition and nutrient needs. Infusion of intravenous nutrients immediately changes blood levels of fluids, electrolytes, and other nutrients and, therefore, requires vigilant attention to the individual's responses.

parenteral nutrition: delivery of nutrient solutions directly into a vein, bypassing the intestines.
para = outside
enteron = intestine

intravenous (IV): through a vein.
intra = within
vena = vein

INTRAVENOUS SOLUTIONS

A variety of nutrient solutions can be administered by vein. These IV solutions may contain any or all of the essential nutrients: water, amino acids, carbohydrate, fat, vitamins, and minerals. Skilled pharmacists can compound individualized IV solutions to meet a client's specific needs.

Amino Acids   Intravenous amino acid solutions usually contain both essential and nonessential amino acids to meet the body's need for protein. Special products that contain only essential amino acids or large amounts of certain amino acids and small amounts of others are available for specific medical conditions. Products designed for liver failure, for example, may contain more branched-chain amino acids and fewer aromatic amino acids (see Chapter 26).

A nonessential amino acid may be omitted from standard solutions because it does not mix well or is not stable. For example, glutamine, which may be a conditionally essential amino acid for some clients, is not stable in IV solutions. Providing glutamine as a dipeptide solves the instability problem, and studies suggest that short-chain peptides can be digested to free amino acids by enzymes bound to cell membranes.[2]

Glutamine may be a conditionally essential amino acid following intestinal resections (see Highlight 22) and during recovery from stress (see Chapter 25).

Carbohydrate   Standard IV solutions provide carbohydrate as dextrose (glucose). Because the form of dextrose in IV solutions contains some water, dextrose solutions provide only 3.4 kcalories per gram, whereas glucose provides 4.

dextrose monohydrate: a form of glucose that contains water and is stable in IV solutions. Dextrose solutions provide 3.4 kcal/g, whereas glucose provides 4 kcal/g.

IV lipid emulsions are made from egg phospholipids (see p. 151) and plant-derived oils.

A 10% IV fat emulsion provides 1.1 kcal/ml, so a 500 ml bottle delivers 550 kcal.

A 20% IV fat emulsion provides 2 kcal/ml, so a 500 ml bottle delivers 1000 kcal.

bilirubin: a pigment in the bile whose concentration in the blood may rise as a result of some disorders.

Hyperlipidemia and atherosclerosis are discussed in Chapter 28. Liver disorders are the subject of Chapter 26.

Lipid   Intravenous lipid emulsions are the vehicle for fat in IV solutions. Intravenous fats are provided either daily or periodically (two or three times a week). If provided daily, IV fat serves as a concentrated source of energy; if offered less often, it serves primarily as a source of essential fatty acids.

Intravenous fat emulsions are contraindicated for newborns with markedly elevated bilirubin levels, people with some types of hyperlipidemia, people with severe liver disease, and those with severe egg allergies. Cautious use of IV lipids is recommended for people with atherosclerosis, moderate liver disease, blood coagulation disorders, pancreatitis, and some types of lung problems. After long-term administration, brown pigments may accumulate in certain liver cells, but these pigments disappear after parenteral therapy is discontinued; their effects on liver function are unknown. Prolonged IV lipid use may also enlarge the liver and spleen and reduce the number of blood platelets and white blood cells.

Micronutrients   Vitamins, electrolytes (minerals), and trace elements may be used in IV solutions. Currently available IV multivitamin solutions for adults meet the recommendations of the Nutrition Advisory Group of the American Medical Association, which do not include a recommendation for vitamin K.[3] Vitamin K must be added separately or given by injection. Pediatric multivitamin solutions contain vitamin K.

Some electrolytes (particularly calcium and phosphorus) can precipitate with other IV solution components, posing life-threatening problems. As an indication of the seriousness of this problem, the Food and Drug Administration recently alerted health care professionals that a precipitate of calcium phosphate might have been responsible for at least two deaths and two cases of respiratory distress.[4] A skilled pharmacist knows how to mix solutions to minimize the risk of precipitation.

Other Additives   Intravenous medications are sometimes added directly to the solution or infused into it through a separate port. Common examples include heparin, insulin, cimetidine, ranitidine, and famotidine. Providing medications along with the IV solution saves time and avoids the need for a separate infusion site. Interactions between medications and IV solutions, however, can and do occur. Deliver medications along with the IV solution only if they have been proven physically compatible with, and biochemically stable in, the solution. When drugs are added directly to the IV solution, the health care team must remember that if the total volume of solution is not infused, then the client may not receive the full dose of medication. Conversely, if the medication is not noted on the drug record, the physician may inadvertently reorder the drug, and the client may suffer potentially severe consequences.

TYPES OF INTRAVENOUS FEEDINGS

Intravenous solutions can be provided in different ways. The method used depends on the person's immediate medical and nutrient needs, nutrition status, and anticipated length of time on IV nutrition support.

Simple IV Solutions   Simple IV solutions are used routinely in hospitals to provide water, dextrose, and electrolytes to maintain the body's fluid and electrolyte and acid-base balances. Most people are expected to be able to eat within

Intravenous fat emulsions provide energy and essential fatty acids and can be easily identified by their milky white color.

How to Calculate the Nutrient Content of IV Solutions

You can have confidence in IV solutions if you know what they contain. The basic thing to remember is that the percentage of a substance in solution tells you how many grams of that substance are present in 100 milliliters. For example, a 5 percent dextrose solution contains 5 grams of dextrose per 100 milliliters. A 3.5 percent amino acid solution contains 3.5 grams of amino acids per 100 milliliters. A 0.9 percent normal saline solution contains 0.9 grams of sodium chloride per 100 milliliters.

Suppose a person is receiving 3 liters of an intravenous solution containing 1500 milliliters of 50 percent dextrose and 1500 milliliters of 7 percent amino acids. For dextrose, the person would get:

$$\frac{50 \text{ g dextrose}}{100 \text{ ml}} = \frac{x \text{ g dextrose}}{1500 \text{ ml}}.$$

$$\frac{50 \text{ g} \times 1500 \text{ ml}}{100 \text{ ml}} = 750 \text{ g dextrose.}$$

And for amino acids:

$$\frac{7 \text{ g amino acids}}{100 \text{ ml}} = \frac{x \text{ g amino acids}}{1500 \text{ ml}}.$$

$$\frac{7 \text{ g} \times 1500 \text{ ml}}{100 \text{ ml}} = 150 \text{ g amino acids.}$$

To calculate the total kcalories in 3000 milliliters of the solution, simply multiply by kcalories per gram:

$$750 \text{ g dextrose} \times 3.4 \text{ kcal/g} = 2550 \text{ kcal}$$
$$105 \text{ g amino acids} \times 4.0 \text{ kcal/g} = \underline{420 \text{ kcal}}$$
$$\text{Total} = 2970 \text{ kcal}$$

a few days following surgery, trauma, or illness, and simple IV solutions usually meet their needs satisfactorily.

Total Parenteral Nutrition Simple IV solutions fall short of meeting total nutrient needs. People who cannot use their GI tracts for a long time, those who are malnourished, and those who have high nutrient requirements need complete parenteral nutrition support. The box above explains how to calculate the nutrient content of IV solutions.

Highly concentrated dextrose and amino acid solutions cannot be infused into the small-diameter peripheral veins, such as those in the forearm and on the back of the hand, because they become irritated and eventually collapse. To deliver all the nutrients needed using less-concentrated solutions would typically require more than 12 liters of solution a day, a volume far greater than the body could safely handle. Two options remain: peripheral parenteral nutrition or central parenteral nutrition.

Simple IV solutions typically contain 5% dextrose and normal saline. Other electrolytes or salts may be added as needed. Often 3 liters of the solution are provided daily and deliver about 150 g glucose, or about 510 kcal per day.

peripheral veins: the small-diameter veins that bring blood to the extremities (arms and legs).

peripheral parenteral nutrition (PPN): the use of the peripheral veins to provide a solution that meets nutrient needs.

A typical PPN solution contains 10% dextrose and 5% amino acids. Often 3 liters of the solution are provided daily along with one 500 ml bottle of a 20% fat emulsion.

IV catheter: a thin tube inserted into a vein through which nutrient solutions or medications can be given directly.

central total parenteral nutrition (TPN): a method for meeting all nutrient needs by infusing formula into a large-diameter central vein.

central veins: the large-diameter veins located close to the heart (see Figure 24–1).

Peripheral Parenteral Nutrition (PPN)　For some people, nutrient needs can be met using the peripheral veins to deliver IV solutions that provide dextrose, amino acids, IV fat, vitamins, minerals, and trace elements—*peripheral parenteral nutrition (PPN)*. A typical PPN solution delivers about 2500 kcalories per day and provides about 150 grams of amino acids; IV lipid emulsions contribute more than half of the total kcalories. Intravenous lipid emulsions make it possible to deliver needed nutrients by peripheral vein because they provide a concentrated source of kcalories in a form that is isotonic to blood and less irritating to the blood vessels than highly concentrated dextrose solutions.

Peripheral parenteral solutions best suit people with normal renal function who need only short-term nutrition support (about 7 to 14 days), people who need additional nutrients temporarily to supplement an oral diet or tube feeding, or those in whom inserting an IV catheter into a central vein might be difficult.[5] People with very high energy requirements, people with weak peripheral veins that collapse easily, and those with fluid restrictions are not candidates for PPN.

Total Parental Nutrition (TPN) by Central Vein　Another method for meeting all nutrient needs by vein is central total parenteral nutrition, or TPN for short. In TPN, the tip of the IV catheter is either placed directly in a large-diameter central vein (see Figure 24–1) or threaded into a central vein through a peripheral vein. Almost a gallon of blood rushes through one such central vein, the superior vena cava, each minute, so highly concentrated solutions quickly become diluted. By the time these solutions reach the peripheral veins, they are no longer concentrated enough to irritate the blood vessels.

Figure 24–1

The Veins Used for TPN

❶　Traditionally, TPN catheters enter the circulation at the right subclavian vein and are threaded into the superior vena cava with the tip of the catheter lying close to the heart. Sometimes catheters are threaded into the superior vena cava from the left subclavian vein, the internal jugular veins, or the external jugular veins.

❷　Peripherally-inserted central catheters usually enter the circulation at the basilic or cephalic vein and are guided up toward the heart so that the catheter tip rests in a central vein, often the superior vena cava.

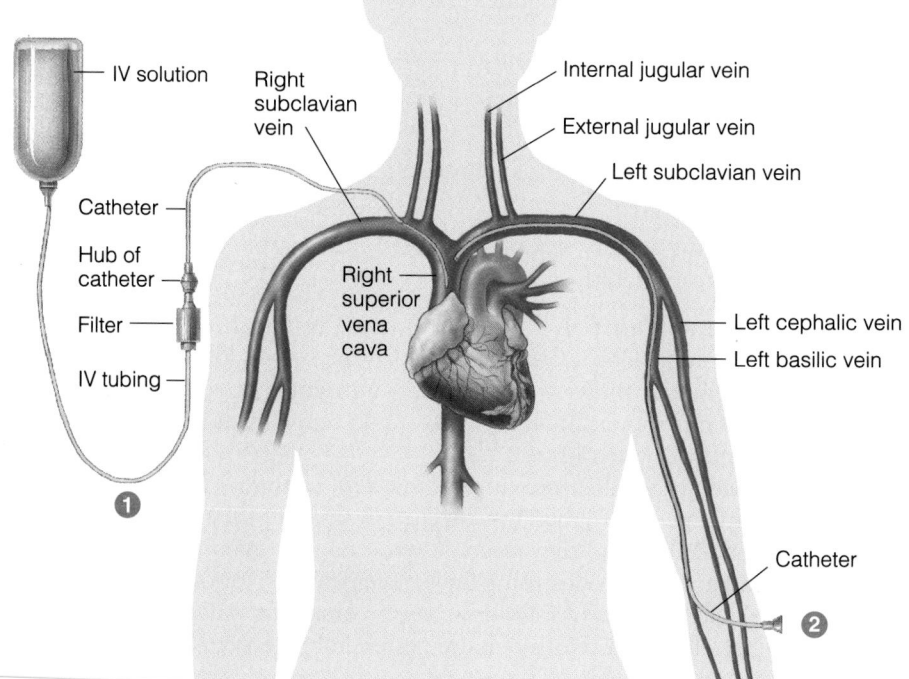

Table 24–1

Possible Indications for TPN by Central Vein

Acquired immune deficiency syndrome (AIDS)

Extensive small bowel resections

Radiation enteritis (inflammation of intestine caused by radiation)

Intractable diarrhea

Intractable vomiting

Severe GI tract obstructions

Bone marrow transplants

Severe acute pancreatitis

Severe malnutrition if surgical or intensive medical intervention is necessary

Hypermetabolic disorders, or major surgery, when it is anticipated that the GI tract will be unusable for more than 2 weeks

High-output enterocutaneous fistulas

Severe nausea and vomiting associated with pregnancy (hyperemesis gravidarum) when they last for more than 14 days

Low birthweight with necrotizing enterocolitis (severe GI inflammatory disease) or bronchopulmonary dysplasia (chronic lung disease)

When it is anticipated that adequate enteral nutrition cannot be established within 14 days of hospitalization

Note: If short-term parenteral nutrition support is anticipated (less than 14 days), PPN is preferred.

Source: Adapted from A.S.P.E.N. Board of Directors, Guidelines for the use of parenteral and enteral nutrition in adult and pediatric patients, *Journal of Parenteral and Enteral Nutrition* (supplement) 17 (1993): 1–49.

TPN is indicated whenever long-term parenteral nutrition will be required, when nutrient requirements are high, or when people are severely malnourished (see Table 24–1). People who need TPN for weeks or months, but risk serious complications if a catheter is inserted directly into a central vein, may be candidates for peripherally inserted central catheters.[6]

Regardless of how the catheter is placed, TPN should be initiated before nutrition status is severely compromised. It is much easier to maintain nutrition status than to try to replenish lost nutrient stores.

Composition of TPN Solutions   The actual concentrations of amino acids, dextrose, and lipids that compose the final TPN solution are determined by each person's unique nutrient needs. TPN solutions meet energy needs primarily from dextrose. Providing too much dextrose, however, can result in hyperglycemia, a common metabolic complication associated with TPN. Clinicians recommend that the solution provide not more than 4 to 5 milligrams of dextrose per minute per kilogram of body weight.[7]

If additional energy is needed, IV lipids can be used. Intravenous fat can provide about 50 to 60 percent of the total daily energy requirement for an adult who is not severely stressed.[8] During stress, clinicians frequently restrict fat to 30 percent of the total daily energy requirement (see Chapter 25).[9]

peripherally inserted central catheter (PICC): a catheter inserted into a peripheral vein and advanced into a central vein.

To prevent hyperglycemia, provide no more than 4 to 5 mg dextrose/min/kg body weight.

One liter of a typical central TPN solution contains 25% dextrose and 3.5% amino acids. Often 3 liters of the solution are given daily and provide about 3000 kcal and 105 g protein.

respiratory acidosis: a condition of too much acid in the blood caused by failure of the lungs to expel carbon dioxide properly. Excess carbon dioxide is normally released from the lungs during exhalation; diseased lungs, however, are unable to perform this function rapidly enough.

Providing energy from fat helps to minimize hyperglycemia in people who are sensitive to high glucose loads. Providing more energy from fat may also help prevent respiratory acidosis in people with respiratory failure, because they are unable to expel carbon dioxide efficiently, and fat oxidation produces less carbon dioxide than glucose oxidation does. If lipids are not used as an energy source, essential fatty acid requirements may be met by giving IV lipid periodically (two to three times per week).

Researchers are actively working to identify the best types and amounts of amino acids, carbohydrates, and lipid for TPN solutions, as well as the factors affecting the bioavailability of vitamins, minerals, trace minerals, and drugs. Many of these studies are particularly relevant for clients with severe stresses and will be described in Chapter 25.

Nutrient solutions delivered by vein are called intravenous or parenteral solutions and typically contain all or a combination of the essential nutrients. Sometimes drugs are added to the solution as well. Simple IV solutions provide water, dextrose, and electrolytes; they support well-nourished people with average nutrient needs for a short time. Other people need complete parenteral nutrition, delivered either by peripheral vein (PPN) or central vein (TPN).

Intravenous Nutrition Techniques

Intravenous solutions are like tube feedings in that careful attention to selection, preparation, and delivery helps support nutrition status while minimizing the risks of complications. To prevent bacterial contamination and ensure the stability of IV solutions, they should be shielded from light and refrigerated until used. As Table 24–2 shows, many of the risks associated with IV nutrition are more serious than those associated with enteral nutrition.

INSERTION AND CARE OF THE CATHETER

Insertion of a catheter for PPN is the same as for simple IV solutions. Skilled nurses can place peripherally inserted central catheters for TPN, but a catheter for direct central access is inserted surgically by a qualified physician either at bedside or in an operating room. The client is often awake for the procedure, but is given a local anesthetic. Unnecessary apprehension can be avoided by explaining the procedure to the client.

Maintaining the integrity of peripheral veins is often a problem with PPN. Veins may become inflamed and sometimes infected. Often the infusion catheter must be removed and reinserted at a new site; consequently, long-term feedings are difficult and rarely indicated. Peripherally inserted central catheters are less irritating to the veins and can be in place longer than catheters for PPN.

The presence of disease-causing bacteria in the blood is called sepsis—a major complication of TPN.

Infections can develop at the catheter site in both PPN and central TPN. Compared with peripherally inserted catheters (for either PPN or TPN), though, central TPN presents a greater risk of introducing disease-causing microorganisms into the bloodstream, because the catheter is inserted so near the heart. Health care workers must inspect the catheter site regularly and change the dressing frequently to keep the site clean.

Table 24–2

Complications Associated with TPN

Catheter- or Care-Related Complications

Fluid in the chest (hydrothorax)

Air or gas in the chest (pneumothorax)

Blood in the chest (hemothorax)

Catheter tip broken off, obstructing blood flow (catheter embolism)

Air leaking into catheter, obstructing blood flow (air embolism)

Hole or tear in heart made by catheter tip (myocardial perforation)

Catheter inadvertently placed in subclavian artery (arterial puncture)

Improperly positioned catheter tip

Sepsis

Blood clot (thrombosis)

Infusion pump malfunctions

Metabolic or Nutrition-Related Complications

Elevated blood glucose (hyperglycemia)

Low blood glucose (hypoglycemia)

Dehydration

Fluid overload

Coma from excessive glucose load (hyperosmolar, hyperglycemic, nonketotic coma)

Electrolyte imbalances

Essential fatty acid deficiency

Vitamin and mineral deficiencies

Trace element deficiencies

High blood ammonia levels (hyperammonemia)

Acid-base imbalances

Elevated liver enzymes

Fatty liver

Bone demineralization

ADMINISTRATION OF THE TPN SOLUTION

Just as a tube feeding is started slowly to allow the GI tract time to adapt to the formula, a central TPN feeding is started slowly to allow the blood time to adapt to the high glucose concentration and osmolality of the TPN solution. Typically, 1 liter of TPN solution is infused at a constant rate (about 40 milliliters per hour) during the first 24 hours. An infusion pump ensures an accurate and steady delivery rate. Electrolytes and blood glucose are monitored periodically. If tests indicate electrolyte imbalances or unacceptably high blood glucose, the causes are investigated and treated. After the first 24 hours, the infusion rate is increased by 1 liter a day until the desired volume of solution is being given every 24 hours.

Rapid changes in the infusion rate can cause severe hyperglycemia and hypoglycemia, which can lead to coma, convulsions, or even death, so all changes must be made gradually and cautiously. Problems are more likely to occur in peo-

Recall from Chapter 23 that infusion pumps may seem like toys to young children and must be kept at a safe distance from the bed so that the child will not change the flow rate or topple the pump or IV pole.

ple with organ dysfunction or in infants with immature organ systems. When the administration of solution gets behind or ahead of schedule, the drip rate should be adjusted to the correct hourly infusion rate, but no attempt should be made to speed up or slow down the drip rate to meet the originally ordered volume. When a person is being taken off TPN, the infusion rate of the solution must be tapered off gradually to prevent hypoglycemia. Table 24–3 provides guidelines for monitoring clients on TPN.

Peripheral TPN Infusion   Unlike central TPN solutions, peripheral TPN does not have to be increased gradually when feedings are initiated or tapered off gradually when feedings are discontinued. Peripheral TPN solutions do not have the high concentrations of glucose or the high osmolality of central TPN solutions and do not present the associated problems.

IV Lipid Infusion   Traditionally, IV lipid emulsions are infused separately from the TPN solution containing dextrose, amino acids, and micronutrients (see the photo on p. 784). Occasionally, people experience adverse reactions to IV lipid emulsions, particularly when the IV lipids are given in large amounts or administered too rapidly. Immediate reactions may include fever, warmth, chills, backache, chest pain, allergic reactions, palpitations, rapid breathing, wheezing, cyanosis, nausea, and an unpleasant taste in the mouth. To guard against adverse reactions, the client receives only small amounts of lipid emulsion over the first 15 to 30 minutes. After that time, the rate can be increased.

When IV lipid emulsions are used as an energy source, they are often added directly to the base solution and infused along with it. The use of total nutrient admixtures for clients in the hospital as well as at home has grown dramati-

TPN solutions that contain all nutrients, including fat, are called total nutrient admixtures, 3-in-1 admixtures, or all-in-one admixtures.

Table 24–3

Guidelines for Monitoring People on TPN

Before starting TPN:	Complete nutrition assessment.
	Confirm placement of catheter tip by X ray.
	Check blood glucose, electrolytes, chemical profile, and complete blood count.
Every 4 to 6 hours:	Check blood glucose.
	Monitor vital signs.
	Check pump infusion rate.
Daily:	Monitor weight changes.
	Record intake and output.
	Check urine specific gravity.
Daily until stable, and then 2 to 3 times weekly:	Monitor serum electrolytes, calcium, magnesium, phosphorus, and blood urea nitrogen.
Weekly:	Reassess nutrition status.
	Monitor serum proteins, ammonia, and triglycerides.
	Check the complete blood count.

cally.[10] Total nutrient admixtures must be compounded carefully, refrigerated prior to use, and mixed gently before they are infused.

Cyclic Infusion   A person on cyclic parenteral nutrition receives the TPN solution at a constant rate for 8 to 12 hours a day. Because the infusion can be given during the night to allow freedom for routine daytime activities, cyclic parenteral nutrition is often used for long-term TPN. When a person receives a TPN solution continuously, insulin levels stay high. As a result, the person cannot mobilize fat stores for energy or for essential fatty acids; eventually, fat may be deposited in the liver. Cyclic TPN reverses these problems.[11] Additionally, fewer kcalories seem to be necessary to maintain nitrogen balance, probably because the person uses body fat for energy. Some people, however, cannot tolerate the delivery of a day's volume of solution over a short period of time.

Careful attention to the selection, preparation, and delivery of parenteral solutions minimizes the risks of complications (review Table 24–2). Table 24–3 presents a schedule for monitoring people on TPN.

cyclic parenteral nutrition: the continuous administration of TPN solutions for 8 to 12 hours with time periods when no nutrients are infused.

From Parenteral to Enteral Feedings

Once the problem causing the need for IV nutrition resolves, the client can gradually shift to an enteral diet while the volume of the IV solution is tapered off. The transition requires careful planning. During long periods of disuse, the intestinal villi shrink and lose some of their function. Reintroducing nutrients to the GI tract at the appropriate rate and volume will stimulate the progressive restoration of the villi's normal structure and function and prevent malabsorption and other GI discomforts.

Transitional Feedings   The transition from IV feeding to an enteral diet can be accomplished in different ways and often involves a combination of feeding methods. One way is to start an oral diet while the person is still on IV nutrition. The diet is often progressive, beginning with liquids provided in small amounts. If the person cannot eat enough food to meet at least 50 percent of daily nutrient needs within a few days, and intake does not seem to be improving, tube feedings should be considered.[12]

Whether a person is given a tube feeding initially or provided an oral diet and then switched to a tube feeding, the volume of the IV solution is reduced as the volume of tube feeding is increased. The person who cannot tolerate large volumes of tube feeding can still rely on TPN to meet nutrient needs. Parenteral nutrition can be discontinued when at least 60 percent of estimated energy needs are being met by oral intake, tube feeding, or a combination of the two.[13] Chapter 23 described the transition from tube feedings to table foods.

Psychological Effects   Returning to oral intake after having been fed either intravenously or by tube can have a variety of psychological effects. Some people may be extremely eager to eat again, and food can be an important morale booster. Others may be apprehensive about eating, particularly if they have had extensive GI problems. Appetite may be slow to return for some. In such circumstances, all members of the health care team can support the successful

Nutrition Assessment Checklist

For People on Parenteral Nutrition Support

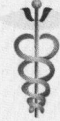 **Medical**   Review the client's medical record for information necessary to select the appropriate feeding site (peripheral versus central), insertion method (PPN, peripherally inserted central catheter, or central TPN catheter), and IV solution. The development of undesirable symptoms related to IV fluids requires prompt treatment.

 Drug   Assure that drugs delivered along with IV solutions are physically compatible with the solution and that drug activity will not be adversely affected. Remember that all of the drug dosage will not be delivered if the drug has been added to the solution and the infusion is stopped for any reason.

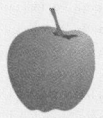 **Nutrient Intake**   Ensure that IV solutions are being delivered as prescribed. For clients beginning enteral nutrition, determine the degree to which nutrient needs are being met by enteral formulas (orally or by tube) or by table foods, and reduce the volume of nutrient IV solutions accordingly.

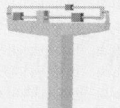 **Anthropometric**   Assess the client's weight daily to make sure that nutrient goals are being met.

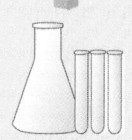 **Laboratory**   Monitor serum and urine lab values for signs of glucose intolerance and fluid and electrolyte imbalances. Check serum protein levels to ensure that they are rising or being maintained. When available, assess nitrogen balance to determine if the IV solution is meeting the client's protein needs.

 Physical   Inspect catheter insertion sites for signs of infection or inflammation. Check the infusion pump drip rate as needed. Assess blood pressure, temperature, pulse, and respiration about every 4 hours. Look for physical signs of malnutrition and dehydration.

reintroduction of food. Recognize the person's concerns, and provide reassurances that you will be there to help throughout the process.

A gradual transition from an IV feeding to an oral diet helps to prevent GI problems. During the transition, the client may experience various psychological effects ranging from apprehension to eagerness.

The many decisions surrounding the provision of TPN require careful consideration. The nutrition assessment checklist reviews the areas of nutrition assessment that require attention in people on IV nutrition support, and the case study presents an example for your review.

Case Study   Mail Carrier Requiring Parenteral Nutrition

Mr. Rossi, a 37-year-old mail carrier has been admitted to the hospital for Crohn's disease (see Chapter 22). He has been steadily losing weight and appears emaciated. A thorough examination indicates that Mr. Rossi needs surgery as soon as possible to remove a portion of his small intestine. In the meantime, he cannot be placed on enteral feedings. The nutrition assessment reveals severe protein-energy malnutrition.

Mr. Rossi is placed on central TPN before surgery. He progresses well, gains weight, and undergoes surgery one week after admission.

What factors in Mr. Rossi's history indicate the need for central TPN? How would you explain the need for TPN to Mr. Rossi?

Describe the components of a typical TPN solution. Calculate the energy and protein that 1 liter of this solution provides.

Consider some of the physiological and psychological problems Mr. Rossi might face when enteral nutrition is reintroduced. How will the health care team know when it will be safe to take Mr. Rossi off central TPN? Describe the different ways the transition from TPN to enteral feedings can be accomplished.

Specialized Nutrition Support at Home

Occasionally, a client must continue to receive specialized nutrition support (tube feedings or parenteral nutrition) after the primary medical condition has stabilized. In such a case, continuing nutrition support at home may be an option.

Since the first report of a person sent home successfully on TPN in 1969,[14] the use of nutrition support at home has expanded rapidly. Since 1992, the number of people on home parenteral nutrition has grown from 17,000 to 40,000, while the number of people on home enteral nutrition has grown from 48,000 to 150,000.[15] As the number of people on home nutrition programs continues to grow, health care professionals who work with these programs are gaining valuable experience and improving the quality of home nutrition support. Medical supply companies provide the equipment, formulas, and services necessary to support home nutrition care.

THE BASICS OF HOME PROGRAMS

As with tube feedings and TPN in the hospital, the main objective of home enteral and parenteral nutrition is to maintain or achieve adequate nutrition status. Nutrition support at home, however, has an added dimension: it permits the person to receive nutrition care in familiar surroundings. If you have ever been in the hospital, or taken a long trip for that matter, you probably remember the comfort you experienced when you returned to your own bed, knew where things were, and could get things when you needed them. Certainly, a home nutrition support program has a big impact on the person's lifestyle, but clients report that they feel their lives have improved with home nutrition therapy.[16] Many people who require nutrition support at home can also eat some foods by mouth, and some resume activities, such as going to work, driving, and playing sports.

Cost Savings   When the responsibilities formerly performed by hospital staff are assumed by the client or caregiver, the costs of nutrition support decline dramatically. One institution reports a cost savings of $1.5 million a year for ten clients maintained on home TPN versus TPN in the hospital.[17] Costs for home care are rising, however, because of the increasingly complex care available for home clients and the strict regulation of the home care industry.[18] As a result, more skilled professionals and additional time are required, and both increase costs.

Candidates for Home Nutrition Support   The nutrition support team most frequently decides whether a client is a candidate for home enteral or parenteral nutrition. In addition to medical considerations, the candidate for home nutrition support and those who care for that person must have rational, stable personalities so they can successfully handle any problems that may arise. They must be capable of learning the necessary techniques and of dealing with complications. They must have adequate financial resources and access to the equipment, supplies, and professional support that are integral components of a successful home program.

Roles of Health Care Professionals   Once a home nutrition program is initiated, a nurse visits the client at home, and the person also sees a physician at regular intervals. In some programs, dietitians also make home visits. A qualified nurse, dietitian, or physician must be available to answer questions and handle problems as they arise.

HOME ENTERAL NUTRITION

People on home enteral nutrition programs most commonly have cancer or swallowing disorders. Gastrostomies, and sometimes jejunostomies, usually provide access to the GI tract for long-term tube feedings (see Chapter 23). Some people learn to use transnasal tubes, which they insert at each feeding. Others have a transnasal tube inserted by a health care professional. When possible, intermittent feeding schedules are arranged so that clients are free to move around between meals. Clients on continuous feedings who must use pumps can obtain small pumps that are easily concealed and allow more freedom of movement.

The person on a home program usually purchases commercially prepared, premixed formulas. Most clients prefer these, and such formulas should certainly be used whenever a person's ability to mix the formula safely and appropriately is questionable.

HOME PARENTERAL NUTRITION

People on home TPN often have acquired immune deficiency syndrome (AIDS), cancer, Crohn's disease, or other intestinal disorders. Different types of home TPN programs are currently in use. Ideally, clients assume as much responsibility for their own care as they can handle. For example, a client who is capable of changing the catheter dressing is trained to do so. Typically, caregivers also learn the procedures so that they can assist as needed.

Special catheters, designed for long-term use, often are inserted for home TPN. The day's volume of TPN solution is frequently delivered within 8 to 12

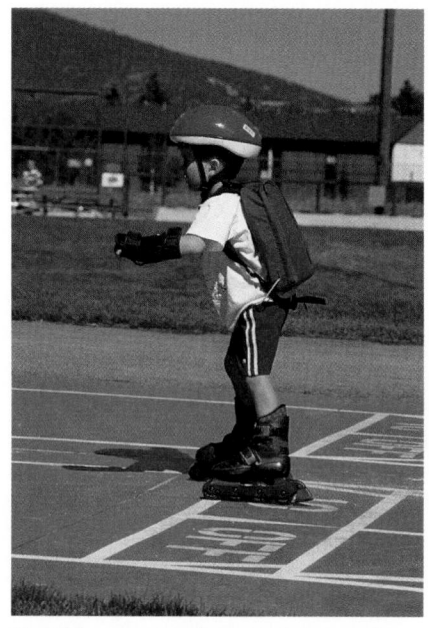

Portable pumps and convenient carrying cases allow clients who require nutrition support at home to move about freely.

hours using an infusion pump. Many clients prefer to infuse the solution while sleeping, so they can move about unencumbered during the rest of the day.

For people who cannot tolerate an 8- to 12-hour infusion rate, nutrients are infused over 24 hours. Those who are ambulatory may use a lightweight carrying case that holds a small pump and IV bags. This system allows the client to move around freely with little inconvenience.

Unquestionably, specialized nutrition support provides life-saving alternatives for nourishing people who cannot eat traditional diets either in the hospital or at home. Such support can be adapted for use in virtually any medical disorder, including those of the GI tract described in Chapters 21 and 22, and in severe stress, described in the next chapter.

Study Questions

1. What are the components of a typical TPN solution? What other additives may be present?
2. Describe the differences between simple IV solutions, PPN solutions, and central TPN solutions. When would each type be used?
3. How have IV lipid emulsions made it possible to meet energy requirements by peripheral vein? When are IV lipids preferable to IV dextrose for meeting energy needs?
4. How are PPN and TPN catheters inserted? Describe how PPN and TPN solutions are started and discontinued, and discuss the reasons for any differences.
5. Describe two ways that lipid emulsions can be delivered. What precautions should be taken when giving IV lipid emulsions?
6. Why is cyclic feeding of TPN solutions preferable to continuous feeding?
7. Describe some ways in which a person on parenteral nutrition can be weaned to ordinary table foods.
8. What are the advantages of home enteral and parenteral nutrition programs over hospital-administered programs?
9. Discuss how a home enteral nutrition program works. Describe some features of TPN that are unique to home programs.

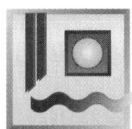 # Clinical Applications

1. The development of technology for feeding people by vein has expanded our knowledge in many areas and has raised important issues as well. Specifically, the ability to meet all nutrient needs by vein has:
   - Spurred appreciation of the role of nutrition in recovery from illness and fostered identification of specific nutrients and other therapies that may aid recovery (Highlight 22 and Chapter 25).
   - Enlightened health care professionals about the importance of the GI tract during stress (see Chapter 25), thus spurring a greater understanding of both parenteral and enteral nutrition.
   - Expanded the home health care industry.

Important issues raised as a result of the increased use of nutrition support techniques include:
   - Formula safety and efficacy. How should formulas be regulated so that their safe use can be assured (Highlight 23)?
   - Cost containment. Do the benefits of specialized nutrition support techniques justify their costs (Highlight 30)?
   - Ethics. When are special feedings appropriate (Highlight 24)?

As you read about these developments and issues in the remaining chapters of this book, reflect on the contributions special nutrition support has made to medical care.

2. One liter of a TPN solution contains 500 milliliters of 50 percent dextrose and 500 milliliters of 8.5 percent amino acids. Determine the daily kcalorie and protein intakes of a person who receives 2 liters of this TPN solution. Calculate the average daily energy intake if the person also receives 500 milliliters of a 10 percent fat emulsion three times a week.

3. Consider what it must be like to be on a home TPN program with no foods allowed by mouth.

What advantages would there be to being at home instead of in the hospital? Think of how you would manage feedings. How would you feel about the time, costs, and commitment required to maintain this therapy? How would you feel about not being able to eat after a long time? How would you handle holidays and special occasions that often center around food?

Notes

1. D. W. Wilmore and S. J. Dudrick, Growth and development of an infant receiving all nutrients exclusively by way of the vein, *Journal of the American Medical Association* 203 (1968): 860–864.

2. M. S. Dahn, Intravenous peptides, *Nutrition in Clinical Practice* 8 (1993): 93–94; J. A. Vazquez, H. Daniel, and S. A. Adibi, Dipeptides in parenteral nutrition: From basic science to clinical applications, *Nutrition in Clinical Practice* 8 (1993): 95–105; P. Fürst and P. Stehle, The potential use of parenteral dipeptides in clinical nutrition, *Nutrition in Clinical Practice* 8 (1993): 106–114.

3. J. D. Anderson, Components and compounding of total parenteral nutrition, *Support Line*, February 1993, pp. 12–15.

4. B. T. McKinnon, FDA safety alert: Hazards of precipitation associated with parenteral nutrition, *Nutrition in Clinical Practice* 11 (1996): 59–65.

5. M. A. Stokes and G. L. Hill, Peripheral parenteral nutrition: A preliminary report on its efficacy and safety, *Journal of Parenteral and Enteral Nutrition* 17 (1993): 145–147.

6. J. Z. Rogers, K. McKee, and E. McDermott, Peripherally inserted central venous catheters, *Support Line*, October 1995, pp. 6–9; S. C. Loughran and M. Borzatta, Peripherally inserted central catheters: A report of 2506 catheter days, *Journal of Parenteral and Enteral Nutrition* 19 (1995): 133–136.

7. D. K. Rosmarin, G. M. Wardlaw, and J. Mirtallo, Hyperglycemia associated with high, continuous infusion rates of total parenteral nutrition dextrose, *Nutrition in Clinical Practice* 11 (1996): 151–156; A.S.P.E.N. Board of Directors, Guidelines for the use of total parenteral nutrition in adult and pediatric patients, *Journal of Parenteral and Enteral Nutrition* (supplement) 17 (1993): 21.

8. A. M. Karch, *Lippincott's Nursing Drug Guide* (Philadelphia: Lippincott-Raven Publishers, 1997), p. 468.

9. R. G. Barton, Nutrition support in critical illness, *Nutrition in Clinical Practice* 9 (1994): 127–139.

10. D. F. Driscoll, Total nutrient admixtures: Theory and practice, *Nutrition in Clinical Practice* 10 (1995): 114–119.

11. L. M. Gramlich and B. Bistrian, Cyclic parenteral nutrition: Considerations of carbohydrates and lipid metabolism, *Nutrition in Clinical Practice* 9 (1994): 49–50.

12. R. S. DeChicco and L. E. Matarese, Selection of nutrition support regimens, *Nutrition in Clinical Practice* 7 (1992): 239–245.

13. M. F. Winkler and coauthors, Transitional feeding: The relationship between nutritional intake and plasma protein components, *Journal of the American Dietetic Association* 89 (1989): 969–970.

14. M. E. Shils and coauthors, Long-term parenteral nutrition through an external arteriovenous shunt, *New England Journal of Medicine* 283 (1970): 341–344.

15. As cited in M. Evans, Home nutrition support materials, *Nutrition in Clinical Practice* 10 (1995): 37–39.

16. M. Malone, Effect of home nutrition support on patient's lifestyle (abstract), *Journal of Parenteral and Enteral Nutrition* (supplement) 19 (1995): 23.

17. E. T. Herfinal and coauthors, Survey of home nutritional support patients, *Journal of Parenteral and Enteral Nutrition* 13 (1989): 255–261.

18. K. S. Crocker, Current status of home infusion therapy, *Nutrition in Clinical Practices* 7 (1992): 256–263.

Ethical Issues in Nutrition Care

Chapters 23 and 24 described how enteral and parenteral feedings can meet nutrient needs and support recovery in many cases. Only in the past few decades have we had the capability of providing nourishment to clients unable to eat by mouth. The technical advances made in the areas of enteral and parenteral nutrition have been life-saving for many people. Like other medical technologies, however, the availability of special nutrition support forces health care professionals and society to face ethical issues. Such treatments can prolong life by merely delaying death; the remaining life may be of low quality. Is it ever morally and legally appropriate to withhold or withdraw nutrition support?

In answering such a question, ethics experts are guided by the following principles:

- *Autonomy*—the client's right to make decisions concerning his or her own well-being.
- *Beneficence* and *maleficence*—the treatment or its withdrawal will do more good than harm, and the caregivers will promote well-being and act without selfish intent.

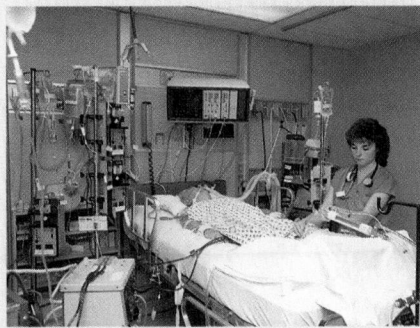

When is it morally and legally appropriate to use special nutrition support?

Glossary

advance directive: the means by which competent adults record their preferences for future medical interventions. The living will and durable power of attorney are types of advance directives.

artificial feeding: parenteral and enteral nutrition; feeding by a route other than the normal ingestion of food.

comatose: in a state of deep unconsciousness from which the person cannot be aroused.

competent: having sufficient mental ability to understand a treatment, weigh its risks and benefits, and comprehend the consequences of refusing or accepting the treatment.

death: permanent cessation of vital functions.

durable power of attorney: a legal document in which one competent adult authorizes another competent adult to make decisions for her or him in the event of incapacitation. The phrase "durable power" means that the agent's authority survives the client's incompetence; "attorney" refers to an attorney-in-fact (not an attorney-at-law).

ethical: in accordance with moral principles or professional standards. Socrates described *ethics* as "how we ought to live."

legal: established by law.

living will: a document signed by a competent adult that specifically states whether the person wishes any heroic measures to be taken in the event of terminal illness or irreversible coma from which the person is not expected to recover.

persistent vegetative state: exhibiting motor reflexes but without the ability to regain cognitive behavior, communicate, or interact purposefully with the environment.

terminal illness: a progressive, irreversible disease that will lead to death in the near future.

- *Justice*—the actions are based on fairness, honesty, and loyalty to agreements.

Ideally, these principles help people find the answers to ethical questions. In reality, though, the answers often lie entangled in personal values, charged emotions, and legal conflict. Answers rarely come easily. This highlight explores some of the ethical questions that surround the use of special nutrition support; the accompanying glossary defines related terms.

A LOOK AT THE PROBLEMS

To put the problems into perspective, consider the circumstances under which health care professionals make their decisions to feed clients. Most often, they readily provide whatever form of nutrition is necessary to support all clients who have any chance of recovering from a disease. Clearly, health care professionals cannot rightfully withhold nutrition support because of poor judgment or negligence. If a client were to die because nourishment was withheld, the staff and facility would be held responsible, and in all likelihood, a malpractice lawsuit would result. A discipline known as "medical ethics" has developed out of the need to discuss and solve problems of this nature.

The decision of whether to feed a client becomes less clear, however, when the client is not expected to recover. How aggressively do we support the person who is terminally ill or in a persistent vegetative state? How do we respond to elderly or physically disabled people who refuse special nutrition support because they feel the quality of their lives is so poor that they do not wish to be sustained? Do we (as a society) allow them such choices? Are health care professionals morally and legally obligated to comply with, or to deny, requests to discontinue feedings? Furthermore, when clients are incompetent and unable to speak for themselves, who, if anyone, should be allowed to make such life-and-death decisions?

These unanswered questions are but a few that have evolved along with the technology of special nutrition support. Occasionally, they spark intense controversy and give rise to court cases. Then the courts define the questions more clearly and lay down rules to answer them. Much more often, though, families and physicians work out their own answers to these questions. This highlight reviews the court decisions that have resolved some of the legal issues raised by these questions and also reports on how people are resolving the same questions in daily life.

NANCY CRUZAN AND THE COURTS' DECISIONS

Nancy Cruzan was a young woman who suffered permanent and irre-versible brain damage after a car crash in 1983. For eight years, she was in a persistent vegetative state—awake but unaware. Her physicians and parents held no hope for recovery. They knew that few people who have had traumatic injuries recover consciousness after a year; those who do remain severely disabled.[1] Yet given food and water, Cruzan might have lived for another 30 years. Her parents requested permission to discontinue tube feeding, but their request was rejected by the Missouri Supreme Court in 1987. The court held that Cruzan never definitively stated her "right to die" wishes and that Cruzan's parents had no legal right to make such a request for her. The court said that preserving life, no matter its quality, takes precedence over all other considerations.

Unsatisfied with the Missouri Supreme Court decision, the Cruzans took further legal action. In 1989 the U.S. Supreme Court agreed to hear the *Cruzan* case. Several professional organizations—including the American Medical Association, American Academy of Family Physicians, American Association of Neurological Surgeons, American College of Surgeons, American College of Physicians, and American Society for Parenteral and Enteral Nutrition—filed briefs with the Supreme Court in support of the Cruzans.

The Cruzans tried to convince the Supreme Court that their once independent and vivacious daughter would not want to live in a vegetative state. Their lawyer argued that Cruzan had a right to be free from medical intervention. No one questioned that Cruzan's parents knew their daughter's wishes better than anyone and had the highest and most loving motives. The question for the Court was whether families (or anyone) can make life-and-death decisions on behalf of incompetent persons.

The Supreme Court recognized that competent adults have the right to stop life-sustaining treatments. But, in a 5-to-4 decision, the Court held that life-sustaining treatment could not be withdrawn without "clear and convincing" evidence that the incompetent person would refuse treatment.[2] Cruzan's statements to her roommate and family about her desire to live or die under certain conditions were insufficient to convince the Court. In making its decision, the Supreme Court entrusted state legislatures with the task of enacting laws that address the issue of whether families (or other third parties) can authorize the withdrawal of life-sustaining treatment on behalf of incompetent persons in the absence of exacting evidence.

After another round of court battles in which additional evidence did convince the Missouri trial court of Nancy Cruzan's wishes, her feeding tube was removed. She died from dehydration two weeks later. The financial and emotional costs of supporting Cruzan were enormous. In terms of money, health care costs to support her ran about $130,000 per year (paid by the state). The emotional costs are more difficult to calculate, of course. Cruzan's parents first faced the initial shock of their daughter's accident. Then, for several years, they maintained hope that with continued care she would survive and regain consciousness. Finally, they endured court battles over their child's fate—a fate that meant grief whichever way the courts decided.

Some 30,000 other families of people who live in a persistent vegetative state face similar struggles. No doubt, the Supreme Court's decision had widespread implications for these people and the health professionals who care for them. In fact, this decision touches all of us, because it influences the extent to which our society views life-sustaining treatment as optional not only for our clients, but for ourselves and our families.[3] It decides how we may be allowed to die.[4]

INDIVIDUAL RIGHTS

The emerging ethical, medical, and legal consensus seems to support the view that individual rights outweigh those of the state. Competent individuals have a legal right to refuse medical treatment—including nourishment and hydration—even when medical experts consider that treatment necessary to sustain life. In other words, even when treatment is life-saving and its refusal may bring an earlier death, clients' rights remain paramount.

Many people will agree that competent adults have the right to accept or refuse medical treatment.[5] The controversy heightens, however, when the adult is comatose, incompetent, or otherwise unable to refuse or accept medical treatment—especially when the person's wishes are not known. Without clear and convincing evidence of an incompetent person's wishes, a court must decide in favor of protecting and preserving the client's life. For many families such as the Cruzans, it becomes their burden to provide such evidence; the Supreme Court rejected the argument that families have a constitutional right to speak on behalf of their incompetent relatives.

Several court cases over the years have raised the question of whether there is a distinction between providing "extraordinary" medical care such as ventilators and providing "ordinary" care such as nourishment and hydration.[6] Some people have suggested that "pulling the plug" on a life-support machine is acceptable, but that denying food and water—the basics of life—is inhumane. The courts have defined special nutrition support as a medical procedure, and in reviewing the Cruzan case, the Supreme Court did not distinguish between nutrition and other life-saving treatments. Nor did the Court recognize a moral or legal difference between not starting life support and discontinuing it.

INFORMED CONSENT

How can people protect their rights to retain or refuse treatment in the event of incompetency? How can health care professionals provide treatment in accordance with their clients' wishes? The answers rest with the attending health care professionals, the clients, and the clients' families.

Health care professionals should initiate discussions about advance directives as part of their routine care.[7] They should encourage their competent clients to express ahead of time their preferences for medical treatments, including artificial feedings, should terminal illness or coma develop. These professionals can be a valuable source of information, but they must be careful not to project their personal views onto their clients. Each client's preferences should be noted in the medical records.

The rights and personal beliefs of both the client and health care professionals must be respected. Any health care professional who is uncomfortable or unwilling to abide by the client's stated preferences should arrange for continuing care by an equally qualified professional and then withdraw from that client's care.[8] The law does not force health care professionals to withdraw or provide treatment that is contrary to their personal beliefs or professional standards. Clients should expect that health care professionals and facilities will comply with their preferences and not merely tolerate them grudgingly.

In addition to informing their physicians, clients can state their preferences in legal documents known as living wills (see Form H24–1). A living will allows a competent adult to express clear directions regarding medical treatment in the event that the person is unable to make the necessary decisions at that time. The living will may specify that no extraordinary treatments should be administered, or alternatively it may declare that every effort should be made to maintain life. Some people regard the providing of nourishment and hydration as ordinary care, and they consider withholding or withdrawing nutrition support for any reason to be unjustified. Others consider artificial nutrition support intrusive and believe the refusal of nutrition support is justified for people who want no heroic measures taken to sustain life.[9] People who prefer that nourishment and hydration be continued or discontinued need to write this specification into their living wills to ensure that their wishes will be carried out. Physicians seem more likely to comply with a *specific* living will than with a standard one.[10]

Most states have statutes regarding the use of living wills; health care professionals should be aware of these regulations. Some states'

Form H24–1
An Example of a Living Will

DECLARATION TO MY FAMILY, MY PHYSICIAN, MY LAWYER, AND MY SPIRITUAL ADVISER

If the time arrives when I can no longer take part in decisions for my own future, this statement and Declaration shall stand as the expression of my wishes.

I recognize that death is as much a reality as birth, growth, maturity, and old age. It is but one phase in the cycle of life and is the only certainty. I do not fear death as much as I fear there is no reasonable expectation of my recovery from physical or mental disability, I wish to be allowed to die and not to be kept alive by artificial means or heroic measures, but wish only that drugs be mercifully administered to me for terminal suffering, even if they hasten the moment of my death.

I recognize that my wishes place a heavy burden of responsibility upon you, and I therefore make the following declaration with the intention of sharing this responsibility and this decision with you and of mitigating any feelings of guilt that you may have:

THIS DECLARATION is made this _____ day of _____, 19 ____ .

I, _____ , willfully and voluntarily make known my desire that my dying not be artificially prolonged under the circumstances set forth below, and I do hereby declare:

If at any time I should have a terminal condition and if my attending physician has determined that there can be no recovery from such condition and that my death is imminent, I direct that life-prolonging procedures be withheld or withdrawn when the application of such procedures would serve only to prolong artificially the process of dying, and that I be permitted to die naturally with only the administration of medication or the performance of any medical procedures deemed necessary to provide me with comfort care or to alleviate pain. I desire that nutrition and hydration (food and water) be withheld or withdrawn when the application of such procedures would serve only to prolong artificially the process of dying.

In the absence of my ability to give directions regarding the use of such life-prolonging procedures, it is my intention that this declaration be honored by my family and physician as the final expression of my legal right to refuse medical or surgical treatment and to accept the consequences for such refusal.

I understand the full import of this declaration, and I am emotionally and mentally competent to make this declaration.

_____
(signature)

The declarant is known to me, and I believe him/her to be of sound mind.

_____
Witness

_____
Witness

The foregoing instrument was acknowledged before me this _____ day of _____, 19 ____ , by _____ .

_____
Notary Public

laws allow withdrawal of nutrition support; others specifically prohibit it; and still others do not mention it.[11] Form H24–1 shows how a living will might begin, and Appendix F provides an address for obtaining additional information. People should make their wishes known in writing to their attending physicians and family. Unfortunately, only one out of five adults has taken such steps.

Although most health care professionals advocate the use of living wills and agree that clients' wishes

Form H24–2
Durable Power of Attorney

I, _____ now residing at _____ hereby constitute and appoint _____ as my true and lawful attorney-in-fact for me and in my name, place and stead, giving and granting unto my said attorney full power and authority to do and perform every act as fully as I might do if personally present, with full power of substitution and revocation. I hereby ratify and confirm all that my attorney shall lawfully do or cause to be done pursuant to this power.

This Power includes, but is not limited to, the right to encumber, assign or convey realty, including homestead realty. In addition, my attorney-in-fact is authorized to arrange for and consent to medical, therapeutical and surgical procedures for me as principal, including the administration of drugs.

I have executed this Power while in command of my faculties and with knowledge of the consequences, both legal and practical.

This Durable Power of Attorney shall not be affected by my disability as principal except as provided by statute.

IN WITNESS WHEREOF, I have hereunto set my hand and seal this _____ day of _____, 19 ___.

WITNESSES:

_____ _____ (SEAL)

_____

STATE OF _____
COUNTY OF _____

I HEREBY CERTIFY that on this day, before me, a Notary Public duly authorized in the State and County named above to take acknowledgments, personally appeared _____ to me known to be the person described in and who executed the foregoing DURABLE POWER OF ATTORNEY, and said individual acknowledged before me that execution of this instrument was for the uses and purposes herein expressed.

WITNESS my hand and official seal in the State and County named above this _____ day of _____, 19 ___.

(SEAL)

_____
NOTARY PUBLIC

should be honored, actual medical care may not always reflect these beliefs. In practice, physicians are more likely to follow family directives concerning tube feedings and other life support than the instructions in a living will.[12] If people wish to ensure that they receive medical care consistent with their individual wishes, they need to discuss their living wills and hypothetical scenarios with family members before medical conditions arise that will necessitate others making decisions for them.

In many states, the durable power of attorney offers clients a way to ensure that their wishes will be carried out (see Form H24–2). Some states have enacted statutes authorizing the use of durable powers of attorney specifically for health care.[13] A durable power of attorney allows a competent adult to designate another competent adult (usually a relative or close friend) as an agent to make health care decisions in the event of incapacitation. In essence, it says, "I give this person the right to make health care deci-

sions on my behalf should I become unable to make them."

Ideally, the person representing the client will make decisions that reflect the client's health care preferences. In reality, though, when faced with hypothetical situations, clients and those who would have to decide for them agree on treatment only 70 percent of the time.[14] Such discrepancy is natural because each views the other's experience as most important when making decisions. Clients want to avoid burdening their families, and families want

801

to provide any treatment that offers a possible cure or relief from pain.

The person who plans ahead for future care in the case of a terminal illness or irreversible state of unconsciousness relieves others of the guilt and some of the anxiety of having to make decisions. Imagine the anguish a family member goes through in directing the health care team to stop nutrition support, knowing its cessation will hasten death. That decision is a little easier if the family member knows that it is what the individual would want or, better yet, if a legal document takes the decision out of the family's hands altogether.

When the person's wishes regarding life-sustaining measures are unknown, life support can be discontinued only if the burden of providing it clearly and markedly outweighs the benefits to the individual. Providers must also consider the pain caused by withdrawing the treatment in weighing the benefits against the negative aspects of treatment.

The questions raised in this highlight have no easy answers, yet decisions must be made. Each case must be carefully decided individually. Most hospitals have established ethics committees to deal with problems such as those presented here. Health care professionals should ensure that their disciplines are represented on such committees and become familiar with their profession's ethics policies and guidelines.[15] In addition, education programs designed to help professionals develop the analytical skills needed to resolve ethical dilemmas can be most beneficial.[16] Education enables professionals to make informed decisions and promote greater public awareness of these issues.[17]

NOTES

1. The Multi-Society Task Force on PVS, Medical aspects of the persistent vegetative state, *New England Journal of Medicine* 330 (1994): 1572–1579.

2. *Cruzan v. Director, Missouri Department of Health,* __ U.S. __, 110 S.Ct. 2841, 111 L.Ed.2d 224 (1990).

3. M. Angell, Prisoners of technology: The case of Nancy Cruzan, *New England Journal of Medicine* 322 (1990): 1226–1228; B. Lo, F. Rouse, and L. Dornbrand, Family decision making on trial—Who decides for incompetent patients? *New England Journal of Medicine* 322 (1990): 1228–1232.

4. The Court and Nancy Cruzan, *Hastings Center Report,* January/February 1990, pp. 38–50.

5. R. Burck, Feeding, withdrawing, and withholding: Ethical perspectives, *Nutrition in Clinical Practice* 11 (1996): 243–253.

6. T. W. Mayo, Forgoing artificial nutrition and hydration: Legal and ethical considerations, *Nutrition in Clinical Practice* 11 (1996): 254–264.

7. *Advance Directives: The Role of Health Care Professionals* (Columbus, Ohio: Ross Products Division, Abbott Laboratories, 1996).

8. C. R. Gallagher-Allred, Managing ethical issues in nutrition support of terminally ill patients, *Nutrition in Clinical Practice* 6 (1991): 113–116.

9. G. Chapman, An oncology patient's choice to forgo novolitional nutrition support: Ethical considerations, *Nutrition in Clinical Practice* 11 (1996): 265–268.

10. J. W. Ely and coauthors, The physician's decision to use tube feedings: The role of the family, the living will, and the *Cruzan* decision, *Journal of the American Geriatrics Society* 40 (1992): 471–475.

11. H. Brody and M. B. Noel, Dietitians' role in decisions to withhold nutrition and hydration, *Journal of the American Dietetic Association* 91 (1991): 580–585.

12. Ely and coauthors, 1992.

13. A. M. Capron, The implications of the *Cruzan* decision for clinical nutrition teams, *Nutrition in Clinical Practice* 6 (1991): 89–94.

14. J. Hare, C. Pratt, and C. Nelson, Agreement between patients and their self-selected surrogates on difficult medical decisions, *Archives of Internal Medicine* 152 (1992): 1049–1054.

15. American Dietetic Association, Position of The American Dietetic Association: Legal and ethical issues in feeding permanently unconscious patients, *Journal of the American Dietetic Association* 95 (1995): 231–234; American Academy of Pediatrics Committee on Bioethics, Guidelines on forgoing life-sustaining medical treatment, *Pediatrics* 93 (1994): 532–536; A.S.P.E.N. Board of Directors, Ethical and legal issues in specialized nutrition support, *Journal of Parenteral and Enteral Nutrition* (supplement) 17 (1993): 50–52; American Dietetic Association, Position of The American Dietetic Association: Issues in feeding the terminally ill adult, *Journal of the American Dietetic Association* 92 (1992): 996–1005.

16. S. Edelstein and S. Anderson, Bioethics and dietetics: Education and attitudes, *Journal of the American Dietetic Association* 91 (1991): 546–548.

17. M. G. Wall and coauthors, Feeding the terminally ill: Dietitians' attitudes and beliefs, *Journal of the American Dietetic Association* 91 (1991): 549–552.

Chapter 25

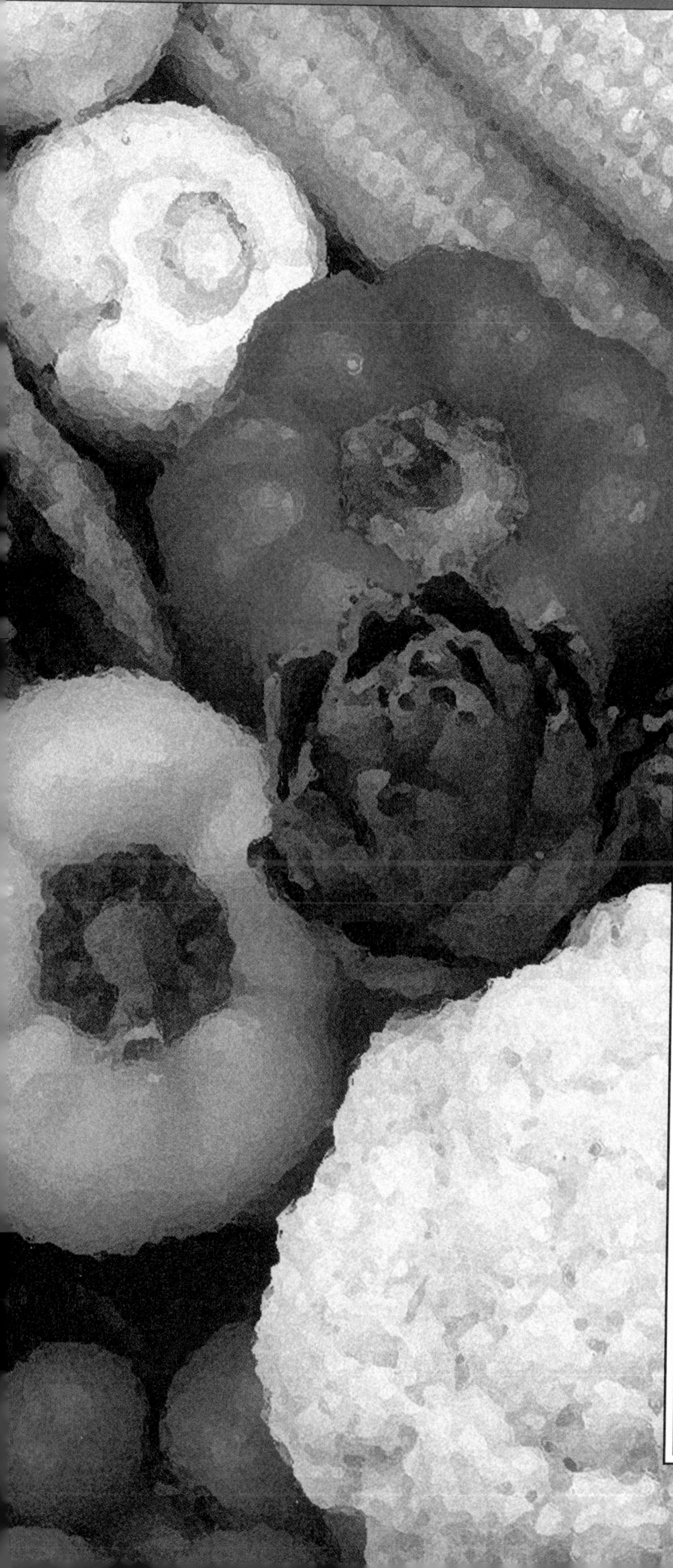

Nutrition and Severe Stress

CONTENTS

The Body's Response to Stress
  Metabolic Responses to Severe Stress
  Effects on Nutrition Status
  Effects on GI Tract Immune Function
  Secondary Effects of Stress and Illness on Nutrition Status
Nutrition Support during Stress
  Nutrient Needs
  Delivering Nutrients during Stress
HIGHLIGHT: **Food and Foodservice in the Hospital**

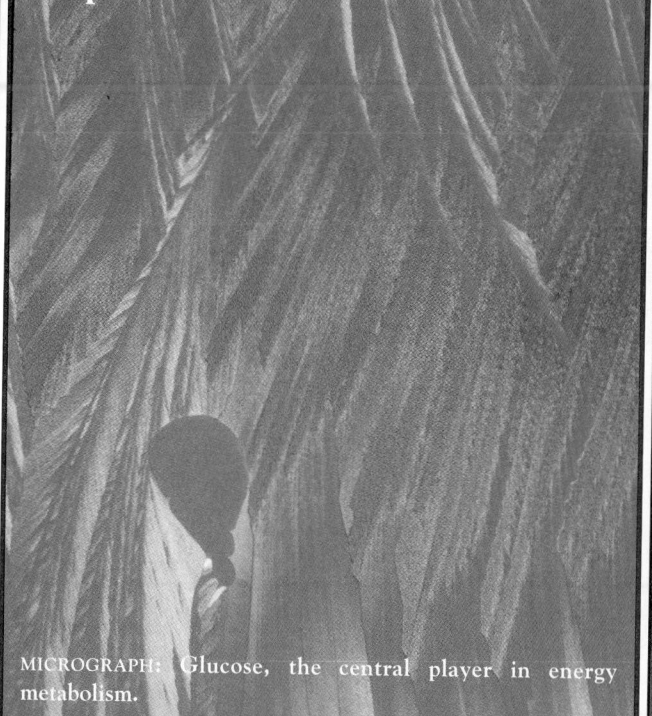

MICROGRAPH: Glucose, the central player in energy metabolism.

803

Reminder: Any threat to a person's well-being is a *stress*. Some stresses fall within the body's normal and healthy functioning and are known **physiological stresses**. Outside these limits, additional stresses imposed by disease or trauma are **pathological stresses**. The term **severe stresses** is used here to refer to pathological stresses that rapidly and markedly raise the body's metabolic rate and significantly upset its normal internal balance.

trauma: physical insult to the body that causes tissue damage including fractures, wounds, burns, or surgery.

Reminder: The *stress response* is an elaborate series of metabolic events orchestrated by the body in response to *stressors* such as severe infections, extensive surgery, major burns, serious or multiple fractures, and deep, penetrating wounds such as gunshot wounds, fistulas, and surgical incisions. These stressors lead to tissue injury or necrosis (death), inflammation, or shock.

inflammatory response: the changes that occur in tissues when they are injured by such forces as blows, wounds, foreign bodies (chemicals, microorganisms), heat, cold, electricity, or radiation.

The fluid containing plasma proteins, electrolytes, and immune factors that leaks out through the capillaries is called the **exudate**.

exudare = to sweat out

During an infection, the body is invaded by disease-causing microorganisms or viruses. An infection may remain localized in one area and form an abscess or granuloma, or it may enter the bloodstream and, thereby, the whole body. The presence of microorganisms or their poisonous products in the bloodstream is known as **sepsis** or **septicemia** (sep-tih-SEE-me-ah).

C hapters 21 and 22 described how diseases of the GI tract can compromise nutrition status by interfering with the intake, digestion, or absorption of nutrients. This chapter focuses on severe stresses that can alter nutrition status by markedly and rapidly raising the body's metabolic rate and upsetting its internal balances. Severe stresses include serious infections, major tissue damage, extensive surgery, and severe burns. Special attention to nutrition during severe stress can help preserve nutrition status and promote recovery.

The Body's Response to Stress

All illnesses can threaten the body and impair nutrition status to some extent, but the burden of severe stresses is exceptionally great. Such stresses require that the body employ complicated mechanisms to reestablish its balance. These mechanisms, which are collectively called the stress response, constitute an adaptation that is sustained for as long as is necessary or until the body can no longer sustain them and exhaustion leads to death.

METABOLIC RESPONSES TO SEVERE STRESS

In response to severe stresses, the body speeds up its metabolic rate (hypermetabolism) and mobilizes nutrients into glucose and amino acid pools, so that it can synthesize the special factors it needs to limit and repair damage and to regain homeostasis. These metabolic responses are mediated by immune, inflammatory, and hormonal factors.

The exact factors the body makes depends on the type of stress. Mending a broken bone requires different factors than does healing a wound or fighting an infection. Researchers are working to elucidate the complex and interrelated mechanisms of the stress response in order to find new approaches to promote recovery.

Immune System and Inflammatory Responses   The body's natural defense against pathogens—the immune system—enables the body to fight off infectious agents. The immune system defends the body so alertly and silently that most healthy people are unaware that thousands of microbes mount attacks against them every day. Occasionally, though, an infection succeeds in making a person ill, and the immune system must then mount a counterattack. Of all severe stresses, serious infections most intensely tax the immune system, and if the system fails, death may follow.

In other severe stresses, the immune system plays a key, although less obvious, role. Tissue damage renders the body vulnerable to invading organisms. The body's inflammatory response to tissue injury inactivates invaders, removes foreign particles, and repairs tissue damage. At the site of injury, the capillaries dilate and become more permeable, allowing blood, blood proteins, and immune system factors to flow into the injured area. The accumulation of fluid in the interstial space causes edema. Eventually, blood flow to the injured tissue slows, and clots form around the injured area, sealing it off from the rest of the body and limiting the spread of invaders. Meanwhile, immune system factors at the injury site begin to attack and neutralize the foreign substances. If the immune factors fail, the infection may remain localized and form an abscess or granuloma, or it may spread throughout the body. When infectious microorganisms or their poisonous by-products invade the bloodstream, sepsis develops. Critically ill people who develop sepsis may experience progressive failure of multiple organ systems. Such a combination is the most common cause of serious complications and death in critically ill people.

The immune and inflammatory responses to stressors result in redness, swelling, heat, and pain at the injury site. Body temperature, heart rate, and respiratory rate increase; blood concentrations of iron and zinc fall; and anorexia develops. All of these changes are believed to assist the immune system in fighting infection. In some responses, particularly if a bacterial infection is involved, white blood cell production increases. Among the hundreds of factors that mediate the body's complex response to inflammation are the *cytokines*, factors believed to contribute to the hypermetabolism, GI tract changes, anorexia, fever, and malaise that accompany the inflammatory response.[1]

Hormonal Factors   Hormonal changes characteristic of the immediate stress response drive catabolism by shifting the balance between insulin, which promotes the storage of carbohydrate and lipid and the synthesis of protein, and the counterregulatory hormones, which promote the breakdown of glycogen, the mobilization of fatty acids from lipids, and the synthesis of glucose from protein (see Table 25–1). As a result, the metabolic rate rises, and the body mobilizes energy stores and elevates blood glucose at the expense of protein tissue. Other

Reminder: An abscess is an accumulation of pus and may contain immune system cells and foreign bodies. Treatment involves draining the abscess.

Reminder: A granuloma is a granular growth that contains foreign bodies surrounded by immune system cells and covered with a fibrous coat; the body may retain live bacteria in the form of a granuloma for years without exhibiting symptoms of infection.

The changes that result from the activation of immune and inflammatory factors during stress are sometimes called the **systemic inflammatory response syndrome (SIRS)**

cytokines (SIGH-toe-kynes): immune system factors that help regulate the inflammatory response. During infections, the cytokine *interleukin-1* (in-ter-LOO-kin) causes fever-induced anorexia, the cytokine *cachetin* (ka-KEK-tin) also induces anorexia, and the cytokine *gamma-interferon* (in-ter-FEAR-on) induces fever and malaise.

Reminder: The metabolic breakdown of large molecules into smaller ones is *catabolism*. Catabolic reactions usually release energy.

counterregulatory hormones: hormones such as glucagon, cortisol, and catecholamines that oppose insulin's actions and promote catabolism.

Table 25–1
Hormonal Changes That Occur during Severe Stress

Hormone	Alteration	Metabolic Effect
Catecholamines	Increase	Glucagon release increases.
		Insulin-to-glucagon ratio decreases.[a]
		Glycogen breakdown increases.
		Glucose production from amino acids increases.
		Mobilization of free fatty acids increases.
Cortisol	Increases	Mobilization of free fatty acids increases.
		Glucose production from amino acids increases.
Glucagon	Increases	Insulin-to-glucagon ratio decreases.[a]
		Glucose production from amino acids increases.
		Glycogen breakdown increases.
		Storage of glucose, amino acids, and fatty acids decreases.
Antidiuretic hormone	Increases	Retention of water increases.
Aldosterone	Increases	Retention of sodium increases.

Note: These changes are part of the immediate stress response. As adaptation occurs and recovery is in progress, hormone levels gradually return to normal.
[a]The net effect of a decrease in the ratio of insulin to glucagon is that catabolism predominates.

The acute, or flow, phase of the stress response is the catabolic period immediately following the onset of stress. During the adaptive phase, the body adjusts to the stress to minimize losses. If adaptation succeeds, recovery follows. If adaptation fails, exhaustion follows.

Not all amino acids can be used to make glucose. The most important amino acids in glucose production are alanine and glutamine; they are synthesized in the body from the branched-chain amino acids.

Reminder: *Ketone bodies* are compounds formed during the incomplete oxidation of fatty acids.

hormones promote the retention of water and sodium and the excretion of potassium. With recovery, hormones gradually return to normal. To understand the impact of severe stress on nutrient stores, it is helpful to compare the body's response to simple fasting and severe stress.

Response to Simple Fasting   Fasting (see pp. 239–244) and severe stresses both require the body to use its stored carbohydrate and fat for energy and to mobilize amino acids to make glucose. The body adapts to simple starvation by reducing its use of glucose, thus conserving its vital proteins. The liver begins to produce an alternate energy source from fat—ketone bodies. At the same time, the metabolic rate and body temperature fall, reducing the body's need for energy from any source. The person feels fatigued and uses less energy.

Response to Severe Stress   In contrast to simple fasting, severe stress raises the metabolic rate for an extended time. Carbohydrate continues to be oxidized for energy, but despite high blood glucose levels, amino acids continue to be used for glucose synthesis. Fat metabolism increases as well, but the high insulin levels suppress the mobilization of fat from body stores. Plasma levels of essential fatty acids fall dramatically, and clinical signs of deficiency may develop in as few as 10 days.[2] Figure 25–1 illustrates the metabolic differences between simple fasting and severe stress.

Figure 25–1

Metabolic Responses to Fasting and Stress

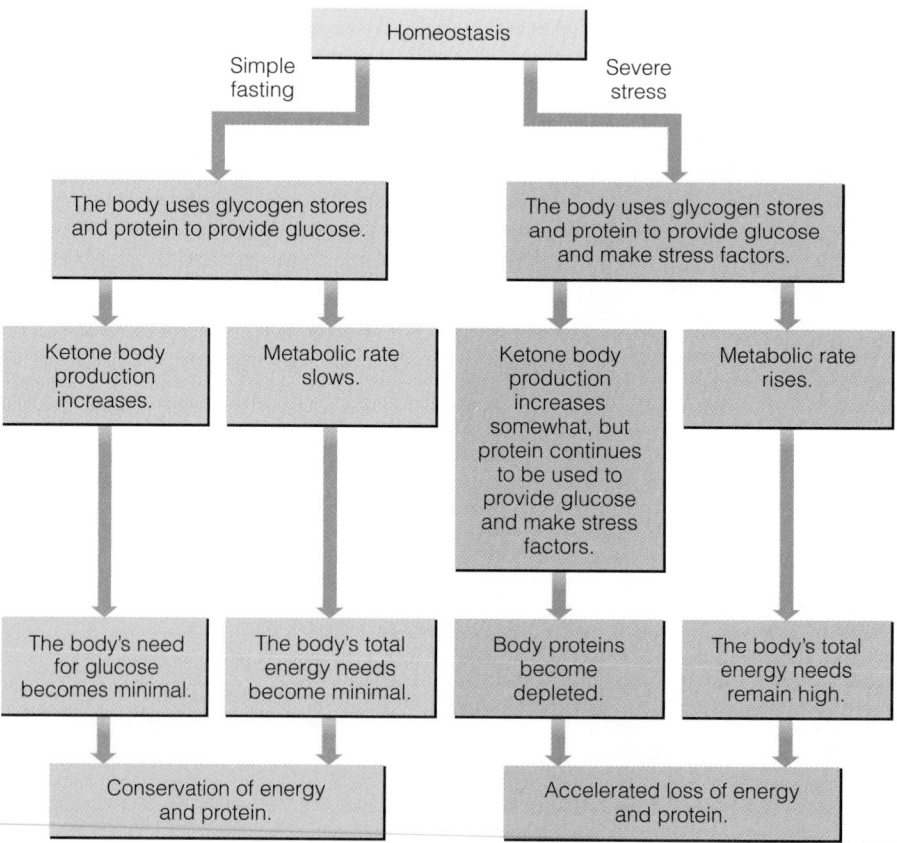

Generally, hypermetabolism peaks at about 3 to 4 days and subsides in about 7 to 10 days.[3] Clinical findings typical of the stress response—elevated blood glucose (hyperglycemia), negative nitrogen balance, elevated blood urea nitrogen (from protein catabolism), increased retention of fluid and sodium, and increased excretion of potassium—gradually return to normal as the stress resolves.

EFFECTS ON NUTRITION STATUS

The effects of hypermetabolic illnesses and protein-energy malnutrition (PEM) show astonishing similarities. Both deplete energy reserves, cause the breakdown of protein tissue, impair nutrient absorption, and tax the immune system.

Unlike glucose and fat, protein is not held in reserve in case the body needs it. All of the body's proteins are already in use as skeletal muscle, cell structures, enzymes, hormones, immune system factors, and other blood proteins and body components. During stress, the body needs extra protein to synthesize additional hormones to orchestrate metabolism, immune factors to fight infection, collagen to rebuild damaged tissue and bone, muscle cells to maintain the physical work of taxed organ systems, and many more vital tissue constituents. Without adequate protein, the body loses its ability to adapt, and it becomes vulnerable and defenseless.

Acute Malnutrition　In a previously healthy person, extreme or prolonged stress can trigger a dramatic and immediate form of acute malnutrition. The rerouting of nutrients to make stress response factors leaves the body unable to meet its regular protein and energy needs. The body is effectively "starved" for these nutrients. In addition, the body's organs and cells have not had time to adapt to conserving protein by using fat (ketone bodies) for energy. That adaptation is also made more difficult by stress. Providing adequate nutrition support to the client with acute malnutrition precipitated by stress is extremely difficult.

Chronic Malnutrition　People with chronic PEM do not have the nutrient reserves to successfully mount a stress response. They require immediate nutrition support and generally respond well when the stress is not too severe. The person's body has adapted to limited energy and protein intake over a prolonged period by conserving lean body mass to the greatest extent possible and depending on fat stores for energy.

Mixed Malnutrition　When the person with chronic malnutrition is faced with an extreme or prolonged stress, or when adequate nutrients are not provided, the person experiences the deficits of both conditions. Likewise, the person with acute malnutrition may progress to mixed malnutrition. Table 25–2 shows the clinical findings that distinguish the different forms of malnutrition.

Nutrient Absorption　Organs that undergo rapid cell replacement—such as the GI tract—are among the first to suffer the consequences of protein losses, whether they occur due to stress or to malnutrition. The intestinal microvilli gradually shrink and become nonfunctional; up to 90 percent of them can be lost.

Gastric Motility　Severe stress reduces blood flow to the GI tract and slows gastric motility, prohibiting the use of oral diets in the early poststress period. But

Figure 25–2

Stress, Malnutrition, and Immunity

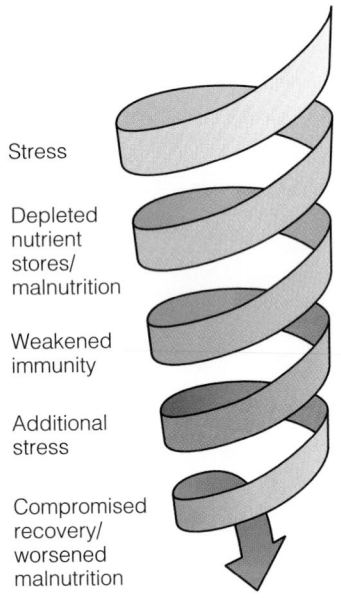

Stress

Depleted
nutrient
stores/
malnutrition

Weakened
immunity

Additional
stress

Compromised
recovery/
worsened
malnutrition

Regardless of where a person enters the spiral, the effects of stress, malnutrition, and impaired immunity can interact to worsen malnutrition and compromise recovery.

To understand the relationship of PEM to severe stress, think of energy stores and protein status as money in the bank. Severe stress can be compared to a major expense that arises unexpectedly. The person who has saved enough money can pay off the expense without too much difficulty. If more and more expenses arise, however, the money may run out. The person with little or no savings is unable to pay even a small expense.

Table 25–2

Clinical Findings Used to Distinguish Different Types of PEM

	Weight and Fat Stores	Blood Protein, Internal Organs, and Immune Function
Acute Malnutrition (Kwashiorkor)	Excessive or adequate	Depleted/compromised
Chronic Malnutrition (Marasmus)	Low/depleted	Adequate
Mixed Malnutrition	Low/depleted	Depleted/compromised

when people—even healthy people— are fed entirely by vein, their intestinal tracts undergo structural and functional changes.[4] Lack of enteral nutrients in the GI tract further contributes to reduced GI blood flow and reduced motility. Thus stress interferes with the person's ability to handle oral nutrients, and even though adequate nutrients are provided, the GI tract will have a compromised ability to absorb them. Consequently, PEM may develop or worsen, and the body may have difficulty providing the extra energy and protein it needs to fight the stress.

Appetite and Eating   As described earlier, immune factors involved in the stress response cause fever, malaise, and pain and interfere with appetite and eating, even when oral diets are possible. The location of an injury may also interfere with eating. A person with burned hands, for example, may be unable to hold eating utensils. A person with a surgical incision near the waist may find sitting up to eat uncomfortable.

Other GI Effects   Some severe stresses further impair GI tract function. Wounds or trauma to the GI tract, including surgical resections, can interfere with nutrient intake and aggravate malabsorption and nutrient losses.

Left unattended, PEM can interact with stress in a deadly cycle: stress worsens malnutrition, and malnutrition hinders the stress response (see Figure 25–2). Malnutrition renders the body vulnerable to infections and markedly interferes with the ability to recover.

EFFECTS ON GI TRACT IMMUNE FUNCTION

The significant role of the GI tract in preventing foreign invaders from entering the body has only recently received the attention it deserves. A protective coating of mucus lines the entire GI tract. The mucus contains antimicrobial chemicals and enzymes to destroy foreign bodies and forms a slippery coat that prevents invaders from attaching to the lining of the GI tract. To reach the intestine, invaders must also avoid destruction by the highly acidic contents of the stomach. Invaders that enter the intestine directly (through breaks in tissue) or avoid destruction by mucus or gastric acidity encounter other formidable obstacles in the intestinal tract.

Intestinal Barrier Function   Healthy intestinal villi are crowded close together, forming a physical barrier that prevents anything from passing between them. Damaged cells allow substances to cross the intestinal cells' membranes and enter the body.

Immune System Cells   Interspersed among the villi are mucus-secreting cells and lymph tissue that houses immune cells to fend off invaders. To appreciate the vast importance of the intestinal lymph tissue in fighting foreign invaders, consider that of all the body's immunologic-secreting cells, 70 to 80 percent of them are located in the intestine.[5]

Bacterial Flora   The large intestine also supports a bacterial population that inhibits the growth of harmful bacteria by competing with them for nutrients and space. The normal bacterial flora also produce short-chain fatty acids (see Highlight 22) that prevent harmful bacteria from sticking to the intestinal surface.

Bacterial Translocation   Conditions that compromise the GI tract's barrier, alter the normal bacterial flora, or compromise the function of the immune system may allow infectious agents to cross the intestinal barrier and enter the body—a process called translocation.[6] Table 25–3 lists conditions that may increase the likelihood of translocation; many of these conditions exist during severe stress or malnutrition. In small amounts, the translocation of infectious

Recall from Chapter 22 that disorders or drug therapies that significantly raise gastric pH may result in bacterial overgrowth and malabsorption.

translocation: the passage of infectious agents into the body through the intestinal tract.

Table 25–3

Conditions That Increase the Likelihood of Translocation

Altered structure and function of GI tract barrier
   Prolonged fasting or lack of enteral nutrients
   Injury to the GI tract
   Inflammatory responses
   Malnutrition
Changes in bacterial flora
   Lack of enteral nutrients
   Decreased GI tract motility
   Use of broad-spectrum antibiotics
Compromised function of immune factors
   Malnutrition
   Hypermetabolism

Source: Adapted from M. T. DeMeo, The role of enteral nutrition in maintaining the structural and functional integrity of the GI tract, in *Enteral Nutrition Support,* Report of the First Ross Conference on Enteral Devices, Ross Laboratories 1996, pp. 4–8.

agents may stimulate the immune system, but extensive translocation may cause serious infection and even death.

Research suggests that translocation may be a major factor in the development of sepsis and multiple organ failure.[7] Frequently, multiple organ failure does not occur until days or weeks after the initial stress. Regardless of the type of stress, the typical course of multiple organ failure is remarkably similar in all people, suggesting that common factors may be involved. People with multiple organ failure develop sepsis, and the first organs to fail are the lungs, followed by the liver and kidneys. Some of the infectious agents associated with multiple organ failure arise from the intestinal tract.[8] Clinical evidence to support a role for intestinal translocation as a primary factor, or even one of the factors, leading to sepsis and multiple organ failure following severe stress is lacking, and the theory remains unproven.[9] In practice, however, measures to support intestinal integrity including early enteral nutrition (described later) are widely accepted and utilized by clinicians.

SECONDARY EFFECTS OF STRESS AND ILLNESS ON NUTRITION STATUS

Some effects of stress or illness on nutrition status arise not from the stress itself, but rather from its consequences or treatment. A person suffering from anxiety and psychological stress associated with an injury, for example, may lose all interest in eating.

Immobility and Pressure Sores   Stresses often necessitate bed rest and immobility. Immobility further compromises nutritional health. Without the muscle tension and weight load incurred by normal activity, the muscles and bones are not stimulated to maintain themselves and begin to lose nitrogen and calcium, respectively. In prolonged immobilization, blood and urinary calcium may rise so high that calcium stones form in the bladder and kidneys.

Immobility, severe stress, and poor food intake are all associated with the development of pressure sores.[10] Pressure sores can form whenever there is constant pressure on the skin. The elderly and people who are unable to respond to pain or change body positions are at great risk for developing pressure sores. These sores can be extremely painful and are an open invitation to infections, which can further contribute to stress and tax nutrient stores.

Diagnostic Tests and Medical Procedures   Diagnostic tests and medical procedures may require special diets or no food by mouth in order to obtain accurate test results or to protect health. Such restrictions further interfere with a person's ability to receive adequate nourishment.

Nutrient-Drug Interactions   Drug therapy, critical in the treatment of many stresses and illnesses, may further tax nutrition status. When people who are severely stressed or malnourished are given multiple drugs, the likelihood of drug-nutrient interactions increases, and serious deficiencies may result. Furthermore, the intestinal changes associated with both stress and malnutrition can hinder the absorption of both drugs and nutrients.

Severe stresses and malnutrition can also interfere with the metabolism and excretion of drugs. Many drugs are transported in the blood bound to serum pro-

pressure sores: the breakdown of skin and underlying tissues due to constant pressure and lack of oxygen to the affected area; often called decubitus (dee-CUE-bih-tis) ulcers or bedsores.

  PRESCRIPTION PAD

Drugs used in the treatment of severe stresses may include:

- Analgesics
- Antidiarrheals
- Anti-infective agents
- Anti-inflammatory agents
- Antiulcer agents
- Immunosuppressants

See Appendix E for timing with meals and nutrition-related side effects.

teins such as albumin, and low serum albumin is a symptom of both stress and PEM. Without sufficient carriers, drugs may be slow to reach their sites of action. Once drugs do arrive at their target cells, the lack of carriers may delay the drugs' transport to the liver and kidneys, where many drugs are detoxified and excreted. Thus drugs may take a long time to work and then may remain active for a longer time, making side effects more likely.

In summary, severe stresses spark a series of hormonal and metabolic responses to reestablish balance. These changes demand energy and drain nutrient stores, which can lead a well-nourished body rapidly into PEM and send a malnourished body perilously close to death.

Nutrition Support during Stress

Following stress, the immediate concerns are to restore blood flow and maintain oxygen transport and to prevent or treat infection. Possible measures include giving transfusions, providing IV solutions to correct fluid and electrolyte imbalances, removing dead tissues, draining abscesses, and administering antibiotics. Nutrition support following stress helps to prevent acute malnutrition, preserve organ function, maintain immune defenses, and minimize nutrient losses—all of which aid the client's recovery. Restoring nutrient deficits before the hypermetabolism that initially accompanies stress subsides is difficult, however. Once hypermetabolism does subside, nutrition support can promote positive nitrogen balance and weight gain.

Nourishment must be introduced cautiously to the stressed person with PEM. If nutrients are introduced too rapidly, severe complications, including malabsorption, cardiac insufficiency, respiratory distress, congestive heart failure, convulsions, coma, and even death, can result. Collectively, these complications are called the refeeding syndrome.

NUTRIENT NEEDS

Health professionals caring for severely stressed individuals face a challenge. Providing enough nourishment, but not too much, is critical to recovery.

Fluids and Electrolytes People experiencing severe stress often lose fluids and electrolytes through bleeding, wounds, vomiting, diarrhea, and fever. To restore blood volume and prevent dehydration and electrolyte imbalances, the medical team must act quickly to stabilize the body's fluid and electrolyte balances.

The physician determines the person's fluid needs based on clinical measures such as blood pressure, heart rate, respiratory rate, urinary output, level of consciousness, and body temperature. Serum electrolytes are closely monitored and adjustments are made as necessary.

With catabolism, electrolytes normally concentrated in the intracellular fluids (potassium, phosphorus, magnesium, and calcium) rise and disrupt the body's chemical balances. Once hypermetabolism subsides, these intracellular electrolytes move into the cells along with glucose and amino acids to begin rebuilding tissue. Without careful attention to replacement, circulating levels of these electrolytes can plummet, resulting in life-threatening complications.

When a sudden drop in the blood volume disrupts the supply of oxygen to the tissues and the return of blood to the heart, shock results. Shock is a critical event that must be corrected immediately. Many severe stresses can lead to shock through massive bleeding or severe dehydration.

The removal of dead tissue resulting from burns and other wounds, called debridement (dee-BREED-ment), speeds healing and helps prevent infection.

Chapter 22 described dietary modifications beneficial in treating malabsorption. Dietary therapy for other organ system failures is described in later chapters: liver failure (Chapter 26), heart failure (Chapter 28), respiratory failure (Chapter 28), and kidney failure (Chapter 29).

refeeding syndrome: a set of physiologic and metabolic complications associated with reintroducing adequate nutrition too rapidly for a person with severe PEM. These complications can include malabsorption, cardiac insufficiency, respiratory distress, congestive heart failure, convulsions, coma, and possibly death.

Table 25–4

The Harris-Benedict Equation for Estimating Energy Needs

Harris-Benedict equation for estimating basal energy expenditure (BEE):[a]

Women:

$$BEE = 655 + (9.6 \times wt^b \text{ in } kg^c) + (1.7 \times ht \text{ in } cm^c) - (4.7 \times age \text{ in } yr)$$

Men:

$$BEE = 66 + (13.7 \times wt^b \text{ in } kg^c) + (5 \times ht \text{ in } cm^c) - (6.8 \times age \text{ in } yr)$$

Add to BEE for activity:

20% Sedentary

35% Moderately active

50% Active

Add to BEE for stress:

10–15% Uncomplicated elective surgery

20–40% Complicated surgery or fractures

50–100% Major burn

Add to BEE for fever (if present):

13% per degree centigrade over normal body temperature (37°C)[c]

Add to BEE to promote weight gain (if necessary):

5% if weight loss is moderate

10–15% if weight loss is severe

For people with a %IBW greater than 125, adjust the weight used in the BEE equation by following this equation:[d]

(Actual body weight − IBW) × 25%[e] + IBW = Adjusted body weight

[a]Basal metabolic rate (BMR, described on p. 262) and BEE express the same thing: basal energy need. The equation for BMR is traditionally used in physiology and fitness laboratories; that for BEE, in hospitals. The two equations yield slightly different results, each suitable for the purposes intended. Adjustments for activity used in the hospital differ from those on p. 264 for similar reasons. All are approximations; all require judgment in their application.
[b]Use actual body weight, not ideal body weight.
[c]See Appendix D for equations to convert pounds to kilograms, inches to centimeters, and degrees Fahrenheit to degrees centigrade.
[d]From J. M. Karkeck, Adjustment for obesity, *American Dietetic Association Renal Practice Group Newsletter*, Winter, 1984.
[e]Approximately 25 percent of body fat tissue is metabolically active.

Reminder: Indirect calorimetry is the estimation of energy output from measures of the amount of oxygen used and carbon dioxide eliminated.

Energy Energy needs during severe stress depend on both the type and severity of the stress, organ function, and the individual's metabolic state and nutrition status. Energy requirements may double for clients with severe burns, for example.[12] When measurements are carefully taken and cautiously interpreted, indirect calorimetry provides an accurate assessment of energy needs during severe stress.[11] Many facilities lack the equipment necessary to perform this measurement, however, so clinicians often rely on various other estimates of energy needs. The Harris-Benedict equation shown in Table 25–4 is frequently used.* Alternatively, some clinicians simply provide minimally stressed clients

*Several studies suggest that the Harris-Benedict equation overestimates energy needs during severe stress.

with 25 to 30 nonprotein kcalories per kilogram of body weight per day. (Note: kcalories from protein are not counted as meeting part of the energy needs when this formula is used.) The box on p. 814 shows how to estimate energy and protein needs during severe stress. Clinical judgment and continual monitoring of nutrition status are always necessary to confirm that energy needs are being met without overfeeding.

Supplying too much energy contributes to an elevated metabolic rate, which increases the use of oxygen and the production of carbon dioxide. Then the heart and lung muscles, already working hard as a consequence of stress, must work even harder to keep the body's gases in balance. If these vital organs are weakened by malnutrition, they may not be able to respond to the additional insult. Supplying too little energy compromises recovery.

Fever, a frequent consequence of stress, is associated with an elevated basal metabolic rate (BMR) of approximately 13 percent for each degree centigrade (7 percent for each degree Fahrenheit) that the temperature rises above normal (98.6° Fahrenheit; 37° centigrade). Thus a person with a fever of 4 degrees (Fahrenheit)—that is, a temperature of 102.6°F—will have a BMR that is running about a fourth faster than normal (4 degrees × 7 percent = 28 percent). Since the BMR requires some 1000 to 2000 kcalories a day (recall from Chapter 8), this person may need an additional 300 to 600 kcalories a day.

Reports suggest that people who are obese and mildly to moderately stressed may be able to attain positive nitrogen balance and recover while receiving about half of their estimated energy needs, provided that protein needs are met.[13] Obese people who are severely stressed, however, need no less energy during the hypermetabolic phase than people of normal weight.[14] Energy restriction is not appropriate, and weight-loss efforts should wait until recovery is well under way.

Protein   The greater the stress, the more body protein is broken down (up to the limit of the body's capabilities), the more nitrogen is excreted in the urine, and the greater the need for protein. Only after the hypermetabolic stage of stress subsides can negative nitrogen balance be fully corrected. Clinicians can use nitrogen balance studies to determine how much dietary protein the stressed person needs. Alternatively, they can estimate protein needs by providing 1 to 2 grams of protein per kilogram of body weight per day. People with severe burns may require up to 3 grams of protein per kilogram of body weight per day.[15] As always, adequate energy from nonprotein kcalories is necessary to spare protein use for energy.

Amino Acids   In recent years, increasing attention has been placed on supplying higher amounts of specific amino acids during stress, rather than simply supplying protein. Research has been far from conclusive, but some studies suggest that supplementing branched-chain amino acids (leucine, isoleucine, and valine) may minimize negative nitrogen balance.

Another amino acid receiving wide attention in relation to stress is glutamine. As Highlight 22 described, glutamine provides fuel for intestinal cells and helps maintain their structure and function. During stress, glutamine may become a conditionally essential amino acid. Most enteral and parenteral formulas lack glutamine because it is unstable in solution. Studies to determine whether supplemental glutamine helps to minimize negative nitrogen balance,

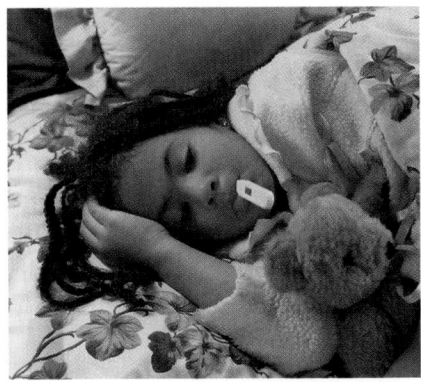

The energy needs of a child with a fever (a mild stress) are elevated, but not nearly as high as those of a person with extensive burns (a severe stress).

A *fever* is an elevation of body temperature above normal. A person who is *febrile* (FEE-brile) has a fever; *afebrile* (AY-fee-brile) means "without fever."

Reminder: Branched-chain amino acids and glutamine participate in gluconeogenesis. Glutamine and arginine may help augment the immune system.

How to Estimate Energy and Protein Needs Following Severe Stress

Bernadette is a 39-year-old female, who is 5 feet 3 inches tall and weighs 130 pounds. She recently underwent extensive surgery and currently has a temperature of 101°F. Her energy needs can be estimated using the Harris-Benedict equation as follows:

$$\text{Weight in kilograms} = 130 \text{ lb} \div 2.2 \text{ kg} = 59 \text{ kg.}$$

$$\text{Height in centimeters} = 63 \text{ in} \times 2.54 \text{ cm} = 160 \text{ cm.}$$

$$\text{BEE} = 655 + (9.6 \times \text{wt in kg}) + (1.7 \times \text{ht in cm}) - (4.7 \times \text{age in yr}).$$

$$655 + (9.6 \times 59 \text{ kg}) + (1.7 \times 160 \text{ cm}) - (4.7 \times 39) = 655 + 566 + 272 - 183 = 1310 \text{ kcal.}$$

Next add 20–40% × BEE for surgery (see Table 25–4 on p. 812):

$$1310 \text{ kcal} \times 20\% = 262 \text{ kcal.}$$

$$1310 \text{ kcal} \times 40\% = 524 \text{ kcal.}$$

$$1310 + 262 = 1572 \text{ kcal.}$$

$$1310 + 524 = 1834 \text{ kcal.}$$

Bernadette needs between 1572 and 1834 kcalories to meet her BEE and additional energy needs due to surgery.

To determine additional energy needs for fever, you must first convert degrees Fahrenheit to degrees centigrade (see Appendix D):

$$°C = \tfrac{5}{9}(°F - 32°).$$

$$°C = \tfrac{5}{9}(101° - 32°) = \tfrac{5}{9}(69°) = 38°C.$$

Normal body temperature is 37°C, so Bernadette has a body temperature elevation of 1°C.

To determine the percentage of the BEE needed due to fever:

$$1° \times 13\% = 13\%.$$

Add 13% BEE for fever:

$$1310 \times 13\% = 170 \text{ kcal.}$$

Add fever needs to energy needs:

$$1572 \text{ kcal} + 170 \text{ kcal} = 1742 \text{ kcal.}$$

$$1834 \text{ kcal} + 170 \text{ kcal} = 2004 \text{ kcal.}$$

Bernadette's estimated energy needs range from about 1750 to 2000 kcalories; clinicians monitor weight changes to determine if actual needs are higher or lower. Her energy needs will change as stress resolves.

Protein needs for Bernadette can be estimated at 1 to 2 grams of protein per kilogram of body weight per day. Use her weight of 59 kilograms to make the calculation:

$$59 \text{ kg} \times 1 \text{ g/kg} = 59 \text{ g protein.}$$

$$59 \text{ kg} \times 2 \text{ g/kg} = 118 \text{ g protein.}$$

Bernadette needs an estimated 59 to 118 grams of protein daily. Clinicians can monitor serum proteins (see Chapter 16) or use nitrogen balance studies to determine if the estimate is meeting actual protein needs.

protect the structure and function of the intestinal tract, and enhance the immune system have produced promising, yet inconclusive results.[16] Whether these effects can prevent translocation also remains to be proven.

Other nitrogen-containing substances, including arginine and nucleotides, may be important following severe stress. Studies suggest that supplemental arginine may help minimize negative nitrogen balance, improve wound healing, and stimulate the immune system. Nucleotides may help improve the function of certain immune cells. Studies are sparse, however, and their results have been variable.

Carbohydrate and Fat   Nonprotein energy sources spare protein, so the amount of carbohydrate and fat to recommend has ramifications for stressed people. Carbohydrate provides a readily usable source of energy, but the body can only metabolize a fixed amount (about 500 grams per day) of glucose during stress. Excess glucose may contribute to hyperglycemia and its consequences.[17] Fat provides essential fatty acids and energy, but given in excess, it can also tax metabolic functions and hamper immune responses. Clinicians often supply nonprotein kcalories through a mixture of 70 to 75 percent glucose and 25 to 30 percent lipids.[18] For clients with burns, restricting fat further (15 to 20 percent of the nonprotein kcalories) appears to be beneficial.

Fatty Acids   Intravenous lipid emulsions and enteral formulas are rich sources of omega-6 fatty acids. When given in excess of essential fatty acid requirements, however, omega-6 fatty acids may impair immune function and, therefore, may be inappropriate for severely stressed clients.[19] Alternate lipid sources such as fish oils (a rich source of omega-3 fatty acids) are currently under investigation. Triglycerides chemically modified to contain both long- and medium-chain fatty acids may also be advantageous during stress.[20] Highlight 22 described short-chain fatty acids and their potential benefits.

Micronutrients   Vitamin and mineral needs during stress are highly variable, and specific requirements are unknown. The need for many B vitamins increases when energy and protein intakes increase. Some micronutrients act as cofactors in the many metabolic reactions that are occurring, so their levels dwindle quickly. Other micronutrients play specific roles in healing wounds and mending broken bones. Levels of antioxidant nutrients fall, and although research is lacking, supplementing these nutrients is believed to be of value.[21] Other vitamins and minerals are frequently supplemented at levels above the RDA as well.

Stress Formulas   Clinicians eager to improve a client's outcome often rely on enteral formulas designed to meet nutrient needs during stress. Many such formulas are high in kcalories and protein. Some contain extra vitamins A and C, zinc, and other nutrients designed to promote wound healing. Formulas designed to preserve immune function often contain added glutamine, arginine, nucleotides, and omega-3 fatty acids. Although such formulas appear to be beneficial for specific situations, further research is necessary to determine their impact on recovery.[22]

Growth Hormone and Insulinlike Growth Factor   Researchers have begun to study nondietary factors that might improve nitrogen balance and lessen the

nucleotides: nitrogen-containing components of RNA and DNA. Nucleotides can be synthesized in the body and therefore are not essential in the diets of healthy individuals. In severely stressed individuals, however, a dietary source may be beneficial.

Nutrition Assessment Checklist
For People with Swallowing Disorders

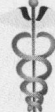

Medical Use the medical record to determine the degree and type of stress and to help estimate prestress nutrition status.

Drug Assess the client's drug history for drug-nutrient interactions that might alter nutrient needs.

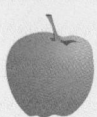

Nutrient Intake Calculate nutrient intake from parenteral and enteral formulas and oral diets to determine if intake is meeting calculated needs. If not, investigate the cause and take corrective actions, when possible. For severely stressed clients, indirect calorimetry may provide a more accurate assessment of energy needs. For clients on oral diets, a careful history of food preferences will be invaluable in encouraging adequate oral intake.

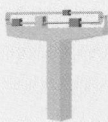

Anthropometric Interpret anthropometrics cautiously in the immediate poststress period. Weights may reflect the infusion of fluids or edema and can be deceptively high. The location of injuries may make anthropometric measurements impossible.

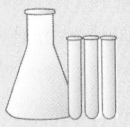

Laboratory Anticipate low serum protein in stressed clients, especially those with burns or severe wounds. (Remember that plasma proteins leak through the capillaries to the injury site.) Use nitrogen balance studies for a more accurate assessment of protein needs for severely stressed clients when necessary. Check blood glucose at regular intervals and treat hyperglycemia according to the hospital's protocol or physician's orders. Monitor electrolytes to replace losses immediately after stress and to prevent metabolic complications once hypermetabolism subsides.

Physical Check for physical signs of nutrient deficiencies, energy level, and emotional state. Regular assessment of blood pressure, pulse, and intake and output records can help prevent dehydration or overhydration.

impact of severe stress on the host. Highlight 22 described two such factors, growth hormone and insulinlike growth factor-1 (IGF-1), which stimulate the growth of intestinal cells. Although research is limited, growth hormone has been shown to improve nitrogen balance in both animals and people.[23] Similarly, IGF-1 improves nitrogen balance in animals.[24]

DELIVERING NUTRIENTS DURING STRESS

Selecting the appropriate amounts and types of nutrients to help people recover from stress is only part of diet therapy. Just as important is supplying nutrients in a form that best serves the body's ability to recover.

Oral Diets Well-nourished clients who are expected to eat within a few days following a mild-to-moderate stress receive simple IV solutions to maintain fluid and electrolyte balances and provide minimal kcalories. Once GI motility returns, they begin an oral diet that often progresses from clear liquids to full liquids and on to soft and then regular foods as tolerated (see Chapter 22). Highlight 25 describes how foods are prepared and delivered to meet clients' needs while hospitalized.

Case Study Journalist with a Third-Degree Burn

Mr. Sampson, a 48-year-old journalist, has been admitted to the emergency room. He suffered a severe burn covering over 40 percent of his body when he was trapped in a building fire. His height on admission was 6 feet, and he weighed 175 pounds. The physician ordered lab work, including serum proteins; the results are not back yet.

Identify Mr. Sampson's immediate postinjury needs. How can these needs be met?

Do you have enough information to determine Mr. Sampson's preinjury, preburn nutrition status? If not, what information would be useful? Is information about preburn nutrition status important in this case? Why or why not?

Considering Mr. Sampson's condition, what problems might the dietitian encounter in getting information from him about his preburn nutrition status?

Calculate Mr. Sampson's energy and protein needs to support burn healing (use 2 × the BEE for energy and 2 to 3 grams of protein per kilogram of body weight). What other nutrients must be considered?

Describe the possible benefits of early enteral nutrition to Mr. Sampson. How might these benefits be particularly important following a severe burn injury?

Specialized Nutrition Support   People with severe malnutrition, those who undergo severe stresses, and those who are not expected to be able to eat within 10 days benefit from parenteral nutrition or tube feedings. Oral or gastric feedings have to wait until gastric motility is restored to prevent abdominal distention, nausea, vomiting, and the possible aspiration of foods or formula into the lungs. Peristalsis returns more quickly to the small intestine than to the stomach, however, and feeding formula directly into the small intestine through a tube is not only possible, but provides advantages over parenteral nutrition.[25] Early feeding (initiated within about 36 hours following stress) stimulates intestinal blood flow, function, and adaptation and may minimize hypermetabolism and help prevent translocation. Most significantly, however, early enteral feeding improves recovery following stress by reducing septic complications.[26] Early enteral feeding following major trauma, head injuries, extensive burns, and surgery improves clinical outcomes. Early enteral feedings are not possible in cases where blood flow to the intestine is severely disrupted, however. Additionally, some clients may need both enteral feedings and parenteral nutrition until they are able to meet all nutrient needs orally.

Once hypermetabolism subsides and oral feeding is possible, clients can begin to receive enteral formulas or table foods. Chapters 23 and 24 described the different ways that clients can be weaned from tube feedings or parenteral nutrition. The box on p. 757 described ways to encourage oral intake. The nutrition assessment checklist summarizes the important information necessary to monitor the nutrition care of stressed clients. The accompanying case study of a client with burns tests your knowledge of nutrition and severe stress.

The stresses of surgery, infections, and burns can place tremendous demands on the body. The body uses all of its resources to fight the battle to survive and regain health. Recovery depends, in part, on the body's receiving the energy and nutrients required to mount a defense, repair damaged tissues, and replenish nutrient reserves. The next chapter describes the ways liver diseases affect nutrition status.

Study Questions

1. What is the stress response, and what does it achieve?
2. How do immune system factors and hormones mediate the stress response?
3. How do acute and chronic PEM relate to stress? Describe the effect of nutrition status on the body's ability to respond to stress. How can stress rapidly lead to PEM?
4. How do stress and PEM affect vital organ systems, gastric motility, and GI tract absorptive and immune functions?
5. Describe how nutrient needs change during severe stress. Describe precautions that must be taken when feeding the acutely or chronically malnourished person with stress.
6. Why might enteral nutrition be preferable to parenteral nutrition after a severe stress? Why can enteral nutrients be delivered by tube into the small intestine but not be taken by mouth in the early poststress period? When are enteral feedings inappropriate?

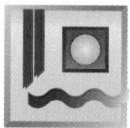 # Clinical Applications

1. Returning to Bernadette from the box on p. 814, recalculate her energy needs using the estimate of 25 to 30 nonprotein kcalories per kilogram of body weight per day. Now add the kcalories to meet protein needs. Compare these results with those obtained using the Harris-Benedict equation. Are the estimates similar?
2. Assuming that Bernadette can tolerate an intact enteral formula, find at least three formulas in Appendix K that meet her energy and protein needs and supply at least 100 percent of the RDA for vitamins and minerals.
3. Susan Griff is a 28-year-old woman admitted to the hospital following a car accident in which she broke several bones, ruptured a portion of her small intestine, and suffered a severe burn. Aside from the nutrient demands imposed by these stresses, describe how the following factors can impair her nutrition status:

- Susan's injuries are painful.
- Susan's medications cause extreme drowsiness.
- Susan is depressed.
- Susan is often out of her room for X rays and other diagnostic tests when her food trays arrive.
- Susan's food intake is often restricted for diagnostic tests she will be receiving.

How might these problems be resolved to improve Susan's ability to eat?

Notes

1. R. G. Barton, Nutrition support in critical illness, *Nutrition in Clinical Practice* 9 (1994): 127–139.
2. Barton, 1994.
3. J. D. Anderson, F. A. Moore, and E. E. Moore, Enteral feeding in the critically injured patient, *Nutrition in Clinical Practice* 7 (1992): 117–122.
4. A. L. Buchman and coauthors, Parenteral nutrition is associated with intestinal morphologic and functional changes in humans, *Journal of Parenteral and Enteral Nutrition* 19 (1995): 453–460.
5. P. Brandtzaeg and coauthors, Immunobiology and immunopathology of human gut mucosa: Humoral immunity and intraepithelial lymphocytes, *Gastroenterology* 97 (1989): 1562–1584.
6. M. T. DeMeo, The role of enteral nutrition in maintaining the structural and functional integrity of the gastrointestinal tract, in *Enteral Nutrition Support,* Report of the First Ross Conference on Enteral Devices, Ross Laboratories, 1996, pp. 4–8.
7. DeMeo, 1996; E. V. Shronts, Enteral versus parenteral nutrition: A clinical review, *Support Line,* June 1996, pp. 10–13; K. A. Kudsk, Clinical applications of enteral nutrition, *Nutrition in Clinical Practice* 9 (1994): 165–171.
8. Shronts, 1996.

9. T. O. Lipman, Bacterial translocation and enteral nutrition in humans: An outsider looks in, *Journal of Parenteral and Enteral Nutrition* 19 (1995): 156–165.

10. B. J. Braden, Using the Braden Scale for predicting pressure sore risk, *Support Line*, August 1996, pp. 14–17.

11. C. Porter and N. H. Cohen, Indirect calorimetry in critically ill patients: Role of the clinical dietitian in interpreting results, *Journal of the American Dietetic Association* 96 (1996): 49–54.

12. W. W. Souba, Nutritional support, *New England Journal of Medicine* 336 (1997): 41–48.

13. J. C. Burge and coauthors, Efficacy of hypocaloric total parenteral nutrition in hospitalized obese patients: A prospective, double-blind randomized trial, *Journal of Parenteral and Enteral Nutrition* 18 (1994): 203–207.

14. P. Amato and coauthors, Formulaic methods of estimating calorie requirements in mechanically ventilated obese patients: A reappraisal, *Nutrition in Clinical Practice* 10 (1995): 229–232.

15. D. J. Rodriguez, Nutrition in major burn patients: State of the art, *Support Line*, August 1995, pp. 1–8.

16. T. R. Ziegler, Glutamine supplementation in catabolic illness, *American Journal of Clinical Nutrition* 64 (1996): 645–647.

17. D. K. Rosmarin, G. M. Wardlaw, and J. Mirtallo, Hyperglycemia associated with high, continuous infusion rates of total parenteral nutrition dextrose, *Nutrition in Clinical Practice* 11 (1996): 151–156, A.S.P.E.N. Board of Directors, Guidelines for the use of total parenteral nutrition in adult and pediatric patients, *Journal of Parenteral and Enteral Nutrition* (supplement) 17 (1993): 21.

18. M. M. Gottschlich, Selection of optimal lipid sources in enteral and parenteral nutrition, *Nutrition in Clinical Practice* 7 (1992): 152–165; R. H. Bower, Nutritional and metabolic support of critically ill patients, *Journal of Parenteral and Enteral Nutrition* (supplement) 14 (1990): 257–259; G. L. Blackburn, In search of the "preferred fuel," *Nutrition in Clinical Practice* 4 (1989): 3–5; F. Negro and F. Cerra, Nutritional monitoring in the ICU: Rational and practical application, *Critical Care Clinics* 4 (1988): 34–47.

19. A. Hyltander, R. Sandström, and K. Lundholm, Metabolic effects of structured triglycerides in humans, *Nutrition in Clinical Practice* 10 (1995): 91–97.

20. Hyltander, Sandström, and Lundholm, 1995; E. Pscheidi and coauthors, Effects of chemically defined structured lipid emulsions on reticuloendothelial system function and morphology of liver and lung in a continuous low-dose endotoxin rat model, *Journal of Parenteral and Enteral Nutrition* 19 (1994): 33–40.

21. V. Sardesai, Role of antioxidants in health maintenance, *Nutrition in Clinical Practice* 10 (1995): 19–25.

22. R. G. Barton, Immune-enhancing enteral formulas: Are they beneficial in critically ill patients? *Nutrition in Clinical Practice* 12 (1997): 51–62.

23. K. Takagi and coauthors, Recombinant human growth hormone and protein metabolism of burned rats and esophagectomized patients, *Nutrition* 11 (1995): 22–26.

24. T. Inaba and coauthors, Effects of growth hormone and insulin-like growth factor-1 (IGF-1) treatments on the nitrogen metabolism and hepatic IGF-1–messenger RNA expression in postoperative parenterally fed rats, *Journal of Parenteral and Enteral Nutrition* 20 (1996): 325–331.

25. Souba, 1997; Shronts, 1996; Kudsk, 1994.

26. K. A. Kudsk, Immunologic support: Enteral vs parenteral feeding, in *Enteral Nutrition Support*, Report of the First Ross Conference on Enteral Devices, Ross Laboratories 1996, pp. 70–74.

Food and Foodservice in the Hospital

People who suffer severe stresses, as well as many others, require a level of care that necessitates hospitalization. These people often have illnesses that interfere with appetite either directly or through the psychological stress of the illness or the hospitalization itself. The hospital's dietary department, under the direction of management dietitians and foodservice managers, faces a challenge in planning, producing, and delivering meals designed to accommodate dozens of special diets and food preferences. This highlight explores the problems health care professionals must resolve when feeding clients in the hospital and describes how hospital foodservice systems work. Although this discussion focuses on hospitals, much of the discussion applies to any health care facility that serves meals to large groups of people, including nursing homes, assisted living centers, and residential mental health care facilities. While people in hospitals may eat poorly, they can make up for nutrient deficits by eating well when they return home. The resident of a long-term care facility does not have this option. For this reason, dietary departments in long-term care facilities must make even greater efforts to ensure that their clients receive nutritious and appealing foods.

THE CLIENT'S PERSPECTIVE

What comes to mind when you see or hear the words "hospital food"? What are your own experiences with hospital food or the experiences of someone close to you? Viewing hospital food from a client's perspective will add to your understanding of nutrition care.

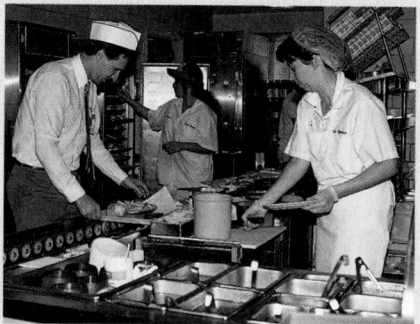

Dietary departments prepare foods to accommodate dozens of special diets and hundreds of food preferences.

Most people generally look forward to eating, and in the hospital, eating may become even more enjoyable than usual, for it offers clients familiarity in an otherwise strange environment. It is also one of the few experiences in the hospital where clients have a choice. Consider that clients usually cannot choose when they will receive tests, how much blood will be drawn, what nurse will care for them, or what time they will have surgery. But they usually can select their meals, and they can also exercise some control: they can eat or refuse to eat!

Clients may complain about hospital food. Complaining may have little to do with the food itself, but serves instead as a way to vent fear, frustration, anger, and physical pain. Clients need opportunities to express their feelings, and often you may find that a problem can be resolved simply by listening and providing emotional support.[1] Actual food problems need to be corrected by the dietary department as soon as possible.

Problems with foodservice unrelated to a client's physical or mental state can interfere with appetite. For one, the hospital does not cook food the same way a client does at home—a considerable problem when the client must eat three meals a day for many days in the hospital. Unfortunately, hot foods may not be hot and cold foods may not be cold by the time they arrive in the client's room. In addition, the client receives meals at specified times regardless of hunger and often must eat without companionship in bed, which can be more of a chore than a pleasurable experience. Meals may be unwelcome if they follow painful treatments. Food is so important to most people that a bad experience with it in the hospital can make both the client and those who work with the client agitated and angry.

All of this is not to say that every person in the hospital has a problem with meals. The majority of clients will eat adequate amounts of food, even though they complain about it. If their intakes decrease somewhat, the deficit will be easy to correct once they are at home eating familiar foods.

Suggestions for helping people to eat were provided in the box on p. 757. In some cases, the solution to a problem can be handled directly by the person caring for the client. In other cases, the dietary department must be contacted to solve a food-related problem. Understanding how the foodservice system works will help you deal with problems more efficiently.

HOW FOODSERVICE SYSTEMS WORK

The responsibility of budgeting, planning, preparing, and serving food in

Figure H25–1

Sample Lunch Menus

Lunch

REGULAR   **SUNDAY**

Meats
Baked chicken♥   Fried fish
Hamburger on bun with chips
(with lettuce and tomato)

Starchy Vegetables
Cornbread dressing   Parsleyed potatoes♥

Vegetables
Baby carrots♥   Stewed tomatoes

Soup/Salad/Juice   **Dressings**
Coleslaw   French
Clam chowder   Thousand Island
Gelatin   Italian
Tossed salad♥   Diet Thousand Island♥

Desserts
Apple pie   Butterscotch pudding
Fresh fruit♥

Breads
Dinner roll   Bran bread♥
White bread   Crackers
Wheat bread

Beverages & Condiments
Coffee   Sugar
Decaf. coffee   Sugar substitute
Hot tea   Herb seasoning
Decaf. hot tea   Creamer
Iced tea   Lemon
Whole milk   Mustard
Buttermilk   Mayonnaise
2% milk   Catsup
Skim milk♥   Margarine
Chocolate milk

PLEASE DO NOT LEAVE MENU ON THE TRAY

NAME _____ ROOM _____

Lunch

SOFT/BLAND/LOW RESIDUE   **SUNDAY**

Meats
Baked chicken   Baked fish (cod)
Hamburger on bun

Starchy Vegetables
Rice   Boiled potatoes

Vegetables
Baby carrots   Green beans

Soup/Salad/Juice   **Dressings**
Gelatin   Mayonnaise
Lemonade   Catsup
Tomato soup

Desserts
Apple pie   Pears

Breads
Dinner roll   Crackers
White bread

Beverages & Condiments
Decaf. coffee   Sugar
Decaf. hot tea   Sugar substitute
Decaf. iced tea   Creamer
Hot chocolate   Lemon
Whole milk   Margarine
2% milk
Buttermilk
Skim milk

NO PEPPER
PLEASE DO NOT LEAVE MENU ON TRAY

NAME _____ ROOM _____

Lunch

KCALORIE RESTRICTED, DIABETIC
1200 CALORIES   **SUNDAY**

LF = Low Fat   LSLF = Low Sodium, Low Fat

Meat Exchange (Select _1_)
LSLF Baked chicken (2 oz)   LSLF Baked fish (2 oz)
LSLF Hamburger on bun (with lettuce and
tomato, 2 oz meat) omit 2 starches

Starch Exchange (Select _1_)
Clam chowder (1 c)   LF Dinner roll (1)
LSLF Rice (1/3 c)   White bread (1 slice)
LSLF Boiled potatoes (1/2 c) Wheat bread (1 slice)
Angel food cake   Bran bread (1 slice)
(1" slice)   Crackers (6)

Vegetable Exchange (Select _2_)
LSLF Baby carrots   LSLF Green beans
(1/2 c)   (1/2 c)

Fruit Exchange (Select _1_)
Diet pears (1/2 c)   Fresh fruit

Milk Exchange (Select _1_)
Whole milk (1 c) omit 2 fats   Buttermilk (1 c)
2% milk (1 c) omit 1 fat   Skim milk (1 c)

Fat Exchange (Select _1_)
Margarine (1 tsp)   Creamer (1 = 1/2 fat)
Diet mayonnaise (1/2 oz)

Calorie-free Foods
Coffee   LSLF Coleslaw (1/2 c)
Decaf. coffee   Tossed salad (1 c)
Hot tea   Diet gelatin (1/2 c)
Decaf. hot tea   Diet French
Iced tea   Diet Thousand Island
Sugar substitute   Diet Italian
Lemon   Mustard
Herb seasoning   Diet catsup

PLEASE DO NOT LEAVE MENU ON THE TRAY

NAME _____ ROOM _____

People on regular diets select the foods of their choice. The regular menu may also be used for high-kcalorie, high-protein diets. The menu items marked with a heart guide people in selecting foods that are lower in fat, cholesterol, sodium, and caffeine or higher in fiber than other menu choices.

Foods for soft/bland/low-residue diets are similar to those for regular diets. Foods from the regular menu that are not appropriate have been eliminated from the menu, and substitutes have been made. For clients on bland diets, decaffeinated coffee and tea would be crossed off the menu.

For kcalorie-restricted and diabetic diets, the number of exchanges allowed is written on the menu beforehand. (This example uses a 1200-kcalorie diet.) Note that the meat exchange is written in 2-ounce portions so that 1 serving = 2 exchanges. (Chapter 17 describes the exchange system.)

the hospital rests with either a chief administrative dietitian or a foodservice manager. In some hospitals, foodservice companies from outside the hospital perform these duties.

Clinical dietitians work directly with clients to assess their nutrition status, plan appropriate diets, and provide nutrition education. In some hospitals, dietetic techni-

cians assist dietitians in both administrative and clinical responsibilities. Other dietary employees include clerks, aides, cooks, porters, and other assistants. Keep in mind that only dietitians have extensive formal training in nutrition. Other dietary employees do not have such training, and their ability to interpret diet orders or

provide accurate information may be limited.

Menu Procedures

Most hospitals provide menus from which clients can select their meals. A client who must follow a special diet receives menus that list only foods specified in the hospital's diet

821

Figure H25–1

(continued)

Lunch

LOW-FAT/LOW CHOLESTEROL/
CARDIAC   **SUNDAY**

LF = Low Fat   LSLF = Low Sodium, Low Fat

Meats

LSLF Baked chicken   LSLF Baked fish (cod)
LSLF Hamburger on bun
(with lettuce and tomato)

Starchy Vegetables

LSLF Rice   LSLF Boiled potatoes

Vegetables

LSLF Baby carrots   LSLF Green beans

Soup/Salad/Juice	Dressings
LSLF Coleslaw	Diet French
Gelatin	Diet Thousand Island
Tomato soup	Diet Italian
LS Chicken broth	
Tossed salad	

Desserts

Pears	Angel food cake
	Fresh fruit

Breads

LF Dinner roll	Bran bread
White bread	Crackers
Wheat bread	LS Crackers

Beverages & Condiments

Coffee	Creamer
Decaf. coffee	Sugar
Hot tea	Sugar substitute
Decaf. hot tea	Herb seasoning
Iced tea	Lemon
Buttermilk	Margarine
Skim milk	Mustard
	Diet mayonnaise
	Catsup

PLEASE DO NOT LEAVE MENU ON THE TRAY

NAME _____ ROOM _____

Lunch

LOW SODIUM   **SUNDAY**

LF = Low Fat   LSLF = Low Sodium, Low Fat

Meats

LSLF Baked chicken   LSLF Baked fish (cod)
LSLF Hamburger on bun
(with lettuce and tomato)

Starchy Vegetables

LSLF Rice   LSLF Boiled potatoes

Vegetables

LSLF Baby carrots   LSLF Green beans

Soup/Salad/Juice	Dressings
LSLF Coleslaw	Diet French
LS Chicken broth	Diet Thousand Island
Apple juice	Diet Italian
Tossed salad	

Desserts

Angel food cake	Pears
	Fresh fruit

Breads

Dinner roll	Bran bread
White bread	LS Crackers
Wheat bread	

Beverages & Condiments

Coffee	Sugar
Decaf. coffee	Sugar substitute
Hot tea	Creamer
Decaf. hot tea	Lemon
Iced tea	Herb seasoning
Whole milk	Margarine
2% milk	Diet mustard
Skim milk	Diet mayonnaise
	Diet catsup

NO SALT
PLEASE DO NOT LEAVE MENU ON TRAY

NAME _____ ROOM _____

Lunch

RENAL   **SUNDAY**

LF = Low Fat   LSLF = Low Sodium, Low Fat

Meats (2 oz)

LSLF Baked chicken   LSLF Baked fish
LSLF Hamburger on bun (with lettuce)

Starchy Vegetables

LSLF Rice   LSLF Dialyzed potatoes

Vegetables

LSLF Baby carrots   LSLF Green beans

Soup/Salad/Juice	Dressings
Lemonade	Diet French
LSLF Coleslaw	Diet Thousand Island
Tossed salad	Diet Italian
(no tomato)	

Desserts

Pears	Apple pie

Breads

Dinner roll	Bran bread
White bread	LS Crackers
Wheat bread	

Beverages & Condiments

Coffee	Sugar
Decaf. coffee	Sugar substitute
Hot tea	Creamer
Decaf. hot tea	Lemon
Iced tea	Margarine
	Diet mustard
	Mayonnaise

NO SALT
PLEASE DO NOT LEAVE MENU ON THE TRAY

NAME _____ ROOM _____

People on low-fat, low-cholesterol diets who also need kcalorie restriction receive a kcalorie-restricted menu to control portion sizes and number of servings. Both menus provide low-fat, low-cholesterol foods. Foods not appropriate for a low-fat, low-cholesterol diet, such as whole milk, would be crossed off the menu beforehand.

Low-sodium menus are similar to those provided for low-fat, low-cholesterol diets, but they eliminate high-sodium foods, such as tomato soup. The person on a low-sodium, low-fat, low-cholesterol diet selects foods from a low-fat menu with high-sodium foods crossed off beforehand. If the person is also on a low-kcalorie diet, foods would be selected from a low-kcalorie menu with high-sodium foods crossed off the menu beforehand.

Renal diets must be highly individualized and the person checking the menu has to carefully consider the client's selections and make appropriate changes when necessary.

manual for that diet. By allowing a choice, this system helps to ensure that clients receive foods they enjoy and will eat. An added advantage for people on special diets is that they become familiar with their diets by marking the appropriate menus.

Although procedures vary somewhat between hospitals, generally dietary employees deliver menus to each client's room early in the day and pick them up again later in the day. Each menu shows the client's name and room number as well as the name of the meal, the type of diet, and the day the menu will be served. Generally, the client makes selections for the next day or for the next few days to give the dietary department time to collect the menus and estimate the amount of food to prepare. Menus are usually color coded by diet. Color coding helps ensure that foodservice employees put the right foods on a client's tray and helps the person delivering the tray to quickly determine whether the client has received the right diet. Figure H25–1 shows lunch menus from several different diet menus and explains how each menu might be used.

Clients typically select one or more items from each food category on the menu. Clients may not receive foods they enjoy if they fail to mark the appropriate selections. If menus are not marked or if a menu is lost, the client receives meals preselected by the dietary department. Menus may not be marked for several reasons:

- Clients may have trouble seeing, reading, understanding, or physically marking the menus.
- Clients may not understand that their selections will be for the *next* (or another) day.
- Clients may be out of their rooms (for tests, procedures, or exercise) or asleep when the menus arrive; when the clients return or wake up, they may not see the menus or may have missed the menu pickup time.
- Clients may be too ill or too disinterested in food to make menu selections.

Occasional problems with menu selections can usually be corrected simply by explaining the menu system to clients or taking extra time to help them mark the menus. If clients continue to complain about food selections, the dietitian should be contacted.

Once food selections have been made, menus are often checked by a member of the dietary staff (often a registered dietetic technician) to make sure selections are appropriate. Completed menus can provide valuable clues about a client's food habits or understanding of a modified diet. In checking menus, the technician may notice that one person on a regular diet is selecting very little or that another is selecting too much. In another case, the technician may see that a person on a low-kcalorie diet is not selecting the appropriate number of servings from each exchange list. Such problems suggest the need for intervention by a dietitian.

Some hospitals do not offer selective menus. Instead, they serve a standard house diet, adjusting the menu for individual food preferences or special diets when necessary. For example, clients can request simple changes, such as the substitution of one vegetable for another. Similarly, if the regular menu offers fried fish, a person on a low-fat or low-kcalorie diet would receive baked fish.

Food Preparation and Delivery

The logistics of preparing foods tailored to each modified diet can be overwhelming. For this reason, foodservice departments use special systems designed to limit costs and keep errors to a minimum. Foods prepared for regular and soft/bland/low-residue diets are prepared with some fat and salt, because these dietary components are not restricted on such diets. Note that the other diet menus in Figure H25–1 provide a number of low-fat (LF) or low-sodium, low-fat (LSLF) foods.

If the dietary department were to prepare a food (baked chicken, for example) for each different diet, it would have to prepare regular baked chicken, low-fat baked chicken, low-sodium baked chicken, and low-sodium, low-fat baked chicken, Using the system illustrated in the menus of Figure H25–1, only two types of baked chicken need to be prepared, one with some fat and salt, the other without fat or salt.

Keep in mind that baked chicken is only one of many menu items in a day, and you can see why preparing individual foods for each diet is not feasible. Instead, clients can add allowed items to their foods. For example, the person on a low-salt diet could add margarine to a serving of vegetables; the person on a low-fat diet could add salt to a serving of rice.

Sometimes foods are prepared in a main kitchen, assembled on trays, and heated in areas close to the clients' rooms. In other cases, foods are delivered directly to the floor from the main kitchen. In either case, dietary personnel deliver the food carts directly to the nursing unit. Once at the unit, nursing or dietary personnel take a tray to each client. Efficient delivery of foods to the nursing unit and then to the clients' rooms helps ensure that clients receive foods at the appropriate temperature.

Once a client has finished eating, the tray is returned to the food cart. Dietary personnel pick up the carts and return them to the dietary department.

Working with the System

You can help your clients greatly—and save yourself needless aggravation and time—by learning about the foodservice system in the health care facility where you work. Better yet, ask to spend a few hours or a day working with a dietary employee to see firsthand how the department operates. If that is not possible, learn the facility's procedure for ordering diets, making diet changes, reporting problems with a client's tray, or making special requests. Remember that requests are not simply made by one individual to another. Often many people are involved in processing even a simple request, and the number of requests made during a short period can be considerable. Translating requests (for example, requesting a diet change or another tray) takes time, and delays are often unavoidable.

One of the most important things to know about your facility's foodservice system is the time when meals are actually assembled, so that you can call in any requests before that time. Once tray assembly begins, dietary employees are extremely busy, and requests will be difficult to process.

With so many people and steps involved in the delivery of food and so many clients with individual dietary needs and food preferences, it is easy to see many opportunities for problems to arise regarding food in the hospital. Once you understand how the dietary department operates, you can use the system to tackle problems efficiently and avoid needless frustration for your client and yourself.

NOTES

1. M. Bélanger and L. Dubé, The emotional experience of hospitalization: Its moderators and its role in patient satisfaction with foodservices, *Journal of the American Dietetic Association* 96 (1996): 354–360.

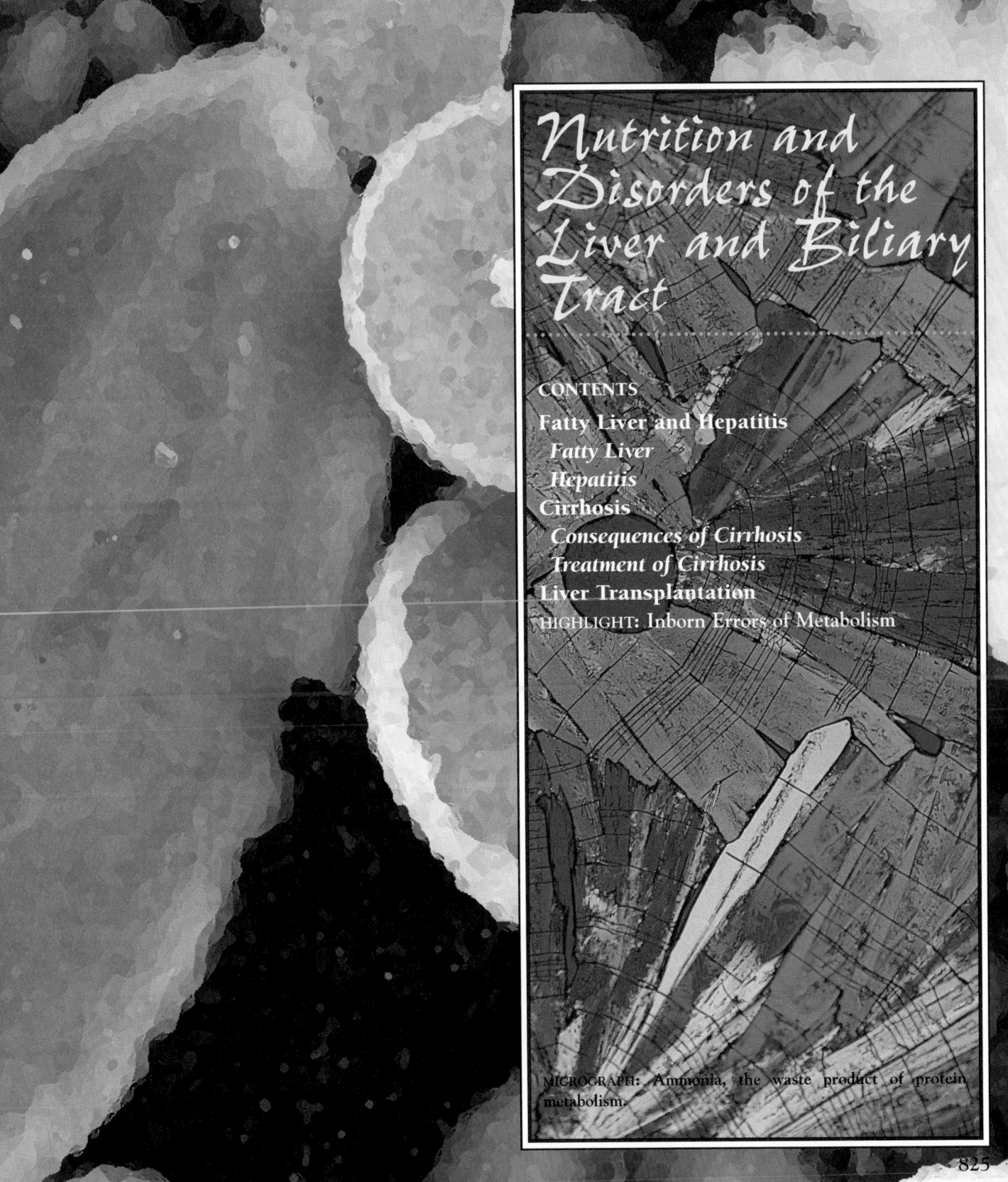

Chapter 26

Nutrition and Disorders of the Liver and Biliary Tract

CONTENTS

Fatty Liver and Hepatitis
Fatty Liver
Hepatitis
Cirrhosis
Consequences of Cirrhosis
Treatment of Cirrhosis
Liver Transplantation
HIGHLIGHT: Inborn Errors of Metabolism

MICROGRAPH: Ammonia, the waste product of protein metabolism.

hepatic (he-PAT-ik): of, like, or pertaining to the liver.

*D*uring severe stress, hypermetabolism necessitates that the liver work diligently to synthesize stress factors and provide glucose. Indeed, the liver is the metabolic crossroad of the body, and its health is crucial to every body function. The liver receives nutrients and metabolizes, packages, stores, or ships them out for use by the other organs. It manufactures bile, which the body uses to emulsify fat in preparation for digestion and absorption. The liver also detoxifies drugs, prepares waste products for excretion, and participates in iron recycling and the manufacture of red blood cells. No wonder hepatic disorders can profoundly affect both nutrition and general health status. Figure 26–1 shows the liver, its circulatory system, and the biliary tract.

Liver disease can be caused by a variety of conditions, including alcohol abuse, congenital disorders, poisoning by toxins, infections, biliary tract obstructions, and heart disease. This chapter describes several types of liver disorders for which dietary management is appropriate.

Figure 26–1
• • • • • • • • • • • • • •

The Liver, Biliary Tract, and Associated Blood Vessels

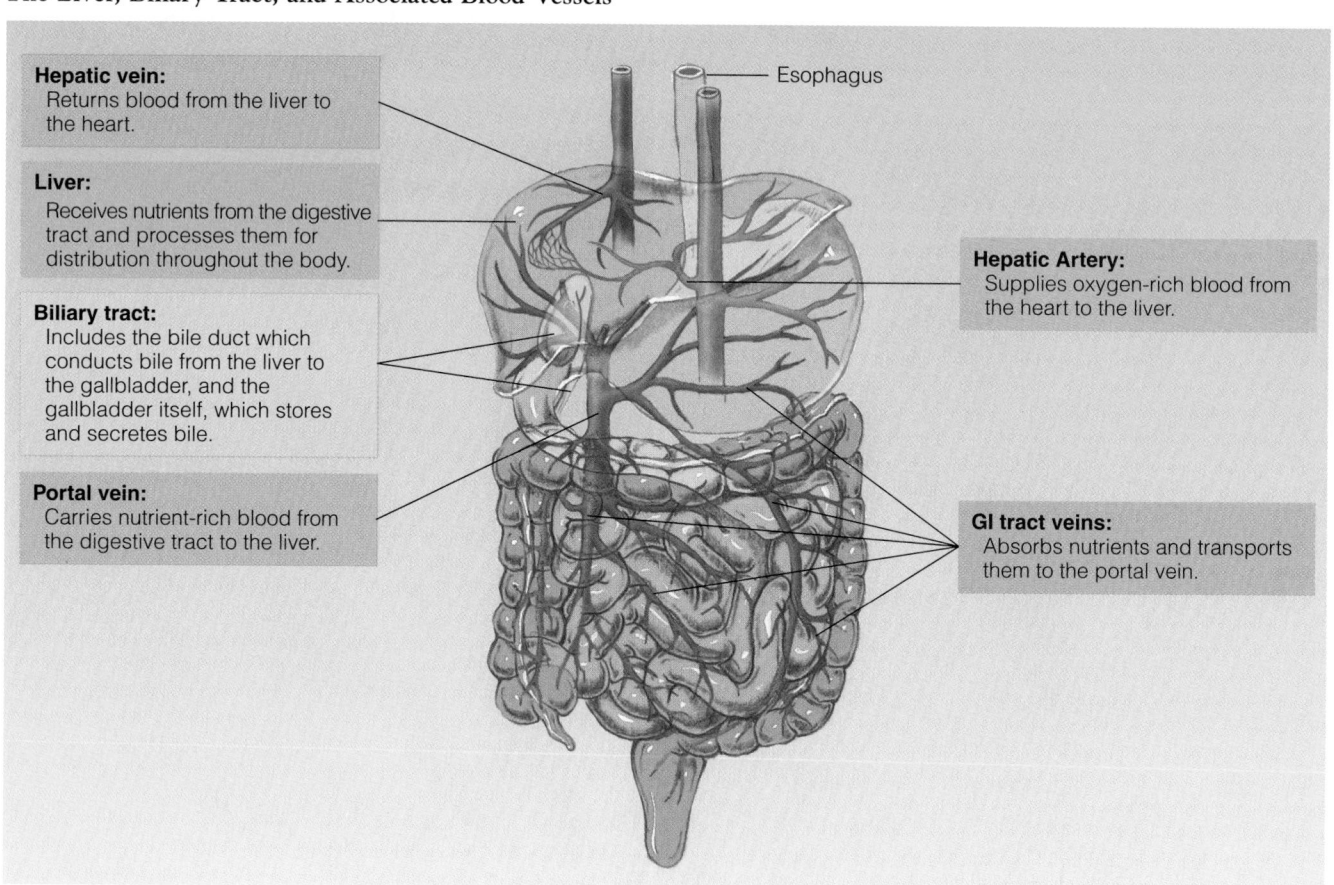

Hepatic vein:
Returns blood from the liver to the heart.

Liver:
Receives nutrients from the digestive tract and processes them for distribution throughout the body.

Biliary tract:
Includes the bile duct which conducts bile from the liver to the gallbladder, and the gallbladder itself, which stores and secretes bile.

Portal vein:
Carries nutrient-rich blood from the digestive tract to the liver.

Esophagus

Hepatic Artery:
Supplies oxygen-rich blood from the heart to the liver.

GI tract veins:
Absorbs nutrients and transports them to the portal vein.

CONSEQUENCES OF CIRRHOSIS

Unlike healthy liver tissue, which is soft and flexible, scar tissue is unyielding. This difference leads to major consequences, as shown in Figure 26–2 and described in the following paragraphs.

Portal Hypertension   The portal vein (see Figure 26–1) and the hepatic artery carry 1½ quarts of blood every minute to the miles of intermeshed capillaries within the liver. This huge volume of blood cannot pulse easily through the scarred tissue of a cirrhotic liver. Consequently, blood backs up and pressure in the portal vein rises sharply, causing portal hypertension.

Esophageal Varices   With normal blood flow through the liver blocked, pressure forces some of the blood to take a detour through smaller vessels around the liver. These collaterals, or shunts, often develop in the area around the esophagus. Frequently, high pressure enlarges the collaterals so that they bulge into the lumen of the esophagus much as varicose veins in the legs do, creating

Reminder: The *portal vein* is the blood vessel that carries nutrients from the GI tract to the liver. The *hepatic vein* returns blood from the liver to the heart. The *hepatic artery* delivers oxygen-rich blood from the heart back to the liver.

portal hypertension: elevated blood pressure in the portal vein caused by obstructed blood flow through the liver.

Figure 26–2

The Consequences of Cirrhosis

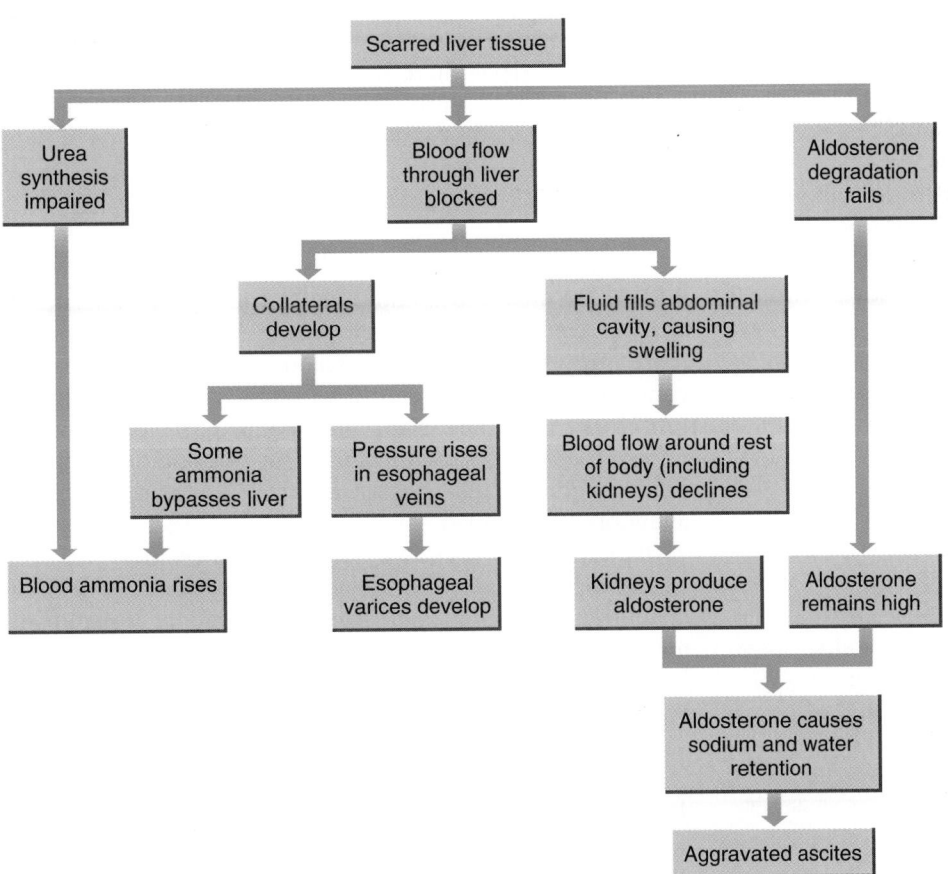

collaterals: small blood vessels that develop to divert blood flow away from an obstructed organ; also called shunts.

   shunt = to avoid

esophageal varices (ee-SOFF-ah-GEE-al VAIR-ih-seez): tangles of distended blood vessels that protrude into the esophagus.

ascites (ah-SIGH-teez): a type of edema characterized by the accumulation of fluid in the abdominal cavity.

An elevated blood ammonia level is called hyperammonemia. Normal blood ammonia levels are less than 50 μg/100 ml.

hepatic coma: a state of unconsciousness that results from severe liver disease; also called hepatic encephalopathy or portal systemic encephalopathy.

Phenylalanine and tyrosine are the aromatic amino acids; they are characterized by a ringlike structure.

Leucine, isoleucine, and valine are the branched-chain amino acids, so named because their side chains have a branched structure.

The odor that may develop in people with impending hepatic coma is called fetor hepaticus.

flapping tremor: uncontrolled movement of the muscle group that causes the outstretched arm and hand to flap like a wing; occurs in hepatic coma and other diseases that cause encephalopathy; also called asterixis (AS-ter-ICK-sis).

esophageal varices. Eventually, the thin esophageal lining that covers the varices may wear away, and massive bleeding follows. Bleeding esophageal varices tend to recur, and people can bleed to death.

Ascites   The rising pressure in the portal vein forces plasma out of the liver's blood vessels into the abdominal cavity, causing the abdomen to swell. This accumulation of fluid in the abdominal cavity is called ascites. Ascites tends to be a self-aggravating condition. Because less blood reaches the kidneys, the body responds by making more aldosterone, the hormone that expands the body's blood volume by triggering the retention of sodium and water. As a result of the sodium and water retention, ascites worsens and edema spreads to all body compartments. To make matters worse, the diseased liver cannot dispose of aldosterone as it normally does, so aldosterone levels remain high.

Elevated Blood Ammonia Levels   Normally, the healthy liver removes ammonia from circulation and converts it to urea, but a severely diseased liver fails at this task, and blood ammonia rises. Even if the liver does handle the ammonia it receives, some ammonia-laden blood bypasses the liver by way of the collaterals. Elevated blood ammonia levels disrupt central nervous system function, compounding the risk of hepatic coma. Thus therapy aims to control ammonia production.

Hepatic Coma   Hepatic coma is a dangerous complication of liver failure. Its exact cause remains elusive; high blood ammonia plays an important role, but the degree of elevation does not correlate with the severity of coma. A possible explanation for this poor correlation is that *blood* ammonia levels do not parallel *brain* ammonia concentration. When brain ammonia is elevated, the body produces greater quantities of two substances (glutamine and ketoglutarate), and the degree of their elevation tends to correlate with the degree of coma. Other nitrogen-containing compounds may also be involved.

Blood amino acid patterns also change in hepatic coma. The liver fails to break down aromatic amino acids, so their blood concentrations rise. Hormonal changes that accompany liver disease (specifically, elevated insulin levels) promote the uptake of branched-chain amino acids by muscle cells, so the blood concentrations of these amino acids fall. The resulting high ratio of aromatic to branched-chain amino acids interferes with the formation of certain neurotransmitters (dopamine and norepinephrine) and causes the production of substances that may contribute to hepatic coma.[2] Altered amino acid metabolism also adds ammonia to the blood.

Typically, the person with impending hepatic coma exhibits mental disturbances such as changes in judgment, personality, or mood. The person may be unable to draw even a simple shape, such as a star. A sweet, musty, or pungent odor may develop on the breath. Flapping tremor may also develop in the precoma state. Just before passing into coma, the person becomes very difficult to arouse.

TREATMENT OF CIRRHOSIS

Treatment of cirrhosis includes diet and drugs to preserve remaining organ function to the greatest extent possible, to control clinical manifestations of the disorder, and to prevent hepatic coma. When liver failure has progressed to a severe stage, liver transplantation becomes an option.

How to Adjust Diets for Liver Disease

Health care professionals adjust diets in liver disease to meet each client's medical needs. The following guidelines help to determine nutrient needs for liver failure:

Energy: 35 to 45 kcalories per kilogram of actual body weight.

Protein in cirrhosis: 1.0 to 1.5 grams of protein per kilogram of body weight.

Protein in impending coma: 40 to 60 grams per day from foods; additional protein to meet needs can be supplied from special formulas.

Protein in hepatic coma: Protein from all sources may need to be restricted. Tolerances are determined individually; protein intake is gradually increased as the condition improves.

Sodium and fluids: 1000 to 2000 milligrams of sodium per day and 1500 to 2000 milliliters of fluid per day if ascites has developed; intake is increased as liver function improves.

As noted earlier, therapy seeks to limit blood ammonia levels. The GI tract produces about two-thirds of the body's ammonia. Intestinal bacteria make ammonia from undigested proteins (including dietary proteins, proteins from shed mucosal cells, and protein from GI tract bleeding). Digestive enzymes also produce ammonia as they dismantle proteins. Thus diet and drug therapy also aim to control intestinal ammonia production.

Drug Therapy   Drug therapy for cirrhosis often includes broad-spectrum antibiotics to limit the growth of intestinal bacteria and laxatives to speed intestinal transit time, thus limiting the time available for bacteria to produce ammonia. In addition, diuretics are frequently given to reduce fluid retention and prevent ascites.

Energy and Protein   In providing diet therapy for cirrhosis, health care professionals must pay attention to clients' intakes of energy, protein, sodium, and fluid. Adequate carbohydrate and fat prevent the catabolism of protein for energy, which would further raise blood ammonia. Dietary protein should be sufficient to regenerate liver cells and prevent infections, but not so excessive as to aggravate ammonia buildup and induce hepatic coma. A diet adequate in energy and restricted, but not low, in protein is the cornerstone of cirrhosis treatment. The accompanying box shows how diets are adjusted to meet nutrient needs for different stages of liver failure. (Note that protein needs actually exceed the RDA of 0.8 grams of protein per kilogram of body weight per day.)

A person who shows signs of impending coma requires additional dietary modifications. Protein intake must be restricted to 40 to 60 grams of high-quality protein per day. Restricting protein reduces the risk of coma, but may threaten protein status. Although research is limited and controversial, many clinicians recommend special enteral or parenteral formulas that are low in aromatic amino acids and high in branched-chain amino acids to meet the demand for additional protein.[3] If coma ensues, some people may be able to tolerate these special formulas, but for others, both dietary protein and special formulas may be restricted.[4] As the client's neurological status improves, protein can gradually be increased.

 PRESCRIPTION PAD

Drugs used in the treatment of liver failure may include:

- Antibiotics
- Diuretics
- Laxatives (lactulose)

See Appendix E for timing with meals and nutrition-related side effects.

Avoiding hypermetabolism is critical for a person with compromised liver function. The impaired liver is already taxed in maintaining homeostasis. The added demands of stress factor synthesis and gluconeogenesis can easily overwhelm the liver and lead to death.

Appendix K includes enteral formulas for hepatic insufficiency.

People with liver disease may tolerate vegetable and dairy proteins better than meat proteins, perhaps because vegetables contain fewer ammonia-forming constituents and aromatic amino acids and more branched-chain amino acids than meats. In addition, diets high in plant foods contain more fiber, which speeds up intestinal transit time and reduces the time available for ammonia absorption from the gut.

Fat   Because fat helps make foods more appetizing and delivers energy efficiently, it serves an important role in the diet of a person with cirrhosis. Fat needs to be restricted only if the cirrhotic person develops steatorrhea, a clear sign of fat malabsorption. Even then, the body can usually handle MCT fat (see Chapter 22, p. 729).

Fluid and Sodium   For people with ascites, the diet often restricts fluid and sodium (see the box on p. 831 for details). To assess changes in fluid balance, health care professionals monitor weight changes and measure abdominal girth. Rapid weight gain indicates fluid retention; sudden weight loss indicates successful fluid excretion. To measure abdominal girth, the assessor places a tape measure around the back and over the person's abdomen directly over the umbilicus. A decreasing abdominal girth indicates fluid mobilization; an increasing abdominal girth signifies worsening ascites. Table 26–1 shows diet patterns for two levels of sodium restriction. The menu on p. 834 provides sample protein- and sodium-restricted meals.

Alcohol   To protect the liver from further injury, clients with cirrhosis must completely abstain from alcohol use. A cirrhotic liver exposed to the toxic effects of alcohol cannot function.

Vitamins   The liver's central role in the metabolism and storage of vitamins and minerals, combined with coexisting conditions (such as malabsorption, alcoholism, and malnutrition), explains why nutrient deficiencies commonly occur in people with liver disorders. Virtually all people with advanced liver disease require supplementation of some vitamins, minerals, and trace elements. Physicians determine which nutrients to supplement by monitoring serum levels and by checking for clinical signs of deficiencies.

The B vitamins serve as coenzymes for the liver's many metabolic reactions and repair work; deficiencies of thiamin, vitamin B_6, riboflavin, and folate are common. Fat-soluble vitamins may be malabsorbed if steatorrhea develops. If the diseased liver fails to synthesize adequate amounts of retinol-binding protein, body tissues may not receive the vitamin A they need. Vitamin D nutrition status may suffer if the impaired liver fails to activate vitamin D for the body's use. Vitamin K deficiencies can prolong the time blood takes to clot, a dangerous complication that increases the risk of massive bleeding from esophageal varices or other areas of the GI tract.

One laboratory test that evaluates the time it takes for blood to clot is called the **prothrombin time.** Both vitamin K deficiency and liver disease can prolong prothrombin time.

Minerals   Calcium deficiencies can develop from three causes: steatorrhea, low serum albumin (albumin, which carries calcium in the blood, is manufactured in the liver), and impaired vitamin D metabolism. Fluid and electrolyte imbalances and ascites may necessitate that diuretics be used, and these may lead to deficiencies of potassium, magnesium, and zinc.

Table 26–1

One- and Two-Gram Sodium-Restricted Diets

Foods Restricted	Number of Servings[a]		Serving Size	Sodium per Serving (mg)
	1 gram (1000 mg) sodium	2 grams (2000 mg) sodium		
Regular breads and cooked cereals	3	4	1 slice	125
Fresh, frozen, or canned vegetables without salt: artichokes; beets; carrots; celery; beet, collard, dandelion, mustard, and turnip greens; kale; swiss chard; white turnips; low-sodium vegetable juice	3 per week	Avoid excessive use	½ cup	50
Canned or frozen vegetables with salt; frozen corn, lima beans, mixed vegetables, and peas	0	2	½ cup	250
Regular nonfat, whole, and evaporated milk and milk products	2	2	8 oz	120
Fresh and fresh frozen meats, poultry, and freshwater fish; low-sodium canned meats and fish, peanut butter, cheese; unsalted soybeans, textured vegetable protein, and cottage cheese	8	8	1 oz	25
Eggs	1	1	1	70
Regular butter and margarine	0	6	1 tsp	50

Foods Allowed

1. Low-sodium breads, bread products, and cereals; bread products made without salt and with low-sodium baking powder; puffed rice and wheat and shredded wheat cereals; rice; pasta.
2. Fresh, unsalted frozen, and low-sodium canned vegetables (except those listed above); low-sodium tomato juice.
3. All fruits and fruit juices.
4. Unsalted butter, margarine, nuts, and gravy; low-sodium salad dressings and mayonnaise; shortening.
5. Low-sodium catsup, mustard, and tabasco sauce.
6. Soups, casseroles, and recipes made with allowed foods and food ingredients.

Foods Not Allowed (Unless Calculated Into the Diet)

1. Table, celery, garlic, and onion salts; reduced-sodium salts; regular catsup, mustard, and tabasco sauce; monosodium glutamate; Worcestershire, barbeque, and soy sauces; baking powder and soda.
2. Instant and quick-cooking hot cereals; commercial bread products made from self-rising flour or cornmeal, salt, baking powder, or baking soda; salted snack foods such as potato chips, corn chips, tortilla chips, popcorn, and pretzels.
3. Sauerkraut, pickles, and salted vegetable juices.
4. Maraschino cherries; crystallized or glazed fruits, and dried fruits with sodium sulfite added.
5. Buttermilk, chocolate milk, instant milk mixes, regular cheeses, and prepared pudding mixes; commercial ice cream, sherbet, and frozen desserts.
6. Cured, canned, salted, or smoked meats, poultry and fish such as bacon, luncheon meats, corned beef, kosher meats, and canned tuna and salmon; imitation fish products; salted textured vegetable protein; regular peanut butter; salted nuts.
7. Salt pork and bacon fat; commercial salad dressings and mayonnaise; olives; regular gravy.
8. Regular canned soups and bouillon.

[a]Number of servings daily, except as noted.

Sample Protein-Restricted (60 g), Sodium-Restricted (1000 mg) Diet Menu

Foods on this low-sodium menu are cooked without salt. To raise sodium intake, add salt to foods. To reduce sodium, use unsalted margarine and low-sodium milk. The kcalories provided by this menu depend on how much fat is used in cooking. To raise energy intake, encourage the liberal use of fats and sugars from foods that do not contain protein (for example, margarine and table sugar).

Menu

Breakfast	Lunch	Supper
Orange juice	Sandwich with	2 oz baked chicken
½ c oatmeal	2 oz roast beef,	½ c mashed potatoes
½ c milk	2 slices bread, lettuce,	Broccoli
1 egg	and mayonnaise	1 low-sodium dinner roll
Margarine	Cole slaw	Margarine
Coffee	Cinnamon applesauce	Fruit cocktail
Cream	½ c milk	½ c milk
Sugar		

Diet Planning   Dietitians face a challenge in devising a diet plan that is low in sodium, supplies adequate energy and nutrients, and also stimulates the appetite. Many high-quality protein foods (for example, eggs, meat, and milk) also contain significant amounts of sodium. To circumvent this problem, planners recommend special supplements and milk products that are low in sodium. Diet offers critical support in the care of liver failure, and health professionals should make every effort to solve food-related problems.

Offer encouragement and work closely with clients and their caregivers to individualize the diet and serve foods attractively. Try the tactics suggested in Chapter 23 to encourage clients to eat.

Enteral and Parenteral Nutrition   If the person with cirrhosis cannot take enough food or formula by mouth, health care professionals should promptly begin tube feedings or TPN. As mentioned earlier, enteral and parenteral formulas designed for liver failure provide fewer aromatic and more branched-chain amino acids than standard formulas. Both types of special nutrition support have been used successfully in people with cirrhosis.

People with bleeding esophageal varices will be unable to consume food by mouth and are often given simple IV solutions to maintain fluid and electrolyte balances. Parenteral nutrition should be considered if the person is malnourished or unable to resume oral intake for an extended period of time. The accompanying box presents a case study on cirrhosis. Use your clinical knowledge and judgment in answering the questions presented.

Liver Transplantation

When liver failure progresses to a severe and irreversible stage, liver transplantation may become an option. Surgeons remove the diseased liver, replace it with

Case Study   Carpenter with Cirrhosis

Mr. Sloan, a 48-year-old carpenter, has been hospitalized many times. He recognizes his problem with alcohol abuse and has entered alcohol rehabilitation programs several times over the last few years. Nevertheless, he is still drinking. Mr. Sloan was recently admitted to the hospital, and a diagnosis of alcoholic cirrhosis has been confirmed. At 5 feet 7 inches tall, Mr. Sloan, who once weighed 150 pounds, now weighs 120 pounds. He looks thin, although his abdomen is distended with ascites, and his skin is yellow. He has advanced liver disease and is showing signs of impending hepatic coma. Laboratory findings include elevated AST, ALT, alkaline phosphatase, and blood ammonia. Compare these findings with Table 26–2 to determine if they are consistent with liver disease.

Can you explain to Mr. Sloan what cirrhosis is and what its consequences are? From the limited information available, what can you determine about Mr. Sloan's nutrition status? What medical problem makes it difficult to interpret Mr. Sloan's actual weight? How can his weight measurements help determine if his condition is improving?

What dietary changes do clients with cirrhosis generally receive? How will Mr. Sloan's diet be altered now that he is in a precoma state? What signs suggest that a person is in a precoma state?

Why is Mr. Sloan's abdomen distended? Explain the development of ascites in liver disease and how diet is adjusted.

Would you expect Mr. Sloan's blood ammonia levels to be high? Why or why not?

Describe portal hypertension, jaundice, and esophageal varices. How would Mr. Sloan's diet be changed if he were found to have esophageal varices?

---

a donor liver, and reconnect the blood vessels and the biliary tract. In some liver transplant cases, the graft fails to function, and retransplantation forestalls an otherwise inevitable death.

Nutrition before Transplantation   In severe liver failure, malnutrition has often progressed for some time. Clinicians report malnutrition in over 70 percent of liver transplant recipients and note that malnutrition increases the risk of

Table 26–2

Standards for Tests Used to Diagnose and Monitor Liver Disease

Test	Normal Values	Values in Liver Disease
Albumin	3.5–5.0 g/100 ml	Decreased
Alkaline phosphatase	Varies[a]	Normal or elevated
ALT (formerly SGPT)[b]	Varies[a]	Elevated
Ammonia	<50 µg/100 ml	Elevated
AST (formerly SGOT)[b]	Varies[a]	Elevated
Bilirubin (direct)	0.1–0.3 mg/100 ml	Elevated
Prothrombin time		Prolonged

Note: To convert albumin (g/100 ml) to standard international (SI) units, multiply by 10; to convert ammonia (µg/100 ml) to SI units, multiply by 0.5872; to convert bilirubin (mg/100 ml) to SI units (µmol/L) multiply by 17.10
[a]Reference ranges vary depending on the test used. Consult laboratory report for normal ranges.
[b]ALT = alanine transaminase; SGPT = serum glutamic pyruvic transaminase; AST = aspartate transaminase; SGOT = serum glutamic oxaloacetic transaminase.

Nutrition Assessment Checklist
For People with Liver Disorders

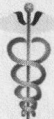

Medical   Review the medical record to determine the type and cause of liver disease, as well as any history of alcohol abuse, hepatitis, or biliary tract obstruction. Recognize that the effects of advanced liver disease and malnutrition are often difficult to distinguish.

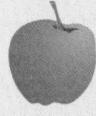

Nutrient Intake   Obtain an accurate diet history to determine nutrition status, calculate nutrient requirements, and identify inadequate nutrient intake. Assess current intake to help pinpoint tolerance for protein in people with advanced liver disease. People who abuse alcohol normally derive much of their daily energy intake from alcohol. Without that energy source, as occurs during hospitalization, special care must be taken to ensure that the diet supplies sufficient energy.

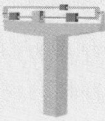

Anthropometric   Interpret anthropometric data cautiously in people with edema and ascites. In advanced liver disease, weight is measured daily to assess changes in fluid status. Abdominal girth measurements are also useful for assessing fluid status.

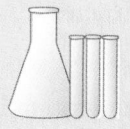

Laboratory   Anticipate low serum protein levels in people with advanced liver diseases. Many laboratory tests, including serum albumin, reflect liver function as well as nutrition status. Supplying adequate protein may fail to raise serum proteins if the liver is unable to synthesize them. AST, ALT, ammonia, and bilirubin levels increase with deteriorating liver function.

Physical   Note physical signs of altered liver function including ascites, edema, and jaundice. Gynecomastia (abnormally large mammary tissue) and testicular atrophy may be present in men with liver failure. Other physical signs of liver dysfunction include angiomas (masses of dilated capillaries and arterioles) and distended abdominal blood vessels. Flapping tremor suggests impending hepatic coma.

complications and death following a liver transplant.[5] A liver transplant candidate must often wait for a liver donor before surgery is possible. Wise health care professionals use this time to identify and correct nutrient imbalances whenever possible. Often TPN is used to provide nutrients prior to a transplant. The person equipped with adequate nutrient stores faces the transplant better prepared to fight infections, heal wounds, and mount a stress response.

Difficulties arise in assessing nutrition status in liver transplant candidates because the metabolic effects of liver disease and those of malnutrition are difficult to distinguish. Edema may mask weight loss and alter other anthropometric measurements. Low serum protein may reflect liver disease itself, rather than nutrition status.

Nutrition following Transplantation   Following liver transplantation, liver function determines nutrient needs. All people are hypermetabolic after surgery, and energy needs must be met. Immunosuppressant drugs given to prevent tissue rejection can contribute to nutrient imbalances by causing nausea, vomiting, diarrhea, and mouth sores. The client has an increased susceptibility to infection, and if an infection does occur, nutrient stores are further taxed. The nutrition support team often uses indirect calorimetry to estimate energy needs and carefully monitors clinical and laboratory data to make specific nutrient recommendations.

Although TPN has been the traditional source of nutrients in the posttransplant period, researchers report equal success with intestinal tube feedings.[6] Early enteral nutrition support may reduce the incidence of infection, a particularly important consideration for people with suppressed immune systems.[7]

The complications of cirrhosis outlined in Figure 26–2 all result from the scar tissue that forms within the liver. Dietary and drug treatment aims to preserve liver function and prevent hepatic coma. Perhaps the greatest dietary challenge is providing enough protein to heal, but not so much as to generate ammonia.

The recovery of people with disorders of the liver depends in large part on attention to nutrition and nutrition assessment parameters. The accompanying nutrition assessment checklist reviews important points to keep in mind when assessing the nutrition status of people with liver diseases.

Without a doubt, liver disorders wreak havoc on the body's metabolic work. Equally disturbing to the body's homeostasis are disorders that alter blood glucose concentrations, the topic of the next chapter.

Study Questions

1. What is fatty liver, and what are its causes? What diet modifications, if any, are useful for the treatment of fatty liver?
2. What is hepatitis, and what nutrition concerns arise in the person suffering from hepatitis?
3. Discuss cirrhosis, and describe how it leads to portal hypertension, esophageal varices, ascites, formation of collaterals, and elevated blood ammonia levels.
4. Describe the dietary treatment of the person with cirrhosis and hepatic coma. Consider special dietary concerns of the person with ascites and esophageal varices.
5. How does nutrition status influence recovery from a liver transplant?

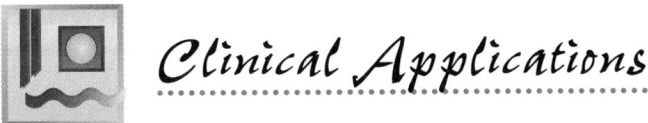 *Clinical Applications*

1. Think about the problems a person might have in receiving adequate energy from a diet restricted to 40 grams of protein. On such a diet, the total protein allowance could be used up on just one scrambled egg, 3 ounces of meat, a cup of milk, and two slices of bread. Using Figure 17–1 on pp. 572–573

for reference, write down the exchange lists that contain no protein, and add enough of these foods to the diet to meet energy needs (assume an energy need of 2000 kcalories).

Now compare the results with the Daily Food Guide on pp. 42–43. Which food groups have you offered in the recommended quantities? Which food groups are in short supply? Which nutrients might be low? How might fats and sugars be useful in such a diet?

2. The more restrictive a diet is, the harder it usually is to comply with it. The person given the diet in question 1, for example, may miss eating large amounts of meat or meat alternates, breads and grains, or milk and milk products. What effect might additional restrictions, such as fluid and sodium restrictions, have on dietary compliance? Consider, in addition, how much more difficult compliance might be for an alcohol abuser, who must also abstain from alcohol.

Notes

1. Springhouse Corporation, *Diseases,* 2nd ed. (Springhouse, Pa.: Springhouse Corporation, 1997), p. 933.
2. J. E. Fischer, Branched-chain-enriched amino acid solutions in patients with liver failure: An early example of nutritional pharmacology, *Journal of Parenteral and Enteral Nutrition* (supplement) 14 (1990): 249–256.
3. A. Fabri and coauthors, Overview of randomized clinical trials of oral branched-chain amino acid treatment in chronic hepatic encephalopathy, *Journal of Parenteral and Enteral Nutrition* 20 (1996): 159–164.
4. A.S.P.E.N. Board of Directors, Practice guidelines: Liver failure, *Journal of Parenteral and Enteral Nutrition* (supplement) 17 (1993): 14–15; E. P. Shronts and coauthors, Nutrition support of the adult liver transplant candidate, *Journal of the American Dietetic Association* 87 (1987): 441–451.
5. J. Hasse, Nutrition and transplantation, *Nutrition in Clinical Practice* 8 (1993): 3–4; J. Pikul and coauthors, Degree of preoperative malnutrition is predictive of postoperative morbidity and mortality in liver transplant recipients, *Transplantation* 57 (1994): 469–472.
6. C. Wicks and coauthors, Comparison of enteral feeding and total parenteral nutrition after liver transplantation, *Lancet* 344 (1994): 837–840; J. M. Hasse, Early enteral nutrition support in patients undergoing liver transplantation, *Journal of Parenteral and Enteral Nutrition* 19 (1995): 437–443.
7. Hasse, 1995.

Inborn Errors of Metabolism

The discussion in Chapter 26 of the metabolic consequences of liver disorders sets the stage for a closer look at metabolic disorders caused by genetic errors in protein synthesis. When the body makes certain proteins in an insufficient quantity or with an abnormal structure, body functions that depend on those proteins, such as metabolic reactions and transports, cannot proceed. If an enzyme that converts compound A to compound B is missing or malfunctioning in the metabolic pathway, then compound A accumulates and compound B becomes deficient. Both the excess of compound A and the lack of compound B can lead to a variety of problems and, in many cases, to death. Furthermore, this imbalance creates excesses and deficiencies in other metabolic pathways that present another array of problems. The diseases that result

from inherited biochemical blocks in normal metabolic pathways are known as inborn errors of metabolism. The accompanying glossary defines related terms.

In some instances, the accumulated compound is not toxic and the deficient compound is not essential, so individuals experience no problem. In all likelihood, they will never know about the error. In other cases, however, inborn errors have severe consequences, including possible mental retardation. Without proper diagnosis and treatment, they can be lethal. As is true of most medical disorders, the earlier the diagnosis and treatment, the better the prognosis.

The primary treatment for many inborn errors of metabolism is nutrition intervention. With an understanding of the biochemical path-

way involved, a clinician can often manipulate the diet to compensate for excesses and inadequacies. Management involves restricting dietary precursors that occur prior to the error in the metabolic pathway, replacing needed products that fail to be produced, or both. The goal of therapy is to:

- Prevent the accumulation of toxic metabolites.
- Replace essential nutrients that are deficient as a result of the defective metabolic pathway.
- Provide a diet that supports normal growth, development, and maintenance.

Meeting these three objectives is a major challenge that was previously unattainable. New knowledge about the body's many biochemical pathways, coupled with current technol-

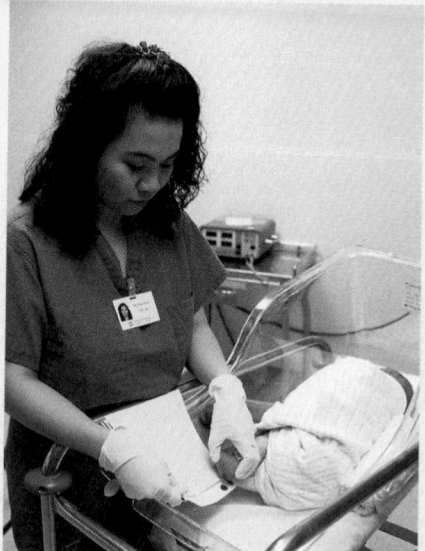

A simple blood test screens newborns for PKU—the most common inborn error of metabolism.

Glossary

carrier: an individual who possesses one dominant and one recessive gene for a recessive trait, such as an inborn error of metabolism. Such a person may show no signs of the trait but can pass it on.

dominant gene: a gene that has an observable effect on an organism even when it is paired with a normal gene; see also *recessive gene*.

galactosemia (ga-LAK-toe-SEE-me-ah): an inborn error of metabolism in which galactose cannot be metabolized normally to compounds the body can handle and an alternative metabolite accumulates in the tissues, causing damage.

genes: the basic units of hereditary information, made of DNA, that are passed from parent to offspring in the chromosomes. Each gene codes for a protein.

inborn error of metabolism: an inherited flaw evident as a metabolic disorder or disease present from birth.

mutation: an alteration in a gene such that an altered protein is produced.
   muta = change

PKU, phenylketonuria (FEN-el-KEY-toe-NEW-ree-ah): an inborn error of metabolism in which phenylalanine, an essential amino acid, cannot be converted to tyrosine. Alternative metabolites of phenylalanine (phenylketones) accumulate in the tissues, causing damage, and overflow into the urine.

recessive gene: a gene that has no observable effect on an organism as long as it is paired with a normal gene that can produce a normal product. In this case, the normal gene is said to be *dominant*.

ogy for synthesizing formulas of specific nutrient compositions, has greatly enhanced the treatment of inborn errors.

CLASSIC PHENYLKETONURIA

This discussion focuses primarily on the most common inborn error of metabolism—phenylketonuria (PKU). PKU is only one of several inborn errors that affect amino acid metabolism. Other disorders affect not only amino acid metabolism but also carbohydrate, lipid, and vitamin metabolism. The number of possible inborn errors is limited only by the number of possible gene mutations, for genes carry the codes to make the enzymes in the body.

PKU affects approximately 1 out of every 10,000 newborns in the United States each year. The ability to detect and treat PKU has saved and significantly improved the lives of many people. The achievements in this area offer hope to those suffering from other inborn errors.

Classic PKU results from a deficiency of the enzyme phenylalanine hydroxylase, which converts the essential amino acid phenylalanine to tyrosine (see Figure H26–1). Without the enzyme, abnormally high concentrations of phenylalanine and other related compounds accumulate and damage the developing nervous system. Simultaneously, the body cannot make tyrosine or other compounds (such as the neurotransmitter epinephrine) that normally derive from tyrosine. Under these conditions, tyrosine becomes an essential amino acid; that is, the body cannot make it, and therefore the diet must supply it.

PKU is a hidden disease that cannot be seen at birth, yet diagnosis and treatment beginning in the first few days of life can prevent its devastating effects. For these reasons, and because PKU is the most common inborn error of metabolism, all newborns in the United States receive a screening test for PKU.[1] The test must be conducted after the infant has consumed several meals containing protein (usually after 24 hours and before seven days). Before screening became routine, an infant with PKU would suffer the dire consequences of uncorrected high phenylalanine concentrations. At first, the only signs are a skin rash and light skin pigmentation. Between three and six months,

Figure H26–1
. . . .

The Biochemical Pathway in PKU

Normal:

Normally, the amino acid phenylalanine follows two pathways, one in the liver, the other in the kidneys. In the liver, the enzyme phenylalanine hydroxylase adds a hydroxyl group (OH) to produce the amino acid tyrosine. Tyrosine, in turn, produces melanin, the pigmented compound found in skin and brain cells; the neurotransmitters epinephrine and norepinephrine; and the hormone thyroxin. In the kidneys, enzymes convert phenylalanine to by-products that are excreted.

In the liver:

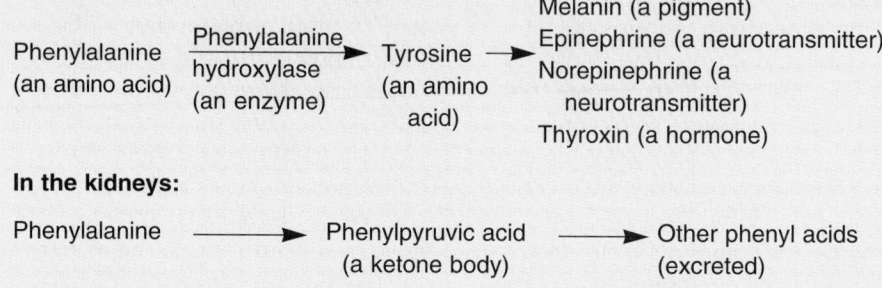

In the kidneys:

Phenylalanine ——————▶ Phenylpyruvic acid ——————▶ Other phenyl acids
                        (a ketone body)   (excreted)

In PKU:

Individuals with PKU lack the liver enzyme phenylalanine hydroxylase, impairing conversion of phenylalanine to tyrosine. Phenylalanine accumulates in the liver and blood, reaching the kidneys in abnormally high concentrations. In the kidneys, an aminotransferase enzyme converts phenylalanine to the ketone body phenylpyruvic acid, which spills into the urine—thus the name phenylketonuria.

In the liver:

Phenylalanine   Phenylalanine hydroxylase   Tyrosine
(accumulates) ————————————(deficient)————————————————▶ (deficient)

In the kidneys:

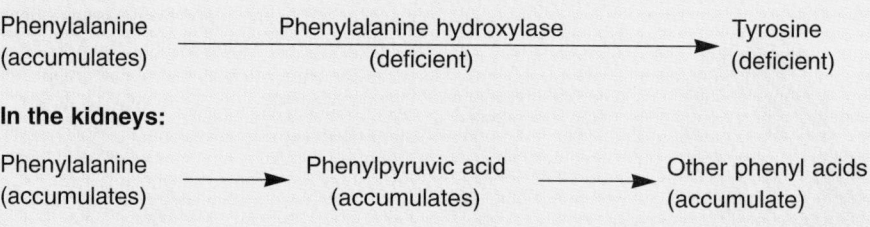

signs of developmental delay begin to appear. The infant becomes irritable and frantic and is unable to sleep restfully. By one year, irreversible brain damage is clearly evident, and the child will score poorly on developmental and intellectual tests.

Nutrition Therapy

The effect of nutrition intervention in PKU is remarkable. In almost every case, dietary management can prevent the devastating array of symptoms described. Essentially, the diet restricts phenylalanine and supplements tyrosine to maintain blood concentrations within a safe range. As most dietitians can attest, the diet is more easily described than designed.

Because phenylalanine is an essential amino acid, the diet cannot exclude it completely. If phenylalanine intake is too low, children suffer bone, skin, and blood disorders; growth and mental retardation; and death. Therefore, the diet must strike a balance, providing enough phenylalanine to support normal growth and health but not enough to cause harm. The problem is not that children with PKU require less phenylalanine than other children, but that they cannot handle excesses without detrimental effects. To ensure that blood phenylalanine and tyrosine concentrations remain within an acceptable range, children with PKU receive blood tests periodically and alterations in their diets when necessary. With a controlled phenylalanine intake, children with PKU can lead normal, healthy lives.

To control phenylalanine intake requires strict dietary management that was impossible prior to 1958, when a special low-phenylalanine

Sample Phenylalanine-Restricted Menu for a Child with PKU

Note: Lofenalac is a special low-phenylalanine formula that is commercially available.

Menu

Breakfast
2 tbs raisins
5 tbs cream of rice
2 tsp sugar
8 oz Lofenalac

Lunch
½ small banana
2 tbs tomato soup (without milk)
3 tbs rice
1½ tsp margarine
8 oz Lofenalac

Supper
2 tbs instant potatoes (without milk)
3 tbs green beans
4 tbs vegetable and beef broth
1½ tsp margarine
¾ c sliced peaches
8 oz Lofenalac

Midmorning Snack
4 oz orange juice

Afternoon Snack
4 oz Lofenalac
5 round butter crackers

Bedtime Snack
2 tbs raisins
4 oz Lofenalac

formula became commercially available. Low-phenylalanine formulas are now the primary source of energy and protein for children with PKU. Their diets exclude high-protein foods such as meat, fish, poultry, cheese, eggs, milk, nuts, and dried beans and peas. Also excluded are commercial breads and pastries made from regular flour, which has a high phenylalanine content. Basically, the diet allows foods that contain some phenylalanine, such as fruits, vegetables, and cereals, and those that contain none, such as fats, sugars, jellies, and some candies. Clearly, it is impossible to create such a diet using only whole, natural foods, but children who depend primarily on a formula for their nourishment risk multiple trace mineral deficiencies.[2] Health care professionals monitor trace mineral status and supplement as needed. The accompanying menu

provides a sample phenylalanine-restricted diet for a child with PKU.

Infants receive a special casein hydrolysate formula with a low-phenylalanine content. It does not contain all the phenylalanine an infant requires, so parents supplement it with measured quantities of milk, rice cereal, and baby foods as the infant develops. Other formulas and products are available that provide a synthetic mixture of amino acids without phenylalanine. This enables older children to receive their entire phenylalanine quota from foods.

People with PKU must also be aware of the phenylalanine in products containing the sweetener aspartame (see Table H4–1 on p. 134) and use these products only with guidance from their physicians or dietitians. For adolescents on phenylalanine-restricted diets, occasional diet beverages appear to cause no harm.[3]

Perhaps one of the hardest aspects of this diet is the children's sense of social isolation. From birth, children with PKU are on a "special diet" and cannot eat the foods that other children are eating. Some low-protein cookies and other products containing very little, if any, phenylalanine are commercially available and allow children to share treats with others. Teachers, friends, and family members must understand that they cannot offer foods to children with PKU without permission from the children's parents. Until the children are old enough to know their dietary restrictions, parents must teach them to ask before eating any food. Parents who have learned positive and creative problem-solving skills can effectively resolve situations involving dietary decisions. Consequently, their children are more likely to eat appropriate foods and maintain phenylalanine levels within normal ranges than children of parents without such skills.[4] Routine blood tests and the threat of possible brain damage motivate children and their parents to adhere to the diet.

During the early years of central nervous system development, prompt nutrition intervention is clearly critical to preventing irreversible mental retardation in the young PKU child. Less clear is the length of time the nervous system is vulnerable to the PKU defect. Until the late 1970s, researchers assumed that the child with PKU could abandon the special diet after the first few years of life when the central nervous system had completed its development. They realized that with a regular diet, phenylalanine and associated metabolite concentrations would rise, but thought perhaps these high levels would not be

damaging. Unfortunately, elevated phenylalanine concentrations in the older child do cause problems such as short attention span, poor short-term memory, and poor eye-to-hand coordination, although the damage is less severe than at an earlier age. In general, children with PKU who have discontinued their controlled diet experience problems in school performance, mood, and behavior. For these reasons, clinicians now encourage children to continue the low-phenylalanine diet indefinitely. Convincing adolescents to return to the phenylalanine-restricted diet after several years of an unrestricted diet requires intense education and reinforcement. Even then the effort is quite often unsuccessful. Reinstitution of a controlled diet, however, does improve blood phenylalanine concentrations, behavior, and IQ scores.

Therapy for inborn errors goes beyond nutrition to include psychological counseling for the people who are affected and their families. A genetic disorder is a lifelong problem that affects the entire family. All family members are at high risk for being carriers, and they inevitably become involved in the care and management of the person with the inborn error. Therefore, families must learn how to handle the impact such a diagnosis has on their relationships.

Maternal PKU

PKU, like all inborn errors, is a recessive disorder; that is, it appears only when a person inherits two defective genes—one from each parent. This can occur even if neither parent has PKU, because both may be carriers (see Figure H26–2). A carrier is a person who inherits one defective gene and one normal

gene. The carrier may be unaware of having a defective gene, for the symptoms are usually mild or absent.

Before the development of routine metabolic screenings, special formulas, and restricted diets, children with PKU died young. Now that people with PKU are living longer and reaching reproductive age, the chances of women with PKU conceiving children have increased significantly. The chance that a mother with PKU will have a child with PKU is about 1 out of 120.[5]

The risks for a PKU mother primarily affect her baby. When a woman is off the diet as an adult, her blood phenylalanine concentrations are high. When she becomes pregnant, her fetus's blood concentrations rise even higher than hers, and fetal development is impaired. The mother may experience a spontaneous abortion; or her infant is likely to suffer mental retardation, microcephaly, congenital heart disease, and low birthweight.[6]

Dietary control of maternal PKU may protect the fetus, at least in part, if implemented early enough.[7] Dietary control does not ensure a successful outcome of pregnancy, but the children of women who follow a low-phenylalanine diet from at least one to two months prior to conception and continue it throughout pregnancy are more likely to have higher birthweights, larger head circumferences, fewer malformations, and higher scores on intelligence tests than the children of women who begin diet therapy during their pregnancy or not at all.[8]

As mentioned, many physicians recommend adherence to a restricted diet throughout life. Resuming a low-phenylalanine diet is not easy. Special formulas that meet the energy, protein, vitamin, and mineral needs of pregnant PKU women are now available. These special formulas are costly and may be inconvenient and unpalatable to an adult who has been eating foods freely. Many women have forgotten that they were ever on a special diet as a child or may never have understood why.

Given the genetic risks and fetal abnormalities associated with a poorly controlled PKU pregnancy, a woman with PKU needs genetic and medical counseling. She must consider the possible consequences of pregnancy, her ability to follow the special diet, and the options of contraception to prevent pregnancy and adoption if she wants children.

Before closing this discussion, it is appropriate to briefly describe another inborn error of metabolism to illustrate the similarities and differences between these types of disorders. To this point, the discussion has focused on PKU, an example of a defect in amino acid metabolism. The following paragraphs describe a defect in carbohydrate metabolism—galactosemia.

Figure H26–2

The Inheritance of PKU

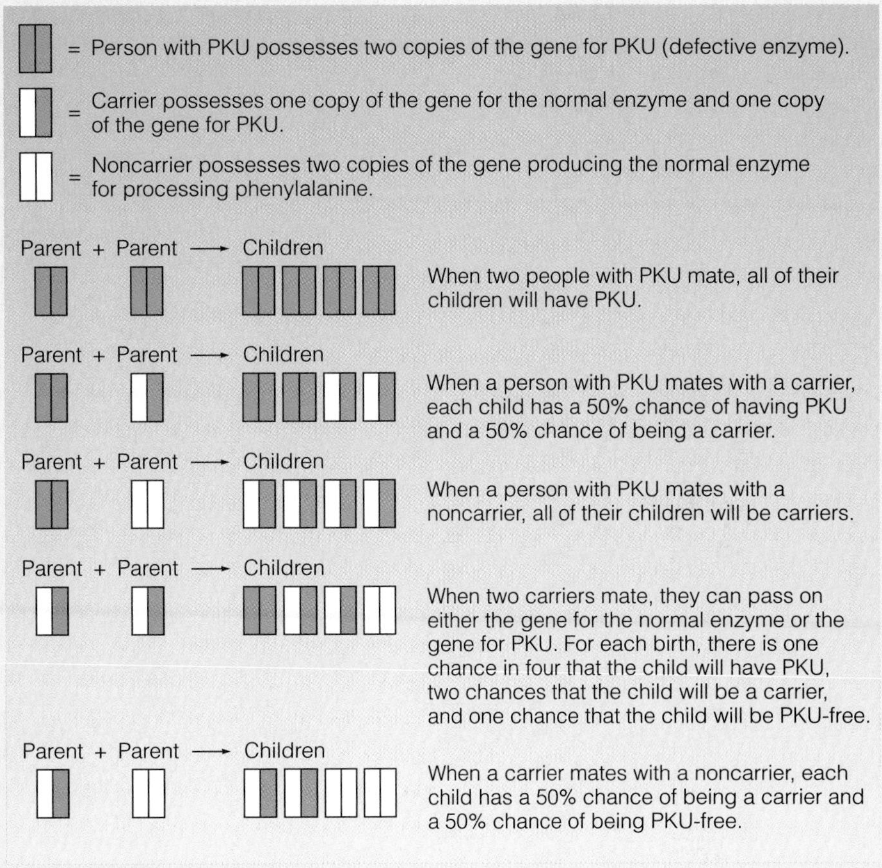

= Person with PKU possesses two copies of the gene for PKU (defective enzyme).

= Carrier possesses one copy of the gene for the normal enzyme and one copy of the gene for PKU.

= Noncarrier possesses two copies of the gene producing the normal enzyme for processing phenylalanine.

Parent + Parent → Children

When two people with PKU mate, all of their children will have PKU.

Parent + Parent → Children

When a person with PKU mates with a carrier, each child has a 50% chance of having PKU and a 50% chance of being a carrier.

Parent + Parent → Children

When a person with PKU mates with a noncarrier, all of their children will be carriers.

Parent + Parent → Children

When two carriers mate, they can pass on either the gene for the normal enzyme or the gene for PKU. For each birth, there is one chance in four that the child will have PKU, two chances that the child will be a carrier, and one chance that the child will be PKU-free.

Parent + Parent → Children

When a carrier mates with a noncarrier, each child has a 50% chance of being a carrier and a 50% chance of being PKU-free.

GALACTOSEMIA

Galactosemia is an inborn error of carbohydrate metabolism in which the body cannot use the monosaccharide galactose. Three enzymes are required for the conversion of galactose to glucose; in galactosemia, at least one of those enzymes is missing or defective. When infants with galactosemia are given standard infant formula or breast milk (which contains a galactose unit in each molecule of lactose), they vomit and have diarrhea. The unmetabolized product accumulates and follows an alternative metabolic pathway to form an abnormal product that causes growth failure, liver enlarge-

ment, and other neurological abnormalities that lead to coma and death. Early introduction of a galactose-restricted diet prevents or minimizes most of these symptoms. However, it may not prevent ovarian damage, some visual and speech problems, and other neurological abnormalities.

Dietary adjustment in galactosemia is simpler than in PKU for a couple of reasons. First, unlike phenylalanine, galactose is not an essential nutrient. The PKU diet is a balancing act between providing enough phenylalanine for normal growth and development on the

one hand and assuring that not enough is left over to be toxic on the other. The galactosemia diet needs only to exclude galactose. Second, galactose occurs primarily in lactose (the sugar in milk), so treatment depends chiefly on the careful restriction of milk and all milk products. This is not to say that the diet is easy to follow; many commercially prepared products contain milk. Still, milk is less widespread in the diet than the amino acid phenylalanine, which appears in all proteins.

As scientific understanding of human genetics and biochemistry

843

increases, more and more inborn errors affecting enzyme function are being recognized. Understanding the roles of enzymes in metabolism makes it possible to compensate for these defects of metabolism that otherwise would destroy the quality of life. Diet cannot always be tailored to prevent the defects of inborn errors, but in many such diseases diet can make a dramatic difference in people's lives.

NOTES

1. Committee on Genetics, Newborn screening fact sheet, *Pediatrics* 98 (1996): 473–501.

2. C. Reilly and coauthors, Trace element nutrition status and dietary intake of children with phenylketonuria, *American Journal of Clinical Nutrition* 52 (1990): 159–165.

3. L. C. Wolf-Novak and coauthors, Aspartame ingestion with and without carbohydrate in phenylketonuric and normal subjects: Effect on plasma concentrations of amino acids, glucose, and insulin, *Metabolism* 39 (1990): 391–396.

4. A. M. B. Fehrenbach and L. Peterson, Parental problem-solving skills, stress, and dietary compliance in phenylketonuria, *Journal of Consulting and Clinical Psychology* 57 (1989): 237–241.

5. Committee on Genetics, Maternal phenylketonuria, *Pediatrics* 88 (1991): 1284–1285.

6. P. B. Acosta, Phenylketonuria—Impact of nutrition support on reproductive outcomes, *Nutrition Today,* January/February 1991, pp. 43–47.

7. The Maternal Phenylketonuria Collaborative Study: A status report, *Nutrition Reviews* 52 (1994): 390–393.

8. Committee on Genetics, 1991; Acosta, 1991.

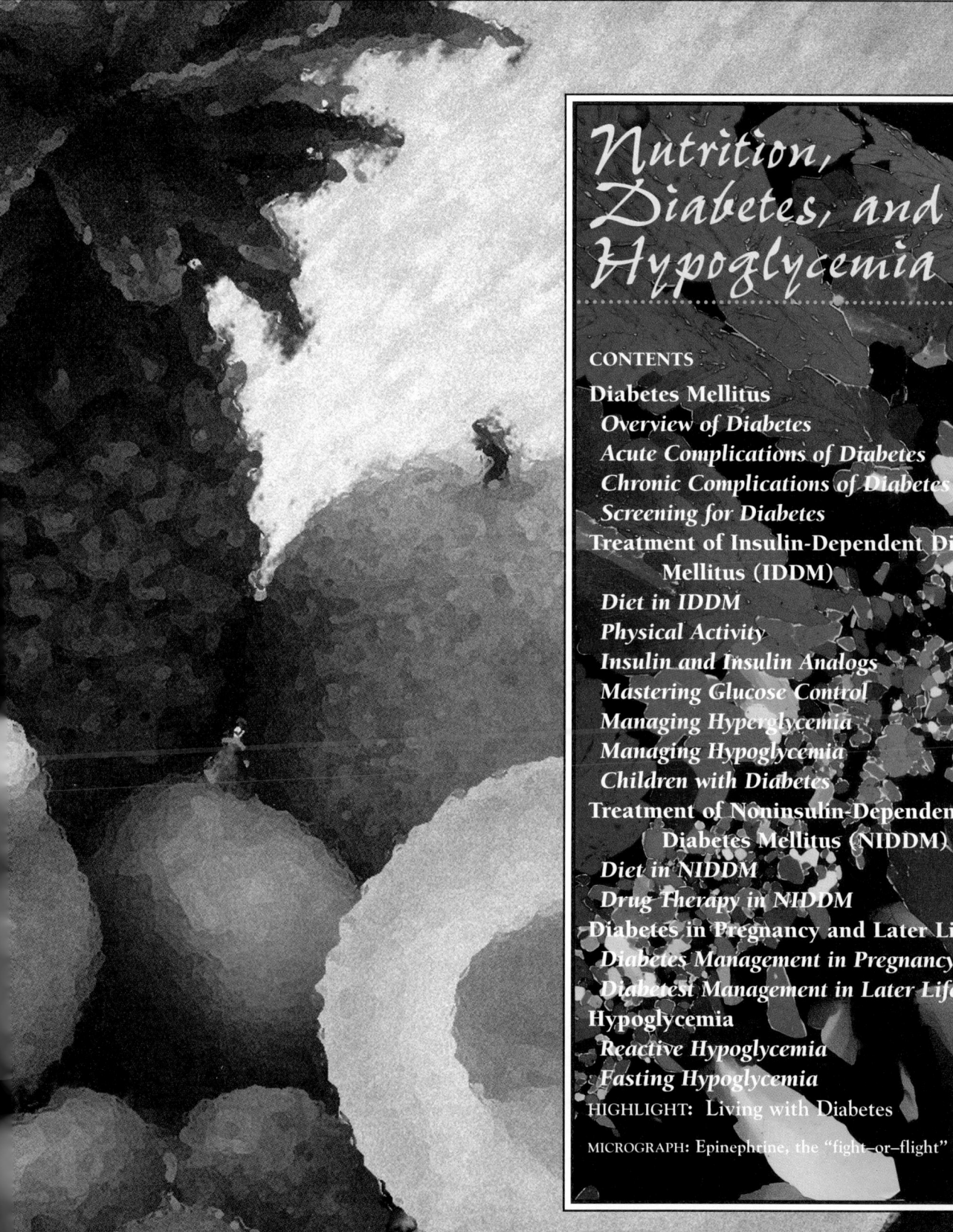

Chapter 27

Nutrition, Diabetes, and Hypoglycemia

CONTENTS

Diabetes Mellitus
Overview of Diabetes
Acute Complications of Diabetes
Chronic Complications of Diabetes
Screening for Diabetes
Treatment of Insulin-Dependent Diabetes Mellitus (IDDM)
Diet in IDDM
Physical Activity
Insulin and Insulin Analogs
Mastering Glucose Control
Managing Hyperglycemia
Managing Hypoglycemia
Children with Diabetes
Treatment of Noninsulin-Dependent Diabetes Mellitus (NIDDM)
Diet in NIDDM
Drug Therapy in NIDDM
Diabetes in Pregnancy and Later Life
Diabetes Management in Pregnancy
Diabetes Management in Later Life
Hypoglycemia
Reactive Hypoglycemia
Fasting Hypoglycemia
HIGHLIGHT: Living with Diabetes

MICROGRAPH: Epinephrine, the "fight–or–flight" hormone.

*t*he body's metabolic work is so vital to survival that metabolic disturbances, such as those imposed by severe stresses and liver dysfunction, are often severe and even fatal. Likewise, diabetes mellitus, a disorder of energy metabolism, and hypoglycemia, a symptom of altered glucose metabolism, can lead to serious consequences. Medical nutrition therapy for both conditions serves not only to maintain nutrition status, but also to control symptoms and prevent complications associated with each disorder.

Diabetes Mellitus

diabetes (DYE-uh-BEET-eez) mellitus (MELL-ih-tus or mell-EYE-tus): a metabolic disorder characterized by altered blood glucose regulation and utilization, usually caused by insufficient or relatively ineffective insulin.

diabetes = passing through (the body)
mellitus = honey-sweet (sugar)

Diabetes mellitus is a chronic disorder characterized by elevated blood glucose and altered energy metabolism caused by an absolute deficiency of insulin or ineffective insulin. About 8 million people in the United States have been diagnosed with diabetes, and estimates suggest that another 8 million people have the disorder but remain undiagnosed.[1] Still others have the first signs that they may develop diabetes later; the prevalence increases with age.

OVERVIEW OF DIABETES

Diabetes ranks among the leading causes of death in the United States. It is a major cause of blindness, kidney failure, infections necessitating leg amputations, and birth defects. In addition, people with diabetes are twice as likely to develop cardiovascular problems as those without diabetes. Table 27–1 shows the distinguishing features of the two main forms of diabetes, which are described next. Both forms appear to develop as a consequence of both hereditary and environmental factors.

Insulin-Dependent Diabetes Mellitus   Insulin, which signals the body to store energy fuels following meals, is produced by the islets of Langerhans—the

Table 27–1

Features of IDDM and NIDDM

	IDDM	NIDDM
Other names	Type I diabetes	Type II diabetes
	Juvenile-onset diabetes	Adult-onset diabetes
	Ketosis-prone diabetes	Ketosis-resistant diabetes
	Brittle diabetes	Lipoplethoric diabetes
		Stable diabetes
Age of onset	<20 (mean age, 12)	>40
Associated conditions	Viral infection	Obesity
Insulin required?	Yes	Sometimes
Cell response to insulin	Normal	Resistant
Symptoms	Relatively severe	Relatively moderate
Prevalence in diabetic population	5 to 10%	90 to 95%

endocrine cells of the pancreas. The pancreatic islets consist of several cell types including the beta cells, which produce insulin, and the alpha cells, which produce glucagon. In insulin-dependent diabetes (IDDM), the less common type of diabetes (about 5 to 10 percent of all diagnosed cases), the pancreas cannot synthesize insulin. Without insulin, the body's energy metabolism is dramatically altered with such serious consequences that people with IDDM cannot survive unless they obtain insulin from another source.

IDDM most frequently develops in people younger than 20, although the incidence peaks again in individuals over 40 who initially develop noninsulin-dependent diabetes and later become insulin dependent. Researchers believe that the individual with IDDM may have inherited a defect in which immune cells mistakenly attack and destroy insulin-producing pancreatic cells. IDDM frequently develops following exposure to certain viruses, further suggesting an immune system connection. Indeed, the detection of antibodies to the insulin-producing pancreatic cells indicates the destruction of such cells and predicts the subsequent development of IDDM.[2] Diabetes can develop secondary to other disorders, such as pancreatitis and cystic fibrosis (discussed in Chapter 22), or as a result of exposure to certain drugs or chemicals.

Noninsulin-Dependent Diabetes Mellitus   The predominant type of diabetes mellitus (90 to 95 percent of all cases), and the type likely to go undiagnosed, is called noninsulin-dependent diabetes mellitus (NIDDM). Although the exact cause of NIDDM remains unknown, high blood glucose and insulin resistance are the hallmarks of the disorder. In the initial stages, the pancreas produces insulin, but the cells become less and less sensitive to its effects. As blood glucose rises, the pancreas makes more insulin, and blood insulin rises to abnormally high levels (hyperinsulinemia). The chronic demand for insulin exhausts the beta cells, and finally insulin production falters as the disease progresses. NIDDM develops most often in people over 40 and appears to be associated with obesity (often of long duration), abdominal fat, and physical inactivity.[3] As body fat increases, body tissues become less able to respond to insulin. Thus NIDDM appears to be a self-aggravating condition.

Diabetes-Related Risk Disorders   A nationwide multicenter study (the Diabetes Prevention Program) is currently under way to determine whether early interventions for people with impaired glucose metabolism can prevent NIDDM.[4] People with impaired glucose tolerance have mild hyperglycemia without the symptoms of diabetes. Those most likely to develop impaired glucose tolerance include people from certain ethnic groups (Native Americans, Hispanic Americans, and African Americans); people who are obese, are over age 45 (especially those over 65), and have close relatives with diabetes; and women who have given birth to babies weighing more than 9 pounds or have developed hyperglycemia while pregnant—gestational diabetes (described in a later section).

Consequences of Diabetes   To appreciate the problems caused by either insufficient or ineffective insulin, recall that insulin enhances cellular uptake of glucose and fatty acids and stimulates protein synthesis, glycogen synthesis, and fat synthesis. Disruption of energy metabolism and exposure of the tissues to high glucose concentrations result in both acute and chronic complications. The accompanying glossary defines diabetes-related symptoms and complications.

insulin-dependent diabetes mellitus (IDDM): the less common type of diabetes in which the person produces no insulin at all.

The immune system disorders in which the body destroys its own tissues are called **autoimmune disorders.**

noninsulin-dependent diabetes mellitus (NIDDM): the more common type of diabetes that develops gradually and is associated with insulin resistance. A type of NIDDM that develops during the teen years has been termed **maturity-onset diabetes in the young (MODY).**

insulin resistance: the condition in which a set amount of insulin produces a subnormal effect.

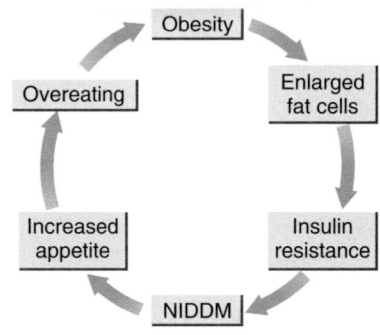

glucose tolerance: the ability of the body to regulate its blood glucose concentration to either the intake of dietary carbohydrate or the release of glucose from cells during fasting or metabolic stress.

Glossary of Diabetes-Related Symptoms and Complications

acetone breath: a distinctive fruity odor that can be detected on the breath of a person who is experiencing ketosis.

diabetic coma: unconsciousness precipitated by hyperglycemia, dehydration, ketosis, and acidosis in uncontrolled IDDM.

gangrene: death of tissue due to a deficient blood supply and/or infection.

gastroparesis: delayed gastric emptying.

glycosuria (GLY-ko-SUE-ree-ah) or glucosuria (GLUE-ko-SUE-ree-ah): glucose in the urine, which generally occurs when blood glucose exceeds 180 mg/100 ml.

hyperglycemia: elevated blood glucose.

hyperosmolar hyperglycemia nonketotic coma: coma that occurs in uncontrolled NIDDM precipitated by the presence of hypertonic blood and dehydration.

hypoglycemia: low blood glucose.

ketonemia: ketones in the blood.

ketonuria: ketones in the urine.

macroangiopathies: disorders of the large blood vessels.

microangiopathies: disorders of the capillaries.

nephropathy: a disorder of the kidneys.

neuropathy: a disorder of the nerves.

polydipsia (POLL-ee-DIP-see-ah): excessive thirst.

polyphagia (POLL-ee-FAY-gee-ah): excessive eating.

polyuria (POLL-ee-YOU-ree-ah): excessive urine production.

retinopathy: a disorder of the retina.

ACUTE COMPLICATIONS OF DIABETES

Figure 27–1 presents an overview of the metabolic changes and acute complications that occur in uncontrolled diabetes. The metabolic consequences of IDDM are more immediate and severe than those of NIDDM because in IDDM no glucose enters the cells.

Hyperglycemia, Dehydration, and Glycosuria With insufficient or ineffective insulin, blood glucose rises and hyperglycemia results. High blood glucose creates an osmotic effect, drawing water from tissues into the blood. Then the high blood concentration of glucose overwhelms the kidneys' ability to reabsorb glucose (the renal threshold). The excess glucose "spills" into the urine along with fluid and electrolytes. Glycosuria generally occurs when blood glucose exceeds 180 milligrams per 100 milliliters. As a result of hyperglycemia, both the intracellular and the extracellular fluid compartments become depleted, leading to severe dehydration. This series of events explains why the person with uncontrolled diabetes produces excessive urine (polyuria) and exhibits excessive thirst (polydipsia).

Ketosis and Coma in IDDM IDDM continuously deprives cells of the energy fuels they need. Amino acids and glucose may abound in the body fluids, but the cells have limited access to them. Consequently, the body mobilizes fat for energy. The liver responds to the mobilization of fatty acids by producing ketone bodies, which accumulate in the blood (ketonemia). A fruity odor on the

Symptoms of hyperglycemia:
- Intense thirst and hunger.
- Increased urination.
- Weight loss.
- Blurred vision.
- Fatigue.
- Acetone breath.
- Glycosuria.
- Labored breathing.

renal threshold: the point at which blood glucose rises so high that the kidneys cannot reabsorb it.

Figure 27–1

Metabolic Consequences and Acute Clinical Manifestations of Untreated IDDM and NIDDM

As you can see, when glucose cannot enter the cells, a cascade of metabolic changes follows. In NIDDM, some glucose enters the cells. Because the cells are not "starved" for glucose, the body does not shift into the metabolism of fasting (losing weight and producing ketones).

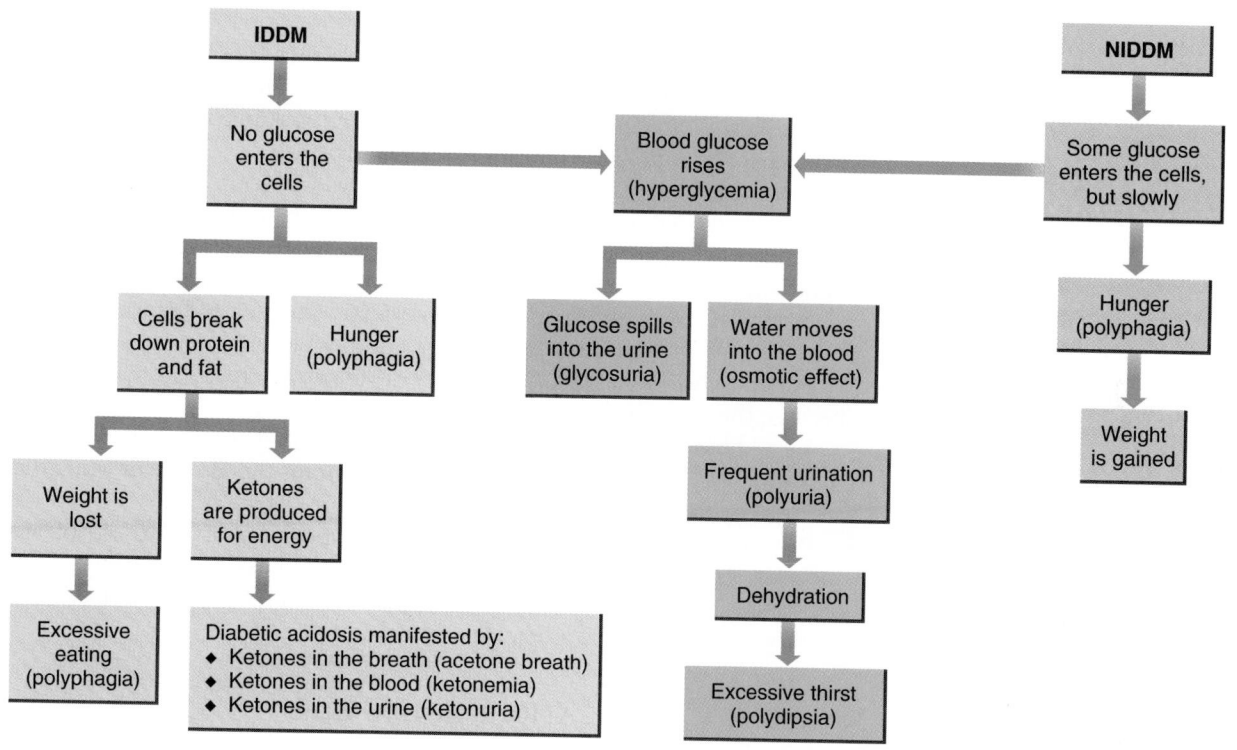

breath of a person with uncontrolled IDDM reflects the presence of the ketone acetone. Ketone bodies in the blood lower its pH (acidosis) because they contain acid groups. Ketone bodies also begin to appear in the urine (ketonuria). In addition, the kidneys excrete sodium and potassium along with the ketone bodies in a way that worsens acidosis. When acidosis becomes severe enough, a potentially fatal coma may follow.

Nonketotic Coma in NIDDM   People with NIDDM generally are not prone to ketosis and acidosis, but they can develop another kind of coma caused by extremely high blood glucose. This problem is common in the elderly because they may not recognize thirst and drink enough water to compensate for high blood glucose levels. Logically, this kind of coma is termed hyperosmolar hyperglycemic nonketotic coma.

Weight Loss in IDDM   With the loss of glucose and ketone bodies (both energy sources) in the urine, combined with protein breakdown, serious weight loss follows. The person with poorly controlled IDDM is likely to be thin despite eating excessively (polyphagia).

Reminder: *Ketone bodies* are produced by the incomplete breakdown of fat when glucose is not available in the cells.

Weight Gain in NIDDM NIDDM also deprives cells of the energy fuels they need, not continuously, but enough to make the cells hungry. As a result, people with NIDDM often overeat. Then the insulin they do have slowly takes effect, and the body ends up storing fat from the excess energy consumed. This explains why the person with NIDDM is likely to remain overweight and also why ketone bodies do not accumulate in the blood and urine.

Hypoglycemia Hypoglycemia is a consequence, not of untreated diabetes, but rather of inappropriate management. It can result from too much insulin or glucose-lowering drugs, strenuous physical activity, skipped meals, delayed meals, inadequate food intake, vomiting, or severe diarrhea.

Left untreated, severe hypoglycemia can lead to loss of consciousness, brain damage, and even death. Some research suggests that repeated episodes of hypoglycemia might permanently impair cognitive function.[5] Mental confusion and shakiness may make it difficult for the person to recognize symptoms of hypoglycemia (see the margin) and to take corrective measures. Recovery from severe hypoglycemia requires the assistance of another person.

Adults who have had diabetes for a long time risk severe hypoglycemia because the warning signs become less noticeable over time. People who tightly manage their blood glucose levels (intensive therapy) are more likely to develop hypoglycemia than others with diabetes. Symptoms can also occur while the person is sleeping, making hypoglycemia difficult to detect.

Notice that many of the symptoms of hypoglycemia are those of alcohol intoxication. If the true problem goes unrecognized, the person may die. To prevent such a tragic mistake, advise every person with IDDM to wear medical identification in the form of a bracelet or necklace.

CHRONIC COMPLICATIONS OF DIABETES

Chronic hyperglycemia damages the structures of the blood vessels and nerves. Circulation becomes poor and nerve function falters. Infections are more likely to occur due to poor circulation coupled with glucose-rich blood and urine. People with diabetes must pay special attention to hygiene and keep alert for early signs of infection.

Cardiovascular Diseases Atherosclerosis (see Chapter 28) tends to develop early, progress rapidly, and be more severe in people with diabetes. More than 80 percent of people with diabetes die as a consequence of cardiovascular diseases, especially heart attacks. If nerve function is also impaired, the person may have a heart attack and not even realize it.

Microangiopathies Disorders of the small blood vessels (capillaries) may also develop and lead to loss of kidney function and retinal degeneration with accompanying loss of vision. About 85 percent of people with diabetes have nephropathy, retinopathy, or both (see the glossary on p. 848). Consequently, as mentioned earlier, diabetes is a leading cause of both kidney failure and blindness.

Neuropathy Nerve tissues may also deteriorate, resulting in neuropathy. Neuropathy may express itself at first as a painful prickling sensation, often in the arms and legs. Later, the person loses sensation in the hands and feet. Injuries to

Symptoms of hypoglycemia:
- Hunger.
- Headache.
- Sweating.
- Shakiness.
- Nervousness.
- Confusion.
- Disorientation.
- Slurred speech.

Disorders of the large blood vessels, including atherosclerosis, are called macroangiopathies.

macro = large
angio = blood vessel
pathy = disease

A heart attack that goes unnoticed is called a silent heart attack.

Disorders of the small blood vessels are called microangiopathies.

micro = small

these areas may go unnoticed, and infections can progress rapidly. With loss of both circulation and nerve function, undetected injury and infection may lead to death of tissue (gangrene), necessitating amputation of the limbs (most often the legs or feet). People with neuropathy are advised to take conscientious care of their feet and visit a podiatrist regularly.

Neuropathy can also delay gastric emptying. When the stomach empties slowly after a meal, the person may experience a premature feeling of fullness, bloating, nausea, vomiting, weight loss, and poor blood glucose control due to irregular nutrient absorption.

SCREENING FOR DIABETES

A major multicenter clinical trial, the Diabetes Control and Complications Trial (DCCT), showed that carefully controlling blood glucose in a near-normal range can reduce the risks of chronic complications in IDDM by 50 to 80 percent.[6] Evidence that similar results might be possible in NIDDM is mounting. Recognizing that many people may have diabetes and not know it, and that early treatment might reduce the risk of serious complications, efforts are under way to screen for diabetes.

Because the lifetime risk of developing NIDDM is one in five, screening all people over age 30 for the early detection of diabetes would be ideal.[7] The American Diabetes Association recommends that all people over the age of 45 be tested for diabetes every three years.[8] Those at high risk for diabetes (see p. 847) need screening at earlier ages or more frequently.

Blood tests help identify people with diabetes or impaired glucose tolerance. Most commonly, high fasting blood glucose on two occasions suggests diabetes. Fasting blood glucose higher than normal, but not high enough to confirm diabetes, indicates impaired glucose tolerance. Health care professionals often advise people with impaired glucose tolerance to begin diet therapy for diabetes. Some physicians prefer to test a person's fasting blood glucose and then retest several times more after glucose is given orally—a procedure called a glucose tolerance test.

Diabetes mellitus is characterized by elevated blood glucose caused by either an absolute deficiency of insulin (IDDM) or ineffective insulin (NIDDM). Table 27–1 summarizes the distinguishing features of IDDM and NIDDM, and Figure 27–1 shows their metabolic consequences and symptoms. Long-term complications of diabetes include cardiovascular diseases, kidney failure, blindness, and nerve damage. Screening for diabetes through blood and urine tests allows for early detection and early treatment, which helps to minimize complications.

Major risk factors for NIDDM:
- Obesity.
- Family history.
- High-risk ethnic background.
- Gestational diabetes or mother giving birth to a baby weighing over 9 lb.

Interpretation of fasting blood glucose:
 Normal: <110 mg/100 ml.
 Impaired glucose tolerance: 110–126 mg/100 ml.
 Diabetes: >126 mg/100 ml.

Impaired glucose tolerance is sometimes called borderline diabetes.

Treatment of Insulin-Dependent Diabetes Mellitus (IDDM)

A diagnosis of IDDM can be devastating. The parents of a young child with IDDM may feel overwhelmed, angry, anxious, and even guilty. A teenager may feel that it is the end of the world. A person of any age may fear the prospect of daily insulin injections, possible complications, and the new diet. To control blood glucose successfully, the person must master the complex task of

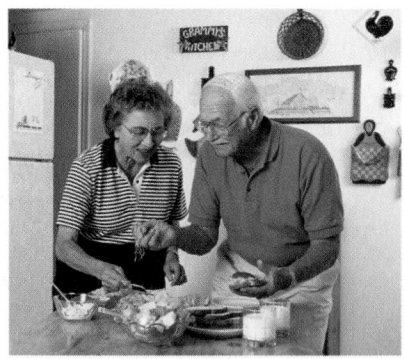

The diet for diabetes emphasizes a consistent intake of carbohydrate spaced evenly throughout the day.

coordinating diet, physical activity, and insulin. On the bright side, however, is that with such mastery the person can live a full and active life and significantly reduce the risk of chronic complications. Highlight 27 describes how health care professionals can assist in this process.

The goals of medical and nutrition therapy for diabetes are to maintain blood glucose within a fairly normal range, achieve optimal blood lipid levels, control blood pressure, support health and well-being, and treat complications. The most important of these goals is to maintain blood glucose control.

To the student reading about diabetes today, such a goal may seem obvious: of course, blood glucose should be maintained at or near levels observed in people without diabetes. Only recently, however, have improvements in the technology for monitoring blood levels at home made such tight control possible. Only recently, too, have the benefits of tight control been clearly demonstrated. (A later section describes blood glucose monitoring in more detail.)

Assessment is important in diabetes: an accurate history enables the health care team to work out acceptable goals for a diet, physical activity, and insulin program. To promote success, the health care team plans and adjusts therapy for the client's medical needs, motivational level, educational ability, and lifestyle. Successful diabetes education takes time and must be flexible to accommodate changing needs.

DIET IN IDDM

The diet for diabetes parallels a healthy diet for all people in both amounts and types of nutrients. It differs from a regular diet in that carbohydrate intake must be consistent from day to day and at each meal and snack, or adjustments must be made in insulin administration. The actual distribution of nutrients for each client depends on medical needs and current food habits.

Energy   The diet for IDDM first focuses on providing adequate food energy to achieve or maintain a healthy and realistic body weight and to support growth in children and pregnant women. To determine whether energy intake is appropriate, the planner uses the RDA for energy as a guide, takes height and weight measures periodically, and adjusts the diet as necessary.

Carbohydrate   Carbohydrate-containing foods provide energy and directly affect blood glucose. The more carbohydrate a person eats in a meal, the higher blood glucose rises, but the diet for IDDM does not restrict carbohydrate intake. Carbohydrate is necessary to maintain a steady supply of glucose. Typically, diet plans provide from 45 to 60 percent of the total kcalories from carbohydrate. Eating about the same amount of carbohydrate at about the same time each day helps the person avoid hyperglycemia and hypoglycemia and eases the task of coordinating insulin doses and food intake.

Encourage clients to select foods rich in complex carbohydrates: whole-grain breads and cereals, legumes, fruits, and vegetables. In addition to carbohydrates, these foods provide vitamins and minerals and offer many health benefits (see Chapter 4).

Recall that authorities recommend 20 to 35 g of dietary fiber a day.

Traditionally, concentrated sweets were strictly excluded from the diet for diabetes, but now they are restricted only to the same extent as they are for all people. Health care professionals recognize that the *total* carbohydrate is of greater concern in diabetes than the *type* of carbohydrate.[9] The person with diabetes can use concentrated sweets as a limited part of a healthy diet, as long as they are counted as part of the carbohydrate allowance. Artificial sweeteners that contain minimal kcalories, and products made from them, can be used in place of sugar.

Carbohydrate Replacement for Missed Meals   A person with IDDM who misses a meal needs to eat about 15 to 30 grams of complex carbohydrate to forestall hypoglycemia. If appetite is poor, people can use juice, flavored gelatin, soft drinks, or frozen juice bars to meet their carbohydrate needs. In the hospital, if a person with IDDM misses a meal, different procedures may be employed. One procedure provides at least half the prescribed carbohydrate and kcalories within three hours of the missed meal. If this cannot be done, the physician may change the insulin schedule, give IV dextrose, or change the diet prescription to include more simple carbohydrates.

Carbohydrate from Enteral and Parenteral Formulas   When people with diabetes require enteral or parenteral formulas, adjustments may need to be made for the large amount of carbohydrates the formulas contain. Often health care professionals adjust insulin doses to meet the higher carbohydrate load.[10] If additional insulin fails to control hyperglycemia, people on parenteral nutrition may need to receive less energy from dextrose and more from IV fat emulsions (see Chapter 24). People who cannot tolerate the carbohydrate in standard enteral formulas may benefit from specially designed formulas that contain less total carbohydrate (see Appendix K).

Protein   Protein provides about 10 to 20 percent of the total kcalories in the diet for diabetes. Providing adequate, but not excessive, protein may help delay the onset or progression of kidney disease (see Chapter 29). At the first sign of kidney disease, people with diabetes may need to restrict protein to 0.8 grams per kilogram of body weight per day (same as the RDA).[11]

An early sign of impending kidney disease is elevated albumin in the urine or microalbuminuria (see Chapter 29).

Fat   People with diabetes who have normal blood lipids benefit from a fat intake consistent with the *Dietary Guidelines for Americans* (30 percent or less of total kcalories from fat and less than 10 percent from saturated fat). Those who need to lose weight may need to restrict fat further. People with diabetes and elevated LDL may need to restrict saturated fat to 7 percent or less of total kcalories and cholesterol to less than 200 milligrams daily (see Chapter 28). To lower fat and cholesterol intakes, clients can use low-fat and nonfat milk and lean meats, among other strategies (see p. 168).

Sodium   People with diabetes frequently develop hypertension and are likely to be salt sensitive. Practitioners generally advise all clients with diabetes to limit sodium to less than 3000 milligrams per day.[12] People with diabetes and hypertension may need to restrict sodium to 2400 milligrams or less per day. Chapter 12 (p. 421) describes strategies to lower sodium intake.

One drink is defined as 1½ oz liquor or 5 oz wine or 12 oz beer. Note: light beer contains the same amount of alcohol as regular beer, with half the carbohydrate. When counting kcalories, 1 drink = 2 fat exchanges.

Alcohol   The person whose blood glucose is well controlled can usually include some alcoholic beverages with the consent of the physician. Because alcohol can cause hypoglycemia in any person, however, people with IDDM are advised to take only moderate amounts (no more than two drinks a day), with meals, and in addition to the usual meal plan. Remember, too, that the person with hypoglycemia may appear to be intoxicated, and alcohol use can add confusion to a potentially dangerous situation.

Alcohol intake is discouraged for people with a history of alcohol abuse; those with pancreatitis, abnormal blood lipids, or neuropathy; and pregnant women. Alcohol use is also discouraged for people who are overweight; if it is used, alcohol should be substituted for fat exchanges. Drinks that contain simple sugars (mixers, sweet wines, and liqueurs) are best avoided. If they are used, the person must count their carbohydrate contents as part of the daily carbohydrate allowance.

Timing and Composition of Meals   In diabetes, consistent timing and composition of meals and snacks from day to day improve glucose control. An evening snack is especially important because it helps sustain the person's blood glucose through the night. A person with a regular physical activity program who takes a prescribed dose of insulin at a set time and then eats about the same amount of carbohydrate at about the same time each day knows that glucose and insulin will be available to the body when they are needed. Meal patterns and physical activity programs that change dramatically from day to day require careful blood glucose monitoring and insulin adjustments to help maintain control. People who find a set schedule difficult to maintain need to work with skilled health care professionals to learn how to adjust their insulin doses to fit their food intakes and physical activity schedules.

Diet-related behaviors that may improve blood glucose control include:

- Adherence to the meal plan.
- Appropriate treatment of hypoglycemia.
- Prompt treatment of hyperglycemia.
- Consistent and appropriate bedtime snacking.[13]

Dietitians teach the diet in stages, starting first with simple concepts and progressing to more difficult ones as the client's abilities and needs dictate.

Appendix G includes the U.S. Exchange System, and Appendix I shows the Canadian Exchange System.

Meal-Planning Strategies   No single approach to diet therapy meets everyone's needs, and diet planners use several approaches to help clients achieve blood glucose control. Some diet strategies teach clients to use food guides or simple menus to plan diets. Traditionally, however, diet planners use the exchange patterns described in Chapter 17 (see pp. 570–575). Recall that the foods within each list of the exchange system are similar in food energy and in carbohydrate, protein, and fat per serving. The person using this system learns that the food portions on any one list can be exchanged freely for one another. For example, a person who needs a starch exchange might select one slice of bread or ½ cup of bran cereal or one small (3 ounce) baked potato. The accompanying box shows how to plan a diet for diabetes using exchange lists.

A strategy gaining wide use, called *carbohydrate counting*, teaches clients to focus mainly on the carbohydrate contents of foods. Clients can use food composition tables, food labels, and exchange lists to determine the carbohydrate contents of the foods they eat. Clients using this system learn to eat consistent amounts of carbohydrates at meals and snacks. They must have the motivation to weigh or measure portion sizes and the ability to perform the mathematical operations necessary to calculate their carbohydrate intakes. Regardless of the

How to Plan a Diet for Diabetes Using Exchange Lists

The dietitian most often plans the diet for a client with diabetes. In doing so, the dietitian carefully considers the client's lifestyle and medical needs. Planning a diet using exchange lists takes time, but with practice, a dietitian can learn to plan diets quickly. This box describes a simplified diet plan.

Dietitians begin by assessing each individual to determine what weight is reasonable and how many kcalories are necessary to achieve or maintain that body weight. Chapter 16 described ways of estimating desirable body weights, and the box on p. 265 in Chapter 8 showed how to estimate energy needs based on body weight and physical activity levels. Chapter 9 described kcalorie needs for safe weight loss (see p. 302) and weight gain (see p. 310). The growth charts in Appendix E can be used to estimate desirable weights for children, and Chapter 19 (see p. 638) described their energy needs. Remember, though, that desirable weights and calculated energy needs are estimates only.

For this example, we will use a man who is 6 feet tall and is comfortable with the weight of 178 pounds that he has maintained throughout his adult life. From an assessment of food intake, the dietitian estimates that the man has maintained his weight on about 2900 kcalories per day with 25 percent of kcalories from protein, 45 percent from carbohydrate, and 30 percent from fat.

1. The first step is to determine the grams of protein, carbohydrate, and fat recommended for a diet for diabetes.

   - 10 to 20% of the kcalories from protein.
   - 45 to 60% of the kcalories from carbohydrate.
   - 30% or less of the kcalories from fat.

   For 2900 kcalories, this division of nutrients translates into grams as follows:

   - Protein:

     $$10\% \times 2900 \text{ kcal} = 290 \text{ kcal.} \qquad 290 \text{ kcal} \div 4 \text{ kcal/g} = 73 \text{ g.}$$
     $$20\% \times 2900 \text{ kcal} = 580 \text{ kcal.} \qquad 580 \text{ kcal} \div 4 \text{ kcal/g} = 145 \text{ g.}$$

   Thus the man needs between 73 and 145 g protein.

   - Carbohydrate:

     $$45\% \times 2900 \text{ kcal} = 1305 \text{ kcal.} \qquad 1305 \text{ kcal} \div 4 \text{ kcal/g} = 326 \text{ g.}$$
     $$60\% \times 2900 \text{ kcal} = 1740 \text{ kcal.} \qquad 1740 \text{ kcal} \div 4 \text{ kcal/g} = 435 \text{ g.}$$

   Thus the man needs between 326 and 435 g carbohydrate.

   - Fat:

     $$30\% \times 2900 \text{ kcal} = 870 \text{ kcal.} \qquad 870 \text{ kcal} \div 9 \text{ kcal/g} = 97 \text{ g.}$$

   Thus the man needs about 97 g fat or less.

2. The dietitian recognizes that the client will need to make dietary changes to conform to a healthy eating plan. To minimize the changes the client must make, the dietitian decides to plan the diet to include 20 percent protein or 580 kcalories. Thus 80 percent or 2320 kcalories remain for carbohydrate and fat. After reviewing information about the man's blood lipids, which are within acceptable limits, the dietitian plans the diet to keep fat at the current level of 30 percent (870 kcalories). This means that 50 percent of the kcalories (1450 kcalories) remain for carbohydrate.

   $$2900 \text{ total kcal} - 580 \text{ protein kcal} - 870 \text{ fat kcal} = 1450 \text{ carbohydrate kcal.}$$

3. To translate the kcalories from fat and carbohydrate to grams:

   $$870 \text{ fat kcal} \div 9 \text{ kcal/g} = 96.6 \text{ g (round down to 96 to limit fat).}$$

How to Plan a Diet for Diabetes Using Exchange Lists (continued)

1450 carbohydrate kcal ÷ 4 kcal/g = 362.5 g (round up to 363).

Thus the diet will provide 2900 kcalories with a distribution of 20 percent protein (145 grams or 580 kcalories), 50 percent carbohydrate (363 grams or 1450 kcalories), and 30 percent fat (96 grams or 870 kcalories).

4. Now it is time to translate the diet prescription into a meal plan. Table 17–2 on p. 571 shows the grams of carbohydrate, protein, and fat and the energy value in each serving on an exchange list. Using this table and the client's food intake record as a guide, the dietitian first plans servings of foods that contain carbohydrate, then protein, and finally fat, trying to match foods as closely as possible to the client's usual food intake. This process takes practice and requires some adjusting based on trial and error. Most often, the final result does not fit the meal plan exactly, but comes close. Table 27–2 shows how the dietitian might plan a day's exchanges for the man in this example. Note that the plan falls within the guidelines of the Daily Food Guide on p. 42. The plan uses nonfat milk and lean meat exchanges for calculations. Lower-fat foods are encouraged. If the client occasionally chooses to use another type of milk or meat, the number of fat servings must be adjusted accordingly. For example, if the client eats 4 ounces of a high-fat meat (32 grams of fat) instead of lean meat (12 grams of fat), he must then use four fewer fat exchanges during the day (20 grams of fat). The plan shown in Table 27–2 does not include the "other carbohydrates" list; starches and other foods (described later) can be substituted for foods on this list.

5. Distribute foods into meals that fit the client's usual eating patterns. Table 27–3 shows how the day's exchanges might be divided for the man in this example. With this information in hand, the dietitian and client can begin to fill in the plan with real foods to create a sample menu such as the one shown on p. 858. The client is reminded to eat about the same amount of carbohydrate at about the same time each day.

6. Teach clients how to tailor the diet to meet their own preferences. For example, foods from the starch, fruit, milk, and other carbohydrate lists contain similar amounts of energy and carbohydrate and can be substituted for one another from time to time. Regular substitution is discouraged, however, because each list makes unique contributions to other nutrient needs. A client who regularly substitutes fruit for milk, for example, may not be getting enough calcium. The client who regularly substitutes milk for a starch or fruit may not be getting enough fiber.[a]

Several servings of free foods can be used as long as their use is spread throughout the day. Free foods contain up to 20 kcalories and 5 grams of carbohydrate per serving.

---

[a]M. Wheeler, M. J. Franz, and P. Barrier, Helpful hints: Using the 1995 exchange lists for meal planning, *Diabetes Spectrum* 8 (1995): 325–326.

diet strategy, all clients receive instructions on planning well-balanced and healthy meals, eating consistent amounts of foods at regular times, and maintaining a desirable weight.

PHYSICAL ACTIVITY

Fitness programs confer benefits on the cardiovascular system that people with diabetes especially need. People with IDDM must take certain precautions when engaging in physical activity, however.

Physical Activity and Blood Glucose in IDDM   For the person without diabetes, blood glucose generally varies little during physical activity unless the activity is intense and of very long duration, such as marathon running. This is

Table 27–2

A Day's Exchanges for a Sample 2900-kCalorie Diet

Exchange Group/List	Number of Exchanges	Carbohydrate (g)	Protein (g)	Fat[a] (g)
Carbohydrate Group[b]				
Starch	13	195	39	0
Fruit	7	105	—	—
Milk	3	36	24	0
Vegetable	6	30	12	—
Meat and Meat Substitutes Group				
Lean	10	—	70	30
Fat Group	13	—	—	65
Total grams		366	145	95
Total kcalories		1464	580	855
% kcalories		50.5	20	29.5

[a]To ease calculation, exchanges from the carbohydrate groups are assumed to have 0 grams fat. If the client uses a fat-containing exchange, the fat can be deducted from the daily fat allowance.
[b]Foods from the "other carbohydrates" list can be substituted for a starch, fruit, or milk list exchange. Any fat in the selected food is then deducted from the daily fat allowance.

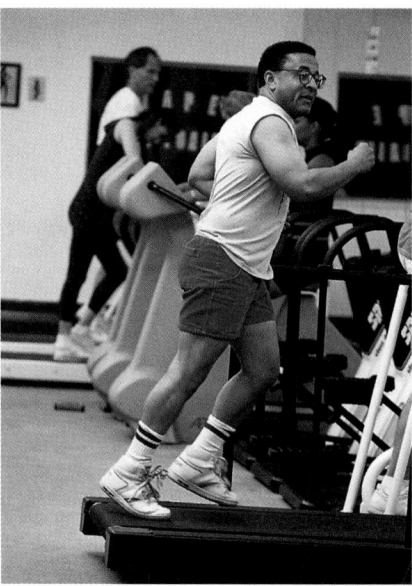

Physical activity plays an important role in the management of diabetes.

not the case in IDDM, where blood glucose can vary markedly with exercise. People with IDDM who have mild hyperglycemia may experience a *fall* in blood glucose during physical activity, whereas those with marked hyperglycemia may experience a still greater *rise* in blood glucose. For this reason, people with IDDM check their blood glucose prior to exercise and refrain from vigorous physical activity if their blood glucose levels are too high (greater than 300 milligrams per 100 milliliters).

Table 27–3

Translating a Day's Exchanges into Meals

Exchange Group/List	Number of Exchanges[a]	Breakfast	Lunch	Midafternoon Snack	Supper	Bedtime Snack
Carbohydrate Group						
Starch	13	3	3	2	3	2
Fruit	7	2	1	1	1	2
Milk	3	1	1		1	
Vegetable	6		3		3	
Meat and Meat Substitutes Group						
Lean	10		3	1	4	2
Fat Group	13	3	3	2	3	2

[a]From Table 27–2.

with insulin treatment and relief from the constant hyperglycemia of uncontrolled diabetes, the insulin-producing cells of the pancreas become able to function normally again—but only temporarily. Tight control of blood glucose—whether by diet, insulin, or hypoglycemic agents—helps prolong the "honeymoon."

multiple daily injections (MDI): delivery of different types of insulin by injection three or more times daily.

Insulin Delivery   People with IDDM inject insulin or use pumps to deliver the insulin they need. The person with IDDM who chooses injections often receives a mixture of two or more types of insulin, three or more times daily; single injections are seldom effective.

External pumps, about the size of a pager, hold enough insulin to meet needs for two to three days. From the pump, the insulin enters the body through tubing and a needle that has been inserted into the abdominal area. Personal preferences, motivational level, and financial considerations guide clients in deciding which delivery system works best for them.

Researchers continue to search for better and more comfortable methods of delivering insulin. Although not yet commercially available, researchers report promising results using implantable pumps that automatically deliver scheduled doses of insulin.[15] Each pump is approximately the size of a hockey puck and holds a three-month supply of insulin. Once the pump is surgically implanted in the abdomen, the client can release extra doses of insulin as needed by sending signals to the pump with a transmitter. The pump can be refilled as needed at the physician's office. Researchers are also working to develop glucose sensors that will continuously monitor blood glucose and adjust insulin delivery as needed.

Insulin and Food Intake   Insulin delivery is timed to mimic the body's normal insulin action as closely as possible. Normally, the body secretes a constant, baseline amount of insulin at all times and secretes more as blood glucose rises following meals. The person with IDDM often receives NPH (intermediate-acting) insulin to meet baseline needs and regular (rapid-acting) insulin or insulin analogs to process energy nutrients following meals. The physician initially prescribes the types and dosages of insulin based on individual needs. Although these needs vary greatly, as a rule of thumb, a total of about 0.5 to 1.0 unit of insulin is given per kilogram of body weight per day. The health care team teaches people with IDDM to adjust their insulin doses to accommodate changes in eating patterns, physical activity, or health status.

Insulin and Physical Activity   Generally, insulin should be taken more than an hour before physical activity. Vigorous physical activity and warm temperatures speed blood flow, increase the rate of insulin absorption, and set the stage for a hypoglycemic reaction, which may even occur after several hours. Reducing the insulin doses before and after the activity by up to 30 percent, or even 50 percent, can help to prevent this sequence of events.

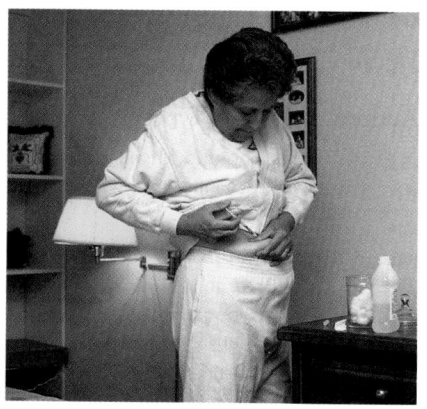
Injections are one option for delivering insulin for people with diabetes.

Pancreas Transplants   Pancreas transplants in people with IDDM have been successful in providing functional, insulin-producing cells. People with IDDM who are candidates for pancreas transplants often are those who encounter serious problems managing their diseases with insulin. Otherwise, the risks associated with the surgery and the need for immunosuppressant drugs would outweigh the benefits of the transplant. Most often, however, a pancreas transplant is combined with a kidney transplant. For the person with IDDM who needs a kidney transplant, the addition of a pancreas transplant can enhance the quality of life.[16] One year after surgery, 75 percent of people who received a simultaneous pancreas-kidney transplant do not need insulin.[17] For people undergoing a pancreas transplant only, 50 percent do not need insulin after one year.

MASTERING GLUCOSE CONTROL

Motivated clients who keep accurate records of food intake, physical activity, blood glucose measurements, and insulin doses learn how to control their blood glucose even when they change their usual eating habits or activity schedule. The health care team determines acceptable fasting and after-meal blood glucose goals for each client. People with IDDM on intensive therapy receive insulin three or four times a day, either through injections or from an external pump. They test their blood glucose levels about four times daily and have monthly medical checkups that include measurement of hemoglobin A_{1c} (described below). People on standard therapy receive insulin one or two times a day, monitor blood glucose once a day, and have medical checkups that include measurement of hemoglobin A_{1c} three or four times a year. The team uses the client's records to make sure goals are being met; if not, the team investigates the reasons and suggests solutions.

Blood Glucose Monitoring   To test blood glucose at home, the client pricks a finger to get a blood sample (the same method used to determine hematocrit) and transfers the blood to a strip. Most clients today rely on computerized meters that measure the blood glucose concentration from the blood sample. Less accurate and less costly are paper strips that change to different colors, depending on the blood glucose concentration.

At first, the person performs blood tests at least seven times during the day: before each meal, two hours after each meal, and at bedtime. During this time, clients who conscientiously adhere to a consistent diet and physical activity program learn how their blood glucose levels respond to diet, physical activity, and insulin. Once people learn to control their blood glucose levels, they can test blood glucose less often.

Glycated Hemoglobin   In addition to blood glucose records, physicians monitor blood glucose control by evaluating hemoglobin A_{1c}. As blood glucose rises, small glucose molecules spontaneously attach to an amino acid on each hemoglobin. The glucose molecules remain attached to the hemoglobin molecules until the cells die (about 120 days). Therefore, hemoglobin A_{1c} reflects diabetes control over the past two to three months, whereas a single blood glucose test reflects diabetes control just prior to the test.

Urinary Ketones   Health care professionals often recommend that clients with consistently high blood glucose also monitor ketones in the urine, especially during illness. As described earlier, the individual with diabetes can develop a type of coma associated with high ketone levels.

Other Measures   The health care team also monitors the client's weight, blood lipid levels, blood pressure, and reflexes and checks for early signs of

The Diabetes Control and Complications Trial sought to maintain fasting and pre-meal glucose between 80 and 120 mg/100 ml. In this study, groups receiving intensive treatment achieved an average fasting blood glucose of 155 mg/100 ml.

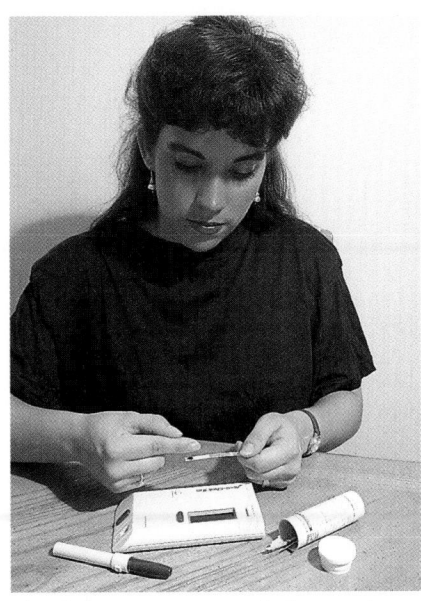

Blood glucose monitoring helps people with diabetes maintain blood glucose in a safe range.

Glycated hemoglobin is also called glycosylated hemoglobin. The type of glycated hemoglobin most commonly measured to screen for diabetes or monitor control of diabetes is hemoglobin A_{1c}, which normally averages <6%.

In the Diabetes Control and Complications Trial, groups receiving intensive treatment achieved an average hemoglobin A_{1c} of 7.2%.

complications. As described earlier, urine tests can help detect the early signs of kidney disease. Eye exams help identify the early signs of retinopathy, and foot exams detect early signs of infection.

At medical appointments, the health care team reviews the client's records to monitor the client's progress and look for patterns that suggest the need for adjustments in the treatment plan. In making recommendations, the team keeps in mind the four factors that influence blood glucose regulation: diet, physical activity, insulin dose, and the level of counterregulatory hormones.

The counterregulatory hormones (including glucagon, cortisol, and catecholamines) oppose insulin's actions.

MANAGING HYPERGLYCEMIA

Table 27–5 on p. 863 summarizes strategies for adjusting treatment plans to correct problems with hyperglycemia and hypoglycemia. Regular detection of hyperglycemia before lunch or dinner in a person with a consistent carbohydrate intake signals the health care professional to look back to the previous meal to make corrections. (Recall that it takes time for food to be digested and absorbed before blood glucose rises.) Treatment may involve adjusting the dose of regular insulin, adding physical activity to the plan, reducing the amount of carbohydrate at the previous meal, or spacing the meals so that the available insulin has time to work. The client's medical needs, lifestyle, and preferences dictate which course is best.

dawn phenomenon: early morning hyperglycemia that develops in response to counterregulatory hormones that act to raise glucose levels during an overnight fast.

Dawn Phenomenon   Early morning (before breakfast) hyperglycemia can occur in people with diabetes as a natural response to an overnight fast. During the night, levels of counterregulatory hormones increase and act to raise blood glucose. Without adequate insulin, glucose fails to enter the cells and hyperglycemia results. Treatment of this form of hyperglycemia may require adjustment of the intermediate-acting insulin given at bedtime. Many clients need more regular insulin to cover their needs in the morning, until counterregulatory hormone levels fall.

rebound hyperglycemia: hyperglycemia resulting from excessive secretion of counterregulatory hormones in response to excessive insulin; also called the Somogyi (so-MOHG-yee) effect.

Rebound Hyperglycemia   A similar but more dramatic and severe form of hyperglycemia can occur when a person uses too much insulin to meet needs. People who take high insulin doses or engage in strenuous physical activity (which reduces insulin needs) are more likely than others with diabetes to experience this form of hyperglycemia. At first, the insulin drives glucose into the cells, and hypoglycemia results. Then, the body reacts by markedly raising the level of counterregulatory hormones, which causes blood glucose levels to rise rapidly. Giving more insulin at this point makes the problem worse, so treatment includes reducing the insulin dose.

Illness   Even a minor illness such as a cold or flu may cause blood glucose to rise dramatically, and the client may require higher insulin doses. Thus a record of illness helps evaluators interpret blood glucose test results. During this precarious time, clients with diabetes should vigilantly monitor blood glucose and urinary ketones and carefully follow insulin and dietary instructions. Physicians may advise clients to reduce total energy and carbohydrate intakes slightly to limit the need for extra insulin. A major concern is the prevention of starvation, dehydration, and vomiting.

Table 27–5

Strategies for Managing Hyperglycemia and Hypoglycemia

Problem	Possible Solutions[a]
HYPERGLYCEMIA	
Before breakfast	• Adjust dose of intermediate-acting insulin at bedtime.[b]
Before lunch	• Adjust morning dose of rapid-acting insulin.[b]
	• Reduce amount of carbohydrate at breakfast.
	• Reduce or omit midmorning snack.
	• Change time of breakfast or midmorning snack.
	• Add physical activity after breakfast.
Before dinner	• Adjust afternoon dose of rapid-acting insulin.[b]
	• Reduce carbohydrate at lunch.
	• Reduce or omit midafternoon snack.
	• Change time of lunch or midafternoon snack.
	• Add physical activity between lunch and dinner.
At bedtime	• Adjust insulin dose before dinner.[b]
	• Reduce amount of carbohydrate at dinner.
	• Reduce or omit evening snack.
	• Add physical activity after dinner.
HYPOGLYCEMIA	
Before breakfast	• Adjust dose of intermediate- or long-acting insulin at bedtime.[b]
	• Add carbohydrate at evening snack.
	• Avoid strenuous activity late in the day.
Before lunch	• Adjust morning dose of rapid-acting insulin.[b]
	• Add carbohydrate at breakfast.
	• Add a morning snack.
	• Change time of breakfast, lunch, or morning snack.
	• Adjust physical activity schedule.
Before dinner	• Adjust afternoon dose of rapid-acting insulin.[b]
	• Add carbohydrate at lunch.
	• Add an afternoon snack.
	• Change time of lunch, dinner, or afternoon snack.
	• Adjust physical activity schedule.
At bedtime	• Adjust insulin dose before dinner.[b]
	• Add carbohydrate at dinner.
	• Add an evening snack.
	• Change time of dinner or evening snack.

[a]Skilled health care professionals gather additional data to find the best solution for problems with blood glucose control. Is the problem an isolated occurrence or a pattern? Has food intake changed? If yes, why? Has the activity level changed? Has illness been a problem? Whenever diet changes might be difficult for the client, insulin is adjusted to correct problems, if possible.
[b]Insulin doses can be adjusted in amount or timing or both.

Severe Hyperglycemia and Ketoacidosis   Severe hyperglycemia and ketoacidosis can occur in untreated IDDM or when the person with IDDM omits an insulin dose, makes an error in the type of insulin taken, overeats without taking additional insulin, experiences rebound hyperglycemia, or suffers a stress (infection, trauma) that causes blood glucose to rise. Severe hyperglycemia and ketoacidosis is a medical emergency that can lead to coma and death. Prevention is the best treatment. Educating the client to follow the treatment plan (including regular blood glucose monitoring) is critical. When prevention fails, a physician treats hyperglycemia and ketoacidosis by carefully administering insulin and correcting fluid and electrolyte and acid-base balances using IV fluids.

MANAGING HYPOGLYCEMIA

Tightly controlling blood glucose reduces the risk of chronic complications, but increases the risk of hypoglycemia. Hypoglycemia in the person with IDDM is also known as an *insulin reaction* or *insulin shock*. An insulin reaction can result from an overdose of insulin, strenuous physical activity, skipped meals, or inadequate food intake. People with IDDM and those who spend time with them need to learn to recognize the symptoms of hypoglycemia (see margin note on p. 850).

Judicious treatment of hypoglycemia prevents overtreatment and thus avoids subsequent hyperglycemia. As soon as the symptoms are observed, the person needs to receive 10 to 15 grams of carbohydrate. Any carbohydrate source that is readily available and easy to eat is a good choice.[18] It is best to avoid carbohydrate sources that also contain fat (such as a candy bar), because fat slows the absorption of carbohydrate. Blood glucose is then checked within 15 to 20 minutes to see if it has risen to an acceptable level. If not, an additional 10 to 15 grams of carbohydrate are given, and blood glucose is rechecked. The procedure continues until blood glucose returns to an acceptable range. Advise clients to carry some convenient source of carbohydrate with them at all times, so that they can act immediately when hypoglycemic symptoms occur.

If the person frequently experiences hypoglycemia, treatment can lead to excessive weight gain. Therefore, repeated episodes of hypoglycemia require investigation, so their causes can be corrected.

Hypoglycemia before Meals   Consistent hypoglycemia before meals suggests the need to reduce the prior insulin dose, increase the prior carbohydrate intake, or eat the next meal earlier. The best solution depends on the person's medical needs and preferences.

Nocturnal Hypoglycemia   Hypoglycemia that occurs during sleep makes symptoms difficult to detect. People prone to nocturnal hypoglycemia may be advised to wake up during the night and test their blood glucose. Nocturnal hypoglycemia may occur more readily in people who engage in strenuous physical activity late in the day. For this reason, strenuous activity should be undertaken earlier in the day, if possible. Other strategies that may help eliminate the problem are to snack consistently at bedtime or reduce the insulin dose following evening activity.

Severe Hypoglycemia   In severe cases, the person may be disoriented, unable to recognize a hypoglycemic reaction, and unable to swallow safely. In

---

insulin reaction: hypoglycemia that results from an overdose of insulin, strenuous physical activity, skipped meals, or inadequate intake of food; also called insulin shock.

Easy-to-eat sources of carbohydrate (10 to 15 g per serving):
- 2 to 3 tsp honey.
- 4 to 5 hard candies (such as Lifesavers).
- 5 to 6 large jelly beans.
- 4 to 6 oz regular soft drink.
- 4 oz orange juice.
- 1 tbs icing from a tube.
- Glucose tablets (check label for amount).

nocturnal hypoglycemia: hypoglycemia that occurs while a person is sleeping.

such cases, the person needs to receive intravenous glucose, the hormone glucagon, or both to counteract the insulin reaction. Without treatment, the person may lapse into shock and die.

CHILDREN WITH DIABETES

The overall approach to diabetes remains the same throughout life, but special problems may become apparent at different stages. Consider some of the problems of children with diabetes. Like those of all children, the energy and nutrient needs of children with diabetes keep changing throughout the growing years. Children's appetites and activities vary widely from day to day. A child may eat like a horse one day and like a mouse the next. A teen may spend hours walking around the mall one day and spend the next day watching TV. Growth and activity influence the needs for food and insulin, and management must adjust to meet those needs.

Meal Plans   To support growth and development, children with IDDM need flexible, balanced meals and snacks that offer wide varieties of foods from each of the food groups. Dietitians often teach children and caregivers carbohydrate counting to provide flexibility from day to day. Concentrated sweets are allowed within the context of a healthy diet. Caregivers need not force children to finish meals, but should encourage them not to skip meals either, because hypoglycemia can result. Meals are best taken at about the same times each day, and children with diabetes can eat the same foods as the rest of the family.

Family Lifestyles   Successful diet management incorporates prescribed meals into existing family lifestyles and eating patterns. Depending on insulin administration and personal preferences, children generally receive three meals with two to three snacks a day. Snacks before bedtime help prevent nocturnal hypoglycemia, especially if the child engages in strenuous activity late in the day. Caregivers should vary snacks to prevent boredom, provide enough to share with friends, and avoid identifying foods as "good" or "bad." Such connotations create unrealistic expectations or fears and invite the development of manipulative eating behaviors. The case study presents a child with IDDM.

The goals of IDDM therapy are to control blood glucose, blood lipids, and blood pressure; support health; and treat complications. To maintain blood glucose within a fairly normal range, people with IDDM need to be consistent in their carbohydrate intake each day. They also need to coordinate their food intake, physical activity, and insulin. Regular glucose monitoring allows clients to make the adjustments necessary to avoid hypoglycemia and hyperglycemia (review Table 27–5).

Treatment of Noninsulin-Dependent Diabetes Mellitus (NIDDM)

The striking results of the Diabetes Control and Complications Trial clearly show the value of tight blood glucose control for preventing long-term complications in IDDM and suggest that similar benefits might be possible for the vast

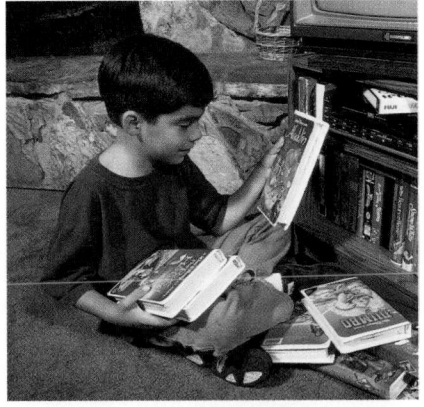

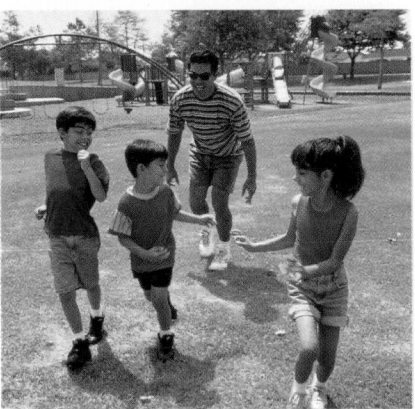

Because a child's activities vary from day to day, food and insulin needs may also change.

Case Study   Child with IDDM

One year ago, Yusuf, a 12-year-old boy, was diagnosed with IDDM. The initial diagnosis was made after Yusuf's parents became concerned when he began to lose weight, urinate excessively, and complain of thirst. Aware of a family history of diabetes, the parents quickly sought medical help. Since that time, Yusuf's diabetes has been well controlled. Recently, however, Yusuf was admitted to the emergency room, complaining of nausea, vomiting, and intense thirst. He had a fever, and his blood glucose records from the previous day showed that his blood glucose was high throughout the day. The physician observed that Yusuf was confused and breathing with difficulty and also noted the smell of acetone on his breath. Urine tests were positive for glycosuria and ketonuria, and Yusuf's blood glucose was 400 milligrams per 100 milliliters. The diagnosis was diabetic ketoacidosis.

Describe the metabolic events that led to the symptoms associated with diabetes (before diagnosis), as well as those associated with diabetic ketoacidosis. Were Yusuf's physical symptoms and laboratory tests consistent with this diagnosis? How can you distinguish between diabetic ketoacidosis and hypoglycemia?

When Yusuf recovers, what advice can you offer him to prevent future incidents of ketoacidosis? Assume that Yusuf had instructions for a diet for diabetes. What dietary modifications would you advise him to make?

Think about and discuss the influence of Yusuf's age on his outlook and ability to cope with diabetes. What problems does his age pose? Consider some ways you might help him deal with these problems. Regarding his future, describe the possible role of diet in preventing the chronic complications of diabetes.

majority of people with diabetes—those with NIDDM.[19] The goals of therapy for NIDDM mimic those for IDDM, namely:

- To achieve and maintain acceptable blood glucose levels, blood lipid concentrations, and blood pressure.
- To prevent the acute and chronic complications associated with diabetes.
- To support quality of life by enabling people to continue the activities they enjoy with the best possible health.

DIET IN NIDDM

The benefits of medical nutrition therapy in NIDDM are receiving increasing attention.[20] The diet for NIDDM is designed to maintain near-normal blood glucose by delivering a balanced nutrient intake with carbohydrates spaced evenly throughout the day. As in IDDM, many approaches can be used to plan diets in NIDDM. The diet's balance typifies healthy eating for all people and is the same as for people with IDDM.

Timing and Distribution of Meals   Providing a consistent carbohydrate intake spaced throughout the day helps people with NIDDM maintain appropriate blood glucose levels and maximizes the effectiveness of drug therapy. Giving too much carbohydrate at one time can raise blood glucose too high, stressing the already-compromised insulin-producing cells. Giving too little carbohydrate can lead to hypoglycemia, especially for people on drug therapy (some oral drugs or insulin).

Altering the distribution of kcalories from carbohydrate and fat may be especially important for controlling blood glucose and lipids for people with NIDDM. Although a low-fat diet might be appropriate in some cases, studies suggest that diets providing 40 percent of kcalories from carbohydrate and 45 percent of kcalories from fat (25 percent monounsaturated, 10 percent polyunsaturated, and 10 percent saturated) result in lower blood glucose and insulin levels following meals and lower day-long blood levels of triglycerides. Results such as these remind practitioners to individualize diet prescriptions.[21]

Chapter 28 provides more information on the associations of different blood lipids to cardiovascular disease.

Weight Control   Weight loss is often prescribed for people with NIDDM. Even moderate weight loss (10 to 20 pounds) can help reverse insulin resistance, improve the blood lipid profile, and reduce blood pressure. Weight-reduction diets that provide at least 10 kcalories per pound of body weight allow a safe and gradual weight loss. In some cases, very-low-kcalorie diets (less than 800 kcalories per day) may help establish blood glucose control, but the value of such diets remains controversial.[22] The person at a healthy weight may not need to limit energy intake, but still needs to follow the principles of the diet for diabetes.

Alcohol   The guidelines for alcohol use in NIDDM are the same as for IDDM (see p. 853). Alcohol use is discouraged for people who are overweight—a kcalorie-restricted diet has little room for high-kcalorie foods of limited nutritional value. Furthermore, the combination of alcohol and some oral antidiabetic agents may cause flushing of the skin and a rapid heartbeat.

oral antidiabetic agents: drugs taken by mouth to lower blood glucose levels. They include sulfonylureas, metformin, acarbose, and troglitazone. Sulfonylureas (sull-FAH-nal-you-RE-ahs) are also called **hypoglycemic agents** because they stimulate insulin secretion.

Physical Activity   A regular program of moderate physical activity improves blood glucose control, contributes to weight loss, improves blood lipid levels, and lowers blood pressure in people with NIDDM. Authorities recommend a program of 20 to 30 minutes of low-impact aerobic activity (such as walking) at least three days a week.[23] Many clinicians believe that 80 to 90 percent of overweight people with NIDDM can achieve metabolic control by following a kcalorie-restricted diet combined with a moderately intense physical activity program. The Diabetes Prevention Program (see p. 847) is studying the effects of diet and physical activity in delaying or preventing the development of NIDDM.[24]

DRUG THERAPY IN NIDDM

People with NIDDM may also monitor their blood glucose to maintain it within an acceptable range. When diet and physical activity fail to control blood glucose adequately, oral drugs called antidiabetic agents may be prescribed to lower blood glucose. Drugs do not replace diet and physical activity; advise clients to continue these therapies as instructed. Physicians select drug therapy based on the client's fasting and after-meal blood glucose, body weight, and response to the current therapy.

Oral Antidiabetic Agents   Sulfonylureas are antidiabetic agents that have been in wide use for many years. Sulfonylureas stimulate the release of insulin from the pancreas, sensitize the insulin-producing cells of the pancreas to glucose, and reduce insulin resistance.[25] Because sulfonylureas raise insulin levels, people taking them may experience hypoglycemia and weight gain.

Caution: People taking sulfonylureas who also consume alcohol may experience hypoglycemia, flushing of the skin, and a rapid heartbeat.

A more recently approved antidiabetic agent is metformin. Metformin suppresses the liver's production of glucose and may reduce insulin resistance; it does not stimulate insulin secretion, however, and therefore does not cause hypoglycemia. Metformin is not associated with weight gain, and it has a further advantage of reducing serum triglycerides and cholesterol and raising HDL.

Another recently approved antidiabetic agent is acarbose, an enzyme inhibitor that reduces the rate of complex carbohydrate and sucrose digestion and the subsequent absorption of glucose from the intestine. Acarbose may be used alone for people with mild NIDDM or in combination with sulfonylureas or metformin in other cases.

Finally, troglitazone, the newest class of oral antidiabetic agents, works primarily by lessening peripheral insulin resistance without stimulating insulin secretion.[26] In addition to lowering blood glucose, troglitazone reduces triglyceride levels and raises HDL. Troglitazone has also been shown to improve insulin resistance and reduce blood pressure in people with impaired glucose tolerance. For these reasons, troglitazone may prove valuable in preventing or delaying the development of NIDDM or complications associated with insulin resistance, and it is being included as an intervention in the Diabetes Prevention Program.[27]

Insulin and Insulin Analogs   Oral antidiabetic agents have a maximum dose; if blood glucose cannot be adequately controlled at the maximum dose, physicians prescribe insulin or insulin analogs, alone or in combination with oral drugs. Diabetes management for a person with NIDDM who is on insulin therapy is the same as for a person with IDDM. The accompanying case study provides practice in working with clients with NIDDM.

The goals of NIDDM therapy are similar to those of IDDM, but the approach differs slightly. Weight loss receives a high priority because of its beneficial effect in reversing insulin resistance, improving blood lipids, and reducing blood pressure. If diet and physical activity cannot control blood glucose, physicians may prescribe oral antidiabetic agents, insulin, insulin analogs, or a combination of these.

Diabetes in Pregnancy and Later Life

All stages of growth and development have unique characteristics that influence nutrient needs and affect nutrition education. An earlier section mentioned some special considerations for children and teenagers who most often have IDDM. Special considerations also apply to pregnant women and to elderly people with diabetes.

DIABETES MANAGEMENT IN PREGNANCY

As Chapter 18 noted, pregnancy elevates blood insulin and alters insulin resistance in all women. Blood insulin begins to rise soon after conception, and the cells respond by storing energy nutrients to provide for the developing fetus. Later in pregnancy, insulin remains high, but the cells become insulin resistant. Hormones that act antagonistically to insulin rise. This hormonal shift signals the body to stop storing energy fuels and allows the fetus to rapidly take up

Because acarbose inhibits sucrose absorption, people taking it who develop hypoglycemia need to use glucose for treatment.

The hormones that oppose the action of insulin during late pregnancy are placental lactogen, cortisol, prolactin, and progesterone.

Case Study   Truck Driver with NIDDM

Mr. Evans, a truck driver, was 52 years old when he was first diagnosed with NIDDM. He visited his physician after experiencing excessive thirst, excessive urination, and excessive appetite. Mr. Evans, who stands 5 feet 11 inches tall and currently weighs 200 pounds, experienced a 30-pound weight gain over the past two years. His fasting blood glucose is 235 milligrams per 100 milliliters. His fasting triglycerides and cholesterol are also elevated.

The diabetes health care team members have evaluated Mr. Evans's case. They are eager to help him achieve the first goal of diabetes management—to bring his blood glucose under control. The team has helped Mr. Evans plan a diet and physical activity program that considers the nature of his job and life on the road.

Mr. Evans is concerned about his health. He is worried that he may need insulin injections and overwhelmed by all the information presented to him over the past few days.

What are the differences between NIDDM and IDDM? Describe the factors in Mr. Evans's history that might have predisposed him to NIDDM. Can you explain to Mr. Evans why he will not need insulin injections at this time?

What will be the primary objective of the diet therapy for Mr. Evans? Determine Mr. Evans's desirable body weight, and describe two diet plans that might help him control both his blood glucose and his lipids. Select one of these diet plans and plan Mr. Evans's diet using the information in the box on pp. 855–856. Suggest some types of physical activities that might be appropriate for Mr. Evans. Remember that he travels frequently and needs a plan he can follow regularly. In what ways do diet and physical activity plans benefit clients with NIDDM?

What alternative treatments might Mr. Evans's physician consider if diet and physical activity fail to control his blood glucose?

Consider Mr. Evans's emotional health. How can the health care team help him during this difficult period?

---

energy nutrients. Because pregnancy stresses the glucose regulatory system in these ways, women with diabetes should expect control to become more difficult during pregnancy.

Risks of Diabetes during Pregnancy   Women with diabetes who are contemplating pregnancy should know that poorly controlled diabetes before and during pregnancy presents risks for both mother and infant.[28] Women face a high infertility rate, and those who do conceive may experience episodes of severe hypoglycemia or hyperglycemia, spontaneous abortion, and pregnancy-induced hypertension. Infants also have increased mortality and morbidity, including macrosomia, congenital abnormalities, and other complications such as severe hypoglycemia or respiratory distress, both of which can be fatal. The greatest risk of fetal malformations from poorly controlled diabetes occurs during the first trimester, a time when the woman with diabetes may not realize she is pregnant. Therefore, women with diabetes should receive preconceptual care, which aims to achieve excellent blood glucose control before conception, and continued prenatal care to maintain blood glucose control during pregnancy.

Gestational Diabetes   Women who never had diabetes or never knew they had it may be diagnosed with diabetes for the first time during pregnancy (see Chapter 18). Gestational diabetes is relatively common, and the American

Reminder: High blood pressure that develops in pregnancy is known as *pregnancy-induced hypertension* and may signal the onset of other complications (see p. 599).

respiratory distress: a disorder of the lung membranes that results in delayed onset of respiration at birth and difficulty in breathing after birth.

Diabetes Association recommends that health care professionals screen all women for diabetes between 24 and 28 weeks gestation.

Blood Glucose Monitoring   Obstetricians recommend blood glucose monitoring for all pregnant women with any type of diabetes. Establishing blood glucose control is important to the health of both mother and infant. Pregnant women with diabetes may also monitor their urine for ketones, either daily or periodically, because ketosis in early pregnancy can lead to congenital malformations, central nervous system disorders, and low measures of intelligence in infants.

Diet Therapy   For the pregnant woman with diabetes, a diet tailored to meet the increased demands of pregnancy and carefully coordinated with insulin therapy (when necessary) is central to therapy. The diet plan aims to provide adequate but not excessive kcalories to support weight gain (see the weight-gain recommendations in the margin on p. 589). Carbohydrate is often provided at lower amounts (40 to 45 percent of kcalories) than in the usual diet for diabetes to keep blood glucose levels from rising too high after meals.[29] Limiting carbohydrate to about 15 to 30 grams at breakfast helps maintain morning blood glucose levels in an acceptable range until counterregulatory hormone levels have diminished (see p. 862). Frequent small meals and snacks help assure an ongoing supply of glucose without inducing hyperglycemia. A bedtime snack is recommended to prevent nocturnal hypoglycemia in the mother and to provide fuel and prevent ketosis in the developing fetus.

Preventive Measures after Gestational Diabetes   For most women with gestational diabetes, glucose tolerance returns to normal after pregnancy. Nevertheless, those with gestational diabetes are likely to develop NIDDM later in life, especially if they are overweight. In women with previous gestational diabetes, being 20 percent or more overweight doubles the risk of NIDDM. For this reason, health care professionals encourage clients with gestational diabetes to avoid excessive weight gain during pregnancy and to achieve or maintain a healthy weight thereafter. Yearly screenings for diabetes are recommended so that treatment can begin promptly and complications avoided.

DIABETES MANAGEMENT IN LATER LIFE

The elderly face special problems in dealing with diabetes. They have greater risks of hyperglycemia and hypoglycemia because of reduced appetite, altered thirst regulation, altered kidney and liver functions, depression or mental deterioration, multiple medications, and other medical conditions.

Many elderly people have NIDDM, and with aging their insulin resistance may progress until they can no longer maintain glucose levels within acceptable ranges with diet and oral drugs. The prospect of daily insulin injections and the need for additional blood glucose monitoring may be overwhelming to the elderly client. Those who have also suffered a loss of vision as a consequence of aging or diabetes may be unable to draw correct insulin doses, give self-injections, or use glucose strips or meters. The inability to perform these necessary tasks may make it impossible for the person to live independently.

The elderly may also lack the financial resources or social support necessary to help them cope with their diabetes. Caring health care professionals address these problems and help elderly clients find solutions.

Poorly controlled diabetes during pregnancy is associated with infertility, spontaneous abortion, and congenital abnormalities. Some women first develop diabetes during pregnancy—gestational diabetes. To minimize complications, women need to control blood glucose levels by carefully coordinating a diet that meets the nutrient needs of pregnancy with insulin therapy (when necessary). Changes that occur with aging present special problems for the management of diabetes.

Hypoglycemia

Strictly speaking, the term *hypoglycemia* simply means "low blood glucose," and it refers not to a disease, but to a symptom of an alteration in carbohydrate metabolism. Ordinarily, blood glucose initially rises and then falls after eating; in healthy people the decline is gradual, blood glucose remains in the normal range, and the transition occurs without notice. In some people, however, blood glucose falls too low as the body shifts from the fed to the fasting state. Hypoglycemia may or may not be accompanied by other symptoms, and the symptoms may or may not be uncomfortable. There are two major types of hypoglycemia, reactive and fasting.

REACTIVE HYPOGLYCEMIA

Reactive hypoglycemia occurs within an hour or two after eating and is triggered by the release of the hormone epinephrine in response to rapidly falling blood glucose. Hypoglycemia may occur, for example, after gastric surgery (see Chapter 21), when central parenteral solutions are discontinued too quickly (see Chapter 24), or early in NIDDM when insulin levels are elevated. In most cases, however, the reason for the rapid decline in blood glucose is unknown. This section describes reactive hypoglycemia of unknown origin.

Symptoms of Reactive Hypoglycemia   The symptoms of reactive hypoglycemia are similar to those of an anxiety attack: weakness, rapid heartbeat, sweating, anxiety, hunger, and trembling. These symptoms are not surprising, as they are caused by the "emergency hormone," epinephrine.

Diagnosis of Reactive Hypoglycemia   True reactive hypoglycemia can be identified by directly testing blood glucose at intervals after a meal. Low blood glucose and the simultaneous presence of symptoms confirm a diagnosis of reactive hypoglycemia. True reactive hypoglycemia is rare, although it is often misdiagnosed and has been the subject of much misguided advice. Many dishonest or ill-informed practitioners "diagnose" hypoglycemia on the basis of their clients' verbal reports alone and prescribe all sorts of "remedies" for it with transparently thin rationale. People also "diagnose" themselves so commonly that physicians have identified a special category for their condition: *non*hypoglycemia.

reactive hypoglycemia: hypoglycemia experienced simultaneously with epinephrine-release symptoms one to three hours after a meal; also called *postprandial hypoglycemia.*

Carbohydrate-Modified Diet for Reactive Hypoglycemia For people who experience true reactive hypoglycemia, a judicious carbohydrate-modified diet may bring relief. Avoiding both low-carbohydrate dieting (see p. 243) and sudden large carbohydrate doses may be all that is required. The remedy, then, is similar to the diet for diabetes: eat a consistent amount of carbohydrate from balanced meals at regular times. If average-sized meals fail to relieve symptoms, smaller meals eaten more frequently may help. A registered dietitian, if consulted, develops a diet plan that is appropriate to achieve or maintain a healthy body weight.

FASTING HYPOGLYCEMIA

fasting hypoglycemia: hypoglycemia that develops gradually and primarily affects the brain and central nervous system.

A person who has symptoms while well advanced into the fasting state (for example, overnight) is experiencing a different kind of hypoglycemia. So is the person whose symptoms occur because insulin has driven too much glucose into the cells. Fasting hypoglycemia arises from medically diverse disorders, such as diabetes or tumors of the pancreas or liver, that interfere with normal blood glucose regulation. Table 27–6 lists the major distinguishing characteristics of fasting and reactive hypoglycemia.

Symptoms of Fasting Hypoglycemia The symptoms of fasting hypoglycemia differ from those of reactive hypoglycemia because they are not related to epinephrine release. Instead, blood glucose falls slowly, and the major effect is on the brain and central nervous system. The symptoms include headache, blurred vision, mental dullness, fatigue, confusion, amnesia, and even seizures and unconsciousness.

Carbohydrate-Modified Diets for Fasting Hypoglycemia Earlier sections of this chapter described how an evenly spaced, consistent carbohydrate intake can help prevent fasting hypoglycemia in people with diabetes and also discussed how

Table 27–6

Characteristics of Reactive and Fasting Hypoglycemia

	Reactive Type	Fasting Type
Onset of symptoms	Sudden; occurs 1 to 3 hours after meals	Gradual
Type of symptoms	Anxiety, weakness, sweating, rapid heartbeat, hunger, trembling	Headache, mental dullness, fatigue, confusion, amnesia, seizures, unconsciousness
Duration of symptoms	Transient	Persistent
Possible causes	Early NIDDM, gastric surgery, TPN	Hormonal imbalance, diabetes, drugs, tumors
Clinical course	Less serious; treat with diet	Can be serious; treat underlying problems

Nutrition Assessment Checklist
For People with Diabetes and Hypoglycemia

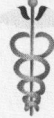

Medical   For people with diabetes, use the medical record to determine the person's type of diabetes, its duration, acute and chronic complications, and other medical conditions that may affect nutrient needs. For people with hypoglycemia, check the medical record for the cause, if known, and for a confirmation of the diagnosis.

Drug   For clients with preexisting diabetes who use insulin, note the types of insulin and schedule of administration. Note drug therapy, if any, for clients with NIDDM. Check for other drug therapy including antilipemics (to lower blood lipids) and antihypertensives (to reduce blood pressure). Note possible nutrient-drug interactions.

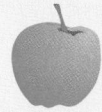

Food Intake   Obtain an accurate diet and physical activity record from the person with diabetes to plan an acceptable plan and to coordinate drug therapy. During reassessment, use food intake and physical activity records along with records of blood glucose monitoring to evaluate the effectiveness of the treatment plan and to help make acceptable adjustments, when necessary. An assessment of food intake for the person with hypoglycemia helps pinpoint foods or amounts of foods that cause undesirable symptoms.

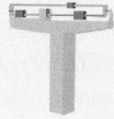

Anthropometric   Take accurate height and weight measurements and determine desirable weight. Initial doses of insulin and calculated energy needs rely on body weight. Food energy intakes may need to be adjusted regularly to account for weight changes, particularly for growing children.

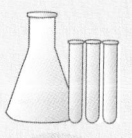

Laboratory   Monitor blood glucose, hemoglobin A_{1c}, and blood lipids regularly for people with diabetes. Check results of urine tests for microalbuminuria when available.

Physical   Check results of eye and foot exams and monitor blood pressure. Look for physical signs of dehydration in elderly people with diabetes.

carbohydrates are used to treat hypoglycemia. Surgery is the primary treatment of fasting hypoglycemia caused by tumors, although carbohydrate-controlled diets (as described for reactive hypoglycemia) may be used temporarily.

Hypoglycemia means low blood glucose and is a symptom of disturbed carbohydrate metabolism. Table 27–6 summarizes the distinguishing features of the two major types of hypoglycemia—reactive and fasting.

Diet therapy has proved to be an essential component of an intensive treatment plan to prevent the complications of diabetes. Although such a plan may be difficult to master, the reward to clients and health care professionals appear to be well worth the effort. The nutrition assessment checklist highlights areas of concern for people with diabetes and hypoglycemia.

Study Questions

1. Name the two major types of diabetes. Which type is more common? Design a table to show the differences between the two types.
2. Give the physiological reasons for the following: hyperglycemia, glycosuria, weight loss, weight gain, dehydration, polyuria, polydipsia, polyphagia, acetone breath, ketosis, diabetic coma, and hyperosmolar hyperglycemic nonketotic coma.
3. List the types of chronic complications that can arise as a result of diabetes.
4. What biochemical tests are used to diagnose diabetes? Why is screening for diabetes important? What risk factors indicate the need for additional screening?
5. What are the goals of therapy for all people with diabetes? Name three aspects of lifestyle that must be coordinated for the person with IDDM.
6. What is the usual distribution of nutrients in the diet in the treatment of IDDM? How does this distribution compare with the healthy diet recommended to all people? What determines the actual distribution of nutrients?
7. Why are the timing and composition of meals important considerations in planning a diet for a person with IDDM?
8. How does physical activity affect blood glucose levels in IDDM? Give general guidelines for adjusting food intake for physical activity (both moderate and vigorous).
9. In what ways does the body normally secrete insulin, and how is commercially available insulin given to simulate these actions? What are the advantages of insulin analogs?
10. How are blood glucose monitoring results used to coordinate insulin, diet, and physical activity plans for people with diabetes? Describe ways that diet, physical activity, and insulin can be adjusted for people with diabetes who experience hyperglycemia or hypoglycemia.
11. How is the diet adjusted to meet the special needs of children with IDDM?
12. What is the primary goal of diet therapy in the person with NIDDM? How does diet therapy for NIDDM differ from that for IDDM? Describe the advantages and disadvantages of different oral antidiabetic drugs.
13. What are the risks of poorly controlled diabetes during pregnancy? How are pregnant women with diabetes managed to control blood glucose?
14. Define gestational diabetes. What preventive measures are important following gestational diabetes?
15. What special concerns arise in elderly people with diabetes?
16. Besides diabetes, what are some other causes of hypoglycemia? What diet is recommended for the treatment of reactive hypoglycemia?

 # Clinical Applications

1. Using the box on pp. 855–856, plan a diet using the exchange lists for a sedentary woman with IDDM who is 5 feet 9 inches tall and weighs 160 pounds. Assume that the distribution of kcalories will be 55 percent from carbohydrate, 20 percent from protein, and 25 percent from fat. Round off kcalories to develop a sample diet pattern.
2. An important part of learning is being able to apply

knowledge and guidelines to real-life situations. Using Table 27–5 as a guide, think about the possible remedies for either hyper- or hypoglycemia. Describe at least one situation when it might be preferable to alter the insulin dose and one situation when it might be preferable to alter the carbohydrate intake.

3. Take a trip to a pharmacy and price these items: blood glucose meter, test strips for the meter selected, glucose test strips for use without a meter, lancets, insulin, and syringes. Determine the approximate cost of insulin injections for a person who uses 14 units of regular insulin and 26 units of NPH insulin daily (don't forget to include the cost of the syringes). Then estimate the cost of testing blood glucose four times daily. How does the cost of using a blood glucose meter compare to the cost of regular blood glucose test strips? How much do lancets add to the total daily cost? Consider how an external pump might affect the total cost of managing diabetes. How does the need for a balanced diet influence the cost of diabetes care? If intensive therapy requires more expenditures for insulin injections, blood glucose testing, and medical checkups than does traditional therapy, how might the added costs be justified?

Notes

1. M. I. Harris, NIDDM: Epidemiology and scope of the problem, *Diabetes Spectrum* 9 (1996): 26–29.
2. R. B. Lyon and D. M. Vinci, Nutrition management of insulin-dependent diabetes mellitus in adults: Review by the Diabetes Care and Education dietetic practice group, *Journal of the American Dietetic Association* 93 (1993): 309–314, 317.
3. Harris, 1996.
4. W. Y. Fujimoto, A national multicenter study to learn whether type II diabetes can be prevented: The Diabetes Prevention Program, *Clinical Diabetes* 15 (1997): 13–15.
5. I. J. Deary, Hypoglycemia-induced cognitive decrements in adults with Type I: A case to answer? *Diabetes Spectrum* 10 (1997): 42–47.
6. The Diabetes Control and Complications Trial Research Group, The effect of intensive treatment of diabetes on the development and progression of long-term complications in insulin-dependent diabetes mellitus, *New England Journal of Medicine* 329 (1993): 977–987.
7. M. C. Riddle and D. M. Karl, Screening for diabetes, *Clinical Diabetes* 14 (1996): 38–40.
8. The Expert Committee on the Diagnosis and Classification of Diabetes Mellitus, Report of the Expert Committee on the diagnosis and classification of diabetes mellitus, *Diabetes Care* 20 (1997): 1183–1197.
9. American Diabetes Association, Nutrition recommendations and principles for people with diabetes mellitus, *Diabetes Care* 17 (1994): 519–522.
10. P. J. Charney, Nutrition support in patients with diabetes mellitus, *Support Line*, April 1993, pp. 1–4.
11. American Diabetes Association, 1994.
12. M. Karlsen, D. Khakpour, and L. L. Thomson, Efficacy of medical nutrition therapy: Are your patients getting what they need? *Clinical Diabetes* 14 (1996): 54–60.
13. American Diabetes Association, 1994.
14. American Diabetes Association, Lispro: A new fast-acting insulin option, *Diabetes Spectrum* 9 (1996): 253.
15. M. Scavini and D. S. Schade, Implantable insulin pumps, *Clinical Diabetes* 14 (1996): 30–35.
16. D. E. Sutherland, The case for pancreas transplantation, *Diabetes Metabolism* 22 (1996): 132–138.
17. J. D. Pirsch and coauthors, Pancreas transplant for diabetes mellitus, *American Journal of Kidney Diseases* 27 (1996): 444–450.
18. M. Franz and coauthors, Who, what, and where—questions from "Maximizing the role of nutrition in diabetes management" continuug education program, *Diabetes Spectrum* 8 (1995): 369–374.
19. American Diabetes Association, Postition statement: Implications of the Diabetes Control and Complications Trial, *Diabetes Care* (supplement) 19 (1996): 50–52.
20. M. J. Franz and coauthors, Outcomes and cost-effectiveness of medical nutrition therapy for non-insulin-dependent diabetes, *Diabetes Spectrum* 9 (1996): 122–127; E. Q. Johnson and S. Valera, Medical nutrition therapy in non-insulin-dependent diabetes improves clinical outcome, *Diabetes Spectrum* 9 (1996): 131–133; M. J. Franz and coauthors, Effectiveness of medical nutrition therapy provided by dietitians in management of non-insulin-dependent diabetes mellitus: A randomized, controlled clinical trial, *Diabetes Spectrum* 9 (1996): 133–135.
21. A. Garg and coauthors, Effects of varying carbohydrate content of diet in patients with non-insulin-dependent diabetes mellitus, *Journal of the American Medical Association* 271 (1994): 1421–1428; L. V. Campbell and coauthors, The high-monounsaturated fat diet as a practical alternative for NIDDM, *Diabetes Care* 17 (1994): 177–182.
22. R. R. Wing, Use of very-low-calorie diets in the treatment of persons with non-insulin-dependent diabetes mellitus, *Journal of the American Dietetic Association* 95 (1995): 569–572.
23. American Diabetes Association, Position statement: Dia-

betes mellitus and exercise, *Diabetes Care* (supplement) 19 (1996): 30.

24. Fujimoto, 1997.

25. J. R. White, The pharmacologic management of patients with type II diabetes in the era of new oral agents and insulin analogs, *Diabetes Spectrum* 9 (1996): 227–234.

26. S. V. Edelman, Troglitazone: A new and unique oral anti-diabetic agent for the treatment of Type II diabetes and the insulin resistance syndrome, *Clinical Diabetes* 15 (1997): 60–65.

27. T. Antonucci and coauthors, Impaired glucose tolerance is normalized by treatment with the thiozolidinedone troglitazone, *Diabetes Care* 20 (1997): 188–193.

28. A. Elixhauser and coauthors, Cost-benefit analysis of preconception care for women with established diabetes mellitus, *Diabetes Care* 16 (1993): 1146–1157.

29. C. Fagen, J. D. King, and M. Erick, Nutrition management in women with gestational diabetes mellitus: A review by ADA's Diabetes Care and Education dietetic practice group, *Journal of the American Dietetic Association* 95 (1995): 460–467.

Living with Diabetes

Ahealthy person goes about daily activities with little thought to how the body will react to everyday routines or disruptions to those routines. If you usually eat breakfast at 8:00 A.M. you may sleep in and choose not to eat breakfast on weekends without a second thought. If your friend asks you to play tennis and the match interferes with dinner, you simply eat later. If you get hungry during the day, you eat a snack. If you're not hungry at your usual dinner hour, you wait and eat later. For people with diabetes, even such simple variations in a daily schedule require thought and adjustment. They need to learn facts, master techniques, and develop new attitudes and behaviors that will provide for a healthy life.

Health care professionals who simply "prescribe" remedies and then expect their clients to comply with those remedies fail to consider the impact that lifestyle changes impose on a person's quality of life. Clients can easily be overwhelmed, and their motivation and compliance may be poor. This highlight describes a different educational approach—client empowerment—that is directed by the client. To use this approach, health care professionals provide clients with the information and skills they need to make decisions about their treatment plans and manage their diseases.

BALANCING MEDICAL NEEDS WITH PERSONAL NEEDS

Some aspects of disease management are critical for survival. Other aspects may be beneficial but less critical. Still other aspects may be ideal but less pressing when consid-

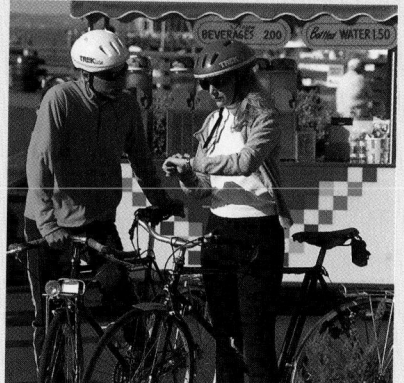

For a person with diabetes, even simple changes in routine require planning and adjustments.

ered in the total context of a treatment plan. The health care team must use clinical judgment in assigning priorities to various treatments. A person with IDDM, for example, must take insulin or face death. The person's goals, motivation, finances, and ability help determine if intensive therapy or traditional therapy is more appropriate. A 30-year-old client with IDDM may be eager to learn intensive therapy, while an 80-year-old client with NIDDM may refuse insulin therapy, even if it means poor blood glucose control. Health care professionals who practice client empowerment explain the ramifications of treatment choices, but respect the individual's right to make health care decisions without judgment.

The health care team uses a similar approach to balancing medical needs and personal needs in planning diet changes. For example, the health care team may agree on a diet plan that encourages a consistent carbohydrate intake at each meal and snack. Once the client has mastered that goal, the next step

may be to work on diet behaviors that improve blood lipid levels or encourage a greater variety of foods. At each step, the health care team balances clinical needs with the individual's goals and motivation.

Health care professionals cannot knowingly encourage clients to practice behaviors that are medically harmful. Nor can they "force" clients to follow advice. With that in mind, the next section describes some of the basic concepts clients with diabetes should ideally learn about their treatment plan.

LEARNING ABOUT DIABETES

Health care professionals encourage their clients to learn about many aspects of diabetes so they can manage their disease and prevent complications:

- *Medication*. Clients need to learn the appropriate type, dose, and schedule. Clients on insulin need to learn how to draw insulin, give themselves an injection, and rotate injection sites. Clients who use external pumps need to know how to operate and maintain them and have them refilled.
- *Blood testing*. Clients need to learn how to administer the tests, record and interpret results, and bring glucose levels within a desirable range.
- *Diet*. Clients need to know how to schedule their meals, distribute carbohydrate throughout the day, and control portion sizes.
- *Changes to accommodate physical activity, missed meals, or illness*. Clients need to know how to meet these demands.
- *Complications associated with diabetes*. Clients need to learn how

to prevent complications and how to recognize and treat them when they occur.

- *Record keeping.* Clients need to learn how to keep accurate food, activity, and insulin administration records so that they can learn how their bodies respond to diabetes and how they can gain control over their disease.

For clients with diabetes and their families, all this new information and simply the time required to manage the disease can be overwhelming. They may find the diagnosis of diabetes and all it entails difficult to grasp and accept. Clients need a great deal of support to cope with their fears, stay motivated when they feel overwhelmed, gain confidence in their abilities to manage the disorder, and live a high-quality life.

Health care professionals facilitate the learning process by working out a highly individualized plan that carefully considers the client's motivation, goals, and ability to grasp new concepts and make lifestyle changes. The plan must be flexible to accommodate changing needs; a person who is highly motivated at one point, for example, may become totally discouraged at another time and need to restructure goals temporarily. The combined expertise of many health care professionals including physicians, nurses, dietitians, counselors, and physical therapists or exercise physiologists enhances diabetes management. Along with the client, these professionals form the health care team. Throughout this discussion, keep in mind that the client is the central member of the team.

PROMOTING DIABETES MANAGEMENT

Health care professionals recognize that all newly diagnosed clients and their families need intensive diabetes care training and counseling and that the learning process takes time. Even highly motivated clients who listen attentively need several counseling sessions to learn the basics of diabetes management. Inevitably, efforts at in-depth, short-term counseling will meet with failure. Diabetes education is a continuous process that is a routine part of diabetes management.

Health care professionals can help clients make lifestyle changes by using a stepwise process that includes assessment, goal setting, intervention, and evaluation.[1] As Chapter 27 describes, a complete assessment serves as the first step in formulating a treatment plan.[2] The more detailed the assessment, the more closely the plan can be tailored to meet the individual's needs and the better the chances for success. Using assessment data, the health care team sets long-term medical goals to provide the health care team and the client with a tool to measure the success of therapy; therefore, they are stated in terms of measurable outcomes such as target ranges for blood glucose, blood lipids, and body weight.

Health care professionals also work with the client to negotiate short-term goals geared toward making lifestyle adjustments. To be successful, short-term goals consider clients' personal views of their health goals and the steps they are willing and ready to take to reach these goals. Let's look at an example. After a complete nutrition assessment of a 55-year-old woman newly diagnosed with NIDDM, the dietitian may find that in addition to the elevated blood glucose, blood lipids are also elevated; the client is 30 pounds overweight, does not have a regular physical activity plan, skips breakfast, has a large dinner, eats many fried and high-fat foods and snacks, and seldom eats vegetables. The dietitian recognizes that several dietary changes are warranted, but works with the client to find an acceptable treatment goal. The client tells the dietitian that she wants to lose weight, but she feels very stressed and doesn't know how to get started. With the guidance of the dietitian, the woman sets these goals: she will eat a consistent amount of carbohydrate three times a day, with careful attention to portion sizes, and begin a physical activity program. By involving the client in goal setting, the dietitian improves the chances for success and encourages the client to take responsibility for her health.

Once goals have been set, the next step is intervention. What specific activities can help the client meet goals? Returning to our example, the dietitian and client might discuss a diet plan that includes appropriate portion sizes for breakfast, lunch, and dinner; review several menu options; practice weighing and measuring foods; and develop a physical activity plan in which the client agrees to walk after dinner for 20 minutes three times a week. The dietitian would like records of food, activity, and blood glucose, but the client feels she cannot handle that task right now. Instead, she will monitor blood glucose as instructed by the nurse.

Once the client tries the plan, the next step is evaluation.[3] Which strategies were successful and which were not? Suppose the client in our example returns for her next appointment. She has been successful at eating breakfast, inconsistent about reducing her portion sizes at lunch and dinner, and has managed to walk for 20 minutes only once or twice a week. From the client's records, the dietitian sees that her blood glucose levels have improved somewhat and that she has lost half a pound. The dietitian reinforces the value of the positive changes the client has made and praises her efforts. At this point, the dietitian, keeping in mind the client's medical goals, must reassess the client's motivation and decide what steps to take next. The client may want to continue the plan and agree to renew her commitment to control portion sizes and to walk more frequently. Alternatively, she may be so pleased with how she is feeling that she is ready to do more. She may then agree to keep up with her original plan, but also keep food and activity records and limit servings of fried foods to two a week, for example.

To help people adjust to the physiological demands imposed by diabetes, health care professionals guide clients through management plans with measurable goals set by the client. Clients' responses to the interventions and level of motivation dictate future actions. Health care professionals who are aware of the psychological burdens associated with diabetes are better equipped to support their clients' emotional health—an important factor in diabetes management.

COPING WITH DIABETES

Consider that in the example just discussed, the plan focused only on the nutrition component of diabetes education. Clients have many other diabetes-related tasks to master. In addition, they have responsibilities related to work, family, and community. It should come as little surprise that even when clients know what

to do and why they should do it, they may be unable to carry out the plan at times.[4] Many people with diabetes report feeling overwhelmed and frustrated by the multitude of self-care demands.[5] In the words of one diabetes educator: "No one but another person who has diabetes can fully appreciate the demands of diabetes. It is 24 hours a day, 365 days a year (except on Leap Year when you get an extra day of diabetes). It involves all manner of imposition and deprivation. And even when you do everything right, there are no guarantees."[6]

People with diabetes often feel that health care professionals, family, and friends "blame" them for diabetes-related problems and complications.[7] They may feel guilt and remorse because their efforts at diabetes control were not good enough.[8] Health care professionals are wise to remain nonjudgmental when working with clients with diabetes and to recognize that diabetes control must be balanced with quality of life. Clients also need to know that they may experience complications even when they are doing everything possible. Expecting perfection can only meet with failure.

Teenagers often have intense difficulty accepting the initial diagnosis of diabetes. At a time when they are striving to develop their identity with a group and to be as similar to their peers as possible, they are faced with an unwelcome diagnosis and new rules they are expected to follow; their response may be denial and refusal to cooperate. Yet their refusal to cooperate might result in serious consequences. The person who appreciates a teen's special views on life is best prepared to help with the adjustment. Adolescents especially need to know that they can manage the disease them-

selves—that it won't turn them back into dependent children.

Parents and other family members also face the challenge of living with diabetes. The intensity of the situation can either reinforce or disrupt family unity. Parents may resent the demands of caring for a child with a chronic illness and also may experience guilt for having those feelings. They may feel anxious and be reluctant to allow their child to follow the diabetes care plan without their constant assistance. Especially in the case of an older child, they may press their care and control on a child who needs to develop autonomy and self-care. Parents may also become emotionally upset when they see their child feeling anxious, depressed, or withdrawn. Parents need time to work through these feelings. They might want to attend meetings for parents of children with diabetes.* Such meetings offer opportunities to share feelings, ideas, and frustrations with others in similar situations. Sometimes just knowing that you're not alone helps.

OTHER RESOURCES

After an initial introduction to the world of diabetes, clients may benefit from educational programs designed to expand their knowledge and promote independence.[9] Some programs encourage clients to bring friends, which makes the experience more comfortable and fun. Some programs are designed specifically for parents, grandparents, and other caregivers.

---

*The American Diabetes Association provides information about the disease and referrals to local support groups. See Appendix F for the address and phone numbers.

Children can combine education and summer vacation at camps designed especially for children with diabetes. These camps offer the chance to learn more about diabetes while "living" the lifestyle with companions under supervision. Children trade snack ideas, try new recipes, and help prepare meals. Older children assist younger ones, and all benefit.

The results of the Diabetes Control and Complications Trial clearly show that tightly managing diabetes can dramatically reduce the complications associated with it. Helping clients with diabetes make the necessary adjustments in a continuous process that balances medical and individual needs.

Many chronic diseases require diet and other lifestyle changes to ensure health. Even relatively minor diet changes can be important to the individual. A person with a hiatal hernia, for example, may be unwilling to give up coffee, even though the consequences include the pain of heartburn and worsening esophagitis. The biggest change the person may be willing to make may be to reduce coffee intake from 6 cups to 2 cups a day or to agree to drink coffee only along with foods. Clients with extremely serious disorders who lack motivation to change their lifestyles may benefit from professional counseling along with the encouragement of health care professionals, family, and friends, but in the end, only the client can determine the course that he or she can accept.

NOTES

1. American Diabetes Association and the American Dietetic Association, *Facilitating Lifestyle Change: A Resource Manual* (Alexandria, Va.: American Diabetes Association, 1996).

2. J. G. Pastors, Nutrition assessment for diabetes medical nutrition therapy, *Diabetes Spectrum* 9 (1996): 99–103.

3. M. Peyrot, Evaluation of patient education programs: How to do it and how to use it, *Diabetes Spectrum* 9 (1996): 86–93.

4. M. M. Funnell and R. M. Anderson, Judge not: Lessons learned from simulated diabetes regimens, *Diabetes Spectrum* 8 (1995): 328–329.

5. W. H. Polonsky, Listening to our patients' concerns: Understanding and addressing diabetes-specific emotional distress, *Diabetes Spectrum* 9 (1996): 8–11.

6. R. R. Rubin, Life's work they have *not* chosen, *Diabetes Spectrum* 8 (1995): 308.

7. K. F. McFarland, The power of words, *Diabetes Spectrum* 8 (1995): 308.

8. J. Betschart, Neither good nor bad, *Diabetes Spectrum* 8 (1995): 309.

9. G. L. Grossan and M. L. Uster, Islet pilots— An educational program for children with diabetes, *Journal of the American Dietetic Association* 88 (1988): 471.

Nutrition and Disorders of the Blood Vessels, Heart, and Lungs

CONTENTS
Atherosclerosis
  Consequences of Atherosclerosis
  Risk Factors for CHD
  Prevention and Treatment of Atherosclerosis
Hypertension
  Blood Pressure Regulation and
    Hypertension
  Treatment of Hypertension
Heart Attacks, Heart Failure, and Strokes
  Heart Attacks
  Congestive Heart Failure
  Strokes
Disorders of the Lungs
  Acute Respiratory Failure
  Chronic Obstructive Pulmonary Disease
    (COPD)
HIGHLIGHT: Diet and Protection against CHD

MICROGRAPH: Prostaglandin, the hormone-like substance that helps regulate blood pressure, blood lipids, and blood clot formation.

33. J. Horner and E. W. Massey, Silent aspiration following stroke, *Neurology* 38 (1988): 317–319.

34. A.S.P.E.N. Board of Directors, Practice guidelines: Respiratory failure, *Journal of Parenteral and Enteral Nutrition* (supplement) 17 (1993): 16–17; C. S. Ireton-Jones, K. R. Borman, and W. W. Turner, Nutrition considerations in the management of ventilator-dependent patients, *Nutrition in Clinical Practice* 8 (1993): 60–64.

35. Ireton-Jones, Borman, and Turner, 1993; R. A. Landon and E. A. Young, Role of magnesium in regulation of lung function, *Journal of American Dietetic Association* 93 (1993): 674–677.

36. T. Petty, Building a national strategy for the prevention and management of and research in chronic obstructive pulmonary disease, *Journal of the American Medical Association* 277 (1997): 246–253.

37. Petty, 1997.

Diet and Protection against CHD

In general, experts agree that lowering LDL cholesterol reduces complications and mortality from CHD, but the value of lowering LDL to *prevent* CHD is less clear.[1] What is obvious is that there is much to learn about how cardiovascular diseases develop and what yet-to-be-defined factors might be protective. Furthermore, as Chapter 28 noted, the current dietary recommendations to reduce CHD risk, which include reducing total fat and saturated fat and maintaining a healthy weight, may not be as effective as other measures at lowering LDL. Such findings have led researchers to explore other avenues for pieces of the puzzle. A good deal of that research continues to focus on dietary factors; those that appear most promising are featured in this highlight.

THE ANTIOXIDANT NUTRIENTS

A discussion of dietary factors to reduce CHD risk must include the antioxidant nutrients—a hot topic in both the popular press and scientific journals today. Highlight 11 describes the antioxidant nutrients in detail and explains how they attack free radicals and protect against heart disease. Evidence continues to mount that antioxidant nutrients, particularly vitamin E, may be protective against CHD by preventing the toxic effects of free radicals. Vitamin E may also slow the progression of plaques that have already formed in the arteries or may lower the risk of developing a heart attack in people with existing CHD.[2]

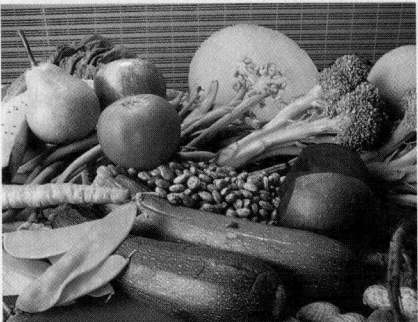

Eating a variety of fruits and vegetables may confer special protection against CHD.

The amount of vitamin E that appears to be protective against CHD exceeds the RDA and is difficult to consume from a standard diet, particularly from a diet that obtains less than 30 percent of its energy from fat. (The most frequently consumed dietary sources of vitamin E are vegetable oils, polyunsaturated margarines, some nuts, and wheat germ.) Therefore, vitamin E supplements may be necessary to maximize its effects. When provided in large amounts, vitamin E may have pharmacological, rather than nutritional, effects. Before such supplements can be recommended, large-scale studies (and several are under way) are needed to rule out whether other dietary factors or lifestyle behaviors are actually responsible for the protective effects attributed to vitamin E.[3] The safety of the long-term use of high doses of vitamin E also requires further investigation.

DIETARY FIBER

Soluble fiber lowers blood cholesterol, especially in those with high blood cholesterol.[4] A recent study of more than 43,000 male health care professionals found that men who had the highest fiber intakes (about 29 grams per day) had the lowest rate of heart attacks.[5] Similarly, a Finnish study of more than 21,000 male smokers found that those with high-fiber intakes (over 25 grams per day) had fewer heart attacks than those with lower-fiber intakes (about 16 grams a day). People with diabetes (NIDDM) showed improved blood glucose control and an improved ratio of LDL to HDL with a diet that provided 18 grams of fiber from breads made from oat bran concentrates.[6]

As Chapter 4 noted (see pp. 126–128), the reasons why high-fiber diets may be protective are difficult to determine. High-fiber diets tend to be lower in fat and cholesterol and higher in vitamins (including folate, discussed later) and other nonnutrient compounds (phytochemicals). These properties may actually account for some of the findings. Regardless, consuming from 20 to 35 grams of fiber daily seems a prudent health measure with few risks and possible protection from CHD.

HOMOCYSTEINE AND FOLATE

As Chapter 6 noted (see p. 202), elevated blood levels of the amino acid homocysteine may be a risk factor for cardiovascular disease.[7] For many years researchers have recognized that people with homocysteinuria, a genetic disorder characterized by markedly elevated blood and urine levels of homocysteine, show characteristic patterns of accelerated atherosclerosis, blood clots, and emboli.

Researchers have also suspected a link between moderately elevated homocysteine and cardiovascular disease, but early studies failed to show whether cardiovascular disease itself was the cause of elevated homocysteine or elevated homocysteine was the cause of cardiovascular disease.[8] More recently, several prospective studies of people who entered the study without preexisting heart disease have shown a positive association between elevated blood homocysteine and risk of cardiovascular disease.[9] How elevated homocysteine contributes to heart disease remains unclear, but researchers speculate that it may structurally change the blood vessels to promote plaque formation, increase the likelihood of clot formation, and interfere with the metabolism of cholesterol in the liver.[10]

What causes elevated homocysteine in people without homocysteinuria? Again, the answer is not always clear. In many cases, elevated homocysteine is associated with suboptimal concentrations of the B vitamins involved in the metabolism of homocysteine. Most commonly, a suboptimal dietary intake of folate is to blame, but an optimal intake has yet to be defined. Some research suggests that folate intakes that meet the current RDA may be insufficient to prevent elevated homocysteine.[11] In people with low folate intakes, supplementation brings homocysteine back to desirable levels.[12] Supplementation may not be necessary, though, if rich sources of folate are selected daily.[13]

The question that remains to be answered is whether providing adequate dietary folate to reduce homocysteine also reduces the risk of cardiovascular disease.[14] One study followed more than 5000 men and women for 15 years and found that those with the lowest serum folate had a significantly higher risk of dying from cardiovascular disease.[15] As noted earlier, foods high in folate (fruits, vegetables, and legumes) also tend to be high in other nutrients, nonnutrients, and fiber; further research may help to define exactly which factors provide protective effects.

For most people, selecting at least five servings of folate-rich fruits and vegetables daily should be sufficient to normalize homocysteine concentrations. The Food and Drug Administration's recent decision to require folate fortification of grain products in an effort to reduce the incidence of birth defects will also increase folate intakes.[16] Whether folate fortification confers an added benefit of reducing CHD risks remains to be seen.

FISH OIL

From the dietary factors described up to now and the information presented in Chapter 28, it seems logical to assume that diets low in saturated fats and cholesterol that include abundant fruits and vegetables would be protective against heart disease. Yet the Inuit peoples of Alaska and Greenland, who eat a diet consisting almost entirely of meat (rich in saturated fat) and fish (rich in cholesterol and relatively rich in saturated fat), have a remarkably low incidence of heart disease. In searching for factors that might account for the low incidence of CHD, researchers discovered that compared to other populations, the Inuit had lower blood triglycerides, their platelets contained higher amounts of omega-3 fatty acids, and their blood took longer to clot.

Early research regarding fish oil suggested that its protective effects were related to blood clotting, which is under the control of certain hormonelike substances (eicosanoids), the prostaglandins and thromboxanes. Thromboxanes, which the body makes from the omega-6 fatty acids abundant in vegetable oils, *promote* platelet aggregation (sticking together). Prostaglandins, which the body makes from the omega-3 fatty acids abundant in fish oil, *inhibit* platelet aggregation. Although a diet rich in omega-3 fatty acids can limit clot formation by changing the balance between the prostaglandins and thromboxanes, researchers have found that only large amounts of fish oils are effective. Yet the protective effects of fish oils have been seen even in cases where people consume only one or two fish meals per week, suggesting that a different mechanism is involved.[17] Furthermore, the effects of fish oils on platelet function are modest when compared to even tiny doses of aspirin, which is known to significantly reduce clot formation.[18]

A recent, large, carefully conducted study failed to show a correlation between fish oil and CHD risk.[19] The authors noted, however, that very few men in the study group ate no fish at all, and eating one or two fish meals per week may confer the same benefits as eating five to six fish meals per week.

Fish oils may help prevent cardiac arrhythmias (irregular heartbeats that can lead to a sudden and fatal heart attack) and sudden death in people with CHD.[20] When men with no known heart disease who suffered a heart attack were compared to a matched control group, researchers found that men who ate about one fish meal per week had a 50 percent lower incidence of heart attacks and a 29 percent reduction in two-year mortality from all causes.[21]

Eating one or two fish meals per week may be beneficial and is certainly safe. Fish oil supplements are unnecessary and may be toxic; people who dislike fish may want to review the warnings on p. 169 before choosing a fish oil supplement.

ALCOHOL

Research suggests that a *moderate* consumption of alcohol may reduce the risk of heart disease by raising HDL cholesterol and preventing blood clot formation.[22] These benefits are more apparent in people over age 50, in those with other risk factors, and in those with high LDL.[23] Researchers speculate that when LDL levels are high, alcohol may cause changes that reduce the likelihood of clot formation.[24] Early studies suggested that red wine was more effective than other alcoholic beverages in reducing CHD risk, indicating that perhaps something other than alcohol was responsible for the protective effect. A review of studies to date, however, found that alcohol from any source—red or white wine, beer, or liquor—appears to be equally effective, and that alcohol itself may be the protective factor.[25]

These findings pose a dilemma for health care professionals who are well aware of the potentially damaging effects of alcohol on many body systems (see Highlight 7). Any benefits that alcohol may confer on cardiovascular health must be weighed against the risks of raising complications and mortality from other causes.[26] The question to answer is how much alcohol is protective, and how much is harmful? Early studies suggested that total mortality was

reduced in people who drank 1 to 2 drinks per day as compared to abstainers, but in larger amounts (more than 3 drinks per day), alcohol was associated with increased mortality.[27] More recent studies suggest that the beneficial effects of alcohol occur at lower intakes. In one study, researchers examined alcohol intake and mortality over a ten-year period in more than 22,000 male physicians with no history of heart attacks, strokes, transient ischemic attacks, or cancer.[28] Men who consumed 2 to 6 drinks per *week* had the lowest mortality risk, and those who consumed 2 or more drinks per *day* had the highest mortality risk. The lower mortality risks found in men who consumed some alcohol were largely the result of a reduced risk of death from cardiovascular causes. Studies of Danish adults found the lowest mortality risk in people who drank 1 to 6 drinks per week.[29] Among British male physicians, researchers found that 5 to 9 drinks per week were protective.[30] The amount of alcohol that exerts a positive effect on CHD risk for women may be lower still. A study of more than 85,000 women found the most beneficial alcohol consumption level to be no more than 1 to 3 drinks per week.[31]

The advice clinicians offer clients regarding the use of alcohol to lower CHD risks rests largely on clinical judgment.[32] The number of deaths attributed to alcohol is greatest for people between the ages of 15 and 44—and their risk of heart disease is relatively minor. Clearly, for these people, the benefits do not outweigh the risks. Additionally, people with a personal or family history of alcohol abuse and those with medical conditions complicated by alcohol use (liver and pancreatic disorders, for example) should not

use alcohol. Clients who do use alcohol should be cautioned to avoid alcohol use during times when clear judgment is important, such as when they are driving, working, or operating potentially dangerous equipment. These clients should also be evaluated periodically to assure that alcohol intake has not become excessive or problematic.

CONFOUNDING FACTORS

As this discussion has pointed out, diets are complex and foods that contain one protective factor for CHD may contain several. Is one factor responsible or is it the combination of factors?

Furthermore, groups of people with low risks of CHD may have lifestyle habits or genetic characteristics that explain the low risks. The native people of Alaska (described early) may have a low incidence of CHD, but their lifestyles differ significantly from other populations, and many do not live to a very old age.[33] Certainly, major lifestyle factors and other characteristics account for some differences in CHD risks.

In making decisions regarding the value of dietary changes to protect against CHD, one must weigh the potential benefits against the potential risks. Certainly, including plenty of fruits, vegetables, and legumes would be safe and may offer the beneficial effects of antioxidant nutrients, phytochemicals, fiber, and folate. With respect to vitamin E supplements, the issues become somewhat complicated. Research regarding vitamin E's protective effects is inconclusive, and because vitamin E must be taken in large doses, it may prove to have some adverse effects. The issues surrounding alcohol's protective effects are clearly the most complex. While alcohol may have a protective effect against CHD, its potential for abuse and its damaging effects on many body systems limit its usefulness as a protective factor. Clinicians must use clinical judgment in helping clients decide if alcohol consumption is warranted.

NOTES

1. J. B. Ubbink, Homocysteine—An atherogenic and a thromogenic factor? *Nutrition Reviews* 53 (1995): 323–326.

2. H. N. Hodis and coauthors, Serial coronary angiographic evidence that antioxidant vitamin intake reduces progression of coronary artery atherosclerosis, *Journal of the American Medical Association* 273 (1995): 1849–1854; N. G. Stephens and coauthors, Randomised controlled trial of vitamin E in patients with coronary disease: Cambridge Heart Antioxidant Study (CHAOS), *Lancet* 347 (1996): 781–786.

3. J. M. Gaziano, Antioxidants in cardiovascular disease: Randomized trials, *Nutrition Reviews* 54 (1996): 175–184.

4. C. Dubois and coauthors, Chronic oat bran intake alters post-prandial lipemia and lipoproteins in healthy adults, *American Journal of Clinical Nutrition* 61 (1995): 325–333; S. R. Glore and coauthors, Soluble fiber and serum lipids: A literature review, *Journal of the American Dietetic Association* 94 (1994): 425–436; C. M. Ripsin and coauthors, Oat products and lipid lowering, *Journal of the American Medical Association* 267 (1992): 3317–3325.

5. E. B. Rimm and coauthors, Vegetable, fruit, and cereal fiber intake and risk of coronary heart disease among men, *Journal of the American Medical Association* 275 (1996): 447–451.

6. M. E. Pick and coauthors, Oat bran concentrate bread products improve long-term control of diabetes: A pilot study, *Journal of the American Dietetic Association* 96 (1996): 1254–1261.

7. J. Selhub and coauthors, Association between plasma homocysteine concentrations and extracranial carotid-artery stenosis, *New England Journal of Medicine* 332 (1995): 286–289; E. Arnesen and coauthors, Serum total homocysteine and coronary heart disease, *International Journal of Epidemiology* 24 (1995): 704–709; K. Robinson and coauthors, Hyperhomocysteinemia and low pyridoxal phosphate: Common and independent reversible risk factors for coronary artery disease, *Circulation* 92 (1995): 2825–2830.

8. P. Verhoef and M. J. Stampfer, Prospective studies of homocysteine and cardiovascular disease, *Nutrition Reviews* 53 (1995): 283–288.

9. M. J. Stampfer and coauthors, A prospective study of plasma homocyst(e)ine and risk of myocardial infarction in US physicians, *Journal of the American Medical Association* 268 (1992): 877–880; Arnesen and coauthors, 1995; P. Verhoef and coauthors, A prospective study of plasma homocyst(e)ine and risk of ischemic stroke, *Stroke* 25 (1994): 1924–1930.

10. J. S. Stamler and A. Slivka, Biological chemistry of thiols in the vasculature and in vascular-related disease, *Nutrition Reviews* 54 (1996): 1–30.

11. J. Selhub and coauthors, Vitamin status and intake as primary determinants of homocysteinemia in an elderly population, *Journal of the American Medical Association* 270 (1993): 2693–2698.

12. J. B. Ubbink, P. J. Becker, and W. J. H. Vermaak, Will an increased dietary folate intake reduce the incidence of cardiovascular disease? *Nutrition Reviews* 54 (1996): 213–216.

13. J. B. Ubbink, Vitamin nutrition status and homocysteine: An atherogenic risk factor, *Nutrition Reviews* 52 (1994): 383–393; Ubbink, Becker, and Vermaak, 1996.

14. M. J. Stampfer and E. B. Rimm, Folate and cardiovascular disease, *Journal of the American Medical Association* 276 (1996): 1929–1930.

15. H. I. Morrison and coauthors, Serum folate and risk of fatal coronary heart disease, *Journal of the American Medical Association* 275 (1996): 1893–1896.

16. J. Foulke, Folic acid to fortify U.S. food products to prevent birth defects, Food and Drug Administration press release, February 29, 1996.

17. M. B. Katan, Fish and heart disease: What is the real story? *Nutrition Reviews* 53 (1995): 228–229.

18. N. W. Schoene and G. A. Fitzgerald, Thromogenic potential of dietary long-chain polyunsaturated fatty acids: Session summary, *American Journal of Clinical Nutrition* (supplement) 56 (1992): 977–982.

19. A. Ascherio and coauthors, Marine *n*-3 fatty acids, fish intake, and the risk of coronary disease among men, *New England Journal of Medicine* 332 (1995): 977–982.

20. A. Sellmayer and coauthors, Effects of dietary fish oil on VPC's, *American Journal of Cardiology* 76 (1995): 974–977; D. S. Siscovick and coauthors, Fish intake and risk of primary cardiac arrest, *Journal of the American Medical Association* 274 (1995): 1363–1367.

21. Siscovick and coauthors, 1995.

22. J. M. Gaziano and coauthors, Moderate alcohol intake, increased levels of high-density lipoprotein and its subfractions, and decreased risk of myocardial infarction, *New England Journal of Medicine* 329 (1993): 1829–1834; P. R. Ridker and coauthors, Association of moderate alcohol consumption and plasma concentration of endogenous tissue-type plasminogen activator, *Journal of the American Medical Association* 272 (1994): 929–933.

23. C. S. Fuchs and coauthors, Alcohol consumption and mortality among women, *New England Journal of Medicine* 332 (1995): 1245–1250; H. O. Hein, P. Suadicani, and F. Gyntelberg, Alcohol consumption, serum low density lipoprotein cholesterol concentration, and risk of ischaemic heart disease: Six year follow up in the Copenhagen male study, *British Medical Journal* 312 (1996): 736–741.

24. Hein, Suadicani, and Gyntelberg, 1996.

25. E. B. Rimm and coauthors, Review of moderate alcohol consumption and reduced risk of coronary heart disease: Is the effect due to beer, wine, or spirits? *British Medical Journal* 312 (1996): 731–736.

26. G. D. Friedman and A. L. Klatsky, Is alcohol good for your health? *New England Journal of Medicine* 329 (1993): 1882–1883.

27. T. A. Pearson and P. Terry, What to advise patients about drinking alcohol, *Journal of the American Medical Association* 272 (1994): 967–968.

28. C. A. Camargo and coauthors, Prospective study of moderate alcohol consumption and mortality in US male physicians, *Archives of Internal Medicine* 137 (1997): 79–85.

29. N. Grønbaek and coauthors, Influence of sex, age, body mass index, and smoking on alcohol intake and mortality, *British Medical Journal* 308 (1994): 302–306.

30. R. Doll and coauthors, Mortality in relation to consumption of alcohol, *British Medical Journal* 309 (1994): 911–918.

31. Fuchs and coauthors, 1995.

32. Pearson and Terry, 1994.

33. Katan, 1995.

Chapter 29

Nutrition and Disorders of the Kidneys

CONTENTS

The Nephrotic Syndrome
Consequences of Nephrotic Syndrome
Treatment of Nephrotic Syndrome
Acute Renal Failure
Consequences of Acute Renal Failure
Treatment of Acute Renal Failure
Chronic Renal Failure
Consequences of Chronic Renal Failure
Treatment of Chronic Renal Failure
Kidney Transplants and Diet
HIGHLIGHT: **Kidney Stones—Treatments and Prevention**

MICROGRAPH: Urea, the body's vehicle for eliminating excess nitrogen.

The kidneys:

- Help maintain fluid, electrolyte, and acid-base balances.
- Eliminate metabolic waste products.
- Help regulate blood pressure.
- Produce a hormone that stimulates red blood cell production.
- Activate vitamin D.

nephrotic syndrome: the complex of symptoms that occur when glomerular function fails; it includes proteinuria and albuminuria.

The loss of protein in the urine is called proteinuria, and the loss of the protein albumin in the urine is called albuminuria. Sensitive laboratory tests allow clinicians to detect microalbuminuria, the loss of albumin in the urine in quantities that are greater than normal but not enough to precipitate symptoms. Tests for microalbuminuria are routinely performed in people are high risk for renal disease.

renal failure: failure of the kidneys to maintain normal function.

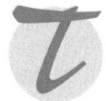 he kidneys certainly illustrate the adage that good things come in small packages. Within each kidney, which is only about the size of a fist, the nephrons selectively eliminate or reabsorb fluids and blood components to maintain the body's acid-base, fluid, and electrolyte balances. The kidneys also help to regulate blood pressure, stimulate red blood cell production, and maintain bone structure. The accompanying glossary reviews terms related to the kidneys and their functions. Figure 29–1 illustrates the kidneys and the urinary tract, and Figure 3–8 (on page 88) shows how the nephrons filter wastes from the blood. This chapter describes disorders that disrupt renal function, including nephrotic syndrome and kidney failure. Highlight 29 discusses kidney stones, which can lead to complications that affect the kidneys.

The Nephrotic Syndrome

The nephrotic syndrome is not a disease, but rather a distinct cluster of symptoms including proteinuria, low serum albumin, edema, and elevated blood lipids. Causes of nephrotic syndrome include damage to the kidneys from infections, blood clots in the renal veins, metabolic disorders (including diabetes mellitus), and some drugs and toxins. As a consequence, the permeability of the glomerular capillaries increases, and plasma proteins, which are normally retained in the blood, escape into the urine instead. Nephrotic syndrome is sometimes an early sign of renal failure, especially in people with diabetes (see page 853). In other cases, treatment of the underlying condition can correct the disorder before renal failure develops.

Figure 29–1

The Kidneys and Urinary Tract

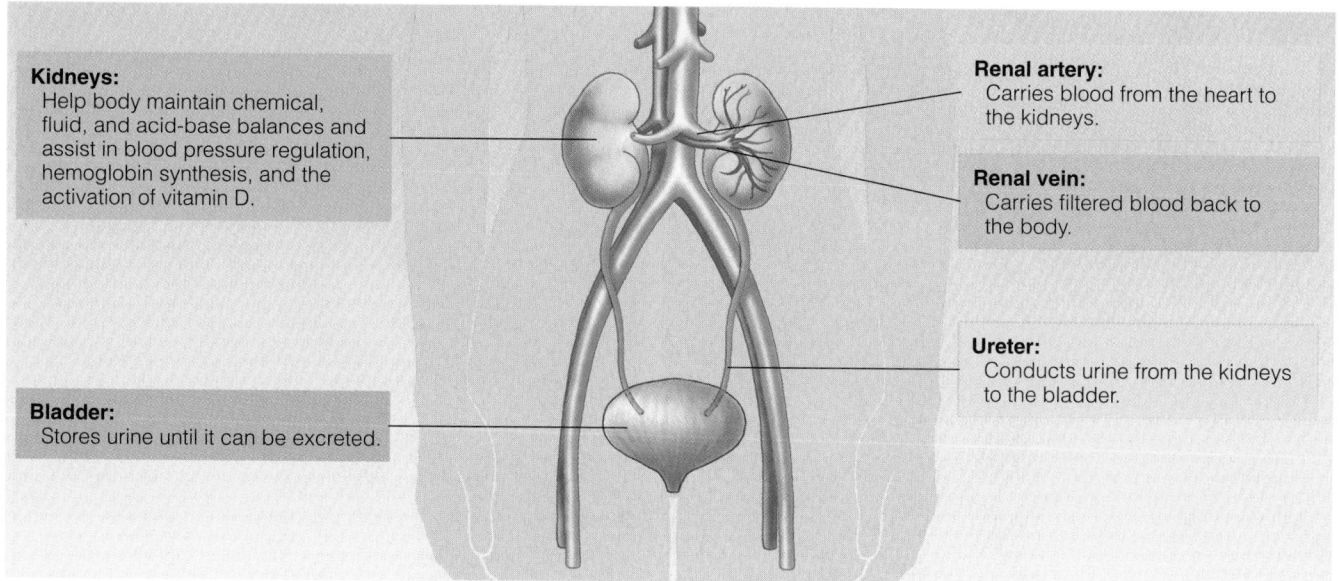

Kidneys:
Help body maintain chemical, fluid, and acid-base balances and assist in blood pressure regulation, hemoglobin synthesis, and the activation of vitamin D.

Renal artery:
Carries blood from the heart to the kidneys.

Renal vein:
Carries filtered blood back to the body.

Ureter:
Conducts urine from the kidneys to the bladder.

Bladder:
Stores urine until it can be excreted.

Glossary of Kidney-Related Terms

active vitamin D: the 1,25-dihydroxy form of vitamin D that promotes calcium balance and bone mineralization. Figure 11–8 (on p. 387) shows how the kidneys participate in the final conversion of vitamin D to its most active form.

erythropoietin (eh-REE-throw-POY-eh-tin): a hormone secreted by the kidneys in response to oxygen depletion or anemia that stimulates the bone marrow to produce red blood cells.
erythro = red (blood cell)
poiesis = creating (like poetry)

filtrate: in the kidneys, the fluid that passes from the blood through the capillary walls of the glomeruli, eventually forming urine.

glomerular filtration rate (GFR): the rate at which the kidneys form filtrate. Normally, the GFR is between 90 and 120 ml/min.

glomerulus (glow-MARE-you-lus): a cup-shaped membrane enclosing a tuft of capillaries within a nephron. (The plural is *glomeruli*.)

nephrons (NEF-rons): the working units of the kidneys; each consists of a glomerulus and a tubule.

renal: pertaining to the kidneys.

renin: an enzyme secreted by the kidneys in response to a reduced blood flow that triggers the release of the hormone aldosterone from the adrenal glands. Aldosterone, in turn, signals the kidneys to retain sodium and water.

tubule: a tube like structure that surrounds the glomerulus and descends through the nephron. A pressure gradient between the glomerular capillaries and the tubule returns needed materials to the blood and moves wastes into the tubule to be sent to the bladder.

CONSEQUENCES OF NEPHROTIC SYNDROME

The major consequences of nephrotic syndrome include protein-energy malnutrition (PEM), infection, blood coagulation disorders, occlusion of blood vessels from clots in the lungs and legs, and accelerated atherosclerosis. Many of the consequences of the disorder are the same as those of malnutrition, which is not surprising because both alter protein status (see Figure 29–2). If nephrotic syndrome progresses to renal failure, the person develops other complications, as a later section describes.

Blood Proteins Fall and Malnutrition Develops As plasma proteins are lost in the urine, blood proteins fall sharply. Albumin, the major plasma protein, is also the major protein lost in the urine, and its blood level is markedly reduced. Among the other blood proteins lost are immunoglobulins, transferrin, and the vitamin D–binding protein. Losses of immunoglobulins render the person prone to infections, which can further compromise health and nutrition status. Loss of transferrin, the iron-carrying protein, may lead to anemia. When the vitamin D–binding protein is lost in the urine, vitamin D deficiency may develop, which impairs calcium absorption. Some calcium is also lost directly along with the albumin that carries it. Consequently, rickets may develop as a result of the nephrotic syndrome, particularly in children. If protein loss continues without replacement, lean body tissues break down, and PEM and general malnutrition follow.

Figure 29–2

Consequences of Urinary Protein Losses in the Nephrotic Syndrome

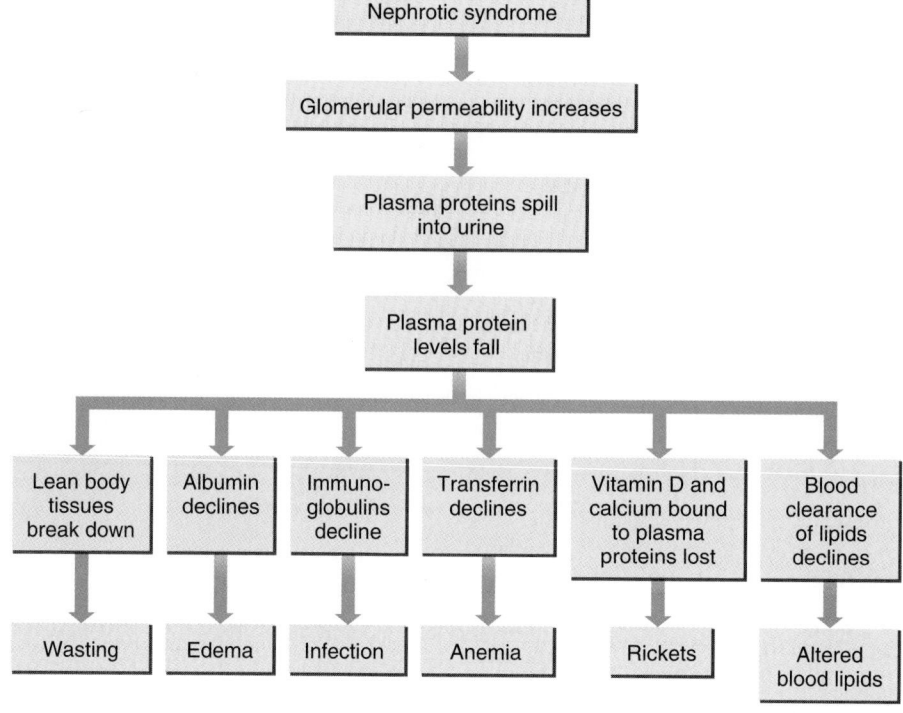

Edema Develops   Low blood protein contributes to edema by failing to exert enough pressure to keep fluids from moving into the interstitial spaces. As fluids enter the interstitial spaces, blood volume diminishes, and the kidneys respond by retaining sodium and fluid, further aggravating edema.

Blood Lipids Change   Elevated cholesterol, triglycerides, LDL, and VLDL and low HDL are characteristics of nephrotic syndrome. This lipid pattern increases the risk of cardiovascular disease and stroke and may damage the kidneys further.[1]

Exactly why blood lipids increase in nephrotic syndrome remains unknown, but the defective clearance of lipids by the kidneys may be partially to blame. Animal studies suggest that these lipid changes occur as a consequence of urinary protein loss.[2]

TREATMENT OF NEPHROTIC SYNDROME

Medical treatment first requires treatment of the underlying disorder and then drug and diet therapy to resolve the nephrotic syndrome. Corticosteroids are sometimes used in the treatment of nephrotic syndrome, but they must be used judiciously because they can contribute to nutrient imbalances (see Appendix E). Diet is central to preventing protein malnutrition and alleviating edema.

Energy   A diet adequate in energy sustains desirable weight and spares protein. Additional kcalories may be appropriate if the person loses weight or devel-

 PRESCRIPTION PAD

Drugs used in the treatment of nephrotic syndrome may include:

- Antibiotics
- Anti-inflammatory agents
- Antilipemics
- Diuretics
- Immunosuppressants

See Appendix E for timing with meals and nutrition-related side effects.

ops an infection or fever. Obese people with nephrotic syndrome may be advised to reduce their energy intakes to help control blood lipid levels.

Protein   In the past, high-protein diets (about 120 grams per day) were often prescribed for people with nephrotic syndrome, stemming from the belief that protein intakes would compensate for protein losses. High-protein diets do accelerate albumin synthesis, but they also produce greater urinary losses of albumin as well.[3] Furthermore, extra dietary protein may accelerate deterioration of renal function.[4] For these reasons, protein is provided in amounts consistent with the RDA.

Fat   A low-fat diet such as the plan shown in Chapter 28 (see p. 893) can help control the elevated blood lipids associated with nephrotic syndrome. Such a diet limits total fat, saturated fat, and cholesterol. Often, however, people with nephrotic syndrome are unable to control blood lipids adequately using diet alone, and physicians must prescribe drugs.

Sodium   Because the body avidly retains sodium in nephrotic syndrome, sodium must be restricted. Early treatment combines a diet very low in sodium (250 milligrams) with diuretics to help mobilize the accumulated fluid from the interstitial spaces.

Hidden sources of sodium can undermine severely restricted diets. If the local water has a high-sodium concentration and is used for preparing and cooking foods, it can significantly contribute to sodium intake. (Health departments can supply information on the sodium content of local water supplies.) Medications such as antacids, antibiotics, cough medicines, laxatives, pain relievers, and sedatives may also contain sodium. Some toothpaste and mouthwashes also contain large amounts of sodium; people should not swallow these compounds and should rinse thoroughly after brushing their teeth or using a mouthwash.

Once edema is resolved and sodium balance is achieved, sodium restriction relaxes, but is still fairly stringent. Chapter 26 provides more information on sodium-restricted diets. Clients on thiazide or loop diuretics should be encouraged to select foods rich in potassium.

The kidneys maintain the body's acid-base, fluid, and electrolyte balances, eliminate waste products, regulate blood pressure, stimulate red blood cell production, and activate vitamin D. Damage to the kidneys can lead to nephrotic syndrome, a disorder characterized by protein losses, fluid imbalances (edema), and elevated blood lipids. Because nephrotic syndrome alters protein status in the same way malnutrition does , the consequences are similar (review Figure 29–2). Treatment includes a diet adequate in energy and protein, with less than 30 percent of the total kcalories from fat, and low in saturated fat, cholesterol, and sodium (see the box on p. 914).

Acute Renal Failure

In acute renal failure, the nephrons suddenly lose function and are unable to maintain homeostasis. The degree of renal dysfunction varies among individuals and can range from mild to severe. With prompt treatment, acute renal failure may be reversible, but in some cases, the damage is permanent.

Chronic renal failure [is like] a downhill course for your patient; acute renal failure is like seeing him go over a cliff no one quite knew was there.

—J. L. Stark

How to Modify the Diet for Nephrotic Syndrome

- Energy: Adequate to maintain a healthy body weight (about 35 kcalories per kilogram of body weight per day).
- Protein: 0.8 to 1.0 gram per kilogram of body weight per day.
- Fat: Less than 30 percent of the total kcalories, low in saturated fat and cholesterol.
- Sodium: 250 to 1500 milligrams per day.

Reduced blood flow to the kidneys is a **prerenal** cause of acute renal failure.

A urinary tract obstruction is a **postrenal** cause of acute renal failure. The kidneys can make urine, but the urine cannot be excreted.

Damage to the kidneys' cells is an **intrarenal** cause of acute renal failure.

Abnormal accumulation of nitrogen-containing substances in the blood is called **uremia** (you-REE-me-ah) or **azotemia** (AZE-oh-TEE-me-ah). Normal BUN levels are 10 to 20 mg/dL. A BUN of 50 to 150 mg/dL indicates serious impairment of renal function. BUN may rise as high as 150 to 250 mg/dL in end-stage renal disease.

hyperkalemia: an excessive amount of potassium in the blood.

The early phase of acute renal failure, when urine volume is reduced, is the **oliguric phase**; the phase characterized by large fluid and electrolyte losses in the urine is the **diuretic phase**; the gradual return of renal function marks the **recovery phase**.

Acute renal failure frequently develops when blood flow to the kidneys suddenly drops, often as a result of a severe stress such as heart failure, shock, or severe blood loss following surgery or trauma. Less than normal amounts of blood reach the kidneys, less blood is filtered, and less urine is produced. Urinary tract obstructions can also precipitate acute renal failure. In this case, the kidneys can make urine initially, but the urine cannot be excreted. In still other cases, infections, toxins, and some drugs directly damage the kidney's cells.

CONSEQUENCES OF ACUTE RENAL FAILURE

Acute renal failure is characterized by a sudden and precipitous drop in the glomerular filtration rate (GFR) and urine output. As the nephrons fail, the composition of the blood and urine changes.

Waste Products Accumulate   When the kidneys fail to function, the body's principal nitrogen-containing metabolic waste products—blood urea nitrogen (BUN), creatinine, and uric acid—accumulate in the blood. Clinicians evaluate renal function by performing laboratory tests to measure blood levels of these waste products and urinary clearance tests to measure the GFR.

Potassium Rises   Blood potassium rises as renal function deteriorates because the kidneys can no longer excrete it. A severe stress taxes the kidneys further as the body's cells break down and intracellular fluids release potassium. Blood potassium rises sharply (hyperkalemia) and can result in sudden heart failure.

Blood Volume Changes   In the early stages of acute renal failure, the kidneys fail to excrete fluids, and blood pressure may rise to dangerously high levels. During this stage, clients, particularly elderly clients, may develop fluid overload, which may lead to pulmonary edema.

Later in the course of acute renal failure, the kidneys cannot conserve water, and the person begins to excrete large amounts of fluids and electrolytes. If recovery occurs, kidney function gradually normalizes.

Clinical Symptoms Develop   As toxic waste products build up, the person may experience uremic syndrome—a wide array of symptoms in virtually every body system. Hemorrhages may be visible on the skin, and GI bleeding sometimes occurs. In advanced stages, seizures and coma may ensue.

TREATMENT OF ACUTE RENAL FAILURE

The primary goal in acute renal failure is to treat the underlying disorder in order to prevent permanent or further damage to the kidneys. For example, a blood transfusion may be given to restore blood volume in the case of severe blood loss. Diet therapy, drug therapy, and dialysis may be undertaken to restore fluid and electrolyte balance and minimize blood concentrations of toxic waste products. Health care professionals diligently monitor indices of renal function to determine the best treatment plan.

Energy   The person in acute renal failure is often unable to obtain enough energy to meet needs. Without sufficient energy to fuel hypermetabolism, proteins break down and blood urea and potassium concentrations rise even higher—all taxing the kidneys further. Thus wasting and malnutrition complicate recovery. The person's energy needs depend on the rate of catabolism; usually 30 to 50 kcalories per kilogram of body weight will meet these needs.

Protein   The protein needs of people with acute renal failure depend on the degree of renal function, the metabolic rate, and nutrition status. People who are not on dialysis (described later in this section) receive about 0.6 to 1.0 gram of protein per kilogram of body weight per day.[5] Complicating factors must also be considered, however. Impaired wound healing, infections, muscle wasting, and negative nitrogen balance are commonly seen in individuals with acute renal failure, and these complications may prove to be fatal. Accordingly, some practitioners consider it most important to prevent negative nitrogen balance and its possible consequences; they prefer to provide a higher protein intake, even if it necessitates dialysis. If dialysis is instituted, a more liberal protein intake is indicated because some amino acids are lost during the procedure. Depending on the type of dialysis, people receive from 1.1 to 2.5 grams of protein per kilogram of body weight per day.[6]

Fluids   Fluid balances are carefully restored in clients who are either overhydrated or dehydrated. Thereafter, health care professionals determine fluid needs by measuring urine output and then adding about 500 milliliters to account for water lost through the skin, lungs, and perspiration. The person who is vomiting, has diarrhea, has a high fever, or otherwise loses fluids has greater fluid needs. In the oliguric stage, the person needs small amounts of fluids. In the diuretic stage, urine volume may increase significantly, and large amounts of fluids may have to be provided.

Electrolytes   Sodium may be restricted (to 500 to 1000 milligrams) in the oliguric phase, but this may change as the person enters the diuretic phase. Likewise, potassium is often restricted to less than 2 grams per day in the oliguric phase, but may need to be supplemented in the diuretic phase.

uremic (you-REE-mic) **syndrome:** the many symptoms that accompany the buildup of toxic waste products in the blood. Symptoms include:

- Fatigue.
- Weakness.
- Diminished mental alertness.
- Agitation.
- Muscular twitches.
- Muscle cramps.
- Anorexia.
- Nausea.
- Vomiting.
- Stomatitis.
- Unpleasant taste in the mouth.
- Diarrhea.

Take a moment to consider the high energy needs of an 80 kg (176 lb) person: 2400 to 4000 kcal/day.

Enteral and Parenteral Nutrition   Because clients with acute renal failure are often severely stressed, they frequently receive their nutrients from tube feedings or TPN. Special enteral and parenteral formulas meet nutrient needs in small volumes. Compared with standard enteral formulas, renal formulas have less protein, fewer electrolytes, and more kcalories per milliliter (see Appendix K). TPN formulas are compounded with mixtures of both nonessential and essential amino acids at lower concentrations and dextrose at higher concentrations than in standard TPN solutions. Electrolytes are added in appropriate amounts.

The carbohydrate-dense enteral and parenteral formulas used for acute renal failure may exacerbate the hyperglycemia that frequently accompanies both hypermetabolic disorders and renal failure. Fat can be used to add kcalories, reduce the need for carbohydrate, and limit the glucose load. Insulin may be provided to lower blood glucose.

Drug Therapy   In the oliguric phase of acute renal failure, diuretics may be used to mobilize fluids. Drugs called exchange resins may be used to treat hyperkalemia. These drugs, provided by mouth or through an enema, cause sodium to be exchanged for potassium in the colon, and the potassium is then excreted in the stool.

As mentioned, insulin may be provided to help lower blood glucose. Insulin also temporarily lowers blood potassium in two ways. First, as insulin moves glucose into the cells, potassium follows. Second, as an anabolic hormone, insulin minimizes tissue breakdown and, consequently, retains potassium in the cells.

Dialysis   Dialysis removes excess fluids and wastes from the blood by employing the principles of simple diffusion and osmosis across a semipermeable membrane. In so doing, dialysis reduces the symptoms of uremia, but the hormonal functions of the kidneys are not restored. The two major types of dialysis are hemodialysis and peritoneal dialysis.

In acute renal failure, the nephrons suddenly fail to maintain homeostasis, most often because of an abrupt decline in blood flow to the kidneys. Waste products accumulate, blood potassium rises, blood volume changes, and the clinical symptoms of uremic syndrome develop. Energy and protein needs are high, but those not on dialysis may need to restrict their protein intake. In the early oliguric stage, treatment includes small amounts of fluids, a diet restricted in sodium and potassium, and diuretics to mobilize fluids. In the later diuretic phase, treatment provides large amounts of fluids and may supplement potassium. The accompanying box provides a case study of a client with acute renal failure. Take a moment to review the many parameters health care professionals must consider when treating such clients.

Chronic Renal Failure

Most often chronic renal failure develops gradually from disorders that progressively and permanently damage the kidneys. Some of these disorders include nephritis, renal artery obstruction, kidney stones (see Highlight 29), renal tubular disorders, diabetic nephropathy (Chapter 27), hypertension (Chapter 28), and atherosclerosis (Chapter 28). Recall that nephrotic syndrome sometimes

---

Rx   PRESCRIPTION PAD

Drugs used to treat acute renal failure may include:

- Diuretics
- Exchange resins (sodium polystyrene)
- Insulin

See Appendix E for timing with meals and nutrition-related side effects.

---

dialysis (dye-AL-ih-sis): removal of waste from the blood using the principles of simple diffusion and osmosis through a semipermeable membrane.

In hemodialysis (HE-mo-dye-AL-ih-sis), a blood vessel is tapped, and the blood is routed through a dialysis machine where excess fluids and wastes are removed. Blood is then returned from the machine to the body.

In peritoneal (PERR-ee-toe-NEE-al) dialysis, excess fluids and wastes are removed from the blood using the peritoneum as a semipermeable membrane.

nephritis (nef-RYE-tis): inflammation of the kidneys.

Impairment of renal blood flow because of renal artery damage is called nephrosclerosis (NEF-ro-skle-ROH-sis). It can be caused by hypertension or atherosclerosis.

Common nephropathies include pyelonephritis (PIE-eh-loh-neh-FRY-tis), an inflammation of the kidneys and bladder, and glomerulonephritis (glo-MARE-you-loh-neh-FRY-tis), an inflammation of the glomerular capillaries.

Case Study   Store Manager with Acute Renal Failure

Mrs. Calley is a 35-year-old woman admitted to the hospital's intensive care unit. She was first seen in the emergency room after she sustained multiple and severe injuries in an auto accident. She had lost so much blood she almost died before reaching the hospital. Her injuries include a fractured leg, broken ribs, a collapsed lung, and internal bleeding. Following emergency surgery to stop the internal bleeding and repair injuries, she developed acute renal failure. Mrs. Calley is 5 feet 3 inches tall and weighs 125 pounds.

Mrs. Calley has a urine volume of less than 50 ml/day and a BUN of 75 mg/dL. A test of GFR could not be performed due to the low volume of urine she was excreting.

Describe the most probable reason why Mrs. Calley developed acute renal failure. What other problems can cause acute renal failure? Describe the phases of acute renal failure.

What are Mrs. Calley's dietary needs in the early phase? What waste products and electrolytes are of greatest concern? Why? What factors do you have to keep in mind in determining Mrs. Calley's energy and protein needs during acute renal failure? How will these needs change if dialysis is begun?

How will Mrs. Calley's nutrient needs change as she progresses to the second stage of acute renal failure? Why?

progresses to chronic renal failure. In a few cases, chronic renal failure develops from a disorder that rapidly causes irreversible kidney damage, as may occur following acute renal failure.

CONSEQUENCES OF CHRONIC RENAL FAILURE

Chronic renal failure progresses in stages. In the early stages, the body compensates for the loss of some nephron function by enlarging the remaining functional nephrons. The hypertrophied nephrons work so efficiently that the GFR may fall to 75 percent of its normal rate before symptoms appear. This efficiency explains why renal failure is often advanced before its presence is detected.

The body eventually exhausts the overworked nephrons, and renal function deteriorates further. (This effort is similar to the pancreatic cells in NIDDM, which at first produce more and more insulin in response to high blood glucose and later become exhausted and unable to produce adequate insulin.) In end-stage renal disease, the GFR drops below 20 percent of normal.

Blood Chemistry Alterations   As renal function deteriorates, nitrogen-containing waste products accumulate in the blood, and the uremic syndrome (described on p. 915) develops. The skin becomes dry and scaly, and the person may itch uncomfortably. Skin hemorrhages may be visible. In later stages, urea (which can be excreted through sweat) may crystallize on the skin, a symptom known as uremic frost.

Normal metabolic processes generate more acid than base, and in healthy people, the kidneys excrete this excess acid. Lacking this ability, the person with chronic renal failure easily develops acidosis.

In addition to nitrogen-containing compounds, the body retains excess fluids and electrolytes that are normally excreted in the urine. The retention of fluids and sodium causes edema and stresses the cardiovascular and pulmonary systems. Elevated blood potassium can trigger arrhythmias (irregular heartbeats) that

The capacity of the kidneys to function despite loss of some nephrons is referred to as **renal reserve.**

end-stage renal disease: the severe stage of renal failure in which dialysis or a kidney transplant is necessary to sustain life.

Reminder: The nitrogen-containing waste products that accumulate in renal failure include blood urea nitrogen (BUN), creatinine, and uric acid.

uremic frost: the appearance of urea crystals on the skin.

Reminder: The condition of having above-normal acidity in the blood and body fluids is *acidosis.*

further stress the heart and lead to heart failure. Elevated phosphorus alters bone metabolism (described later).

Uremia, together with altered hormonal activity, upsets the body's homeostasis and frequently leads to hypertension, hyperglycemia, elevated blood lipids (especially triglycerides), low serum albumin levels, and altered bone metabolism. All of these conditions further impair health.

Cardiovascular Complications   Accelerated atherosclerosis and cardiovascular disease frequently accompany renal failure. Retention of fluid, sodium, and potassium, together with elevated blood lipids, hormonal changes, and hyperglycemia, can lead to hypertension, congestive heart failure, heart attacks, and pulmonary edema (see Chapter 28). In addition, some people with renal failure have elevated homocysteine levels, which may be an independent risk factor for cardiovascular disease (see Highlight 28).[7] Whether lowering homocysteine levels in people with renal disease can reduce their risk of cardiovascular disease remains to be determined. Cardiovascular disease is the cause of death in about a third of people with end-stage renal failure.[8]

Bone Disease   The blood's normal balance between calcium and phosphorus prevents the two minerals from precipitating and forming calcium phosphate salts. When blood phosphorus rises too high because the kidneys are unable to excrete it, however, the excess phosphorus forms salts with calcium, which are then deposited in soft tissues such as eyes, skin, lungs, heart, and blood vessels. As calcium phosphate salts precipitate, serum levels of both phosphorus and calcium fall. As serum calcium, which were not elevated to begin with, falls, low calcium levels trigger the release of parathormone (PTH), which promotes excretion of phosphorus from the kidneys.

For a while, PTH effectively restores calcium and phosphorus balance, but as the GFR progressively declines, more PTH is needed to promote phosphorus excretion. Eventually, serum phosphorus remains high and calcium remains low despite markedly elevated levels of PTH (hyperparathyroidism).

To compound these problems, the diseased kidneys are unable to effectively activate vitamin D, which normally responds to low blood calcium by increasing calcium absorption from the GI tract. With lower levels of active vitamin D available, less calcium is absorbed. Besides all this, renal diets tend to be low in calcium as well. Hence the body is forced to draw calcium from bone tissue to raise blood calcium.

For all these reasons, bone disorders are common in chronic renal failure as evidenced by bone pain, diminished bone mass, soft (demineralized) bones, and fractures. Figure 29–3 summarizes the events leading to renal osteodystrophy.

Gastrointestinal Disturbances   Nausea, vomiting, diarrhea, and constipation commonly accompany the uremic syndrome. Gastritis and GI bleeding are also prevalent. All of these conditions can reduce food intake and increase nutrient losses.

Growth Failure and Wasting Syndrome   Both children and adults with chronic renal disease frequently develop wasting and PEM. Nutrition status becomes more difficult to maintain as renal failure progresses. Taking multiple drugs over long periods of time further compromises nutrition status. Table 29–1

The deposition of phosphorus and calcium salts in soft tissue is called metastatic (MET-ah-STAT-ik) calcification.

Reminder: Parathormone (PTH) is a hormone secreted by the parathyroid glands that regulates calcium and phosphorus metabolism; also known as parathyroid hormone.

renal osteodystrophy (OS-tee-oh-DIS-tro-fee): bone disorders resulting from calcium and phosphorus imbalances in renal disease. In osteopenia, bone mass is reduced; in osteomalacia (see p. 388), bones soften and fracture easily.

A type of renal osteodystrophy that results from hyperparathyroidism and is characterized by kidney stones, decalcification and softening of bones, and, sometimes, formation of cysts and tumors is called osteitis (os-tee-EYE-tis) fibrosis.

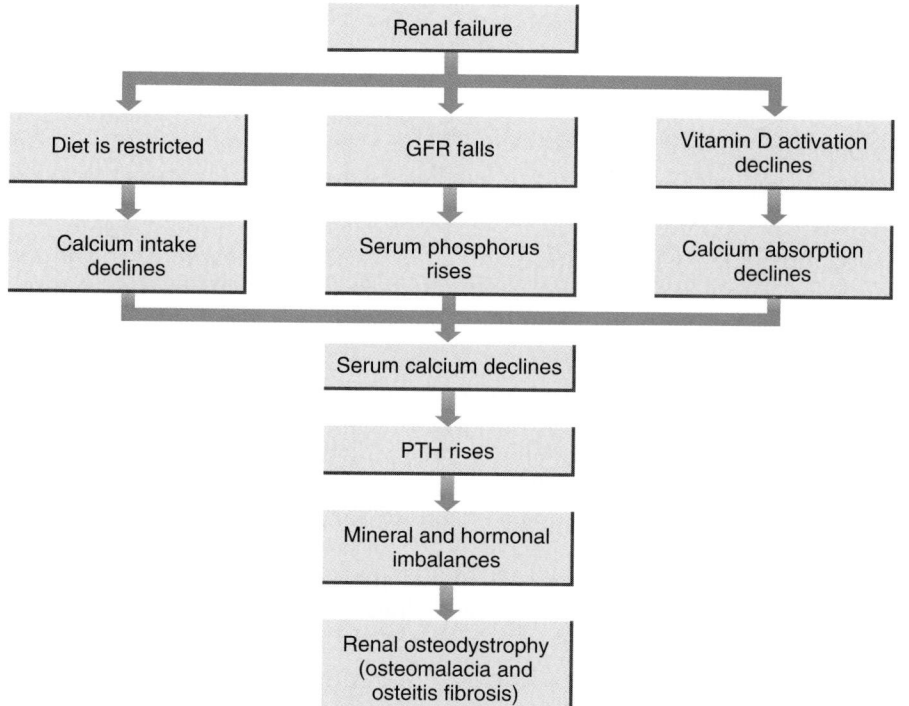

Figure 29–3

Events Leading to Renal Osteodystrophy

summarizes the causes of wasting associated with renal failure. Children with renal disease need nutrition intervention before the end of puberty if they are to make up growth deficits. Adults with renal disease can maintain or restore nutrition status, avoid complications, and improve quality of life by conscientiously attending to their diets as well.

Anemia   People with functional kidneys respond to any type of anemia by increasing their production of erythropoietin, a hormone that stimulates hemoglobin and red blood cell synthesis. Depressed erythropoietin synthesis by the

Table 29–1

Possible Causes of Wasting in Renal Failure

Reduced Nutrient Intake	Excessive Nutrient Losses	Raised Nutrient Needs
Anorexia	Dialysis	Drugs
Drugs	Diarrhea	Hormonal alterations
Fatigue	Drugs	Infection
Nausea	GI bleeding	
Pain	Numerous blood tests	
Restrictive diet	Poor absorption	
Taste alterations	Vomiting	

damaged kidneys often results in anemia. Other factors that contribute to iron-deficiency anemia in renal failure include:

- Limited iron intake from the restrictive diet.
- Impaired intestinal absorption of iron.
- Blood (and iron) losses from hemodialysis, frequent blood tests, and GI bleeding.

When the kidneys fail, the effects are felt throughout the entire body, and the consequences are severe. Although renal failure is fatal without intervention, proper treatment can help sustain life and improve its quality.

TREATMENT OF CHRONIC RENAL FAILURE

Treatment for chronic renal failure includes diet, drugs, dialysis, and kidney transplants. Treatments aim to delay the progression of renal failure, prevent the buildup of toxic metabolic products and associated complications, maintain nutrition status, and alleviate symptoms to improve the client's well-being.

Diet therapy is highly individualized and changes as renal disease progresses from renal insufficiency to end-stage renal disease. Table 29–2 summarizes nutrient needs for renal insufficiency and shows how these needs change for hemodial-

renal insufficiency: reduced renal function but not to the degree that requires dialysis or a kidney transplant.

Table 29–2
Nutrient Needs in Chronic Renal Failure

Nutrients	Renal Insufficiency (Predialysis)	Hemodialysis	Peritoneal Dialysis
Energy (kcal/kg)	35–40	30–35	25–35
Protein (g/kg)	0.6–0.8	1.2–1.4	1.2–1.5
Fluid (ml)	Typically not restricted	500–750 plus daily urine output, or 1000 if anuric	≥2000
Sodium (g)	2–4	2–3	2–4
Potassium (g/kg)	Typically not restricted	3–4	Typically not restricted
Phosphorus (mg/g protein)	10–12[a]	12–15[a]	12–15[a]
Supplements			
Calcium (mg)	1000–1500	1000–1500	1000–1500
Folate (mg)	1	1	1
Vitamin B$_6$ (mg)	5	10	10
Other water-soluble vitamins	RDA	RDA	RDA
Vitamin D	As appropriate	As appropriate	As appropriate

Note: The actual amounts of these nutrients in the diet must be highly individualized based on each person's responses. For example, calcium supplementation may be as high as 3000 milligrams per day.

[a]The extent of phosphorus restriction depends on serum phosphorus. The goal is to maintain serum phosphorus between 4.5 and 6.0 milligrams per deciliter. Often, phosphate binders are useful for this purpose.

Sources: Adapted from Meeting the challenge of the renal diet: A preview of the 'National Renal Diet' educational series, *Journal of the American Dietetic Association* 93 (1993): 637–639; J. A. Beto, Which diet for which renal failure: Making sense of the options, *Journal of the American Dietetic Association* 95 (1995): 898–903.

ysis and peritoneal dialysis. The complexity of the renal diet, as well as its crucial role in the treatment of renal disease, underscores the need for a specialist, a renal dietitian, to educate clients and provide diet plans. Other health care professionals need not know the specifics of diet therapy, but they must understand the general concepts in order to communicate effectively with clients.

Energy   All people with renal failure need adequate food energy to achieve or maintain a desirable body weight and to prevent protein catabolism. Diet restrictions and the nausea associated with uremia may make it difficult for people with renal insufficiency to eat enough food. Most adults need at least 35 kcalories per kilogram of body weight per day. People on peritoneal dialysis, however, may need to restrict food intake because they absorb a significant amount of energy as glucose from the dialysate. For children, 100 or even more kcalories per kilogram of body weight per day is desirable, but 80 kcalories per kilogram of body weight per day is considered a reasonable intake. At the minimum, energy intake should meet the RDA.[9]

To evaluate dialysis and guide diet therapy, renal teams often use a mathematical model that takes into account the kidneys' ability to clear urea and the person's protein catabolic rate. The technique is called urea kinetic modeling.

Protein   Providing the right amount of protein in renal failure is like walking a tightrope. Too little protein, and the person develops malnutrition. Too much protein, and blood urea (the toxic waste product of protein metabolism) rises. For people with renal insufficiency, restricting protein may help protect the remaining nephrons, but human studies have not clearly demonstrated a beneficial effect.[10] Because dietary protein is limited, the diet emphasizes high-quality protein sources such as eggs, milk, meat, poultry, and fish.

A diet that includes protein from both animal and plant sources may be best because it combines the high quality of animal proteins with the low saturated fat and low cholesterol of plant proteins. As renal failure progresses, some clinicians prescribe very-low-protein diets supplemented with essential amino acids or their precursors (keto acids). Once the client begins dialysis, protein restrictions can be relaxed somewhat because dialysis incurs protein losses, peritoneal dialysis more so than hemodialysis.

People at high risk for developing chronic renal failure (such as those with diabetes) are often advised to limit protein intake to about the RDA.

Lipid   The ideal renal diet restricts total fat, saturated fat, and cholesterol to help control elevated blood lipids and reduce the risk of cardiovascular disease. A later section describes the difficulties of meeting this dietary goal.

Carbohydrate   A diet rich in complex carbohydrate helps to minimize the elevated blood glucose and triglycerides commonly seen in people with chronic renal failure. People on peritoneal dialysis may need to further restrict the intake of total carbohydrate, and especially simple carbohydrates, because they absorb a considerable amount of glucose from the dialysate.

Sodium and Fluids   As renal failure progresses, the person excretes less urine and cannot handle even normal amounts of sodium and fluids. At this point, limiting sodium and fluids helps to prevent hypertension, edema, and heart failure. Individual needs for sodium and fluids are determined by carefully monitoring each person's weight, blood pressure, urine output, and blood electrolyte levels. A rise in body weight and blood pressure suggests that the person is retaining sodium and fluid; conversely, a decline in body weight and blood pressure (a desirable outcome of dialysis) represents fluid loss.

Minimal urine volume is oliguria; no urine excretion is anuria.

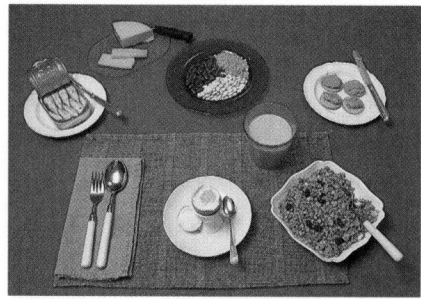

Foods such as milk and milk products, cheese, peanut butter, bran cereal, sardines, and legumes are high in phosphorus and so must be restricted in a renal diet. See Appendix H for other foods high in phosphorus.

Caution: People with renal failure who must restrict potassium must avoid using low-sodium products and salt substitutes that contain potassium.

People with renal failure should avoid aluminum- and magnesium-containing antacids and laxatives or enemas containing magnesium; aluminum toxicity or serious hypermagnesemia can result.

The active form of supplemental vitamin D, or calcitriol, can be given orally or intravenously. A new, experimental form of active vitamin D called 22 oxa calcitriol is associated with a less marked rise in serum calcium than calcitriol.

Fluids are not restricted in renal insufficiency until urine output decreases. For the person who is neither dehydrated nor overhydrated, daily fluid needs amount to the daily urine output plus about 500 to 750 milliliters to provide for insensible water losses.

Once a person is on dialysis, sodium and fluid intake is controlled to allow a weight gain of about 2 pounds (of fluid) between dialysis treatments, although larger weight gains are common.[11] Typical renal diets provide from 2 to 4 grams of sodium and 500 to 3000 milliliters (about ½ to 3 quarts) of fluids daily. Table 29–3 lists foods considered part of the fluid allowance.

Potassium   Most people with renal insufficiency and those on peritoneal dialysis can handle typical intakes of potassium.[12] People on hemodialysis, however, may experience elevated potassium levels between dialysis treatments. When hyperkalemia is a problem, potassium may be moderately restricted to about 2 to 3 grams per day. Figure 12–7 on p. 425 lists the potassium contents of commonly eaten foods; the person who must restrict potassium limits potassium-rich foods. Remember, however, that individual needs vary. People with renal disease who are taking potassium-wasting diuretics may need to adjust their potassium intakes accordingly.

Phosphorus   Dietary phosphorus restrictions help control rising phosphorus levels and may help slow the progression of renal failure. Fortunately, when a client follows a protein-restricted diet, phosphorus is restricted as well. In addition, the person must limit foods high in phosphorus, such as those shown in the margin photo.

Physicians may also prescribe drugs that bind phosphorus in the GI tract, thus making it unavailable for absorption. These phosphate binders must be taken with meals. Calcium salts—calcium carbonate and calcium acetate—are the preferred phosphate binders for people with end-stage renal disease. Aluminum and magnesium salts also bind phosphate, but they carry a risk of toxicity and are therefore avoided.

Calcium Supplements   As mentioned, impaired calcium absorption due to the lack of active vitamin D and limited calcium intake may contribute to bone disease in people with renal failure. Most people with renal disease need calcium supplements; some, however, develop hypercalcemia. The renal team monitors serum calcium closely to prevent both low and high blood calcium. Calcium-containing phosphate binders provide some calcium, but the absorption of calcium from these products varies widely.

Water-Soluble Vitamins   People with renal failure frequently develop vitamin B_6 and folate deficiencies because of the restrictive diet, loss of vitamins during dialysis, drug therapy, and altered metabolism. For these reasons, clients receive generous amounts of vitamin B_6 and folate, along with RDA amounts of the other water-soluble vitamins. Intakes of vitamin C from both the diet and supplements should be limited to less than 100 milligrams per day to prevent the formation of oxalate stones (see Chapter 22 p. 728).[13]

Fat-Soluble Vitamins   Supplemental vitamin D in its active form can help maintain blood calcium and prevent bone disease. The dosages and methods of administering vitamin D supplements must be carefully adjusted for each client to maintain serum calcium levels within the normal range. Supplementation of the other fat-soluble vitamins is usually not necessary.

Trace Minerals   The administration of human erythropoietin along with the iron needed to synthesize hemoglobin is effective in treating iron-deficiency anemia, once a common and persistent problem in people with chronic renal disease. Poor iron absorption and the GI side effects of iron supplements may make it difficult for clients to fully meet their iron needs. Clients should be cautioned to avoid iron supplements that also contain vitamin C.

People on dialysis frequently complain of anorexia and altered taste perceptions (dysgeusia), symptoms typical of zinc deficiency. Clients with these symptoms may need supplements if their serum zinc levels are inadequate.

Enteral and Parenteral Nutrition   Enteral and parenteral nutrition can provide nutrients to people with chronic renal failure who are unable to eat adequate amounts of foods. If the GI tract is functional, health care professionals first try to supplement the diet with enteral formulas orally. Glucose polymer powders may be used to add food energy without requiring clients to eat extra food or use their fluid allowances. In addition, formulas designed for use with renal failure (as described earlier on p. 916) can be given by tube (see Appendix K). Parenteral formulas are also available.

Diet Planning   The ideal renal diet presents a challenge: provide adequate energy, but restrict protein, fat, and, sometimes, simple carbohydrate. Complex carbohydrates, which might appear to be the ideal energy source, are rich sources of electrolytes, which are also restricted on the renal diet. Complex carbohydrates are also rich sources of fiber; and because fibers absorb fluids, which are often restricted, they must be used cautiously. Diet planners must accept that under such circumstances, no diet is truly ideal. They must recognize that the need to meet protein and electrolyte requirements outweighs the need to restrict fats and simple carbohydrates.

To help meet energy needs, clients include as many complex carbohydrate foods as their diet plans allow. They supplement their meals with formulas high in kcalories but restricted in protein and electrolytes (see Appendix K) and use foods such as sugars (glucose polymers, hard candy, and jelly) and fats (margarine, oil) freely. The person with elevated blood lipids may be advised to restrict fat and modify the type of fat if possible. The person with diabetes or hyperglycemia is advised to maintain a consistent carbohydrate intake at regular intervals and to adjust insulin to cover carbohydrate intake.

To help individuals on renal diets find foods they will accept and enjoy, food lists similar to the exchange system are available. Whereas the exchange system for diabetes groups foods by their energy, carbohydrate, protein, and fat contents, renal food lists group foods by their energy, protein, sodium, potassium, and phosphorus contents. The box on p. 924 provides suggestions to ease the task of complying with a renal diet. A sample renal diet menu is shown on p. 925.

Diet Compliance   The challenges dietitians face in designing renal diets pale in comparison to those encountered by clients and caregivers who must follow a complicated medical care plan of which diet is only one part. Successful

Table 29–3

Substances Controlled on Fluid-Restricted Diets

Foods
Cream
Frozen yogurt
Fruit ice
Gelatin
Ice cream
Ice milk
Popsicles
Sherbet
Soup

Other
Ice
Liquid medications

Note: All foods contain some water, but these foods contain considerable amounts of water and, therefore, must be considered part of the fluid allowance on a fluid-restricted diet.

How to Help Clients Comply with a Renal Diet

The following suggestions can assist clients in complying with the renal diet:

1. To keep track of fluid intake:

   - Fill a container with an amount of water equal to your total fluid allowance. Each time you use a liquid food or beverage, discard an equivalent amount of water from the container. The amount remaining in the container will show you how much fluid you have left for the day.
   - Be sure to save enough fluid to take medications.

2. To help control thirst:

   - Chew gum or suck hard candy.
   - Freeze fluids so they take longer to consume.
   - Add lemon juice to water to make it more refreshing.
   - Gargle with refrigerated mouthwash.

3. To prevent the diet from becoming monotonous:

   - Experiment with new combinations of allowed foods.
   - Use favorite foods whenever possible.
   - Substitute nondairy products for regular dairy products. Nondairy products are lower in protein, phosphorus, and potassium than regular dairy foods, and they can substitute for milk and add energy to the diet.
   - Add zest to foods by seasoning with garlic, onion, chili, curry powder, oregano, pepper, or lemon juice.
   - Consult a dietitian when you want to eat restricted foods. Many restricted foods can be used occasionally and in small amounts if the diet is carefully adjusted.

Psychosocial factors include:
- Knowledge.
- Attitude.
- Support.
- Satisfaction.
- Self-perception of success.

Behavioral factors include:
- Self-monitoring of protein intake.
- Provision of feedback by a dietitian.

treatment hinges on compliance with the medical plan. To help clients understand medical plans and support their efforts, the health care team must effectively communicate with their clients and, just as important, listen to them. Within a tangled web of abnormal metabolic processes, dialysis lines, and toxic waste products is a person, often a frightened or discouraged one. All of the members of the health care team need to understand the plan if they are to offer the most effective support.

A nutrition education approach that emphasizes self-management appears to be a useful strategy for helping clients comply with a renal diet.[14] This approach (described in Highlight 27) guides clients in identifying goals, selecting strategies to meet their goals, and evaluating their progress. Both psychosocial and behavioral factors play key roles in helping clients adhere to protein-restricted diets.[15]

Menu

Breakfast
1 egg, fried with
   1 tbs margarine
1 slice toast
2 tsp margarine
Jelly
½ c grape juice
Coffee
Nondairy creamer
Sugar

Snacks
Hard candy, gum drops,
   marshmallows
Carbonated beverages

Lunch
Sandwich with
   2 oz turkey
   2 slices bread
1 tbs mayonnaise
Lettuce leaf
1 c green beans
2 tsp margarine
½ c strawberries
2 tbs whipping cream
Sugar
½ c milk

Supper
3 oz roast beef
½ c rice
2 tsp margarine
½ c mushrooms sautéed
   in 2 tsp olive oil and
   seasonings
½ c applesauce
Iced tea
2 tsp sugar

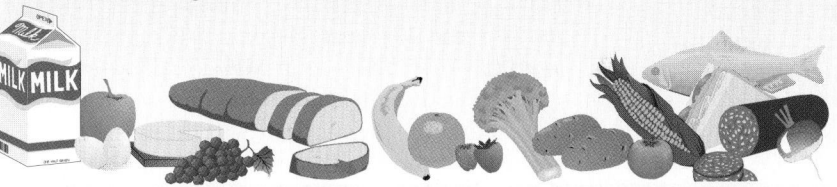

Sample Renal Diet Menu

This diet menu provides 60 grams of protein and controls phosphorus, potassium, and sodium intake. To increase the kcalories in this diet, prepare food with oil or unsalted margarine (regular margarine, if allowed) and use additional fat, sugar, or syrup whenever possible. For example, canned fruit packed in heavy syrup, rather than juice, adds kcalories.

KIDNEY TRANSPLANTS AND DIET

A preferable alternative to dialysis in end-stage renal disease is a kidney transplant. Kidney transplants can successfully restore kidney function and normal growth. For this reason, transplants are particularly desirable in children. Given a choice, many would prefer transplants, but suitable kidney donors cannot always be found.

Immunosuppressant Drug Therapy   After receiving a new kidney, the person must take very large doses of immunosuppressants to prevent rejection (see Table E–1 in Appendix E for nutrient-drug interactions). Muscular weakness, GI bleeding, protein catabolism, carbohydrate intolerance, sodium retention, fluid retention, hypertension, weight gain, and a characteristic puffy-faced appearance commonly accompany immunosuppressant therapy. Infections and increased susceptibility to malignant tumors are also common. Diuretics are frequently prescribed to promote the excretion of sodium and fluid and prevent hypertension. The kidney may be rejected or fail to function, in which case dialysis must be reinstituted either temporarily until another kidney can be found or permanently.

Dietary Interventions   Immediately following a kidney transplant, enough energy and protein are provided to limit catabolism and preserve organ function and nutrition status. Once recovery is underway, the degree of renal function guides diet therapy. Typical post-transplant diet modifications appear in Table 29–4. Dietary protein is provided in amounts adequate to prevent the protein catabolism that immunosuppressants may incur, but not too much to tax renal function. Because blood lipids are frequently elevated, clients are advised to follow a low-fat diet. Sodium restrictions help prevent fluid

Table 29–4

Dietary Guidelines Following Kidney Transplant

Energy: Adequate to achieve or maintain desirable body weight.

Protein: 1g per kg body wt. (Adjust based on renal function tests.)

Fat: ≤30 percent of total kcal; ≤300 mg cholesterol.

Sodium: 3 to 4 g per day.

Potassium: Adjust according to diuretic therapy.

Source: Adapted from J. A. Beto, Which diet for which renal failure: Making sense of the options, *Journal of the American Dietetic Association* 95 (1995): 898–903.

Case Study   Child with Chronic Renal Failure

Jason is a nine-year-old child who developed chronic glomerulonephritis several months after suffering from a streptococcal infection (strep throat). Jason's renal function has declined steadily over the last three years. His mother consulted his pediatrician because the boy had been very tired, unable to eat, and complaining of stomach cramps and unpleasant taste sensations. Laboratory tests revealed the following information:

- GFR: 4 ml/min (below normal).
- BUN: 102 mg/dL (above normal).

Jason was admitted to the hospital, and after further testing, dialysis was instituted, and a search for a suitable kidney donor was begun. Jason is 4 feet 3 inches tall and weighs 55 pounds. Before coming to the hospital, he was following a fluid-, sodium-, potassium-, and phosphorus-restricted diet that allowed 30 grams of protein. His typical energy intake is 1100 kcalories per day.

Describe chronic renal failure. Are the symptoms Jason complained of typical of renal failure? Why did his GFR fall, and why did his BUN levels rise?

Look closely at Jason's height and weight. How do they compare with the height and weight of other children of the same age? (Use the growth charts in Appendix E.) Discuss reasons why growth may be compromised in the child with renal failure.

Think about Jason's diet before he came to the hospital. Describe the reasons why protein, fluid, sodium, potassium, and phosphorus were restricted. Calculate Jason's energy range, and compare this estimate with his actual energy intake. Consider the effect of Jason's energy intake on his growth.

Describe ways Jason's nutrient needs will change when he begins hemodialysis. How will his needs change if he receives a kidney transplant?

Discuss some diet strategies you can suggest to Jason and his parents to help him comply with his diet. Consider the impact of renal disease on Jason, his family, and his interactions with friends. How can all members of the health team help support Jason and his family during this difficult time?

retention and hypertension. Depending on the type of diuretic prescribed, potassium intakes may have to be adjusted as well.

As mentioned, people with kidney transplants may reject their new kidneys either temporarily or permanently. During these times, they must return to the prescribed diet for renal failure. Clients may find this regression difficult to accept and need to be prepared for the possibility before it occurs. The accompanying case study helps direct your thoughts toward the special needs of a client with chronic renal failure.

Chronic renal failure develops gradually from any disorder that progressively and permanently damages the kidneys. At first, the nephrons compensate for the loss of function, making detection in the early stages difficult. Eventually, end-stage renal disease will dramatically affect every body system and compromise nutrition status. Diet plans control fluid, energy, protein, sodium, potassium, and phosphorus intakes; plans differ depending on the degree of renal insufficiency, the type of dialysis, and the success of a transplant. Use the nutrition assessment checklist to review assessment findings of concern in renal failure.

Nutrition Assessment Checklist
For People with Renal Diseases

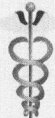

Medical   Use the medical record to evaluate the cause of renal insufficiency or renal failure and the treatment plan. Determine what other conditions such as severe stress, hyperlipidemia, hypertension, congestive heart disease, or diabetes may alter nutrient needs.

Drug   Review the client's drug therapy for possible drug-nutrient interactions, particularly for clients with chronic renal diseases that will require long-term use of various drugs including antilipemics, antihypertensives, diuretics, and immunosuppressants. Assess the client's over-the-counter drug use for sources of electrolytes.

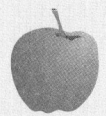

Food Intake   Assess food intake to evaluate usual intake of energy, protein, fluids, sodium, potassium, phosphorus, calcium, vitamins, and minerals. Use food records to assess the client's compliance with diet therapy and to make additional suggestions.

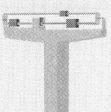

Anthropometric   Monitor changes in height and weight in children and weight in adults. Interpret anthropometric measurements cautiously in people with oliguria, anuria, or edema because anthropometrics may be deceptively normal or high due to fluid retention. For people on dialysis, the weight measured immediately after a treatment most accurately reflects the person's true weight and is sometimes called the "dry weight." Rapid weight gain between dialysis treatments often reflects fluid retention. Weight loss should be expected following dialysis treatment.

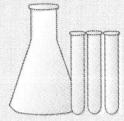

Laboratory   Check serum protein levels, which are often low in people with nephrotic syndrome and renal failure and may be even lower if malnutrition complicates renal disease. Review laboratory measurements of GFR, electrolytes, BUN, and creatinine, which are commonly used to determine dietary and medical treatments. Note whether serum lipids are elevated, as frequently occurs in people with nephrotic syndrome, renal failure, and kidney transplants.

Physical   Check for physical signs of fluid retention or dehydration, iron deficiency (pale skin and conjunctiva), uremia (fatigue, mental confusion, dry itchy skin, skin hemorrhages, nausea, vomiting, altered taste perceptions), osteodystrophy (bone pain, fractures, and bowed legs in children), hyperkalemia (arrhythmias and muscle weakness), and zinc deficiencies (altered taste perceptions). Record blood pressure and vital signs.

Study Questions

1. What functions do the kidneys perform? What roles do they play in maintaining chemical homeostasis?
2. What is nephrotic syndrome? What are its consequences? What are the energy and protein needs of the person with nephrotic syndrome? Why is a low-fat, low-cholesterol diet important in nephrotic syndrome? What are the fluid and electrolyte needs of these individuals?
3. Describe acute renal failure and list some of its causes. What symptoms are associated with the buildup of toxic metabolic products in the blood? What are the consequences of acute renal failure?
4. What are the nutrient needs of the person in the oliguric phase of acute renal failure? How do these needs change as the person progresses to the diuretic phase?
5. Can tube feedings and TPN be used safely for the person with renal failure? What special considerations are involved in selecting an enteral or parenteral formula for the person with acute renal failure?
6. What are the causes of chronic renal failure? Why is it often difficult to detect in the early stages? What happens in the end stage of renal failure?
7. What are the objectives of dietary treatment of chronic renal failure? When is a special diet instituted in the course of renal failure? When is dialysis or a kidney transplant considered for the person with renal failure?
8. What are the energy needs of adults with chronic renal failure? Of children? What are the consequences of providing too little energy in the diet of the person with chronic renal failure?
9. Why is the protein (nitrogen) intake of the person with chronic renal failure a particular concern? How does dialysis affect protein needs?
10. What fluid and electrolyte modifications are made to the diet of the person with chronic renal failure? What modifications are made concerning phosphorus, calcium, and vitamin D? Why?
11. What other vitamins and minerals need special consideration in the diet of the person with chronic renal failure? Describe why each of the nutrients you list may be a problem.
12. Discuss the nutrient needs of the person with a kidney transplant.

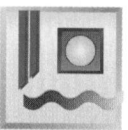

Clinical Applications

1. Chapter 25 described severe stresses and discussed how the combination of severe stress, hypermetabolism, and malnutrition can lead to multiple organ failure. The sequence of multiple organ failure often begins with respiratory failure (Chapter 28), followed by liver failure (Chapter 26), and then renal failure. Design a table with four columns: severe stress, respiratory failure, liver failure, and renal failure. Make the following rows: energy, protein, fat, fluid, and other nutrients. Fill the appropriate block with a brief description if there is a need for consideration: Which nutrient modifications are common to all four disorders? Do some of the necessary modifications for one disorder conflict with those for another? If yes, describe how the final decision might be made for the most appropriate diet.
2. Using the box on p. 924 as a guide, suggest ways to help people adjust to different aspects of their renal diets.

Notes

1. J. D. Dwyer, Vegetarian diets for treating nephrotic syndrome, *Nutrition Reviews* 51 (1993): 44–56; G. A. Kaysen, Nutritional management of nephrotic syndrome, *Journal of Renal Nutrition* 2 (1992): 50–58.

2. R. W. Davies and coauthors, Proteinuria, not altered albumin metabolism, affects hyperlipidemia in the nephrotic rat, *Journal of Clinical Investigations* 86 (1990): 600–605.

3. R. Rodrigo and M. Pino, Proteinuria and albumin homeostasis in the nephrotic syndrome: Effect of dietary protein intake, *Nutrition Reviews* 54 (1996): 337–347.

4. Kaysen, 1992.

5. J. D. Kopple, Nutrition management of the patient with acute renal failure, *Journal of Parenteral and Enteral Nutrition* 20 (1996): 3–12.

6. Kopple, 1996.

7. J. A. Friedman and J. T. Dwyer, Hyperhomocysteinemia as a risk factor for cardiovascular disease in patients undergoing hemodialysis, *Nutrition Reviews* 53 (1995): 197–201.

8. K. W. Ma, G. L. Greene, and L. Raij, Cardiovascular risk factors in chronic renal failure and hemodialysis populations, *American Journal of Kidney Diseases* 19 (1992): 505–513.

9. A.S.P.E.N. Board of Directors, Practice guidelines: Kidney failure—Pediatric, *Journal of Parenteral and Enteral Nutrition* (supplement) 17 (1993): 43.

10. The Modification of Diet in Renal Disease Study Group, The effects of dietary protein restriction and blood pressure control on the progression of chronic renal disease, *New England Journal of Medicine* 330 (1994): 877–884.

11. J. A. Beto, Which diet for which renal failure: Making sense of the options, *Journal of the American Dietetic Association* 95 (1995): 898–903.

12. Beto, 1996.

13. Beto, 1996.

14. B. P. Gillis and coauthors, Nutrition intervention program of the Modification of Diet in Renal Disease Study: A self-management approach, *Journal of the American Dietetic Association* 95 (1995): 1288–1294.

15. N. C. Milas and coauthors, Factors associated with adherence to the dietary protein intervention in the Modification of Diet in Renal Disease Study, *Journal of the American Dietetic Association* 95 (1995): 1295–1300; T. Coyne and coauthors, Dietary satisfaction correlated with adherence in the Modification of Diet in Renal Disease Study, *Journal of the American Dietetic Association* 95 (1995): 1301–1306.

Kidney Stones—Treatments and Prevention

Kidney stones affect 10 to 20 percent of the U.S. population, with about one in a thousand people requiring hospitalization for this painful, although rarely fatal, condition. Most people with kidney stones are men over age 25, and although they may have recurrences, many report only a single episode. Kidney stones are prevalent in certain geographical locations, particularly in the southeastern United States. These findings suggest that kidney stones may be preventable. The glossary on p. 931 defines terms related to kidney stones.

KIDNEY STONES

Kidney stones may form anywhere in the urinary tract, but most often they form in the area just above the ureter called the renal pelvis (review Figure 29–1 on p. 910). Kidney stones vary in size, and a person may form a single stone or multiple stones. Kidney stones form when stone constituents become concentrated in the urine and form crystals that grow. Stone constituents vary, but most stones are composed of calcium oxalate. The incidence of calcium oxalate kidney stones has climbed steadily in affluent countries.[1] Less commonly, stones are composed of calcium phosphate, uric acid, the amino acid cystine, or magnesium ammonium phosphate (known as struvite). Table H29–1 on p. 931 lists some conditions associated with stone formation.

Consequences of Kidney Stones

In most cases, kidney stones pose no problems, especially when they are

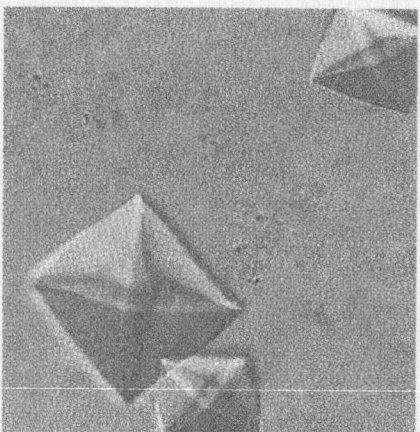

Most kidney stones are formed from calcium oxalate crystals, shown here.

few and small. Small stones (less than one-fifth of an inch in diameter) may pass readily through the ureters and out of the body via the urine with minimal treatment. Large stones, on the other hand, cannot pass easily through the ureter. When a large stone or a large piece of a stone enters a ureter, it produces a sharp, stabbing pain, called *renal*

colic. Typically, the pain starts suddenly in the back and intensifies as the stone follows the course down the abdomen toward the groin. The intense pain is often accompanied by nausea and vomiting. When the stone reaches the bladder, the pain subsides abruptly. Large stones that fail to pass through the ureter may cause a urinary tract obstruction or infection and serious bleeding. Symptoms may include frequent urination, urgency of urination, painful urination (dysuria), and bloody urine (hematuria).

Treatment of Kidney Stones

Clinicians analyze the chemical composition of urine, blood, and stones (when available) to determine the composition of the stone and its cause. Whenever the cause can be determined, treatment depends on resolving the underlying condition.[2]

Clients with small kidney stones may more readily pass the stone if

Glossary

cystinuria (SIS-te-NEW-ree-ah): the presence of cystine in the urine; the symptom of an inherited metabolic disorder in which large amounts of the amino acids cystine, lysine, arginine, and ornithine are excreted in the urine. Cystinuria commonly results in kidney stone formation.

dysuria (dis-YOU-ree-ah): painful or difficult urination.

gout: a metabolic disorder that results in excess uric acid in the blood and sometimes in the urine; characterized by acute arthritis and inflammation of the joints.

hematuria (HEME-at-YOU-ree-ah): blood in the urine.

hypercalciuria (HIGH-per-kal-see-YOU-ree-ah): excessive urinary excretion of calcium. When not related to a known underlying medical condition, it is known as idiopathic hypercalciuria.

renal colic: the severe pain that accompanies the movement of a kidney stone from the kidney through the ureter to the bladder.

struvite: crystals of magnesium ammonium phosphate.

Table H29–1

Conditions Associated with Kidney Stones

Cystinuria

Fat malabsorption

Glucocorticoid excess

Gout

Hyperparathyroidism

Hyperthyroidism

Immobilization

Malignancies (some types)

Osteoporosis

Paget's disease

Recurrent urinary tract infections

Renal tubular acidosis

Vitamin D toxicity

they drink plenty of fluids (more than 3 liters a day). They may also need antimicrobials if an infection is present and may sometimes need diuretics to help maintain urine output so that stones do not have a chance to form or enlarge. Large stones that block the flow of urine or cause an infection require removal either surgically or, more commonly, by using shock waves to break the stone into pieces small enough to pass readily through the urinary tract.

PREVENTION OF KIDNEY STONES

Treatment of the underlying medical condition is necessary to help prevent recurrences of kidney stones. Dietary measures vary according to the composition of the stone, but prevention of all stones includes this advice: increase fluid intake to dilute the urine. People who have had kidney stones need to drink enough fluid (mostly water)

to maintain a urine volume of at least 2 liters a day. This level of output requires an intake of 3 or 4 liters of fluids throughout the day. People who are physically active or who live in warm climates may need additional fluids. People with fevers, diarrhea, or vomiting also need additional fluids until these conditions resolve.

Dietary therapies for specific types of stones are described next. Phosphate stones are not responsive to diet and are treated with drugs or surgery.

Calcium Stones

About half of all people with calcium stones excrete normal amounts of calcium in the urine, and the other half excrete excess calcium (hypercalciuria). People with hypercalciuria are either more efficient at absorbing calcium from the intestine or more wasteful in their excretion of calcium than most people. Diet therapy for people with hypercalciuria limits calcium intake to the RDA appropriate for age and sex. It is important that the diet not fall below the RDA, however. Those with hypercalciuria who follow a low-calcium diet generally excrete more calcium than they ingest, indicating that they are losing calcium from their bones.

Oxalate-Restricted Diets Calcium restriction increases urinary oxalate excretion (see p. 728), which poses a problem for people with calcium oxalate stones. Hyperoxaluria increases the likelihood of calcium oxalate stone formation even more than hypercalciuria does.

People with calcium oxalate stones, including people with fat malabsorption, are advised to limit

their intakes of foods high in oxalate—spinach, rhubarb, beets, nuts, chocolate, tea, wheat bran, and strawberries.[3] Some clinicians report that for most people, only nuts (and peanut butter) need to be restricted.[4]

Most of the oxalate in the urine, however, comes from the body's synthesis of oxalate. One of the pathways of oxalate synthesis in the body begins with vitamin C. Consequently, megadoses of vitamin C can raise urinary oxalate concentrations. People at risk for oxalate stones are therefore advised to avoid vitamin C supplements.

Sodium-Restricted Diets In addition to calcium and oxalate, attention to salt intake may be important in preventing calcium oxalate stones. Studies suggest that excess salt increases urinary calcium excretion in all people, but causes a proportionately greater amount of calcium to be excreted in people with hypercalciuria.[5] Thus people who form calcium oxalate stones and who have hypercalciuria may benefit by moderately restricting salt. Further research is necessary to determine if such a restriction can prevent calcium stones from forming.[6]

People with calcium stones may be treated with thiazide diuretics, which effectively reduce the excretion of calcium and increase the excretion of fluids, thus reducing the likelihood of stone formation. A high salt intake can offset the beneficial effects of thiazide diuretics and can cause excessive potassium excretion. Thus people taking thiazide diuretics have an additional reason to lower their salt intake. Potassium-rich foods are recommended. Potassium supplements may also be prescribed.

Uric Acid Stones

Uric acid stones are frequently associated with gout, a metabolic disorder characterized by elevated levels of uric acid in the blood and urine. Uric acid stones form when the urine becomes persistently acid, contains excessive uric acid, or both. Purine-restricted diets are commonly prescribed to prevent uric acid stones. A purine-restricted diet limits red meats, particularly organ meats, anchovies, sardines, and meat extracts. The benefits of such a diet are unproven, but avoiding excessive protein may be useful; health care professionals recommend a diet limited to 100 grams of protein per day. Alcohol intake is also limited. Drug therapy (allopurinol) is often prescribed to inhibit uric acid production, reducing both uric acid levels and urinary acidity.

Cystine Stones

Cystine stones form when an inherited disorder of amino acid metabolism (cystinuria) causes an abnormally high urinary excretion of cystine. For cystine stones, health care professionals recommend a diet restricted in the amino acid methionine, because the body makes cystine from methionine. Drug therapy to reduce urinary acidity may also be beneficial.

Struvite Stones

Struvite stones, sometimes called "infection stones," form when the urinary tract becomes infected with a specific type of microorganism that hydrolyzes urea, creating an ammonia-rich, alkaline urine. (You may want to review the discussion of how the body disposes of excess nitrogen on p. 234.) Unlike most stones, struvite stones are about twice as prevalent in women as in men. Effective treatment includes removal of the stones and antimicrobial drugs.

Many people experience kidney stones during the course of their lives, and the incidence of kidney stones is increasing. Modifying dietary and other risk factors for kidney stones has the potential to save many people from the pain and possible complications of kidney stones.

NOTES

1. L. K. Massey, Dietary salt, urinary calcium, and kidney stone risk, *Nutrition Reviews* 53 (1995): 131–139.
2. F. L. Coe, J. H. Parks, and J. R. Asplin, The pathogenesis and treatment of kidney stones, *New England Journal of Medicine* 327 (1992): 1141–1152.
3. L. K. Massey, H. Roman-Smith, and R. A. L. Sutton, Effect of dietary oxalate and calcium on urinary oxalate and risk of formation of calcium oxalate kidney stones, *Journal of the American Dietetic Association* 93 (1993): 901–906.
4. C. L. Smith, M. Davis, and R. O. Berkseth, Dietary factors in calcium nephrolithiasis, *Journal of Renal Nutrition* 2 (1992): 146–153.
5. W. J. Burtis and coauthors, Dietary hypercalciuria in patients with calcium oxalate kidney stones, *American Journal of Clinical Nutrition* 60 (1994): 424–429.
6. Massey, 1995.

Chapter 30

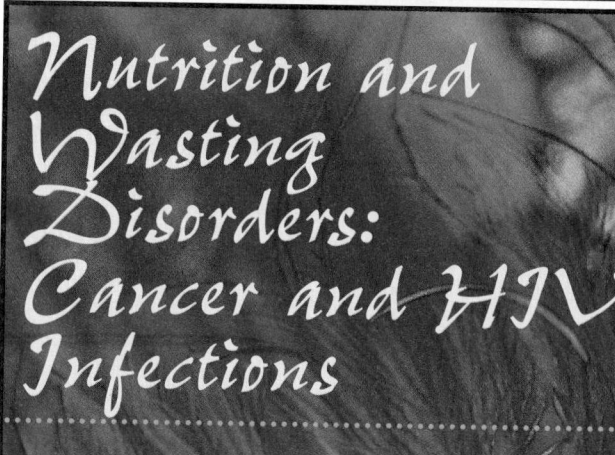

Nutrition and Wasting Disorders: Cancer and HIV Infections

CONTENTS

Cancer
How Cancer Develops
Dietary Guidelines to Reduce Cancer Risks
Nutrition Consequences of Cancer
Treatments for Cancer
Nutrition Support for People with Cancer
Human Immunodeficiency Virus (HIV) Infection and Acquired Immune Deficiency Syndrome (AIDS)
How AIDS Develops
Treatments for HIV Infection
The HIV Wasting Syndrome
Nutrition Support for People with HIV Infection
HIGHLIGHT: Cost-Conscious Health Care

MICROGRAPH: AZT, the drug that inhibits the replication of the human immunodeficiency virus.

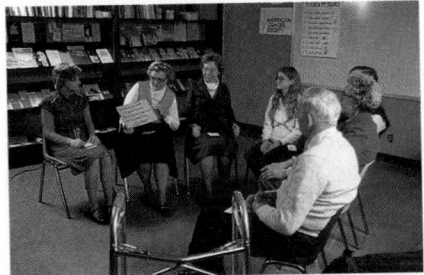

People with cancer take comfort from the support of others and from the knowledge that medical science is waging an unrelenting battle in their defense.

cancers: diseases that result from the unchecked growth of malignant tumors.

tumor: a new growth of tissue forming an abnormal mass with no function; also called a neoplasm (NEE-oh-plazm). Tumors that multiply out of control, threaten health, and require treatment are malignant (ma-LIG-nant). Tumors that stop growing without intervention or can be removed surgically and pose no threat to health are benign (bee-NINE).

  malignus = of bad kind

  benign = mild

Cancers are classified by the tissues or cells from which they develop:

- Adenomas (ADD-eh-NO-mahz) arise from glandular tissues.
- Carcinomas (KAR-see-NO-mahz) arise from epithelial tissues.
- Gliomas (gly-OH-mahz) arise from glial cells of the central nervous system.
- Leukemias (loo-KEY-mee-ahz) arise from the white blood cells.
- Lymphomas (lim-FOE-mahz) arise from lymph tissue.
- Melanomas (MEL-ah-NO-mahz) arise from pigmented skin cells.
- Sarcomas (sar-KO-mahz) arise from muscle, bone, or connective tissues.

A cancer that spreads from one part of the body to another is said to metastasize (me-TAS-tah-size).

revious chapters have shown that malnutrition accompanies and complicates many disorders. Acute stresses place substantial and immediate demands on nutrient stores, and chronic stresses such as liver diseases, renal diseases, and malabsorption syndromes drain nutrient stores over time. Both types of stress can lead to severe protein-energy malnutrition (PEM) and further tax health. This chapter describes the impact of cancer and human immunodeficiency virus (HIV) infection on nutrition status. Highlight 30 reviews issues of rising health care costs—a topic of great importance in the treatment of prolonged diseases like cancer and HIV infections that incur considerable costs.

From a nutrition standpoint, cancer and HIV infection present many similarities. Both affect many organ systems. Both involve symptoms that limit nutrient intake. Both are associated with wasting, and in both, the wasting is caused not only by the diseases themselves but also by their treatments. In both cases, malnutrition aggravates the symptoms, impairs the quality of life, and shortens life expectancy. A diagnosis of cancer or HIV infection alerts health care professionals to potential nutrition problems so that remedial steps can be taken to improve the quality of life and prevent early death.

Cancer

The thought of cancer often strikes fear in people. Indeed, cancer ranks just below cardiovascular disease as a cause of death, and thus many people have personal experiences with cancer. As with cardiovascular diseases, however, the prognosis for cancer today is far brighter than in the past. Identification of risk factors, new detection techniques, and innovative therapies offer hope and encouragement.

Cancer is not a single disorder. There are many *cancers*, that is, many different kinds of malignancies. They have different characteristics, occur in different locations in the body, take different courses, and require different treatments.

HOW CANCER DEVELOPS

The genes in a healthy body work together regulating cell division to ensure that each new cell is a replica of the parent cell. In this way, the healthy body grows, replacing dead cells and repairing damaged ones. Cancers develop from mutations in the genes that regulate cell division. The mutations silence the genes that ordinarily monitor replicating DNA for chemical errors. The affected cells seemingly have no built-in brakes to halt cell division. As the abnormal mass of cells, called a malignant *tumor* or *neoplasm*, grows, blood vessels form to supply the tumor with the nutrients it needs to support its growth. Eventually, the tumor invades healthy tissue and may spread. Clinicians describe cancers by their size and extent, specifically noting if the tumor has spread to surrounding lymph nodes or to distant sites in the body. Figure 30–1 illustrates tumor formation.

Genetic Factors Some cancers appear to have a genetic component. A person with a family history of breast cancer, for example, has a greater risk of developing breast cancer than a person without such a genetic predisposition. This does not mean, however, that the person *will* develop cancer, only that the risk is greater.

Figure 30–1

Tumor Formation

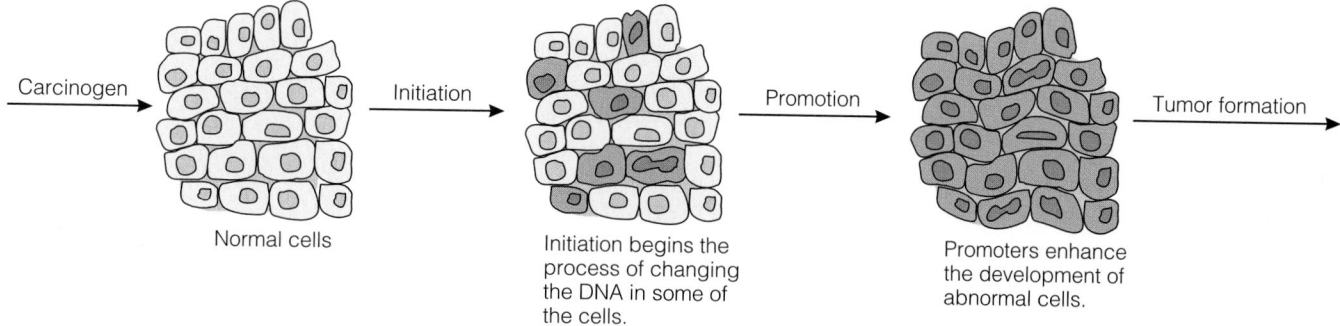

Carcinogen →

Normal cells

Initiation →

Initiation begins the process of changing the DNA in some of the cells.

Promotion →

Promoters enhance the development of abnormal cells.

Tumor formation →

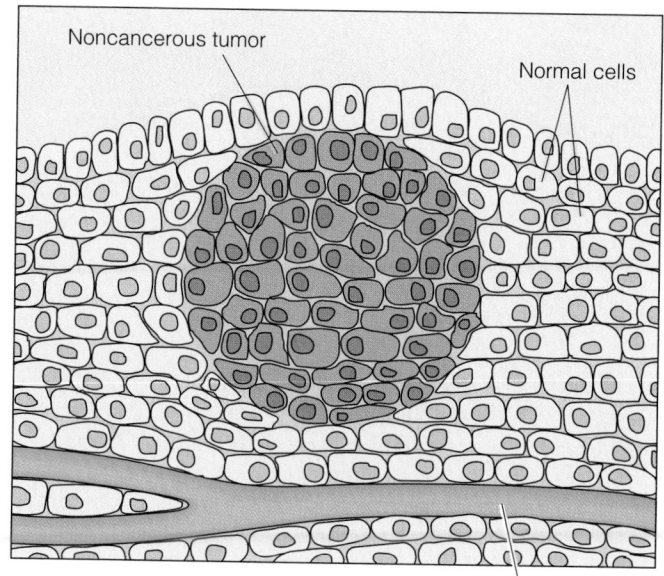

Noncancerous tumor

Normal cells

Blood vessel

A noncancerous (benign) tumor usually grows within a self-contained capsule. It does not invade nearby tissue, nor does it spread.

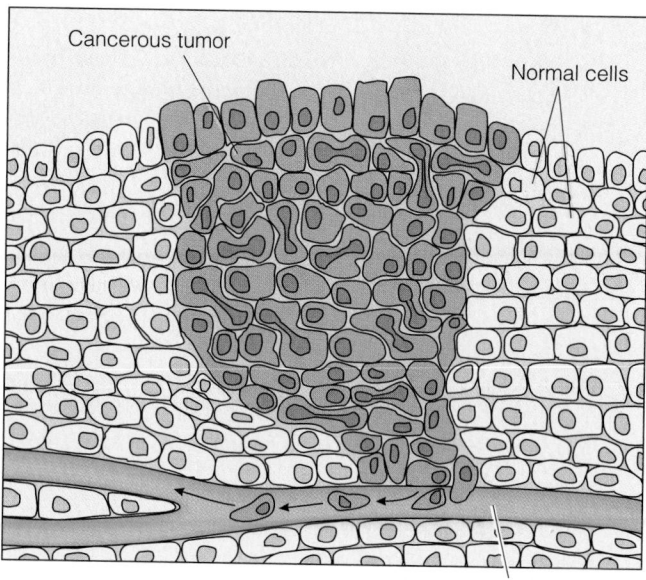

Cancerous tumor

Normal cells

Blood vessel

A cancerous (malignant) tumor usually grows out of control and may spread to other parts of the body through the blood or lymph systems.

Immune Factors   A healthy immune system recognizes foreign cells and destroys them. Researchers theorize that an ineffective immune system may interfere with the recognition of tumor cells as foreign, thus allowing tumor growth. Aging affects immune function, and the incidence of cancer increases with age. Medications that suppress the immune system and viral infections (including HIV infection) and other disorders that severely tax the immune system may increase the risk of cancer.

Environmental Factors   Among environmental factors exposure to radiation and sun, water and air pollution, and smoking are known to cause cancer. As Table 30–1 shows, dietary constituents are also associated with an increased

Table 30–1

Factors Associated with Cancer at Specific Sites

Cancer Sites	High Incidence Associated with:	Protective Effect Associated with:
Esophageal cancer	High alcohol use, tobacco use, and especially combined use; use of preserved foods (such as pickles); low intakes of vitamins and minerals; high intakes of vitamin A supplements	
Stomach cancer	High intakes of salt-preserved foods (such as dried, salted fish); low intakes of fresh fruits and vegetables	Fresh fruit and vegetables
Colorectal cancer	High intakes of fat (particularly saturated fat), meat, and alcohol (especially beer); low intakes of fiber, folate, and vegetables; inactivity	High intake of vegetables
Liver cancer	Infection with hepatitis B or aflatoxins; high intakes of alcohol; iron overload	
Pancreatic and lung cancer	No dietary risk factors have been established; correlated primarily with cigarette smoking	Fruits and vegetables, especially green and yellow ones
Breast cancer	High intakes of food energy and alcohol; little or no association with dietary fat specifically	Fruits and vegetables, especially green and yellow ones
Ovarian cancer	No dietary risk factors have been established; inversely correlated with oral contraceptive use	Fruits and vegetables, especially green and yellow ones
Cervical cancer	Folate deficiency	
Endometrial cancer	No dietary risk factors have been established; associated with estrogen therapy, obesity, hypertension, and diabetes (NIDDM)	
Bladder cancer	*Possible* associations with coffee, artificial sweeteners, and alcohol; associated with cigarette smoking	Fruits and vegetables, especially green and yellow ones
Prostate cancer	High fat intake, especially saturated fats from meats	Fruits and vegetables, especially green and yellow ones

Note: Findings based on epidemiological studies.
Sources: Committee on Diet and Health, *Diet and Health: Implications for Reducing Chronic Disease Risk* (Washington, D.C.: National Academy Press, 1989), pp. 594–600; J. H. Weisburger, Nutritional approach to cancer prevention with emphasis on vitamins, antioxidants, and carotenoids, *American Journal of Clinical Nutrition* (supplement) 53 (1991): 226–237; R. G. Ziegler, Vegetables, fruits, and carotenoids and the risk of cancer, *American Journal of Clinical Nutrition* (supplement) 53 (1991): 251–259; Potential mechanisms for food-related carcinogens and anticarcinogens: A scientific status summary by the Institute of Food Technologists' Expert Panel on Food Safety and Nutrition, *Food Technology* 47 (1993): 105–118.

Factors such as radiation and carcinogens (car-SIN-oh-jenz) which cause mutations that give rise to cancer are called initiators.

Factors that favor the development of cancer once it has begun are called promoters.

Factors that oppose the development of cancer are called antipromoters.

risk of certain cancers. Some dietary factors may initiate cancer development, others may promote cancer development once it has started, and still others may protect against the development of cancer.

Dietary Factors—Cancer Initiators   We do not know to what extent diet contributes to cancer development, although some experts estimate that diet may be responsible for a third or more of all cases. Many people think that certain foods are carcinogenic, especially those that contain additives or pesticides. As Chapter 14 explained, however, our food supply is one of the safest in the world. Additives that have been approved for use in foods are not carcinogenic. Some pesticides are carcinogenic at high doses, but not at the concentrations allowed on fruits and vegetables.[1]

The incidence of cancers, especially stomach cancers, is high in parts of the world where people eat a lot of heavily smoked, pickled, or salt-cured foods that produce carcinogenic nitrosamines. Most commercial manufacturers in the United States use different preservative methods, and all are carefully controlled to minimize carcinogenic contamination.

Alcohol has also been associated with a high incidence of some cancers, especially of the mouth and throat. Beverages such as beer and scotch may contain damaging nitrosamines as well as alcohol.[2] The amounts of these compounds found in alcoholic beverages currently on the market are not considered harmful—assuming consumption in moderate amounts. These findings illustrate clearly why any potential benefit of moderate alcohol consumption on cardiovascular disease (see Highlight 28) must be weighed against potential dangers.

Dietary Factors—Cancer Promoters   Unlike carcinogens, which initiate cancers, some dietary components may accelerate cancers that have already begun to develop. Studies suggest that certain dietary fats eaten in excess may promote cancer, in part by contributing to obesity. More specifically, linoleic acid, the omega-6 fatty acid of vegetable oils, has been implicated in enhancing cancer development in rats.[3] (In contrast, omega-3 fatty acids from fish oils appear to delay cancer development.)

Dietary Factors—Antipromoters   It seems apparent that, besides promoters, foods may contain antipromoters. Almost without exception, epidemiological studies find a link between eating plenty of fruits and vegetables and a low incidence of cancers.[4] The fiber in fruits and vegetables helps to protect against some cancers by speeding up the transit time of all materials through the colon so that the colon walls are not exposed to cancer-causing substances for long. In addition to fiber, fruits and vegetables contain both nutrients and nonnutrients that protect against cancer. By acting as scavengers of oxygen-derived free radicals, the antioxidant nutrients beta-carotene, vitamin C, and vitamin E may help to prevent cell and tissue damage that can give rise to cancer. Phytochemicals common to many vegetables, especially those of the cabbage family, can activate enzymes that are capable of destroying carcinogens. (Highlight 11 describes the cancer preventive properties of antioxidants and phytochemicals in more detail.)

DIETARY GUIDELINES TO REDUCE CANCER RISKS

On the basis of current knowledge and available evidence, the following dietary guidelines are recommended for cancer prevention:

- Control weight and prevent obesity.
- Reduce consumption of total fat to 30 percent or less of total food energy.
- Increase fiber intake to 20 to 30 grams per day.
- Include a variety of vegetables and fruits in the daily diet.
- Minimize consumption of salt-cured, salt-pickled, and smoked foods.
- Consume alcoholic beverages in moderation, if at all.

One additional recommendation is in order: *vary food choices*. This last suggestion is based on an important concept—dilution. Switching from food to food dilutes the negative qualities of a food. For example, it is safe to eat *some* salt-cured or smoked meats, but not all the time. Combine such foods with a variety of others so that any carcinogens that may be present will be diluted in the total diet.

Some dietary factors, such as alcohol and heavily smoked or salted foods, may initiate cancer development; others, such as dietary fat, may promote cancer once it has gotten started; and still others, such as fiber and antioxidant nutrients and nonnutrients, may serve as antipromoters that protect against the development of cancer. Eating many green, yellow, and orange vegetables, including high-fiber foods, and reducing fat intake offer the best possible nutrition at the lowest possible risk.

NUTRITION CONSEQUENCES OF CANCER

Once cancer has developed, its consequences depend on its severity, location, and treatment. An isolated, nonspreading type of skin cancer may be removed in a physician's office with no observable effect on nutrition status, but a pancreatic cancer may seriously impair the person's ability to digest and absorb nutrients. Similarly, cancers of the gastrointestinal tract can severely affect nutrition status. The following sections describe the kinds of nutrition problems that often occur in certain types of cancers.

Cancer Cachexia   Just as cardiac cachexia describes the PEM associated with heart failure, cancer cachexia describes the PEM associated with cancer. Loss of appetite, weight loss, and depletion of lean body mass and serum proteins typify the cancer cachexia syndrome, which affects about two-thirds of people with cancer. It is often evident at the time of diagnosis. The combination of poor appetite, accelerated and abnormal metabolism, and the diversion of nutrients to support tumor growth simultaneously reduces the supply of energy and nutrients and increases the demand for them.

People who develop cachexia swiftly fall into a downward spiral. Poor food intake paired with heightened nutrient demands leads to muscle wasting and general poor health, which diminishes intake further. The body is unable to respond to this reduced nutrient supply as it does during uncomplicated fasting, so it continues to deplete its nutrient stores at an accelerated rate. The resulting malnutrition compromises the quality of life and may lead to complications and early death. Figure 30–2 summarizes some of the many known causes of the cancer cachexia syndrome.

Mechanisms of Cachexia   Altered metabolism begins early in tumor development, even before weight loss occurs. Cachexia appears to be tumor derived; that is, the tumor itself causes the changes that lead to cachexia, and removal of the tumor can reverse the cachexia. Cytokines, secreted by the host's immune system in response to tumors, appear to be important mediators of the cancer cachexia syndrome.[5] They induce anorexia and alter metabolism. Current research into the roles of various cytokines and possible ways to block their actions holds promise for treating cachexia.

cancer cachexia (ka-KEKS-ee-ah) syndrome: a syndrome that frequently accompanies many types of cancer; characterized by anorexia, inadequate intake of food, malnutrition, accelerated metabolism and wasting, and general ill health.

Reminder: *Cytokines* are proteins secreted as part of the immune response (see Chapter 25). Some of the cytokines identified as mediators of cancer cachexia include tumor necrosis factor (cachectin), interleukin-1 alpha and beta, interleukin-6, interferon-τ, and differentiation factor.

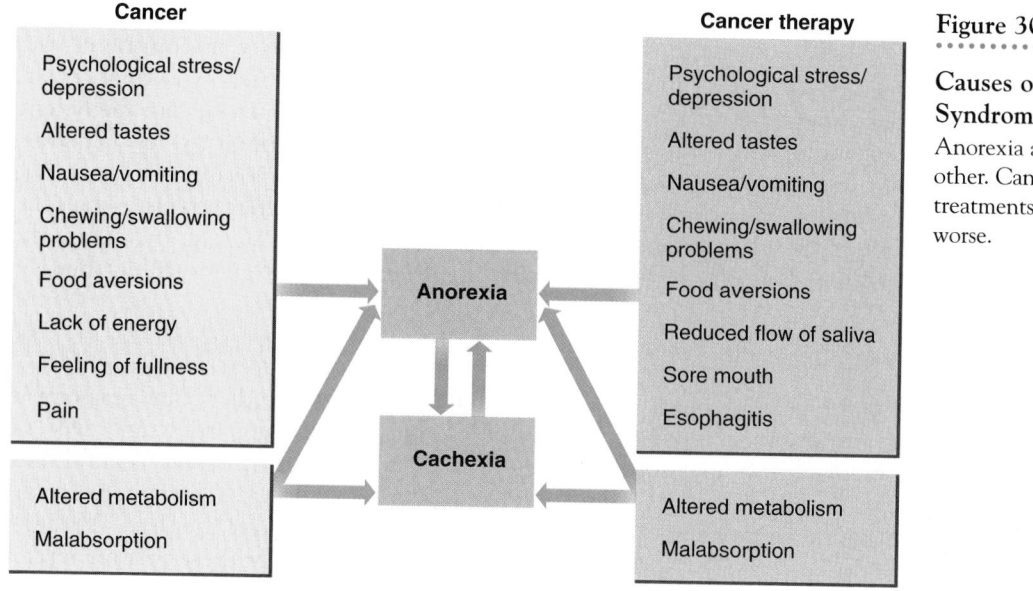

Figure 30–2

Causes of the Cancer Cachexia Syndrome
Anorexia and cachexia contribute to each other. Cancer itself and the available treatments for it make both problems worse.

Anorexia and Inadequate Nutrient Intake   Anorexia is widely recognized as the major precipitating event in cancer cachexia. Factors contributing to anorexia in the person with cancer include:

- *Early satiety and nausea.* A premature feeling of fullness after eating small amounts of food or nausea may interfere with the appetite.

- *Fatigue.* People with cancer often tire easily and lack energy to prepare meals and eat.

- *Pain.* People in pain may have little interest in food, particularly if eating aggravates the pain.

- *Psychological stress.* The very diagnosis of cancer as well as its treatment can cause so much anxiety that eating becomes unimportant.

- *Obstructions.* A tumor may partially or completely obstruct any portion of the GI tract and interfere with chewing and swallowing; cause delayed gastric emptying, nausea, or vomiting; or make oral diets impossible.

Nutrient Losses   Excessive nutrient losses in the person with cancer can contribute to deteriorating nutrition status. Depending on the location and type of cancer as well as its treatments, the person may experience nutrient losses due to inadequate digestion, malabsorption, vomiting, and diarrhea.

Maldigestion and malabsorption frequently accompany cancer of the pancreas (which depletes digestive enzymes) or liver (which depletes bile salts). Tumors of the small intestine can cause malabsorption, as does a tumor that obstructs the upper small intestine, creating a blind loop (see Chapter 22). Some tumors directly cause severe vomiting, diarrhea, or both, and electrolyte imbalances and dehydration may result. (Later sections describe the nutrient losses associated with various cancer treatments.)

Cancer-induced causes of nutrient losses include:
- Inadequate digestion.
- Malabsorption.
- Vomiting.
- Diarrhea.

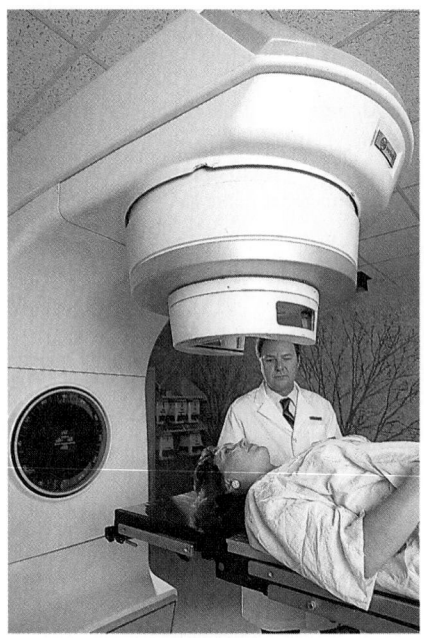

Radiation therapy is one of several weapons in the fight against cancer.

Metabolic Alterations   Some people with cancer are hypermetabolic while others are not. In all cases, metabolic pathways are altered and nutrients used inefficiently. In comparison to the metabolic pathways used by normal cells to derive most of their energy, the pathways used by tumor cells are inefficient, demanding extra energy nutrients and wasting vital protein tissues. Fat stores are also mobilized. Many people with cancer develop insulin resistance and hyperglycemia, which interferes with the availability of energy fuels to the cells. In addition, cancer and its treatments tax the immune system, increasing the likelihood of infections, which raise energy and nutrient needs still further.

TREATMENTS FOR CANCER

Unlike diabetes, heart disease, and renal failure, in which diet plays a major role in treatment, nutrition therapy in cancer is only supportive and will be described in a later section. The primary cancer treatments aim to annihilate cancer cells, relieve pain, and prevent further tumor growth. They include radiation therapy, chemotherapy, surgery, or any combination of the three. Through their use, cancer can sometimes be arrested, but ironically, these treatments can also threaten health and nutrition status. Table 30–2 summarizes the nutrition-related side effects of radiation and chemotherapy, and Table 30–3 shows how various cancer surgeries can affect nutrition status.

Table 30–2

Possible Causes of Wasting Associated with Radiation and Chemotherapy

	Reduced Nutrient Intake	**Accelerated Nutrient Losses**	**Altered Metabolism**
Radiation	Anorexia	Chronic blood loss from intestine and bladder	Secondary effects of malnutrition or infection
	Damage to teeth and jaws	Diarrhea	
	Esophagitis	Fistula formation	
	Mouth ulcers	Intestinal obstructions	
	Nausea	Malabsorption	
	Reduced salivary secretions	Vomiting	
	Taste alterations		
	Thick salivary secretions		
	Vomiting		
Chemotherapy	Abdominal pain	Diarrhea	Fluid and electrolyte imbalances
	Anorexia	Intestinal ulcers	Hyperglycemia
	Mouth ulcers	Malabsorption	Interference with vitamins or other metabolites
	Nausea	Vomiting	Negative nitrogen and calcium balance
	Taste alterations		Secondary effects of malnutrition or infection
	Vomiting		

Table 30–3
. . . .

Possible Effects of Surgery for Cancer on Nutrition Status

Head and Neck Resection	
Difficulty in chewing/swallowing	Inability to chew/swallow
Esophageal Resection	
Diarrhea	Reduced gastric motility
Fistula formation	Steatorrhea (fat malabsorption)
Reduced gastric acid secretion	Stenosis (constriction)
Gastric Resection	
Dumping syndrome	Lack of gastric acid
General malabsorption	Vitamin B_{12} malabsorption
Hypoglycemia	
Intestinal Resection	
Blind loop syndrome	General malabsorption
Diarrhea	Hyperoxaluria
Fluid and electrolyte imbalance	Steatorrhea
Pancreatic Resection	
Diabetes mellitus	General malabsorption

Radiation Therapy   Radiation therapy disrupts DNA replication and, consequently, cell division. In doing so, radiation damages all actively dividing cells—normal body cells as well as tumor cells. Treatment is often effective because cancer cells divide more rapidly than normal cells, they are damaged more severely by radiation, and they are slower to recover from its effects. Therapists must carefully administer radiation treatments in doses that target tumor cells and minimize damage to normal cells.

Radiation therapy can cause fatigue, anorexia, nausea, vomiting, and diarrhea. Radiation may inflame tissues in the mouth and esophagus, lead to the development of mouth ulcers, interfere with the flow of saliva, and damage teeth and the bones of the jaws—all of which can make chewing and swallowing painful and difficult. The person may develop food aversions if certain foods are associated with the radiation therapy. Radiation therapy to the small intestine can alter the structure of the intestinal cells (radiation enteritis) and result in malabsorption, chronic blood loss, and fluid and electrolyte imbalances. The intestinal wall may become thick and fibrotic, narrowing the intestinal lumen and increasing the likelihood that an intestinal obstruction or a fistula will develop. Small blood vessels may become so inflamed that blood flow to some sections of the bowel may be blocked. Any of these events can be fatal. Intestinal function may return after radiation therapy ends, but for some, the changes are permanent.

Chemotherapy   Medications can also be used to interrupt cell division, but like radiation, they have undesirable side effects. Chemotherapeutic agents

radiation therapy: the use of radiation to arrest or destroy cancer cells.

The cells of the GI tract, bone marrow, hair, and skin are actively dividing and are often affected by cancer treatments.

radiation enteritis: radiation damage to intestine.

chemotherapy: the use of drugs to arrest or destroy cancer cells. Drugs used for chemotherapy are called **chemotherapeutic** or **antineoplastic agents.**
    chemo = chemical

include some antibiotics, alkaloids, alkylating agents, antimetabolites, steroids, and others. The current trend in chemotherapy is to use high doses of several chemotherapeutic agents together in cycles. This method helps ensure that malignant cells will be destroyed. Although these treatments are often effective, they frequently intensity undesirable side effects.

Chemotherapy can dramatically reduce food intake by causing nausea, vomiting, altered taste perceptions, mouth ulcers, reduced flow of saliva, and food aversions. Additionally, chemotherapy may cause diarrhea, malabsorption, and peptic ulcers that aggravate nutrient losses. Chemotherapy using vitamin antagonists interferes with normal metabolic pathways, further compromising nutrition status.

Other Drug Therapy   Depending on which organ systems are affected by cancer and by the side effects of treatment, many other medications may also be used in treatment. Medications commonly used to treat symptoms of cancers include antinausea agents, antidiarrheals, analgesics, and sedatives.

Several medications may be useful in the treatment of wasting.[6] The most promising medication, megestrol acetate, stimulates the appetite and promotes weight gain (primarily as body fat). Preliminary studies suggest that growth hormone and insulin-like growth factor can promote weight gain, particularly a gain in lean body mass. Dronabinol (a medication containing the principal psychoactive ingredient in marijuana) works as both an appetite stimulant and an antiemetic and may be useful in some cases.

Surgery   Often surgery is necessary to remove the tumor. The side effects of surgery depend on the location of the tumor and its size (see Table 30–3). Surgery is often followed by radiation or chemotherapy to prevent new tumor growth.

Surgery can also cause anorexia, nausea, and vomiting. Some surgeries, such as a partial or total removal of the tongue, resection of the muscles of the mouth, esophagus, or salivary glands, and removal of the jaw, invariably create extensive problems with chewing and swallowing. Surgeries may also aggravate nutrient losses through diarrhea, malabsorption, and blood loss. Surgery also accelerates metabolism because it initiates the stress response.

Bone Marrow Transplants   The use of bone marrow transplants to treat certain cancers and blood disorders has grown markedly.[7] During a bone marrow transplant, the individual's diseased bone marrow is replaced with healthy bone marrow from a donor, usually a close relative. Before the bone marrow transplant is performed, the recipient is treated with high doses of chemotherapy and sometimes whole-body radiation therapy. In addition, immunosuppressants are given before and after the procedure. Although these procedures effectively kill abnormal cells and help prevent tissue rejection, they also render the individual defenseless against infections. Antibiotics are frequently prescribed.

Graft-versus-host disease (GVHD), a serious complication of bone marrow transplants, develops when the recipient's body mounts an immune system attack against healthy donor cells, which it recognizes as foreign. Most often, the skin, liver, and GI tract are affected. Acute GVHD develops within a few months of transplantation; chronic GVHD may develop later.

The preparatory procedures for a bone marrow transplant frequently result in anorexia, taste alterations, nausea, vomiting, and inflammation of mucous mem-

PRESCRIPTION PAD

Drugs used in the treatment of cancer may include:

- Analgesics
- Antidiarrheals
- Anti-inflammatory agents
- Antinauseants
- Antineoplastics
- Appetite stimulants
- Sedatives

See Appendix E for timing with meals and nutrition-related side effects.

bone marrow transplant: the replacement of diseased bone marrow in a recipient with healthy bone marrow from a donor; used as a treatment for breast cancer, leukemia, and other blood disorders.

Bone marrow transplants may be a treatment for leukemia, lymphomas, and certain blood disorders.

graft-versus-host disease (GVHD): destruction of healthy donor cells by the recipient's immune system, which recognizes the donor cells as foreign.

branes of the GI tract. Following transplantation, severe diarrhea and malabsorption, with fluid losses often exceeding 10 liters per day, signal acute GVHD.[8] Immunosuppressive drugs used to help treat or prevent GVHD can lead to negative nitrogen and calcium balances, sodium and fluid retention, muscular weakness, osteoporosis, and glucose intolerance.

Other Treatments   Researchers continue to search for more effective ways of treating people with cancer. One such treatment, immunotherapy, provides antigens to bolster the immune system so that it can recognize and attack cancer cells. Another treatment being investigated uses highly specific antibodies to deliver chemotherapy directly to the cancer site, thus leaving healthy cells unaffected. The overall effectiveness of these therapies remains undetermined at present.

Alternative Therapies   People who feel they are making little progress in their fight against cancer or think conventional medicine offers little hope of recovery may try alternative therapies. (Highlight 20 provides a perspective on alternative therapy.) Fortunately, most people with cancer rely on traditional medical treatments, although they may supplement them with alternative therapies.[9]

Health care professionals should be alert to alternative therapies that include nutrition components. Potentially harmful practices include:

- Discontinuing prescribed therapy to adhere to an unproven remedy.
- Following a diet that eliminates or severely restricts specific food groups.
- Taking vitamins or minerals that can be toxic in large doses.
- Using herbal preparations that may be contaminated.

Cancer and its treatments lead to cachexia—a combination of anorexia, accelerated nutrient losses, and altered metabolism. In fact, many people with cancer die from cachexia rather than the cancer itself.[10] Providing optimal nutrition care supports recovery and improves quality of life.

NUTRITION SUPPORT FOR PEOPLE WITH CANCER

Prior to the widespread use of tube feedings and TPN, the deteriorating nutrition status that accompanies cancer was largely accepted. Without a way to feed people who simply could not eat, many practitioners believed that emaciation and physical debilitation were inevitable. Others believed that if you fed the client, you also fed the tumor, so to "starve the tumor," they would almost starve the client.

The Scope of Nutrition Support for Cancer   Nutrition cannot cure cancer, nor is it a primary treatment. Whether nutrition support directly prolongs survival or improves tolerance for chemotherapy or radiation therapy has not been proven.[11] The wide variety of cancers and their various stages of development make proving a beneficial effect difficult. In some malnourished people with cancer, nutrition support has proven to be beneficial.[12] Attention to diet can help prevent or reverse poor nutrition status and its associated complications, and in this way, nutrition plays a supportive role in cancer therapy. Compared with the malnourished person, the person in good nutrition status:

- Feels better.
- Functions better.
- Is more active.
- Is stronger.
- Eats more.
- Resists infections better.
- Enjoys a better quality of life.

Although it is sometimes hard to quantify these benefits, they are of great importance to the person with cancer.[13]

Dietary Interventions   Considering the many adverse effects that threaten the appetite of a person with cancer, health care professionals face an enormous challenge in helping these individuals maintain nutrition status. Every bit of nutrition knowledge and interpersonal skill helps, beginning with the professional's awareness of the client's predicament. Oral food intake can often be improved once the individual's specific problems are addressed. The box on pp. 946–947 is long and detailed, reflecting both the complexity and the importance of offering specific suggestions to deal with specific problems.

Energy and Protein Needs   Actual nutrient needs vary depending on the type and severity of the cancer, its treatment, and the person's nutrition status. Table 30–4 shows diet modifications that may be necessary for different types of cancer. Often clinicians aim to provide about 1.5 times the basal energy expenditure and 1.5 to 2.0 grams of protein per kilogram of body weight per day.

Women diagnosed with breast cancer often gain, rather than lose, weight, and this weight gain can be distressing.[14] Health care professionals serve these clients best by helping them avoid unnecessary weight gain.

To review calculations of basal energy expenditure, see Table 25–3 on p. 809.

Vitamins and Minerals   Vitamin and mineral needs are highly variable depending on the specific treatment and the presence and severity of complications such as vomiting and malabsorption. The individual must be carefully monitored for early signs of nutrient deficiencies to prevent the development of serious deficiencies.

Tube Feedings and TPN   Because studies have failed to confirm that aggressive nutrition support directly benefits survival and response to cancer treatment, tube feedings or TPN are not routinely recommended for adequately nourished or mildly malnourished people with cancer who must undergo surgery, chemotherapy, or radiation therapy.[15] Special nutrition support may be indicated, however, when anorexia persists or when a person is severely malnourished, particularly during and immediately after other cancer treatments. As is true whenever special nutrition support is indicated, tube feedings are preferred to TPN when the GI tract is functional. People requiring head and neck resections may need long-term tube feedings and may need to continue tube feedings at home. People with severe radiation enteritis may require home TPN.

Table 30–4

Dietary Considerations for Various Cancers

Cancer Sites	Dietary Considerations
Brain	Physical feeding disabilities (see Highlight 21); chewing and swallowing problems see (Chapter 21).
Head/neck	Chewing and swallowing problems.
Mouth/esophagus	Chewing and swallowing problems; if obstructed, tube feeding below the obstruction may be necessary.
Stomach	Nausea, vomiting; if obstructed, tube feeding below the obstruction or TPN may be necessary; if resection is performed, a postgastrectomy diet (see Chapter 21) may be needed; nutrient deficiencies due to bacterial overgrowth (Chapter 22) may occur.
Intestine	If obstructed, tube feeding or TPN may be necessary; resections or inflammation may cause multiple nutrition problems (see Chapter 22); fat- and lactose-restricted diet may be useful.
Liver	Protein-, sodium-, and fluid-restricted diet may be necessary (see Chapter 26).
Pancreas	Fat-restricted diet and enzyme replacements may be necessary (see Chapter 22); diabetic diet may be necessary if insulin production is affected (see Chapter 27).
Kidneys	Protein-, electrolyte-, and fluid-controlled diet may be necessary (see Chapter 29).

Note: The considerations listed here are specific to the type of cancer; they do not include other nutrition-related concerns, such as anorexia, nausea, and vomiting.

Ethical Issues   Every malnourished person with cancer who cannot consume an adequate diet orally is a potential candidate for aggressive nutrition support. Before tube feeding or parenteral nutrition is undertaken, some important questions should be considered. What is the prognosis if the cachexia can be reversed and progressive wasting can be arrested? Will the person survive longer? Will the quality of life improve? Will therapy be more successful? Does the client want aggressive nutrition support? Special nutrition support should be undertaken only if it can provide direct benefits and the client is in agreement. For the person with little hope of recovery, the as yet unproven benefits of specialized nutrition support may not be worth the cost and discomfort involved. Making this decision requires good clinical judgment from the health care team as well as consideration of the client's feelings about the goals of nutrition therapy. (Highlight 24 describes these and other ethical issues that must be considered when people receive tube feedings or TPN.)

Nutrition Support before Bone Marrow Transplants   Because the GI tract is severely compromised by the preparatory procedure for a bone marrow transplant, TPN is routinely provided. Although not extensively studied, tube

How to Help Clients Handle Food-Related Problems

For each problem, find a solution using these suggestions.

1. *To improve nutrient intake:*

   - Explain why eating is important.
   - Encourage clients to eat the most when they feel the best.
   - Encourage people to eat extra food between chemotherapy or radiation treatments.
   - Suggest that clients eat nutrient-dense foods first.
   - Recommend indulging in favorite foods throughout the day.
   - Encourage clients to eat with family and friends.
   - Recommend smaller, more frequent meals.
   - Advise clients to avoid drinking large amounts of liquids with meals.
   - Work out a medication schedule that allows the client to take pain or antinausea medications at times when they will be effective during meals.
   - Provide a pleasant and relaxed environment.
   - Serve foods attractively.
   - Reassess clients regularly to solve problems as they arise.

2. *To save energy for eating:*

   - Recommend that others prepare foods.
   - Suggest foods that are easy to prepare and eat.
   - Encourage the use of time-saving appliances for food preparation.

3. *To combat bitter or metallic taste perceptions:*

   - Advise clients to brush their teeth or use a mouthwash before eating.
   - Recommend adding sauces and seasonings to meats.
   - Suggest that meats be served cold or at room temperature.
   - Encourage clients to try using eggs, fish, poultry, and dairy products instead of meats.
   - Encourage clients to try new foods and experiment with herbs and spices.

4. *To control nausea and vomiting:*

   - Give antinausea drugs at times when they will be effective during meals.
   - Recommend small, frequent meals.
   - Advise clients to avoid spicy and high-fat foods.
   - Suggest that clients avoid food odors that cause nausea. It may help to have others prepare meals, if possible.
   - Encourage clients to save most liquids for after meals. Clear liquids or popsicles after meals help prevent dehydration.
   - Suggest that clients get fresh air, loosen tight clothing, or rest after meals.

5. *To prevent food aversions:*
   - Suggest that clients save favorite foods for time when they are feeling relatively good.
   - Advise clients not to eat their favorite foods during the times of day when they usually experience nausea or vomiting.
   - Suggest that clients maintain a food-free "window" of an hour or so before and after treatment times, if the treatments cause nausea or vomiting.

6. *To alleviate problems with chewing and swallowing:*
   - Work with clients to find the consistency of food that will be easiest to handle. Thin liquids, true solids, and sticky foods are often difficult to swallow.
   - Recommend that clients add sauces and gravies to dry foods.
   - Provide fluids with meals to ease chewing and swallowing.
   - Advise clients with mouth sores to try foods at cooler temperatures. They are often soothing.
   - Recommend that clients with mouth ulcers avoid foods that are spicy, acidic, or coarse; foods that contain seeds that can be trapped in an ulcer; or sticky foods such as peanut butter that may be difficult to swallow.
   - Recommend that clients experiment with tilting the head forward and backward to see if swallowing is easier with the head positioned differently.
   - Suggest a straw for drinking.
   - Encourage clients who suffer from a reduced flow of saliva to rinse the mouth frequently. Artificial saliva from the pharmacy can also help. Sour candy or gum can stimulate the flow of saliva.
   - Encourage good oral and dental hygiene to prevent cavities and oral infections.

7. *To add kcalories and protein:*
   - Add milk powder to liquid milk, meat loafs, casseroles, soups, puddings, and cereals.
   - Add ground meats, chicken, fish, or grated cheeses to sauces, soups, casseroles, or vegetables.
   - Eat peanut butter on fruit, celery, or crackers.
   - Use plenty of butter, margarine, mayonnaise, cream cheese, oil, and salad dressings on breads, sandwiches, potatoes, vegetables, salads, pasta, and rice.
   - Use yogurt, sour cream, or a sour cream dip with vegetables.
   - Add whipping cream to deserts and hot chocolate, or use it to lighten coffee.
   - Have snacks available at all times.
   - Add nuts and dried fruits such as raisins to desserts, cereals, or salads.
   - Use cream instead of milk with cereal.
   - Try commercially available liquid supplements or instant breakfast mixes for milk shakes, meals, or between-meal snacks.
   - Use whole milk instead of low-fat or nonfat milks.

feedings have also proven effective in providing nutrition support for bone marrow transplant recipients.[16] Appropriate nutrition support helps to heal the GI tract and support the immune system. Glutamine added to the TPN solution may be particularly beneficial for people undergoing bone marrow transplants (see Highlight 22). Researchers have found that adding glutamine to TPN solutions results in fewer infections and shorter hospital stays for bone marrow transplant recipients.[17]

Nutrition Support after Bone Marrow Transplants   After a bone marrow transplant, the person usually continues TPN until GI function returns. As the person begins to receive food orally, parenteral nutrition is gradually tapered off (see Chapter 24). The nutrition-related side effects of the bone marrow transplant procedure make oral intake difficult, and the individual needs encouragement from all members of the health care team. Early oral feedings often start with lactose-free, low-residue, low-fat liquids to maximize absorption and minimize nausea, vomiting, and steatorrhea. Gradually, solid foods are introduced. For about three months after a transplant, the diet excludes most fresh fruits and vegetables, undercooked meats, poultry and eggs, and ground meats to minimize the risk of food-borne bacterial infections. Fiber and lactose are gradually added to the diet as individual tolerances allow. Additional fat is given if steatorrhea is not evident.

After a bone marrow transplant, nutrition complications can be severe and debilitating, especially for people with gastrointestinal GVHD. Because the bone marrow recipient must take immunosuppressants following the procedure, recommendations include a high-protein, high-calcium diet. In addition, physicians often prescribe calcium and vitamin D supplements. Individuals with persistent diarrhea are encouraged to eat high-potassium foods (see Figure 12–7 on p. 425). The accompanying box provides a case study for cancer.

Human Immunodeficiency Virus (HIV) Infection and Acquired Immune Deficiency Syndrome (AIDS)

For many years, the devastating effects of infection by the human immunodeficiency virus (HIV), the infection that eventually causes acquired immune deficiency syndrome (AIDS), seemed unstoppable. And although the disease still has no cure, remarkable progress has been made in understanding and treating HIV infections, giving rise to a renewed hope that a cure may be possible. Without a cure, however, the best course is prevention. Transmission of the virus requires sexual activity, direct blood contact, or passage of the infection from a mother to her infant during pregnancy, birth, or breastfeeding. Table 30–5 on p. 950 presents strategies for preventing HIV transmission.

Once a person has been infected with HIV, it takes about 6 to 12 weeks before laboratory tests can confirm a diagnosis. Because people remain symptom-free in the early stages of infection, however, they may not even be tested for HIV for several years following infection. Thus early detection to prevent the spread of HIV infection and to ensure early treatment for the person infected is an important health goal.

human immunodeficiency virus (HIV): the virus that causes AIDS. The infection progresses to become an immune system disorder that leaves its victims defenseless against numerous infections.

acquired immune deficiency syndrome (AIDS): the end stage of HIV infection, in which severe complications are manifested.

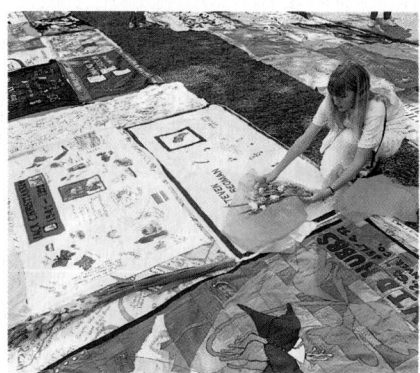

The countless lives touched by AIDS serve as a potent reminder of the need to continue the search for a cure.

Case Study   Retired Newscaster with Cancer

Mr. Bustamante is a retired newscaster who first visited his doctor when he noticed that he was losing weight rapidly and was easily fatigued. He also had a lesion in his mouth that wouldn't heal. Mr. Bustamante smokes a pack of cigarettes a day and has a history of alcohol abuse. After he was admitted to the hospital, tests confirmed a diagnosis of cancer of the mouth. The doctor would like to prepare Mr. Bustamante nutritionally before proceeding with radiation therapy. Radical surgery is a possibility. A thorough nutrition assessment reveals that Mr. Bustamante is suffering from severe mixed PEM. His height is 5 feet 10 inches, and he weighs 125 pounds.

What is Mr. Bustamante's ideal weight? His %IBW? What other anthropometric measurements would you expect to see affected?

Given his PEM status, what lab test results would you expect to find? How might Mr. Bustamante's past history have affected his nutrition status before he developed cancer?

In what ways can cancer affect his nutrition status? How can radiation therapy affect his nutrition status? Discuss the possible impact of radical head and neck surgery on his nutrition status.

Describe cancer cachexia. What are some of its causes? What are the benefits of preventing or correcting it?

If Mr. Bustamante is able to take food by mouth, what suggestions will you give him for dealing with poor appetite, nausea and vomiting, dry and sore mouth, and chewing and swallowing problems?

If Mr. Bustamante is unable to eat an oral diet, is aggressive nutrition support indicated? Why or why not?

HOW AIDS DEVELOPS

HIV infection attacks the immune system and leaves its victims defenseless against opportunistic infections and disorders from which most people are protected. The disorder begins with infection by the virus and progresses in stages. The virus gradually destroys cells with a specific protein called CD4+ on their surfaces. Among the cells most affected are CD4+ T-lymphocytes, essential components of the immune system. At first, CD4+ lymphocytes decline gradually, and the HIV-infected individual remains symptom-free. As the infection progresses, though, depletion of CD4+ lymphocytes greatly impairs immune function. Early symptoms may include fatigue, skin rashes, fevers, diarrhea, muscle pain, night sweats, weight loss, oral lesions and infections, and other opportunistic infections that are not life-threatening. In the final stages, frequent and often fatal complications arise, such as severe weight loss; tuberculosis; recurrent bacterial pneumonia; serious infections of the central nervous system, GI tract, and skin; cancers; and severe diarrhea. On average, it takes about 10 years for an HIV infection to progress to AIDS. Clinicians monitor the progress of HIV infection by measuring the concentrations of CD4+ lymphocytes and the circulating virus (viral load).

People with AIDS frequently experience severe PEM and wasting. The wasting often begins early in the progression of the disease and becomes worse. People with AIDS may lose up to 34 percent of their ideal body weight in the four to five months before death, a degree of wasting similar to that seen in people who die from starvation.[18] Such findings prompt clinicians to speculate that severe wasting alone causes the death of some individuals with AIDS.[19] Even

opportunistic infections: infections from microorganisms that normally do not cause disease in the general population but can cause great harm in people once their immune systems are compromised (as in HIV infection).

CD4+ T-lymphocyte: a type of circulating white blood cell that has the CD4+ protein on its surface and is a necessary component of the immune system.

The cluster of mild symptoms that sometimes occur early in the course of AIDS is called AIDS-related complex (ARC).

Table 30–5

Strategies to Prevent HIV Transmission

> HIV is transmitted from one person to another by direct contact with contaminated body fluids, most often through sexual intercourse, through contaminated needles or blood products, or from mother to infant during pregnancy or lactation. To prevent the transmission of HIV infection:
>
> - Avoid sexual contact with anyone with an HIV infection.
> - Use a latex condom and a spermicidal agent during sexual contact unless you are in a monogamous relationship with a person who is free from AIDS and whose sexual history you know.
> - Do not share toothbrushes, razors, or other implements that could be contaminated with blood.
> - Exercise caution when undergoing procedures such as acupuncture, tattooing, or ear piercing, in which needles might be contaminated.
> - If you are an IV drug user, seek help for your addiction. Meanwhile, use only sterile, unused needles and dispose of them so that others will not use them. Avoid unprotected sexual contact with others.

when other complications ultimately cause death, malnutrition appears to be an important cofactor. Studies suggest that for people with AIDS, malnutrition contributes to disease-related complications and morbidity.[20] Finally, although direct evidence is lacking, the effects of PEM on the immune system, combined with those of HIV infection, may hasten the course of the disease. A later section describes the wasting associated with HIV infection.

TREATMENTS FOR HIV INFECTION

Treatments for HIV infection focus on improving the individual's comfort and quality of life by slowing the course of the infection and controlling its symptoms. Clinical trials of new drug treatments for HIV infection have yielded encouraging results and have expanded the array of medications available for treatment.

Drug therapy often includes a combination of AZT (zidovudine) and other medications called protease inhibitors that prevent the virus from replicating. Studies are underway to determine if providing combinations of medications in the earliest stages of infection might destroy the virus. In addition to drugs targeted to destroy the HIV virus, other medications are used to treat the symptoms and complications of HIV infection. The medications described on p. 942 can also be used to prevent wasting due to HIV infection. Diet therapy, which plays a supportive role in the treatment of HIV infection, is described in a later section.

THE HIV WASTING SYNDROME

The wasting associated with HIV infection occurs in the later stages and shares many similarities with the wasting associated with cancer. In both, the causes of malnutrition are related to the disease, its complications, and its treatments. Both result in inadequate nutrient intake, excessive nutrient losses, and hyper-

The antiviral drugs used in the treatment of HIV infection include zidovudine (AZT), didanosine (ddl), zalcitabine (ddC), stavudine (d4T), lamivudine (3TC), nevirapine, indinavir, ritonavir, and saquinavir.

 PRESCRIPTION PAD

Drugs used in the treatment of HIV infection may include:

- Analgesics
- Antidiarrheals
- Anti-infectives
- Antinauseants
- Antineoplastics
- Appetite stimulants

See Appendix E for timing with meals and nutrition-related side effects.

metabolism. As is true for cancer cachexia, the cytokines appear to play an important role in HIV wasting. Slow, progressive weight loss is usually associated with reduced food intake and gastrointestinal complications, whereas rapid weight loss is most often associated with infections.[21] The strongest predictors of weight loss and depletion of lean body mass and fat in people with HIV infection include anorexia, diarrhea, and other infections.[22] Table 30–6 lists the many factors that lead to progressive wasting from HIV infection.

Anorexia and Inadequate Nutrient Intake   People with AIDS have inadequate nutrient intakes for reasons similar to those of people with cancer. Clinicians report that the oral intakes of hospitalized people with AIDS meet only 70 percent of their *basal* energy needs and 65 percent of their protein needs.[23] These percentages would be even lower if the extra energy and protein needs imposed by hypermetabolism and activity were taken into account. Indeed, another group of investigators found that HIV-infected people with additional infections did not consume adequate energy to meet their high metabolic needs.[24]

HIV-related causes of anorexia include:

- *Psychological stress and pain.* Depression over the HIV diagnosis, progression, and prognosis and the medical, personal, and financial problems that lie ahead, as well as the pain associated with the disorder, can destroy the appetite.

- *Oral infections.* Infections and fever cause anorexia. In addition, oral infections associated with HIV cause further problems. Thrush, a common oral infection associated with HIV infection, can alter taste sensitivity, reduce the flow of

HIV-related causes of anorexia include:
- Depression.
- Fever.
- Pain.
- Mouth blindness.
- Dry mouth.
- Difficulty swallowing.
- Mouth ulcers.
- Esophageal lesions and obstructions.
- Use of oxygen masks.
- Drug therapy.
- Lethargy.
- Dementia.

Table 30–6

Possible Causes of Wasting in HIV Infection

Reduced Food Intake	
Altered taste perceptions	Infections
Cancer/cancer therapy	Lack of energy to eat
Difficulty chewing/swallowing	Mouth blindness
Drug therapy	Nausea/vomiting
Dry mouth	Oral lesions
Esophageal lesions/obstructions	Pain
Fear, depression, and dementia	Use of oxygen masks
Fever	

Accelerated Nutrient Losses	Altered Metabolism
Cancer/cancer therapy	Cancer
Diarrhea	Drug therapy
Drug or other therapy	Infections
Infections	
Malabsorption	
PEM	

thrush: a fungal infection of the mouth and esophagus caused by *Candida albicans*; the technical term for this infection is candidiasis. Thrush is characterized by a thick white coating of the tongue that alters taste sensations and causes pain on chewing and swallowing.

herpes virus: a virus that can lead to mouth lesions and may also affect the lower GI tract, causing diarrhea.

Kaposi's (cap-OH-seez) sarcoma: a type of cancer rare in the general population but common in people with HIV infection.

AIDS-induced causes of nutrient losses include:
- HIV infection.
- GI tract infections.
- Cancer.
- Cancer therapy.
- Anti-infective drugs.
- Megadoses of vitamins.
- Home remedies for AIDS.
- Reduced gastric acid secretion.
- Bacterial overgrowth.
- Malnutrition.

The diarrhea and malabsorption associated with AIDS for which no known cause has been identified are called AIDS enteropathies.

saliva, and cause pain on swallowing. Oral infections caused by the herpes virus can cause painful mouth ulcers that interfere with chewing and swallowing.

- *Respiratory infections.* Pneumonia and tuberculosis cause fever and pain that contribute to anorexia. The person who uses an oxygen mask may find eating difficult.
- *GI tract complications and altered organ function.* In addition to the problems associated with oral infections, people with HIV may experience belching, gastric reflux, and heartburn that may interfere with eating. Intestinal complications and altered organ function contribute to anorexia, early satiety, and food aversions.[25]
- *Cancer.* As previously described, cancer leads to anorexia. Kaposi's sarcoma, a cancer associated with HIV infection, can cause lesions and obstructions in the esophagus that make eating very painful.
- *Medical treatments.* Drugs used to treat HIV infection, associated infections, and cancer often cause anorexia, nausea, and vomiting that reduce food intake. Food aversions associated with medical treatments can also arise.
- *Lethargy and dementia.* In the later stages of AIDS, lethargy and dementia become common problems that interfere with food intake. The individual may be chronically exhausted and may not care or even remember to eat.

Nutrient Losses   In addition to anorexia, AIDS and its complications and treatments accelerate nutrient losses and contribute to wasting. From 50 to 90 percent of people with AIDS experience chronic or recurrent diarrhea and malabsorption, often associated with GI tract infections (see Table 30–7). Foods may serve as a source of infectious agents, and people with advanced HIV infection are highly susceptible to food-borne illness. Diarrhea may be severe and unresponsive to drug therapy—the person may lose from 10 to 15 liters of diarrheal fluids daily.

Nutrient losses may also arise when advanced HIV infection suppresses gastric acid secretion. A high gastric pH limits the absorption of iron and calcium

Table 30–7

Causes of GI Infections in AIDS

Bacterial	Protozoan
Clostridium dificile	*Cryptosporidium* species
Mycobacterium avium-intracellulare	*Giardia lamblia*
Mycobacterium tuberculosis	*Isosporia belli*
Salmonella species	*Microsporidium* species
Fungal	*Pneumocystitis carinii*
Candida albicans	*Toxoplasma gondii*
Cryptococcus neoformans	**Viral**
Parasitic	AIDS enteropathy
Nonpathogenic amoeba	*Cytomegalovirus* species
Entamoeba histolytica	Epstein-Barr
	Herpes simplex

and allows bacteria to grow in the upper GI tract. Bacterial overgrowth can lead to fat malabsorption and vitamin B_{12} and folate deficiencies (see Chapter 22).

Treatments common among HIV-infected individuals, especially anti-infective agents, chemotherapy, and radiation therapy, can accelerate nutrient losses due to vomiting, diarrhea, and malabsorption. Megadoses of vitamin C and other home remedies that some people with HIV infection use may also cause diarrhea. Once malnutrition is underway, it, too, contributes to malabsorption.

Metabolic Alterations   The accelerated metabolism associated with repeated infections significantly taxes nutrition status in people with HIV infection (see Chapter 25). Metabolic alterations associated with cancer also affect people with HIV infection who have cancer.

NUTRITION SUPPORT FOR PEOPLE WITH HIV INFECTION

In an era of improved treatments and prolonged survival for people with HIV infection, measures that improve the quality of life assume great importance. Attention to nutrition cannot change the ultimate outcome of an HIV infection, but it can offer an improved quality of life and possibly slow disease progression. Good nutrition status may also improve a person's response to drug therapy, reduce duration of hospital stays, and promote physical independence.[26] At a minimum, meeting nutrient needs eliminates the additional stresses imposed by malnutrition.

Benefits of Early Nutrition Support   Nutrition intervention takes a high priority from the moment an individual receives a positive diagnosis for HIV infection. The initial nutrition assessment evaluates the individual's current nutrition status and establishes baseline parameters from which to monitor changes. Nutrition therapy may be most effective in the early stages of HIV infection when reduced food intake is more likely to lead to malnutrition than in the later stages when repeated infections and hypermetabolism quickly deplete nutrient stores.[27] Clinicians can begin to encourage gradual improvements in eating habits before the person becomes debilitated and the task becomes monumental.

Oral Diets   Nutrition counseling for clients with HIV infection often includes recommendations for high-energy, high-protein diets; strategies for avoiding food-borne illnesses; and suggestions for alleviating anorexia, altered taste sensations, nausea and vomiting, and difficulty with chewing and swallowing (see the box on pp. 946–947). Often clinicians recommend that clients take daily vitamin and mineral supplements that provide at least 100 percent of the RDA. Health care professionals remind clients that supplements are intended to augment dietary sources, not to replace them.

Provided early in the course of HIV infection, nutrition counseling, a standard high-energy, high-protein diet, and oral supplements have been successful in halting weight loss and restoring weight in people without secondary infections.[28] Limited research suggests that immune-enhancing formulas that include omega-3 fatty acids, arginine, and nucleotides (see p. 815) may improve nutrition status early in the course of HIV infection, possibly by modulating the effects of tumor necrosis factor, a cytokine associated with wasting.[29] Other

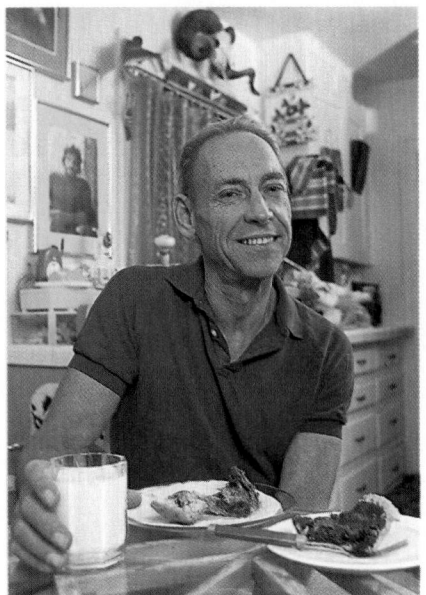

Nutrition provides an edge in maintaining quality of life and encouraging independence.

Energy and protein needs for people with HIV infection depend on the stage of the infection and the complications associated with each case. Typical diets provide 1.5 times the basal energy expenditure (see Chapter 25) and at least 1.5 g of protein per kilogram of body weight per day.

researchers report that supplementing the diet with hydrolyzed protein and fish oil (rich in omega-3 fatty acids) may help prevent weight loss and reduce the frequency of hospitalizations in the early stages of HIV infection.[30] Whether special formulas confer benefits over regular high-energy, high-protein foods and formulas in the early stages of HIV infection remains to be proven. Because special formulas are quite expensive and people with HIV infection face an enormous financial burden in treating their disorders, standard formulas (see Chapter 23) may be appropriate for people with weight loss related to poor food intake. Special formulas, however, may be beneficial for people who develop malabsorption or secondary infections.[31]

Treatment of Diarrhea   Treatment of HIV-associated diarrhea depends on its cause and the extent to which the intestine is affected. Although diarrhea is sometimes unresponsive to therapy, often a pathogen can be identified. Appropriate drug therapy along with the provision of adequate fluids and electrolytes is at the core of treatment. Drinking plenty of fluids is essential. The liberal use of table salt, salty broths, and high-potassium foods and juices can help replace electrolytes. Oral rehydration formulas (see Chapter 22) may be useful for severe cases of diarrhea. Other dietary modifications may include lactose and fat restrictions.

Susceptibility to food-borne illnesses requires that the individual with HIV infection be given written and oral instructions on the safe handling of foods. Table 14–1 on p. 488 summarizes food-borne illnesses and describes ways to prevent them.

Tube Feedings and Parenteral Nutrition   Individuals unable to consume adequate oral diets to prevent nutrition complications and unintentional weight loss need aggressive nutrition support. Both enteral and parenteral nutrition support have been shown to be effective in repleting lean body mass and promoting weight gain in some people with AIDS.[32] As a guideline, aggressive nutrition support should be considered when:

- The individual loses 5 percent of body weight within one month.
- The individual loses more than 10 percent of body weight over the past six months.[33]
- It can provide direct benefits and the client is in agreement.

As always, tube feedings are preferred to parenteral feeding. Tube feedings given at night can supplement oral diets during the day. If pain or obstructions in the upper GI tract make nasogastric passage of the feeding tube difficult or painful, gastrostomy or jejunostomy feedings are indicated. Preventing bacterial contamination of the formula is particularly important because of the susceptibility of HIV-infected individuals to GI infections.

TPN is generally reserved for people with HIV infection who are unable to tolerate enteral nutrition, but need to maintain their nutrition status while undergoing a therapy that is expected to improve their condition. TPN may be more useful in repleting the body mass of people whose primary problems are reduced food intake or malabsorption than in supporting those who have other

Case Study Travel Agent with HIV Infection

Mr. Sands, a travel agent, sought medical help at age 34 when he began feeling run-down and developed a painful white coating over his mouth and tongue. The presence of thrush and anemia alerted Mr. Sands's physician to the possibility of an HIV infection. When Mr. Sands tested positive for an HIV infection, he and his family and friends were devastated by the news. Fortunately, those closest to him have been supportive during this difficult time, and he has a strong desire to live out his life as independently as possible.

Four months after the diagnosis of HIV infection, Mr. Sands developed a serious, continuous diarrhea that required hospitalization to classify and control.

Since the diagnosis of HIV infection was made, Mr. Sands has lost 10 pounds. At 6 feet tall, he currently weighs 158 pounds.

Describe how HIV infection can lead to reduced food intake, nutrient losses, and hypermetabolism.

From the limited information given here, what factors could have contributed to Mr. Sands's weight loss? Is his weight loss significant? What is Mr. Sands's %IBW? What steps could prevent further weight loss?

Discuss nutrition strategies for dealing with thrush and diarrhea.

What additional nutrition consequences might be anticipated if Mr. Sands develops cancer?

---

systemic diseases.[34] People with GI tract obstructions, severe vomiting, or GI infections affecting the entire small bowel may benefit from TPN.

The concern for infection when receiving TPN is magnified in people with AIDS because their immune systems are already compromised. Data are scarce, but seem to indicate that TPN can be used safely and effectively in AIDS treatment.[35] The accompanying box presents a case study on HIV infection.

Wasting and severe malnutrition are commonly associated with both cancer and HIV infection. Health care professionals who work with people with these disorders serve their clients best by identifying nutrition problems early (see the nutrition assessment checklist) and offering solutions before nutrition status seriously deteriorates.

This chapter brings to a close your introduction to normal and clinical nutrition. Congratulations! You have received an abundance of information since you first turned to page 1. The normal nutrition chapters of this text provided you with current recommendations to promote optimal health. You learned how the body transforms food into nutrients and how those nutrients support the body's growth and well-being. The clinical chapters of the text addressed you as a future health care professional, concerned not only with your own health, but also with the well-being of others throughout the life cycle and during times of illness. They provided guidelines on diet for a variety of disorders. Along the way, you learned about tube feedings, parenteral nutrition, and a variety of modified diets.

We hope that this text has served you well and that when selecting food for yourself or making recommendations for others, you will remember to honor the body. It is a prized possession. Nourish it well.

systemic: affecting the whole body rather than one part or organ system.

Nutrition Assessment Checklist
For People with Cancer and HIV Infection

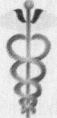

Medical   Check the client's medical history for the type of cancer or stage of HIV infection, associated complications, medical therapy, and symptoms. A diagnosis of cancer or HIV infection alerts health care professionals to the need for a thorough nutrition assessment.

Drug   Record the client's drug therapy for possible drug-nutrient interactions and nutrient-related complications. Antineoplastic agents, antiviral agents, anti-inflammatory agents, and antimicrobial agents can significantly and adversely affect nutrition status. Medications used to treat wasting can promote weight gain. Ask clients if they are using alternative therapies, including megadoses of vitamins and herbal preparations.

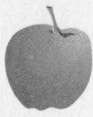

Food Intake   Determine if anorexia or nutrition-related complications are interfering with the client's ability to eat. Aggressively work with clients to improve nutrient intake and preserve nutrition status in the early stages of cancer or HIV infection. For clients with pain or nausea, check the timing of the administration of analgesics and antinausea agents to be sure they are given at times when they will improve appetite.

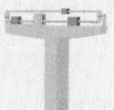

Anthropometric   Measure height and weight at regular intervals to detect wasting early.

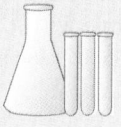

Laboratory   Assess laboratory data for changes in nutrition status, fluid and electrolyte balance, organ function, and response to therapy. Low serum protein levels are common in both cancer and advanced HIV infection.

Physical   Check for physical signs of nutrient deficiencies, dehydration (especially for those with fever, diarrhea, or vomiting), and mouth ulcers.

Study Questions

1. What is cancer? What events are believed to lead to its development?
2. What roles may dietary factors play in cancer development or cancer prevention? What dietary advice might be most effective in reducing the risk of cancer?
3. What is cancer cachexia? What factors contribute to its development?
4. Describe the anorexia that is associated with cancer. How does it differ from anorexia in other disease states? Discuss how cancer and its therapies contribute to anorexia.

5. How can cancer result in excessive nutrient losses, and how do these losses contribute to the cancer cachexia syndrome?
6. Describe the metabolic changes that occur in the person with cancer, and discuss their role in the cancer cachexia syndrome.
7. What are some of the treatments for cancer, and how do they work? In what ways can each treatment for cancer contribute to malnutrition?
8. Discuss strategies for combating anorexia, bitter or metallic tastes in the mouth, nausea and vomiting, problems with mouth ulcers, reduced flow of saliva, or other problems with chewing or swallowing.

9. What are the recommended uses for tube feedings and parenteral nutrition for people with cancer?
10. What is HIV infection? What are the consequences of HIV infection? What is the HIV wasting syndrome?
11. Describe factors that can lead to reduced nutrient intake, excessive nutrient losses, and altered metabolism in people with HIV infection.
12. In what ways might good nutrition status possibly alter the course of HIV infection?
13. Why are people with HIV infection highly susceptible to food-borne illness?

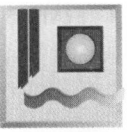

Clinical Applications

1. Many disorders can lead to wasting. For some of these, such as renal disease, diet is a cornerstone of treatment. For others, such as cancer and HIV infection, nutrition plays a supportive role. What determines whether nutrition plays a major or supportive role in the treatment of a disorder? Review the effects of PEM on pp. 199–202 and p. 551. Carefully consider how severe malnutrition can further debilitate people with cancer and advanced HIV infection.
2. Consider problems associated with nutrition in a 36-year-old woman with a malignant brain tumor affecting her ability to move the right side of her body (including the tongue) and to speak coherently. She has an expected length of survival of six months and is taking a pain medication that makes her nauseated and sleepy. What would be a realistic goal of nutrition support? If she is right-handed, how can her impairment interfere with eating? What suggestions might you have for overcoming this problem? How might nutrition be affected by her speech problems? Describe ways that the medications she is taking can affect her nutrition status. Would tube feedings or TPN be appropriate for this woman? Why or why not?

Notes

1. Council on Scientific Affairs, American Medical Association, Report of the Council on Scientific Affairs, Diet and cancer: Where do matters stand? *Archives of Internal Medicine* 153 (1993): 50–56.
2. H. Hwang, J. Dwyer, and R. M. Russel, Diet *Heliobacter pylori* infection, food preservation and gastric cancer risk: Are there new roles for preventative factors? *Nutrition Reviews* 52 (1994): 75–83.
3. R. A. Karmali, Fatty acid metabolism and biochemical mechanisms in cancer, in *Health Effects of Dietary Fatty Acids*, ed.

G. J. Nelson (Champaign, Ill.: American Oil Chemists Society, 1991), pp. 150–156.
4. Y. Kim and J. B. Mason, Nutrition chemoprevention of gastrointestinal cancers: A critical review, *Nutrition Reviews* 54 (1996): 259–279.
5. T. C. Hardin, Cytokine mediators of malnutrition: Clinical implications, *Nutrition in Clinical Practice* 8 (1993): 55–59.
6. A. M. Herrington, J. D. Herrington, and C. A. Church, Pharmacologic options for the treatment of cachexia, *Nutrition in Clinical Practice* 12 (1997): 101–113.

7. T. Duell and coauthors, Health and functional status of long-term survivors of bone marrow transplantation. EBMT Working Party on Late Effects and EULEP Study Group on Late Effects. European Group for Blood and Marrow Transplantation, *Annals of Internal Medicine* 126 (1997): 184–192.

8. K. Ringwald-Smith, R. Krance, and L. Stricklin, Enteral nutrition support in a child after bone marrow transplantation, *Nutrition in Clinical Practice* 10 (1995): 140–143.

9. B. R. Cassileth and C. C. Chapman, Alternative and complementary cancer therapies, *Cancer* 77 (1996): 1026–1034.

10. C. Grunfeld, Therapy for treatment of the wasting syndrome in cancer and AIDS: What can we do and what should we do? *Nutrition in Clinical Practice* 12 (1997): 99–100.

11. W. W. Souba, Nutritional support, *New England Journal of Medicine* 336 (1997): 41–48.

12. A. M. B. Hunter, Nutrition management of patients with neoplastic disease of the head and neck treated with radiation therapy, *Nutrition in Clinical Practice* 11 (1996): 157–169.

13. D. F. Cella, Overcoming difficulties in demonstrating health outcome benefits, *Journal of Parenteral and Enteral Nutrition* (supplement) 16 (1992): 106–111.

14. W. Demark-Wahnefried, B. K. Rimer, and E. Winer, Weight gain in women diagnosed with breast cancer, *Journal of the American Dietetic Association* 97 (1997): 519–526, 529.

15. A.S.P.E.N. Board of Directors, Practice guidelines: Cancer, *Journal of Parenteral and Enteral Nutrition* (supplement) 17 (1993): 12–13.

16. Ringwald-Smith, Krance, and Stricklin, 1995.

17. T. R. Ziegler and coauthors, Clinical and metabolic efficacy of glutamine-supplemented parenteral nutrition after bone marrow transplantation, *Annals of Internal Medicine* 116 (1992): 821–828; P. R. Schloerb and M. Amare, Total parenteral nutrition with glutamine in bone marrow transplantation and other clinical applications (randomized, double-blind study), *Journal of Parenteral and Enteral Nutrition* 17 (1993): 407–413.

18. D. P. Kotler and coauthors, Magnitude of body-cell-mass depletion and the timing of death from wasting in AIDS, *American Journal of Clinical Nutrition* 50 (1989): 444–447.

19. D. O. Jacobs, Bioelectrical impedance analysis: A way to assess changes in body cell mass in patients with acquired immunodeficiency syndrome? *Journal of Parenteral and Enteral Nutrition* 17 (1993): 401–402.

20. U. Süttmann and coauthors, Incidence and prognostic value of malnutrition and wasting in human immunodeficiency virus–infected outpatients, *Journal of Acquired Immune Deficiency Syndromes and Human Retrovirology* 8 (1995): 239–246.

21. D. C. Macallan and coauthors, Prospective analysis of patterns of weight change in stage IV human immunodeficiency virus infection, *American Journal of Clinical Nutrition* 58 (1993): 417–424.

22. A. Schwenk and coauthors, Clinical risk factors for malnutrition in HIV-1-infected patients, *AIDS* 7 (1993): 1213–1219.

23. E. B. Trujillo and coauthors, Assessment of nutritional status, nutrient intake, and nutrition support in AIDS patients, *Journal of the American Dietetic Association* 93 (1993): 477–478.

24. C. Grunefeld, M. Pange, and L. Shimizu, Resting energy expenditure, caloric intake, and short-term change in HIV infection and AIDS, *American Journal of Clinical Nutrition* 55 (1992): 455–460.

25. C. Fields-Gardner, A review of mechanisms of wasting in HIV disease, *Nutrition in Clinical Practice* 10 (1995): 167–176.

26. Federation of American Societies for Experimental Biology, Nutrition and HIV infection: A review and evaluation of the extant knowledge of the relationship between nutrition and HIV infection, *Nutrition in Clinical Practice* (supplement) 6 (1991): 46–48.

27. J. A. Stack and coauthors, High-energy, high-protein, oral, liquid, nutrition supplementation in patients with HIV infection: Effect on weight status in relation to incidence of secondary infection, *Journal of the American Dietetic Association* 96 (1996): 337–341.

28. Stack and coauthors, 1996.

29. Süttmann and coauthors, 1995.

30. R. T. Chelowski and coauthors, Long-term effects of early nutrition support with new enterotropic peptide-based formula vs. standard enteral formula in HIV-infected patients: Randomized prospective study, *Nutrition* 9 (1993): 507–512.

31. Stack and coauthors, 1996.

32. A.S.P.E.N. Board of Directors, Acquired immune deficiency syndrome, *Journal of Parenteral and Enteral Nutrition* (supplement) 17 (1993): 13–14; P. Singer and coauthors, Risks and benefits of home parenteral nutrition in the acquired immunodeficiency syndrome, *Journal of Parenteral and Enteral Nutrition* 15 (1991): 75–79.

33. Department of Continuing Education in Health Sciences, UCLA Extension, 1989.

34. D. P. Kotler and coauthors, Effect of home total parenteral nutrition on body composition in patients with acquired immunodeficiency syndrome, *Journal of Parenteral and Enteral Nutrition* 14 (1990): 454–458.

35. Singer and coauthors, 1991.

Cost-Conscious Health Care

*D*ecades of medical research have resulted in an explosion of knowledge and technologies to diagnose and treat diseases. This astounding progress, however, has come at a tremendous financial cost. Anyone who has paid an insurance premium or needed medical attention recently has felt the effects of skyrocketing health care costs. The United States spends more money on health care than any other nation, yet some citizens go without needed care. Without attention to cost containment, the health status of the nation is threatened; sophisticated medical services do little good if people cannot use them.

To address this problem, government officials, health care professionals, and insurance executives look for ways to cut costs without sacrificing quality and to make health care affordable to all people in the United States. Thus the medical community, which once embodied the idealistic approach of sparing no cost when it came to health care, has embraced the reality that cost is an element of quality.[1]

The full implications of cost containment and its impact on the nation's health remain to be seen. In the words of one clinician, "Our American society is in the midst of the most far reaching and profoundly disturbing uncontrolled study in the history of health care. We are experiencing major changes in the way we practice and pay for health care with very little evidence that these changes will achieve the desired outcome."[2] To address all of the ramifications of cost containment for health care delivery and payment systems is beyond the

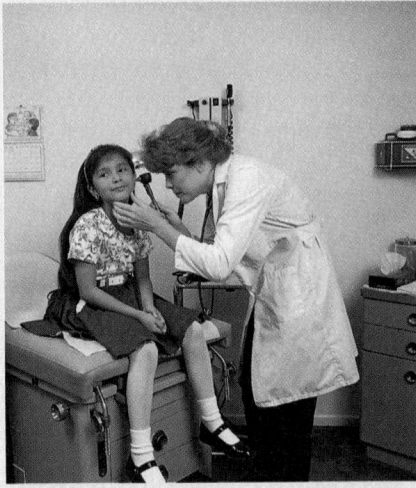

Health care professionals work diligently to deliver high-quality health care while controlling costs.

scope of this highlight. Instead, this highlight focuses on how cost containment affects nutrition services and how attention to nutrition might help reduce health care costs. As you read, keep in mind that as new strategies are implemented and studied, some will prove successful and others will not.

OUTCOME-ORIENTED CARE

Among other things, efforts to control health care costs aim at eliminating duplication of services, limiting access to unnecessary services, and reducing the number of hours or professionals involved in client care. Spurred by changes in the government insurance program (Medicare), which successfully lowered health costs by limiting reimbursement for services, traditional fee-for-service medical insurance is increasingly being replaced by managed care systems. (The glossary defines insurance-related and other terms.) Managed care organizations, which were rare just 15 years ago, now account for over 40 percent of the insurance provided by employers, and that percentage appears to be rising.[3] Managed care, which includes health maintenance organizations (HMOs) and preferred provider organizations (PPOs), is a health care delivery system that strives to control the use of resources to achieve the best health outcomes at tolerable costs.[4]

Glossary

health maintenance organization (HMO): a form of managed care that limits the subscriber's choice of health care professionals and controls access to services by directing care through a primary care physician.

indemnity insurance: traditional insurance that pays a fee for service.

managed care: a health care delivery system that is directed at providing quality health care at tolerable costs by coordinating services.

preferred provider organization (PPO): a form of managed care that encourages subscribers to select health care providers from a group that has contracted with the organization to provide services at lower costs.

Implicit in managed care and any effort to reduce medical costs is the need to identify which services provide the best outcomes at the lowest costs. The more expensive the procedure or test, the more critical justifying its costs becomes. For example, the clinical benefits of highly technical, costly, and potentially hazardous nutrition services, such as tube feedings and parenteral nutrition, are justified only when they have a reasonable chance of improving the client's outcome. Examples of desirable outcomes include the person's ability to function independently (the more care a person needs, the more expenses incurred), reduced hospital stays, prevention of complications, and extended survival time. For a person with cancer, the costs of tube feedings or parenteral nutrition might be justified if the person's inability to eat, rather than the cancer itself, is interfering with treatment or quality of life.[5] In other cases, the ability of tube feedings or parenteral nutrition to improve outcomes remain unproven; thus their associated costs are difficult to justify.

In representing nutrition professionals, the American Dietetic Association takes the position that managed care organizations and integrated health delivery systems should provide medical nutrition therapy as an essential component of health care and that it should be provided by qualified nutrition professionals.[6] Nutrition professionals must keep abreast of changing health care delivery systems and document how their unique knowledge and skills provide cost-effective care.[7]

Nutrition advocates continue to respond to the challenge of cost containment by documenting the proper use of nutrition services, improved outcomes associated with medical nutrition therapy, and innovative ways to reduce costs associated with nutrition therapy.[8] In one analysis of data from several sources, researchers report that early attention to malnutrition in hospitalized clients may result in cost savings of approximately $8300 per hospital bed per year.[9]

The speed at which cost containment measures are sweeping through the medical community suggests that there is little time to hesitate. Without data to support the costs of valuable health services such as nutrition, third-party payers (insurers) may opt to exclude services that might ultimately improve the quality of health care. Trying to implement changes later will be far more difficult. The rest of this highlight describes specific strategies nutrition professionals have begun to use to control costs and ensure the inclusion of their services.

CLINICAL PATHWAYS

To ensure that people's nutrition needs are addressed in the changing health care environment, nutrition professionals must be actively involved in the development of outcome measures and standards of care that guide health care. One such example, clinical pathways, is described here. Clinical pathways, also called *critical pathways* or *care maps*, are used to provide coordinated, outcome-oriented, cost-effective care. Clinical pathways are charts or tables that map out a plan of care for a specific diagnosis, procedure, or treatment. The plan defines a time frame for each intervention with a goal of providing the best outcome at the lowest cost. The development of a clinical pathway requires a multidisciplinary approach that focuses on the goal of the pathway, rather than on individual professional interests.[10]

The health care team develops each clinical pathway after careful study of their unique client population. Once in place, each pathway must be reassessed by studying unexpected outcomes or variances from the expected plan. When necessary, the pathway is improved.

To ensure that clients' nutrition needs are addressed in clinical pathways, nutrition professionals must actively participate in the multidisciplinary teams that develop the pathways and monitor their effectiveness. To be successful, nutrition professionals must educate themselves in areas beyond nutrition; they need to understand how to manage data, resources, programs, finances, and people.[11] They must develop skill in balancing nutrition needs with other medical needs and in making compromises that will not jeopardize the overall quality of care.[12]

HOME CARE

Another change in health care delivery, spurred by rising health care costs, is a shift from hospital care to home care. Early discharges lower hospital costs. Because clients may be discharged before they have regained health, however, they may require additional medical care at home. By teaching clients and caregivers to perform many of the procedures formerly performed by hospital staff, health care costs can be reduced. Some home care clients receive therapeutic diets as part of their treatment plans; others continue tube feedings and parenteral nutrition programs at home (see Chapter 24).

Nutrition professionals seek to ensure that nutrition services are included in home health care delivery systems. With their specialized knowledge and skills, nutrition professionals are uniquely qualified to assess nutrition status and to implement measures to prevent or correct malnutrition. They are also uniquely qualified to resolve eating problems (such as anorexia or nausea) and to evaluate the best feeding method (such as oral diet, tube feedings, or TPN) and composition of the diet (such as high protein or low sodium). The task for nutrition professionals is to document how these nutrition services improve outcomes and save money.[13] Dietitians in home health care need business and marketing skills to ensure that their nutrition services will be available to clients and that their position in the market will be secure.[14]

Clearly, health care professionals need to work within the health care system to provide cost-effective nutrition care without sacrificing quality. Suggestions for providing cost-saving, yet appropriate, nutrition care include:

- Use a qualified professional (registered dietitian) to complete a nutrition assessment and determine the most appropriate nutrition care plan for each person.
- Identify nutrition interventions that can prevent or treat disease and document the positive effects

and cost savings of these services.
- Recommend the most cost-effective method of feeding people (oral, enteral, or parenteral).

Whatever the final direction of health care delivery, one thing is certain. Health care professionals must continue to provide high-quality nutrition care in a cost-effective manner. In doing so, they help to ensure that quality, affordable health care will be available to all.

NOTES

1. A. Bothe, Consensus: We should not lower quality to cut costs, *Nutrition in Clinical Practice* (supplement) 10 (1995): 1–7.

2. J. R. Wesley, Managing the future of nutrition support, *Journal of Parenteral and Enteral Nutrition* 20 (1996): 383–384.

3. J. K. Iglehart, The American health care system: Introduction, *New England Journal of Medicine* 326 (1992): 962–967; D. A. August, Creation of a specialized nutrition support outcomes research consortium: If not now, when? *Journal of Parenteral and Enteral Nutrition* 20 (1996): 394–400.

4. A. W. Wojner and A. Hedberg, Incorporating nutrition care into critical pathways for improved outcomes, in *Integrating Nutrition Care into Critical Pathways*, Report of the Fifteenth Ross Roundtable on Medical Issues (Columbus, Ohio: Ross Laboratories, 1995), pp. 1–8.

5. W. W. Souba, Nutritional support, *New England Journal of Medicine* 336 (1997): 41–48.

6. American Dietetic Association, Position of The American Dietetic Association: Nutrition services in managed care, *Journal of the American Dietetic Association* 96 (1996): 391–395.

7. August, 1996; R. Chernoff, Managing managed care—A mission impossible? *Journal of the*

American Dietetic Association 96 (1996): 715.

8. E. L. Johnson and S. Valera, Medical nutrition therapy in non-insulin-dependent diabetes mellitus improves clinical outcomes, *Journal of the American Dietetic Association* 95 (1995): 700–701; B. R. Dahl and M. H. Read, Effect of a nutrition education program on the reduction of serum cholesterol level in Veterans Administration outpatients, *Journal of the American Dietetic Association* 95 (1995): 702–703; M. R. Gallagher-Allred and coauthors, Malnutrition and clinical outcomes: The case for medical nutrition therapy, *Journal of the American Dietetic Association* 96 (1996): 361–369; D. B. Schwartz, Enhanced enteral and parenteral nutrition practice and outcomes in an intensive care unit with a hospital-wide performance improvement process, *Journal of the American Dietetic Association* 96 (1996): 484–489; M. A. Puangco, H. L. Nguyen, and M. J. Sheridan, Computerized PN ordering optimizes timely nutrition therapy in a neonatal intensive care unit, *Journal of the American Dietetic Association* 97 (1997): 258–261; J. Maurer and coauthors, Reducing the inappropriate use of parenteral nutrition in an acute care teaching hospital, *Journal of Parenteral and Enteral Nutrition* 20 (1996): 272–274.

9. H. N. Tucker and S. G. Miguel, Cost containment through nutrition intervention, *Nutrition Reviews* 54 (1996): 111–121.

10. L. Wolf, Integrating nutrition care into critical pathways: An example, in *Integrating Nutrition Care into Critical Pathways*, Report of the Fifteenth Ross Roundtable on Medical Issues (Columbus, Ohio: Ross Laboratories, 1995) pp. 28–31.

11. Chernoff, 1996.

12. Wolf, 1995.

13. T. Byars, Dietetics professionals are paving new paths in home care, *Support Line*, December 1996, pp. 1–4.

14. A. Arkin, Marketing nutrition services to home health care: A client-focused, three-step marketing strategy, *Support Line*, December 1996, pp. 11–13.

Appendixes

CONTENTS

Appendix A   Cells, Hormones, and Nerves

Appendix B   Basic Chemistry Concepts

Appendix C   Biochemical Structures and Pathways

Appendix D   Aids to Calculation

Appendix E   Nutrition Assessment

Appendix F   Nutrition Resources

Appendix G   United States: Recommendations and Exchanges
World Health Organization: Recommendations

Appendix H   Table of Food Composition

Appendix I   Canada: Recommendations, Choices, and Labels

Appendix J   Measures of Protein Quality

Appendix K   Enteral Formulas

MICROGRAPH: Vitamin E, the fat-soluble vitamin that acts as an antioxidant

Contents

The Cell

The Hormones

The Nervous System

Putting It Together

CELLS, HORMONES, AND NERVES

◆

*T*his appendix is offered as an optional chapter for readers who want to enhance their understanding of the body's ways of coordinating its activities. The text presents a brief summary of the structure and function of the body's basic working unit (the cell) and of the body's two major regulatory systems (the hormonal system and the nervous system).

THE CELL

◆

The body's organs are made up of millions of cells and of materials produced by them. Each cell is specialized to perform its organ's functions, but all cells have common structures (see Figure A–1). Every cell is contained within a cell membrane. The cell membrane assists in moving materials into and out of the cell, and some of its special proteins act as "pumps" (described in Chapter 6). Some features of cell membranes, such as microvilli (Chapter 3), permit cells to interact with other cells and with their environments in highly specific ways.

Inside the membrane lies the cytoplasm, or cell "fluid." The cytoplasm contains much more than just fluid, though. It is a highly organized system of fibers, tubes, membranes, particles, and subcellular organelles as complex as a city. These parts intercommunicate, manufacture and exchange materials, package and prepare materials for export, and maintain and repair themselves.

Within each cell is another membrane-enclosed body, the nucleus. Inside the nucleus are the chromosomes, which contain the genetic material, DNA. The DNA encodes all the instructions for carrying out the cell's activities. The role of DNA in coding for cell proteins is summarized in Chapter 6, Figure 6–6. Chapter 6 also describes the variety of proteins produced by cells and the ways they perform the body's work.

Among the organelles within a cell are ribosomes, mitochondria, and lysosomes. Figure 6–6 briefly refers to the ribosomes; they assemble amino acids into proteins, following directions conveyed to them by RNA copies from the DNA in the chromosomes.

The mitochondria are made of intricately folded membranes that bear thousands of highly organized sets of enzymes on their inner and outer surfaces. Although mentioned only briefly in this book's chapters, their presence is implied whenever the enzymes of the TCA cycle and electron transport chain are mentioned because

---

cell: the basic unit of life, of which all living things are composed. Every cell is surrounded by a membrane and contains cytoplasm, within which are organelles and a nucleus; the cell nucleus contains chromosomes.

cell membrane: the membrane that surrounds the cell and encloses its contents; made primarily of lipid and protein.

cytoplasm (SIGH-toe-plazm): the cell contents, except for the nucleus.
 cyto = cell
 plasm = a form

nucleus: a major membrane-enclosed body within every cell, which contains the cell's genetic material, DNA, embedded in chromosomes.
 nucleus = a kernel

chromosomes: a set of structures within the nucleus of every cell that contain the cell's genetic material, DNA, associated with other materials (primarily proteins).

organelles: subcellular structures such as ribosomes, mitochondria, and lysosomes.
 organelle = little organ

ribosomes: protein-making organelles in cells; composed of RNA and protein.
 ribo = containing the sugar ribose (in RNA)
 some = body

mitochondria (my-toe-KON-dree-uh); singular **mitochondrion:** the cellular organelles responsible for producing ATP aerobically; made of membranes (lipid and protein) with enzymes mounted on them.
 mitos = thread (referring to their slender shape)
 chondros = cartilage (referring to their external appearance)

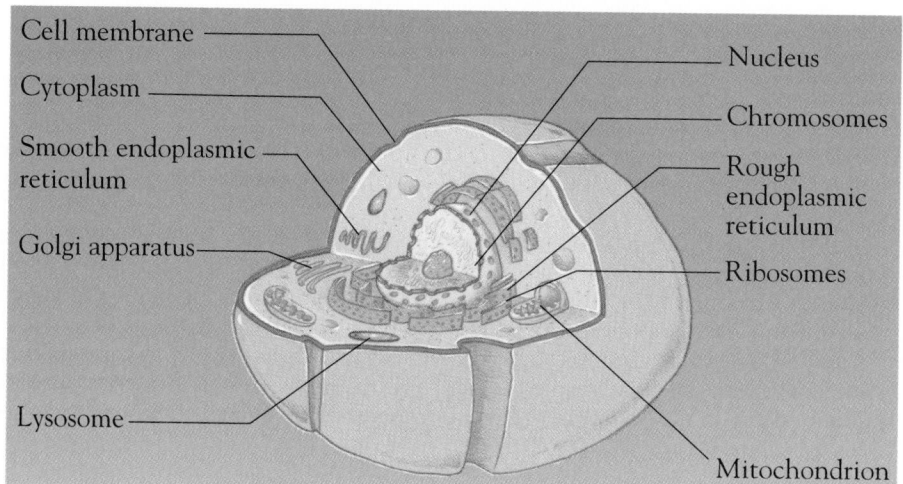

Cell membrane
Cytoplasm
Smooth endoplasmic reticulum
Golgi apparatus
Lysosome
Nucleus
Chromosomes
Rough endoplasmic reticulum
Ribosomes
Mitochondrion

Figure A–1
The Structure of a Typical Cell
The cell shown might be one in a gland (such as the pancreas) that produces secretory products (enzymes) for export (to the intestine). The rough endoplasmic reticulum with its ribosomes produces the enzymes; the smooth reticulum conducts them to the Golgi region; the Golgi membranes merge with the cell membrane, where the enzymes can be released into the extracellular fluid.

the mitochondria house all these enzymes.* Mitochondria are therefore crucial to aerobic metabolism, described in Chapter 7, and muscles conditioned to work aerobically are packed with them.

The lysosomes are membranes that enclose degradative enzymes. When a cell needs to self-destruct or to digest materials in its surroundings, its lysosomes free their enzymes. Lysosomes are active when tissue repair or remodeling is taking place—for example, in cleaning up infections, healing wounds, shaping embryonic organs, and remodeling bones.

Besides these and other cellular organelles, the cell's cytoplasm contains a highly organized system of membranes, the endoplasmic reticulum. The ribosomes may either float free in the cytoplasm or be mounted on these membranes. A membranous surface dotted with ribosomes looks speckled under the microscope and is called "rough" endoplasmic reticulum; such a surface without ribosomes is called "smooth." Some intracellular membranes are organized into tubules that collect cellular materials, merge with the cell membrane, and discharge their contents to the outside of the cell; these membrane systems are named the Golgi apparatus, after the scientist who first described them. The rough and smooth endoplasmic reticula and the Golgi apparatus are continuous with one another, so secretions produced deep in the interior of the cell can be efficiently transported to the outside and released. These and other cell structures enable cells to perform the multitudes of functions for which they are specialized.

The actions of cells are coordinated by both hormones and nerves, as the next sections show. Among the types of cellular organelles are receptors for the hormones delivering instructions that originate elsewhere in the body. Some hormones penetrate the cell and its nucleus and attach to receptors on chromosomes, where they activate certain genes to initiate, stop, speed up, or slow down synthesis of certain proteins as needed. Other hormones attach to receptors on the cell surface and transmit their messages from there. The hormones are described in the next section; the nerves, in the one following.

lysosomes: cellular organelles; membrane-enclosed sacs of degradative enzymes.
  lysis = dissolution

rough endoplasmic reticulum (en-doh-PLAZ-mic reh-TIC-you-lum): intracellular membrane dotted with ribosomes, where protein synthesis takes place.
  endo = inside
  plasm = the cytoplasm

smooth endoplasmic reticulum: smooth intracellular membrane bearing no ribosomes.

Golgi (GOAL-gee) **apparatus:** a set of membranes within the cell where secretory materials are packaged for export.

The study of hormones and their effects is **endocrinology**.

*For the reactions of glycolysis, the TCA cycle, and the electron transport chain, see Chapter 7 and Appendix C. The reactions of glycolysis take place in the cytoplasm; the end product acetyl CoA moves into the mitochondria; and the TCA and electron transport reactions take place there. The mitochondria then release carbon dioxide, water, and ATP as their end products.

THE HORMONES

◆

hormone: a chemical messenger. Hormones are secreted in response to altered conditions by a variety of endocrine glands in the body. Each hormone travels to one or more specific target tissues or organs, where it elicits a specific response.

A hormonal message originates in a gland and travels as a chemical compound—a hormone—in the bloodstream. The hormone flows everywhere in the body, but only its target organs respond to it, because only they possess the receptors to receive it.

The hormones, the glands they originate in, and their target organs and effects are described in this section. Many of the hormones you might be interested in are included, but only a few are discussed in detail. Figure A–2 identifies the glands that produce the hormones discussed in this section.

The hormonal system is a complex system in which many of the parts interact with one another. For example, several hormones are produced in the anterior pituitary gland in the brain. All of these hormones are regulated by other hormones

**Figure A–2
The Endocrine System**

These organs and glands release hormones that regulate body processes.

endocrine: with reference to a gland, one that secretes its product directly into (*endo*) the blood; for example, the pancreas cells that produce insulin. An **exocrine** gland secretes its product(s) out (*exo*) of the gland through a duct into a cavity; the sweat glands of the skin and the enzyme-producing glands of the pancreas are both examples. The pancreas is therefore both an endocrine and an exocrine gland.

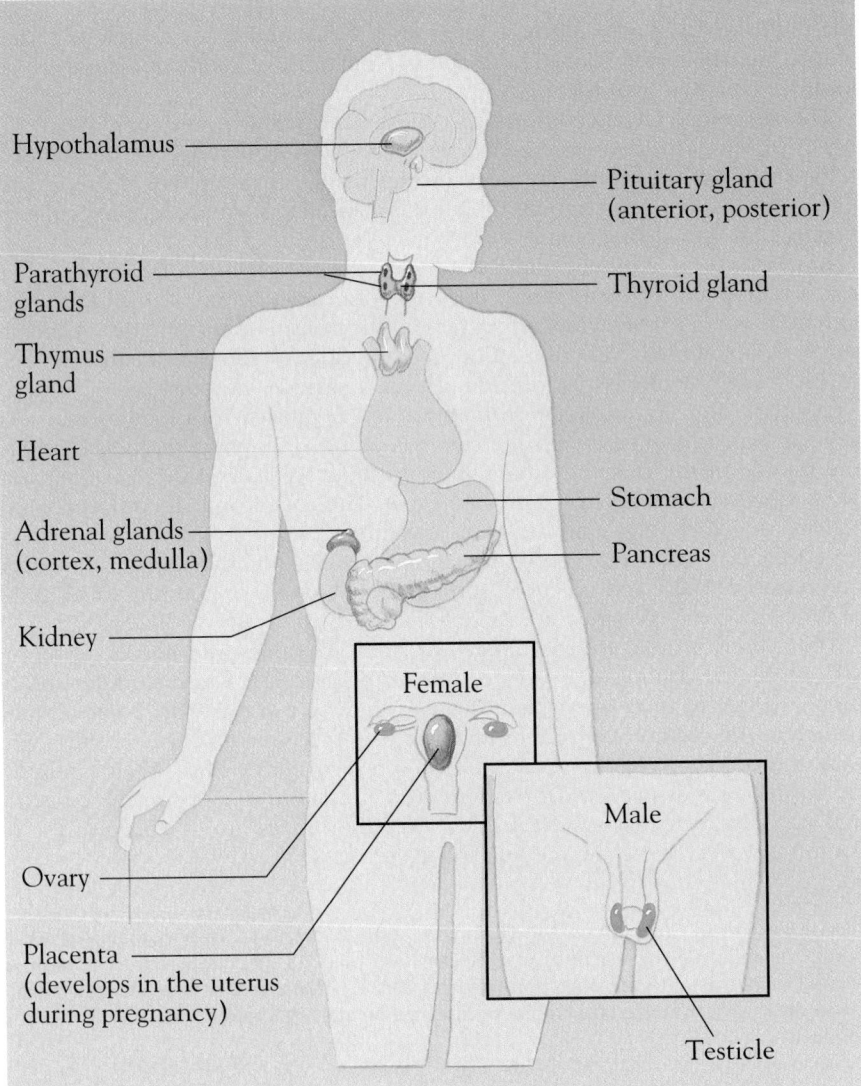

produced in another part of the brain, the hypothalamus. Furthermore, each of the pituitary gland hormones has effects on the production of compounds elsewhere in the body. Some of these compounds are also hormones that will affect still other body parts. A hormone may travel far from its point of origin and ultimately have profound, even unexpected, effects.

hypothalamus: a brain region (see Figure A–2) that is connected by a channel to the pituitary and can produce many hormones in response to signals from it or from other body conditions.
hypo = below
thalamus = another brain region

HORMONES OF THE PITUITARY GLAND AND HYPOTHALAMUS

The anterior pituitary gland produces the following hormones, each of which acts on one or more target organs and elicits a characteristic response:

The **pituitary** gland in the brain has two parts—the **anterior** (front) and the **posterior** (hind) parts.

◆ Adrenocorticotropin (ACTH) acts on the adrenal cortex, promoting the making and release of its hormones.

adrenocorticotropin: so named because it stimulates (*trope*) the adrenal cortex. The adrenal gland, like the pituitary, has two parts, in this case an outer portion (*cortex*) and an inner core (*medulla*).

◆ Thyroid-stimulating hormone (TSH) acts on the thyroid gland, promoting the making and release of thyroid hormone.

◆ Growth hormone (GH) works on all tissues, promoting growth, fat breakdown, and the formation of antibodies.

◆ Follicle-stimulating hormone (FSH) works on the ovaries in the female, promoting their maturation, and on the testicles in the male, promoting sperm formation.

follicle (ovarian): that part of the female reproductive system where the ovary lies and eggs are produced.

◆ Luteinizing hormone (LH) also acts on the ovaries, advancing their maturation, the making of progesterone and estrogens, and ovulation; and on the testicles, promoting the making and release of androgens (male hormones).

luteinizing: so called because the follicle turns orange as it matures.
lutein = an orange pigment

◆ Prolactin, secreted in the female during pregnancy and after she has borne a baby, acts on the mammary glands to stimulate their growth and the making of milk.

prolactin: so named because it promotes (*pro*) the production of milk (*lacto*).

◆ Melanocyte-stimulating hormone (MSH) acts on the pigment cells, promoting the making and dispersal of pigment.

melanocyte (MEL-an-oh-cite)**:** a cell containing the pigment melanin.
cyte = cell

The controls over this array of actions are sensitive and specific. Each of these seven hormones has one or more signals that turn it on and another (or others) that turns it off. Among the controlling signals are several hormones from the hypothalamus:

Hormones that are turned off by their own effects are said to be regulated by **negative feedback.** For example, when a pituitary gland hormone has caused the release of a substance from a target organ, that substance itself switches off the original hormone signal (that is, it feeds back negatively).

◆ Corticotropin-releasing hormone (CRH), which promotes release of ACTH, is turned on by stress and turned off by ACTH when enough has been released.

◆ TSH-releasing hormone (TRH), which promotes release of TSH, is turned on by large meals or low body temperature.

◆ GH-releasing hormone (GRH), which stimulates the release of GH, is turned on by insulin.

◆ GH-inhibiting hormone (GIH or somatostatin), which inhibits the release of GH and interferes with the release of TSH, is turned on by hypoglycemia and/or exercise and is rapidly destroyed by body tissues so that it does not accumulate.

somatostatin (GIH): a hormone that inhibits the release of growth hormone; the opposite of **somatotropin (GH).**
somato = body
stat = keep the same
tropin = make more

◆ FSH/LH–releasing hormone (FSH/LH–RH) is turned on in the female by nerve messages or low estrogen and in the male by low testosterone.

◆ Prolactin-inhibiting hormone (PIH) is turned on by high prolactin levels and off by estrogen, testosterone, and suckling (by way of nerve messages).

◆ MSH-inhibiting hormone (MIH) is turned on by the hormone melatonin.

Let's examine some of these controls. PIH, for example, responds to high prolactin levels (remember, prolactin promotes the making of milk). High prolactin levels ensure that milk is made and—by calling forth PIH—ensure that prolactin levels don't get too high. But when the infant is suckling—and creating a demand for milk—PIH is not allowed to work (suckling turns off PIH). The consequence: prolactin remains high, and milk manufacture continues. Demand from the infant thus directly adjusts the infant's supply of milk. This example not only shows how the need is met but also illustrates the cooperation between nerves and hormones that achieves this effect.

As another example, consider CRH. Stress, perceived in the brain and relayed to the hypothalamus, switches on CRH. On arriving at the pituitary, CRH switches on ACTH. Then ACTH acts on its target organ, the adrenal cortex, which responds by producing and releasing stress hormones, and the stress response is under way. Events cascading from there involve every body cell and many other hormones.

The numerous steps required to set the stress response in motion make it possible for the body to fine-tune the response; control can be exerted at each step. These two examples illustrate what the body can do in response to two different stimuli—producing milk in response to an infant's need and gearing up for action in an emergency.

Two hormones produced by the posterior pituitary gland are:

◆ Antidiuretic hormone (ADH), or vasopressin.

◆ Oxytocin.

ADH promotes contraction of arteries and acts on the kidney to prevent water from being excreted. It is turned on whenever the blood volume is depleted, the blood pressure is low, or the salt concentration of the blood is too high (see Chapter 12). It is turned off by the return of these conditions to normal. Oxytocin is produced in response to reduced progesterone levels, suckling, or the stretching of the cervix and acts on two target organs. One, the uterus, contracts, thus inducing labor; the other, the mammary glands, release milk.

antidiuretic hormone (ADH): the hormone that prevents water loss in urine (also **vasopressin**).
anti = against
di = through
ure = urine
vaso = blood vessels
pressin = pressure

oxytocin: the hormone of childbirth.
oxy = quick
tocin = childbirth

cervix: the circular muscle that guards the opening of the uterus. When a baby is about to be born, the cervix begins to stretch.
cervic = neck

HORMONES THAT REGULATE ENERGY METABOLISM

Hormones produced by a number of different glands have effects on energy metabolism:

◆ Insulin from the pancreas beta cells.

◆ Glucagon from the pancreas alpha cells.

◆ Thyroxin from the thyroid gland.

◆ Norepinephrine and epinephrine from the adrenal medulla.

◆ Growth hormone (GH) from the anterior pituitary (already mentioned).

◆ Glucocorticoids from the adrenal cortex.

Insulin is turned on by many stimuli, including raised blood glucose. It acts on cells to increase glucose and amino acid uptake into them and to promote the secretion of GRH. Glucagon responds to low blood glucose and acts on the liver to promote the breakdown of glycogen to glucose, the conversion of amino acids to glucose, and the release of glucose. Thyroxin responds to TSH and acts on many cells to increase their metabolic rate, growth, and heat production. The hormones norepinephrine and epinephrine respond to stimulation by sympathetic nerves and produce reactions in many cells that facilitate the body's readiness for fight or flight: increased heart activity, blood vessel constriction, breakdown of glycogen and glucose, raised blood glucose levels, and fat breakdown. Norepinephrine and epinephrine also influence the secretion of the many hormones from the hypothalamus that

Norepinephrine and epinephrine were formerly called noradrenalin and adrenalin.

glucocorticoid: a hormone from the adrenal cortex that affects the body's management of glucose.
gluco = glucose
corticoid = from the cortex

exert control on the body's other systems. The glucocorticoid hormones become active during times of stress and carbohydrate metabolism.

Every body part is affected by these hormones. Each different hormone has unique effects; and hormones that oppose each other are produced in carefully regulated amounts, so each can respond to the exact degree that is appropriate to the condition.

HORMONES THAT ADJUST OTHER BODY BALANCES

Hormones are involved in moving calcium into and out of the body's storage deposits in the bones:

◆ Calcitonin (CT) from the thyroid gland.

◆ Parathormone (parathyroid hormone or PTH) from the parathyroid gland.

◆ Vitamin D from the kidneys.

One of calcitonin's target tissues is the bones, which respond by storing calcium from the bloodstream whenever blood calcium rises above the normal range. Calcitonin also acts on the kidneys to increase excretion of both calcium and phosphorus in the urine. Parathormone responds to the opposite condition—lowered blood calcium—and acts on three targets: the bones, which release stored calcium into the blood; the kidneys, which slow the excretion of calcium; and the intestine, which increases calcium absorption. Vitamin D acts with parathormone and is essential for the absorption of calcium in the intestine. Figure 12–9 in Chapter 12 diagrams the ways vitamin D, and the hormones calcitonin and parathormone, regulate calcium homeostasis.

Another hormone has effects on blood-making activity:

◆ Erythropoietin from the kidneys.

Erythropoietin is responsive to oxygen depletion of the blood and to anemia. It acts on the bone marrow to stimulate the making of red blood cells.

Another hormone, special for pregnancy, is:

◆ Relaxin from the ovary.

This hormone, which is secreted in response to the raised progesterone and estrogen levels of late pregnancy, acts on the cervix and pelvic ligaments to allow them to stretch so that they can accommodate the birth process without strain.

Other agents help regulate blood pressure:

◆ Renin (an enzyme), from the kidneys, in cooperation with angiotensin in the blood.

◆ Aldosterone, a hormone from the adrenal cortex.

Renin responds to a reduced blood supply experienced by the kidneys and acts in several ways. Encountering the inactive form of angiotensin in the bloodstream, renin converts this molecule to active angiotensin I and then to the very active angiotensin II. The angiotensins constrict the blood vessels, thus raising the blood pressure. They also stimulate thirst, leading to increased water intake, another way of raising the blood pressure. The angiotensins also cause the kidneys to retain water and salt. Thus the angiotensins increase blood pressure by several means at once.

Renin and angiotensin also stimulate the adrenal cortex to secrete the hormone aldosterone. This hormone's target is also the kidneys, which respond by excreting less sodium and with it, less water. The effect is to retain more water in the bloodstream—thus, again, raising the blood pressure. Figure 12–1 in Chapter 12 provides more details.

---

calcitonin: so called because it regulates (tones) the calcium level.

parathyroid: named for their location, the four parathyroid glands nestle in the surface layers of the two thyroid lobes in the neck.
 para = beside, next to

Vitamin D is sometimes viewed as a hormone because it is produced in one body organ and regulates others.

erythropoietin (eh-REE-throw-POY-eh-tin): named for its red blood cell–making function.
 erythro = red (blood cell)
 poiesis = creating (like poetry)

relaxin: the hormone of late pregnancy.

renin (REN-in): an enzyme from the kidneys, which works by activating angiotensin.
 ren = kidney

angiotensin: a hormone involved in blood pressure regulation.
 angio = blood vessels
 tensin = pressure

aldosterone: a hormone from the adrenal gland involved in blood pressure regulation.
 aldo = aldehyde

THE GASTROINTESTINAL HORMONES

Several hormones are produced in the stomach and intestines in response to the presence of food or the components of food:

◆ Gastrin from the stomach and duodenum.

◆ Cholecystokinin from the duodenum.

◆ Secretin from the duodenum.

◆ Gastric-inhibitory peptide from the duodenum and jejunum.

Gastrin stimulates the stomach to make and release its acid and digestive juices and to move and churn its contents actively. Cholecystokinin signals the gallbladder and pancreas to release their contents into the intestine to aid in digestion. Secretin calls forth acid-neutralizing bicarbonate from the pancreas into the intestine and slows the action of the stomach and its secretion of acid and digestive juices. Gastric-inhibitory peptide inhibits the secretion of gastric acid and slows the process of digestion. These hormones are presented in more detail in Chapter 3.

THE SEX HORMONES

The three major sex hormones are:

◆ Testosterone from the testicles.

◆ Estrogens from the ovary.

◆ Progesterone from the ovary's corpus luteum in preparation for, and during, pregnancy.

testosterone: a steroid hormone from the testicles, or testes. The steroids, as explained in Chapter 5, are chemically related to, and some are derived from, the lipid cholesterol.
sterone = a steroid hormone

estrogens: hormones responsible for the menstrual cycle and other female characteristics.
oestrus = the egg-making cycle
gen = gives rise to

progesterone: the hormone of gestation (pregnancy).
pro = promoting
gest = gestation (pregnancy)
sterone = a steroid hormone

Reminder: A *prostaglandin* is a hormonelike compound, derived from the polyunsaturated fatty acids.

In the male, testosterone is released in response to LH (described earlier). It acts on all the tissues that are involved in male sexuality and promotes their development and maintenance. Estrogens, released in response to both FSH and LH, act similarly in females. Progesterone, released in response to raised LH and prolactin, acts on the uterus and mammary glands, stimulating them to grow and develop.

THE PROSTAGLANDINS

The prostaglandins are a group of hormonelike substances produced by many different body organs. They perform a multitude of diverse functions including the regulation of blood vessel contractions, nerve impulses, and hormone responses. They don't have descriptive names but are designated by letters and numbers: E_1, E_2, and so forth. The prostaglandins are all derived from the polyunsaturated fatty acids and account in part for the necessity for these fatty acids in the diet.

This brief description of the hormones and their functions should suffice to provide an awareness of the enormous impact these compounds have on body processes. The other overall regulating agency is the nervous system.

THE NERVOUS SYSTEM

◆

central nervous system: the central part of the nervous system, the brain and spinal cord.

peripheral (puh-RIFF-er-ul) **nervous system:** the peripheral (outermost) part of the nervous system, the vast complex of wiring that extends from the central nervous system to the body's outermost areas. It contains both somatic and autonomic components (defined next).

The nervous system has a central control system—a sort of computer—that can evaluate information about conditions within and outside the body, and a vast system of wiring that receives information and sends instructions. The control unit is the brain and spinal cord, called the central nervous system; and the vast complex of wiring between the center and the parts is the peripheral nervous system. The smooth functioning that results from the system's adjustments to changing conditions is homeostasis.

The nervous system has two general functions: it controls voluntary muscles in response to sensory stimuli from them, and it controls involuntary, internal muscles and glands in response to nerve-borne and chemical signals about their status. In fact, the nervous system is best understood as two systems that use the same or similar pathways to receive and transmit their messages. The somatic nervous system controls the voluntary muscles; the autonomic nervous system controls the internal organs.

When scientists were first studying the autonomic nervous system, they noticed that when something hurt one organ of the body, some of the other organs reacted as if in sympathy for the afflicted one. They therefore named the nerve network they were studying the sympathetic nervous system. The term is still used today to refer to that branch of the autonomic nervous system that responds to pain and stress. The other branch is called the parasympathetic nervous system. (Think of the sympathetic branch as the responder when homeostasis needs restoring and the parasympathetic branch as the commander of function during normal times.) Both systems transmit their messages through the brain and spinal cord. Nerves of the two branches travel side by side along the same pathways to transmit their messages, but they oppose each other's actions (see Figure A–3).

An example will show how the sympathetic and parasympathetic nervous systems work to maintain homeostasis. When you go outside in cold weather, your skin's temperature receptors send ''cold'' messages to the spinal cord and brain. Your conscious mind may intervene at this point to tell you to zip your jacket, but let's say

somatic (so-MAT-ick) **nervous system:** the division of the nervous system that controls the voluntary muscles, as distinguished from the autonomic nervous system, which controls involuntary functions.
soma = body

autonomic nervous system: the division of the nervous system that controls the body's automatic responses. Its two branches are the **sympathetic** branch, which helps the body respond to stressors from the outside environment, and the **parasympathetic** branch, which regulates normal body activities between stressful times.
autonomos = self-governing

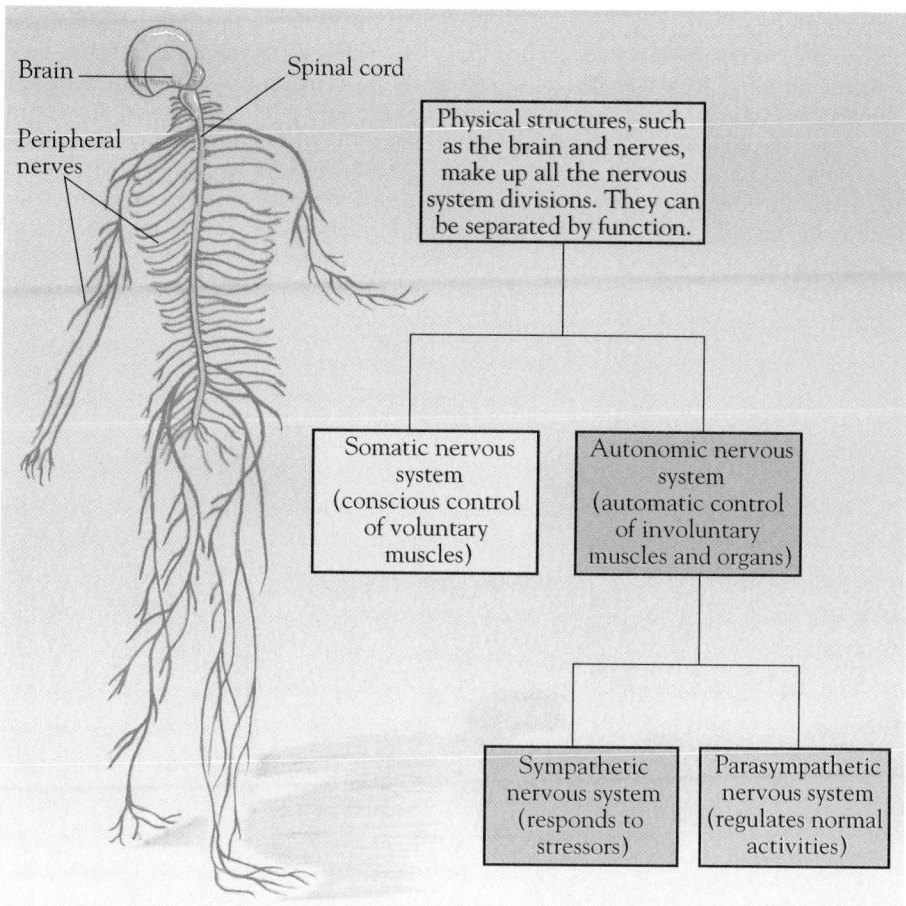

Brain — Spinal cord

Peripheral nerves

Physical structures, such as the brain and nerves, make up all the nervous system divisions. They can be separated by function.

Somatic nervous system (conscious control of voluntary muscles)

Autonomic nervous system (automatic control of involuntary muscles and organs)

Sympathetic nervous system (responds to stressors)

Parasympathetic nervous system (regulates normal activities)

Figure A–3
The Organization of the Nervous System

The brain and spinal cord evaluate information about conditions within and outside the body, and the peripheral nerves receive information and send instructions.

you have no jacket. Your sympathetic nervous system reacts to the external stressor, the cold. It signals your skin-surface capillaries to shut down so your blood will circulate deeper in your tissues, where it will conserve heat. Your sympathetic nervous system also signals involuntary contractions of the small muscles just under the skin surface. The product of these muscle contractions is heat, and the visible result is goose bumps. If these measures do not raise your body temperature enough, then the sympathetic nerves signal your large muscle groups to shiver; the contractions of these large muscles produce still more heat. All of this activity adds up to a set of adjustments that maintain your homeostasis (with respect to temperature) under conditions of external extremes (cold) that would throw it off balance. The cold was a stressor; the body's response was resistance.

Now let's say you come in and sit by a fire and drink hot cocoa. You are warm and no longer need all that sympathetic activity. At this point, your parasympathetic nerves take over; they signal your skin-surface capillaries to dilate again, your goose bumps to subside, and your muscles to relax. Your body is back to normal. This is recovery.

PUTTING IT TOGETHER

◆

The hormonal and nervous systems coordinate body functions by transmitting and receiving messages. The point-to-point messages of the nervous system travel through a central switchboard (the spinal cord and brain), whereas the messages of the hormonal system are broadcast over the airways (the bloodstream), and any organ with the appropriate receptors can pick them up. Nerve impulses travel faster than hormonal messages do—although both are remarkably swift. Whereas your brain's command to wiggle your toes reaches the toes within a fraction of a second and stops as quickly, a gland's message to alter a body condition may take several seconds or minutes to get started and may fade away equally slowly.

Together, the two systems possess every characteristic a superb communication network needs: varied speeds of transmission, along with private communication lines or public broadcasting systems, depending on the needs of the moment. The hormonal system, together with the nervous system, integrates the whole body's functioning so that all parts act smoothly together.

BASIC CHEMISTRY CONCEPTS

◆

Contents

Matter: The Properties of Atoms

Chemical Bonding

Formation of Ions

Water, Acids, and Bases

Chemical Reactions

Formation of Free Radicals

*T*his appendix is intended to provide the background in basic chemistry that you need to understand the nutrition concepts presented in this book. Chemistry is the branch of natural science that is concerned with the description and classification of matter, the changes that matter undergoes, and the energy associated with these changes. Matter is anything that takes up space and has mass. Energy is the ability to do work.

MATTER: THE PROPERTIES OF ATOMS

◆

Every substance has characteristics or properties that distinguish it from all other substances and thus give it a unique identity. These properties are both physical and chemical. The physical properties include such characteristics as color, taste, texture, and odor, as well as the temperatures at which a substance changes its state (from a solid to a liquid or from a liquid to a gas) and the weight of a unit volume (its density). The chemical properties of a substance have to do with how it reacts with other substances or responds to a change in its environment so that new substances with different sets of properties are produced.

A physical change does not change a substance's chemical composition. For example, the three states ice, water, and steam all consist of two hydrogen atoms and one oxygen atom bound together. However, a chemical change occurs if an electric current passes through water. The water disappears and two different substances are formed: hydrogen gas, which is flammable, and oxygen gas, which supports life. Chemical changes are also referred to as chemical reactions.

SUBSTANCES: ELEMENTS AND COMPOUNDS

Molecules are one or more atoms of the same element or two or more atoms of different elements joined by chemical bonds. They constitute the smallest part of a substance that can exist separately without losing its physical and chemical properties. If a molecule is composed of atoms that are alike, the substance is an element (for example, O_2). If a molecule is composed of two or more different kinds of atoms, the substance is a compound (for example, H_2O).

Just over 100 elements are known, and these are listed in Table B–1. A familiar example is hydrogen, whose molecules are composed only of hydrogen atoms linked together in pairs (H_2). On the other hand, over a million compounds are known. An example is the sugar glucose. Each of its molecules is composed of 6 carbon, 6 oxygen, and 12 hydrogen atoms linked together in a specific arrangement (as described in Chapter 4).

THE NATURE OF ATOMS

Atoms themselves are made of smaller particles. Within the atomic nucleus are protons (positively charged particles), and surrounding the nucleus are electrons (negatively charged particles). The number of protons (+) in the nucleus of an atom determines the number of electrons (−) around it. The positive charge on a proton is equal to the negative charge on an electron, so the charges cancel each other out and leave the atom neutral to its surroundings.

The nucleus may also include neutrons, subatomic particles that have no charge. Protons and neutrons are of equal mass, and together they give an atom its weight. Electrons bond atoms together to make molecules, and they are involved in chemical reactions.

Table B–1
Chemical Symbols for the Elements

Number of Protons (Atomic Number)	Element	Number of Electrons in Outer Shell	Number of Protons (Atomic Number)	Element	Number of Electrons in Outer Shell
1	Hydrogen (H)	1	52	Tellurium (Te)	6
2	Helium (He)	2	53	Iodine (I)	7
3	Lithium (Li)	1	54	Xenon (Xe)	8
4	Beryllium (Be)	2	55	Cesium (Cs)	1
5	Boron (B)	3	56	Barium (Ba)	2
6	Carbon (C)	4	57	Lanthanum (La)	2
7	Nitrogen (N)	5	58	Cerium (Ce)	2
8	Oxygen (O)	6	59	Praseodymium (Pr)	2
9	Fluorine (F)	7	60	Neodymium (Nd)	2
10	Neon (Ne)	8	61	Promethium (Pm)	2
11	Sodium (Na)	1	62	Samarium (Sm)	2
12	Magnesium (Mg)	2	63	Europium (Eu)	2
13	Aluminum (Al)	3	64	Gadolinium (Gd)	2
14	Silicon (Si)	4	65	Terbium (Tb)	2
15	Phosphorus (P)	5	66	Dysprosium (Dy)	2
16	Sulfur (S)	6	67	Holmium (Ho)	2
17	Chlorine (Cl)	7	68	Erbium (Er)	2
18	Argon (Ar)	8	69	Thulium (Tm)	2
19	Potassium (K)	1	70	Ytterbium (Yb)	2
20	Calcium (Ca)	2	71	Lutetium (Lu)	2
21	Scandium (Sc)	2	72	Hafnium (Hf)	2
22	Titanium (Ti)	2	73	Tantalum (Ta)	2
23	Vanadium (V)	2	74	Tungsten (W)	2
24	Chromium (Cr)	1	75	Rhenium (Re)	2
25	Manganese (Mn)	2	76	Osmium (Os)	2
26	Iron (Fe)	2	77	Iridium (Ir)	2
27	Cobalt (Co)	2	78	Platinum (Pt)	1
28	Nickel (Ni)	2	79	Gold (Au)	1
29	Copper (Cu)	1	80	Mercury (Hg)	2
30	Zinc (Zn)	2	81	Thallium (Tl)	3
31	Gallium (Ga)	3	82	Lead (Pb)	4
32	Germanium (Ge)	4	83	Bismuth (Bi)	5
33	Arsenic (As)	5	84	Polonium (Po)	6
34	Selenium (Se)	6	85	Astatine (At)	7
35	Bromine (Br)	7	86	Radon (Rn)	8
36	Krypton (Kr)	8	87	Francium (Fr)	1
37	Rubidium (Rb)	1	88	Radium (Ra)	2
38	Strontium (Sr)	2	89	Actinium (Ac)	2
39	Yttrium (Y)	2	90	Thorium (Th)	2
40	Zirconium (Zr)	2	91	Protactinium (Pa)	2
41	Niobium (Nb)	1	92	Uranium (U)	2
42	Molybdenum (Mo)	1	93	Neptunium (Np)	2
43	Technetium (Tc)	1	94	Plutonium (Pu)	2
44	Ruthenium (Ru)	1	95	Americium (Am)	2
45	Rhodium (Rh)	1	96	Curium (Cm)	2
46	Palladium (Pd)	—	97	Berkelium (Bk)	2
47	Silver (Ag)	1	98	Californium (Cf)	2
48	Cadmium (Cd)	2	99	Einsteinium (Es)	2
49	Indium (In)	3	100	Fermium (Fm)	2
50	Tin (Sn)	4	101	Mendelevium (Md)	2
51	Antimony (Sb)	5	102	Nobelium (No)	2

Key:
Elements found in energy-yielding nutrients, vitamins, and water.
Major minerals.
Trace minerals.

B

Each type of atom has a characteristic number of protons in its nucleus. The hydrogen atom (symbol H) is the simplest of all. It possesses a single proton, with a single electron associated with it:

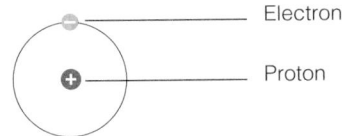

Hydrogen atom (H), atomic number 1.

Just as hydrogen always has one proton, helium always has two, lithium three, and so on. The atomic number of each element is the number of protons in the nucleus of that atom, and this never changes in a chemical reaction; it gives the atom its identity. The atomic numbers for the known elements are listed in Table B–1.

Besides hydrogen, the atoms most common in living things are carbon (C), nitrogen (N), and oxygen (O), whose atomic numbers are 6, 7, and 8, respectively. Their structures are more complicated than that of hydrogen, but each of them possesses the same number of electrons as there are protons in the nucleus. These electrons are found in orbits, or shells:

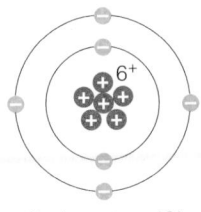

Carbon atom (C),
atomic number 6.

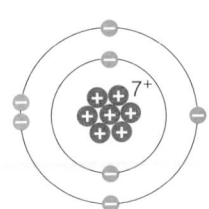

Nitrogen atom (N),
atomic number 7.

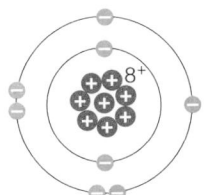

Oxygen atom (O),
atomic number 8.

In these and all diagrams of atoms that follow, only the protons and electrons are shown. The neutrons, which contribute only to atomic weight, not to charge, are omitted.

The most important structural feature of an atom for determining its chemical behavior is the number of electrons in its outermost shell. The first, or innermost, shell is full when it is occupied by two electrons; so an atom with two or more electrons has a filled first shell. When the first shell is full, electrons begin to fill the second shell.

The second shell is completely full when it has eight electrons. A substance that has a full outer shell tends not to enter into chemical reactions. Atomic number 10, neon, is a chemically inert substance because its outer shell is complete. Fluorine, atomic number 9, has a great tendency to draw an electron from other substances to complete its outer shell, and thus it is highly reactive. Carbon has a half-full outer shell, which helps explain its great versatility; it can combine with other elements in a variety of ways to form a large number of compounds.

Atoms seek to reach a state of maximum stability or of lowest energy in the same way that a ball will roll down a hill until it reaches the lowest place. An atom achieves a state of maximum stability:

◆ By gaining or losing electrons to either fill or empty its outer shell.

◆ By sharing its electrons through bonding together with other atoms and thereby completing its outer shell.

The number of electrons determines how the atom will chemically react with other atoms. Hence the atomic number, not the weight, is what gives an atom its chemical nature.

CHEMICAL BONDING

◆

Atoms often complete their outer shells by sharing electrons with other atoms. In order to complete its outer shell, a carbon atom requires four electrons. A hydrogen atom requires one. Thus, when a carbon atom shares electrons with four hydrogen atoms, each completes its outer shell (as shown on the next page).

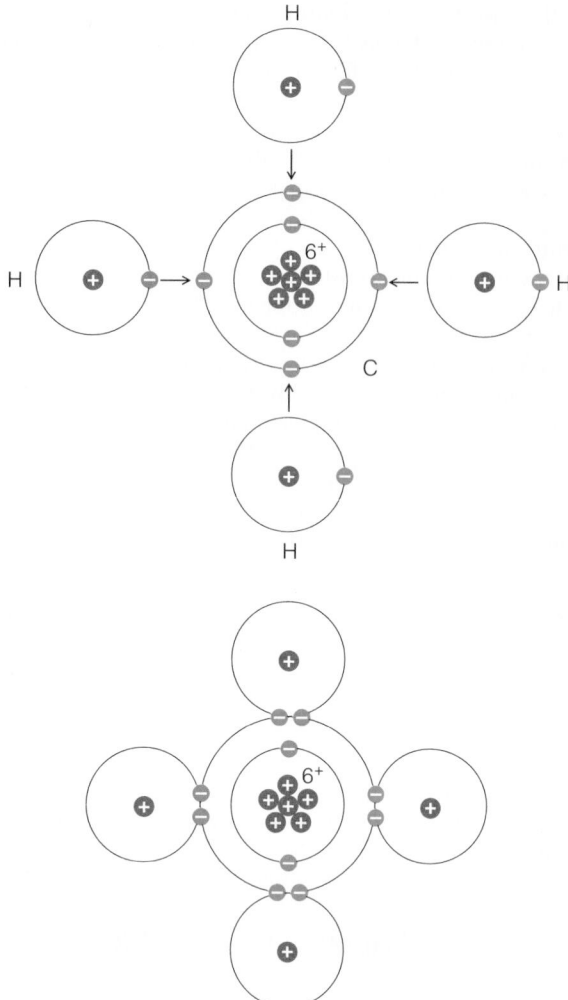

Methane molecule. The chemical formula for methane is CH_4. Note that by sharing electrons, every atom achieves a filled outer shell.

Electron sharing binds the atoms together and satisfies the conditions of maximum stability for the molecule. The outer shell of each atom is complete, since hydrogen effectively has the required two electrons in its first (outer) shell, and carbon has eight electrons in its second (outer) shell; and the molecule is electrically neutral, with a total of ten protons and ten electrons.

Bonds that involve the sharing of electrons, like the bond between carbon and hydrogen, are the most stable kind of association that atoms can form with one another. They are sometimes called covalent bonds, and the resulting combinations of atoms are called molecules. A single pair of shared electrons forms a single bond. A simplified way to

represent a single bond is with a single line. Thus the structure of methane (CH_4) could be represented like this (ignoring the inner-shell electrons, which do not participate in bonding):

$$
\begin{array}{c}
\text{H} \\
| \\
\text{H--C--H} \\
| \\
\text{H}
\end{array}
$$

Methane (CH_4).

Similarly, one nitrogen atom and three hydrogen atoms can share electrons to form one molecule of ammonia (NH_3):

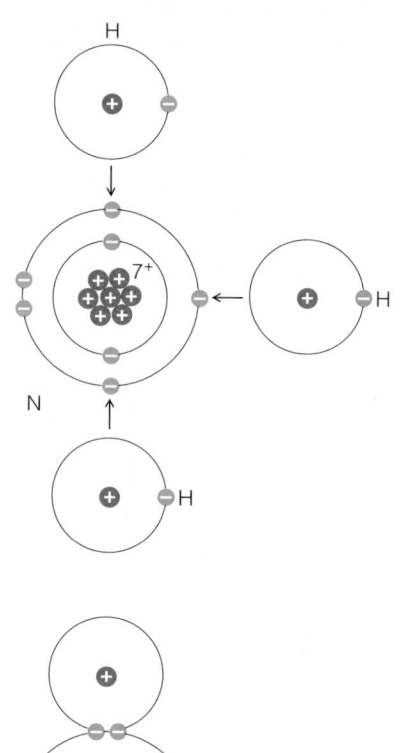

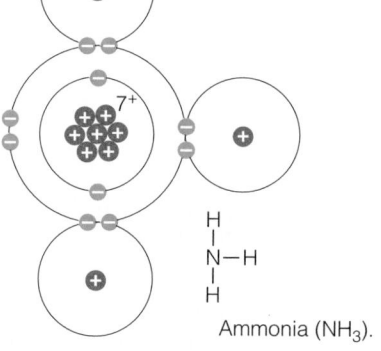

$$
\begin{array}{c}
\text{H} \\
| \\
\text{N--H} \\
| \\
\text{H}
\end{array}
$$

Ammonia (NH_3).

Ammonia molecule (NH_3). Count the electrons in each atom's outer shell to confirm that it is filled.

One oxygen atom may be bonded to two hydrogen atoms to form one molecule of water (H_2O):

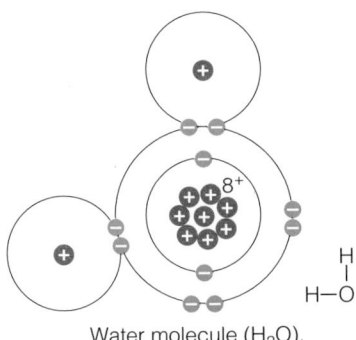

Water molecule (H_2O).

When two oxygen atoms form a molecule of oxygen, they must share two pairs of electrons. This double bond may be represented as two single lines:

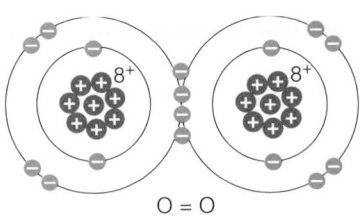

O = O

Oxygen molecule (O_2).

Small atoms form the tightest, most stable bonds. H, O, N, and C are the smallest atoms capable of forming one, two, three, and four electron-pair bonds (respectively). This is the basis for the statement in Chapter 4 that in drawings of compounds containing these atoms, hydrogen must always have one, oxygen two, nitrogen three, and carbon four bonds radiating to other atoms:

$$H- \quad -O- \quad -\overset{|}{N}- \quad -\overset{|}{\underset{|}{C}}-$$

The stability of the associations between these small atoms and the versatility with which they can combine make them very common in living things. Interestingly, all cells, whether they come from animals, plants, or bacteria, contain the same elements in very nearly the same proportions. The atomic elements commonly found in living things are shown in Table B–2.

Table B–2
Elemental Composition of Living Cells

Element	Chemical Symbol	Composition by Weight (%)
Oxygen	O	65
Carbon	C	18
Hydrogen	H	10
Nitrogen	N	3
Calcium	Ca	1.5
Phosphorus	P	1.0
Sulfur	S	0.25
Sodium	Na	0.15
Magnesium	Mg	0.05
Total		99.30[a]

[a]The remaining 0.70 percent by weight is contributed by the trace elements: copper (Cu), zinc (Zn), selenium (Se), molybdenum (Mo), fluorine (F), chlorine (Cl), iodine (I), manganese (Mn), cobalt (Co), and iron (Fe). Cells may also contain variable traces of some of the following: lithium (Li), strontium (Sr), aluminum (Al), silicon (Si), lead (Pb), vanadium (V), arsenic (As), bronium (Br), and others.

FORMATION OF IONS

◆

An atom such as sodium (Na, atomic number 11) cannot easily fill its outer shell by sharing. Sodium possesses a filled first shell of two electrons and a filled second shell of eight; there is only one electron in its outermost shell:

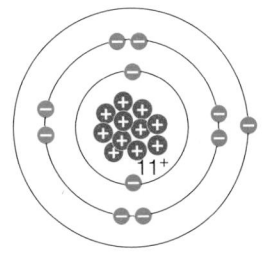

Sodium atom (Na)
11 + charges
11 − charges

0 net charge with one reactive electron in the outer shell

Loss of 1 electron

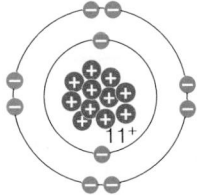

Sodium ion (Na^+)
11 + charges
10 − charges

1 + net charge and a filled outer shell

B

If sodium loses this electron, it satisfies one condition for stability: a filled outer shell (now its second shell counts as the outer shell). However, it is not electrically neutral. It has 11 protons (positive) and only 10 electrons (negative). It therefore has a net positive charge. An atom or molecule that has lost or gained one or more electrons and so is electrically charged is called an ion.

An atom such as chlorine (Cl, atomic number 17), with seven electrons in its outermost shell, can share electrons to fill its outer shell, or it can gain one electron to complete its outer shell and thus give it a negative charge:

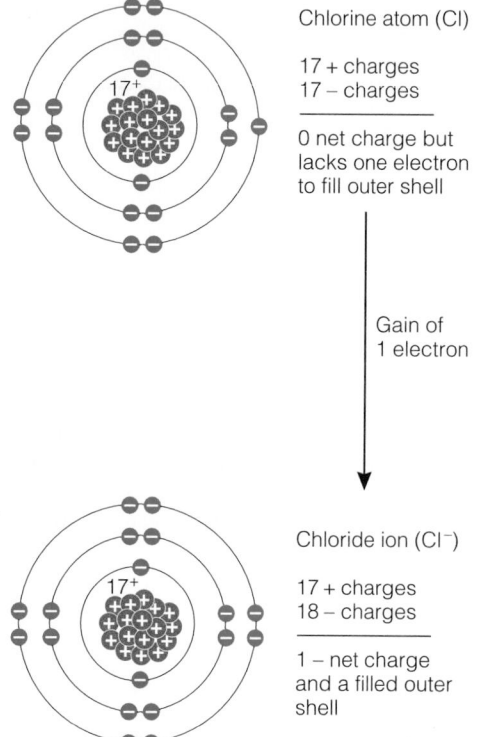

Chlorine atom (Cl)

17 + charges
17 − charges
―――――――――
0 net charge but
lacks one electron
to fill outer shell

Gain of
1 electron

Chloride ion (Cl⁻)

17 + charges
18 − charges
―――――――――
1 − net charge
and a filled outer
shell

A positively charged ion such as sodium ion (Na^+) is called a cation; a negatively charged ion such as a chloride ion (Cl^-) is called an anion. Cations and anions attract one another to form salts:

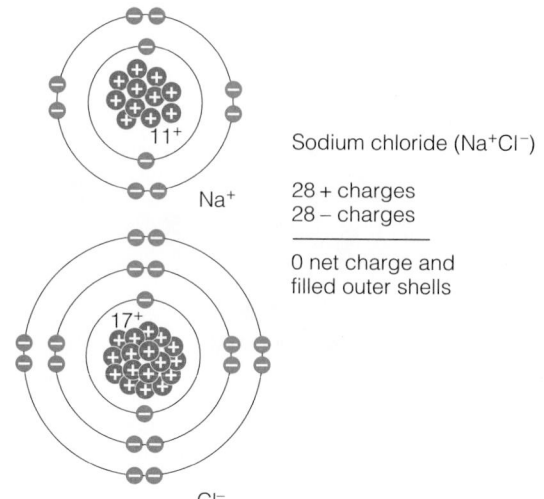

Sodium chloride (Na^+Cl^-)

28 + charges
28 − charges
―――――――――
0 net charge and
filled outer shells

Na^+

Cl^-

With all its electrons, sodium is a shiny, highly reactive metal; chlorine is the poisonous greenish-yellow gas that was used in World War I. But after sodium and chlorine have transferred electrons, they form the stable white salt familiar to you as table salt, or sodium chloride (Na^+Cl^-). The dramatic difference illustrates how profoundly the electron arrangement can influence the nature of a substance. The wide distribution of salt in nature attests to the stability of the union between the ions. Each meets the other's needs (a good marriage).

When dry, salt exists as crystals; its ions are stacked very regularly into a lattice, with positive and negative ions alternating in a three-dimensional checkerboard structure. In water, however, the salt quickly dissolves, and its ions separate from one another, forming an electrolyte solution in which they move about freely. Covalently bonded molecules rarely dissociate like this in a water solution. The most common exception is when they behave like acids and release H^+ ions, as discussed in the next section.

An ion can also be a group of atoms bound together in such a way that the group has a net charge and enters into reactions as a single unit. Many such groups are active in the fluids of the body. The bicarbonate ion is composed of five atoms—one H, one C, and three O—and has a net charge of −1 (HCO_3^-). Another important ion of this type is a phosphate ion with one H, one P, and four O, and a net charge of -2 (HPO_4^{-2}).

Whereas many elements have only one configuration in the outer shell and thus only one way to bond with other elements, some elements have the possibility of varied configurations. Iron is such an element. Under some conditions iron loses two electrons, and under other circumstances it loses three. If iron loses two electrons, it then has a net charge of $+2$, and we call it ferrous iron (Fe^{++}). If it donates three electrons to another atom, it becomes the $+3$ ion, or ferric iron (Fe^{+++}).

Ferrous iron (Fe^{++}) (had 2 outer-shell electrons but has lost them)	Ferric iron (Fe^{+++}) (had 3 outer-shell electrons but has lost them)
26 + charges	26 + charges
24 − charges	23 − charges
2 + net charge	3 + net charge

It is important to remember that a positive charge on an ion means that negative charges—electrons—have been lost and not that positive charges have been added to the nucleus.

WATER, ACIDS, AND BASES

◆

Water The water molecule is electrically neutral, having equal numbers of protons and electrons. However, when a hydrogen atom shares its electron with oxygen, that electron will spend most of its time closer to the positively charged oxygen nucleus. This leaves the positive proton (nucleus of the hydrogen atom) exposed on the outer part of the water molecule. We know, too, that the two hydrogens both bond toward the same side of the oxygen. These two facts explain why water molecules are polar: they have regions of more positive and more negative charge.

Polar molecules like water are drawn to one another by the attractive forces between the positive polar areas of one and the negative poles of another. These attractive forces, sometimes known as polar bonds or hydrogen bonds, occur among many molecules and also within the different parts of single large molecules. Although very weak in comparison with covalent bonds, polar bonds may occur in such abundance that they become exceedingly important in determining the structure of such large molecules as proteins and DNA.

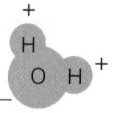

This diagram of the polar water molecule shows displacement of electrons toward the O nucleus; thus the negative region is near the O and the positive regions are near the Hs.

Water molecules have a slight tendency to ionize, separating into positive (H^+) and negative (OH^-) ions. In pure water, a small but constant number of these ions is present, and the number of positive ions exactly equals the number of negative ions.

Acids An acid is a substance that releases H^+ ions (protons) in a water solution. Hydrochloric acid (HCl) is such a substance because it dissociates in a water solution into H^+ and Cl^- ions. Acetic acid is also an acid because it dissociates in water to acetate ions and free H^+:

$$H-\overset{\overset{\textstyle H}{|}}{\underset{\underset{\textstyle H}{|}}{C}}-\overset{\overset{\textstyle O}{\|}}{C}-O-H \longrightarrow H-\overset{\overset{\textstyle H}{|}}{\underset{\underset{\textstyle H}{|}}{C}}-\overset{\overset{\textstyle O}{\|}}{C}-O^- + H^+$$

Acetic acid dissociates into an acetate ion and a hydrogen ion.

The more H^+ ions released, the stronger the acid.

pH Chemists define degrees of acidity by means of the pH scale, which runs from 0 to 14. The pH expresses the concentration of H^+ ions: a pH of 1 is extremely acidic, 7 is neutral, and 13 is very basic. There is a tenfold difference in the concentration of H^+ ions between points on this scale. A solution with pH 3, for example, has *ten times* as many H^+ ions as a solution with pH 4. At pH 7, the concentrations of free H^+ and OH^- are exactly the same—1/10,000,000 moles per liter (10^{-7} moles per liter).* At pH 4, the concentration of free H^+ ions is 1/10,000 (10^{-4}) moles per liter. This is a higher concentration of H^+ ions, and the solution is therefore acidic.

---

*A mole is a certain number (about 6×10^{23}) of molecules. The pH of a solution is defined as the negative logarithm of the hydrogen ion concentration of the solution. Thus, if the concentration is 10^{-2} (moles per liter), the pH is 2; if 10^{-8}, the pH is 8; and so on.

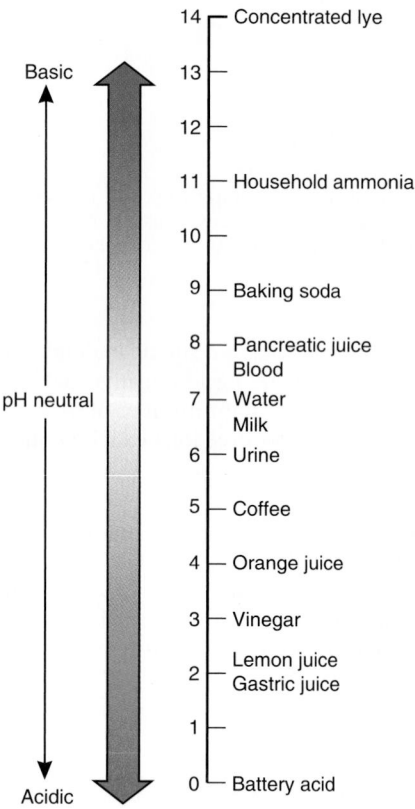

The pH scale.

Note: Each step is ten times as concentrated in base ($^1/_{10}$ as much acid, H^+) as the one below it.

Bases A base is a substance that can soak up, or combine with, H^+ ions, thus reducing the acidity of a solution. The compound ammonia is such a substance. The ammonia molecule has two electrons that are not shared with any other atom; a hydrogen ion (H^+) is just a naked proton with no shell of electrons at all. The proton readily combines with the ammonia molecule to form an ammonium ion; thus a free proton is withdrawn from the solution and no longer contributes to its acidity. Many compounds containing nitrogen are important bases in living systems. Acids and bases neutralize each other to produce substances that are neither acid nor base.

$$
\begin{array}{cc}
\text{H} & \phantom{\text{H--N}}\text{H} \\
| & \phantom{\text{H--N}}| \\
:\text{N--H} + \text{H}^+ \longrightarrow & \text{H--N}^+\text{--H} \\
| & \phantom{\text{H--N}}| \\
\text{H} & \phantom{\text{H--N}}\text{H}
\end{array}
$$

Ammonia captures a hydrogen ion from water. The two dots here represent the two electrons not shared with another atom. These are ordinarily not shown in chemical structure drawings. Compare this with the earlier diagram of an ammonia molecule (p. B-4).

CHEMICAL REACTIONS

◆

A chemical reaction, or chemical change, results in the breakdown of substances and the formation of new ones. Almost all such reactions involve a change in the bonding of atoms. Old bonds are broken, and new ones are formed. The nuclei of atoms are never involved in chemical reactions—only their outer-shell electrons take part. At the end of a chemical reaction, the number of atoms of each type is always the same as at the beginning. For example, two hydrogen molecules ($2H_2$) can react with one oxygen molecule (O_2) to form two water molecules ($2H_2O$). In this reaction two substances (hydrogen and oxygen) disappear, and a new one (water) is formed, but at the end of the reaction there are still four H atoms and two O atoms, just as there were at the beginning. Because the atoms are now linked in a different way, their characteristics or properties have changed.

In many instances chemical reactions involve not the re-linking of molecules but the exchanging of electrons or protons among them. In such reactions the molecule that gains one or more electrons (or loses one or more hydrogen ions) is said to be reduced; the molecule that loses electrons (or gains protons) is oxidized. A hydrogen ion is equivalent to a proton. Oxidation and reduction take place simultaneously because an electron or proton that is lost by one molecule is accepted by another. The addition of an atom of oxygen is also oxidation because oxygen (with six electrons in the outer shell) accepts two electrons in becoming bonded. Oxidation, then, is loss of electrons, gain of protons, or addition of oxygen (with six electrons); reduction is the opposite—gain of electrons, loss of protons, or loss of oxygen. The addition of hydrogen atoms to oxygen to form water can thus be described as the reduction of oxygen *or* the oxidation of hydrogen.

If a reaction results in a net increase in the energy of a compound, it is called an endergonic, or "uphill," reaction (energy, *erg*, is added into, *endo*, the compound). An example is the chief result of photosynthesis, the making of sugar in a plant from carbon dioxide and water using the energy of sunlight. Conversely, the oxidation of sugar to carbon dioxide and water is an exergonic, or "downhill," reaction because the end products have less energy than the starting products. Oftentimes, but not always, reduction reactions are endergonic, resulting in an increase in the energy of the products. Oxidation reactions often, but not always, are exergonic.

Chemical reactions tend to occur spontaneously if the end products are in a lower energy state and therefore are more stable than the reacting compounds. These reactions often give off energy in the form of heat as they occur. The generation of heat by wood burning in a fireplace and the maintenance of human body warmth both depend on energy-

Diagrams:

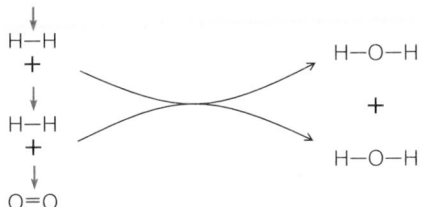

Hydrogen   Oxygen

Water

Structures:

H—H
+
H—H   H—O—H
+   +
H—H   H—O—H
+
O=O

Formulas:

$$2H_2 + O_2 \longrightarrow 2H_2O$$

Hydrogen and oxygen react to form water.

yielding chemical reactions. These downhill reactions occur easily, although they may require some activation energy to get them started, just as a ball requires a push to start rolling downhill.

Uphill reactions, in which the products contain more energy than the reacting compounds started with, do not occur until an energy source is provided. An example of such an energy source is the sunlight used in photosynthesis, where carbon dioxide and water (low-energy compounds) are combined to form the sugar glucose (a higher-energy compound). Another example is the use of the energy in glucose to combine two low-energy compounds in the body into the high-energy compound ATP (see Chapter 7). The energy in ATP may be used to power many other energy-requiring, uphill reactions. Clearly, any of many different molecules can be used as a temporary storage place for energy.

Energy change as reaction occurs

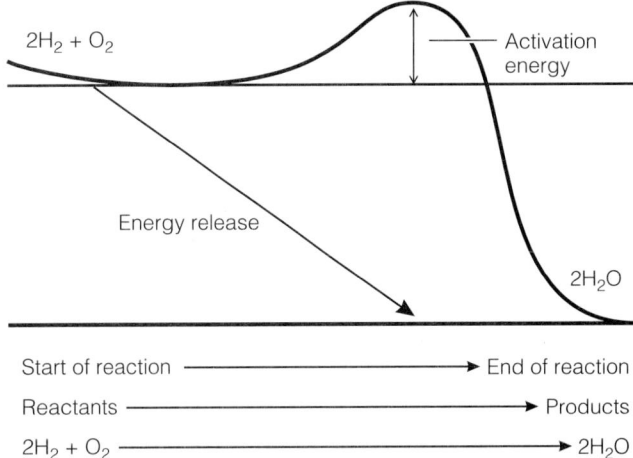

Neither downhill nor uphill reactions occur until something sets them off (activation) or until a path is provided for them to follow. The body uses enzymes as a means of providing paths and controlling chemical reactions (see Chapter 6). By controlling the availability and the action of its enzymes, the body can "decide" which chemical reactions to prevent and which to promote.

FORMATION OF FREE RADICALS
◆

Normally, when a chemical reaction takes place, bonds break and re-form with some redistribution of atoms and rearrangement of bonds to form new, stable compounds. Normally, bonds don't split in such a way as to leave a molecule with an odd, unpaired electron. However, weak bonds can split this way, and when they do, free radicals are formed. Free radicals are highly unstable and quickly react with other compounds, forming more free radicals in a chain reaction.

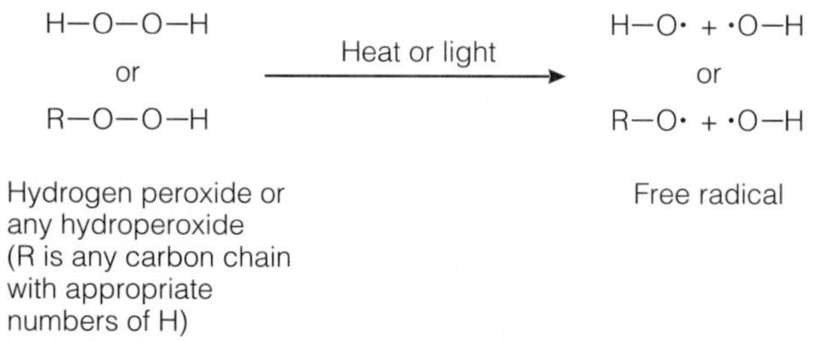

$$H-O-O-H$$

or

$$R-O-O-H$$

Heat or light ⟶

$$H-O\cdot + \cdot O-H$$

or

$$R-O\cdot + \cdot O-H$$

Hydrogen peroxide or
any hydroperoxide
(R is any carbon chain
with appropriate
numbers of H)

Free radical

Free radicals are formed. The dots represent single electrons that are available for sharing (the atom needs another electron to fill its outer shell).

A physical event such as the arrival of an energy-carrying particle of light or other radiation starts the process by breaking a weak bond so that free radicals are formed. A cascade may ensue in which many highly reactive radicals are generated, resulting finally in the disruption of a living structure such as a cell membrane.

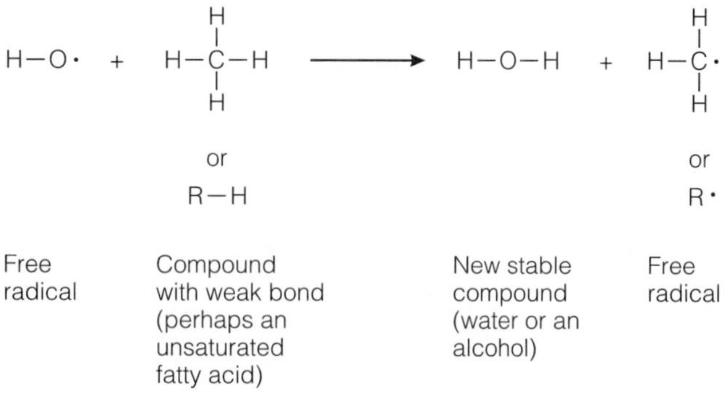

$$H-O\cdot \ + \ H-\overset{\overset{\displaystyle H}{|}}{\underset{\underset{\displaystyle H}{|}}{C}}-H \ \longrightarrow \ H-O-H \ + \ H-\overset{\overset{\displaystyle H}{|}}{\underset{\underset{\displaystyle H}{|}}{C}}\cdot$$

or

$$R-H$$

or

$$R\cdot$$

| Free radical | Compound with weak bond (perhaps an unsaturated fatty acid) | New stable compound (water or an alcohol) | Free radical |

Destruction of biological compounds by free radicals. The free radical attacks a weak bond in a biological compound, disrupting it and forming a new stable molecule and another free radical. This can attack another biological compound, and so on.

Oxidation of some compounds can be induced by air at room temperature in the presence of light. Such reactions are thought to take place through the formation of compounds called peroxides:

Peroxides:

$$H-O-O-H$$ Hydrogen peroxide

$$R-O-O-H$$ Hydroperoxides (R is any carbon chain with appropriate numbers of H)

$$R-O-O-R$$ Peroxide

Some peroxides readily disintegrate into free radicals, initiating chain reactions like those just described.

Free radicals are of special interest in nutrition because the antioxidant properties of vitamins A, C, and E as well as the mineral selenium are thought to protect against the destructive effects of these free radicals (see Highlight 11). For example, vitamin E on the surface of the lungs reacts with, and is destroyed by, free radicals, thus preventing the radicals from reaching underlying cells and oxidizing the lipids in their membranes.

BIOCHEMICAL STRUCTURES AND PATHWAYS

◆

Contents

Carbohydrates

Lipids

Protein: Amino Acids

Vitamins and Coenzymes

Glycolysis

The TCA Cycle

The Electron Transport Chain

Alcohol's Interference with Energy Metabolism

The Urea Cycle

Formation of Ketone Bodies

*T*he diagrams of nutrients presented here are meant to enhance your understanding of the most important organic molecules in the human diet. The names used are those agreed on by the American Institute of Nutrition and other scientific organizations in 1987.[1] Following the diagrams of nutrients are sections on the major metabolic pathways mentioned in Chapter 7—glycolysis, the TCA cycle, and the electron transport chain—and a description of how alcohol interferes with these pathways. Discussions of the urea cycle and the formation of ketone bodies complete the appendix.

CARBOHYDRATES

◆

MONOSACCHARIDES

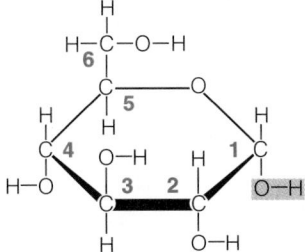

Glucose (alpha form). The ring would be at right angles to the plane of the paper. The bonds directed upward are above the plane; those directed downward are below the plane. This molecule is considered an alpha form because the OH on carbon 1 points downward.

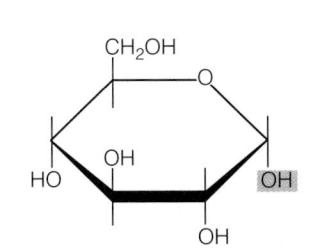

Glucose (alpha form) shorthand notation. This notation, in which the carbons in the ring and single hydrogens have been eliminated, will be used throughout this appendix.

Glucose (beta form). The OH on carbon 1 points upward.
Fructose, galactose: see Chapter 4.

C

DISACCHARIDES

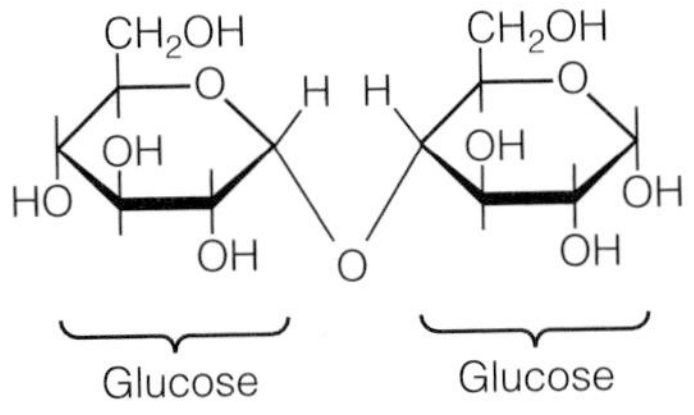

Maltose.

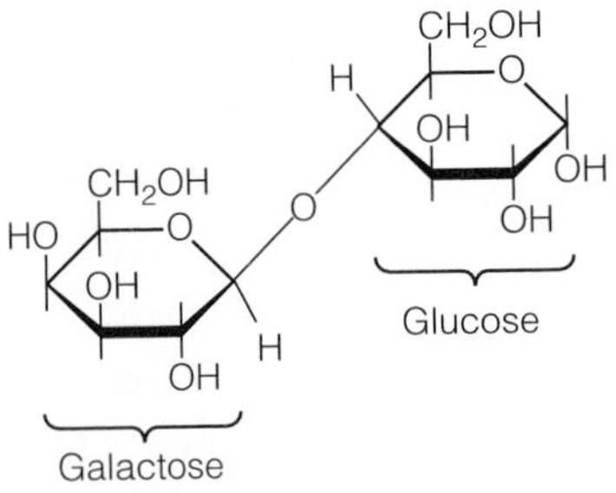

Glucose   Glucose

Galactose

Lactose (alpha form).

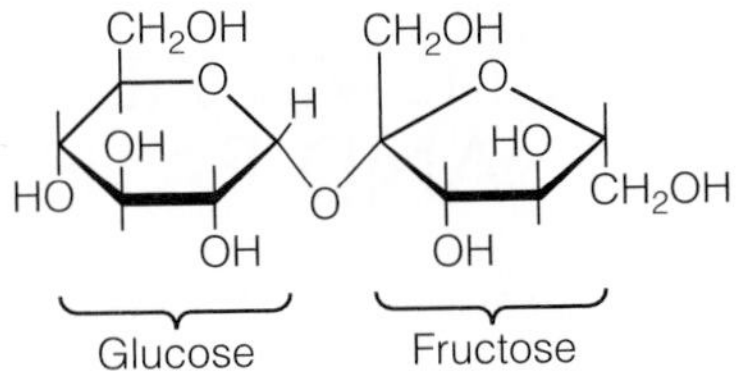

Glucose

Glucose   Fructose

Sucrose.

POLYSACCHARIDES

As described in Chapter 4, starch, glycogen, and cellulose are all long chains of glucose molecules covalently linked together.

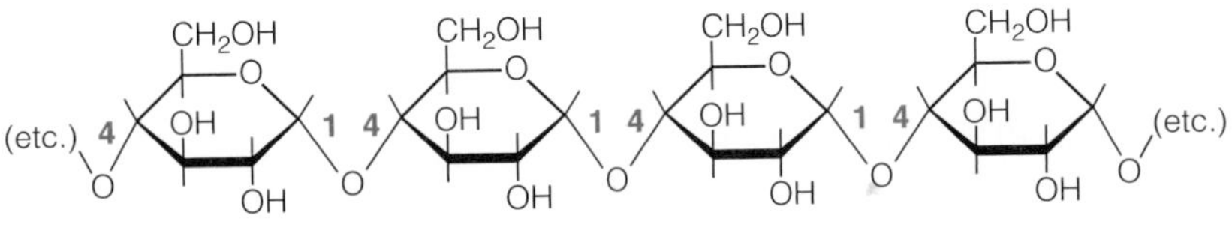

Amylose (unbranched starch)

Starch. Two kinds of covalent linkages occur between glucose molecules in starch, giving rise to two kinds of chains. Amylose is composed of straight chains, with carbon 1 of one glucose linked to carbon 4 of the next (α-1,4 linkage). Amylopectin is made up of straight chains like amylose but has occasional branches arising where the carbon 6 of a glucose is also linked to the carbon 1 of another glucose (α-1,6 linkage).

Glycogen. The structure of glycogen is like amylopectin but with many more branches.

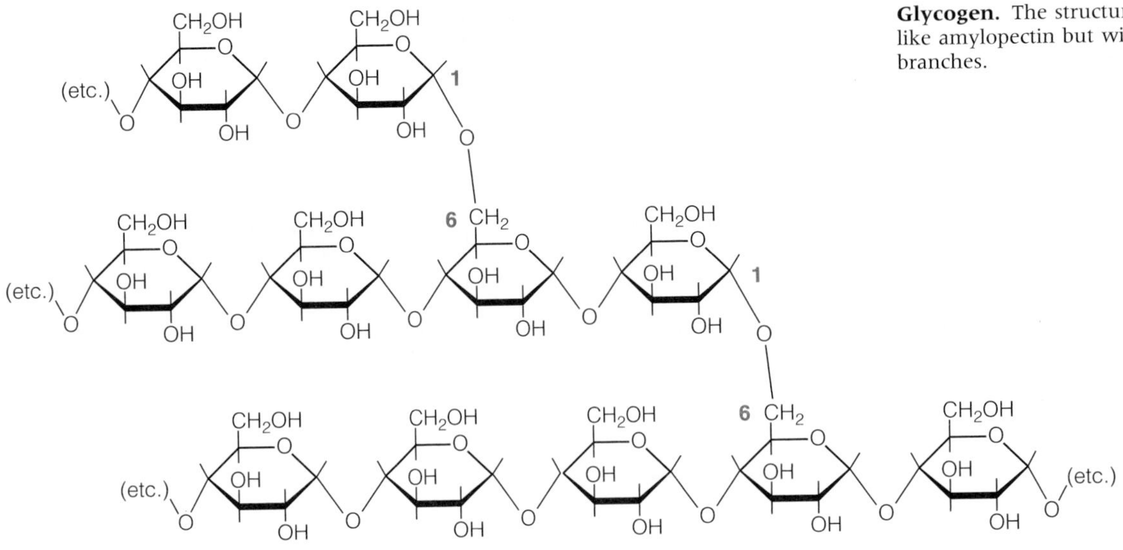

Amylopectin (branched starch)

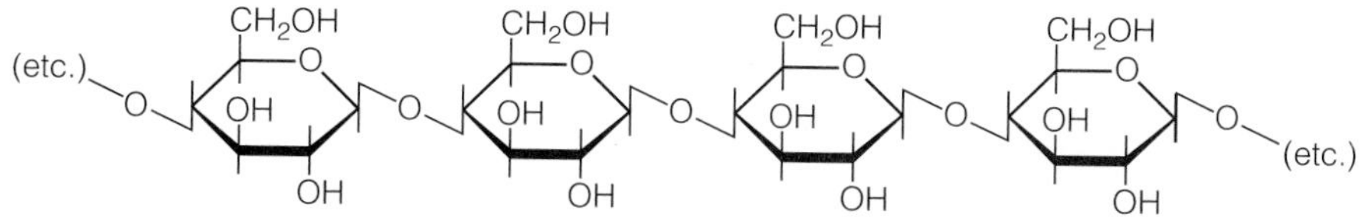

Cellulose. Like starch and glycogen, cellulose is also made of chains of glucose units, but there is an important difference: in cellulose, the OH on carbon 1 is in the beta position (see p. C-1). When carbon 1 of one glucose is linked to carbon 4 of the next, it forms a β-1, 4 linkage, which cannot be broken by digestive enzymes in the human GI tract.

Monosaccharides in backbone chain

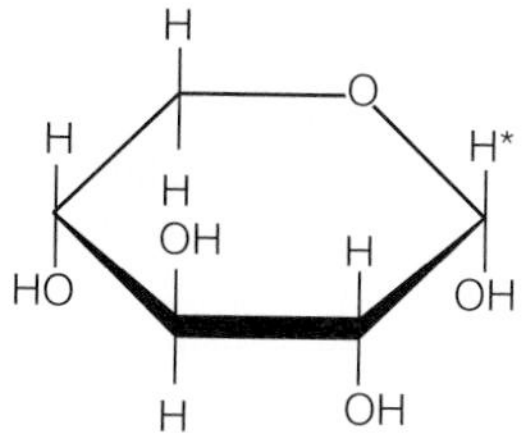

xylose

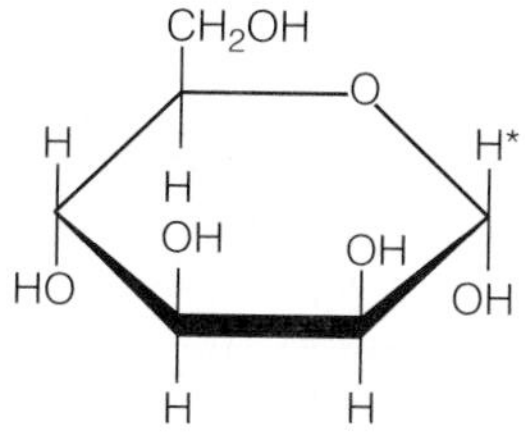

mannose

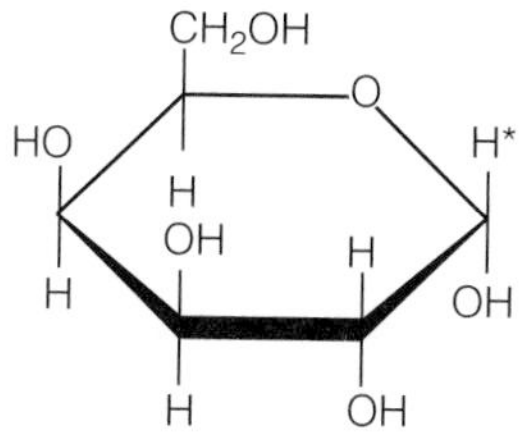

galactose

Monosaccharides in side chains

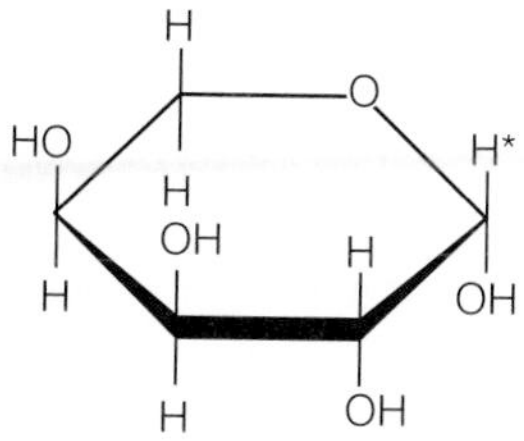

arabinose

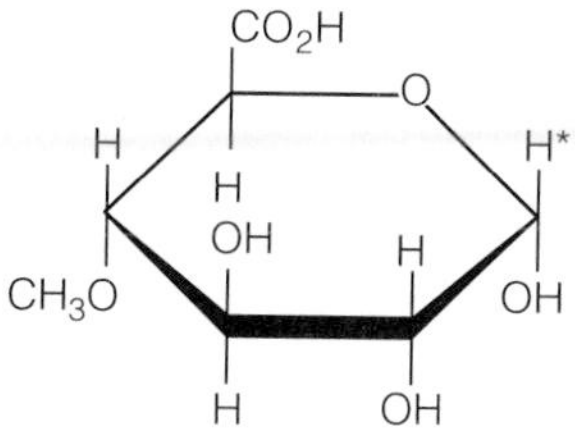

glucuronic acid

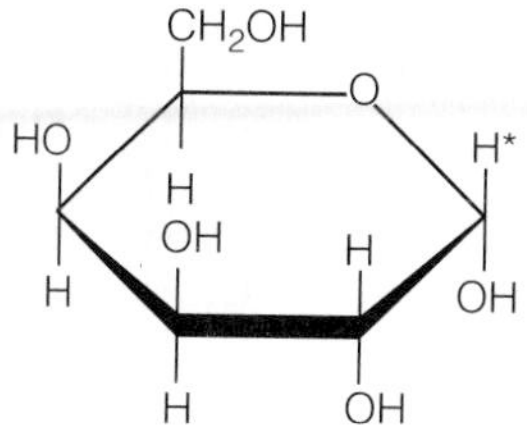

galactose

Hemicelluloses. The most common hemicelluloses are composed of a backbone chain of xylose, mannose, and galactose, with branching side chains of arabinose, glucuronic acid, and galactose.

---

*These structures are shown in the alpha form with the H on the carbon pointing upward and the OH pointing downward, but they may also appear in the beta form with the H pointing downward and the OH upward.

LIPIDS

◆

Table C–1
Saturated Fatty Acids Found in Natural Fats

Saturated Fatty Acids	Chemical Formulas	Number of Carbons	Food Source
Butyric	C_3H_7COOH	4	Butterfat
Caproic	$C_5H_{11}COOH$	6	Butterfat
Caprylic	$C_7H_{15}COOH$	8	Coconut oil
Capric	$C_9H_{19}COOH$	10	Palm oil
Lauric	$C_{11}H_{23}COOH$	12	Coconut oil
Myristic[a]	$C_{13}H_{27}COOH$	14	Coconut oil, butterfat
Palmitic[a]	$C_{15}H_{31}COOH$	16	Animal and vegetable fat
Stearic[a]	$C_{17}H_{35}COOH$	18	Animal and some vegetable fat
Arachidic	$C_{19}H_{39}COOH$	20	Peanut oil

[a]Most common saturated fatty acids.

Table C–2
Unsaturated Fatty Acids Found in Natural Fats

Unsaturated Fatty Acids	Chemical Formulas	Number of Carbons	Number of Double Bonds	Standard Notation[b]	Omega Notation[b]	Food Source
Palmitoleic	$C_{15}H_{29}COOH$	16	1	16:1;9	16:1ω7	Butterfat
Oleic	$C_{17}H_{33}COOH$	18	1	18:1;9	18:1ω9	Olive oil
Linoleic	$C_{17}H_{31}COOH$	18	2	18:2;9,12	18:2ω6	Linseed oil
Linolenic	$C_{17}H_{29}COOH$	18	3	18:3;9,12,15	18:3ω3	Linseed oil
Arachidonic	$C_{19}H_{31}COOH$	20	4	20:4;5,8,11,14	20:4ω6	Lecithin
Eicosapentanoic	$C_{18}H_{29}COOH$	20	5	20:5;5,8,11,14,17	20:5ω3	Fish oils

Note: A fatty acid has two ends; designated the methyl (CH_3) end and the carboxyl, or acid (COOH), end.

[a]Standard chemistry notation begins counting carbons at the acid end. The number of carbons the fatty acid contains comes first, followed by a colon and another number that indicates the number of double bonds; next comes a semicolon followed by a number or numbers indicating the positions of the double bonds. Thus the notation for linoleic acid, an 18-carbon fatty acid with two double bonds between carbons 9 and 10 and between carbons 12 and 13, is 18:2;9,12.

[b]Because fatty acid chains are lengthened by adding carbons at the acid end of the chain, chemists use the omega system of notation to ease the task of identifying them. The omega system begins counting carbons at the methyl end. The number of carbons the fatty acid contains comes first, followed by a colon and the number of double bonds; next comes the omega symbol (ω) and number indicating the position of the double bond nearest the methyl end. Thus linoleic acid with its first double bond at the sixth carbon from the methyl end would be noted 18:2ω6 in the omega system.

PROTEIN: AMINO ACIDS

◆

The common amino acids may be classified into the seven groups listed on the next page.[2] Amino acids marked with an asterisk (*) are essential because human beings cannot synthesize them.

1. Amino acids with aliphatic side chains, which consist of hydrogen and carbon atoms (hydrocarbons):

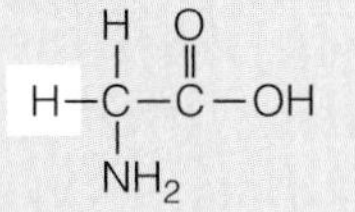

Glycine (Gly)

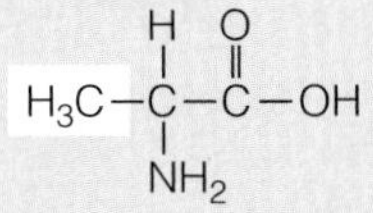

Alanine (Ala)

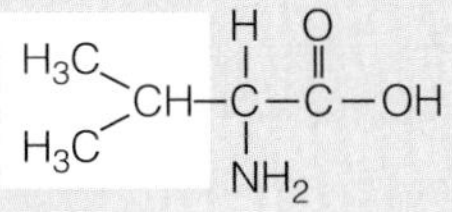

Valine* (Val)

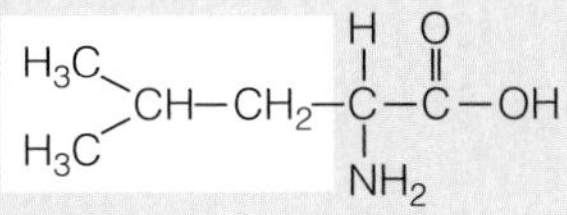

Leucine* (Leu)

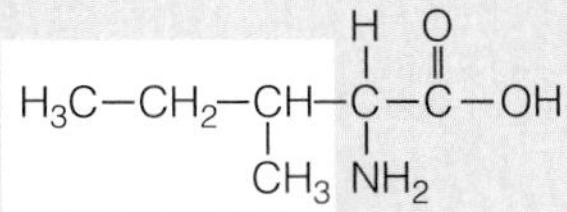

Isoleucine* (Ile)

2. Amino acids with hydroxyl (OH) side chains:

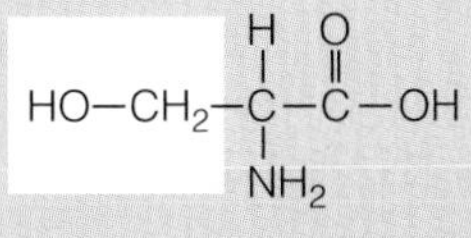

Serine (Ser)

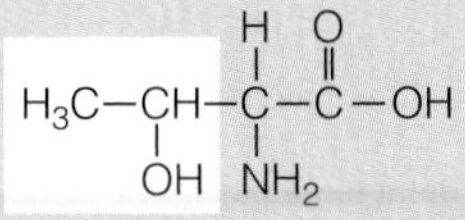

Threonine* (Thr)

3. Amino acids with side chains containing acidic groups or their amides, which contain the group NH$_2$:

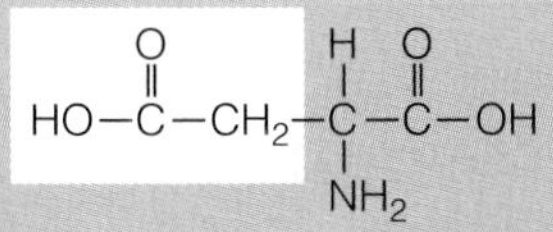

Aspartic acid (Asp)

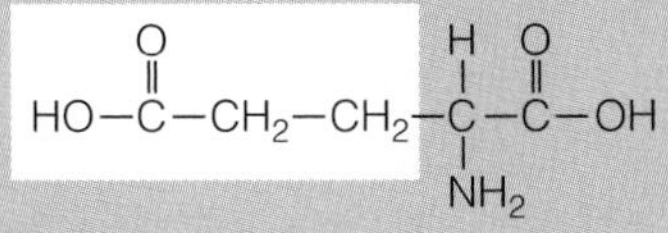

Glutamic acid (Glu)

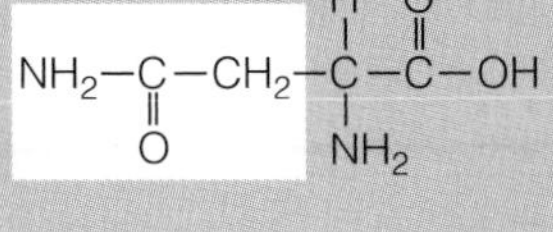

Asparagine (Asn)

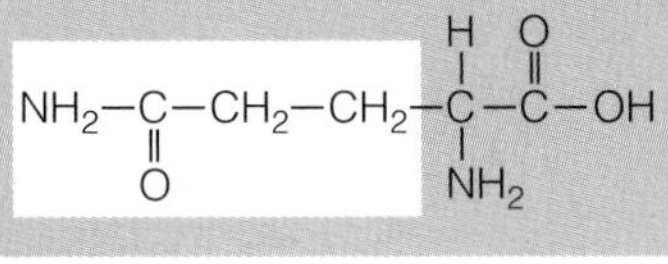

Glutamine (Gln)

4. Amino acids with basic side chains:

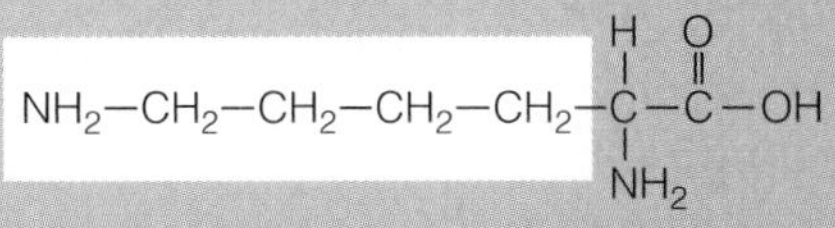

Lysine* (Lys)

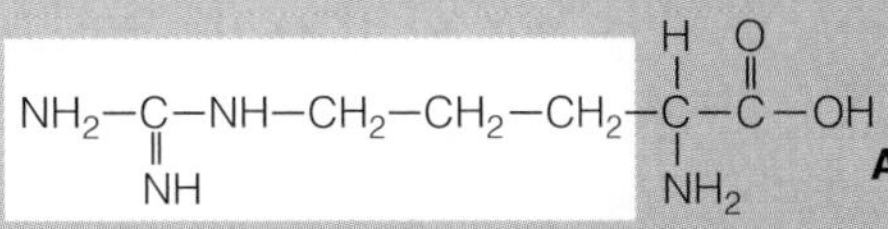

Arginine (Arg)

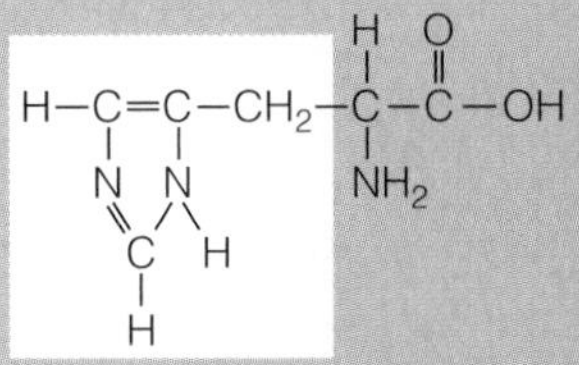

Histidine* (His)

5. Amino acids with aromatic side chains, which are characterized by the presence of at least one ring structure:

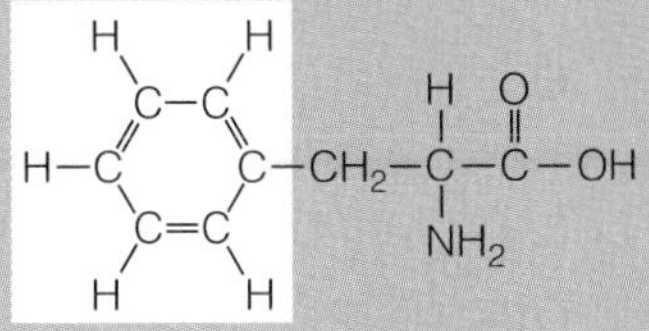

Phenylalanine* (Phe)

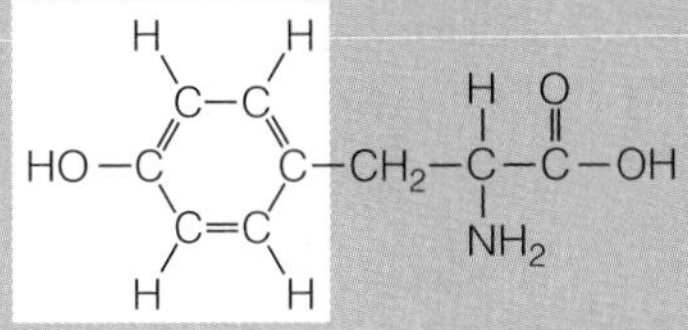

Tyrosine (Tyr)

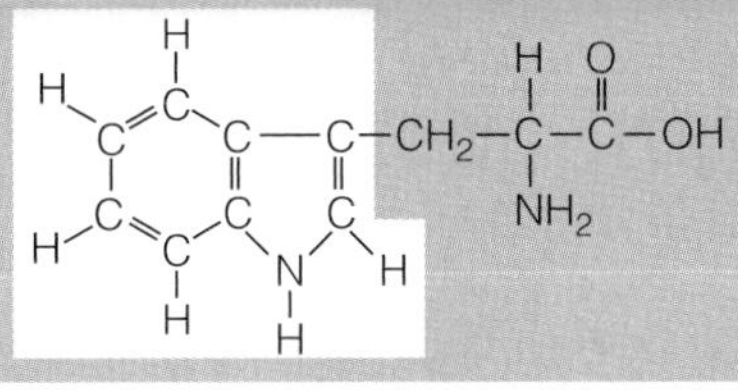

Tryptophan* (Trp)

6. Amino acids with side chains containing sulfur atoms:

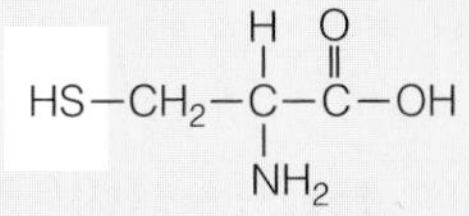

Cysteine (Cys)

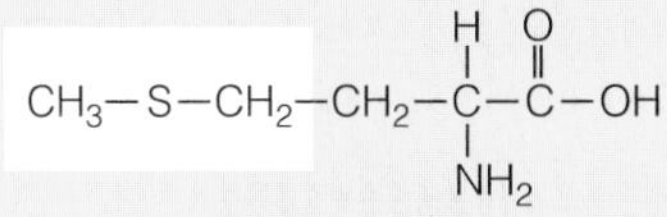

Methionine* (Met)

7. Imino acid:

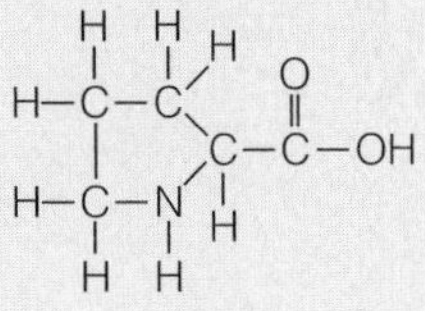

Proline (Pro)[a]

[a]Proline has the same H$_2$N–C–COOH structure as the other amino acids, but its amino group has given up a hydrogen to form a ring.

C

VITAMINS AND COENZYMES

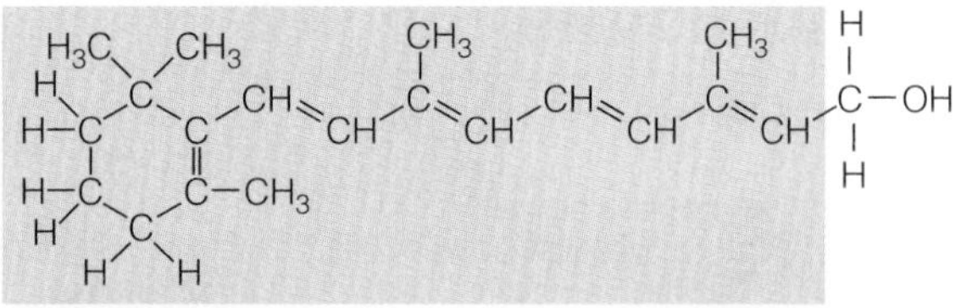

◆

Vitamin A: retinol.

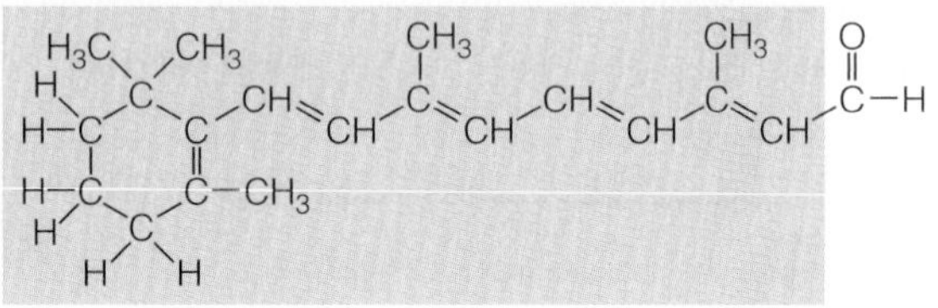

Vitamin A: retinal.

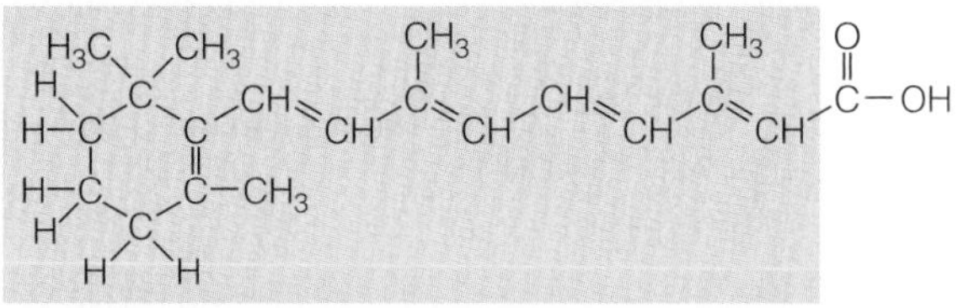

Vitamin A: retinoic acid.

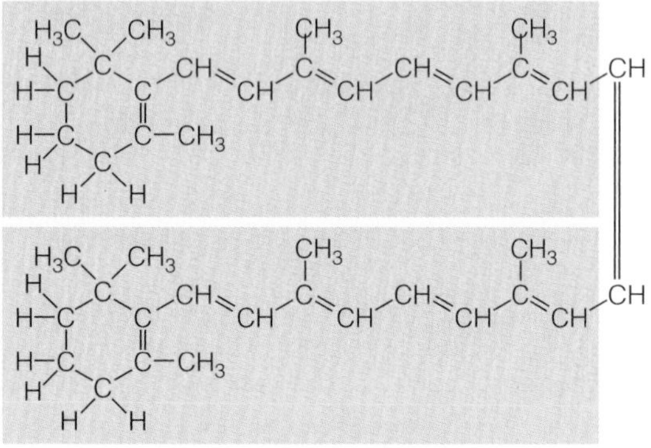

Vitamin A precursor: beta-carotene.

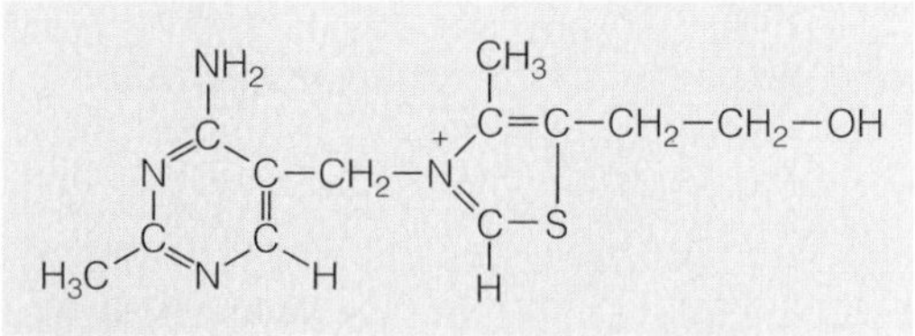

Thiamin. This molecule is part of the coenzyme thiamin pyrophosphate (TPP).

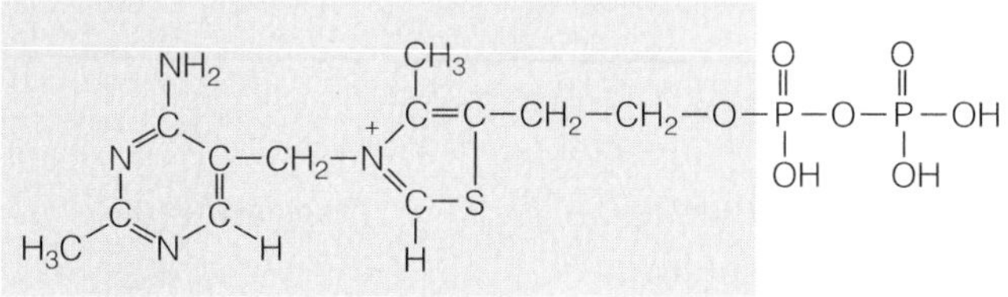

Thiamin pyrophosphate (TPP). TPP is a coenzyme that includes the thiamin molecule as part of its structure.

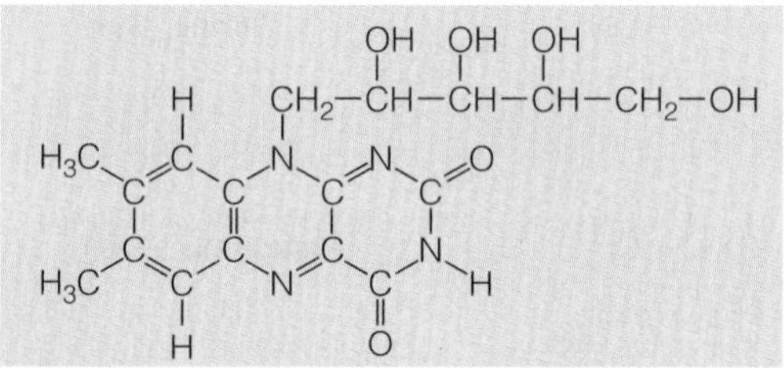

Riboflavin. This molecule is a part of two coenzymes—flavin mononucleotide (FMN) and flavin adenine dinucleotide (FAD).

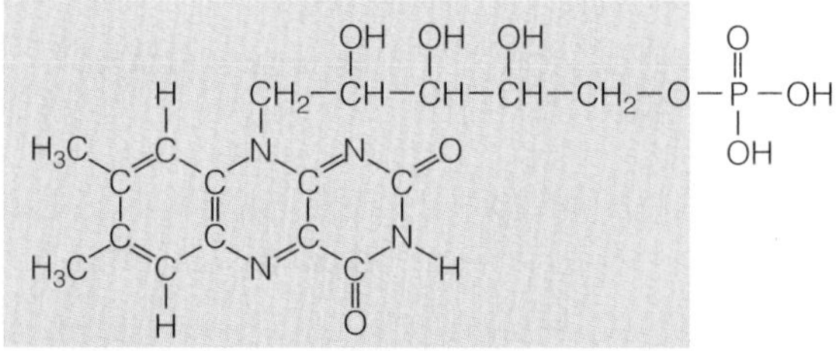

Flavin mononucleotide (FMN). FMN is a coenzyme that includes the riboflavin molecule as part of its structure.

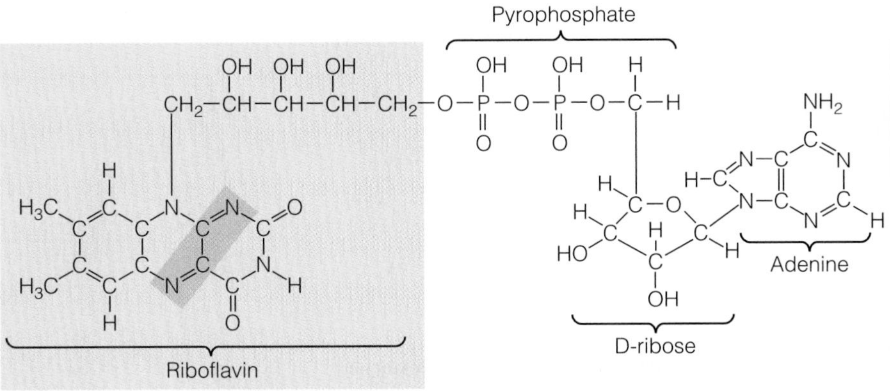

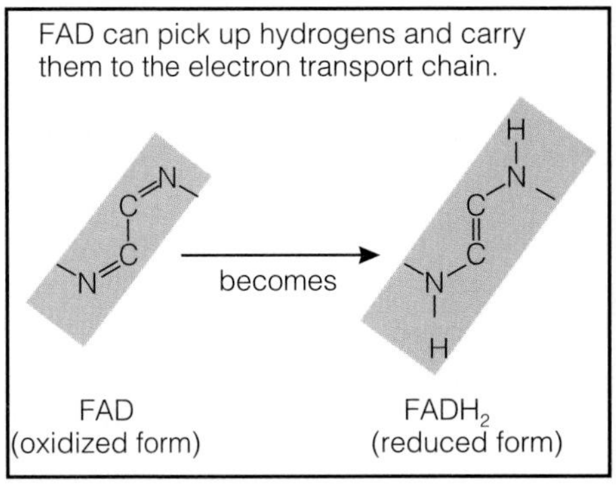

Pyrophosphate

FAD can pick up hydrogens and carry them to the electron transport chain.

becomes

FAD (oxidized form)

FADH$_2$ (reduced form)

Riboflavin

Adenine

D-ribose

Flavin adenine dinucleotide (FAD). FAD is a coenzyme that includes the riboflavin molecule as part of its structure.

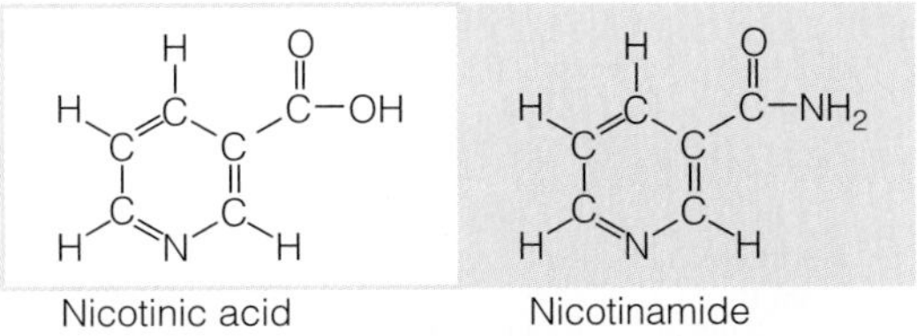

Nicotinic acid

Nicotinamide

Niacin (nicotinic acid and nicotinamide). These molecules are a part of two coenzymes—nicotinamide adenine dinucleotide (NAD$^+$) and nicotinamide adenine dinucleotide phosphate (NADP$^+$).

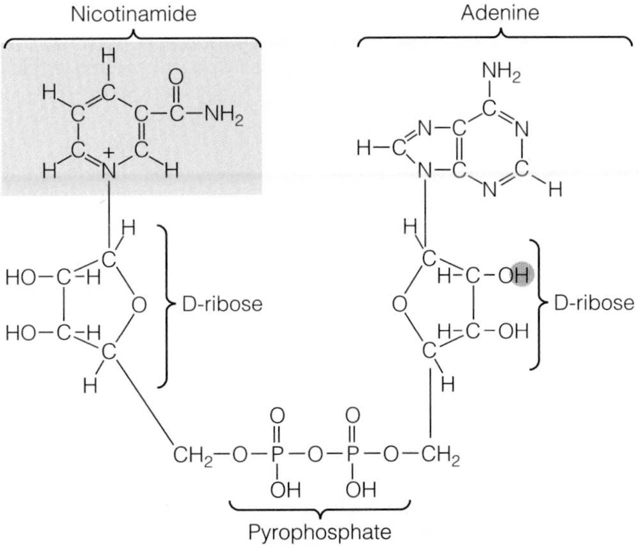

Nicotinamide

Adenine

D-ribose

D-ribose

Pyrophosphate

Nicotinamide adenine dinucleotide (NAD$^+$) and nicotinamide adenine dinucleotide phosphate (NADP$^+$). NADP has the same structure as NAD but with a phosphate group attached to the O instead of the H.

C

Reduced NAD⁺ (NADH). When NAD^+ is reduced by the addition of H^+ and two electrons, it becomes the coenzyme NADH. (The dots on the H entering this reaction represent electrons—see Appendix B.)

Pyridoxine   Pyridoxal   Pyridoxamine

Vitamin B_6 (a general name for three compounds—pyridoxine, pyridoxal, and pyridoxamine). These molecules are a part of two coenzymes—pyridoxal phosphate and pyridoxamine phosphate.

Pyridoxal phosphate   Pyridoxamine phosphate

Pyridoxal phosphate (PLP) and pyridoxamine phosphate. These coenzymes are necessary for transamination and other important processes.

Vitamin B$_{12}$ (cyanocobalamin). The arrows in this diagram indicate that the spare electron pairs on the nitrogens attract them to the cobalt.

Folate (folacin or folic acid). This molecule consists of a double ring combined with a single ring and at least one glutamate (a nonessential amino acid marked in the box).

Tetrahydrofolic acid, the active coenzyme form of folate. This active form has four added hydrogens. An intermediate form, dihydrofolate, has two added hydrogens.

Pantothenic acid

Coenzyme A (CoA). This molecule is made up in part of pantothenic acid.

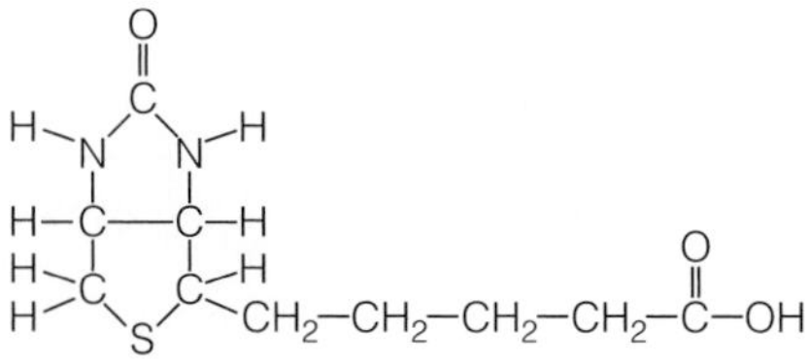

Biotin.

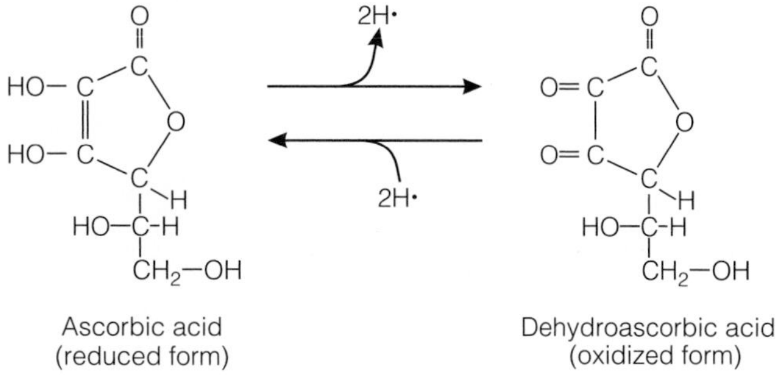

Ascorbic acid
(reduced form)

Dehydroascorbic acid
(oxidized form)

Vitamin C. The dots on the H indicate that two hydrogen atoms, complete with their electrons, are lost when ascorbic acid is oxidized and gained when it is reduced again.

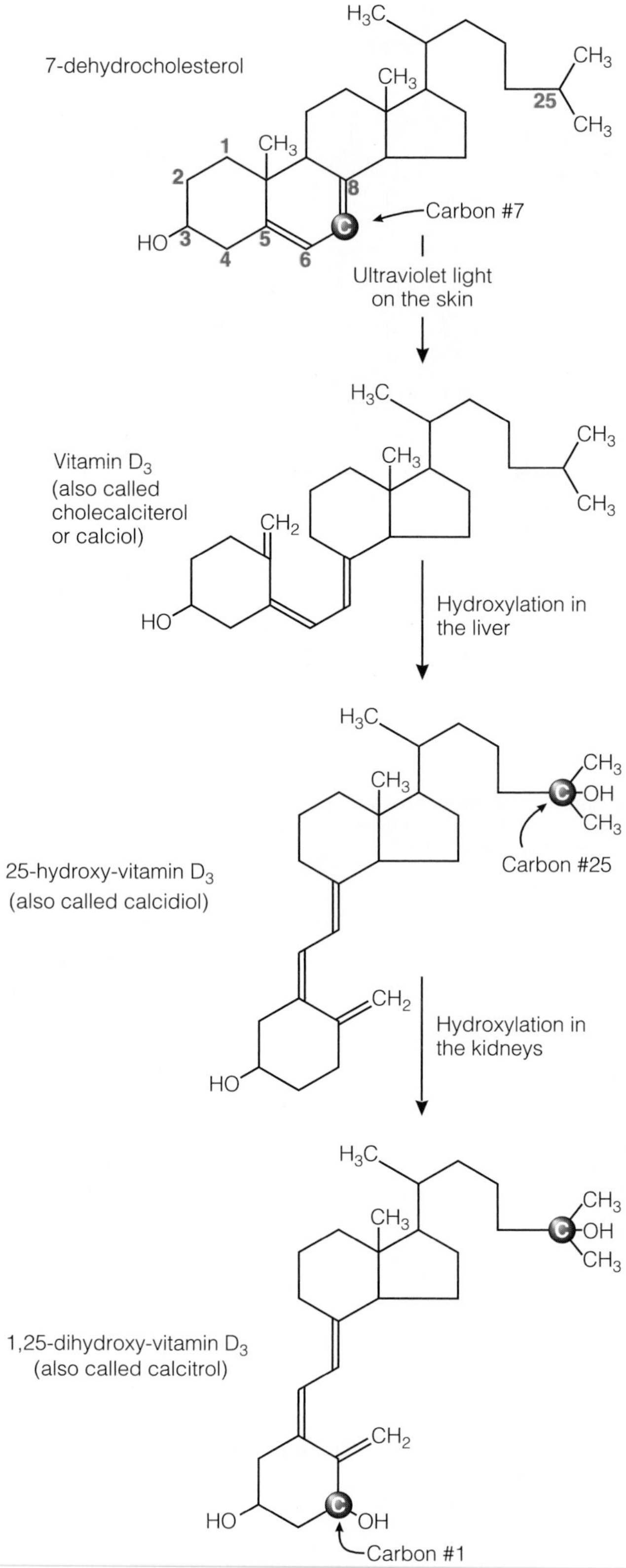

7-dehydrocholesterol

Carbon #7

Ultraviolet light on the skin

Vitamin D_3
(also called cholecalciterol or calciol)

Hydroxylation in the liver

25-hydroxy-vitamin D_3
(also called calcidiol)

Carbon #25

Hydroxylation in the kidneys

1,25-dihydroxy-vitamin D_3
(also called calcitrol)

Carbon #1

Active vitamin D and its precursors, beginning with 7-dehydrocholesterol. (The carbon atoms at which changes occur are numbered.)

Tocotrienols contain double bonds here.

Vitamin E (alpha-tocopherol). The number and position of the methyl groups (CH_3) bonded to the ring structure differentiate among the tocopherols.

Vitamin K, a naturally occurring compound.

Menadione, a synthetic compound that has the same activity as natural vitamin K.

Adenosine triphosphate (ATP), the energy carrier. The cleavage point marks the bond that is broken when ATP splits to become ADP + P.

Adenosine diphosphate (ADP).

GLYCOLYSIS

◆

Figure C–1 (on the next page) depicts the events of glycolysis. First, a phosphate is attached to glucose at the carbon that chemists call number 6. The product is called, logically enough, glucose-6-phosphate.

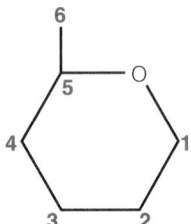

This is the way chemists number the carbons in a glucose molecule.

In the next couple of steps, glucose-6-phosphate is rearranged by an enzyme, and a phosphate is added in another coupled reaction with ATP. (A coupled reaction is a chemical event in which an enzyme complex catalyzes two reactions simultaneously. It often involves the breakdown of one compound and the synthesis of another.)

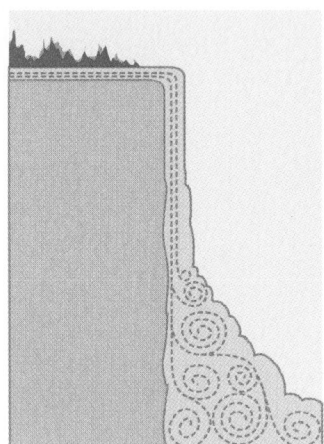

Falling water produces energy that is dissipated without doing work.

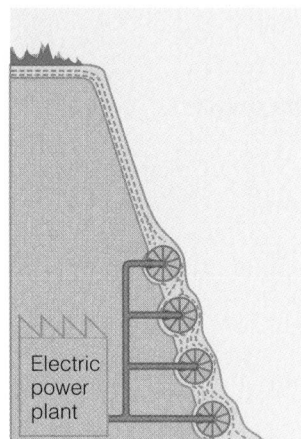

With the addition of a power plant (analogous to an enzyme), the energy of the falling water is coupled with a series of water wheels and turns them, producing energy.

A physical analogy of a coupled reaction. A coupled reaction often involves the breakdown of one compound and the synthesis of another. For example, the breakdown of glucose is coupled with the making of ATP, and the breakdown of ATP is coupled with the activation of glucose, or the making of glucose-P.

The product this time is fructose-1,6-diphosphate. At this point the six-carbon sugar has a phosphate group on its first and sixth carbons and is ready to break apart. Two ATP molecules have been used to accomplish this.

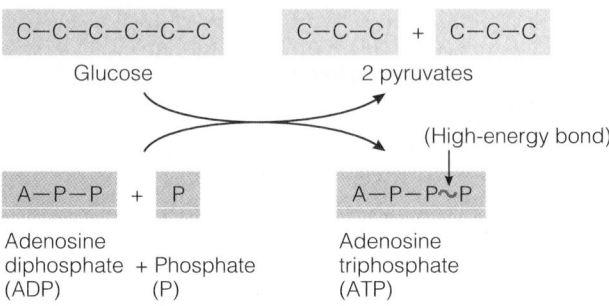

The breakdown of glucose is coupled with the making of ATP (simplified). Actually two ATP are used to prepare glucose for the reactions, and four ATP are gained in the breakdown of one glucose molecule to two molecules of pyruvate.

(From this point to the production of pyruvate, we will use letters in place of compound names. The names are in Figure C–1, for those who wish to know them.)

When fructose-1,6-diphosphate breaks in half, the two three-carbon compounds (A and A′) are not identical. Each has a phosphate group attached, but only one converts directly to pyruvate. The other compound, however, converts easily to the first. (Compound A′ is usually ignored, except for its role as the point of entry for the synthesis of glycerol; we say that two molecules of compound A are derived from one glucose molecule.)

In the step from compound A to compound B, enough energy is released to convert NAD^+ to $NADH + H^+$. Also, in the steps from B to C and from E to pyruvate, ATP is regenerated. Remember that in effect two molecules of compound A are produced from glucose; therefore, four ATP molecules are generated from each glucose molecule. Two ATP were needed to get the sequence started, so the net gain at this point is two ATP and two molecules of $NADH + H^+$.

So far, no oxygen has been used; the process has been anaerobic. But at this point, oxygen is needed. If oxygen is not immediately available, pyruvate converts to lactic acid to soak up the hydrogens from the $NADH + H^+$ that was generated. Lactic acid accumulates until oxygen becomes available. However, in the energy path from glucose to carbon dioxide, this side step usually is not necessary. As you will see later, each $NADH + H^+$ moves to the electron transport chain to unload its hydrogens onto oxygen. The associated energy produces two ATP, making a total yield of eight ATP for the process from glucose to pyruvate.

Figure C–1
Glycolysis

Notice that galactose and fructose enter at different places but all continue on the same pathway. Two molecules of compound A are produced (because compound A' converts to A), and therefore two molecules of each succeeding compound.

- ◆ A = glyceraldehyde-3-phosphate.
- ◆ A' = dihydroxyacetone phosphate.
- ◆ B = 1,3-diphosphoglyceric acid.
- ◆ C = 3-phosphoglyceric acid.
- ◆ D = 2-phosphoglyceric acid.
- ◆ E = phosphoenol pyruvic acid.

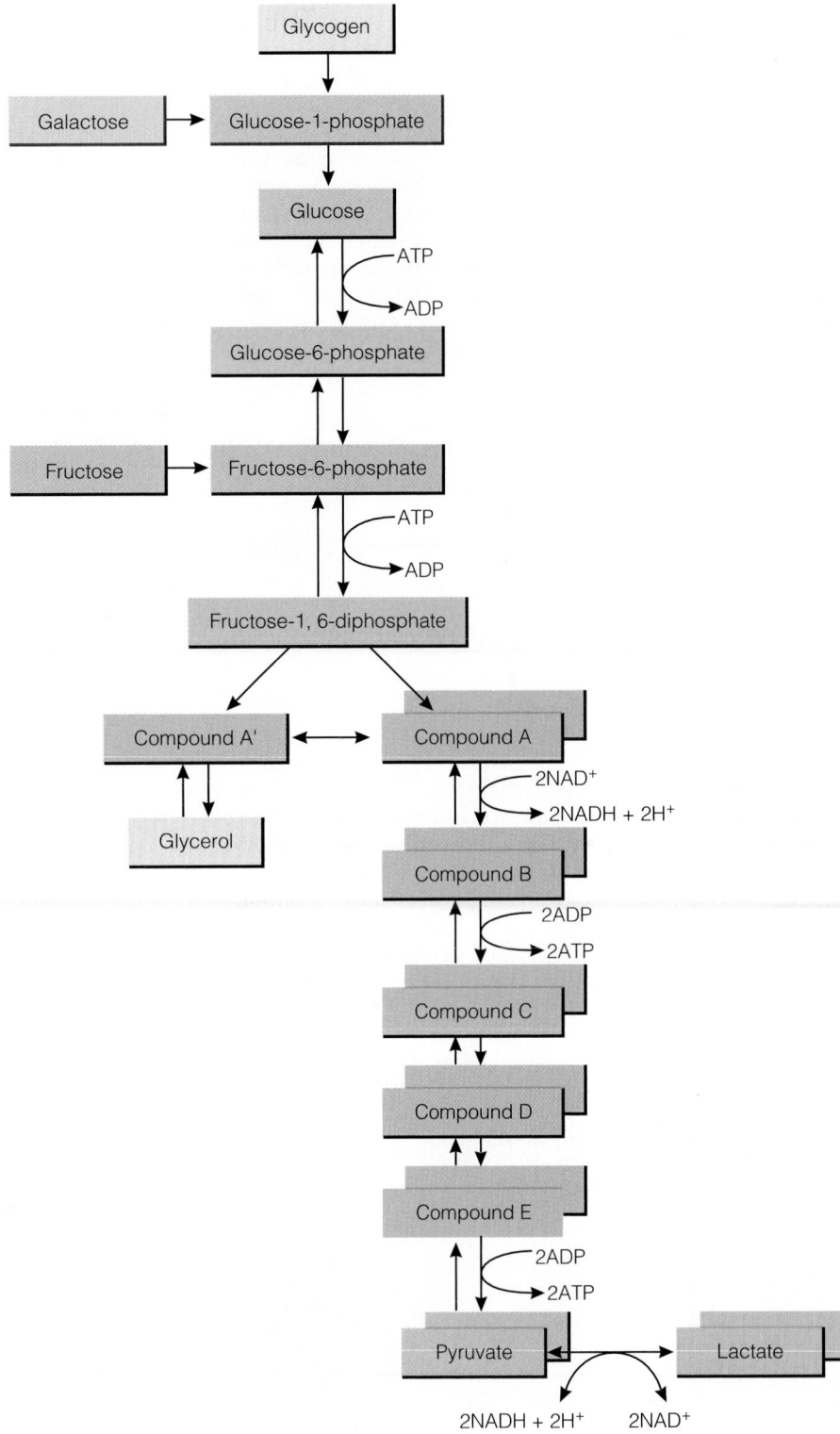

THE TCA CYCLE

◆

The tricarboxylic acid, or TCA, cycle (Figure C–2 on p. C-15) is the name given to the set of reactions involving oxygen and leading from acetyl CoA to carbon dioxide (and water). To link glycolysis to the TCA cycle, pyruvate loses a carbon group and bonds with a molecule of CoA to become acetyl CoA. The TCA cycle is not restricted to the metabolism of carbohydrate. It also includes fat and protein. Any substance that can be converted to acetyl CoA directly, or indirectly through pyruvate, may enter the cycle.

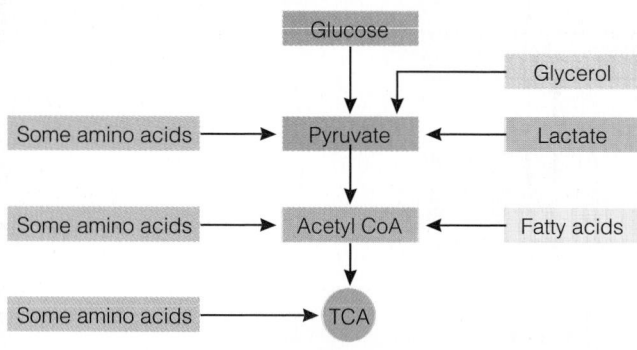

The step from pyruvate to acetyl CoA is exceedingly complex. We have included only those substances that will help you understand the transfer of energy from the nutrients. In the presence of oxygen, pyruvate loses a carbon

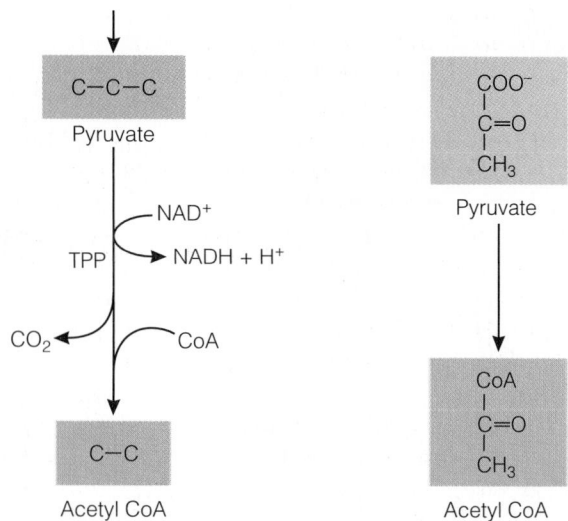

The step from pyruvate to acetyl CoA. (TPP and NAD are coenzymes containing the B vitamins thiamin and niacin, respectively.)

to carbon dioxide and is attached to a molecule of CoA. In the process, NAD^+ picks up two hydrogens with their associated energy, becoming $NADH + H^+$.

As the acetyl CoA breaks down to carbon dioxide and water, its energy is captured in ATP. Let's follow the steps by which this occurs (see Figure C–2).

1. The two-carbon acetyl CoA combines with a four-carbon compound, oxaloacetate. The CoA comes off, and the product is a six-carbon compound, citrate.
2. The atoms of citrate are rearranged to form isocitrate.
3. Now NAD^+ reacts with isocitrate. Two H and two electrons are removed from the isocitrate. One H becomes attached to the NAD^+ with the two electrons; the other H is released as H^+. Thus NAD^+ becomes $NADH + H^+$. (Remember this $NADH + H^+$. It is carrying the H and the energy released from the last reaction. But let's follow the carbons first.) A carbon is combined with two oxygens, forming carbon dioxide (which diffuses away into the blood and is exhaled). What is left is the five-carbon compound alpha-ketoglutarate.
4. Now two compounds interact with alpha-ketoglutarate —a molecule of CoA and a molecule of NAD^+. In this complex reaction, a carbon and two oxygens are removed (forming carbon dioxide); two hydrogens are removed and go to NAD^+ (forming $NADH + H^+$); and the remaining four-carbon compound is attached to the CoA, forming succinyl CoA. (Remember this $NADH + H^+$ also. You will see later what happens to it.)
5. Now two molecules react with succinyl CoA—a molecule called GDP and one of phosphate (P). The CoA comes off, the GDP and P combine to form the high-energy compound GTP (similar to ATP), and succinate remains. (Remember this GTP.)
6. In the next reaction, two H with their energy are removed from succinate and are transferred to a molecule called FAD (an electron-hydrogen receiver like NAD^+) to form $FADH_2$. The product that remains is fumarate. (Remember this $FADH_2$.)
7. Next a molecule of water is added to fumarate, forming malate.
8. A molecule of NAD^+ reacts with the malate; two H with their associated energy are removed from the malate and form $NADH + H^+$. The product that remains is the four-carbon compound oxaloacetate. (Remember this $NADH + H^+$.)

We are back where we started. The oxaloacetate formed in this process can combine with another molecule of acetyl CoA (step 1), and the cycle can begin again. The whole scheme is shown in Figure C–2.

**Figure C–2
The TCA Cycle**

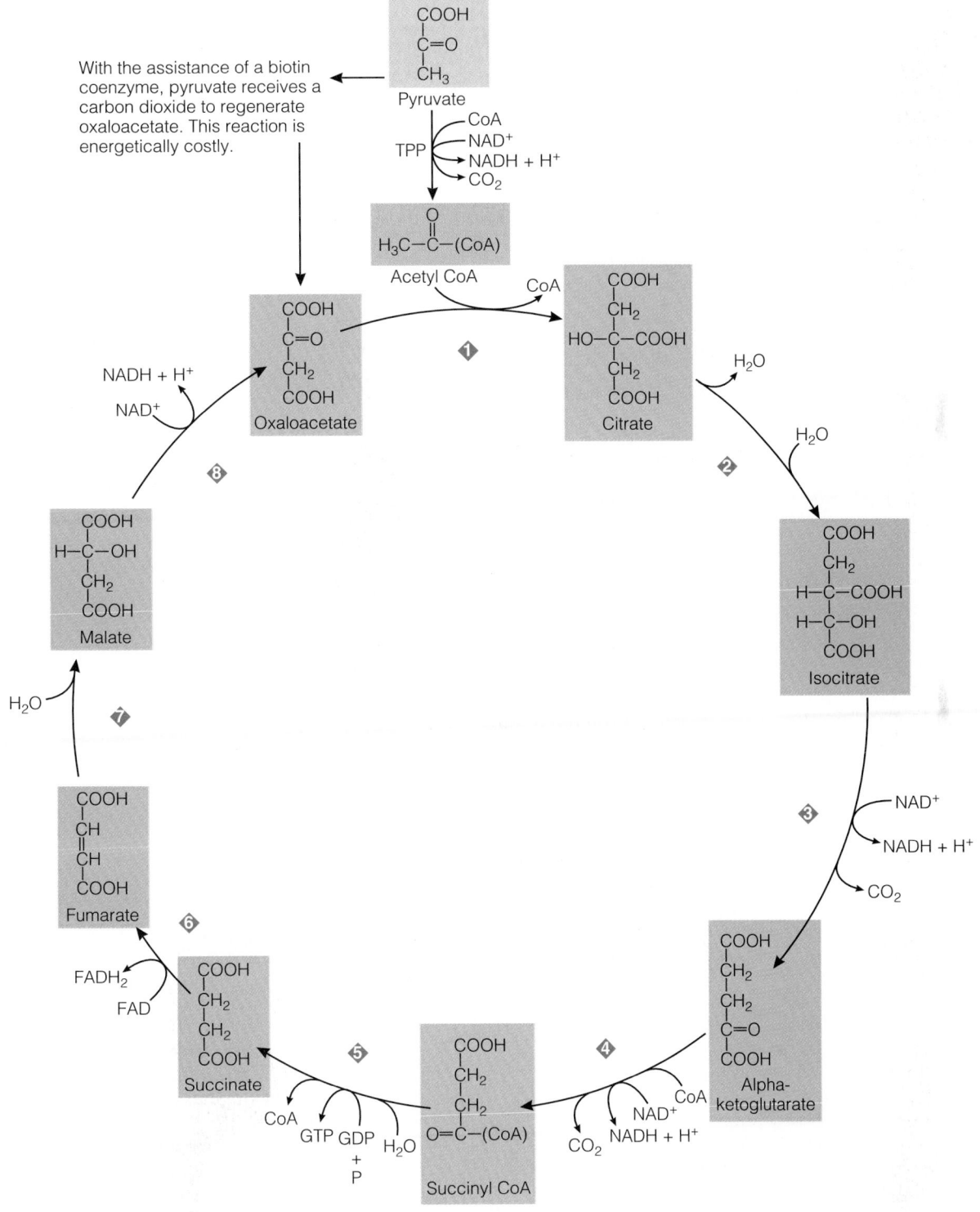

So far, we have seen two carbons brought in with acetyl CoA and two carbons ending up in carbon dioxide. But where are the energy and the ATP we promised?

Each time a pair of hydrogen atoms is removed from one of the compounds in the cycle, it includes a pair of electrons. Then the energy from this chemical bond is captured in the compound to which the H become attached. A review of the eight steps of the cycle shows that energy is transferred in this way into other compounds in steps 3, 4, 6, and 8. In step 5, energy is stored when GDP and P are bound together to form GTP. Thus the compounds NADH + H$^+$ (three molecules), FADH$_2$, and GTP store energy originally found in acetyl CoA. To see how this energy ends up in ATP, we must follow the electrons further. Let us take those attached to NAD$^+$ as an example.

THE ELECTRON TRANSPORT CHAIN
◆

The six reactions described here are those of the electron transport chain, which is shown in Figure C–3. Since oxygen is required for these reactions, and ADP and P are combined to form ATP in several of them (ADP is phosphorylated), these reactions are also called oxidative phosphorylation.

An important concept to remember at this point is that an electron is not a fixed amount of energy. The electrons that bond the H to NAD$^+$ in NADH have a relatively large amount of energy. In the series of reactions that follow, they lose this energy in small amounts, until at the end they are attached (with H) to oxygen (O) to make water (H$_2$O). In some of the steps, the energy they lose is captured into ATP in coupled reactions.

1. In the first step of the electron transport chain, NADH reacts with a molecule called a flavoprotein, losing its electrons (and their H). The products are NAD$^+$ and reduced flavoprotein. A little energy is lost as heat in this reaction.
2. The flavoprotein passes on the electrons to a molecule called coenzyme Q. Again they lose some energy as heat, but ADP and P bond together and form ATP, storing much of the energy. This is a coupled reaction: ADP + P → ATP.
3. Coenzyme Q passes the electrons to cytochrome b. Again the electrons lose energy.
4. Cytochrome b passes the electrons to cytochrome c in a coupled reaction in which ATP is formed: ADP + P → ATP.
5. Cytochrome c passes the electrons to cytochrome a.
6. Cytochrome a passes them (with their H) to an atom of oxygen (O), forming water (H$_2$O). This is a coupled reaction in which ATP is formed: ADP + P → ATP.

Figure C–3
The Electron Transport Chain

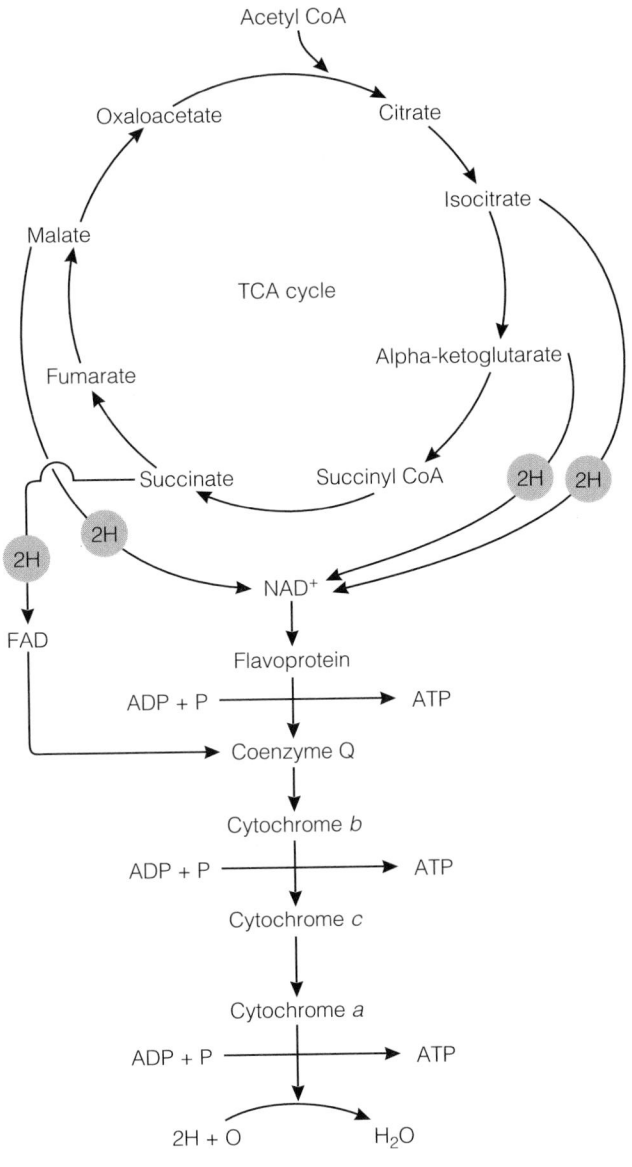

As Figure C–3 shows, each time NADH is oxidized (loses its electrons) by this means, the energy it loses is parceled out into three ATP molecules. When the electrons are passed on to water at the end, they are much lower in energy than they were originally. This completes the story of the electrons from NADH.

As for FADH$_2$, its electrons enter the electron transport chain at coenzyme Q. From coenzyme Q to water, ATP is generated in only two steps. Therefore, FADH$_2$ coming out of the TCA cycle yields just two ATP molecules.

Table C-3
Balance Sheet for Glucose Metabolism

	Expenditures	Income
Glycolysis:		
1 glucose	2 ATP	4 ATP
1 fructose-1,6-diphosphate		2 NADH + H$^+$
2 pyruvate		2 NADH + H$^+$
TCA cycle:		
2 isocitrate		2 NADH + H$^+$
2 alpha-ketoglutarate		2 NADH + H$^+$
2 succinyl CoA		2 GTP
2 succinate		2 FADH$_2$
2 malate		2 NADH + H$^+$
Total ATP collected:		
From glycolysis	2 ATP	4 ATP
From 2 NADH + H$^+$		4–6 ATP[a]
From 8 NADH + H$^+$		24 ATP
From 2 GTP		2 ATP
From 2 FADH$_2$		4 ATP
Totals:	2 ATP	38–40 ATP
Balance on hand from		
1 molecule of glucose:		36–38 ATP

[a]Each NADH + H$^+$ from glycolysis can yield 2 or 3 ATP. See the accompanying text.

One energy-receiving compound of the TCA cycle (GTP) does not enter the electron transport chain but gives its energy directly to ADP in a simple phosphorylation reaction. This reaction yields one ATP.

It is now possible to draw up a balance sheet of glucose metabolism (see Table C–3). Glycolysis has yielded 4 NADH + H$^+$ and 4 ATP molecules and has spent 2 ATP. The 2 acetyl CoA going through the TCA cycle have yielded 6 NADH + H$^+$, 2 FADH$_2$, and 2 GTP molecules. After the NADH + H$^+$ and FADH$_2$ have gone through the electron transport chain, there are 34 ATP. Added to these are the 4 ATP from glycolysis and the 2 ATP from GTP, making the total 40 ATP generated from one molecule of glucose. After

the expense of 2 ATP is subtracted, there is a net gain of 38 ATP.*

The TCA cycle and the electron transport chain are the body's major means of capturing the energy from nutrients in ATP molecules. Other means, such as anaerobic glycolysis, contribute, but the aerobic processes are the most efficient. Biologists and chemists understand much more about these processes than has been presented here.

ALCOHOL'S INTERFERENCE WITH ENERGY METABOLISM

♦

Highlight 7 provides an overview of how alcohol interferes with energy metabolism. With an understanding of the TCA cycle, a few more details may be appreciated. During alcohol metabolism, the enzyme alcohol dehydrogenase oxidizes alcohol to acetaldehyde while it simultaneously reduces a molecule of NAD$^+$ to NADH + H$^+$. The related enzyme acetaldehyde dehydrogenase reduces another NAD$^+$ to NADH + H$^+$ while it oxidizes acetaldehyde to acetyl CoA, the compound that enters the TCA cycle to generate energy. Thus whenever alcohol is being metabolized in the body, NAD$^+$ diminishes, and NADH + H$^+$ accumulates. Chemists say that the body's "redox state" is altered, because NAD$^+$ can oxidize, and NADH + H$^+$ can reduce, many other body compounds. During alcohol metabolism, NAD$^+$ becomes unavailable for the multitude of reactions for which it is required.

As the previous sections just explained, for glucose to be completely metabolized, the TCA cycle must be operating, and NAD$^+$ must be present. If these conditions are not met (and when alcohol is present, they may not be), the pathway will be blocked, and traffic will back up—or an alternate route will be taken. Think about this as you follow the pathway shown in Figure C–4 on p. C-18.

In each step of alcohol metabolism in which NAD$^+$ is converted to NADH + H$^+$, hydrogen ions accumulate, resulting in a dangerous shift of the acid-base balance toward acid (Chapter 12 explains acid-base balance). The accumulation of NADH + H$^+$ depresses TCA cycle activity, so pyruvate and acetyl CoA build up. This condition favors the conversion of pyruvate to lactic acid, which serves as a temporary storage place for hydrogens from NADH + H$^+$. The conversion of pyruvate to lactic acid restores some NAD$^+$, but a lactic acid buildup has serious consequences of its own. It adds to the body's acid burden and interferes with the excretion of uric acid, causing goutlike symptoms. Molecules of acetyl CoA become building blocks for fatty acids or ketone bodies. The making of ketone bodies consumes acetyl CoA and generates NAD$^+$; but some ketone bodies are acids, so they push the acid-base balance further toward acid.

---

*The total may sometimes be 36 or 37, rather than 38, ATP. The NADH + H$^+$ generated in the cytoplasm during glycolysis pass their electrons on to shuttle molecules, which move them into the mitochondria. One shuttle, malate, contributes its electrons to the electron transport chain before the first site of ATP synthesis, yielding 3 ATP. Another, glycerol phosphate, adds its electrons into the chain beyond that first site, yielding 2 ATP. Thus sometimes 3, and sometimes only 2, ATP result from the NADH + H$^+$ that arise from glycolysis. The amount depends on the cell.

Figure C–4
Ethanol Enters the Metabolic Path

This is a simplified version of the glucose-to-energy pathway showing the entry of ethanol. The coenzyme NAD (which is the active form of the B vitamin niacin) is the only one shown here; however, many others are involved.

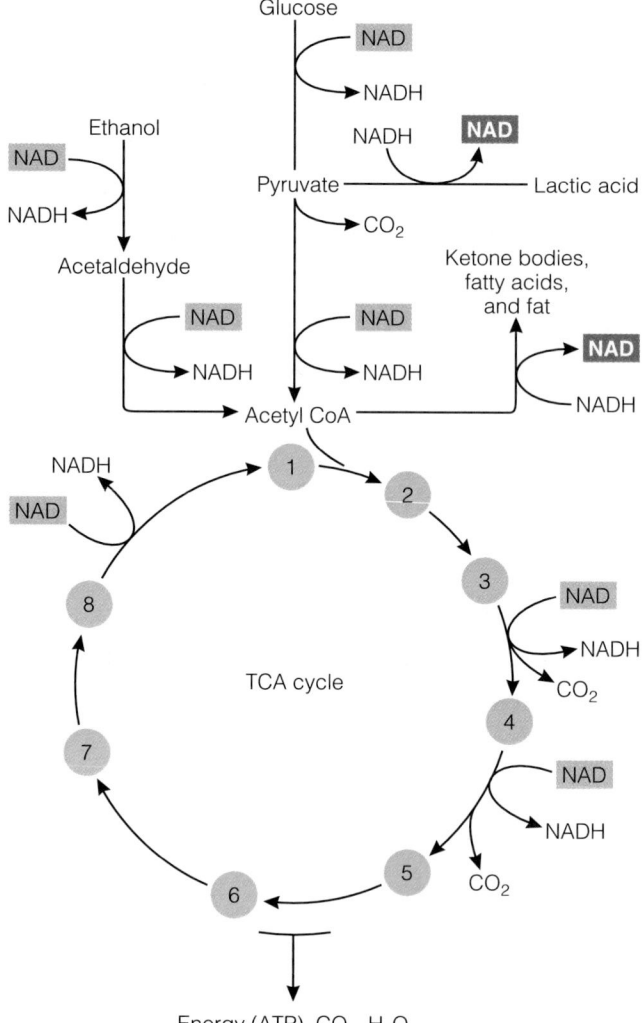

Thus alcohol cascades through the metabolic pathways, wreaking havoc along the way. These consequences have physical effects, which Highlight 7 describes.

THE UREA CYCLE

◆

Chapter 7 sums up the process by which waste nitrogen is eliminated from the body by stating that ammonia molecules combine with carbon dioxide to produce urea. This is true, but it is not the whole story. Urea is produced in a multistep process within the cells of the liver.

Ammonia, freed from an amino acid or other compound during metabolism anywhere in the body, arrives at the liver by way of the bloodstream and is taken into a liver cell. There, it is first combined with carbon dioxide and a phosphate group from ATP to form carbamyl phosphate:

$$CO_2 \ + \ NH_3 \ \xrightarrow{\text{2 ATP} \quad \text{2 ADP + P}} \ H_2N\!-\!\overset{\displaystyle O}{\overset{\|}{C}}\!-\!O\!-\!\overset{\displaystyle O}{\underset{\underset{O^-}{|}}{\overset{\|}{P}}}\!-\!O^-$$

Carbon dioxide Ammonia

Carbamyl phosphate Phosphate group

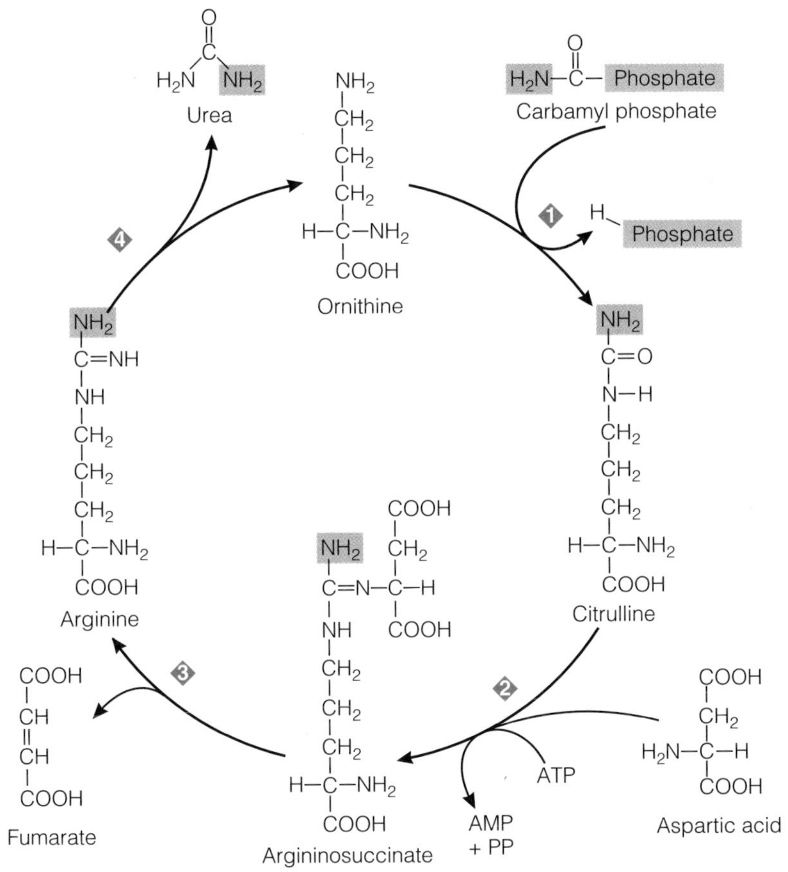

**Figure C–5
The Urea Cycle**

C

Figure C–5 shows the cycle of four reactions that follow. In the first step, carbamyl phosphate combines with the amino acid ornithine, losing its phosphate group. The compound formed is citrulline.

In the second step, citrulline combines with the amino acid aspartic acid, to form argininosuccinate. The reaction requires energy from ATP. (ATP was shown earlier losing one phosphorus atom in a phosphate group, P, to become ADP. In this reaction, it loses two phosphorus atoms joined together, PP, and becomes adenosine monophosphate, AMP.)

In the third step, argininosuccinate is split, forming another acid, fumarate, and the amino acid arginine.

In the fourth step, arginine loses its terminal carbon with two attached amino groups and picks up an oxygen from water. The end product is urea, which the kidneys excrete in the urine. The compound that remains is ornithine, identical to the ornithine with which this series of reactions began, and ready to react with another molecule of carbamyl phosphate and turn the cycle again.

FORMATION OF KETONE BODIES

◆

Normally, fatty acid oxidation proceeds all the way to carbon dioxide and water. However, in ketosis (discussed in Chapter 7), an intermediate is formed from the condensation of two molecules of acetyl CoA: acetoacetyl CoA. Figure C–6 shows the formation of ketone bodies from that

Figure C–6
Formation of Ketone Bodies

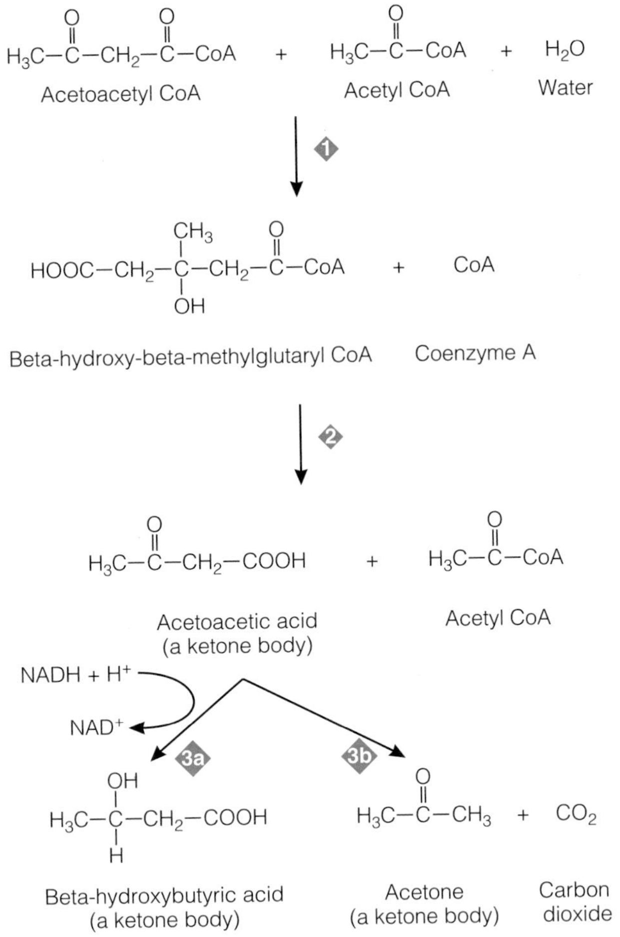

$$H_3C-\overset{\overset{O}{\parallel}}{C}-CH_2-\overset{\overset{O}{\parallel}}{C}-CoA \quad + \quad H_3C-\overset{\overset{O}{\parallel}}{C}-CoA \quad + \quad H_2O$$

Acetoacetyl CoA   Acetyl CoA   Water

①

$$HOOC-CH_2-\overset{\overset{\displaystyle CH_3}{|}}{\underset{\displaystyle OH}{C}}-CH_2-\overset{\overset{O}{\parallel}}{C}-CoA \quad + \quad CoA$$

Beta-hydroxy-beta-methylglutaryl CoA   Coenzyme A

②

$$H_3C-\overset{\overset{O}{\parallel}}{C}-CH_2-COOH \quad + \quad H_3C-\overset{\overset{O}{\parallel}}{C}-CoA$$

Acetoacetic acid   Acetyl CoA
(a ketone body)

NADH + H$^+$

NAD$^+$

3a   **3b**

$$H_3C-\overset{\overset{\displaystyle OH}{|}}{\underset{\displaystyle H}{C}}-CH_2-COOH \qquad\qquad H_3C-\overset{\overset{O}{\parallel}}{C}-CH_3 \quad + \quad CO_2$$

Beta-hydroxybutyric acid   Acetone   Carbon
(a ketone body)   (a ketone body)   dioxide

---

intermediate. In step 1, acetoacetyl CoA condenses with another acetyl CoA to form a six-carbon intermediate, beta-hydroxy-beta-methylglutaryl CoA. In step 2, this intermediate is cleaved to acetyl CoA and acetoacetic acid. This product can be metabolized either to beta-hydroxybutyric acid (step 3a) or to acetone (3b).

Acetoacetic acid, beta-hydroxybutyric acid, and acetone are the so-called ketone bodies of ketosis. Two are real ketones (they have a C=O group between two carbons); the other is an alcohol that has been produced during ketone formation—hence the term *ketone bodies,* rather than ketones, to describe the three of them. There are many other ketones in nature; these three are characteristic of ketosis in the body.

NOTES

◆

1. Nomenclature policy: Generic descriptors and trivial names for vitamins and related compounds, *Journal of Nutrition* 117 (1987): 7–14; Nomenclature policy: Abbreviated designations of amino acids, *Journal of Nutrition* 117 (1987): 15.
2. A discussion of the designated abbreviations for the common amino acids presented here is found in Nomenclature policy: Abbreviated designations of amino acids, *Journal of Nutrition* 117 (1987): 15.

AIDS TO CALCULATION

◆

Contents

Conversion Factors

Percentages

Ratios

Weights and Measures

many mathematical problems have been worked out as examples at appropriate places in the text. This appendix aims to help with the use of the metric system and with problems not fully explained elsewhere.

CONVERSION FACTORS

◆

Conversion factors are useful mathematical tools in everyday calculations, including those encountered in the study of nutrition. Skill in the use of conversion factors is especially desirable as the United States "goes metric."

A conversion factor is a fraction in which the numerator (top) and the denominator (bottom) express the same quantity in different units. For example, 2.2 pounds (lb) and 1 kilogram (kg) are equivalent; they express the same weight. The conversion factor used to change pounds to kilograms or vice versa is:

$$\frac{2.2 \text{ lb}}{1 \text{ kg}} \text{ or } \frac{1 \text{ kg}}{2.2 \text{ lb}} .$$

Because both factors equal 1, measurements can be multiplied by the factor without changing the value of the measurement. Thus the units can be changed.

To perform a conversion, use the factor with the unit you are seeking in the numerator (top) of the fraction. Following are two examples of problems commonly encountered in nutrition study; they illustrate the usefulness of conversion factors.

Example 1 Convert the weight of 130 pounds to kilograms.

1. Choose the conversion factor in which the unit you are seeking is on top:

$$\frac{1 \text{ kg}}{2.2 \text{ lb}} .$$

2. Multiply 130 pounds by the factor:

$$130 \text{ lb} \times \frac{1 \text{ kg}}{2.2 \text{ lb}} = \frac{130 \text{ kg}}{2.2} =$$

59 kg (rounded off to the nearest whole number).

Example 2 How many grams (g) of saturated fat are contained in a 3-ounce (oz) hamburger?

1. Consider a 4-ounce hamburger that contains 7 grams of saturated fat. You are seeking grams of saturated fat; therefore, the conversion factor is:

$$\frac{7 \text{ g saturated fat}}{4 \text{ oz hamburger}} .$$

2. Multiply 3 ounces of hamburger by the conversion factor:

$$3 \text{ oz hamburger} \times \frac{7 \text{ g saturated fat}}{4 \text{ oz hamburger}} =$$

$$\frac{3 \times 7}{4} = \frac{21}{4}$$

$$= 5 \text{ g saturated fat (rounded off to the nearest whole number).}$$

PERCENTAGES

◆

A percentage is a comparison between a number of items (perhaps your intake of energy) and a standard number (perhaps the number of kcalories recommended for your age and sex—your energy RDA). The standard number is the number you divide by. The answer you get after the division must be multiplied by 100 to be stated as a percentage (*percent* means "per 100").

Example 3 What percentage of the RDA for energy is your energy intake?

1. Find your energy RDA (inside front cover, left). We'll use 2200 kcalories to demonstrate.
2. Total your energy intake for a day—for example, 1500 kcalories.
3. Divide your kcalorie intake by the RDA kcalories:

   1500 kcal (your intake) ÷ 2200 kcal (RDA) = 0.68.

4. Multiply your answer by 100 to state it as a percentage:

   $$0.68 \times 100 = 68 = 68\%.$$

In some problems in nutrition, the percentage may be more than 100. For example, suppose your daily intake of vitamin A is 3200 RE and your RDA (male) is 1000 RE. Your intake as a percentage of the RDA is more than 100 percent (that is, you consume more than 100 percent of your vitamin A RDA). The following calculations show your vitamin A intake as a percentage of the RDA:

$$3200 \div 1000 = 3.2.$$
$$3.2 \times 100 = 320\% \text{ of RDA.}$$

Sometimes the comparison is between a part of a whole (for example, your kcalories from protein) and the total amount (your total kcalories). In this case, the total number is the one you divide by.

Example 4 What percentages of your total kcalories for the day come from protein, fat, and carbohydrate?

1. Using Appendix H and your diet record, find the total grams of protein, fat, and carbohydrate you consumed—for example, 60 grams protein, 80 grams fat, and 310 grams carbohydrate.
2. Multiply the number of grams by the number of kcalories from 1 gram of each energy nutrient (conversion factors):

$$60 \text{ g protein} \times \frac{4 \text{ kcal}}{1 \text{ g protein}} = 240 \text{ kcal.}$$

$$80 \text{ g fat} \times \frac{9 \text{ kcal}}{1 \text{ g fat}} = 720 \text{ kcal.}$$

$$310 \text{ g carbohydrate} \times \frac{4 \text{ kcal}}{1 \text{ g carbohydrate}} = 1240 \text{ kcal.}$$

$$240 + 720 + 1240 = 2200 \text{ kcal.}$$

3. Find the percentage of total kcalories from each energy nutrient (see Example 3):

◆ Protein: 240 ÷ 2200 = 0.109 × 100 = 10.9 = 11% of kcal.

◆ Fat: 720 ÷ 2200 = 0.327 × 100 = 32.7 = 33% of kcal.

◆ Carbohydrate: 1240 ÷ 2200 = 0.563 × 100 = 56.3 = 56% of kcal.

◆ 11% + 33% + 56% = 100% of kcal (total).

The percentages total 100 percent, but sometimes they total 99 or 101 because of rounding off. This is a reasonable error.

RATIOS

◆

A ratio is a comparison of two or three values in which one of the values is reduced to 1. A ratio compares identical units and so is expressed without units. For example, Figure 12–6 in Chapter 12 compares the milligrams of potassium to the milligrams of sodium in selected foods.

Example 5 Find the potassium-to-sodium ratio of your diet.

1. Using Appendix H and your diet record, find how many milligrams of potassium and sodium you consumed, say, 3000 milligrams potassium and 2500 milligrams sodium.
2. Divide the potassium milligrams by the sodium milligrams:

   3000 mg potassium ÷ 2500 mg sodium = 1.2.

3. The potassium-to-sodium ratio is usually expressed as correct to one decimal point: 1.2.

The potassium-to-sodium ratio of your diet is 1.2:1 (read as "one point two to one" or simply "one point two"). A ratio greater than 1 means that the first value (in this case, milligrams of potassium) is greater than the second (sodium). When the second value is larger, the ratio is less than 1.

WEIGHTS AND MEASURES

◆

Length

1 inch (in) = 2.54 centimeters (cm).
1 foot (ft) = 30.48 centimeters.
1 meter (m) = 39.37 inches.

Temperature

Steam — 100°C 212°F — Steam
Body temperature — 37°C 98.6°F — Body temperature
Ice — 0°C 32°F — Ice

Celsius*   Fahrenheit

To find degrees Fahrenheit (t_F) when you know degrees Celsius (t_C), multiply by 9/5 and then add 32:

$$(9/5 \times t_C) + 32 = t_F.$$

To find degrees Celsius (t_C) when you know degrees Fahrenheit (t_F), multiply by 5/9 after subtracting 32:

$$5/9 \ (t_F - 32) = t_C.$$

Volume

1 liter (L) = 1.06 quarts (qt) or 0.85 imperial quart.
1 liter = 1000 milliliters (mL).
1 milliliter = 0.03 fluid ounces.
30 milliliters = 1 fluid ounce.
1 gallon = 3.79 liters.
1 quart = 0.95 liter or 32 fluid ounces.

_____

*Also known as *centigrade*.

1 cup (c) = 8 fluid ounces or about 250 milliliters.
1 tablespoon (tbs) = 15 milliliters.
3 teaspoons (tsp) = 1 tablespoon.
1 teaspoon = about 5 g or 5 mL.
16 tablespoons = 1 cup.
4 cups = 1 quart.

Weight

1 ounce (oz) = approximately 28 grams (g).
16 ounces = 1 pound (lb).
1 pound = 454 grams.
1 kilogram (kg) = 1000 grams or 2.2 pounds.
1 gram = 1000 milligrams (mg).
1 milligram = 1000 micrograms (μg).

Energy units

1 kcalorie (kcal) = 4.2 kilojoules (kJ).
1 millijoule (mJ) = 240 kcal.
1 kJ = 0.24 kcal.
1 g carbohydrate = 4 kcal = 17 kJ.
1 g fat = 9 kcal = 37 kJ.
1 g protein = 4 kcal = 17 kJ.
1 g alcohol = 7 kcal = 29 kJ.

International Units (IU)

To convert IU to:

◆ μg RE, divide by 3.33 for retinol and by 10 for beta-carotene.
◆ μg vitamin D, divide by 40 or multiply by 0.025.
◆ mg α-TE, divide by 1.5.

D

Contents

Drug History: Nutrition and Drug
Interactions

Growth Charts and
Anthropometric Data

Laboratory Tests of Nutrition
Status

NUTRITION ASSESSMENT: SUPPLEMENTAL INFORMATION

◆

*C*hapters 15 and 16 described the nutrition assessment techniques health
care professionals commonly use to determine clients' nutrition status.
From this assessment, they identify clients' nutrition needs and develop
care plans for meeting those needs. This appendix provides additional
details and alternative methods of assessing nutrition status to support a complete
nutrition assessment.

DRUG HISTORY: NUTRITION AND DRUG INTERACTIONS

◆

Chapter 15 described nutrient-drug interactions and Chapters 21 through 30
provided a series of "prescription pads," listing drugs used in the treatment of the
specific diseases being discussed. Table E–1 provides examples of selected drugs,
describes nutrition-related factors that affect drug administration, and lists the most
common nutrition-related side effects.

Table E-1
Administration and Common Nutrition-Related Side Effects of Selected Drugs

Drug Classification and Examples	Administration	Common Nutrition-Related Side Effects[a]
Analgesics Narcotic: codeine, merperidine, morphine sulfate	Give with food to reduce GI distress.	N/V, GI distress, reduced GI motility, constipation, lethargy.
Nonnarcotic (also act as nonsteroidal anti-inflammatory agents): aspirin, ibuprofen, naproxen		N/V, GI distress, GI bleeding, constipation. Aspirin may lower blood folate and vitamin C.
Antacids	Give with fluids between meals or at bedtime.	
Al-containing (also act as phosphate binders): Al carbonate, Al hydroxide, Al phosphate	Give with meals when used as phosphate binder.	Constipation, phosphorus deficiency. Long-term use in renal failure may cause Al toxicity.
Ca-containing (also act as phosphate binders and Ca supplements): Ca carbonate and Ca gluconate	When used as a phosphate binder or supplement, give with meals and separately from foods high in fiber, oxalate, or phytate and iron or fluoride supplements.	Constipation, chalky taste. Concurrent use with vitamin D supplements may lead to elevated blood Ca.
Mg-containing (also act as laxatives): Mg hydroxide, Mg oxide, and Mg citrate	Give separately from iron and folate supplements.	Diarrhea, chalky taste. Long-term use in renal failure may lead to Mg toxicity.
Antianginals Amyl nitrate, isosorbide dinitrate, nitroglycerin (see also *Antihypertensives*)	Give oral forms on an empty stomach. Limit alcohol.	Nutrition-related side effects are uncommon.
Antianxiety Agents Alprazolam, chlordiazepoxide	Give with food to reduce GI distress. Avoid alcohol.	Increased appetite, weight gain, nausea, drowsiness.
Diazepam, lorazepam, oxazepam	Limit caffeine and avoid alcohol.	Constipation, diarrhea, dry mouth, drowsiness.
Meprobamate	Avoid alcohol.	N/V, diarrhea, drowsiness.
Anticoagulants, oral Ticlopidine	Give with food to improve drug absorption and reduce GI distress.	N/V, GI pain, diarrhea.
Warfarin	Maintain consistent vitamin K intake, avoid high doses of vitamins A and E, which can reduce the anticoagulant effect. Avoid high doses of vitamin C, which can reduce drug absorption.	Nausea.
Anticonvulsants Phenytoin	Give with meals to reduce GI distress. Tube feedings may interfere with drug absorption (see Chapter 23).	N/V, swollen gums. May cause folate-deficiency anemia. Increases metabolism of vitamins D and K.

[a]Note that many other medications not listed in this table also have nutrition-related side effects. In addition, nutrition-related side effects other than those listed may occur. For example, almost all medications cause nausea in some people. In this table, nausea is only listed as a side effect if it occurs with relative frequency or does not resolve with time. More detailed texts should be consulted for the medications you routinely encounter in clinical practice.

Abbreviations: N/V = nausea/vomiting; Al = aluminum; Ca = calcium; Mg = magnesium; K = potassium; GERD = gastroesophageal reflux disease; ACE = angiotensin-converting enzyme; H2 = histamine$_2$.

Table E–1

Administration and Common Nutrition-Related Side Effects of Selected Drugs (continued)

Drug Classification and Examples	Administration	Common Nutrition-Related Side Effects[a]
Anticonvulsants		
Primidone	Avoid alcohol.	N/V. May cause folate-deficiency anemia.
Valproic acid	Do not take tablets with milk or liquid form with carbonated beverages.	N/V, GI pain.
Antidepressants		
MAO inhibitors: phenelzine, tranylcypromine	Give with food to reduce GI distress. Avoid foods high in tyramine (see Chapter 15), alcohol, and tryptophan supplements. Limit caffeine.	Weight changes, dry mouth, constipation.
Tricyclic: amitriptyline, clomipramine, doxepin, imipramine, protriptyline	Give with food to reduce GI distress. Avoid alcohol and limit caffeine and high-fiber foods.	Dry mouth, constipation. Stimulates appetite, especially for sweets.
Other:		
bupropion	Give with food to reduce GI distress. Avoid alcohol.	Dry mouth, constipation.
fluoxetine	Give in morning without regard to food. Avoid tryptophan supplements.	Anorexia, weight loss, dry mouth, N/V, diarrhea.
nefazone	Food reduces drug absorption and bioavailability.	Dry mouth, N/V, constipation.
sertraline	Give at same time each day without regard to food. Avoid alcohol.	Dry mouth, N/V, constipation.
Antidiabetics		
Acarbose	Give at the start of each meal.	GI pain, flatulence, diarrhea, hypoglycemia.
Glipizide	Give 30 min before breakfast. Limit alcohol.	Hypoglycemia. GI side effects uncommon.
Glyburide	Give with breakfast. Limit alcohol.	Hypoglycemia. GI side effects uncommon.
Metformin	Give with meals to reduce GI distress. Limit alcohol.	N/V, bloating, flatulence, diarrhea. Lowers blood glucose, cholesterol, LDL, and triglycerides and raises HDL.
Troglitazone[c]	Give with meals.	Risk of hypoglycemia increases when used in combination with other antidiabetic agents. GI side effects uncommon.
Antidiarrheals		
Loperamide	Give without regard to food.	Nutrition-related side effects are uncommon.
Opium and paregoric	Give without regard to food.	N/V, constipation, sedation.

[a]Note that many other medications not listed in this table also have nutrition-related side effects. In addition, nutrition-related side effects other than those listed may occur. For example, almost all medications cause nausea in some people. In this table, nausea is only listed as a side effect if it occurs with relative frequency or does not resolve with time. More detailed texts should be consulted for the medications you routinely encounter in clinical practice.

Abbreviations: N/V = nausea/vomiting; Al = aluminum; Ca = calcium; Mg = magnesium; K = potassium; GERD = gastroesophageal reflux disease; ACE = angiotensin-converting enzyme; H2 = histamine$_2$.

[c]*Source:* Product advertisement in *Diabetes Care,* August 1977.

Table E–1

Administration and Common Nutrition-Related Side Effects of Selected Drugs (continued)

Drug Classification and Examples	Administration	Common Nutrition-Related Side Effects[a]
Antihypertensives	Avoid natural licorice.	
ACE inhibitors:		
benazepril, enalapril, lisopril, ramipril	Limit alcohol and avoid salt substitutes. Monitor use of K supplements.	May elevate blood K.
captopril	Give 1 hr before or 2 hr after meals. Limit alcohol and avoid salt substitutes. Monitor use of K supplements.	Mouth ulcers. May elevate blood K.
fosinopril	Give separately from Ca or Mg supplements. Limit alcohol and avoid salt substitutes. Monitor use of K supplements.	May elevate blood K.
Alpha-adrenergic blockers: doxazosin, prazosin, terazosin	Limit alcohol.	Weight gain, fatigue.
Beta-blockers (also act as antiarrythmics and antianginals):		May mask signs of hypoglycemia.
atenolol	Give with food to reduce GI distress. Give separately from Ca supplements or antacids.	Nausea, dizziness.
metoprolol	Give with food to enhance bioavailability.	Diarrhea, confusion, dizziness.
nadolol	Limit alcohol.	Nutrition-related side effects are uncommon.
propranolol	Give with food to enhance bioavailability. Avoid alcohol and give separately from Ca supplements or antacids.	Dizziness, drowsiness, weakness.
Ca-channel blockers (also act as antianginals):		
amlopidine, isradipine	Give without regard to food.	Edema, headache.
dilitiazem	Give tablets or extended release capsules before meals.	Edema, dizziness.
felopidine	Do not give with grapefruit juice.	Edema, headache.
nicarpidine, nisoldipine	Do not give with high-fat foods or grapefruit juice.	Edema, headache, dizziness.
Other:		
clonidine	Avoid alcohol.	Dry mouth, constipation, edema, drowsiness, dizziness.

[a]Note that many other medications not listed in this table also have nutrition-related side effects. In addition, nutrition-related side effects other than those listed may occur. For example, almost all medications cause nausea in some people. In this table, nausea is only listed as a side effect if it occurs with relative frequency or does not resolve with time. More detailed texts should be consulted for the medications you routinely encounter in clinical practice.

Abbreviations: N/V = nausea/vomiting; Al = aluminum; Ca = calcium; Mg = magnesium; K = potassium; GERD = gastroesophageal reflux disease; ACE = angiotensin-converting enzyme; H2 = histamine$_2$.

E

Table E–1
Administration and Common Nutrition-Related Side Effects of Selected Drugs (continued)

Drug Classification and Examples	Administration	Common Nutrition-Related Side Effects[a]
Antihypertensives (continued)		
guanfacine	Limit alcohol.	Dry mouth, constipation, drowsiness.
hydralazine	Give with food to enhance bioavailability. Limit alcohol.	Anorexia, N/V, edema, headache. Pyridoxine supplements correct drug-induced peripheral neuropathy.
methyldopa	Avoid alcohol. Do not give drug within 2 hr of giving iron supplements.	Dry mouth, headache, drowsiness, edema. High doses increase vitamin B_{12} and folate needs.
minoxidil		Bloating, edema.
Anti-Infectives		
Antibiotics:		
amoxicillin	Give without regard to food.	Diarrhea.
ampicillin	Give with 8 oz of water 1 hr before or 2 hr after meals.	Diarrhea.
cefaclor, cefoperazone, cefotaxime	Give parenterally. Avoid alcohol while using and for 3 days afterward. Give foods high in vitamin K or a vitamin K supplement with long-term use.	May interfere with bacterial vitamin K synthesis in intestine.
chloramphenicol	Give with 8 oz water 1 hr before or 2 hr after meals. Avoid alcohol. Limit use of iron supplements.	Increases risk of iron overload. Delays response to iron, folate, or vitamin B_{12}.
erythromycin	Give with 8 oz water 1 hr before or 2 hr after meals. Food decreases absorption of some forms (base and stearate), but may be given to reduce GI distress.	Epigastric pain, abdominal cramps.
ethambutol	Give with food to reduce GI distress.	Nutrition-related side effects are uncommon.
penicillin	Give penicillin K without regard to meals; penicillin G 1 hr before or 2 hr after meals. Use K supplements cautiously with penicillin K.	N/V, epigastric distress, mouth sores, diarrhea.
tetracycline	Give with water 1 hr before or 2 hr after meals. Separate the administration of Ca, iron, Mg, zinc, Al, or vitamin-mineral supplements or Al-, Ca-, or Mg-containing antacids by 3 hr.	N/V, diarrhea, cramps, dizziness.

[a]Note that many other medications not listed in this table also have nutrition-related side effects. In addition, nutrition-related side effects other than those listed may occur. For example, almost all medications cause nausea in some people. In this table, nausea is only listed as a side effect if it occurs with relative frequency or does not resolve with time. More detailed texts should be consulted for the medications you routinely encounter in clinical practice.

Abbreviations: N/V = nausea/vomiting; Al = aluminum; Ca = calcium; Mg = magnesium; K = potassium; GERD = gastroesophageal reflux disease; ACE = angiotensin-converting enzyme; H2 = histamine$_2$.

Table E–1

Administration and Common Nutrition-Related Side Effects of Selected Drugs (continued)

Drug Classification and Examples	Administration	Common Nutrition-Related Side Effects[a]
Anti-Infectives (continued)		
Antifungals:		
amphotericin	Give parenterally and encourage fluids.	Anorexia, N/V, weight loss, stomach pain, fever, headache, soreness.
clotrimazole	Dissolve lozenge slowly in mouth over 15–30 min.	N/V.
flucytosine	Give capsules slowly over 15 min to reduce GI distress.	N/V, diarrhea, lethargy, dizziness.
ketoconazole	Give with foods to enhance absorption. Give Ca or Mg separately by 2 hr.	N/V.
Antivirals:		
acyclovir	Encourage fluids.	Headache.
famciclovir	Give without regard to food.	Headache.
foscarnet	Give parenterally and encourage fluids.	Anorexia, N/V, abdominal pain, diarrhea, fever, headache, weakness, dizziness.
ganciclovir	Give with food and encourage fluids.	N/V, abdominal pain, headache, fever, weakness.
lamivudine (3TC)	Give without regard to food.	Nausea, GI pain, diarrhea, headache, fever.
saquinavir	Give within 2 hr of a full meal.	Nausea, GI pain, diarrhea, headache.
stavudine (d4T)	Give without regard to food.	N/V, diarrhea, fever.
zalcitabine (DDC)	Give on empty stomach, if possible, to enhance absorption.	Anorexia, weight loss, N/V, mouth ulcers.
zidovudine (AZT)	Give without regard to food.	Anorexia, N/V, headache, anemia.
Anti-Inflammatory Agents		
Corticosteroids (also act as immunosuppressants): cortisone, dexamethasone, hydrocortisone, prednisone	Give with food to reduce GI distress. Encourage high-protein, low-sodium diet. Avoid alcohol. May need supplements of or diets high in K, Ca, and phosphorus; vitamins A, C, and D; and pyridoxine and folate.	Edema, osteoporosis. Increase appetite and weight. Induce negative nitrogen and Ca balances.
Diclofenac	Give with food, milk, or water to reduce GI distress. Avoid alcohol.	Nausea, GI pain, constipation, diarrhea, headache, edema.
Diflunisal	Give with food or milk to reduce GI distress. Avoid alcohol.	Nausea, GI pain, diarrhea, headache.
Mesalamine, olsalazin	Give with food and 8 oz water.	Nutrition-related side effects are uncommon.
Salsalate	Give with food, milk or water. Limit alcohol and caffeine.	Nausea, dizziness.

[a]Note that many other medications not listed in this table also have nutrition-related side effects. In addition, nutrition-related side effects other than those listed may occur. For example, almost all medications cause nausea in some people. In this table, nausea is only listed as a side effect if it occurs with relative frequency or does not resolve with time. More detailed texts should be consulted for the medications you routinely encounter in clinical practice.

Abbreviations: N/V = nausea/vomiting; Al = aluminum; Ca = calcium; Mg = magnesium; K = potassium; GERD = gastroesophageal reflux disease; ACE = angiotensin-converting enzyme; H2 = histamine$_2$.

Table E–1
Administration and Common Nutrition-Related Side Effects of Selected Drugs (continued)

Drug Classification and Examples	Administration	Common Nutrition-Related Side Effects[a]
Anti-Inflammatory Agents (continued)		
Sulfasalazine (See also *Analgesics, nonnarcartic*)	Give with 8 oz water or food to reduce GI distress. Give folate supplement and encourage fluids.	Anorexia, N/V, GI pain, diarrhea, headache, dizziness. Lowers blood folate.
Antilipemics		
Cholestyramine	Give before meals. Mix powder form with water or fluids; never give dry or with carbonated beverages.	Nausea, belching, dyspepsia, constipation. May decrease absorption of fat, fat-soluble vitamins, folate, Ca, iron, zinc, and Mg.
Clofibrate	Give with food or milk to reduce GI distress.	Nausea, anemia.
Fluvastatin	Give without regard to food.	Nutrition-related side effects are uncommon.
Gemfibrozil	Give ½ hr before meals.	Taste alterations, dyspepsia, abdominal pain.
Lovastatin	Give with meals to enhance absorption. Give fiber, pectin, or oat bran separately by several hr. Avoid high doses of niacin and limit alcohol.	Constipation, headache.
Pravastatin, simvastatin	Avoid high doses of niacin and limit alcohol.	Nutrition-related side effects are uncommon.
Antinauseants, Antiemetics		
Dronabinol (marijuana derivative)	Give before lunch and dinner.	Stimulates appetite and causes weight gain. Euphoria.
Granisetron	Give without regard to food.	Constipation, headache, weakness.
Meclizine	Give without regard to food	Nutrition-related side effects are uncommon.
Metoclopramide	Give ½ hr before meals and at bedtime.	Nausea, diarrhea, lethargy.
Ondansetron	Give without regard to food.	Abdominal pain, constipation, headache, weakness.
Prochlorperazine	Give with food or milk. Avoid alcohol and limit caffeine.	Dry mouth, constipation. Stimulates appetite and causes weight gain. Increases urinary excretion of riboflavin.
Antineoplastics		
Aldesleukin	Give parenterally.	Anorexia, N/V, mouth inflammation, diarrhea, mental changes, dizziness, anemia, impaired renal function, fever, edema, infection.

[a]Note that many other medications not listed in this table also have nutrition-related side effects. In addition, nutrition-related side effects other than those listed may occur. For example, almost all medications cause nausea in some people. In this table, nausea is only listed as a side effect if it occurs with relative frequency or does not resolve with time. More detailed texts should be consulted for the medications you routinely encounter in clinical practice.

Abbreviations: N/V = nausea/vomiting; Al = aluminum; Ca = calcium; Mg = magnesium; K = potassium; GERD = gastroesophageal reflux disease; ACE = angiotensin-converting enzyme; H2 = histamine$_2$.

Table E-1

Administration and Common Nutrition-Related Side Effects of Selected Drugs (continued)

Drug Classification and Examples	Administration	Common Nutrition-Related Side Effects[a]
Antineoplastics (continued)		
Bleomyin	Give parenterally.	Anorexia, N/V, mouth inflammation, weight loss, fever, respiratory impairment.
Carboplatin	Give parenterally with adequate fluids to maintain hydration.	Anorexia, N/V, mouth inflammation, GI pain, diarrhea, constipation, weakness, infections, anemia. Lowers blood levels of sodium, K, Ca, and Mg.
Carmustine	Give parenterally with adequate fluids to maintain hydration.	N/V, mild liver impairment.
Cisplatin	Give parenterally with adequate fluids to maintain hydration.	Severe N/V, taste alterations, diarrhea, infections, impaired renal function, anemia. Lowers blood levels of sodium, K, Ca, phosphorus, Mg, and zinc.
Cyclophosphamide	Give oral forms with food only if GI distress occurs. Encourage fluids.	Anoerxia, N/V, mouth inflammation, delayed wound healing.
Cytarbine	Give parenterally and provide adequate liquids.	Anorexia, N/V, mouth inflammation, diarrhea, anal ulcers, weight loss, infection. Lowers blood levels of K and Ca.
Dactinomycin	Give parenterally and provide adequate fluids. Encourage high-kcalorie foods. Raises vitamin B_{12} needs.	Anorexia, severe N/V, dry mouth, mouth and tongue inflammation, taste alterations, severe esophagitis, dysphagia, GI pain, diarrhea, weight loss, fatigue, anemia. Reduces absorption of fat, Ca, and iron.
Daunorubicin, doxorubicin, idarubicin	Give parenterally and provide adequate fluids.	Anorexia, N/V, weight loss, dry mouth, mouth and esophageal inflammation, anemia.
Estramustine	Store capsules in refrigerator.	Anorexia, N/V, diarrhea, edema, lethargy, Impairs glucose tolerance.
Etoposide, teniposide	Give parenterally or orally (etoposide).	Anorexia, N/V, mouth inflammation, diarrhea.
Floxuridine	Give parenterally.	Anorexia, N/V, diarrhea, weakness, lethargy.
Fluorouracil	Give parenterally.	Anorexia, severe N/V, mouth and esophageal inflammation, taste alterations, intestinal inflammation, diarrhea, weakness, anemia. May increase pyridoxine needs.
Interferon alfa 2a and 2b	Give parenterally and provide adequate liquids.	Anorexia, N/V, dry mouth, taste alterations, mouth inflammation, abdominal pain, diarrhea, weight loss, dizziness, headache, fatigue.

[a]Note that many other medications not listed in this table also have nutrition-related side effects. In addition, nutrition-related side effects other than those listed may occur. For example, almost all medications cause nausea in some people. In this table, nausea is only listed as a side effect if it occurs with relative frequency or does not resolve with time. More detailed texts should be consulted for the medications you routinely encounter in clinical practice.

Abbreviations: N/V = nausea/vomiting; Al = aluminum; Ca = calcium; Mg = magnesium; K = potassium; GERD = gastroesophageal reflux disease; ACE = angiotensin-converting enzyme; H2 = histamine$_2$.

Table E-1
Administration and Common Nutrition-Related Side Effects of Selected Drugs (continued)

Drug Classification and Examples	Administration	Common Nutrition-Related Side Effects[a]
Antineoplastics (continued)		
Leuprolide	Give parenterally.	Anorexia, N/V, constipation, edema, headache, weakness, anemia.
Levamisole	Give without regard to food.	Nausea, taste alterations, diarrhea, fatigue.
Lomustine	Give on empty stomach to reduce GI distress. Provide adequate fluids.	N/V, anemia.
Mechlorethamine	Give adequate fluids.	Anorexia, severe N/V, anemia.
Megestrol acetate (see *Appetite Stimulants*)		
Melphalan	Give adequate fluids. Divide single daily dose if GI distress occurs (food reduces drug bioavailability).	Nutrition-related side effects are uncommon, but may include mild N/V and diarrhea.
Mercaptopurine	Give adequate fluids.	Anorexia, mild N/V, anemia.
Methotrexate	Give adequate fluids.	Anorexia, N/V, mouth and gum inflammation, weight loss, infection.
Mithramycin, plicamycin	Give parenterally.	Anorexia, N/V, mouth inflammation, diarrhea.
Mitomycin	Give parenterally.	Anorexia, N/V, weight loss, fever, weakness.
Mitoxantrone	Give parenterally.	N/V, mouth inflammation, GI bleeding, abdominal pain, diarrhea, fever.
Paclitaxel	Give parenterally.	N/V, mouth and esophageal inflammation, diarrhea, edema, fatigue, anemia.
Pegasparagase	Give parenterally.	N/V, fever, weakness.
Porfimer	Give parenterally.	N/V, dysphagia, abdominal pain, constipation, fever.
Streptozocin	Give parenterally.	N/V, renal and liver impairment.
Tamoxifen citrate	Give Ca and Mg supplements separately from enteric-coated tablet by 2 hr.	N/V.
Tretinoin	Give with meals. Do not give vitamin A supplements. Limit alcohol and fat.	N/V, abdominal pain, GI bleeding, respiratory impairment, elevated blood lipids, fever.
Antipsychotics		
Chlorpromazine (also acts as an antinauseant)	Give with food, milk, or water to reduce GI distress. Dilute oral concentrate in a 4 oz drink or soft food. Give Mg separately by 2 hr. Avoid alcohol.	Dry mouth, constipation, drowsiness, dizziness. May reduce vitamin B_{12} absorption.

[a]Note that many other medications not listed in this table also have nutrition-related side effects. In addition, nutrition-related side effects other than those listed may occur. For example, almost all medications cause nausea in some people. In this table, nausea is only listed as a side effect if it occurs with relative frequency or does not resolve with time. More detailed texts should be consulted for the medications you routinely encounter in clinical practice.

Abbreviations: N/V = nausea/vomiting; Al = aluminum; Ca = calcium; Mg = magnesium; K = potassium; GERD = gastroesophageal reflux disease; ACE = angiotensin-converting enzyme; H2 = histamine$_2$.

Table E-1
Administration and Common Nutrition-Related Side Effects of Selected Drugs (continued)

Drug Classification and Examples	Administration	Common Nutrition-Related Side Effects[a]
Antipsychotics (continued)		
Fluphenazine, perphenazine, trifluoperazine	Give with food to reduce GI distress. Do not mix concentrates with caffeinated drinks, tea, or apple juice. Avoid alcohol.	Stimulate appetite. Weight gain, dry mouth, constipation, drowsiness. May increase riboflavin needs.
Haloperidol	Give with food or milk to reduce GI distress. Do not mix concentrates with coffee, tea, or fruit juice. Avoid alcohol.	Stimulates appetite. Weight gain, dry mouth, constipation, drowsiness.
Loxapine	Give with food, milk, or water to reduce GI distress. Dilute concentrate with orange or grapefruit juice.	Dry mouth, drowsiness.
Prochlorperazine (see *Antinauseants*)		
Resperidone	Avoid alcohol.	Stimulates appetite. Weight gain, drowsiness.
Thioridazine	Give with food, milk, or water. Dilute concentrate in orange or grapefruit juice.	Stimulates appetite. Weight gain, dry mouth, constipation, drowsiness, dizziness. May increase riboflavin needs.
Antiulcer Agents		
Antisecretory agents (also act as anti-GERD): lanisoprazole, omeprazole	Give before a meal. Swallow capsules whole.	May reduce absorption of iron and vitamin B_{12}.
H2 blockers (also act as anti-GERD): cimetidine	Give iron supplements 1 hr before giving drug. Give Ca or Mg supplements separately by 2 hr. Limit caffeine, xanthine, and alcohol. Liquid form not compatible with tube feedings.	May reduce vitamin B_{12} absorption.
famotidine, nizatidine, rantidine	Limit caffeine, xanthine, and alcohol.	May reduce vitamin B_{12} absorption.
Other: sucralfate	Give with water on an empty stomach 1 hr before meals or at bedtime. Give Ca or Mg supplement separately by 30 min. Limit alcohol.	Nutrition-related side effects are uncommon. May cause Al-toxicity in people with end-stage renal failure.
Appetite Stimulants		
Dronabinol (see *Antinauseants*)		
Megestrol acetate, medroxy progesterone acetate	May take with food to reduce GI distress.	Increases appetite. Weight gain, edema. May increase blood sodium.
Appetite Suppressants		
Dexfenfluramine, fenfluramine, mazindol, phendimetrazine, phentermine	Give on empty stomach 1 hr before meals. Instruct client to follow a low-kcalorie diet.	Nausea, taste alterations, dry mouth, dizziness, drowsiness.

[a]Note that many other medications not listed in this table also have nutrition-related side effects. In addition, nutrition-related side effects other than those listed may occur. For example, almost all medications cause nausea in some people. In this table, nausea is only listed as a side effect if it occurs with relative frequency or does not resolve with time. More detailed texts should be consulted for the medications you routinely encounter in clinical practice.

Abbreviations: N/V = nausea/vomiting; Al = aluminum; Ca = calcium; Mg = magnesium; K = potassium; GERD = gastroesophageal reflux disease; ACE = angiotensin-converting enzyme; H2 = histamine$_2$.

E

Table E–1

Administration and Common Nutrition-Related Side Effects of Selected Drugs (continued)

Drug Classification and Examples	Administration	Common Nutrition-Related Side Effects[a]
Cardiac Glycosides		
Digitoxin, digoxin, digitalis	Give separately from high-fiber, high-pectin foods. Encourage low-salt, high-K diet. Mg supplements may decrease drug absorption. Avoid natural licorice and give Ca or vitamin D supplements cautiously. Hypokalemia, hypomagnesemia, hypoalbuminemia, and hypercalcemia increase drug effects.	Anorexia, N/V, weight loss, diarrhea.
Diuretics		
K–losing (thiazide, thiazide-related, and loop diuretics):		
bendroflumethiazide, chlorothalidone, chlorothiazide, hydrochlorothiazide, methyclothiazide, metolazone, quinethazone	Give with food or milk to reduce GI distress. Avoid natural licorice and limit alcohol. May need K or Mg supplements. Carefully monitor use of Ca and vitamin D supplements.	Lowers blood sodium, K, chloride, Mg. Raises blood Ca and glucose.
indapamide	Same as above.	Headache, dizziness, fatigue. Lowers blood K, sodium, chloride, Mg, and phosphorus. Raises blood Ca and glucose.
ethacrynic acid, furosemide	Give with food or milk to reduce GI distress. Avoid natural licorice and limit alcohol. May need K or Mg supplements.	Lowers blood K, sodium, chloride, Ca, Mg, and zinc. Raises blood glucose.
K-sparing:		
amiloride	Give with food or milk to reduce GI distress. Avoid natural licorice and alcohol. Avoid foods high in K, K supplements, and salt substitutes.	Anorexia, N/V. Lowers blood sodium and chloride. Raises blood K.
spironolactone	Same as above.	N/V, cramps, diarrhea. Lowers blood sodium and chloride. Raises blood K and Mg.
triamterene	Same as above.	Decreases the metabolism of folate. Lowers blood sodium, Mg, and folate. Raises blood K.
Immunosuppressants		
Azathioprine	Give with food to reduce GI distress.	N/V.

[a]Note that many other medications not listed in this table also have nutrition-related side effects. In addition, nutrition-related side effects other than those listed may occur. For example, almost all medications cause nausea in some people. In this table, nausea is only listed as a side effect if it occurs with relative frequency or does not resolve with time. More detailed texts should be consulted for the medications you routinely encounter in clinical practice.

Abbreviations: N/V = nausea/vomiting; Al = aluminum; Ca = calcium; Mg = magnesium; K = potassium; GERD = gastroesophageal reflux disease; ACE = angiotensin-converting enzyme; H2 = histamine$_2$.

Table E-1
Administration and Common Nutrition-Related Side Effects of Selected Drugs (continued)

Drug Classification and Examples	Administration	Common Nutrition-Related Side Effects[a]
Immunosuppressants (continued)		
Corticosteroids (see *Anti-Inflammatory Agents*)		
Cyclosporine	Mix liquid with milk or orange juice at room temperature; no grapefruit juice. Avoid K supplements or salt substitutes.	N/V, diarrhea, swollen gums, headache, impaired renal function, elevated blood pressure, elevated blood glucose. May raise blood K and lower Mg.
Muromonab-cd3	Give parenterally.	N/V, diarrhea, fever, infection.
Mycophenolate	Give with food to reduce GI distress.	N/V, diarrhea, constipation, impaired liver function, impaired kidney function, anemia, infection.
Tacrolimus	Give with food to reduce GI distress.	N/V, diarrhea, constipation, impaired liver function, impaired kidney function, headache.
Laxatives		
Bisacodyl	Give on empty stomach with water or juice. Encourage use of high-fiber foods and fluids.	Laxative dependency and low blood K and Ca with long-term use.
Docusate	Give syrup with milk or juice to mask taste. Encourage use of high-fiber foods and fluids.	Nausea, throat irritation. Long-term use may raise blood glucose and lower K.
Lactulose	Give with juice, milk, or water, or sweet food to improve palatability. Encourage use of high-fiber foods and fluids. Do not give to clients on lactose- or galactose-restricted diets. Dilute before using with tube feeding.	Belching, cramps, flatulence.
Magnesium salts (see *Antacids, Mg-containing*)		
Methycellulose	Give with fluids. Encourage use of high-fiber foods and fluids.	Increased peristalsis.
Mineral oil	Give 2 hr before or after eating. Encourage use of high-fiber foods and fluids.	May reduce absorption of fat-soluble vitamins.
Psyllium	Mix powder in water, juice, or milk. Encourage use of high-fiber foods and fluids.	Reduces blood cholesterol and LDL.
Senna	Give with water or juice. Encourage use of high-fiber foods and fluids.	Nausea, cramps.

[a]Note that many other medications not listed in this table also have nutrition-related side effects. In addition, nutrition-related side effects other than those listed may occur. For example, almost all medications cause nausea in some people. In this table, nausea is only listed as a side effect if it occurs with relative frequency or does not resolve with time. More detailed texts should be consulted for the medications you routinely encounter in clinical practice.

Abbreviations: N/V = nausea/vomiting; Al = aluminum; Ca = calcium; Mg = magnesium; K = potassium; GERD = gastroesophageal reflux disease; ACE = angiotensin-converting enzyme; H2 = histamine$_2$.

Table E–1

Administration and Common Nutrition-Related Side Effects of Selected Drugs (continued)

Drug Classification and Examples	Administration	Common Nutrition-Related Side Effects[a]
Phosphate Binders Al carbonate, Al hydroxide, Ca acetate, Ca carbonate, Ca citrate (see *Antacids, Al- and Ca-containing*)		
Miscellaneous		
Calcitonin (Ca regulator)	Give at bedtime to reduce GI distress.	N/V. Lowers blood Ca and phosphorus.
Calcitriol (Ca regulator)	Do not give with vitamin D, Mg supplements, or Mg–containing antacids. Avoid high-phosphorus foods.	Raises blood Ca levels.
Colchicine (antigout)	Give with low-purine diet during acute attacks of gout.	N/V, GI pain, diarrhea.
Dextroamphetamine (stimulant)	Limit caffeine.	Anorexia, weight loss, dizziness, headache, confusion.
Epoetin alfa (erythropoietin)	May need iron, folate, or vitamin B_{12} supplement.	Raises hemoglobin and hematocrit.
Lithium carbonate (antimanic)	Give with meals to reduce GI distress. Consistent sodium intake helps maintain drug levels. Give adequate fluids. Do not use syrup form with tube feedings.	N/V, thirst, weight gain, dry mouth, fatigue, weakness, edema, dizziness. Raises blood Ca, phosphorus, and Mg.
Oral contraceptives (hormone)	Give with food. Give foods high in folate, pyridoxine, and vitamin B_{12} and vitamin C supplements. Limit caffeine.	N/V, weight changes, appetite changes, bone loss, edema. Lowers blood folate, pyridoxine, and vitamin B_{12}.
Sodium polystyrene sulfonate (K exchange resin)	Mix powder with cool water or sorbitol. Mix with sorbitol-containing syrup to combat constipation. Avoid K supplements. Do not give Ca-containing supplements or antacids for at least several hours.	Anorexia, constipation. Lowers blood K, Ca, and Mg.

[a]Note that many other medications not listed in this table also have nutrition-related side effects. In addition, nutrition-related side effects other than those listed may occur. For example, almost all medications cause nausea in some people. In this table, nausea is only listed as a side effect if it occurs with relative frequency or does not resolve with time. More detailed texts should be consulted for the medications you routinely encounter in clinical practice.

Abbreviations: N/V = nausea/vomiting; Al = aluminum; Ca = calcium; Mg = magnesium; K = potassium; GERD = gastroesophageal reflux disease; ACE = angiotensin-converting enzyme; H2 = histamine₂.

Sources: Z. M. Pronsky, *Food Medication Interactions*, 9th ed. (Pottstown, Pa.: Food Medication Interactions, 1993); *Nursing Drug Guide* (Philadelphia: Lippincott-Raven Publishers, 1997).

GROWTH CHARTS AND ANTHROPOMETRIC DATA

◆

Growth charts, shown in Figures E–1 through E–6, allow health care professionals to evaluate the growth and development of children from birth to 18 years of age. The assessor follows these steps to plot a weight measurement on a percentile graph:

◆ Select the appropriate chart based on age and gender. (When length is measured, use the chart for birth to 36 months; when height is measured, use the chart for 2 to 18 years.)

◆ Locate the child's age along the horizontal axis on the bottom or top of the chart.

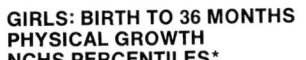

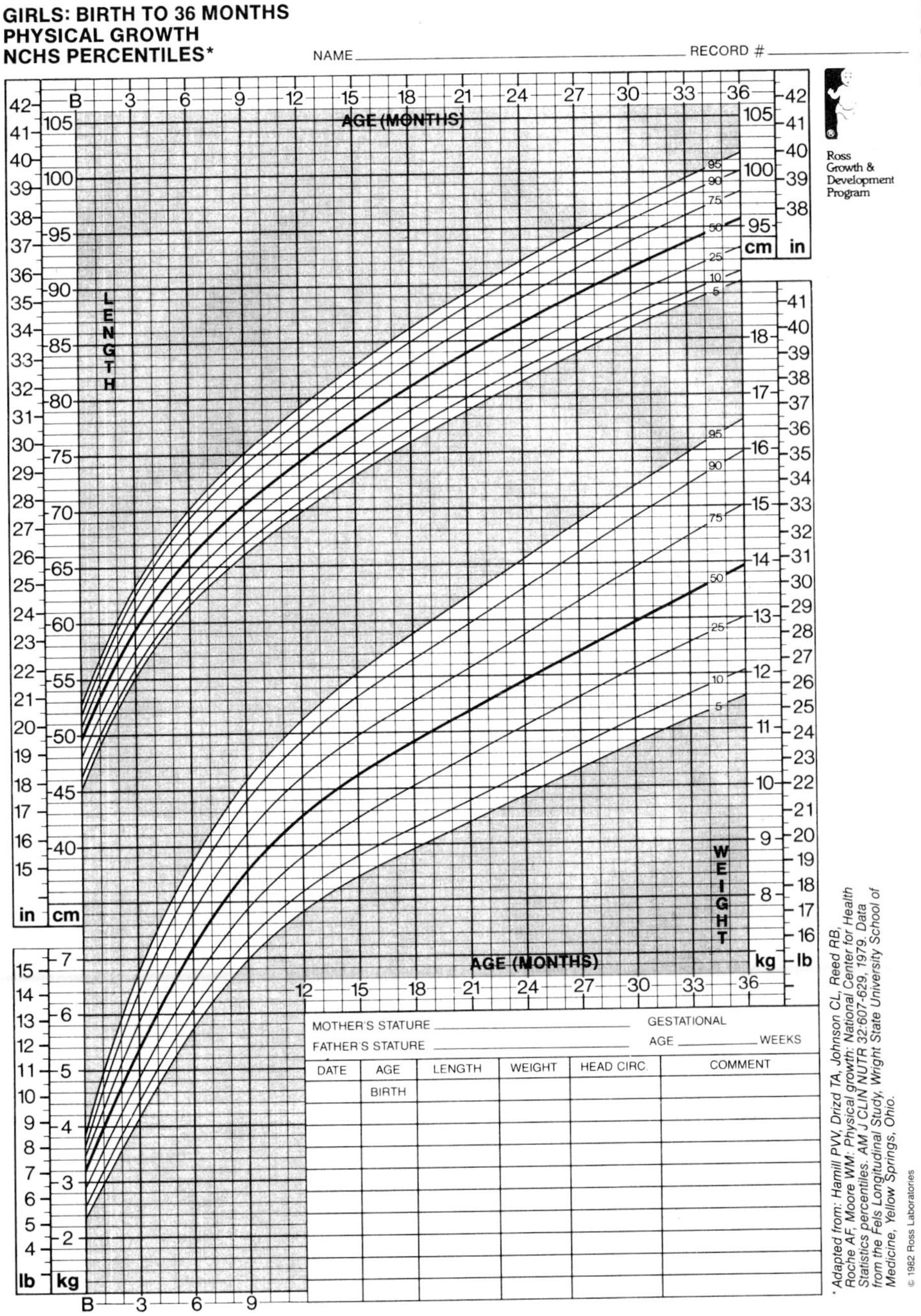
GIRLS: BIRTH TO 36 MONTHS
PHYSICAL GROWTH
NCHS PERCENTILES*
NAME
RECORD #
AGE (MONTHS)
LENGTH
WEIGHT
in
cm
lb
kg
Ross Growth & Development Program
MOTHER'S STATURE
FATHER'S STATURE
GESTATIONAL AGE
WEEKS
DATE
AGE
LENGTH
WEIGHT
HEAD CIRC
COMMENT
BIRTH
*Adapted from: Hamill PVV, Drizd TA, Johnson CL, Reed RB, Roche AF, Moore WM: Physical growth: National Center for Health Statistics percentiles. AM J CLIN NUTR 32:607-629, 1979. Data from the Fels Longitudinal Study, Wright State University School of Medicine, Yellow Springs, Ohio.
© 1982 Ross Laboratories

Figure E-1A
Girls: Birth to 36 Months Physical Growth NCHS Percentiles—Length and Weight for Age

- Locate the child's weight in pounds or kilograms along the vertical axis on the lower left or right side of the chart.
- Mark the chart where the age and weight lines intersect. Read the percentile.

To assess length, height, or head circumference, the assessor follows the same procedure, using the appropriate chart. Head circumference percentile should be similar to the child's height and weight percentiles.

**Figure E–1B
Girls: Birth to 36 Months Physical
Growth NCHS Percentiles—Head
Circumference for Age and Weight
for Length**

E

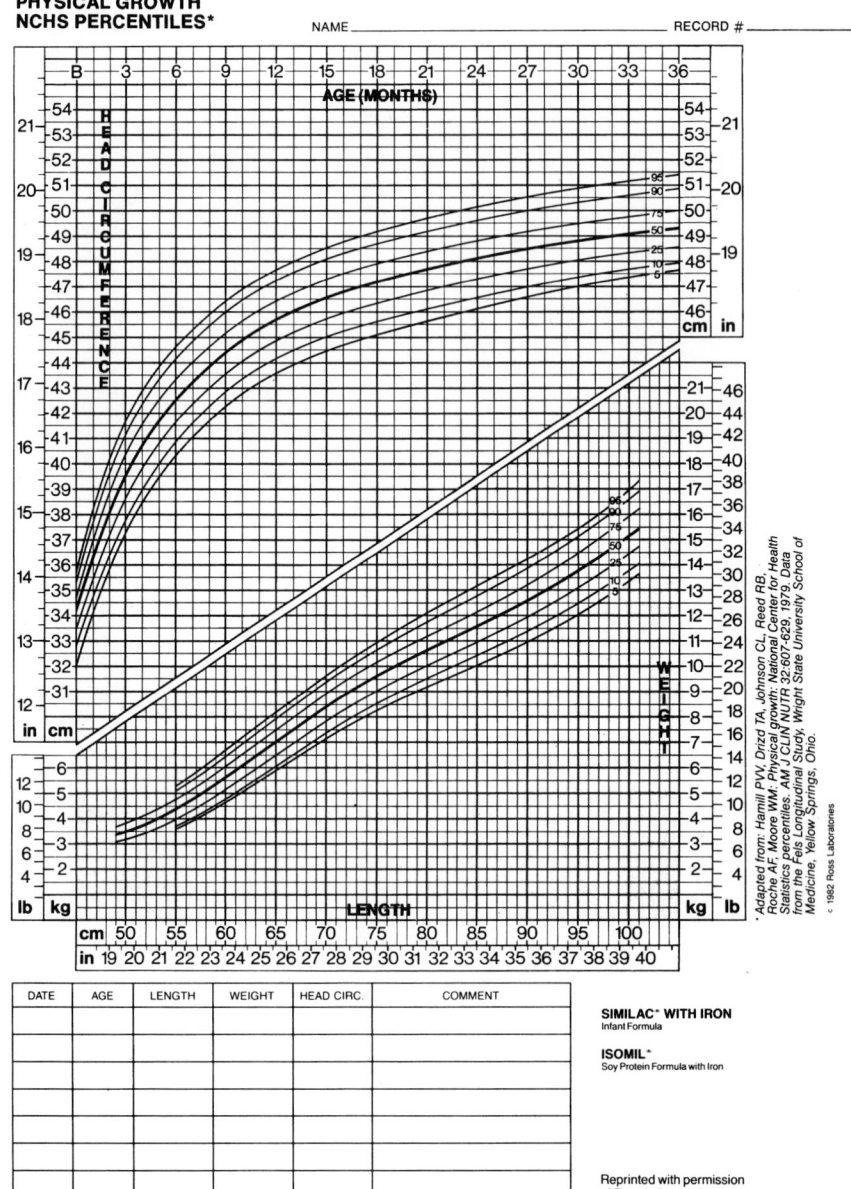

GIRLS: BIRTH TO 36 MONTHS
PHYSICAL GROWTH
NCHS PERCENTILES*

NAME _____ RECORD # _____

*Adapted from: Hamill PVV, Drizd TA, Johnson CL, Reed RB, Roche AF, Moore WM. Physical growth: National Center for Health Statistics percentiles. AM J CLIN NUTR 32:607-629, 1979. Data from the Fels Longitudinal Study, Wright State University School of Medicine, Yellow Springs, Ohio.
© 1982 Ross Laboratories

DATE	AGE	LENGTH	WEIGHT	HEAD CIRC.	COMMENT

SIMILAC® WITH IRON
Infant Formula

ISOMIL®
Soy Protein Formula with Iron

Reprinted with permission
of Ross Laboratories

With height, weight, and head circumference measures plotted on growth percentile charts, a skilled clinician can begin to interpret the data. Percentile charts divide the measures of a population into 100 equal divisions. Thus half of the population falls above the 50th percentile, and half falls below. The use of percentile measures allows for comparisons among people of the same age and gender. For example, a six-month-old female infant whose weight is at the 75 percentile weighs more than 75 percent of the female infants her age.

(continued on p. E–19)

**BOYS: BIRTH TO 36 MONTHS
PHYSICAL GROWTH
NCHS PERCENTILES***

**Figure E–2A
Boys: Birth to 36 Months Physical
Growth NCHS Percentiles—Length
and Weight for Age**

Ross
Growth &
Development
Program

NAME _____ RECORD # _____

*Adapted from: Hamill PVV, Drizd TA, Johnson CL, Reed RB, Roche AF, Moore WM: Physical growth: National Center for Health Statistics percentiles. AM J CLIN NUTR 32:607-629, 1979. Data from the Fels Longitudinal Study, Wright State University School of Medicine, Yellow Springs, Ohio.

© 1982 Ross Laboratories

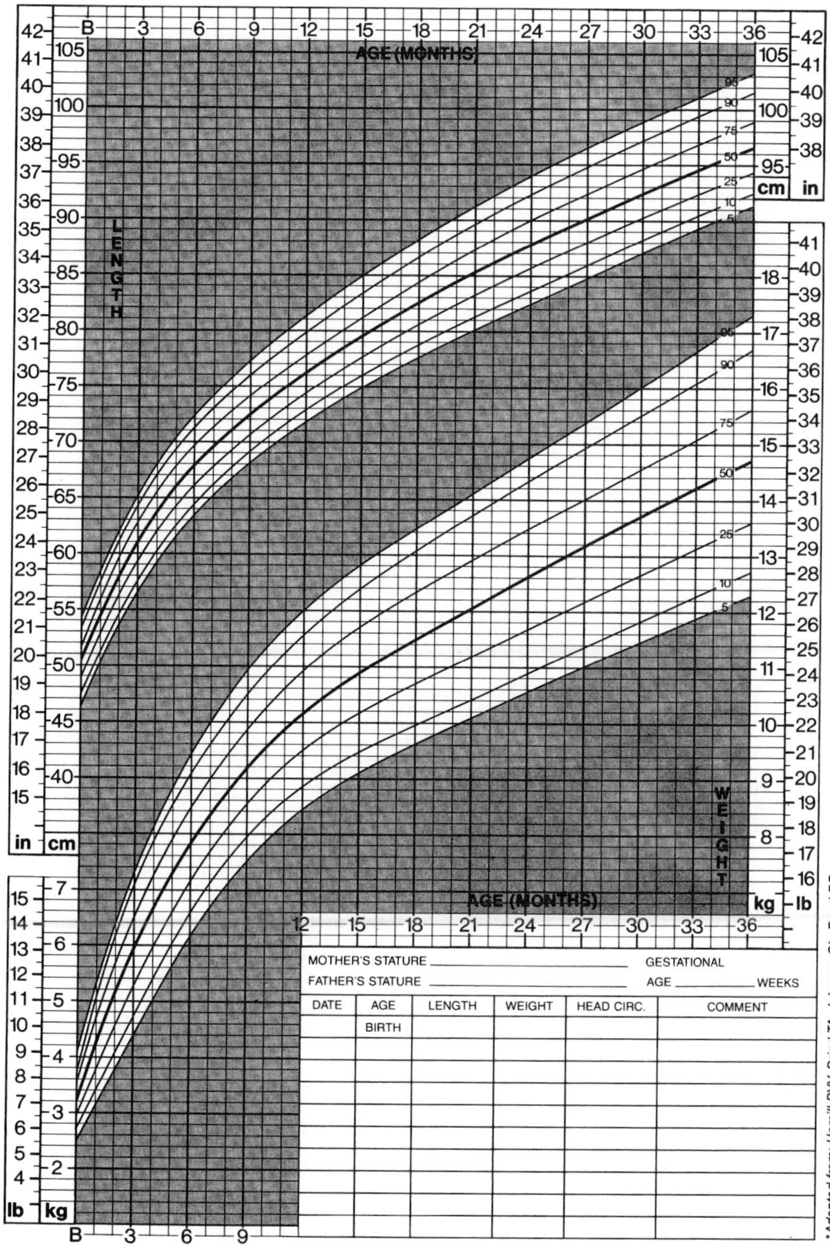

MOTHER'S STATURE _____ GESTATIONAL
FATHER'S STATURE _____ AGE _____ WEEKS

DATE	AGE	LENGTH	WEIGHT	HEAD CIRC.	COMMENT
	BIRTH				

E

Figure E-2B
Boys: Birth to 36 Months Physical
Growth NCHS Percentiles—Head
Circumference for Age and Weight
for Length

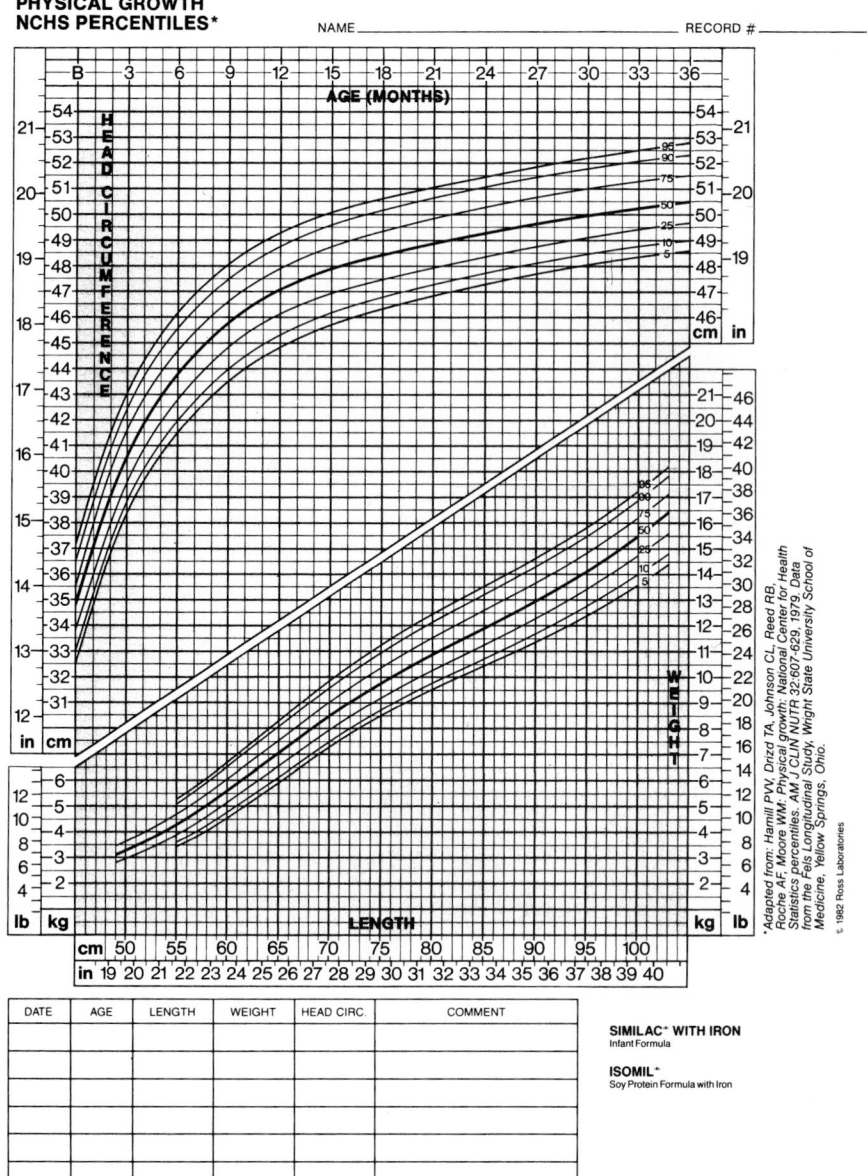

BOYS: BIRTH TO 36 MONTHS
PHYSICAL GROWTH
NCHS PERCENTILES*

NAME_____ RECORD #_____

DATE	AGE	LENGTH	WEIGHT	HEAD CIRC.	COMMENT

SIMILAC® WITH IRON
Infant Formula

ISOMIL®
Soy Protein Formula with Iron

Reprinted with permission
of Ross Laboratories

*Adapted from: Hamill PVV, Drizd TA, Johnson CL, Reed RB,
Roche AF, Moore WM: Physical growth: National Center for Health
Statistics percentiles. AM J CLIN NUTR 32:607-629, 1979. Data
from the Fels Longitudinal Study, Wright State University School of
Medicine, Yellow Springs, Ohio.

© 1982 Ross Laboratories

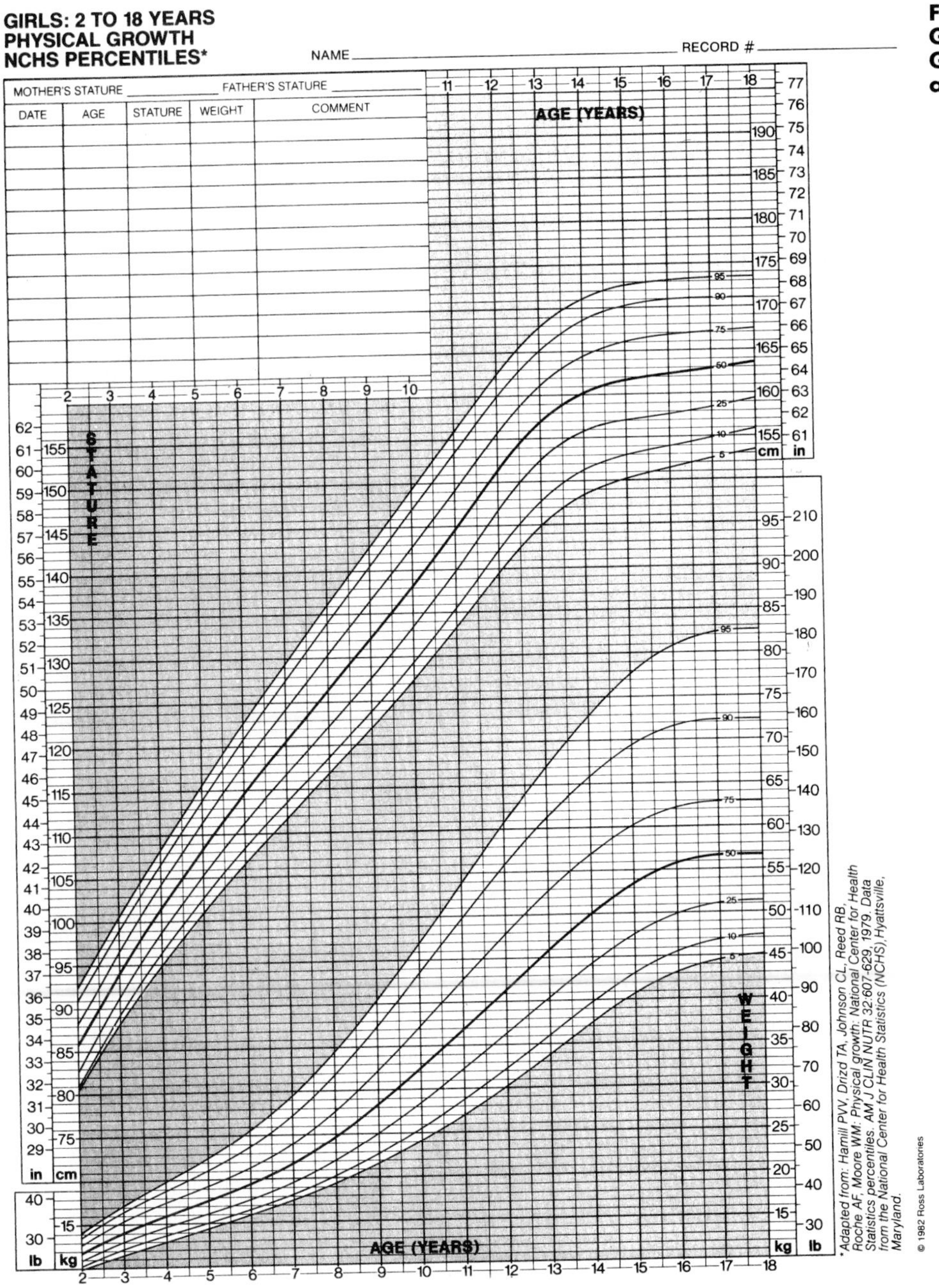
GIRLS: 2 TO 18 YEARS
PHYSICAL GROWTH
NCHS PERCENTILES*
NAME
RECORD #
MOTHER'S STATURE
FATHER'S STATURE
DATE
AGE
STATURE
WEIGHT
COMMENT
AGE (YEARS)
STATURE
WEIGHT
in
cm
kg
lb
*Adapted from: Hamill PVV, Drizd TA, Johnson CL, Reed RB, Roche AF, Moore WM: Physical growth: National Center for Health Statistics percentiles. AM J CLIN NUTR 32:607-629, 1979. Data from the National Center for Health Statistics (NCHS), Hyattsville, Maryland.
© 1982 Ross Laboratories

Figure E-3
Girls: 2 to 18 Years Physical Growth NCHS Percentiles—Height and Weight for Age

E

**Figure E–4
Boys: 2 to 18 Years Physical
Growth NCHS Percentiles—Height
and Weight for Age**

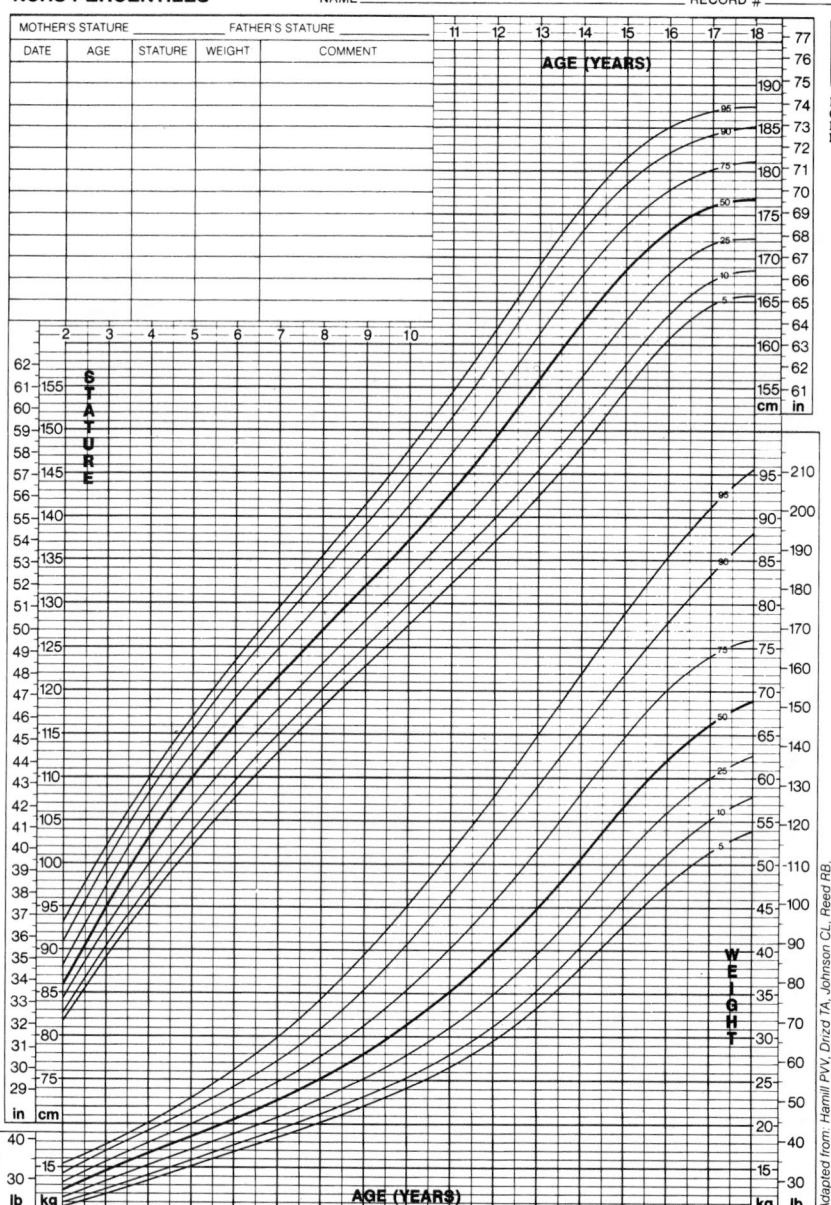

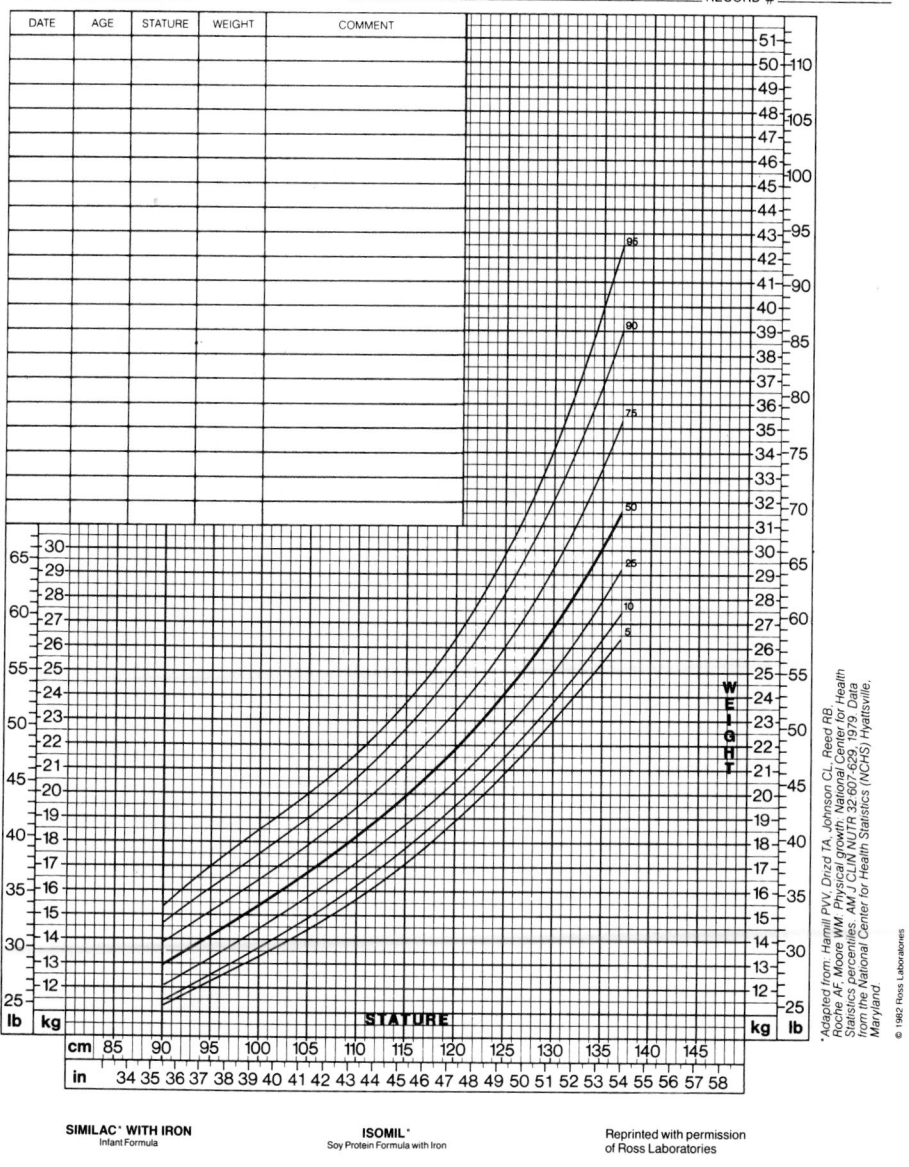

Figure E-5
Girls: Prepubescent Physical Growth
NCHS Percentiles—Weight for Height

Chapter 8 described how assessors use the body mass index (BMI) to evaluate weight in adults. Assessors can also evaluate weight for height by comparing measures with population standards. To use the height-weight tables to assess body weight in adults, the assessor must determine the client's frame size. Figure E-7 shows how to measure the wrist to determine frame size (see Table E-2). Table E-3 (see p. E-21) presents another method of determining frame size, and Table E-4 shows the metropolitan height and weight standards. As noted, the BMI can also be used to assess body weight in adults. Figure E-8 on p. E-22 presents a nomogram for BMI. Figure E-9 on p. E-23 shows normal weight gains related to duration of pregnancy in weeks for women who start their pregnancies at normal weight, underweight, or overweight.

Figure E–6
Boys: Prepubescent Physical Growth NCHS Percentiles—Weight for Height

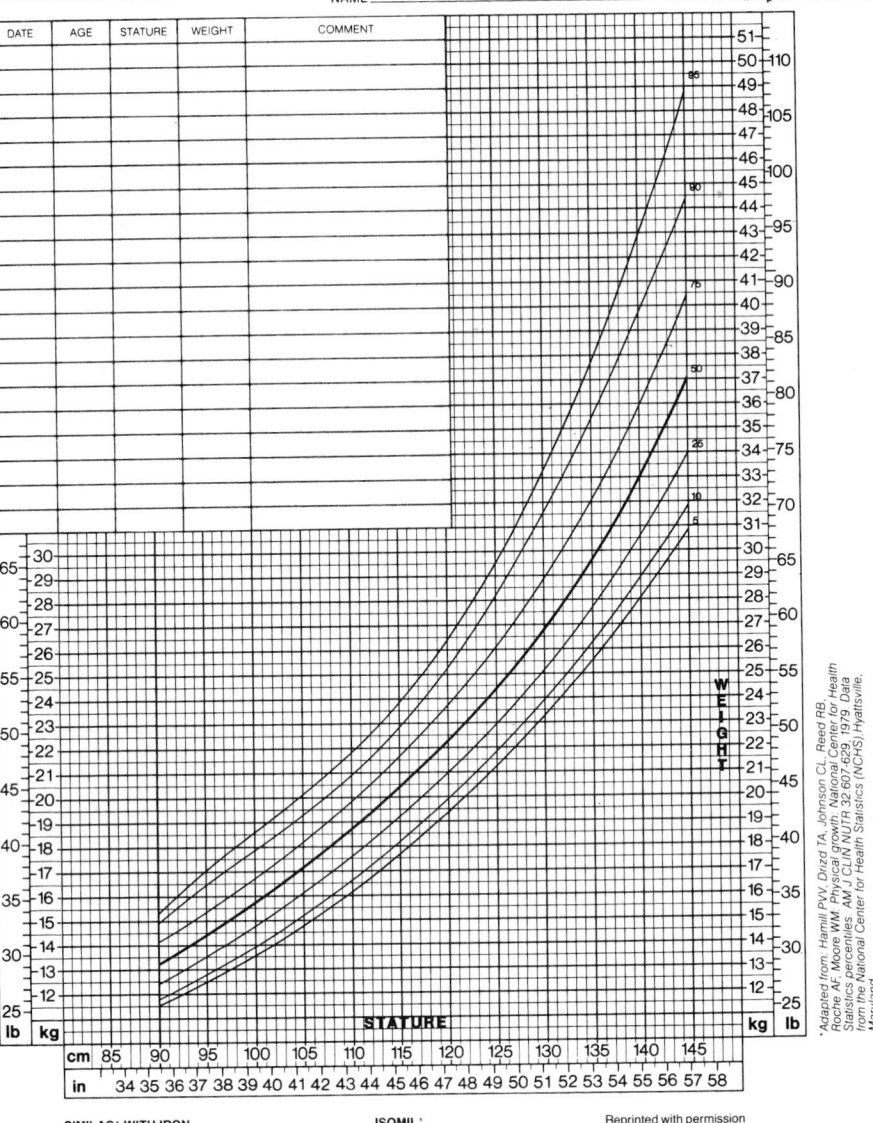

BOYS: PREPUBESCENT PHYSICAL GROWTH NCHS PERCENTILES*

NAME _____   RECORD # _____

DATE	AGE	STATURE	WEIGHT	COMMENT

SIMILAC® WITH IRON
Infant Formula

ISOMIL®
Soy Protein Formula with Iron

Reprinted with permission of Ross Laboratories

*Adapted from: Hamill PVV, Drizd TA, Johnson CL, Reed RB, Roche AF, Moore WM. Physical growth: National Center for Health Statistics percentiles. AM J CLIN NUTR 32:607-629, 1979. Data from the National Center for Health Statistics (NCHS), Hyattsville, Maryland.

© 1982 Ross Laboratories

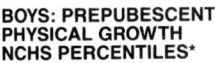

**Figure E–7
Wrist Circumference**

Place tape here

Styloid process ("wristbone")

Table E–2
Frame Size from Height-Wrist Circumference Ratios (r)[a]

Frame Size	Male r Values	Female r Values
Small	>10.4	>11.0
Medium	9.6–10.4	10.1–11.0
Large	<9.6	<10.1

[a]$r = \dfrac{\text{height (cm)}}{\text{wrist circumference (cm)}}$. The wrist is measured where it bends (distal to the styloid process), on the right arm (see Figure E–7).

Table E–3
How to Determine Body Frame by Elbow Breadth

To make a simple approximation of frame size, do the following: Extend the arm, and bend the forearm upward at a 90° angle. Keep the fingers straight, and turn the inside of the wrist away from the body. Place the thumb and index finger on the two prominent bones on *either side* of the elbow. Measure the space between the fingers against a ruler or a tape measure.[a] Compare the measurements with the following standards.

These standards represent the elbow measurements for medium-framed men and women of various heights. Measurements smaller than those listed indicate a small frame, and larger measurements indicate a large frame.

Men

HEIGHT IN 1-INCH HEELS	ELBOW BREADTH
5 ft 2 in to 5 ft 3 in	2½ to 2⅞ in
5 ft 4 in to 5 ft 7 in	2⅝ to 2⅞ in
5 ft 8 in to 5 ft 11 in	2¾ to 3 in
6 ft 0 in to 6 ft 3 in	2¾ to 3⅛ in
6 ft 4 in and over	2⅞ to 3¼ in

Women

HEIGHT IN 1-INCH HEELS	ELBOW BREADTH
4 ft 10 in to 4 ft 11 in	2¼ to 2½ in
5 ft 0 in to 5 ft 3 in	2¼ to 2½ in
5 ft 4 in to 5 ft 7 in	2⅜ to 2⅝ in
5 ft 8 in to 5 ft 11 in	2⅜ to 2⅝ in
6 ft 0 in and over	2½ to 2¾ in

[a]For the most accurate measurement, measure elbow breadth with a caliper.

Source: Metropolitan Life Insurance Company.

Table E–4
1983 Metropolitan Height and Weight Tables

Men Height FEET	INCHES	SMALL	MEDIUM	LARGE	Women Height FEET	INCHES	SMALL	MEDIUM	LARGE
5	2	128–134	131–141	138–150	4	10	102–111	109–121	118–131
5	3	130–136	133–143	140–153	4	11	103–113	111–123	120–134
5	4	132–138	135–145	142–156	5	0	104–115	113–126	122–137
5	5	134–140	137–148	144–160	5	1	106–118	115–129	125–140
5	6	136–142	139–151	146–164	5	2	108–121	118–132	128–143
5	7	138–145	142–154	149–168	5	3	111–124	121–135	131–147
5	8	140–148	145–157	152–172	5	4	114–127	124–138	134–151
5	9	142–151	148–160	155–176	5	5	117–130	127–141	137–155
5	10	144–154	151–163	158–180	5	6	120–133	130–144	140–159
5	11	146–157	154–166	161–184	5	7	123–136	133–147	143–163
6	0	149–160	157–170	164–188	5	8	126–139	136–150	146–167
6	1	152–164	160–174	168–192	5	9	129–142	139–153	149–170
6	2	155–168	164–178	172–197	5	10	132–145	142–156	152–173
6	3	158–172	167–182	176–202	5	11	135–148	145–159	155–176
6	4	162–176	171–187	181–207	6	0	138–151	148–162	158–179

Note: To use the table, add an inch to your barefoot height (you are assumed to be wearing shoes with 1-inch heels), and adjust for clothing (the tables assume 5 pounds for clothes for men and 3 pounds for women). Weights are at age 25 to 29 based on lowest mortality, in pounds according to frame size.

Source: Reproduced courtesy of Metropolitan Life Insurance Company. Source of basic data: Society of Actuaries and Association of Life Insurance Medical Directors of America, *1979 Build Study,* 1980.

Figure E–8
Nomogram for Body Mass Index (BMI)

Weights and heights are without clothing. With clothes, add 5 pounds for men or 3 pounds for women, and 1 inch in height for shoes. Draw a straight line, or place a ruler, from your height (left) to your weight (right). At the point where it crosses the BMI line, read your BMI. The accompanying table in the margin indicates the BMI used to define the cutoff points in the graphs on the inside back covers.

	Men	Women
Underweight	<20.7	<19.1
Acceptable weight	20.7 to 27.8	19.1 to 27.3
Overweight	≥27.8	≥27.3
Severe overweight	≥31.1	≥32.3
Morbid obesity	≥45.4	≥44.8

Source: From the 1983 Metropolitan Life Insurance Company tables, designed by B. T. Burton and W. R. Roster, Health implications of obesity, and NIH Consensus Development Conference, *Journal of the American Dietetic Association* 85 (1985): 1117–1121.

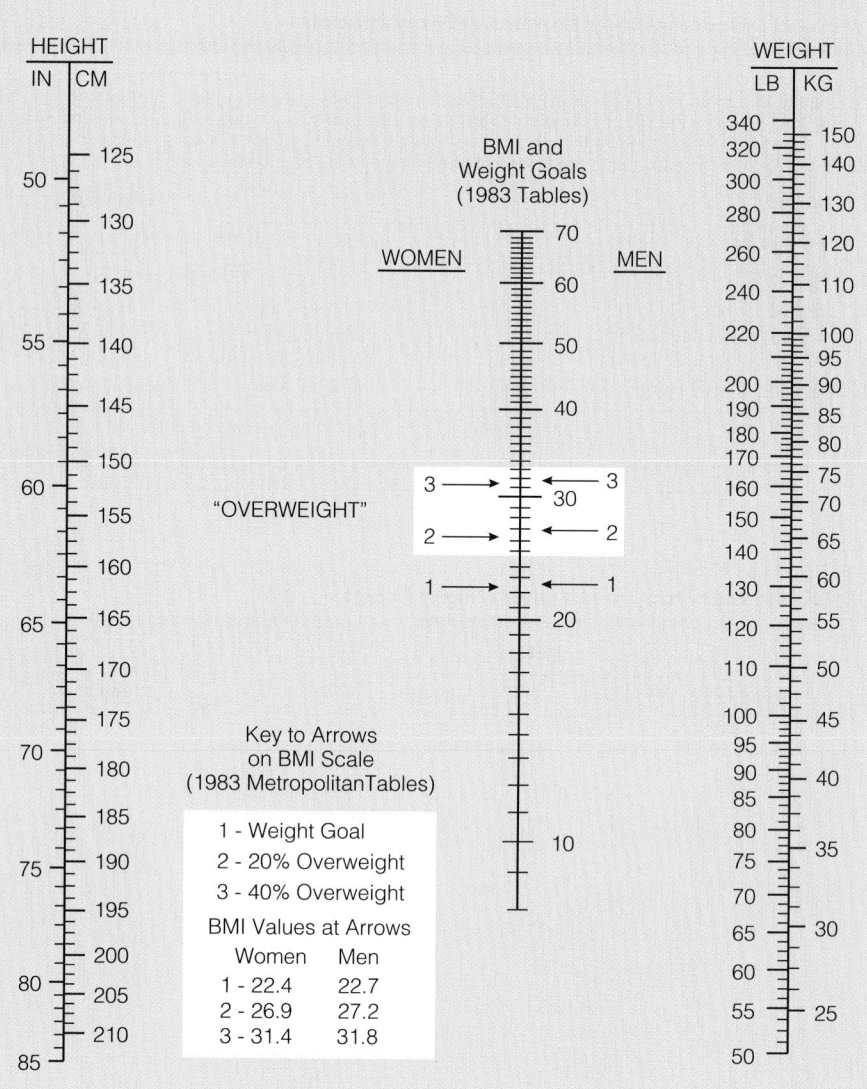

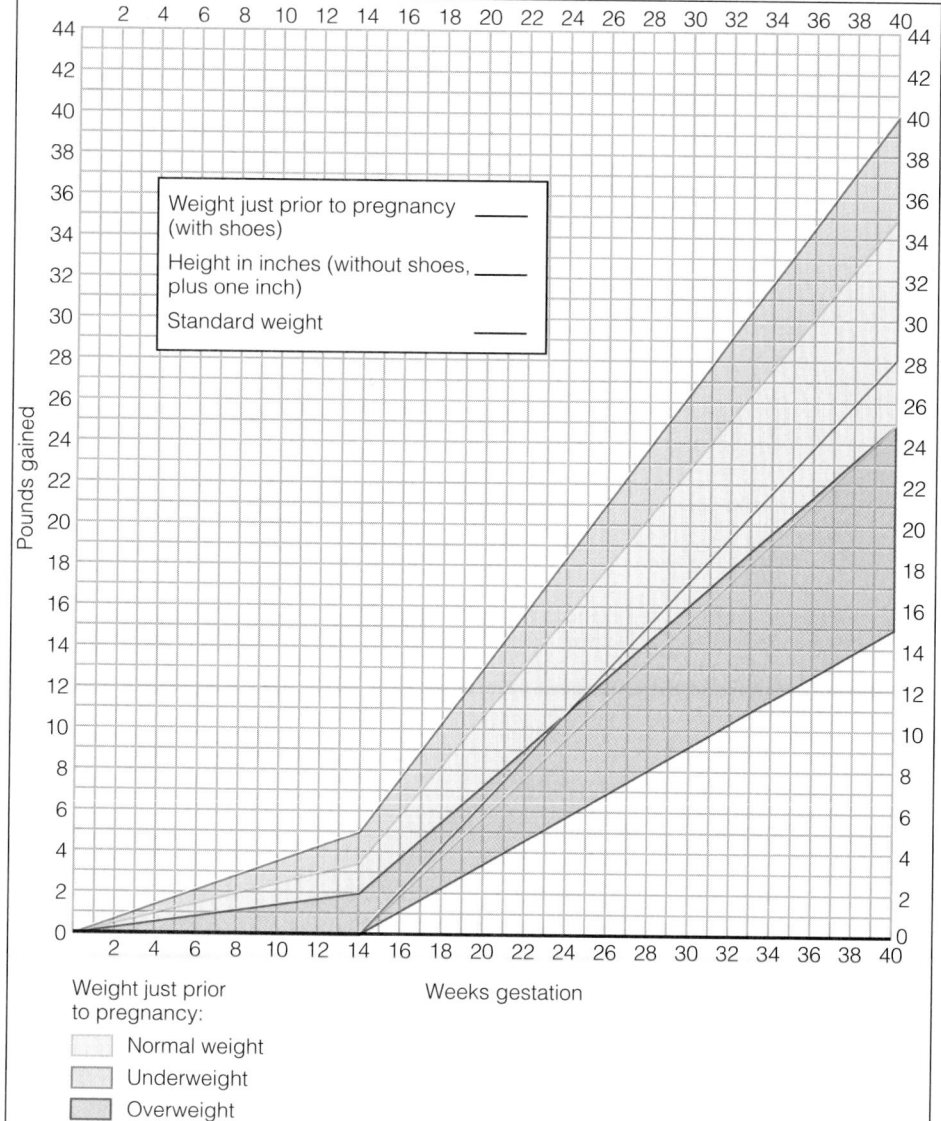

Figure E–9
Prenatal Weight-Gain Grid

A prenatal weight-gain grid plots the rate of weight gain during pregnancy. Normal-weight women should gain about 3 1/2 pounds in the first trimester and just under 1 pound/week thereafter, achieving a total gain of 25 to 35 pounds by term; underweight women should gain about 5 pounds in the first trimester and just over 1 pound/week thereafter, achieving a total gain of 28 to 40 pounds by term; and overweight women should gain about 2 pounds in the first trimester and 2/3 pound/week thereafter, achieving a total gain of 15 to 25 pounds.

Fatfold measurements (see Figure E–10 on p. E–24) assist health care professionals in evaluating the composition of body weight. As already explained in Chapter 16, a lean tissue measure can be computed from the triceps fatfold measurement together with the midarm circumference measurement: the midarm muscle circumference (see Figures E–11 and E–12 on pp. E–24 and E–25). Table E–5 (p. E–25) gives triceps fatfold percentile standards. Table E–6 on p. E–26 shows the midarm muscle circumference percentile standards, and Figure E–13 (p. E–27) illustrates a nomogram method for determining midarm muscle circumference from these two measures.

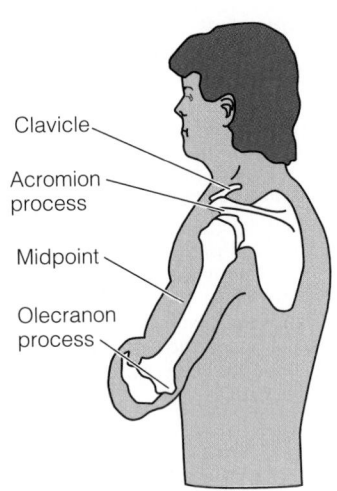

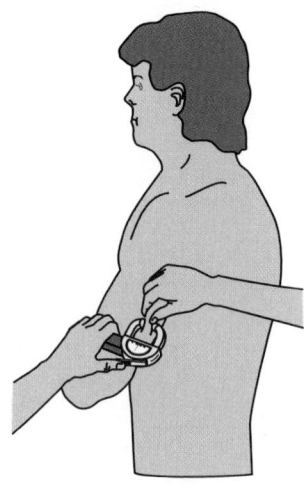

Figure E-10
How to Measure the Triceps Fatfold

A. Find the midpoint of the arm:

1. Ask the subject to bend his or her arm at the elbow and lay the hand across the stomach. (If he or she is right-handed, measure the left arm, and vice versa.)

2. Feel the shoulder to locate the acromion process. It helps to slide your fingers along the clavicle to find the acromion process. The olecranon process is the tip of the elbow.

3. Place a measuring tape from the acromion process to the tip of the elbow. Divide this measurement by 2, and mark the midpoint of the arm with a pen.

B. Measure the fatfold:

1. Ask the subject to let his or her arm hang loosely to the side.

2. Grasp the fold of skin and subcutaneous fat between the thumb and forefinger slightly above the midpoint mark. Gently pull the skin away from the underlying muscle. (This step takes a lot of practice. If you want to be sure you don't have muscle as well as fat, ask the subject to contract and relax the muscle. You should be able to feel if you are pinching muscle.)

3. Place the calipers over the fatfold at the midpoint mark, and read the measurement to the nearest 1.0 millimeter in two to three seconds. (If using plastic calipers, align pressure lines, and read the measurement to the nearest 1.0 millimeter in two to three seconds.)

4. Repeat steps 2 and 3 twice more. Add the three readings, and then divide by 3 to find the average.

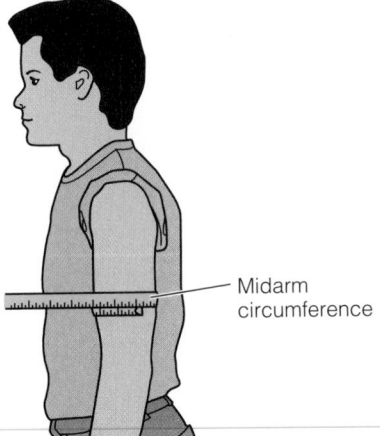

Figure E-11
How to Measure the Midarm Circumference

Ask the subject to let his or her arm hang loosely to the side. Place the measuring tape horizontally around the arm at the midpoint mark. This measurement is the midarm circumference.

Figure E–12
How to Derive the Midarm Muscle Circumference

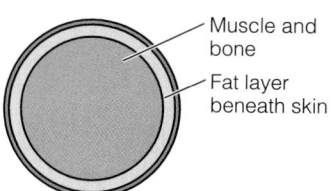

Muscle and bone

Fat layer beneath skin

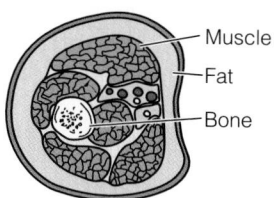

Muscle

Fat

Bone

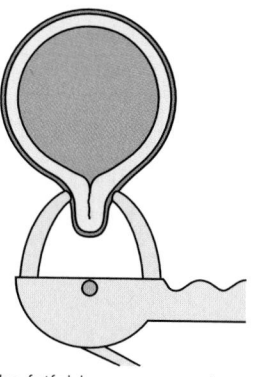

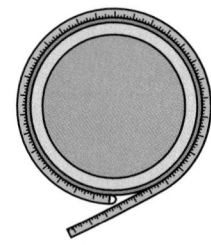

The arm is visualized as an inner circle of muscle and bone surrounded by an outer layer of fat and skin.

In reality, the arm is not circular, and there is some bone and blood vessels, but the simplified picture is approximately correct.

The fatfold measurement equals two times the thickness of the fat and skin.

The midarm circumference measures the size of the arm and all of its components.

The following equation then derives the *circumference of the muscle*, an index of the body's total skeletal mass:
Midarm muscle circumference (cm) = midarm circumference (cm) – [0.314[a] × triceps fatfold (mm)].
[a]This factor converts the fatfold measurement to a circumference measurement and millimeters to centimeters.

Table E–5
Triceps Fatfold Percentiles (Millimeters)

Age	Male					Female				
	5TH	25TH	50TH	75TH	95TH	5TH	25TH	50TH	75TH	95TH
1–1.9	6	8	10	12	16	6	8	10	12	16
2–2.9	6	8	10	12	15	6	9	10	12	16
3–3.9	6	8	10	11	15	7	9	11	12	15
4–4.9	6	8	9	11	14	7	8	10	12	16
5–5.9	6	8	9	11	15	6	8	10	12	18
6–6.9	5	7	8	10	16	6	8	10	12	16
7–7.9	5	7	9	12	17	6	9	11	13	18
8–8.9	5	7	8	10	16	6	9	12	15	24
9–9.9	6	7	10	13	18	8	10	13	16	22
10–10.9	6	8	10	14	21	7	10	12	17	27
11–11.9	6	8	11	16	24	7	10	13	18	28
12–12.9	6	8	11	14	28	8	11	14	18	27
13–13.9	5	7	10	14	26	8	12	15	21	30
14–14.9	4	7	9	14	24	9	13	16	21	28
15–15.9	4	6	8	11	24	8	12	17	21	32
16–16.9	4	6	8	12	22	10	15	18	22	31
17–17.9	5	6	8	12	19	10	13	19	24	37
18–18.9	4	6	9	13	24	10	15	18	22	30
19–24.9	4	7	10	15	22	10	14	18	24	34
25–34.9	5	8	12	16	24	10	16	21	27	37
35–44.9	5	8	12	16	23	12	18	23	29	38
45–54.9	6	8	12	15	25	12	20	25	30	40
55–64.9	5	8	11	14	22	12	20	25	31	38
65–74.9	4	8	11	15	22	12	18	24	29	36

Note: If measurements fall between the percentiles shown here, the percentile can be estimated from the information in this table. For example, a measurement of 7 millimeters for a 27-year-old male would be about the 20th percentile.

Source: Adapted from A. R. Frisancho, New norms of upper limb fat and muscle areas for assessment of nutritional status. *American Journal of Clinical Nutrition* 34 (1981): 2540–2545.

Table E–6
Midarm Muscle Circumference Percentiles (Centimeters)

Age	Male					Female				
	5TH	25TH	50TH	75TH	95TH	5TH	25TH	50TH	75TH	95TH
1–1.9	11.0	11.9	12.7	13.5	14.7	10.5	11.7	12.4	13.9	14.3
2–2.9	11.1	12.2	13.0	14.0	15.0	11.1	11.9	12.6	13.3	14.7
3–3.9	11.7	13.1	13.7	14.3	15.3	11.3	12.4	13.2	14.0	15.2
4–4.9	12.3	13.3	14.1	14.8	15.9	11.5	12.8	13.6	14.4	15.7
5–5.9	12.8	14.0	14.7	15.4	16.9	12.5	13.4	14.2	15.1	16.5
6–6.9	13.1	14.2	15.1	16.1	17.7	13.0	13.8	14.5	15.4	17.1
7–7.9	13.7	15.1	16.0	16.8	19.0	12.9	14.2	15.1	16.0	17.6
8–8.9	14.0	15.4	16.2	17.0	18.7	13.8	15.1	16.0	17.1	19.4
9–9.9	15.1	16.1	17.0	18.3	20.2	14.7	15.8	16.7	18.0	19.8
10–10.9	15.6	16.6	18.0	19.1	22.1	14.8	15.9	17.0	18.0	19.7
11–11.9	15.9	17.3	18.3	19.5	23.0	15.0	17.1	18.1	19.6	22.3
12–12.9	16.7	18.2	19.5	21.0	24.1	16.2	18.0	19.1	20.1	22.0
13–13.9	17.2	19.6	21.1	22.6	24.5	16.9	18.3	19.8	21.1	24.0
14–14.9	18.9	21.2	22.3	24.0	26.4	17.4	19.0	20.1	21.6	24.7
15–15.9	19.9	21.8	23.7	25.4	27.2	17.5	18.9	20.2	21.5	24.4
16–16.9	21.3	23.4	24.9	26.9	29.6	17.0	19.0	20.2	21.6	24.9
17–17.9	22.4	24.5	25.8	27.3	31.2	17.5	19.4	20.5	22.1	25.7
18–18.9	22.6	25.2	26.4	28.3	32.4	17.4	19.1	20.2	21.5	24.5
19–24.9	23.8	25.7	27.3	28.9	32.1	17.9	19.5	20.7	22.1	24.9
25–34.9	24.3	26.4	27.9	29.8	32.6	18.3	19.9	21.2	22.8	26.4
35–44.9	24.7	26.9	28.6	30.2	32.7	18.6	20.5	21.8	23.6	27.2
45–54.9	23.9	26.5	28.1	30.0	32.6	18.7	20.6	22.0	23.8	27.4
55–64.9	23.6	26.0	27.8	29.5	32.0	18.7	20.9	22.5	24.4	28.0
65–74.9	22.3	25.1	26.8	28.4	30.6	18.5	20.8	22.5	24.4	27.9

Source: Adapted from A. R. Frisancho, New norms of upper limb fat and muscle areas for assessment of nutritional status, *American Journal of Clinical Nutrition* 34 (1981): 2540–2545.

LABORATORY TESTS OF NUTRITION STATUS

◆

As Chapter 16 pointed out, urine and blood tests provide valuable information in a nutrition assessment. Two urine tests—creatinine excretion and urine urea nitrogen—require a 24-hour urine collection and, therefore, are not routinely used.

Collecting a 24-hour urine sample presents many problems. Much effort is wasted if everyone involved does not conscientiously follow proper techniques. The collection of urine and recording of food intake data require client cooperation. The client must receive thorough instructions on how to collect and save all urine samples and must be advised to call for help if needed. Each urine sample is added to the collection container and refrigerated until the collection is complete. If even one urine sample is spilled or discarded, the test is invalid.

Most hospitals have a standard time for beginning urinary collections (often, between 6:00 A.M. and 6:00 P.M.). For nitrogen balance studies, food intake must also be recorded during the exact same time period. All nurses caring for the client on all shifts must record, or ensure that the client records, food intake data carefully.

To calculate the creatinine-height index (CHI) from the measured urinary creatinine and the client's height, use the following equation:

$$\text{CHI} = \frac{\text{measured urinary creatinine (24-hour sample)}}{\text{standard creatinine excretion for height and sex}} \times 100.$$

For example, to calculate the CHI in a man of medium frame, 5 feet 8 inches tall, who excretes 1090 milligrams of creatinine in 24 hours, follow these steps:

◆ Look up the standard creatinine excretion (Table E–7 on p. E–28).

In this example, the standard creatinine excretion is 1.56 grams or 1560 milligrams.

Figure E–13
Nomograms for Determination of Midarm Muscle Circumference

To obtain arm muscle circumference using either nomogram, lay a ruler between values of arm circumference and fatfold, and read off arm muscle circumference.

Source: Reproduced with permission from J. Gurney and D. Jelliffe, Arm anthropometry in nutritional assessment; nomogram for rapid calculation of muscle circumference and cross-sectional muscle and fat areas. *American Journal of Clinical Nutrition* 26 (1973): 912, as adapted by A. Grant, *Nutritional Assessment Guidelines,* 2nd ed., 1979.

♦ Complete the CHI equation: $\text{CHI} = \dfrac{1090 \text{ mg}}{1560 \text{ mg}} \times 100 = 70\%.$

Based on the CHI, the man in this example has a skeletal muscle mass 70 percent of that considered typical for a man of his height. Table E–8 (p. E–28) shows the standard creatinine excretions for women.

Table E-7
Creatinine-Height Index Standards for Men

Height		Small Frame			Medium Frame			Large Frame		
		Ideal Weight	Creatinine		Ideal Weight	Creatinine		Ideal Weight	Creatinine	
in	cm	(kg)	(g/24 h)	(mmol/d)	(kg)	(g/24 h)	(mmol/d)	(kg)	(g/24 h)	(mmol/d)
61	154.9	52.7	1.21	10.7	56.1	1.29	11.4	60.7	1.40	12.4
62	157.5	54.1	1.24	11.0	57.7	1.33	11.8	62.0	1.43	12.6
63	160.0	55.4	1.27	11.2	59.1	1.36	12.0	63.6	1.46	12.9
64	162.5	56.8	1.31	11.6	60.4	1.39	12.3	65.2	1.50	13.3
65	165.1	58.4	1.34	11.8	62.0	1.43	12.6	66.8	1.54	13.6
66	167.6	60.2	1.39	12.3	63.9	1.47	13.0	68.9	1.59	14.1
67	170.2	62.0	1.43	12.6	65.9	1.52	13.4	71.1	1.64	14.5
68	172.7	63.9	1.47	13.0	67.7	1.56	13.8	72.9	1.68	14.9
69	175.3	65.9	1.52	13.4	69.5	1.60	14.1	74.8	1.72	15.2
70	177.8	67.7	1.56	13.8	71.6	1.65	14.6	76.8	1.77	15.6
71	180.3	69.5	1.60	14.1	73.6	1.69	14.9	79.1	1.82	16.1
72	182.9	71.4	1.64	14.5	75.7	1.74	15.4	81.1	1.87	16.5
73	185.4	73.4	1.69	14.9	77.7	1.79	15.8	83.4	1.92	17.0
74	187.9	75.2	1.73	15.3	80.0	1.85	16.4	85.7	1.97	17.4
75	190.5	77.0	1.77	15.6	82.3	1.89	16.7	87.7	2.02	17.9

Note: To convert urinary creatinine measures (g/24 h) to standard international units (mmol/d) multiply by 8.840.

Source: A. Grant and S. DeHoog, *Nutritional Assessment and Support,* 3rd ed., 1985.

Table E-8
Creatinine-Height Index Standards for Women

Height		Small Frame			Medium Frame			Large Frame		
		Ideal Weight	Creatinine		Ideal Weight	Creatinine		Ideal Weight	Creatinine	
in	cm	(kg)	(g/24 h)	(mmol/d)	(kg)	(g/24 h)	(mmol/d)	(kg)	(g/24 h)	(mmol/d)
56	142.2	43.2	0.79	7.0	46.1	0.83	7.3	50.7	0.91	8.0
57	144.8	44.3	0.80	7.1	47.3	0.85	7.5	51.8	0.93	8.2
58	147.3	45.4	0.82	7.2	48.6	0.88	7.8	53.2	0.96	8.5
59	149.8	46.8	0.84	7.4	50.0	0.90	8.0	54.5	0.98	8.7
60	152.4	48.2	0.87	7.7	51.4	0.93	8.2	55.9	1.01	8.9
61	154.9	49.5	0.89	7.9	52.7	0.95	8.4	57.3	1.03	9.1
62	157.5	50.9	0.92	8.1	54.3	0.98	8.7	58.9	1.06	9.4
63	160.0	52.3	0.94	8.3	55.9	1.01	8.9	60.6	1.09	9.6
64	162.5	53.9	0.97	8.6	57.9	1.04	9.2	62.5	1.13	10.0
65	165.1	55.7	1.00	8.8	59.8	1.08	9.5	64.3	1.16	10.3
66	167.6	57.5	1.04	9.2	61.6	1.11	9.8	66.1	1.19	10.5
67	170.2	59.3	1.07	9.5	63.4	1.14	10.1	67.9	1.22	10.8
68	172.7	61.4	1.11	9.8	65.2	1.17	10.3	70.0	1.26	11.1
69	175.2	63.2	1.14	10.1	67.0	1.21	10.7	72.0	1.30	11.5
70	177.8	65.0	1.17	10.3	68.9	1.24	11.0	74.1	1.33	11.8

Note: To convert urinary creatinine measures (g/24 h) to standard international units (mmol/d) multiply by 8.840.

Source: A. Grant and S. DeHoog, *Nutritional Assessment and Support,* 3rd ed., 1985.

Table E–9
Biochemical Tests Useful for Assessing Vitamin and Mineral Status

Nutrient	Assessment Tests
Vitamins	
Vitamin A	Retinol-binding protein, serum carotene
Thiamin	Erythrocyte (red blood cell) transketolase activity, urinary thiamin
Riboflavin	Erythrocyte glutathione reductase activity, urinary riboflavin
Vitamin B_6	Urinary xanthurenic acid excretion after tryptophan load test, urinary vitamin B_6, erythrocyte transaminase activity
Niacin	Urinary metabolites NMN (N-methyl nicotinamide) or 2-pyridone, or preferably both expressed as a ratio
Folate	Free folate in the blood, erythrocyte folate (reflects liver stores), urinary formiminoglutamic acid (FIGLU), vitamin B_{12} status (folate assessment tests alone do not distinguish between the two deficiencies)
Vitamin B_{12}	Serum vitamin B_{12}, erythrocyte vitamin B_{12}, urinary methyl-malonic acid synthesis or DUMP test (from the abbreviation for the chemical name of DNA's raw material, deoxyuridine monophosphate) Schilling test
Biotin	Serum biotin, urinary biotin
Vitamin C	Serum or plasma vitamin C[a], leukocyte vitamin C, urinary vitamin C
Vitamin D	Serum alkaline phosphatase
Vitamin E	Serum tocopherol, erythrocyte hemolysis
Vitamin K	Blood clotting time (prothrombin time)
Minerals	
Potassium	Serum potassium
Magnesium	Serum magnesium
Iron	Hemoglobin, hematocrit, serum ferritin, total iron-binding capacity (TIBC), protoporphyrin, mean corpuscular volume (MCV), serum iron
Iodine	Serum protein-bound iodine, radioiodine uptake
Zinc	Plasma zinc, hair zinc

[a]Vitamin C shifts unpredictably between the plasma and the while blood cells known as leukocytes; thus a plasma or serum determination may not accurately reflect the body's pool. The appropriate clinical test may be a measurement of leukocyte vitamin C. A combination of both tests may be more reliable than either one alone.

Source: Adapted from A. Grant and S. DeHoog. *Nutritional Assessment and Support,* 3rd ed., 1985.

Table E–9 shows laboratory tests that help assess vitamin and mineral status. Some vitamin and mineral deficiencies, notably folate, vitamin B_{12}, and iron, can lead to anemia. Anemia, defined as a reduced number of red blood cells, can also result from many medical conditions unrelated to nutrition. Table E–10 shows the tests that help to define anemia and to distinguish among its major nutrition-related causes. Tables E–11 through E–15 provide standards for hemoglobin, hematocrit, serum ferritin, serum iron, percent transferrin saturation, and folate concentrations.

Table E–10
Laboratory Tests Useful in Evaluating Nutrition-Related Anemias

Test or Test Result	What It Reflects
General Tests for Anemia	
Hemoglobin (Hg)	Total amount of hemoglobin in the red blood cells (RBC)
Hematocrit (Hct)	Percentage of RBC in the total blood volume
Red blood cell (RBC) count	Number of RBC
Mean corpuscular volume (MCV)	RBC size; helps to determine if anemia is microcytic (iron deficiency) or macrocytic (folate or vitamin B_{12} deficiency)
Mean corpuscular hemoglobin concentration (MCHC)	Hemoglobin concentration within the average RBC; helps to determine if anemia is hypochromic (iron deficiency) or normochromic (folate or vitamin B_{12} deficiency)
Bone marrow aspiration	The manufacture of blood cells in different developmental states
Early Stages of Iron Deficiency	
↓ Serum ferritin	Early deficiency state with depleted iron stores
↓ Transferrin saturation	Progressing deficiency state with diminished transport iron
↑ Erythrocyte protoporphyrin	Later deficiency state with limited hemoglobin production
Folate-Deficiency Anemia	
↓ Serum Folate	Progressing deficiency state
↓ RBC Folate	Later deficiency state
Vitamin B_{12}–Deficiency Anemia	
↓ Serum vitamin B_{12}	Progressing deficiency state
Schilling test	Whether or not vitamin B_{12} is being absorbed

Table E–11
Standards for Hemoglobin Test Results

Age (yr)	Sex	Deficient (g/100 ml)	Acceptable (g/100 ml)
<2	M–F	<9.0	10.0 or >
2–5	M–F	<10.0	11.0 or >
6–12	M–F	<10.0	11.5 or >
13–16	M	<12.0	13.0 or >
	F	<10.0	11.5 or >
>16	M	<12.0	14.0 or >
	F	<10.0	12.0 or >
Pregnancy, 2nd trimester	F	<9.5	11.0 or >
Pregnancy, 3rd trimester	F	<9.0	10.5 or >

Note: To convert hemoglobin values (g/100 ml) to international standard units (g/L), multiply by 10.

Table E–12
Standards for Hematocrit Test Results

Age (yr)	Sex	Deficient (%)	Acceptable (%)
<2	M–F	<28	31 or >
2–5	M–F	<30	34 or >
6–12	M–F	<30	36 or >
13–16	M	<37	40 or >
	F	<31	36 or >
>16	M	<37	44 or >
	F	<31	38 or >
Pregnancy, 2nd trimester	F	<30	35 or >
Pregnancy, 3rd trimester	F	<30	33 or >

Note: To convert hematocrit values (%) to standard units, multiply by 0.01.

Table E–13
Standards for Serum Ferritin

Group	Deficient (ng/ml)
Children (3–14 years of age)	<10
Adolescents and adults	<12
Pregnant women	<10

Table E–14
Standards for Serum Iron

Age (yr)	Sex	Deficient (µg/100 ml)	Deficient (µmol/L)	Acceptable (µg/100 ml)	Acceptable (µmol/L)
<2	M–F	<30	<5.3	30 or >	5.3 or >
2–5	M–F	<40	<7.1	40 or >	7.1 or >
6–12	M–F	<50	<8.9	50 or >	8.9 or >
<12	M	<60	<10.7	60 or >	10.7 or >
	F	<40	<7.1	40 or >	7.1 or >

Note: To convert mg/100 ml to international units, multiply by 0.1791.

Table E–15
Standards for Percent Transferrin Saturation

Age (yr)	Sex	Deficient %	Acceptable %
<2	M–F	<15	15 or >
2–12	M–F	<20	20 or >
≥13	M	<20	20 or >
	F	<15	15 or >

Table E–16
Standards for Folate Concentrations

Measurement	Deficient (ng/ml)	Borderline (ng/ml)	Acceptable (ng/ml)
Serum folate	<3.0	3.0–6.0	>6.0
Erythrocyte folate	<140	140–160	>160

Note: To convert folate values (ng/ml) to international standard units (nmol/L), multiply by 2.266.

NUTRITION RESOURCES

◆

Contents

Books

Journals

Addresses

*P*eople interested in nutrition often want to know where they can find reliable nutrition information. Wherever you live, there are several sources you can turn to:

◆ The Department of Health may have a nutrition expert.

◆ The local extension agent is often an expert.

◆ The food editor of your local paper may be well informed.

◆ The dietitian at the local hospital had to fulfill a set of qualifications before he or she became an RD (see Highlight 1).

◆ There may be knowledgeable professors of nutrition or biochemistry at a nearby college or university.

In addition, you may be interested in building a nutrition library of your own. Books you can buy, journals you can subscribe to, and addresses you can write to for general information are given below.

BOOKS

◆

For students seeking to establish a personal library of nutrition references, the authors of this text recommend the following books:

◆ *Present Knowledge in Nutrition,* 7th ed. (Washington, D.C.: International Life Sciences Institute—Nutrition Foundation, 1996).

This 646-page paperback has a chapter on each of 64 topics, including energy, obesity, each of the nutrients, several diseases, malnutrition, growth and its assessment, immunity, alcohol, fiber, exercise, drugs, and toxins. Watch for an update; new editions come out every few years.

◆ M. E. Shils, J. A. Olson, and M. Shike, eds., *Modern Nutrition in Health and Disease,* 8th ed. (Philadelphia: Lea & Febiger, 1994).

This two-volume set is a major technical reference book on nutrition topics. It contains encyclopedic articles on the nutrients, foods, the diet, metabolism, malnutrition, age-related needs, and nutrition in disease.

◆ Food and Nutrition Board, *Recommended Dietary Allowances,* 10th ed. (Washington, D.C.: National Academy Press, 1989).

This book reviews the function of each nutrient, dietary sources, and deficiency and toxicity symptoms as well as recommendations for intakes. The Canadian equivalent is *Nutrition Recommendations,* available by mail from the Canadian Government Publishing Centre, Supply and Services Canada, Ottawa, Ontario K1A OS9, Canada.

◆ Food and Nutrition Board, *Diet and Health: Implications for Reducing Chronic Disease Risk* (Washington, D.C.: National Academy Press, 1989).

This 749-page book presents the integral relationship between diet and chronic disease prevention. Its nutrient chapters provide evidence on how diet influences disease development, and its disease chapters review the dietary patterns implicated in each chronic disease.

◆ E. M. N. Hamilton and S. A. S. Gropper, *The Biochemistry of Human Nutrition: A Desk Reference* (St. Paul, Minn.: West, 1987).

This 324-page paperback presents the biochemical concepts necessary for an understanding of nutrition. It is a handy reference book for those who have forgotten the basics of biochemistry or for those who are learning biochemistry for the first time.

We also recommend three of our own books that explore current topics in nutrition, health, and the life span:

◆ E. N. Whitney, C. B. Cataldo, L. K. DeBruyne, and S. R. Rolfes, *Nutrition for Health and Health Care* (St. Paul, Minn.: West, 1995).

◆ F. S. Sizer and E. N. Whitney, *Nutrition: Concepts and Controversies,* 7th ed. (Belmont, Calif.: West/Wadsworth, 1997).

◆ S. R. Rolfes, L. K. DeBruyne, and E. N. Whitney, *Life Span Nutrition: Conception through Life* (St. Paul, Minn.: West, 1990).

JOURNALS
◆

Nutrition Today is an excellent magazine for the interested layperson. It makes a point of raising controversial issues and providing a forum for conflicting opinions. Six issues per year are published. Order from Williams and Wilkins, 428 East Preston Street, Baltimore, MD 21202.

The *Journal of the American Dietetic Association,* the official publication of the ADA, contains articles of interest to dietitians and nutritionists, news of legislative action on food and nutrition, and a very useful section of abstracts of articles from many other journals of nutrition and related areas. There are twelve issues per year, available from the American Dietetic Association (see "Addresses," later).

Nutrition Reviews, a publication of the International Life Sciences Institute, does much of the work for the library researcher, compiling recent evidence on current topics and presenting extensive bibliographies. Twelve issues per year are available from Springer-Verlag New York, 175 Fifth Avenue, New York, NY 10010.

Nutrition and the M.D. is a monthly newsletter that provides up-to-date, easy-to-read, practical information on nutrition for health care providers. It is available from PM, Inc., 7100 Hayven Hurst Avenue, Suite 107, Van Nuys, CA 91406.

Other journals that deserve mention here are *Food Technology, Journal of Nutrition, American Journal of Clinical Nutrition, Nutrition Research,* and *Journal of Nutrition Education. FDA Consumer,* a government publication with many articles of interest to the consumer, is available from the Food and Drug Administration (see "Addresses," below). Many other journals of value are referred to throughout this book.

ADDRESSES
◆

Many of the organizations listed below will provide publication lists free on request.

U.S. GOVERNMENT

◆ Federal Trade Commission (FTC)
Public Reference Branch
(202) 326-2222
Internet address: http://www.ftc.gov

◆ Food and Drug Administration (FDA)
Office of Consumer Affairs
5600 Fishers Lane, HFE 88 Room 16–63
Rockville, MD 20857
(301) 443-3170 1 PM–3:30 PM EST
Internet address: http://www.fda.gov

◆ FDA Office of Food Labeling (HFS-150)
200 C Street SW
Washington, DC 20204
(202) 205-4561; fax: (202) 205-4564

◆ FDA Office of Plant and Dairy Foods
and Beverages (HFS-300)
200 C Street SW
Washington, DC 20204
(202) 205-4064; fax: (202) 205-4422

◆ FDA Office of Special Nutritionals (HFS-450)
200 C Street SW
Washington, DC 20204
(202) 205-4168; fax: (202) 205-5295

◆ Food and Nutrition Information Center
National Agricultural Library, Room 304
10301 Baltimore Blvd.
Beltsville, MD 20705-2351
(301) 504-5719; fax: (301) 504-6409
Internet address: http://www.nal.usda.gov/fnic

◆ Food Research and Action Center
1875 Connecticut Avenue, NW, Suite 540
Washington, DC 20009
(202) 986-2200

◆ Superintendent of Documents
Government Printing Office
Washington, DC 20402

◆ U.S. Department of Agriculture (USDA)
14th Street SW and Independence Avenue
Washington, DC 20250
(202) 720-2791
Internet address: http://www.usda.gov

◆ USDA Center for Nutrition Policy and Promotion
1120 20th Street, NW, Suite 200, North Lobby
Washington, DC 20036
(202) 418-2321

◆ U.S. Department of Education (DOE)
Accreditation Agency Evaluation Branch
7th and D Street SW, Building 3, Room 336
Washington, DC 20202
(202) 708-7417

◆ U.S. Environmental Protection Agency (EPA)
Public Information Center, 3404
401 M Street SW
Washington, DC 20460
(202) 260-2080

F

◆ U.S. Public Health Service Public Affairs Office
Hubert H. Humphrey Building, Room 725–H
200 Independence Avenue SW
Washington, DC 20201
(202) 245-6867

CANADIAN GOVERNMENT

◆ Bureau of Nutritional Sciences, Food Directorate
Health Protection Branch, Health Canada
Sir Frederick Banting Research Centre
Tunney's Pasture
Ottawa, Ontario K1A 0L2, Canada

◆ Food Production and Inspection Branch
Agriculture and Agri-Food Canada
59 Camelot Drive
Nepean, Ontario K1A 0Y9, Canada
Internet address: http//aceis.agr.ca

◆ Nutrition Programs Unit
Healthy Living and Disease Prevention Directorate
Health Promotion and Services Branch
Health Canada
Jeanne Mance Building
Tunney's Pasture
Ottawa, Ontario K1A 1B4, Canada
Internet address: http://hwc.ca

◆ Nutrition Specialist, Health Support Services
Indian and Northern Health Services
Health Canada
11th Flood, Jeanne Mance Building
Tunney's Pasture
Ottawa, Ontario K1A 0L3, Canada

INTERNATIONAL AGENCIES

◆ Food and Agriculture Organization of the United
Nations (FAO), Liaison Office for North America
1001 22nd Street NW
Washington, DC 20437
(202) 653-2400

◆ World Health Organization (WHO)
Regional Office
525 23rd Street NW
Washington, DC 20037
(202) 861-3200
Internet address: http://www.who.ch

◆ International Food Information Council Foundation
Internet address: http://ificinfo.health.org

CONSUMER ORGANIZATIONS

◆ Center for Science in the Public Interest (CSPI)
1875 Connecticut Avenue NW, Suite 300
Washington, DC 20009

◆ Choice in Dying, Inc.
200 Varick Street, Suite 1001
New York, NY 10014
(212) 366-5540; fax: (212) 366-5337

◆ Consumer Information Center
Pueblo, CO 81009
Internet address: http://www.pueblo.gsa.gov

◆ Consumers Union of US Inc.
101 Truman Avenue
Yonkers, NY 10703–1057
(914) 378-2000

◆ National Council Against Health Fraud, Inc.
P.O. Box 1276
Loma Linda, CA 92354
Internet address: http://www.primenet.com/~nachf

FOOD SAFETY

◆ Alliance for Food & Fiber
Food Safety Hotline
(800) 266-0200

◆ FDA Seafood Hotline
(800) FDA-4010

◆ National Lead Information Center
(800) LEAD-FYI (532-3394)
(800) 424-LEAD (424-5323)

◆ National Pesticide Telecommunications Network
Oregon State University
Agricultural Chemistry Extension
Weniger Hall 333
Corvallis, OR 97331-6502

◆ USDA Meat and Poultry Hotline
(800) 535-4555

◆ U.S. EPA Safe Drinking Water Hotline
(800) 426-4791

INFANCY AND CHILDHOOD

◆ American Academy of Pediatrics
141 Northwest Point Boulevard
P.O. Box 927
Elk Grove Village, IL 60009–0927

◆ Association of Birth Defect Children, Inc.
827 Irma Street
Orlando, FL 32803
(407) 245-7035

◆ Canadian Pediatric Society
410 Smyth Road
Ottawa, Ontario K1H 8L1, Canada

◆ National Center for Education in Maternal & Child Health
2000 15th Street North, Suite 701
Arlington, VA 22201-2617
(703) 524-7802

◆ National Maternal and Child Health Clearinghouse
8201 Greensboro Drive
Suite 600
McLean, VA 22102
(703) 821-8955, Ext. 254 or 255

◆ Nurture/Center to Prevent Childhood Malnutrition
1840 18th Street, NW
Washington, DC 20009
(202) 797-9244; fax: (202) 797-9257

PROFESSIONAL NUTRITION ORGANIZATIONS

◆ American Dietetic Association (ADA)
216 West Jackson Boulevard, Suite 800
Chicago, IL 60606–6995
(312) 899-0040
Internet address: http://www.eatright.org

◆ ADA, National Center for Nutrition and Dietetics
(800) 366-1655

◆ American Institute of Nutrition
Internet address: http://www.nutrition.org/nutrition

◆ American Society for Clinical Nutrition
9650 Rockville Pike
Bethesda, MD 20814-3998
Internet address: http://www.faseb.org/ascn

◆ Dietitians of Canada
480 University Avenue, Suite 601
Toronto, Ontario M5G 1V2, Canada
(416) 596-0857

◆ National Academy of Sciences/National Research Council (NAS/NRC)
2101 Constitution Avenue NW
Washington, DC 20418

◆ National Institute of Nutrition
302-265 Carling Avenue
Ottawa, Ontario K1S 2E1, Canada

◆ Nutrition Foundation, Inc. (INACG)
1126 Sixteenth Street NW, Suite 111
Washington, DC 20036

◆ Nutrition Information Service
University of Alabama at Birmingham
Room 447 Webb Building
UAB Station
Birmingham, AL 35294-3360

◆ Society for Nutrition Education
2001 Killebrew Drive, Suite 340
Minneapolis, MN 55425-1882
(612) 854-6721
Internet address: http://www.uidaho.edu/~mswanson/sne.html

ALCOHOL AND DRUG ABUSE

◆ Al-Anon Family Group Headquarters
P.O. Box 862, Midtown Station
New York, NY 10018–0862
(800) 356-9996

◆ Alateen
1600 Corporate Landing Parkway
Virginia Beach, VA 23454
(800) 356-9996

◆ Alcohol & Drug Abuse Information Line
(800) 252-6465

◆ Alcoholics Anonymous (AA)
475 Riverside Drive
New York, NY 10115
(212) 870-3400

◆ Narcotics Anonymous (NA)
P.O. Box 9999
Van Nuys, CA 91409-9999
(818) 780-3951

◆ National Clearinghouse for Alcohol and Drug Information (NCADI)
P.O. Box 2345
Rockville, MD 20847-2345
(800) 729-6686

◆ National Council on Alcoholism and Drug Dependence, Inc.
12 West 21st Street
New York, NY 10010
(800) NCA-CALL

WEIGHT CONTROL AND EATING DISORDERS

◆ American Anorexia & Bulimia Association, Inc.
418 East 76th Street
New York, NY 10021
(212) 734-1114

◆ Anorexia Nervosa and Related Eating Disorders, Inc.
P.O. Box 5102
Eugene, OR 97405
(503) 344-1144

◆ National Association of Anorexia Nervosa and Associated Disorders, Inc. (ANAD)
P.O. Box 7
Highland Park, IL 60035
(708) 831-3438

◆ National Eating Disorder Information Centre
200 Elizabeth Street, College Wing 1-328
Toronto, Ontario M5G 2C4, Canada

◆ Overeaters Anonymous (OA)
383 Van Ness Avenue, Suite 1610
Torrance, CA 90501

F

F

◆ TOPS (Take Off Pounds Sensibly)
P.O. Box 07360
Milwaukee, WI 53207
(800) 932-8677

FITNESS

◆ American College of Sports Medicine
P.O. Box 1440
Indianapolis, IN 46204
(317) 637-9200

◆ President's Council on Physical Fitness and Sports
701 Pennsylvania Avenue NW
Suite 250
Washington, DC 20004
(202) 272-3421

◆ Sport Medicine and Science Council of Canada
1600 James Naismith Drive
Gloucester, Ontario K1B 5N4

PREGNANCY AND LACTATION

◆ American College of Obstetricians and Gynecologists
409 12th Street SW
Washington, DC 20024-2188
(202) 638-5577

◆ La Leche League International, Inc.
1400 N. Meacham Rd.
P.O. Box 4079
Schaumburg, IL 61068-4079
(847) 519-7730

◆ March of Dimes Birth Defects Foundation
(National Headquarters)
1275 Mamaroneck Avenue
White Plains, NY 10605

TRADE AND INDUSTRY ORGANIZATIONS

◆ Ralcorp Holdings, Inc.
Beech-Nut Nutrition Corporation
800 Market Street
St. Louis, MO 63106
(800) 523-6633

◆ Borden Farm Products, Product Publicity
180 East Broad Street
Columbus, OH 43215

◆ Campbell Soup Company, Food Service Division
Campbell Place
Camden, NJ 08103-1799

◆ Elan Pharma, Nutrition Division
2 Thurber Blvd.
Smithfield, RI 02917

◆ Kraft Foods
Consumer Response and Information Center
One Kraft Court
Glenview, Illinois 60025

◆ General Mills, Inc., Nutrition Department
Number One General Mills Boulevard
Minneapolis, MN 55426

◆ Kellogg Company
P.O. Box CAMB
Battle Creek, MI 49016-1986

◆ Mead Johnson Nutritionals
2400 West Lloyd Expressway
Evansville, IN 47721

◆ Nabisco Consumer Affairs
100 DeForest Avenue
East Hanover, NJ 07936
(800) 932-7800; (800) NABISCO

◆ National Dairy Council
10255 West Higgins Road, Suite 900
Rosemond, IL 60018

◆ The NutraSweet Company
P.O. Box 830
1751 Lake Cook Road
Deerfield, IL 60015-5239
(800) 323-5316

◆ Pillsbury Company, Consumer Relations
P.O. Box 550
Minneapolis, MN 55440-9843

◆ Procter and Gamble Company
One Procter and Gamble Plaza
Cincinnati, OH 45202

◆ Ross Laboratories, Abbot Laboratory
625 Cleveland Avenue
Columbus, OH 43216

◆ Sherwood Medical
1915 Olive Street
St. Louis, MO 63103

◆ Sunkist Growers, Consumer Affairs
P.O. Box 7888
Van Nuys, CA 91409-7888

◆ United Fresh Fruit and Vegetable Association
727 North Washington Street
Alexandria, VA 22314
(703) 836-3410

◆ USA Rice Council
P.O. Box 740121
Houston, TX 77274

◆ Vitamin Nutrition Information Service (VNIS)
Hoffmann-LaRoche, Inc.
340 Kingsland Street
Nutley, NJ 07110

◆ Weight Watchers® Food Company
Consumer Affairs Department
P.O. Box 10
Boise, ID 83707–0010

WORLD HUNGER

◆ Bread for the World
1100 Wayne Ave., Ste 1000
Silver Spring, MD 20910

◆ Center on Hunger, Poverty and Nutrition Policy
Tufts University School of Nutrition
11 Curtis Avenue
Medford, MA 02155
(617) 627-3956

◆ Freedom from Hunger
P.O. Box 2000
1644 DaVinci Court
Davis, CA 95617
(916) 758-6200

◆ Oxfam America
115 Broadway
Boston, MA 02116

◆ SEEDS Magazine
P.O. Box 6170
Waco, TX 76706
(817) 755-7745

◆ Worldwatch Institute
1776 Massachusetts Avenue NW
Washington, DC 20036

HEALTH AND DISEASE

◆ Alzheimer's Association
919 North Michigan Avenue, Suite 1000
Chicago, IL 60611
(800) 272-3900

◆ Alzheimer's Disease Education and Referral Center
P. O. Box 8250
Silver Spring, Maryland 20907-8250
(800) 438-4380

◆ American Academy of Allergy, Asthma, and Immunology
611 East Wells Street
Milwaukee, WI 53202
(414) 272-6071; fax: (414) 276-3349

◆ American Cancer Society Information Center
2200 Lake Blvd.
Atlanta, GA 30319
(800) ACS-2345
Internet address: http://www.cancer.org

◆ American Council on Science and Health
1995 Broadway, 2nd Floor
New York, NY 10023-5860

◆ American Dental Association
Division of Communications
211 East Chicago Avenue
Chicago, IL 60611-2678

◆ American Diabetes Association
1660 Duke Street
Alexandria, VA 22314
(703) 549-1500; (800) 232-3472
Internet address: http://www.diabetes.org

◆ American Heart Association
Box BHG, National Center
7320 Greenville Avenue
Dallas, TX 75231
(800) 242-8721
Internet address: http://www.amhrt.org

◆ American Institute for Cancer Research
1759 R Street NW
Washington, DC 20009
Internet address: http://www.aicr.org

◆ American Medical Association
515 North State Street
Chicago, IL 60610
(312) 464-5000
Internet address: http://www.ama-assn.org

◆ American Public Health Association
1015 Fifteenth Street NW
Washington, DC 20005
Internet address: http://www.apha.org

◆ American Red Cross AIDS Education Office
1730 D Street NW
Washington, DC 20006
(202) 737-8300

◆ Canadian Diabetes Association
15 Toronto Street, Suite 1001
Toronto ON M5C 2E3
(416) 363-0177; fax: (416) 363-3393

◆ Canadian Public Health Association
Publications, Suite 400
1565 Carling Avenue
Ottawa, Ontario K1Z 8R1, Canada

◆ Centers for Disease Control (CDC)
Information Hotline
(404) 332-4555
Internet address: http://www.cdc.gov

◆ Disease Prevention and Health Promotion's National Health Information Center
(800) 336-4797

◆ The Food Allergy Network
10400 Eaton Place, Suite 107
Fairfax, VA 22030-5647
(703) 691-3179
(800) 929-4040

F

◆ National AIDS Hotline (CDC)
(800) 342-AIDS (English)
(800) 344-SIDA (Spanish)
(800) 2437-TTY (Deaf)
(900) 820-2437

◆ National Cancer Institute
31 Center Drive MSC 2580
Building 31, Room 10A16
Bethesda, MD 20892-2580
(800) 4–CANCER; (800) 422-6237
Internet address: http://www.nci.nih.gov

◆ National Digestive Disease Information Clearinghouse
2 Information Way
Bethesda, MD 20892-3570
(301) 654-3810

◆ National Heart, Lung, and Blood Institute
National High Blood Pressure Education Program
P.O. Box 30105
Bethesda, MD 20824-0105
(301) 951-3260

◆ National Institute of Allergy and Infectious Diseases
Office of Communications, Building 31, Room 7A50
31 Center Drive, MSC 2520
Bethesda, MD 20892-2520
(301) 496-5717
Internet address: http://www.niaid.nih.gov

◆ National Institute of Dental Research (NIDR)
Building 31, Room 2C35
31 Center Drive, MSC 2290
Bethesda, MD 20892
(301) 496-4261

◆ National Institutes of Health (NIH)
9000 Rockville Pike
Bethesda, MD 20892
(301) 496-2433
Internet address: http://www.nih.gov

◆ National Osteoporosis Foundation
1150 17th Street NW, Suite 500
Washington, DC 20036
(202) 223-2226

◆ Smoking and Health Office (CDC)
Mail Stop K-12
1600 Clifton Road NE
Atlanta, GA 30333

UNITED STATES: RECOMMENDATIONS AND EXCHANGES

◆

WORLD HEALTH ORGANIZATION: RECOMMENDATIONS

◆

Contents

RDA

U.S. RDA and Daily Values

Healthy People 2000

Exchange Lists for Meal Planning

Nutrition Recommendations from WHO

*C*hapters 1 and 2 introduced Recommended Dietary Allowances (RDA), Daily Values, Healthy People 2000, and exchange systems. This appendix provides additional details. (See Appendix I for Canada's nutrition recommendations and exchange system.)

RDA

◆

Some of the U.S. recommendations for nutrient intakes appear in the RDA table on the inside front cover, left. The remaining RDA are here, in Tables G–1, G–2, and G–3.

U.S. RDA AND DAILY VALUES

◆

Food labels use another set of standards that derive from the RDA. From the late 1960s to the early 1990s, the set of standards used on food labels was called the U.S. RDA. The U.S. RDA were derived from the 1968 RDA and were established by the Food and Drug Administration (FDA) so that labels could express the nutrient contents of foods as percentages of those standards (see Table G–4). The intent was to help consumers evaluate the nutrient contents of foods for themselves and at the same time to spare them the burden of learning the different units in which nutrient amounts are expressed. Thus all nutrient amounts in a food, whether originally measured in micrograms, milligrams, grams, or RE, could be expressed as "percent of U.S. RDA."

With the new labeling regulations came a name change. The revised set of standards used on food labels—the Daily Values—are discussed fully in Chapter 2. With the exception of protein, the current Daily Values continue to use the same values as the old U.S. RDA. The FDA continues to consider their revision.

Table G–1
Estimated Safe and Adequate Daily Dietary Intakes of Additional Selected Vitamins and Minerals (United States)[a]

Age (yr)	Vitamins		Trace Elements[b]				
	Biotin (μg)	Pantothenic Acid (mg)	Chromium (μg)	Molybdenum (μg)	Copper (mg)	Manganese (mg)	Fluoride (mg)
Infants							
0–0.5	10	2	10–40	15–30	0.4–0.6	0.3–0.6	0.1–0.5
0.5–1	15	3	20–60	20–40	0.6–0.7	0.6–1.0	0.2–1.0
Children							
1–3	20	3	20–80	25–50	0.7–1.0	1.0–1.5	0.5–1.5
4–6	25	3–4	30–120	30–75	1.0–1.5	1.5–2.0	1.0–2.5
7–10	30	4–5	50–200	50–150	1.0–2.0	2.0–3.0	1.5–2.5
11+	30–100	4–7	50–200	75–250	1.5–2.5	2.0–5.0	1.5–2.5
Adults	30–100	4–7	50–200	75–250	1.5–3.0	2.0–5.0	1.5–4.0

[a]Less information is available on which to base allowances for these nutrients. Therefore, they are not included in the main table of the RDA, and the figures provided here are in the form of ranges of recommended intakes.
[b]The toxic levels for many trace elements may be only several times usual intakes, so the upper levels for the trace elements given in this table should not be habitually exceeded.
Source: Recommended Dietary Allowances, © 1989 by the National Academy of Sciences, National Academy Press, Washington, D.C.

Table G–2
Estimated Minimum Requirements of Sodium, Chloride, and Potassium

Age (yr)	Weight (kg)	Sodium[a] (mg)	Chloride (mg)	Potassium[b] (mg)
Infants				
0.0–0.5	4.5	120	180	500
0.5–1.0	8.9	200	300	700
Children				
1	11.0	225	350	1000
2–5	16.0	300	500	1400
6–9	25.0	400	600	1600
Adolescents	50.0	500	750	2000
Adults	70.0	500	750	2000

[a]Sodium requirements are based on estimates of needs for growth and for replacement of obligatory losses. They cover a wide variation of physical activity patterns and climatic exposure but do not provide for large, prolonged losses from the skin through sweat.
[b]Dietary potassium may benefit the prevention and treatment of hypertension, and recommendations to include many servings of fruits and vegetables would raise potassium intakes to about 3500 milligrams per day.
Source: Recommended Dietary Allowances, © 1989 by the National Academy of Sciences, National Academy Press, Washington, D.C.

G

Table G–3
Median Heights and Weights and Recommended Energy Intakes (United States)

Age (yr)	Weight		Height		Average Energy Allowance			
	kg	lb	cm	in	REE[a] (kcal/day)	MULTIPLES OF REE[b]	kcal/kg	kcal/day[c]
Infants								
0.0–0.5	6	13	60	24	320		108	650
0.5–1.0	9	20	71	28	500		98	850
Children								
1–3	13	29	90	35	740		102	1300
4–6	20	44	112	44	950		90	1800
7–10	28	62	132	52	1130		70	2000
Males								
11–14	45	99	157	62	1440	1.70	55	2500
15–18	66	145	176	69	1760	1.67	45	3000
19–24	72	160	177	70	1780	1.67	40	2900
25–50	79	174	176	70	1800	1.60	37	2900
51+	77	170	173	68	1530	1.50	30	2300
Females								
11–14	46	101	157	62	1310	1.67	47	2200
15–18	55	120	163	64	1370	1.60	40	2200
19–24	58	128	164	65	1350	1.60	38	2200
25–50	63	138	163	64	1380	1.55	36	2200
51+	65	143	160	63	1280	1.50	30	1900
Pregnant (2nd and 3rd trimesters)								+300
Lactating								+500

[a]REE (resting energy expenditure) represents the energy expended by a person at rest under normal conditions.

[b]Recommended energy allowances assume light-to-moderate activity and were calculated by multiplying the REE by an activity factor.

[c]Average energy allowances have been rounded.

Source: Recommended Dietary Allowances, © 1989 by the National Academy of Sciences, National Academy Press, Washington, D.C.

G

Table G–4
U.S. Recommended Daily Allowances (U.S. RDA)

Nutrient	Adults and Children over 4 Years	Infants	Children under 4 Years	Pregnant or Lactating Women
Protein (g)	45[a]	18[a]	20[a]	
Vitamin A (RE)	1000	300	500	1600
Vitamin D[b] (IU)	400	400	400	400
Vitamin E[b] (IU)	30	5.0	10	30
Vitamin C (mg)	60	35	40	60
Folate (mg)	0.4	0.1	0.2	0.8
Thiamin (mg)	1.5	0.5	0.7	1.7
Riboflavin (mg)	1.7	0.6	0.8	2.0
Niacin (mg)	20	8	9	20
Vitamin B_6[b] (mg)	2.0	0.4	0.7	2.5
Vitamin B_{12}[b] (μg)	6.0	2.0	3.0	8.0
Biotin[b] (mg)	0.3	0.5	0.15	0.3
Pantothenic acid[b] (mg)	10	3	5	10
Calcium (g)	1.0	0.6	0.8	1.3
Phosphorus[b] (g)	1.0	0.5	0.8	1.3
Iodine[b] (μg)	150	45	70	150
Iron (mg)	18	15	10	18
Magnesium[b] (mg)	400	70	200	450
Copper[b] (mg)	2.0	0.6	1.0	2.0
Zinc[b] (mg)	15	5	8	15

Note: Four sets of U.S. RDA were developed for different groups of people—infants, children, adults, and pregnant and lactating women. The most commonly used set was the U.S. RDA for adults. The one for infants was used for formulas. Supplements designed for children and for pregnant and lactating women used the U.S. RDA for these groups on their labels.

[a]If protein efficiency ratio of protein is equal to or better than that of casein.

[b]Optional for adults and children 4 years or over in vitamin and mineral supplements.

Source: U.S. Department of Health and Human Services, Public Health Service, Food and Drug Administration, Office of Public Affairs, 5600 Fishers Lane, Rockville, Maryland 20857, HHS publication no. (FDA) 81–2146, revised March 1981.

HEALTHY PEOPLE 2000

◆

In 1990, the U.S. Department of Health and Human Services established a set of almost 300 health objectives for the nation called *Healthy People 2000*.[1] The 21 objectives that have a nutrition component were presented throughout this text wherever their topic was discussed. Table G–5 presents them in full.

Table G–5
Healthy People 2000 Nutrition Objectives

Health-Related Objectives
- Reduce coronary heart disease deaths to no more than 100 per 100,000 people.
- Reverse the rise in cancer deaths to achieve a rate of no more than 130 per 100,000 people.
- Reduce overweight to a prevalence of no more than 20% among people aged 20 years and older and maintain prevalence at no more than 15% among adolescents aged 12 through 19 years.
- Reduce growth retardation among low-income children aged five years and younger to less than 10%.

Nutrient Intake Objectives
- Reduce dietary fat intake to an average of 30% of energy or less and average saturated fat intake to less than 10% of energy among people aged two years and older.
- Increase complex carbohydrate and fiber-containing foods in the diets of adults to five or more daily servings for vegetables (including legumes) and fruits and to six or more daily servings for grain products.
- Increase to at least 50% the proportion of overweight people aged 12 years and older who have adopted sound dietary practices combined with regular physical activity to attain an appropriate body weight.
- Increase calcium intake, so that at least 50% of youth aged 12 through 24 years and 50% of pregnant and lactating women consume three or more servings of calcium-rich foods daily and at least 50% of people aged 25 years and older consume two or more servings of calcium-rich foods daily.
- Decrease salt and sodium intake so at least 65% of home meal preparers prepare foods without adding salt, at least 80% of people avoid using salt at the table, and at least 40% of adults regularly purchase foods modified or lower in sodium.
- Reduce iron deficiency to less than 3% among children aged 1 to 4 and women of childbearing age.
- Increase to at least 75% the proportion of mothers who breastfeed their babies in the early weeks and to at least 50% the proportion who continue breastfeeding until their babies are five to six months old.
- Increase to at least 75% the proportion of parents and caregivers who use feeding practices that prevent nursing bottle tooth decay.
- Increase to at least 85% the proportion of people aged 18 and older who use food labels to make nutritious food selections.

Services and Information Objectives
- Achieve useful and informative nutrition labeling for virtually all processed foods and at least 40% of fresh meats, poultry, fish, fruits, vegetables, baked goods, and ready-to-eat carry-away foods.
- Increase to at least 5000 brand items the number of processed food products that are reduced in fat and saturated fat.
- Increase to at least 90% the proportion of restaurants and institutional foodservice operations that offer identifiable low-fat, low-kcalorie food choices, consistent with the *Dietary Guidelines for Americans.*
- Increase to at least 90% the proportion of school lunch and breakfast services and increase to at least 50% the proportion of child care foodservices with menus that are consistent with the nutrition principles in the *Dietary Guidelines for Americans.*
- Increase to at least 80% the receipt of home foodservices by people aged 65 and older who have difficulty in preparing their own meals or are otherwise in need of home-delivered meals.
- Increase to at least 75% the proportion of the nation's schools that provide nutrition education from preschool through grade 12, preferably as part of quality school health education.
- Increase to at least 50% the proportion of worksites with 50 or more employees that offer nutrition education and/or weight management programs for employees.
- Increase to at least 75% the proportion of primary care providers who provide nutrition assessment and counseling and/or referral to qualified nutritionists or dietitians.

G

The U.S. exchange system groups together foods that have about the same amount of carbohydrate, protein, fat, and kcalories. Then any food on a list can be "exchanged" for any other food on that same list. Chapter 2 introduced the exchange lists and Tables G–6 through G–14 present the lists in detail.

Table G–6

U.S. Exchange System: Starch List

1 starch exchange = 15 g carbohydrate, 3 g protein, 0–1 g fat, and 80 kcal
Note: In general, a starch serving is ½ c cereal, grain, pasta, or starchy vegetable; 1 oz of bread; ¾ to 1 oz snack food.

Serving Size	Food	Serving Size	Food
Bread		½ c	Plantains
½ (1 oz)	Bagels	1 small (3 oz)	Potatoes, baked or boiled
2 slices (1½ oz)	Bread, reduced-kcalorie	½ c	Potatoes, mashed
1 slice (1 oz)	Bread, white (including French and Italian), whole-wheat, pumpernickel, rye	1 c	Squash, winter (acorn, butternut)
		½ c	Yams, sweet potatoes, plain
2 (⅔ oz)	Bread sticks, crisp, 4" x ½"	**Crackers and Snacks**	
½	English muffins	8	Animal crackers
½ (1 oz)	Hot dog or hamburger buns	3	Graham crackers, 2½" square
½	Pita, 6" across	¾ oz	Matzoh
1 (1 oz)	Plain rolls, small	4 slices	Melba toast
1 slice (1 oz)	Raisin bread, unfrosted	24	Oyster crackers
1	Tortillas, corn, 6" across	3 c	Popcorn (popped, no fat added or low-fat microwave)
1	Tortillas, flour, 7–8" across	¾ oz	Pretzels
1	Waffles, 4½" square, reduced-fat	2	Rice cakes, 4" across
Cereals and Grains		6	Saltine-type crackers
½ c	Bran cereals	15–20 (¾ oz)	Snack chips, fat-free (tortilla, potato)
½ c	Bulgur, cooked		
½ c	Cereals, cooked	2–5 (¾ oz)	Whole-wheat crackers, no fat added
¾ c	Cereals, unsweetened, ready-to-eat	**Dried Beans, Peas, and Lentils**	
3 tbs	Cornmeal (dry)	½ c	Beans and peas, cooked (garbanzo, lentils, pinto, kidney, white, split, black-eyed)
⅓ c	Couscous		
3 tbs	Flour (dry)		
¼ c	Granola, low-fat	⅔ c	Lima beans
¼ c	Grape nuts	3 tbs	Miso ✎
½ c	Grits, cooked	**Starchy Foods Prepared with Fat**	
½ c	Kasha	**Count as 1 starch + 1 fat exchange.**	
¼ c	Millet	1	Biscuit, 2½" across
¼ c	Muesli	½ c	Chow mein noodles
½ c	Oats	1 (2 oz)	Corn bread, 2" cube
½ c	Pasta, cooked	6	Crackers, round butter type
1½ c	Puffed cereals	1 c	Croutons
½ c	Rice milk	16–25 (3 oz)	French-fried potatoes
⅓ c	Rice, white or brown, cooked	¼ c	Granola
½ c	Shredded wheat	1 (1½ oz)	Muffin, small
½ c	Sugar-frosted cereal	2	Pancake, 4" across
3 tbs	Wheat germ	3 c	Popcorn, microwave
Starchy Vegetables		3	Sandwich crackers, cheese or peanut butter filling
⅓ c	Baked beans		
½ c	Corn	⅓ c	Stuffing, bread (prepared)
1 (5 oz)	Corn on cob, medium	2	Taco shell, 6" across
1 c	Mixed vegetables with corn, peas, or pasta	1	Waffle, 4½" square
		4–6 (1 oz)	Whole-wheat crackers, fat added
½ c	Peas, green		

✎ = 400 mg or more of sodium per serving.

Table G–7
U.S. Exchange System: Fruit List

1 fruit exchange = 15 g carbohydrate and 60 kcal
Note: In general, a fruit serving is 1 small to medium fresh fruit; ½ c canned or fresh fruit or fruit juice; ¼ c dried fruit.

Serving Size	Food	Serving Size	Food
1 (4 oz)	Apples, unpeeled, small	½ (8 oz) or 1 c cubes	Papayas
½ c	Applesauce, unsweetened	1 (6 oz)	Peaches, medium, fresh
4 rings	Apples, dried	½ c	Peaches, canned
4 whole (5½ oz)	Apricots, fresh	½ (4 oz)	Pears, large, fresh
8 halves	Apricots, dried	½ c	Pears, canned
½ c	Apricots, canned	¾ c	Pineapple, fresh
1 (4 oz)	Bananas, small	½ c	Pineapple, canned
¾ c	Blackberries	2 (5 oz)	Plums, small
¾ c	Blueberries	½ c	Plums, canned
⅓ melon (11 oz) or 1 c cubes	Cantaloupe, small	3	Prunes, dried
		2 tbs	Raisins
12 (3 oz)	Cherries, sweet, fresh	1 c	Raspberries
½ c	Cherries, sweet, canned	1¼ c whole berries	Strawberries
3	Dates	2 (8 oz)	Tangerines, small
1½ large or 2 medium (3½ oz)	Figs, fresh	1 slice (13½ oz) or 1¼ c cubes	Watermelon
1½	Figs, dried	**Fruit Juice**	
½ c	Fruit cocktail	½ c	Apple juice/cider
½ (11 oz)	Grapefruit, large	⅓ c	Cranberry juice cocktail
¾ c	Grapefruit sections, canned	1 c	Cranberry juice cocktail, reduced-kcalorie
17 (3 oz)	Grapes, small		
1 slice (10 oz) or 1 c cubes	Honeydew melon	⅓ c	Fruit juice blends, 100% juice
		⅓ c	Grape juice
1 (3½ oz)	Kiwi	½ c	Grapefruit juice
¾ c	Mandarin oranges, canned	½ c	Orange juice
½ (5½ oz) or ½ c	Mangoes, small	½ c	Pineapple juice
1 (5 oz)	Nectarines, small	⅓ c	Prune juice
1 (6½ oz)	Oranges, small		

Table G–8
U.S. Exchange System: Milk List

Serving Size	Food	Serving Size	Food
Nonfat and Very Low-Fat Milk		**Low-Fat Milk**	
1 nonfat/low-fat milk exchange = 12 g carbohydrate, 8 g protein, 0–3 g fat, 90 kcal		1 low-fat milk exchange = 12 g carbohydrate, 8 g protein, 5 g fat, 120 kcal	
1 c	Nonfat milk	1 c	2% milk
1 c	½% milk	¾ c	Plain low-fat yogurt
1 c	1% milk	1 c	Sweet acidophilus milk
1 c	Nonfat or low-fat buttermilk	**Whole Milk**	
½ c	Evaporated nonfat milk	1 whole milk exchange = 12 g carbohydrate, 8 g protein, 8 g fat, 150 kcal	
⅓ c dry	Dry nonfat milk		
¾ c	Plain nonfat yogurt	1 c	Whole milk
1 c	Nonfat or low-fat fruit-flavored yogurt sweetened with aspartame or with a nonnutritive sweetener	½ c	Evaporated whole milk
		1 c	Goat's milk
		1 c	Kefir

Table G–9
U.S. Exchange System: Other Carbohydrates List

1 other carbohydrate exchange = 15 g carbohydrate, or 1 starch, or 1 fruit, or 1 milk exchange

Food	Serving Size	Exchanges per Serving
Angel food cake, unfrosted	1/12 cake	2 carbohydrates
Brownies, small, unfrosted	2″ square	1 carbohydrate, 1 fat
Cake, unfrosted	2″ square	1 carbohydrate, 1 fat
Cake, frosted	2″ square	2 carbohydrates, 1 fat
Cookie, fat-free	2 small	1 carbohydrate
Cookies or sandwich cookies	2 small	1 carbohydrate, 1 fat
Cupcakes, frosted	1 small	2 carbohydrates, 1 fat
Cranberry sauce, jellied	¼ c	2 carbohydrates
Doughnuts, plain cake	1 medium, (1½ oz)	1½ carbohydrates, 2 fats
Doughnuts, glazed	3¾″ across (2 oz)	2 carbohydrates, 2 fats
Fruit juice bars, frozen, 100% juice	1 bar (3 oz)	1 carbohydrate
Fruit snacks, chewy (pureed fruit concentrate)	1 roll (¾ oz)	1 carbohydrate
Fruit spreads, 100% fruit	1 tbs	1 carbohydrate
Gelatin, regular	½ c	1 carbohydrate
Gingersnaps	3	1 carbohydrate
Granola bars	1 bar	1 carbohydrate, 1 fat
Granola bars, fat-free	1 bar	2 carbohydrates
Hummus	⅓ c	1 carbohydrate, 1 fat
Ice cream	½ c	1 carbohydrate, 2 fats
Ice cream, light	½ c	1 carbohydrate, 1 fat
Ice cream, fat-free, no sugar added	½ c	1 carbohydrate
Jam or jelly, regular	1 tbs	1 carbohydrate
Milk, chocolate, whole	1 c	2 carbohydrates, 1 fat
Pie, fruit, 2 crusts	⅙ pie	3 carbohydrates, 2 fats
Pie, pumpkin or custard	⅛ pie	1 carbohydrate, 2 fats
Potato chips	12–18 (1 oz)	1 carbohydrate, 2 fats
Pudding, regular (made with low-fat milk)	½ c	2 carbohydrates
Pudding, sugar-free (made with low-fat milk)	½ c	1 carbohydrate
Salad dressing, fat-free 🖉	¼ c	1 carbohydrate
Sherbet, sorbet	½ c	2 carbohydrates
Spaghetti or pasta sauce, canned 🖉	½ c	1 carbohydrate, 1 fat
Sweet roll or danish	1 (2½ oz)	2½ carbohydrates, 2 fats
Syrup, light	2 tbs	1 carbohydrate
Syrup, regular	1 tbs	1 carbohydrate
Syrup, regular	¼ c	4 carbohydrates
Tortilla chips	6–12 (1 oz)	1 carbohydrate, 2 fats
Yogurt, frozen, low-fat, fat-free	⅓ c	1 carbohydrate, 0–1 fat
Yogurt, frozen, fat-free, no sugar added	½ c	1 carbohydrate
Yogurt, low-fat with fruit	1 c	3 carbohydrates, 0–1 fat
Vanilla wafers	5	1 carbohydrate, 1 fat

🖉 = 400 mg or more sodium per exchange.

Table G–10

U.S. Exchange System: Vegetable List

1 vegetable exchange = 5 g carbohydrate, 2 g protein, 25 kcal
Note: In general, a vegetable serving is ½ c cooked vegetables or vegetable juice; 1 c raw vegetables. Starchy vegetables such as corn, peas, and potatoes are on the starch list.

Artichokes
Artichoke hearts
Asparagus
Beans (green, wax, Italian)
Bean sprouts
Beets
Broccoli
Brussels sprouts
Cabbage
Carrots
Cauliflower
Celery
Cucumbers
Eggplant
Green onions or scallions
Greens (collard, kale, mustard, turnip)
Kohlrabi
Leeks
Mixed vegetables (without corn, peas, or pasta)

Mushrooms
Okra
Onions
Pea pods
Peppers (all varieties)
Radishes
Salad greens (endive, escarole, lettuce, romaine, spinach)
Sauerkraut ✐
Spinach
Summer squash (crookneck)
Tomatoes
Tomatoes, canned
Tomato sauce ✐
Tomato/vegetable juice ✐
Turnips
Water chestnuts
Watercress
Zucchini

✐ = 400 mg or more sodium per exchange.

Note: In general, a meat serving is 1 oz meat, poultry, or cheese; ½ c dried beans (weigh meat and poultry and measure beans after cooking).

Serving Size	Food	Serving Size	Food
Very Lean Meat and Substitutes		1 oz	Cheeses with ≤ 3 g fat/oz
1 very lean meat exchange = 7 g protein, 0–1 g fat, 35 kcal			Other:
1 oz	Poultry: Chicken or turkey (white meat, no skin), Cornish hen (no skin)	1½ oz	Hot dogs with ≤ 3 g fat/oz
1 oz	Fish: Fresh or frozen cod, flounder, haddock, halibut, trout; tuna, fresh or canned in water	1 oz	Processed sandwich meat with ≤ 3 g fat/oz (turkey pastrami or kielbasa)
1 oz	Shellfish: Clams, crab, lobster, scallops, shrimp, imitation shellfish	1 oz	Liver, heart (high in cholesterol)
1 oz	Game: Duck or pheasant (no skin), venison, buffalo, ostrich	**Medium-Fat Meat and Substitutes**	
	Cheese with ≤ 1 g fat/oz:	1 medium-fat meat exchange = 7 g protein, 5 g fat, and 75 kcal	
¼ c	Nonfat or low-fat cottage cheese	1 oz	Beef: Most beef products (ground beef, meatloaf, corned beef, short ribs, Prime grades of meat trimmed of fat, such as prime rib)
1 oz	Fat-free cheese		
	Other:	1 oz	Pork: Top loin, chop, Boston butt, cutlet
1 oz	Processed sandwich meats with ≤ 1 g fat/oz (such as deli thin, shaved meats, chipped beef 🖊, turkey ham)	1 oz	Lamb: Rib roast, ground
		1 oz	Veal: Cutlet (ground or cubed, unbreaded)
2	Egg whites	1 oz	Poultry: Chicken dark meat (with skin), ground turkey or ground chicken, fried chicken (with skin)
¼ c	Egg substitutes, plain		
1 oz	Hot dogs with ≤ 1 g fat/oz	1 oz	Fish: Any fried fish product
1 oz	Kidney (high in cholesterol)		Cheese with ≤ 5 g fat/oz:
1 oz	Sausage with ≤ 1 g fat/oz 🖊	1 oz	Feta
Count as one very lean meat and one starch exchange:		1 oz	Mozzarella
½ c	Dried beans, peas, lentils (cooked)	¼ c (2 oz)	Ricotta
Lean Meat and Substitutes			Other:
1 lean meat exchange = 7 g protein, 3 g fat, 55 kcal		1	Egg (high in cholesterol, limit to 3/week)
1 oz	Beef: USDA Select or Choice grades of lean beef trimmed of fat (round, sirloin, and flank steak); tenderloin; roast (rib, chuck, rump); steak (T-bone, porterhouse, cubed), ground round	1 oz	Sausage with ≤ 5 g fat/oz
		1 c	Soy milk
		¼ c	Tempeh
		4 oz or ½ c	Tofu
1 oz	Pork: Lean pork (fresh ham); canned, cured, or boiled ham; Canadian bacon 🖊; tenderloin, center loin chop	**High-Fat Meat and Substitutes**	
		1 high-fat meat exchange = 7 g protein, 8 g fat, 100 kcal	
		1 oz	Pork: Spareribs, ground pork, pork sausage
1 oz	Lamb: Roast, chop, leg	1 oz	Cheese: All regular cheeses (American 🖊, cheddar, Monterey Jack, swiss)
1 oz	Veal: Lean chop, roast		
1 oz	Poultry: Chicken, turkey (dark meat, no skin), chicken white meat (with skin), domestic duck or goose (well-drained of fat, no skin)		Other:
		1 oz	Processed sandwich meats with ≤ 8 g fat/oz (bologna, pimento loaf, salami)
	Fish:	1 oz	Sausage (bratwurst, Italian, knockwurst, Polish, smoked)
1 oz	Herring (uncreamed or smoked)		
6 medium	Oysters	1 (10/lb)	Hot dog (turkey or chicken) 🖊
1 oz	Salmon (fresh or canned), catfish	3 slices (20 slices/lb)	Bacon
2 medium	Sardines (canned)		
1 oz	Tuna (canned in oil, drained)	Count as one high-fat meat plus one fat exchange:	
1 oz	Game: Goose (no skin), rabbit	1 (10/lb)	Hot dog (beef, pork, or combination) 🖊
	Cheese:	2 tbs	Peanut butter (contains unsaturated fat)
¼ c	4.5%-fat cottage cheese		
2 tbs	Grated Parmesan		

🖊 = 400 mg or more sodium per exchange.

Table G–12
U.S. Exchange System: Fat List

1 fat exchange = 5 g fat, 45 kcal
Note: In general, a fat serving is 1 tsp regular butter, margarine, or vegetable oil; 1 tbs regular salad dressing. Many fat-free and reduced fat foods are on the Free Foods List.

Serving Size	Food
Monounsaturated Fats	
⅛ medium (1 oz)	Avocadoes
1 tsp	Oil (canola, olive, peanut)
8 large	Olives, ripe (black)
10 large	Olives, green, stuffed 🖊
6 nuts	Almonds, cashews
6 nuts	Mixed nuts (50% peanuts)
10 nuts	Peanuts
4 halves	Pecans
2 tsp	Peanut butter, smooth or crunchy
1 tbs	Sesame seeds
2 tsp	Tahini paste
Polyunsaturated Fats	
1 tsp	Margarine, stick, tub, or squeeze
1 tbs	Margarine, lower-fat (30% to 50% vegetable oil)
1 tsp	Mayonnaise, regular
1 tbs	Mayonnaise, reduced-fat
4 halves	Nuts, walnuts, English
1 tsp	Oil (corn, safflower, soybean)
1 tbs	Salad dressing, regular
2 tbs	Salad dressing, reduced-fat
2 tsp	Mayonnaise type salad dressing, regular 🖊
1 tbs	Mayonnaise type salad dressing, reduced-fat
1 tbs	Seeds: pumpkin, sunflower
Saturated Fats*	
1 slice (20 slices/lb)	Bacon, cooked
1 tsp	Bacon, grease
1 tsp	Butter, stick
2 tsp	Butter, whipped
1 tbs	Butter, reduced-fat
2 tbs (½ oz)	Chitterlings, boiled
2 tbs	Coconut, sweetened, shredded
2 tbs	Cream, half and half
1 tbs (½ oz)	Cream cheese, regular
2 tbs (1 oz)	Cream cheese, reduced-fat
	Fatback or salt pork**
1 tsp	Shortening or lard
2 tbs	Sour cream, regular
3 tbs	Sour cream, reduced-fat

🖊 = 400 mg or more sodium per exchange
*Saturated fats can raise blood cholesterol levels.
** Use a piece 1″ × 1″ × ¼″ if you plan to eat the fatback cooked with vegetables.
Use a piece 2″ × 1″ × ½″ when eating only the vegetables with the fatback removed.

G

Table G–13
U.S. Exchange System: Free Foods List

Note: A serving of free food contains less than 20 kcalories; those with serving sizes should be limited to three servings a day whereas those without serving sizes can be eaten freely.

Serving Size	Food	Serving Size	Food
Fat-Free or Reduced-Fat Foods			Bouillon or broth, low-sodium
1 tbs	Cream cheese, fat-free		Carbonated or mineral water
1 tbs	Creamers, nondairy, liquid	1 tbs	Cocoa powder, unsweetened
2 tsp	Creamers, nondairy, powdered		Coffee
1 tbs	Mayonnaise, fat-free		Club soda
1 tsp	Mayonnaise, reduced-fat		Diet soft drinks, sugar-free
4 tbs	Margarine, fat-free		Drink mixes, sugar-free
1 tsp	Margarine, reduced-fat		Tea
1 tbs	Mayonnaise type salad dressing, nonfat		Tonic water, sugar-free
1 tsp	Mayonnaise type salad dressing, reduced-fat	**Condiments**	
	Nonstick cooking spray	1 tbs	Catsup
1 tbs	Salad dressing, fat-free		Horseradish
2 tbs	Salad dressing, fat-free, Italian		Lemon juice
¼ c	Salsa		Lime juice
1 tbs	Sour cream, fat-free, reduced-fat		Mustard
2 tbs	Whipped topping, regular or light	1½ large	Pickles, dill 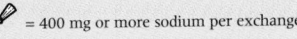
			Soy sauce, regular or light
Sugar-Free or Low-Sugar Foods		1 tbs	Taco sauce
1 piece	Candy, hard, sugar-free		Vinegar
	Gelatin dessert, sugar-free	**Seasonings**	
	Gelatin, unflavored		Flavoring extracts
	Gum, sugar-free		Garlic
2 tsp	Jam or jelly, low-sugar or light		Herbs, fresh or dried
	Sugar substitutes		Pimento
2 tbs	Syrup, sugar-free		Spices
Drinks			Hot pepper sauces
	Bouillon, broth, consommé		Wine, used in cooking
			Worcestershire sauce

 = 400 mg or more sodium per exchange.

Table G–14
U.S. Exchange System: Combination Foods List

Food	Serving Size	Exchanges per Serving
Entrees		
Tuna noodle casserole, lasagna, spaghetti with meatballs, chili with beans, macaroni and cheese 🖉	1 c (8 oz)	2 carbohydrates, 2 medium-fat meats
Chow mein (without noodles or rice)	2 c (16 oz)	1 carbohydrate, 2 lean meats
Pizza, cheese, thin crust 🖉	¼ of 10" (5 oz)	2 carbohydrates, 2 medium-fat meats, 1 fat
Pizza, meat topping, thin crust 🖉	¼ of 10" (5 oz)	2 carbohydrates, 2 medium-fat meats, 2 fats
Pot pie 🖉	1 (7 oz)	2 carbohydrates, 1 medium-fat meat, 4 fats
Frozen entrees		
Salisbury steak with gravy, mashed potato	1 (11 oz)	2 carbohydrates, 3 medium-fat meats, 3–4 fats
Turkey with gravy, mashed potato, dressing 🖉	1 (11 oz)	2 carbohydrates, 2 medium-fat meats, 2 fats
Entree with less than 300 kcalories 🖉	1 (8 oz)	2 carbohydrates, 3 lean meats
Soups 🖉		
Bean 🖉	1 c	1 carbohydrate, 1 very lean meat
Cream (made with water) 🖉	1 c (8 oz)	1 carbohydrate, 1 fat
Split pea (made with water) 🖉	½ c (4 oz)	1 carbohydrate
Tomato (make with water) 🖉	1 c (8 oz)	1 carbohydrate
Vegetable beef, chicken noodle, or other broth-type 🖉	1 c (8 oz)	1 carbohydrate
Fast Foods		
Burritos with beef 🖉	2	4 carbohydrates, 2 medium-fat meats, 2 fats
Chicken nuggets 🖉	6	1 carbohydrate, 2 medium-fat meats, 1 fat
Chicken breast and wing, breaded and fried 🖉	1	1 carbohydrate, 4 medium-fat meats, 2 fats
Fish sandwich/tartar sauce 🖉	1	3 carbohydrates, 1 medium-fat meat, 3 fats
French fries, thin	20–25	2 carbohydrates, 2 fats
Hamburger, regular	1	2 carbohydrates, 2 medium-fat meats
Hamburger, large 🖉	1	2 carbohydrates, 3 medium-fat meats, 1 fat

G

Table G–14 (continued)
U.S. Exchange System: Combination Foods List

Food	Serving Size	Exchanges per Serving
Hot dog with bun 🖋	1	1 carbohydrate, 1 high-fat meat, 1 fat
Individual pan pizza 🖋	1	5 carbohydrates, 3 medium-fat meats, 3 fats
Soft serve cone 🖋	1 medium	2 carbohydrates, 1 fat
Submarine sandwich 🖋	1 (6″)	3 carbohydrates, 1 vegetable, 2 medium-fat meats, 1 fat
Taco, hard shell 🖋	1 (6 oz)	2 carbohydrates, 2 medium-fat meats, 2 fats
Taco, soft shell 🖋	1 (3 oz)	1 carbohydrate, 1 medium-fat meat, 1 fat

🖋 = 400 mg or more sodium per exchange.

NUTRITION RECOMMENDATIONS FROM WHO

◆

Like the Committee on Diet and Health in the United States, the World Health Organization (WHO) has also assessed the relationships between diet and the development of chronic diseases.[2] Their recommendations are expressed in average daily ranges that represent the lower and upper limits:

◆ Total energy: sufficient to support normal growth, physical activity, and body weight (body mass index = 20–22).
◆ Total fat: 15 to 30 percent of total energy.
  ◆ Saturated fatty acids: 0 to 10 percent total energy.
  ◆ Polyunsaturated fatty acids: 3 to 7 percent total energy.
  ◆ Dietary cholesterol: 0 to 300 milligrams per day.
◆ Total carbohydrate: 55 to 75 percent total energy.
  ◆ Complex carbohydrates: 50 to 75 percent total energy.
  ◆ Dietary fiber: 27 to 40 grams per day.
  ◆ Refined sugars: 0 to 10 percent total energy.
◆ Protein: 10 to 15 percent total energy.
◆ Salt: upper limit of 6 grams/day (no lower limit set).

NOTES

◆

1. The Exchange Lists are the basis of a meal planning system designed by a committee of the American Diabetes Association and The American Dietetic Association. While designed primarily for people with diabetes and others who must follow special diets, the Exchange Lists are based on principles of good nutrition that apply to everyone. Copyright © 1995 by American Diabetes Association, Inc., and The American Dietetic Association.
2. *Healthy People 2000: National Health Promotion and Disease Prevention Objectives* (Washington, D.C.: U.S. Department of Health and Human Services, 1990).
3. Diet, nutrition and the prevention of chronic diseases: A report of the WHO Study Group on Diet, Nutrition and Prevention of Noncommunicable Diseases, *Nutrition Reviews* 49 (1991): 291–301.

TABLE OF FOOD COMPOSITION

◆

*T*his edition of the table of food composition contains more complete values for several nutrients than any comparable table.[1] These include dietary fiber; saturated, monounsaturated, and polyunsaturated fat; vitamin B_6; vitamin E; folate; magnesium; and zinc. The table includes a wide variety of foods from all food groups and is updated yearly to reflect current food patterns. For example, this edition includes many new nonfat items; several new ethnic items such as adzuki beans, tahitian taro, and gai choy chinese mustard; and a new selection of baby foods.

Sources of Data To achieve a complete and reliable listing of nutrients for all the foods, over 1200 sources of information are researched. Government sources are the primary base for all data for most foods. In addition to USDA data (from Release 11 and surveys), provisional USDA information—both published and unpublished—is included.

Even with all the government sources available, however, some nutrient values are still missing; and as the USDA updates various data, it sometimes reports conflicting values for the same items. To fill in the missing values and resolve discrepancies, other reliable sources of information are used. These sources include refereed journal articles, food composition tables from Canada and England, information from other nutrient data banks and publications, unpublished scientific data, and manufacturers' data.

---

1. This food composition table has been prepared for West Publishing Company and is copyrighted by ESHA Research in Salem, Oregon—the developer and publisher of the Food Processor®, Genesis® R·D, and Computer Chef® nutrition software systems. The major sources for the data from the U.S. Department of Agriculture are supplemented by more than 1200 additional sources of information. Because the list of references is so extensive, it is not provided here, but it is available from the publisher.

The selection of brand foods are included as provided by the food manufacturers and the food chain restaurants. This information changes often because recipes and formulations are modified to meet consumer preferences, and the data is usually limited to those nutrients required for food labels. To provide more complete information, values for several nutrients have been estimated based on known values for major ingredients.

Accuracy The energy and nutrients in recipes and combination foods vary widely, depending on the ingredients. The amounts of various fatty acids and cholesterol are influenced by the type of fat used (the specific type of oil, vegetable shortening, butter, margarine, etc.).

Estimates of nutrient amounts for foods and nutrients include all possible adjustments in the interest of accuracy. When multiple values are reported for a nutrient, the numbers are averaged and weighted with consideration of the original number of analyses in the separate sources. Whenever water percentages are available, estimates of nutrient amounts are adjusted for water content. When no water is given, water percentage is assumed to be that shown in the table. Whenever a reported weight appeared inconsistent (cooked eggplant and collards, for example), many kitchen tests were made, and the average weight of the typical product was given as tested.

When estimates of nutrient amounts in cooked foods are derived from reported amounts in raw foods, published retention factors are applied. Data for combination foods are modified to include newer data for major ingredients.

Considerable effort has been made to report the most accurate data available and to eliminate missing values. The table is updated annually, and the authors welcome any suggestions or comments for future editions.

Average Values It is important to know that many different nutrient values can be reported for foods, even by reliable sources. Many factors influence the amounts of nutrients in foods, including the mineral content of the soil, the method of processing, genetics, the diet of the animal or the fertilizer of the plant, the season of the year, methods of analysis, the difference in moisture content of the samples analyzed, the length and method of storage, and methods of cooking the food.

Although each nutrient is presented as a single number, each number is actually an average of a range of data. More detailed reports from the USDA, for example, indicate the number of samples and the standard deviation of the data. One can also find different reported values for foods as older data is replaced with newer data from more recent publications and newer analytical techniques. Therefore, nutrient data should be viewed and used only as a guide, a close approximation of nutrient content.

Dietary Fiber   There can be many different reported values for dietary fiber in foods, because information is dependent on the type of analytical technique used. The data in this table are primarily from the USDA/ARS Human Nutrition Information Service in Hyattsville, Maryland; Composition of Foods by Southgate and Paul (England); and many journal articles.

Vitamin A   Vitamin A is reported in retinol equivalents. The amount of this vitamin can vary by the season of the year and the maturity of the plant. Reported values in both dairy products and plants are higher in summer and early fall than in winter. The values reported here represent year-round averages. The organ meats of all animal products (liver especially) contain large amounts of vitamin A, which vary widely, depending on the background of the animal. The vitamin is also present in very small amounts in regular meat and is often reported as a trace.

Vitamin E   Vitamin E values are newly added to this Composition of Foods Table, reflecting the importance of this vitamin in human health. Vitamin E is actually a combination of various forms of this nutrient, and the measure of alpha tocopherol equivalents (α-TE) summarizes the activity of the various types of tocopherols and tocotrienols into on measure.

Fats   Total fats, as well as the breakdown of total fats to saturated, monounsaturated, and polyunsaturated fats, are listed in the table. The fatty acids seldom add up to the total. This is due to rounding, to other fatty acid components that are not included in these basic categories, *trans*-fatty acids and glycerol. Trans-fatty acids can comprise a large share of the total fat in margarine and shortening (hydrogenated oils) and in any foods that include them as ingredients.

Brand Name Foods from Manufacturers   The information for brand name foods from manufacturers will change from time to time as recipes and formulations change to meet consumer preferences. In addition, the data provided is usually limited to those nutrients required to meet label requirements. Additional values for magnesium, phosphorus, zinc, thiamin, riboflavin, niacin, vitamin B6, folate, some of the fatty acids, and percent water are estimates calculated from known values for major ingredients.

Niacin   Niacin values are for preformed niacin and do not include additional niacin that may form in the body from the conversion of tryptophan.

Using the Table   The items in this table have been organized into several categories, which are listed at the head of each right-hand page. As the key shows, each group has been color-coded to make it easier to find individual items.

In an effort to conserve space, the following abbreviations have been used in the food descriptions and nutrient breakdowns:

◆ diam = diameter
◆ ea = each
◆ enr = enriched
◆ f/ = from
◆ g = grams
◆ liq = liquid
◆ pce = piece
◆ pkg = package
◆ w/ = with
◆ w/o = without
◆ t = trace
◆ 0 = zero (no nutrient value)
◆ — = information not available

Caffeine Sources   Caffeine occurs in several plants, including the familiar coffee bean, the tea leaf, and the cocoa bean from which chocolate is made. Most human societies use caffeine regularly, most often in beverages, for its stimulant effect and flavor. Caffeine contents of beverages vary depending on the plants they are made from, the climates and soils where the plants are grown, the grind or cut size, the method and duration of brewing, and the amounts served. The accompanying table shows that in general, a cup of coffee contains the most caffeine; a cup of tea, less than half as much; and cocoa or chocolate, less still. As for cola beverages, they are made from kola nuts which contain caffeine, but most of their caffeine is added, using the purified compound obtained from decaffeinated coffee beans.

The FDA lists caffeine as a multipurpose GRAS substance that may be added to foods and beverages. Drug industries in developed countries use caffeine in many kinds of drugs: stimulants, pain relievers, cold remedies, diuretics, and weight-loss aids.

1. This food composition table has been prepared for West Publishing Company and is copyrighted by ESHA Research in Salem, Oregon—the developer and publisher of the Food Processor®, Genesis® R&D and the Computer Chef® nutrition software systems. The major sources for the data are from the USDA, supplemented by more than 1100 additional sources of information. Because the list of references is so extensive, it is not provided here, but is available from the publisher.

Caffeine Content of Beverages, Foods, and Over-the-Counter Drugs

Beverages and Foods	Average (mg)	Range(mg)
Coffee (5-oz cup)		
Brewed, drip method	130	110–150
Brewed, percolator	94	64–124
Instant	74	40–108
Decaffeinated, brewed or instant	3	1–5
Tea (5-oz cup)		
Brewed, major U.S. brand	40	20–90
Brewed, imported brands	60	25–110
Instant	30	25–50
Iced (12-oz can)	70	67–76
Soft drinks (12-oz can)		
Dr. Pepper		40
Colas and cherry cola		
Regular		30–46
Diet		2–58
Caffeine-free		0–trace
Jolt		72
Mountain Dew, Mello Yello		52
Fresca, Hires Root Beer, 7-Up, Sprite, Squirt, Sunkist Orange		0
Cocoa beverage (5-oz cup)	4	2–20
Chocolate milk beverage (8 oz)	5	2–7
Milk chocolate candy (1 oz)	6	1–15
Dark chocolate, semisweet (1 oz)	20	5–35
Baker's chocolate (1 oz)	26	26
Chocolate flavored syrup (1 oz)	4	4

Drugs[a]

	Average (mg)	Range(mg)
Cold remedies (standard dose)		
Dristan	0	
Coryban-D, Triaminicin	30	
Diuretics (standard dose)		
Aqua-ban, Permathene H_2Off	200	
Pre-Mens Forte	100	
Pain relievers (standard dose)		
Excedrin	130	
Midol, Anacin	65	
Aspirin, plain (any brand)	0	
Stimulants		
Caffedrin, NoDoz, Vivarin	200	
Weight-control aids (daily dose)		
Prolamine	280	
Dexatrim, Dietac	200	

Note: A pharmacologically active dose of caffeine is defined as 200 milligrams.

[a]Because products change, contact the manufacturer for an update on products you use regularly.

H

Table H–1
Food Composition

Computer Code Number	Food Description	Measure	Wt (g)	H₂O (%)	Ener (kcal)	Prot (g)	Carb (g)	Dietary Fiber (g)	Fat (g)	Fat Breakdown (g)		
										Sat	Mono	Poly
BEVERAGES												
	Alcoholic:											
	Beer:											
1	Regular (12 fl oz)	1½ c	356	92	146	1	13	3	0	0	0	0
2	Light (12 fl oz)	1½ c	354	95	99[1]	1	5	1	0	0	0	0
1506	Nonalcoholic (12 fl oz)	1 ea	360	98	32	1	5	0	0	0	0	0
	Gin, rum, vodka, whiskey:											
3	80 proof	1½ fl oz	42	67	97	0	0	0	0	0	0	0
4	86 proof	1½ fl oz	42	64	105	0	<1	0	0	0	0	0
5	90 proof	1½ fl oz	42	62	110	0	0	0	0	0	0	0
	Liqueur:											
1359	Coffee liqueur, 53 proof	1½ fl oz	52	31	175	<1	24	0	<1	.1	<.1	.1
1360	Coffee & cream liqueur, 34 proof	1½ fl oz	47	46	154	1	10	0	7	4.5	2.1	.3
1361	Crème de menthe, 72 proof	1½ fl oz	50	28	186	0	21	0	<1	<.1	<.1	.1
	Wine:											
6	Dessert (4 fl oz)	½ c	118	72	181[2]	<1	14	0	0	0	0	0
7	Red	3½ fl oz	103	88	74	<1	2	0	0	0	0	0
8	Rosé	3½ fl oz	103	89	73	<1	1	0	0	0	0	0
9	White medium	3½ fl oz	103	90	70	<1	1	0	0	0	0	0
1592	Nonalcoholic	1 c	232	98	14	1	3	0	0	0	0	0
1593	Nonalcoholic light	1 c	251	98	15	1	3	0	0	0	0	0
1409	Wine cooler, bottle (12 fl oz)	1½ c	340	90	169	<1	20	<1	<1	<.1	<.1	<.1
1595	Wine cooler, cup	1 c	227	90	113	<1	13	<1	<1	<.1	<.1	<.1
	Carbonated:[3]											
10	Club soda (12 fl oz)	1½ c	355	100	0	0	0	0	0	0	0	0
11	Cola beverage (12 fl oz)	1½ c	370	89	152	0	38	0	0	0	0	0
12	Diet cola w/aspartame (12 fl oz)	1½ c	355	100	4	<1	<1	0	0	0	0	0
13	Diet cola w/saccharin (12 fl oz)	1½ c	355	100	0	0	<1	0	0	0	0	0
14	Ginger ale (12 fl oz)	1½ c	366	91	124	0	32	0	0	0	0	0
15	Grape soda (12 fl oz)	1½ c	372	89	160	0	42	0	0	0	0	0
16	Lemon-lime (12 fl oz)	1½ c	368	90	147	0	38	0	0	0	0	0
17	Orange (12 fl oz)	1½ c	372	88	179	0	46	0	0	0	0	0
18	Pepper-type soda (12 fl oz)	1½ c	368	89	151	0	38	0	<1	.1	0	0
19	Root beer (12 fl oz)	1½ c	370	89	152	0	39	0	0	0	0	0
20	Coffee,[3] brewed	1 c	240	99	5[4]	<1	1	0	<1	t	0	t
21	Coffee,[3] prepared from instant	1 c	240	99	5[4]	<1	1	0	<1	t	0	0
	Fruit drinks, noncarbonated:[5]											
22	Fruit punch drink, canned	½ c	126	88	59	0	15	0	<1	0	0	0
1358	Gatorade	1 c	240	94	60	0	15	0	0	0	0	0
23	Grape drink, canned	½ c	125	87	63	<1	16	<1	0	0	0	0
1304	Kool-Aid, with sugar	1 c	240	90	89	0	23	0	<1	<.1	<.1	<.1
1356	Kool-Aid, with NutraSweet	1 c	240	95	43	0	11	0	0	0	0	0

[1] kCalories can vary from 78 to 131 for 12 fl. oz.

[2] Values are for sweet dessert wine. Dry dessert wines contain 149 kcal and 5 g of carbohydrate.

[3] Mineral content varies depending on water source.

[4] kCalorie values vary from 1 to 5 kcal per cup.

[5] Usually less than 10% fruit juice.

(Computer code number is for West Diet Analysis program)

H

TABLE OF FOOD COMPOSITION

◆ **H-5**

PAGE KEY: H–4 = BEV H–6 = DAIRY H–12 = EGGS H–14 = FAT/OIL H–18 = FRUIT H–26 = BAKERY H–36 = GRAIN H–44 = FISH
H–48 = MEATS H–50 = POULTRY H–54 = SAUSAGE H–56 = MIXED/FAST H–64 = NUTS/SEEDS H–68 = SWEETS H–70 = VEG/LEG
H–84 = MISC H–88 = SOUPS/SAUCES H–90 = FAST H–106 = FRZN ENTREE H–112 = BABY FOODS

Chol (mg)	Calc (mg)	Iron (mg)	Magn (mg)	Pota (mg)	Sodi (mg)	Zinc (mg)	VT-A (RE)	Thia (mg)	VT-E (α-TE)	Ribo (mg)	Niac (mg)	V-B6 (mg)	Fola (μg)	VT-C (mg)
0	18	.11	21	89	18	.07	0	.04	0	.11	1.60	.18	21	0
0	18	.14	18	64	11	.11	0	.04	0	.11	1.38	.11	15	0
0	25	.04	32	90	18	.04	0	.02	0	.09	1.63	.18	22	0
0	0	.02	0	1	<1	.02	0	<.01	0	0	0	0	0	0
0	0	.02	0	1	<1	.02	0	<.01	0	0	0	0	0	0
0	0	.02	0	1	<1	.02	0	<.01	0	0	0	0	0	0
0	1	.03	2	16	4	.02	0	<.01	0	.01	.07	0	0	0
7	8	.06	1	15	43	.08	20	0	.09	.03	.04	.01	0	0
0	0	.04	0	0	3	.02	0	0	0	0	<.01	0	0	0
0	9	.28	11	108	11	.08	0	.02	0	.02	.25	0	<1	0
0	8	.44	13	116	5	.09	0	.01	0	.03	.08	.03	2	0
0	8	.39	10	102	5	.06	0	0	0	.02	.07	.02	1	0
0	9	.33	10	83	5	.07	0	0	0	.01	.07	.01	<1	0
0	21	.93	23	204	16	.19	0	0	0	.02	.23	.05	2	0
0	23	1	25	221	18	.2	0	0	0	.03	.25	.05	3	0
0	19	.92	18	152	29	.2	<1	.02	.02	.02	.15	.04	4	6
0	13	.61	12	102	19	.13	<1	.01	.02	.02	.10	.03	3	4
0	18	.04	4	7	75	.36	0	0	0	0	0	0	0	0
0	11	.11	4	4	15	.04	0	0	0	0	0	0	0	0
0	14	.11	4	0	21[6]	.28	0	.02	0	.08	0	0	0	0
0	14	.14	4	7	57	.18	0	0	0	0	0	0	0	0
0	11	.66	4	4	26	.18	0	0	0	0	0	0	0	0
0	11	.3	4	4	56	.26	0	0	0	0	0	0	0	0
0	7	.26	4	4	40	.18	0	0	0	0	.06	0	0	0
0	19	.22	4	7	45	.37	0	0	0	0	0	0	0	0
0	11	.15	0	4	37	.15	0	0	0	0	0	0	0	0
0	19	.19	4	4	48	.26	0	0	0	0	0	0	0	0
0	5	.12	12	130	5	.05	0	0	0	0	.53	0	<1	0
0	7	.12	10	86	7	.07	0	0	0	<.01	.68	0	0	0
0	10	.26	3	32	28	.15	2	0	0	.03	.03	0	2	37
0	0	.12	2	26	96	.05	0	.01	0	0	0	0	0	0
0	4	.13	5	44	1	.04	0	.01	0	.01	.13	.03	1	20
0	38	.12	2	2	34	.07	0	0	0	<.01	<.01	0	<1	28
0	17	.65	5	50	50	.26	2	.02	0	.05	.05	0	5	77

[6] Value for product sweetened with aspartame only; sodium is 32 mg if a blend of aspartame and sodium saccharin is used.

(For purposes of calculations, use "0" for t, <1, <.1, <.01, etc.)

Table H–1
Food Composition

Computer Code Number	Food Description	Measure	Wt (g)	H₂O (%)	Ener (kcal)	Prot (g)	Carb (g)	Dietary Fiber (g)	Fat (g)	Fat Breakdown (g)		
										Sat	Mono	Poly
	BEVERAGES—Cont.											
	Fruit drinks, noncarbonated—Cont.											
26	Lemonade, frozen concentrate (6-oz can)	¾ c	219	52	396	1	103	1	<1	.1	t	.1
27	Lemonade, from concentrate	1 c	248	89	99	<1	26	<1	<1	t	t	t
28	Limeade, frozen concentrate (6-oz can)	¾ c	218	50	408	<1	107	1	<1	t	t	.1
29	Limeade, from concentrate	1 c	247	89	101	0	27	<1	<1	0	0	t
24	Pineapple grapefruit, canned	1 c	250	88	118	<1	29	<1	<1	t	t	.1
25	Pineapple orange, canned	1 c	250	87	125	3	30	<1	0	0	0	0
	Fruit and vegetable juices: see Fruit and Vegetable sections											
	Slim Fast:[1]											
1612	Chocolate malt with nonfat milk	1 c	273	82	190	14	32	2	1	.3	.1	<.1
1613	Strawberry with nonfat milk	1 c	273	82	190	14	32	2	1	.3	.1	<.1
1611	Vanilla with nonfat milk	1 c	273	82	190	14	32	2	1	.3	.1	<.1
	Ultra Slim Fast:[1]											
1616	Chocolate with nonfat milk	1 c	278	81	200	14	36	5	1	.3	.1	<.1
1614	French vanilla with nonfat milk	1 c	278	81	190	14	36	4	1	.3	.1	<.1
1615	Strawberry Supreme with nonfat milk	1 c	278	81	190	14	36	4	1	.3	.1	t
1357	Water, bottled: Perrier (6½ fl oz)	1 ea	192	100	0	0	0	0	0	0	0	0
1594	Water, bottled: Tonic water	1½ c	366	91	124	0	32	0	0	0	0	0
	Tea:[2]											
30	Brewed, regular	1 c	240	100	2	0	1	0	<1	t	0	t
1662	Brewed, herbal	¾ c	178	100	2	0	<1	0	<1	<.1	<.1	<.1
32	From instant, sweetened	1 c	262	91	89	<1	22	0	<1	t	0	t
31	From instant, unsweetened	1 c	237	100	2	<1	<1	0	0	0	0	0
	DAIRY											
	Butter: see Fats and Oils, #158,159,160											
	Cheese, natural:											
33	Blue	1 oz	28	42	100	6	1	0	8	5.3	2.2	.2
34	Brick	1 oz	28	41	105	7	1	0	8	5.3	2.4	.2
35	Brie	1 oz	28	48	95	6	<1	0	8	4.9	2.3	.2
36	Camembert	1 oz	28	52	85	6	<1	0	7	4.3	2	.2
37	Cheddar:	1 oz	28	37	114	7	<1	0	9	6	2.7	.3
38	1" cube	1 ea	17	37	69	4	<1	0	6	3.6	1.6	.2
39	Shredded	1 c	113	37	455	28	1	0	37	24	10.6	1.1
1406	Low fat, low sodium	1 oz	28	65	49	7	1	0	2	1.3	0.6	.1
	Cottage:											
984	Low sodium, low fat	1 c	225	84	162	28	6	0	2	1.4	.6	.1
40	Creamed, large curd	1 c	225	79	232	28	6	0	10	6.4	2.9	.3
41	Creamed, small curd	1 c	210	79	216	26	6	0	9	6	2.7	.3
42	With fruit	1 c	226	72	280	22	30	0	8	4.9	2.2	.2
43	Low fat 2%	1 c	226	79	203	31	8	0	4	2.8	1.2	.1
44	Low fat 1%	1 c	226	82	164	28	6	0	2	1.5	.7	.1
46	Cream	1 oz	28	54	99	2	1	0	10	6.2	2.8	.4
983	Cream, low fat	1 oz	28	64	65	3	2	0	5	3.1	1.6	.2
47	Edam	1 oz	28	42	101	7	<1	0	8	5	2.3	.2
48	Feta	1 oz	28	55	75	4	1	0	6	4.2	1.3	.2

[1] See Chapter 9 for healthy weight loss strategies. The formulas for these products change periodically; these data reflect nutrient values as of our publication date.

[2] Mineral content varies depending on water source.

Chol (mg)	Calc (mg)	Iron (mg)	Magn (mg)	Pota (mg)	Sodi (mg)	Zinc (mg)	VT-A (RE)	Thia (mg)	VT-E (α-TE)	Ribo (mg)	Niac (mg)	V-B6 (mg)	Fola (µg)	VT-C (mg)
0	15	1.58	11	146	9	.18	22	.06	0	.21	.16	.05	22	39[3]
0	7	.4	5	37	7	.1	5	.01	0	.05	.04	.01	5	10[3]
0	11	.22	9	128	0	.09	0	.02	0	.02	.22	0	9	26
0	7	.07	2	32	5	.05	0	0	0	0	.05	0	2	7
0	18	.78	15	152	35	.15	9	.08	0	.04	.67	.1	26	115
0	13	.68	15	115	7	.15	13	.08	0	.05	.52	.12	27	56
4	450	6.3	140	690	230	5.25	350	.53	5	.59	7	.7	120	21
4	450	6.3	140	720	220	5.25	350	.53	5	.59	7	.7	120	21
4	450	6.31	140	721	220	5.24	350	.53	5	.59	7	.7	120	21
<1	450	6.3	140	800	230	5.25	350	.53	10	.59	7	.7	120	21
<1	450	6.3	140	730	250	5.25	350	.53	10	.59	7	.7	120	21
<1	450	6.3	140	710	250	5.25	350	.52	10	.59	7	.7	120	21
0	27	0	0	0	2	0	0	0	0	0	0	0	0	0
0	4	.04	0	0	15	.37	0	0	0	0	0	0	0	0
0	0	.05	7	89	7	.05	0	0	0	.03	0	0	12	0
0	4	.14	2	16	2	.07	0	.02	0	.01	0	0	1	0
0	5	.05	5	50	8	.08	0	0	0	.05	.09	.01	10	0
0	5	.05	5	47	7	.07	0	0	0	<.01	.09	0	1	0
21	150	.09	6	73	395	.75	65	.01	.18	.11	.29	.05	10	0
27	191	.12	7	39	159	.74	86	0	.14	.1	.03	.02	6	0
28	52	.14	6	43	178	.67	52	.02	.18	.15	.11	.07	18	0
20	110	.09	6	53	239	.67	71	.01	.18	.14	.18	.06	18	0
30	204	.19	8	28	176	.88	86	.01	.1	.11	.02	.02	5	0
18	123	.12	5	17	106	.53	51	0	.06	.06	.01	.01	3	0
119	815	.77	31	111	702	3.51	342	.03	.41	.43	.09	.08	21	0
6	197	.2	8	32	6	.87	17	.01	.05	.01	.03	.02	5	0
9	137	.32	11	194	29	.86	25	.05	.25	.36	.3	.16	27	0
33	135	.32	12	190	911	.83	108	.05	.28	.37	.28	.15	27	0
31	126	.29	11	177	851	.78	101	.04	.26	.34	.26	.14	26	0
25	108	.25	9	151	915	.65	81	.04	.21	.29	.23	.12	22	0
19	155	.36	14	217	918	.95	45	.05	.13	.42	.33	.17	30	0
10	138	.32	12	193	918	.86	25	.05	.25	.37	.29	.15	28	0
31	23	.34	2	34	84	.15	124	0	.26	.06	.03	.01	4	0
16	32	.47	2	47	83	.22	62	.01	.13	.08	.04	.02	5	0
25	207	.12	8	53	274	1.07	72	.01	.21	.11	.02	.02	5	0
25	140	.18	5	18	316	.82	36	.04	.01	.24	.28	.12	9	0

[3]Vitamin C can range from 5 to 72 mg in a small can of frozen concentrate, and from 1 to 18 mg in 1 c of prepared lemonade.

(For purposes of calculations, use "0" for t, <1, <.1, <.01, etc.)

Table H–1
Food Composition

Computer Code Number	Food Description	Measure	Wt (g)	H$_2$O (%)	Ener (kcal)	Prot (g)	Carb (g)	Dietary Fiber (g)	Fat (g)	Fat Breakdown (g) Sat	Mono	Poly
	DAIRY—Cont.											
	Cheese—Cont.											
49	Gouda	1 oz	28	42	101	7	1	0	8	5	2.2	.2
50	Gruyère	1 oz	28	33	117	8	<1	0	9	5.4	2.8	.5
51	Gorgonzola	1 oz	28	39	111	7	0	0	9	5.5	2.4	.5
52	Liederkranz	1 oz	28	53	87	5	<1	0	8	5.3	2.2	.2
1676	Limburger	1 oz	28	48	92	6	<1	0	8	4.7	2.4	.1
53	Monterey Jack	1 oz	28	41	106	7	<1	0	9	5.4	2.5	.3
54	Mozzarella, whole milk	1 oz	28	54	80	6	1	0	6	3.7	1.9	.2
55	Mozzarella, part-skim milk, low moisture	1 oz	28	49	79	8	1	0	5	3.1	1.4	.1
56	Muenster	1 oz	28	42	104	7	<1	0	9	5.4	2.5	.2
1399	Nonfat (Kraft Singles)	1 oz	28	61	44	6	4	0	0	0	0	0
	Parmesan, grated:											
57	Cup, not pressed down	1 c	100	18	456	42	4	0	30	20	8.7	.7
58	Tablespoon	1 tbs	5	18	23	2	<1	0	2	1	.4	t
59	Ounce	1 oz	28	18	128	12	1	0	8	5.5	2.4	.2
60	Provolone	1 oz	28	41	100	7	1	0	8	4.9	2.1	.2
61	Ricotta, whole milk	1 c	246	72	428	28	7	0	32	20.4	8.9	1
62	Ricotta, part-skim milk	1 c	246	74	339	28	13	0	19	12.1	5.7	.6
63	Romano	1 oz	28	31	109	9	1	0	8	4.8	2.2	.2
64	Swiss	1 oz	28	37	107	8	1	0	8	5	2.1	.3
976	Swiss, low fat	1 oz	28	60	50	8	1	0	1	.9	.4	<.1
	Pasteurized processed cheese products:											
65	American	1 oz	28	39	106	6	<1	0	9	5.6	2.5	.3
66	Swiss	1 oz	28	42	94	7	1	0	7	4.6	2	.2
67	American cheese food, jar	1 oz	28	43	93	6	2	0	7	4.4	2	.2
68	American cheese spread	1 oz	28	48	82	5	2	0	6	3.8	1.8	.2
982	Velveeta cheese spread, low fat, low sodium	1 oz	28	63	51	7	1	0	2	1.3	0.6	0.1
69	Cream, sweet:	1 c	242	81	315	7	10	0	28	17.3	8	1
	Half & half (cream & milk):											
70	Tablespoon	1 tbs	15	81	19	<1	1	0	2	1.1	.5	.1
71	Light, coffee or table:	1 c	240	74	468	6	9	0	46	28.8	13.4	1.7
72	Tablespoon	1 tbs	15	74	29	<1	1	0	3	1.8	.8	.1
73	Light whipping cream, liquid:[1]	1 c	239	64	698	5	7	0	74	46.1	21.7	2.1
74	Tablespoon	1 tbs	15	64	44	<1	<1	0	5	2.9	1.4	.1
75	Heavy whipping cream, liquid:[1]	1 c	238	58	821	5	7	0	88	54.7	25.5	3.3
76	Tablespoon	1 tbs	15	58	52	<1	<1	0	6	3.4	1.6	.2
77	Whipped cream, pressurized:	1 c	60	61	154	2	8	0	13	8.3	3.8	.5
78	Tablespoon	1 tbs	4	61	10	<1	<1	0	1	.6	.3	t
79	Cream, sour, cultured:	1 c	230	71	492	7	10	0	48	29.9	13.9	1.8
80	Tablespoon	1 tbs	14	71	30	<1	1	0	3	1.8	.8	.1
	Cream products—imitation and part dairy:											
81	Coffee whitener, frozen or liquid	1 tbs	15	77	20	<1	2	0	2	1.4	t	0
82	Coffee whitener, powdered	1 tsp	2	2	11	<1	1	0	1	.6	t	t
83	Dessert topping, frozen, nondairy:	1 c	75	50	239	1	17	0	19	16.4	1.2	.4
84	Tablespoon	1 tbs	5	50	16	<1	1	0	1	1.1	.1	t
85	Dessert topping, mix with whole milk:	1 c	80	67	151	3	13	0	10	8.6	.7	.2
86	Tablespoon	1 tbs	5	67	9	<1	1	0	1	.5	t	t

[1]For whipped cream, (non-pressurized), double the liquid cream volume of codes 73, 74 or 75, 76. One tablespoon liquid cream becomes 2 tablespoons when "whipped."

(Computer code number is for West Diet Analysis program)

PAGE KEY: H–4 = BEV   H–6 = DAIRY   H–12 = EGGS   H–14 = FAT/OIL   H–18 = FRUIT   H–26 = BAKERY   H–36 = GRAIN   H–44 = FISH
H–48 = MEATS   H–50 = POULTRY   H–54 = SAUSAGE   H–56 = MIXED/FAST   H–64 = NUTS/SEEDS   H–68 = SWEETS   H–70 = VEG/LEG
H–84 = MISC   H–88 = SOUPS/SAUCES   H–90 = FAST   H–106 = FRZN ENTREE   H–112 = BABY FOODS

Chol (mg)	Calc (mg)	Iron (mg)	Magn (mg)	Pota (mg)	Sodi (mg)	Zinc (mg)	VT-A (RE)	Thia (mg)	VT-E (α-TE)	Ribo (mg)	Niac (mg)	V-B6 (mg)	Fola (μg)	VT-C (mg)
32	198	.07	8	34	232	1.11	49	.01	.1	.09	.02	.02	6	0
31	286	.05	10	23	95	1.11	85	.02	.1	.08	.03	.02	3	0
25	149	.12	8	26	512	.57	103	.01	.22	.09	.2	.04	9	0
21	110	.12	7	68	389	.7	91	.01	.21	.18	.1	.04	34	0
25	140	.04	6	36	224	.6	89	.02	.18	.14	.04	.02	16	0
25	211	.2	8	23	152	.85	72	0	.1	.11	.03	.02	5	0
22	146	.05	5	19	105	.63	68	0	.1	.07	.02	.02	2	0
15	207	.07	7	27	149	.89	54	.01	.13	.1	.03	.02	3	0
27	203	.12	8	38	178	.8	90	0	.13	.09	.03	.02	3	0
4	221	0	–	81	427	–	126	–	0	.10	–	–	–	0
79	1375	.95	51	107	1861	3.19	173	.04	.8	.39	.31	.1	8	0
4	69	.05	3	5	93	.16	9	0	.04	.02	.02	.01	<1	0
22	385	.27	14	30	521	.9	48	.01	.22	.11	.09	.03	2	0
20	215	.15	8	39	249	.92	75	.01	.1	.09	.04	.02	3	0
124	509	.93	28	258	206	2.85	330	.03	.86	.48	.26	.11	30	0
76	669	1.08	36	308	308	3.3	278	.05	.53	.45	.19	.05	32	0
30	302	.22	12	25	341	.73	40	.01	.2	.1	.02	.02	2	0
26	273	.05	10	31	74	1.1	72	.01	.14	.1	.03	.02	2	0
10	269	.05	10	31	73	1.11	18	.01	.05	.1	.03	.02	2	0
27	175	.11	6	46	406	.85	82	.01	.13	.1	.02	.02	2	0
24	219	.17	8	61	389	1.03	65	0	.19	.08	.01	.01	2	0
18	163	.24	9	79	338	.85	62	.01	.2	.13	.04	.04	2	0
16	159	.09	8	69	380	.73	54	.01	.2	.12	.04	.03	2	0
10	191	.12	7	50	2	.93	18	.01	.14	.11	.02	.02	3	0
89	254	.17	25	315	98	1.23	259	.08	.27	.36	.19	.09	6	2
6	16	.01	2	19	6	.08	16	.01	.02	.02	.01	.01	<1	<1
158	231	.1	21	293	95	.65	437	.08	.36	.35	.14	.08	6	2
10	14	.01	1	18	6	.04	27	.01	.02	.02	.01	0	<1	<1
265	166	.07	17	231	82	.6	705	.06	1.43	.3	.1	.07	9	1
17	10	0	1	15	5	.04	44	.01	.09	.02	.01	.01	1	<1
326	154	.07	17	179	89	.55	1001	.05	1.5	.26	.09	.06	9	1
21	10	0	1	11	6	.03	63	0	.1	.02	.01	0	1	<1
46	61	.03	6	88	78	.22	124	.02	.36	.04	.04	.02	2	0
3	4	0	<1	6	5	.01	8	0	.02	0	0	0	<1	0
102	267	.14	26	331	123	.62	449	.08	1.3	.34	.15	.04	25	2
6	16	.01	2	20	7	.04	27	0	.45	.02	.01	0	2	<1
0	1	<.01	<1	29	12	0	1	0	.24	0	0	0	0	0
0	<1	.02	<1	16	4	.01	<1	0	.01	0	0	0	0	0
0	5	.09	1	14	19	.02	64[2]	0	.14	0	0	0	0	0
0	<1	.01	<1	1	1	0	4[2]	0	.01	0	0	0	0	0
8	72	.03	8	120	53	.22	39[2]	.02	.11	.09	.05	.02	3	1
<1	5	0	<1	8	3	.01	2[2]	0	.01	.01	0	0	<1	<1

[2] Vitamin A value is from beta-carotene used for coloring.

(For purposes of calculations, use "0" for t, <1, <.1, <.01, etc.)

Table H–1
Food Composition

Computer Code Number	Food Description	Measure	Wt (g)	H$_2$O (%)	Ener (kcal)	Prot (g)	Carb (g)	Dietary Fiber (g)	Fat (g)	Fat Breakdown (g)		
										Sat	Mono	Poly
DAIRY—Cont.												
88	Dessert topping, pressurized:	1 c	70	60	185	1	11	0	16	13.3	1.3	.2
87	Tablespoon	1 tbs	4	60	11	<1	1	0	1	.8	.1	t
91	Sour cream, imitation:	1 c	230	71	478	6	15	0	45	40.9	1.3	.1
92	Tablespoon	1 tbs	14	71	29	<1	1	0	3	2.5	.1	t
89	Sour dressing, part dairy:	1 c	235	75	418	8	11	0	39	31.3	4.6	1.1
90	Tablespoon	1 tbs	15	75	27	<1	1	0	2	2	.3	.1
	Milk, fluid:											
93	Whole milk	1 c	244	88	150	8	11	0	8	5.1	2.7	.3
94	2% low-fat milk	1 c	244	89	121	8	12	0	5	2.9	1.4	.2
95	2% milk solids added[1]	1 c	245	89	125	9	12	0	5	2.9	1.4	.2
96	1% low-fat milk	1 c	244	90	102	8	12	–	3	1.6	.8	.1
97	1% milk solids added[1]	1 c	245	90	104	9	12	0	2	1.5	.7	.1
98	Nonfat milk, vitamin A added	1 c	245	91	86	8	12	0	<1	.3	.12	t
99	Nonfat milk solids added[1]	1 c	245	90	90	9	12	0	1	.4	.2	t
100	Buttermilk, nonfat	1 c	245	90	99	8	12	0	2	1.3	.6	.1
	Milk, canned:											
101	Sweetened condensed	1 c	306	27	982	24	166	0	27	16.8	7.4	1
103	Evaporated, nonfat	1 c	255	79	199	19	29	0	1	.3	.2	t
	Milk, dried:											
104	Buttermilk, sweet	1 c	120	3	464	41	59	0	7	4.3	2	.3
105	Instant, nonfat, envelope[2]	1 ea	91	4	325	32	47	0	1	.4	.2	t
106	Instant nonfat, cup	1 c	68	4	243	24	35	0	<1	.3	.1	t
107	Goat milk	1 c	244	87	167	9	11	0	10	6.5	2.7	.4
108	Kefir, 2% milkfat[3]	1 c	233	82	122	9	9	0	5	2.9	1.2	.1
	Milk beverages and powdered mixes:											
	Chocolate:											
109	Whole	1 c	250	82	208	8	26	2	8	5.3	2.5	.3
110	2% fat	1 c	250	83	178	8	26	1	5	3.1	1.5	.2
111	1% fat	1 c	250	85	157	9	26	3	3	1.5	.8	.1
	Chocolate-flavored beverages:											
112	Powder containing nonfat dry milk:	1 oz	28	2	102	3	22	<1	1	.7	.4	t
113	Prepared with water	¾ c	206	86	100	4	23	<1	1	.7	.4	t
114	Powder without nonfat dry milk:	¾ oz	22	1	76	1	20	1	1	.4	.2	t
115	Prepared with whole milk	1 c	266	81	226	9	31	1	9	5.5	2.6	.3
116	Eggnog, commercial	1 c	254	74	343	10	34	0	19	11.3	5.7	.9
974	2% low-fat eggnog	1 c	254	85	189	12	17	0	8	3.8	2.7	.7
1027	Instant Breakfast, envelope, powder only:	1 ea	37	7	131	7	24	<1	1	.3	.1	<.1
1028	Prepared with whole milk	1 c	281	77	280	15	36	<1	9	5.4	2.5	.3
1029	Prepared with 2% milk	1 c	281	78	252	15	36	<1	5	3.3	1.5	.2
1283	Prepared with 1% milk	1 c	281	80	215	16	36	<1	1	.7	.3	<.1
1284	Prepared with nonfat milk	1 c	281	80	215	16	36	<1	1	.7	.3	<.1
117	Malted milk, chocolate, powder:	¾ oz	21	1	79	1	18	<1	1	.5	.2	.1
118	Prepared with whole milk	1 c	265	81	228	9	30	<1	9	5.5	2.6	.4
1661	Ovaltine with whole milk	1 c	265	81	225	9	29	<1	9	5.5	2.6	.4
119	Malted mix powder, natural	¾ oz	21	2	87	2	16	<1	2	.9	.4	.3
121	Milk shakes, chocolate (10 fl oz)	1¼ c	283	72	359	10	58	2	10	6.5	3.1	.4

[1]Milk solids added, label claims less than 10 g protein per cup.

[2]Yields 1 qt fluid milk when reconstituted according to package directions.

[3]Most values provided by product labeling.

(Computer code number is for West Diet Analysis program)

Chol (mg)	Calc (mg)	Iron (mg)	Magn (mg)	Pota (mg)	Sodi (mg)	Zinc (mg)	VT-A (RE)	Thia (mg)	VT-E (α-TE)	Ribo (mg)	Niac (mg)	V-B6 (mg)	Fola (μg)	VT-C (mg)
0	4	.01	1	13	43	.01	33[4]	.0	.12	0	0	0	0	0
0	<1	0	<1	1	2	0	2[4]	0	.01	0	0	0	0	0
0	6	.9	15	370	235	2.71	0	0	.34	0	0	0	0	0
0	<1	.05	1	23	14	.16	0	0	.02	0	0	0	0	0
13	266	.07	23	381	113	.87	5[4]	.09	.29	.38	.17	.04	28	2
1	17	0	1	24	7	.06	<1[4]	.01	.02	.02	.01	0	2	<1
33	290	.12	33	371	120	.93	76	.09	.24	.39	.2	.1	12	2
18	298	.12	33	376	122	.95	139	.09	.17	.4	.21	.1	12	2
18	311	.12	35	397	128	.98	140	.1	.17	.42	.22	.11	13	2
10	300	.12	34	381	123	.95	144	.09	.1	.41	.21	.1	12	2
10	314	.12	35	397	128	.98	145	.1	.1	.42	.22	.11	13	2
4	301	.1	28	407	126	.98	149	.09	.1	.34	.22	.1	13	2
5	316	.12	35	419	130	1	149	.1	.1	.43	.22	.11	13	2
9	284	.12	27	370	257	1.03	20	.08	.15	.38	.14	.08	12	2
104	869	.58	79	1135	389	2.88	248	.27	.65	1.27	.64	.16	34	8
9	740	.74	69	847	293	2.29	298	.11	.01	.79	.44	.14	22	3
83	1421	.36	132	1910	620	4.82	65	.47	.48	1.9	1.05	.41	57	7
17	1119	.28	106	1551	500	4.01	646[5]	.38	.02	1.58	.81	.31	45	5
12	836	.21	80	1159	373	3	483[5]	.28	.01	1.18	.61	.23	34	4
28	327	.12	34	498	122	.73	137	.12	.22	.34	.68	.11	1	3
10	350	.5	28	205	50	.9	155	.45	.12	.44	.3	.09	23	<1
30	280	.6	33	418	149	1.03	73	.09	.23	.41	.31	.1	12	2
17	285	.6	33	423	151	1.03	143	.09	.13	.41	.32	.1	12	2
7	288	.6	33	425	152	1.03	148	.09	.07	.42	.32	.1	12	2
1	93	.34	24	202	143	.41	1	.03	.04	.16	.17	.03	0	1
1	89	.28	23	223	139	1.25	1	.03	.08	.17	.18	.04	3	1
0	8	.68	21	128	45	.33	<1	.01	.09	.03	.11	<.01	1	<1
32	301	.8	53	497	165	1.28	77	.1	.22	.43	.32	.1	12	2
149	330	.51	47	419	138	1.17	203	.09	.58	.48	.27	.13	2	4
194	270	.71	32	367	155	1.26	197	.11	1.01	.55	.21	.15	30	2
4	106	4.74	84	350	143	3.16	554	.31	5.31	.07	5.27	.42	106	28
38	396	4.86	117	719	262	4.09	630	.41	5.51	.47	5.46	.52	118	31
23	401	4.86	118	726	264	4.12	693	.41	5.41	.48	5.46	.53	118	31
9	406	4.82	112	752	267	4.13	701	.4	5.28	.42	5.45	.52	118	31
9	406	4.82	112	752	267	4.13	701	.4	5.28	.42	5.47	.52	118	31
1	13	.48	15	129	53	.17	4	.04	.08	.04	.42	.03	4	<1
34	305	.61	48	498	172	1.09	80	.13	.27	.44	.62	.13	16	3
34	385	4	53	620	244	1.17	901	.74	.32	1.26	10.9	1.02	32	34
4	63	.15	20	159	104	.21	18	.11	.08	.19	1.1	.09	10	1
37	320	.88	48	566	275	1.16	65	.16	.19	.69	.46	.14	10	1

[4]Vitamin A value is from beta-carotene used for coloring.

[5]With added vitamin A.

(For purposes of calculations, use "0" for t, <1, <.1, <.01, etc.)

H

Table H–1
Food Composition

Computer Code Number	Food Description	Measure	Wt (g)	H$_2$O (%)	Ener (kcal)	Prot (g)	Carb (g)	Dietary Fiber (g)	Fat (g)	Fat Breakdown (g) Sat	Mono	Poly
DAIRY—Cont.												
122	Milk shakes, vanilla (10 fl oz)	1¼ c	283	75	314	10	51	1	8	5.3	2.4	.3
	Milk desserts:											
134	Custard, baked	1 c	265	79	278	14	28	0	12	6.2	4	1
1548	Low-fat frozen dessert bars	1 ea	81	72	89	2	18	0	1	.2	.1	.4
	Ice cream, vanilla (about 10% fat):											
123	Hardened: ½ gallon	1 ea	1064	61	2138	37	251	0	117	72.4	33.8	4.4
124	Cup	1 c	133	61	267	5	31	0	15	9	4.2	.6
125	Fluid ounces	3 oz	50	61	100	2	12	0	6	3.4	1.6	.2
126	Soft serve	1 c	173	60	372	7	38	0	22	12.9	6	.8
	Ice cream, rich vanilla (16% fat):											
127	Hardened: ½ gallon	1 ea	1188	60	2554	49	264	0	154	88.9	41.5	5.5
128	Cup	1 c	148	57	357	5	33	0	24	14.8	6.9	.9
1724	Ben & Jerry's	½ c	106	64	226	4	21	0	17	10	–	–
	Ice milk, vanilla (about 4% fat):											
129	Hardened: ½ gallon	1 ea	1048	68	1456	40	238	0	45	27.7	12.9	1.7
130	Cup	1 c	131	68	182	5	30	0	6	3.5	1.6	.2
131	Soft serve (about 3% fat)	1 c	175	70	221	9	38	0	5	2.8	1.3	.2
	Pudding, canned (5-oz can = .55 cup):											
135	Chocolate	1 ea	142	69	189	4	32	1	6	1	2.4	2
136	Tapioca	1 ea	142	74	169	3	27	<1	5	.9	2.2	1.9
137	Vanilla	1 ea	142	71	185	3	31	<1	5	.8	2.2	1.9
	Puddings, dry mix with whole milk:											
138	Chocolate, instant	1 c	260	75	289	8	49	3	8	4.8	2.4	.5
139	Chocolate, regular, cooked	½ c	130	74	144	4	23	1	4	2.7	1.3	.2
140	Rice, cooked	½ c	132	72	161	4	28	<1	4	2.3	1.1	.2
141	Tapioca, cooked	½ c	130	74	148	4	25	0	4	2.3	1.1	.1
142	Vanilla, instant	½ c	130	74	148	4	26	0	4	2.3	1.1	.2
143	Vanilla, regular, cooked	½ c	130	75	144	4	24	0	4	2.4	1.1	.2
132	Sherbet (2% fat): ½ gallon	1 ea	1542	66	2127	17	469	8	31	17.9	8.3	1.2
133	Cup	1 c	193	66	266	2	59	1	4	2.2	1	.2
144	Soy milk	1 c	240	93	79	7	4	3	5	.7	1	3.6
2301	Soy milk, fortified, fat free[2]	1 c	240	88	110	6	22	1	0	0	0	0
1584	Yogurt, frozen, low-fat	½ c	87	65	138	3	21	0	5	3	1.4	.2
1512	Scoop	1 ea	79	74	78	4	16	0	<1	.1	<.1	0
	Yogurt, low-fat:											
1172	Fruit added with low-calorie sweetener	1 c	241	86	122	12	19	1	<1	.2	.1	<.1
145	Fruit added[1]	1 c	227	75	232	10	43	<1	2	1.6	.7	.1
146	Plain	1 c	227	85	144	12	16	0	4	2.3	1	.1
147	Vanilla or coffee flavor	1 c	227	79	194	12	31	0	3	1.8	.8	.1
148	Yogurt, made with nonfat milk	1 c	227	85	127	14	17	0	<1	.3	.1	t
149	Yogurt, made with whole milk	1 c	227	88	139	9	11	0	7	4.8	2	.2
EGGS												
	Raw, large:											
150	Whole, without shell	1 ea	50	75	74	6	1	0	5	1.5	1.9	.7
151	White	1 ea	33	88	17	3	<1	0	0	0	0	0
152	Yolk	1 ea	17	49	61	3	<1	0	5	1.6	1.9	.7

[1]Carbohydrate and kcalories vary widely—consult label if more precise values are needed.

[2]Nutrients will vary according to manufacturer—consult label.

Chol (mg)	Calc (mg)	Iron (mg)	Magn (mg)	Pota (mg)	Sodi (mg)	Zinc (mg)	VT-A (RE)	Thia (mg)	VT-E (α-TE)	Ribo (mg)	Niac (mg)	V-B6 (mg)	Fola (μg)	VT-C (mg)
31	345	.25	34	492	232	1.02	91	.13	.17	.52	.52	.15	9	2
231	297	.79	37	405	204	1.4	159	.09	.64	.6	.22	.13	27	1
1	82	.07	10	111	47	.26	38	.03	.07	.11	.06	.03	3	1
468	1362	.96	149	2117	851	7.34	1245	.44	0	2.55	1.23	.51	53	6
59	170	.12	19	265	106	.92	156	.05	0	.32	.15	.06	7	1
22	64	.04	7	100	40	.34	59	.02	0	.12	.06	.02	3	<1
157	227	.36	21	306	106	.9	266	.08	.64	.31	.16	.08	16	1
1081	1556	2.49	143	2102	725	6.18	1829	.58	4.4	2.16	1.13	.57	107	10
90	173	.07	16	235	83	.59	272	.06	0	.24	.12	.06	7	1
93	147	.36	–	–	54	–	225	–	0	–	–	–	–	0
147	1457	1.05	157	2211	891	4.61	493	.61	0	2.78	.94	.68	63	8
18	182	.13	20	276	111	.58	62	.08	0	.35	.12	.08	8	1
21	275	.1	25	387	123	.93	51	.09	0	.35	.21	.08	11	2
4	128	.72	30	256	183	.6	16	.04	.18	.22	.49	.04	4	3
1	119	.33	11	148	168	.38	0	.03	.13	.14	.44	.14	6	1
10	125	.18	11	160	192	.35	9	.03	.18	.2	.36	.02	0	0
29	265	.75	47	432	738	1.09	55	.09	.16	.37	.25	.1	10	2
16	144	.47	20	212	134	.58	34	.04	.08	.23	.13	.05	5	1
15	136	.5	17	165	140	.6	26	.1	.07	.18	.6	.04	5	1
16	135	.08	16	172	157	.44	35	.04	.1	.18	.09	.05	5	1
14	131	.09	16	166	372	.43	33	.04	.08	.18	.1	.05	5	1
16	139	.06	17	177	208	.45	35	.04	.08	.18	.1	.04	5	1
77	833	2.16	123	1480	709	7.4	216	.39	.88	1.05	1.48	.52	62	66
10	104	.27	15	185	89	.93	27	.05	.11	.13	.18	.07	8	8
0	10	1.39	46	338	29	.55	7	.39	.02	.17	.35	.1	4	0
0	400	1.44	46	20	60	.5	0	.075	.02	.102	3	.1	4	0
2	124	.26	12	184	76	.36	50	.03	.04	.19	.25	.07	5	1
1	137	.07	13	175	53	.67	1	.03	<.01	.16	.09	.04	8	1
3	370	.61	41	550	140	1.83	6	.1	.17	.45	.5	.11	32	26
10	345	.16	33	443	133	1.68	25	.08	.07	.4	.22	.09	21	2
14	415	.18	40	531	159	2.02	36	.1	.1	.49	.26	.11	25	2
11	388	.16	37	497	149	1.88	30	.09	.08	.46	.24	.1	24	2
4	452	.2	43	579	174	2.2	5	.11	.01	.53	.28	.12	28	2
29	275	.11	26	352	105	1.34	68	.07	.2	.32	.17	.07	17	1
213	25	.72	5	61	63	.55	96	.03	.53	.25	.04	.07	24	0
0	2	.01	4	47	54	0	0	<.01	0	.15	.03	0	1	0
218	23	.6	2	16	7	.52	99	.03	.54	.11	<.1	.06	25	0

H

(For purposes of calculations, use "0" for t, <1, <.1, <.01, etc.)

Table H–1
Food Composition

Computer Code Number	Food Description	Measure	Wt (g)	H₂O (%)	Ener (kcal)	Prot (g)	Carb (g)	Dietary Fiber (g)	Fat (g)	Fat Breakdown (g) Sat	Mono	Poly
EGGS—Cont.												
	Cooked:											
153	Fried in margarine	1 ea	46	69	92	6	1	0	7	1.9	2.8	1.3
154	Hard-cooked, shell removed	1 ea	50	75	78	6	1	0	5	1.6	2	.7
155	Hard-cooked, chopped	1 c	136	75	211	17	2	0	14	4.5	5.6	1.9
156	Poached, no added salt	1 ea	50	75	75	6	1	0	5	1.6	1.9	.7
157	Scrambled with milk & margarine	1 ea	61	73	101	7	1	0	7	2.2	2.9	1.3
1681	Egg substitute, liquid	½ c	126	83	106	17	1	0	4	.8	1.1	2
1254	Egg Beaters, Fleischmann's	¼ c	61	–	30	6	1	0	0	0	0	0
1262	Eggs, Second Nature, prepared	⅓ c	69	80	66	9	1	0	3	.5	.7	1.3
FATS and OILS												
158	Butter: Stick	½ c	113	16	810	1	<1	0	92	57.2	27.1	3.4
159	Tablespoon	1 tbs	14	16	100	<1	<1	0	11	7.1	3.4	.4
160	Pat (about 1 tsp)[1]	1 ea	5	16	36	<1	<1	0	4	2.5	1.2	.2
1682	Whipped	1 tsp	3	16	22	<1	<1	0	2	1.5	.7	.1
	Fats, cooking:											
1363	Bacon fat	1 tbs	14	0	125	<1	0	0	14	6.4	5.9	1.1
1362	Beef fat/tallow	1 c	205	0	1849	0	0	0	205	103	87.3	8.2
1364	Chicken fat	1 c	205	<1	1845	0	0	0	205	61.1	91.6	42.8
161	Vegetable shortening:	1 c	205	0	1812	0	0	0	205	52.1	91.2	53.5
162	Tablespoon	1 tbs	13	0	115	0	0	0	13	3.3	5.8	3.4
163	Lard:	1 c	205	0	1849	0	0	0	205	80.4	92.5	28
164	Tablespoon	1 tbs	13	0	117	0	0	0	13	5.1	5.5	1.8
	Margarine:											
165	Imitation (about 40% fat), soft:	1 c	227	58	783	1	1	0	88	14.5	33	37
166	Tablespoon	1 tbs	14	58	49	<1	<1	0	6	1	2.2	2
167	Regular, hard (about 80% fat):	½ c	113	16	812	1	1	0	91	14.8	42	29.6
168	Tablespoon	1 tbs	14	16	101	<1	<1	0	11	1.8	5	3.6
169	Pat	1 ea	5	16	36	<1	<1	0	4	.8	1.8	1.3
170	Regular, soft (about 80% fat):	1 c	227	16	1625	2	1	0	183	30.7	83	61
171	Tablespoon	1 tbs	14	16	100	<1	<1	0	11	1.9	4	4.8
2056	Saffola, unsalted	1 tbs	14	20	100	0	0	0	11	2	3	4.5
2057	Saffola, reduced fat	1 tbs	14	37	60	0	0	0	8	1.3	2.7	4.4
172	Spread (about 60% fat), hard:	½ c	113	37	610	1	0	0	69	15.9	29.4	20.5
173	Tablespoon	1 tbs	14	37	76	<1	0	0	9	2	3.6	2.5
174	Pat[1]	1 ea	5	37	27	<1	0	0	3	.7	1.2	1
175	Spread (about 60% fat), soft:	1 c	227	37	1226	1	0	0	138	29.3	71.5	31.3
176	Tablespoon	1 tbs	14	37	76	<1	0	0	9	1.8	4.4	1.9
2160	Touch of Butter (47% fat)	1 tbs	14	36	60	0	0	0	7	1.5	3.1	1.5
	Oils:											
1585	Canola:	1 c	218	0	1927	0	0	0	218	15.5	128	64.5
1586	Tablespoon	1 tbs	14	0	124	0	0	0	14	1	8.2	4.1
177	Corn:	1 c	218	0	1927	0	0	0	218	29.4	54.1	130.8
178	Tablespoon	1 tbs	14	0	124	0	0	0	14	1.8	3.5	8.4

[1]Pat is 1" square, ⅛" thick; about 1 tsp; 90 per lb.

TABLE OF FOOD COMPOSITION

◆ **H-15**

PAGE KEY: H–4 = BEV   H–6 = DAIRY   H–12 = EGGS   H–14 = FAT/OIL   H–18 = FRUIT   H–26 = BAKERY   H–36 = GRAIN   H–44 = FISH
H–48 = MEATS   H–50 = POULTRY   H–54 = SAUSAGE   H–56 = MIXED/FAST   H–64 = NUTS/SEEDS   H–68 = SWEETS   H–70 = VEG/LEG
H–84 = MISC   H–88 = SOUPS/SAUCES   H–90 = FAST   H–106 = FRZN ENTREE   H–112 = BABY FOODS

Chol (mg)	Calc (mg)	Iron (mg)	Magn (mg)	Pota (mg)	Sodi (mg)	Zinc (mg)	VT-A (RE)	Thia (mg)	VT-E (α-TE)	Ribo (mg)	Niac (mg)	V-B6 (mg)	Fola (μg)	VT-C (mg)
211	25	.72	5	61	162	.55	114	.03	.75	.24	.04	.07	17	0
212	25	.59	5	63	62	.53	84	.03	.53	.26	.03	.06	22	0
577	68	1.62	14	171	169	1.43	228	.09	1.43	.7	.09	.17	60	0
212	25	.72	5	60	140	.55	95	.02	.53	.22	.03	.06	18	0
215	43	.73	7	84	171	.61	119	.03	.8	.27	.05	.07	18	<1
1	67	2.65	11	416	223	1.64	272	.14	.61	.38	.14	<.01	19	0
0	40	1.08	–	85	100	–	–	–	.3	–	–	–	–	–
1	42	1.65	7	260	139	1.02	170	.07	.38	.22	.08	<.01	9	0
247	27	.18	2	29	933[2]	.06	852[3]	.01	1.79	.04	.05	<.01	3	0
31	3	.02	<1	4	117[2]	.01	107[3]	<.01	.22	<.01	.01	0	<1	0
11	1	.01	<1	1	41[2]	<.01	38[3]	0	.08	<.01	<.01	0	<1	0
7	1	<.01	<1	1	25[2]	<.01	23[3]	<.01	.05	<.01	<.01	0	<1	0
14	<1	<.01	<1	<1	76	<.01	0	0	.31	0	0	0	0	0
224	0	0	0	<1	<1	0	0	0	3.08	0	0	0	0	0
174	0	0	0	0	0	0	351	0	5.54	0	0	0	0	0
0	0	0	0	0	0	0	0	0	17	0	0	0	0	0
0	0	0	0	0	0	0	0	0	1.08	0	0	0	0	0
195	<1	0	<1	<1	<1	.23	0	0	2.46	0	0	0	0	0
12	<1	0	<1	<1	<1	.01	0	0	.16	0	0	0	0	0
0	40	0	4	57	800	0	1814[4]	.01	5.29	.05	.03	.01	2	<1
0	3	0	<1	4	136	0	114[4]	<.01	.33	<.01	<.01	<.01	<1	<1
0	34	0	3	48	1065	.23	903[4]	.01	14.5	.04	.03	.01	1	<1
0	4	0	<1	6	132	.03	112[4]	<.01	1.8	<.01	<.01	<.01	<1	<1
0	2	0	<1	2	47	.01	40[4]	<.01	.64	<.01	<.01	0	<1	<1
0	60	0	5	86	2447	0	1814[4]	.02	27.2	.07	.04	.02	2	<1
0	4	0	<1	5	151	0	112[4]	<.01	1.68	<.01	<.01	<.01	<1	<1
–	0	0	–	–	0	–	51	–	–	–	–	–	–	0
–	0	0	–	–	115	–	51	–	.14	–	–	–	–	0
0	24	0	2	34	1123	.17	903[4]	.01	5.65	.03	.02	.01	1	<1
0	3	0	<1	4	139	0	112[4]	<.01	.7	<.01	<.01	<.01	<1	<1
0	1	0	<1	1	50	0	40[4]	0	.25	<.01	<.01	0	<1	<1
0	47	0	4	68	2256	0	1814[4]	.02	20.5	.06	.04	.01	2	<1
0	3	0	<1	4	139	0	112[4]	<.01	1.26	<.01	<.01	<.01	<1	<1
0	0	0	<1	0	110	0	100	<.01	1.27	<.01	<.01	<.01	<1	<.1
0	0	0	0	0	0	0	0	0	45.8	0	0	0	0	0
0	0	0	0	0	0	0	0	0	2.94	0	0	0	0	0
0	0	0	0	0	0	0	0	0	46	0	0	0	0	0
0	0	0	0	0	0	0	0	0	2.95	0	0	0	0	0

H

[2] For salted butter, unsalted butter contains 12 mg sodium per stick or ½ c, 1.5 mg/tbs, or .5 mg/pat.

[3] Values for vitamin A are a year-round average.

[4] Based on average vitamin A content of fortified margarine. Federal specifications require a minimum of 15,000 IU/lb.

(For purposes of calculations, use "0" for t, <1, <.1, <.01, etc.)

Table H–1
Food Composition

Computer Code Number	Food Description	Measure	Wt (g)	H₂O (%)	Ener (kcal)	Prot (g)	Carb (g)	Dietary Fiber (g)	Fat (g)	Fat Breakdown (g) Sat	Mono	Poly
	FATS and OILS—Cont.											
	Oils—Cont.											
179	Olive:	1 c	216	0	1909	0	0	0	216	29.4	159	21.3
180	Tablespoon	1 tbs	14	0	124	0	0	0	14	1.9	10.3	1.4
1683	Olive, extra virgin	1 tbs	14	<1	126	0	0	0	14	1.96	10.8	1.3
181	Peanut:	1 c	216	0	1909	0	0	0	216	40	99.8	71.3
182	Tablespoon	1 tbs	14	0	124	0	0	0	14	2.6	6.5	4.6
183	Safflower:	1 c	218	0	1927	0	0	0	218	19.8	26.4	162
184	Tablespoon	1 tbs	14	0	124	0	0	0	14	1.3	1.7	10.4
185	Soybean:	1 c	218	0	1927	0	0	0	218	32	50.8	126
186	Tablespoon	1 tbs	14	0	124	0	0	0	14	2.1	3.3	8.1
187	Soybean/cottonseed:	1 c	218	0	1927	0	0	0	218	40	64.3	105
188	Tablespoon	1 tbs	14	0	124	0	0	0	14	2.5	4.1	6.7
189	Sunflower:	1 c	218	0	1927	0	0	0	218	25	42.5	143
190	Tablespoon	1 tbs	14	0	124	0	0	0	14	1.6	2.7	9.2
	Salad dressings/sandwich spreads:											
191	Blue cheese, regular	1 tbs	15	32	75	1	1	<1	8	1.5	1.9	4.4
1040	Low calorie	1 tbs	15	80	15	1	<1	<1	1	.2	.5	.4
1684	Caesar's	1 tbs	12	36	55	1	<1	<1	5	.9	3.7	.5
192	French, regular	1 tbs	16	38	67	<1	3	<1	9	1.5	1.2	3.4
193	Low calorie	1 tbs	16	71	21	<1	3	0	1	.1	.2	.5
194	Italian, regular	1 tbs	15	38	70	<1	1	<1	9	1	1.6	4.1
195	Low calorie	1 tbs	15	82	8	<1	1	<1	1	.1	.1	.2
	Kraft, Deliciously Right											
2150	1000 Island	2 tbs	32	–	70	0	8	0	4	1	–	–
2153	Bacon & tomato	2 tbs	31	–	60	1	3	0	5	1	–	–
2154	Cucumber ranch	2 tbs	31	–	60	0	2	0	5	1	–	–
2151	French	2 tbs	32	–	50	0	6	0	3	.5	–	–
2152	Ranch	2 tbs	31	–	100	0	5	0	9	1.5	–	–
199	Mayo type, regular	1 tbs	15	40	58	<1	4	0	5	.8	1.4	2.7
1030	Low calorie	1 tbs	15	54	39	<1	4	0	3	.4	.8	1.5
	Mayonnaise:											
197	Imitation, low calorie	1 tbs	15	63	35	<1	2	0	3	.5	.7	1.6
196	Regular (soybean)	1 tbs	14	17	100	<1	<1	0	11	1.7	3.1	5.7
1488	Regular, low calorie, low sodium	1 tbs	14	63	32	<1	2	0	3	.5	.6	1.4
1493	Regular, low calorie	1 tbs	16	63	37	<1	3	0	3	.5	.7	1.7
198	Ranch, regular	½ c	119	35	436	4	5	0	45	6.7	19.4	17
2251	Low calorie	2 tbs	28	70	60	0	2	0	5	1	–	–
1685	Russian	1 tbs	15	35	74	<1	2	0	8	1.1	1.8	4.4
1502	Salad dressing, low calorie, oil free	1 tbs	15	88	4	<1	1	<1	<1	<.1	0	<.1
1605	Salad dressing, no cholesterol (Miracle Whip)	1 tbs	15	57	48	0	2	0	4	1.1	1.1	2.1
203	Salad dressing, from recipe, cooked[1]	1 tbs	16	69	25	1	2	<1	2	.5	.6	.3
200	Tartar sauce, regular	1 tbs	14	34	74	<1	1	<1	8	1.5	2.6	4.1
1503	Low calorie	1 tbs	14	63	31	<1	2	<1	2	.4	.6	1.3
201	Thousand island, regular	1 tbs	16	46	60	<1	2	<1	6	1	1.3	3.2
202	Low calorie	1 tbs	15	69	25	<1	3	<1	2	.2	.4	.9
204	Vinegar & oil	1 tbs	16	47	72	0	<1	0	8	1.5	2.4	3.9

[1]Fatty acid values apply to product made with regular margarine.

Chol (mg)	Calc (mg)	Iron (mg)	Magn (mg)	Pota (mg)	Sodi (mg)	Zinc (mg)	VT-A (RE)	Thia (mg)	VT-E (α-TE)	Ribo (mg)	Niac (mg)	V-B6 (mg)	Fola (µg)	VT-C (mg)
0	<1	.82	<1	0	<1	.13	0	0	26.8	0	0	0	0	0
0	<1	.05	<1	0	<1	.01	0	0	1.74	0	0	0	0	0
0	–	–	–	–	–	–	0	0	1.74	0	0	0	0	0
0	<1	.06	<1	<1	<1	.02	0	0	27.9	0	0	0	0	0
0	<1	0	<1	0	<1	0	0	0	1.81	0	0	0	0	0
0	0	0	0	0	0	0	0	0	94	0	0	0	0	0
0	0	0	0	0	0	0	0	0	6.03	0	0	0	0	0
0	<1	.04	<1	0	0	0	0	0	39.7	0	0	0	0	0
0	<1	<.01	<1	0	0	0	0	0	2.55	0	0	0	0	0
0	0	0	0	0	0	0	0	0	61.5	0	0	0	0	0
0	0	0	0	0	0	0	0	0	3.95	0	0	0	0	0
0	0	0	0	0	0	0	0	0	110	0	0	0	0	0
0	0	0	0	0	0	0	0	0	7.08	0	0	0	0	0
3	12	.03	0	6	164	0	10	<.01	1.4	.02	.02	.01	1	<1
<1	13	.08	1	1	180	.04	<1	<.01	.14	.02	.01	<.01	<1	<1
12	22	.19	3	20	203	.12	6	<.01	.7	.02	.49	.01	2	1
9	2	.06	1.6	2	188	.01	3	<.01	1.63	<.01	<.01	<.01	1	0
0	2	.06	0	13	126	.03	21	0	.19	0	0	0	0	0
0	2	.03	<1	5	118	.02	4	<.01	1.56	<.01	0	<.01	1	0
0	<1	.03	0	2	120	.02	0	0	.68	0	0	0	0	0
5	0	0	–	55	320	–	0	–	.38	–	–	–	–	0
3	0	0	–	40	300	–	0	–	1.45	–	–	–	–	0
0	0	0	–	20	450	–	0	–	1.41	–	–	–	–	0
0	0	0	–	15	260	–	100	–	.85	–	–	–	–	0
0	0	0	–	10	320	–	0	–	2.54	–	–	–	–	0
4	2	.03	<1	1	107	.03	13	<.01	.6	<.01	<.01	<.01	1	0
4	2	.03	<1	1	107	.03	10	<.01	.65	<.01	0	<.01	1	0
4	<1	0	<1	2	75	.02	0	0	.97	0	0	0	0	0
8	3	.07	<1	5	80	.02	12	0	1.7	0	<.01	.08	1	0
3	0	0	0	1	15	.02	1	0	.53	<.01	0	0	<1	0
4	<1	0	<1	2	80	02	0	0	1.03	0	0	0	0	0
47	119	.31	12	158	522	.44	86	.04	4.76	.17	.08	.05	6	1
10	20	0	–	–	240	–	0	–	1.41	–	–	–	–	0
3	3	.1	.23	24	130	.06	31	.01	1.53	.01	.1	<.01	1.59	1
0	1	.04	2	7	256	<.01	<1	<.01	<.01	<.01	<.01	<.01	<1	<1
0	0	<.01	0	0	102	0	2	0	.65	0	0	0	0	0
9	13	.08	0	19	117	0	20	.01	.3	.02	.04	0	0	<1
7	3	.13	<1	11	99	.02	9	<.01	2.24	<.01	0	.01	1	<1
3	2	.09	<1	5	83	.02	2	<.01	.83	<.01	.01	<.01	<1	<1
4	2	.09	<1	18	110	.02	15	<.01	1.14	<.01	<.01	<.01	1	<1
2	2	.09	<1	17	153	.02	14	<.01	1.19	<.01	<.01	<.01	1	<1
0	0	0	0	1	<1	0	0	0	1.41	0	0	0	0	0

H

(For purposes of calculations, use "0" for t, <1, <.1, <.01, etc.)

Table H–1
Food Composition

Computer Code Number	Food Description	Measure	Wt (g)	H₂O (%)	Ener (kcal)	Prot (g)	Carb (g)	Dietary Fiber (g)	Fat (g)	Fat Breakdown (g)		
										Sat	Mono	Poly
FATS and OILS—Cont.												
	Salad dressings/sandwich spreads—Cont.											
	Wishbone											
2180	Creamy Italian, lite	1 tbs	15	–	26	<1	2	–	2	.4	–	.7
2166	Italian, lite	1 tbs	16	79	6	0	1	–	<1	0	–	.1
FRUITS and FRUIT JUICES												
	Apples:											
	Fresh, raw, with peel:											
205	2 ¾" diam (about 3 per lb w/cores)	1 ea	138	84	81	<1	21	3	<1	.1	t	.1
206	3 ¾" diam (about 2 per lb w/cores)	1 ea	212	84	125	<1	32	6	1	.1	t	.2
207	Raw, peeled slices	1 c	110	85	63	<1	16	2	<1	.1	t	.1
208	Dried, sulfured	10 ea	64	32	155	1	42	6	<1	t	t	.1
209	Apple juice, bottled or canned	1 c	248	88	116	<1	29	<1	<1	<1	t	<.1
210	Applesauce, sweetened	1 c	255	80	193	<1	51	3	<1	.1	t	.1
211	Applesauce, unsweetened	1 c	244	88	104	<1	28	3	<1	<1	t	t
	Apricots:											
212	Raw, w/o pits (about 12 per lb w/pits)	3 ea	106	86	51	1	12	3	<1	t	.2	.1
	Canned (fruit and liquid):											
213	Heavy syrup	1 c	258	78	214	1	55	4	<1	t	.1	t
214	Halves	3 ea	85	78	70	<1	18	1	<1	t	t	t
215	Juice pack	1 c	248	87	119	2	30	4	<1	t	t	t
216	Halves	3 ea	84	87	40	1	10	1	<1	t	t	t
217	Dried, halves	10 ea	35	31	83	1	22	3	<1	t	.1	t
218	Dried, cooked, unsweetened, w/liquid	1 c	250	76	212	3	55	8	<1	t	.2	.1
219	Apricot nectar, canned	1 c	251	85	140	1	36	2	<1	t	.1	t
	Avocados, raw, edible part only:											
220	California (2 lb with refuse)	1 ea	173	73	306	4	12	8	30	4.5	19.6	3.5
221	Florida (1 lb with refuse)	1 ea	304	80	340	5	27	16	27	5.3	14.8	4.5
222	Mashed, fresh, average	1 c	230	74	370	5	17	12	35	5.6	22.1	4.5
	Bananas, raw, without peel:											
223	Whole, 8¾" long (175 g w/peel)	1 ea	114	74	104	1	27	3	1	.2	t	.1
224	Slices	1 c	150	74	137	2	35	4	1	.3	.1	.1
1285	Bananas, dehydrated slices	1 oz	28	3	97	1	25	2	1	.2	<.1	.1
225	Blackberries, raw	1 c	144	86	75	1	18	8	1	<.1	.1	.3
	Blueberries:											
226	Fresh	1 c	145	85	81	1	20	4	1	t	.1	.2
227	Frozen, sweetened	10 oz	284	77	230	1	62	6	<1	t	.1	.2
228	Frozen, thawed	1 c	230	77	186	1	50	5	<1	t	t	.1
	Cherries:											
229	Sour, red pitted, canned water pack	1 c	244	90	88	2	22	3	<1	.1	.1	.1
230	Sweet, red pitted, raw	10 ea	68	81	49	1	11	2	1	.1	.2	.2
231	Cranberry juice cocktail	1 c	253	85	144	0	36	<1	<1	t	t	.1
1411	Cranberry juice, low calorie	¾ c	178	95	34	0	8	<1	0	0	0	0
232	Cranberry-apple juice	1 c	253	83	169	<1	43	<1	0	0	0	0

(Computer code number is for West Diet Analysis program)

PAGE KEY: H-4 = BEV   H-6 = DAIRY   H-12 = EGGS   H-14 = FAT/OIL   H-18 = FRUIT   H-26 = BAKERY   H-36 = GRAIN   H-44 = FISH   H-48 = MEATS   H-50 = POULTRY   H-54 = SAUSAGE   H-56 = MIXED/FAST   H-64 = NUTS/SEEDS   H-68 = SWEETS   H-70 = VEG/LEG   H-84 = MISC   H-88 = SOUPS/SAUCES   H-90 = FAST   H-106 = FRZN ENTREE   H-112 = BABY FOODS

Chol (mg)	Calc (mg)	Iron (mg)	Magn (mg)	Pota (mg)	Sodi (mg)	Zinc (mg)	VT-A (RE)	Thia (mg)	VT-E (α-TE)	Ribo (mg)	Niac (mg)	V-B6 (mg)	Fola (μg)	VT-C (mg)
<1	0	0	–	–	148	–	–	0	.56	0	0	–	–	0
0	1	0	–	–	255	–	–	0	.24	0	0	–	–	.2
0	10	.25	7	159	0	.05	7	.02	.44	.02	.11	.07	4	8
0	15	.38	11	244	0	.08	11	.04	.68	.03	.16	.1	6	12
0	4	.08	3	124	0	.04	4	.02	.09	.01	.1	.05	<1	4
0	9	.9	10	288	56	.13	4	0	.35	.1	.59	.08	0	2
0	17	.92	7	295	7	.07	<1	.05	.03	.04	.25	.07	<1	2
0	10	.89	8	155	8	.1	3	.03	.03	.07	.48	.07	2	4[1]
0	7	.29	7	183	5	.07	7	.03	.02	.06	.46	.06	1	3[1]
0	15	.57	8	313	1	.28	277	.03	.94	.04	.64	.06	9	11
0	23	.77	18	361	10	.28	317	.05	2.3	.06	.97	.14	4	8
0	8	.25	6	119	3	.09	105	.02	.76	.02	.32	.05	1	3
0	30	.74	25	409	10	.27	419	.04	2.21	.05	.85	.13	4	12
0	10	.25	8	139	3	.09	142	.01	.75	.02	.29	.04	1	4
0	16	1.65	16	482	4	.26	253	<.01	.53	.05	1.05	.05	4	1
0	40	4.18	42	1222	8	.66	590	.01	1.25	.07	2.36	.28	0	4
0	18	.95	13	286	8	.23	331	.02	.20	.03	.65	.05	3	2[2]
0	19	2.04	71	1096	21	.73	106	.19	2.32	.21	3.32	.48	113	14
0	33	1.61	103	1483	15	1.28	185	.33	2.37	.37	5.84	.85	162	24
0	25	2.34	90	1377	23	.97	140	.25	3.08	.28	4.42	.64	142	18
0	7	.35	33	451	1	.18	9	.05	.31	.11	.62	.66	22	10
0	9	.46	43	594	2	.24	12	.07	.41	.15	.81	.87	29	14
0	6	.33	30	418	1	.17	9	.05	0	.07	.79	.12	4	2
0	46	.82	29	282	0	.39	23	.04	1.02	.06	.58	.08	49	30
0	9	.25	7	129	9	.16	15	.07	1.45	.07	.52	.05	9	19
0	17	1.11	6	170	3	.17	11	.06	2.02	.15	.72	.17	19	3
0	14	.9	5	138	2	.14	9	.05	1.63	.12	.58	.14	15	2
0	27	3.34	15	239	17	.17	183	.04	.32	.1	.43	.11	19	5
0	10	.26	7	152	0	.04	14	.03	.09	.04	.27	.02	3	5
0	8	.38	5	45	5	.18	1	.02	0	.02	.09	.05	1	90[3]
0	16	.07	4	39	5	.04	1	.02	0	.02	.06	.03	<1	57
0	18	.15	5	68	5	.1	1	.01	0	.05	.15	.05	1	81[3]

[1] Value based on products without added vitamin C. Bottled apple juice with added vitamin C usually contains 41.6 mg/100 g, or 103 mg per cup. Check label for specific vitamin C values.

[2] Without added vitamin C. Products with added vitamin C contain 136 mg per cup. Check label.

[3] Nutrient added.

(For purposes of calculations, use "0" for t, <1, <.1, <.01, etc.)

Table H–1
Food Composition

Computer Code Number	Food Description	Measure	Wt (g)	H₂O (%)	Ener (kcal)	Prot (g)	Carb (g)	Dietary Fiber (g)	Fat (g)	Fat Breakdown (g) Sat	Fat Breakdown (g) Mono	Fat Breakdown (g) Poly
FRUITS and FRUIT JUICES—Cont.												
233	Cranberry sauce, canned, strained	1 c	277	61	418	1	108	3	<1	t	<.1	.2
234	Dates, whole, without pits	10 ea	83	22	228	2	61	6	<1	.2	.1	t
235	Dates, chopped	1 c	178	22	490	4	130	13	1	.3	.3	<.1
236	Figs, dried	10 ea	187	28	477	6	122	17	2	.4	.5	1
	Fruit cocktail, canned, fruit and liq:											
237	Heavy syrup pack	1 c	255	80	186	1	48	3	<1	t	t	.1
238	Juice pack	1 c	248	87	114	1	30	2	<1	t	t	t
	Grapefruit:											
	Raw 3¾" diam (half w/rind = 241 g)											
239	Pink/red, half fruit, edible part	1 ea	123	91	37	1	9	2	<1	t	t	t
240	White, half fruit, edible part	1 ea	118	90	39	1	10	1	<1	t	t	t
241	Canned sections with light syrup	1 c	254	84	152	1	39	1	<1	t	t	.1
	Grapefruit juice:											
242	Fresh, raw	1 c	247	90	96	1	23	<1	<1	t	t	.1
243	Canned, unsweetened	1 c	247	90	94	1	22	<1	<1	t	t	.1
244	Sweetened	1 c	250	87	115	1	28	<1	<1	t	t	.1
	Frozen concentrate, unsweetened:											
245	Undiluted, 6-fl-oz can	¾ c	207	62	302	4	71	1	1	.1	.1	.2
246	Diluted with 3 cans water	1 c	247	89	101	1	24	<1	<1	.1	t	.1
	Grapes, raw European (adherent skin):											
247	Thompson seedless	10 ea	50	81	35	<1	9	<1	<1	.1	t	.1
248	Tokay/Emperor, seeded types	10 ea	57	81	40	<1	10	<1	<1	.1	t	.1
	Grape juice:											
249	Bottled or canned	1 c	253	84	154	1	38	2	<1	.1	t	.1
	Frozen concentrate, sweetened:											
250	Undiluted, 6-fl-oz can	¾ c	216	54	387	1	96	<1	1	.2	t	.2
251	Diluted with 3 cans water	1 c	250	87	127	<1	32	<1	<1	.1	t	.1
1410	Low calorie	1 c	250	84	153	1	38	<1	<1	.1	t	.1
252	Kiwi fruit, raw, peeled (88 g with peel)	1 ea	76	83	46	1	11	3	<1	t	t	.2
253	Lemons, raw, without peel and seeds (about 4 per lb whole)	1 ea	58	89	17	1	5	2	<1	t	t	.1
	Lemon juice:											
254	Fresh:	1 c	244	91	61	1	21	1	0	0	0	0
255	Tablespoon	1 tbs	15	91	4	<1	1	<1	0	0	0	0
256	Canned or bottled, unsweetened:	1 c	244	93	51	1	16	1	1	.1	t	.2
257	Tablespoon	1 tbs	15	93	3	<1	1	<1	<1	t	t	t
258	Frozen, single strength, unsweetened:	1 c	244	92	54	1	16	1	1	.1	t	.2
2298	Tablespoon	1 tbs	15	92	3	<1	1	<1	<1	t	t	t
	Lime juice:											
260	Fresh:	1 c	246	90	66	1	22	1	<1	t	t	.1
261	Tablespoon	1 tbs	15	90	4	<1	1	<1	<1	t	t	t
262	Canned or bottled, unsweetened	1 c	246	93	52	1	16	1	1	.1	.1	.2
263	Mangoes, raw, edible part (300 g w/skin & seeds)	1 ea	207	82	134	1	35	4	1	.1	.2	.1

Chol (mg)	Calc (mg)	Iron (mg)	Magn (mg)	Pota (mg)	Sodi (mg)	Zinc (mg)	VT-A (RE)	Thia (mg)	VT-E (α-TE)	Ribo (mg)	Niac (mg)	V-B6 (mg)	Fola (μg)	VT-C (mg)
0	11	.61	8	72	80	.14	6	.04	.28	.06	.28	.04	2	6
0	27	.95	29	541	2	.24	4	.07	.08	.08	1.83	.16	10	0
0	57	2.05	62	1160	5	.52	9	.16	.18	.18	3.92	.34	22	0
0	269	4.17	110	1331	21	.95	24	.13	9.35	.16	1.3	.42	14	2
0	15	.74	13	224	15	.2	51	.05	.74	.05	.95	.13	7	5
0	20	.52	17	235	10	.22	77	.03	.5	.04	1	.13	6	7
0	14	.15	10	159	0	.09	32[1]	.04	.31	.02	.23	.05	15	47
0	14	.07	11	175	0	.08	0	.04	.3	.02	.32	.05	12	39
0	36	1.02	25	328	5	.2	2	.1	.64	.05	.62	.05	22	54
0	23	.49	30	400	2	.12	2[2]	.1	.12	.05	.49	.11	25	94
0	17	.49	25	378	2	.22	2	.1	.12	.05	.57	.05	26	72
0	20	.9	25	405	5	.15	0	.1	.13	.06	.8	.05	26	67
0	56	1.01	79	1001	6	.37	6	.3	.37	.16	1.6	.32	26	248
0	20	.35	27	336	2	.12	2	.1	.12	.05	.54	.11	9	83
0	6	.13	3	92	1	.03	3	.05	.35	.03	.15	.05	2	5
0	6	.15	3	105	1	.03	4	.05	.4	.03	.17	.06	2	6
0	23	.61	25	334	8	.13	3	.07	0	.09	.66	.16	7	<1
0	28	.78	32	159	15	.28	6	.11	.38	.2	.93	.32	9	179[3]
0	10	.25	10	52	5	.1	3	.04	.13	.06	.31	.1	3	60[3]
0	23	.6	25	330	8	.13	3	.07	0	.09	.66	.16	7	<1
0	20	.31	23	252	4	.13	14	.01	.85	.04	.38	.07	29	74
0	15	.35	5	80	1	.03	2	.02	.14	.01	.06	.05	6	31
0	17	.07	15	303	2	.12	5	.07	.22	.02	.24	.12	31	112
0	1	0	1	19	<1	.01	<1	0	.01	0	.01	.01	2	7
0	27	.32	19	249	51	.15	5	.1	.22	.02	.48	.1	25	60
0	2	.02	1	15	3	.01	<1	.01	.01	0	.03	.01	2	4
0	19	.29	19	217	2	.12	2	.14	.22	.03	.33	.15	23	77
0	1	.02	1	13	<1	.01	<1	.01	.01	<.01	.02	.01	1	5
0	22	.07	15	268	2	.15	2	.05	.22	.02	.25	.11	20	72
0	1	0	1	16	<1	.01	<1	0	.01	0	.01	.01	1	4
0	29	.57	17	184	39[4]	.15	5	.08	.07	.01	.4	.07	19	16
0	21	.27	19	323	4	.08	805	.12	2.32	.12	1.21	.28	29	57

[1] Vitamin A in Texas red grapefruit would be 74 RE.

[2] This is vitamin A for white grapefruit juice; pink or red grapefruit juice = 109 RE per cup.

[3] With added vitamin C (ascorbic acid).

[4] Sodium benzoate and sodium bisulfite added as preservatives.

(For purposes of calculations, use "0" for t, <1, <.1, <.01, etc.)

H

Table H–1
Food Composition

Computer Code Number	Food Description	Measure	Wt (g)	H$_2$O (%)	Ener (kcal)	Prot (g)	Carb (g)	Dietary Fiber (g)	Fat (g)	Fat Breakdown (g)		
										Sat	Mono	Poly
	FRUITS and FRUIT JUICES—Cont.											
	Melons, raw, without rind and contents:											
264	Cantaloupe, 5" diam (2⅓ lb whole with refuse), orange flesh	½ ea	267	90	93	2	22	2	1	.2	t	.3
265	Honeydew, 6½" diam (5¼ lb whole with refuse), slice = ⅒ melon	1 pce	129	90	45	1	12	1	<1	t	t	t
266	Nectarines, raw, w/o pits, 2½" diam	1 ea	136	86	67	1	16	2	1	.1	.2	.3
	Oranges, raw:											
267	Whole w/o peel and seeds, 2⅝" diam (180 g with peel and seeds)	1 ea	131	87	62	1	15	3	<1	t	t	t
268	Sections, without membranes	1 c	180	87	85	2	21	4	<1	t	t	t
	Orange juice:											
269	Fresh, all varieties	1 c	248	88	112	2	26	<1	<1	.1	.1	.1
270	Canned, unsweetened	1 c	249	89	105	1	25	<1	<1	t	.1	.1
271	Chilled	1 c	249	88	110	2	25	<1	1	.1	.1	.2
	Frozen concentrate:											
272	Undiluted (6-oz can)	¾ c	213	58	339	5	81	2	<1	.1	.1	.1
273	Diluted w/3 parts water by volume	1 c	249	88	112	2	27	<1	<1	t	t	t
1345	Orange juice, from dry crystals	1 c	248	88	114	0	29	0	0	0	0	0
274	Orange and grapefruit juice, canned	1 c	247	89	106	1	25	<1	<1	t	t	t
	Papayas, raw:											
275	½" slices	1 c	140	89	54	1	14	3	<1	.1	.1	t
276	Whole, 3½" diam by 5⅛" w/o seeds and skin (1 lb w/refuse)	1 ea	304	89	118	2	30	5	<1	.1	.1	.1
1031	Papaya nectar, canned	1 c	250	85	143	<1	36	2	<1	.1	.1	.1
	Peaches:											
277	Raw, whole, 2½" diam, peeled, pitted (about 4 per lb whole)	1 ea	87	88	37	1	10	2	<1	t	t	t
278	Raw, sliced	1 c	170	88	73	1	19	3	<1	t	.1	.1
	Canned, fruit and liquid:											
279	Heavy syrup pack:	1 c	256	79	189	1	51	3	<1	t	.1	.1
280	Half	1 ea	81	79	60	<1	16	1	<1	t	t	t
281	Juice pack:	1 c	248	88	109	2	29	3	<1	t	t	t
282	Half	1 ea	77	88	34	<1	9	1	<1	t	t	t
283	Dried, uncooked	10 ea	130	32	311	5	80	11	1	.1	.4	.5
284	Dried, cooked, fruit and liquid	1 c	258	78	198	3	51	7	1	.1	.2	.3
	Frozen, slice, sweetened:											
285	10-oz package	1 ea	284	75	267	2	68	5	<1	t	.1	.2
286	Cup, thawed measure	1 c	250	75	235	2	60	5	<1	t	.1	.2
1032	Peach nectar, canned	1 c	249	86	135	1	35	1	<1	t	t	t
	Pears:											
	Fresh, with skin, cored:											
287	Bartlett, 2½" diam (about 2½ per lb)	1 ea	166	84	98	1	25	4[1]	1	t	.1	.2
288	Bosc, 2 1/5" diam (about 3 per lb)	1 ea	141	84	83	1	21	3[1]	1	t	.1	.1
289	D'Anjou, 3" diam (about 2 per lb)	1 ea	200	84	118	1	30	5[1]	1	t	.2	.2
	Canned, fruit and liquid:											
290	Heavy syrup pack:	1 c	255	80	188	1	49	4[1]	<1	t	.1	.1
291	Half	1 ea	79	80	58	<1	15	1[1]	<1	t	t	t
292	Juice pack:	1 c	248	86	124	1	32	4[1]	<1	t	t	t
293	Half	1 ea	77	86	38	<1	10	1[1]	<1	t	t	t

[1]Dietary fiber data vary 2.4 to 3.4 g/100 g for fresh pears; 1.6 to 2.6 g/100 g for canned pears.

(Computer code number is for West Diet Analysis program)

TABLE OF FOOD COMPOSITION
◆ H–23

PAGE KEY: H–4 = BEV   H–6 = DAIRY   H–12 = EGGS   H–14 = FAT/OIL   H–18 = FRUIT   H–26 = BAKERY   H–36 = GRAIN   H–44 = FISH   H–48 = MEATS   H–50 = POULTRY   H–54 = SAUSAGE   H–56 = MIXED/FAST   H–64 = NUTS/SEEDS   H–68 = SWEETS   H–70 = VEG/LEG   H–84 = MISC   H–88 = SOUPS/SAUCES   H–90 = FAST   H–106 = FRZN ENTREE   H–112 = BABY FOODS

Chol (mg)	Calc (mg)	Iron (mg)	Magn (mg)	Pota (mg)	Sodi (mg)	Zinc (mg)	VT-A (RE)	Thia (mg)	VT-E (α-TE)	Ribo (mg)	Niac (mg)	V-B6 (mg)	Fola (μg)	VT-C (mg)
0	29	.56	29	825	24	.43	860	.1	.4	.06	1.53	.31	45	113
0	8	.09	9	350	13	.1	5	.1	.19	.02	.77	.08	8	32
0	7	.2	11	288	0	.12	101	.02	1.21	.06	1.35	.03	5	7
0	52	.13	13	237	0	.09	28	.11	.31	.05	.37	.08	40	70
0	72	.18	18	326	0	.13	38	.16	.43	.07	.51	.11	54	96
0	27	.5	27	496	2	.12	50	.22	.22	.07	.99	.1	75	124
0	20	1.1	27	436	5	.17	45	.15	.22	.07	.78	.22	45	86
0	25	.42	27	473	3	.1	20[2]	.19	.47	.28	.05	.7	45[2]	82[2]
0	68	.75	72	1435	6	.38	60	.6	.68	.14	1.53	.33	330	294
0	22	.25	25	473	3	.12	20	.2	.47	.04	.5	.11	109	97
0	62	.2	2	50	12	.1	551	<.01	0	.04	0	0	143	121
0	20	1.14	25	390	7	.17	30	.14	.17	.07	.83	.06	35	72
0	34	.14	14	360	4	.1	39	.04	1.6	.04	.47	.03	53	86
0	73	.3	30	781	9	.21	85	.08	3.4	.1	1.03	.06	115	187
0	25	.85	8	78	13	.38	28	.01	.05	.01	.38	.02	5	8
0	4	.1	6	171	0	.12	47	.01	.61	.04	.86	.02	3	6
0	8	.19	12	335	0	.24	92	.03	1.2	.07	1.68	.03	6	11
0	8	.69	13	235	15	.23	84	.03	2.28	.06	1.57	.05	8	7
0	2	.22	4	74	5	.07	27	.01	.72	.02	.5	.01	3	2
0	15	.67	17	317	10	.27	94	.02	3.72	.04	1.44	.05	8	9
0	5	.21	5	99	3	.08	29	.01	1.2	.01	.45	.01	3	3
0	36	5.28	55	1293	9	.74	281	<.01	0	.28	5.69	.09	<1	6
0	23	3.38	33	825	5	.46	52	.01	0	.05	3.92	.1	<1	10
0	9	1.05	14	369	17	.14	80	.04	2.53	.1	1.85	.05	9	267[3]
0	8	.92	12	325	15	.12	70	.03	2.23	.09	1.63	.04	8	236[3]
0	12	.47	10	100	17	.2	65	.01	.2	.03	.72	.02	3	13
0	18	.41	10	208	0	.2	3	.03	.83	.07	.17	.03	12	7
0	16	.35	8	176	0	.17	3	.03	.71	.06	.14	.02	10	6
0	22	.5	12	250	0	.24	4	.04	1	.08	.2	.04	15	8
0	13	.56	10	165	13	.2	0	.03	1.28	.06	.62	.04	3	3
0	4	.17	3	51	4	.06	0	.01	.4	.02	.19	.01	1	1
0	22	.72	17	238	10	.22	2	.03	1.24	.03	.5	.03	3	4
0	7	.22	5	74	3	.07	1	.01	.39	.01	.15	.01	1	1

[2]Values for juice from California oranges indicate the following values for 1 c: 36 RE of vitamin A, 72 μg of folate, and 106 mg of vitamin C.

[3]With added vitamin C (ascorbic acid).

(For purposes of calculations, use "0" for t, <1, <.1, <.01, etc.)

Table H–1
Food Composition

Computer Code Number	Food Description	Measure	Wt (g)	H₂O (%)	Ener (kcal)	Prot (g)	Carb (g)	Dietary Fiber (g)	Fat (g)	Fat Breakdown (g) Sat	Mono	Poly	
	FRUITS and FRUIT JUICES—Cont.												
294	Dried halves	10 ea	175	27	459	3	121	13	1	.1	.2	.3	
1033	Pear nectar, canned	1 c	250	84	150	<1	40	2	<1	t	t	t	
	Pineapple:												
295	Fresh chunks, diced	1 c	155	87	76	1	19	2	1	t	.1	.2	
	Canned, fruit and liquid:												
	Heavy syrup pack:												
296	Crushed, chunks, tidbits	⅓ c	84	79	65	<1	17	1	<1	t	t	t	
297	Slices	1 ea	58	79	45	<1	12	<1	<1	t	t	t	
298	Juice pack, crushed, chunks, tidbits	1 c	250	84	150	1	39	2	<1	t	t	.1	
299	Juice pack, slices	1 ea	58	84	35	<1	9	<1	<1	t	t	t	
300	Pineapple juice, canned, unsweetened	1 c	250	86	140	1	35	<1	<1	t	t	.1	
	Plantains, without peel:												
301	Raw slices (whole = 179 g w/o peel)	1 c	148	65	181	2	47	3¹	1	.2	t	.1	
302	Cooked, boiled, sliced	1 c	154	67	179	1	48	4	<1	.1	t	.1	
	Plums:												
303	Fresh, medium, 2⅛" diam	1 ea	66	85	36	1	9	1	<1	t	.3	.1	
304	Fresh, small, 1½" diam	1 ea	28	85	15	<1	4	<1	<1	t	.1	t	
	Canned, purple, with liquid:												
305	Heavy syrup pack:	1 c	258	76	229	1	60	3	<1	t	.2	.1	
306	Plums	3 ea	110	76	98	<1	26	1	<1	t	.1	t	
307	Juice pack:	1 c	252	84	146	1	38	3	<1	t	t	t	
308	Plums	3 ea	95	84	55	<1	14	1	<1	t	t	t	
1698	Pomegranate, fresh	1 ea	154	81	105	1	27	1	<1	.1	.1	.1	
	Prunes, dried, pitted:												
309	Uncooked (10 = 97 g w/pits, 84 g w/o pits)	10 ea	84	32	200	2	53	6²	<1	t	.3	.1	
310	Cooked, unsweetened, fruit & liq (250 g w/pits)	1c	212	70	227	2	60	14	<1	t	.3	.1	
311	Prune juice, bottled or canned	1c	256	81	182	2	45	3	1	t	.5	t	
	Raisins, seedless:												
312	Cup, not pressed down	1 c	145	15	435	5	115	5	1	.2	t	.2	
313	One packet, ½ oz	½ oz	14	15	42	<1	11	1	<1	t	t	t	
	Raspberries:												
314	Fresh	1 c	123	87	60	1	14	8	1	t	.1	.4	
315	Frozen, sweetened:	10 oz	284	73	293	2	74	13	<1	t	t	.3	
316	Cup, thawed measure	1 c	250	73	258	2	66	11	<1	t	t	.2	
317	Rhubarb, cooked, added sugar	1 c	240	68	278	1	75	5	<1	t	t	.1	
	Strawberries:												
318	Fresh, whole, capped	1 c	149	92	45	1	10	3	1	t	.1	.3	
	Frozen, sliced, sweetened:												
319	10-oz container	10 oz	284	73	272	2	74	5	<1	t	.1	.2	
320	Cup, thawed measure	1 c	255	73	244	1	66	5	<1	t	t	.2	
	Tangerines, without peel and seeds:												
321	Fresh (2⅜" whole) 116 g w/refuse	1 ea	84	88	37	1	9	2	<1	t	t	t	
322	Canned, light syrup, fruit and liquid	1 c	252	83	153	1	41	2	<1	t	t	t	
323	Tangerine juice, canned, sweetened	1 c	249	87	124	1	30	<1	<1	t	t	.1	

[1]Dietary fiber value partially derived from data for bananas.

[2]Dietary fiber data can vary between 6 and 13 g for 10 prunes.

(Computer code number is for West Diet Analysis program)

H

Chol (mg)	Calc (mg)	Iron (mg)	Magn (mg)	Pota (mg)	Sodi (mg)	Zinc (mg)	VT-A (RE)	Thia (mg)	VT-E (α-TE)	Ribo (mg)	Niac (mg)	V-B6 (mg)	Fola (μg)	VT-C (mg)
0	59	3.68	58	933	10	.68	1	.01	0	.25	2.4	.13	0	12
0	13	.65	8	33	10	.18	<1	<.01	.25	.03	.32	.04	3	3
0	11	.57	22	175	2	.12	3	.14	.16	.06	.65	.13	16	24
0	12	.32	13	87	1	.1	1	.08	.08	.02	.24	.06	4	6
0	8	.22	9	60	1	.07	1	.05	.06	.01	.17	.04	3	4
0	35	.7	35	305	3	.25	10	.24	.25	.05	.71	.18	12	24
0	8	.16	8	71	1	.06	3	.05	.06	.01	.16	.04	3	6
0	42	.65	32	335	3	.27	1	.14	.05	.05	.64	.24	58	27[3]
0	4	.89	55	739	6	.21	167[4]	.08	.4	.08	1.02	.44	33	27
0	3	.89	49	716	8	.2	140	.07	.22	.08	1.16	.37	40	17
0	3	.07	5	113	0	.07	21	.03	.4	.06	.33	.05	1	6
0	1	.03	2	48	0	.03	9	.01	.17	.03	.14	.02	1	3
0	23	2.17	13	234	49	.18	67	.04	1.81	.1	.75	.07	6	1
0	10	.92	5	100	21	.08	29	.02	.77	.04	.32	.03	3	<1
0	25	.86	20	388	3	.28	255	.06	1.76	.15	1.19	.07	7	7
0	10	.32	8	146	1	.1	96	.02	.67	.06	.45	.03	2	3
0	5	.46	5	399	5	.18	0	.05	.85	.05	.46	.16	9	9
0	43	2.08	38	625	3	.44	167	.07	1.22	.14	1.65	.22	3	3
0	49	2.35	42	708	4	.51	66	.05	<.01	.21	1.53	.46	<1	6
0	31	3	36	707	10	.54	1	.04	.03	.18	2	.56	1	11
0	71	3.02	48	1088	17	.39	1	.23	1.02	.13	1.19	.36	5	5
0	7	.29	5	105	2	.04	<1	.02	.1	.01	.11	.03	<1	<1
0	27	.7	22	186	0	.57	16	.04	.55	.11	1.11	.07	32	31
0	43	1.85	37	324	3	.51	17	.05	1.28	.13	.65	.1	74	47
0	37	1.63	32	285	3	.45	15	.05	1.13	.11	.57	.08	65	41
0	348	.5	29	230	2	.19	17	.04	.48	.05	.48	.05	13	8
0	21	.57	15	247	1	.19	4	.03	.21	.1	.34	.09	26	84
0	31	1.68	20	278	9	.17	6	.04	.4	.14	1.14	.08	42	117
0	28	1.51	18	250	8	.15	5	.04	.4	.13	1.02	.08	38	105
0	12	.08	10	132	1	.2	77	.09	.2	.02	.13	.06	17	26
0	18	.93	20	196	15	.6	212	.13	.9	.11	1.12	.11	12	50
0	45	.5	20	443	3	.07	105	.15	.22	.05	.25	.08	11	55

[3]If vitamin C is added, it contains 96 mg per cup.

[4]Vitamin A values range from 1.5 RE for white-fleshed varieties to 178 RE for yellow-fleshed varieties.

(For purposes of calculations, use "0" for t, <1, <.1, <.01, etc.)

Table H–1
Food Composition

Computer Code Number	Food Description	Measure	Wt (g)	H₂O (%)	Ener (kcal)	Prot (g)	Carb (g)	Dietary Fiber (g)	Fat (g)	Fat Breakdown (g) Sat	Mono	Poly
	FRUITS and FRUIT JUICES—Cont.											
	Watermelon, raw, without rind & seeds:											
324	Piece, 1" by 10" diam (2 lb w/refuse or 926 g)	1 pce	482	91	154	3	35	1	2	.2	.5	.1
325	Diced	1 c	160	91	51	1	11	1	1	.1	.2	.2
	BAKED GOODS: BREADS, CAKES, COOKIES, CRACKERS, PIES											
326	Bagels, plain, enriched, 3½" diam	1 ea	68	33	187	7	36	2	1	.1	.1	.5
1663	Bagel, oat bran	1 ea	71	33	181	8	38	3	1	.1	.2	.3
	Biscuits:											
327	From home recipe	1 ea	28	29	100	2	13	<1	5	1.2	2	1.2
328	From mix	1 ea	28	29	95	2	14	1	3	.8	1.2	1.2
329	From refrigerated dough	1 ea	20	27	75	1	9	<1	4	2	1	.1
330	Bread crumbs, dry, grated (see #364, 365 for soft crumbs)	1 c	100	6	395	13	73	2	5	1.3	2.1	1.6
2087	Bread sticks, brown & serve	1 ea	57	34	150	7	28	1	2	.5	.5	.5
	Breads:											
331	Boston brown, canned, 3¼" slice	1 pce	45	47	88	2	19	2	1	.1	.1	.3
332	Cracked wheat (¼ cracked-wheat & ¾ enr wheat flour): 1-lb loaf	1 ea	454	36	1180	39	225	25	18	4.2	8.6	3.1
333	Slice (18 per loaf)	1 pce	25	36	65	2	12	1	1	.2	.5	.2
334	Slice, toasted	1 pce	21	30	59	2	11	1	1	.2	.4	.2
335	French/Vienna, enriched: 1-lb loaf	1 ea	454	34	1243	40	236	14	14	2.9	5.5	3.1
337	Slice, 4¾ x 4 x ½"	1 pce	25	34	68	2	13	1	1	.2	.3	.2
336	French, slice, 5 x 2½"	1 pce	35	34	96	3	18	1	1	.2	.4	.2
	French toast: see Mixed Dishes, and Fast Foods, #691											
2083	Honey Wheatberry	1 pce	39	3	100	3	18	2	2	0	.5	0
338	Italian, enriched: 1-lb loaf	1 ea	454	36	1230	40	227	12	16	3.9	3.7	6.3
339	Slice, 4½ x 3¼ x ¾"	1 pce	30	36	81	3	15	1	1	.3	.2	.4
340	Mixed grain, enriched: 1-lb loaf	1 ea	454	38	1135	45	211	29	17	3.7	6.9	4.2
341	Slice (18 per loaf)	1 pce	25	38	62	3	12	2	1	.2	.4	.2
342	Slice, toasted	1 pce	23	32	63	3	12	2	1	.2	.4	.2
343	Oatmeal, enriched: 1-lb loaf	1 ea	454	37	1221	38	220	18	20	3.2	7.2	7.7
344	Slice (18 per loaf)	1 pce	25	37	67	2	12	1	1	.2	.4	.4
345	Slice, toasted	1 pce	23	31	67	2	12	1	1	.2	.4	.4
346	Pita pocket bread, enr, 6½" round	1 ea	60	32	165	5	33	1	1	.1	.1	.3
347	Pumpernickel (⅔ rye & ⅓ enr wheat flour): 1-lb loaf	1 ea	454	38	1135	40	216	30	14	2	4.2	5.6
348	Slice, 5 x 4 x ⅜"	1 pce	32	38	80	3	15	2	1	.1	.3	.4
349	Slice, toasted	1 pce	29	32	80	3	15	2	1	.1	.3	.4
350	Raisin, enriched: 1-lb loaf	1 ea	454	34	1244	36	237	20	20	4.9	10.5	3.1
351	Slice (18 per loaf)	1 pce	25	34	68	2	13	1	1	.3	.6	.2
352	Slice, toasted	1 pce	21	28	62	2	12	1	1	.2	.5	.2
353	Rye, light (⅓ rye & ⅔ enr wheat flour): 1-lb loaf	1 ea	454	37	1177	39	219	26	15	2.9	6	3.6
354	Slice, 4¾ x 3¾ x 7⁄16"	1 pce	25	37	65	2	12	1	1	.2	.3	.2
355	Slice, toasted	1 pce	22	31	62	2	12	1	1	.2	.3	.2

PAGE KEY: H–4 = BEV   H–6 = DAIRY   H–12 = EGGS   H–14 = FAT/OIL   H–18 = FRUIT   H–26 = BAKERY   H–36 = GRAIN   H–44 = FISH
H–48 = MEATS   H–50 = POULTRY   H–54 = SAUSAGE   H–56 = MIXED/FAST   H–64 = NUTS/SEEDS   H–68 = SWEETS   H–70 = VEG/LEG
H–84 = MISC   H–88 = SOUPS/SAUCES   H–90 = FAST   H–106 = FRZN ENTREE   H–112 = BABY FOODS

Chol (mg)	Calc (mg)	Iron (mg)	Magn (mg)	Pota (mg)	Sodi (mg)	Zinc (mg)	VT-A (RE)	Thia (mg)	VT-E (α-TE)	Ribo (mg)	Niac (mg)	V-B6 (mg)	Fola (μg)	VT-C (mg)
0	39	.82	53	559	10	.34	178	.39	.72	.1	.96	.69	11	46
0	13	.27	18	186	3	.11	59	.13	.24	.03	.32	.23	4	15
0	50	2.42	20	69	363	.6	0	.37	.02	.21	3.1	.03	15	0
0	9	2.2	40	145	360	1.48	<1	.24	.17	.24	2.1	.14	33	<1
1	67	.82	5	34	165	.15	6	.1	.67	.09	.84	.01	3	<1
1	53	.58	7	53	271	.17	7	.1	.11	.1	.86	.02	2	<1
1	24	.44	2	23	158	.08	7	.07	.12	.05	.44	.01	2	0
0	227	6.12	46	221	862	1.22	<1	.76	.88	.43	6.85	.1	25	0
0	60	2.7	–	–	290	–	0	.225	–	.102	1.6	–	–	0
<1	31	.95	28	143	284	.22	5	.01	.13	.05	.5	.04	3	0
0	195	12.8	236	804	2442	5.62	0	1.63	2.6	1.09	16.7	1.38	177	0
0	11	.7	13	44	135	.31	0	.09	.14	.06	.92	.08	10	0
0	10	.64	12	40	123	.28	0	.07	.13	.05	.75	.06	6	0
0	341	11.5	123	513	2766	3.95	0	2.36	1.07	1.49	21.6	.19	141	0
0	19	.63	7	28	152	.22	0	.13	.06	.08	1.19	.01	8	0
0	26	.89	9	40	213	.3	0	.18	.08	.11	1.66	.01	11	0
0	20	.72	–	–	200	–	0	.12	.24	.07	.8	–	–	0
0	354	13.3	123	499	2651	3.9	0	2.15	1.26	1.33	19.9	.22	136	0
0	23	.88	8	33	175	.26	0	.14	.08	.09	1.31	.01	9	0
0	413	15.8	241	926	2210	5.76	0	1.85	2.79	1.55	19.8	1.51	218	1
0	23	.87	13	51	122	.32	0	.1	.15	.09	1.09	.08	12	<1
0	23	.87	13	51	122	.32	0	.08	.15	.08	.98	.07	9	<1
0	300	12.3	168	645	2724	4.63	9	1.81	1.56	1.09	14.3	.31	123	2
0	17	.68	9	36	150	.26	<1	.1	.09	.06	.78	.02	7	<1
0	17	.68	9	35	150	.26	<1	.08	.09	.05	.71	.01	5	<1
0	52	1.57	16	72	322	.5	0	.36	.02	.2	2.78	.02	14	0
0	309	13	245	944	3046	6.72	0	1.48	2.3	1.38	14	.57	155	0
0	22	.92	17	67	215	.47	0	.1	.16	.1	.99	.04	11	0
0	22	.91	17	66	214	.47	0	.08	.17	.09	.89	.04	8	0
0	300	13.2	118	1030	1770	3.27	<1	1.54	3.44	1.81	15.8	.31	154	2
0	17	.73	7	57	98	.18	0	.08	.19	.1	.87	.02	9	<1
0	15	.66	6	52	89	.16	<1	.06	.173	.08	.71	.01	5	<1
0	331	12.8	182	754	2996	5.17	2	1.97	2.51	1.52	17.3	.34	232	1
0	18	.71	10	42	165	.29	<1	.11	.14	.08	.95	.02	13	<1
0	18	.68	9	40	160	.28	0	.08	.13	.07	.83	.02	9	<1

H

(For purposes of calculations, use "0" for t, <1, <.1, <.01, etc.)

Table H–1
Food Composition

Computer Code Number	Food Description	Measure	Wt (g)	H₂O (%)	Ener (kcal)	Prot (g)	Carb (g)	Dietary Fiber (g)	Fat (g)	Fat Breakdown (g)		
										Sat	Mono	Poly
	BAKED GOODS: BREADS, CAKES, COOKIES, CRACKERS, PIES—Cont.											
356	Wheat (enr wheat & whole-wheat flour):[1] 1-lb loaf	1 ea	454	37	1160	43	213	25	19	3.9	7.3	4.5
357	Slice (18 per loaf)	1 pce	25	37	64	2	12	1	1	.2	.4	.2
358	Slice, toasted	1 pce	23	32	65	2	12	1	1	.2	.4	.2
359	White, enriched: 1-lb loaf	1 ea	454	37	1210	38	222	12	18	5.6	6.5	4.2
360	Slice (18 per loaf)	1 pce	25	37	67	2	12	1	1	.3	.4	.2
361	Slice, toasted	1 pce	22	30	69	2	13	1	1	.2	.3	.1
362	Slice (22 per loaf)	1 pce	20	37	53	2	10	1	1	.2	.3	.2
363	Slice, toasted	1 pce	17	24	53	2	10	<1	1	.2	.2	.1
364	White bread cubes, soft	1 c	30	36	81	3	15	1	1	.4	.5	.2
365	White bread crumbs, soft	1 c	45	36	121	4	23	1	2	.6	.8	.4
366	Whole-wheat: 1-lb loaf	1 ea	454	38	1116	44	209	31	19	4.2	7.6	4.6
367	Slice (16 per loaf)	1 pce	28	38	69	3	13	2	1	.3	.5	.3
368	Slice, toasted	1 pce	25	30	69	3	13	2	1	.3	.5	.3
	Bread stuffing, prepared from mix:											
369	Dry type	1 c	140	65	249	5	30	4	12	2.4	5.3	3.6
370	Moist type, with egg and margarine	1 c	203	65	341	8	45	4	15	3	6.5	4.3
	Cakes, prepared from mixes:[1]											
	Angel food:											
371	Whole cake, 9¾" diam tube	1 ea	635	33	1638	38	367	10	5	.8	.5	2.3
372	Piece, ½ of cake	1 pce	53	33	137	3	31	1	<1	.1	t	.2
373	Boston cream pie, ⅛ of cake	1 pce	120	45	302	3	52	2	10	3	5.3	1.2
	Coffee cake:											
374	Whole cake, 7¾ x 5⅛ x 1¼"	1 ea	430	31	1367	24	227	5	41	8	16.7	13.6
375	Piece, ⅙ of cake	1 pce	72	31	229	4	38	1	7	1.3	2.8	2.3
	Devil's food, chocolate frosting:											
376	Whole cake, 2 layer, 8 or 9" diam	1 ea	1107	23	4062	45	604	31	182	52	99.6	21.1
377	Piece, 1/16 of cake	1 pce	69	23	253	3	38	2	11	3.2	6.2	1.3
378	Cupcake, 2½" diam	1 ea	42	23	154	2	23	1	7	2	3.8	.8
	Gingerbread:											
379	Whole cake, 8" square	1 ea	570	33	1764	23	289	7	58	14.9	32	7.6
380	Piece, ⅛ of cake	1 pce	63	33	195	3	32	1	6	1.6	3.5	.8
	Yellow, chocolate frosting, 2 layer:											
381	Whole cake, 8 or 9" diam	1 ea	1108	22	4199	42	613	20	193	53	107	23.2
382	Piece, 1/16 of cake	1 pce	69	22	262	3	38	1	12	3.3	6.7	1.4
	Cakes from recipes w/enr flour:											
	Carrot cake, cream cheese frosting:[2]											
383	Whole, 9 x 13" cake	1 ea	1536	21	6696	71	725	18	406	75.1	100	209
384	Piece, 1/16 of cake, 2¼ x 3¼" slice	1 pce	112	21	488	5	53	1	30	5.5	7.3	15.2
	Fruitcake, dark:											
386	Piece, 1/32 of cake, ⅔" arc	1 pce	43	25	139	1	26	2	4	.5	1.8	1.4
	Sheet, plain, no frosting:[3]											
387	Whole cake, 9" square	1 ea	777	23	2828	35	434	3	108	30	51.8	25.6
388	Piece, ⅛ of cake	1 pce	86	23	313	4	48	<1	12	3.3	5.7	2.8

[1] Excepting angel food cake, cakes were made from mixes containing vegetable shortening, and frostings were made with margarine. All mixes use enriched flour.

[2] Made with vegetable oil.

[3] Cake made with vegetable shortening.

(Computer code number is for West Diet Analysis program)

PAGE KEY: H–4 = BEV   H–6 = DAIRY   H–12 = EGGS   H–14 = FAT/OIL   H–18 = FRUIT   H–26 = BAKERY   H–36 = GRAIN   H–44 = FISH
H–48 = MEATS   H–50 = POULTRY   H–54 = SAUSAGE   H–56 = MIXED/FAST   H–64 = NUTS/SEEDS   H–68 = SWEETS   H–70 = VEG/LEG
H–84 = MISC   H–88 = SOUPS/SAUCES   H–90 = FAST   H–106 = FRZN ENTREE   H–112 = BABY FOODS

Chol (mg)	Calc (mg)	Iron (mg)	Magn (mg)	Pota (mg)	Sodi (mg)	Zinc (mg)	VT-A (RE)	Thia (mg)	VT-E (α-TE)	Ribo (mg)	Niac (mg)	V-B6 (mg)	Fola (μg)	VT-C (mg)
0	572	15.8	209	627	2447	4.77	0	2	3	1.45	20.5	.5	204	0
0	32	.87	12	50	135	.26	0	.11	.17	.08	1.13	.03	11	0
0	26	.83	12	50	132	.26	0	.08	.14	.06	.93	.02	7	0
5	572	12.9	95	508	2334	2.81	0	2.13	1.3	1.4	17	.15	159	
<1	32	.71	5	28	129	.15	0	.12	.07	.09	.99	.01	9	0
<1	22	.73	5	28	130	.16	0	.08	.04	.06	.84	.01	9	0
<1	25	.57	4	22	103	.12	0	.09	.06	.06	.75	.01	7	0
<1	17	.56	4	21	101	.12	0	.06	.03	.05	.67	.01	7	0
<1	25	.84	6	32	151	.19	0	.12	.05	.1	1	.01	10	0
1	38	1.3	9	48	227	.28	0	.18	.08	.11	1.5	.15	16	0
0	327	15	390	1144	2382	8.8	0	1.59	4.72	.93	17.4	.81	227	0
0	20	.94	24	72	150	.55	0	.1	.29	.06	1.09	.05	14	0
0	20	.93	24	71	148	.55	0	.08	.23	.05	.97	.05	10	0
0	45	1.53	17	104	760	.39	113	.19	1.96	.15	2.07	.06	24	0
0	130	3.33	30	266	936	.65	140	.34	2.44	.29	3.23	.11	35	3
0	889	3.3	76	591	4756	.44	0	.65	.64	3.12	5.61	.2	19	0
0	74	.28	6	49	397	.04	0	.05	.05	.26	.47	.02	2	0
44	28	.46	7	47	173	.19	28	.49	1.27	.32	.23	.03	10	<1
211	585	6.15	77	482	1810	1.94	172	.72	7.14	.75	6.54	.21	52	1
35	98	1.03	13	81	303	.32	29	.12	1.2	.13	1.09	.04	9	<1
509	476	24.3	376	2214	3697	7.64	310	.3	18.7	1.47	6.39	.34	89	1
32	30	1.52	23	138	231	.48	19	.02	1.7	.09	.4	.02	6	<1
19	18	.93	14	84	140	.29	12	.01	.71	.06	.24	.01	3	<1
200	393	18.9	91	1373	2615	2.34	91	1.08	7.81	1.06	8.89	.22	57	1
22	43	2.09	10	152	289	.26	10	.12	.73	.12	.98	.02	6	<1
609	410	23.1	332	1972	3733	6.87	299	1.33	29.9	1.74	13.9	.32	89	1
38	25	1.44	21	123	233	.43	19	.08	1.86	.11	.86	.02	6	<1
829	384	19.2	276	1720	3778	7.53	5898	2.09	64.8	2.4	15.5	1.17	184	17
60	28	1.4	20	125	276	.55	480	.15	4.73	.17	1.13	.08	13	1
2	14	.89	7	66	116	.12	8	.02	1.34	.04	.34	.02	1	<1
505	497	11.7	108	613	2331	2.75	373	1.24	11.03	1.4	10.1	.26	54	2
56	55	1.3	12	68	258	.3	41	.14	1.22	.15	1.12	.03	6	<1

(For purposes of calculations, use "0" for t, <1, <.1, <.01, etc.)

Table H–1
Food Composition

Computer Code Number	Food Description	Measure	Wt (g)	H_2O (%)	Ener (kcal)	Prot (g)	Carb (g)	Dietary Fiber (g)	Fat (g)	Fat Breakdown (g) Sat	Mono	Poly
	BAKED GOODS: BREADS, CAKES, COOKIES, CRACKERS, PIES—Cont.											
	Sheet, plain, uncooked white frosting:[1]											
389	Whole cake, 9" square	1 ea	1096	22	4088	39	644	4	159	26.2	67.5	56.1
390	Piece, ⅛ of cake	1 pce	121	22	451	4	71	<1	18	2.9	7.4	6.2
	Cakes, commercial:											
	Cheesecake:											
401	Whole cake, 9" diam	1 ea	1110	46	3540	61	283	5	250	128	86	15.3
402	Piece, 1/12 of cake	1 pce	92	46	295	5	23	<1	21	10.6	7.1	1.3
	Pound cake:											
393	Loaf, 8½ x 3½ x 3"	1 ea	500	25	1948	27	244	2	99	56	27.9	5.4
394	Slice, 1/17 of loaf, 2" slice	1 pce	29	25	113	2	14	<1	6	3.2	1.6	.3
	Snack: 2 small cakes per package											
395	Chocolate w/creme filling (Ding Dong)	1 ea	28	20	107	1	17	<1	4	1.8	1.6	.4
396	Sponge w/creme filling (Twinkie)	1 ea	42	20	153	1	27	<1	5	1.1	1.9	1.5
1677	Sponge cake, 1/12 of 12" cake	1 pce	38	30	110	2	23	<1	1	.3	.4	.2
1678	Strawberry shortcake, fresh	1 ea	254	74	327	5	40	4	17	10.1	4.9	1
	White, white frosting, 2 layer:											
397	Whole cake, 8 or 9" diam	1 ea	1140	20	4272	38	718	11	154	68.4	60	15.5
398	Piece, 1/16 of cake	1 pce	71	20	266	2	45	1	10	4.3	3.8	1
	Yellow, chocolate frosting, 2 layer:											
399	Whole cake, 8 or 9" diam	1 ea	1108	22	4196	42	614	20	193	53	107	23.2
400	Piece, 1/16 of cake	1 pce	69	22	262	3	38	1	12	3.3	6.7	1.4
1332	Bagel chips	5 pce	70	3	298	6	52	6	7	1.3	2.1	3.4
2225	Bagel chips, onion garlic, toasted	½ oz	14	–	55	2	9	1	2	.5	1.5	0
1035	Cheese puffs/Cheetos	1 oz	28	2	155	2	15	<1	10	1.9	5.7	1.3
	Cookies made with enriched flour:											
	Brownies with nuts:											
403	Commercial w/frosting, 1½ x 1¾ x ⅞"	1 ea	25	14	101	1	16	1	4	1.1	2.1	.6
404	Home recipe, 1¾ x 1¾ x ⅞"[2]	1 ea	20	13	93	1	10	<1	6	1.5	2.2	1.9
1902	Fat free fudge, Entenmann's	1 pce	40	24	110	2	27	1	0	0	0	0
	Chocolate chip:											
405	Commercial, 2¼" diam	4 ea	42	12	192	2	25	1	10	3.1	5.5	1.1
406	Home recipe, 2¼" diam	4 ea	40	6	195	2	23	1	11	3.2	4.2	3.4
407	From refrigerated dough, 2¼" diam	4 ea	48	13	213	2	29	1	10	3.3	4.9	1
408	Fig bars	4 ea	56	16	195	2	40	3	4	.7	2.2	.7
2052	Fruit bar, no fat	1 ea	28	–	90	2	21	0	0	0	0	0
2162	Fudge, fat free, Snackwell	1 ea	16	14	53	1	12	<1	<1	.1	.1	<.1
409	Oatmeal raisin, 2⅝" diam	4 ea	52	6	226	3	36	2	8	1.7	3.6	2.6
410	Peanut butter, home recipe, 2⅝" diam[3]	4 ea	48	6	228	4	28	1	11	2.1	5.2	3.5
411	Sandwich-type, all	4 ea	40	2	189	2	28	1	8	1.7	4.7	1.1
412	Shortbread, commercial, small	4 ea	32	4	161	2	21	1	8	2	4.3	1
413	Shortbread, home recipe, large[4]	2 ea	28	3	155	2	16	<1	9	5.8	2.7	.4

(1)Made with margarine.
(2)Made with vegetable oil.
(3)Made with vegetable shortening.
(4)Made with butter.

(Computer code number is for West Diet Analysis program)

TABLE OF FOOD COMPOSITION ◆ **H–31**

PAGE KEY: H–4 = BEV   H–6 = DAIRY   H–12 = EGGS   H–14 = FAT/OIL   H–18 = FRUIT   H–26 = BAKERY   H–36 = GRAIN   H–44 = FISH   H–48 = MEATS   H–50 = POULTRY   H–54 = SAUSAGE   H–56 = MIXED/FAST   H–64 = NUTS/SEEDS   H–68 = SWEETS   H–70 = VEG/LEG   H–84 = MISC   H–88 = SOUPS/SAUCES   H–90 = FAST   H–106 = FRZN ENTREE   H–112 = BABY FOODS

Chol (mg)	Calc (mg)	Iron (mg)	Magn (mg)	Pota (mg)	Sodi (mg)	Zinc (mg)	VT-A (RE)	Thia (mg)	VT-E (α-TE)	Ribo (mg)	Niac (mg)	V-B6 (mg)	Fola (µg)	VT-C (mg)
614	680	11.7	66	581	3770	2.74	208	1.1	20.8	.77	5.48	.38	99	2
68	75	1.31	7	64	416	.3	23	.12	2.3	.08	.6	.04	11	<1
611	566	6.99	122	999	2297	5.66	1787	.31	11.7	2.14	2.16	.58	167	7
51	47	.58	10	83	190	.47	148	.03	.97	.18	.18	.05	14	1
1105	175	6.9	55	595	1983	2.3	779	.68	3.29	1.15	6.55	.17	55	1
64	10	.4	3	34	115	.13	45	.04	.19	.07	.38	.01	3	<1
5	21	.95	12	35	121	.16	1	.06	.56	.08	.69	.01	2	<1
7	19	.54	3	38	153	.13	2	.06	.82	.06	.51	.01	2	<1
39	27	1	4	38	93	.19	18	.09	.17	.1	.73	.02	5	0
53	209	2.33	29	359	510	.57	172	.29	.73	.33	2.26	.13	40	95
91	547	9.12	60	661	2668	1.77	369	1.14	20.5	1.48	10.3	.16	64	1
6	34	.57	4	41	166	.11	23	.07	1.28	.09	.64	.01	4	<1
609	410	23	332	1972	3734	6.87	299	1.33	29.9	1.74	13.9	.32	89	1
38	25	1.44	21	123	233	.43	19	.08	1.86	.11	.86	.02	6	<1
0	9	1.38	41	167	419	.9	0	.1	.47	.12	1.57	.19	58	0
0	0	.72	–	–	140	–	0	.11	<.01	.07	1	–	–	0
1	16	.66	5	47	294	.11	10	.07	1.43	.1	.9	.04	34	<1
4	7	.56	8	37	78	.18	5	.06	.53	.05	.43	.01	3	<1
15	11	.37	11	35	69	.19	40	.03	.58	.04	.2	.02	3	<1
0	0	1.08	–	90	140	–	0	–	.01	–	–	–	–	0
0	6	1.01	15	39	137	.19	<1	.05	1.22	.08	.68	.07	2	0
13	16	.98	22	90	144	.37	66	.07	1.16	.07	.54	.03	5	<1
11	12	1.08	11	86	100	.24	8	.09	.98	.09	.95	.02	4	0
0	36	1.62	15	116	196	.22	2	.09	.39	.12	1.05	.04	6	<1
0	0	.36	–	–	95	–	0	–	.01	–	–	–	–	0
0	3	.29	5	26	71	.08	–	.02	<.01	.02	.26	<.01	–	0
17	52	1.38	22	124	280	.45	85	.13	1.3	.09	.65	.04	6	<1
15	19	1.07	19	111	249	.39	75	.11	1.82	.1	1.68	.04	9	<1
0	10	1.56	18	70	242	.32	0	.03	1.21	.07	.83	.01	2	0
6	11	.88	5	32	146	.17	4	.11	.98	.1	1.07	.01	3	0
25	5	.74	4	20	132	.12	86	.1	.22	.07	.83	.01	3	0

(For purposes of calculations, use "0" for t, <1, <.1, <.01, etc.)

H

Table H–1
Food Composition

Computer Code Number	Food Description	Measure	Wt (g)	H$_2$O (%)	Ener (kcal)	Prot (g)	Carb (g)	Dietary Fiber (g)	Fat (g)	Fat Breakdown (g) Sat	Mono	Poly
	BAKED GOODS: BREADS, CAKES, COOKIES, CRACKERS, PIES—Cont.											
414	Sugar, from refrigerated dough, 2" diam	4 ea	48	5	232	2	31	<1	11	2.8	6.2	1.4
1874	Vanilla sandwich, Snackwell's	2 ea	26	4	109	1	21	1	2	.5	.8	.2
415	Vanilla wafers	10 ea	40	5	176	2	29	1	6	1.4	2.4	1.5
416	Corn chips	1 oz	28	1	153	2	16	1	9	1.3	2.7	4.7
	Crackers:[1]											
1034	Armenian cracker bread	4 pce	28	4	115	5	19	4	2	.4	.7	1
417	Cheese	10 ea	10	3	50	1	6	<1	3	.9	.9	.5
418	Cheese with peanut butter	4 ea	30	4	145	4	17	<1	7	1.5	3.6	1.3
	Fat Free:											
2161	Cracked pepper, Snackwell	1 ea	15	2	60	2	13	<1	<1	.1	<.1	.1
2159	Wheat, Snackwell	7 ea	15	1	60	2	12	1	<1	.1	.1	.1
2075	Whole wheat, herb seasoned	½ oz	14	5	50	2	11	2	0	0	0	0
2077	Whole wheat, onion	½ oz	14	5	50	2	11	2	0	0	0	0
419	Graham	2 ea	14	4	59	1	11	<1	1	.4	.7	.2
420	Melba toast, plain	1 pce	5	5	19	1	4	<1	<1	<.1	<.1	<.1
1514	Rice cakes, unsalted	2 ea	18	6	70	1	15	<1	1	.1	.2	.2
421	Rye wafer, whole grain	2 ea	14	5	47	1	11	3	<1	<.1	<.1	<.1
422	Saltine®[2]	4 ea	12	4	52	1	9	<1	1	.3	.8	.2
1971	Saltine®, Unsalted Tops	2 ea	6	–	25	1	4	0	1	0	0	0
423	Snack-type, round like Ritz	3 ea	9	3	45	1	5	<1	2	.4	1	.7
424	Wheat, thin	4 ea	8	3	35	1	5	1	1	.5	.5	.4
425	Whole-wheat wafers	2 ea	8	3	35	1	5	1	1	.2	.8	.2
426	Croissants, 4½ x 4 x 1¾"	1 ea	57	23	231	5	26	1	12	6.7	3.2	.7
1699	Croutons, seasoned	½ c	15	4	53	2	11	<1	0	0	0	0
	Danish pastry:											
427	Packaged ring, plain, 12 oz	1 ea	340	21	1349	19	181	1	65	13.5	40.9	6.4
428	Round piece, plain, 4¼" diam, 1" high	1 ea	57	21	226	3	30	<1	11	2.3	6.9	1.1
429	Ounce, plain	1 oz	28	21	111	2	15	<1	5	1.1	3.4	.5
430	Round piece with fruit	1 ea	65	29	231	3	31	–	11	2.3	7	1.1
	Desserts, 3 x 3" piece:											
1348	Apple crisp	1 pce	78	62	127	1	25	–	3	.6	1.2	.9
1353	Apple cobbler	1 pce	104	57	200	2	35	2	6	1.2	2.8	2
1349	Cherry crisp	1 pce	138	77	146	2	24	1	5	1	2.5	1.8
1352	Cherry cobbler	1 pce	129	66	198	2	34	1	6	1.2	2.8	1.9
1350	Peach crisp	1 pce	139	75	155	2	27	2	5	1	2.4	1.7
1351	Peach cobbler	1 pce	130	64	204	3	36	2	6	1.2	2.8	1.9
	Doughnuts:											
431	Cake type, plain, 3¼" diam	1 ea	50	21	211	3	25	1	11	1.9	4.8	4.1
432	Yeast-leavened, glazed, 3¾" diam	1 ea	60	25	242	4	27	1	14	3.5	7.7	1.7
	English muffins:											
433	Plain, enriched	1 ea	57	42	134	4	26	2	1	.2	.2	.5
434	Toasted	1 ea	50	37	128	4	25	1	1	.1	.2	.5
1504	Whole wheat	1 ea	50	46	102	4	20	3	1	.2	.3	.4
1414	Granola bar, soft	1 ea	42	6	187	3	29	2	7	3	1.6	2.2
1415	Granola bar, hard	1 ea	28	4	132	3	18	1	6	.7	1.2	3.4

[1]Crackers made with enriched white (wheat) flour except for rye wafers and whole-wheat wafers.

[2]Made with lard.

Chol (mg)	Calc (mg)	Iron (mg)	Magn (mg)	Pota (mg)	Sodi (mg)	Zinc (mg)	VT-A (RE)	Thia (mg)	VT-E (α-TE)	Ribo (mg)	Niac (mg)	V-B6 (mg)	Fola (µg)	VT-C (mg)
15	43	.88	4	78	225	.13	5	.09	1.54	.06	1.16	.01	3	0
<1	17	.61	5	28	95	.16	–	.05	–	.07	.69	.01	–	0
23	19	.95	6	39	125	.14	7	.11	.54	.13	1.24	.03	4	0
0	36	.37	21	40	179	.36	3	.01	.38	.04	.33	.07[3]	6	<1
0	21	.44	40	76	140	.89	1	.06	1.11	.04	1.04	.03	12	2
1	15	.48	4	15	100	.11	3	.06	.1	.04	.47	.05	3	0
2	24	.88	17	73	298	.33	11	.12	1.33	.1	1.96	.45	8	0
<1	26	.73	4	19	148	.14	–	.05	–	.06	.78	.01	–	<1
<1	28	.58	7	43	169	.21	–	.04	–	.07	.73	.02	–	0
0	–	.36	–	70	80	–	100	.06	–	–	.4	–	–	2
0	–	.36	–	70	80	–	500	.06	–	–	.4	–	–	2
0	3	.52	4	19	85	.11	0	.03	.27	.04	.58	.01	2	0
0	5	.19	3	10	41	.1	0	.02	.01	.01	.21	<.01	1	0
0	2	.27	24	52	5	.54	1	.01	.02	.03	1.4	.03	4	0
0	6	.83	17	69	111	.39	<1	.06	.28	.04	.22	.04	6	<1
0	14	.65	3	15	156	.09	0	.07	.2	.05	.63	<.01	4	0
0	–	.36	–	5	50	–	–	–	.1	–	–	–	–	–
0	11	.32	2	12	76	.06	2	.03	.4	.03	.36	<.01	1	0
1	3	.25	6	17	69	.24	0	.04	.3	.03	.4	.01	3	0
0	4	.25	8	24	53	.17	0	.02	.31	.01	.36	.01	2	0
43	21	1.16	9	67	424	.43	78	.22	.25	.14	1.25	.03	16	<1
<1	15	.81	6	20	195	.16	1	.07	.24	.11	.9	<.01	<1	0
105	143	6.94	54	371	1261	1.87	20	.99	3.06	.75	8.5	.2	54	10
18	24	1.16	9	62	211	.31	3	.16	.51	.12	1.43	.03	9	2
9	12	.57	4	31	104	.16	2	.08	.25	.06	.7	.02	4	1
13	15	.97	10	76	230	.33	17	.2	.59	.14	1.24	.04	10	1
0	22	.59	5	76	142	.12	24	.07	–	.06	.6	.03	4	2
1	22	.79	6	106	288	.16	76	.1	1.1	.09	.74	.04	3	<1
0	26	2.14	11	154	74	.16	150	.06	.93	.08	.59	.06	11	3
1	28	1.81	9	133	294	.2	135	.1	1.01	.11	.85	.05	9	2
0	20	.95	1	189	70	.2	108	.06	1.13	.05	1.06	.03	6	5
1	24	.91	10	159	291	.23	105	.09	1.16	.09	1.19	.03	6	3
18	22	.98	10	63	273	.27	9	.11	1.73	.12	.92	.03	4	<1
4	26	1.22	13	65	205	.46	6	.22	1.75	.13	1.71	.03	13	0
0	99	1.43	12	75	265	.4	0	.25	.07	.16	2.21	.02	21	<1
0	94	1.36	11	71	252	.38	0	.19	.06	.14	1.9	.02	15	<1
0	133	1.23	36	105	319	.8	0	.15	.35	.07	1.71	.08	25	0
<1	44	1.08	31	137	117	.63	0	.12	.51	.07	.22	.04	10	0
0	17	.83	27	94	82	.57	4	.07	.37	.03	.44	.02	6	<1

[3] Vitamin B$_6$ values vary between brands. Check the label.

(For purposes of calculations, use "0" for t, <1, <.1, <.01, etc.)

Table H–1
Food Composition

Computer Code Number	Food Description	Measure	Wt (g)	H$_2$O (%)	Ener (kcal)	Prot (g)	Carb (g)	Dietary Fiber (g)	Fat (g)	Fat Breakdown (g)		
										Sat	Mono	Poly
	BAKED GOODS: BREADS, CAKES, COOKIES, CRACKERS, PIES—Cont.												
	Granola bar, fat free:												
1985	Blueberry	1 ea	43	11	143	2	36	3	0	0	0	0
2012	Chocolate chip	1 ea	43	11	143	2	36	3	0	0	0	0
1983	Date almond	1 ea	43	11	143	2	36	3	0	0	0	0
1984	Raisin	1 ea	43	11	143	2	36	3	0	0	0	0
2011	Strawberry	1 ea	43	11	143	2	36	3	0	0	0	0
	Muffins, 2½" diam, 1½" high:												
	From home recipe												
435	Blueberry[1]	1 ea	45	39	131	3	18	1	5	1.1	1.2	2.4
436	Bran, wheat[2]	1 ea	45	35	130	3	19	3	6	1.2	1.4	2.8
437	Cornmeal	1 ea	45	32	144	3	20	2	6	1.2	1.4	2.8
	From commercial mix:												
438	Blueberry	1 ea	45	36	135	2	22	<1	4	.7	1.6	1.4
439	Bran, wheat	1 ea	45	35	124	3	21	2	4	1.1	2.1	.6
440	Cornmeal	1 ea	45	30	144	3	22	1	5	1.3	2.4	.6
	Nabisco Newtons, fat free:												
1864	Cranberry	1 ea	23	–	69	1	16	–	0	0	0	0
1867	Fig	1 ea	23	–	69	1	16	–	0	0	0	0
1865	Raspberry	1 ea	23	–	69	1	16	–	0	0	0	0
1868	Strawberry	1 ea	23	–	69	1	16	–	0	0	0	0
	Pancakes, 4" diam:												
441	Buckwheat, from mix w/ egg and milk	1 ea	27	54	56	2	8	1	2	.5	.5	.8
442	Plain, from home recipe	1 ea	27	53	61	2	8	<1	3	.6	.7	1.2
443	Plain, from mix; egg, milk, oil added	1 ea	27	53	52	1	10	<1	1	.1	.2	.2
1468	Pan dulce, sweet roll w/topping	1 ea	79	21	291	5	48	1	9	2	3.9	2.7
	Piecrust, with enriched flour, vegetable shortening, baked:												
444	Home recipe, 9" shell	1 ea	180	10	949	12	85	3	62	15.5	27.4	16.4
	From mix:												
445	For 2-crust pie	1 ea	320	10	1686	21	152	5	111	27.6	48.6	29.2
446	1 pie shell	1 ea	180	11	902	12	91	3	55	13.9	31.1	6.9
	Pies, 9" diam; crust made with vegetable shortening, enriched flour:												
447	Apple: Whole pie	1 ea	945	52	2239	18	321	15	104	19.9	56.1	19.8
448	Piece, ⅙ of pie	1 pce	158	52	374	3	54	3	17	3.3	9.4	3.3
449	Banana cream: Whole pie	1 ea	1188	48	3195	52	391	8	162	44.7	68	39.2
450	Piece, ⅙ of pie	1 pce	198	48	533	9	65	1	27	7.4	11.3	6.5
451	Blueberry: Whole pie	1 ea	945	51	2315	25	317	13	112	27.6	48.4	29.1
452	Piece, ⅙ of pie	1 pce	158	51	387	4	53	2	19	4.6	8.1	4.9
453	Cherry: Whole pie	1 ea	945	46	2551	26	364	14	115	28.3	50.2	30.7
454	Piece, ⅙ of pie	1 pce	158	46	427	4	61	2	19	4.7	8.4	5.1
455	Chocolate cream:[3] Whole pie	1 ea	1194	63	2150	47	281	12	97	35	38	18.6
456	Piece, ⅙ of pie	1 pce	199	63	358	8	47	2	16	5.9	6.4	3.1
457	Custard:[3] Whole pie	1 ea	910	61	1911	50	189	15	106	25.3	52.4	17.5
458	Piece, ⅙ of pie	1 pce	152	61	319	8	32	2	18	4.2	8.8	2.9
459	Lemon meringue: Whole pie	1 ea	840	42	2251	13	396	10	73	13.1	30.5	24.3
460	Piece, ⅙ of pie	1 pce	140	42	375	2	66	2	12	2.2	5.1	4
461	Peach: Whole pie	1 ea	945	45	2546	22	377	13	111	26.4	47	31.8

[1] Made with vegetable shortening.
[2] Made with vegetable oil.
[3] Values based on recipe: pie crust, cooked chocolate pudding, whipped cream topping.

(Computer code number is for West Diet Analysis program)

PAGE KEY: H–4 = BEV   H–6 = DAIRY   H–12 = EGGS   H–14 = FAT/OIL   H–18 = FRUIT   H–26 = BAKERY   H–36 = GRAIN   H–44 = FISH   H–48 = MEATS   H–50 = POULTRY   H–54 = SAUSAGE   H–56 = MIXED/FAST   H–64 = NUTS/SEEDS   H–68 = SWEETS   H–70 = VEG/LEG   H–84 = MISC   H–88 = SOUPS/SAUCES   H–90 = FAST   H–106 = FRZN ENTREE   H–112 = BABY FOODS

Chol (mg)	Calc (mg)	Iron (mg)	Magn (mg)	Pota (mg)	Sodi (mg)	Zinc (mg)	VT-A (RE)	Thia (mg)	VT-E (α-TE)	Ribo (mg)	Niac (mg)	V-B6 (mg)	Fola (μg)	VT-C (mg)
0	0	3.7	–	120	5	–	512	.03	–	.07	.4	–	–	0
0	0	1.1	–	120	5	–	102	.03	–	.07	.4	–	–	0
0	0	3.7	–	120	5	–	102	.03	–	.07	.4	–	–	0
0	0	3.7	–	120	5	–	102	.03	–	.07	.4	–	–	0
0	20	1.1	–	120	5	–	102	.03	–	.07	.4	–	–	0
18	85	1.02	7	55	198	.24	13	.12	.81	.13	.99	.02	5	1
16	84	1.89	35	143	265	1.24	108	.15	1.04	.2	1.81	.14	23	4
20	116	1.18	10	65	263	.27	18	.14	.86	.14	1.07	.04	8	<1
21	11	.51	5	35	197	.17	10	.07	.63	.14	1.01	.03	5	<1
31	14	1.14	26	66	210	.51	14	.09	.68	.11	1.29	.08	7	0
28	34	.88	9	59	358	.29	20	.11	.68	.12	.94	.05	5	<1
–	–	–	–	–	77	–	–	–	–	–	–	–	–	–
–	–	–	–	–	77	–	–	–	–	–	–	–	–	–
–	–	–	–	–	77	–	–	–	–	–	–	–	–	–
–	–	–	–	–	77	–	–	–	–	–	–	–	–	–
18	69	.51	15	63	144	.32	18	.05	.56	.07	.36	.04	5	<1
16	59	.49	4	36	119	.15	15	.05	.26	.08	.42	.01	3	<1
3	34	.42	5	47	170	.1	2	.06	.23	.06	.46	.03	2	<1
26	13	1.82	10	57	140	.35	88	.23	1.35	.21	1.98	.04	22	<1
0	18	5.2	25	121	976	.79	0	.7	9.94	.5	5.96	.04	20	0
0	32	9.24	45	214	1734	1.41	0	1.25	17.7	.89	10.6	.08	35	0
0	108	3.87	27	112	1312	.7	0	.54	9.94	.33	4.27	.1	22	0
0	104	4.25	66	614	2513	1.51	284	.26	15.6	.25	2.49	.36	38	30
0	17	.71	11	103	420	.25	47	.04	2.61	.04	.42	.06	6	5
606	891	12.4	190	1960	2851	5.7	832	1.65	17.5	2.46	12.5	1.58	131	19
101	149	2.06	32	327	475	.95	139	.27	2.91	.41	2.08	.26	22	3
0	66	11.6	76	473	1748	1.89	38	1.45	19.8	1.25	11.2	.32	47	7
0	11	1.94	13	79	292	.32	6	.24	3.32	.21	1.88	.05	8	1
0	94	17.5	85	728	1804	1.89	454	1.4	18	1.18	12.1	.32	66	9
0	16	2.92	14	122	302	.32	76	.23	3	.2	2.02	.05	11	2
108.6	1028	8.8	170	1705	2085	4.9	235	1	11.4	2.4	7.34	.37	59	6
18	171	1.47	28	284	347.5	.82	39	.17	1.89	.4	1.22	.06	10	1
300	728	5.28	100	965	2184	4.73	455	.35	10.8	1.89	2.66	.44	182	3
50	122	.88	17	161	365	.79	76	.06	1.81	.32	.44	.07	30	<1
378	470	5.12	126	748	1226	4.12	437	.52	12	1.76	5.45	.25	67	27
63	78	.85	21	125	204	.69	73	.09	2	.29	.91	.04	11	4
0	50	10	68	891	1722	1.59	328	1.2	22.3	1	12.97	.17	49	501

(For purposes of calculations, use "0" for t, <1, <.1, <.01, etc.)

H

Table H–1
Food Composition

Computer Code Number	Food Description	Measure	Wt (g)	H_2O (%)	Ener (kcal)	Prot (g)	Carb (g)	Dietary Fiber (g)	Fat (g)	Fat Breakdown (g) Sat	Mono	Poly
	BAKED GOODS: BREADS, CAKES, COOKIES, CRACKERS, PIES—Cont.											
462	Piece, ⅙ of pie	1 pce	158	45	426	4	63	3	19	4.4	7.9	5.3
463	Pecan: Whole pie	1 ea	825	19	3400	34	486	30	157	32	91.8	25.5
464	Piece, ⅙ of pie	1 pce	138	19	552	6	79	5	26	5.2	14.9	4.1
465	Pumpkin: Whole pie	1 ea	1240	58	2604	48	339	33	118	25	62.1	19.8
466	Piece, ⅙ of pie	1 pce	206	58	433	8	56	6	20	4.2	10.3	3.3
467	Pies, fried, commercial: Apple	1 ea	85	40	266	2	33	2	14	6.5	5.8	1.2
468	Pies, fried, commercial: Cherry	1 ea	85	40	269	3	36	2	14	2	6	4.6
	Pretzels, made with enriched flour:											
469	Thin sticks, 2¼" long	10 ea	3	3	11	<1	2	<1	<1	t	t	t
470	Dutch twists, 2¾ x 2⅝"	1 ea	16	3	61	1	13	<1	1	.1	.2	.2
471	Thin twists, 3¼ x 2¼ x ¼"	10 ea	60	3	229	5	48	2	2	.4	.8	.7
	Rolls & buns, enriched, commercial:											
472	Cloverleaf rolls, 2½" diam, 2" high	1 ea	28	32	85	2	14	1	2	.5	1.1	.3
473	Hot dog buns	1 ea	40	34	114	3	20	1	2	.5	1	.4
474	Hamburger buns	1 ea	45	34	129	4	23	1	2	.5	1.1	.4
475	Hard roll, white, 3¾" diam, 2" high	1 ea	50	31	147	5	26	1	2	.3	.6	.9
476	Submarine rolls/hoagies, 11½ x 3 x 2½"	1 ea	135	31	392	12	75	4	4	.9	1.3	1.4
	Rolls & buns, enriched, home recipe:											
477	Dinner rolls 2½" diam, 2" high	1 ea	35	29	112	3	19	1	3	.7	1.1	.7
	Sports/fitness bar:											
2043	Forza energy bar	1 ea	70	18	231	11	45	4	1	–	–	–
2042	Power bar	1 ea	65	21	230	10	45	3	3	–	–	–
2041	Tiger sports bar	1 ea	65	17	229	11	40	4	2	–	–	–
478	Toaster pastries, fortified (Poptarts)	1 ea	54	12	212	3	38	1	6	.8	2.2	2.1
2132	Toaster strudel pastry—cream cheese	1 ea	53	32	184	3	24	<1	9	2.7	–	–
2134	Toaster strudel pastry—french toast	1 ea	53	31	184	3	24	<1	9	2.8	–	–
	Tortilla chips:											
1271	Plain	1 oz	28	7	140	2	18	2	7	1.4	4.3	1
1036	Nacho flavor	1 oz	28	2	139	2	17	1	7	1.4	4.3	1
1037	Taco flavor	1 oz	28	2	134	2	18	1	7	1.3	4	1
	Tortillas:											
479	Corn, enriched, 6" diam	1 ea	30	44	67	2	14	2	1	.1	.2	.3
480	Flour, 8" diam	1 ea	35	27	115	3	20	1	3	.4	1	1
1301	Flour, 10" diam	1 ea	57	27	185	5	32	2	4	.6	1.6	1.6
481	Taco shells	1 ea	14	4	63	1	9	1	3	.4	1.5	.6
	Waffles, 7" diam:											
482	From home recipe	1 ea	75	42	218	6	25	1	11	2.1	2.6	5.1
483	From mix, egg/milk added	1 ea	75	42	218	5	26	1	10	1.7	2.7	5.2
1510	Whole grain, prepared from frozen	1 ea	39	43	107	4	13	1	5	1.6	1.9	1
	GRAIN PRODUCTS: CEREAL, FLOUR, GRAIN, PASTA and NOODLES, POPCORN											
484	Barley, pearled, dry, uncooked	1 c	200	10	704	20	155	31	2	.5	.3	1.1
485	Barley, pearled, cooked	1 c	157	69	193	4	44	6	1	.1	.1	.3
	Breakfast bars, fat free:											
2009	Apple	1 ea	38	25	110	2	26	3	0	0	0	0
2005	Chocolate	1 ea	38	23	81	2	19	3	0	0	0	0
2003	Strawberry	1 ea	38	25	110	2	26	3	0	0	0	0

(Computer code number is for West Diet Analysis program)

PAGE KEY: H–4 = BEV   H–6 = DAIRY   H–12 = EGGS   H–14 = FAT/OIL   H–18 = FRUIT   H–26 = BAKERY   H–36 = GRAIN   H–44 = FISH   H–48 = MEATS   H–50 = POULTRY   H–54 = SAUSAGE   H–56 = MIXED/FAST   H–64 = NUTS/SEEDS   H–68 = SWEETS   H–70 = VEG/LEG   H–84 = MISC   H–88 = SOUPS/SAUCES   H–90 = FAST   H–106 = FRZN ENTREE   H–112 = BABY FOODS

Chol (mg)	Calc (mg)	Iron (mg)	Magn (mg)	Pota (mg)	Sodi (mg)	Zinc (mg)	VT-A (RE)	Thia (mg)	VT-E (α-TE)	Ribo (mg)	Niac (mg)	V-B6 (mg)	Fola (µg)	VT-C (mg)
0	8	1.7	11	149	288	.27	55	.2	3.73	.17	2	.03	8	84
272	145	8.84	153	629	3604	4.8	400	.77	20.9	1.03	2.12	.18	51	9
44	23	1.45	25	102	585	.79	65	.13	3.49	.17	.34	.03	8	2
248	744	9.8	186	1909	3496	5.58	5951	.68	20	1.9	2.32	.71	186	19
41	124	1.63	31	317	581	.93	989	.11	3.32	.31	.38	.12	31	3
13	13	.88	8	51	325	.17	8	.1	.37	.08	.98	.03	4	2
0	19	1.03	9	55	318	.19	14	.1	.37	.09	1.2	.03	3	1
0	1	.13	1	4	51	.03	0	.01	.01	.02	.16	<.01	2	0
0	6	.69	6	23	274	.14	0	.07	.03	.1	.84	.02	13	0
0	22	2.59	21	88	1029	.51	0	.28	.13	.37	3.15	.07	50	0
<1	34	.89	6	38	148	.22	0	.14	.22	.09	1.14	.01	9	<1
0	56	1.27	8	56	224	.25	0	.19	.19	.12	1.57	.02	11	0
0	63	1.43	9	63	252	.28	0	.22	.21	.14	1.77	.02	12	0
0	48	1.64	14	54	272	.47	0	.24	.09	.17	2.12	.03	8	0
0	122	3.78	27	122	783	.85	0	.54	.1	.33	4.47	.05	41	0
13	21	1.04	7	53	145	.24	28	.14	.35	.14	1.21	.02	15	<1
0	300	6.3	160	220	65	5.25	–	1.5	20	1.7	20	2	400	60
–	300	5.4	140	150	110	5.25	–	1.5	–	1.7	20	2	400	60
–	349	4.5	140	279	100	–	50	1.5	20	1.7	20	2	400	60
0	14	1.89	10	60	226	.36	57[1]	.16	1	.2	2.13	.21	43	<1
12	12	.95	–	–	213	–	17	–	.99	–	–	–	–	0
12	12	.95	–	–	213	–	17	–	.99	–	–	–	–	0
0	43	.43	25	55	148	.43	6	.02	.38	.05	.36	.08	3	0
1	41	.4	23	60	198	.34	11	.04	.38	.05	.4	.08	4	1
1	44	.57	25	61	220	.36	25	.07	.38	.06	.56	.08	6	<1
0	52	.42	20	46	48	.28	7	.03	.05	.02	.45	.07	5	0
0	44	1.17	9	46	169	.25	0	.19	.44	.1	1.26	.02	4	0
0	71	1.88	15	74	273	.4	0	.3	.72	.17	2.03	.03	7	0
0	35	.35	15	34	25	.18	6	.04	.58	.02	.24	.04	4	0
52	191	1.74	14	119	383	.51	49	.2	1.73	.26	1.55	.04	11	<1
52	93	1.23	15	134	458	.35	20	.15	1.5	.2	1.23	.08	9	<1
39	84	.7	15	91	150	.46	25	.08	.53	.13	.75	.05	7	<1
0	58	5	158	560	18	4.26	4	.38	.26	.23	9.22	.52	46	0
0	17	2.09	34	146	5	1.29	2	.13	.08	.1	3.23	.18	25	0
0	20	.72	–	160	25	–	20	.09	–	.03	.4	–	–	1
0	20	1.3	–	160	22	–	74	.09	–	.03	.4	–	–	0
0	20	.72	–	160	25	–	20	.09	–	.03	.4	–	–	1

[1]Vitamin A values from label declarations vary.

(For purposes of calculations, use "0" for t, <1, <.1, <.01, etc.)

Table H–1
Food Composition

Computer Code Number	Food Description	Measure	Wt (g)	H₂O (%)	Ener (kcal)	Prot (g)	Carb (g)	Dietary Fiber (g)	Fat (g)	Fat Breakdown (g) Sat	Mono	Poly
	GRAIN PRODUCTS: CEREAL, FLOUR, GRAIN, PASTA and NOODLES, POPCORN—Cont.											
	Breakfast bar, Snackwell											
2165	Apple-cinnamon	1 ea	37	16	119	1	29	1	<1	0.1	<.1	.1
2164	Blueberry	1 ea	37	16	121	1	29	1	<1	<.1	<.1	.1
2163	Strawberry	1 ea	37	16	120	1	29	1	<1	<.1	<.1	.1
	Breakfast cereals, hot, cooked:											
	Corn grits (hominy) enriched:											
486	Regular and quick, prepared, yellow	1 c	242	85	145	3	31	5	<1	.1	.1	.2
487	Instant, prepared from packet, white	1 ea	137	82	89	2	21	1	<1	t	t	<.1
	Cream of wheat:											
488	Regular, quick, instant	1 c	244	87	132	5	27	1	<1	.1	.1	.2
489	Mix and eat, plain, packet	1 ea	142	82	102	3	21	<1	<1	t	t	.1
1664	Farina cereal, cooked	½ c	117	87	59	2	12	2	<1	<.1	<.1	<.1
490	Malt-O-Meal	1 c	240	88	122	4	26	1	<1	t	t	.1
494	Maypo	1 c	242	83	172	6	32	6	2	.4	.8	.1
	Oatmeal or rolled oats:											
491	Regular, quick, instant, nonfort	1 c	234	85	145	6	25	4	2	.4	.7	.9
	Instant, fortified:											
492	Plain, from packet	¾ c	177	85	104	5	18	3	2	.3	.6	.7
493	Flavored, from packet	¾ c	164	76	160	5	31	3	2	.3	.7	.8
	Breakfast cereals, ready to eat:											
495	All-Bran	⅓ c	28	4	77	4	21	10	1	.2	.2	.6
1306	Alpha Bits	1 c	28	1	110	2	24	1	1	.1	.2	.2
1307	Apple Jacks	1 c	28	3	108	1	25	1	<1	.1	.1	.2
1308	Bran Buds	1 c	84	3	232	8	67	34	2	.3	.4	1.3
1305	Bran Chex	1 c	49	2	156	5	39	8	1	.2	.3	.7
1309	Honey BucWheat Crisp	¾ c	28	5	109	3	23	2	1	.2	.2	.4
1310	C. W. Post, plain	1 c	97	2	421	9	73	7	13	1.7	6	4.7
1311	C. W. Post, with raisins	1 c	103	4	446	9	74	14	15	11	1.7	1.4
496	Cap'n Crunch	1 c	37	2	147	2	32	1	2	.5	.4	.3
1312	Cap'n Crunchberries	1 c	38	2	152	2	33	1	2	.5	.4	.3
1313	Cap'n Crunch, peanut butter	1 c	38	2	158	3	30	1	3	.7	1.2	.7
497	Cheerios	1 c	23	3	84	2	18	2	1	.3	.5	.2
1314	Cocoa Krispies	1 c	36	2	140	2	32	<1	1	.1	.2	.2
1316	Cocoa Pebbles	1 c	31	2	127	1	27	<1	2	1	.4	.1
1315	Corn Bran	1 c	36	3	120	2	30	6	1	.3	.3	.4
1317	Corn Chex	1 c	28	2	110	2	25	<1	1	.1	.2	<.1
498	Corn Flakes, Kellogg's	1¼ c	28	3	102	2	24	1	<1	t	t	t
499	Corn Flakes, Post Toasties	1¼ c	28	3	108	2	24	1	<1	t	t	t
1340	Corn Pops	1 c	28	3	107	1	26	<1	<1	.1	.1	<.1
1318	Cracklin' Oat Bran	1 c	60	4	245	5	44	7	8	3.2	3.5	.8
1038	Crispy Wheat `N Raisins	1 c	43	7	150	3	35	3	1	.1	.1	.2
1319	Fortified Oat Flakes	1 c	48	3	181	8	36	1	1	.2	.3	.4
500	40% Bran Flakes, Kellogg's	1 c	39	3	127	4	31	6	1	.1	.1	.5
501	40% Bran Flakes, Post	1 c	47	3	152	5	37	9	1	.12	.1	.3
502	Froot Loops	1 c	28	2	111	1	25	1	1	.3	.2	.2
518	Frosted Flakes	1 c	35	3	132	1	32	1	<1	t	t	t
1320	Frosted Mini-Wheats	4 ea	31	5	105	3	26	3	<1	.1	.1	.3
1321	Frosted Rice Krispies	1 c	28	3	106	1	25	<1	<1	.1	.1	.1
1324	Fruit & Fibre w/dates	½ c	28	9	95	2	21	4	1	.2	.6	.5
1325	Fruitful Bran	¾ c	34	1	111	3	27	5	<1	<.1	<.1	.1

TABLE OF FOOD COMPOSITION ◆ **H–39**

PAGE KEY: H–4 = BEV   H–6 = DAIRY   H–12 = EGGS   H–14 = FAT/OIL   H–18 = FRUIT   H–26 = BAKERY   H–36 = GRAIN   H–44 = FISH   H–48 = MEATS   H–50 = POULTRY   H–54 = SAUSAGE   H–56 = MIXED/FAST   H–64 = NUTS/SEEDS   H–68 = SWEETS   H–70 = VEG/LEG   H–84 = MISC   H–88 = SOUPS/SAUCES   H–90 = FAST   H–106 = FRZN ENTREE   H–112 = BABY FOODS

Chol (mg)	Calc (mg)	Iron (mg)	Magn (mg)	Pota (mg)	Sodi (mg)	Zinc (mg)	VT-A (RE)	Thia (mg)	VT-E (α-TE)	Ribo (mg)	Niac (mg)	V-B6 (mg)	Fola (μg)	VT-C (mg)
<1	17	5	6	68	103	3.88	–	.39	–	.44	5.2	.52	–	<1
<1	14	4.83	5	44	107	3.85	–	.39	–	.44	5.2	.52	–	<1
<1	14	4.82	6	47	102	3.83	–	.39	–	.44	5.2	.52	–	2
0	0	1.55[1]	10	53	0[2]	.17	15[3]	.24[1]	.12	.14[1]	1.96[1]	.06	2	0
0	8	8.19[1]	11	29	289	.21	0	.15[1]	.03	.08[1]	1.3[1]	.05	1	0
0	51[1]	10.5[1]	12	46	141[4]	.34	0	.24[1]	.03	0[1]	1.46[1]	.03	10	0
0	20[1]	8.09[1]	7	38	241[5]	.24	376[1]	.43[1]	.02	.28[1]	4.97[1]	.57	101	0
0	2	.59	2	15	0[5]	.08	0	.09	.02	.06	.64	.01	2	0
0	5	9.6[1]	5	31	2[5]	.17	0	.48[1]	.03	.24[1]	5.76[1]	.02	5	0
0	126	8.47	51	213	261	1.5	709	.73	1.7	.73	9.44	.97	10	29
0	19	1.59	56	131	2[5]	1.15	5	.26	.23	.05	.3	.05	9	0
0	162[1]	6.3[1]	42	99	285[1]	.87	453[1]	.53[1]	.21	.28[1]	5.47[1]	.74	150	0
0	168[1]	7[1]	51	137	254[1]	1	460[1]	.53[1]	.21	.38[1]	5.9[1]	.76	150	0
0	100	4.26[1]	122	284	261	3.6	213[1]	.37[1]	.52	.39[1]	5[1]	.48	100	14[1]
0	8	2.7	17	54	178	1.48	371	.37	.02	.42	5	.5	99	0
0	3	4.2	8	23	125	3.5	210	.37	.05	.39	5	.48	99	14
0	56	12.6	234	755	559	18.06	631	1.09	1.33	1.2	14.03	1.43	252	42
0	29	14	69	216	346	6.5	11	.64	.56	.26	8.62	.88	173	26
0	40	8.12	32	105	266	.5	673	.67	6.62	.76	9	1.4	8	27
<1	47	15.4	67	198	167	1.64	1284	1.26	.68	1.46	17.1	1.75	342	0
<1	50	16.4	74	261	161	1.64	1363	1.34	.72	1.55	18.1	1.85	363	0
0	7	6.18[1]	13	47	285	5	5[1]	.5[1]	.18	.58[1]	6.85[1]	1	137	0
0	10	6.6	14	54	278	5.85	7	.55	.27	.62	7.3	.73	146	<1
0	4	6	26	87	287	5.28	5	.53	.21	.6	7.03	.7	141	0
0	42	6.2[1]	25	68	218	2.87	288	.28[1]	.16	.33[1]	3.84[1]	.38	77	12[1]
0	5	2.09	13	70	244	1.7	261	.43	.17	.5	5.8	.58	108	17
0	5	1.95	13	51	175	1.64	410	.4	.04	.47	5.5	.56	109	0
0	27	10	19	75	338	5	5	.1	.19	.6	6.7	.67	134	0
0	3	8	4	23	306	.1	14	.37	.07	.07	5	.5	99	15
0	1	8.68[1]	3	25	298	.16	210[1]	.36[1]	.03	.39[1]	4.68[1]	.48	99	15[1]
0	1	.74[1]	4	32	293	.08	371[1]	.36[1]	.07	.42[1]	4.93[1]	.5	99	0
0	2	1.7	2	20	111	1.4	210	.36	.03	.39	5	.48	99	14
0	27	2.2	83	278	213	1.8	276	.5	.4	.5	6.12	.6	167	18
0	54	3.52	33	180	223	.85	293	.29	.45	.33	3.9	.39	78	0
0	68	13.7	58	228	220	2.5	636	.62	.34	.72	8.45	.86	169	0
0	19	11[1]	81	236	304	5.03	488[1]	.51[1]	7.22	.58[1]	6.7[1]	.66	138	20
0	21	13.44[1]	102	251	431	2.49	622[1]	.61[1]	.54	.7[1]	8.27[1]	.85	166	0
0	3	4[1]	8	30	133	3.55	200[1]	.37[1]	.1	.4[1]	5[1]	.48	85	13[1]
0	1	5.25[1]	3	23	228	.18	263[1]	.45[1]	.05	.49[1]	5.85[1]	.6	124	18[1]
0	11	9.15	31	103	1	.84	0	.2	.28	.25	2.8	.28	58	0
0	2	1.93	7	22	205	.34	243	.39	.03	.45	5	.53	112	16
0	15	5	40	165	132	1.48	356	.37	.65	.42	5	.5	99	0
0	18	4	52	212	203	1	208	.35	.61	.4	5	.46	92	<1

[1] Nutrient added (values sometimes based on label declaration).

[2] Cooked without salt. If salt is added according to label recommendation, sodium content is 540 mg.

[3] Value for yellow corn grits; cooked white corn grits contain 0 RE of vitamin A.

[4] Values for quick cereal.

[5] Cooked without salt. If added according to label recommendations, sodium content is 390 mg for Cream of Wheat; 324 mg for Malt-O-Meal; 374 mg for oatmeal; 385 mg for Farina.

(For purposes of calculations, use "0" for t, <1, <.1, <.01, etc.)

H

Table H–1
Food Composition

Computer Code Number	Food Description	Measure	Wt (g)	H₂O (%)	Ener (kcal)	Prot (g)	Carb (g)	Dietary Fiber (g)	Fat (g)	Fat Breakdown (g) Sat	Mono	Poly
GRAIN PRODUCTS: CEREAL, FLOUR, GRAIN, PASTA and NOODLES, POPCORN—Cont.												
Breakfast cereals, ready to eat—Cont.												
1322	Fruity Pebbles	1 c	32	3	130	1	28	<1	2	1.4	.1	.1
503	Golden Grahams	1 c	39	3	150	2	33	1	1	.2	.4	.2
504	Granola, homemade	½ c	61	5	285	9	32	6	15	2.9	4.8	6.5
1670	Granola, low fat, commercial	½ c	47	5	173	4	37	3	2	1	1	1
505	Grape Nuts	½ c	57	3	203	7	47	6	<1	t	t	.1
1326	Grape Nuts Flakes	1 c	32	3	118	4	26	3	1	.1	.1	.2
1665	Heartland Natural with raisins	1 c	101	5	429	10	70	6	14	3.7	3.9	5.7
1327	Honey & Nut Corn Flakes	1 c	38	4	154	3	32	1	2	.3	.7	.6
506	Honey Nut Cheerios	1 c	33	2	128	3	27	2	1	.3	.5	.2
1328	HoneyBran	1 c	35	3	119	3	29	4	1	.3	.1	.3
1329	HoneyComb	1 c	22	1	86	1	20	<1	<1	.2	.1	.1
1330	King Vitaman	1 c	19	2	73	1	16	1	1	.2	.3	.2
1039	Kix	1 c	19	2	73	1	16	<1	<1	.1	.1	<.1
1331	Life	1 c	43	4	163	4	34	3	2	.3	.6	.8
507	Lucky Charms	1 c	32	2	124	2	27	1	1	.2	.4	.2
1323	Mueslix Five Grain	1 c	82	5	279	7	63	7	3	.5	1	1.2
1416	Granola, low-fat	⅓ c	31	3	119	3	25	2	2	0	–	–
508	Nature Valley Granola	1 c	113	4	510	12	74	7	20	2.6	13	3.8
1666	Nutri Grain Almond Raisin	⅔ c	40	6	147	3	31	3	3	.1	1	1.2
1333	Nutri-Grain—corn	1 c	42	3	160	3	35	3	1	.1	.5	.2
1336	100% Bran	1 c	66	3	178	8	48	20	3	.6	.6	1.9
509	100% Natural cereal, plain	½ c	57	3	252	6	39	4	9	4	4.1	1.2
1337	100% Natural with apples & cinnamon	1 c	104	2	477	11	70	7	20	15.5	1.8	1.3
1338	100% Natural with raisins & dates	1 c	110	3	496	11	72	7	20	13.6	3.7	1.7
510	Product 19	1 c	33	4	121	3	28	1	<1	t	.1	.2
1339	Quisp	1 c	30	3	121	2	25	<1	2	.5	.4	.2
511	Raisin Bran, Kellogg's	1 c	49	9	158	5	38	6	1	.12	.1	.3
512	Raisin Bran, Post	1 c	56	9	172	5	42	8	1	.2	.1	.5
1667	Raisin Squares	½ c	28	10	95	2	22	3	1	.1	.1	.3
1041	Rice Chex	¾ c	19	3	75	1	17	<1	1	<.1	.2	<.1
513	Rice Krispies, Kellogg's	1 c	29	2	114	2	26	<1	<1	t	t	t
514	Rice, puffed	1 c	14	4	53	1	12	<1	<1	t	t	t
515	Shredded Wheat	1 c	43	5	154	5	34	4	1	.1	.1	.4
516	Special K	1 c	21	3	78	4	15	1	<1	t	t	.1
517	Super Golden Crisp	1 c	33	1	123	3	30	<1	<1	t	t	.1
519	Honey Smacks	1 c	38	3	144	2	33	1	1	.4	.1	.3
1341	Tasteeos	1 c	24	2	94	3	19	3	1	.2	.2	.2
1342	Team	1 c	42	4	164	3	36	<1	1	.1	.2	.3
520	Total, wheat, with added calcium	1 c	33	3	116	3	26	3	1	.1	.1	.1
521	Trix	1 c	28	2	114	1	24	<1	2	.4	.9	.3
1344	Wheat Chex	1 c	46	2	169	5	38	4	1	.2	.1	.5

H

(Computer code number is for West Diet Analysis program)

PAGE KEY: H–4 = BEV   H–6 = DAIRY   H–12 = EGGS   H–14 = FAT/OIL   H–18 = FRUIT   H–26 = BAKERY   H–36 = GRAIN   H–44 = FISH   H–48 = MEATS   H–50 = POULTRY   H–54 = SAUSAGE   H–56 = MIXED/FAST   H–64 = NUTS/SEEDS   H–68 = SWEETS   H–70 = VEG/LEG   H–84 = MISC   H–88 = SOUPS/SAUCES   H–90 = FAST   H–106 = FRZN ENTREE   H–112 = BABY FOODS

Chol (mg)	Calc (mg)	Iron (mg)	Magn (mg)	Pota (mg)	Sodi (mg)	Zinc (mg)	VT-A (RE)	Thia (mg)	VT-E (α-TE)	Ribo (mg)	Niac (mg)	V-B6 (mg)	Fola (μg)	VT-C (mg)
0	4	2.02	9	24	178	1.7	424	.42	.03	.48	5.6	.58	113	0
0	19	5.86[1]	12	69	357	4.88	293[1]	.49[1]	.29	.55[1]	6.5[1]	.7	130	19[1]
0	49	2.56[1]	109	328	15	2.47	2	.45	7.87	.17	1.25	.2	52	1
0	21	1.65	39	133	106	2.96	176	.28	4.74	.33	3.9	.38	94	0
0	5	16[1]	38	190	396	1.25	755[1]	.74[1]	.14	.85[1]	10.03[1]	1.03	201	0
0	13	9.15	35	114	181	.64	424	.42	.08	.48	5.6	.58	113	0
0	61	3.7	129	381	207	2.6	6	.29	.71	.13	1.41	.18	40	1
0	4	3.12	3	41	256	.27	159	.27	.1	.3	3.46	.34	76	10
0	23	5	33	95	288	4.17	250[1]	.42[1]	.34	.5[1]	5.57[1]	.6	111	17[1]
0	16	5.57	46	151	202	.9	463	.46	.81	.53	6.16	.63	23	19
0	4	2.09	7	25	124	1.17	291	.29	.09	.33	3.87	.4	78	0
0	2	5.36	16	52	159	2.39	192	.24	1.29	.27	3.2	.32	64	8
0	28	5.13	6	26	167	2.34	238	.24	.05	.27	3.17	.32	63	10
0	131	12	42	106	234	5.4	2	.54	.22	.61	7.2	.71	144	0
0	35	4.79[1]	21	58	217	4	240	.4[1]	.14	.45[1]	5.34[1]	.53	107	16[1]
0	38	8.94	82	369	107	7.46	747	.75	8.94	.84	9.84	.99	197	1
0	–	1.8	24	94	60	3.72	149	.37	4.99	.42	4.96	.5	100	–
0	85	3.53	107	375	183	2.27	0	.4	7.97	.12	1.25	.16	17	0
0	122	1	9	143	142	2.72	0	.28	4	.32	4	.36	80	0
0	1	.89	27	98	276	5.54	556	.55	11.1	.63	7.39	.76	148	22
0	46	8.12	312	652	457	5.74	0	1.58	1.53	1.78	20.9	2.11	47	63
<1	55	1.7	60	281	15	1.36	<1	.2	.65	.09	1	.1	14	<1
1	157	2.9	72	514	52	2	6	.33	.73	.57	1.87	.11	17	1
1	159	3.12	124	537	47	2.11	6	.31	.77	.65	2.09	.16	45	0
0	3	20[1]	14	57	310	16.5	248[1]	1.65[1]	24.4	1.88[1]	22[1]	2.21	466	66[1]
0	6	5.1	15	40	216	4.26	4	.42	.16	.48	5.67	.56	113	0
0	32	4[1]	72	281	314	3	200[1]	.34[1]	.45	.39[1]	4.46[1]	.44	91	0
0	26	8.9[1]	95	355	365	2.97	741[1]	.73[1]	1.3	.84[1]	9.86[1]	1.01	197	0
0	10	8.6[1]	24	132	2	.78	0	.2	.15	.22	3	.3	56	0
0	3	5.4[1]	5	22	159	.26	1	.25	.02	.01	3.34	.34	67	10
0	5	.73[1]	12	28	213	.49	384[1]	.54[1]	.03	.6[1]	7.16[1]	.72	143	15[1]
0	1	.4[1]	4	16	<1	.15	0	.01[1]	.01	.01[1]	.38[1]	0	1	0
0	16	1.8	57	155	4	1.41	0	.11	.23	.12	2.26	.11	22	0
0	3	5.69[1]	12	37	196	2.5	153[1]	.35[1]	.05	.39[1]	4.75	.48	63	10[1]
0	7	2.08[1]	20	48	51	1.75	437[1]	.43[1]	.12	.49[1]	5.81[1]	.59	117	0
0	4	2.53[1]	22	59	71	.49	316[1]	.53[1]	.2	.6	7[1]	.72	140	21[1]
0	11	6.86[1]	26	71	182	.69	318	.31	.17	.36	4.22	.43	85	13
0	6	12[1]	12	71	260	.58	556	.55	.1	.63	7.39	.76	7	22
0	284	20[1]	35	107	219	16.5	413[1]	1.65[1]	25.8	1.87[1]	22.1	2.2	440	66
0	30	4.2[1]	3	17	184	3.49	210[1]	.35[1]	.56	.39[1]	5[1]	.47	93	14[1]
0	18	13.16[1]	58	173	308	1.23	0	.6	.17	.17	8.1	.83	162	24

[1]Nutrient added (values sometimes based on label declaration).

(For purposes of calculations, use "0" for t, <1, <.1, <.01, etc.)

H

Table H–1
Food Composition

Computer Code Number	Food Description	Measure	Wt (g)	H₂O (%)	Ener (kcal)	Prot (g)	Carb (g)	Dietary Fiber (g)	Fat (g)	Fat Breakdown (g) Sat	Mono	Poly
	GRAIN PRODUCTS: CEREAL, FLOUR, GRAIN, PASTA and NOODLES, POPCORN—Cont.											
1043	Wheat cereal, puffed, fortified	1 c	12	4	44	2	10	1	<1	<.1	<.1	.1
522	Wheaties	1 c	29	3	106	3	23	2	1	.1	.2	.1
	Buckwheat flour:											
523	Dark	1 c	98	11	328	12	69	10	3	.7	.9	.9
524	Light	1 c	98	12	340	6	78	6	1	.2	.4	.4
525	Buckwheat, whole grain, dry	1 c	175	10	600	23	125	18	6	1.3	1.8	1.8
526	Bulgar, dry, uncooked	1 c	140	9	479	17	106	26	2	.3	.2	.8
527	Bulgar, cooked	1 c	182	78	151	6	34	8	<1	<.1	<.1	.2
	Cornmeal:											
528	Whole-ground, unbolted, dry	1 c	122	10	442	10	94	10	4	.6	1.2	2
529	Bolted, nearly whole, dry	1 c	122	10	441	10	94	12	4	.6	1.2	2
530	Degermed, enriched, dry	1 c	138	12	505	12	107	10	2	.3	.6	1
531	Degermed, enriched, cooked	1 c	240	78	209	5	44	4	1	.1	.2	.4
	Macaroni, cooked:											
532	Enriched	1 c	140	66	197	7	40	2	1	.1	.1	.4
533	Whole wheat	1 c	140	67	174	7	37	4	1	.1	.1	.3
534	Vegetable, enriched	1 c	134	68	172	6	36	2	<1	t	t	.1
535	Millet, cooked	½ c	120	71	143	4	28	2	1	.2	.2	.6
	Noodles (see also Pasta and Spaghetti)											
1507	Cellophane noodles, cooked	1 c	190	79	160	<1	39	<1	<1	<.1	<.1	<.1
1995	Cellophane noodles, dry	½ c	70	13	246	<1	60	<1	<1	<.1	<.1	<.1
537	Chow mein, dry	1 c	45	1	237	4	26	2	14	2	3.5	7.8
536	Egg noodles, cooked, enriched	1 c	160	69	213	8	40	2	2	.5	.7	.7
538	Spinach noodles, dry	3½ oz	100	8	372	13	75	11	2	.2	.2	.6
1343	Oat bran, dry	¼ c	23	7	57	4	15	4	2	.3	.6	.6
	Pasta, cooked:											
1418	Fresh	2 oz	57	69	75	3	14	1	1	.1	.1	.2
1417	Linguini	1 c	140	66	197	7	40	4	1	.1	.1	.4
1598	Rotini	1 c	140	66	197	7	40	2	1	.1	.1	.4
	Popcorn:											
539	Air popped, plain	1 c	8	4	31	1	6	1	<1	<.1	.1	.2
1042	Microwaved, low fat, low sodium	1 c	6	3	24	1	4	1	1	.1	.2	.3
540	Popped in vegetable oil/salted	1 c	11	2	55	1	6	1	3	.5	.9	1.5
541	Sugar-syrup coated	1 c	35	2	151	1	28	2	4	1.3	1	1.6
	Rice:											
542	Brown rice, cooked	1 c	195	73	216	5	45	4	2	.4	.6	.6
2215	Mexican rice, cooked	½ c	113	–	410	8	90	3	15	2	.1	.1
2216	Spanish rice, cooked	½ c	123	85	65	2	14	1	1	–	–	–
	White, enriched, all types:											
543	Regular/long grain, dry	1 c	185	11	675	13	148	2	1	.3	.4	.3
544	Regular/long grain, cooked	1 c	205	68	267	6	58	1	<1	.2	.2	.2
545	Instant, prepared without salt	1 c	165	76	161	3	35	1	<1	.1	.1	.1

TABLE OF FOOD COMPOSITION

◆ **H–43**

PAGE KEY: H–4 = BEV H–6 = DAIRY H–12 = EGGS H–14 = FAT/OIL H–18 = FRUIT H–26 = BAKERY H–36 = GRAIN H–44 = FISH H–48 = MEATS H–50 = POULTRY H–54 = SAUSAGE H–56 = MIXED/FAST H–64 = NUTS/SEEDS H–68 = SWEETS H–70 = VEG/LEG H–84 = MISC H–88 = SOUPS/SAUCES H–90 = FAST H–106 = FRZN ENTREE H–112 = BABY FOODS

Chol (mg)	Calc (mg)	Iron (mg)	Magn (mg)	Pota (mg)	Sodi (mg)	Zinc (mg)	VT-A (RE)	Thia (mg)	VT-E (α-TE)	Ribo (mg)	Niac (mg)	V-B6 (mg)	Fola (μg)	VT-C (mg)
0	3	.57	17	44	1	.37	<.1	.05	.08	.03	1.4	.02	4	0
0	53	7.83[1]	31	101	215	.69	218[1]	.36[1]	.36	.41[1]	4.8[1]	.48	97	15[1]
0	40	3.98	246	566	11	3.06	0	.41	1.01	.19	6.03	.57	53	0
0	11	1	47	314	1	2.56	0	.09	.5	.05	.47	.09	100	0
0	31	3.85	404	805	2	4.2	0	.18	1.8	.74	12.3	.37	52	0
0	49	3.44	230	574	24	2.7	0	.32	.22	.16	7.15	.48	38	0
0	18	1.75	58	124	9	1.04	0	.1	.05	.05	1.82	.15	33	0
0	7	4.21	155	350	43	2.22	57	.47	.82	.24	4.43	.37	31	0
0	7	4.21	154	350	43	2.22	57	.37	.96	.1	2.3	.37	31	0
0	7	5.7	55	224	4	.99	57	.99	.46	.56	6.94	.35	66	0
0	3	2.35	22	91	1	.41	23	.3	.21	.21	2.42	.12	22	0
0	10	1.96	25	43	1	.74	0	.29	.04	.14	2.34	.05	10	0
0	21	1.48	42	62	4	1.13	0	.15	.14	.06	.99	.11	7	0
0	15	.66	25	42	8	.59	7	.15	.05	.08	1.43	.03	8	0
0	4	.76	53	74	2	1.09	0	.13	.22	.1	1.6	.13	23	0
0	14	1	3	5	9	.23	0	.07	.06	0	.09	.02	1	0
0	18	1.52	2	7	7	.29	0	.11	.09	0	.14	.04	1	0
0	18	2.13	23	54	198	.63	4	.26	.07	.19	2.7	.05	10	0
53	19	2.54	30	45	11	.99	10	.3	.08	.13	2.38	.06	11	0
0	58	2.13	174	376	36	2.76	46	.37	.04	.2	4.55	.32	48	0
0	13	1.27	54	130	1	.72	0	.27	.39	.05	.22	.04	12	0
19	3	.65	10	14	3	.32	3	.12	.09	.09	.56	.02	4	0
0	10	1.96	25	43	1	.74	0	.29	.08	.14	2.34	.05	10	0
0	10	1.96	25	43	1	.74	0	.29	.04	.14	2.34	.05	10	0
0	1	.21	11	24	<1	.27	2	.02	.01	.02	.15	.02	2	0
0	1	.14	9	14	29	.22	1	.02	.06	.01	.12	.01	1	0
0	1	.31	12	25	97	.29	2	.01	.03	.01	.17	.02	2	<1
2	15	.61	12	38	72	.2	4	.02	.42	.02	.77	.01	1	0
0	20	.82	84	84	10	1.23	0	.19	5.3	.05	2.98	.28	8	0
0	150	4.5	–	–	1350	–	–	–	–	–	–	–	–	48
0	–	.36	–	–	670	–	–	–	–	–	–	–	–	–
0	52	8	46	213	9	2.02	0	1.07	.24	.09	7.75	.3	15	0
0	20	2.46	25	72	2	1	0	.33	.1	.03	3.03	.19	6	0
0	13	1.04	8	7	5[2]	.4	0	.12	.08	.08	1.45	.02	7	0

[1]Nutrient added (values sometimes based on label declaration).

[2]If prepared with salt according to label recommendation, sodium would be 608 mg.

(Computer code number is for West Diet Analysis program)

H

Table H–1
Food Composition

Computer Code Number	Food Description	Measure	Wt (g)	H₂O (%)	Ener (kcal)	Prot (g)	Carb (g)	Dietary Fiber (g)	Fat (g)	Fat Breakdown (g)		
										Sat	Mono	Poly
	GRAIN PRODUCTS: CEREAL, FLOUR, GRAIN, PASTA and NOODLES, POPCORN—Cont.											
	Parboiled/converted rice:											
546	Raw, dry	1 c	185	10	686	13	151	3	1	.3	.3	.3
547	Cooked	1 c	175	73	200	4	43	1	<1	.1	.1	.1
1486	Sticky rice (glutinous), cooked	1 c	241	77	234	5	51	2	<1	.1	.2	.2
548	Wild rice, cooked	1 c	164	73	166	7	35	3	1	.1	.1	.4
1700	Rice and pasta (Rice-a-Roni), cooked	½ c	109	72	133	3	23	1	3	.6	1.2	1
549	Rye flour, medium	1 c	102	10	361	10	79	15	2	.2	.2	.8
1044	Soy flour, low-fat	1 c	88	2	325	45	30	9	6	.9	1.3	3.3
	Spaghetti pasta:											
550	Without salt, enriched	1 c	140	66	197	7	40	4	1	.1	.1	.4
551	With salt, enriched	1 c	140	66	197	7	40	2	1	.1	.1	.4
552	Whole-wheat spaghetti, cooked	1 c	140	67	174	7	37	6	1	.1	.1	.3
1302	Tapioca, pearl, dry	1 c	152	11	544	<1	134	1	<1	.01	.01	.01
553	Wheat bran, crude	½ c	30	10	65	5	19	13	1	.2	.2	.7
554	Wheat germ, raw	1 c	100	11	360	23	52	13	10	1.7	1.4	6
555	Wheat germ, toasted	1 c	113	5	432	33	56	15	12	2.1	1.7	7.5
1669	Wheat germ, with brown sugar & honey	½ c	57	3	212	15	33	6	4	.8	.6	2.8
556	Rolled wheat, cooked	1 c	240	83	149	5	33	4	1	.1	.1	.5
557	Whole-grain wheat, cooked	⅓ c	50	86	28	1	7	1	<1	t	t	.1
	Wheat flour (unbleached):											
	All-purpose white, enriched:											
558	Sifted	1 c	115	11	419	12	88	3	1	.2	.1	.5
559	Unsifted	1 c	125	11	455	13	95	3	1	.2	.1	.5
560	Cake or pastry, enriched, sifted	1 c	96	12	348	8	75	2	1	.1	.1	.4
561	Self-rising, enriched, unsifted	1 c	125	11	443	12	93	3	1	.2	.1	.5
562	Whole wheat, from hard wheats	1 c	120	10	406	16	87	15	2	.4	.3	.9
	MEATS: FISH and SHELLFISH											
1045	Bass, baked or broiled	4 oz	113	69	165	27	0	0	5	1.4	1.5	2.3
1046	Bluefish, baked or broiled	4 oz	113	63	180	29	0	0	6	1.4	2	2.7
1047	Bluefish, fried in bread crumbs	4 oz	113	61	232	26	5	<1	11	2.4	4.9	2.8
1686	Catfish, breaded/flour fried	4 oz	113	49	325	21	14	1	20	5	9	5
	Clams:											
563	Raw meat only	4 oz	113	81	84	14	3	0	1	.2	.3	.5
564	Canned, drained	4 oz	113	72	168	29	6	0	2	.5	.6	1.1
1290	Steamed, meat only	20 ea	90	64	133	23	5	0	2	.4	.5	.8
	Cod:											
565	Baked with butter	4 oz	113	75	150	26	0	0	4	.4	.3	.6
566	Batter fried	4 oz	113	76	196	20	8	<1	9	2.2	3.6	2.6
567	Poached, no added fat	4 oz	113	77	116	25	0	0	1	.2	.1	.3
	Crab, meat only:											
1048	Blue crab, cooked	4 oz	113	77	115	23	0	0	2	.3	.3	.8
1049	Dungeness crab, cooked	4 oz	113	73	124	25	1	0	1	.2	.2	.5
568	Blue crab, canned	4 oz	113	76	112	23	0	0	1	.3	.2	.5
1587	Crab, imitation, from surimi	4 oz	113	74	115	14	12	0	1	.3	.2	.8
569	Fish sticks, breaded pollock	2 ea	57	46	155	9	14	<1	7	1.8	2.9	1.8
	Flounder/sole, baked w/lemon juice:											
570	With butter	4 oz	113	73	160	21	<1	0	8	4.3	2	.7
571	With margarine	4 oz	113	73	160	21	<1	0	8	1.6	3.1	2.5

(Computer code number is for West Diet Analysis program)

PAGE KEY: H–4 = BEV   H–6 = DAIRY   H–12 = EGGS   H–14 = FAT/OIL   H–18 = FRUIT   H–26 = BAKERY   H–36 = GRAIN   H–44 = FISH
H–48 = MEATS   H–50 = POULTRY   H–54 = SAUSAGE   H–56 = MIXED/FAST   H–64 = NUTS/SEEDS   H–68 = SWEETS   H–70 = VEG/LEG
H–84 = MISC   H–88 = SOUPS/SAUCES   H–90 = FAST   H–106 = FRZN ENTREE   H–112 = BABY FOODS

Chol (mg)	Calc (mg)	Iron (mg)	Magn (mg)	Pota (mg)	Sodi (mg)	Zinc (mg)	VT-A (RE)	Thia (mg)	VT-E (α-TE)	Ribo (mg)	Niac (mg)	V-B6 (mg)	Fola (μg)	VT-C (mg)
0	111	6.6	57	222	9	1.78	0	1.1	.24	.13	6.71	.65	31	0
0	33	1.98	21	65	5	.54	0	.44	.09	.03	2.45	.03	7	0
0	5	.34	12	24	12	.99	0	.05	.1	.03	.7	.06	2	0
0	5	.98	52	166	5	2.2	0	.08	.38	.14	2.12	.22	43	0
1	9	1.02	13	46	619	.31	0	.13	.15	.08	1.94	.11	8	<1
0	24	2.16	76	347	3	2.03	0	.29	1.4	.12	1.76	.27	19	0
0	165	5.27	201	2261	16	1.04	4	.33	.2	.25	1.9	.46	361	0
0	10	1.96	25	43	1	.74	0	.29	.08	.14	2.34	.05	10	0
0	10	1.96	25	43	140	.74	0	.29	.38	.14	2.34	.05	10	0
0	21	1.48	42	62	4	1.13	0	.15	.07	.06	.99	.11	7	0
0	30	2.4	2	17	2	.18	0	.01	0	0	0	.01	6	0
0	22	3.18	183	355	1	2.18	0	.16	.7	.17	4.08	.39	24	0
0	39	6.26	239	892	12	12.3	0	1.88	18	.5	6.81	1.3	281	0
0	51	10.3	362	1070	5	18.8	0	1.89	20.5	.93	6.32	1.11	398	7
0	29	4.59	155	550	6	7.92	6	.76	12.54	.39	2.7	.29	190	0
0	17	1.49	53	170	0	1.15	0	.17	.48	.12	2.14	.17	26	0
0	3	.29	12	33	<1	.24	0	.04	.1	.01	.5	.03	4	0
0	17	5.34	25	123	2	.8	0	.9	.07	.57	6.79	.05	30	0
0	19	5.8	27	133	2	.87	0	.98	.08	.62	7.38	.05	32	0
0	13	7	15	101	2	.6	0	.36	.06	.4	6.5	.03	18	0
0	422	5.84	24	155	1588	.77	0	.84	.08	.52	7.29	.06	53	0
0	41	4.66	166	486	6	3.52	0	.54	1.48	.26	7.64	.41	53	0
98	116	2.16	43	515	102	.94	40	.1	.84	.1	1.72	.16	19	2
86	10	.7	47	539	87	1.18	156	.08	.71	.11	8.19	.52	2	0
68	9	.6	42	468	76	1.02	136	.07	2.6	.09	6.22	.41	2	<1
92	41	1.44	34	376	598	1.03	33	.4	2.48	.19	3.4	.21	19	1
38	52	15.9	10	355	63	1.54	102	.09	1.13	.24	2	.07	18	15
76	104	31.6	20	712	127	3.1	194	.17	2.15	.48	3.79	.12	33	25
60	83	25.2	16	565	101	2.46	154	.13	1.8	.38	3.02	.1	26	20
68	23	.56	48	277	254	.66	34	.1	.41	.09	2.85	.32	11	<1
64	43	.9	36	443	124	.61	17	.12	.92	.13	2.58	.23	10	1
61	23	.54	41	496	69	.64	14	.09	.32	.08	2.48	.28	8	1
113	118	1.03	37	367	315	4.79	2	.11	1.13	.06	3.74	.2	57	4
86	67	.49	66	461	427	6.21	35	.06	1.3	.23	4.11	.2	47	4
100	114	.95	44	423	376	4.56	2	.09	1.13	.09	1.55	.17	48	3
23	15	.44	49	102	951	.37	23	.04	.12	.03	.2	.03	2	0
64	11	.42	14	149	331	.38	18	.07	.78	.1	1.21	.03	10	0
91	21	.37	67	363	193	.71	72	.09	2.5	.13	2.47	.27	13	1
73	21	.37	67	364	201	.71	92	.09	3.12	.13	2.47	.27	13	1

(For purposes of calculations, use "0" for t, <1, <.1, <.01, etc.)

H

Table H-1
Food Composition

Computer Code Number	Food Description	Measure	Wt (g)	H₂O (%)	Ener (kcal)	Prot (g)	Carb (g)	Dietary Fiber (g)	Fat (g)	Fat Breakdown (g) Sat	Mono	Poly
MEATS: FISH and SHELLFISH—Cont.												
572	Without added fat	4 oz	113	73	133	27	0	0	2	.5	.4	.9
1599	Grouper, baked or broiled	4 oz	113	73	133	28	0	0	1	.4	.4	.6
573	Haddock, breaded, fried[1]	4 oz	113	55	264	22	14	1	13	3.2	5.4	3.3
1050	Haddock, smoked	4 oz	113	72	131	28	0	0	1	.3	.3	.5
	Halibut:											
574	Baked with butter & lemon juice	4 oz	113	69	186	29	0	0	7	2.7	2.1	1.1
1051	Smoked	1 oz	28	49	63	6	0	0	4	.7	1.3	1.9
1054	Raw	4 oz	113	78	124	24	0	0	3	.7	.8	1.1
575	Herring, pickled	3 oz	85	55	223	12	8	0	15	3.3	8.3	3.6
1052	Lobster meat, cooked w/moist heat	1 c	145	76	142	30	2	0	1	.2	.2	.5
1687	Ocean perch, baked/broiled	4 oz	113	73	137	27	0	0	2	.4	1	.7
576	Ocean perch, breaded/fried	4 oz	113	59	249	22	9	<1	13	3.2	5.7	3.4
1056	Octopus, raw	4 oz	113	80	93	17	3	0	1	.3	.2	.3
	Oysters:											
577	Raw, Eastern	1 c	248	85	169	17	10	0	6	2	.9	2.9
578	Raw, Pacific	1 c	248	82	201	23	12	0	6	1.3	.9	2.2
	Cooked:											
579	Eastern, breaded, fried, medium	6 ea	88	65	173	8	10	<1	11	3.2	2	5.6
580	Western, simmered	4 oz	113	64	184	21	11	0	5	1.7	.8	2.4
581	Pollock, baked or broiled	4 oz	113	74	128	27	0	0	1	.3	.2	.6
1055	Pollock, moist heat, poached	4 oz	113	74	128	27	0	0	1	.3	.2	.6
	Salmon:											
582	Canned pink, solids and liquid	4 oz	113	69	157	22	0	0	7	1.7	2.1	2.3
583	Broiled or baked	4 oz	113	62	244	31	0	0	12	2.2	6	2.7
584	Smoked	4 oz	113	72	132	21	0	0	5	1	2.3	1.1
585	Atlantic sardines, canned, drained, 2 = 24 g	4 oz	113	60	235	28	0	0	13	1.9	4.4	6.4
586	Scallops, breaded, cooked from frozen	6 ea	93	58	199	17	9	<1	10	2.1	2.5	5.3
1588	Scallops, imitation, from surimi	4 oz	113	74	112	14	12	0	<1	.1	.1	.3
1688	Scallops, steamed/boiled	½ c	60	76	64	10	1	0	2	.3	.7	.6
	Shrimp:											
587	Cooked, boiled, 2 large = 11 g	16 ea	86	77	76	16	0	0	1	.2	.2	.4
588	Canned, drained	½ c	64	73	77	15	1	0	1	.3	.3	.7
589	Fried, 2 large = 15 g[1]	12 ea	90	53	218	19	10	<1	11	2	3	5.9
1057	Raw, large, about 7 g each	14 ea	100	76	106	20	1	0	2	.3	.4	1
1589	Shrimp, imitation, from surimi	4 oz	113	75	114	14	10	0	2	.3	.2	1
1053	Snapper, baked or broiled	4 oz	113	70	145	30	0	0	2	.4	.4	.7
1060	Squid, fried in flour[2]	4 oz	113	65	198	20	9	0	8	2.1	3.1	2.4
1590	Surimi[3]	4 oz	113	76	112	17	8	0	1	.2	.2	.6
1058	Swordfish, raw	4 oz	113	76	137	22	0	0	5	1.3	1.8	1
1059	Swordfish, baked or broiled	4 oz	113	69	175	29	0	0	6	1.7	2.2	1.3
590	Trout, baked or broiled	4 oz	113	71	170	26	0	0	7	1.8	2	2.2
	Tuna, light, canned, drained solids:											
591	Oil pack	3 oz	85	60	168	25	0	0	7	1.3	2.5	2.5
592	Water pack	3 oz	85	75	99	22	0	0	1	.2	.1	.3
1061	Bluefin tuna, fresh	4 oz	113	68	163	26	0	0	6	1.4	1.8	1.6

[1] Dipped in egg, bread crumbs, and flour; fried in vegetable shortening.
[2] Recipe is 94.6% squid, 4.9% flour, and 0.6% salt.
[3] Surimi is processed from Walleye (Alaska) pollock. Also see Imitation crab, shrimp, scallops.

Chol (mg)	Calc (mg)	Iron (mg)	Magn (mg)	Pota (mg)	Sodi (mg)	Zinc (mg)	VT-A (RE)	Thia (mg)	VT-E (α-TE)	Ribo (mg)	Niac (mg)	V-B6 (mg)	Fola (μg)	VT-C (mg)
77	20	.39	66	390	119	.72	13	.09	2.6	.13	2.47	.27	10	2
53	24	1.29	42	537	60	.58	57	.09	.71	.01	.43	.4	12	0
96	63	1.93	46	346	524	.59	33	.08	1.56	.14	4.51	.28	19	<1
87	55	1.58	61	469	862	.57	25	.05	.57	.06	5.75	.45	17	0
54	66	1.17	116	636	112	.57	93	.08	1.27	.1	7.69	.43	16	5
28	13	.24	23	126	134	.12	13	.01	.27	.02	1.64	.09	1	<1
36	53	.95	94	509	61	.48	53	.07	.96	.08	6.62	.39	14	0
11	65	1.04	7	59	740	.45	219	.03	1.4	.12	2.81	.14	2	0
104	88	.57	51	510	551	4.23	38	.01	2.1	.1	1.55	.11	16	0
61	155	1	44	396	109	.7	16	.15	1.8	.15	2.76	.31	12	1
71	136	1.58	38	324	432	.67	23	.14	2.41	.18	2.69	.24	15	1
54	60	6.01	34	396	260	1.9	51	.03	1.36	.04	2.37	.41	18	6
131	112	16.5	117	387	523	225	74	.25	1.98	.24	3.42	.15	25	9
124	20	12.6	55	417	263	41.2	201	.17	2.11	.58	4.98	.12	25	20
71	55	6.12	51	214	367	76.6	79	.13	2.01	.18	1.45	.06	12	3
113	18	10.4	50	341	240	37.5	165	.14	2	.5	4.1	.1	17	14
109	7	.32	83	439	132	.68	26	.08	.32	.09	1.87	.08	4	0
109	7	.32	83	437	132	.68	26	.08	.32	.09	1.87	.08	4	0
62	241[4]	.95	38	368	626	1.04	19	.03	1.53	.21	7.42	.34	17	0
98	8	.62	35	425	75	.58	71	.24	1.42	.19	7.56	.25	6	0
26	12	.96	20	198	886	.35	29	.03	1.53	.11	5.33	.31	2	0
160	433[4]	3.3	44	449	571	1.5	76	.09	.34	.26	5.93	.19	13	0
57	39	.76	55	310	432	.99	20	.04	1.77	.1	1.4	.13	17	2
25	9	.35	49	116	898	.37	23	.01	.12	.02	.35	.03	2	0
19	15	.15	33	168	246	.55	27	.01	.81	.04	.6	.08	7	1
150	30	2.37	26	140	172	1.2	51	.02	.66	.03	1.99	.09	3	2
111	38	1.75	26	134	108	.8	12	.02	.6	.02	1.76	.07	1	1
159	60	1.13	36	203	310	1.24	50	.12	1.35	.12	2.76	.09	7	1
152	52	2.41	37	185	148	1.11	54	.03	.82	.03	2.55	.1	3	2
41	21	.68	49	101	797	.37	23	.03	.12	.04	.19	.03	2	0
53	45	.27	42	590	64	.5	40	.06	.7	<.01	.39	.52	7	2
294	44	1.14	43	315	346	1.97	12	.06	2.1	.52	2.94	.07	6	5
34	10	.29	49	127	162	.37	23	.02	.28	.02	.25	.03	2	0
44	5	.92	31	325	102	1.3	41	.04	.57	.11	11	.37	2	1
57	7	1.18	38	417	130	1.67	46	.05	.71	.13	13.3	.43	3	1
78	97	.43	35	506	63	.58	17	.17	.57	.11	6.52	.39	21	2
15	11	1.18	26	176	301	.77	20	.03	1.02	.1	10.5	.09	5	0
26	9	1.3	23	202	287	.65	14	.03	.45	.06	11.3	.3	3	0
43	9	1.15	57	285	44	.68	740	.27	1.13	.28	9.78	.51	2	0

[4]If bones are discarded, calcium value is greatly reduced.

(For purposes of calculations, use "0" for t, <1, <.1, <.01, etc.)

H

Table H–1
Food Composition

Computer Code Number	Food Description	Measure	Wt (g)	H$_2$O (%)	Ener (kcal)	Prot (g)	Carb (g)	Dietary Fiber (g)	Fat (g)	Fat Breakdown (g)		
										Sat	Mono	Poly
	MEATS: BEEF, LAMB, PORK, and others											
	BEEF, cooked:[1]											
	Braised, simmered, pot roasted:											
	Relatively fat, choice chuck blade:											
593	Lean and fat, piece 2½ x 2½ x ¾"	4 oz	113	47	393	31	0	0	29	13	14.8	1.2
594	Lean only	4 oz	113	55	297	35	0	0	16	7.3	8.2	.7
	Relatively lean, like choice round:											
595	Lean and fat, pce 4⅛ x 2½ x ¾"	4 oz	113	52	311	32	0	0	19	8.6	9.7	.8
596	Lean only	4 oz	113	57	249	36	0	0	11	4.8	5.4	.5
	Ground beef, broiled, patty 3 x ⅝":											
597	Extra lean, about 16% fat	4 oz	113	54	300	32	0	0	18	8	9.1	.8
598	Lean, 21% fat	4 oz	113	53	316	32	0	0	20	8.9	10.1	.8
	Roasts, oven cooked, no added liquid:											
	Relatively fat, prime rib:											
601	Lean and fat, pce 4⅛ x 2¼ x ½"	4 oz	113	46	425	25	0	0	35	15.8	17.9	1.5
602	Lean only	4 oz	113	58	271	31	0	0	16	7	7.9	.7
	Relatively lean, choice round:											
603	Lean and fat, pce 2½ x 2½ x ¾"	4 oz	113	59	272	30	0	0	16	7.1	8.1	.7
604	Lean only	4 oz	113	65	198	33	0	0	6	2.9	3.3	.3
1701	Steak, rib, broiled, lean	4 oz	113	58	250	32	0	0	13	5.7	6.4	.5
	Steak, broiled, relatively lean, choice sirloin:											
606	Lean only	4 oz	113	62	228	34	0	0	9	4	4.6	.4
	Steak, broiled, relatively fat, choice T-bone:											
1063	Lean and fat	4 oz	113	53	349	26	0	0	26	11.8	13.3	1.1
1064	Lean only	4 oz	113	62	232	30	0	0	11	5.1	5.8	.5
	Variety meats:											
1086	Brains, panfried	4 oz	113	71	222	14	0	0	18	6.7	7	3.9
599	Heart, simmered	4 oz	113	64	198	33	<1	0	6	2.9	1.5	1.5
600	Liver, fried	4 oz	113	56	245	30	9	0	9	3	1.8	1.9
1062	Tongue, cooked	4 oz	113	56	320	25	<1	0	23	10.1	11	.9
607	Beef, canned, corned	4 oz	113	58	283	31	0	0	17	7.5	8.5	.7
608	Beef, dried, cured	1 oz	28	57	46	8	<1	0	1	.5	.5	.1
	LAMB, domestic, cooked:											
	Chop, arm, braised (5.6 oz raw w/bone):											
609	Lean and fat	1 ea	70	44	242	21	0	0	17	7.8	7.3	1.4
610	Lean only	1 ea	55	49	154	20	0	0	8	3.6	3.4	.6
	Chop, loin, broiled (4.2 oz. raw w/bone):											
611	Lean and fat	1 ea	64	52	202	16	0	0	15	6.8	6.4	1.2
612	Lean only	1 ea	46	61	99	14	0	0	4	2.1	2	.4
1067	Cutlet, avg of lean cuts, cooked	4 oz	113	54	330	28	0	0	23	10.9	10.2	2
	Leg, roasted, 3 oz = 4⅛ x 2¼ x ½":											
613	Lean and fat	4 oz	113	58	292	29	0	0	19	8.7	8.1	1.6
614	Lean only	4 oz	113	64	216	32	0	0	9	4.1	3.8	.7
615	Rib, roasted, lean and fat	4 oz	113	48	406	24	0	0	34	15.7	14.7	2.8
616	Rib, roasted, lean only	4 oz	113	60	262	30	0	0	15	7	6.6	1.3
1065	Shoulder, roasted, lean and fat	4 oz	113	56	312	25	0	0	23	10.5	9.9	1.9

[1]Outer layer of fat removed to about ½" of the lean. Deposits of fat within the cut remain.

(Computer code number is for West Diet Analysis program)

Chol (mg)	Calc (mg)	Iron (mg)	Magn (mg)	Pota (mg)	Sodi (mg)	Zinc (mg)	VT-A (RE)	Thia (mg)	VT-E (α-TE)	Ribo (mg)	Niac (mg)	V-B6 (mg)	Fola (µg)	VT-C (mg)
112	11	3.46	22	275	67	7.57	0	.08	.26	.27	3.54	.32	10	0
120	15	4.16	26	297	80	11.6	0	.09	.16	.32	3.02	.33	7	0
109	7	3.53	25	319	57	5.55	0	.08	.21	.27	4.22	.37	11	0
109	6	3.91	28	348	58	6.19	0	.08	.2	.29	4.61	.41	12	0
112	10	3.14	28	417	93	7.27	0	.08	.2	.36	6.61	.36	12	0
114	14	2.77	27	394	101	7.01	0	.07	.23	.27	6.77	.34	12	0
96	12	2.61	21	335	71	5.92	0	.08	.27	.19	3.8	.26	8	0
92	11	2.95	28	425	84	7.84	0	.09	.14	.24	4.64	.34	9	0
81	7	2.07	27	406	67	4.87	0	.09	.23	.18	3.92	.4	7	0
78	6	2.2	31	446	70	5.36	0	.1	.12	.19	4.24	.43	8	0
90	15	3	31	445	78	8	0	.11	.16	.25	5.42	.45	9	0
101	12	3.8	36	455	75	7.37	0	.15	.16	.33	4.84	.51	11	0
76	9	3.01	26	363	72	5.3	0	.1	.24	.24	4.64	.37	8	0
67	7	3.6	32	427	80	6.12	0	.12	.16	.28	5.23	.44	9	0
2254	10	2.51	17	400	179	1.53	0	.15	2.37	.29	4.27	.44	7	4
218	7	8.49	28	263	71	3.54	0	.16	.81	1.74	4.6	.24	2	2
545	12	7.1	26	411	120	6.16	12123[2]	.24	.72	4.68	16.3	1.62	249	26
121	8	3.83	19	203	68	5.42	0	.03	.4	.4	2.44	.18	6	1
97	14	2.35	16	154	1136	4.03	0	.02	.17	.17	2.75	.15	10	0
12	2	1.26	9	124	972	1.47	0	.02	.04	.06	1.53	.1	3	3
84	18	1.67	18	214	50	4.26	0	.05	.11	.18	4.67	.08	13	0
67	14	1.49	16	186	42	4.01	0	.04	.1	.15	3.48	.07	12	0
64	13	1.16	15	209	49	2.23	0	.06	.08	.16	4.54	.08	12	0
44	9	.92	13	173	39	1.9	0	.05	.07	.13	3.15	.07	11	0
110	12	2.26	25	340	77	4.68	0	.13	.15	.32	7.48	.16	19	0
105	12	2.24	27	354	75	4.97	0	.11	.17	.31	7.45	.17	23	0
101	9	2.4	29	382	77	5.6	0	.12	.2	.33	7.16	.19	26	0
110	25	1.81	23	306	82	3.94	0	.1	.11	.24	7.63	.12	17	0
99	24	2	24	356	92	5.05	0	.1	.17	.26	6.96	.17	25	0
104	23	2.23	26	284	75	5.91	0	.1	.16	.27	6.95	.15	24	0

[2]Value varies widely.

(For purposes of calculations, use "0" for t, <1, <.1, <.01, etc.)

Table H–1
Food Composition

Computer Code Number	Food Description	Measure	Wt (g)	H₂O (%)	Ener (kcal)	Prot (g)	Carb (g)	Dietary Fiber (g)	Fat (g)	Sat	Mono	Poly
										Fat Breakdown (g)		
MEATS: BEEF, LAMB, PORK, and others—Cont.												
1066	Shoulder, roasted, lean only	4 oz	113	63	231	28	0	0	12	5.7	5.3	1.1
	Variety meats:											
1069	Brains, panfried	4 oz	113	76	164	14	0	0	12	4.4	3.7	1.9
1068	Heart, braised	4 oz	113	64	209	28	2	0	9	3.9	2.7	1.1
1070	Sweetbreads, cooked	4 oz	113	60	264	26	0	0	17	8.2	6.6	1.4
1071	Tongue, cooked	4 oz	113	58	311	24	0	0	23	8.9	11.7	1.4
	PORK, cured, cooked (see also #669–672):											
617	Bacon, medium slices	3 pce	19	13	109	6	<1	0	9	3.3	4.5	1.1
1087	Breakfast strips, cooked	2 pce	23	27	106	7	<1	0	8	2.9	3.7	1.3
618	Canadian-style bacon	2 pce	47	62	87	11	1	0	4	1.3	1.9	.4
	Ham, roasted:											
619	Lean and fat, 2 pces 4⅛ x 2¼ x ¼"	4 oz	113	65	202	26	0	0	10	3.5	5.1	1.7
620	Lean only	4 oz	113	68	164	24	2	0	6	2	3	.6
621	Ham, canned, roasted, 8% fat	4 oz	113	69	154	24	1	0	6	1.8	2.8	.5
	PORK, fresh, cooked:											
	Chops, loin (cut 3 per lb with bone):											
1291	Braised, lean and fat	1 ea	71	58	170	19	0	0	10	3.6	4.3	1
1292	Braised, lean only	1 ea	55	61	112	16	0	0	5	1.9	2.3	.4
622	Broiled, lean and fat	1 ea	87	58	209	25	0	0	11	4.2	5	.9
623	Broiled, lean only	1 ea	72	61	146	22	0	0	6	2	2.6	.4
624	Panfried, lean and fat	1 ea	89	53	247	27	0	0	15	5.4	6.3	1.7
625	Panfried, lean only	1 ea	67	59	161	17	0	0	10	3.5	4	1.3
626	Leg, roasted, lean and fat	4 oz	113	55	310	30	0	0	20	7	9	2
627	Leg, roasted, lean only	4 oz	113	61	234	35	0	0	9	3	4	1
628	Rib, roasted, lean and fat	4 oz	113	56	289	31	0	0	17	6.7	7.9	1.5
629	Rib, roasted, lean only	4 oz	113	59	253	33	0	0	13	4.9	6	1
630	Shoulder, braised, lean and fat	4 oz	113	48	373	32	0	0	26	9.6	11.8	2.6
631	Shoulder, braised, lean only	4 oz	113	54	281	37	0	0	14	4.7	6.6	1.3
1088	Spareribs, cooked, yield from 1 lb raw with bone	4 oz	113	40	450	33	0	0	34	12.6	15	3
1095	Rabbit, roasted (1 cup meat = 140 g)	4 oz	113	61	223	33	0	0	9	4	2	3
	VEAL, cooked:											
632	Cutlet, braised or broiled, 4⅛ x 2¼ x ½"	4 oz	113	52	322	34	0	0	20	7.6	7.6	1.3
633	Rib roasted, lean, 2 pieces 4⅛ x 2¼ x ¼"	4 oz	113	60	259	27	0	0	16	6.1	6.2	1.1
634	Liver, panfried	4 oz	113	67	187	25	3	0	8	3.3	1.9	2.2
1096	Venison (deer meat), roasted	4 oz	113	65	179	34	0	0	4	1.4	1	.7
MEATS: POULTRY and POULTRY PRODUCTS												
	CHICKEN, cooked:											
	Fried, batter dipped:[1]											
635	Breast (5.6 oz with bones)	1 ea	140	52	364	35	13	<1	19	5	7.6	4.3
636	Drumstick (3.4 oz with bones)	1 ea	72	53	193	16	6	<1	11	3	4.7	2.7
637	Thigh	1 ea	86	52	238	19	8	<1	14	3.8	5.9	3.4
638	Wing	1 ea	49	46	159	10	5	<1	11	2.9	4.5	2.5
	Fried, flour coated:[1]											
639	Breast (4.2 oz with bones)	1 ea	98	57	218	31	2	<1	9	2.5	3.5	1.9

[1]Fried in vegetable shortening.

(Computer code number is for West Diet Analysis program)

PAGE KEY: H–4 = BEV   H–6 = DAIRY   H–12 = EGGS   H–14 = FAT/OIL   H–18 = FRUIT   H–26 = BAKERY   H–36 = GRAIN   H–44 = FISH
H–48 = MEATS   H–50 = POULTRY   H–54 = SAUSAGE   H–56 = MIXED/FAST   H–64 = NUTS/SEEDS   H–68 = SWEETS   H–70 = VEG/LEG
H–84 = MISC   H–88 = SOUPS/SAUCES   H–90 = FAST   H–106 = FRZN ENTREE   H–112 = BABY FOODS

Chol (mg)	Calc (mg)	Iron (mg)	Magn (mg)	Pota (mg)	Sodi (mg)	Zinc (mg)	VT-A (RE)	Thia (mg)	VT-E (α-TE)	Ribo (mg)	Niac (mg)	V-B6 (mg)	Fola (μg)	VT-C (mg)
99	21	2.42	28	301	77	6.85	0	.1	.2	.29	6.53	.17	28	0
2309	14	1.91	16	232	152	1.54	0	.12	1.73	.27	2.8	.12	6	14
281	16	6.26	27	213	71	4.17	0	.19	.79	1.35	4.94	.34	2	8
452	14	2.4	21	328	59	3.04	0	.02	.77	.24	2.9	.06	15	23
213	11	2.99	18	179	76	3.39	0	.09	.36	.48	4.18	.19	3	8
16	2	.31	5	92	303	.62	0	.13	.1	.05	1.39	.05	1	0
24	3	.45	6	107	483	.83	0	.17	.08	.08	1.72	.08	1	0
27	5	.38	10	183	726	.8	0	.39	.16	.09	3.25	.21	2	0
67	9	1.52	25	464	1701	2.8	0	.83	.45	.37	6.97	.35	3	0
60	9	1.68	16	326	1364	3.3	0	.86	.29	.23	4.56	.45	3	0
34	7	1	24	395	1287	2.6	0	1.2	.29	.28	5.55	.51	6	0
57	15	.76	13	266	34	1.7	2	.43	.24	.18	3	.26	2	<1
43	10	.62	11	213	28	1.4	1	.36	.21	.15	2.52	.21	2	<1
71	29	.7	22	312	50	2	3	.93	.28	.25	4.56	.37	5	<1
59	22	.61	19	270	43	1.7	2	.83	.3	.22	3.99	.34	4	<1
82	24	.81	26	378	71	2	2	1	.37	.27	5	.4	5	<1
55	15	.7	17	245	52	2.6	1	.49	.32	.24	3.03	.27	3	<1
107	16	1.15	25	399	68	3.36	3	.72	.34	.35	5.18	.46	11	<1
109	8	1.29	33	443	74	3.41	3	.91	.46	.4	5.58	.38	3	<1
83	32	1.01	24	477	52	2.34	2	.82	.41	.34	7	.37	3	<1
81	30	1.11	25	496	53	2.4	2	.86	.55	.36	7	.39	3	<1
124	20	1.83	22	418	100	4.7	3	.61	.5	.35	6	.4	5	<1
129	9	2.21	25	459	116	5.64	3	.68	.59	.41	6.74	.47	6	<1
137	53	2.1	27	363	106	5.22	3	.46	.52	.43	6.2	.4	5	0
93	22	2.57	24	434	53	2.57	0	.1	.96	.24	9.56	.53	13	0
134	32	1.24	27	318	91	4.12	0	.05	.45	.34	10.24	.3	16	0
125	13	1.1	25	335	104	4.64	0	.06	.4	.31	7.92	.28	15	0
636	8	2.97	22	233	60	10.8	9127[2]	.15	.42	2.2	9.62	.56	861	35
127	8	5.07	27	380	61	3.12	0	.2	.28	.68	7.61	.43[3]	5[3]	0
119	28	1.75	34	281	385	1.33	28	.16	1.48	.2	14.7	.6	8	0
62	12	.97	14	134	194	1.68	19	.08	.88	.16	3.67	.19	7	0
80	16	1.25	18	165	247	1.75	25	.1	1.05	.2	4.92	.22	8	0
39	10	.63	8	68	157	.68	17	.05	.52	.08	2.58	.15	3	0
87	16	1.17	29	254	75	1.08	15	.08	.56	.13	13.43	.57	4	0

[2]Value varies widely.

[3]Values estimated from other game meat.

(For purposes of calculations, use "0" for t, <1, <.1, <.01, etc.)

H

Table H–1
Food Composition

Computer Code Number	Food Description	Measure	Wt (g)	H₂O (%)	Ener (kcal)	Prot (g)	Carb (g)	Dietary Fiber (g)	Fat (g)	Fat Breakdown (g) Sat	Mono	Poly
	MEATS: POULTRY and POULTRY PRODUCTS—Cont.											
	CHICKEN—Cont.											
1212	Breast, without skin	1 ea	86	60	161	29	<1	<1	4	1.1	1.6	.9
640	Drumstick (2.6 oz with bones)	1 ea	49	57	120	13	1	<1	7	1.8	2.7	1.6
641	Thigh	1 ea	62	54	162	17	2	<1	9	2.5	3.7	2.1
1099	Thigh, without skin	1 ea	52	59	113	15	1	<1	5	1.4	2	1.3
642	Wing	1 ea	32	49	103	8	1	<1	7	2	2.9	1.6
	Roasted:											
643	All types of meat	1 c	140	64	266	41	0	0	10	2.9	3.9	2.4
644	Dark meat	1 c	140	63	287	38	0	0	14	3.7	5	3.2
645	Light meat	1 c	140	65	242	43	0	0	6	1.8	2.2	1.4
646	Breast, without skin	1 ea	86	65	142	27	0	0	3	.9	1.1	.7
647	Drumstick	1 ea	44	67	76	13	0	0	3	.7	.8	.6
1703	Leg, without skin	1 ea	95	65	163	26	0	0	5	1.4	2	1
648	Thigh	1 ea	62	59	153	15	0	0	10	2.7	3.8	2.1
1100	Thigh, without skin	1 ea	52	63	108	13	0	0	6	1.6	2.2	1.3
649	Stewed, all types:	1 c	140	67	248	38	0	0	9	2.6	3.3	2.2
656	Canned, boneless chicken	4 oz	113	69	187	25	0	0	9	2.5	3.6	2
1102	Gizzards, simmered	3 ea	66	67	101	18	1	0	2	.7	.6	.7
1101	Hearts, simmered	8 ea	25	65	45	6	<1	0	2	.6	.5	.6
2300	Liver, simmered: Ounce	3 oz	85	68	133	21	1	0	5	1.6	1.1	.8
1098	Liver, simmered: Piece = 20 g	6 ea	120	68	188	29	1	0	7	2.2	1.6	1.1
	DUCK, roasted:											
1293	Meat with skin, about 2.7 cups	½ ea	382	52	1288	73	0	0	109	37	49.3	13.9
651	Meat only, about 1.5 cups	½ ea	221	64	444	52	0	0	25	9.2	8.2	3.2
	GOOSE, domesticated, roasted:											
1294	Meat only, 4.2 cups	½ ea	591	57	1407	173	0	0	75	23.6	40	10.9
1295	Meat with skin, about 5.5 cups	½ ea	774	52	2360	195	0	0	170	53.2	80.5	24.8
	TURKEY:											
	Roasted, meat only:											
652	Dark meat	4 oz	113	63	212	33	0	0	8	2.7	1.9	2.5
653	Light meat	4 oz	113	66	178	34	0	0	4	1.2	.6	1
654	All types, chopped or diced	1 c	140	65	238	42	0	0	7	2.3	1.5	2
655	All types, sliced	4 oz	113	65	193	34	0	0	6	1.9	1.2	1.6
1103	Ground, cooked	4 oz	113	59	267	31	0	0	15	4.2	5.6	3.7
1106	Gizzard, cooked	2 ea	134	65	218	39	1	0	5	1.5	1	1.5
1107	Heart, cooked	4 ea	64	64	113	17	1	0	4	1.1	.8	1.1
1108	Liver, cooked	1 ea	75	66	127	18	3	0	5	1.4	1.1	.8
	POULTRY FOOD PRODUCTS (see also items in Sausages and Lunchmeats section):											
1567	Chicken patty, breaded, cooked	1 ea	75	49	213	12	11	<1	13	4	6	1.7
659	Turkey and gravy, frozen package	3 oz	85	85	57	5	4	<1	2	.8	.8	.4
	Turkey breast, Louis Rich:											
1104	Barbecued	2 oz	57	40	58	12	2	0	1	.2	.2	.1
1943	Hickory smoked	1 pce	80	–	80	16	2	0	1	0	–	–

(Computer code number is for West Diet Analysis program)

TABLE OF FOOD COMPOSITION ◆ **H-53**

PAGE KEY: H–4 = BEV   H–6 = DAIRY   H–12 = EGGS   H–14 = FAT/OIL   H–18 = FRUIT   H–26 = BAKERY   H–36 = GRAIN   H–44 = FISH
H–48 = MEATS   H–50 = POULTRY   H–54 = SAUSAGE   H–56 = MIXED/FAST   H–64 = NUTS/SEEDS   H–68 = SWEETS   H–70 = VEG/LEG
H–84 = MISC   H–88 = SOUPS/SAUCES   H–90 = FAST   H–106 = FRZN ENTREE   H–112 = BABY FOODS

Chol (mg)	Calc (mg)	Iron (mg)	Magn (mg)	Pota (mg)	Sodi (mg)	Zinc (mg)	VT-A (RE)	Thia (mg)	VT-E (α-TE)	Ribo (mg)	Niac (mg)	V-B6 (mg)	Fola (µg)	VT-C (mg)
78	14	.98	27	237	68	.93	6	.07	.36	.11	12.7	.55	3	0
44	6	.66	11	112	44	1.42	12	.04	.41	.11	2.96	.17	4	0
60	9	.92	16	147	55	1.56	18	.06	.52	.15	4.31	.2	5	0
53	7	.76	14	135	49	1.45	11	.05	.3	.13	3.7	.2	5	0
26	5	.4	6	57	25	.56	12	.02	.18	.04	2.14	.13	1	0
125	21	1.69	35	340	120	2.94	22	.1	.58	.25	12.8	.66	8	0
130	21	1.86	32	336	130	3.92	31	.1	.81	.32	9.17	.5	11	0
119	21	1.48	38	346	108	1.72	13	.09	.37	.16	17.4	.84	6	0
73	13	.89	25	220	64	.86	5	.06	.33	.1	11.8	.52	3	0
41	5	.57	11	108	42	1.4	8	.03	.26	.1	2.68	.17	4	0
88	11	1.26	23	234	90	3.03	18	.07		.22	5.8	.35	9	0
58	7	.83	14	137	52	1.46	30	.04		.13	3.95	.19	4	0
49	6	.68	12	123	46	1.34	10	.04		.12	3.39	.18	4	0
116	20	1.64	29	252	98	2.79	21	.07		.23	8.55	.36	8	0
70	16	1.79	14	155	570	1.6	39	.02		.15	7.18	.4	5	2
128	7	2.74	13	118	44	2.89	37	.02		.16	2.63	.08	35	1
61	5	2.22	5	33	12	1.8	2	.01		.18	.69	.08	20	<1
536	12	7.23	18	119	42	3.68	4177	.13		1.49	3.78	.5	655	13
757	17	10.2	25	168	61	5.21	5895	.18	2.04	2.1	5.34	.7	924	19
321	42	10.3	61	779	225	7.1	241	.67	2.5	1.03	18.45	.69	23	0
197	27	5.97	44	557	144	5.75	51	.57	1.55	1.04	11.3	.55	22	0
568	83	17	148	2293	449	18.7	71	.54	9.16	2.3	24.1	2.78	71	0
704	101	21.9	170	2547	542	20.3	163	.6	13.47	2.5	32.3	2.86	16	0
96	36	2.64	27	329	90	5.06	0	.07	.95	.28	4.14	.41	10	0
78	22	1.53	32	346	73	2.31	0	.07	.12	.15	7.76	.61	7	0
106	35	2.49	36	417	98	4.34	0	.09	.59	.25	7.62	.64	10	0
86	28	2.02	29	338	79	3.52	0	.07	.48	.21	6.17	.52	8	0
116	28	2.2	27	306	121	3.24	0	.06	.45	.19	5.47	.44	8	0
311	20	7.29	26	283	72	5.57	74	.04	.27	.44	4.11	.16	70	2
145	8	4.4	14	117	35	3.37	5	.05	.13	.57	2.08	.2	51	1
470	8	5.85	11	146	48	2.32	2805	.04	2.41	1.07	4.46	.39	500	1
45	12	.94	15	185	399	.78	23	.07	1.46	.1	5.04	.23	8	<1
15	12	.79	7	52	472	.6	11	.02	.3	.11	1.53	.09	3	0
25	14	.6	16	178	608	.6	0	.02	–	.06	5.45	.22	2	0
35	0	.72	–	–	1060	–	0	–	–	–	–	–	–	0

(For purposes of calculations, use "0" for t, <1, <.1, <.01, etc.)

H

Table H–1
Food Composition

Computer Code Number	Food Description	Measure	Wt (g)	H₂O (%)	Ener (kcal)	Prot (g)	Carb (g)	Dietary Fiber (g)	Fat (g)	Fat Breakdown (g) Sat	Mono	Poly
MEATS:	**POULTRY and POULTRY PRODUCTS**											
	TURKEY—Cont.											
1947	Honey roasted	1 pce	80	–	80	16	3	0	1	.5	–	–
1945	Oven roasted	1 pce	80	–	70	16	–	0	1	.0	–	–
661	Turkey patty, breaded, fried	2 oz	57	50	161	8	9	<1	10	2.7	4.2	2.7
662	Turkey, frozen, roasted, seasoned	4 oz	113	68	176	25	4	0	7	2.2	1.4	1.9
1704	Turkey roll, light meat	1 pce	28	72	41	5	<1	0	2	.6	.7	.5
MEATS:	**SAUSAGES and LUNCHMEATS** (see also Poultry Food Products)											
1072	Beerwurst/beer salami, beef	1 oz	28	53	93	4	<1	0	9	3.7	4	.3
1074	Beerwurst/beer salami, pork	1 oz	28	62	68	4	1	0	5	1.8	2.6	.7
1075	Berliner sausage	1 oz	28	61	65	4	1	0	5	1.7	2.3	.5
	Bologna:											
1297	Beef	1 pce	23	55	72	3	<1	0	7	2.8	3.2	.3
2115	Beef, light, Oscar Mayer	1 pce	28	65	56	3	2	0	4	1.6	2	.1
663	Beef & pork	1 pce	28	54	90	3	1	0	8	3	3.8	.7
2155	Healthy Favorites	2 ea	46	–	45	7	2	0	1	0	–	–
1298	Pork	1 pce	23	61	57	4	<1	0	5	1.6	2.3	.5
2114	Regular, light, Oscar Mayer	1 pce	28	65	56	3	2	0	4	1.6	2.1	.4
664	Turkey	1 pce	28	65	56	4	<1	0	4	1.4	1.4	1.2
1970	Turkey, Louis Rich	1 pce	28	67	58	3	1	0	5	1.5	1.8	1.3
665	Braunschweiger sausage	2 pce	57	48	205	8	2	0	18	6.2	8.5	2.1
1073	Bratwurst, link	1 ea	70	51	226	10	2	0	20	7	9.3	2
666	Brown & serve sausage links, cooked	2 ea	26	45	102	4	1	0	10	3.4	4.4	1
1089	Cheesefurter/cheese smokie	2 ea	86	53	281	12	1	0	25	9	11.8	2.6
2157	Chicken breast, Healthy Favorites	4 pce	52	–	40	9	1	0	0	0	0	0
1556	Chorizo, pork & beef	3 oz	85	32	387	22	2	0	33	12.2	15.6	2.9
1950	Coldcuts, fat free, deli thin	1 pce	13	77	11	2	1	0	<1	t	t	t
1090	Corned beef loaf, jellied	1 pce	28	69	43	7	0	0	2	.7	.8	.1
	Frankfurters:											
1077	Beef, large link, 8/package	1 ea	57	55	180	7	1	0	16	6.9	7.9	.8
1078	Beef and pork, large link, 8/package	1 ea	57	54	182	6	1	0	17	6.2	8	1.6
667	Beef and pork, small link, 10/pkg	1 ea	45	54	144	5	1	0	13	4.9	6.3	1.2
668	Turkey frankfurter, 10/package	1 ea	45	63	102	6	1	0	8	2.7	2.5	2.3
1968	Turkey/chicken frank 8/pkg	1 ea	43	–	80	6	1	0	6	2	–	–
	Ham:											
669	Ham lunchmeat, canned, 3 x 2 x ½"	1 pce	21	52	70	3	<1	0	6	2.3	3	.8
670	Chopped ham, packaged	2 pce	42	64	96	7	0	0	7	2.4	3	.8
2156	Honey ham, Healthy Favorites	4 pce	52	73	55	9	2	0	2	.5	–	.1
2113	Oscar Mayer lower sodium ham	1 pce	21	46	23	4	1	0	1	.3	.4	.1
673	Turkey ham lunchmeat	2 pce	57	71	73	11	<1	0	3	1	.7	.9
1091	Kielbasa sausage	1 pce	26	54	81	4	1	0	7	2.6	3.4	.8
1092	Knockwurst sausage, link	1 ea	68	56	210	8	1	0	19	6.9	8.7	2
1093	Mortadella lunchmeat	2 pce	30	52	93	5	1	0	8	2.9	3.4	.9
1097	Olive loaf lunchmeat	2 pce	57	58	134	7	5	<.01	9	3.3	4.5	1.1

(Computer code number is for West Diet Analysis program)

Chol (mg)	Calc (mg)	Iron (mg)	Magn (mg)	Pota (mg)	Sodi (mg)	Zinc (mg)	VT-A (RE)	Thia (mg)	VT-E (α-TE)	Ribo (mg)	Niac (mg)	V-B6 (mg)	Fola (μg)	VT-C (mg)
35	0	.72	–	–	940	–	0	–	–	–	–	–	–	0
35	0	–	–	–	910	–	0	–	–	–	–	–	–	0
35	8	1.25	9	156	454	.82	6	.06	1.4	.11	1.3	.11	5	0
60	6	1.85	25	338	771	2.88	0	.05	.43	.19	7.11	.31	6	0
12	11	.36	5	70	137	.44	0	.02	.04	.06	1.96	.09	1	0
17	3	.43	3	49	291	.69	0	.02	.05	.03	.96	.05	1	0
17	2	.22	4	72	352	.49	0	.16	.06	.05	.92	.1	1	0
13	3	.33	4	80	368	.7	0	.11	.06	.06	.88	.06	1	0
13	3	.38	3	36	226	.5	0	.01	.04	.03	.55	.04	1	0
13	4	.34	4	44	314	.53	0	–	–	–	–	–	–	0
16	3	.43	3	51	289	.55	0	.05	.06	.04	.73	.05	1	0
15	–	.36	–	–	510	–	–	–	–	–	–	–	–	–
14	3	.18	3	65	272	.47	0	.12	.06	.04	.9	.06	1	0
15	14	.39	6	46	312	.45	0	–	–	–	–	–	–	0
28	24	.43	4	56	249	.49	0	.02	.15	.05	1	.06	2	0
22	34	.45	5	52	242	.57	0	.02	–	.05	1.08	.05	–	0
89	5	5.34	6	113	652	1.6	2405	.14	.2	.87	4.77	.19	25	0
44	34	.72	11	197	779	1.47	0	.18	.19	.16	2.31	.09	4	0
16	2	.62	4	70	248	.3	0	.21	.06	.09	.96	.06	1	0
58	50	.93	11	177	931	1.94	33	.21	.27	.14	2.5	.11	3	0
25	–	.72	–	–	620	–	–	–	–	–	–	–	–	–
75	7	1.35	15	338	1049	2.9	0	.54	.19	.26	4.36	.45	2	0
4	1	.15	4	27	155	.11	0	–	–	–	–	–	–	0
13	3	.58	3	29	270	1.16	0	0	.05	.03	.5	.03	2	0
35	11	.81	2	95	585	1.24	0	.03	.11	.06	1.38	.07	2	0
29	6	.66	6	95	638	1.05	0	.11	.14	.07	1.5	.07	2	0
23	5	.52	5	75	504	.83	0	.09	.11	.05	1.18	.06	2	0
48	48	.83	6	81	642	1.4	0	.02	.28	.08	1.86	.1	4	0
40	60	1.08	–	–	480	–	0	–	–	–	–	–	–	0
13	1	.15	2	45	271	.31	0	.08	.06	.04	.66	.04	1	<1
21	3	.35	7	134	576	.8	0	.27	.11	.09	1.63	.15	<1	0
24	6	.7	18	144	635	1.02	–	–	–	–	–	–	–	0
9	1	.3	5	197	175	.42	0	–	–	–	–	–	–	0
32	6	1.57	9	185	568	1.68	0	.03	.37	.14	2.01	.14	3	0
17	11	.38	4	71	280	.53	0	.06	.06	.06	.75	.05	1	0
40	8	.62	7	135	687	1.13	0	.23	.39	.1	1.86	.12	1	0
17	5	.42	3	49	374	.63	0	.04	.07	.05	.8	.04	1	0
22	62	.31	11	169	846	.79	11	.17	.14	.15	1.05	.13	1	0

(For purposes of calculations, use "0" for t, <1, <.1, <.01, etc.)

H

Table H–1
Food Composition

Computer Code Number	Food Description	Measure	Wt (g)	H₂O (%)	Ener (kcal)	Prot (g)	Carb (g)	Dietary Fiber (g)	Fat (g)	Fat Breakdown (g) Sat	Fat Breakdown (g) Mono	Fat Breakdown (g) Poly
MEATS: SAUSAGES and LUNCHMEATS (see also Poultry Food Products)—Cont.												
1952	Turkey breast, fat free	1 pce	28	77	22	4	1	0	<1	<.1	<.1	<.1
1080	Turkey pastrami	2 pce	57	71	80	11	1	0	4	1	1.2	.9
1969	Turkey salami	1 pce	28	72	41	4	<1	0	3	1	1	.8
1081	Pepperoni sausage	2 pce	11	27	55	2	<1	0	5	1.8	2.3	.5
1094	Pickle & pimento loaf	2 pce	57	57	149	7	3	<.01	12	4.5	5.5	1.5
1082	Polish sausage	1 oz	28	53	92	4	<1	0	8	2.9	3.9	.9
674	Pork sausage, cooked,[1] link, small	2 ea	26	45	96	5	<1	0	8	2.8	4	1
1079	Pork sausage, cooked, patty	4 oz	113	45	418	22	1	0	35	12.2	17.8	3.3
675	Salami, pork and beef	2 pce	57	60	142	8	1	0	11	4.6	5.2	1.1
676	Salami, turkey	2 pce	57	66	112	9	<1	0	8	2.3	2.6	2
677	Beef & pork, dry	3 pce	30	35	125	7	1	0	10	3.7	5.1	1
	Sandwich spreads:											
1300	Ham salad spread	1 c	240	63	518	21	26	0	37	12.2	17.3	6.5
678	Pork and beef	2 tbs	30	60	71	2	4	<1	5	1.8	2.3	.8
1296	Chicken/turkey	2 tbs	26	66	52	3	2	0	4	.9	.8	1.6
1084	Smoked link sausage, beef and pork	1 ea	68	52	229	9	1	0	21	7.2	9.7	2.2
1083	Smoked link sausage, pork	1 ea	68	39	265	15	1	0	22	7.7	9.9	2.6
1085	Summer sausage	2 pce	46	51	154	7	<1	0	14	5.5	6	.6
1076	Turkey breakfast sausage	1 pce	28	60	65	6	0	0	5	1.6	1.8	1.2
679	Vienna sausage, canned	2 ea	32	60	89	3	1	0	8	3	4	.5
MIXED DISHES and FAST FOODS												
MIXED DISHES:												
1445	Almond chicken	1 c	242	77	275	20	18	4	14	2	5.3	5.9
1981	Baked beans, fat free, honey	½ c	120	74	110	7	24	7	0	0	0	0
1454	Bean cake	1 ea	32	23	130	2	16	1	7	1	2.9	2.6
680	Beef stew w/ vegetables, homemade	1 c	245	82	218	16	15	2	11	5	4.5	.5
1109	Beef stew w/ vegetables, canned	1 c	245	83	194	14	17	3	8	2.5	3.1	.4
1116	Beef, macaroni, tomato sauce casserole	1 c	226	76	255	16	26	3	10	3.8	4.1	.5
2295	Beef fajita	1 ea	189	63	347	14	39	3	15	4.3	6.4	3.3
1265	Beef flauta	1 ea	113	49	360	17	13	2	27	4.9	11.6	9.1
681	Beef pot pie, homemade[2]	1 pce	210	55	517	21	40	3	31	8.4	14.7	7.4
1898	Broccoli, batter fried	1 c	85	74	123	3	9	2	9	1.3	2.2	4.9
1462	Buffalo wings/spicy chicken wings	2 ea	32	53	98	8	<1	<1	7	1.8	2.8	1.6
1675	Carrot raisin salad	½ c	88	58	204	1	21	2	14	2	3.9	7.3
2248	Cheeseburger deluxe	1 ea	219	53	563	28	38	–	33	15	12.6	2
682	Chicken à la king, homemade	1 c	245	68	468	27	12	1	34	12.7	14.3	6.2
683	Chicken & noodles, homemade	1 c	240	71	367	22	26	2	19	5.9	7.1	3.5
684	Chicken chow mein, canned	1 c	250	89	95	7	18	2	1	0	.1	.8
685	Chicken chow mein, homemade	1 c	250	78	255	31	10	1	10	2.4	4.3	3.1
1266	Chicken fajitas	1 ea	223	61	405	22	50	4	13	2.5	6	3.5
1264	Chicken flauta	1 ea	113	53	343	14	13	2	27	4.3	11.1	9.6
686	Chicken pot pie, homemade (⅓)	1 pce	232	57	545	23	43	4	31	10.9	14.5	5.8
1672	Chili con carne	½ c	127	77	128	12	11	2	4	1.7	1.7	.3
1112	Chicken salad with celery	½ c	78	53	268	11	3	<1	25	3.1	4.5	15.8
1382	Chicken teriyaki, breast	1 pce	128	67	176	26	7	<1	4	.9	1	.9
687	Chili with beans, canned	1 c	255	76	286	15	30	11	14	6	6	.9
1479	Chinese pastry	1 oz	28	46	67	1	13	<1	2	.2	.4	.8
688	Chop suey with beef & pork	1 c	250	63	483	25	35	4	28	5.7	9.8	10.5

[1]Cooked weight is half the weight of raw sausage.

[2]Crust made with vegetable shortening and enriched flour.

(Computer code number is for West Diet Analysis program)

TABLE OF FOOD COMPOSITION ◆ **H–57**

PAGE KEY: H–4 = BEV   H–6 = DAIRY   H–12 = EGGS   H–14 = FAT/OIL   H–18 = FRUIT   H–26 = BAKERY   H–36 = GRAIN   H–44 = FISH   H–48 = MEATS   H–50 = POULTRY   H–54 = SAUSAGE   H–56 = MIXED/FAST   H–64 = NUTS/SEEDS   H–68 = SWEETS   H–70 = VEG/LEG   H–84 = MISC   H–88 = SOUPS/SAUCES   H–90 = FAST   H–106 = FRZN ENTREE   H–112 = BABY FOODS

Chol (mg)	Calc (mg)	Iron (mg)	Magn (mg)	Pota (mg)	Sodi (mg)	Zinc (mg)	VT-A (RE)	Thia (mg)	VT-E (α-TE)	Ribo (mg)	Niac (mg)	V-B6 (mg)	Fola (μg)	VT-C (mg)
9	3	.34	8	59	387	.24	0	–	–	–	–	–	–	0
31	5	.95	8	148	596	1.23	0	.03	.12	.14	2.01	.15	3	0
21	11	.35	6	61	281	.65	0	–	–	–	–	–	–	0
9	1	.15	2	38	224	.28	0	.03	.02	.04	.55	.03	<1	0
21	54	.58	10	194	792	.8	4	.17	.14	.15	1.17	.11	3	0
20	3	.41	4	67	248	.55	0	.14	.07	.04	.98	.05	1	<1
22	8	.32	4	94	336	.65	0	.19	.07	.07	1.18	.09	<1	<1
94	36	1.42	19	409	1467	2.85	0	.84	.3	.29	5.13	.37	2	2
37	7	1.51	9	112	604	1.21	0	.14	.13	.21	2.01	.12	1	0
47	11	.92	9	139	572	1.03	0	.04	.33	.1	2.01	.14	2	0
24	2	.45	5	113	558	.97	0	.18	.08	.09	1.46	.15	<1	0
89	19	1.42	24	360	2188	2.64	0	1.04	4.18	.29	5.04	.36	2	0
11	4	.24	2	33	304	.31	3	.05	.52	.04	.52	.04	<1	0
8	3	.16	3	48	98	.27	11	.01	.57	.02	.43	.03	1	<1
48	7	.99	8	129	643	1.44	0	.18	.15	.12	2.2	.12	1	0
46	20	.79	13	229	1020	1.92	0	.48	.17	.18	3.08	.24	3	1
35	6	1.17	6	125	571	1.18	0	.07	.1	.15	1.98	.12	1	0
23	5	.52	6	76	191	.97	0	.03	.14	.08	1.42	.08	1	0
17	3	.28	2	32	305	.51	0	.03	.07	.03	.51	.04	1	0
35	81	2	59	551	615	1.54	76	.09	2.64	.19	8.59	.4	32	11
0	40	2.7	–	–	135	–	900	–	–	–	–	–	–	14
0	3	.67	6	58	55	.16	0	.07	1.14	.05	.49	.02	9	0
64	29	2.94	40	613	292	5.29	568	.15	.49	.17	4.66	.28	37	17
34	29	2.21	39	426	1006	4.24	262	.07	.34	.12	2.45	.2	31	7
39	26	2.7	40	522	862	3.14	97	.22	.57	.22	4.31	.29	20	14
22	64	3	32	362	721	2	44	.39	1.77	.26	4	.27	21	24
45	50	2.15	29	292	187	4.18	15	.07	4.01	.15	2.13	.25	10	14
44	29	3.78	6	334	596	3.17	519	.29	3.78	.29	4.83	.24	29	6
16	67	.94	20	242	62	.38	102	.08	2.1	.13	.75	.11	43	53
26	5	.4	6	59	61	.56	17	.01	.24	.04	2.06	.13	1	<1
10	26	.75	14	317	118	.19	1462	.08	5.03	.05	.64	.22	9	5
88	206	4.67	44	445	1108	5	129	.39	1.18	.46	7.4	.29	29	8
186	127	2.45	20	404	760	1.8	272	.1	.98	.42	5.39	.23	11	12
96	26	2.16	26	149	600	1.53	10	.05	–	.17	4.32	.19	10	0
8	45	1.25	14	418	725	1.3	28	.05	.05	.1	1	.09	12	13
78	58	2.5	28	473	718	2.12	50	.08	.75	.23	4.25	.41	19	10
41	83	3.7	51	532	439	1.77	56	.48	2.05	.37	6.6	.35	41	22
37	53	.97	28	243	189	1.18	22	.05	4.06	.1	3.21	.22	8	14
72	70	3.02	25	343	594	2	735	.33	3.25	.33	4.87	.46	29	5
67	34	2.6	23	347	505	1.8	84	.06	.81	.57	1.25	.17	15	<1
48	16	.62	11	138	201	.8	31	.03	6.27	.07	3.28	.34	9	1
80	27	1.76	36	309	1866	1.94	16	.08	.35	.2	8.69	.46	13	3
43	120	8.75	115	931	1331	5.1	87	.12	1.87	.27	.91	.34	58	4
0	8	.51	6	28	3	.2	<1	.04	.26	<.01	.42	.02	1	0
52	45	4.7	61	586	930	4	153	.42	2.07	.42	6.4	.51	50	23

(For purposes of calculations, use "0" for t, <1, <.1, <.01, etc.)

H

Table H–1
Food Composition

Computer Code Number	Food Description	Measure	Wt (g)	H₂O (%)	Ener (kcal)	Prot (g)	Carb (g)	Dietary Fiber (g)	Fat (g)	Sat	Mono	Poly
										Fat Breakdown (g)		
MIXED DISHES and FAST FOOD—Cont.												
	MIXED DISHES—Cont.											
690	Coleslaw[1]	1 c	120	74	178	2	16	2	13	2	2.9	7.8
689	Corn pudding[2]	1 c	250	76	273	11	32	4	13	6.3	4.3	1.8
1110	Corned beef hash, canned	1 c	220	67	398	19	24	1	25	11.9	10.9	.9
1255	Deviled egg (½ egg + filling)	1 ea	31	69	63	4	<1	0	5	1.24	1.8	1.5
	Egg foo yung patty:											
1467	Meatless	1 ea	86	78	113	6	3	<1	8	1.9	3.4	2.1
1458	With beef	1 ea	86	74	129	9	3	<1	9	2.2	3.2	2.4
1465	With chicken	1 ea	86	74	130	9	4	<1	9	2.1	3.1	2.5
1602	Egg roll, meatless	1 ea	64	70	102	3	10	1	6	1.3	2.5	1.6
1550	Egg roll, with meat	1 ea	64	66	115	5	9	1	6	1.5	2.8	1.6
1113	Egg salad	1 c	183	57	586	17	3	0	57	10.6	17.4	24.2
691	French toast w/wheat bread, homemade[3]	1 pce	65	54	151	5	16	<1	7	2	3	1.7
1355	Green pepper, stuffed	1 ea	172	75	229	11	20	2	12	5.1	4.9	.5
1487	Hot & sour soup (Chinese)	1 c	244	88	133	12	5	<1	6	2	2.5	1.2
2242	Hamburger deluxe	1 ea	110	49	279	13	27	–	14	4.1	5.3	2.6
1997	Hummous/hummus	¼ c	62	65	106	3	13	3	5	.8	2.2	2
	Lasagna:											
1346	With meat, homemade	1 pce	245	67	382	22	39	3	15	7.8	5	.9
1111	Without meat, homemade	1 pce	218	70	298	15	39	3	9	5.4	2.5	.6
1117	Frozen entree	1 pce	205	75	235	15	25	3	9	4	3.3	.5
1606	Lo mein, meatless	1 c	200	82	134	6	27	3	1	.1	.1	.3
1607	Lo mein, with meat	1 c	200	70	285	17	32	2	10	1.9	2.9	4.5
692	Macaroni & cheese, canned[4]	1 c	240	80	228	9	26	1	10	4.2	3.1	1.4
693	Macaroni & cheese, homemade[5]	1 c	200	58	430	17	40	1	22	8.9	8.8	3.6
1115	Macaroni salad, no cheese	1 c	177	60	461	5	28	2	37	4.1	6.1	25.5
1120	Meat loaf, beef	1 pce	87	63	182	16	4	<1	11	4	4.7	.5
1119	Meat loaf, beef and pork (⅓)	1 pce	87	60	205	15	5	<1	14	5.2	6.3	.9
1303	Moussaka (lamb & eggplant)	1 c	250	82	236	16	13	4	13	4.6	5.4	1.9
1899	Mushrooms, batter fried	5 ea	70	66	148	2	8	1	12	2.1	3	6.4
715	Potato salad with mayonnaise and eggs[6]	½ c	125	76	179	3	14	2	10	1.8	3.1	4.7
1674	Pizza, combination, ½ of 12" round	1 pce	53	48	123	9	14	–	4	1	1.7	.6
1673	Pizza, pepperoni, ½ of 12" round	1 pce	47	47	121	7	13	–	5	1.5	2.1	.8
694	Quiche Lorraine, ⅛ of 8" quiche[7]	1 pce	176	54	508	20	20	1	39	18	13.8	4.9
1449	Ramen noodles, cooked	1 c	227	82	156	6	29	3	2	.4	.5	.5
1671	Ravioli, meat	½ c	125	76	122	14	19	1	4	1	2.3	1
1597	Fried rice (meatless)	1 c	166	68	264	5	34	1	12	1.7	3	6.3
2142	Roast beef hash	½ c	95	66	187	8	9	1	13	5.7	4.7	2.6
	Spaghetti (enriched) in tomato sauce:											
	With cheese:											
695	Canned	1 c	250	80	190	6	39	3	2	0	.4	.5
696	Homemade	1 c	250	77	260	9	37	3	9	2	5.4	1.2

[1]Recipe: 41% cabbage; 12% celery; 12% table cream; 12% sugar; 7% green pepper; 6% lemon juice; 4% onion; 3% pimento; 3% vinegar; 2% each for salt, dry mustard, and white pepper.

[2]Recipe: 55% yellow corn, 23% whole milk, 14% egg, 4% sugar, 3% salt, and 1% pepper.

[3]Recipe: 35% whole milk, 32% white bread, 29% egg, and cooked in 4% margarine.

[4]Made with corn oil.

[5]Made with margarine.

[6]Recipe: 62% potatoes; 12% egg; 8% mayonnaise; 7% celery; 6% sweet pickle relish; 2% onion; 1% each for green pepper, pimento, salt, and dry mustard.

[7]Crust made with vegetable shortening and enriched flour.

(Computer code number is for West Diet Analysis program)

Chol (mg)	Calc (mg)	Iron (mg)	Magn (mg)	Pota (mg)	Sodi (mg)	Zinc (mg)	VT-A (RE)	Thia (mg)	VT-E (α-TE)	Ribo (mg)	Niac (mg)	V-B6 (mg)	Fola (μg)	VT-C (mg)
6[8]	41	.88	11	215	324	.24	60	.05	4.8	.04	.1	.13	47	10
250	100	1.4	38	403	138	1.25	90	1.03	.53	.32	2.47	.3	63	7
73	29	4.4	36	440	1188	3.3	0	.02	.48	.2	4.62	.43	20	0
121	15	.35	3	37	94	.3	49	.02	.86	.14	.02	.05	13	0
184	31	1.1	12	118	310	.7	86	.05	1.57	.26	.44	.1	30	5
180	26	1.1	12	145	184	1.16	92	.05	1.79	.24	.74	.16	22	3
182	28	.85	12	145	187	.81	95	.05	1.87	.25	.96	.13	23	3
30	12	.76	9	98	306	.25	15	.08	.81	.11	.81	.06	13	3
37	13	.78	10	124	304	.5	14	.17	.79	.13	1.31	.1	9	2
574	74	1.8	13	180	666	1.42	260	.08	8.87	.66	.09	.47	62	0
76	64	1.09	11	87	311	.44	81	.13	.31	.21	1.06	.05	15	<1
34	16	1.77	21	233	201	2.3	44	.15	.75	.1	2.74	.3	17	55
23	29	1.83	27	351	1562	1.17	2	.19	.12	.22	4.58	.15	12	1
26	63	2.63	22	227	504	2	9	.23	.83	.2	3.7	.12	18.7	2
0	31	.97	18	108	151	.68	1	.06	.62	.03	.25	.25	37	5
57	258	3.22	50	461	745	3.25	158	.23	1.15	.33	4	.21	19	16
31	252	2.5	44	375	714	1.77	156	.23	1.07	.27	2.49	.17	17	15
33	158	2.08	39	453	496	2.23	149	.16	2.08	.23	3.06	.2	17	25
0	48	2.06	33	389	623	.92	130	.23	.35	.24	2.83	.19	49	13
30	25	2.11	40	246	276	1.63	6	.37	1.51	.24	4.25	.28	41	8
24	199	.96	31	139	730	1.2	73	.12	.14	.24	.96	.02	8	<1
42	362	1.8	37	240	1086	1.2	234	.2	.12	.4	1.8	.05	10	1
27	31	1.56	20	170	352	.53	44	.18	10.31	.1	1.43	.33	21	4
84	29	1.61	14	187	145	3.23	24	.05	.31	.22	2.61	.15	11	1
84	34	1.42	14	213	381	2.68	24	.2	.32	.22	2.68	.17	10	1
97	68	1.79	40	556	431	2.55	105	.15	.81	.31	4.13	.23	45	6
14	54	.77	8	180	121	.42	10	.07	.92	.22	1.65	.05	8	1
85	24	.81	19	318	661	.39	41	.1	2.33	.08	1.11	.18	8	13
14	68	1.02	12	119	255	.74	68	.14	1.05	.12	1.31	.06	18	1
10	43	.62	6	102	178	.35	36	.09	1.09	.16	2.03	.04	35	1
205	201	1.9	27	271	549	1.66	243	.23	1.91	.44	4.71	.2	17	3
38	20	1.89	24	51	1349	.77	204	.22	.09	.1	1.75	.06	9	<1
88	23	1.17	23	306	498	.76	22	.1	–	.09	1.9	.16	12	7
42	30	1.84	24	134	286	.89	21	.21	2.46	.11	2.25	.15	22	4
32	8	.73	18	294	564	2.43	0	.08	–	.1	1.89	.25	10	0
8	40	2.75	21	303	955	1.12	120	.35	2.13	.28	4.5	.13	6	10
8	80	2.25	26	408	955	1.3	140	.25	2.75	.18	2.25	.2	8	13

[8]From dairy cream in recipe.

(For purposes of calculations, use "0" for t, <1, <.1, <.01, etc.)

H

Table H–1
Food Composition

Computer Code Number	Food Description	Measure	Wt (g)	H₂O (%)	Ener (kcal)	Prot (g)	Carb (g)	Dietary Fiber (g)	Fat (g)	Fat Breakdown (g) Sat	Mono	Poly
	MIXED DISHES and FAST FOODS—Cont.											
	MIXED DISHES—Cont.											
	With meatballs:											
697	Canned	1 c	250	78	258	12	29	6	10	2.2	3.9	3.9
698	Homemade	1 c	248	70	332	19	39	8	12	3.3	6.3	2.2
716	Spinach soufflé[1]	1 c	136	74	219	12	3	4	20	9.6	5.7	2.2
1553	Sweet & sour pork	1 c	226	77	231	15	25	1	8	2.2	2.9	2.5
1263	Sweet & sour chicken breast	1 ea	131	79	117	8	15	1	3	.6	.8	1.5
1515	Three bean salad	1 ea	340	82	316	9	31	7	19	2.8	4.3	11.1
717	Tuna salad[2]	1 c	205	63	383	33	19	0	19	3.2	5.9	8.5
1121	Tuna noodle casserole, homemade	1 c	202	75	238	17	26	1	7	1.9	1.5	3.2
1270	Waldorf salad	1 c	137	58	408	4	13	2	40	4.2	7.3	27
	FAST FOODS and SANDWICHES (see end of this appendix for additional Fast Foods):											
699	Burrito,[3] beef & bean	1 ea	175	52	385	17	50	4	14	6.3	5.3	.9
700	Burrito, bean	1 ea	174	53	358	11	57	7	11	5.5	3.8	1
2106	Burrito, chicken con queso	1 ea	306	77	280	12	53	5	6	1.5	–	–
701	Cheeseburger with bun, regular	1 ea	112	55	261	13	21	–	15	6.7	5.2	1.1
702	Cheeseburger with bun, 4-oz patty	1 ea	194	51	487	25	41	–	25	10.2	9.1	3.1
703	Chicken patty sandwich	1 ea	157	47	444	21	33	1	25	7.4	9	7.2
704	Corndog	1 ea	111	47	292	11	35	–	12	3.3	5.8	2.2
1922	Corndog, chicken	1 ea	113	59	271	13	26	–	13	–	–	–
705	Enchilada	1 ea	230	63	451	14	40	–	27	15	8.9	1.2
706	English muffin with egg, cheese, bacon	1 ea	138	49	362	19	30	1	19	8.6	6.4	2
	Fish sandwich:											
707	Regular, with cheese	1 ea	140	45	400	16	36	<1	22	6.2	6.8	7.2
708	Large, no cheese	1 ea	170	47	464	18	44	<1	25	5.6	8.3	8.9
709	Hamburger with bun, regular	1 ea	98	46	252	13	30	1	9	3.2	3.4	1.6
710	Hamburger with bun, 4-oz patty	1 ea	174	51	466	26	31	–	26	9.7	11.4	2.3
711	Hot dog/frankfurter with bun	1 ea	85	54	210	9	16	–	13	4.4	5.9	1.5
	Lunchables:											
2129	Bologna & American cheese	1 ea	128	–	450	18	19	0	34	15	–	–
2130	Ham & cheese	1 ea	128	–	320	22	19	0	17	8	–	–
2117	Honey ham & Amer. w/choc pudding	1 ea	176	–	390	18	34	<1	20	9	–	–
2118	Honey turkey & cheddar w/Jello	1 ea	163	–	320	17	27	1	16	9	–	–
2131	Pepperoni & American cheese	1 ea	128	–	480	20	19	0	36	17	–	–
2125	Salami & American cheese	1 ea	128	–	430	18	18	0	32	15	–	–
2127	Turkey & cheddar cheese	1 ea	128	–	360	20	20	1	22	11	–	–
712	Pizza, cheese, ⅛ of 15" round[4]	1 pce	120	49	268	15	39	2	6	2.9	1.9	.9
	SANDWICHES:											
	Avocado, cheese, tomato, & lettuce:											
1276	On white bread, firm	1 ea	210	58	478	15	41	5	29	8.7	11.3	7.3
1278	On part whole wheat	1 ea	201	59	444	15	35	7	29	8.6	11.4	7.4
1277	On whole wheat	1 ea	214	58	468	16	40	8	30	8.7	11.6	7.5

[1]Recipe: 29% whole milk, 26% spinach, 13% egg white, 13% cheddar cheese, 7% egg yolk, 7% butter, 4% flour, 1% salt and pepper.

[2]Made with drained chunk light tuna, celery, onion, pickle relish, and mayonnaise-type salad dressing.

[3]Made with a 10½"-diameter flour tortilla.

[4]Crust made with vegetable shortening and enriched flour.

(Computer code number is for West Diet Analysis program)

Chol (mg)	Calc (mg)	Iron (mg)	Magn (mg)	Pota (mg)	Sodi (mg)	Zinc (mg)	VT-A (RE)	Thia (mg)	VT-E (α-TE)	Ribo (mg)	Niac (mg)	V-B6 (mg)	Fola (µg)	VT-C (mg)
23	53	3.25	20	245	1220	2.39	100	.15	1.5	.18	2.25	.12	5	5
74	124	3.72	40	665	1009	2.45	159	.25	1.64	.3	3.97	.2	10	22
184	230	1.35	38	201	763	1.29	675	.09	1.22	.3	.48	.12	62	3
38	28	1.36	34	390	1219	1.5	28	.55	.62	.21	3.6	.41	11	20
23	16	.8	21	187	732	.66	20	.06	.39	.08	3.06	.18	6	13
0	80	3.21	57	508	1164	1.22	52	.16	4.43	.21	.91	.1	120	10
27	35	2.05	39	365	824	1.15	55	.06	1.95	.14	13.7	.17	15	5
41	34	2.3	31	183	776	1.21	13	.18	1.19	.15	7.82	.2	10	1
21	43	.89	39	270	234	.63	40	.1	8.67	.05	.36	.37	27	6
37	81	3.71	63	497	1011	2.91	49	.4	1.05	.63	4.1	.28	56	1
4	91	3.62	70	524	790	1.22	26	.5	1.39	.49	3.25	.24	94	2
10	40	.72	–	–	600	–	40	–	–	–	–	–	–	15
38	132	1.93	19	167	710	1.9	51	.24	.97	.17	4.64	.11	16	2
70	200	4	35	392	1228	4.07	76	.41	–	.33	9.41	.21	27	2
52	52	4.04	30	305	826	1.62	27	.28	.47	.2	5.87	.17	25	8
50	64	3.92	11	167	617	.83	23	.18	.44	.44	2.64	.06	38	0
64	–	–	–	–	668	–	–	–	–	–	–	–	–	–
62	458	1.86	71	338	1106	3.54	262	.12	2.07	.6	2.69	.55	48	1
221	196	3.11	32	202	741	1.71	149	.46	.57	.5	3.71	.15	41	1
52	141	2.67	28	270	718	.9	74	.35	1.4	.32	3.23	.08	24	2
60	90	2.81	36	366	661	1.07	32	.36	.94	.24	3.66	.12	48	3
39	47	2.25	21	197	517	1.88	12	.24	.39	.29	4.3	.12	16	2
84	75	4.49	37	426	600	4.7	4	.28	1.31	.33	5.45	.3	37	1
38	20	2.01	11	124	581	1.72	0	.2	.24	.24	3.16	.04	26	<1
85	300	2.7	–	–	1620	–	60	–	–	–	–	–	–	0
60	300	1.8	–	–	1770	–	80	–	–	–	–	–	–	–
55	250	2.7	–	–	1540	–	–	–	–	–	–	–	–	–
50	20	6	–	–	1360	–	–	–	–	–	–	–	–	–
95	250	2.7	–	–	1840	–	–	–	–	–	–	–	–	–
80	250	2.7	–	–	1740	–	60	–	–	–	–	–	–	–
70	300	1.8	–	–	1650	–	60	–	–	–	–	–	–	–
18	222	1.1	30	209	640	1.55	140	.35	–	.31	4.73	.08	112	2
34	294	3.06	54	581	550	1.7	140	.37	4.55	.39	3.77	.32	80	11
31	291	3.1	67	617	525	1.91	140	.35	4.55	.39	3.94	.35	80	11
31	281	3.53	102	679	593	2.68	140	.36	4.17	.37	4.3	.42	92	11

H

(For purposes of calculations, use "0" for t, <1, <.1, <.01, etc.)

Table H-1
Food Composition

Computer Code Number	Food Description	Measure	Wt (g)	H₂O (%)	Ener (kcal)	Prot (g)	Carb (g)	Dietary Fiber (g)	Fat (g)	Fat Breakdown (g) Sat	Mono	Poly
	FAST FOODS and SANDWICHES (see end of this appendix for additional Fast Foods)—Cont.											
	SANDWICHES—Cont.											
	Bacon, lettuce & tomato:											
1137	On white bread, soft	1 ea	124	53	308	10	28	2	18	4.5	6.1	6.1
1139	On part whole wheat	1 ea	124	54	303	11	27	4	18	4.3	6.2	6.1
1138	On whole wheat	1 ea	137	53	328	12	32	5	18	4.4	6.5	6.3
	Cheese, grilled:											
1140	On white bread, soft	1 ea	118	37	399	18	30	1	24	13.1	7.5	2
1142	On part whole wheat	1 ea	118	37	394	18	28	3	24	12.9	7.5	2.07
1141	On whole wheat	1 ea	132	38	421	20	33	4	25	13.1	7.9	2.2
1596	Chicken fillet	1 ea	182	47	515	24	39	1	30	8.5	10.4	8.4
	Chicken salad:											
1143	On white bread, soft	1 ea	110	40	369	11	31	1	23	3.7	6	12
1145	On part whole wheat	1 ea	110	41	364	11	29	4	23	4	6	12
1144	On whole wheat	1 ea	123	41	387	13	35	5	24	3.6	6.4	12
1146	Corned beef & swiss on rye	1 ea	154	49	420	28	22	<1	26	9.4	7.4	6.3
	Egg salad:											
1147	On white bread, soft	1 ea	116	43	379	10	31	1	25	4.4	6.8	12
1149	On part whole wheat	1 ea	116	43	374	10	29	3	25	4.1	6.8	12.1
1148	On whole wheat	1 ea	130	43	400	12	35	5	25	4.3	7.1	12.2
	Ham:											
1279	On rye bread	1 ea	150	60	283	22	21	<1	14	2.4	3.8	6
1151	On white bread, soft	1 ea	156	55	333	22	30	1	14	3	4.4	5.9
1153	On part whole wheat	1 ea	156	55	328	22	28	3	14	2.7	4.4	6
1152	On whole wheat	1 ea	169	54	352	24	34	5	15	2.9	4.7	6.1
	Ham & cheese:											
1280	On white bread, soft	1 ea	156	49	402	23	30	1	22	8.4	5.9	6.1
1282	On part whole wheat	1 ea	156	50	397	23	28	3	22	8.1	5.9	6.2
1281	On whole wheat	1 ea	170	49	423	24	34	5	22	8.3	6.2	6.3
1150	Ham & swiss on rye	1 ea	150	54	339	22	22	<1	19	6.5	5.1	6
	Ham salad:											
1154	On white bread, soft	1 ea	131	47	362	11	37	1	20	4.8	6.8	7.4
1156	On part whole wheat	1 ea	131	48	357	11	35	3	20	4.6	6.8	7.5
1155	On whole wheat	1 ea	144	47	380	13	40	5	20	4.7	7.1	7.6
1157	Patty melt: Ground beef & cheese on rye	1 ea	182	46	561	37	22	3	37	13.3	11.7	8.4
	Peanut butter & jelly:											
1158	On white bread, soft	1 ea	101	26	351	12	47	3	15	3.1	6.7	3.9
1160	On part whole wheat	1 ea	101	27	346	12	45	5	15	2.9	6.7	4
1159	On whole wheat	1 ea	114	29	370	13	50	6	16	3	7	4.1
1161	Reuben, grilled: Corned beef, swiss cheese, sauerkraut on rye	1 ea	237	64	461	28	25	2	29	9.9	9.5	7.1
	Roast beef:											
713	On a bun	1 ea	150	49	374	23	36	—	15	3.9	7.4	1.9
1162	On white bread, soft	1 ea	156	46	403	29	34	1	17	3.4	4.2	8.2
1164	On part whole wheat	1 ea	156	47	398	29	32	3	17	3.2	4.3	8.3
1163	On whole wheat	1 ea	169	46	422	31	38	4	17	3.3	4.5	8.4
	Tuna salad:											
1165	On white bread, soft	1 ea	122	46	327	14	35	2	15	2.5	3.8	7.9
1167	On part whole wheat	1 ea	122	47	322	14	33	4	15	2.2	3.9	8

(Computer code number is for West Diet Analysis program)

PAGE KEY: H–4 = BEV   H–6 = DAIRY   H–12 = EGGS   H–14 = FAT/OIL   H–18 = FRUIT   H–26 = BAKERY   H–36 = GRAIN   H–44 = FISH
H–48 = MEATS   H–50 = POULTRY   H–54 = SAUSAGE   H–56 = MIXED/FAST   H–64 = NUTS/SEEDS   H–68 = SWEETS   H–70 = VEG/LEG
H–84 = MISC   H–88 = SOUPS/SAUCES   H–90 = FAST   H–106 = FRZN ENTREE   H–112 = BABY FOODS

Chol (mg)	Calc (mg)	Iron (mg)	Magn (mg)	Pota (mg)	Sodi (mg)	Zinc (mg)	VT-A (RE)	Thia (mg)	VT-E (α-TE)	Ribo (mg)	Niac (mg)	V-B6 (mg)	Fola (μg)	VT-C (mg)
22	52	1.99	18	234	590	.96	31	.35	2.34	.19	3.2	.14	34	12
20	63	2.27	33	283	604	1.2	31	.37	2.7	.21	3.62	.17	37	12
20	55	2.68	64	342	670	1.9	31	.4	2.36	.2	4	.24	48	12
55	398	1.81	25	154	1139	2.05	211	.24	1.13	.34	1.91	.06	24	<1
53	410	2.11	39	208	1154	2.3	211	.25	1.52	.36	2.38	.1	28	<1
54	403	2.55	73	271	1229	3.08	212	.26	1.15	.35	2.74	.17	40	<1
60	60	4.68	35	353	957	1.88	31	.33	.55	.24	6.81	.2	29	9
32	60	2.04	18	139	460	.8	24	.25	6.16	.18	3.7	.25	26	<1
31	73	2.35	33	195	475	1.06	24	.26	6.57	.2	4.2	.29	30	<1
30	63	2.79	68	259	543	1.85	24	.27	6.14	.19	4.5	.36	42	<1
82	268	3.11	28	225	1391	3.64	81	.19	2.58	.33	2.7	.17	19	1
157	70	2.17	16	113	524	.74	76	.26	4.51	.31	1.97	.2	37	0
155	83	2.47	31	170	539	1	76	.27	4.91	.33	2.45	.23	41	0
155	74	2.92	66	234	611	1.8	76	.28	4.53	.32	2.82	.3	53	0
47	48	2.3	26	364	1566	2.11	8	.99	2.36	.31	5.45	.48	15	23
47	60	2.39	29	367	1615	2.04	8	1.02	2.34	.33	5.98	.47	24	22
45	72	2.68	43	421	1630	2.29	8	1.03	2.7	.35	6.45	.5	27	22
45	62	3.1	77	483	1696	3.05	8	1.04	2.34	.33	6.78	.57	39	22
60	232	2.28	30	314	1616	2.34	90	.76	2.53	.36	4.63	.36	25	15
59	244	2.58	45	368	1630	2.59	90	.77	2.93	.39	5.09	.39	28	15
59	235	3.01	79	431	1702	3.36	90	.78	2.55	.37	5.45	.46	40	15
57	258	2.25	29	344	1602	2.59	79	.72	2.52	.36	4.06	.35	16	15
31	56	2.07	19	160	921	1.06	8	.51	3.29	.22	3.26	.17	22	4
29	69	2.4	34	216	936	1.32	8	.52	3.69	.24	3.74	.21	26	4
29	59	2.82	69	279	1001	2.11	8	.53	3.29	.23	4.1	.28	38	4
113	222	4.19	36	391	701	7.11	123	.25	3.5	.46	6.14	.35	25	<1
2	60	2.25	56	245	293	1.07	<1	.27	.12	.17	5.33	.13	40	<1
0	72	2.55	71	299	308	1.32	<1	.28	.51	.19	5.8	.17	44	<1
0	63	2.97	104	361	375	2.09	<1	.29	.14	.17	6.14	.24	56	<1
80	288	4.24	38	361	1945	3.72	130	.21	4.45	.34	3	.27	38	13
56	59	4.56	33	341	855	3.66	23	.41	.21	.33	6.33	.29	44	2
45	60	3.97	28	431	1592	3.77	12	.29	3.3	.3	6.38	.39	30	12
43	62	4.3	43	485	1607	4.02	12	.31	3.69	.32	6.84	.42	34	12
43	62	4.7	77	547	1672	4.79	12	.31	3.31	.31	7.18	.49	46	12
16	60	2.24	23	161	567	.67	22	.25	2.72	.18	5.53	.12	25	1
13	73	2.55	37	217	582	.93	22	.26	3.12	.2	6.01	.16	29	1

(For purposes of calculations, use "0" for t, <1, <.1, <.01, etc.)

H

Table H–1
Food Composition

Computer Code Number	Food Description	Measure	Wt (g)	H$_2$O (%)	Ener (kcal)	Prot (g)	Carb (g)	Dietary Fiber (g)	Fat (g)	Fat Breakdown (g) Sat	Fat Breakdown (g) Mono	Fat Breakdown (g) Poly
	FAST FOODS and SANDWICHES (see end of this appendix for additional Fast Foods)—Cont.											
1166	On whole wheat	1 ea	135	46	346	16	39	5	16	2.4	4.1	8.1
	Turkey:											
1168	On white bread, soft	1 ea	156	54	346	24	29	1	15	2.4	3.2	8.3
1170	On part whole wheat	1 ea	156	54	341	25	27	3	15	2.2	3.2	8.3
1169	On whole wheat	1 ea	169	53	365	26	33	4	15	2.3	3.5	8.5
	Turkey ham:											
1272	On rye bread	1 ea	150	60	280	21	20	<1	14	2.5	2.8	6.9
1273	On white bread, soft	1 ea	156	55	331	21	30	1	14	3	3.4	6.8
1275	On part whole wheat	1 ea	156	56	326	22	28	3	14	3	4.2	5.6
1274	On whole wheat	1 ea	169	55	350	23	33	5	15	2.9	3.7	7
714	Taco	1 ea	78	58	169	9	12	–	9	5.2	3	.4
	Tostada:											
1114	With refried beans	1 ea	157	66	243	11	29	8	11	5.9	3.3	.8
1118	With beans & beef	1 ea	192	70	284	14	25	3	15	9.8	3	.5
1354	With beans & chicken	1 ea	156	68	248	20	18	3	11	5.3	3.9	1.6
	Vegetarian foods:											
1511	Baked beans, canned	½ c	127	73	118	6	26	6	1	.2	t	.3
1175	Breakfast links	1 ea	34	60	31	6	1	1	2	.4	.5	.96
1171	Nuteena	1 pce	67	58	198	7	7	2	16	6.3	7.1	2.1
1173	Redi-burger	1 pce	68	59	88	13	4	4	8	1.2	1.9	4.6
1174	Vege-burger	½ c	108	71	130	21	5	4	3	.9	1.2	1
	Vegetarian foods, Worthington											
1846	Chik slices, canned	2 pce	60	78	62	6	<1	<1	4	.6	.9	.2.3
1833	Chili, canned	½ c	106	73	136	9	10	4	7	1.1	1.7	4.1
1835	Choplets, canned slices	2 pce	92	72	94	17	3	2	2	.9	.3	.3
1831	Country stew, canned	1 c	240	73	208	13	20	5	9	1.6	2.3	4.9
1838	Numete, canned slices	1 pce	68	58	164	8	6	4	12	2.9	5.4	3.3
1839	Prime stakes, canned	1 pce	92	71	136	9	4	4	9	1.4	2.9	4.9
1840	Protose, canned slices	1 pce	76	53	181	18	7	4	9	1.3	4.2	3.3
1842	Saucettes, canned links	2 pce	67	62	152	10	2	2	11	1.9	2.8	6.7
1844	Savory slices, canned	2 pce	56	66	97	7	4	2	6	2.4	2.6	1.1
1847	Turkee slices, canned	2 pce	63	64	129	9	2	1	9	1.6	3.6	4
	NUTS, SEEDS, and PRODUCTS											
	Almonds:											
1365	Dry roasted, salted	1 c	138	3	810	23	33	19	71	6.8	46.2	14.9
718	Slivered, packed, unsalted	1 c	135	4	795	27	28	15[1]	71	6.7	45.8	14.9
719	Whole, dried, unsalted:	1 c	142	4	836	28	29	16[1]	74	7	48.1	15.6
720	Ounce	1 oz	28	4	165	6	6	3[1]	15	1.4	9.5	3.1
721	Almond butter	1 tbs	16	1	101	2	3	<1	10	.9	6.1	2
722	Brazil nuts, dry (about 7)	1 oz	28	3	184	4	4	2	19	4.5	6.4	6.8
	Cashew nuts, salted:											
723	Dry roasted:	1 c	137	2	786	21	45	4	64	12.8	37.4	10.7
724	Ounce	1 oz	28	2	161	4	9	1	13	2.6	7.6	2.2

[1]Values reported for dietary fiber in almonds vary from 7.0 to 14.3 g/100 g.

(Computer code number is for West Diet Analysis program)

H

Chol (mg)	Calc (mg)	Iron (mg)	Magn (mg)	Pota (mg)	Sodi (mg)	Zinc (mg)	VT-A (RE)	Thia (mg)	VT-E (α-TE)	Ribo (mg)	Niac (mg)	V-B6 (mg)	Fola (μg)	VT-C (mg)
13	63	2.98	73	280	649	1.72	22	.27	2.71	.19	6	.23	41	1
45	56	2.01	29	302	1585	1.33	12	.26	3.46	.23	9	.4	24	0
43	68	2.3	43	356	1600	1.58	12	.27	3.85	.25	9.44	.44	28	0
43	59	2.73	77	418	1665	2.35	12	.28	3.47	.23	9.77	.51	40	0
55	51	4.06	25	342	1185	3	8	.22	2.8	.33	4.3	.29	17	<1
55	62	4.09	28	346	1248	2.9	8	.27	2.75	.35	4.87	.28	25	0
53	74	4.37	42	400	1262	3.15	8	.28	3.57	.37	5.34	.32	29	0
53	65	4.81	76	462	1329	3.91	8	.29	2.76	.35	5.68	.39	41	0
26	101	1.1	32	216	366	1.79	67	.07	.86	.2	1.47	.11	11	1
33	229	2.06	64	440	592	2.07	93	.11	1.26	.36	1.44	.17	82	1
63	161	2.09	58	419	743	2.71	148	.08	1.54	.42	2.44	.21	83	4
53	168	1.79	47	365	433	2.28	86	.11	1.87	.2	4.52	.32	54	4
0	64	.37	41	376	504	1.78	22	.19	.67	.08	.54	.17	30	4
1	11	1.62	12	44	255	.27	0	5.25	–	.16	3.92	.25	9	0
0	11	.33	40	202	145	.56	0	.13	–	.43	1.27	.55	60	0
<1	10	.85	13	97	364	.88	0	.11	–	.24	1.52	.41	17	0
0	15	.98	24	59	224	1.1	0	.39	–	.49	1.52	.61	29	0
<1	9	.73	–	111	257	.26	0	.06	–	.05	.37	.08	–	0
0	20	1.5	–	196	523	.57	0	.02	–	.03	1.04	.31	–	0
0	6	.37	–	40	500	.65	0	.05	–	.06	0	.06	–	0
2	51	5.09	–	270	826	1.03	432	1.85	–	.29	4.22	.86	–	0
0	12	1.39	–	192	337	.69	0	.1	–	.08	.67	.25	–	0
2	12	.4	–	82	445	.38	0	.12	–	.13	2	.38	–	0
<1	1	2.55	–	69	391	.99	0	.24	–	.18	1.85	.33	–	0
1	16	2.03	–	44	361	.46	0	1.05	–	.13	.17	.23	–	0
1	1	.94	–	27	357	.17	0	.16	–	.11	.96	.21	–	0
1	5	.91	–	31	388	.21	0	2.2	–	.1	.74	.16	–	0
0	389	5.24	420	1062	1076	6.76	0	.18	7.66	.83	3.89	.1	88	1
0	359	4.94	400	988	15	3.94	0	.29	32.4	1.05	4.54	.15	79	1
0	378	5.2	420	1039	16[2]	4.15	0	.3	34.08	1.11	4.77	.16	83	1
0	75	1.03	83	205	3[2]	.82	0	.06	6.72	.22	.94	.03	16	<1
0	43	.59	49	121	2[3]	.49	0	.02	3.25	.1	.46	.01	10	<1
0	49	.95	63	168	1	1.3	0	.28	2.13	.03	.45	.07	1	<1
0	62	8.22	356	774	877[4]	7.67	0	.27	.78	.27	1.92	.35	95	0
0	13	1.7	73	158	179[4]	1.59	0	.06	.16	.06	.4	.07	19	0

[2] Salted almonds contain 1108 mg sodium per cup, 221 mg per ounce.

[3] Salted almond butter contains 72 mg sodium per tablespoon.

[4] Dry-roasted cashews without salt contain 21 mg sodium per cup, or 4 mg per ounce.

(For purposes of calculations, use "0" for t, <1, <.1, <.01, etc.)

Table H–1
Food Composition

Computer Code Number	Food Description	Measure	Wt (g)	H₂O (%)	Ener (kcal)	Prot (g)	Carb (g)	Dietary Fiber (g)	Fat (g)	Fat Breakdown (g) Sat	Mono	Poly
	NUTS, SEEDS, and PRODUCTS—Cont.											
725	Oil roasted:	1 c	130	4	749	23	37	5	63	12.6	36.9	10.6
726	Ounce	1 oz	28	4	161	5	8	1	14	2.7	8	2.3
1366	Cashew nuts, unsalted, dry roasted	1 c	137	2	786	21	45	6	64	12.8	37.4	10.7
1367	Cashew nuts, unsalted, oil roasted	1 c	130	4	749	21	37	5	63	12.6	36.9	10.6
727	Cashew butter, unsalted	1 tbs	16	3	94	3	4	1	8	1.6	4.7	1.3
728	Chestnuts, European, roasted (1 cup = approx 17 kernels)	1 c	143	41	350	5	76	7	3	.6	1.1	1.2
	Coconut, raw:											
729	Piece 2 x 2 x ½"	1 pce	45	47	159	2	7	4	15	13.6	.6	.2
730	Shredded/grated, unpacked[1]	½ c	40	47	142	2	6	4	13	12	.6	.2
	Coconut, dried, shredded/grated:											
731	Unsweetened	1 c	78	3	515	6	19	13	50	45.1	2.2	.6
732	Sweetened	1 c	93	13	466	3	44	4	33	29.6	1.4	.4
733	Filberts/hazelnuts, chopped:	1 c	115	5	727	15	18	7	72	5.3	56.5	6.9
734	Ounce	1 oz	28	5	177	4	4	2	18	1.3	13.8	1.7
735	Macadamias, oil roasted, salted:	1 c	134	2	962	10	17	13	103	15.4	80.9	1.8
736	Ounce	1 oz	28	2	201	2	4	3	21	3.2	16.9	.4
1368	Macadamias, oil roasted, unsalted	1 c	134	2	962	10	17	13	103	15.4	80.9	1.8
	Mixed nuts:											
737	Dry roasted, salted	1 c	137	2	814	24	35	12	71	9.5	43	14.8
738	Oil roasted, salted	1 c	142	2	876	24	30	13	80	12.4	45	18.9
1369	Oil roasted, unsalted	1 c	142	2	876	27	30	14	80	12.4	45	18.9
	Peanuts:											
1370	Oil roasted, unsalted	1 c	144	2	837	38	27	10	71	9.9	35.3	22.5
741	Dried, salted:	1 c	146	2	854	35	31	12	73	10.1	36.1	22.9
742	Ounce	1 oz	28	2	164	7	6	2	14	1.9	6.9	4.4
1371	Peanut butter	2 tbs	32	1	190	8	6	2	16	3.6	7.8	4.4
744	Pecan halves, dried, unsalted:	1 c	108	5	720	9	20	8	73	5.9	45.6	18
745	Ounce	1 oz	28	5	187	2	5	2	19	1.5	11.8	4.7
1372	Pecan halves, dry roasted, salted	¼ c	28	1	185	2	6	3	18	1.5	11.3	4.5
746	Pine nuts/piñons, dried	1 oz	28	6	176	3	5	3	17	2.6	6.4	7.2
747	Pistachios, dried, shelled	1 oz	28	4	162	6	7	3	14	1.8	9.2	2.1
1373	Pistachios, dry roasted, salted, shelled	1 c	128	2	776	19	35	14	68	8.8	45.7	10.2
748	Pumpkin kernels, dried, unsalted	1 oz	28	7	152	7	5	1	13	2.4	4	5.9
1374	Pumpkin kernels, roasted, salted	1 c	227	7	1184	75	30	9	96	18.1	29.7	43.6
749	Sesame seeds, hulled, dried	¼ c	38	5	223	10	4	4	21	2.9	7.9	9.1
	Sunflower seed kernels:											
750	Dry	¼ c	36	5	205	8	7	4	18	1.9	3.4	11.8
751	Oil roasted	¼ c	34	3	209	7	5	2	20	2.1	3.7	12.9
752	Tahini (sesame butter)	1 tbs	15	3	91	3	3	1	9	1.2	3.2	3.7
1334	Trail Mix w/chocolate chips	1 c	146	7	707	21	66	8	47	9.3	19.8	16.5
753	Black walnuts, chopped:	1 c	125	4	759	31	15	6	71	4.8	15.9	46.9

[1]½ cup packed = 65 g.

TABLE OF FOOD COMPOSITION ♦ **H–67**

PAGE KEY: H–4 = BEV H–6 = DAIRY H–12 = EGGS H–14 = FAT/OIL H–18 = FRUIT H–26 = BAKERY H–36 = GRAIN H–44 = FISH
H–48 = MEATS H–50 = POULTRY H–54 = SAUSAGE H–56 = MIXED/FAST H–64 = NUTS/SEEDS H–68 = SWEETS H–70 = VEG/LEG
H–84 = MISC H–88 = SOUPS/SAUCES H–90 = FAST H–106 = FRZN ENTREE H–112 = BABY FOODS

Chol (mg)	Calc (mg)	Iron (mg)	Magn (mg)	Pota (mg)	Sodi (mg)	Zinc (mg)	VT-A (RE)	Thia (mg)	VT-E (α-TE)	Ribo (mg)	Niac (mg)	V-B6 (mg)	Fola (μg)	VT-C (mg)
0	53	5.33	332	689	814²	6.18	0	.55	2.03	.23	2.34	.33	88	0
0	12	1.15	71	148	175²	1.33	0	.12	.44	.05	.5	.07	19	0
0	62	8.22	356	774	22	7.67	0	.27	.78	.27	1.92	.35	95	0
0	53	5.33	332	689	22	6.18	0	.55	2.03	.23	2.34	.33	88	0
0	7	.8	41	87	2³	.83	0	.05	.25	.03	.26	.04	11	0
0	42	1.3	47	847	3	.82	3	.35	1.72	.25	1.92	.71	100	37
0	6	1.09	14	160	9	.5	0	.03	.33	.01	.24	.02	12	2
0	6	.97	13	142	8	.44	0	.03	.29	.01	.22	.02	11	1
0	20	2.59	70	424	29	1.57	0	.05	1.05	.08	.47	.23	7	1
0	14	1.79	47	313	244	1.69	0	.03	1.26	.02	.44	.25	8	1
0	216	3.76	328	512	4	2.76	8	.58	27.49	.13	1.31	.7	83	1
0	53	.92	80	125	1	.67	2	.14	6.69	.03	.32	.17	20	<1
0	60	2.41	157	441	348⁴	1.47	1	.29	.55	.15	2.71	.27	21	0
0	13	.5	33	92	73⁴	.31	<1	.06	.12	.03	.57	.06	4	0
0	60	2.41	157	441	9	1.47	1	.29	.55	.15	2.71	.27	21	0
0	96	5.07	308	818	917⁵	5.21	1	.27	8.22	.27	6.44	.41	69	1
0	153	4.56	334	825	926⁵	7.21	3	.71	8.52	.32	7.19	.34	118	1
0	153	4.56	334	825	16	7.21	3	.71	8.52	.32	7.19	.34	118	1
0	127	2.64	266	982	9	9.55	0	.36	10.67	.16	20.6	.37	181	0
0	79	3.3	257	961	1186	4.83	0	.64	10.82	.14	19.7	.37	212	0
0	15	.63	49	184	228	.93	0	.12	2.08	.03	3.78	.07	41	0
0	12	.59	51	214	149⁶	.93	0	.03	3.2	.03	4.29	.15	24	0
0	39	2.3	138	423	1⁷	5.91	14	.92	3.35	.14	.96	.2	42	2
0	10	.6	36	110	<1⁷	1.53	4	.24	.87	.04	.25	.05	11	1
0	10	.61	37	104	218	1.59	4	.09	.84	.03	.26	.06	11	1
0	2	.86	66	176	20	1.2	1	.35	.98	.06	1.22	.03	16	1
0	38	1.9	44	306	2⁸	.38	6	.23	1.46	.05	.3	.07	16	2
0	90	4.06	166	1241	998	1.74	31	.54	8.26	.32	1.81	.33	76	9
0	12	4.2	150	226	5⁹	2.09	11	.06	.28	.09	.49	.06	16	1
0	98	33.8	1212	1829	1305	16.9	86	.48	2.27	.72	3.95	.2	130	4
0	50	2.96	132	155	15	3.91	3	.27	.86	.03	1.78	.06	37	0
0	42	2.44	127	248	1¹⁰	1.82	2	.82	18.11	.09	1.62	.28	82	1
0	19	2.28	43	164	1¹⁰	1.77	2	.11	17.1	.1	1.4	.27	80	<1
0	21	.95	53	69	<1	1.58	1	.24	.34	.02	.85	.02	15	0
5.84	159	4.95	235	946	177	4.58	7	.6	15.62	.33	6.44	.38	95	2
0	73	3.84	253	655	1	4.28	38	.27	3.28	.14	.86	.69	82	4

(2) Oil-roasted cashews without salt contain 22 mg sodium per cup, or 5 mg per ounce.
(3) Salted cashew butter contains 98 mg sodium per tablespoon.
(4) Macadamia nuts without salt contain 9 mg sodium per cup, or 2 mg per ounce.
(5) Mixed nuts without salt contain about 15 mg sodium per cup.
(6) Peanut butter without added salt contains 3 mg sodium per tablespoon.
(7) Salted pecans contain 816 mg sodium per cup, or 214 mg per ounce.
(8) Salted pistachios contain approx 221 mg sodium per ounce.
(9) Salted pumpkin/squash kernels contain approximately 163 mg sodium per ounce.
(10) Unsalted sunflower seeds contain 1 mg sodium per ¼ cup.

(For purposes of calculations, use "0" for t, <1, <.1, <.01, etc.)

H

Table H–1
Food Composition

Computer Code Number	Food Description	Measure	Wt (g)	H₂O (%)	Ener (kcal)	Prot (g)	Carb (g)	Dietary Fiber (g)	Fat (g)	Fat Breakdown (g)		
										Sat	Mono	Poly
	NUTS, SEEDS, and PRODUCTS—Cont.											
754	Ounce	1 oz	28	4	170	7	3	1	16	1.1	3.6	10.5
755	English walnuts, chopped:	1 c	120	4	770	17	22	6	74	7.2	17	46.9
756	Ounce	1 oz	28	4	180	4	5	1	17	1.7	4	11
	SWEETENERS and SWEETS (see also Dairy [milk desserts] and Baked Goods)											
757	Apple butter	2 tbs	35	52	64	<1	17	<1	<1	t	t	t
1124	Butterscotch topping	2 tbs	41	32	103	1	27	<1	<1	t	t	0
1125	Caramel topping	2 tbs	41	32	103	1	27	<1	<1	t	t	0
	Cake frosting, creamy vanilla:											
1127	Canned	2 tbs	31	13	130	<1	22	<1	5	1.5	2.7	.7
1123	From mix	2 tbs	31	12	131	<1	22	<1	5	1	2.1	1.8
	Cake frosting, lite:											
2061	Milk chocolate	1 tbs	29	18	105	<1	21	1	2	.7	–	–
2062	Vanilla	1 tbs	29	15	110	0	22	<1	2	.6	–	–
	Candy:											
1128	Almond Joy candy bar	1 oz	28	8	130	1	16	1	8	4.7	1.5	.7
2069	Butterscotch morsels	¼ c	43	1	246	0	29	0	13	12.5	–	–
758	Caramel, plain or chocolate	1 oz	28	8	107	1	22	<1	2	1.9	.2	.1
1961	Chewing gum, sugarless	1 pce	3	–	5	0	2	–	0	–	0	0
	Chocolate (see also #784, 785, 971):											
	Milk chocolate:											
759	Plain	1 oz	28	1	144	2	17	1	9	5.2	2.8	.3
760	With almonds	1 oz	28	2	147	3	15	2	10	4.8	3.8	.6
761	With peanuts	1 oz	28	1	155	5	12	2	12	3.4	5.1	2.6
762	With rice cereal	1 oz	28	2	139	2	18	1	7	4.5	2.4	.2
763	Semisweet chocolate chips	1 c	170	1	814	7	107	10	51	30.3	17	1.7
764	Sweet dark chocolate (candy bar)	1 oz	28	1	133	1	17	2	9	4.8	2.8	.3
1133	SKOR English toffee candy bar	1 ea	32	4	169	1	18	<1	11	7.1	2.5	.3
765	Fondant candy, uncoated (mints, candy corn, other)	1 oz	28	7	100	0	26	0	0	0	0	0
1697	Fruit Roll-up (small)	1 ea	14	11	49	<1	12	<1	<1	t	t	.1
766	Fudge, chocolate	1 oz	28	10	107	<1	22	<1	2	1.5	.7	.1
767	Gumdrops	1 oz	28	1	108	0	28	0	0	0	0	0
768	Hard candy, all flavors	1 oz	28	1	104	0	28	0	0	0	0	0
769	Jellybeans	1 oz	28	6	103	0	26	0	<1	t	t	t
1134	M&M's plain chocolate candy	1 pkg	48	2	236	2	34	1	10	6	3	.3
1135	M&M's peanut chocolate candy	1 pkg	47	2	243	5	28	2	12	4.8	5.2	2
1130	Mars almond bar	1 ea	50	5	234	4	31	1	12	2.7	5.6	2.8
1129	Milky Way candy bar	1 ea	60	6	254	3	43	1	10	4.7	3.6	.4
1708	Milk chocolate-coated peanuts	½ c	85	2	441	11	42	4	29	12.4	11.1	3.7
1709	Peanut brittle, recipe	½ c	74	2	335	6	51	2	14	3.7	6.3	3.5
1132	Reese's peanut butter cup	2 ea	45	6	222	5	22	2	14	6.4	4.4	1.8
1131	Snickers candy bar (2.2oz)	1 ea	61	6	292	5	36	2	15	5.5	6.4	3
1482	Fruit juice bar (2.5 fl oz)	1 ea	77	78	63	1	16	0	<1	t	0	t
771	Gelatin dessert/Jello, prepared	½ c	120	85	71	2	17	0	0	0	0	0
1702	SugarFree	½ c	113	98	8	1	1	0	0	0	0	0
772	Honey:	1 c	339	17	1030	1	279	<1	0	0	0	0
773	Tablespoon	1 tbs	21	17	64	<1	17	<1	0	0	0	0

(Computer code number is for West Diet Analysis program)

PAGE KEY: H–4 = BEV   H–6 = DAIRY   H–12 = EGGS   H–14 = FAT/OIL   H–18 = FRUIT   H–26 = BAKERY   H–36 = GRAIN   H–44 = FISH
H–48 = MEATS   H–50 = POULTRY   H–54 = SAUSAGE   H–56 = MIXED/FAST   H–64 = NUTS/SEEDS   H–68 = SWEETS   H–70 = VEG/LEG
H–84 = MISC   H–88 = SOUPS/SAUCES   H–90 = FAST   H–106 = FRZN ENTREE   H–112 = BABY FOODS

Chol (mg)	Calc (mg)	Iron (mg)	Magn (mg)	Pota (mg)	Sodi (mg)	Zinc (mg)	VT-A (RE)	Thia (mg)	VT-E (α-TE)	Ribo (mg)	Niac (mg)	V-B6 (mg)	Fola (μg)	VT-C (mg)
0	16	.86	57	147	<1	.96	8	.06	.73	.03	.2	.16	18	1
0	113	2.93	203	602	12	3.28	14	.46	3.14	.18	1.25	.67	79	4
0	26	.68	47	141	3	.76	3	.11	.73	.04	.29	.16	19	1
0	2	.05	1	32	0	.02	0	<.01	.01	<.01	.03	.01	0	1
<1	22	.08	3	34	143	.08	11	<.01	0	.04	.02	.01	1	<1
<1	22	.08	3	34	143	.08	11	<.01	0	.04	.02	.01	1	<1
0	1	.03	<1	15	28	0	70	0	.62	<.01	<.01	0	0	0
0	3	.07	1	7	69	.03	33	.01	.62	.01	.11	<.01	0	0
0	3	.44	–	–	72	–	0	–	–	–	–	–	–	0
0	1	.03	–	–	53	–	0	–	–	–	–	–	–	0
1	22	.34	19	104	38	.22	1	.01	.63	.04	.13	.02	2	<1
0	0	0	–	80	46	–	0	.03	–	.04	.03	–	–	0
2	39	.04	5	61	69	.12	2	<.01	–	.05	.07	.01	1	<1
–	–	–	–	0	0	–	–	–	–	–	–	–	–	–
6	54	.39	17	108	23	.39	15	.02	.35	.08	.09	.01	2	<1
5	63	.46	25	124	21	.38	4	.02	.53	.12	.21	.01	3	<1
3	32	.52	35	150	11	.69	6	.08	1.3	.05	2.12	.05	23	0
5	48	.21	14	96	41	.31	3	.02	.35	.08	.13	.02	3	<1
0	54	5.32	196	621	19	2.75	3	.09	2.02	.15	.73	.06	5	0
0	5	.59	32	95	3	.42	1	.01	.28	.07	.19	.01	1	0
20	36	.13	11	76	74	.24	22	.01	.44	.11	.03	.01	2	<1
0	1	.02	<1	5	11	.01	0	<.01	0	<.01	<.01	<.01	0	0
0	5	.14	3	41	9	.03	2	<.01	.04	<.01	.01	.04	1	<1
4	12	.13	7	29	17	.11	13	<.01	.03	.02	.03	<.01	1	<1
0	1	.11	<1	1	12	0	0	0	0	<.01	<.01	0	0	0
0	1	.08	1	1	11	<.01	0	<.01	0	<.01	<.01	<.01	0	0
0	1	.31	1	10	7	.01	0	0	0	0	0	0	0	0
7	50	.53	20	128	29	.46	25	.03	.41	.1	.11	.01	2	<1
4	48	.54	29	162	23	.63	11	.07	1.01	.1	.95	.04	20	<1
5	84	.55	36	163	85	.56	23	.02	.3	.16	.47	.03	7	1
8	78	.46	20	145	144	.43	34	.02	.39	.13	.21	.03	5	1
8	88	1.11	77	427	35	1.6	0	.1	2.17	.15	3.61	.18	7	0
10	22	1.02	37	154	335	.72	35	.14	1.21	.04	2.59	.08	52	0
5	35	.5	38	180	131	.63	8	.02	.6	.1	1.79	.04	13	<1
8	57	.46	42	206	162	.9	24	.13	.93	.1	2.23	.07	45	<1
0	4	.15	3	41	3	.04	2	.01	0	.01	.12	.02	5	7
0	2	.04	1	1	50	.04	0	0	0	<.01	<.01	<.01	0	0
0	2	.01	1	0	54	.03	0	0	0	<.01	<.01	<.01	0	0
0	20	1.42	7	176	14	.75	0	0	0	.13	.41	.08	7	2
0	1	.09	<1	11	1	.05	0	0	0	.01	.03	.01	<1	<1

(For purposes of calculations, use "0" for t, <1, <.1, <.01, etc.)

H

Table H–1
Food Composition

Computer Code Number	Food Description	Measure	Wt (g)	H$_2$O (%)	Ener (kcal)	Prot (g)	Carb (g)	Dietary Fiber (g)	Fat (g)	Sat	Mono	Poly
										Fat Breakdown (g)		
SWEETENERS and SWEETS (see also Dairy [milk desserts] and Baked Goods)—Cont.												
774	Jams or preserves:	1 tbs	20	29	54	<1	14	<1	<1	0	t	t
775	Packet	1 ea	14	35	34	<1	9	<1	<1	t	t	0
776	Jellies:	1 tbs	18	28	49	<1	13	<1	<1	t	t	t
777	Packet	1 ea	14	28	38	<1	10	<1	<1	t	t	t
1136	Marmalade	2 tbs	40	33	98	<1	27	0	0	0	0	0
770	Marshmallows	4 ea	28	16	89	1	23	<1	<1	t	t	t
1126	Marshmallow creme topping	3 tbs	50	18	155	1	40	<1	<1	t	t	t
778	Popsicle/ice pops	1 ea	95	80	68	0	18	0	0	0	0	0
	Sugars:											
779	Brown sugar	1 c	220	2	827	0	214	0	0	0	0	0
780	White sugar, granulated:	1 c	200	0	774	0	200	0	0	0	0	0
781	Tablespoon	1 tbs	12	0	46	0	12	0	0	0	0	0
782	Packet	1 ea	6	0	23	0	6	0	0	0	0	0
783	White sugar, powdered, sifted	1 c	100	<1	389	0	100	0	<1	t	t	t
	Sweeteners:											
1711	Equal, packet	1 ea	1	12	4	<1	1	0	t	t	t	t
1712	Sweet 'N Low, packet	1 ea	1	<1	4	0	1	0	0	0	0	0
	Syrups:											
	Chocolate:											
785	Hot fudge type	2 tbs	38	22	132	2	22	<1	5	2.2	1.4	1.2
784	Thin type	2 tbs	38	29	93	1	25	1	<1	.3	.2	<.1
786	Molasses, blackstrap[1]	2 tbs	40	29	94	0	24	0	0	0	0	0
1710	Light cane	1 tbs	21	24	53	0	14	0	0	0	0	0
787	Pancake table syrup (corn and maple)	¼ c	79	24	227	0	60	0	0	0	0	0
VEGETABLES and LEGUMES												
788	Alfalfa sprouts	1 c	33	91	10	1	1	1	<1	t	t	.1
1815	Amaranth leaves, raw, chopped	1 c	28	92	7	1	1	<1	<1	<.1	<.1	<.1
1816	Amaranth leaves, raw, each	1 ea	14	92	4	<1	1	<1	<1	<.1	<.1	<.1
1817	Amaranth leaves, cooked	1 c	132	92	28	3	5	2	<1	.1	.1	.1
1987	Arugula, raw, chopped	5 ea	10	92	3	<1	<1	<1	<.1	<.1	<.1	<.1
789	Artichokes, cooked globe (300 g w/refuse)	1 ea	120	84	60	4	13	7	<1	t	t	.1
1177	Artichoke hearts, cooked from frozen	9 oz	240	87	108	8	22	11	·1	.3	t	.5
1176	Artichoke hearts, marinated	6 oz	170	59	168	4	13	8	14	2	3	7.7
2021	Artichoke hearts, in water	⅔ c	101	87	44	2	10	6	<1	<.1	<.1	.1
	Asparagus, green, cooked:											
	From fresh:											
790	Cuts and tips	½ c	90	92	22	2	4	1	<1	.1	t	.1
791	Spears, ½" diam at base	6 ea	90	92	22	2	4	1	<1	.1	t	.1
	From frozen:											
792	Cuts and tips	½ c	90	91	25	3	4	1	<1	.1	t	.2
793	Spears, ½" diam at base	6 ea	90	91	25	3	4	1	<1	.1	t	.2
794	Canned, spears, ½" diam at base	6 ea	120	94	23	3	3	2	1	.2	t	.3
795	Bamboo shoots, canned, drained slices	1 c	131	94	25	2	4	2	1	.1	t	.2
1795	Bamboo shoots, raw slices	1 c	151	91	41	4	8	3	<1	.1	<.1	.2
1798	Bamboo shoots, cooked slices	1 c	120	96	14	2	2	1	<1	.1	<.1	.1

[1]Light molasses would contain about 66 mg calcium, 2.1 mg iron, 18 mg magnesium, and 366 mg potassium for 2 tbsp.

(Computer code number is for West Diet Analysis program)

TABLE OF FOOD COMPOSITION ◆ H-71

PAGE KEY: H–4 = BEV   H–6 = DAIRY   H–12 = EGGS   H–14 = FAT/OIL   H–18 = FRUIT   H–26 = BAKERY   H–36 = GRAIN   H–44 = FISH
H–48 = MEATS   H–50 = POULTRY   H–54 = SAUSAGE   H–56 = MIXED/FAST   H–64 = NUTS/SEEDS   H–68 = SWEETS   H–70 = VEG/LEG
H–84 = MISC   H–88 = SOUPS/SAUCES   H–90 = FAST   H–106 = FRZN ENTREE   H–112 = BABY FOODS

Chol (mg)	Calc (mg)	Iron (mg)	Magn (mg)	Pota (mg)	Sodi (mg)	Zinc (mg)	VT-A (RE)	Thia (mg)	VT-E (α-TE)	Ribo (mg)	Niac (mg)	V-B6 (mg)	Fola (µg)	VT-C (mg)
0	4	.2	1	18	2	.01	<1	<.01	.02	<.01	.04	<.01	2	<1
0	3	.07	1	11	6	.01	<1	0	0	<.01	.01	<.01	5	1
0	1	.04	1	12	7	.01	<1	<.01	0	<.01	.01	<.01	<1	<1
0	1	.03	1	9	5	.01	<1	<.01	0	<.01	.01	<.01	<1	<1
0	15	.06	1	15	22	.02	2	<.01	0	<.01	.02	.01	14	2
0	1	.06	1	1	13	.01	<1	<.01	0	<.01	.02	<.01	<1	0
0	2	.11	1	3	23	.02	<1	<.01	0	<.01	.04	<.01	1	0
0	0	0	1	4	11	.02	0	0	0	0	0	0	0	0
0	187	4.2	64	761	86	.4	0	.02	0	.02	.18	.06	2	0
0	2	.12	0	4	2	.06	0	0	0	.04	0	0	0	0
0	<1	.01	0	<1	<1	<.01	0	0	0	<.01	0	0	0	0
0	<1	<.01	0	<1	<1	<.01	0	0	0	<.01	0	0	0	0
0	1	.06	0	2	1	.03	0	0	0	0	0	0	0	0
0	<1	<.01	<1	<1	<1	0	0	0	0	0	0	0	0	0
0	0	0	<1	3	4	–	0	0	–	0	–	0	–	0
5	38	.46	18	82	49	.3	8	.01	0	.08	.08	.01	2	<1
0	5	.5	25	183	58	.28	494	<.01	.01	.31	.13	<.01	2	<1
0	344[1]	7[1]	86[1]	997[1]	22	.4	0	.01	0	.02	.43	.28	<1	0
0	35	.9	51	193	3	.06	0	.02	0	.01	.04	.14	0	0
0	1	.07	2	2	66	.03	0	.01	0	.01	.02	0	0	0
0	11	.32	9	26	2	.3	5	.03	.01	.04	.16	.01	12	3
0	60	.65	15	171	6	.25	82	.01	.22	.04	.18	.05	24	12
0	30	.33	8	86	3	.13	41	<.01	.11	.02	.09	.03	12	6
0	276	2.98	73	846	28	1.16	366	.03	.66	.18	.74	.23	75	54
0	16	.15	5	37	3	.05	24	<.01	.04	.01	.03	.01	10	2
0	54	1.55	72	425	114	.59	22	.08	.23	.08	1.2	.13	61	12
0	50	1.34	74	634	127	.86	39	.15	.46	.38	2.2	.21	286	12
0	39	1.62	48	439	899	.54	28	.06	1.87	.17	1.38	.15	149	52
0	40	1.36	40	266	66	.3	15	.06	.2	.05	.6	.09	45	8
0	18	.66	9	144	10	.38	49	.11	.34	.11	.97	.11	131	10
0	18	.66	9	144	10	.38	49	.11	.34	.11	.97	.11	131	10
0	21	.58	12	196	4	.5	74	.06	1.13	.09	.94	.02	122	22
0	21	.58	12	196	4	.5	74	.06	1.13	.09	.94	.02	122	22
0	19	2.2	12	206	344[2]	.48	64	.07	.52	.12	1.15	.13	115	22
0	11	.42	5	105	9	.85	1	.03	.5	.03	.18	.18	4	1
0	20	.76	5	805	6	1.66	3	.23	1.51	.11	.91	.36	11	6
0	14	.29	4	640	5	.56	0	.02	.8	.06	.36	.12	3	0

[2]Low sodium pack contains 3 mg sodium.

(For purposes of calculations, use "0" for t, <1, <.1, <.01, etc.)

H

Table H–1
Food Composition

Computer Code Number	Food Description	Measure	Wt (g)	H$_2$O (%)	Ener (kcal)	Prot (g)	Carb (g)	Dietary Fiber (g)	Fat (g)	Fat Breakdown (g) Sat	Mono	Poly
	VEGETABLES AND LEGUMES—Cont.											
	Beans (see also alphabetical listing in this section):											
1990	Adzuki beans, cooked	½ c	115	66	147	9	29	1	<1	.04	.01	.02
796	Black beans, cooked	½ c	86	66	114	8	20	8	<1	.1	t	.2
	Canned beans (white/navy):											
803	With pork and tomato sauce	½ c	126	73	124	7	24	6	1	.5	.6	.2
804	With sweet sauce	1 c	253	71	281	13	53	11	4	1.4	1.6	.5
805	With frankfurters	1 c	253	69	359	17	39	18	17	6	7.2	2.1
	Lima beans:											
797	Thick seeded (Fordhooks), cooked from frozen	½ c	85	74	85	5	16	5	<1	.1	t	.1
798	Thin seeded (Baby), cooked from frozen	½ c	90	72	95	6	18	5	<1	.1	t	.1
799	Cooked from dry, drained	½ c	94	70	108	7	20	7	<1	.1	t	.2
1998	Red Mexican, cooked f/dry	1 c	224	70	252	16	47	18	1	.2	.2	.3
	Snap bean/green string beans cuts and french style:											
800	Cooked from fresh	½ c	62	89	22	1	5	2	<1	t	t	.1
801	Cooked from frozen	½ c	67	91	19	1	4	2	<1	t	t	.1
802	Canned, drained	½ c	67	93	13	1	3	1	<1	t	t	t
1713	Snap bean, yellow, cooked f/fresh	½ c	63	89	22	1	5	2	<1	t	t	.1
	Bean sprouts (mung):											
806	Raw	1 c	104	90	31	3	6	2	<1	.1	t	.1
807	Cooked, stir-fried	1 c	124	84	62	5	13	2	<1	.1	.1	.1
808	Cooked, boiled, drained	1 c	124	93	26	3	5	1	<1	t	t	t
1788	Canned, drained	1 c	125	96	15	2	3	1	<1	<.1	<.1	<.1
	Beets, cooked from fresh:											
809	Sliced or diced	½ c	85	87	37	1	9	2	<1	t	t	.1
810	Whole beets, 2" diam	2 ea	100	87	44	2	10	2	<1	t	t	.1
	Beets, canned:											
811	Sliced or diced	½ c	85	91	26	1	6	2	<1	t	t	t
812	Pickled slices	½ c	114	82	74	1	19	2	<1	t	t	t
813	Beet greens, cooked, drained	½ c	72	89	19	2	4	2	<1	t	t	.1
	Broccoli, raw:											
817	Chopped	1 c	88	91	25	3	5	3	<1	.1	t	.2
818	Spears	1 ea	151	91	42	5	8	5	1	.1	t	.3
	Broccoli, cooked from fresh:											
819	Spears	1 ea	180	91	50	5	9	5	1	.1	t	.3
820	Chopped	1 c	156	91	44	5	8	5	1	.1	t	.3
	Broccoli, cooked from frozen:											
821	Spear, small piece	3 ea	90	91	25	3	5	3	<1	t	t	.1
822	Chopped	1 c	184	91	52	6	10	6	<1	t	t	.1
1603	Broccoflower, steamed	3½ oz	100	90	32	3	6	3	<1	t	t	.1
823	Brussels sprouts, cooked from fresh	½ c	78	87	30	2	7	3	<1	.1	t	.2
824	Brussels sprouts, cooked from frozen	½ c	77	87	32	3	6	3	<1	.1	t	.2
	Cabbage, common varieties:											
825	Raw, shredded or chopped	1 c	70	92	18	1	4	2	<1	t	t	.1

(Computer code number is for West Diet Analysis program)

PAGE KEY: H–4 = BEV   H–6 = DAIRY   H–12 = EGGS   H–14 = FAT/OIL   H–18 = FRUIT   H–26 = BAKERY   H–36 = GRAIN   H–44 = FISH
H–48 = MEATS   H–50 = POULTRY   H–54 = SAUSAGE   H–56 = MIXED/FAST   H–64 = NUTS/SEEDS   H–68 = SWEETS   H–70 = VEG/LEG
H–84 = MISC   H–88 = SOUPS/SAUCES   H–90 = FAST   H–106 = FRZN ENTREE   H–112 = BABY FOODS

Chol (mg)	Calc (mg)	Iron (mg)	Magn (mg)	Pota (mg)	Sodi (mg)	Zinc (mg)	VT-A (RE)	Thia (mg)	VT-E (α-TE)	Ribo (mg)	Niac (mg)	V-B6 (mg)	Fola (μg)	VT-C (mg)
0	32	2.3	60	612	9	2	1	.13	.12	.07	.83	.11	139	0
0	23	1.81	60	305	1	.96	1	.21	.07	.05	.43	.06	128	0
9	71	4.13	44	378	554	7.4	15	.07	.68	.06	.63	.09	28	4
18	154	4.23	86	673	850	3.82	29	.12	–	.15	.89	.22	95	8
15	121	4.38	71	595	1087	4.73	38	.15	1.19	.14	2.28	.12	76	6
0	19	1.16	29	347	45	.37	16	.06	.25	.05	.91	.1	18	11
0	25	1.76	50	370	26	.5	15	.06	.58	.05	.69	.1	14	5
0	16	2.25	40	478	2	.89	0	.15	.17	.05	.4	.15	78	0
0	84	3.72	96	738	481	1.74	1	.27	.16	.13	.75	.23	188	4
0	29	.79	16	185	2	.22	42	.05	.09	.06	.38	.03	21	6
0	33	.59	16	84	6	.32	27	.02	.09	.06	.26	.04	15	3
0	17	.6	9	73	176	.19	24	.01	.09	.04	.14	.03	21	3
0	29	.8	16	188	2	.23	5	.05	.18	.06	.39	.04	21	6
0	14	.95	22	155	6	.43	2	.09	.03	.13	.78	.09	63	14
0	16	2.36	41	272	11	1.12	4	.17	.02	.22	1.49	.16	86	20
0	15	.81	17	125	12	.58	1	.06	.01	.13	1.01	.07	36	14
0	18	.54	11	34	175	.35	3	.04	.01	.09	.28	.04	12	<1
0	14	.67	20	259	66	.3	3	.02	.26	.03	.28	.06	68	3
0	16	.79	23	305	77	.35	4	.03	.3	.04	.33	.07	80	4
0	13	1.55	15	126	165	.18	1	.01	.26	.03	.13	.05	26	4
0	13	.47	17	169	301	.3	1	.01	.15	.06	.29	.06	30	3
0	82	1.37	49	655	174	.36	367	.08	.22	.21	.36	.1	10	18
0	42	.77	22	286	24	.35	136[1]	.06	1.46	.1	.56	.14	63	82
0	73	1.33	38	491	41	.6	233[1]	.1	2.51	.18	.96	.24	107	141
0	83	1.51	43	526	47	.68	250[1]	.1	3.04	.2	1.03	.26	90	134
0	73	1.31	37	456	41	.59	217[1]	.09	2.64	.18	.9	.22	78	116
0	46	.55	18	162	22	.27	170[1]	.05	.93	.07	.41	.12	27	36
0	94	1.12	37	331	44	.55	348[1]	.1	3.04	.15	.84	.24	104	74
0	32	.7	20	322	23	.5	7	.07	.3	.1	.76	.18	49	63
0	28	.94	16	247	16	.26	56	.08	.66	.06	.47	.14	47	48
0	19	.57	19	250	18	.28	45	.08	.45	.09	.41	.22	78	35
0	33	.41	11	172	13	.13	9	.04	.07	.03	.21	.07	30	23

[1]Vitamin A for whole plant: leaves are 1600 RE/100 g raw; flower clusters are 300/100 g raw; stalks are 40 RE/100 g raw.

H

(For purposes of calculations, use "0" for t, <1, <.1, <.01, etc.)

Table H–1
Food Composition

Computer Code Number	Food Description	Measure	Wt (g)	H₂O (%)	Ener (kcal)	Prot (g)	Carb (g)	Dietary Fiber (g)	Fat (g)	Fat Breakdown (g)		
										Sat	Mono	Poly
	VEGETABLES AND LEGUMES—Cont.											
826	Cooked, drained	1 c	150	94	33	2	7	4	1	.1	t	.3
	Cabbage, Chinese:											
1178	Bok choy, raw, shredded	1 c	70	95	9	1	2	1	<1	t	t	.1
827	Bok choy, cooked, drained	1 c	170	96	20	3	3	3	<1	t	t	.1
1937	Kim chee style	1 c	150	92	31	3	6	2	<1	<.1	<.1	.2
828	Pe tsai, raw, chopped	1 c	76	94	12	1	3	2	<1	t	t	.1
1796	Pe tsai, cooked	1 c	119	95	17	2	3	3	<1	<.1	<.1	.1
	Cabbage, red, coarsely chopped:											
829	Raw	1 c	70	92	19	1	4	1	<1	t	t	.1
830	Cooked, drained	½ c	75	94	16	1	4	2	<1	t	t	.1
831	Cabbage, savoy, coarsely chopped, raw	1 c	70	91	19	1	4	2	<1	t	t	t
1785	Cabbage, savoy, cooked	1 c	145	92	35	3	8	4	<1	<.1	<.1	.1
1896	Capers	1 tsp	5	86	0	0	0	0	0	–	–	–
	Carrots, raw:											
832	Whole, 7½ x 1⅛"	1 ea	72	88	31	1	7	2	<1	t	t	.1
833	Grated	½ c	55	88	24	1	6	2	<1	t	t	t
	Carrots, cooked, sliced, drained:											
834	From fresh	½ c	78	87	35	1	8	3	<1	t	t	.1
835	From frozen	½ c	73	90	26	1	6	3	<1	t	t	t
836	Carrots, canned, sliced, drained	½ c	73	93	17	<1	4	1	<1	t	t	.1
837	Carrot juice, canned	½ c	123	89	49	1	11	1	<1	t	t	.1
	Cauliflower, flowerets:											
838	Raw	½ c	50	92	13	1	3	1	<1	t	t	.1
839	Cooked from fresh, drained	½ c	62	93	14	1	3	2	<1	.1	t	.1
840	Cooked, from frozen, drained	½ c	90	94	17	1	3	2	<1	t	t	.1
	Celery, pascal type, raw:											
841	Large outer stalk, 8 x 1½" (root end)	1 ea	40	95	6	<1	2	1	<1	t	t	t
842	Diced	1 c	120	95	19	1	4	2	<1	t	t	.1
1789	Celeriac/celery root, cooked	3½ oz	99	92	25	1	6	1	<1	<.1	<.1	.1
1179	Chard, swiss, raw, chopped	1 c	36	93	7	1	1	1	<1	t	t	t
1180	Chard, swiss, cooked	1 c	175	93	35	3	7	4	<1	t	t	.1
1855	Chayote fruit, raw	1 ea	203	93	49	2	11	6	1	.1	.1	.3
1856	Chayote fruit, cooked	1 c	160	93	38	1	8	5	1	.2	.1	.3
	Chickpeas (see Garbanzo Beans #854)											
	Collards, cooked, drained:											
843	From fresh	½ c	64	92	17	1	4	2	<1	t	t	.1
844	From frozen	½ c	85	89	31	3	6	3	<1	.1	t	.2
	Corn, cooked, drained:											
845	From fresh, on cob, 5" long	1 ea	77	73	72	3	17	2	1	.1	.2	.3
846	From frozen, on cob, 3½" long	1 ea	63	73	59	2	14	2	<1	.1	.1	.2
847	Kernels, cooked from frozen	½ c	82	77	66	2	16	2	<1	.1	.1	.2
	Corn, canned:											
848	Cream style	½ c	128	79	92	2	23	3	1	.1	.2	.3
849	Whole kernel, vacuum pack	½ c	105	77	83	3	20	2	1	.1	.2	.3
	Cowpeas (see Black-eyed peas #814–816)											
850	Cucumber slices with peel	7 pce	28	96	4	<1	1	<1	<1	t	t	t
1948	Cucumber, kim chee style	1 c	150	91	32	2	7	2	<1	.1	0	.1

TABLE OF FOOD COMPOSITION ◆ **H–75**

PAGE KEY: H–4 = BEV   H–6 = DAIRY   H–12 = EGGS   H–14 = FAT/OIL   H–18 = FRUIT   H–26 = BAKERY   H–36 = GRAIN   H–44 = FISH
H–48 = MEATS   H–50 = POULTRY   H–54 = SAUSAGE   H–56 = MIXED/FAST   H–64 = NUTS/SEEDS   H–68 = SWEETS   H–70 = VEG/LEG
H–84 = MISC   H–88 = SOUPS/SAUCES   H–90 = FAST   H–106 = FRZN ENTREE   H–112 = BABY FOODS

Chol (mg)	Calc (mg)	Iron (mg)	Magn (mg)	Pota (mg)	Sodi (mg)	Zinc (mg)	VT-A (RE)	Thia (mg)	VT-E (α-TE)	Ribo (mg)	Niac (mg)	V-B6 (mg)	Fola (μg)	VT-C (mg)
0	47	.26	12	146	12	.14	20	.09	.16	.08	.42	.17	30	30
0	74	.56	13	176	46	.13	210	.03	.08	.05	.35	.14	46	32
0	158	1.77	19	631	58	.29	437	.05	.2	.11	.73	.28	69	44
0	145	1.28	28	375	995	.35	426	.07	.24	.1	.76	.34	88	80
0	59	.24	10	181	7	.18	91	.03	.09	.04	.3	.18	60	21
0	38	.36	12	268	11	.21	115	.05	.14	.05	.6	.21	64	19
0	36	.34	11	144	8	.15	3	.04	.07	.02	.21	.15	15	40
0	28	.26	8	105	6	.11	2	.03	.09	.02	.15	.1	10	26
0	25	.28	20	161	20	.19	70	.05	.07	.02	.21	.13	56	22
0	44	.55	35	267	35	.33	129	.07	.15	.03	.04	.22	67	25
0	2	.05	–	–	105	–	1	–	–	–	–	–	–	0
0	19	.36	11	233	25	.14	2025	.07	.33	.04	.67	.11	10	7
0	15	.28	8	178	19	.11	1547	.05	.25	.03	.51	.08	8	5
0	24	.48	10	177	52	.23	1914	.03	.33	.04	.4	.19	11	2
0	20	.34	7	115	43	.18	1292	.02	.31	.03	.32	.09	8	2
0	18	.47	6	131	177[1]	.19	1005	.01	.31	.02	.4	.08	7	2
0	30	.57	17	359	36	.22	3167	.11	.01	.07	.5	.27	5	11
0	11	.22	8	152	15	.14	1	.03	.02	.03	.26	.11	29	23
0	10	.2	6	88	9	.11	1	.03	.03	.03	.25	.11	27	28
0	15	.37	8	125	16	.12	2	.03	–	.05	.28	.08	37	28
0	16	.16	4	115	35	.05	5	.02	.14	.02	.13	.03	11	3
0	48	.48	13	344	104	.16	16	.06	.43	.05	.39	.1	34	8
0	26	.43	12	171	60	.2	0	.03	.2	.04	.42	.1	3	4
0	18	.65	29	136	77	.13	119	.01	.68	.03	.14	.04	5	11
0	102	3.96	151	961	313	.58	550	.06	3.31	.15	.63	.15	15	32
0	39	.81	28	305	8	.71	12	.06	.24	.08	1.02	.27	56	22
0	21	.35	19	277	2	.5	8	.04	.19	.06	.67	.19	29	13
0	15	.1	5	84	10	.07	175	.01	.56	.03	.19	.03	4	8
0	179	.95	26	213	43	.23	508	.04	.43	.1	.54	.1	65	22
0	2	.47	22	193	3	.49	16[2]	.13	.07	.05	1.17	.17	24	4
0	2	.38	18	158	3	.4	13[2]	.11	.06	.04	.96	.14	19	3
0	3	.29	16	121	4	.33	18[2]	.07	.07	.06	1.07	.11	25	3
0	4	.49	22	172	365[3]	.68	13[2]	.03	.12	.07	1.23	.08	57	6
0	5	.44	24	195	286[4]	.48	25[2]	.04	.1	.08	1.23	.06	52	9
0	4	.07	3	40	1	.06	6	.01	.02	.02	.06	.02	4	2
0	14	7.23	12	176	1531	.77	50	.05	.24	.05	.69	.17	35	5

[1]Low sodium pack contains 31 mg sodium.

[2]For yellow varieties; white varieties contain only a trace of vitamin A.

[3]Low sodium pack contains 4 mg sodium per ½ cup.

[4]Low sodium pack contains 6 mg sodium per cup.

(For purposes of calculations, use "0" for t, <1, <.1, <.01, etc.)

Table H–1
Food Composition

Computer Code Number	Food Description	Measure	Wt (g)	H$_2$O (%)	Ener (kcal)	Prot (g)	Carb (g)	Dietary Fiber (g)	Fat (g)	Fat Breakdown (g)		
										Sat	Mono	Poly
	VEGETABLES AND LEGUMES—Cont.											
	Dandelion greens:											
851	Raw	1 c	55	86	25	2	5	2	<1	.1	t	.2
852	Chopped, cooked, drained	1 c	105	90	35	2	7	3	1	.2	t	.3
853	Eggplant, cooked	1 c	160	92	45	1	11	4	<1	.1	t	.2
1714	Endive, fresh, chopped	¼ c	13	94	2	<1	<1	<1	<1	t	t	t
856	Escarole/curly endive, chopped	1 c	50	94	9	1	2	2	<1	t	t	t
854	Garbanzo beans (chickpeas), cooked	1 c	164	60	269	15	45	13	4	.4	1	1.9
1939	Grape leaves, raw	10 g	10	79	7	<1	1	–	<1	–	–	–
855	Great northern beans, cooked	1 c	177	69	209	15	37	12	1	.3	t	.3
857	Jerusalem artichoke, raw slices	1 c	150	78	114	3	26	2	<1	0	t	t
1794	Jicama	1 c	120	90	46	1	11	6	<1	<.1	<.1	.1
	Kale, cooked, drained:											
858	From fresh	½ c	65	91	21	1	4	1	<1	t	t	.1
859	From frozen	½ c	65	91	20	2	3	1	<1	t	t	.2
860	Kidney beans, canned	1 c	256	77	218	13	40	16	1	.1	.1	.5
1181	Kohlrabi, raw slices	1 c	140	91	38	2	9	5	<1	t	t	.1
861	Kohlrabi, cooked	1 c	165	90	48	3	11	2	<1	t	t	.1
1183	Leeks, raw, chopped	1 c	104	83	63	2	15	2	<1	t	t	.2
1182	Leeks, cooked, chopped	½ c	52	91	16	<1	4	<1	<1	t	t	.1
862	Lentils, cooked from dry	½ c	99	70	115	9	20	9	<1	.1	.1	.2
1288	Lentils, sprouted, stir-fried	4 oz	113	69	114	10	24	4	1	.1	.1	.2
1289	Lentils, sprouted, raw	1 c	77	67	82	7	17	3	<1	t	.1	.2
	Lettuce:											
	Butterhead/Boston types:											
863	Head, 5" diameter	¼ ea	41	96	5	1	1	<1	<1	t	t	.1
864	Leaves, inner or outer	4 ea	30	96	4	<1	1	<1	<1	t	t	t
	Iceberg/crisphead:											
865	Head, 6" diameter	¼ ea	135	96	16	1	3	2	<1	t	t	.1
866	Wedge, ¼ head	1 ea	135	96	16	1	3	2	<1	t	t	.1
867	Chopped or shredded	1 c	56	96	7	1	1	1	<1	t	t	.1
868	Looseleaf, chopped	½ c	28	94	5	<1	1	<1	<1	t	t	t
869	Romaine, chopped	½ c	28	95	5	<1	1	<1	<1	t	t	t
870	Romaine, inner leaf	3 ea	30	95	5	<1	1	<1	<1	t	t	t
1930	Luffa, cooked (Chinese okra)	1 c	178	89	57	3	13	6	<1	.1	.1	.1
	Mushrooms:											
871	Raw, sliced	½ c	35	92	9	1	2	<1	<1	t	t	.1
872	Cooked from fresh, pieces	½ c	78	91	21	2	4	2	<1	t	t	.1
1962	Stir fried, shitake slices	1 c	145	84	80	2	21	3	<1	.1	.1	<.1
873	Canned, drained	½ c	78	91	19	2	4	2	<1	t	t	.1
1951	Mushroom caps, pickled	8 ea	47	92	11	1	2	1	<1	<.1	<.1	.1
	Mustard greens:											
874	Cooked from fresh	½ c	70	95	11	2	2	1	<1	t	.1	t
875	Cooked from frozen	½ c	75	94	14	2	2	2	<1	t	.1	t
876	Navy beans, cooked from dry	1 c	182	63	258	16	48	12	1	.3	.1	.5
	Okra, cooked:											
877	From fresh pods	8 ea	85	90	27	2	6	2	<1	t	t	t
878	From frozen slices	½ c	92	91	34	2	5	3	<1	.1	.1	.1
1236	Batter fried from fresh	1 c	92	69	175	3	12	2	13	2.1	3.5	7.2
1930	Chinese, (Luffa), cooked	1 c	178	89	57	3	13	6	<1	.1	.1	.1

(Computer code number is for West Diet Analysis program)

H

TABLE OF FOOD COMPOSITION

◆ **H–77**

PAGE KEY: H–4 = BEV   H–6 = DAIRY   H–12 = EGGS   H–14 = FAT/OIL   H–18 = FRUIT   H–26 = BAKERY   H–36 = GRAIN   H–44 = FISH
H–48 = MEATS   H–50 = POULTRY   H–54 = SAUSAGE   H–56 = MIXED/FAST   H–64 = NUTS/SEEDS   H–68 = SWEETS   H–70 = VEG/LEG
H–84 = MISC   H–88 = SOUPS/SAUCES   H–90 = FAST   H–106 = FRZN ENTREE   H–112 = BABY FOODS

Chol (mg)	Calc (mg)	Iron (mg)	Magn (mg)	Pota (mg)	Sodi (mg)	Zinc (mg)	VT-A (RE)	Thia (mg)	VT-E (α-TE)	Ribo (mg)	Niac (mg)	V-B6 (mg)	Fola (µg)	VT-C (mg)
0	103	1.71	20	218	42	.23	770	.11	1.38	.14	.44	.14	15	19
0	147	1.89	25	244	46	.29	1228	.14	2.63	.18	.54	.17	13	19
0	10	.56	21	397	5	.24	10	.12	.48	.03	.96	.14	23	2
0	7	.10	2	41	3	.1	27	.01	.06	.01	.05	<.01	19	1
0	26	.42	8	157	11	.4	103	.04	.22	.04	.2	.01	71	3
0	80	4.74	79	477	12	2.51	5	.19	.57	.1	.86	.23	282	2
0	72	.69	–	26	2	–	270	.02	–	.01	.12	–	–	1
0	120	3.77	89	692	4	1.56	<1	.28	.53	.1	1.21	.21	181	2
0	21	5.1	26	644	6	.18	3	.3	.29	.09	1.95	.12	20	6
0	14	.72	14	180	5	.19	2	.02	5.48	.04	.24	.05	14	24
0	47	.59	12	148	15	.16	481	.04	.55	.05	.33	.09	9	27
0	90	.61	12	209	10	.12	413	.03	.12	.07	.44	.06	9	16
0	61	3.23	72	658	873	1.41	0	.27	.13	.23	1.17	.06	130	3
0	34	.56	27	490	28	.04	6	.07	.67	.03	.56	.21	23	87
0	41	.66	31	561	35	.51	7	.07	2.76	.03	.64	.25	20	89
0	61	2.18	29	187	21	.13	10	.06	.96	.03	.42	.24	67	13
0	16	.57	7	45	5	.03	3	.01	.32	.01	.1	.06	13	2
0	19	3.3	36	365	2	1.26	1	.17	.11	.07	1.05	.18	179	2
0	16	3.5	40	321	11	1.81	5	.25	.1	.1	1.36	.19	76	14
0	19	2.47	29	248	9	1.16	4	.18	.07	.1	.87	.15	77	13
0	13	.12	5	105	2	.07	40	.03	.18	.03	.12	.02	30	3
0	10	.09	4	77	2	.05	29	.02	.13	.02	.09	.02	22	2
0	26	.68	12	213	12	.3	45	.06	.38	.04	.25	.05	76	5
0	26	.68	12	213	12	.3	45	.06	.38	.04	.25	.05	76	5
0	11	.28	5	89	5	.12	19	.03	.16	.02	.1	.02	31	2
0	19	.39	3	74	3	.08	53	.01	.12	.02	.11	.02	14	5
0	10	.31	2	81	2	.07	73	.03	.12	.03	.14	.01	38	7
0	11	.33	2	87	2	.08	78	.03	.13	.03	.15	.01	41	7
0	112	.8	101	570	420	.97	103	.23	1.22	.1	1.54	.33	81	29
0	2	.43	4	130	1	.26	0	.04	.04	.16	1.44	.03	7	1
0	5	1.36	9	278	2	.68	0	.06	.09	.23	3.48	.07	14	3
0	4	.64	20	170	6	1.93	0	.05	.17	.25	2.18	.23	30	.44
0	9	.62	12	101	332	.56	0	.07	.09	.02	1.24	.05	10	0
0	2	.5	5	139	95	.28	0	.03	.05	.16	1.42	.03	6	1
0	52	.49	11	141	11	.08	212	.03	1.41	.04	.3	.07	51	18
0	76	.84	10	104	19	.15	335	.03	1.31	.04	.19	.08	52	10
0	127	4.51	107	670	2	1.93	<1	.37	.73	.11	.97	.3	255	2
0	54	.38	49	274	4	.47	49	.11	.59	.05	.74	.16	39	14
0	88	.62	47	215	3	.57	47	.09	.64	.11	.72	.04	134	11
15	104	.77	37	214	137	.5	43	.13	3.09	.1	.75	.13	38	10
0	112	.8	101	570	420	.97	103	.23	1.22	.1	1.54	.33	81	29

(For purposes of calculations, use "0" for t, <1, <.1, <.01, etc.)

H

Table H–1
Food Composition

Computer Code Number	Food Description	Measure	Wt (g)	H₂O (%)	Ener (kcal)	Prot (g)	Carb (g)	Dietary Fiber (g)	Fat (g)	Fat Breakdown (g) Sat	Mono	Poly
	VEGETABLES AND LEGUMES—Cont.											
	Onions:											
879	Raw, chopped	1 c	160	90	61	2	14	3	<1	<.1	<.1	.1
880	Raw, sliced	1 c	115	90	44	1	10	2	<1	<.1	<.1	.1
881	Cooked, drained, chopped	½ c	105	88	46	1	11	1	<1	<.1	<.1	.1
882	Dehydrated flakes	¼ c	14	4	45	1	12	1	<1	<.1	<.1	<.1
1934	Onions, pearl, cooked	1 c	185	87	81	3	19	3	<1	.1	.1	.1
	Spring/green onions, chopped:											
883	Bulb and top	½ c	50	90	16	1	4	1	<1	<.1	<.1	<.1
1185	Green tops only	1 c	100	92	34	2	6	3	<1	.1	.1	.2
1184	White part only	½ c	50	92	25	1	5	1	<1	<.1	<.1	<.1
884	Onion rings, breaded, heated f/frozen	2 ea	20	29	81	1	8	<1	5	1.7	2.2	1
1917	Palm hearts, cooked slices	1 c	146	70	150	4	39	2	<1	.1	.1	<.1
	Parsley:											
885	Raw, chopped	½ c	30	88	11	1	2	1	<1	<.1	.1	<.1
886	Raw, sprigs	5 ea	5	88	2	<1	<1	<1	<1	<.1	<.1	<.1
888	Parsnips, sliced, cooked	½ c	78	78	63	1	15	3	<1	<.1	.1	<.1
	Peas:											
	Black-eyed, cooked:											
814	From dry, drained	½ c	85	70	99	7	18	3	<1	.1	<.1	.2
815	From fresh, drained	½ c	82	76	80	3	17	4	<1	.1	<.1	.1
816	From frozen, drained	½ c	85	66	112	7	20	5	1	.1	.1	.2
889	Edible pod peas, cooked	1 c	160	89	67	5	11	4	<1	.1	<.1	.2
890	Green, canned, drained	½ c	85	82	59	4	11	3	<1	.1	<.1	.1
891	Green, cooked from frozen	½ c	80	80	62	4	11	4	<1	t	t	.1
1786	Snow peas, raw	1 c	145	89	61	4	11	4	<1	.1	<.1	.1
1787	Snow peas, raw	10 ea	29	89	12	1	2	1	<1	<.1	<.1	<.1
892	Split, green, cooked from dry	½ c	98	70	116	8	21	3	<1	.1	.1	.2
1187	Peas & carrots, cooked from frozen	½ c	80	86	38	2	8	3	<1	.1	t	.2
1186	Peas & carrots, canned w/liquid	½ c	128	88	49	3	11	4	<1	.1	t	.2
	Peppers, hot:											
893	Hot green chili, canned	½ c	68	93	14	1	4	1	<1	t	t	t
894	Hot green chili, raw	1 ea	45	88	18	1	4	1	<1	t	t	.1
1715	Hot red chili, raw, diced	1 tbs	9	88	4	<1	1	<1	<1	t	t	t
1988	Jalapeno, raw	2 oz	57	90	25	–	–	–	–	–	–	–
895	Jalapeno, chopped, canned	½ c	68	90	16	1	3	1	<1	<.1	<.1	.2
1918	Jalapeno wheels, in brine (Ortega)	2 tbs	29	90	10	<1	2	1	<1	<.1	<.1	.1
	Peppers, sweet, green:											
896	Whole pod (90 g with refuse), raw	1 ea	74	92	20	1	5	1	<1	t	t	.1
897	Cooked, chopped (1 pod cooked = 73 g)	½ c	68	92	19	1	5	1	<1	t	t	.1
	Peppers, sweet, red:											
1286	Raw, chopped	1 c	100	92	27	1	6	2	<1	t	t	.1
1807	Raw, each	1 ea	74	92	20	1	5	2	<1	<.1	<.1	.1
1287	Cooked, chopped	½ c	68	92	19	1	5	1	<1	t	t	.1
	Peppers, sweet, yellow:											
1872	Raw, large	1 ea	186	92	50	2	12	2	<1	<.1	<.1	.2
1873	Strips	10 pce	52	92	14	1	3	1	<1	<.1	<.1	.1
898	Pinto beans, cooked from dry	½ c	85	64	117	7	22	7	<1	t	.1	.2

TABLE OF FOOD COMPOSITION

◆ **H–79**

PAGE KEY: H–4 = BEV   H–6 = DAIRY   H–12 = EGGS   H–14 = FAT/OIL   H–18 = FRUIT   H–26 = BAKERY   H–36 = GRAIN   H–44 = FISH
H–48 = MEATS   H–50 = POULTRY   H–54 = SAUSAGE   H–56 = MIXED/FAST   H–64 = NUTS/SEEDS   H–68 = SWEETS   H–70 = VEG/LEG
H–84 = MISC   H–88 = SOUPS/SAUCES   H–90 = FAST   H–106 = FRZN ENTREE   H–112 = BABY FOODS

Chol (mg)	Calc (mg)	Iron (mg)	Magn (mg)	Pota (mg)	Sodi (mg)	Zinc (mg)	VT-A (RE)	Thia (mg)	VT-E (α-TE)	Ribo (mg)	Niac (mg)	V-B6 (mg)	Fola (µg)	VT-C (mg)
0	32	.35	16	251	5	.3	0	.07	.21	.03	.24	.19	30	10
0	23	.25	12	181	3	.22	0	.05	.15	.02	.17	.13	22	7
0	23	.25	12	174	3	.22	0	.04	.14	.02	.17	.14	16	5
0	36	.22	13	227	3	.26	0	.07	.19	.01	.14	.22	23	11
0	41	.44	20	305	433	.39	0	.08	.24	.04	.30	.24	28	10
0	36	.74	10	138	8	.2	20	.03	.07	.04	.26	.03	32	9
0	56	2.2	21	260	7	.22	40	.07	.3	.1	.6	0	80	51
0	20	.45	8	115	4	.13	<1	.03	.06	.02	.17	.05	18	13
0	6	.34	4	26	75	.08	5	.06	.14	.03	.72	.01	3	<1
0	26	2.47	15	2637	20	5.45	10	.07	.73	.25	1.25	1.06	30	10
0	41	1.86	15	166	17	.32	156	.03	.54	.03	.39	.03	46	40
0	7	.31	2	27	2	.04	26	<.01	.09	<.01	.04	<.01	9	5
0	29	.45	23	286	8	.2	0	.06	.78	.04	.56	.07	45	10[1]
0	20	2.13	45	236	3	1.1	2	.17	.24	.05	.42	.09	177	<1
0	105	.92	43	343	3	.85	65	.08	.18	.12	1.15	.05	104	2
0	20	1.8	43	319	4	1.21	7	.22	.33	.05	.62	.08	120	2
0	67	3.15	42	384	6	.59	21	.2	.62	.12	.86	.23	47	77
0	17	.81	14	147	214[2]	.6	65	.1	.32	.07	.62	.05	38	8
0	19	1.26	23	134	70	.75	54	.23	.14	.08	1.18	.09	47	8
0	62	3.02	35	290	6	.39	20	.22	.57	.12	.87	.23	61	87
0	13	.6	7	58	1	.08	4	.04	.11	.02	.17	.05	12	17
0	14	1.26	35	355	2	.98	1	.19	.38	.05	.87	.05	64	<1
0	18	.75	13	126	54	.36	621	.18	.26	.05	.92	.07	21	6
0	29	.96	18	128	332	.74	739	.09	.54	.07	.74	.11	23	8
0	5	.34	10	127	798	.12	42[3]	.01	.47	.03	.54	.1	7	46
0	8	.54	11	153	3	.14	35[3]	.04	.31	.04	.43	.13	11	109
0	2	.11	2	31	1	.03	97	.01	.06	.01	.09	.03	2	22
—	—	—	—	3	3	—	39	—	.47	—	—	—	—	66
0	18	1.9	8	93	995	.13	116	.02	.47	.03	.34	.14	9	9
0	8	.8	4	55	390	—	49	.01	.2	.01	.14	.06	4	21
0	7	.34	7	131	2	.09	47	.05	.51	.02	.38	.18	16	66
0	6	.31	7	113	1	.08	40	.04	.47	.02	.32	.16	11	51
0	9	.46	10	177	2	.12	570	.07	.69	.03	.51	.25	22	190
0	7	.34	7	131	2	.09	422	.05	.51	.02	.38	.18	16	141
0	6	.31	7	113	1	.08	256	.04	.47	.02	.32	.16	11	116
0	21	.86	22	394	4	.32	45	.05	1.28	.05	1.66	.31	48	342
0	6	.24	6	110	1	.09	13	.02	.36	.01	.46	.09	14	96
0	41	2.22	47	398	2	.92	<1	.16	.8	.08	.34	.13	146	2

[1] Value for Vitamin C is highest right after harvest and drops after that.

[2] Low sodium pack contains 1.7 mg sodium.

[3] Data is for green chili peppers; red varieties contain 809 RE vitamin A per ½ cup; 484 RE per whole pepper.

(For purposes of calculations, use "0" for t, <1, <.1, <.01, etc.)

H

Table H–1
Food Composition

Computer Code Number	Food Description	Measure	Wt (g)	H₂O (%)	Ener (kcal)	Prot (g)	Carb (g)	Dietary Fiber (g)	Fat (g)	Fat Breakdown (g) Sat	Mono	Poly
	VEGETABLES AND LEGUMES—Cont.											
1191	Poi, two finger	¼ c	60	72	67	<1	16	<1	<1	<.1	<.1	<.1
	Potatoes:[1]											
	Baked in oven, 4¾" x 2⅓" diam:											
899	With skin	1 ea	202	71	220	5	51	5	<1	.1	<.1	.1
900	Flesh only	1 ea	156	75	145	3	34	2	<1	<.1	<.1	.1
901	Skin only	1 ea	58	47	115	2	27	5	<1	<.1	<.1	<.1
	Baked in microwave, 4¾" x 2⅓" diam:											
902	With skin	1 ea	202	72	212	5	49	5	<1	.1	<.1	.1
903	Flesh only	1 ea	156	74	156	3	36	2	<1	<.1	<.1	.1
904	Skin only	1 ea	58	64	77	3	17	3	<1	<.1	<.1	<.1
	Boiled, about 2½" diam:											
905	Peeled after boiling	1 ea	136	77	118	3	27	2	<1	<.1	<.1	.1
906	Peeled before boiling	1 ea	135	78	116	2	27	2	<1	<.1	<.1	.1
	French fried, strips 2–3½" long:											
907	Oven heated	10 pce	50	35	167	2	20	2	9	3	5.7	.7
908	Fried in vegetable oil	10 ea	50	40	155	2	19	2	8	2.5	4	1.2
1188	Fried in veg and animal oil	10 ea	50	38	158	2	20	2	8	1.9	4.7	.7
909	Hashed browns from frozen	1 c	156	56	340	5	44	3	18	7	8	2.1
	Mashed:											
910	Home recipe with whole milk[2]	½ c	105	79	81	2	18	2	1	.4	.2	.1
911	Home recipe with milk and marg	½ c	105	76	111	2	18	2	4	1.1	1.9	1.3
912	Prepared from flakes; water, milk, margarine, salt added	½ c	110	76	124	2	17	3	6	1.6	2.5	1.7
	Potato products, prepared:											
	Au gratin:											
913	From dry mix	½ c	122	79	114	3	16	1	5	3.5	1.4	.2
914	From home recipe[3]	½ c	122	74	161	7	14	2	9	4.8	3.2	1.3
	Scalloped:											
915	From dry mix	½ c	122	79	114	3	16	1	5	3.2	1.5	.2
916	From home recipe[4]	½ c	122	81	105	4	13	2	5	1.7	1.7	.9
	Potato salad (see Mixed Dishes #715)											
1192	Potato puffs, cooked from frozen	½ c	62	53	138	2	19	2	7	3.2	2.7	.5
918	Pumpkin, cooked from fresh, mashed	1 c	245	94	49	2	12	4	<1	.1	<.1	<.1
919	Pumpkin, canned	½ c	123	90	42	1	10	4	<1	.2	<.1	<.1
1891	Radicchio, raw, shredded	½ c	20	93	5	<1	1	<1	<1	<.1	<.1	<.1
1894	Radicchio, raw, leaf	10 ea	80	93	18	1	4	<1	<1	<.1	<.1	<.1
920	Red radishes	10 ea	45	95	8	<1	2	<1	<1	<.1	<.1	<.1
1793	Daikon radishes (Chinese) raw	½ c	44	95	8	<1	2	1	<1	<.1	<.1	<.1
921	Refried beans, canned	½ c	126	76	118	7	20	7	2	.6	.7	.2
1375	Rutabaga, cooked cubes	½ c	85	89	33	1	7	2	<1	<.1	<.1	.1
922	Sauerkraut, canned with liquid	½ c	118	93	22	1	5	3	<1	<.1	<.1	.1
923	Seaweed, kelp, raw	1 oz	28	82	12	<1	3	<1	<1	.1	<.1	<.1
924	Seaweed, spirulina, dried	1 oz	28	5	81	16	7	1	2	.7	.2	.6
1866	Shallots, raw, chopped	1 tbs	10	80	7	<1	2	<1	<1	<.1	<.1	<.1

(1) Vitamin C varies with length of storage. After 3 months of storage approximately two-thirds of the ascorbic acid remains; after 6 to 7 months, about one-third remains.

(2) Recipe: 84% potatoes, 15% whole milk, 1% salt.

(3) Recipe: 55% potatoes, 30% whole milk, 9% cheddar cheese, 3% butter, 2% flour, 1% salt.

(4) Recipe: 59% potatoes, 36% whole milk, 2% butter, 2% flour, 1% salt.

TABLE OF FOOD COMPOSITION ◆ **H–81**

PAGE KEY: H–4 = BEV   H–6 = DAIRY   H–12 = EGGS   H–14 = FAT/OIL   H–18 = FRUIT   H–26 = BAKERY   H–36 = GRAIN   H–44 = FISH
H–48 = MEATS   H–50 = POULTRY   H–54 = SAUSAGE   H–56 = MIXED/FAST   H–64 = NUTS/SEEDS   H–68 = SWEETS   H–70 = VEG/LEG
H–84 = MISC   H–88 = SOUPS/SAUCES   H–90 = FAST   H–106 = FRZN ENTREE   H–112 = BABY FOODS

Chol (mg)	Calc (mg)	Iron (mg)	Magn (mg)	Pota (mg)	Sodi (mg)	Zinc (mg)	VT-A (RE)	Thia (mg)	VT-E (α-TE)	Ribo (mg)	Niac (mg)	V-B6 (mg)	Fola (μg)	VT-C (mg)
0	10	.53	14	110	7	.13	1	.08	.11	.02	.66	.16	13	2
0	20	2.75	55	844	16	.65	0	.22	.1	.07	3.33	.7	22	26[1]
0	8	.55	39	610	8	.45	0	.16	.06	.03	2.18	.47	14	20[1]
0	20	4.08	25	332	12	.28	0	.07	.02	.06	1.78	.36	13	8[1]
0	22	2.5	55	903	16	.73	0	.24	.1	.06	3.45	.69	24	31[1]
0	8	.64	39	641	11	.51	0	.2	.06	.04	2.54	.5	19	24[1]
0	27	3.45	21	377	9	.3	0	.04	.02	.04	1.29	.29	10	9[1]
0	7	.42	30	515	5	.41	0	.14	.07	.03	1.96	.41	14	18[1]
0	11	.42	27	443	7	.36	0	.13	.07	.03	1.77	.36	12	10[1]
0	6	.83	12	270	307	.2	0	.04	.25	.02	1.34	.11	11	3
0	8	.68	17	356	82	.26	1	.07	.25	.02	1.14	.12	17	3
7	10	.38	17	366	108	.19	0	.09	.25	.01	1.63	.12	15	5
0	23	2.36	27	680	53	.5	0	.17	.3	.03	3.78	.2	10	10
2	27	.28	19	314	318	.3	6	.09	.05	.04	1.18	.24	9	7[1]
2[5]	27	.27	19	304	310	.28	21	.09	.32	.04	1.13	.24	8	6[1]
4[5]	54	.24	20	256	365	.2	23	.12	.77	.06	.74	.01	8	11
18	101	.39	18	267	536	.29	38	.02	1.5	.1	1.15	.05	8	4
18[6]	145	.78	24	483	528	.84	46	.08	.64	.14	1.21	.21	10	12
13	44	.47	17	248	416	.31	26	.02	.18	.07	1.26	.05	12	4
7[7]	70	.7	23	461	409	.49	23	.08	.4	.11	1.28	.22	11	13
0	19	.97	12	236	463	.19	1	.12	.03	.04	1.3	.14	10	4
0	37	1.4	22	564	2	.56	2651	.08	2.6	.19	1.01	.11	21	12
0	32	1.71	28	253	6	.21	2713	.03	1.3	.07	.45	.07	15	5
0	4	.11	3	60	4	.12	1	<.01	.45	.01	.05	.01	12	2
0	15	.45	10	242	18	.5	2	.01	1.81	.02	.2	.05	48	6
0	9	.13	4	104	11	.14	<1	<.01	<.01	.02	.14	.03	12	10
0	12	.18	7	100	9	.07	0	.01	<.01	.01	.09	.02	12	10
10	44	2.09	42	336	377	1.47	0	.03	.39	.02	.4	.18	14	8
0	41	.45	20	277	17	.3	48	.07	.13	.03	.61	.09	13	16
0	35	1.74	15	201	780	.22	2	.02	.12	.03	.17	.15	28	17
0	47	.8	34	25	65	.34	3	.01	.24	.04	.13	<.01	50	1
0	34	8	55	382	293	.56	16	.67	1.4	1.03	3.6	.1	26	3
0	4	.12	2	33	1	.04	125	.01	.01	<.01	.02	.03	3	1

[5] Data is for margarine; if butter is used, cholesterol = 25 mg for 29 total mg.

[6] Data is for butter; if margarine is used, cholesterol = 37 mg.

[7] Data is for butter; if margarine is used cholesterol = 15 mg.

(For purposes of calculations, use "0" for t, <1, <.1, <.01, etc.)

H

Table H–1
Food Composition

Computer Code Number	Food Description	Measure	Wt (g)	H$_2$O (%)	Ener (kcal)	Prot (g)	Carb (g)	Dietary Fiber (g)	Fat (g)	Fat Breakdown (g) Sat	Mono	Poly
	VEGETABLES AND LEGUMES—Cont.											
1557	Snow peas, stir-fried	1 c	165	89	69	5	12	4	<1	.1	<.1	.1
925	Soybeans, cooked from dry	½ c	86	63	149	15	9	5	8	1.1	1.7	4.4
1996	Soybeans, dry roasted	½ c	86	1	387	34	28	7	19	2.7	4.1	10.6
	Soybean products:											
	Soy milk, see Dairy											
926	Miso	½ c	138	46	282	16	39	7	8	1.2	1.9	4.7
927	Tofu (soybean curd, regular)	½ c	124	85	94	10	2	1	6	.9	1.3	3.4
	Spinach:											
928	Raw, chopped	1 c	56	92	12	2	2	2	<1	<.1	<.1	.1
929	Cooked, from fresh, drained	½ c	90	91	21	3	3	2	<1	<.1	<.1	.1
930	Cooked from frozen (leaf)	½ c	95	90	27	3	5	3	<1	<.1	<.1	.1
931	Canned, drained solids	½ c	107	92	25	3	4	3	1	.1	<.1	.2
	Spinach soufflé (see Mixed Dishes)											
	Squash, summer varieties, cooked:											
932	Varieties averaged	½ c	90	94	18	1	4	1	<1	.1	<.1	.1
933	Crookneck	½ c	90	94	18	1	4	2	<1	.1	<.1	.1
934	Zucchini	½ c	90	95	14	1	4	1	<1	<.1	<.1	<.1
	Squash, winter varieties, cooked:											
	Average of all varieties, baked:											
935	Mashed	1 c	245	89	96	2	21	7	2	.3	.1	.6
936	Cubes	1 c	205	89	80	2	18	6	1	.3	.1	.5
937	Acorn, baked, mashed	½ c	122	83	68	1	18	5	<1	<.1	<.1	.1
1218	Acorn, boiled, mashed	½ c	122	90	41	1	11	3	<1	<.1	<.1	<.1
	Butternut:											
938	Baked cubes	1 c	205	88	82	2	22	6	<1	<.1	<.1	.1
1219	Baked, mashed	½ c	122	88	49	1	13	3	<1	<.1	<.1	<.1
1193	Cooked from frozen	½ c	120	88	47	1	12	3	<1	<.1	<.1	<.1
1194	Hubbard, baked, mashed	½ c	120	85	60	3	13	3	1	.2	.1	.3
1195	Hubbard, boiled, mashed	½ c	118	91	35	2	8	3	<1	.1	<.1	.2
1196	Spaghetti, baked or boiled	½ c	77	92	22	1	5	1	<1	<.1	<.1	.1
1189	Succotash, cooked from frozen	½ c	85	74	79	4	17	4	1	.1	.1	.4
	Sweet potatoes:											
939	Baked in skin, peeled, 5 x 2" diam	1 ea	114	73	117	2	28	3	<1	<.1	<.1	.1
940	Boiled without skin, 5 x 2" diam	1 ea	151	73	159	3	37	4	<1	.1	<.1	.2
941	Candied, 2½ x 2"	1 pce	105	67	144	1	29	3	3	1.4	.7	.2
	Canned:											
942	Solid pack	½ c	128	74	129	3	30	3	<1	.1	<.1	.1
943	Vacuum pack, mashed	½ c	127	76	116	2	27	3	<1	.1	<.1	.1
944	Vacuum pack, 3¾ x 1"	2 pce	80	76	73	1	17	2	<1	<.1	<.1	.1
1940	Taro shoots, cooked slices	1 c	140	95	20	1	4	1	<1	<.1	<.1	<.1
1941	Taro, tahitian, cooked slices	1 c	137	87	60	6	9	1	1	.19	.08	.39
	Tomatillos:											
1877	Raw, each	1 ea	34	92	11	<1	2	1	<1	<.1	.1	.1
1875	Raw, chopped	½ c	66	92	21	1	4	1	1	.1	.1	.3
	Tomatoes:											
945	Raw, whole, 2⅗" diam	1 ea	123	94	26	1	6	1	<1	.1	.1	.2
946	Raw, chopped	1 c	180	94	38	2	8	2	1	.1	.1	.2

(Computer code number is for West Diet Analysis program)

Chol (mg)	Calc (mg)	Iron (mg)	Magn (mg)	Pota (mg)	Sodi (mg)	Zinc (mg)	VT-A (RE)	Thia (mg)	VT-E (α-TE)	Ribo (mg)	Niac (mg)	V-B6 (mg)	Fola (μg)	VT-C (mg)
0	71	3.43	40	330	7	.45	21	.22	.64	.13	.94	.25	55	84
0	88	4.42	74	443	1	.99	1	.13	1.68	.25	.34	.2	46	1
0	232	3.4	196	1173	2	4.1	2	.37	3.96	.65	.91	.19	176	4
0	92	3.76	58	226	5014	4.57	12	.13	.01	.34	1.19	.3	46	0
0	130	6.65	128	150	9	.99	11	.1	.01	.06	.24	.06	19	<1
0	55	1.52	44	313	44	.3	376	.04	1.06	.11	.4	.11	109	16
0	122	3.21	78	419	63	.68	737	.09	.86	.21	.44	.22	131	9
0	139	1.44	66	283	82	.67	739	.06	.91	.16	.4	.14	103	12
0	136	2.46	81	370	29[1]	.49	940	.02	1.39	.15	.42	.11	105	15
0	24	.32	22	173	1	.35	26[2]	.04	.11	.04	.46	.06	18	5
0	24	.32	22	173	1	.35	26[2]	.04	.11	.04	.46	.08	18	5
0	12	.31	20	228	3	.16	22[2]	.04	.11	.04	.39	.07	15	4
0	34	.81	20	1070	2	.64	872	.21	.29	.06	1.72	.18	69	24
0	29	.68	16	896	2	.53	730	.17	.25	.05	1.44	.15	57	20
0	54	1.14	52	533	5	.21	52	.2	.15	.02	1.08	.24	23	13
0	32	.68	32	321	4	.13	32	.12	.15	.01	.65	.14	14	8
0	84	1.23	59	582	8	.27	1435	.15	.35	.03	1.99	.25	39	31
0	50	.73	35	347	5	.16	854	.09	.2	.02	1.19	.15	23	18
0	23	.7	11	160	2	.14	401	.06	.16	.05	.56	.08	20	4
0	20	.56	26	430	10	.18	725	.09	.14	.06	.67	.21	19	11
0	12	.33	15	253	6	.12	473	.05	.14	.03	.39	.12	11	8
0	16	.26	8	90	14	.15	8	.03	.09	.02	.63	.08	6	3
0	13	.76	20	225	38	.38	20	.06	.31	.06	1.11	.08	28	5
0	32	.51	23	397	11	.33	2487	.08	.32	.14	.69	.27	26	28
0	32	.85	15	278	20	.41	2574	.08	.42	.21	.97	.37	17	26
8[3]	27	1.19	12	199	74	.16	440	.02	3.99	.04	.41	.04	12	7
0	38	1.7	31	269	96	.27	1936	.03	.35	.12	1.22	.3	14	7
0	28	1.13	28	396	67	.23	1013	.05	.32	.07	.94	.24	21	34
0	18	.71	18	250	42	.14	638	.03	.2	.05	.59	.15	13	21
0	20	.57	11	482	3	.76	7	.05	1.4	.07	1.13	.16	4	26
0	204	2.14	70	854	74	.14	241	.06	3.7	.27	.66	.16	9.9	52
0	2	.21	7	91	<1	.07	4	.02	.13	.01	.63	.02	2	4
0	5	.41	13	177	1	.15	7	.03	.25	.02	1.22	.04	5	8
0	6	.55	14	273	11	.11	76	.07	.47	.06	.77	.1	18	23[4]
0	9	.81	20	400	16	.16	112	.11	.68	.09	1.13	.14	27	34[4]

[1]Dietary pack contains 58 mg sodium.

[2]Applies to squash including skin; flesh has no appreciable vitamin A value.

[3]For recipe using butter.

[4]Year-round average. From June through October, ascorbic acid is approximately 32 mg and 47 mg, respectively, for one tomato and 1 c chopped tomato. From November through May, market samples average around 12 and 18 mg, respectively.

(For purposes of calculations, use "0" for t, <1, <.1, <.01, etc.)

H

Table H-1
Food Composition

Computer Code Number	Food Description	Measure	Wt (g)	H₂O (%)	Ener (kcal)	Prot (g)	Carb (g)	Dietary Fiber (g)	Fat (g)	Fat Breakdown (g)		
										Sat	Mono	Poly
	HAAGEN DAZS											
1755	Ice cream bar, vanilla almond	1 ea	107	–	371	6	26	–	27	14	10	3
	Sorbet:											
1758	Lemon	½ c	113	–	140	0	35	–	0	0	0	0
1760	Orange	½ c	113	–	140	0	36	–	0	0	0	0
1759	Raspberry	½ c	113	–	110	0	27	–	0	0	0	0
	Yogurt, frozen:											
1753	Chocolate	½ c	98	–	171	8	26	–	4	2	2	0
1754	Strawberry	½ c	98	–	171	6	27	–	4	2	2	0
	Yogurt extra, frozen:											
1752	Brownie nut	½ c	101	–	220	8	29	–	9	4	4	1
1751	Raspberry rendezvous	½ c	101	–	132	4	26	–	2	1	1	0
	HEALTHY CHOICE											
	Entrees:											
2112	Fish, lemon pepper	1 ea	303	78	290	14	47	7	5	1	–	–
1624	Lasagna	1 ea	284	76	289	19	44	7	4	1	–	–
2111	Meatloaf, traditional, entree	1 ea	340	79	320	16	46	7	8	4	–	–
2104	Zucchini lasagna	1 ea	397	80	330	20	58	11	2	1	–	–
	Dinners:											
2110	Pasta shells marinara	1 ea	340	74	360	25	59	5	3	1.5	–	–
	Low-fat ice milk:											
1608	Cookie & cream	½ c	113	62	191	5	33	1	3	2.4	–	0
1621	Vanilla	½ c	113	66	159	5	29	2	3	1	–	0
	Low-fat ice cream:											
973	Brownie	½ c	71	61	120	3	22	2	2	1	–	.7
650	Chocolate chip	½ c	71	62	120	3	21	1	2	1	–	0
259	Butter pecan	½ c	71	61	89	2	16	1	1	.7	–	.5
45	Rocky road	½ c	71	53	140	3	28	2	2	1	–	0
391	Vanilla fudge	½ c	71	62	120	3	21	1	2	1.5	–	.7

Source: ConAgra Frozen Foods, Omaha, NE.

	HEALTH VALLEY											
	Soups, fat-free:											
2001	Beef broth, no salt added	6.9 oz	196	98	15	4	0	0	0	0	0	0
2073	Beef broth, w/salt	6.9 oz	196	98	25	4	2	0	0	0	0	0
2016	Black bean & vegetable	7.5 oz	213	85	98	10	21	11	0	0	0	0
2017	Chicken broth	7.5 oz	213	97	27	5	0	0	0	0	0	0
2018	14 garden vegetable	7.5 oz	213	90	71	5	15	4	0	0	0	0
2015	Lentil & carrot	7.5 oz	213	85	80	9	22	12	0	0	0	0
2014	Split pea & carrot	7.5 oz	213	89	98	7	15	4	0	0	0	0
2013	Tomato vegetable	7.5 oz	213	90	71	5	15	4	0	0	0	0
	LA CHOY											
2100	Egg rolls, mini, chicken	1 svg	106	53	220	8	35	3	6	1.5	–	–
2099	Egg rolls, mini, shrimp	1 svg	106	56	210	7	35	3	4	1	–	–
	LEAN CUISINE											
	Dinners:											
1639	Baked cheese ravioli	1 ea	241	77	250	12	32	4	8	3	2	1

PAGE KEY: H–4 = BEV   H–6 = DAIRY   H–12 = EGGS   H–14 = FAT/OIL   H–18 = FRUIT   H–26 = BAKERY   H–36 = GRAIN   H–44 = FISH
H–48 = MEATS   H–50 = POULTRY   H–54 = SAUSAGE   H–56 = MIXED/FAST   H–64 = NUTS/SEEDS   H–68 = SWEETS   H–70 = VEG/LEG
H–84 = MISC   H–88 = SOUPS/SAUCES   H–90 = FAST   H–106 = FRZN ENTREE   H–112 = BABY FOODS

Chol (mg)	Calc (mg)	Iron (mg)	Magn (mg)	Pota (mg)	Sodi (mg)	Zinc (mg)	VT-A (RE)	Thia (mg)	VT-E (α-TE)	Ribo (mg)	Niac (mg)	V-B6 (mg)	Fola (μg)	VT-C (mg)
90	161	.39	–	222	85	–	161	–	–	.18	–	–	–	–
0	–	–	–	30	20	–	–	–	–	–	–	–	–	7
0	–	–	–	80	20	–	–	–	–	–	–	–	–	20
0	–	–	–	60	15	–	–	–	–	–	–	–	–	7
40	147	.71	–	241	45	–	20	–	–	.17	–	–	–	5
50	147	–	–	141	45	–	20	.03	–	.17	–	–	–	5
55	152	.73	–	250	60	–	20	–	–	.14	–	–	–	–
20	81	–	–	97	25	–	0	–	–	.1	–	–	–	5
25	20	1.08	–	–	360	–	100	–	–	–	–	–	–	30
11	111	2.7	–	37	408	–	74	.2	–	.2	1	–	–	4
35	40	1.8	–	–	460	–	150	–	–	–	–	–	–	54
10	200	2.7	–	–	310	–	250	–	–	–	–	–	–	0
25	400	1.8	–	–	390	–	100	–	–	–	–	–	–	4
4	159	–	–	404	143	–	96	.04	–	.24	–	–	–	4
8	159	–	–	404	80	–	96	.08	–	.36	–	–	–	4
3	80	0	–	268	55	–	40	–	–	–	–	–	–	0
3	100	0	–	240	50	–	40	–	–	–	–	–	–	0
2	74	0	–	156	44	–	30	–	–	–	–	–	–	0
3	100	0	–	168	60	–	40	.03	–	.15	–	–	–	0
3	100	0	–	296	50	–	40	–	–	–	–	–	–	0
0	–	–	–	160	60	–	–	–	–	–	.8	–	–	–
0	–	–	–	160	131	–	0	–	–	–	.8	–	–	4
0	36	3.2	–	600	249	–	1775	.3	–	.1	1.2	.2	120	8
0	18	1.6	–	130	151	–	0	–	–	.03	2.17	–	–	1
0	36	1.6	–	360	222	–	1775	.23	–	.07	2	.16	24	13
0	53	4.8	–	390	195	–	1775	.09	–	.14	5	.4	24	2
0	36	4.8	–	390	204	–	1775	.09	–	.14	5	.4	–	8
0	36	4.8	–	540	213	–	1775	.09	–	.07	2	.12	32	8
5	20	1.44	–	–	460	–	20	–	–	–	–	–	–	0
5	20	1.44	–	–	510	–	20	–	–	–	–	–	–	0
55	200	1.08	42	400	500	1.5	150	.06	–	.26	1.2	.2	48	6

(For purposes of calculations, use "0" for t, <1, <.1, <.01, etc.)

Table I-6
Canadian Choice System: Sugars

1 sugar choice = 10 g carbohydrate (sugar), 167 kJ (40 kcal)

Food	Measure	Mass (Weight)
Beverages		
Condensed milk	15 mL (1 tbs)	
Flavoured fruit crystals*	75 mL (⅓ c)	
Iced tea mixes*	75 mL (⅓ c)	
Regular soft drinks	125 mL (½ c)	
Sweet drink mixes*	75 mL (⅓ c)	
Tonic water	125 mL (½ c)	

*These beverages have been made with water.

Food	Measure	Mass (Weight)
Miscellaneous		
Bubble gum (large square)	1 piece	5 g
Cranberry cocktail	75 mL (⅓ c)	80 g
Cranberry cocktail, light	350 mL (1⅓ c)	260 g
Cranberry sauce	30 mL (2 tbs)	
Hard candy mints	2	5 g
Honey, molasses, corn & cane syrup	10 mL (2 tsp)	15 g
Jelly bean	4	10 g
Licorice	1 short stick	10 g
Marshmallows	2 large	15 g
Popsicle	1 stick (½ popsicle)	
Powdered gelatin mix (Jello®) (reconstituted)	50 mL (¼ c)	
Regular jam, jelly, marmalade	15 mL (1 tbs)	
Sugar, white, brown, icing, maple	10 mL (2 tsp)	10 g
Sweet pickles	2 small	100 g
Sweet relish	30 mL (2 tbs)	

Food	Choices per Serving	Measures	Mass (Weight)
The following food items provide more than 1 sugar exchange:			
Brownie	1 sugar + 1 fat	1	20 g
Clamato juice	1½ sugars	175 mL (⅔ c)	
Fruit salad, light syrup	1 sugar + 1 fruits & vegetables	125 mL (½ c)	130 g
Aero® bar	2½ sugars + 2½ fats	1 bar	43 g
Smarties®	4½ sugars + 2 fats	1 box	60 g
Sherbet	3 sugars + ½ fat	125 mL (½ c)	95 g

Table I–7
Canadian Choice System: Protein Foods

1 protein choice = 7 g protein, 3 g fat, 230 kJ (55 kcal)

Food	Measure	Mass (Weight)
Cheese		
Low-fat cheese, about 7% milk fat	1 slice	30 g
Cottage cheese, 2% milkfat or less	50 mL (¼ c)	55 g
Ricotta, about 7% milkfat	50 mL (¼ c)	60 g
Fish		
Anchovies (see *Extras,* Table I–9)		
Canned, drained (e.g., mackerel, salmon, tuna packed in water)	(⅓ of 6.5 oz can)	30 g
Cod tongues, cheeks	75 mL (⅓ c)	50 g
Fillet or steak (e.g., Boston blue, cod, flounder, haddock, halibut, mackerel, orange roughy, perch, pickerel, pike, salmon, shad, snapper, sole, swordfish, trout, tuna, whitefish)	1 piece	30 g
Herring	⅓ fish	30 g
Sardines, smelts	2 medium or 3 small	30 g
Squid, octopus	50 mL (¼ c)	40 g
Shellfish		
Clams, mussels, oysters, scallops, snails	3 medium	30 g
Crab, lobster, flaked	50 mL (¼ c)	30 g
Shrimp, fresh	5 large	30 g
Frozen	10 medium	30 g
Canned	18 small	30 g
Dry pack	50 mL (¼ c)	30 g
Meat and Poultry (e.g., beef, chicken, goat, ham, lamb, pork, turkey, veal, wild game)		
Back, peameal bacon	3 slices, thin	30 g
Chop	½ chop, with bone	40 g
Minced or ground, lean or extra-lean	30 mL (2 tbs)	30 g
Sliced, lean	1 slice	30 g
Steak, lean	1 piece	30 g
Organ Meats		
Hearts, liver	1 slice	30 g
Kidneys, sweetbreads, chopped	50 mL (¼ c)	30 g
Tongue	1 slice	30 g
Tripe	5 pieces	60 g
Soyabean		
Bean curd or tofu	½ block	70 g
Eggs		
In shell, raw or cooked	1 medium	50 g
Without shell, cooked or poached in water	1 medium	45 g
Scrambled	50 mL (¼ c)	55 g

(continued on the next page)

Table I–7 (continued)
Canadian Choice System: Protein Foods

1 protein choice = 7 g protein, 3 g fat, 230 kJ (55 kcal)

Food	Choices per Serving	Measures	Mass (Weight)
Note: The following choices provide more than 1 protein exchange:			
Cheese			
Cheeses	1 protein + 1 fat	1 piece	25 g
Cheese, coarsely grated (e.g., Cheddar)	1 protein + 1 fat	50 mL (¼ c)	25 g
Cheese, dry, finely grated (e.g., parmesan)	1 protein + 1 fat	45 mL	15 g
Cheese, ricotta, high fat	1 protein + 1 fat	50 mL (¼ c)	55 g
Fish			
Eel	1 protein + 1 fat	1 slice	50 g
Meat			
Bologna	1 protein + 1 fat	1 slice	20 g
Canned lunch meats	1 protein + 1 fat	1 slice	20 g
Corned beef, canned	1 protein + 1 fat	1 slice	25 g
Corned beef, fresh	1 protein + 1 fat	1 slice	25 g
Ground beef, medium-fat	1 protein + 1 fat	30 mL (2 tbs)	25 g
Meat spreads, canned	1 protein + 1 fat	45 mL	35 g
Mutton chop	1 protein + 1 fat	½ chop, with bone	35 g
Paté (see *Fats and Oils* group, Table I–8)			
Sausages, garlic, Polish or knockwurst	1 protein + 1 fat	1 slice	50 g
Sausages, pork, links	1 protein + 1 fat	1 link	25 g
Spareribs or shortribs, with bone	1 protein + 1 fat	1 large	65 g
Stewing beef	1 protein + 1 fat	1 cube	25 g
Summer sausage or salami	1 protein + 1 fat	1 slice	40 g
Weiners, hot dog	1 protein + 1 fat	½ medium	25 g
Miscellaneous			
Blood pudding	1 protein + 1 fat	1 slice	25 g
Peanut butter	1 protein + 1 fat	15 mL (1 tbs)	15 g

Table I-8
Canadian Choice System: Fats and Oils

1 fat choice = 5 g fat, 190 kJ (45 kcal)

Food	Measure	Mass (Weight)	Food	Measure	Mass (Weight)
Avocado*	⅛	30 g	Nuts (continued):		
Bacon, side, crisp*	1 slice	5 g	Sesame seeds	15 mL (1 tbs)	10 g
Butter*	5 mL (1 tsp)	5 g	Sunflower seeds		
Cheese spread	15 mL (1 tbs)	15 g	Shelled	15 mL (1 tbs)	10 g
Coconut, fresh*	45 mL (3 tbs)	15 g	In shell	45 mL (3 tbs)	15 g
Coconut, dried*	15 mL (1 tbs)	10 g	Walnuts	4 halves	10 g
Cream, Half and half			Oil, cooking and salad	5 mL (1 tsp)	5 g
(cereal), 10%*	30 mL (2 tbs)	30 g	Olives, green	10	45 g
Light (coffee), 20%*	15 mL (1 tbs)	15 g	Ripe black	7	57 g
Whipping, 32 to 37%*	15 mL (1 tbs)	15 g	Pâté, liverwurst,	15 mL (1 tbs)	15 g
Cream cheese*	15 mL (1 tbs)	15 g	meat spreads		
Gravy*	30 mL (2 tbs)	30 g	Salad dressing: blue,	10 mL (2 tsp)	10 g
Lard*	5 mL (1 tsp)	5 g	French, Italian,		
Margarine	5 mL (1 tsp)	5 g	mayonnaise,		
Nuts, shelled:			Thousand Island	5 mL (1 tsp)	5 g
Almonds	8	5 g	Salad dressing,	30 mL (2 tbs)	30 g
Brazil nuts	2	10 g	low-calorie		
Cashews	5	10 g	Salt pork, raw	5 mL (1 tsp)	5 g
Filberts, hazelnuts	5	10 g	or cooked*		
Macadamia	3	5 g	Sesame oil	5 mL (1 tsp)	5 g
Peanuts	10	10g	Sour cream		
Pecans	5 halves	5 g	12% milkfat	30 mL (2 tbs)	30 g
Pignolias, pine nuts	25 mL (5 tsp)	10 g	7% milkfat	60 mL (4 tbs)	60 g
Pistachios, shelled	20	10 g	Shortening*	5 mL (1 tsp)	
Pistachios, in shell	20	20 g			
Pumpkin and squash seeds	20 mL (4 tsp)	10 g			

*These items contain higher amounts of saturated fat.

Table I-9
Canadian Choice System: Extras

Extras have no more than 2.5 g carbohydrate, 60 kJ (14 kcal)

Vegetables 125 mL (½ c)
Artichokes
Asparagus
Bamboo shoots
Bean sprouts, mung or soya
Beans, string, green, or yellow
Bitter melon (balsam pear)
Bok choy
Broccoli
Brussels sprouts
Cabbage
Cauliflower
Celery
Chard
Cucumbers
Eggplant
Endive
Fiddleheads
Greens: beet, collard, dandelion, mustard, turnip, etc.
Kale
Kohlrabi
Leeks
Lettuce
Mushrooms
Okra
Onions, green or mature
Parsley
Peppers, green, yellow or red
Radishes
Rapini
Rhubarb
Sauerkraut
Shallots
Spinach
Sprouts: alfalfa, radish, etc.
Tomato wedges
Watercress
Zucchini

Free Foods (may be used without measuring)

Artificial sweetener, such as cyclamate or aspartame
Baking powder, baking soda
Bouillon from cube, powder, or liquid
Bouillon or clear broth
Chowchow, unsweetened
Coffee, clear
Consommé
Dulse
Flavorings and extracts
Garlic
Gelatin, unsweetened
Ginger root
Herbal teas, unsweetened
Horseradish, uncreamed
Lemon juice or lemon wedges
Lime juice or lime wedges
Marjoram, cinnamon, etc.
Mineral water
Mustard
Parsley
Pimentos
Salt, pepper, thyme
Soda water, club soda
Soya sauce
Sugar-free Crystal Drink
Sugar-free Jelly Powder
Sugar-free soft drinks
Tea, clear
Vinegar
Water
Worcestershire sauce

Condiments

Food	Measure
Anchovies	2 fillets
Barbecue sauce	15 mL (1 tbs)
Bran, natural	30 mL (2 tbs)
Brewer's yeast	5 mL (1 tsp)
Carob powder	5 mL (1 tsp)
Catsup	5 mL (1 tsp)
Chili sauce	5 mL (1 tsp)
Cocoa powder	5 mL (1 tsp)
Cranberry sauce, unsweetened	15 mL (1 tbs)
Dietetic fruit spreads	5 mL (1 tsp)
Maraschino cherries	1
Nondairy coffee whitener	5 mL (1 tsp)
Nuts, chopped pieces	5 mL (1 tsp)
Pickles	
unsweetened dill	2
sour mixed	11
Sugar substitutes, granular	5 mL (1 tsp)
Whipped toppings	15 mL (1 tbs)

Table I-10
Canadian Choice System: Combined Food Choices

Food	Choices per serving	Measure	Mass (Weight)
Angel food cake	½ starch + 2½ sugars	1⁄12 cake	50 g
Apple crisp	½ starch + 1½ fruits & vegetables + 1 sugar + 1–2 fats	125 mL (½ c)	
Applesauce, sweetened	1 fruits & vegetables + 1 sugar	125 mL (½ c)	
Beans and pork in tomato sauce	1 starch + ½ fruits & vegetables + ½ sugar + 1 protein	125 mL (½ c)	135 g
Beef burrito	2 starches + 3 proteins + 3 fats		110 g
Brownie	1 sugar + 1 fat	1	20 g
Cabbage rolls*	1 starch + 2 proteins	3	310 g
Caesar salad	2–4 fats	20 mL dressing (4 tsp)	
Cheesecake	½ starch + 2 sugars + ½ protein + 5 fats	1 piece	80 g
Chicken fingers	1 starch + 2 proteins + 2 fats	6 small	100 g
Chicken and snow pea Oriental	2 starches + ½ fruits & vegetables + 3 proteins + 1 fat	500 mL (2 c)	
Chili	1½ starches + ½ fruits & vegetables + 3½ protein	300 mL (1¼ c)	325 g
Chips			
Potato chips	1 starch + 2 fats	15 chips	30 g
Corn chips	1 starch + 2 fats	30 chips	30 g
Tortilla chips	1 starch + 1½ fats	13 chips	
Cheese twist	1 starch + 1½ fats	30 chips	30 g
Chocolate bar			
Aero®	2½ sugars + 2½ fats	bar	43 g
Smarties®	4½ sugars + 2 fats	package	60 g
Chocolate cake (without icing)	1 starch + 2 sugars + 3 fats	1⁄10 of a 8″ pan	
Chocolate devil's food cake (without icing)	2 starches + 2 sugars + 3 fats	1⁄12 of a 9″ pan	
Chocolate milk	2 milks 2% + 1 sugar	250 mL (1 c)	300 g
Clubhouse (triple-decker) sandwich	3 starches + 3 proteins + 4 fats		
Cookies			
chocolate chip	½ starch + ½ sugar + 1½ fats	2	22 g
oatmeal	1 starch + 1 sugar + 1 fat	2	40 g
Donut (chocolate glazed)	1 starch + 1½ sugars + 2 fats	1	65 g
Egg roll	1 starch + ½ protein + 1 fat		75 g
Four bean salad	1 starch + ½ protein + 1 fat	125 mL (½ c)	
French toast	1 starch + ½ protein + 2 fats	1 slice	65 g
Fruit in heavy syrup	1 fruits & vegetables + 1½ sugars	125 mL (½ c)	
Granola bar	½ starch + 1 sugar + 1–2 fats		30 g
Granola cereal	1 starch + 1 sugar + 2 fats	125 mL (½ c)	45 g
Hamburger	2 starches + 3 proteins + 2 fats	junior size	
Ice cream and cone, plain flavour			
Ice cream	½ milk + 2–3 sugars + 1–2 fats		100 g
Cone	½ sugar		4 g
Lasagna			
regular cheese	1 starch + 1 fruits & vegetables + 3 proteins + 2 fats	3″ x 4″ piece	
low-fat cheese	1 starch + 1 fruits & vegetables + 3 proteins	3″ x 4″ piece	

* If eaten with sauce, add ½ fruits & vegetables exchange.

(continued on the next page)

Table I-10 (continued)
Canadian Choice System: Combined Food Choices

Food	Choices per serving	Measure	Mass (Weight)
Legumes			
Dried beans (kidney, navy, pinto, fava, chick peas)	2 starches + 1 protein	250 mL (1 c)	180 g
Dried peas	2 starches + 1 protein	250 mL (1 c)	210 g
Lentils	2 starches + 1 protein	250 mL (1 c)	210 g
Macaroni 'and cheese	2 starches + 2 proteins + 2 fats	250 mL (1 c)	210 g
Minestrone soup	1½ starches + ½ fruits & vegetables + ½ fat	250 mL (1 c)	
Muffin	1 starch + ½ sugar + 1 fat	1 small	45 g
Nuts (dry or roasted without any oil added).			
Almonds, dried sliced	½ protein + 2 fats	50 mL (¼ c)	22 g
Brazil nuts, dried unblanched	½ protein + 2½ fats	5 large	23 g
Cashew nuts, dry roasted	½ starch + ½ protein + 2 fats	50 mL (¼ c)	28 g
Filbert hazelnut, dry	½ protein + 3½ fats	50 mL (¼ c)	30 g
Macadamia nuts, dried	½ protein + 4 fats	50 mL (¼ c)	28 g
Peanuts, raw	1 protein + 2 fats	50 mL (¼ c)	30 g
Pecans, dry roasted	½ fruits & vegetables + 3 fats	50 mL (¼ c)	22 g
Pine nuts, pignolia dried	1 protein + 3 fats	50 mL (¼ c)	34 g
Pistachio nuts, dried	½ fruits & vegetables + ½ protein + 2 ½ fats	50 mL (¼ c)	27 g
Pumpkin seeds, roasted	2 proteins + 2½ fats	50 mL (¼ c)	47 g
Sesame seeds, whole dried	½ fruits & vegetables + ½ protein + 2½ fats	50 mL (¼ c)	30 g
Sunflower kernel, dried	½ protein + 1½ fats	50 mL (¼ c)	17 g
Walnuts, dried chopped	½ protein + 3 fats	50 mL (¼ c)	26 g
Perogies	2 starches + 1 protein + 1 fat	3	
Pie, fruit	1 starch + 1 fruits & vegetables + 2 sugars + 3 fats	1 piece	120 g
Pizza, cheese	1 starch + 1 protein + 1 fat	1 slice (⅛ of a 12″)	50 g
Pork stir fry	½ to 1 fruits & vegetables + 3 proteins	200 mL (¾ c)	
Potato salad	1 starch + 1 fat	125 mL (½ c)	130 g
Potatoes, scalloped	2 starches + 1 milk + 1–2 fats	200 mL (¾ c)	210 g
Pudding, bread or rice	1 starch + 1 sugar +1 fat	125 mL (½ c)	
Pudding, vanilla	1 milk + 2 sugars	125 mL (½ c)	
Raisin bran cereal	1 starch + ½ fruits & vegetables + ½ sugar	175 mL (⅔ c)	40 g
Rice krispie squares	½ starch + 1½ sugars + ½ fat	1 square	30 g
Shepherd's pie	2 starches + 1 fruits & vegetables + 3 proteins	325 mL (1⅓ c)	
Sherbet, orange	3 sugars + ½ fat	125 mL (½ c)	
Spaghetti and meat sauce	2 starches + 1 fruits & vegetables + 2 proteins + 3 fats	250 mL (1 c)	
Stew	2 starches + 2 fruits & vegetables + 3 proteins + ½ fat	200 mL (¾ c)	
Sundae	4 sugars + 3 fats	125 mL (½ c)	
Tuna casserole	1 starch + 2 proteins + ½ fat	125 mL (½ c)	
Yogurt, fruit bottom	1 fruits & vegetables + 1 milk + 1 sugar	125 mL (½ c)	125 g
Yogurt, frozen	1 milk + 1 sugar	125 mL (½ c)	125 g

FOOD LABELS

Consumers can gather a lot of information from a nutrition label. Figure I-1 demonstrates the reading of a food label and Table I-11 defines terms.

Figure I-1

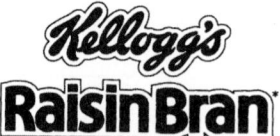

OUR COMMITMENT TO QUALITY

Kellogg's is committed to providing foods of outstanding quality and freshness. If this product in any way falls below the high standards you've come to expect from Kellogg's, please send your comments and both top flaps to:

Consumer Affairs
KELLOGG CANADA INC.
Etobicoke, Ontario M9W 5P2

IF IT DOESN'T SAY *Kellogg's* ON THE BOX,
IT'S NOT *Kellogg's* IN THE BOX.
SI LE NOM *Kellogg's* N'EST PAS SUR LA BOÎTE,
CE N'EST PAS *Kellogg's* DANS LA BOÎTE.

- HIGH IN FIBRE
- LOW IN FAT
- PRESERVATIVE FREE
- SOURCE ÉLEVÉE DE FIBRES
- FAIBLE EN MATIÈRES GRASSES
- SANS AGENT DE CONSERVATION

NUTRITION INFORMATION / APPORT NUTRITIONNEL

	Per 40 g serving cereal (175 mL, ¾ cup) Par ration de 40 g de céréale (175 mL, ¾ tasse)	Per 40 g serving cereal with 125 mL Partly Skimmed Milk (2%) Par ration de 40 g de céréale avec 125 mL de lait partiellement écrémé (2,0 %)	
ENERGY	130Cal 540kJ	195Cal 810kJ	ÉNERGIE
PROTEIN	3.0g	7.3g	PROTÉINES
FAT	0.4g	2.9g	MATIÈRES GRASSES
CARBOHYDRATE	32g	38g	GLUCIDES
SUGARS*	11g	18g	*SUCRES
STARCH	16g	16g	AMIDON
DIETARY FIBRE	4.6g	4.6g	FIBRES ALIMENTAIRES
SODIUM	235mg	300mg	SODIUM
POTASSIUM	240mg	440mg	POTASSIUM

% of Recommended Daily Intake
% de l'apport quotidien conseillé

VITAMIN A	0%	7%	VITAMINE A
VITAMIN D	0%	23%	VITAMINE D
VITAMIN B1	62%	66%	VITAMINE B1
VITAMIN B2	3%	16%	VITAMINE B2
NIACIN	13%	18%	NiACINE
VITAMIN B6	13%	16%	VITAMINE B6
FOLACIN	11%	14%	FOLACINE
VITAMIN B12	0%	25%	VITAMINE B12
PANTOTHENATE	9%	15%	PANTOTHÉNATE
CALCIUM	1%	15%	CALCIUM
PHOSPHORUS	12%	23%	PHOSPHORE
MAGNESIUM	20%	27%	MAGNÉSIUM
IRON	38%	39%	FER
ZINC	16%	22%	ZINC

*Approximately half of the sugars occur naturally in the raisins.
Environ la moitié des sucres se retrouvent à l'état naturel dans les fruits.

Canadian Diabetes Association Food Choice Values:
40 g (175 mL, ¾ cup) cereal. Système des choix d'aliments de l'Association canadienne du diabète : 40 g (175 mL, ¾ tasse)
céréale = 1 [■] + ½ [◗] + ½ [✱] choices/choix

INGREDIENTS / INGRÉDIENTS

WHOLE WHEAT, RAISINS (COATED WITH SUGAR, HYDROGENATED VEGETABLE OIL), WHEAT BRAN, SUGAR/GLUCOSE-FRUCTOSE, SALT, MALT (CORN FLOUR, MALTED BARLEY), VITAMINS (THIAMIN HYDROCHLORIDE, PYRIDOXINE HYDROCHLORIDE, FOLIC ACID, d-CALCIUM PANTOTHENATE), MINERALS (IRON, ZINC OXIDE).

BLÉ ENTIER, RAISINS SECS (ENROBÉS DE SUCRE, D'HUILE VÉGÉTALE HYDROGÉNÉE), SON DE BLÉ, SUCRE/GLUCOSE-FRUCTOSE, SEL, MALT (FARINE DE MAÏS, ORGE MALTÉE), VITAMINES (CHLORHYDRATE DE THIAMINE, CHLORHYDRATE DE PYRIDOXINE, ACIDE FOLIQUE, PANTOTHÉNATE DE d-CALCIUM), MINÉRAUX (FER, OXYDE DE ZINC).

Made by / Produit par
KELLOGG CANADA INC.
ETOBICOKE, ONTARIO
CANADA M9W 5P2
*Registered trademark of /
*Marque déposée de
KELLOGG CANADA INC. © 1994

00094

WHAT YOU WILL FIND ON A LABEL:

Nutrition Claims
- in Canada, it is optional for a company to decide to use claims,
- when claims appear on a label, they must follow government laws

Nutrition Information
- gives detailed nutrition facts about the product, including serving size and core list
- does not have to appear by law on food products in Canada
- refers to the food as packaged, so if you add milk, eggs or other food, the nutritional content of the food you eat can be very different

Serving Size
- the amount of food for which the information is given
- check the serving size: the serving size on the label may not be the same as the serving size you would actually eat (for example, the serving size of cereal may be ¾ cup, much smaller than your regular serving

Core List
- the energy (in Calories and kilojoules), grams of protein, fat and carbohydrate for each serving
- some products break down fat into monounsaturates, polyunsaturates, saturates, and cholesterol (to find out what these mean, look at the Fats & Oils section)
- carbohydrates may include the amount of sugars, starch and fibre, or may list these items separately

Sodium and Potassium (in milligrams)

Vitamins and Minerals (as percent of your recommended daily intake)

Canadian Diabetes Association Food Choice Values and Symbols
- the Values and Symbols are tools to help you fit the food into your meal plan, they are not an endorsement by CDA
- it is up to the food company to decide if they want their foods analyzed and assigned symbols
- when they are on a label, they have been assigned by a dietitian working for CDA, so you can be sure the information is correct

Ingredients
- must be found on all food labels by law
- ingredients are listed in decreasing order by weight, so what you see first is what you get the most of

Table I-11
Terms on Food Labels

Energy

kcalorie reduced: 50% or fewer kcalories than the regular version.
light: term may be used to describe anything (for example, light in colour, texture, flavour, taste, or kcalories); read the label to find out what is "light" about the product.
low kcalorie: kcalorie-reduced and no more than 15 kcalories per serving.

Fat and Cholesterol

low cholesterol: no more than 3 mg of cholesterol per 100 g of the food and low in saturated fat; *does not* always mean low in total fat.
low fat: no more than 3 g of fat per serving; *does not* always mean low in kcalories.
lower fat: at least 25% less fat than the comparison food; be aware that 80% fat-free still means the food is 20% fat.

Carbohydrates: Fibre and Sugar

carbohydrate reduced: not more than 50% of the carbohydrate found in the regular version; *does not* always mean the product is lower in kcalories because other ingredients such as fat may have increased.
source of dietary fibre: a product that provides 2–4 g of fibre.
high source of dietary fibre: a product that provides 4–6 g of fibre.
very high source of fibre: a product that provides 6 g (or more) of fibre.
sugar free: low in carbohydrates and kcalories; can be used as an extra food in the exchange system.
unsweetened or no sugar added: no sugar was added to the product; sugar may be found naturally in the food (for example, fruit canned in its own juice).

MEASURES OF PROTEIN QUALITY

♦

Contents

Amino Acid Scoring

PDCAAS

Biological Value

Net Protein Utilization

Protein Efficiency Ratio

*I*n a world where food is scarce and many people's diets contain marginal or inadequate amounts of protein, it is important to know which foods contain the highest-quality protein. Chapter 6 describes protein quality and the different measures researchers use to assess the quality of a food protein. This appendix provides a few more details.

AMINO ACID SCORING

♦

Amino acid, or chemical, scoring allows researchers to determine the amino acid composition of any protein relatively inexpensively, but unfortunately, it does not always accurately reflect the way the body will use a protein. The advantages of amino acid scoring are that it is simple and inexpensive, it identifies in one step the limiting amino acid, and it can be used to score mixtures of different proportions of two or more proteins mathematically without having to make up a mixture and test it. Its chief weaknesses are that it fails to predict the digestibility of a protein, which may strongly affect the protein's quality; it relies on a chemical procedure in which certain amino acids may be destroyed, making the pattern that is analyzed inaccurate; and it is blind to other features of the protein (such as the presence of substances that may inhibit the digestion or utilization of the protein) that would only be revealed by a test in living animals. Table J–1 shows how to use a reference pattern for the nine essential amino acids.

PDCAAS

♦

PDCAAS (protein-digestibility-corrected amino acid score) takes the amino acid scoring method a step further by correcting for the digestibility of the protein. To calculate the PDCAAS, researchers first determine the amino acid profile of the test protein (in this example, pinto beans). The second column of Table J–2 presents the essential amino acid profile for pinto beans. The third column presents the amino acid requirements of preschool-aged children for comparison. To determine how well the food protein meets human needs, researchers calculate the ratio by dividing the second column by the third column (for example, 30 ÷ 19 = 1.578 or 1.58).

The amino acid with the lowest ratio is the first limiting amino acid—in this case, tryptophan. Its ratio is the amino acid score for the protein—in this case, 80. Remember, though, the amino acid score does not account for digestibility. Protein digestibility, as determined by rat balance studies, yields a value of 79 percent for pinto beans. Together, the amino acid score and the digestibility value determine the PDCAAS:

PDCAAS = protein digestibility × lowest amino acid ratio.
PDCAAS for pinto beans = .79 × .80 = 63%.

Thus the PDCAAS for pinto beans is 63 percent (or 0.63).

The PDCAAS is used to determine the % Daily Value on food labels. To calculate the % Daily Value for protein for canned pinto beans, multiply the number of grams of protein in a standard serving (in this case, 7 grams per ½ cup) by the PDCAAS:

7 g × .63 = 4.41.

This value is then divided by the RDI for protein (for children over age four and adults, the RDI is 50 grams):

4.41 ÷ 50 = 0.088 (or 8.8%).

The food label for this can of pinto beans would declare that one serving provides 7 grams protein, and if the label included a % Daily Value for protein, the value would be 9 percent.

BIOLOGICAL VALUE

♦

To determine the actual value of a protein as it is used by the body, it is necessary to measure both urinary and fecal losses of nitrogen

Table J-1

A Reference Pattern for Amino Acid Scoring of Proteins

Essential Amino Acids	Reference Protein (Whole Egg) Mg Amino Acid per G Nitrogen
Histidine	145
Isoleucine	340
Leucine	540
Lysine	440
Methionine + cystine[a]	355
Phenylalanine + tyrosine[b]	580
Threonine	294
Tryptophan	106
Valine	410
Total	3210

[a]Methionine is essential and is also used to make cystine. Thus the methionine requirement is lower if cystine is supplied.

[b]Phenylalanine is essential and is also used to make tyrosine if not enough of the latter is available. Thus the phenylalanine requirement is lower if tyrosine is also supplied.

Note: To interpret the table, read, "For every 3210 units of essential amino acids, 145 must be histidine, 340 must be isoleucine, 540 must be leucine," and so on. To compare a test protein with the reference protein, the experimenter first obtains a chemical analysis of the test protein's amino acids. Then, taking 3210 units of the amino acids, the experimenter compares the amount of each amino acid to the amount found in 3210 units of essential amino acids in egg protein. For example, suppose the test protein contained (per 3210 units) 360 units of isoleucine; 500 units of leucine; 350 of lysine; and for each of the other amino acids, more units than egg protein contains. The two amino acids that are low are leucine (500 as compared with 540 in egg) and lysine (350 versus 440 in egg). The ratio, amino acid in the test protein divided by amino acid in egg, is 500/540 (or about 0.93) for leucine and 350/440 (or about 0.80) for lysine. Lysine is the limiting amino acid (lowest ratio compared with egg), so the test protein receives a chemical score of 80.

when that protein is actually fed to human beings under test conditions. Even then, small additional losses from sweat, shed skin, hair, and fingernails will be missed. This kind of experiment determines the biological value (BV) of proteins, a measure used internationally.

In a test of biological value, two nitrogen balance studies are done. In the first, no protein is fed, and nitrogen (N) excretions in the urine and feces are measured. It is assumed that under these conditions, N lost in the urine is the amount the body always necessar-

ily loses by filtration into the urine each day, regardless of what protein is fed (endogenous N). The N lost in the feces (called metabolic N in the equation) is the amount the body invariably loses into the intestine each day, whether or not food protein is fed. (To help you remember the terms: endogenous N is "urinary N on a zero-protein diet"; metabolic N is "fecal N on a zero-protein diet.")

In the second study, an amount of protein slightly below the requirement is fed. Intake and losses are measured; then the BV is derived using this formula:

Table J-2

An Example of PDCAAS

Essential Amino Acids	Amino Acid Profile of Pinto Beans (mg/g protein)	Amino Acid Requirements for 2–5 yr (mg/g protein)	Ratio
Histidine	30.0	19	1.58
Isoleucine	42.5	28	1.52
Leucine	80.4	66	1.22
Lysine	69.0	58	1.19
Methionine + cystine	21.1	25	0.84
Phenylalanine + tyrosine	90.5	63	1.44
Threonine	43.7	34	1.28
Tryptophan	8.8	11	0.80
Valine	50.1	35	1.43

$$BV = \frac{\text{food N} - (\text{fecal N} - \text{metabolic N}) - (\text{urinary N} - \text{endogenous N})}{\text{food N} - (\text{fecal N} - \text{metabolic N})} \times 100.$$

The denominator of this equation expresses the amount of nitrogen *absorbed:* food N minus fecal N (excluding the N the body would lose in the feces anyway, even without food). The numerator expresses the amount of N *retained* from the N absorbed: absorbed N (as in the denominator) minus the N excreted in the urine (excluding the N the body would lose in the urine anyway, even without food). Thus it can be more simply expressed:

$$BV = \frac{\text{N retained}}{\text{N absorbed}} \times 100.$$

This method has the advantages of being based on experiments with human beings (it can be done with animals, too, of course) and of measuring actual nitrogen retention. But it is also cumbersome, expensive, and often impractical, and it is based on several assumptions that may not be valid. For example, the physiology, normal environment, or typical food intake of the subjects used for testing may not be similar to those for whom the test protein may ultimately be used. For another example, the retention of protein in the body does not necessarily mean that it is being well utilized. Considerable exchange of protein among tissues (protein turnover) occurs, but is hidden from view when only N intake and output are measured. The test of biological value wouldn't detect if one tissue were shorted.

NET PROTEIN UTILIZATION

◆

Like measurements of BV, determinations of net protein utilization (NPU) involve two balance studies: one on zero nitrogen intake, and the other on submaximal intake. The formula for NPU is:

$$NPU = \frac{\text{food N} - (\text{fecal N} - \text{metabolic N}) - (\text{urinary N} - \text{endogenous N})}{\text{food N}} \times 100.$$

The numerator is the same as it is for BV, but the denominator represents food N intake only—not absorbed N. More simply exprssed:

$$NPU = \frac{\text{N retained}}{\text{N intake}} \times 100.$$

This method offers advantages similar to those of BV determinations and is used more frequently, with animals as the test subjects. A drawback is that if a low NPU is obtained, the test results offer no help in distinguishing between two possible causes: a poor amino acid composition of the test protein or poor digestibility. There is also a limit to the extent to which animal test results can be assumed to be applicable to human beings.

PROTEIN EFFICIENCY RATIO

◆

The protein efficiency ratio (PER) is a widely used procedure for evaluating protein quality. Young rats are fed a measured amount of protein and weighed periodically as they grow. The PER is expressed as:

$$PER = \frac{\text{weight gain (g)}}{\text{protein intake (g)}}.$$

This method has the virtues of economy and simplicity, but it also has many drawbacks. The experiments are time-consuming; the amino acid needs of rats are not the same as those of human beings; and the amino acid needs for growth are not the same as for the maintenance of adult animals (growing animals need more lysine, for example).

ENTERAL FORMULAS

♦

The staggering number of enteral formulas available allows health care professionals to meet a variety of their client's medical needs, but also complicates the process of selecting an appropriate formula. The first step in narrowing the choice of formulas is to determine the client's ability to digest and absorb nutrients. Table K–1 lists examples of intact protein formulas for clients with the ability to digest and absorb nutrients and Table K–2 provides examples of hydrolyzed formulas for clients with limited ability to digest and absorb nutrients. Each formula is listed only once, although the formula may have more than one use. A high-protein formula, for example, may also be a fiber-containing formula. Tables K-3 through K-5 list modular formulas. Although this appendix provides many examples, the list of formulas is not complete. The information reflects the manufacturers literature and does not suggest endorsement by the authors. Be aware that formula composition changes periodically. Consult manufacturer's literature for updates. The following products are listed in this appendix:

- Braun Medical, Inc.[a]
  Hepatic-Aid® II
  Immune-Aid®

- Mead Johnson Nutritionals[b]
  Casec®
  Choice®
  Comply®
  Criticare HN®
  Deliver® 2.0
  Isocal®
  Isocal® HN
  Kindercal®
  Lipisorb®
  MCT Oil®
  Microlipid®
  Moducal®
  Magnacal® Renal
  Protain XL®
  Respalor®
  Sustacal®
  Sustacal® Basic
  Sustacal® with Fiber
  Sustacal® Plus
  Traumacal®
  Ultracal®

- Nestlé Clinical Nutrition[c]
  Crucial®
  Entrition® HN
  Glytrol®
  Nutren ®1.0
  Nutren® 1.0 with Fiber
  Nutren® 1.5
  Nutren® 2.0
  Nutren® Junior
  Nutren® Junior with Fiber
  NutriHep®
  NutriVent®
  Peptamen®
  Peptamen® Junior
  Peptamen® VHP
  ProBalance®
  Reabilan®
  Reabilan® HN
  Replete®
  Replete® with Fiber

- Novartis Nutrition Corporation[d]
  Compleat® Modified
  Compleat® Regular
  Compleat® Pediatric
  DiabetiSource®
  FiberSource®

  FiberSource® HN
  Impact®
  Impact® 1.5
  Impact® with Fiber
  IsoSource® Standard
  IsoSource® HN
  IsoSource® VHN
  IsoSource® 1.5
  Resource® Diabetic
  Resource® Standard
  Resource® Plus
  SandoSource® Peptide
  Tolerex®
  Vivonex® Pediatric
  Vivonex® Plus
  Vivonex® T.E.N.

- Nutrition Medical[e]
  Fiberlan®
  Gluco-PRO®
  Isolan®
  L-Emental®
  L-Emental® Hepatic
  L-Emental® Pediatric
  L-Emental® Plus
  Nitrolan®
  PRO-Peptide®
  PRO-Peptide® for Kids

  PRO-Peptide® VHN
  Ultralan®

- Ross Laboratories[f]
  Advera®
  Alitraq®
  Ensure®
  Ensure® Plus
  Ensure® Plus HN
  Ensure® with Fiber
  Glucerna®
  Jevity®
  Jevity® Plus
  Nepro®
  Osmolite®
  Osmolite® HN
  Osmolite® HN Plus
  PediaSure®
  PediaSure® with Fiber
  Perative®
  Polycose®
  ProMod®
  Promote®
  Promote® with Fiber
  Pulmocare®
  Suplena®
  TwoCal® HN
  Vital® HN

[a]*Enteral Nutrition Products Ready Reference* (provided June, 1997), *Hepatic-Aid II Instant Drink* (1992), and *Immune-Aid* (1992), McGaw Inc., Irvine, CA 92714.

[b]*Enteral Product Handbook* (1994), *Choice* (1995), *Comply* (1996), *Magnacal Renal* (1996), and *Protain XL* (1996), Mead-Johnson Nutritionals, Evansville, IN 47721.

[c]*Enteral Product Reference Guide* (1997), Nestlé Clinical Nutrition, Deerfield, IL 60015.

[d]*Enteral Products Guide* (1995) and *Compleat Pediatric* (1997), Sandoz Nutrition, Minneapolis, MN 55416.

[e]*Enteral Formulary, Gluco-PRO* (1997), *L-Emental* (1994), *L-Emental Hepatic* (1996), *L-Emental Pediatric* (1996), *L-Emental Plus* (1997), *PRO-peptide* (1997), *PRO-Peptide for Kids* (1997), and *PRO-Peptide VHN* (1997), Nutrition Medical, Inc., Minneapolis, MN 55442.

[f]*Ross Medical Nutritional System* (1996), Ross Laboratories, Columbus, OH 43215.

Table K–1
Intact Protein Formulas

Product	Form	Volume to Meet 100% RDI (ml)	Energy (kcal/ml)	Protein or Amino Acids (g/L)	Carbohydrate (g/L)	Fat (g/L)	Osmolality (mOsm/kg)	Notes
Lactose-Free, Isotonic or Near-Isotonic Formulas								
Compleat® Modified	liquid	1500	1.07	43	140	37	300	4.4 g fiber/L
Isocal®	liquid	1890	1.06	34	135	44	270	Low-residue, 20% fat from MCT
Isolan®	liquid	1250	1.06	40	144	36	300	Low-residue
IsoSource Standard®	liquid	1500	1.20	43	170	41	360	Low-residue, 50% fat from MCT
Nutren® 1.0	liquid	1500	1.00	40	127	38	300	Low-residue, 24% fat from MCT
Osmolite®	liquid	1887	1.06	37	151	35	300	Low-residue, 20% fat from MCT
Low- to Moderate-Residue Formulas[a]								
Compleat® Regular	liquid	1500	1.07	43	130	43	450	Blenderized formula, contains lactose, 4.4 g fiber/1000 ml
Ensure®	liquid	948	1.06	37	145	37	555	Lactose-free
Resource® Standard	liquid	1890	1.10	37	140	37	430	Lactose-free
Sustacal Basic®	liquid	1080	1.01	61	140	23	650	Lactose-free
Lactose-Free, Fiber-Containing Formulas								
Ensure® with Fiber	liquid	1391	1.10	40	162	37	480	14 g fiber/L
Fiberlan®	liquid	1250	1.20	50	160	40	310	Near-isotonic 14 g fiber/L
FiberSource®	liquid	1500	1.20	43	170	41	390	10 g fiber/L
Impact® with Fiber	liquid	1500	1.00	56	140	28	375	10 g fiber/L, enriched with arginine, nucleic acids, and omega-3 fatty acids
Jevity®	liquid	1321	1.06	44	154	35	300	Isotonic, 14 g fiber/L
Nutren® 1.0 with Fiber	liquid	1500	1.00	40	127	38	303	Near-isotonic, 14 g fiber/L
ProBalance®	liquid	1000	1.20	45	130	34	350	10 g fiber/L
Promote® with Fiber	liquid	1000	1.00	63	139	28	370	14.4 g fiber/L
Replete® with Fiber	liquid	1000	1.00	63	113	34	300	Isotonic, 14 g fiber/L
Sustacal® with Fiber	liquid	1500	1.06	46	139	35	480	11 g fiber/L
Ultracal®	liquid	1250	1.06	44	123	45	310	Near isotonic, 14.4 g fiber/L
Lactose-Free, High-kCalorie, High-Protein Formulas								
Comply®	liquid	1250	1.50	60	180	61	60	
Ensure® Plus	liquid	1420	1.50	55	200	53	690	
Ensure® Plus HN	liquid	947	1.50	63	200	50	650	
Deliver® 2	liquid	1000	2.00	75	200	102	640	
IsoSource® 1.5 Cal	liquid	933	1.50	68	170	65	650	8.0 g fiber/L
Nutren® 1.5	liquid	1000	1.50	40	113	45	430	50% fat from MCT
Nutren® 2.0	liquid	750	2.00	40	98	53	720	75% fat from MCT

[a]These formulas are frequently used as oral supplements. All formulas listed under "Intact Formulas: Isotonic or Near-Isotonic Formulas" can be used as a low- to moderate-residue formula.

K

Table K-1
Intact Protein Formulas (continued)

Product	Form	Volume to Meet 100% RDI (ml)	Energy (kcal/ml)	Protein or Amino Acids (g/L)	Carbohydrate (g/L)	Fat (g/L)	Osmolality (mOsm/kg)	Notes
Lactose-Free, High-kCalorie, High-Protein Formulas								
Osmolite® HN Plus	liquid	1000	1.20	56	158	39	360	
Resource Plus®	liquid	1400	1.50	55	200	53	600	
Sustacal® Plus	liquid	1180	1.52	61	190	57	670	
TwoCal HN®	liquid	947	2.00	84	217	91	690	20% fat from MCT
Ultralan®	liquid	1000	1.50	60	202	50	540	50% fat from MCT
Lactose-Free, High-Protein Formulas								
Entrition® HN	liquid	1300	1.00	44	114	41	300	Isotonic, low-residue
FiberSource® HN	liquid	1500	1.20	53	160	41	390	7 g fiber/L
Isocal® HN	liquid	1250	1.06	44	123	46	270	Near-isotonic, low residue, 20% fat from MCT
IsoSource® HN	liquid	1500	1.20	53	160	41	330	Near-isotonic, low residue
IsoSource® VHN	liquid	1250	1.00	62	130	29	300	Isotonic, 10g fiber/L
Jevity® Plus	liquid	1000	1.20	56	175	39	450	12.0 g fiber/L
Libisorb®	liquid	1180	1.35	57	161	57	630	85% fat from MCT
Nitrolan	liquid	1250	1.24	60	160	40	310	Near-isotonic, 50% fat from MCT
Osmolite® HN	liquid	1321	1.06	44	144	35	300	Lactose-free, low-residue, 20% fat from MCT
Promote®	liquid	1000	1.00	63	130	26	340	Fat primarily from polyunsaturated and monounsaturated sources, 20% fat from MCT
Replete®	liquid	1500	1.00	63	113	33	350	Near-isotonic, lactose-free, low-residue
Sustacal®	liquid	1080	1.01	61	139	23	650	
Special Use Formulas: Pediatric (1 to 10 years)								
Compleat® Pediatric	liquid	900	1.00	38	126	39	N/A	Blenderized formula, 4.4 g fiber/L
Kindercal®	liquid	946	1.06	32	127	42	N/A	
Nutren Junior™	liquid	1000	1.00	30	128	42	350	
Nutren Junior™ with Fiber	liquid	1000	1.00	30	128	42	350	6.0 g fiber/L
PediaSure®	liquid	1000	1.00	30	110	50	345	
PediaSure® with Fiber	liquid	1000	1.00	30	114	50	345	5.0 g fiber/L
Special Use Formulas: Glucose Intolerance								
Choice dm™	liquid	948	1.06	45	106	51	440	13.6 g fiber/L, 25% kcalories from monounsaturated fat
DiabetiSource™	liquid	1500	1.00	50	90	49	360	4.4 g fiber/L

Table K-1
Intact Protein Formulas (continued)

Product	Form	Volume to Meet 100% RDI (ml)	Energy (kcal/ml)	Protein or Amino Acids (g/L)	Carbohydrate (g/L)	Fat (g/L)	Osmolality (mOsm/kg)	Notes
Special-Use Formulas: Glucose Intolerance								
Glucerna®	liquid	1422	1.00	42	96	54	355	14.4 g fiber/L, high in monounsaturated fat
Gluco-PRO™	liquid	1000	1.06	45	106	51	300	Isotonic, 14.4 g fiber/L
Glytrol®	liquid	1400	1.00	45	100	48	380	15 g fiber/L
Resource® Diabetic	liquid	1890	1.06	63	99	47	450	12 g fiber/L
Special Use Formulas: Immune System Support								
Immun-Aid®	powder	2000	1.00	80	120	22	460	Enriched with arginine, glutamine, branched-chain amino acids, nucleic acids, omega-3 fatty acids, vitamins A, C, E, and B$_6$ and trace elements
Impact®	liquid	1500	1.00	56	130	28	375	Enriched with arginine, nucleic acids, and omega-3 fatty acids
Impact® 1.5	liquid	1250	1.50	80	140	69	550	Same as above
Impact® with Fiber (see Fiber-Containing Formulas)								
Special Use Formulas: Renal Insufficiency								
Magnacal® Renal	liquid	N/A	2.00	75	200	101	570	High in monounsaturated fat, 20% fat from MCT; intended for use once hemodialysis has been instituted
Nepro®	liquid	947	2.00	70	215	96	635	Lactose-free, high-calcium, low phosphorus; intended for use once dialysis has been instituted
Suplena®	liquid	947	2.00	30	255	96	600	Lactose-free, low in electrolytes; intended for use before dialysis is instituted
Special Use Formulas: Respiratory Insufficiency								
NutriVent®	liquid	1000	1.50	68	100	94	450	Lactose-free, 55% kcal from fat, 40% fat from MCT
Pulmocare®	liquid	947	1.50	63	106	93	475	Lactose-free, 55% kcal from fat, 20% fat from MCT, enriched with antioxidant nutrients
Respalor™	liquid	1420	1.52	76	148	71	580	Lactose-free, 41% kcal from fat; 30% fat from MCT; enriched with vitamins C and E, B-complex vitamins, zinc and trace elements

K

Table K-1

Intact Protein Formulas (continued)

Product	Form	Volume to Meet 100% RDI (ml)	Energy (kcal/ml)	Protein or Amino Acids (g/L)	Carbohydrate (g/L)	Fat (g/L)	Osmolality (mOsm/kg)	Notes
Special Use Formulas: Wound Healing								
Protain XL®	liquid	1200	1.00	57	129	30	340	14 g fiber/L, 20% fat from MCT, enriched with vitamins A and C and zinc
Replete®	liquid	1000	1.00	63	113	34	320	Enriched with vitamins A and C and zinc
Replete® with Fiber (see Fiber-Containing Formulas)								
TraumaCal®	liquid	2000	1.50	83	145	69	560	Enriched with vitamins C, B-complex, and E and copper and zinc

Table K-2
Hydrolyzed Protein Formulas

Product	Form	Volume to Meet 100% RDI (ml)	Energy (kcal/ml)	Protein or Amino Acids (g/L)	Carbohydrate (g/L)	Fat (g/L)	Osmolality (mOsm/kg)	Notes
Formulas Containing 40 grams or Less Protein per Liter								
Criticare HN®	liquid	1890	1.06	38	220	5	650	50% free amino acids, 50% small peptides
L-Emental™	powder	N/A	1.00	38	205	3	630	100% free amino acids, enriched with glutamine
Peptamen	liquid	1500	1.00	40	127	39	325	Near-isotonic
PRO-Peptide™	liquid	1500	1.00	40	127	39	270	Isotonic, 70% fat from MCT, enriched with glutamine
Reabilan®	liquid	2000	1.00	32	132	53	350	50% fat from MCT
Tolerex®	powder	3160	1.00	21	230	1.5	550	100% free amino acids
Vivonex® T.E.N.	powder	2000	1.00	38	210	3.0	630	100% free amino acids, enriched with branched-chain amino acids
Formulas Containing More than 40 Grams Protein per Liter								
L-Emental™ Plus	powder	1800	1.00	45	190	7	650	100% free amino acids, enriched with glutamine
Peptamen VHP®	liquid	1500	1.00	63	105	39	365	70% fat from MCT
PRO-Peptide™ VHN	liquid	1500	1.00	62	104	39	300	Isotonic, 70% fat from MCT, enriched with glutamine
Reabilan® HN	liquid	1500	1.33	44	119	41	490	50% fat from MCT
SandoSource® Peptide	liquid	1750	1.00	50	160	17	490	60% free amino acids and small peptides
Vital® HN	powder	1500	1.00	42	185	11	500	87% hydrolyzed proteins, 13% essential amino acids
Special Use Hydrolyzed Formulas: Pediatric (1 to 10 years)								
L-Emental™ Pediatric	powder	1000* 1170**	0.8	24	130	24	360	100% free amino acids, contains glutamine
Peptamin Junior™	liquid	1000	1.0	30	138	39	310	60% fat from MCT
PRO-Peptide™ for Kids	liquid	1000**	1.0	30	138	39	360	40% fat from MCT, enriched with trace elements, taurine, and carnitine
Vivonex® Pediatric	powder	1000* 1170**	0.8	24	130	24	360	100% free amino acids

*Children 1 to 6 years old.
**Children 7 to 10 years old

K

K

Table K-2
Hydrolzed Protein Formulas (continued)

Product	Form	Volume to Meet 100% RDI (ml)	Energy (kcal/ml)	Protein or Amino Acids (g/L)	Carbohydrate (g/L)	Fat (g/L)	Osmolality (mOsm/kg)	Notes
Special Use Hydrolyzed Formulas: Hepatic Insufficiency								
Hepatic Aid® II	powder	—	1.20	44	169	36	560	Free amino acids, high in branched-chain amino acids, low in aromatic amino acids, no added vitamins or electrolytes.
L-Emental™ Hepatic	powder	N/A	1.20	44	169	36	560	Free amino acids, high in branched-chain amino acids, low in aromatic amino acids, contains vitamins and minimal electrolytes
NutriHep®	liquid	1000	1.50	40	290	21	690	Free amino acids, high in branched-chain amino acids, low in aromatic amino acids, contains vitamins and minimal electrolytes
Special Use Hydrolyzed Formulas: HIV Infection or AIDS								
Advera®	liquid	1184	1.28	60	216	23	680	78% hydrolyzed and 22% intact protein, low fat, fiber added, enriched with vitamins E, C, B₆, B₁₂, and folate
Special Use Hydrolyzed Formulas: Immune System Support								
Alitraq®	powder	1500	1.00	53	165	16	575	47% free amino acids, 42% small peptides, enriched with glutamine and arginine
Crucial®	liquid	1000	1.50	63	90	45	490	Enriched with arginine
Perative®	liquid	1155	1.30	67	177	37	385	Enriched with arginine and β-carotene
Vivonex® Plus	powder	1800	1.00	45	190	7	650	100% free amino acids, enriched with glutamine, arginine, and branched-chain amino acids

Table K–3
Protein Modules

Product	Form	Major Protein Source	Energy (kcal/g)	Protein (g/100 g)
Casec®	powder	Calcium caseinate	3.7	88
Pro Mod®	powder	Whey protein	4.2	75.8

Table K–4
Carbohydrate Modules

Product	Form	Major Carbohydrate Source	Energy (kcal/ml or g)
Moducal®	powder	Hydrolyzed corn starch	3.8 kcal/g
Polycose Liquid®	liquid	Hydrolyzed corn starch	2.0 kcal/ml
Polycose Powder®	powder	Hydrolyzed corn starch	3.8 kcal/g

Table K–5
Fat Modules

Product	Form	Major Fat Source	Energy (kcal/ml)	Fat (g/100 ml)
MCT Oil®	liquid	Derived from coconut oil	7.7	87
Microlipid®	liquid	Safflower oil	4.5	50

K

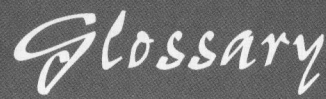

Many medical terms have their origins in Latin or Greek. By learning a few common derivations, you can glean the meaning of words you have never heard of before. For example, once you know that "hyper" means above normal, "glyc" means glucose, and "emia" means blood, you can easily determine that "hyperglycemia" means high blood glucose. The following derivations will help you to learn many terms presented in this glossary.

GENERAL
◆

a or *an* = not or without
anti = against
di = two
dys or *mal* = bad
endo = inside or within
exo or *extra* = outside
genesis = gives rise to, making
homeo = the same

hyper = over, above normal, excessive
hypo = below normal, under, beneath
inter = between, in the midst
intra = within
-itis = infection or inflammation
-lysis = break
macro = large
micro = tiny

mono = one
neo = new
-osis = condition
peri = around
poly = many
pre or *pro* = before
-stasis = staying
tri = three

BODY
◆

arterio = artery
cardiac or *cardio* = heart
cyte = cell
enteron = intestine
gastro = stomach

hemo or *-emia* = blood
hepatic = liver
myo = muscle
osteo = bone
pulmo = lung

renal = kidney
ure or *-uria* = urine
vaso = vessel
vena = vein

CHEMISTRY
◆

-al = aldehyde
-ase = enzyme
-ate = salt

glyc or *gluc* = glucose
hydro or *hydrate* = water
lipo = lipid

-ol = alcohol
-ose = sugar
saccharide = sugar

abscess: an accumulation of pus, caused by a local infection, that builds up and may eventually burst.

absorption: the taking up of nutrients into the intestinal cells.

Acceptable Daily Intake: the amount of a sweetener that individuals can safely consume each day over the course of a lifetime without adverse effect. It includes a 100-fold safety factor.

accredited: approved; in the case of medical centers or universities, certified by an agency recognized by the U.S. Department of Education.

acesulfame potassium: a low-kcalorie sweetener recently approved by the FDA; also known as acesulfame-K, because K is the chemical symbol for potassium. Approved in Canada.

acetaldehyde: an intermediate in alcohol metabolism.

acetone breath: a distinctive fruity odor that can be detected on the breath of a person who is experiencing ketosis.

acetyl CoA: a 2-carbon compound (acetate, or acetic acid) to which a molecule of CoA is attached.

acid-base balance: the equilibrium in the body between acid and base concentrations.

acidosis: above-normal acidity in the blood and body fluids.

acids: compounds that release hydrogen ions in a solution.

acne: a chronic inflammation of the skin's follicles and oil-producing glands, which leads to an accumulation of oils inside the ducts that surround hairs; usually associated with the maturation of young adults.

acquired immune deficiency syndrome (AIDS): the end stage of HIV infection, in which severe complications are manifested.

active vitamin D: the 1,25-dihydroxy form of vitamin D that promotes calcium balance and bone mineralization.

acupuncture: a technique that involves piercing the skin with long thin needles at specific anatomical points to relieve pain or illness. Acupuncture sometimes uses heat, pressure, friction, suction, or electromagnetic energy to stimulate the points.

acute disease: a disease the develops quickly, produces sharp symptoms, and runs a short course.

acute PEM: protein-energy malnutrition caused by recent severe food restriction or hypermetabolism; characterized in children by thinness for height (wasting).

ADA: see American Dietetic Association.

adaptive thermogenesis: adjustments in energy expenditure related to changes in environment such as cold and to physiological events such as overfeeding, trauma, and changes in hormone status.

additives: substances not normally consumed as foods but added to food either intentionally or by accident.

adenomas: cancers that arise from glandular tissues.

adenosine triphosphate: see ATP.

adequacy (dietary): providing all the essential nutrients, fiber, and energy in amounts sufficient to maintain health.

ADH: see antidiuretic hormone.

ADI: see Acceptable Daily Intake.

adipose tissue: the body's fat tissue, which consists of masses of fat-storing cells.

adolescence: the period from the beginning of puberty until maturity.

adrenal glands: glands adjacent to, and just above, each kidney.

advance directive: the means by which competent adults record their preferences for future medical interventions. The living will and durable power of attorney are types of advance directives.

adverse reactions: unusual responses to food (including intolerances and allergies).

aerobic: requiring oxygen.

aflatoxin: potent cancer-causing toxin produced by the mold Aspergillus flavus that infects grains and peanuts. The USDA tests grains and peanuts grown in this country for aflatoxin contamination.

AIDS: see acquired immune deficiency syndrome.

AIDS enteropathies: the diarrhea and malabsorption associated with AIDS for which no known cause has been identified.

AIDS-related complex (ARC): the cluster of mild symptoms that sometimes occur early in the course of HIV infection.

albuminuria: loss of the protein albumin in the urine.

alcohol dehydrogenase: an enzyme that converts ethanol to acetaldehyde; see also MEOS.

alcohol: a class of organic compounds containing hydroxyl (OH) groups.

aldosterone: a hormone secreted by the adrenal glands that stimulates the reabsorption of sodium by the kidneys; aldosterone also regulates chloride and potassium concentrations.

alimentary (or postgastrectomy) hypoglycemia: the type of hypoglycemia that occurs following gastric surgery.

alitame: a compound of two amino acids (alanine and aspartic acid) that is 2000 times sweeter than sucrose; FDA approval pending.

alkalosis: above-normal alkalinity (base) in the blood and body fluids.

alpha-lactalbumin: the chief protein in human breast milk, as opposed to casein, the chief protein in cow's milk.

alpha-tocopherol: the most biologically active vitamin E compound.

alternative therapies: approaches to medical diagnosis and treatment that are not fully accepted by the established medical community; as such, they are not widely taught at U.S. medical schools or practiced in U.S. hospitals; also called adjunctive, unconventional, or unorthodox therapies.

alveoli: air sacs in the lungs; one sac is an alveolus.

Alzheimer's disease: see senile dementia of the Alzheimer's type.

amenorrhea: the absence of or cessation of menstruation. Primary amenorrhea is menarche delayed beyond 16 years of age. Secondary amenorrhea is the absence of three to six consecutive menstrual cycles.

American Dietetic Association: the professional organization of dietitians in the United States. The Canadian equivalent is the Dietitians of Canada (DC), which operates similarly.

amino acids: building blocks of proteins; each contains an amino group, an acid group, a hydrogen atom, and a distinctive side group attached to a central carbon atom.

amino acid scoring: a method of evaluating protein quality by comparing a test protein's amino acid pattern with that of a reference protein; sometimes called chemical scoring.

ammonia: a compound with the chemical formula NH_3; produced during the deamination of amino acids.

amniotic sac: the "bag of waters" in the uterus, in which the fetus floats.

amylase: an enzyme that hydrolyzes amylose (a form of starch). Amylase is a carbohydrase, an enzyme that breaks down carbohydrates.

anabolism: reactions in which small molecules are put together to build larger ones. Anabolic reactions require energy.

anaerobic: not requiring oxygen.

anemia: literally, "too little blood." Anemia is any condition in which too few red blood cells are present, or the red blood cells are immature (and therefore large) or too small or contain too little hemoglobin to carry the normal amount of oxygen to the tissues. It is not a disease itself but can be a symptom of many different disease conditions, including many nutrient deficiencies, bleeding, excessive red blood cell destruction, and defective red blood cell formation.

angina: a painful feeling of tightness or pressure, felt in the area in and around the heart, often radiating to the back, neck, and arms; caused by a lack of oxygen to an area of heart muscle.

angiotensin: a blood protein that helps to raise blood pressure.

angiotensinogen: precursor protein for angiotensin.

anions: negatively charged ions.

anorexia nervosa: an eating disorder characterized by a refusal to maintain a minimally normal body weight and a distortion in perception of body shape and weight, most commonly seen in teenage girls and young women.

antacids: acid-buffering agents used to counter excess acidity in the stomach.

antagonist: a competing factor that counteracts the action of another factor. When a drug displaces a vitamin from its site of action, the drug renders the vitamin ineffective and thus acts as a vitamin antagonist.

anthropometric: relating to measurement of the physical characteristics of the body, such as height and weight.

antibodies: large proteins of the blood and body fluids, produced by the immune system in response to the invasion of the body by foreign molecules (usually proteins called *antigens*); antibodies combine with and inactivate the foreign invaders, thus protecting the body.

antidiarrheal agents: drugs used to treat diarrhea.

antidiuretic hormone (ADH): a hormone produced by the pituitary gland in response to dehydration (or a high sodium concentration in the blood); it stimulates the kidneys to reabsorb more water and therefore to excrete less. This ADH should not be confused with the enzyme alcohol dehydrogenase, which is sometimes also abbreviated ADH.

antigen: a substance that elicits the formation of antibodies or an inflammation reaction from the immune system. A bacterium, a virus, a toxin, and a protein in food that causes allergy are all examples of foreign antigens.

antimicrobial agents: preservatives that prevent microorganisms from growing.

antioxidant: a compound that protects others from oxidation by being oxidized itself. An antioxidant donates electrons to another substance; that substance becomes reduced as the antioxidant simultaneously becomes oxidized. Chemists describe the antioxidant action of vitamin C as maintaining the "oxidation-reduction equilibrium," or "redox state."

antipromoters: factors that oppose the development of cancer.

antiscorbutic factor: the original name for vitamin C.

antisense gene: the chemical opposite of a native gene that adheres to the native working gene and blocks its production of proteins.

anuria: no urine excretion.

anus: the terminal sphincter of the GI tract.

appendix: a narrow blind sac extending from the beginning of the colon; a vestigial organ with no known function.

appetite: the psychological desire to eat or an interest in food; a positive sensation that accompanies the sight, smell, or thought of food.

arachidonic acid: an omega-6 polyunsaturated fatty acid with 20 carbons and four double bonds (20:4); synthesized from linoleic acid.

aroma therapy: a technique that uses oil extracts from plants and flowers (usually applied by massage or baths) to enhance physical, psychological, and spiritual health.

artery: a vessel that carries blood away from the heart.

artesian water: water that is drawn from a well that taps a confined aquifer in which the water level stands above the natural water table.

arthritis: a usually painful inflammation of a joint caused by many conditions, including infections, metabolic disturbances, or injury; joint structure is usually altered, with loss of function.

artificial colors: certified food colors added to enhance appearance. (*Certified* means approved by the FDA.)

artificial feeding: feeding by tube or by vein.

artificial flavors, flavor enhancers: chemicals that mimic natural flavors and those that enhance flavor.

artificial sweeteners: sugar substitutes that provide no energy; sometimes called *nonnutritive sweeteners*.

ascites: a type of edema characterized by the accumulation of fluid in the abdominal cavity.

ascorbic acid: one of the two active forms of vitamin C. Many people refer to vitamin C by this name.

-ase: a word ending denoting an enzyme. Enzymes are often identified by the place they come from and the compounds they work on; *gastric lipase*, for example, is a stomach enzyme that acts on lipids, whereas *pancreatic lipase* comes from the pancreas (and also works on lipids).

aspartame: a compound of two amino acids (phenylalanine and aspartic acid) that tastes like the sugar sucrose but is much sweeter. It provides 4 kcalories per gram, as does protein, but because so little is used, it is virtually kcalorie-free. In powdered form it is sometimes mixed with lactose, however, so a 1-gram packet may provide 4 kcalories. It is used in both the United States and Canada.

aspiration: to draw in by suction, as may occur when food or liquid is sucked into the lungs.

aspiration pneumonia: an infection of the lungs caused by inhaling fluids regurgitated from the stomach. Aspiration pneumonia can be a fatal complication of a tube feeding.

-ate: a word ending denoting a salt of the mineral.

atherosclerosis: a type of artery disease characterized by accumulations of lipid-containing material on the inner walls of the arteries.

atom: the smallest component of an element that has all of the properties of the element.

ATP (adenosine triphosphate): a common high-energy compound composed of a purine (adenine), a sugar (ribose), and three phosphate groups.

atrophic gastritis: chronic inflammation of the stomach accompanied by a diminished size and functioning of the mucosa and glands.

atrophy: of muscles, a decrease in size because of disuse, undernutrition, or wasting diseases.

attention deficit hyperactivity disorder (ADHD): hyperactivity accompanied by an inability to pay attention and poor impulse control.

autoimmune disorders: immune system disorders in which the body destroys its own tissues.

available carbohydrates: carbohydrates such as starch and sugar that human digestive enzymes make available to the body.

avidin: a protein in egg whites that binds biotin.

ayurveda: a traditional Hindu system of improving health by using herbs, diet, meditation, massage, and yoga to stimulate the body to make its own natural drugs.

balance (dietary): providing foods of a number of types in proportion to each other, such that foods rich in some nutrients do not crowd out foods that are rich in other nutrients.

basal metabolic rate (BMR): the rate of energy use for metabolism under basal conditions, usually expressed as kcalories per kilogram body weight per hour.

basal metabolism: the energy needed to maintain life when a body is at complete rest after a 12-hour fast (to exclude the thermic effect of the previous meal).

bases: compounds that accept hydrogen ions in a solution.

beer: an alcoholic beverage brewed by fermenting malt and hops.

behavior modification: the changing of behavior by the manipulation of *antecedents* (cues or environmental factors that trigger behavior), the *behavior* itself, and *consequences* (the penalties or rewards attached to behavior).

beikost: supplemental, or weaning, foods.

belch: the expulsion of gas from the stomach through the mouth.

benign: tumors that stop growing without intervention or can be removed surgically and pose no threat to health.

beriberi: the thiamin-deficiency disease; it pointed the way to discovery of the first vitamin, thiamin.

beta-carotene: an orange pigment and vitamin A precursor found in plants.

BGH: see *bovine growth hormone*.

BHA and **BHT:** preservatives commonly used to slow the development of off-flavors, odors, and color changes caused by oxidation.

bicarbonate: an alkaline secretion of the pancreas, part of the pancreatic juice. (Bicarbonate also occurs widely in all cell fluids.)

bifidus factors: factors in colostrum and breast milk that favor the growth of the "friendly" bacterium *Lactobacillus bifidus* in the infant's intestinal tract, so that other, less desirable intestinal inhabitants will not flourish.

bile: an emulsifier that prepares fats and oils for digestion; an exocrine secretion made by the liver, stored in the gallbladder, and released into the small intestine when needed.

bilirubin: a pigment in the bile whose concentration in the blood may rise as a result of some disorders.

binders: chemical compounds occurring in foods that can combine with nutrients (especially minerals) to form complexes the body cannot absorb. Examples of such binders include *phytic acid* and *oxalic acid*.

bioaccumulation: the accumulation of contaminants in the flesh of animals high on the food chain.

bioavailability: the rate and extent to which a nutrient is absorbed.

bioelectrical impedance: a method for estimating body fat using low-intensity electrical current.

bioelectromagnetic medical applications: the use of electrical energy, magnetic energy, or both to stimulate bone repair, wound healing, and tissue regeneration.

biofeedback: the use of special devices to convey information about heart rate, blood pressure, skin temperature, muscle relaxation, and the like to enable a person to learn how to consciously control these medically important functions.

biofield therapeutics: a manual healing method that directs a healing force from an outside source (commonly God or another supernatural being) through the practitioner and into the client's body; commonly known as "laying on of hands."

biological value (BV): the amount of protein nitrogen that is retained for growth and maintenance, expressed as a percentage of the protein nitrogen that has been digested and absorbed; a measure of protein quality.

biosensor: a genetically altered microbe that provides a rapid, low-cost, and accurate test for the products of spoilage in foods.

biotechnology: the use of biological systems or organisms to create or modify products; also called *biogenetic engineering*.

biotin: a B vitamin that functions as a coenzyme in the metabolism of carbohydrates and fats.

blind experiment: an experiment in which the subjects do not know whether they are members of the experimental group or the control group.

blood lipid profile: results of blood tests that reveal a person's total cholesterol, triglycerides, and various lipoproteins.

BMI: see *body mass index*.

BMR: see *basal metabolic rate*.

body composition: the proportions of muscle, bone, fat, and other tissue that make up a person's total body weight.

body mass index (BMI): an index of a person's weight in relation to height, determined by dividing the weight (in kilograms) by the square of the height (in meters).

bolus: a portion; with respect to food, the amount swallowed at one time.

bolus feeding: delivery of about 300 to 400 ml of a tube feeding over 10 minutes or less.

bomb calorimeter: an instrument that measures the *heat* energy released when foods are burned, thus providing an estimate of the potential energy of foods.

bone density: a measure of bone strength. When minerals fill the bone matrix, they give it strength.

bone marrow transplant: the replacement of diseased bone marrow in a recipient with healthy bone marrow from a donor; used as a treatment for breast cancer, leukemia, and other blood disorders.

borderline diabetes: impaired glucose tolerance.

botulin: the toxin responsible for botulism.

botulism: an often fatal food-borne illness caused by the ingestion of foods containing a toxin produced by bacteria that grow in improperly canned acidic foods.

bovine growth hormone (BGH): a hormone produced naturally in the pituitary gland of a cow that promotes growth and milk production; now produced for agricultural use by transgenic bacteria.

bran: the protective coating around the kernel similar in function to the shell of a nut; rich in nutrients and fiber.

bronchitis: inflammation of the lungs' air passages.

brown sugar: refined white sugar crystals to which manufacturers have added molasses syrup with natural flavor and color; 91 to 96 percent pure sucrose.

buffers: compounds that help keep a solution's acidity or alkalinity constant.

bulimia nervosa: an eating disorder characterized by repeated episodes of binge eating usually followed by self-induced vomiting, misuse of laxatives or diuretics, fasting, or excessive exercise.

calcitonin: a hormone from the thyroid gland that lowers blood calcium by inhibiting its release from bone.

calcitriol: the active form of supplemental vitamin D.

calcium: the most abundant mineral in the body, found primarily in the body's bones and teeth.

calcium-binding protein: a protein in the intestinal cells, made with the help of vitamin D, that facilitates calcium absorption.

calcium rigor: hardness or stiffness of the muscles caused by high blood calcium concentrations.

calcium tetany: intermittent spasm of the extremities due to nervous and muscular excitability caused by low blood calcium concentrations.

calmodulin: an inactive protein that becomes active when bound to calcium; then it becomes a messenger that tells other proteins what to do. The system serves as interpreter for hormone- and nerve-mediated messages arriving at cells.

calorie: a unit by which energy is measured. Food energy is measured in *kilocalories* (1000 calories equal 1 kilocalorie), abbreviated *kcalories* or *kcal* A capitalized version is also sometimes used: *Calories*. One kcalorie is the amount of heat necessary to raise the temperature of 1 kilogram (kg) of water 1°C.

cancer cachexia syndrome: a syndrome that frequently accompanies many types of cancer; characterized by anorexia, inadequate intake of food, malnutrition, accelerated metabolism and wasting, and general ill health.

cancers: diseases that result from the unchecked growth of malignant tumors.

capillary: a small vessel that branches from an artery. Capillaries connect arteries to veins. Exchange of oxygen, nutrients, and waste materials takes place across capillary walls.

carbohydrase: an enzyme that hydrolyzes carbohydrates.

carbohydrate loading: a regimen of exhaustive exercise followed by the consumption of a high-carbohydrate diet that enables muscles to store glycogen beyond their normal capacity; also called *glycogen loading* or *glycogen supercompensation.*

carbohydrates: compounds composed of carbon, oxygen, and hydrogen arranged as monosaccharides or multiples of monosaccharides.

carbonic acid: a compound with the formula H_2CO_3 that results from the combination of carbon dioxide (CO_2) and water (H_2O), of particular importance in the body's buffer system.

carcinogens: agents that can give rise to cancer.

carcinomas: cancers that arise from epithelial tissues.

cardiac cachexia: chronic PEM that develops as a consequence of heart disease.

cardiac sphincter: the sphincter muscle at the junction between the esophagus and the stomach; also called the *lower esophageal sphincter* or the *gastroesophageal sphincter.*

cardiomegaly: enlargement of the heart.

cardiovascular disease (CVD): a general term for all diseases of the heart and blood vessels. Atherosclerosis is the main cause of CVD.

carotene: a vitamin A precursor found in plants; an orange pigment.

carotenoids: pigments commonly found in plants and animals, some of which have provitamin A activity. Carotenoids are among the best-known *phytochemicals*—plant chemicals that are not nutrients but have biological activity in the body.

carotid endartectomy: surgery to restore blood flow through the carotid artery to the brain.

carpal tunnel syndrome: a pinched nerve at the wrist, causing pain or numbness in the hand.

carrier: an individual who possesses one dominant and one recessive gene for a recessive trait, such as an inborn error of metabolism. Such a person may show no signs of the trait but can pass it on.

cartilage therapy: the use of cleaned and powdered connective tissue, such as collagen, to improve health.

cash crops: crops grown for cash, as opposed to crops grown for food; examples include cotton and tobacco.

catabolism: reactions in which large molecules are broken down to smaller ones. Catabolic reactions usually release energy.

catalyst: a compound that facilitates chemical reactions without itself being changed in the process.

cataracts: thickenings of the eye lenses that impair vision and can lead to blindness.

cathartic: a strong laxative.

cations: positively charged ions.

CCK: see *cholecystokinin.*

CDC: see *Centers for Disease Control.*

CD4+ T-lymphocyte: a type of circulating white blood cell that has the CD4+ protein on its surface and is a necessary component of the immune system.

celiac disease: a sensitivity to gliadin that causes flattening of the intestinal villi and generalized malabsorption; also called *gluten-sensitive enteropathy* or *celiac sprue.*

cellulite: supposedly, a lumpy form of fat; actually, a fraud. The lumpy appearance in fatty areas of the body is caused by strands of connective tissue that attach the skin to underlying muscles. These points of attachment may pull tight where the fat is thick, making lumps appear between them. The fat itself is not different from fat anywhere else in the body. So, if the fat in these areas is lost, the lumpy appearance disappears.

Centers for Disease Control: a branch of the Department of Health and Human Services that is responsible for, among other things, monitoring food-borne diseases.

central obesity: excess fat around the trunk of the body; also called *abdominal fat* or *upper-body fat.*

central total parenteral nutrition (TPN): a method for meeting all nutrient needs by infusing formula into a large-diameter central vein.

central veins: the large-diameter veins located close to the heart.

cerebral cortex: the outer surface of the cerebrum.

certification: the process in which a private laboratory inspects shipments of a product for selected chemicals and then, if the product is free of violative levels of those chemicals, issues a guarantee to that effect.

cesarean section: a surgically assisted birth involving removal of the fetus by an incision into the uterus, usually by way of the abdominal wall.

CHD: see *coronary heart disease.*

chelate: a substance that can grasp the positive ions of a metal.

chelation therapy: the use of ethylene diamine tetraacetic acid (EDTA) to bind with metallic ions, thus healing the body by removing toxic metals.

chemical scoring: see *amino acid scoring.*

chemotherapy: the use of drugs to arrest or destroy cancer cells. Drugs used for chemotherapy are called *chemotherapeutic* or *antineoplastic agents.*

CHF: see *congestive heart failure.*

Chinese restaurant syndrome: an intolerance reaction that may occur in 1 to 2 percent of the population 20 minutes after the ingestion of the additive MSG (monosodium glutamate). Symptoms include burning sensations, chest and facial flushing and pain, and throbbing headaches.

chiropractic: a manual healing method of manipulating vertebrae to relieve musculoskeletal pain suspected of causing problems with internal organs.

chloride: the major anion in the extracellular fluids of the body. Chloride is the ionic form of chlorine, Cl^-; see Appendix B for a description of the chlorine-to-chloride conversion.

chlorophyll: the green pigment of plants, which absorbs photons and transfers their energy to other molecules, thereby initiating photosynthesis.

cholecalciferol: vitamin D; also known as vitamin D_3.

cholecystokinin (CCK): a hormone produced by cells of the intestinal wall. Target organ: the gallbladder. Response: release of bile and slowing of GI motility.

cholesterol: one of the sterols.

choline: a nonessential nutrient that can be made in the body from an amino acid. Choline is used to make the phospholipid lecithin and the neurotransmitter acetylcholine.

chronic disease: a disease of long duration that progresses slowly, often characterized by deterioration of the body organs; also called *chronic, noncommunicable diseases (NCD)*. Examples include heart disease, cancer, and diabetes.

chronic obstructive pulmonary disease (COPD): one of several disorders, including emphysema and bronchitis, that interfere with respiration.

chronic PEM: protein-energy malnutrition caused by long-term food deprivation; characterized in children by short height for age (stunting).

chronological age: a person's age in years from his or her date of birth.

chylomicrons: the class of lipoproteins that transport lipids from the intestinal cells into the body.

chyme: the semiliquid mass of partly digested food expelled by the stomach into the duodenum.

cirrhosis: advanced liver disease in which liver cells turn orange, die, and harden, permanently losing their function; often associated with alcoholism.

clinically severe obesity: a BMI of 40 or greater or 100 pounds or more overweight for an average adult. A less preferred term used to describe the same condition is *morbid obesity*.

CoA: coenzyme A; the coenzyme derived from the B vitamin pantothenic acid and central to the energy metabolism of nutrients.

coenzymes: small organic molecules that work with enzymes to facilitate the enzymes' activity. Many coenzymes have B vitamins as part of their structures.

cofactor: a mineral element that, like a coenzyme, works with an enzyme to facilitate a chemical reaction. The cofactor maintains the structural integrity of the enzyme and may also facilitate the enzyme's catalytic activity.

collagen: the protein material from which connective tissues such as scars, tendons, ligaments, and the foundations of bones and teeth are made.

collaterals: small blood vessels that develop to divert blood flow away from an obstructed organ; also called *shunts*.

colon: see *large intestine*.

colonic irrigation: the popular, but potentially harmful practice of "washing" the large intestine with a powerful enema machine.

colostomate: a person who has a surgically formed opening from the colon to the outside of the body (a colostomy).

colostrum: a milklike secretion from the breast, present during the first day or so after delivery before milk appears; rich in protective factors.

comatose: in a state of deep unconsciousness from which the person cannot be aroused.

competent: having sufficient mental ability to understand a treatment, weigh its risks and benefits, and comprehend the consequences of refusing or accepting the treatment.

complementary proteins: two or more proteins whose amino acid assortments complement each other in such a way that the essential amino acids missing from one are supplied by the other.

complete formulas: enteral formulas designed to supply all needed nutrients when given in sufficient volume.

complete protein: a dietary protein containing all the amino acids essential in human nutrition in amounts adequate for human use.

complex carbohydrates (starches and fibers): polysaccharides composed of straight or branched chains of monosaccharides.

compound: a substance composed of two or more different atoms—for example, water (H_2O).

condensation: a chemical reaction in which two reactants combine to yield a larger product.

conditionally essential amino acid: an amino acid that is normally nonessential, but must be supplied by the diet in special circumstances when the need for it exceeds the body's ability to produce it.

cones: the cells of the retina that respond to bright light and are responsible for color vision.

confectioners' sugar: finely powdered sucrose; 99.9 percent pure.

congestive heart failure (CHF): a syndrome in which the heart can no longer adequately pump blood through the circulatory system.

congregate meal sites: nutrition programs that provide food for the elderly in a conveniently located setting such as a community center.

constipation: the condition of having painful or difficult bowel movements (elapsed time between movements is not relevant).

contaminant: a substance that does not normally occur in a food.

contamination iron: iron found in foods as the result of contamination by inorganic iron salts from iron cookware, iron-containing soils, and the like.

control group: a group of individuals similar in all possible respects to the experimental group except for the treatment. Ideally, the control group receives a placebo while the experimental group receives a real treatment.

COPD: see *chronic obstructive pulmonary disease*.

Cori cycle: the path from muscle glycogen to glucose to pyruvate to lactic acid (which travels to the liver) to glucose (which can travel back to the muscle) to glycogen; named after the scientist who elucidated this pathway.

corn sweeteners: corn syrup and sugars derived from corn.

corn syrup: a syrup produced by the action of enzymes on cornstarch; contains mostly glucose. See also *high-fructose corn syrup (HFCS)*.

cornea: the transparent membrane covering the outside of the eye.

coronary artery bypass graft (CABG): surgery to restore blood flow to the heart muscle to prevent a heart attack.

coronary heart disease (CHD): insufficient delivery of oxygen to the heart that occurs when the arteries that carry blood to the heart muscle become occluded.

correlation: the simultaneous increase, decrease, or change of two variables. If A increases as B increases, or if A decreases as B decreases, the correlation is positive. (This does not mean that A causes B or vice versa.) If A increases as B decreases, or if A decreases as B increases, the correlation is negative. (This does not mean that A prevents B or vice versa.) Some third factor may account for both A and B.

correspondence school: a school that offers courses and degrees by mail. Some correspondence schools are accredited; others are *diploma mills*.

cortical bone: the ivorylike outer bone layer that forms a shell surrounding trabecular bone and comprises the shaft of a long bone.

counterregulatory hormones: hormones such as glucagon, cortisol, and catecholamines that oppose insulin's actions and promote catabolism.

coupled reactions: pairs of chemical reactions in which energy released from the breakdown of one compound is used to create a bond in the formation of another compound.

covert: hidden, as if under covers.

cretinism: an iodine-deficiency disease characterized by mental and physical retardation.

critical periods: finite periods during development in which certain events may occur that will have irreversible effects on later developmental stages. In a body organ, a critical period is usually a period of rapid cell division.

Crohn's disease: inflammation and ulceration along the length of the GI tract, often with granulomas; also called *regional ileitis*.

crypts: tubular glands that lie between the intestinal villi and secrete intestinal juices into the small intestine.

cuisine: style of cooking or preparing food.

CVD: see *cardiovascular disease*.

cyanosis: a bluish discoloration of the skin caused by a lack of oxygen.

cyclamate: a 0-kcalorie sweetener; FDA approval pending in the United States; available in Canada on grocery-store shelves but only as a tabletop sweetener, not as an additive.

cystic fibrosis: a hereditary disorder characterized by the production of thick mucus that affects many organs, including the lungs, pancreas, liver, heart, gallbladder, and small intestine.

cystinuria: the presence of cystine in the urine; the symptom of an inherited metabolic disorder in which large amounts of the amino acids cystine, lysine, arginine, and ornithine are excreted in the urine. Cystinuria commonly results in kidney stone formation.

cytokines: immune system factors that help to control the inflammatory response.

D, L: *D* stands for *dextro*, or "right-handed," and *L*, for *levo*, or "left-handed," referring to the shapes of the molecules, which are mirror images of each other.

Daily Reference Values (DRV): a set of standards for nutrients and food components (such as fat and fiber) that have important relationships with health; used on food labels as part of the Daily Values.

Daily Values (DV): reference values developed by the FDA specifically for use on food labels. The Daily Values represent two sets of standards: Reference Daily Intakes (RDI) and Daily Reference Values (DRV).

dawn phenomenon: early morning hyperglycemia that develops in IDDM in response to counterregulatory hormones that act to raise glucose levels during an overnight fast.

deamination: removal of the amino (NH_2) group from a compound such as an amino acid.

death: permanent cessation of vital functions.

debridement: the removal of dead tissue resulting from burns and other wounds; speeds healing and helps prevent infection.

defecate: to move the bowels and eliminate waste.

deficient: the amount of a nutrient below which *almost all healthy people* can be expected, over time, to experience deficiency symptoms.

dehydration: the condition in which body water output exceeds water input.

Delaney Clause: a clause in the Food Additive Amendment to the Food, Drug, and Cosmetic Act that states that no substance that is known to cause cancer in animals or human beings at any dose level shall be added to foods.

denaturation: the change in a protein's shape brought about by heat, acid, base, alcohol, heavy metals, or other agents.

dental caries: decay of teeth.

dextrins: short chains of glucose that result from the breakdown of starch.

dextrose: an older name for glucose.

dextrose monohydrate: the form of glucose used in IV solutions. Dextrose solutions provide 3.4 kcal/g, whereas glucose provides 4 kcal/g.

DHEA (dehydroepiandrosterone): a hormone secreted by the adrenal glands. DHEA is available without prescription and is sold as an anti-aging remedy to improve energy, strength, and immunity. Proof of safety or effectiveness is lacking.

diabetes mellitus: a metabolic disorder characterized by altered blood glucose regulation and utilization, usually caused by insufficient or relatively ineffective insulin.

diabetic coma: unconsciousness precipitated by hyperglycemia, dehydration, ketosis, and acidosis in uncontrolled IDDM.

diagnosis: the disease a person has or is thought to have.

dialysis: removal of waste from the blood using the principles of simple diffusion and osmosis through a semipermeable membrane.

diarrhea: the frequent passage of watery bowel movements.

diet: the foods and beverages a person eats and drinks.

diet history: a record of eating behaviors and the foods a person eats.

diet manual: a book that describes the foods allowed and restricted on a diet, outlines the rationale and indications for use of each diet, and provides sample menus.

diet order: a physician's written statement in the medical record of what diet a client should receive.

Dietary Reference Intakes (DRI): the revised set of dietary recommendations that will replace the RDA; see inside front cover, left.

dietetic technician registered (DTR): a person with an associate's degree and training in nutrition, food science, and diet planning who works under the guidance of an RD (registered dietitian).

dietitian: a person trained in nutrition, food science, and diet planning. See also *registered dietitian*.

differentiation: development of specific functions different from those of the original.

digestion: the process by which food is broken down into absorbable units.

digestive enzymes: proteins found in digestive juices that act on food substances, causing them to break down into simpler compounds.

diglyceride: a molecule of glycerol with two fatty acids attached.

diketopiperazine (DKP): a product to which aspartame breaks down during metabolism.

dioxins: any of 75 structurally related compounds that contain both nitrogen and chlorine.

dipeptide: two amino acids bonded together.

direct calorimetry: the measurement of energy output as heat energy.

disaccharide: a pair of monosaccharides linked together.

dissociation: the physical separation of a compound into ions.

distilled liquor: an alcoholic beverage made by fermenting and distilling grains; sometimes called *distilled spirits* or *hard liquor*.

distilled water: water that has been vaporized and recondensed, leaving it free of dissolved minerals.

diuretics: a drug that promotes water excretion; popularly, a "water pill."

diuretic phase: the phase of renal failure characterized by large fluid and electrolyte losses in the urine.

diverticula: a sac or pouch that develops in the weakened areas of the intestinal wall (like bulges in an inner tube where the tire wall is weak).

diverticulitis: diverticula that have become infected or inflamed and may rupture.

diverticulosis: the condition of having diverticula.

docosahexaenoic acid (DHA): an omega-3 polyunsaturated fatty acid with 22 carbons and six double bonds (22:6); synthesized from linolenic acid.

dominant gene: a gene that has an observable effect on an organism even when it is paired with a normal gene; see also *recessive gene*.

double-blind experiment: an experiment in which neither the subjects nor the researchers know which subjects are members of the experimental group and which are serving as control subjects until after the experiment is over.

Down syndrome: a genetic abnormality that causes mental retardation, short stature, and flattened facial features.

DRI: see *Dietary Reference Intakes.*

drink: a dose of any alcoholic beverage that delivers ½ ounce of pure ethanol.

drug: a substance that can modify one or more of the body's functions.

drug history: a record of all the medications, over-the-counter and prescribed, that a person takes routinely.

DRV: see *Daily Reference Values.*

DTR: see *dietetic technician registered.*

dumping syndrome: the symptoms that result from the rapid emptying of undigested food into the jejunum: sweating, weakness, and diarrhea shortly after eating and hypoglycemia later. Dumping syndrome is common following pyloroplasties, vagotomies, total gastrectomies, and gastric bypass surgery.

duodenum: the top portion of the small intestine (about "12 fingers' breadth" long in ancient terminology).

durable power of attorney: a legal document in which one competent adult authorizes another competent adult to make decisions for her or him in the event of incapacitation. The phrase "durable power" means that the agent's authority survives the client's incompetence; "attorney" refers to an attorney-in-fact (not an attorney-at-law).

DV: see *Daily Values.*

dysentery: an infection of the digestive tract that causes diarrhea.

dyslipidemia: abnormal blood lipids; elevated LDL and low HDL are examples.

dyspepsia: vague abdominal pain; a symptom, not a disease.

dysphagia: difficulty in swallowing.

dysuria: painful or difficult urination.

eating disorder: a disturbance in eating behavior that jeopardizes a person's physical or psychological health.

eclampsia: a condition characterized by convulsions and coma that develops in some women with untreated preeclampsia.

edema: the swelling of body tissue caused by excessive amounts of fluid in the interstitial spaces; seen in protein deficiency (among other conditions).

edentulous: without teeth.

eicosanoids: derivatives of fatty acids; hormonelike compounds that regulate blood pressure, clotting, and other body functions. They include *prostaglandins, thromboxanes,* and *leukotrienes.*

eicosapentaenoic acid (EPA): an omega-3 polyunsaturated fatty acid with 20 carbons and five double bonds (20:5); synthesized from linolenic acid.

electrolyte solutions: solutions that can conduct electricity due to the presence of ions.

electrolytes: salts that dissolve in water and dissociate.

element: a substance composed of atoms that are alike—for example, iron (Fe).

embolism: the obstruction of a blood vessel by a blood clot or foreign substance causing sudden tissue death.

embolus: a blood clot or other undissolved mass traveling in the circulatory system.

embryo: the developing infant from two to eight weeks after conception.

emetic: an agent that causes vomiting.

emphysema: a type of COPD in which the lungs lose their elasticity and the victim has difficulty breathing; often occurs along with bronchitis.

empty-kcalorie food: a popular term used to denote foods that contribute energy but lack protein, vitamins, and minerals. Empty-kcalorie foods are *low–nutrient density foods.* The most notorious empty-kcalorie foods are sugar, fat, and alcohol.

emulsifier: a substance with both water-soluble and fat-soluble portions that promotes the mixing of oils and fats in a watery solution.

endocrine glands: glands that secrete juices "into" the blood.

endogenous: made in the body.

endogenous protein: the protein in the body. In contrast, protein in foods is *exogenous protein.*

endosperm: the bulk of the edible part of the kernel containing starch and proteins.

end-stage renal disease: the severe stage of renal failure in which dialysis or a kidney transplant is necessary to sustain life.

energy: the capacity to do work. The energy in food is chemical energy. The body can convert this chemical energy to mechanical, electrical, or heat energy.

energy metabolism: all the reactions by which the body obtains and spends the energy from food.

energy-yielding nutrients: the nutrients that break down to yield energy the body can use; carbohydrate, fat, protein.

enriched: the addition of nutrients to a food to meet a specified standard; often used interchangeably with *fortified.*

enteral formulas: liquid diets intended for oral use or for tube feedings.

enteric hyperoxaluria: a condition of excess oxalate absorption that comes about because calcium is unable to bind oxalate in the gut; may lead to kidney stone formation.

enterogastrone: a gastrointestinal hormone.

enterohepatic circulation (of bile): the recycling of cholesterol and bile through the intestine and liver.

enteropancreatic circulation: the circulatory route from the pancreas to the intestine and back to the pancreas.

enterostomal therapist (ET): a health care professional specially trained to assist ostomates in learning the proper methods of caring for ostomy sites and adjusting to the ostomy.

enterostomy: a gastric or jejunal opening made surgically or under local anesthesia through which a feeding tube can be passed.

Environmental Protection Agency: a federal agency that is responsible for, among other things, regulating pesticides and establishing water quality standards.

enzyme replacements: extracts of pork or beef pancreatic enzymes that are taken as supplements to help with digestion.

enzymes: proteins that facilitate chemical reactions without being changed in the process; protein catalysts.

EPA: see *Environmental Protection Agency.*

epigastric: the region of the body just above the stomach.

epiglottis: cartilage in the throat that guards the entrance to the trachea and prevents fluid or food from entering it when a person swallows.

epinephrine: a hormone of the adrenal gland that modulates the stress response; formerly called *adrenaline.*

epithelial cells: cells on the surface of the skin and mucous membranes.

epithelial tissues: the layers of the body that serve as selective barriers between the body's interior and the environment (examples are the cornea, the skin, the respiratory lining, and the lining of the digestive tract).

ergocalciferol: the plant version of vitamin D; also known as vitamin D_2.

erythrocyte: red blood cell.

erythrocyte hemolysis: the breaking open of red blood cells; a symptom of vitamin E–deficiency disease in human beings.

erythrocyte protoporphyrin: a precursor to hemoglobin.

erythropoietin: a hormone secreted by the kidneys in response to oxygen depletion or anemia that stimulates the bone marrow to produce red blood cells.

esophageal stricture: narrowing of the esophagus that occurs when scar tissue forms in response to the continuous reflux of gastric juice.

esophageal ulcers: lesions or sores in the lining of the esophagus.

esophageal varices: tangles of distended blood vessels that protrude into the esophagus.

esophagus: the food pipe; the conduit from the mouth to the stomach.

essential amino acids: amino acids that the body cannot synthesize in amounts sufficient to meet physiological needs. Some researchers refer to essential amino acids as *indispensable* and to nonessential amino acids as *dispensable*.

essential fatty acids: fatty acids needed by the body, but not made by the body in amounts sufficient to meet physiological needs.

essential (primary) hypertension: high blood pressure that develops without an identifiable cause.

essential nutrients: nutrients a person must obtain from food because the body cannot make them for itself in sufficient quantity to meet physiological needs; also called *indispensable nutrients*. About 40 nutrients are known to be essential for human beings.

ethanol: a particular type of alcohol found in beer, wine, and distilled spirits; also called *ethyl alcohol*. Ethanol is the most widely used—and abused—drug in our society. It is also the only legal, nonprescription drug that produces euphoria.

ethical: in accordance with moral principles or professional standards. Socrates described *ethics* as "how we ought to live."

ethnic diets: foodways and cuisines typical of national origins, cultural heritages, or geographic locations.

euphoria: a feeling of great well-being, which people often seek through the use of drugs such as alcohol.

exchange lists: diet-planning tools that organize foods by their proportions of carbohydrate, fat, and protein. Foods on any single list can be used interchangeably.

exocrine glands: glands that secrete juices "out" into the digestive tract or onto the surface of the skin.

exogenous: outside the body (from foods).

experimental group: a group of individuals similar in all possible respects to the control group except for the treatment. The experimental group receives the test treatment.

external cue theory: the theory that some people eat in response to such external factors as the presence of food or the time of day rather than to such internal factors as hunger.

exudate: the fluid containing plasma proteins, electrolytes, and immune factors that leaks out through the capillaries in response to injury.

FAE: see *fetal alcohol effects*.

faith healing: healing by invoking divine intervention without the use of medical, surgical, or other traditional therapy.

false negative: a test result indicating that a condition is *not* present (negative) when in fact it is present (therefore false).

false positive: a test result indicating that a condition is present (positive) when in fact it is not (therefore false).

FAO (Food and Agriculture Organization): an international agency (part of the United Nations) that has adopted standards to regulate pesticide use among other responsibilities.

FAS: see *fetal alcohol syndrome*.

fasting hypoglycemia: hypoglycemia that develops gradually and primarily affects the brain and central nervous system.

fat: the lipids in foods or body fat, both of which are composed mostly of triglycerides.

fatfold measure: a clinical estimate of total body fatness in which the thickness of a fold of skin on the back of the arm (over the triceps muscle), below the shoulder blade (subscapular), or in other places is measured with a caliper. (The older, less preferred, term is *skinfold test*.)

fatty acid: an organic compound composed of a carbon chain with hydrogens attached and an acid group (COOH) at one end.

fatty acid oxidation: the metabolic breakdown of fatty acids to acetyl CoA.

fatty liver: a symptom of liver dysfunction seen in several diseases, including kwashiorkor and alcoholic liver disease. Fatty liver is characterized by an accumulation of fat in the liver cells; also called *hepatic steatosis*.

FDA (Food and Drug Administration): a part of the Department of Health and Human Services' Public Health Service that is responsible for ensuring the safety and wholesomeness of all foods sold in interstate commerce except meat, poultry, and eggs (which are under the jurisdiction of the USDA); inspecting food plants and imported foods; and setting standards for food composition.

fermentation: the oxidation of carbohydrate in the absence of atmospheric oxygen, a process that yields alcohol as an end product.

ferric iron: the oxidized form of iron (Fe^{+++}).

ferritin: an iron storage protein.

ferrous iron: the reduced form of iron (Fe^{++}).

fertility: the capacity of a woman to produce a normal ovum periodically and of a man to produce normal sperm; the ability to reproduce.

fetal alcohol effects (FAE): a subclinical version of FAS, with hidden defects including learning disabilities, behavioral abnormalities, and motor impairments; also called *alcohol-related birth defects (ARBD)*.

fetal alcohol syndrome (FAS): the cluster of symptoms seen in an infant or child whose mother consumed excess alcohol during pregnancy, including retarded growth, impaired development of the central nervous system, and facial malformations.

fetor hepaticus: the odor that may develop in people with impending hepatic coma.

fetus: the developing infant from eight weeks after conception until term.

fever: an elevation of body temperatures above normal.

fiber: a general term denoting in plant foods the *nonstarch polysaccharides* that are not digested by *human* digestive enzymes, although some are digested by GI tract bacteria; fibers include cellulose, hemicelluloses, pectins, gums, and mucilages and the nonpolysaccharides lignins, cutins, and tannins.

fibrocystic breast disease: a harmless condition in which the breasts develop lumps, sometimes associated with caffeine consumption. In some, it responds to treatment by abstinence from caffeine; in others, it can be treated with vitamin E.

fibrosis: the condition in which damaged cells lose function and are replaced by fibrous connective tissue cells.

fibrous: composed of fibers.

filtrate: in the kidneys, the fluid that passes from the blood through the capillary walls of the glomeruli, eventually forming urine.

fistula: an abnormal opening between two organs or from an organ to the skin.

fitness: the characteristics that enable the body to perform physical activity; more broadly, the ability to meet routine physical demands with enough reserve energy to rise to a sudden challenge; or the body's ability to withstand stress of all kinds.

flapping tremor: uncontrolled movement of the muscle group that causes the outstretched arm and hand to flap like a wing; occurs in hepatic coma and other diseases that cause encephalopathy; also called *asterixis*.

fluid and electrolyte balance: maintenance of the proper types and amounts of fluid and minerals in each compartment of the body fluids.

fluorapatite: the stabilized form of bone and tooth crystal, in which fluoride has replaced the hydroxyl groups of hydroxyapatite.

fluoridated water: water that has been treated so as to contain at least 0.8 mg fluoride per liter.

fluorosis: discoloration of tooth enamel caused by excess fluoride.

folate: a B vitamin; also known as folic acid, folacin, or pteroylglutamic acid (PGA). The coenzyme forms are DHF (dihydrofolate) and THF (tetrahydrofolate).

food allergies: adverse reactions to foods that involve an immune response; also called *food-hypersensitivity reactions*.

food aversion: a strong desire to avoid a particular food.

food-borne illnesses: illnesses transmitted to human beings through food, caused by either an infectious agent (*food-borne infection*) or a poisonous substance (*food intoxication*); commonly known as *food poisoning*.

food chain: the sequence in which living things depend on other living things for food.

food consumption survey: a survey that measures the amounts and kinds of foods people consume (using diet histories), estimates the nutrient intakes, and compares them with a standard such as the RDA.

food craving: a deep longing for a particular food.

food frequency checklist: a checklist of foods on which a person can record the frequency with which he or she eats different types of foods.

food group plans: diet-planning tools that sort foods of similar origin and nutrient content into groups and then specify that people should eat certain numbers of servings from each group.

food insecurity: intermittent hunger caused by lack of money or lack of control over other resources needed to assure a reliable food supply; the predominant form of hunger in the United States today.

food intolerances: adverse reactions to foods that do not involve the immune system.

food record: an extensive, accurate log of all foods eaten over a period of several days or weeks.

foods: products derived from plants or animals that can be taken into the body to yield nutrients for the maintenance of life and the growth and repair of tissues.

Food Stamp Program: a federal food assistance program. The USDA issues food stamp coupons through state social services or welfare agencies to households—people who buy and prepare food together. The number of stamps a household receives depends on the household's size and income. Recipients may use the coupons like cash to purchase food and seeds, but not to buy tobacco, cleaning items, alcohol, or other nonfood items.

foodways: the sum of the food habits, customs, beliefs, and preferences of a culture.

fortified: the addition to a food of nutrients that were either not originally present or present in insignificant amounts. Fortification can be used to correct or prevent a widespread nutrient deficiency, to balance the total nutrient profile of a food, or to restore nutrients lost in processing.

fossil fuel: coal, oil, and natural gas; these are nonrenewable fuels that pollute. (Renewable or alternative fuels, such as solar and wind energy, pollute less or not at all.)

frame size: the size of a person's bones and musculature. Appendix E describes how to take measures to estimate body frame size and provides tables of standards used in assessment.

fraud or quackery: the promotion, for financial gain, of devices, treatments, services, plans, or products (including diets and supplements) that alter or claim to alter a human condition without proof of safety or effectiveness. (The word *quackery* comes from the term *quacksalver*, meaning a person who quacks loudly about a miracle product—a lotion or a salve.)

free radical: an atom or molecule that has one or more unpaired electron(s) in the outer orbital (see Appendix B for a review of basic chemistry concepts). This electron imbalance makes free radicals unstable and highly reactive. Radicals typically arise during oxidation reactions and readily attack other molecules with which they come in contact.

fructose: a monosaccharide; sometimes known as fruit sugar or levulose, fructose is found abundantly in fruits, honey, and saps.

galactose: a monosaccharide; part of the disaccharide lactose.

galactosemia: an inborn error of metabolism in which galactose cannot be metabolized normally to compounds the body can handle and an alternative metabolite accumulates in the tissues, causing damage.

gallbladder: the organ that stores and concentrates bile. When it receives the signal that fat is present in the duodenum, the gallbladder contracts and squirts bile through the bile duct into the duodenum.

galvanized: a term referring to metals that have been treated with a zinc-containing coating to prevent rust.

gangrene: death of tissue due to a deficient blood supply and/or infection.

garlic oil: extract of garlic; proof of effectiveness is lacking.

gastric glands: exocrine glands in the stomach wall that secrete gastric juice into the stomach.

gastric-inhibitory peptide: a hormone produced by the intestine. Target organ: the stomach. Response: slowing of the secretion of gastric juices and of GI motility.

gastric juice: the digestive secretion of the gastric glands of the stomach.

gastric partitioning: a surgical procedure used to treat clinically severe obesity. The operation limits food intake by reducing the size of the stomach and delays gastric emptying by restricting the outlet.

gastric residual: the volume of formula that remains in the stomach from a previous feeding. It is measured by gently withdrawing the gastric contents through the feeding tube using a syringe. If the measured gastric residual is acceptable, the residual is returned to the client through the feeding tube.

gastrin: a hormone secreted by cells in the stomach wall. Target organ: the stomach. Response: secretion of gastric juice.

gastritis: inflammation of the stomach lining.

gastrointestinal tract: see *GI tract*.

gastroparesis: delayed gastric emptying.

gastrostomy: an opening in the stomach made surgically or under local anesthesia through which a feeding tube can be passed.

gatekeepers: with respect to nutrition, key people who control other people's access to foods and thereby exert profound impacts on their nutrition. Examples are the spouse who buys and cooks the food, the parent who feeds the children, and the caretaker in a day-care center.

genes: the basic units of hereditary information, made of DNA, that are passed from parent to offspring in the chromosomes. Each gene codes for a protein.

geophagia: clay eating.

germ: the nutrient-rich inner part of a grain. The germ is the seed that grows into a wheat plant, so it is especially rich in vitamins and minerals to support new life.

gestation: the period from conception to birth; for human beings gestation lasts from 38 to 42 weeks.

gestational diabetes: the appearance of abnormal glucose tolerance during pregnancy, with subsequent return to normal postpartum.

GFR: see *glomerular filtration rate*.

GI tract: the gastrointestinal tract or digestive tract; the principal organs are the stomach and intestines.

gland: a cell or group of cells that secretes materials for special uses in the body.

gliadin: a fraction of the gluten protein.

gliomas: cancers that arise from glial cells of the central nervous system.

glomerular filtration rate (GFR): the rate at which the kidneys form filtrate. Normally, the GFR is between 90 and 120 ml/min.

glomerulonephritis: an inflammation of the glomerular capillaries.

glomerulus: a cup-shaped membrane enclosing a tuft of capillaries within a nephron. (The plural is *glomeruli*.)

glucagon: a hormone that is secreted by special cells in the pancreas in response to low blood glucose concentration and elicits release of glucose from storage.

gluconeogenesis: the making of glucose from a noncarbohydrate source.

glucose: a monosaccharide; sometimes known as *blood sugar* or *dextrose*.

glucose tolerance: the ability of the body to regulate its blood glucose concentration to either the intake of dietary carbohydrate or the release of glucose from cells during fasting or metabolic stress.

glucose tolerance factor (GTF): a small organic compound that enhances insulin's action.

glucosuria: see *glycosuria*.

gluten: a vegetable protein found in wheat, oats, rye, barley, and other grains that gives dough its structure and cohesiveness.

glycemic effect: a measure of the extent to which a food, as compared with pure glucose, raises the blood glucose concentration and elicits an insulin response.

glycerol: an alcohol composed of a three-carbon chain, which can serve as the backbone for a triglyceride.

glycogen: an animal polysaccharide composed of glucose; it is manufactured and stored in the liver and muscles as a storage form of glucose. Glycogen is not a significant food source of carbohydrate and is not counted as one of the complex carbohydrates in foods.

glycogen loading: see *carbohhdrate loading*.

glycolysis: the metabolic breakdown of glucose to pyruvate. Glycolysis does not require oxygen (anaerobic).

glycosuria or glucosuria: glucose in the urine, which generally occurs when blood glucose exceeds 180 mg/100 ml.

goblet cells: cells of the GI tract (and lungs) that secrete mucus.

goiter: an enlargement of the thyroid gland due to an iodine deficiency, malfunction of the gland, or overconsumption of a goitrogen. Goiter caused by iodine deficiency is *simple goiter*.

goitrogen: a thyroid antagonist found in food; causes *toxic goiter*. Goitrogens are found in such foods as cabbage, kale, brussels sprouts, cauliflower, broccoli, and kohlrabi.

gout: a metabolic disorder that results in excess uric acid in the blood and sometimes in the urine; characterized by acute arthritis and inflammation of the joints.

graft-versus-host disease (GVHD): destruction of healthy donor cells by the recipient's immune system, which recognizes the donor cells as foreign.

granulated sugar: crystalline sucrose; 99.9 percent pure.

granulomas: granular tumors or growths.

GRAS (generally recognized as safe) list: a list, established by the FDA in 1958, of food additives that had long been in use and were believed safe. The list is subject to revision as new facts become known.

grazing: a popular term to describe eating many small meals and snacks throughout the day.

GTF: see *glucose tolerance factor*.

GVHD: see *graft-versus-host disease*.

hair follicle: a group of cells in the skin from which a hair grows.

hard water: water with a high calcium and magnesium concentration.

hazard: source of danger; used to refer to circumstances in which toxicity is possible under normal conditions of use.

HDL (high-density lipoprotein): the type of lipoprotein that transports cholesterol back to the liver from peripheral cells; composed primarily of protein.

health care team: a group of professionals representing several disciplines who work together to resolve their clients' medical problems.

health claim: any statement that characterizes the relationship between any nutrient or other substance in a food and a disease or health-related condition.

health history: an account of the client's current and past health status and risk factors for disease. Traditionally, the health history has been called the *medical history*. The term *health history* now seems more appropriate, however, since the contents describe the client's health status, and current trends in the medical profession now emphasize health promotion and disease prevention.

health maintenance organization (HMO): a form of managed care that limits the subscriber's choice of health care professionals and controls access to services by directing care through a primary care physician.

Healthy People 2000: a report that sets national objectives in health promotion and disease prevention for the year 2000. The 21 nutrition-related priorities are listed in Appendix G.

heart attacks: sudden tissue death caused by blockages of vessels that feed the heart muscle; also called *myocardial infarction* or *cardiac arrest*.

heartburn: a burning sensation in the chest area caused by backflow of stomach acid into the esophagus.

heat stroke: the dangerous accumulation of body heat with accompanying loss of body fluid.

heavy metal: any of a number of mineral ions such as mercury and lead, so called because they are of relatively high atomic weight. Many heavy metals are poisonous.

Heimlich maneuver: a technique for removing an object from the trachea of a choking person.

hematocrit: measurement of the percentage of the red blood cells in a given volume of blood.

hematuria: blood in the urine.

heme: the iron-holding part of the hemoglobin and myoglobin proteins. About 40 percent of the iron in meat, fish, and poultry is bound into heme; the other 60 percent is nonheme iron.

hemlock: a poisonous herb having finely divided leaves and small white flowers.

hemochromatosis: a hereditary defect in iron metabolism characterized by deposits of iron-containing pigment in many tissues, with tissue damage.

hemodialysis: a method of eliminating waste products in kidney failure whereby a blood vessel is tapped, and the blood is routed through a dialysis machine where excess fluids and wastes are removed. Blood is then returned from the machine to the body.

hemoglobin: the globular protein of the red blood cells that carries oxygen from the lungs to the cells throughout the body.

hemolysis: bursting of red blood cells.

hemophilia: a hereditary disease in which the blood is unable to clot because it lacks the ability to synthesize certain clotting factors.

hemorrhagic disease: a disease characterized by excessive bleeding.

hemorrhoids: painful swelling of the veins surrounding the rectum.

hemosiderin: an iron storage protein.

hemosiderosis: a condition characterized by the deposition of hemosiderin in the liver and other tissues.

hepatic: of, like, or pertaining to the liver.

hepatic coma: a state of unconsciousness that results from severe liver disease; also called *hepatic encephalopathy* or *portal systemic encephalopathy.*

hepatitis: inflammation of the liver caused by a virus, alcohol, drug, or other toxin.

herbal medicine: the use of plants to treat disease or improve health; also known as *botanical medicine* or *phytotherapy.*

herpes virus: a virus that can lead to mouth lesions and may also affect the lower GI tract, causing diarrhea.

hexoses: simple sugars with six atoms of carbon and the formula $C_6H_{12}O_6$.

HFCS: see *high-fructose corn syrup.*

hiatal hernia: a protrusion of a portion of the stomach through the esophageal hiatus of the diaphragm. There are several types of hiatal hernias, but the *sliding hiatal hernia* is the most common.

hiatus: the opening in the diaphragm through which the esophagus passes.

hiccups: repeated cough-like sounds and jerks that are produced when an involuntary spasm of the diaphragm muscle sucks air down the windpipe; also spelled *hiccoughs.*

high-fructose corn syrup (HFCS): a corn-syrup sweetener made especially for use in processed foods and beverages, where it is the predominant sweetener. HFCS is mostly fructose; glucose makes up the balance.

high potency: a nutrient present in a supplement in an amount that provides 100 percent or more of the Daily Value per serving.

high-quality protein: an easily digestible, complete protein.

high-risk pregnancy: a pregnancy characterized by indicators that make it likely the birth will be surrounded by problems such as premature delivery, difficult birth, retarded growth, birth defects, and early infant death.

histamine: a substance produced by cells of the immune system as part of a local immune reaction to an antigen; participates in causing inflammation.

HIV: see *human immunodeficiency virus.*

homeopathic medicine: a practice based on the theory that "like cures like," that is, that substances that cause symptoms in healthy people can cure those symptoms when given in very dilute amounts.

homeostasis: the maintenance of constant internal conditions (such as blood chemistry, temperature, and blood pressure) by the body's control systems. A homeostatic system is constantly reacting to external forces so as to maintain limits set by the body's needs.

honey: sugar (mostly sucrose) formed from nectar gathered by bees. An enzyme splits the sucrose into glucose and fructose. Composition and flavor vary, but honey always contains a mixture of sucrose, fructose, and glucose.

hormones: chemical messengers. Hormones are secreted by a variety of glands in response to altered conditions in the body. Each hormone travels to one or more specific target tissues or organs, where it elicits a specific response to restore normal conditions.

hormone-sensitive lipase: an enzyme inside adipose cells that responds to the body's need for fuel by hydrolyzing triglycerides so that their parts (glycerol and fatty acids) escape into the general circulation and thus become available to other cells as fuel. The signals to which this enzyme responds include epinephrine and glucagon, which oppose insulin.

human immunodeficiency virus (HIV): the virus that causes AIDS. The infection progressively destroys the immune system and leaves its victims defenseless against numerous infections.

hunger: the physiological need to eat, experienced as a drive to obtain food; an unpleasant sensation.

husk: the outer, inedible part of a grain; also called the *chaff.*

hydrochloric acid: an acid composed of hydrogen and chloride atoms (HCl). The gastric glands normally produce this acid.

hydrodensitometry: a method of measuring body density in which the person is first weighed and then submerged in water.

hydrogenation: a chemical process by which hydrogens are added to monounsaturated or polyunsaturated fats to reduce the number of double bonds, making the fats more saturated (solid) and more resistant to oxidation (protecting against rancidity). Hydrogenation produces *trans*-fatty acids.

hydrolysis: a chemical reaction in which a major reactant is split into two products, with the addition of a hydrogen atom (H) to one and a hydroxyl group (OH) to the other (from water, H_2O).

hydrolyzed formula: a liquid diet that contains broken-down molecules of protein, such as amino acids and short peptide chains, and is therefore easy to digest and absorb; also called a *monomeric formula.*

hydrophilic: a term referring to water-loving, or water-soluble, substances.

hydrophobic: a term referring to water-fearing, or non-water-soluble, substances; also known as *lipophilic* (fat loving).

hyperactivity: a condition of excessive activity.

hyperammonemia: an elevated blood ammonia level. Normal blood ammonia levels are less than 50 μg/100 ml.

hypercalcemia: high blood calcium. Hypercalcemia may develop from a variety of disorders, including vitamin D toxicity, but it does *not* develop from a high calcium intake.

hypercalciuria: excessive urinary excretion of calcium.

hyperglycemia: elevated blood glucose.

hyperkalemia: an excessive amount of potassium in the blood.

hyperlipidemia: elevated blood lipids.

hyperosmolar hyperglycemia nonketotic coma: coma that occurs in uncontrolled NIDDM precipitated by the presence of hypertonic blood and dehydration.

hyperplastic obesity: obesity due to an increase in the *number* of fat cells.

hypertension: higher-than-normal blood pressure.

hyperthermia: an above-normal body temperature.

hypertonic formula: a formula with an osmolality higher than that of blood serum.

hypertrophic obesity: obesity due to an increase in the *size* of fat cells.

hypertrophy: of muscles, growing larger; an increase in size in response to use.

hypnotherapy: a technique that uses hypnosis and the power of suggestion to improve health behaviors, relieve pain, and heal.

hypoglycemia: an abnormally low blood glucose concentration.

hypothalamus: a brain center that controls

activities such as maintenance of water balance and regulation of body temperature.

hypothermia: a below-normal body temperature.

hypoxemia: lack of oxygen in the blood.

idopathic hypercalciuria: excessive urinary excretion of calcium not related to a known underlying medical condition.

ileocecal valve: the sphincter separating the small and large intestines.

ileostomate: a person who has a surgically formed opening from the ileum to the outside of the body (an ileostomy).

ileum: the last segment of the small intestine.

illness: as used in this book, any medical condition that alters nutrient needs. Not all such conditions are diseases. For example, major surgery is a metabolic stress that can alter nutrient needs though it is not a disease.

imagery: a technique that guides clients to achieve a desired physical, emotional, or spiritual state by visualizing themselves in that state.

imitation food: a food that substitutes for and resembles another food, but is nutritionally inferior to it with respect to vitamin, mineral, or protein content. If the substitute is not inferior to the food it resembles and if it provides an accurate name for itself, it need not be labeled "imitation."

immunity: the body's ability to recognize and eliminate foreign invaders.

implantation: the stage of development in which the zygote embeds itself in the wall of the uterus and begins to develop; occurs during the first two weeks after conception.

inborn error of metabolism: an inherited flaw evident as a metabolic disorder or disease present from birth.

indemnity insurance: traditional insurance that pays a fee for service.

indirect additives: substances that can get into food as a result of contact with foods during growing, processing, packaging, storing, cooking, or some other stage before the foods are consumed; also called *incidental* or *accidental additives*.

indirect calorimetry: the estimation of energy output from measures of the amount of oxygen used and carbon dioxide eliminated.

induration: a raised, hardened area of skin.

inflammatory response: the changes that occur in tissues when they are injured by such forces as blows, wounds, foreign bodies (chemicals, microorganisms), heat, cold, electricity, or radiation.

initiators: factors such as radiation and carcinogens which cause mutations that give rise to cancer.

inorganic: not containing carbon or pertaining to living things.

inositol: a nonessential nutrient that can be made in the body from glucose. Inositol is used in cell membranes.

insulin: a hormone secreted by special cells in the pancreas in response to (among other things) increased blood glucose concentration. The primary role of insulin is to control the transport of glucose from the bloodstream into the cells.

insulin-dependent diabetes mellitus (IDDM): the less common type of diabetes in which the person produces no insulin at all; also known as *type I diabetes* or *juvenile-onset diabetes* (because it frequently develops in childhood), although some cases arise in adulthood.

insulin–like growth factor (IGF-1): somatomedin–C.

insulin reaction: hypoglycemia that results from an overdose of insulin, strenuous physical activity, skipped meals, or inadequate intake of food; also called *insulin shock*.

insulin resistance: the condition in which a set amount of insulin produces a subnormal effect.

intentional additives: additives intentionally added to foods, such as nutrients, colors, and preservatives.

intermittent claudication: severe calf pain caused by inadequate blood supply; it occurs when walking and subsides during rest.

intermittent feeding: delivery of no more than 250 ml of a tube feeding over 30 minutes.

international units (IU): a measure of vitamin activity, determined by such biological methods as feeding a compound to vitamin-deprived animals and measuring growth. This system was used to measure fat-soluble vitamins before direct chemical analysis was possible.

interstitial fluid: fluid between the cells, usually high in sodium and chloride. Interstitial fluid is a large component of *extracellular fluid* (fluid outside the cells), which also includes plasma and the water of structures such as the skin and bones. Extracellular fluid accounts for approximately one-third of the body's water.

intra-abdominal fat: fat stored within the abdominal cavity in association with the internal abdominal organs, as opposed to the fat stored directly under the skin (subcutaneous fat).

intracellular fluid: fluid within the cells, usually high in potassium and phosphate. Intracellular fluid accounts for approximately two-thirds of the body's water.

intractable diarrhea: severe, chronic diarrhea that does not respond to treatment.

intravenous (IV): through a vein.

intrinsic: inside the system.

intrinsic factor: a glycoprotein (a protein with short polysaccharide chains attached) made in the stomach that aids in the absorption of vitamin B_{12}.

invert sugar: a mixture of glucose and fructose formed by the hydrolysis of sucrose in a chemical process; sold only in liquid form and sweeter than sucrose. Invert sugar is used as a food additive to help preserve freshness and prevent shrinkage.

involuntary activities: the component of a person's daily energy expenditure that occurs independently, without conscious will or knowledge—heart beating, lungs breathing, glands secreting, GI tract muscles contracting, and other activities critical to maintaining life.

iodopsin: the light-sensitive pigment of the cones in the retina. Both rhodopsin and iodopsin contain retinal; the protein portions of the pigments differ.

ions: atoms or molecules that have gained or lost electrons and therefore have electrical charges. Examples include the positively charged sodium ion (Na^+) and the negatively charged chloride ion (Cl^-).

iridology: the study of changes in the iris of the eye and their relationships to disease.

iron deficiency: the state of having depleted iron stores.

iron-deficiency anemia: a blood iron deficiency that results in small, pale, red blood cells.

iron overload: toxicity from excess iron.

isotonic formula: a formula with an osmolality similar to that of blood serum (300 mOsm/kg).

IV catheter: a thin tube inserted into a vein through which nutrient solutions or medications can be given directly.

jaundice: yellowing of the skin, due to spillover of the bile pigments *bilirubin* from the liver into the general circulation; also known as *hyperbilirubinemia*. Jaundice may be caused by obstruction of bile passageways, hemolysis, or dysfunctional liver cells.

jejunostomy: an opening in the jejunum made surgically or under local anesthesia through which a feeding tube can be passed.

jejunum: the first two-fifths of the small intestine beyond the duodenum.

Kaposi's sarcoma: a type of cancer rare in the general population but common in people with HIV infection.

kcalorie (energy) control: management of food energy intake.

keratin: a water-insoluble protein; the normal protein of hair and nails. Keratin-producing cells may replace mucus-producing cells in vitamin A deficiency.

keratinization: accumulation of keratin in a tissue; a sign of vitamin A deficiency.

keratomalacia: softening of the cornea seen in severe vitamin A deficiency that leads to irreversible blindness.

kernicterus: the condition of bile pigments invading the brain.

Keshan disease: a heart disease associated with selenium deficiency that is characterized by heart enlargement and insufficiency; the middle layer of the walls of the heart, which are normally composed of muscle tissue, are replaced with fibrous tissue.

keto acid: an organic acid that contains a carbonyl group (C=O).

ketone bodies: the product of the incomplete breakdown of fat when glucose is not available in the cells.

ketonemia: ketones in the blood.

ketonuria: ketones in the urine.

ketosis: an undesirably high concentration of ketone bodies in the blood and urine.

kosher: foods prepared according to Jewish dietary laws.

kwashiorkor: a form of PEM that results from either inadequate protein intake or, more commonly, from severe stress or infections.

lactase: an enzyme that hydrolyzes lactose.

lactase deficiency: a lack of the enzyme required to digest the disaccharide lactose into its component monosaccharides (glucose and galactose).

lactation: production and secretion of breast milk for the purpose of nourishing an infant.

lactic acid: an acid produced from pyruvate during anaerobic metabolism.

lacto-ovo-vegetarians: people who include milk, milk products, and eggs, but exclude meat, poultry, fish, and seafood from their diets.

lactoferrin: a factor in breast milk that binds iron and keeps it from supporting the growth of the infant's intestinal bacteria.

lactose: a disaccharide composed of glucose and galactose; commonly known as milk sugar.

lactose intolerance: a condition that results from inability to digest the milk sugar lactose; characterized by bloating, gas, abdominal discomfort, and diarrhea. Lactose intolerance differs from milk allergy, which is caused by an immune reaction to the protein in milk

lactovegetarians: people who include milk and milk products, but exclude meat, poultry, fish, seafood, and eggs from their diets.

large intestine (or colon): the lower portion of intestine that completes the digestive process; its segments are the ascending colon, the transverse colon, the descending colon, and the sigmoid colon.

larynx: the voice box.

LBW: see *low birthweight.*

LDL (low-density lipoprotein): the type of lipoprotein derived from very-low-density lipoproteins (VLDL) as cells remove triglycerides from them; composed primarily of cholesterol.

lecithin: one of the phospholipids; a compound of glycerol to which are attached two fatty acids, a phosphate group, and a choline molecule. Both nature and the food industry use lecithin as an emulsifier to combine two ingredients that do not ordinarily mix, such as water and oil.

legal: established by law.

legumes: plants of the bean and pea family. Bacteria in the root nodules of legumes "fix" nitrogen by trapping nitrogen from the air into the soil and then making it a part of the protein in the beans. Thus legumes are rich in high-quality protein compared with other plant-derived foods. Ultimately, the plant leaves more nitrogen in the soil than it takes out (sparing the land). Farmers sometimes plow under legume plants to fertilize the soil.

leukemias: cancers that arise from the white blood cells.

levulose: an older name for fructose.

license to practice: permission under state or federal law, granted on meeting specified criteria, to use a certain title (such as dietitian) and offer certain services. Licensed dietitians may use the initials LD after their names.

life expectancy: the average number of years lived by people in a given society.

life span: the maximum number of years of life attainable by a member of a species.

limiting amino acid: the essential amino acid found in the shortest supply relative to the amounts needed for protein synthesis in the body.

linoleic acid: an essential fatty acid with 18 carbons and two double bonds (18:2).

linolenic acid: an essential fatty acid with 18 carbons and three double bonds (18:3).

lipase: an enzyme that hydrolyzes lipids (fats).

lipids: a family of compounds that includes triglycerides (fats and oils), phospholipids, and sterols.

lipoic acid: a nonessential nutrient.

lipoprotein lipase (LPL): an enzyme mounted on the surface of fat cells (and other cells) that hydrolyzes triglycerides passing by in the bloodstream and directs their parts into the cells, where they can be metabolized or reassembled for storage.

lipoproteins: clusters of lipids associated with proteins that serve as transport vehicles for lipids in the lymph and blood.

liver: the organ that manufactures bile and is the first to receive nutrients from the intestines.

living will: a document signed by a competent adult that specifically states whether the person wishes any heroic measures to be taken in the event of terminal illness or irreversible coma from which the person is not expected to recover.

LPL: see *lipoprotein lipase.*

longevity: long duration of life.

low birthweight (LBW): a birthweight of 5½ pounds (2500 g) or less; indicates probable poor health in the newborn and poor nutrition status in the mother during pregnancy, before pregnancy, or both. Normal birthweight for a full-term baby is 6½ to 8¾ pounds (about 3000 to 4000 g).

low-risk pregnancy: a pregnancy characterized by indicators that make a normal outcome likely.

lumen: the inner open space of a tube or hollow organ (such as the intestine).

lymph: a clear yellowish fluid that resembles blood without the red blood cells; lymph from the GI tract transports fat and fat-soluble vitamins to the bloodstream via lymphatic vessels.

lymphatic system: a loosely organized system of vessels and ducts that convey fluids toward the heart; the GI part of the lymphatic system carries the products of digestion into the bloodstream.

lymphomas: cancers that arise from lymph tissue.

lysosomes: sacs of degradative enzymes.

macroangiopathies: disorders of the large blood vessels, including atherosclerosis.

macrobiotic diets: extremely restrictive diets limited to brown rice, miso soup, sea vegetables, and other traditional Japanese foods; based on metaphysical beliefs and not on nutrition.

macrocytic (or megaloblastic) anemia: large-cell anemia.

magnesium: a cation within the body's cells, active in many enzyme systems.

major minerals: essential mineral nutrients found in the human body in amounts larger than 5 g. The major minerals are calcium, phosphorus, potassium, sodium, chloride, magnesium, and sulfur.

malignant tumors: tumors that multiply out of control, threaten health, and require treatment.

malnutrition: any condition caused by excess or deficient food energy or nutrient intake or by an imbalance of nutrients.

maltase: an enzyme that hydrolyzes maltose.

maltose: a disaccharide composed of two glucose units; sometimes known as *malt sugar*.

managed care: a health care delivery system that is directed at providing quality health care at tolerable costs by coordinating services.

maple sugar: a sugar (mostly sucrose) purified from the concentrated sap of the sugar maple tree.

marasmus: a form of PEM that results from a severe deprivation, or impaired absorption, of energy, protein, vitamins, and minerals.

margin of safety: when speaking of food additives, a zone between the concentration normally used and that at which a hazard exists. For common table salt, for example, the margin of safety is 1/5 (five times the amount normally used would be hazardous).

massage therapy: a healing method in which the therapist manually kneads muscles to reduce tension, increase blood circulation, improve joint mobility, and promote healing of injuries.

mastication: the process of chewing.

matrix: the basic substance that gives form to a developing structure; in the body, the formative cells from which teeth and bones grow.

meat replacement: products formulated to look and taste like meat, fish, or poultry; usually made of textured vegetable protein.

mechanical soft diet: a diet that excludes all foods that are difficult to chew or swallow; also called a *dental soft diet*.

mechanical ventilator: a machine that "breathes" for the person who can't.

medical (or individual) approach: recommendations that urge dietary changes only for people who are known to need them.

medical nutrition therapy: a term intro-

duced by the American Dietetic Association in 1994 to emphasize the role of nutrition in medical care. In this book, the terms *medical nutrition therapy* and *diet therapy* are used interchangeably.

medical record: a continuous written account of a client's health history, diagnosis, therapy, and prognosis.

meditation: a self-directed technique of relaxing the body and calming the mind.

melanomas: cancers that arise from pigmented skin cells.

melatonin: a hormone secreted by the pineal gland believed to help regulate the body's daily rhythms and promote sleep. Proof of safety or effectiveness is lacking.

menadione: a synthetic form of vitamin K.

MEOS (microsomal ethanol-oxidizing system): a system of enzymes in the liver that oxidize not only alcohol, but also several classes of drugs. (The *microsomes* are tiny particles of membranes with associated enzymes that can be collected from broken-up cells.)

metabolism: the sum total of all the chemical reactions that go on in living cells.

metalloenzyme: an enzyme that contains one or more minerals as part of its structure.

metallothionein: a sulfur-rich protein that avidly binds with metals such as zinc.

metastasize: to spread from one part of the body to another.

metastatic calcification: the deposition of phosphorus and calcium salts in soft tissue.

MFP factor: a factor associated with the digestion of meat, fish, and poultry that enhances iron absorption.

micelles: tiny spherical complexes that arise during fat digestion; each carries about 20 fatty acids and/or monoglycerides into intestinal cells.

microalbuminuria: the loss of albumin in the urine in quantities that are greater than normal but not enough to precipitate symptoms.

microangiopathies: disorders of the capillaries.

microcytic hypochromic anemia: small, pale red blood cells common in iron-deficiency anemia.

microvilli: tiny, hairlike projections on each cell of every villus that can trap nutrient particles and transport them into the cells; singular *microvillus*.

milk anemia: iron-deficiency anemia that develops when an excessive milk intake displaces iron-rich foods from the diet.

milliequivalents (mEq): the concentration of electrolytes in a volume of solution. The number of milliequivalents is a useful measure

when considering ions, because the number of charges reveals characteristics about the solution that are not evident when expressed in terms of weight.

mineralization: the process in which calcium, phosphorus, and other minerals crystallize on the collagen matrix of a growing bone, hardening the bone.

minerals: inorganic elements; some minerals are essential nutrients required in small amounts.

mineral water: water from a spring or well that typically contains 250 to 500 ppm of minerals. Minerals give water a distinctive flavor. Many mineral waters are high in sodium.

misinformation: false or misleading information.

moderate exercise: activity that can be sustained comfortably for 60 minutes or so.

moderation: in relation to dietary intake, providing enough but not too much of a substance; in relation to alcohol consumption, not more than two drinks a day for the average-sized man and not more than one drink a day for the average-sized woman.

modified or therapeutic diet: a regular diet that is adjusted to meet special nutrition needs. Such diets can be adjusted in consistency, in level of energy and nutrients, in amount of fluid, in number of meals, or by the elimination of certain foods.

modules: formulas or foods that provide a single nutrient and are designed to be added to other formulas or foods to alter nutrient composition; they can also be combined together to create a highly individualized formula.

molasses: the thick brown syrup produced during sugar refining. Molasses retains residual sugar and other by-products and a few minerals; blackstrap molasses contains significant amounts of calcium and iron—the iron comes from the *machinery* used to process the sugar.

molecule: two or more atoms of the same or different elements joined by chemical bonds. Examples are molecules of the element oxygen, composed of two oxygen atoms (O_2), and molecules of the compound water, composed of two hydrogen atoms and one oxygen atom (H_2O).

molybdenum: a trace element.

monoglyceride: a molecule of glycerol with one fatty acid attached.

monosaccharide: a carbohydrate of the general formula $C_nH_{2n}O_n$ that consists of a single ring.

monounsaturated fatty acid: a fatty acid that lacks two hydrogen atoms and has one double bond between carbons—for example, oleic acid.

mouth ulcers: lesions or sores in the lining of the mouth. Certain drugs, radiation therapy, and some disorders, such as oral herpes virus infections, can cause mouth ulcers.

mucosal ferritin: a protein that holds iron in the cell.

mucosal transferrin: a protein that passes iron from the cell on to *blood transferrin*.

mucous membranes: the membranes, composed of mucus-secreting cells, that line the surfaces of body tissues.

mucus: a slippery substance secreted by goblet cells of the GI lining (and other body linings) that protects the cells from exposure to digestive juices (and other destructive agents). (The noun is *mucus*; the adjective is *mucous*.)

multiple daily injections (MDI): delivery of different types of insulin by injection three or more times daily.

muscle endurance: the ability of a muscle to contract repeatedly without becoming exhausted.

muscle strength: the ability of muscles to work against resistance.

muscular dystrophy: a hereditary disease in which the muscles gradually weaken; its most debilitating effects arise in the lungs.

mutation: an alteration in a gene such that an altered protein is produced.

mutual supplementation: the strategy of combining two protein foods in a meal so that each food provides the essential amino acid(s) lacking in the other. Mutual supplementation is the dietary strategy that brings complementary proteins together in a meal.

myoglobin: the oxygen-holding protein of the muscle cells.

NAD (nicotinamide adenine dinucleotide): the main coenzyme form of the vitamin niacin; its reduced form is NADH.

narcotic: any drug that dulls the senses, induces sleep, and becomes addictive with prolonged use.

nasoduodenal: from the nose to the duodenum.

nasoenteric: from the nose to the stomach or intestine. *Nasoenteric feedings* include nasogastric, nasoduodenal, and nasojejunal feedings. Most clinicians use *nasoenteric* to refer to nasoduodenal and nasojejunal feedings only.

nasogastric: from the nose to the stomach.

nasojejunal: from the nose to the jejunum.

natural water: water obtained from a spring or well that is certified to be safe and sanitary. The mineral content may not be changed, but the water may be treated in other ways such as by filtration or ozonization.

naturopathic medicine: a system that integrates traditional medicine with botanical medicine, clinical nutrition, homeopathy, acupuncture, East Asian medicine, hydrotherapy, and manipulative therapy.

nausea: the feeling that one is about to vomit.

nephritis: inflammation of the kidneys.

nephrons: the working units of the kidneys; each consists of a glomerulus and a tubule.

nephropathy: a disorder of the kidneys.

nephrosclerosis: impairment of renal blood flow because of renal artery damage. It can be caused by hypertension or atherosclerosis.

nephrotic syndrome: the complex of symptoms that occur when glomerular function fails; it includes proteinuria and albuminuria.

net protein utilization (NPU): the amount of protein nitrogen that is retained from a given amount of protein nitrogen eaten; a measure of protein quality.

neuron: a nerve cell; the structural and functional unit of the nervous system. Neurons initiate and conduct nerve transmissions.

neuropathy: a disorder of the nerves.

neurotransmitters: chemicals that are released at the end of a nerve cell when a nerve impulse arrives there; they diffuse across the gap to the next cell and alter the membrane of that second cell to either inhibit or excite it.

niacin: a B vitamin. Niacin can be eaten preformed or made in the body from its precursor, tryptophan, one of the amino acids. The active coenzyme forms are NAD (nicotinamide adenine dinucleotide) and NADP (the phosphate form of NAD).

niacin equivalents: the amount of niacin present in food, including the niacin that can theoretically be made from its precursor, tryptophan, present in the food.

night blindness: slow recovery of vision after flashes of bright light at night or an inability to see in dim light; an early symptom of vitamin A deficiency.

nitrates: salts that are converted to nitrites by bacteria.

nitrites: salts added to food to prevent botulism; one example is sodium nitrite, which is used to preserve meats.

nitrogen balance: the amount of nitrogen consumed (N in) as compared with the amount of nitrogen excreted (N out) in a given period of time.

nitrosamines: derivatives of nitrites that may be formed in the stomach when nitrites combine with amines; nitrosamines are carcinogenic in animals.

nocturnal hypoglycemia: hypoglycemia that occurs while a person is sleeping.

noninsulin-dependent diabetes mellitus (NIDDM): the more common type of diabetes that develops gradually and is associated with insulin resistance; also called *type II diabetes* or *adult-onset diabetes*. NIDDM is usually milder than IDDM and progresses more slowly. A type of NIDDM that develops during the teen years has been termed *maturity-onset diabetes in the young (MODY)*.

nonnutrients: compounds in foods with no known nutritional value.

nonnutritive sweetners: sweetners that provide no energy.

NPO: an order to give a client nothing orally (including food, beverages, and medications): NPO stands for *nil per os*, which means "nothing by mouth."

nucleotides: nitrogen-containing components of RNA and DNA. Nucleotides can be synthesized in the body and therefore are not essential in the diets of healthy individuals. In severely stressed individuals, however, a dietary source may be beneficial.

nursing bottle tooth decay: extensive tooth decay due to prolonged tooth contact with formula, milk, fruit juice, or other carbohydrate-rich liquid offered to an infant in a bottle.

nutraceuticals: substances that supposedly provide medical and health benefits; a term not recognized by the FDA.

nutrient additives: vitamins and minerals added to improve nutritive value.

nutrient density: a measure of the nutrients a food provides relative to the energy it provides. The more nutrients and the fewer kcalories, the higher the nutrient density.

nutrients: substances obtained from food and used in the body to provide energy and structural materials and to regulate growth, maintenance, and repair of the body's tissues; nutrients may also reduce the risks of some chronic diseases.

nutrition assessment: the evaluation of many factors that influence or reflect nutritional health; the tools used for nutrition assessment include historical information, physical examinations, anthropometric findings, and biochemical analyses.

nutrition care plan: a plan that translates nutrition assessment data into a strategy for meeting a client's nutrient and nutrition education needs.

nutrition care process: an organized approach to nutrition intervention that consists of five steps (assessing, analyzing, planning, implementing, and evaluating). The nutrition care process parallels the *nursing care process* except that it focuses on nutrition concerns.

nutrition screening: the use of routine nutrition assessment procedures to identify people who are malnourished or are at risk for malnutrition.

nutrition status survey: a survey that evaluates people's nutrition status using diet histories, anthropometric measures, physical examinations, and laboratory tests.

nutritional yeast: a preparation of yeast cells grown especially as a nutrient supplement, particularly for vegetarian diets. The type of yeast used is brewer's yeast, not baker's yeast. Different species of yeasts produce different compounds; yeast cells used in brewing produce alcohol, proteins, and B vitamins as they grow. The nutrients are removed from beer and wine in the filtering process. Yeast cells used in baking produce mostly carbon dioxide, which causes bread dough to rise.

nutritionist: a person who specializes in the study of nutrition. Some nutritionists are registered dietitians, whereas others are self-described experts whose training is questionable. In states with responsible legislation, the term applies only to people who have MS or PhD degrees from properly accredited institutions.

nutritive sweeteners: sweeteners that yield energy, including both sugars and sugar alcohols.

obligatory water excretion: the amount of water the body has to excrete each day to dispose of its wastes—about 500 ml, or a pint.

oligopeptide: an intermediate-length string of four to nine amino acids.

oliguria: minimal urine volume.

oliguric phase: the early phase of acute renal failure, when urine volume is reduced.

omega: the last letter of the Greek alphabet (ω), used by chemists to refer to the position of the endmost double bond in a fatty acid.

omega-3 fatty acid: a polyunsaturated fatty acid in which the first double bond is three carbons away from the methyl (CH_3) end of the carbon chain.

omega-6 fatty acid: a polyunsaturated fatty acid in which the first double bond is six carbons from the methyl (CH_3) end of the carbon chain.

omnivores: people who have no formal restriction on the eating of any foods.

opportunistic infections: infections from microorganisms that normally do not cause disease in the general population but can cause great harm in people once their

immune systems are compromised (as in HIV infection).

opsin: the protein portion of the visual pigment molecule.

oral antidiabetic agents: drugs taken by mouth to lower blood glucose levels. They include sulfonylureas, metformin, and acarbose. Sulfonylureas are also called *hypoglycemic agents* because they stimulate insulin secretion.

oral rehydration therapy (ORT): the administration of a simple solution of sugar, salt, and water, taken by mouth, to treat dehydration caused by diarrhea.

organic: a substance or molecule containing carbon-carbon bonds or carbon-hydrogen bonds. Some farmers call their produce "organic" if it was grown without manufactured fertilizers and pesticides, but by the definition given here, all foods are organic.

organic halogen: an organic compound containing one or more atoms of a *halogen*—fluorine, chlorine, iodine, or bromine.

orogastric: from the mouth to the stomach. This method is often used to tube feed infants because they breathe through their noses, and tubes inserted through the nose can hinder the infant's breathing.

ORT: see oral rehydration therapy.

orthomolecular medicine: the use of large doses of vitamins to treat chronic disease.

osmolality: the concentration of particles in a solution, expressed as the number of milliosmoles (mOsm) per kilogram.

osmotic diarrhea: diarrhea that results from an increase in the osmolarity of the intestinal contents due to unabsorbed water and electrolytes.

osmotic pressure: the pressure that develops when two solutions of different concentrations are separated by a membrane that permits water, but not the solutes, to cross. Water flows *toward* the side of the membrane on which the solutes are more concentrated.

osteitis fibrosis: a type of renal osteodystrophy that results from hyperparathyroidism and is characterized by kidney stones, decalcification and softening of bones, and, sometimes, formation of cysts and tumors.

osteoblasts: cells that build bone.

osteoclasts: cells that destroy bone during growth.

osteomalacia: a bone disease characterized by softening of the bones; symptoms include bending of the spine and bowing of the legs. The disease occurs most often in adult women.

osteopenia: a metabolic bone disease characterized by reduced bone mass common

in preterm infants; also called *rickets of prematurity.*

osteoporosis: a condition of older persons in which the bones become porous and fragile due to a loss of minerals; also called *adult bone loss.*

ostomate: a person who has a surgically formed opening from the bowel to the outside of the body, bypassing the anus.

overnutrition: excess energy or nutrients.

overt: out in the open and easy to observe.

overweight: body weight above some standard of acceptable weight that is usually defined in relation to height (such as the weight-for-height tables).

ovum: the female reproductive cell, capable of developing into a new organism upon fertilization; commonly referred to as an *egg.*

oxidant: a compound (such as oxygen itself) that oxidizes other compounds. Compounds that prevent oxidation are called *antioxidants,* whereas those that encourage it are called *prooxidants.*

oxidation: the process of a substance combining with oxygen.

oxidative stress: damage to biological systems caused by free-radical formation.

ozone therapy: the use of ozone gas to enhance the body's immune system.

pagophagia: ice craving.

palatability: pleasing taste. When tasting foods, the tongue presses them against the *palate,* or roof of the mouth.

pancreas: a gland that secretes digestive enzymes and juices into the duodenum.

pancreatic juice: the exocrine secretion of the pancreas, containing enzymes for the digestion of carbohydrate, fat, and protein as well as bicarbonate, a neutralizing agent.

pancreatitis: inflammation of the pancreas.

pantothenic acid: a B vitamin; the principal active form is part of coenzyme A, commonly called "CoA" in metabolism.

parathormone: a hormone from the parathyroid gland that raises blood calcium; also called parathyroid hormone.

parenteral formulas: formulas given by vein.

parenteral nutrition: delivery of nutrient solutions directly into a vein, bypassing the intestines.

pasteurization: a process of heating milk sufficiently to kill many disease-causing microbes commonly transmitted through milk; not a sterilization process. Pasteurized milk retains bacteria that cause milk spoilage. Unpasteurized ("certified" raw) milk transmits many food-borne diseases to people each year.

pathogens: microorganisms or substances capable of producing disease.

pathological stresses: stresses imposed by disease or trauma.

PCM: see *protein-energy malnutrition.*

peak bone mass: the highest attainable bone density for an individual, developed during the first three decades of life.

peer review: a process in which a panel of scientists rigorously evaluates a research study to assure that the scientific method was followed.

PEG: see *percutaneous endoscopic gastrostomy.*

PEJ: see *percutaneous endoscopic jejunostomy.*

pellagra: the niacin-deficiency disease.

PEM: see *protein-energy malnutrition.*

pepsin: a gastric protease.

pepsinogen: a precursor protein that is activated by stomach acid to form the enzyme pepsin.

peptic ulcer: an erosion in the mucous membrane of either the stomach (a gastric ulcer) or the duodenum (a duodenal ulcer). Ulcers may also develop in the mouth, esophagus, and intestines and on the skin.

peptidase: a digestive enzyme that hydrolyzes peptide bonds. *Tripeptidases* cleave tripeptides; *dipeptidases* cleave dipeptides. *Endopeptidases* cleave peptide bonds *within* the chain to create smaller fragments, whereas *exopeptidases* cleave bonds at the *ends* to release free amino acids.

peptide bond: a bond that connects the acid end of one amino acid with the amino end of another, forming a link in a protein chain.

percutaneous endoscopic gastrostomy (PEG): a gastrostomy created under local anesthesia.

percutaneous endoscopic jejunostomy (PEJ): a misnomer that refers to a feeding tube insertion technique in which a feeding tube is guided into the jejunum from a gastrostomy created using a nonsurgical procedure.

peripheral parenteral nutrition: the use of the peripheral veins to provide a solution that meets nutrient needs.

peripheral resistance: resistance to the flow of blood by the vessels at the periphery of the body—the smallest arteries and capillaries.

peripheral veins: the small-diameter veins that bring blood to the extremities (arms and legs).

peripherally inserted central catheter (PICC): a catheter inserted into a peripheral vein and advanced into a central vein.

peristalsis: wavelike muscular contractions of the GI tract that push its contents along.

peritoneal dialysis: a method of eliminating excess fluids and wastes from the blood in kidney failure using the peritoneum as a semipermeable membrane.

pernicious anemia: a blood disorder that reflects a vitamin B_{12} deficiency caused by lack of intrinsic factor and characterized by a deficit of red blood cells, muscle weakness, and neurological disturbances.

peroxidation: the production of unstable molecules containing more than the usual amount of oxygen. Hydrogen peroxide, H_2O_2, for example, may be produced from water, H_2O.

persistence: stubborn or enduring continuance; with respect to food contaminants, the quality of persisting, rather than breaking down, in the bodies of animals and human beings.

persistent vegetative state: exhibiting motor reflexes but without the ability to regain cognitive behavior, communicate, or interact purposefully with the environment.

pesticides: chemicals used to control insects, diseases, weeds, fungi, and other pests on plants, vegetables, fruits, and animals. Used broadly, the term includes herbicides (to kill weeds), insecticides (to kill insects), and fungicides (to kill fungi).

pH: the unit of measure expressing a substance's acidity or alkalinity (pH 7 is neutral). The lower the pH below 7, the stronger the acid. A pH above 7 is alkaline, or base.

pharmacological effect: the body's response to a large dose of a nutrient (two to ten times greater than the RDA) that overwhelms some body system and acts like a drug.

phenylketonuria (PKU): an inborn error of metabolism in which phenylalanine, an essential amino acid, cannot be converted to tyrosine. Alternative metabolites of phenylalanine (phenylketones) accumulate in the tissues, causing damage, and overflow into the urine.

phospholipid: a compound similar to a triglyceride but having choline (or another nitrogen-containing compound) and a phosphate group (a phosphorus-containing salt) in place of one of the fatty acids.

phosphorus: a major mineral found mostly in the body's bones and teeth.

photon: a unit of light energy. Depending on its wavelength, a photon conveys different colors of light.

photosynthesis: the process by which green plants make carbohydrates from carbon dioxide and water using the green pigment chlorophyll to trap the sun's energy.

physiological age: a person's age as estimated from her or his body's health and probable life expectancy.

physiological effect: the body's response to a normal dose of a nutrient (levels commonly found in foods and not exceeding 150 percent of the RDA) that provides a normal blood concentration.

physiological fuel value: the number of kcalories that the human body derives from a food, as contrasted with the kcalories determined by calorimetry.

physiological stresses: stresses that fall within the body's normal and healthy functioning.

phytic acid: a nonnutrient component of plant seeds; also called *phytate.* Phytic acid occurs in the husks of grains, legumes, and seeds and is capable of binding minerals such as zinc, iron, calcium, magnesium, and copper in insoluble complexes in the intestine, which the body excretes unused.

phytochemicals: nonnutrient compounds in plant-derived foods that have biological activity in the body.

pica: a craving for nonfood substances.

pigment: a molecule capable of absorbing certain wavelengths of light, so that it reflects only those that we perceive as a certain color.

PKU: see *phenylketonuria.*

placebo: an inert, harmless medication given to provide comfort and hope; a sham treatment used in controlled research studies.

placebo effect: the healing effect that faith in medicine, even inert medicine, often has.

placenta: the organ that develops inside the uterus early in pregnancy, in which maternal and fetal blood circulate in close proximity so that materials can be exchanged between them. The fetus receives nutrients and oxygen across the placenta; the mother's blood picks up carbon dioxide and other waste products to be excreted.

plaque, atheromatous: mounds of lipid material, mixed with smooth muscle cells and calcium, which develop in the artery walls in atherosclerosis.

plaque, dental: a gummy mass of bacteria that grows on teeth and can lead to dental caries and gum disease.

plasma: the fluid that remains when unclotted blood is centrifuged.

platelets: tiny, disc-shaped bodies in the blood, important in blood clot formation.

point of unsaturation: the double bond of a fatty acid, where hydrogen atoms can easily be added to the structure.

polar: a neutral molecule that has opposite charges spatially separated within the molecule; see Appendix B for more details.

polydipsia: excessive thirst.

polypeptide: many (ten or more) amino acids bonded together.

polyphagia: excessive eating.

polysaccharide: many monosaccharides linked together.

polyunsaturated fatty acid (PUFA): a fatty acid that lacks four or more hydrogen atoms and has two or more double bonds between carbons—for example, linoleic acid (two double bonds) and linolenic acid (three double bonds). A *polyunsaturated fat* is composed of triglycerides containing a high percentage of PUFA.

polyuria: excessive urine production.

portal hypertension: elevated blood pressure in the portal vein caused by obstructed blood flow through the liver.

post term (infant): an infant born after the 42nd week of pregnancy.

postgastrectomy diet: a carbohydrate-controlled diet given to prevent the symptoms of dumping syndrome and hypoglycemia that sometimes follow gastric surgery.

postpartum amenorrhea: the normal temporary absence of menstrual periods immediately following childbirth.

potable water: water that is suitable for drinking.

potassium: the principal cation within the body's cells; critical to the maintenance of fluid balance, nerve transmissions, and muscle contractions.

precursors: substances that precede others; with regard to vitamins, compounds that can be converted into active vitamins; also known as *provitamins.*

preeclampsia: a condition characterized by hypertension, fluid retention, and protein in the urine.

preferred provider organization (PPO): a form of managed care that encourages subscribers to select health care providers from a group that has contracted with the organization to provide services at lower costs.

preformed vitamin A: dietary vitamin A in its active form.

pregnancy-induced hypertension (PIH): high blood pressure that develops in the second half of pregnancy.

preservatives: antimicrobial agents, antioxidants, and other additives that retard spoilage or maintain desired qualities, such as softness in baked goods.

pressure sores: the breakdown of skin and underlying tissues due to constant pressure and lack of oxygen to the affected area; often called *decubitus ulcers* or *bedsores.*

preterm (infant): an infant born prior to the 38th week of pregnancy; also called a *premature* infant.

preventive (or population) approach: recommendations that urge all people to make dietary changes believed to forestall or prevent disease.

primary deficiency: a nutrient deficiency caused by inadequate dietary intake of a nutrient.

proenzyme: the inactive form or an enzyme.

prognosis: the predicted course and outcome of a disease.

promoters: factors that favor the development of cancer once it has begun.

proof: a way of stating the percentage of alcohol in distilled liquor. Liquor that is 100 proof is 50 percent alcohol; 90 proof is 45 percent, and so forth.

protease: an enzyme that hydrolyzes proteins.

protein digestibility: a measure of the amount of amino acids absorbed from a given protein intake.

protein digestibility–corrected amino acid score (PDCAAS): a measure of protein quality assessed by comparing the amino acid balance of a food protein with the amino acid requirements of preschool-age children and then correcting for the true digestibility of the protein; recommended by the FAO/WHO and used to establish protein quality of foods for Daily Value percentages on food labels.

protein efficiency ratio (PER): a measure of protein quality assessed by determining how well a given protein supports weight gain in growing rats; used to establish the protein quality for infant formulas and baby foods.

protein-energy malnutrition (PEM): a deficiency of both protein and energy; the world's most widespread malnutrition problem, including kwashiorkor, marasmus, and instances in which they overlap; also called *protein-kcalorie malnutrition (PCM).*

protein isolate: a protein that has been separated from a food. Examples include casein from milk and albumin from egg.

protein-losing enteropathy: the intestinal loss of serum proteins.

proteins: compounds composed of carbon, hydrogen, oxygen, and nitrogen atoms, arranged into amino acids linked in a chain. Some amino acids also contain sulfur atoms.

protein-sparing action: the action of carbohydrate (and fat) in providing energy that allows protein to be used for other purposes.

protein turnover: the degradation and synthesis of endogenous protein.

proteinuria: loss of protein in the urine.

prothrombin time: a laboratory test that evaluates the time it takes for blood to clot.

puberty: the period in life in which a person becomes physically capable of reproduction.

public health nutritionist: a dietitian who specializes in public health nutrition.

public water: water from a municipal or county water system that has been treated and disinfected.

PUFA: see *polyunsaturated fatty acids.*

pulmonary: of or pertaining to the lungs.

pureed foods: foods that have been strained and blenderized to a thickened, near-liquid consistency.

purgative: a strong laxative.

purified water: water that has been processed through distillation, deionization, or reverse osmosis and meets U.S. Pharmacopoeia standards for medical and research purposes.

pyelonephritis: an inflammation of the kidneys and bladder.

pyloric sphincter: the circular muscle that separates the stomach from the small intestine and regulates the flow of partially digested food into the small intestine; also called *pylorus* or *pyloric valve.*

pyruvate: pyruvic acid, a 3-carbon compound that, in metabolism, can be derived from glucose, certain amino acids, or glycerol.

radiation: ionizing rays used to sterilize and protect food.

radiation enteritis: damage to the intestine caused by radiation therapy.

radiation therapy: the use of radiation to arrest or destroy cancer cells.

radiolytic products: chemicals formed during the irradiation of food.

randomization: a process of choosing the members of the experimental and control groups without bias.

raw sugar: the first crop of crystals harvested during sugar processing. Raw sugar cannot be sold in the United States because it contains too much filth (dirt, insect fragments, and the like). Sugar sold as "raw sugar" domestically has actually gone through over half of the refining steps.

RBP: see *retinol-binding protein.*

RD: see *registered dietitian.*

RDA: see *Recommended Dietary Allowances.*

RDI: see *Reference Daily Intakes.*

RE (retinol equivalent): a measure of vitamin A activity; the amount of retinol that the body will derive from a food containing preformed retinol or its precursor beta-carotene.

reactive hypoglycemia: hypoglycemia experienced simultaneously with epinephrine-release symptoms one to three hours after a meal; also called *postprandial hypoglycemia.*

rebound hyperglycemia: hyperglycemia resulting from excessive secretion of counterregulatory hormones in response to excessive insulin; also called the *Somogyi effect.*

rebound scurvy: vitamin C deficiency resulting from the sudden withdrawal of excessive doses of vitamin C.

recessive gene: a gene that has no observable effect on an organism as long as it is paired with a normal gene that can produce a normal product. In this case, the normal gene is said to be *dominant.*

recombinant DNA technology: methods of joining (recombining) pieces of the genetic material DNA in order to change the proteins produced by the altered DNA.

Recommended Dietary Allowances (RDA): the amounts of selected nutrients considered adequate to meet the known nutrient needs of practically all healthy people.

rectum: the muscular terminal part of the intestine, extending from the sigmoid colon to the anus.

refeeding syndrome: a set of physiologic and metabolic complications associated with reintroducing adequate nutrition too rapidly for a person with severe PEM. These complications can include malabsorption, cardiac insufficiency, respiratory distress, congestive heart failure, convulsions, coma, and possibly death.

Reference Daily Intakes (RDI): a set of standards for protein, vitamins, and minerals used on food labels as part of the Daily Values; previously known as the U.S. RDA.

reference protein: a standard against which to measure the quality of other proteins.

refined: the process by which the coarse parts of a food are removed. When wheat is refined into flour, the bran, germ, and husk are removed, leaving only the endosperm.

reflux: a backward flow.

reflux esophagitis: the backflow or regurgitation of gastric contents from the stomach into the esophagus, causing inflammation of the esophagus; also called *gastroesophageal reflux, gastric reflux,* or *acid indigestion.*

registered dietitian (RD): a dietitian who has graduated from a university or college after completing a program of dietetics that has been accredited by the American Dietetic Association (or Dietitians of Canada), has served in an internship or coordinated program to practice the necessary skills, has passed the association's registration examination, and maintains competency through continuing education. Many states require licensing for practicing dietitians.

registration: with respect to health professionals, listing with a professional organization that requires specific course work, experience, and passing of an examination.

remodeling: the dismantling and re-formation of a structure, in this case, bone.

renal: pertaining to the kidneys.

renal colic: the severe pain that accompanies the movement of a kidney stone from the kidney through the ureter to the bladder.

renal failure: failure of the kidneys to maintain normal function.

renal insufficiency: reduced renal function but not to the degree that requires dialysis or a kidney transplant.

renal osteodystrophy: bone disorders resulting from calcium and phosphorus imbalances in renal disease.

renal reserve: the capacity of the kidneys to function despite loss of some nephrons.

renal threshold: the point at which blood glucose rises so high that the kidneys cannot reabsorb it.

renin: an enzyme secreted by the kidneys in response to a reduced blood flow that triggers the release of the hormone aldosterone from the adrenal glands. Aldosterone, in turn, signals the kidneys to retain sodium and water.

rennin: an enzyme that coagulates milk; found in the gastric juice of cows, but not human beings.

replication: repeating an experiment and getting the same results.

requirement: the amount of a nutrient that will maintain normal biochemical and physiological functions and prevent the development of specific deficiency signs; distinguished from the RDA, which is a recommended and generous allowance that provides for variability among individuals.

residue: whatever remains. In the body, the total amount of material in the GI tract, including dietary fiber and also undigested food, intestinal secretions, bacterial cell bodies, and cells shed from the intestinal mucosa. In agriculture, the amounts of pesticides that remain on or in foods when people buy and use them.

resistant starch: starch that is not absorbed in the small intestine of healthy people.

respiratory acidosis: a condition of too much acid in the blood caused by failure of the lungs to adequately expel carbon dioxide during exhalation.

respiratory distress: a disorder of the lung membranes that results in delayed onset of respiration at birth and difficulty in breathing after birth.

respiratory failure: failure of the lungs to exchange gases; also known as *adult respiratory distress syndrome (ARDS).*

respiratory quotient (RQ): the ratio of carbon dioxide produced to oxygen consumed. Clinicians used the RQ to estimate total energy needs and the appropriate mix of carbohydrate and fat to meet those needs.

retina: the layer of light-sensitive nerve cells lining the back of the inside of the eye; consists of rods and cones.

retinal: the aldehyde form of vitamin A, active in the eye.

retinoic acid: the acid form of vitamin A.

retinoids: chemically related compounds with biologic activity similar to retinol; metabolites of retinol.

retinol: the alcohol form of vitamin A.

retinol-binding protein (RBP): the specific protein responsible for transporting retinol.

retinopathy: a disorder of the retina.

rheumatic heart disease: heart damage (often affecting the heart valves) that follows rheumatic fever (caused by a systemic bacterial infection).

rhodopsin: the light-sensitive pigment of the rods in the retina; it contains the retinal form of vitamin A.

riboflavin: a B vitamin; the coenzyme forms are FMN (flavin mononucleotide) and FAD (flavin adenine dinucleotide).

rickets: the vitamin D–deficiency disease in children characterized by inadequate mineralization of bone (manifested in bowed legs or knock-knees, outward-bowed chest, and knobs on ribs). A rare type of rickets, *not* caused by vitamin D deficiency, is known as *vitamin D–refractory rickets.*

risk: a measure of the probability and severity of harm.

risk factors: factors associated with an elevated frequency of a disease but not proven to be causal.

rods: the cells of the retina that respond to dim light and convey black-and-white vision.

saccharin: a 0-kcalorie sweetener used in the United States but available in Canada only in pharmacies and only as a sweetener, not as an additive.

safety: a judgment that considers the risks acceptable.

saliva: the secretion of the salivary glands; its principal enzyme begins carbohydrate digestion.

salivary glands: exocrine glands that secrete saliva into the mouth.

salts: compounds composed of a positive ion other than H^+ and a negative ion other than OH^-. An example is sodium chloride (Na^+Cl^-).

sarcomas: cancers that arise from muscle, bone, or connective tissues.

satiety: the feeling of satisfaction and fullness that food brings.

saturated fatty acid: a fatty acid carrying the maximum possible number of hydrogen atoms—for example, stearic acid. A *saturated fat* is composed of triglycerides in which all or virtually all of the fatty acids are saturated.

science of nutrition: the study of the nutrients in foods and of the body's handling of them (including ingestion, digestion, absorption, transport, metabolism, interaction, storage, and excretion). A broader definition includes the study of the environment and of human behavior as it relates to food.

scurvy: the vitamin C–deficiency disease.

secondary deficiency: a nutrient deficiency caused by something other than diet, such as a disease condition that reduces absorption, accelerates use, hastens excretion, or destroys the nutrient.

secondary hypertension: high blood pressure that is caused by a specific disorder such as kidney disease.

secretin: a hormone produced by cells in the duodenum wall. Target organ: the pancreas. Response: secretion of bicarbonate-rich pancreatic juice.

secretory diarrhea: diarrhea that results from an accelerated movement of fluids and electrolytes from the intestinal capillaries into the lumen of the intestine.

sedentary: physically inactive (literally, "sitting down a lot").

segmentation: a periodic squeezing or partitioning of the intestine at intervals along its length by its circular muscles.

selenium: a trace element.

semivegetarians: people who include some, but not all, groups of animal-derived foods in their diets; they usually exclude red meat, but may occasionally include poultry and seafood; sometimes called *partial vegetarians*.

senile dementia: the loss of brain function beyond the normal loss of physical adeptness and memory that occurs with aging.

senile dementia of the Alzheimer's type (SDAT): a degenerative disease of the brain involving memory loss and major structural changes in neuron networks; also known as *primary degenerative dementia of senile onset* or *chronic brain syndrome*, but often simply called *Alzheimer's disease*.

sepsis (or septicemia): the presence of microorganisms or their poisonous products in the bloodstream.

serotonin: a neurotransmitter important in sleep and sensory perception; it is synthesized from the amino acid tryptophan with the help of vitamin B_6.

serum: the watery portion of the blood that remains after removal of the cells and clot-forming material.

set point: the point at which controls are set (for example, on a thermostat). The set-point theory proposes that the body tends to maintain a certain weight by means of its own internal controls.

severe stresses: pathological stresses that rapidly and markedly raise the body's metabolic rate and significantly upset its normal internal balance.

shock: a critical event that occurs when a sudden drop in the blood volume disrupts the supply of oxygen to the tissues and the return of blood to the heart.

short-bowel or short-gut syndrome: severe malabsorption that may occur when the absorptive surface of the small bowel is reduced, resulting in diarrhea, weight loss, bone disease, hypocalcemia, hypomagnesemia, and anemia.

sickle-cell anemia: a hereditary form of anemia characterized by abnormal sickle- or crescent-shaped red blood cells. Sickled cells interfere with oxygen transport and blood flow. Symptoms include hemolytic anemia (red blood cells burst), fever, and severe pain in the joints and abdomen; they are precipitated by dehydration and insufficient oxygen (as may occur at high altitudes).

SIDS: see *sudden infant death syndrome*.

silent heart attack: a heart attack that goes unnoticed.

simple carbohydrates (sugars): monosaccharides and disaccharides.

sitophobia: fear of eating.

SMA (simultaneous multiple analysis): the measurement of several blood components during a single blood test. SMA is followed by a number (for example, SMA-12) that indicates how many tests will be run.

small intestine: a 10-foot length of small-diameter intestine that is the major site of digestion of food and absorption of nutrients; its segments are the duodenum, jejunum, and ileum.

socioeconomic history: a record of a person's social and economic background, including such factors as education, income, and ethnic identity.

sodium: the principal cation in the extracellular fluids of the body, critical to the maintenance of fluid balance, nerve transmissions, and muscle contractions.

soft water: water with a high sodium concentration.

solanine: a poisonous narcotic-like substance present in potato peels and sprouts. Physical symptoms of solanine poisoning include headache, vomiting, abdominal pain, diarrhea, and fever; neurological symptoms include apathy, restlessness, drowsiness, confusion, stupor, hallucinations, and visual disturbances.

solutes: the substances that are dissolved in a solution.

sperm: the male reproductive cell, capable of fertilizing an ovum.

sphincter: a circular muscle surrounding, and able to close, a body opening.

spring water: water originating from an underground spring or well. It may be carbonated or not ("flat" or "still"). Brand names such as "Spring Pure" do not necessarily mean that the water comes from a spring.

standard diet: a *regular diet*—that is, one that includes all foods and meets the nutrient needs of normal, healthy individuals.

standard formula: a liquid diet that contains complete molecules of proteins; also called *intact* or *polymeric formulas*.

starch: a plant polysaccharide composed of glucose that is digestible by human beings.

steatorrhea: fatty diarrhea characteristic of fat malabsorption; stools are loose, foamy, and foul smelling.

sterile: free of microorganisms, such as bacteria.

sterol: a compound composed of C, H, and O atoms arranged in rings, like those of cholesterol, with any of a variety of side chains attached.

stoma: a surgically formed opening, as in a gastrostomy jejunostomy, ileostomy, or colostomy.

stomach: a muscular, elastic, saclike portion of the digestive tract that grinds and churns swallowed food, mixing it with acid and enzymes to form chyme.

stools: waste matter discharged from the colon; also called *feces*.

stress: any threat to a person's well-being; a demand placed on the body to adapt.

stress eating: eating in response to arousal.

stress fractures: bone damage or breaks caused by stress on bone surfaces during exercise.

stress response: the body's response to stress, mediated initially by both nerves and hormones; begins with an *alarm reaction,* proceeds through a stage of *resistance,* and then leads to *recovery* or, if prolonged, to *exhaustion.* This three-stage response has also been termed the *general adaptation syndrome.*

stressor: an environmental element, physical or psychological, that causes stress.

stroke: an event in which the blood flow to a part of the brain is cut off; also called a *cerebrovascular accident (CVA).*

struvite: crystals of magnesium ammonium phosphate.

subclinical deficiency: a deficiency in the early stages, before the outward signs have appeared.

substitute food: a food that is designed to replace another.

subtotal (or partial) gastrectomy: removal of a portion of the stomach.

sucralose: a 0-kcalorie sweetener that is 600 times sweeter than sucrose; FDA approval pending in the United States; approved in Canada.

sucrase: an enzyme that hydrolyzes sucrose.

sucrose: a disaccharide composed of glucose and fructose; commonly known as table sugar, beet sugar, or cane sugar. Sucrose also occurs in many fruits and some vegetables and grains.

sudden infant death syndrome (SIDS): the unexpected and unexplained death of an apparently well infant; the most common cause of death of infants between the second week and the end of the first year of life; also called *crib death.*

sugar alcohols: sugarlike compounds that can be derived from fruits or commercially produced from dextrose; also called *polyols.* Like sugars, sugar alcohols are sweet to taste and yield 4 kcalories per gram, but they are absorbed more slowly and metabolized differently than other sugars in the human body, and are not readily utilized by ordinary mouth bacteria. Examples are *maltitol, mannitol, sorbitol,* and *xylitol.*

sulfites: salts containing sulfur that are added to foods to prevent spoilage.

sulfur: a mineral present in the body as part of some amino acids.

supplements: pills, liquids, or powders that contain purified nutrients, or foods with puri-fied nutrients added in amounts per serving greater than 50 percent above a standard considered sufficient for all healthy people.

sushi: vinegar-flavored rice and seafood, typically wrapped in seaweed and stuffed with colorful vegetables. Some sushi is stuffed with raw fish; other varieties contain only cooked ingredients.

sustainable: able to continue indefinitely. Here, the term means the use of resources at such a rate that the earth can keep on replacing them—for example, cutting trees no faster than new ones grow and producing pollutants at a rate with which the environment and human cleanup efforts can keep pace, so that no net accumulation of pollution occurs.

syndrome X: the combination of insulin resistance, glucose intolerance, hypertension, elevated blood lipids, and obesity frequently observed in people with cardiovascular disease.

synthetase: an enzyme that enables two or more substances to form a more complex structure.

systemic: affecting the whole body rather than one part or organ system.

systemic inflammatory response syndrome (SIRS): the changes that result from the activation of immune and inflammatory factors during stress.

tachycardia: a rapid heart rate.

TEF: see *thermic effect of food.*

tempeh: a fermented soybean food, rich in protein and fiber.

tension-fatigue syndrome: apparent hyperactivity produced in a child by the combination of lack of sleep, overstimulation, and anxiety.

teratogenic: causing abnormal fetal development and birth defects.

term (infant): an infant born between the 38th and 42nd week of pregnancy.

terminal illness: a progressive, irreversible disease that will lead to death in the near future.

textured vegetable protein: processed soybean protein used in vegetarian products such as soy burgers.

thermic effect of food (TEF): an estimation of the energy required to process food (digest, absorb, transport, metabolize, and store ingested nutrients); also called *diet-induced thermogenesis (DIT),* the *specific dynamic effect (SDE)* of food, or the *specific dynamic activity (SDA)* of food.

thermogenesis: the generation of heat; used in physiology and nutrition studies as an index of how much energy the body is spending.

thiamin: a B vitamin; the coenzyme form is TPP (thiamin pyrophosphate).

thirst: a conscious desire to drink.

thrombosis: the formation of a blood clot that may obstruct a blood vessel, causing gradual tissue death.

thrombus: a blood clot that obstructs a blood vessel or a cavity of the heart.

thrush: a fungal infection of the mouth and esophagus caused by *Candida albicans;* the technical term for this infection is *candidiasis.* Thrush is characterized by a thick white coating of the tongue that alters taste sensations and causes pain on chewing and swallowing.

tocopherol: a general term for several chemically related compounds, most of which have vitamin E activity.

tocopherol equivalents (TE): the units in which vitamin E activity is measured. One TE equals the amount of vitamin E activity in 1 mg of D-alpha-tocopherol.

tofu: a curd made from soybeans, rich in protein and often fortified with calcium; used in many Asian and vegetarian dishes in place of meat.

tolerance level: the maximum amount of a residue permitted in a food when a pesticide is used according to label directions.

total gastrectomy: removal of the entire stomach.

toxicity: the ability of a substance to harm living organisms. All substances are toxic if high enough concentrations are used.

total parenteral nutrition (TPN): the delivery of all nutrient needs by vein.

trabecular bone: the lacy inner structure of calcium crystals that supports the bone's structure and provides a calcium storage bank.

trace minerals: essential mineral nutrients found in the human body in amounts less than 5 g. The trace minerals are iron, iodine, zinc, chromium, selenium, fluoride, molybdenum, copper, and manganese.

trachea: the windpipe; the passageway from the mouth and nose to the lungs.

***trans*-fatty acids:** fatty acids with an unusual configuration around the double bond.

transamination: the transfer of an amino group from one amino acid to a keto acid, producing a new nonessential amino acid and a new keto acid.

transgenic organism: an organism that grows from an embryonic, stem, or germ cell into which a gene is inserted; the organism then carries the new gene in all of its cells.

transient ischemic attack (TIA): a temporary reduction in blood flow to the brain that causes temporary symptoms that depend on the part of the brain that is affected. Some common symptoms include light-headedness, visual disturbances, paralysis, staggering, numbness, or dysphagia.

translocation: the passage of infectious agents into the body through the intestinal tract.

transnasal: through the nose. A *transnasal feeding tube* is one that is inserted through the nose.

trauma: physical insult to the body that causes tissue damage including fractures, wounds, burns, or surgery.

triglycerides: the chief form of fat in the diet and the major storage form of fat in the body; composed of a molecule of glycerol with three fatty acids attached; also called *triacylglycerols.*

trimester: a three-month period, often used to describe a time during pregnancy.

tripeptide: three amino acids bonded together.

tube feedings: delivering nutrient solutions via a tube into the stomach or intestine.

tubule: a tubelike structure that surrounds the glomerulus and descends through the nephron. A pressure gradient between the glomerular capillaries and the tubule returns needed materials to the blood and moves wastes into the tubule to be sent to the bladder.

tumor: a new growth of tissue forming an abnormal mass with no function; also called a *neoplasm.*

turbinado sugar: sugar produced using the same refining process as white sugar, but without the bleaching and anti-caking treatment; traces of molasses give turbinado its sandy color.

24-hour recall: a record of foods eaten by a person for one 24-hour period.

type I osteoporosis: osteoporosis characterized by rapid bone losses, primarily of trabecular bone.

type II osteoporosis: osteoporosis characterized by gradual losses of both trabecular and cortical bone.

ulcer: an erosion in the topmost, and sometimes underlying, layers of cells in an area; see also *peptic ulcer.*

ulcerative colitis: inflammation and ulceration of the colon; see also *Crohn's disease.*

ultrahigh temperature (UHT) treatment: sterilizing a food by short-time exposure to temperatures above those normally used.

umbilical cord: the ropelike structure through which the fetus's veins and arteries reach the placenta; the route of nourishment and oxygen into the fetus and the route of waste disposal from the fetus.

umbilicus: the scar in the middle of the abdomen that marks the former attachment of the umbilical cord; commonly known as the "belly button."

unavailable carbohydrates: carbohydrates such as fibers that human digestive enzymes cannot break down.

unbleached flour: a tan-colored endosperm flour with texture and nutritive qualities that approximate those of regular white flour.

undernutrition: deficiency of energy or nutrients.

underweight: body weight below some standard of acceptable weight that is usually defined in relation to height (such as the weight-for-height tables).

unsaturated fatty acid: a fatty acid that lacks hydrogen atoms and has at least one double bond between carbons (includes monounsaturated and polyunsaturated fatty acids). An *unsaturated fat* is composed of triglycerides in which some of the fatty acids are unsaturated.

upper safe: the amount of a nutrient that appears safe for *most healthy people* and beyond which there is concern that some people will experience toxicity symptoms.

urea: the principal nitrogen-excretion product of metabolism. Two ammonia fragments are combined with carbon dioxide to form urea.

urea kinetic modeling: a technique used to evaluate dialysis and guide diet therapy that takes into account the kidneys' ability to clear urea and the person's protein catabolic rate.

uremia (or azotemia): abnormal accumulation of nitrogen-containing substances in the blood.

uremic syndrome: the many symptoms that accompany the buildup of toxic waste products in the blood.

uremic frost: the appearance of urea crystals on the skin.

urethra: the tube through which urine from the bladder passes out of the body.

USDA (U.S. Department of Agriculture): the federal agency responsible for enforcing standards for the wholesomeness and quality of meat, poultry, and eggs produced in the United States; conducting nutrition research; and educating the public about nutrition.

uterus: the muscular organ within which the infant develops before birth; the womb.

vagotomy: surgery that severs the nerves to the stomach that stimulate gastric acid secretion.

validity: having the quality of being founded on fact or evidence.

variable: a factor that changes. A variable may depend on another variable (for example, a child's height depends on his age), or it may be independent (for example, a child's height does not depend on the color of her eyes). Sometimes both variables correlate with a third variable (a child's height and eye color both depend on genetics).

variety (dietary): eating a wide selection of foods within and among the major food groups (the opposite of monotony).

vasoconstrictor: a substance that constricts or narrows the blood vessels.

vegans: people who exclude all animal-derived foods (including meat, poultry, fish, eggs, and dairy products) from their diets; also called *pure vegetarians*, *strict vegetarians*, or *total vegetarians.*

vegetarians: a general term used to describe people who exclude meat, poultry, fish, or other animal-derived foods from their diets.

vein: a vessel that carries blood back to the heart.

villi: fingerlike projections from the folds of the small intestine; singular *villus.*

vitamin A activity: a term useful for referring to both the preformed vitamin A and the carotene contents of foods without distinguishing between them.

vitamin B_6: a family of compounds—pyridoxal, pyridoxine, and pyridoxamine; the primary active coenzyme form is PLP (pyridoxal phosphate).

vitamin B_{12}: a B vitamin characterized by the presence of cobalt; the active forms of coenzyme B_{12} are methylcobalamin and deoxyadenosylcobalamin.

vitamins: organic, essential nutrients required in small amounts by the body for health. The water-soluble vitamins are vitamin C and the eight B vitamins: thiamin, riboflavin, niacin, vitamins B_6 and B_{12}, folate, biotin, and pantothenic acid. The fat-soluble vitamins are vitamins A, D, E, and K.

VLDL (very-low-density lipoprotein): the type of lipoprotein made primarily by liver cells to transport lipids to various tissues in the body; composed primarily of triglycerides.

voluntary activities: the component of a person's daily energy expenditure that involves conscious and deliberate muscular work—walking, lifting, climbing, or other physical activity.

vomiting: expulsion of the contents of the

stomach up through the esophagus to the mouth.

water balance: the balance between water intake and output (losses). Water balance = intake − output.

water intoxication: the condition in which body water contents are too high.

water-miscible vitamins: fat-soluble vitamins that readily mix with water and can be absorbed without fat.

wean: to gradually replace one form of feeding with another, such as replacing breast milk or infant formula with semi-solid foods, parenteral nutrition with enteral nutrition, or enteral formulas with table foods.

weight cycling: repeated cycles of weight loss and gain. The weight-cycling pattern is popularly called the *ratchet effect* or *yo-yo effect* of dieting.

well water: water drawn from groundwater by tapping into an aquifer.

Wernicke-Korsakoff syndrome: symptoms commonly seen in malnourished alcohol abusers that are similar to those seen in thiamin deficiency and that can be treated with thiamin supplements.

wheat flour: any flour made from wheat, including white flour.

white flour: an endosperm flour that has been refined and bleached for maximum softness and whiteness.

white sugar: pure sucrose or "table sugar," produced by dissolving, concentrating, and recrystallizing raw sugar.

WHO (World Health Organization): an international agency that has adopted standards to regulate pesticide use among other responsibilities.

whole grain: a grain milled in its entirety (all but the husk), not refined.

whole-wheat flour: flour made from whole-wheat kernels; a whole-grain flour.

wine: an alcoholic beverage made by fermenting grape juice.

xanthophylls: pigments found in plants; responsible for the color changes seen in autumn leaves.

xerophthalmia: progressive blindness caused by vitamin A deficiency.

xerosis: drying of the cornea; a sign of vitamin A deficiency.

Zollinger-Ellison syndrome: marked hypersecretion of gastric acid and consequent peptic ulcers caused by a tumor of the pancreas, which releases gastrin.

zygote: the product of the union of ovum and sperm; so-called for the first two weeks after fertilization.

Abdominal distention, tube feeding and, 773t
Abdominal fat, **272**
Abdominal girth, in ascites, 836
Abdominal thrusts, in choking victim, 95
Abscess, **732,** 804-805
Absorption, 81, **83**-86, *84, 85*
  alcohol, 247
  calcium, 429, 430t
  calcium supplement, 446, 447
  carbohydrate, 113, 114, *114,* 120-121
  drug-nutrient interactions and, 526-528, 527t
  enteral formula and, 760
  fat, 157-158, *158*
  folate, *345*
  glucose, 114, 120-121
  illness and, 523
  iron, 452-455, *455,* 461
  iron supplement, 463
  of medium-chain triglycerides, 730
  nutrient release after, 86
  olestra effects on, 178
  optimal, 92-93
  protein, 184, 186
  regulation of, 90-93
  stress effects on, 807
  vitamin B₁₂, 349
  vitamins, 327
  zinc, 464
  see also Digestion; Malabsorption; *specific nutrients*
Abstracts, indexes of, 34
Acarbose, diabetes and, 868
Acceptable Daily Intake (ADI), for artificial sweeteners, **135,** 137
Accidental additives, **503,** 507-508
Accreditation, credentials and, 31
Accredited, **30**
Accredited Institutions of Postsecondary Education Programs Candidates, 31n
Accutane, 384
Acesulfame potassium (acesulfame-K), 133, 134t, **135,** 136
Acetaldehyde, **246**
  malnutrition and, 252
  vitamin B₆ and, 340
Acetaldehyde dehydrogenase, 248
Acetic acid, 113n, 142, *142*
Acetone breath, **848**
Acetyl CoA, **224**
  in alcohol metabolism, 248, *248,* 249
  in energy metabolism, 225, *226,* 226-228, *227*
Acetylcholine, Alzheimer's disease and, 678-679
Acid, **191,** B-7
Acid-base balance, **117,** 191, 416-417, *417*
  alcohol metabolism and, 249
  buffers in regulation of, 416
  chloride and, 423
  chronic renal failure, 917
  excretion in regulation of, 416-417
  kidneys in regulation of, 417, 419n
  proteins in regulation of, 191-192
  sodium and, 419n
  see also pH
"Acid indigestion," 99, **700**

Acidity
  contamination iron and, 461
  food interactions with nicotine gum and, 527-528
  gastric, 79-80
  see also pH
Acidophilus milk, lactose intolerance and, 115
Acidosis, **191**
  chronic renal failure and, 917
  respiratory, **788**
Acne, **384**
Acorn squash
  potassium in, *425*
  thiamin in, *332*
  vitamin B₆ in, *344*
Acquired immune deficiency syndrome. *See* AIDS
Acrodermatitis enteropathica, 467n
ACSM (American College of Sports Medicine), 278, F-5
ACTH (adrenocorticotropin), A-3, A-4
Actinium, B-2t
Active transport, 83, *85. See also* Transport
Active vitamin D, **911**
Activism, hunger and, 621-622, 623t
Activity. *See* Athletes; Exercise; Physical activity
Acupuncture, 296, **689**
Acute, **2**
Acute disease
  chronic disease vs., 2
  see also specific diseases
Acute gastritis, 704
Acute malnutrition, 199, 807, 808t
Acute PEM, **199**
Acute phase (stress response), **806**
Acute renal failure, 913-916
Acute respiratory failure, 898-900
ADA. *See* American Dietetic Association
Adaptation, after bowel resection, 741, 752-754
Adaptive thermogenesis, **265**
Added (on labels), 60t
Addiction. *See* Alcohol; Drug(s); *specific substance*
Additives, 503-513
  accidental, **503**
  antioxidant, 146, 505, 506
  artificial sweeteners, 133-138, 503-504
  incidental, **503**
  indirect, **503,** 507-508
  intentional, **503,** 505-507, *505-507*
  in intravenous solutions, 784
  iron absorption and, 455
  on labels, 54
  nutrient, **505,** 507
  phosphorus in, 434
  regulations governing, 503-505
  sugar as, 121
Adenine, 221
Adenomas, **934**
Adenosine diphosphate (ADP), 221
Adenosine monophosphate (AMP), 221
Adenosine triphosphate. *See* ATP
Adequacy (dietary), **37,** 495
  dietary balance and, 38

  during weight loss, 302
Adequate energy, protein intake and, 204
ADH (antidiuretic hormone), 191t, **246, 411,** **A-4**
  alcohol and, 250
  stress and, 805t
  water retention and, 411
ADHD (attention deficit hyperactivity disorder), **642**
ADI. *See* Acceptable Daily Intake
Adipose tissue, **160**
  brown vs. white, 289
  composition, 257
  see also Fat cells
Adjunctive therapies, **689**
Admixtures, TPN solutions, 790
Adolescents/adolescence, **650**-655
  cholesterol values, 661t
  diabetes in, 879
  drug abuse in, 652-654
  eating disorders in, 322-323. *See also* Eating disorders
  energy and nutrient needs, 651
  food choices and health habits of, 652
  growth and development, 650-651
  iron deficiency in, 456
  milk intake recommendations, 430
  pregnancy in, 600
  see also Children/childhood; Puberty
ADP (adenosine diphosphate), 221
Adrenal glands, **411**
  hormones, A-4 to A-5
Adrenaline, 119. *See also* Epinephrine
Adrenocorticotropin (ACTH), **A-3,** A-4
Adult bone loss, **433.** *See also* Osteoporosis
Adult-onset diabetes. *See* Noninsulin-dependent diabetes mellitus (NIDDM)
Adult respiratory distress syndrome (ARDS), **898**
Adult rickets. *See* Osteomalacia
Adults/adulthood
  with cystic fibrosis, 735
  height and weight tables, 546
  milk intake recommendations, 430
  older. *See* Older adults
Adverse reactions, **644**-645
Aerobic, **225**
Aerobic metabolism, 226
  fat use and, 282, *282*
Aerobic training, benefits, 279, 888-889
Afebrile, **813**
Aflatoxin, **201**
African Americans
  bone metabolism and, 443
  lactose intolerance in, 115
African cuisine, 65-66
AGA (appropriate for gestational age), **598**
Age/aging
  basal metabolic rate and, 263t, 265t
  bone development and, 441, *442*
  calcium recommendations and, 445
  chronological, **667**
  physiological, **667**
  pregnancy and, 596t, 601
  process, 668-670
  weight standards and, 268, 269t

This index lists primarily topics that received significant mention in the text. Inclusive pages (for example, 53–56) indicate major discussions; pages in **boldface** refer to defined terms; pages in *italics* refer to figures, diagrams, or chemical structures; pages followed by a "t" refer to tables; pages followed by an "n" refer to notes; letter-number combinations (such as C-24) refer to appendixes.

NOTE: This index covers *Understanding Normal and Clinical Nutrition,* Fifth Edition. Some pages referred to are not included in the present volume.

see also Adolescents; Children; Infant(s);
   Older adults
Agencies. *See specific agencies*
Agriculture, pesticides, 499-502
Agriculture, U.S. Department of. *See* USDA
AIDS (acquired immune deficiency syndrome),
   948
   development, 949-950
   see also Human immunodeficiency virus
      (HIV)
AIDS enteropathies, **952**
AIDS-related complex (ARC), **949**
Air, swallowing, 98
Air pollution, hunger and, 618
Alanine, 134t, 181t, 806
   chemical structure, 180, *181*
Alanine transaminase, 552t, 827
Alar, 500
Alarm reaction, 668
Alaskans
   native diet of, 66
   see also Inuits
Albumin
   Crohn's disease and, 737
   tests, 552t
   zinc transport by, 464-465
Albuminuria, **910**
Alcohol, *245*, 245-254, **246**
   adolescent abuse, 654
   in beverages, 245-247
   in body, 247
   brain and, 249-251, *250*, 251t
   in breast milk, 608-609
   cancer and, 937
   cirrhosis and, 828, 832
   in Daily Food Guide, 39, *43*, 44
   in diabetes, 853-854, 867
   doses and blood levels, 251t
   excess energy from, 9
   folate deficiency and, 343, 345
   French cuisine and, 63-64
   health effects, 253t, 541t
   and heart disease risk, 907
   hepatitis and, 827
   hypertension and, 893
   illness or death related to, *25*
   interference with energy metabolism, C-17
      to C-18
   iron overload and, 459
   kcalories in, 8, 251, 252t, 258
   kilojoules in, 8n
   liver and, 247-249, 253t, 827, 828, 836
   long-term effects, 253
   magnesium deficiency and, 435
   malnutrition and, 251-252, 253t
   in Mediterranean diet, 214
   metabolism, 247-249, *248*
   moderate intake, 893, 907
   myths concerning, 254t
   oral antidiabetic agents and, 867
   osteoporosis and, 444
   paternal use and fetal development, 603
   in pregnancy, 253, 253t, 601-604
   raw seafood and, 493
   recommendations, 27t, 253-254
   resources on abuse, F-4
   short-term effects, 252-253
   sugar, **135**, 138, 138t
   triglycerides and, 887
   ulcers and, 252
   water and, 411

weight loss and, 303
Wernicke-Korsakoff syndrome and, 329
Alcohol dehydrogenase, **246**, 247-248
Alcohol-related birth defects (ARBD), **601**
Aldicarb, 500
Aldosterone, **411, A-5**
   ascites and, 830
   sodium retention and, 411
   stress and, 805t
Alimentary hypoglycemia, **708**
Alitame, 133, 134t, **135**, 136
Alka Seltzer, sodium in, 529
Alkaline phosphatase, 389t, 463n
   serum, 552t
Alkalinity
   pancreatic juice, 80
   see also pH
Alkalosis, **191, 423**
   metabolic, 423n
   milk alkali syndrome, 446t
All-in-one admixtures, **790**
Allergy
   insulin, **858**
   milk, 115
   see also Food allergies
Allyl sulfides, 406t
Almonds, calcium in, *432*
Alpha-carotene, 406n
Alpha cells (pancreas), 119n
Alpha-lactalbumin, **629**
Alpha-linolenic acid. *See* Linolenic acid
Alpha-tocopherol, **391**. *See also* Vitamin E
Alpha-tocotrienol, 393n
Alternative therapies, 688-693, **689**
   cancer and, 943
   fields of alternative medicine, 688t
   risk-benefit relationships, 690, *691*
Aluminum, B-2t
   Alzheimer's disease and, 679
Aluminum salts, calcium supplements with,
      446, 446t, 447t
Alveoli, **899**
Alzheimer's disease, 678-679
Amenorrhea, **316**, 383t, 597
   in anorexia nervosa, 317
   in athletes, 317, *317*, 442
   bone loss and, 442
   postpartum, **609**
   primary, **316**
   secondary, **316**
American Academy of Pediatrics (AAP)
   on breast milk vs. infant formula, 622
   on infant formula, 631
American College of Sports Medicine
      (ACSM), 278, F-5
American Council on Education, 31n
American Diabetes Association, booklets on
      ethnic foodways, 69n
American Dietetic Association (ADA),
      30, F-4
   on accreditation for dietetics degree, 31n
   on artificial sweeteners, 137
   booklets on ethnic foodways, 69n
   on breastfeeding, 622
   on fiber intake, 128
   hotline for registered dietitians, 30n
   hunger and, 622
   on managed care, 960
   on nutrition education in medical schools,
      29
   registered dietitian examination of, 30

on *trans*-fatty acids, 165
American Heart Association
   on butter vs. margarine, 165
   on eggs, 153
   on salt, 420
American Institute of Nutrition, F-4
American Journal of Clinical Nutrition, 34
American Psychiatric Association, 321
American Society for Bone and Mineral
      Research, 447
American Society for Clinical Nutrition, 29-
      30, F-4
Americans with Disabilities Act, obesity and,
      293
Americium, B-2t
Amino acid(s), **180,** 181t
   in aspartame, 135, *136*
   B vitamins in metabolism of, 328
   branched-chain, 830
   carbons in, 224n
   catabolism, 231, *232*
   chelates, 446, **447t**
   conditionally essential, **181**
   deamination, 195, 231
   essential, **181,** 181t
   fat and, 195, 233
   glucogenic, 195n, 226, 232-233
   in hepatic coma, 830
   inborn errors of metabolism, 839-844
   intravenous solutions, 783
   ketogenic, 195n, 226
   limiting, **196**
   nonessential, 180-181, 181t
   role in metabolism, 231-234, *232-235*
   scoring, **197**, J-1, J-2t
   sequences, 183, 186-188
   sequencing errors, 186-188
   side groups, 180
   stress response, 806, 813, 815
   structures, *180-182*, C-4 to C-5
   supplements, 184, 205-206, 296
   supplements in athletes, 370t
   transamination, **233**-234, *234*
   use as ergogenic aid, 370t
   using for energy, 194-195
   using to make other compounds, 194
   using to make proteins or nonessential
      amino acids, 194
   vitamin B_6 and metabolism of, 340
   see also Protein; *specific amino acids*
Aminopeptidases, in protein digestion, *185*
Ammonia, **233**
   deamination and, 195, 233, *233*
   elevated blood levels in cirrhosis, 830
   hepatic coma and, 830
   molecule, *B-4*
   in urea synthesis, 234
Amniotic sac, **585**
AMP (adenosine monophosphate), 221
Amphetamines
   fetal effects, 604
   food intake and, 526
   weight loss and, 297
Amylase, **113**
   in digestion, *112*, 113
   pancreatitis and, 732
   serum, 552t
Amylopectin, 108
Amylose, 108
Anabolism, **189, 219**-220, *220*
Anaerobic, **225**

Anaerobic activity, benefits, 279
Analgesics, E-1t
"Android" obesity, 272
Anemia, **346**
  assessment, E-30, E-30t to E-31t
  in chronic renal failure, 919-920, 923
  folate-deficiency, 346, 347t
    after gastrectomy, 711
    goat's milk, 633
  iron-deficiency, **456**-457. *See also* Iron-
      deficiency anemia
  lead poisoning and, 482
  macrocytic (megaloblastic), **346,** 350, 351t
  microcytic, 342t, 360t
  microcytic hypochromic, **456**
  milk, **637**
  pernicious, **349**-350, *350,* 351t
  sickle-cell, **188**
  in ulcerative colitis, 744
Anencephaly, **345**
Angina, **883**
Angioplasty, 887
Angiotensin, **411, A-5**
  blood vessel constriction and, 411
Angiotensinogen, **411**
Animal foods. *See* Fish; Meat(s); Poultry;
  Seafood
Animal studies, 11
Anion(s), **413,** 413t, B-6. *See also specific*
  anions
Anorexia
  in cancer, 939
  in hepatitis, 828
  HIV-related, 951-952
Anorexia nervosa, 311, 315-319, **316**
  diagnostic criteria, 317t
  health effects of, 316-317
  treatment, 318t, 318-319
  see also Eating disorders
Antacids, 99, **447t,** 529-530, **702,** E-1t
  as calcium supplements, 446, 446t, 447t,
    529-530
  folate and, 346
Antagonist(s), **340**
  in vitamin/mineral supplements, 369
Antecedents, in behavior modification, 305,
  306
Anterior, **A-3**
Anthropometric, 21
Anthropometric measurements, 273-274, **544,**
  E-13 to *E-27*
  in nutrition assessment, 21, 544-550, 546t,
    548t, *550*
Antianginals, E-1t
Antianxiety agents, E-1t
Antibody(ies), **193**
  in cancer treatment, 943
  proteins as, 192-193
  see also Immune system
Anticoagulants, E-1t
  in atherosclerosis, 889
  vitamin C interactions with, 361n
  vitamin K interactions with, 396
Anticonvulsants, E-1t to E-2t
Antidepressants, E-2t
Antidiabetic agents, oral, **867,** E-2t
Antidiarrheal agents, **724,** E-2t
Antidiuretic hormone. *See* ADH
Antigen, **193**
Antigen skin testing, protein-energy malnutri-
  tion and, 550

Anti-GERD, **702**
Antihypertensive agents, 893-894, E-3t to E-4t
Anti-infectives, E-4t to E-5t
Anti-inflammatory drugs, E-5t to E-6t
  peptic ulcer due to, 99, 705
Antilipemic agents, E-6t
Antimicrobial agents, **505**
  additives, 505-506
  see also specific agents
Antimony, B-2t
Antinauseants, E-6t
Antineoplastic agents, E-6t to E-8t
Antioxidant(s), **146, 357, 402,** B-10
  additives, 146, **505,** 506
  beta-carotene, 379, 402, 403
  cancer and, 402-403, 405, 406t
  cataracts and, 677
  in disease prevention, *400,* 400-405, *401,*
    405, 406t
  in fat processing, 146
  food sources, 404-405
  heart disease and, 403-404, 905
  LDL and, 403
  lutein, 405
  nonnutrient, 405, 406t
  selenium as, 471
  supplements, 372, 405
  supplements vs. food sources, 404
  vitamin C, 357, 402, 506
  vitamin E, 391-392, 402, 506
  see also specific antioxidants
Antipromoters (cancer), **936,** 937
Antipsychotics, E-8t to E-9t
Antiscorbutic factor, 356
Antisecretory agents, **702**
Antisense gene, **512,** 513
Antiulcer agents, **702,** E-9t
Antiviral drugs, for HIV infection, 950
Anuria, **921**
Anus, *74, 75,* 78
Apnea, sleep, 274
Appendicitis, fiber and, 127
Appendix, 73, *74, 75*
Appetite, **259**
  activity effects on, 304
  determinants, 260
  drugs and, 297, 526, 527t
  illness and, 523
  improvement in cancer, 946
  for nonfood substances. *See* Pica
  stress and, 808
  suppression in starvation, 242
  see also Anorexia nervosa; Hunger
Appetite stimulants, E-9t
Appetite suppressants, E-9t
"Apple" vs. "pear" body-fat distribution, 272
Apples, H
Appropriate for gestational age (AGA), **598**
Apricots
  carotenoids in, 406t
  cyanogens in pits, 498
  nutrients in, 124t
Arabinose, 109n
Arachidic acid, C-4t
Arachidonic acid, **148,** C-4t
  food sources, 150t
ARBD (alcohol-related birth defects), **601**
ARC (AIDS-related complex), **949**
ARDS (adult respiratory distress syndrome),
  898
Arginine, 181t

Argon, B-2t
Ariboflavinosis, 334t
Aroma therapy, **689**
Arousal, eating in response to, 261
Arsenic, 450, 477, B-2t
  calcium supplements and, 446t, 447t
Arteriosclerosis, **882**
Artery(ies), **86**-88. *See also specific arteries*
  hepatic, 829
Artesian water, **516**
Arthritis, **677**
  alcohol and, 253t
Artichoke
  iron in, *462*
  magnesium in, *436*
  potassium in, *425*
Artificial colors, **505,** 506, *507*
Artificial feeding, **797**
Artificial flavors, **505,** 507
Artificial sweeteners, 133-138, **135,** 503-504
  PKU and, 841
  in pregnancy, 605
Ascites, **830**
  abdominal girth in, 836
  cirrhosis and, 830
  fluids and sodium in, 832
Ascorbic acid, **357.** *See also* Vitamin C
  -ase, **79,** 152
Asian Americans
  ethnic cuisine of, 67-69. *See also*
    Monosodium glutamate (MSG)
  lactose intolerance in, 115
Asians
  osteoporosis risk in, 443
  sodium intake in, 420-421
  use of stock prepared from bones, 432
Asparagine, 181t
Asparagus, folate in, 348
Aspartame, 133-136, 134t, **135,** 137
  ADI, 137
  chemical structure, *136*
  food sources, 137t
  metabolism, 135-136, *136*
  PKU and, 841
Aspartate transaminase, 552t, 827, 894
Aspartic acid, 134t, 135, *136,* 181t
  chemical structure, *181*
Aspergillus flavus, 201
Aspiration, **697**
  dysphagia and, 697-698
Aspiration pneumonia, 698
  tube feeding and, 773t
Aspirin
  in atherosclerosis, 889
  folate and, 346, 528
  food and, 528
  in preeclampsia, 600
  pregnancy and, 600, 604
  vitamin C and, 529
Assessment. *See* Nutrition assessment
Assistance programs. *See* Food assistance pro-
  grams
Astatine, B-2t
Astemizole (Hismanal), 526
Asterixis, **830**
Asymptomatic allergy, **645**
-ate, **224,** 414
Atheromatous plaque, **883**
Atherosclerosis, **154,** 164, 882, 883-889
  consequences, 883
  development, 658-660, *659*

prevention and treatment, 887t, 887-889, 888t
renal failure and, 918
see also Cardiovascular disease (CVD); Cholesterol; Coronary heart disease
Athletes
amenorrhea and bone loss in, 316-317, 442
eating disorders in, 315, 316-317. *See also* Eating disorders; *specific disorders*
fluid replacement for, 284-285, 285t
meals before and after competition, 285-286
protein recommendations for, 284
protein supplements in, 205
supplements and ergogenic aids used by, 205, 369, 370t-371t
triad of problems in women, 317, *317*
see also Exercise; Physical activity
Atom(s), **5**
bonding by, 102-103, *103. See also* Bonding/bonds
ion formation, B-5 to B-7
properties, B-1 to B-3, B-2t
ATP (adenosine triphosphate), **221**
energy expenditure and, 261
energy from fat and, 238
glycolysis and, 225n
iron and, 451
magnesium and, 434
roles in body, *221*
sodium-potassium pump and, 414
Atpamezole, 297n
Atrophic gastritis, **349,** 669, 705
Atrophy (muscle), **282**
Attention deficit hyperactivity disorder (ADHD), **642**
Attitudes
societal, eating disorders and, 315, 321-322
weight loss and, 307
Autoimmune disorders, **847**
Autonomic nervous system, **A-7**
Autonomy principle, 797
Available carbohydrates, **108**
Aversion. *See* Food aversion
Avidin, **339**
Avocado, 67, H
potassium in, *425*
vitamin E in, *395*
Ayurveda, **689**
Azotemia, **914**
AZT (zidovudine), 950

B vitamins, 328t, 328-356
alcohol and, 252
cirrhosis and, 832
coenzymes, 222, 328, *328,* 329
coenzymes in metabolism, 352, *353*
deficiencies, 354-356
food sources, 356
interactions, 354
pregnancy and, 592-594
supplements, 354-355
toxicities, 356
see also specific B vitamins
Baby foods
commercial, 636
pureed foods vs., 697
Bacon, H
nitrites in, 506
Bacteria
in blind loop syndrome, 710, 738-739
cross-contamination, 492

in drinking water, 516
food-borne illnesses, 487-489, 488t-489t. *See also* Food-borne illnesses
overgrowth causing malabsorption, 738-739, *739*
translocation, 809t, **809**-810
ulcers and, 99, 705
see also Food poisoning; Infection(s); Intestinal flora
"Bad" cholesterol, 160. *See also* LDL (low-density lipoprotein)
Bagels, 69, H
Baked goods
BHA and BHT in, 506
fat in, 170
iodine in, 470-471
Baker's yeast, 333, H
Balance (dietary), **37**-38
Balkan peninsula, bone fracture rates, 443
Balloon angioplasty, **887**
Balloons, gastric, 299
Banana, H
potassium in, *425*
vitamin B_6 in, *344*
Barbiturates, fetal effects, 604
Barium, 477, B-2t
Barley, H
Basal energy expenditure (BEE), 812t, 814
Basal metabolic rate (BMR), **262**
activity effects on, 304
estimation, 265t, 265-266, 267
factors affecting, 263t
Basal metabolism, **262**-263
Basal thermogenesis, **261**
Base, 191, B-8
Beans. *See* Legumes; Vegetables; *specific type*
Bedside rounds, professional communication and, 579, 583
Bedsores, **810**
BEE (basal energy expenditure), 812t, 814
Bee pollen, 370t
Beef
protein in, 198
zinc in, 469
see also Meat(s)
Beef liver
iron in, *462*
vitamin A in, *386*
Beef tallow, 146, 164
Beer, 246, 252t
nitrosamines in, 506
see also Alcohol
Beet sugar. *See* Sucrose
Behavior
child, 640-644, 643t
hunger and, 640-641
infant mealtimes and, 637-638
iron deficiency and, 458
nutrient deficiencies and, 641-642, 643t
sugar and, 125
Behavior modification, **305**
nutrition education and, 576, 578
for weight loss, 305-309, *306*
Beikost, **634**
Belch/belching, **96,** 98
Bell peppers, vitamin C in, *363*
Beneficence principle, 797
Benign, **934**
Benzocaine, weight loss and, 297
Beriberi, **329,** *329,* 329-330, 354
Berkelium, B-2t

Beryllium, B-2t
Beta-carotene, **375,** 406t
as antioxidant, 379, 402, 403
cancer and, 403
chemical structure, *376*
food sources, 382t
in smokers, 655
supplements, 404
vitamin E interactions with, 369
see also Vitamin A
Beta cells (pancreas), 118n
Beta-cryptoxanthin, 406n
Beta-tocopherol, 393n
Beverages, H
alcoholic, 245-247. *See also* Alcohol
aspartame content, 137t
cola, 114, 124t, 644
diuretic effects, 411
fruit juices, 50
milk "drinks," 40
mixers, 252t
safety while traveling, 494
tyramine-containing, 529t
weight gain and, 311
see also Coffee; Water
BGH (bovine growth hormone), **509**-510
BHA (butylated hydroxyanisole), **506**
BHT (butylated hydroxytoluene), 402, **506**
Bicarbonate, **78**
extracellular concentration, 413t
intracellular concentration, 413t
ion, 413t
pancreatic release of, 91
Bifidus factors, **631**
Bile, **78,** 81t, 153
components, *156*
constipation and, 97
in digestive process, 80, 92
enterohepatic circulation, *157*
in fat digestion, 156, *156*
fibers and, 110
hepatitis and, 828
regulation of release, 92
Bile acid, 156
Bile duct, 74
Biliary cirrhosis, **828**
Biliary tract, 826
Bilirubin, 396, **784**
Binders, **419,** 429
Binge drinking, **252**-253
Binge-eating disorder, 321
diagnostic criteria, 322t
see also Bulimia nervosa
Bioaccumulation, **495,** 496
Bioavailability, **342**
supplements and, 368-369
variability among minerals, 419
zinc, 464
Biochemical analyses, 550-555, 552t, E-26 to E-31t
Bioelectrical impedance, 273-**274,** *274,* 548
Bioelectromagnetic medical applications, **689**
Biofeedback, **689**
Biofield therapeutics, **689**
Bioflavonoids, 351
Biological Abstracts, 34
Biological value (BV), **197**-198, J-1 to J-3
Biosensor, **493**-494
Biotechnology, **511**-513, *512*
food safety and, 493-494, 512-513
regulation, 512-513

Biotin, **337**, 339, 339t
  deficiency, 339, 339t
  food sources, 339
  RDI, 55t
  recommendations, 337, 339t, 368t
Birth control pills. *See* Oral contraceptives
Birth defects
  alcohol-related, **601**
  folate deficiency and, 345-346, 587-588
  neural tube, 586-587
  vitamin A toxicity and, 384
Birthweight, 598
  maternal caffeine and, 605
  maternal smoking and, 604
  maternal zinc and, 595
Bismuth, 99, B-2t
Bitot's spots, 382t
Black Americans. *See* African Americans
Black beans, iron in, *462*
Black-eyed peas
  folate in, *348*
  magnesium in, *436*
Blackstrap molasses, 122, 124t, H
  calcium in, *431*
Bladder, 88
  cancer, 133, 936t
Bland diet, liberal, 705t
Blind experiment, **12, 13**
Blind loop syndrome, 710, 738-739, *739*
Blindness
  night, **378,** 381
  vitamin A deficiency and, 382, 382t
  see also Eyes
Blood
  acid-base balance, 191-192
  alcohol levels, 251t
  ammonia levels, 830
  analysis of. *See* specific tests
  circulation. *See* Circulatory system(s)
  clotting. *See* Blood clotting
  iron losses in, 455-456
  very-low-kcalorie diet side effects in, 300t
Blood cholesterol. *See* Cholesterol (blood)
Blood clotting, 396
  atherosclerosis and, 883
  vitamin K and, 394
Blood donation, iron loss with, 456
Blood glucose, 107n, 552t
  acute renal failure and, 916
  alcohol and, 253t
  constancy, 118-121, *119*
  exercise and, 856-857
  fasting, 851
  normal range, 118, 120
  pregnancy and, 870
Blood lipid profile, **164**
Blood-making activity, erythropoietin and, A-5
Blood pressure
  atherosclerosis and, 660, 883
  calcium and, 600
  hormones regulating, A-5
  normal, 890
  potassium and, 424
  during pregnancy, 599-600
  regulation, 890, 890-892, A-5
  salt and, 420
  vegetarian diet and, 210
  water balance and, 411-412, *412*
  see also Hypertension
Blood sugar, 104. *See also* Blood glucose
Blood transferrin, 452

iron transport and, 455
Blood urea nitrogen (BUN), 552t, 914, 917
Blood vessels. *See* Cardiovascular system; Vascular system
Blood volume
  acute renal failure and, 914
  losses at birth, 594
  shock and, 811
  water balance and, 411-412, *412*
Blue sclera, 457t
Blueberries, caffeic acid in, 406t
Bluefish, niacin in, *338*
BMI. *See* Body mass index
BMR. *See* Basal metabolic rate
Body
  composition. *See* Body composition
  density, 273, 548
  energy budget, 238-244, *239, 241, 242*
  fluids. *See* Fluid(s)
  lead effects in, 480, *481. See also* Lead
  mass index (BMI), 546, *E-22,* inside back cover
  mineral handling, 418
  nutrient composition, 4-5
  response to stress, 804-811
  shape in children, 638
  temperature, D-3
Body composition, **266,** 268, *268,* 548-550, *550*
  aging and, 669
  BMR and, 263t
  energy balance and, 257-258
  fat intake and, 303
  measurement of, *273, 273-274, 274*
  see also Fat/lipids (in body); Frame size; Water; Weight
Body fat. *See* Body composition; Fat/lipids (in body)
Body fluids. *See* Fluid(s)
Body image, food choices related to, 3
Body mass index (BMI), *270,* **270**-271, 271t
  disease risks and, *274,* 274-275
  overweight defined by, 270, 288n
  underweight defined by, 308
Body temperature
  stored fat and, 148
  see also Fever; Hyperthermia; Hypothermia; Temperature
Body weight. *See* Weight
Body wraps, 296
Bok choy, calcium in, *432*
Bolus, **73,** 113
Bolus feeding, **768**
Bomb calorimeter, **258,** *259*
Bonding/bonds (of atoms), B-3 to B-5t
  amino acid, 180
  fatty acid, 142, 143n
  number formed by various atoms, 102-103, *103*
  peptide, *182*
Bone(s)
  adolescent calcium needs and, 651
  boron and, 477
  calcium and, 427, *427*
  calcium balance in, *428,* 428-429
  calcium content with age, 441
  calcium deficiency and, 432-433
  calcium in stock prepared from, 432
  in childhood malnutrition, 643t
  in chronic renal failure, 918
  cortical, **439,** 440

fetal development, 594
  fluoride and, 474, 475
  hormones affecting, A-5
  magnesium in, 434
  in nutrition assessment, 537t
  osteoporosis and, 203, 439-447. *See also* Osteoporosis
  peak mass, 432, *442*
  phases of development throughout life, 441, *442*
  postgastrectomy disease, 711
  powdered, 446, **447t**
  preterm infants and, 634
  remodeling, **379**
  stress fractures, **316**
  trabecular, *439,* 439-440, *440*
  vitamin A and, 382t
  vitamin C and, 360t
  vitamin D and, 387-388, 389t
  vitamin K and, 394
  zinc and, 467t
Bone density, **439**
Bone marrow, in iron transport, 455
Bone marrow transplant, **942**-943
  nutrition support before, 945, 948
Bone marrow transplants, nutrition support after, 948
Bone meal, 446, 446t, **447t**
Book recommendations, F-1 to F-2
Borderline diabetes, **851**
Boron, 370t, 450, 477, B-2t
Botanical medicine, **689**
Bottle feeding. *See* Infant formulas
Bottled water, 517
Botulinum toxin, **487**
Botulism, **487,** 489t, **636**
  danger signs, 487
  honey and, 636
  infant, 491
  in infants, 636
Bovine growth hormone (BGH), **509**-510
Brain
  aging effects on, 678-680, 679t
  alcohol effects on, 249-251, *250,* 251t
  cancer, 945t
  glucose and, 240-241, 641
  iron deficiency and, 641-642
  nutrient deficiencies and, 679t, 679-680
Brain stem, *250*
Bran, **45**
  irritable bowel syndrome and, 729
  muffins, 126, H
  rice, 110
Branched-chain amino acids, in hepatic coma, 830
Breads, H
  calcium-fortified, 432
  calcium in, 432
  choices, 45, *45,* 48-50
  in exchange lists, G-6t
  fat intake and, 168
  in food group plans, 41, *42*
  iron-enriched, 460-461
  nutrients in, *49*
  unleavened, 466n
  whole wheat, 124t
  see also Cereals; Grains
Breast cancer, 166, 936t
  antioxidants and, 403
Breast disease, fibrocystic, **393**
Breast milk

alcohol in, 608-609
environmental contaminants in, 610
flavor changes due to particular foods, 608
infant formula vs., 622, 624, *631, 632t*
nutrients in, *629, 629-630, 631, 632t*
smoking effects on, 609
see also Breastfeeding; Lactation
Breastfeeding, 606-607
contraception during, 609
infants with cystic fibrosis and, 735
mothers' concerns about, 608-610
preterm infants and, 634
see also Breast milk; Lactation
Breath, acetone, **848**
Breath tests, diet and, 560
Brewer's yeast, 333, H
use as ergogenic aid, 370t
see also Yeast
Broccoflower, H
Broccoli, H
calcium in, *431, 432*
folate in, *348*
iron in, *462*
magnesium in, *436*
natural toxicants in, 498
nutrients in, 124t
phytochemicals in, 406t
potassium in, *425*
riboflavin in, *335*
vitamin A in, *386*
vitamin B$_6$ in, *344*
vitamin C in, *363*
vitamin E in, *395*
zinc in, *469*
Bromine, B-2t
Bronchitis, **900**
Brown fat, 289
Brown sugar, **122,** 129
Brussels sprouts, H
calcium in, *432*
natural toxicants in, 498
vitamin C in, *363*
Buffers, **191, 416**
Bulimia nervosa, 96, **316,** 319-321, *320*
binge-eating disorder vs., 321
diagnostic criteria, 319t
health effects of, 320
treatment, 320-321, 321t
see also Eating disorders
Bulk food purchases, 682-683
BUN (blood urea nitrogen), 552t, 914, 917
Butter, *145, 146*
calcium in, 430
cholesterol in, 153t
margarine vs., 165
Butternut squash, vitamin A in, *386*
Butylated hydroxyanisole (BHA), **506**
Butylated hydroxytoluene (BHT), 402, **506**
Butyric acid, 113n, C-4t
BV (biological value), **197-**198, J-1 to J-3
Bypass, coronary artery, 887

Cabbage, H
natural toxicants in, 498
CABG (coronary artery bypass graft), **887**
Cachectin, **805**
Cachexia
cancer, **938**
cardiac, **896**
Cadmium, 477, B-2t
calcium supplements and, 446t, 447t

in drinking water, 516
Caffeic acid, 406t
Caffeine
alcohol and, 254
basal metabolic rate and, 263t
breastfeeding and, 609
child behavior and, 643-644
fibrocystic breast disease and, 393
methylene chloride in removal from coffee, 508
osteoporosis and, 444
pregnancy and, 605
recommendations, 27t
water needs and beverages containing, 411
Cahling, Andreas, 268
Cajun cuisine, 64
Calciferol, 389t
Calcification, metastatic, **918**
Calcitonin, 191t, **428,** 441n, **A-5,** E-12t
Calcitriol, **922,** E-12t
Calcium, **426**-433, B-2t, B-5t
absorption, 429, 430t
absorption from different supplement forms, 446
absorption in pregnancy, 429, 594
absorption with age, 441
adolescent needs, 651
age and amount in bone, 441, *442*
amount in body, *418*
in antacids, 446, 446t, 447t, 529-530
balance, *428,* 428-429
blood, 552t
and blood pressure during pregnancy, 600
in body fluids, 427
in bone, 427, *427,* 432-433, 441, *442*
in breast milk, 630
in children, 429
chronic renal failure and, 918, 920t, 922
cirrhosis and, 832
crystals in trabecular bone, *439*
deficiency, 427t, 429, 432-433
in disease prevention, 427-428
extracellular concentration, 413t
fat malabsorption and, 728
food labels and, 55, 61
food sources, 38, 427t, 430-432, *431, 432*
hormones adjusting balance, A-5
hypertension and, 427-428
intracellular concentration, 413t
ion, 413t
iron interactions with, 37-38, 369, 446t
magnesium interactions with, 369, 434, 446t
nonmilk sources, 432, *432*
older adults and, 674-675
osteoporosis and, 59, 203, 433, 439-447
pregnancy and, 429, 594, 600
preterm infants and, 634
problems arising from supplementation, 446t
RDI, 55t
recommendations, 27t, 368t, 427t, 429-430, 445
roles in body, *427,* 427t, 427-429, *428*
supplements, 367, 445-447, 446t, 447t, 922
tetracycline and, 527
toxicity, 427t, 429, 446t
in vegetarian diet, 213
vitamin B$_6$ interactions with, 354
vitamin D and, 387-388, 428, 429, 441, 446t
in water, 435
zinc interactions with, 369
Calcium-binding protein, **429**

Calcium carbonate, 5n, 446
Calcium citrate, 446
Calcium cyclamate, 134t
Calcium gluconate, 446
Calcium lactate, 446
Calcium malate, 446
Calcium oxalate, kidney stones composed of, 930, 931
Calcium phosphate, 446
Calcium phosphate dibasic, 446t
Calcium rigor, **429**
Calcium tetany, **429**
Calculations, D-1 to D-3
Californium, B-2t
Calmodulin, 427, **428**
Calorie(s), 6-**7.** *See also* kCalorie(s)
Calorimetry
direct, **258,** *259,* **261**
indirect, **258,** **261,** 812
Campylobacter jejuni, 487, 488t
Campylobacteriosis, 488t
Canada
amino acid supplements, 205n
choice system, I-2 to I-14t
government nutrition resources, F-3
Guidelines for Healthy Eating, 39t
Nutrition Recommendations, 26, 27t
Nutrition Recommendations, I-0t to I-2t
Recommended Nutrient Intakes. *See* RNI
Canada's Food Guide to Healthy Eating, 44-45, *46-47*
Canadian Pesticide Information Line, 502n
Cancer, **934**-948
alcohol and, 253t
antioxidants and, 402-403, 405, 406t
artificial sweeteners and, 133, 136
beta-carotene and, 403
calcium and, 428
chlorinated water and, 515
development, 934-937, *935,* 936t
fat and, 59, 61, 165-166
fiber and, 61, 127
folate and risk of, 346
fruits and vegetables and, 61
HIV infection and, 952
iron and, 460
laetrile and, 351, 498
nutrition consequences, 938-940, *939*
nutrition support in, 943-948, 945t
obesity and, 275
phytochemicals and, 405, 406t
protein-energy malnutrition and, 201
protein intake and, 203
protein-sparing therapy in, 244
risk factors, 165
risk reduction, 937-938
selenium and, 471-472
therapy and folate deficiency, 346
treatment, 940t, 940-943, 941t
underweight and, 274
vegetarian diet and, 210
vitamin A and, 384, 403
vitamin C and, 403
vitamin E and, 403, 404
vitamin supplements and, 404
see also specific location
Cancer cachexia, **938**
Candida albicans, **952**
Candy, 129, H. *See also* Sweeteners/sweets
Cane sugar. *See* Sucrose
Canned foods

safety, 483, 489, 491
see also specific foods
Canola oil, *146*, H
vitamin E in, *395*
Cantaloupe, H
carotenoids in, 406t
Capillaries, 86-88
Capric acid, C-4t
Caproic acid, C-4t
Caprylic acid, C-4t
Carbohydrase, 79
Carbohydrate(s) (in body), 102-135
available, **108**
chemistry of, 102-111
conversion to fat, 118
digestion and absorption, *82*, 91, 111-116, *112, 114*. *See also* Absorption; Digestion
galactosemia and, 843
metabolism. *See* Carbohydrate metabolism
simple, 103-107
structure, *C-1* to *C-3*
unavailable, **108**
see also Complex carbohydrates; Fiber(s); Sugar(s)
Carbohydrate(s) (in diet), H
acute renal failure and, 916
athletes and, *280*, 281-282, 285, 286
chemical composition, 5
chronic renal failure and, 924
Daily Reference Value, 56t
Daily Value, 128
diabetic diet and, 852-853
excess of, 239
in exchange lists, 570, 571t, *572-573*, G-8t
fasting hypoglycemia and, 872-873
fat metabolism and, 162
gas production and, 98
glucose metabolism and, 117
health and, 122-128
hypoglycemia and, 864
intravenous solutions, 783
kcalories in, *7, 8,* 258
kilojoules in, 8n
postgastrectomy, 708, 709, 710t
reactive hypoglycemia and, 872
recommendations, 16, 27t, 56t, 128-130, 233
recommendations during stress, 815
recommendations for older adults, 673
weight loss and, 126, 303
Carbohydrate-based fat replacements, 176, 177t
Carbohydrate counting, 854
Carbohydrate loading, **282**
Carbohydrate metabolism, 116-121, 148, 843
liver in, 223t
Carbohydrate modules, K-8t
Carbon(s), 5, *5*, B-2t, B-3, B-5t
chain, in fatty acids, *142*, 148n
energy metabolism and, 9, 224
number of bonds formed by, 102, *103*
triglyceride, *231*
Carbon dioxide, 5n
acid-base balance and, 416
energy metabolism and, 9
exchanged in vascular system, 86
produced during metabolism, 226-227, *227*
tests, 552t
Carbonated soda, 129. *See also* Cola beverages
Carbonic acid, 416
Carbonic anhydrase, 463n
Carboxypeptidases, in protein digestion, *185*

Carcinogen(s), **936**
Delaney Clause and, 503-504
Carcinomas, **934**. *See also* Cancer
Cardiac cachexia, **896**
Cardiac cirrhosis, **828**
Cardiac glycosides, E-10t
Cardiac sphincter, 73, *74, 75,* 77, **701**
heartburn and, 98
substances relaxing, 702t
Cardiomegaly, **896**
Cardiovascular disease (CVD), **164, 882-901**
assessment in childhood, 662t
chronic renal failure and, 917-918
development in childhood, 658-660
in diabetes, 850, 885
fat and, 164-165
obesity and, *275*, 884t
prevention in children, 645
risk factors, 164
see also Atherosclerosis; Cholesterol; Heart disease; Hypertension
Cardiovascular system, 882
in childhood malnutrition, 643t
modified diet for conditions affecting, 569t
in nutrition assessment, 537t
very-low-kcalorie diet side effects in, 300t
see also Cardiovascular disease (CVD); Vascular system
Care maps, 960
Caries. *See* Dental caries
Carnitine, 351
use by athletes, 370t
Carotene, **385**
Carotenoids, **375**, 406t
cataracts and, 677
olestra and, 178
Carotid endarterectomy, **887**
Carpal tunnel syndrome, **341**
vitamin B_6 and, 341
Carrageenan, 110
Carrier, **839**
Carrots, H
carotenoids in, 406t
potassium in, *425*
vitamin A in, *386*
Cartilage therapy, **689**
Carver, George Washington, 65
Case-control studies, 11
Casein, 433, **629**
lactose intolerance and, 116
zinc and, 464
Casein hydrolysate formula, in PKU, 841
Cash crops, **614**
Cashews
magnesium in, *436*
vitamin E in, *395*
Catabolism, **189, 220,** *220,* 805
amino acid, 231, *232*
final steps, 234-238, 236t, *236-238*
glucose, 224-228
Catalyst, **79**
Cataracts, **676**-677
Catecholamines, stress and, 805t
Cathartic(s), **316**
in bulimia nervosa, 320
Catheter
insertion and care in TPN, 788
IV, **786**
peripherally inserted central, **787**
Cation(s), **413,** 413t, *B-6*
exchange, fibers and, 110

see also specific cations
Catsup, H
sugar in, 129
Caucasians, lactose intolerance in, 115
Cauliflower
calcium in, *432*
natural toxicants in, 498
CCK. *See* Cholecystokinin
CD4+ T-lymphocyte, **949**
CDC (Centers for Disease Control), **486**
on aspartame safety, 136
Celiac disease, **741**-742, 743t
Celiac sprue, **741**
Cell(s), **A-0** to *A-1*
alpha, 119n
beta, 118n
elemental composition, B-5t
epithelial, **378**
fat, 162, *162,* 239
fluids and, 190-191, *191,* 412
folate and, 346
goblet, **79,** 379, 383
immune system, 809
intestinal, 83-86, *85*
metabolism in, 222, *222*
nucleus, A-0
vitamin A in differentiation, 378-379
zinc and, 467t
see also Red blood cells
Cell division, B vitamins in, 328-329, 346
Cell membrane, **A-0**
phospholipids in, *152*
selectively permeable, 412
Cell salts, 370t
Cellulite, **298**
Cellulose, 109
molecular structure, *109*
Centers for Disease Control. *See* CDC
Centimeters (cm), 7
Central Americans. *See* Hispanics
Central nervous system, **A-6**. *See also* Brain; Nerves/nervous system
Central obesity, **272**
diabetes and, 275
Central total parenteral nutrition, 786, **786**-787, 787t
Central veins, **786**
catheter advanced from peripheral vein into, 787
indications for TPN by, 787, 787t
used for TPN, 786
Cereals, H
choices, 45, 48-50
fat intake and, 168
folate in, 348
in food group plans, 41, *42*
fortified, 49-50
iron-enriched, 460-461
niacin in, *338*
riboflavin in, *335*
sodium in, 421
thiamin in, *332*
vitamin A in, *386*
vitamin B_6 in, *344*
see also Breads; Grains
Cerebellum, *250*
Cerebral cortex, **678**
Cerebral palsy, 721
Cerebrovascular accident (CVA), **897**
Cerebrum, *250*
Cerium, B-2t

Certification (pesticide inspections), **500**
Certified lactation consultants, 606
Ceruloplasmin, 472n
Cervical cancer, 936t
Cervix, **A-4**
Cesarean section, **589,** 594
Cesium, B-2t
Chaff, **45**
Chaparral, 370t
Charts. *See* Medical record
CHD. *See* Coronary heart disease
CHEC (Consumer Health Education Council), 367
Cheddar cheese, calcium in, *431*
Cheese, H
    cholesterol in, 152, 153t
    fat in, 168
    in food group plans, 40, 43
    lactose intolerance and, 115
    safety, 491
    tyramine-containing, 529t
    see also Milk and milk products; *specific type*
Cheilosis, 334t, 342t
Chelate(s), **463**
    amino acid, 446, **447t**
Chelating agent, **447t**
    EDTA, 455n
Chelation therapy, **689**
Chemical reactions, B-8 to B-9
    in body, 219-223
Chemical scoring (protein quality), **197,** J-1, J-2t
Chemistry, B-1 to B-10
    of aspartame, 135, *136*
    blood, 552t
    of carbohydrates, 102-111
    chemical structures, depiction of, 102-103, *103*
    of lipids, 141-154
    of nutrients, *5*
    of proteins, *180-182*, 180-183, 181t
    see also Laboratory tests; *specific substances*
Chemotherapy, **941**-942
    wasting and, 940t, 941-942
Chewing
    alleviation of problems in cancer, 947
    difficulties, 695t-697
Chewing gum
    for heartburn, 99
    nicotine, 527-528
Chewing tobacco, pregnancy and, 605
CHF (congestive heart failure), **895**-897
Chicken, H. *See also* Poultry
Child Care Food Program, 649
Children/childhood
    adverse reactions to foods, 644-645
    aspartame and, 135, 137
    behavior of, nutrition and, 125, 640-644, 643t
    calcium absorption in, 429
    cardiovascular disease assessment in, 662t
    cardiovascular disease development in, 658-660, *659*
    choking prevention in, 94
    cholesterol status in, 660, 661t, 661-662
    cow's milk introduction for, 634, 637
    with cystic fibrosis, 735
    diabetes in, 865, 866
    dietary recommendations for desirable weight, 662-663
    with disabilities, 721

eating habits of, 645-648, 647t
energy/nutrient needs, 638-639
fat intake, 660
food assistance programs for, 648t, 648-649. *See also* WIC (Special Supplemental Food Program for Women, Infants, and Children)
growth and development, 638. *See also* Growth
growth charts, 627
growth retardation, 546
head circumference, 545, 546
height measurement, 544-545
infusion pump and, 769, 789
iodine deficiency in, 470
iron absorption in, 455
iron deficiency in, 456, 457-458, 481-482
iron poisoning in, 460
iron-rich foods for, 641t
lead toxicity in, *480*, 480-484, 481t, *482*, 642
malnutrition in, 481-482, 640-642
meal planning for, 639, 640t
milk intake recommendations, 430
nutrition resources, F-3 to F-4
obesity and chronic disease development in, 658-663
PEM in. *See* Protein-energy malnutrition (PEM)
physical activity and weight, 660-661
with PKU, 841
protein RDI, 198n
smoking prevention in, 663
television's influence on, 292
toxicity from supplements in, 367
vegetarian, 211
vitamin A and, 380-381, 384
vitamin D and, 388, 389t
weight measurement, 545
weight trends, 660
zinc deficiency in, 466, *466*
see also Adolescents; Infant(s)
China/Chinese
    cuisine, 67-68
    hypertension in, 421
    selenium deficiency in, 471
    see also Asian Americans; Asians
Chinese restaurant syndrome, **507**
Chiropractic, **689**
Chloride, **423**
    amount in body, *418*
    deficiency, 423, 424t
    extracellular concentration, 413t
    food sources, 424t
    imbalance, 416
    intracellular concentration, 413t
    ion, 412, 413, 413t
    RDI, 55t
    recommendations, 423, 424t
    roles in body, 423, 424t
    sodium-depleting conditions and, 423
    tests, 552t
    toxicity, 423, 424t
Chlorine, 423, B-2t
    ion, B-6
    water treatment with, 515-516
Chlorocitric acid, 297n
Chlorophyll, **385**
Chocolate, 164
Choice system, Canadian, I-2 to I-14t
Choking, 94, *94, 95*

dysphagia and, 698, 699
infant risk of, 636-637
prevention in children, 646
Cholecalciferol, **387,** 389t
    IU conversion to micrograms of, 390
Cholecystokinin (CCK), 90n, **92**
    in fat digestion, 156
    malabsorption and, 709
Cholecystokinin-octapeptide, 297n
Cholesterol (blood), **152,** 158, 552t
    atherosclerosis and, 660, 884t
    "bad," 160. *See also* LDL (low-density lipoprotein)
    bile excretion and, 157
    calcium and, 428
    chemical structure, 152
    coronary heart disease risk and, 884t, 885
    desirable level, 164
    dietary cholesterol and, 153
    endogenous vs. exogenous, 154
    fiber and, 126-127, 157
    "good," 153. *See also* HDL (high-density lipoprotein)
    heart disease and, 164
    niacin and, 336
    screening for children, 661t, 661-662
    television and, 644
    trans-fatty acids and, 164
    see also Atherosclerosis; Cardiovascular disease (CVD); Fat; Heart disease
Cholesterol (dietary)
    Daily Reference Value, 56t
    effects on blood cholesterol, 153
    food sources, 152-153, 153t, H
    health and, 59, 61
    recommendations, 167, 169
Cholesterol-free (on labels), 57, 60t
Choline, **151,** 350-**351**
    toxicity, 351
Christians, dietary traditions, 69
Chromium, 450, 475-476, 476t, B-2t
    deficiency, 476, 476t
    food sources, 475-476, 476t
    RDI, 55t
    recommendations, 475-476, 476t
    roles in body, 475, 476t
    toxicity, 476t
Chromium picolinate, 370t
Chromosomes, **A-0.** *See also* Genetics/genes
Chronic, **2**
Chronic brain syndrome, **678**
Chronic diseases, **24,** *25*
    acute disease vs., 2
    childhood obesity and early development of, 658-663
    diet/lifestyle risk factors and, 24, 539-540, *540,* 541t
    see also Disease(s); *specific diseases*
Chronic gastritis, 704-705
Chronic malnutrition, 199, 807, 808t
Chronic obstructive pulmonary disease (COPD), **900**-901
Chronic pancreatitis, 733
Chronic PEM, **199**
Chronic renal failure, 916-927
    consequences, 917-920, *919,* 919t
    treatment, 920t, 920-927, 923t
Chronological age, **667**
Chylomicrons, 86, **159,** *161*
    in lipid transport, 158, *159*
Chyme, **73,** 76, 91

Chymotrypsin, in protein digestion, *185*
Cigarette smoking. *See* Smoking
Circulatory system(s)
  carbohydrate absorption and, 114
  enteropancreatic circulation, **464**
  folate and, 346, 347t
  liver, *826*
  in nutrient transport, 83, 86-90, *87-89*
  thiamin and, 330t
  vitamin A and, 382t
  vitamin B$_6$ and, 342t
  vitamin C and, 360t
  vitamin D and, 389t
  zinc and, 467t
  see also Lymphatic system
Cirrhosis, **246,** 828-834
  biliary, **828**
  cardiac, **828**
  consequences, *829,* 829-830
  diet therapy, 830-834, *833,* 833t
  drug therapy, 831
  Laennec's, **828**
  nutrition assessment in, 836-837
  postnecrotic, **828**
Cis-fatty acid, *147*
Citrus fruits, phytochemicals in, 406t
Clams
  canned, iron in, *462*
  riboflavin in, *335*
Classic phenylketonuria, *840,* 840-843
Claudication, intermittent, **393**
Clay eating. *See* Pica
Clear-liquid diets, 728t
Clients
  with feeding disabilities. *See* Feeding
    disabilities
  helping to accept oral formulas, 762
  helping to live with diabetes, 877-880
  helping to meet needs with ordinary foods,
    757
  perspective on hospital foodservice, 820
Climate, hunger and, 618
Clinical dietitian, responsibilities, 30, 31t
Clinical pathways, 960
Clinical trials, 11
Clinically severe obesity, **298**
Clostridium botulinum, 487, 489t, 636n
Clostridium perfringens, 488t
Clotting. *See* Blood clotting
cm (centimeter), 7
CoA (coenzyme A), **224**
  in metabolism, 224-231, *226-230,* 352, *353*
  see also Pantothenic acid
Coagulation. *See* Blood clotting
Cobalamin. *See* Vitamin B$_{12}$
Cobalt, B-2t
  vitamin B$_{12}$ and, 477, *477*
Cocaine
  in adolescence, 654
  pregnancy and, 604
Cocoa butter, 164
Coconut oil, 146, *146*
Cod
  potassium in, *425*
  vitamin E in, *395*
  see also Fish
Coenzyme(s), **222, 329**
  B vitamin, *328,* 328, 329, 352, *353. See also*
    specific vitamins
  folate, 342
  niacin, 334

riboflavin, 330, *333*
  structures, C-6 to *C-11*
  thiamin, 329
Coenzyme A. *See* CoA
Coenzyme Q$_{10}$ (ubiquinone), 351, 370t
Cofactor, **358**
  calcium as, 427
  iron as, 451
  manganese as, 473
  zinc as, 463
Coffee
  decaffeinated, 508
  iron absorption and, 455
  peptic ulcer and, 99
  see also Caffeine
Cola beverages, 114
  child behavior and, 644
  kcalories in, 252t
  nutrients in, 124t
  see also Caffeine; Carbonated soda
Colchicine, E-12t
Colds, vitamin C and, 11-13, 358-359
Colitis, ulcerative, 736, **744-745**
Collagen, **188,** 193
  bone formation and, 427
  copper and, 472
  in growth, 188
  tooth formation and, *427, 427*
  vitamin C in formation, 357-358, *358*
Collagenase, in protein digestion, *185*
Collaterals, 829-**830**
Colloid, hydrophilic, **727**
Colon (large intestine), *74,* **75,** 76
  adaptation after bowel resection, 752-754
  cancer. *See* Colon cancer
  in digestive process, 73, 76, *77, 81, 82*
  disorders, 742-749
  diverticular disease, *127, 128,* 742-744, *745*
  in fat digestion, *155*
  in fiber digestion, *112, 113*
  resections, 745-749, *746*
  residue, 759
Colon cancer, 403, 945t
  fiber and, 127
  methane gas production and, 98
  vegetarian diet and, 210
Colonic irrigation, **96,** 97
Color additives, 505, *506, 507*
Colorectal cancer, 936t
Colostomate, **747**
Colostomy, 745-749, *746,* **747**
Colostrum, **630**-631
Coma
  diabetic, **848,** 848-849
  hepatic, **830,** 831
  hyperosmolar hyperglycemic nonketotic,
    848, 849
Comatose, **797**
Combination foods, in exchange lists, G-13t to
    G-14t
Comfrey, 370t
Commercial baby foods, 636
  pureed foods vs., 697
Committee on Diet and Health, 14, 18
  dietary recommendations for health, 26, 27t
Committee on Dietary Allowances, 14, 15, 16,
    18
  carbohydrate recommendations, 128
  chloride recommendations, 423, 424t
  potassium recommendations, 424, 426t
  sodium recommendations, 419-420

Committee on Dietary Intakes, calcium recom-
    mendations, 445
Common cold, vitamin C and, 11-13, 358-359
Communication, professional, 578-579, 583
Community programs, hunger problems and,
    616t
Competent, **797**
"Complementary medicine," 693
Complementary proteins, **196**-197
Complete formulas, **757**
Complete protein, **196**
Complex carbohydrates, 27t, 102t, 107-111
  missed meals in IDDM and, 853
  weight loss and, 303
  see also Carbohydrate(s)
Compliance, dietary
  diagnostic tests and, 560
  renal diet, 923-925
Compound(s), **5,** B-1
  organic, 5
Concentration gradient, 414
Conception
  maternal weight prior to, 588-589
  nutrition prior to, 587-588, 597
Condensation, **105**
  disaccharide formation by, 105, *106*
  ketosis and, 242
  protein formation by, *182*
  triglyceride formation by, 142, *143*
Conditionally essential amino acids, **181**
Cones (of retina), **378**
Confectioners' sugar, **122**
Congestive heart failure (CHF), **895**-897
Congregate meal sites, 681, **683**
Consensus Conference on Osteoporosis, 447
Consent, informed, 799-802, *800, 801*
Consequences, in behavior modification, 305,
    306
Constipation, **96**-97
  diarrhea alternating with, 726
  iron supplementation and, 463
  during pregnancy, 595
  tube feeding and, 773t
Consumer(s), 51, 53
  concerns about foods, 486-513
  concerns about public water, 515-516
  education about labels, 61
  life-threatening misinformation about sup-
    plements, 367-369
  organizations, F-3
Consumer bill of rights, weight-loss, 294t
Consumer Health Education Council (CHEC),
    367
Contaminant(s), **495**-498
  aflatoxin, 201
  in bottled water, 517
  in breast milk, 610
  in calcium supplements, 446t
  dietary variety and, 38-39
  dioxins, 508, 516
  in drinking water, 516
  examples, 495-498
  harmfulness, 495, *496, 497*
  in herbal remedies, 692
  infant formula, 631, 633
  lead. *See* Lead
  pesticides, 499-502
  pregnancy and, 605
  see also Toxicity(ies)
Contamination
  cross-, 490, **492**

food-borne illnesses, 487-489, 488t-489t. *See also* Food-borne illnesses
water, 481, 516, 517
see also Contaminant(s)
Contamination iron, **461**
Contamination zinc, 468
Contraception
lactation and, 609
see also Oral contraceptives
Control group, 11-**12,** 13
Conversion factors, D-1
Cooking/food preparation
contamination iron and, 461
environmentally conscious, 623t
fat intake and, 168, 170
folate and, 347
in hospital, 823
niacin and, 337
safety and, *490,* 490-494, *492, 493,* 494t
thiamin and, 330
vitamin B$_6$ and, 342
vitamin C and, 362
vitamin E and, 394
COPD (chronic obstructive pulmonary disease), **900-901**
Copper, 450, 472-473, 473t, B-2t
amount in body, *418*
deficiency, 473, 473t
food sources, 473, 473t
RDI, 55t
recommendations, 473, 473t
roles in body, 472, 473t
toxicity, 473, 473t
zinc interactions, 369, 465-466, 468, 473
Cori cycle, 107n, **226**
Corn, H
biotechnology, 512, *512*
oil, H
protein in, 198
Corn flakes. *See* Cereals
Corn oil, *146*
vitamin E in, 394, *395*
Corn sweeteners, **122,** 129
Corn syrup, 105, **122,** 129
botulism and, 636
Cornea, **378**
Coronary artery bypass graft (CABG), **887**
Coronary heart disease (CHD), **164,** 882
dietary protection against, 905-908
fat and, 59, 61
fiber and, 61
physical activity and, 888-889
risk factors, 883-886, 884t
vegetarian diet and, 210
see also Atherosclerosis; Hypertension
Correlation (research), **12,** 13
Correspondence school, **30,** 31
accreditation, 31n
Cortical bone, **439,** 440
osteoporosis and, 440, 440t. *See also* Osteoporosis
Corticotropin-releasing hormone (CRH), A-3, A-4
Cortisol, stress and, 805t
Cost
alternative therapies and, 690-691
consideration for singles, 682
consideration in food choices, 3
consideration in supplement choices, 372
enteral formula, 759

home nutrition support and, 794
of obesity-related illnesses, 274
Cost-conscious health care, 959-961
Cottonseed oil, *123, 146*
Coughing, dysphagia and, 698
Coumadin. *See* Warfarin
Council on Postsecondary Accreditation, 31n
Counseling. *See* Nutrition education
Counterregulatory hormones, **805,** 862
Coupled reactions, **220**
Covert, **23**
Cow's milk
introduction in children, 634, 637
nutrients in, 632t
zinc absorption and, 464
see also Milk and milk products
Crab, zinc in, 469
"Crack" cocaine
adolescent use, 654
fetal effects, 604
Cramps, tube feeding and, 773t
Cravings
for nonfood substances. *See* Pica
pregnancy and, 596
Cream, calcium in, 430
Creatine phosphokinase, 552t, 894
Creatinine
accumulation in renal failure, 914, 917
serum, 552t
urinary excretion, 554-555
Creatinine-height index, 554, E-26, E-28t
Cretinism, **470**
CRH (corticotropin-releasing hormone), A-3, A-4
Crib death, **605**
Criminal behavior, sugar and, 125
Critical pathways, 960
Critical periods, **586-588,** *588*
Crohn's disease, **736-738**
Cross-contamination, **492**
prevention, 490
Cruciferous vegetables
phytochemicals in, 406t
see also Vegetables; *specific vegetables*
Cruzan, Nancy, 798-799
Crypts, **83,** *84*
Cues, in behavior modification for weight loss, 308-309
Cuisine, **64**
Cultural background. *See* Race/ethnicity
Cup (measure), 6
Curium, B-2t
CVA (cerebrovascular accident), **897**
CVD. *See* Cardiovascular disease
Cyanogens, 498
Cyanosis, **899**
Cyclamate, 133, 134t, **135,** 136
Cyclamic acid, 134t
Cyclic parenteral nutrition, **791**
Cysteine, 180n, 181t
in disulfide bridges, *182,* 435
sulfur in, 435
Cystic fibrosis, **733-736**
Cystine, 180n, 435
kidney stones composed of, 930, 932
Cystinuria, **930,** 932
Cytochrome C oxidase, 472n
Cytochromes, 451n
Cytokines, **805**
cancer cachexia and, 938
Cytoplasm, A-0

D (dextro), **393**
D-alpha-tocopherol, 393
Daily Food Guide, 40-44, 41t, *42-43*
adjustments for children, *43*
carbohydrates in, 129
energy intake for weight loss and, 302, 302t
for pregnant and lactating women, 593t
protein in, 205
for vegetarians, 211-212, 212t
Daily Reference Values (DRV), **55,** 56, 56t,
Daily Values (DV), **56-57,** G-1
inside front cover (right)
calculation of personal values, 57
for carbohydrates, 128
for fat, 171, 172
for fiber, 128
for protein, 198
see also Daily Reference Values (DRV), Reference Daily Intakes (RDI)
Dairy products. *See* Cheese; Egg(s); Milk and milk products
Dawn phenomenon, **862**
ddC (zalcitabine), 950
ddI (didanosine), 950
DDT, in breast milk, 610
De minimis rule, 504
Deamination, **195,** 231, 233, *233*
Death, **797**
alcohol and, 250
BMI and, *274*
deficiency and, 354
iron poisoning and, 460
leading causes, 24, *25,* 25t, 539t
obesity and, 293
SIDS, 604-605, 635n
Debridement, **811**
Decaffeinated coffee, safety, 508
Decubitus ulcers, **810**
Defecate/defecation, 73, **96.** *See also* Constipation; Diarrhea; Feces
Deficiency(ies), 16, *18,* 20
alcohol and, 251-252
B vitamin, 354-356
behavior and, 641-642, 643t
biotin, 339, 339t
brain function and, 679t, 679-680
calcium, 427t, 429, 432-433
chloride, 423, 424t
chromium, 476, 476t
copper, 473, 473t
Crohn's disease and, 737
development of, *22*
dietary adequacy and, 37
disease and, 540
fatty acid, 150
fluoride, 474t, 475
folate, 251-252, 346, 347t, *528*
iodine, 470, *470,* 471t
iron, 22-23, 37, 455-459, 457t, *458*
magnesium, 434t, 435
manganese, 473, 474t
niacin, 334, 336, 336t, *337,* 354
nickel, 477
older adults and, 670
panthothenic acid, 339, 340t
phosphorus, 433t
physical examination and, 22
potassium, 424, 426, 426t
primary, **22**
protein. *See* Protein-energy malnutrition (PEM)

riboflavin, 333, 334t
secondary, **22**
selenium, 471, 472t
sodium, 420t, 422-423
subclinical, **23**
sugar and, 123-124
supplements in, 366
thiamin, *329*, 329-330, 330t
trace minerals, 450
vitamin, 326
vitamin A, *380*, 380-383, *381*, 382t-383t, *384*
vitamin B$_6$, 341, 342t
vitamin B$_{12}$, 349-350, *350*, 351t
vitamin C, 356, 359-361, 360t
vitamin D, *388*, 388, 389t, 629
vitamin E, 392t, 393
vitamin K, 394, 396, 397t
zinc, 466, 467t, 640
see also specific nutrients
Deficient, **16**
Deforestation, hunger and, 618
Degenerative diseases. *See* Chronic diseases
Dehydration, **410**
alcohol and, 250-251
chloride toxicity and, 423
diabetes and, 848
diarrhea and, 96, 724, 725
oral rehydration therapy in, 416
physical activity and, 284
physical signs, 536t
salt tablets and, 423
tube feeding and, 773t
vomiting and, 95
see also Hydration
Dehydroepiandrosterone (DHEA), 297, **689**
Delaney Clause, **503-504**
Delta-9-tetrahydrocannabinol (THC), 653n
Dementia
HIV infection and, 952
niacin and, 354
senile, **678**
Denaturation, **183,** 184
Dental caries, **124**
fluoridation and, 474-475
magnesium and, 434
prevention, 124-125, 474-475
prevention in children, 647, 647t
sugar and, 124-125
see also Teeth
Dental plaque, **124**
Dental soft diet, **696**-697, *698*
Dentin, 427, *427*
Dentures, 669
Deoxyadenosylcobalamin, 347
Deoxyribonucleic acid. *See* DNA
Deoxythymidine kinase, 463n
Department of Education, 31, F-2
Department of Health and Human Services. *See* DHHS
Dermatitis
niacin and, 336, 336t, *337*, 354
see also Skin
Desiccated liver, 370t
"Devastating *D*s," pellagra and, 354
Developing countries
hunger in, 616-621
infant formula in, 631, 633
iron loss in blood and, 455-456
kwashiorkor and marasmus in, 199, 200
night blindness in, 381
vitamin A deficiency in, 380, 381

Development. *See* Children/childhood; Growth
Dexfenfluramine, weight loss and, 297
Dextrins, **111**
Dextroamphetamine, E-12t
Dextrose, 104, **122.** *See also* Glucose
in intravenous solutions, 783, 785, 787
Dextrose monohydrate, **783**
d4T (stavudine), 950
DHA. *See* Docosahexaenoic acid
DHEA (dehydroepiandrosterone), 297, **689**
DHF (dihydrofolate), 342
DHHS (Department of Health and Human Services), national nutrition assessment and, 23
Diabetes Control and Complications Trial, 861
Diabetes mellitus, 120, **846-871,** 877-880
acute complications, 848-850, *849*
borderline, **851**
calcium and, 428, 445
cardiovascular disease and, 850, 885
in children, 865, 866
chronic complications, 850-851
client education about, 877-880
consequences, 847-851
coping with, 879
disorders related to, 847
gestational, **599,** 869-870
glycemic effect and, 121
hyperglycemia management in, 862-864, 863t
hypoglycemia management in, 863t, 864-865
insulin-dependent, 877-880
insulin-dependent vs. noninsulin-dependent, 846t, 846-847
lactation and, 609
medical vs. personal needs and, 877
nicotinamide and, 336
obesity and, 275
in older adults, 870-871
oxidative stress in, 402
pancreatitis and, 733
physical activity in, 856-858, 859t
preexisting in pregnant woman, 598-599, 868-869, 870
screening for, 851
starch in, 127
sugar alcohols and, 138
treatment, 851-868
vitamin E and, 402
see also Glucose
Diabetic coma, **848,** 848-849
Diagnosis, **578**
Diagnostic tests, nutrition status and, 559-560, 810
Dialysis, 915, **916,** 920t
Diaminozide (Alar), 500
Diaphragm, hiatal hernia and, *700-701*
Diarrhea, **96**
alternating with constipation, 726
causes, 724
dumping syndrome and, 708
in dysentery, 202
HIV-associated, 954
intractable, **724**
lactose intolerance and, 115
niacin and, 354
nutrition care plan and, 563
osmotic, **724**
in ostomates, 747
secretory, **724**
severe, 724-725

traveler's, 489t, 494
treatment, 724-725
tube feeding and, 773t, 774
in ulcerative colitis, 744
in zinc deficiency, 466
Diary, weight loss and, 305, *306*
Didanosine (ddI), 950
Diet(s), **2**
assurance of compliance before diagnostic tests, 560
for athletes, 285-286
bland, 705t
after bone marrow transplant, 948
breath tests and, 560
cancer and, 404, 936-938
constipation and, 97
coronary heart disease protection and, 905-908
disease risk and, 24, 539-540, *540*, 541t, 885
drugs and dietary restrictions, 529
ethnic, 2, 63-69, **64**
fad, 294-295
fat-restricted, 728-729, 729t, 730, 733, 893
fluid-restricted, 923t
gluten-restricted, 742, 743t
glycogen storage and use and, 280
health and, 24-27, 539-540, *540*, 541t
high-carbohydrate, *280*, 281-282
high-fat, 165, 166-167
high-fiber, 127-128, 460, 744
HIV infection and, 953-954
hyperactivity and, 643-644
illness or death related to, 25
individual approach, 26-27
intestinal adaptation and, 752-753
lactose-restricted, 115-116
liquid, 728t. *See also* Enteral formulas
low-carbohydrate, 243
low-fat, 170, 303, 888t
low-phenylalanine, 841-843
low-potassium, 424
low-sodium, 833t
macrobiotic, **210, 689**
mechanical soft, **696**-697, 698
Mediterranean, 64-65, 213-216
modified, **567,** 568t-569t
nutrition status affected by, 531t
oxalate-restricted, 931
peptic ulcer and, 99
physical endurance and, 280, *280*
population approach, 26, 27t
postgastrectomy, **708**-709, 710t
protein-restricted, 177
protein use during activity and, 283
purine-restricted, 932
reflux esophagitis and, 701-702
renal, 920-925
standard, **567**
tyramine-controlled, 529t
urinary creatinine excretion and, 554
vegetarian. *See* Vegetarian diets
very-low-kcalorie, 299-301, 300t
weight-loss, 605
see also Diet therapy
Diet aids
ineffective, 298n
see also Weight loss; *specific type*
Diet and Health recommendations, 26, 27, 27t
calcium, 447
protein, 203
sodium, 420

Diet history, 21, **531**
  forms for recording, *521, 532, 534-535*
  liver disorders and, 836
  in nutrition assessment, 520t, 531-536
  overeating and, 291
  upper GI tract disorders and, 713
Diet-induced thermogenesis, **261,** 265
Diet manual, **567**
Diet order, **566**-567
Diet planning, 37-59, 567, 570-575
  chronic renal failure and, 923, 924
  diabetes and, 854-856, 857t
  dietary guidelines and, 39t, 39-40
  exchange lists in, 574t, 574-575, 575t
  fat malabsorption and, 730
  food group plans, *40-44,* **40**-45, 46-47
  grocery shopping and, 45, 48-51
  for obesity treatment, 301-303, 302t
  perceptions vs. actual intakes and, 44
  principles, 37-39
  vegetarian, 211-213, 212t
Diet therapy, 519
  for atherosclerosis, 887, 887t, 888t
  for cancer, 944-948, 945t
  for chronic obstructive pulmonary disease, 900
  for chronic renal failure, 920-925
  for cirrhosis, 830-834, *833,* 833t
  for congestive heart failure, 896-897
  for Crohn's disease, 737-738
  for diabetes (IDDM), 852-856, 857t, 858
  for diabetes (NIDDM), 866-867
  for diabetes in pregnancy, 870
  for dysphagia, 699
  for galactosemia, 843
  after gastric partitioning, 711-712
  after heart attack, 895
  for hepatitis, 828
  in hospital, 820-824, *821-822*
  for hypoglycemia, 872-873
  for indigestion and reflux esophagitis, 701-702
  for kidney stones, 931-932
  after kidney transplant, 925t, 925-926
  for nausea, 703, 704
  for nephrotic syndrome, 912-913, 914
  for pancreatitis, 733
  for PKU, 841-842
  for respiratory failure, 899
  for severe diarrhea, 724-725
  during stress, 811-817
  after stroke, 897-898
  for ulcerative colitis, 745
  for vomiting, 703
  see also Medical nutrition therapy
Dietary adequacy, **37,** 495
  balance and, 38
  during weight loss, 302
Dietary balance, **37**-38
Dietary Guidelines for Americans, 39t, 39-40
  on fat, 170
Dietary moderation, **38**
  alcohol and, 246-247
Dietary Reference Intakes. *See* DRI
Dietary Supplement Health and Education Act of 1994, 372, 691
Dietary variety, **38**-39
  nutrient absorption and, 92-93
Dietetic technician registered (DTR), **30,** 31
Dietitian(s), **30**
  clinical, 30, 31t

on health care team, 581, 582, 583
  nutrition education planning by, 562-563
  registered, **21, 30,** 30n, 961
  responsibilities, 30-31, 31t
  responsibility for nutrition education, 576
Dietitians of Canada, F-4
Differentiation (cell), **378**
  vitamin A in, 378-379
Diffusion, 83, 85, 114n
Digestibility, protein, **197**
Digestion, **72**-93, *82*
  absorption and. *See* Absorption
  of carbohydrates, 82, 91, 111-116, *112, 114*
  common problems, 94, 94-100, *95*
  conditions for optimal functioning, 92-93
  energy required for, 265
  enteral formula and, 760
  of fats, 82, 91-92, 154-157, *155-157*
  of fiber, 81, 82
  final stage in process, 80-81
  illness and, 523
  in intestines, 80, *82*
  in mouth, 79, *82*
  muscular action of, 76-78, *77*
  organs involved in, 72-76, *74*
  of proteins, *82,* 184, *185*
  rate of, 92
  regulation of, 90-93
  secretions of, 78-80, *79, 80,* 81t
  in stomach, 79-80, *82*
  transport and. *See* Transport
  see also GI (gastrointestinal) tract
Digestive enzymes, *79,* 80
  pancreatic release of, 91-92
Digestive juices, 79-80, 91-92. *See also* Gastric juice
Diglyceride, **154**
Dihydrofolate (DHF), 342
Dihydroxy vitamin D, 389t
Dihydroxyphenyl isatin, 97n
Diketopiperazine (DKP), **135,** 136
Dioxins, **508**
  chlorinated water and, 516
Dipeptidases, **184**
Dipeptide, **182.** *See also* Protein/amino acids (in body)
Direct calorimetry, **258,** *259,* **261**
Disabilities. *See* Feeding disabilities
Disaccharides, 102t, 103, **105**-107
  structure, C-2
Disease(s)
  acute, 2
  antioxidants in prevention, *400,* 400-405, *401, 405,* 406t
  belching as sign of, 98
  BMI values and risks of, *274,* 274-275
  body fat distribution and, 272
  in breastfeeding mothers, 609
  calcium in prevention, 427-428
  chronic, 2, **24,** 25
  diet and, 539-540, *540,* 541t
  dietary recommendations and, 26-27, 27t
  food label claims about, 58-61, 60t
  hereditary susceptibility to, 26-27
  nonnutrients in prevention, 405, 406t
  obesity and, 274-275, 540, 658-663
  during pregnancy, 598-600
  proteins in defense against, 192-193
  resources, F-6 to F-7
  risk factors, 24-26
  risk reduction with supplements, 367

  vitamin C in prevention, 359
  see also Illness; *specific diseases*
Dispensable amino acids, **181**
Dissociation, **412**
  of salt in water, 412-413
Distance Education and Training Council, 31n
Distention, tube feeding and, 773t
Distilled liquor, **246,** 252t
Distilled water, **516**
Disulfide bridges, *182,* 435
Dithiolthiones, 406t
Diuretic(s), **297,** E-10t
  in acute renal failure, 916
  beverages acting as, 411
  in hypertension treatment, 894
  and nutrient excretion, 529
  potassium deficiency and, 426n, 894
  weight loss and, 295-297
Diuretic phase (acute renal failure), **914**
Diverticula, **127,** *128,* 742
Diverticular disease, 742-744, 745
Diverticulitis, **127,** 743
Diverticulosis, **127,** 743, 744
DKP (diketopiperazine), **135,** 136
DNA, 182n
  biotechnology, 512
  heavy metal effects on, 516
  protein synthesis and, 186, *187*
  use as ergogenic aid, 370t
DNA polymerase, 463n
Docosahexaenoic acid (DHA), 148-**149**
  food sources, 150t
Documentation. *See* Medical record
DOE (Department of Education), 31, F-2
Dolomite, 446, **447t**
Dominant gene, **839**
Dose levels, effects of, 341, *343*
Double-blind experiment, **12,** 13
"Dowager's hump," 440, *441*
Down syndrome, **601**
DRI (Dietary Reference Intake), 19, inside front cover (left)
  calcium, 427t, 429-430, 594
  fluoride, 474t
  magnesium, 434t
  phosphorus, 433t
  pregnancy and, 594
  vitamin D, 389t, 594
Dried fruits, contamination iron in, 461
Drink(s)
  alcoholic, **246,** 252t, 853. *See also* Alcohol
  see also Beverages
Drinking water. *See* Water
Driving, alcohol and, 254
Dronabinol, 942
Drug(s), **246**
  abuse by adolescents, 652-654
  for acute renal failure, 916
  administration through feeding tubes, 769-771
  alcohol with, 249
  antihypertensive, 893-894
  for arthritis, 677
  breastfeeding and, 609
  cancer therapy, 940t, 941-942
  in cirrhosis treatment, 831
  food intake and, 526, 527t
  herbs vs., 691-692
  for HIV infection, 950
  immunosuppressant, 925
  lactose in, 116

lipid-lowering, 889
lipid-lowering in children, 663
nutrient interactions with. *See* Drug-nutrient interactions
nutrition problems in abusers of, 654
in peptic ulcer treatment, 99
peptic ulcers due to, 99, 705
pregnancy and, 604
resources on abuse, F-4
in stress treatment, 810-811
weight loss and, 295-298
Drug history, 21, 520t, *521*, **525**-530, E-0
Drug-nutrient interactions, 525-530, E-1t to E-12t
calcium and tetracycline, 446t
classes of medications involved in, 526t
effects on nutrition status, 810-811
enteral formulas and, 769, 770t, 771, 774
folate and, 346, 528, *528*
mechanisms of, 527t
metabolic effects, *528*, 528-529, 529t
mineral oil and, 97
potassium and, 424, 426
vitamin C and anticoagulants, 361n
vitamin E and insulin, 402
vitamin K and anticoagulants, 396
DRV (Daily Reference Values), **55**, 56, 56t
DTR (dietetic technician registered), **30**, 31
Dumping syndrome, 706-708, **707**, *707*
postgastrectomy diet and, 708-709, 710t
Duodenal ulcer, **96**, 99, 705-706
Duodenum, 73, **75**
hormones from, A-6
surgery in obesity treatment, 298, 298-299
Durable power of attorney, **797**, *801*, 801-802
Duration (physical activity)
effect on fat use, 282
effect on glycogen use, 281
effect on protein use, 283
fuels used and, 281t
recommendations for fitness, 278t
recommendations for health, 278t
recommendations to lose fat, 282, 283
DV. *See* Daily Values
Dwarfism, 466
Dynamometer, 550
Dysentery, **202**
Dyspepsia, **699**-702
Dysphagia, **697**-699, 717
cancer and, 947
stroke and, 897
Dysprosium, B-2t
Dysuria, **930**

E. *coli*, 488, 489t
Ear stapling, 296
Earth Summit, 621
Eating disorders, 311, 315-323, **316**
in athletes, 315, 316-317, *317*
resources, F-4 to F-5
societal context of, 315, 321-322
unspecified, 315, 321, 322t
see also Anorexia nervosa; Bulimia nervosa
Eclampsia, **600**
Economic considerations. *See* Cost; Socioeconomic history; Socioeconomic status
Edema, **191**
in ascites, 830
in beriberi, 329
in kwashiorkor, 201
in nephrotic syndrome, 912

in preeclampsia, 599
pulmonary, 899
sodium and, 423
Edentulous, **696**
EDTA (ethylenediamine tetra acetate), 455n, 689
iron absorption and, 455
Education
consumer, 61
dietitian, 31-32
in medical schools, 29
see also Nutrition education
Egg(s), H
cholesterol in, 152, 153, 153t
protein in, 198, 198t
riboflavin in, *335*
safety, 490, 491, 494t
substitutes, 153
Egypt, zinc deficiency in, 466, *466*
Eicosanoids, **148**
Eicosapentaenoic acid (EPA), 148-**149**, C-4t
arthritis and, 677
food sources, 150t
see also Omega-3 fatty acid
Einsteinium, B-2t
Elaidic acid, *147*
Elastase, in protein digestion, 185
Elbow breadth, body frame and, E-21t
Elderly. *See* Older adults
Electric muscle-stimulating (EMS) devices, 296
Electrolyte(s), **413**, 413t
balance, **202**. *See also* Fluid and electrolyte balance
cystic fibrosis and, 735
pancreatitis and, 732
replacement, 416
solutions, **413**
tests, 552t
water attraction by, 413-414, *414*
water following, 414, *415*
see also Mineral(s); *specific electrolytes*
Electron transport chain, **227**, *227*, 235-236, *236*, C-16 to C-17t
cell and, A-1n
iron and, 451
Elements, **5**, B-1, B-2t
composition of living cells, B-5t
inorganic, 418
in nutrients, 5
Ellagic acid, 406t
Embolism, **883**
Embolus, **883**
Embryo, **585**
stages of development, *587*
Emetic(s), **316**
in bulimia nervosa, 320
Emotions
digestion and, 92, 100
food choices and, 3
nutrition status and, 524-525
ostomates and, 748-749
transition from IV feeding and, 791-792
see also Mental disturbances; Psychological problems; Psychological stress
Emphysema, **900**
Empty-kcalorie food, **123**-124
"Empty" kcalories, 38
EMS (eosinophilia myalgia syndrome), 206
EMS (electric muscle-stimulating) devices, 296
Emulsification, process of, *156*
Emulsifiers, **78**

bile, 80, 92, 156, *156. See also* Bile
lecithin as, 151
Encephalopathy
hepatic, **830**
portal systemic, **830**
End-stage renal disease, **917**. *See also* Chronic renal failure
Endocrine, A-2
Endocrine glands, **78**. *See also* Hormone(s)
Endocrine pancreas, modified diet for conditions affecting, 569t
Endocrine system, A-2
Endocrinology, **A-1**
Endogenous cholesterol, **154**
Endogenous protein, **194**
Endometrial cancer, 936t
Endopeptidases, **184**
Endoplasmic reticulum, A-1
Endosperm, **45**
Endurance
aerobic activity and, 279
diet effect on, 280, *280*
muscle, **282**
Enemas, for constipation, 97
Energy, **6**, H
for activities, 263-265, 267, 279-284, *280*, 281t
acute renal failure and, 915
adequate, 204
adolescent needs, 651
amino acids and, 194-195
B vitamins and, 328
balance, *257*, 257-258
in body. *See* Energy metabolism
breaking down of nutrients for, 224-238. *See also* Energy metabolism
budget, 238-244, *239*, *241*, *242*
cancer and, 944
childhood needs, 638-639
chronic renal failure and, 920t, 921
cirrhosis requirements, 831
control, **38**
cystic fibrosis requirements, 734
declining needs with aging, 671-673
deficiency, 20
diabetic diet and, 852
diet patterns for different intakes, 574t
excess, 9, 20, *239*, 239-240, *241*, 540, 541t
exchange lists and, 574t
expenditure. *See* Energy expenditure
fat and, 162-163, 166, 172t
food group plans and, 41, 41t
in foods, 7-8, 258, *261. See also* Energy-yielding nutrients
foods dense in, 310
genetic influences on expenditure, 290
infant requirements, 621
lactation and, 607
longevity and, 668
measures of, 6-7. *See also* kCalorie(s)
needs during stress, 812t, 812-815
nephrotic syndrome and, 912-913
nutrient density and, 38, 41, *42*
nutrition care plan and needs for, 562
for physical activity in iron deficiency, 458
pregnancy and, 591
RDA estimation based on physical activity, 266t
recommendations, 15
recommendations for weight loss, 301-302
respiratory failure and, 899

restriction and longevity, 668
units, D-3
Energy expenditure, 261-266
  body composition and, 274
  components, *262*, 262-265, *263*, 263t, 264t
  energy requirement calculation and, 265t,
    265-266, 267
  estimation, 266t
  genetics and, 290
  physical activity and weight loss, 304
  resting, **262**
  water requirements and, 411
Energy metabolism, 8-9, **219**-244
  alcohol's interference with, C-17 to C-18
  B vitamin coenzymes in, 352, *353*
  central pathways, *237*
  energy budget and, 238-244, *239*, *241*, *242*
  fasting and, 240-244, *241*, *242*
  fat and, 148, 227, *228*, *229*
  feasting and, *239*, 239-240, *241*
  fiber and, 113
  glucose and, 117
  hormones regulating, A-4 to A-5
  phosphorus and, 433
  riboflavin and, 330, 334t
  thiamin and, 329, 330t
  transfer of energy in chemical reactions,
    220-221
  triglycerides and, 148
Energy-yielding nutrients, **6**-10
  activity and, 279-284, *280*, 281t
  in breast milk, 627t, *629*
  in cow's milk, 627t
  in infant formula, 627t, *631*
  metabolism, summarized, 234-238, 236t,
    236-238
Enriched, **45**
Enrichment, grain products, 45, 48-49, 460-461
Enteral formulas, 727, **756**-771, 779-781, K-1,
  K-2t to K-8t
  administration, 767-769
  availability, 761
  caution for using, 758
  complete, 757
  delivery techniques, 768
  distinguishing characteristics, 758-759
  drug absorption and, 771
  drugs incompatible with, 770t
  inappropriate delivery, 774
  inappropriate selection, 772
  potential problems, 779
  preparation, 767
  provided orally, 761
  selection, 760, 760-761
  stress and, 815
  transition to table foods from, 775
  types, 758
  water in, 769
  see also Nutrition formulas; Tube feedings
Enteral nutrition, 756-781
  in acute renal failure, 916
  in chronic renal failure, 923
  in Crohn's disease, 737
  in diabetes, 853
  ethical issues, 797-802, *800*, *801*
  formulas, 727, 756-781, K-1, K-2t to K-8t
  home, 736, 794
  after intestinal surgery, 741
  in pancreatitis, 733
  in respiratory failure, 900
  in severe diarrhea, 725

see also Enteral formulas
Enteric hyperoxaluria, **728**
Enteritis, radiation, **941**
Enterogastrones, **90**-92
Enterohepatic circulation, **157**
Enterokinase, 185n
Enteropancreatic circulation, **464**
Enteropathy
  AIDS, **952**
  gluten-sensitive, **741**-742, 743t
  protein-losing, **737**
Enteropeptidase, in protein digestion, *185*
Enterostomal therapist (ET), **749**
Enterostomy, **764**
Environment
  cancer and, 935-936
  contaminants in. *See* Contaminant(s)
  hunger and, 618-619
Environmental Defense Fund, 483n
Environmental Protection Agency (EPA), **486**
  lead toxicity and, 483-484
  National Pesticide Hotline, 502n
  nutrition resources from, F-2
  pesticides and, 499-500
  water supply and, 483, 516-517
Environmental temperature
  BMR and, 263t
  consistency of fats at room temperature, 145-
    146
  physical activity and, 284
Environmentally conscious foodways, 3, 622,
  623t
Enzyme replacements, **730**
  in cystic fibrosis, 735
  in pancreatitis, 733
Enzymes, **189**
  assisted by zinc, 463
  in carbohydrate digestion, *112*, 113
  copper-requiring, 472
  digestive, *79*, 80, 91-92
  in energy metabolism, 222
  in fat digestion, 156, 157
  hormones vs., 79
  in lactose intolerance management, 115-116
  in liver disease, 827
  magnesium and, 434
  manganese and, 473
  metalloenzymes, 463, 473
  in protein digestion, 184, *185*
  proteins as, *189*, 189-190, *190*
  serum, 552t
  see also specific enzymes
Eosinophilia myalgia syndrome (EMS)
  hotline, 206n
  tryptophan supplements and, 206
EPA. *See* Eicosapentaenoic acid; Environmental Protection Agency
Epidemiological studies, 11
Epigastric, **699**
Epiglottis, 73, *74*, **75**
Epinephrine, **119**, 194, A-4
  in blood glucose regulation, 119
Epithelial cells, **378**
  vitamin A and, 383
Epithelial tissues, **378**
  vitamin A and, 383
Erbium, B-2t
Ergocalciferol, **387**
Ergogenic aids, used by athletes, 205, 369,
  370t-371t
Erythrocyte, **393**. *See also* Red blood cells

Erythrocyte hemolysis, **393**
Erythrocyte protoporphyrin, **456**, E-30t
Erythropoietin, **911**, A-5, E-12t
  and kidney function, 919-920
ESADDI (Estimated Safe and Adequate Daily
  Dietary Intakes), 15
Escherichia coli, 488, 489t
Esophageal stricture, **700**
Esophageal ulcers, **700**
Esophageal varices, **830**
  cirrhosis and, 829-830
  diet therapy in, 834
Esophagitis, reflux, **700**, **700**-702, 702t, 703
Esophagus, **74**, **75**
  cancer, 403, 936t, 945t
  in digestive process, 73, 76
  disorders, 697-702, *701*, 702t
  hiatal hernia, 700-*701*
  hiatus, **701**
Essential amino acids, **181**, 181t. *See also* Pro-
  tein/amino acids; *specific amino acids*
Essential fatty acids, **148**-151, *149*, 150t. *See
  also* Fatty acid(s); *specific acids*
Essential hypertension, **889**
Essential nutrients, **5**, 149
Estimated Safe and Adequate Daily Dietary
  Intakes (ESADDI), 15
Estrogen(s), 441n, A-6
  bone mass and, 442
  calcium requirement and, 445
  cancer and, 275
  phytochemicals and, 406t
ET (enterostomal therapist), **749**
Ethanol, 245, *245*, **246**
  entry into metabolic path, C-18
  see also Alcohol
Ethical, **797**
Ethical issues
  cancer treatment, 945
  nutrition care, 797-802, *800*, *801*
Ethnic diets, 2, 63-69, **64**
  food group plans, 44
  see also Race/ethnicity
Ethyl alcohol, 102-103, *103*, 245, **246**. *See also*
  Alcohol
Ethylenediamine tetra acetate. *See* EDTA
Euphoria, **246**
  drug use and, 654
Europium, B-2t
Excellent source (on labels), 60t
Exchange lists, **45**, **570**-575, 571t
  diabetic diet and, 854, 855-856, 857t
  diet prescriptions using, 574t, 574-575, 575t
  food group plans combined with, 574
  food groupings, 570-571
  food mixtures in, 574, *574*
  meals and, 57t, 575
  portion sizes, 571t, *572-574*
  U.S. system, G-6t to G-14t
  see also Choice system, Canadian
Excretion
  acid-base balance regulation by, 416-417
  drug-nutrient interactions and, 527t, 529
  illness effects on, 524
  vitamin D and, 389t
  see also Urine; *specific substances*
Exercise
  blood glucose and, 856-857
  breastfeeding and, 607
  to build muscles, 311
  cardiovascular benefits, 888-889

moderate, **282**
older adults and, 672-673
passive, 296
before pregnancy, 597
during pregnancy, 590t, 590-591
thermogenesis induced by, 261
see also Athletes; Physical activity
Exercise-induced thermogenesis, **261**
Exhaustion (stress response), 668
Exocrine, **A-2**
Exocrine glands, **78**
Exogenous cholesterol, **154**
Exogenous protein, **194**
Exopeptidases, **184**
Expectations, for weight loss, 301
Experimental group, 11-**12**, 13
External cue theory, **261**
Extra lean (on labels), 60t
Extracellular fluid, **409**, 412
electrolytes in, 413t
Exudate, **804**
Eyes
aging and, 669, 676-677
cataracts, 676-677
in childhood malnutrition, 643t
iron deficiency and, 457t
in nutrition assessment, 537t
riboflavin and, 334t
vitamin A and, 376-378, *377*, 382t
zinc deficiency and, 467t

Face
in childhood malnutrition, 643t
examination in nutrition assessment, 537t
features in fetal alcohol syndrome, *602, 603*
Facilitated diffusion, 83, *85*, 114n
FAD (flavin adenine dinucleotide), **330**, *333*, 352, *353*
Fad diets, 294-295
FAE (fetal alcohol effects), **601**
Faith healing, **689**
Fajita, 67
False negative, **361**
False positive, **361**
Family
anorexia nervosa and, 315-316
bulimia nervosa and, 319
lifestyles, diabetic child and, 975
see also Genetics/genes
Family medical history
nutrition recommendations and, 539, 541t, *542*
see also Genetics/genes
Family tree, medical, *543*
FAO (Food and Agricultural Organization), 20, **486**, F-3
pesticides and, 501
protein-digestibility-corrected amino acid score, 198
reference protein standard, 197
FAS. *See* Fetal alcohol syndrome
Fast foods
adolescents and, 652
hazards, 488
nutrients in, 652t
vitamin A and, 385
Fasting
BMR and, 263t
fat metabolism and, 163
metabolic effects, 240-244, *241, 242,* 806, *806*

protein-sparing, 243-244
responses to stress vs., 806-807
transition from feasting to, 240, *241*
see also Anorexia nervosa
Fasting blood glucose, 851
Fasting hypoglycemia, 872t, **872**-873
Fat (in diet), 145-147, H
alternatives, 176-178, 177t
bile in digestion of, 92
blood cholesterol and, 164
body fat and, 160, 162, *162*, 166-167
in breast milk, 629
cancer and, 59, 61, 165-166
cardiovascular disease and, 59, 61, 164-165
chemistry of, *5*
in choice system, I-11t
chronic renal failure and, 924
cirrhosis and, 832
constipation and, 97
in Daily Food Guide, 39, *43*
Daily Reference Value, 56t
Daily Value, 171, 172
diabetes and, 853
energy intake and, 172t
ethnic cuisines and, 63, 65, 67
excess, 9, 239-240
excessive restriction of, 167
in exchange lists, *570-571, 571t, 573,* G-11t
exercise and, *280,* 282-283
fatty acid compositions, *146*
food labeling and, 60t, 61, 170-171
fried foods and, 170
health effects of, 59, 61, 163-167, *166*
hydrogenation of, 147, *147*
intravenous emulsions, 784, 790-791
kcalories in, 8, 166, *166,* 258
kilojoules in, 8n
in meats, 50, 168, 169
Mediterranean diet and, 213, *214*
nephrotic syndrome and, 912
obesity and, 166-167
oxidation of, *146, 230,* **230**-231, 238
physical activity and, 282
in poultry, 50, 168
processed, 146
rate of digestion, 92
recommendations, 27t, 56t, 149-150, 167-172, 233
recommendations for older adults, 673
replacements, 176-178, 177t
restriction, 728-729, 729t, 730, 733, 893
sources, *166*
Southern cuisine, 65-66
during stress, 815
substitutes, 176-178, 177t
visible vs. invisible, 170
weight gain and, 310
weight loss and, 302
Fat-based fat replacements, 177t, 177-178
Fat cells, 162, *162*
development, 288-289, *289*
enlargement due to feasting, 239
metabolism, 290
Fat-free (on labels), 60t
Fat-free ice cream, 177
Fat/lipids (in body), **141**-172
abdominal, **272**
amino acids and, 195, 233
cellulite and, 298
chemistry of, 141-154
composition, 163n

coronary heart disease risk and, 885
digestion, absorption, and transport, 82, 91-92, 154-160, *155-158. See also* Absorption; Digestion; Transport
distribution, 272
emulsification by bile, 156, *156*
emulsified particles, 158
energy and, 166
exercise and, 281t, 282-283
fasting and, 163
glucose conversion to, 118
high-fat diet and, 166-167
ideal amount, 271-274
intra-abdominal, **272**
kcalories in, 257
ketone bodies and, 117
loss vs. weight loss, 243
measures, 548-550
metabolism. *See* Fat metabolism
nephrotic syndrome and, 912
phosphorus-containing. *See* Phospholipids
physical activity and, 282-283
stress effects on metabolism, 815
structure, C-4t
subcutaneous, 272
upper-body, **272**
see also Atherosclerosis; Body composition; Cardiovascular disease (CVD); Cholesterol; Heart disease; Lipoprotein
Fat malabsorption, 727-731
blind loop syndrome and, 710
diagnosis, 559
treatment of, 728-731, 729t
Fat metabolism, 160-163, *161, 162*
acetyl CoA and, 227, *228, 229*
fasting and, *241*
liver in, 223t
physical activity and, 282-283
zinc toxicity and, 468
Fat modules, K-8t
Fat-soluble vitamins, 327, 375-398
water-miscible, 732
water-soluble vitamins vs., 328t
see also Vitamin(s); *specific vitamins*
Fatfold measures, **273**, *273,* 548-550, E-23 to E-26t
Fatty acid(s), **142**-145, *142-146,* 144t
alcohol and synthesis of, 249
chain length of, 142
chemical structure vs. glucose structure, *238*
chemistry of, 141-151
cis-, 147
deficiencies, 150
degree of saturation, 142-145
dietary fat composition, *146*
essential, **148**-151, *149,* 150t
heart disease and, 164
intestinal adaptation and, 752-753
long-chain, 158
medium-chain, 158
micelles and, 158
role in metabolism, 229-231, *230-231*
roles in nutrition, 148
short-chain, 113n, 158, 752-753
stress and, 815
structure, C-4t
trans-, 147, **147,** 164-165, 170
vitamin E and, 393
see also Fat
Fatty acid oxidation, *230,* **230**-231, 238
Fatty liver, **246,** 249, 827

in kwashiorkor, 201
FDA (Food and Drug Administration), **486**
 additives and, 503-505, 506, 507-508
 artificial sweeteners and, 133, 136, 137
 bottled water and, 517
 fat substitutes and, 176-178
 folate recommendations, 346, 588
 food labeling, 51-61. *See also* Labeling
 food safety concerns, 486
 garlic preparations and, 405
 gastric balloons and, 299
 GRAS list, 176, 405, 503
 herbal remedies and, 691-692
 infant formula and, 628
 lead and, 480
 listing of ineffective diet aids, 298n
 medical food and, 779, 780
 nutrition resources from, F-2
 pesticides and, 499, 500-501
 protein supplements and, 205
 radiation and, 510, 511
 Retin-A and, 384
 Seafood Hotline, 490
 sugar alcohols and, 138
 sulfites and, 506
 supplements and, 372, 404
 trace minerals in supplements and, 450
 weight loss aids and, 297, 298
Feasting, 239, 239-240, 241
 transition to fasting from, 240, 241
 see also Overnutrition
Feces, **81**
 fiber and, 113, 127
 see also Constipation; Diarrhea
Federal agencies. *See specific agencies*
Federal Trade Commission (FTC), F-2
Feedback mechanisms, 91
Feeding(s)
 artificial, **797**
 bolus, **768**
 intermittent, **768**
 selection of method, 756
 transitional after parenteral nutrition, 791
Feeding devices, 719, 720
Feeding disabilities, 716-721, 719, 720t-721t
 assessment, 717, 718t
 conditions leading to, 716t
 independent eating with, 717-720
 stroke and, 897
Feeding tubes, 761
 clogged, 773t
 drug administration through, 769-771
 insertion methods, 762-763
 placement sites, 764, 764-766, 765t
 transnasal, 765-766
 see also Tube feedings
Female athlete triad, 317, 317
Fermentation, **246**
 fiber, 110n, 113
Fermium, B-2
Ferric iron, **451,** B-7
 copper and, 472
Ferritin, **192, 455**
 mucosal, **452**
 serum, E-31t
Ferrous iron, **451,** B-7
 copper and, 472
Ferroxidase II, 472n
Fertility, **597**
 malnutrition and, 597
 underweight and, 274

Ferulic acid, 406t
Feta cheese, riboflavin in, 335
Fetal alcohol effects (FAE), **601**
Fetal alcohol syndrome (FAS), 253t, **601**-604
 facial features, 602, 603
Fetor hepaticus, **830**
Fetus, **586**
 bone development, 594
 cell growth, 593
 critical periods of development, 586-588,
  588
 growth and development, 585-586, 587, 598
 lead toxicity to, 480
 malnutrition and development of, 598
 stages of development, 587
 teratogenic substances and, 601-605
 tooth development, 594
 see also Infant(s); Pregnancy
Fever, **813**
 BMR and, 263t
 energy needs and, 812t, 813, 814
Few (on labels), 60t
Fewer (on labels), 60t
Fiber(s), 9, **108**-111, **759,** H
 blood cholesterol and, 157
 calcium absorption and, 429
 cancer and, 127
 classification, 110-111
 constipation and, 97
 crude, 109n
 Daily Reference Value, 56t
 Daily Value, 128
 dietary, 109n
 digestion, 81, 82, 112, 113
 effects of adequate intake, 129
 excess, 127-128, 129
 fermentation, 110n, 113
 food labels and, 61
 health effects of, 61, 126-128
 heart disease and, 126-127, 905
 insoluble, 110, 111t
 iron absorption and, 453, 455
 mineral absorption and, 92-93, 113
 neutral-detergent, 109n
 physical properties, 110
 recommendations, 16, 56t, 128-130
 soluble, 110, 111t
 sources, 110, 111t, 128-129, 129t
 weight control and, 126
Fiberall, 727
Fibrin, 193
Fibrocystic breast disease, **393**
Fibrosis, 246, **733**
 cystic, **733**-736
 fatty liver and, 249
 osteitis, **918**
Fibrous, **733**
"Fight-or-flight," epinephrine and, 119
Filtrate, **911**
Fish, H
 cardiovascular health and, 165
 choices, 50-51
 in food group plans, 42
 mercury contamination of, 496-497, 498
 MFP factor in, 453, 454
 omega-3 fatty acids in, 149-150, 150
 protein in, 198
 raw, 493
 recommendations, 169
 safety, 493
 smoked, 421

in voluntary labeling program, 52, 53t
 see also specific type
Fish oil
 arthritis and, 677
 heart disease and, 906-907
 supplements, 169, 907
 see also Omega-3 fatty acid
Fisheries, diminishing, 619
Fistula, **732**
 Crohn's disease and, 736-737
 pancreatitis and, 732
Fitness, 278-286, **282**
 aging and, 667
 benefits, 278-279, 279t
 physical activity and, 278t, 278-279
 resources, F-5
 see also Exercise; Physical activity
"Flaky paint" dermatitis, 337
Flapping tremor, **830**
Flavin adenine dinucleotide (FAD), **330, 333,**
  352, 353
Flavin mononucleotide (FMN), **330**
Flavonoids, 405, 406t
Flavor enhancers, **505,** 507. *See also* Spices
Flaxseed, phytochemicals in, 291t
Flora, intestinal. *See* Intestinal flora
Flour, **45**
Flow phase (stress response), **806**
Fluid(s), 409-417
 accumulation in ascites, 830
 blood pressure and exchange of, 890
 calcium in, 427
 chewing difficulties and, 697
 cirrhosis and, 832
 cystic fibrosis and, 735
 dialysis and requirements for, 920t
 extracellular, **409,** 412
 intake for weight gain, 311
 interstitial, **409**
 intracellular, **409,** 412
 in ostomates, 747
 pancreatitis and, 732
 replacement, 416
 replacement in athletes, 284-285, 285t
 retention, 536t
 retention in chronic renal failure, 917
 see also Dehydration; Fluid and electrolyte
  balance; Water
Fluid and electrolyte balance, **190,** 412-415
 acute renal failure and, 915
 in bulimia, 96
 chronic renal failure and, 924-925
 imbalance, 415-416
 maintenance, 414
 in nutrition assessment, 536
 PEM and, 202
 physical activity and, 284-285, 285t
 proteins in regulation of, 190-191, 191, 414
 respiratory failure and, 899
 severe stress and, 811
 tube feeding and, 773t
Fluid ounces, 6
Fluid-restricted diet, 923t
Fluorapatite, **474**
Fluoridated water, 474-475, **516**
Fluoride, 450, 474t, 474-475
 deficiency, 474t, 475
 food sources, 474t, 475
 infant supplements, 630t
 osteoporosis and, 445, 475
 recommendations, 27t, 474t, 475

roles in body, 474, 474t
supplements, 445
teeth and, 427, 474-475, 475, *475*
toxicity, 474t, *475, 475*
Fluorine, B-2t
Fluorosis, 474t, *475*, **475**
Fluoxetine (Prozac), in bulimia nervosa, 321
FMN (flavin mononucleotide), **330**
FNB. *See* Food and Nutrition Board
Folacin. *See* Folate
Folate, 342-343, 345, H
  absorption, *345*
  activation, *345*
  alcohol and, 251-252
  anemia after gastrectomy and, 711
  blind loop syndrome and, 710
  chronic renal failure and, 920t, 922
  concentrations, E-31t
  deficiency. *See* Folate deficiency
  drugs affecting metabolism of, *528*
  food sources, 346, 347t, *348*
  grain products fortified with, 346
  heart disease and, 906
  homocysteine and, 906
  pregnancy and, 345-346, 587-588, 593
  RDA, 347t, 587
  RDI, 55t
  recommendations, 345, 347t, 368t
  supplements, 367
  supplements in pregnancy, 345, 587-588
  toxicity, 347t
  vitamin B_{12} and, 346, 349, 354
  women and, 345-346
Folate deficiency, 346, 347t
  birth defects and, 345-346
  vitamin B_{12} deficiency and, 349
Folic acid. *See* Folate
Follicle, A-3
Follicle-stimulating hormone (FSH), A-3
Follicular hyperkeratosis, *384*
Fontanel, 389t
Food(s), **4**
  additives. *See* Additives
  adverse reactions, 644-645
  agencies monitoring supply, 486
  associations influencing choices in, 3
  availability of, 3
  biotechnology, 493-494, 511-513
  in bone marrow transplant recipients, 948
  breast milk flavor and, 608
  causing diarrhea, 724
  choices, reasons for, 2-4, 63-69
  choices after gastric surgery, 712
  choices during pregnancy, 591, 593t, 596
  choices for adolescents, 652
  choices for children, 645-648, 647t
  choices for infants, 636
  choices for older adults, 681-684
  choices for optimal nutrient absorption, 92-93
  choices for weight gain, 310
  choices for weight loss, 301-303, 302t
  choking risk and, 94
  composition, 4, H
  convenience of, 3
  cooking. *See* Cooking/food preparation
  Crohn's disease and, 737
  digestion of. *See* Digestion
  drug interactions with. *See* Drug-nutrient interactions
  economic factors in choices, 3

effects on laboratory values, 559-560
empty-kcalorie, **123**-124
energy-dense, 310
energy in, 7-8, 258, *261*
energy required to manage digestion, 265
environmentally conscious choices, 3
exchange lists. *See* Exchange lists
fat in, 145-147. *See also* Fat (in diet)
fortification. *See* Fortification
frequency checklist, **532**, 534-535
gas-producing, 98, 725t
helping clients meet needs with, 757
imitation, **51**
intake and activity in IDDM, 858
intake and insulin therapy, 860
intake data analysis, 21, 533-536
intake determinants, 258-261, *260*
intake during drug therapy, 526, 527t
intake during illness, 523
intake history, *532*
intake improvement in cancer, 946-947
introduction in infants, 634-637, 635t
iron-enriched, 460-461
labeling. *See* Labeling
low-fat, 170, 171, 172
low-fat and weight loss, 302
medical, 779, 780
natural toxicants in, 498-499
nutritional adequacy. *See* Dietary adequacy
observation of intake, 533
odors, 493
for ostomates, 746-748
packaging. *See* Packaging
portions for weight gain, 310
preparation of. *See* Cooking/food preparation
processed. *See* Processed foods
production and environmental problems, 618-619
production limitations, 619
pureed, **696**, 697
safety, 486-513, F-3
serotonin in, 559-560
socioeconomic factors in choices, 530t
specific dynamic activity, **265**
specific dynamic effect, **265**
storage for safety, 490, *491, 492*, 494t
storage for vitamin C preservation, 362
storage time in refrigerator, 494t
stroke complications affecting intake, 897
substitute, **51**
thermic effect of, **265**
transition from formulas to, 775
transition from IV feeding to, 791-792
variety. *See* Variety
see also Diet(s); Food sources; Nutrient(s); *specific foods or nutrients*
Food, Drug, and Cosmetic Act, Food Additive Amendment, 503-504
Food allergies, **644**-645
  foods commonly causing, 645
  in infants, 635-636
Food and Agricultural Organization. *See* FAO
Food and Drug Administration. *See* FDA
Food and Nutrition Board (FNB), 15, 19
  on supplements, 404
  see also National Research Council
Food and Nutrition Information Center, F-2
Food assistance programs, 615-616. *See also* WIC (Special Supplemental Food Program for Women, Infants, and Children)
  for children, 648t, 648-649

for older adults, 681, 683
for pregnant women, 597
Food aversion, **596**
  avoidance in cancer, 947
Food-borne illnesses, **487**-494, 488t-489t
  danger signs, 493
  meat and, 490, *490*, 492, *492*, 494t
  precautions against, 493-494
  prevention, 490-491
  relative safety of different foods and, 493
  seafood and, 493
  travel and, 494
Food chain, **495**
  bioaccumulation of toxins in, 495, *496*
"Food combining," myth of, 85-86
Food consumption survey, **23**
Food craving, **596**
Food diary, weight loss and, 305, *306*
Food group plans, **40**-44, *40-45, 46-47*
  exchange lists combined with, 574
  see also Daily Food Guide
Food Guide Pyramid, 40, 41, *43*, 44
Food Guide to Healthy Eating, Canada's, 44-45, *46-47*
Food-hypersensitivity reactions, **644**. *See also* Food allergies
Food industry lobbyists, nutrition recommendations and, 216
Food insecurity, **614**
  identification, 615
Food intolerances, **644**
Food intoxication, **487**, 489t. *See also* Food poisoning
Food myths
  alcohol myths, 254t
  "food combining," 85-86
  sugar and energy, 114
Food poisoning, **487**
  kwashiorkor and, 201
  see also Food-borne illnesses; Toxicity(ies); *specific toxins*
Food records, **533**
Food Research and Action Center, F-2
Food sources
  antioxidants, 404-405, 406t
  arachidonic acid, 150t
  aspartame, 137t
  B vitamin, 356. *See also specific B vitamins*
  beta-carotene, 382t
  biotin, 339
  calcium, 38, 427t, 430-432, *431, 432*
  chloride, 424t
  cholesterol, 152-153, 153t
  chromium, 475-476, 476t
  fat, *166*
  fibers, 110, 111t, 128-129, 129t
  fluoride, 474t, 475
  folate, 346, 347t, *348*
  insoluble fibers, 110, 111t
  iodine, 470, 471t
  iron, 37, 453, *453*, 457t, 460, *462*, 641t
  lactose, 116
  lignin, 110
  magnesium, 434t, *436*
  manganese, 473, 474t
  molybdenum, 476, 476t
  niacin, 336t, 337, *338*
  omega fatty acids, 149-150, 150t
  oxalic acid, 429
  pantothenic acid, 340
  pectin, 109

phospholipids, 152
phosphorus, 433t
phytic acid, 111, 429
phytochemicals, 406t
potassium, 424, *425*, 426t
protein, 44, 196
retinol, 382t
riboflavin, 333, 334t, *335*
selenium, 472t
single nutrients in, 331. *See also specific nutrients*
sodium, 420t, 421-422
soluble fibers, 110, 111t
stearic acid, 164
sulfur, 437t
thiamin, 330, *330*, 330t, *332*
trace minerals, 450
trans-fatty acid, 147
vitamin A, 382t, 384-387, *385*, *386*
vitamin B₆, 341-342, 342t, *344*
vitamin B₁₂, 350, 351t
vitamin C, 360t, *362*, *363*
vitamin D, 389t, *390*
vitamin E, 392t, *394*, *395*
vitamin K, 397, 397t
vitamin solubility and, 327
water, 410, 410t
zinc, 467t, 468, *468*, *469*
Food Stamp Program, **614**, 616
Foodservice
in hospital, 820-824, *821-822*
hunger solutions and, 622
for older adults, 681, 683
Foodways, **64**
environmentally conscious, 3, 622, 623t
ethnic. *See* Ethnic diets
meat-restricted, 209-216. *See also* Vegetarian diets
Formaldehyde, aspartame metabolism and, *136*
Formulas
enteral, **727**. *See also* Enteral formulas
infant. *See* Infant formulas
liquid diet, 299-300
oral rehydration, 725
parenteral, **727**
protein preparations for weight loss, 243-244
for weight gain, 311
Fortified/fortification, **45, 49**
calcium, 432
folate, 588
ready-to-eat breakfast cereals, 49-50
vitamin A, 385
vitamin D, 390
Fossil fuel, **614**
Four Food Group Plan, 40
Foxglove leaves, 692
Fractures
osteoporosis and, 439. *See also* Osteoporosis
stress, **316**
Frame size, **268**, *E-20* to *E-21t*
Francium, B-2t
Fraud, 29, **30**, 31-32, 33-34
Free (on labels), 60t
Free foods, in exchange lists, G-12t
Free radical(s), **402**
antioxidants and, *401*. *See also* Antioxidant(s); *specific antioxidants*
body's defenses and, 400-402, *401*
cataracts and, 677
chain reaction and damage, *401*
formation, 400, *401*, B-9 to B-10

manganese and, 473
oxidative stress due to, 402
oxygen-derived, 400n
French cuisine, 63-64
Frequency (physical activity), recommendations for fitness, 278t
Fresh (on labels), 57
Freshly (on labels), 57
Fried foods, fat in, 170
Frozen foods, safe storage temperature, 490
Fructose, 103, **105**
absorption, 114n
chemical structure, *105*
conversion to glucose, *114*
sucrose and, 106
Fruit(s), H
calcium in, *431*
cancer and, 61, 403, 404-405
in choice system, I-5t to I-7t
choices, 50
dried, 461
in exchange lists, 571t, *572*, G-7t
fat intake and, 168, 169-170
fiber in, 129t
folate in, *348*
in food group plans, 41, *42*, *46*, *47*
health claims on labels and, 61
iron in, *462*
irradiated, 510
lignin in, 110
magnesium in, *436*
niacin in, 338
nonnutrient compounds in, 405, 406t
pesticide residues on, *499*. *See also* Pesticides
phytochemicals in, 406t
potassium in, 424, *425*
riboflavin in, *335*
sugar in, 103. *See also* Fructose
sugar vs., 123
thiamin in, *332*
vitamin A in, *385*, *386*
vitamin B₆ in, *344*
vitamin C in, *362*, *363*
vitamin E in, *395*
in voluntary labeling program, 52, 53t
weight loss and, 302
zinc in, *469*
Fruit seeds, cyanogens in, 315
Fruit sugar, **105**. *See also* Fructose
FSH (follicle-stimulating hormone), A-3
FSH/LH—releasing hormone (FSH/LH—RH), A-3
FTC (Federal Trade Commission), F-2
Fuel, fossil, **614**
Full-liquid diets, 728t
Fungicides, 499-502

g (gram), 6, 7
Gadolinium, B-2t
Galactose, 103, **105**, 109n
chemical structure, *105*
conversion to glucose, *114*
Galactosemia, **839**, 843
Gallbladder, *74*, **75**, 81t. *See also* Bile
Gallium, B-2t
Galvanized, **468**
Gamma-interferon, 805
Gamma-linolenic acid, 148n
Gamma-tocopherol, 393n
Gamma waves, 510n
Gangrene, **848**

diabetes and, 851
Garbanzo beans
folate in, *348*
vitamin E in, *395*
Garlic, 405
phytochemicals in, 406t
Garlic oil, **689**
Gas, 98
foods producing, 98, 725t
ostomates and, 747-748
Gastrectomy, *706*
diet after, 708-709, 710t
dumping syndrome after, 706-708, *707*
malabsorption after, 709-710
Gastric acid, peptic ulcers and, 705
Gastric acidity, 79-80
Gastric balloons, 299
Gastric bypass, *298*
Gastric glands, **78**, 81t
Gastric-inhibitory peptide, 90n, **92**
Gastric juice, **78**, 81t
in digestion, 79-80
reflux esophagitis and, 700, 701
Gastric lipase, **79**
Gastric partitioning, 298-299, 706, 711-712
Gastric residual, **768**
Gastric surgery, 706-712
Gastric ulcer, **96**, 99, **705**-706
Gastrin, **91**, A-6
Gastritis, **704**-705
atrophic, **349**, 669, 705
Gastroesophageal reflux, **700**-702
Gastroesophageal sphincter, **701**. *See also* Cardiac sphincter
Gastrointestinal hormones, 90-92, A-6
Gastrointestinal tract. *See* GI tract
Gastroparesis, **848**
Gastroplasty, *298*
Gastrostomy, **764**, 765t
Gatekeepers, **645**
Gelatin
aspartame content, 137t
use as ergogenic aid, 370t
Gender differences
puberty and, 650-651
see also Men; Women
General adaptation syndrome, **668**
Generally recognized as safe (GRAS) list, 176, 405, **503**
Genetics/genes, **839**
cancer and, 934
dietary recommendations for health and, 26-27
energy expenditure and, 290
food biotechnology and, 511. *See also* Biotechnology
inborn errors of metabolism and, 839-844
nutrient effects and, 4
osteoporosis and, 443
vitamin B₁₂ deficiency and, 349
weight and, 289-290
Geophagia, **458**
Geriatrics. *See* Older adults
Germ, **45**
Germanium, 370t, 691, B-2t
Gestation, **585**
Gestational age, birthweight and, 598
Gestational diabetes, **599**, 869-870
GFR. *See* Glomerular filtration rate
GH (somatotropin), **A-3**. *See also* Growth hormone

GH-inhibiting hormone (GIH), A-3
GH-releasing hormone (GRH), A-3
GI (gastrointestinal) tract, **72**, 696
 aging and, 669
 anatomy, 72-76, *74, 77*
 anorexia nervosa and, 317
 bleeding detection, 559
 calcium supplements and problems in, 446t
 cells in absorptive process, 83-86, *85*
 in childhood malnutrition, 643t
 in chronic renal failure, 918
 disease and iron absorption, 455
 factors in health of, 92-93
 factors influencing function, 90
 fiber and health of, 127, *128*
 in fluid and electrolyte regulation, 415
 folate deficiency and, 343, 345, 347t
 HIV infection and, 952t, 952-953
 hormones, 90-92, A-6
 iron and, 559
 lower GI tract disorders, 723-749
 modified diet for conditions affecting, 568t
 niacin and, 336t
 pantothenic acid and, 340t
 specialization in, 85
 stress effects on, 807-808
 stress effects on immune function, 808-810,
  809t
 upper GI tract disorders, 695-713
 very-low-kcalorie diet side effects in, 300t
 vitamin A and, 383t
 vitamin C and, 360t, 559
 vitamin E toxicity and, 392t
 zinc and, 467t
 see also Digestion; *specific organs*
Giardia lamblia, 488t
Giardiasis, 488t
GIH (somatostatin), **A-3**
Ginseng, 370t
Girth, abdominal, 836
Gland(s), **78**
 in childhood malnutrition, 643t
 in digestion, 78-80, *79, 80,* 81t
 endocrine system, *A-2*
 in nutrition assessment, 537t
 in zinc deficiency, 467t
 see also specific glands
Gliadin, **742**
Gliomas, **934**
Global environment, problems in, 614-622,
  623t. *See also specific problems*
Glomerular filtration rate (GFR), **911**
 in acute renal failure, 914
 in chronic renal failure, 917, 918
Glomerulonephritis, **916**
Glomerulus, 88, **911**
Glossitis, 355
 B vitamin deficiencies and, 355
 folate and, 347t
 niacin and, 336t
 riboflavin and, 334t
 vitamin B_6 and, 342t
 vitamin B_{12} and, 351t
Glucagon, **118**, 191t, A-4
 in blood glucose regulation, 119, *119*
 stress and, 805t
Glucocorticoid, **A-4,** A-5
Glucogenic amino acids, 195n, 226, 232-233
Glucomannan, 296
Gluconeogenesis, **117**, 195, 231, 813
Glucose, 102, 103, **104**

absorption, 114, 120-121
 Alzheimer's disease and, 678
 behavior and, 641
 brain and, 240-241
 catabolism, 224-228
 chemical structure, *104, 105*
 chemical structure vs. fatty acid structure,
  238
 depletion with activity, 281
 disaccharide formation from condensation,
  106
 in energy metabolism, 224-228, *225-229*
 enzymes in breakdown, 189-190
 glycogen and. *See* Glycogen
 metabolism. *See* Glucose metabolism
 physical activity and, 280-282
 retrieval via Cori cycle, 226
 stress response, 806
 sucrose and, 106
 see also Blood glucose; Diabetes mellitus
Glucose control, measurement, 861
Glucose metabolism, 116-121
 B vitamin coenzymes in, 352, *353*
 balance sheet, C-17t
 chromium and, 475, 476t
 conversion to fat, 118
 energy and, 117
 fasting and, 240-241
 fat in, 148
 ketone bodies and, 117
 magnesium and, 434
 physical activity and, 280-282
 protein and, 117
 see also Diabetes mellitus
Glucose tolerance, **847**
 impaired, 851
Glucose tolerance factor (GTF), **475**
Glucose tolerance test, 559
Glucosuria, **848**
Glucuronic acid, 109n
Glutamate, folate and, 342-343
Glutamic acid, 181t
Glutamine, 181t
 bone marrow transplant recipients and, 948
 in enteral formulas, 780
 intestinal adaptation and, 752, 753
 in intravenous solutions, 783
 stress and, 806
Glutathione peroxidase
 selenium and, 471
 vitamin E and, 471
Gluten, **45,** 742
Gluten-restricted diets, 742, 743t
Gluten-sensitive enteropathy, **741**-742, 743t
Glycated hemoglobin, glucose control and, 865
Glycemic effect, **120**-121
 sugar alcohols and, 138
Glycerol, **141**, *141,* 158
 and ethanol compared, 245
 fasting and, 241
 role in metabolism, *229,* 229-230, 231
 in triglyceride formation, 142, *143*
Glycine, 181t
 chemical structure, 180, *181*
 use as ergogenic aid, 370t
Glycogen, 102, **107,** *108,* C-2
 activity duration effect on use, 281
 activity intensity effect on use, 280
 child behavior and, 641
 diet effect on storage and use, 280
 glucose stored as, 104, 116-117. *See also*

Glucose
 training effect on use, 282
Glycolysis, 224-**225,** *225, C-12* to *C-13*
 cell and, A-1n
Glycosuria, **848**
 diabetes and, 848
Glycosylated hemoglobin, **861**
Goat's milk
 folate and, 346
 infant feeding with, 633
Goblet cells, **79**
 vitamin A and, 379, 383
Goiter, **470,** *470*
Goitrogens, **470,** 498
Gold, B-2t
Golgi apparatus, **A-1**
"Good" cholesterol, 153. *See also* HDL (high-
  density lipoprotein)
Good Health Eating Guide (Canada), I-2 to I-14t
Good source of (on labels), 60t
Gout, **246,** 930
 vitamin C and, 360t, 361
Government agencies. *See specific agencies*
Graft-versus-host disease (GVHD), **942**-943
Grains
 calcium in, *431*
 choices, 45, 48-50
 enrichment, 45, 48-49, 460-461
 fat in, 169-170
 fiber in, 129t
 folate in, 346, 348, 588
 in food group plans, 41, *42, 46, 47*
 iron in, 460, *462*
 magnesium in, *436*
 moldy, and kwashiorkor, 201
 niacin in, *338*
 phytochemicals in, 406t
 potassium in, *425*
 riboflavin in, *335*
 thiamin in, *332*
 vitamin A in, *386*
 vitamin B_6 in, *344*
 vitamin C in, *363*
 vitamin E in, 394, *395*
 weight loss and, 302
 whole, **45**
 zinc in, 469
 see also Breads; Cereals
Grams (g), 6, 7
Granulated sugar, **122**
Granulomas, **736,** 804-805
Grapefruit juice
 potassium in, *425*
 vitamin C in, *363*
Grapes
 phytochemicals in, 406t
 sulfites in, 506, *506*
GRAS (generally recognized as safe) list, 176,
  405, **503**
Grazing, **120**
 blood cholesterol and, 154
Greek cuisine, 64-65
Green beans
 calcium in, *431*
 folate in, *348*
 iron in, *462*
 magnesium in, *436*
 potassium in, *425*
 riboflavin in, *335*
 zinc in, *469*
Green peas

thiamin in, *332*
zinc in, *469*
GRH (GH-releasing hormone), A-3
Grip strength, 550
Groundwater, 515
 bottled waters from, 517
Growth
 during adolescence, 650-651
 BMR and, 263t
 charts, *627*, 638, *E-12 to E-20*
 during childhood, 638
 chronic renal failure and, 918-919
 measures, 544-548, 546t, 548t
 nutrient needs during infancy and, 626, 628
 during pregnancy, 585-588, *587*, *588*
 proteins and, 188-189
 retardation, 466, 546, 640
 vitamin A in, 379
 vitamin D in, 387-388
 zinc and, 466
Growth hormone (GH), 191t, A-3, A-4
 aging and, 669n
 intestinal adaptation and, 753
 stress and, 815-816
Growth hormone releasers, 370t
GTF (glucose tolerance factor), **475**
Guar, 110
 gum, as weight-loss product, 298
Guarana, 370t-371t
Gum, chewing
 for heartburn, 99
 nicotine, 527-528
Gum arabic, 110
Gums (food), 110
 blood cholesterol and, 157
Gums (mouth)
 in childhood malnutrition, 643t
 niacin deficiency and, 336t
 in nutrition assessment, 537t
 riboflavin deficiency and, 334t
 vitamin C deficiency and, 360t, *361*
"Gynoid" obesity, 272

Habit
 food choices and, 2
 see also Lifestyle choices
Hafnium, B-2t
Hair
 in childhood malnutrition, 643t
 in nutrition assessment, 537t
Hair follicle, **383**
Halibut
 magnesium in, *436*
 niacin in, *338*
 see also Fish
Halogen, organic, **495**
Ham
 niacin in, *338*
 thiamin in, *332*
 zinc in, *469*
Hamburger
 nutrients in, H
 safety, 490, 492
 see also Meat(s)
Hand grip strength, 550
Hard liquor, **246**, 252t
Hard water, 435, **516**
Harris-Benedict equations
 for BMR determination, 267n
 energy needs during stress and, 812t, 814
Hazard, **486**

HCG (human chorionic gonadotrophin hormone), 296
HCl. *See* Hydrochloric acid
HDL (high-density lipoprotein), **159**-160, *161*
 coronary heart disease risk and, 884t, 885
 desirable blood level, 164
 LDL ratio to, 160, 885
 monounsaturated fats and, 164
 polyunsaturated fats and, 164
Head and neck, cancer, 945t
Head circumference, 545, 546
Health care facilities
 professional communications in, 578-579
 see also Hospital
Health care professionals
 perspective on alternative therapies, 692-693
 role in home nutrition support, 794
Health care system, cost consciousness and,
  959-961
Health care teams, 581-583, *582*
 diabetes and, 877
Health claims (on labels), **58**-61, 60t
 fat and, 171
 foods providing antioxidants, 404-405
 supplements and, 372
Health food stores, misinformation from, 367-
  368
Health history, **522**
 in nutrition assessment, 21, 520t, *521*, 522-
  525
 see also Historical data
Health maintenance organization (HMO), **959**
Health resources, F-6 to F-7
Health status
 diet and, 24-27, 539-540, *540*, 541t
 physical activity and, 278, 278t
 see also Disease(s)
Healthy (on labels), 60t
Healthy People 2000, **23**, G-4, G-5t
 on breastfeeding, 606
 on calcium during adolescence and young
  adulthood, 652
 on calcium during adulthood, 675
 on calcium during pregnancy and lactation,
  594
 on calcium intake, 430
 on complex carbohydrates, 128
 on dietary guidelines, 40
 on fat, 167, 170
 on fiber, 128
 on growth retardation in children, 640
 on home foodservices for older adults, 681
 on iron deficiency in children, 641
 on iron deficiency in women and children,
  456
 on labeling, 52, 61
 on nursing bottle tooth decay, 633
 on nutrition assessment, 23, 24
 on overweight, 288, 301
 on salt and sodium intake, 420
 on school meals, 648
 on school nutrition education, 650
 on worksite programs for nutrition education
  and weight management, 307
Heaney, Robert, 443
Heart, 86, *87*, *882*. *See also* Cardiovascular system
Heart attacks, **894**-895
 magnesium and, 435
 silent, 850
Heart disease

 alcohol and, 253t
 antioxidants and, 403-404
 fiber and, 126-127
 fish oil and, 906-907
 French cuisine and, 63-64
 iron and, 459-460
 lipoproteins and, 160
 magnesium and, 435
 Mediterranean diet and, 64-65
 protein and, 202
 rheumatic, **894**
 risk factors, 164
 selenium deficiency and, 471
 sugar and, 125
 vitamin C and, 403-404
 vitamin E and, 403, 905
 see also Atherosclerosis; Cardiovascular disease (CVD); Cholesterol; Coronary
  heart disease (CHD)
Heart failure, congestive, **895**-897
Heartburn, **96**, 98-99
 during pregnancy, 595-596
 reflux esophagitis and, 701
Heat energy, kcalorie as unit of, 258
Heat stroke, **282**, 284
Heavy metal, **495**
 in drinking water, 516
 see also specific metals
Height, 544-545
 BMI and, 271t
 BMR and, 263t
 creatinine-height index, 554, E-26, E-28t
 loss in osteoporosis, 440, *441*
 metric measurements, 7
 and weight ranges based on BMI, inside back
  cover
 and weight tables/charts, 268-270, 269t, 546,
  547, E-21t to E-23
 zinc deficiency and, 466
Heimlich maneuver, 94, *95*, **96**
Helicobacter pylori, 704
 peptic ulcer and, 99n, 705
Helium, B-2t
Helpers, roles in feeding disabilities, 720-721
Hematocrit, **456**
 in iron deficiency, 456
 tests, 552t
Hematuria, **930**
Heme, **453**
Heme iron, 453, *453*, *455*
 lead and, 480, *481*
 see also Iron
Hemicelluloses, 109
Hemlock, **689**, 691
Hemochromatosis, **459**
Hemodialysis, **916**, 920t
Hemoglobin, **183**, 192
 glycated, 861
 in iron deficiency, 456
 iron in, 451
 in sickle-cell anemia, 188
 tests, 552t
Hemolysis, **393**
 erythrocyte, **393**
Hemophilia, **394**
Hemorrhagic disease, **394**
Hemorrhoids, **96**
 fiber and, 127
 during pregnancy, 595
Hemosiderin, **455**
Hemosiderosis, **459**

Hepatic, **826**
Hepatic artery, 829
Hepatic coma, **830**
   cirrhosis and, 830
   dietary guidelines, 831
   proteins and, 831-832
Hepatic encephalopathy, **830**
Hepatic steatosis, **827**
Hepatic vein, **87,** 87, 829
Hepatitis, **827**-828
   food-borne, 488t
Hepatitis A virus, 488t
Herbal medicine, **689,** 691-692
Herbal steroids, 371t
Herbicides, 499-502
Herbs, as salt alternative, 421
Heredity. *See* Genetics; Genetics/genes
Hernia, hiatal, 700-**701,** *701*
Heroic measures, living wills and, 799
Heroin, fetal effects, 604
Herpes virus, **952**
Hesperidin, 351
Hexoses, **102**
HFCS (high-fructose corn syrup), 105, **122**
5-HIAA (5-hydroxyindoleacetic acid), urinary,
   559-560
Hiatal hernia, 700-**701,** *701*
Hiatus (esophageal), **701**
Hiccups, **96,** 98
High (on labels), 60t
High, drug use and, 654
High blood pressure. *See* Hypertension
High-carbohydrate diet
   athletes and, 280, 281-282, 285, 286
   carbohydrate loading and, 281-282
High-density lipoprotein. *See* HDL
High-fat diet
   cancer and, 165
   in children, 660
   obesity and, 166-167
High fiber (on labels), 60t
High-fiber diet
   complications of, 127-128
   diverticular disease and, 744
   iron and, 460
High-fructose corn syrup (HFCS), 105, **122**
High potency, **372**
High-protein, high-kcalorie formulas, 311
High-quality protein, **197**
High-risk pregnancy, 596t, **596**-605
Hip
   fractures, osteoporosis and, 439. *See also*
      Osteoporosis
   waist ratio to, 273
Hismanal (astemizole), 526
Hispanics
   bone density of, 443
   complementary proteins in diet, 196
   lactose intolerance in, 115
   Mexican cuisine, 66-67
Histamine, **645**
Histidine, 181t
Historical data (in nutrition assessment), 21,
   520t-536
   forms for recording, *521, 532, 534-535*
   overeating and, 291
   risk factors, 522, 524t
HIV. *See* Human immunodeficiency virus
HMO (health maintenance organization), **959**
Holmium, B-2t
Home foodservices, for older adults, 681, 683

Home nutrition support, 793-795, 960-961
   in cystic fibrosis, 736
Home water treatments, 517
Homeopathic medicine, **689**
Homeostasis, **90**
   calcium, *428,* 428-429
   fluids and, 409
   glucose, 118-119, *119*
Homocysteine, heart disease and, 202, 905-906
Honey, **122,** 123, 129
   contamination, 636
   infant botulism and, 491
   nutrients in, 124t
   safety, 491
   sugar vs., 103, 123
"Honeymoon phase" of insulin therapy, 859-
   860
Hormone(s), **90, 191n,** 191t, **A-2** to A-6
   additives, 509-510
   adjusting other body balances, A-5
   aging and, 669
   BMR and, 263t
   bone and calcium metabolism with age and,
      441
   bone mass and, 441-443
   counterregulatory, **805,** 862
   enzymes vs., 79
   gastrointestinal, 90-92, A-6
   hypothalamic, A-3 to A-4
   intestinal adaptation and, 753
   nervous system and, A-8
   pituitary, A-3 to A-4
   proteins as, 190, 191t
   regulating energy metabolism, A-4 to A-5
   sex, 153, A-6
   stress effects on, 805t, 805-806
   very-low-kcalorie diet and, 300t
   zinc deficiency and, 467t
   see also specific hormones
Hormone-sensitive lipase, **162**
Hospital
   foodservice in, 820-824, *821-822*
   see also Health care facilities
Hotlines
   Canadian Pesticide Information, 502n
   eosinophilia myalgia syndrome, 206n
   Meat and Poultry (USDA), 490
   National Center for Nutrition and Dietetics,
      61n
   National Lead Information Center, 484n
   National Pesticide (EPA), 502n
   for registered dietitians (ADA), 30n
   Seafood (FDA), 490
Household measures, 54t
Human chorionic gonadotrophin hormone
   (HCG), 296
Human immunodeficiency virus (HIV), **948**-
   956
   breastfeeding and, 609
   nutrition support in, 953-955
   prevention of transmission, 948, 950t
   treatment of infection, 950
   wasting syndrome, 950-953, 951t, 952t
Human intervention trials, 11
Human milk. *See* Breast milk
Hunger, **259,** 614-622, 616t
   childhood behavior and, 640-641
   determinants, *260*
   nutrition resources, F-6
   overriding signals of, 261
   solutions, 620-622, 623t

in United States, 614-616, 621-622
   world, 616-621
   see also Appetite
Husk, **45**
Hydration
   effect on laboratory findings, 551
   physical activity and, 284-285, 285t
   see also Dehydration; Fluid(s); Water
Hydrochloric acid (HCl), **78**
   atrophic gastritis and, 349
   gastrin and, 91
   protein digestion and, 184, *185*
   vomiting and, 423
Hydrodensitometry, **273,** *273,* 548
Hydrogen, 5, 5, B-2t, B-3, B-5t
   acid-base balance and, 191
   energy metabolism and, 9
   fatty acid saturation and, 142-145
   number of bonds formed by, 102, *103*
   pH and, 80
Hydrogen peroxide, 400n, 402
Hydrogenation, 146, **147**
   of fats, 147
Hydrolysis, **79**
   ATP, 221
   digestive enzymes and, 79
   disaccharide, 106, *106,* 113
   in energy metabolism, 221
   glycogen, 107
   triglyceride, 157, *157*
Hydrolyzed formulas, **735, 758,** K-6t to K-7t
   in Crohn's disease, 737
   for infants with cystic fibrosis, 735
Hydrophilic, **154, 183**
Hydrophilic colloid, **727**
Hydrophilic vitamins. *See* B vitamins; Vitamin
   C; Water-soluble vitamins
Hydrophobic, **154, 183**
Hydrophobic vitamins. *See* Fat-soluble vita-
   mins; Vitamin A; Vitamin D; Vitamin E;
   Vitamin K
Hydroxyapatite, **427**
   in bone formation, 427
   fluoride and, 474
   in tooth formation, 427, *427*
5-Hydroxyindoleacetic acid (5-HIAA), urinary,
   559-560
Hydroxyl (OH) group, 105, *106*
Hydroxyl radical, 400n
Hydroxyproline, 180n
   vitamin C in synthesis, 358, *358*
Hyperactivity, 125, **642-644**
Hyperammonemia, **830**
   hepatic coma and, 830
Hyperbilirubinemia, **396**
   fatty liver and, 827
   hepatitis and, 828
Hypercalcemia, **388**
Hypercalciuria, **930,** 931
Hypercarotenemia, 382t
Hyperglycemia, **848**
   diabetes and, 848
   management, 862-864, 863t
   rebound, **862**
   renal failure and, 916
   severe, 864
   symptoms, 848
   TPN solutions and, 787, 789
   tube feeding and, 773t
Hyperglycemic nonketotic coma, hyperosmolar,
   848, 849

Hyperkalemia, **914.** *See also* Potassium
Hyperkeratinization, *384*
  vitamin A and, 382t
Hyperkeratosis, 384
Hypermetabolism, 804, **804**
  liver disease and, 831
  stress and, 804-807
Hyperosmolar hyperglycemic nonketotic coma, **848,** 849
Hyperoxaluria, 931
  enteric, **728**
Hyperparathyroidism
  chronic renal failure and, 918
Hyperplastic obesity, **288**
Hypersensitivity. *See* Allergy; Food allergies
Hypertension, **165, 889**-894
  alcohol and, 893
  blood pressure regulation and, *890, 890*-892
  calcium and, 427-428, 893
  consequences, 891
  coronary heart disease risk and, 884t, 885
  essential, **889**
  insulin resistance and, 891
  kidneys and, 891
  magnesium and, 435, 893
  obesity and, 275, 891, 892
  physical activity and, 892
  portal, **829**
  potassium and, 424, 893
  preeclampsia and, 599, 600
  preexisting in pregnant woman, 599
  pregnancy-induced, **599,** 869
  prevention, 891-892
  primary, **889**
  risk factors, 891
  secondary, **889**
  sodium and, 59, 420, 423, 892
  treatment, 892-894
Hyperthermia, **282**
  physical activity and, 284
Hypertonic formula, **759**
Hypertrophic obesity, **288**
Hypertrophy (muscle), **282**
Hypervitaminosis A, 382t, 383-384
Hypervitaminosis D, 388, 389t, 390
Hypnotherapy, **689**
Hypoalbuminemia, in Crohn's disease, 737
Hypochromic anemia, microcytic, **456**
Hypoglycemia, **120, 848,** 871-873
  alimentary, **708**
  child behavior and, 641
  diabetes and, 850
  fasting, 872t, **872**-873
  management, 863t, 864-865
  nocturnal, **864**
  postgastrectomy, **708**
  postprandial, **871**
  reactive, **871**-872, 872t
  severe, 864-865
  symptoms, 850
  TPN solutions and, 789-790
Hypoglycemic agents, **867,** E-2t
Hypokalemia. *See* Potassium
Hypothalamus, **410, A-3**
  hormones, A-3 to A-4
Hypothermia, **282**
  physical activity and, 284
Hypotheses, in research, 11
Hypovitaminosis A, *380,* 380-383, *381,* 382t-383t, 384
Hypoxemia, **899**

Ibuprofen
  peptic ulcer due to, 99n
  peptic ulcers due to, 705
  pregnancy and, 604
-ic acid, **224**
Ice craving. *See* Pica
Ice cream/milk
  cholesterol in, 153t
  fat-free, 177
  see also Milk and milk products
Idazoxon, 297n
IDDM. *See* Insulin-dependent diabetes mellitus
Idiopathic hypercalciuria, **930**
IDL (intermediate-density lipoprotein), 159n
IGF-1. *See* Insulin-like growth factor
Ileitis, regional, **736**
Ileocecal valve, *74,* **75,** 78
  resection, 740-741
Ileostomate, **747**
Ileostomy, 746, **747**
Ileum, 73, *75*
Illness, **562**
  alternative therapies for, 688-693
  constipation due to, 97
  diabetes treatment during, 862
  diet modifications for, 568t-569t
  food-borne. *See* Food-borne illnesses
  nutrition status and, 523-524, *525,* 810-811
  see also Disease(s); Stress; *specific type*
Imagery, **689**
Imitation food, **51**
Immobility, and pressure sores, 810
Immune system
  aging and, 669
  AIDS/HIV and. *See* Human immunodeficiency virus (HIV)
  arthritis and, 677
  breastfed infant, 630-631
  cancer and, 935
  folate deficiency and, 347t
  food allergies and. *See* Food allergies
  iron and, 457t
  stress effects on, 804-805
  stress effects on GI tract and, 808-810, 809t
  vitamin A and, 383t
  vitamin C deficiency and, 360t
  vitamin E and, 392
  zinc and, 463, 466, 467t
  see also Immunity
Immunity, **193**
  very-low-kcalorie diet and, 300t
  vitamin A in, 379
  see also Immune system
Immunosuppressants, E-10t to E-11t
  kidney transplant and, 925
Immunotherapy, for cancer, 943
Implantable pumps, insulin delivery using, 860
Implantation, **585**
Inactivity, obesity and, 291-292
Inborn error of metabolism, **839**-844, *840, 843*
Inches, 7
Incidental additives, **503.** *See also* Indirect additives
Indemnity insurance, **959**
Indexes of abstracts, 34
India, vitamin A supplements in, 380
Indigestion, 699-702
  antacids and, 99, 702
Indinavir, 950
Indirect additives, **503,** 507-508
  hormones, 509-510

radiation, 510-511, *511*
Indirect calorimetry, **258, 261,** 812
Indispensable amino acids, **181.** *See also* Protein/amino acids; *specific amino acids*
Indispensable nutrients, 5
Indium, B-2t
Individual approach (to dietary recommendations), **26**-27
  chewing difficulties and, 696-697
  diabetes and, 878
Individual rights, nutrition care and, 798-799
Individual tolerances, and formula selection, 760
Indoles, 406t
Indonesia, vitamin A supplements in, 380
Induration, **550**
Infant(s), 626-638
  birthweight. *See* Birthweight
  botulism in, 491
  breastfeeding. *See* Breastfeeding
  choking in, 95
  with cystic fibrosis, 735
  diarrhea in, 96
  fat digestion in, 154
  feeding tube insertion, 762
  with fetal alcohol syndrome, 601-604
  first foods for, 634-637, 635t
  formulas for. *See* Infant formulas
  growth retardation, 546
  head circumference, 545, 546
  honey precautions for, 491
  iodine deficiency in, 470
  iron deficiency in, 456, 457, 636
  lead toxicity in, 480, 481
  length measurement, 544-545
  maternal drug abuse and, 604
  mealtimes with, 637-638
  nutrients for, 626-627, *628*
  nutrition resources, F-3 to F-4
  of older mothers, 601
  PKU in, 841
  post-term, **589**
  preterm, **588,** 598, 633-634
  protein RDI, 198n
  scurvy in, *361*
  SIDS in, 604-605
  supplements for, 630, 630t
  supplements in, 367
  term, **588**
  vitamin K in, 367, 396
  vomiting in, 95-96
  water recommendation, 411
  weight gain in first five years, 626
  weight measurement, 545
  see also Children/childhood; Pregnancy
Infant formulas, 631-633
  breast milk vs., 627, 629, *631*
  infants with cystic fibrosis and, 735
  lead contamination, 481, 483
  nutrients in, 627t, *631*
  preparations, 626
  preterm infants and, 634
Infection(s)
  abscess, **732**
  breast milk and protection against, 630-631
  food-borne, **487**-489, 488t-489t. *See also* Food-borne illnesses
  immune system and. *See* Immune system
  infant formula and, 631, 633
  intravenous nutrition and, 788
  opportunistic, **949**

PEM and, 199, 202
peptic ulcers due to, 705
stress and, 804-805
vitamin A and, 380-381
see also specific infections
"Infection stones," 932
Infertility. *See* Fertility
Inflammatory response, **804**
severe stress and, 804-805
see also Immune system
Information. *See* Medical record; Nutrition information
Informed consent, 799-802, *800, 801*
Infusion pumps
children and, 769, 789
TPN solution, 789-790
tube feeding, 769
Ingredient list (on labels), 52-54
INH (isonicotinic acid hydrazide), 340-341
Inheritance. *See* Genetics/genes
Initiators (cancer), **936**-937
Injury. *See* Trauma; *specific type*
Inorganic, **5**
Inorganic elements, 418
Inorganic nutrients, elements in, 5
Inosine, 371t
Inositol, **350**-351
Insecticides, 499-502
Insensible water losses, 411n
Insoluble fibers, 110, 111t
Insulin, **118,** 190, 191t, A-4
actions of types, 859
acute renal failure and, 916
aging and, 669
amino acid sequence, *182*
in blood cholesterol regulation, 154
in blood glucose regulation, 118-119, *119*
chromium and, 475
delivery, 860
diabetes treatment with, 858-860, *859,* 868
food intake and, 860
pancreas transplants and, 860-861
physical activity and, 860
vitamin E and, 402
see also Blood glucose; Diabetes mellitus; Hypoglycemia
Insulin allergy, **858**
Insulin analogs, 858-859, 868
Insulin-dependent diabetes mellitus (IDDM), **120,** 846t, **846**-**847**
insulin and insulin analogs in, 858-860, *859*
ketosis and coma in, 848-849
living with, 877-880
treatment, 851-865
weight loss in, 849
see also Diabetes mellitus
Insulin-like growth factor (IGF-1), 554
intestinal adaptation and, 753
stress and, 815-816
Insulin reaction, **864**
Insulin resistance, **847**
hypertension and, 891
Insurance, indemnity, **959**
Intact formula, **758,** K-2t to K-5t
Intensity (physical activity)
effect on fat use, 282
effect on glycogen use, 280
effect on protein use, 283
fuels used and, 281t
recommendations for fitness, 278t
recommendations to lose fat, 282

Intentional additives, **503,** 505-507, *505-507*
Interactions. *See* Drug-nutrient interactions; Nutrient interactions
Interferon, **805**
Interleukin-1, **805**
Intermediate-density lipoprotein (IDL), 159n
Intermittent claudication, **393**
Intermittent feeding, **768**
International agencies, F-3. *See also specific agencies*
International System of Units (SI), 6
International units (IU), **381**
conversion to cholecalciferol micrograms, 390
Interstitial fluid, **409**
Interview, in nutrition assessment, 522-523
Intestinal flora, **80,** 809
short-chain fatty acids and, 753
translocation, 809t, 809-810
vitamin K and, 394, 396
Intestinal gas. *See* Gas
Intestinal glands, 80, 81t
Intestinal juice, 80, 81t
Intestinal motility. *See* Motility
Intestinal villi, 83, *84, 85*
Intestine. *See* Colon; Digestion; GI (gastrointestinal) tract; Small intestine
Intoxication (food), **487,** 489t. *See also* Food poisoning
Intra-abdominal fat, **272**
Intracellular fluid, **409,** 412
electrolytes in, 413t
Intractable diarrhea, **724**
Intrarenal, **914**
Intravenous (IV), **703, 783**
Intravenous (IV) catheter, **786**
Intravenous (IV) nutrition, 783-791
composition, 787-788
feeding methods, 784-788
lipid emulsions, 784, 790-791
nutrient content calculation and, 785
in prolonged vomiting, 703
solutions for, 783-784
during stress, 816-817
see also Parenteral nutrition
Intrinsic, **349**
Intrinsic factor, **349**
gastritis and, 705
lack of, 349
Inuits
bone density of, 443
breast milk contaminants in, 610
lactose intolerance in, 115
see also Alaskans
Invert sugar, **122**
Invisible fat, **170**
Involuntary activities, **263**
Iodide
iodine vs., 468, 470
roles in body, 470, 471t
Iodine, 450, 468, 470-471, B-2t
amount in body, *418*
deficiency, 470, *470,* 471t
food sources, 470, 471t
iodide vs., 468, 470
RDI, 55t
recommendations, 368t, 471, 471t
toxicity, 470, 471t
Iodopsin, **378**
Ion(s), **412**-413
formation, B-5 to B-7

proteins in flow regulation, 414
see also specific ions
Ionizing radiation. *See* Radiation
Iran, zinc deficiency in, 466
Iridium, B-2t
Iridology, **689**
Iron, 450, 451-463, B-2t, H
absorption, 452-455, *455,* 461
adolescent needs, 651
amount in body, *418*
blood content, 456
in breast milk, 630
calcium interactions with, 37-38, 369, 446t
cancer and, 460
chronic renal failure and, 923
contamination, **461**
daily losses, 455
deficiency. *See* Iron deficiency
ferric, **451,** 472, B-7
ferrous, **451,** 472, B-7
fiber and, 453, 455
food labels and, 54
food sources, 37, 453, *453,* 457t, 460, *462*
foods enriched with, 460-461
foods providing for children, 641t
foods providing for infants, 636
GI bleeding and, 559
heart disease and, 459-460
heme and nonheme, 453, *453*
infant formula fortified with, 631
infant supplements, 630t
ionic states, 451
during lactation, 608
lead and, *481,* 481-482
magnesium interactions with, 369
maximization of absorption, 461
metabolism, *452,* 452-455, *453, 455,* 472
phytates and, 453
poisoning in children, 460
during pregnancy, 594-595
pregnancy and, 455, 456
RDI, 55t
recommendations, 368t, 457t, 460, 461
recycling, *452,* 455
roles in body, 451, 457t
serum, E-31t
storage, 455
supplements, 463
tetracycline and, 527
toxicity, 367, 457t, 459-460
transport, 192, 455
in vegetarian diet, 212
vitamin C and, 86, 453, 454, 455, 459
zinc interactions with, 369, 465
Iron cookware, 461, *461*
Iron deficiency, 37, 455-459, **456,** 457t
assessment, 456
behavior and, 458, 641-642
blood losses and, 455-456
in children, 456, 457-458, 481-482, 641-642
in infants, 456, 457, 636
lead poisoning and, 481-482
nutrition assessment in, 22-23
in older adults, 674
pica and, 458-459
prevalence, 457-458
stages, 456
vulnerable stages of life and, 456
Iron-deficiency anemia, **456**-457
in children, 482, 641-642
after gastrectomy, 711

milk, 637
prevalence, 457
red blood cells in, 456, *458*
Iron overload, **459**
Irradiation. *See* Radiation
Irritable bowel syndrome, 725-727
Isoflavones, 406t
Isoleucine, 181t
Isonicotinic acid hydrazide (INH), 340-341
Isothiocyanates, 406t
Isotonic formula, **759**
Italian cuisine, 64, 65
IU. *See* International units
IV. *See* Intravenous

Jam, 129, H
Japan
hypertension in, 421
mercury contamination of fish in, 496-497
see also Asians
Japanese cuisine, 68-69. *See also* Asian Americans; Asians
Jaundice, 383t, **396**
hepatitis and, 828
Jaw wiring, 299
Jejunostomy, **764,** 765t
needle catheter, 771
Jejunum, 73, **75**
dumping syndrome and, 707
surgery in obesity treatment, *298,* 298-299
Jelly, 129, H
Jewish cuisine, 64, 69
Jin Bu Huan, 371t, 691
Joints, arthritis of, 253t, 677
Joule, 6
Journals, *34,* F-2
Judgmental responses, nonjudgmental responses vs., 531
Juice
fresh fruit vs., 50
weight gain and, 311
see also specific type
Juvenile-onset diabetes. *See* Insulin-dependent diabetes mellitus (IDDM)

Kale
calcium in, *432*
natural toxicants in, 498
Kaposi's sarcoma, **952**
kCalorie(s) (kcal), 6-**7**
adding in cancer, 947
in alcohol, 251, 252t, 258
body fat and, 163, 257
in carbohydrates, 7, 8, 258
control, **38**
"empty," *38,* 123
fat and, 166, *166,* 258
muscle building and, 311
nutritional adequacy during weight loss and, 302, 302t
in protein, 258
recommendations for weight loss, 257-258
recommended carbohydrate percentage, 233
recommended fat percentage, 233
recommended protein percentage, 233
as unit of heat energy, 258
weight loss and, 299-301, 300t
see also Energy
kCalorie-free (on labels), 60t
Kelp, 371t
Keratin, **383**

Keratin matrix, in tooth formation, *427*
Keratinization, **383,** *384*
Keratomalacia, **382,** 382t
Kernicterus, **396**
Keshan disease, **471**
Keto acids, **233,** *233,* 242
Ketoacidosis, severe hyperglycemia and, 865
Ketogenic amino acids, 195n, 226
Ketone bodies, **117,** 162, 163, 242
diabetes and, 849
fasting and, 242, 806
formation, 242, *242,* C-19 to C-20
Ketonemia, **242, 848**
Ketones, 242
glucose control and, 861
Ketonuria, **242, 848**
Ketosis, **117,** 162
fasting and, 242
in IDDM, 848-849
kg (kilogram), 6, 7
Kidney(s), 86, 88, *910*
in acid-base balance regulation, 417, 419n
alcohol effects on, 253t
calcium supplements and, 446t
cancer, 945t
disorders, 910-927, 930-932
in fluid and electrolyte regulation, 415, 417
functions, 910
hormones, A-5
in hypertension, 891
modified diet for conditions affecting, 569t
transplants, 925t, 925-926
urea excretion, 234, *235*
zinc and, 467t
Kidney beans, nutrients in, 124t
Kidney stones, 383t, 930-932, 931t
calcium supplements and, 446t
vitamin C and, 360t, 361n
Kilocalories. *See* kCalorie(s)
Kilograms (kg), 6, 7
Kilojoule (kJ), 6, 8n
Kitchen techniques. *See* Cooking/food preparation
Kiwi, vitamin C in, *363*
Kohlrabi, natural toxicants in, 498
Kombucha tea, 691
Korea, hypertension in, 421
Kosher, **64,** 69
Krebs cycle. *See* TCA cycle
Krypton, B-2t
Kwashiorkor, **201,** 808t
marasmus vs., 199, 200, 200t
pellagra vs., *337*
see also Protein-energy malnutrition (PEM)
Kwashiorkor-marasmus mix, 201

L (levo), **393**
L (liter), 6
Labeling, 51-61, I-14 to I-16t
calculation of exchanges and, *574*
carbohydrate in, 130
consumer education about, 61
Daily Values, 55t, 56t, 56-57, inside front cover (right)
descriptive terms, 57-58, 60t
fat in, *170,* 170-171
health claims in, 58-61, 60t, 171, 404-405
ingredient list, 52-54
irradiated foods, 511, *511*
items not requiring, 51-52
Nutrition Facts, 54-55

package size and, 57, 58, 59
protein in, 198-199
required information, 52
serving sizes, 54
sugar in, 125
sulfites in, 506
supplement, 372
terms used in, 60t
voluntary program for fresh foods, 51-52, 53t
Laboratory tests (in nutrition assessment), 22, 550-555, 552t, E-26 to E-31t
anemia and, E-30, E-30t to E-31t
food effects on, 559-560
liver disease and, 835t
malabsorption and, 749t
protein-energy malnutrition and, 553, 553t, 554
upper GI tract disorders and, 713
see also specific tests
Lactase, **113**
deficiency, **115**-116
Lactate
extracellular concentration, 413t
intracellular concentration, 413t
Lactation, 606-610, **607**
alcohol during, 608-609
caffeine during, 609
calcium during, 594
daily food choices during, 593t
energy needs during, 607
medical considerations during, 609-610
milk intake recommendations, 430
protein RDI during, 198n
RDA during, 592
resources, F-5
smoking during, 609
see also Breast milk; Breastfeeding
Lactic acid, **226**
exercise and, 607
physical activity and, 281
Lactic dehydrogenase, 552t, 894
Lacto-ovo-vegetarians, **210**
Lactoferrin, **631**
Lactose, **107**
in breast milk, 629
calcium absorption and, 429
hydrolysis, 113
sources, 116
Lactose intolerance, **115**-116, 726
Lactovegetarians, **210**
Laennec's cirrhosis, **828**
Laetrile, 351, 498
Lamivudine (3TC), 950
Lanthanum, B-2t
Lard, *146*
Large intestine, **75.** *See also* Colon
Larynx, *94,* **96**
cancer, 403
Laser angioplasty, **887**
Latinos. *See* Hispanics
Lauric acid, 164, C-4t
Laxatives, 97, E-11t
bulimia nervosa and, 320
effect on nutrient absorption, 526
hydrophilic colloids, 727
potassium and, 426
"Laying on of hands," **689**
LBW. *See* Low birthweight
LDL (low-density lipoprotein), **159,** *161*
abdominal fat and, 272
antioxidants and, 403

desirable blood level, 164
diet for reduction of, 887, 887t, 888t
HDL ratio to, 160, 885
heart disease and, 160, 164, 884t, 885
iron toxicity and, 459
monounsaturated fats and, 164
polyunsaturated fats and, 164
saturated fats and, 164
Lead, 477, 480-484, B-2t
in body, 480, *481*
calcium supplements and, 446t, 447t
in drinking water, 516
in environment, *480*, 482, *482-483*
iron deficiency and, 481-482, 642
malnutrition and, 481-482, 642
maternal levels during pregnancy, 605
poisoning in children, *480*, 480-484, 481t, *482*, 642
poisoning in infants, 480, 481
protective strategies against, 483-484
symptoms of poisoning, 481t
threshold for poisoning, 480
toxicity, 605
Lean (on labels), 60t
Lean tissue, measures of body fat and, 548-550
Lecithin, **151**, *151*
Alzheimer's disease and, 679
supplements, 152, 679
toxicity, 351
see also Phospholipids
Lecithinase, 152
Lectein, 406n
Legal, **797**
Legumes, **44**
calcium in, *431, 432, 432*
choices, 50
fiber in, 129t
folate in, *348*
iron in, *462*
magnesium in, *435, 436*
as meat alternate, 44
niacin in, *338*
phytochemicals in, 406t
potassium in, *425*
protein in, 198t
riboflavin in, *335*
thiamin in, *332*
vitamin A in, *386*
vitamin B$_6$ in, *344*
vitamin C in, *363*
vitamin E in, *395*
weight loss and, 302
zinc in, *468, 469*
Length measurements, D-3
Lentils
folate in, *348*
zinc in, *469*
Leptin, weight loss and, 297
LES (lower esophageal sphincter), **701**
LeShan, Eda, 323
Less (on labels), 60t
Less cholesterol (on labels), 60t
Less fat (on labels), 60t
Less saturated fat (on labels), 60t
Leucine, 181t, 195n
Leukemias, **934**
Leukotrienes, 148
Levulose, **105, 122.** *See also* Fructose
LH (luteinizing hormone), A-3
Liberal bland diet, 705t
License to practice, **30**

Life cycle nutrition, 585-610, 626-655, 666-684. *See also specific life cycle stages*
Life expectancy, 25, **666**-668
Life span, **666**
Lifestyle choices
constipation and, 96-97
diabetic child and, 865
disease risk and, 24, 25-26
GI tract health and, 92, 99-100
health risk and, 539-540, *540*
after heart attack, 895
longevity and, 667
osteoporosis and, 443-444, 444t
see also specific type
Light (on labels), 60t
Light, riboflavin sensitivity to, 333
Light in sodium (on labels), 60t
Lignans, 406t
Lignin, 109n, 110
sources, 110
Lima beans, cyanogens in, 498
Limestone (dolomite), 446, 447t
Limiting amino acids, **196**
Limonene, 406t
Lind, James, 356
Linoleic acid, 141, **143**, 144t, 148, C-4t
chemical structure, 143-144, *144, 149*
food sources, 150t
see also Omega-6 fatty acid
Linolenic acid, 141, **144**, 144t, 148-149, C-4t
chemical structure, 144, *149*
food sources, 150t
see also Omega-3 fatty acid
Lipase, **79**
in fat digestion, 154, 156
hormone-sensitive, **162**
lipoprotein, **162**
serum, 552t
Lipid(s), **141**-172. *See also* Fat
Lipid-lowering drugs, 889
in children, 663
Lipid peroxidation
arthritis and, 677
free radicals and, 400, 402, 473
Lipid peroxyl radical, *401*
Lipoic acid, 350-**351**
Lipophilic, **154**
Lipoprotein(s), **159**-160, *161*. *See also* Fat; HDL; LDL
Lipoprotein lipase (LPL), **162**
body fat and, 162
fat cell metabolism and, 290
Liposuction, 299
Liqueurs, 252t
Liquid diets, 728t
after gastric partitioning, 711-712
for weight loss, 299-300
see also Enteral formulas
Liquor, distilled, **246**, 252t
Listeria monocytogenes, 488t
Listeriosis, 488, 488t
Lite (on labels), 60t
Liter (L), 6
Literature, F-1 to F-2
Lithium, B-2t
Lithium carbonate, E-12t
Little (on labels), 60t
Liver (body), *74*, **75**, 81t
abdominal fat and, 272
alcohol and, 247-249, 253t
bile acids and, 156

cancer, 936t, 945t
in carbohydrate absorption, 114, *114*
in carbohydrate metabolism, 223t
in cholesterol synthesis, 154
circulatory system, *826*
disorders, 826-837
fasting and, 240
fatty, 201, **246**, 249, 827
glucose and glycogen in, 107, 116-117
in iron recycling, 455
in iron storage, 455
laboratory tests in disease, 835t
in lipid metabolism, 223t
metabolic work of, 222, 223t
in nutrient transport, 87-89, *89*
in protein metabolism, 223t
transplantation, 834-837
in urea synthesis, 234
vitamin A and, 383t
zinc deficiency and, 467t
Liver (food), 152, H
desiccated, 370t
iron in, *462*
niacin in, 338
riboflavin in, *335*
vitamin A in, 385-387, *386*
Living will, **797**, 799-800, *800*
Long-chain fatty acids, 158
Long-chain triglycerides, medium-chain vs., 729-730
Longevity, **666**
genetics and, 666
nutrition and, 666-668
physical activity and, 667
stress and, 668-669
Low (on labels), 60t
Low birthweight (LBW), **598**
maternal smoking and, 604
maternal zinc and, 595
see also Birthweight
Low-carbohydrate diet, metabolic effects of, 243
Low-carbohydrate dieting, **243**
Low cholesterol (on labels), 60t
Low-density lipoprotein. *See* LDL
Low fat (on labels), 60t
Low-fat diet, 170, 303, 888t
Low-fat foods, 170, 171, 172
milk and milk products, 430
weight loss and, 302
Low kcalorie (on labels), 60t
Low-nutrient density foods, 123-124
Low-potassium diet, 424
Low-risk pregnancy, **597**
Low saturated fat (on labels), 60t
Low sodium (on labels), 60t
Low-sodium diet, 833t
Lower esophageal sphincter (LES), **701**. *See also* Cardiac sphincter
Lower gastrointestinal tract, **725**
disorders, 723-749
Lox, 69
LPL. *See* Lipoprotein lipase
Lung(s), 86, *87*, 882
cancer. *See* Lung cancer
cystic fibrosis and, 733-734
disorders, 898-901
magnesium and, 434
marijuana and, 654
modified diet for conditions affecting, 569t
vitamin C and, 358-359

vitamin E and, 392
water loss from, 411
see also Respiratory system
Lung cancer, 936t
antioxidants and, 403, 404
smoking and, 404
Lutein, as antioxidant, 405
Luteinizing, **A-3**
Luteinizing hormone (LH), A-3
Lutetium, B-2t
Lycopene, 406n
Lymph, **90**
Lymphatic system, **90**
in lipid transport, 158
in nutrient transport, 83, *84*, 90
Lymphocytes, protein-energy malnutrition and, 554
Lymphomas, **934**
Lysine, 181t, 196
supplements, 206
Lysosomes, **379, A-1**
Lysyl oxidase, 472n

m (meter), 7
Ma huang, 371t
Macroangiopathies, **848**
in diabetes, 850
Macrobiotic diets, **210, 689**
Macrocytic (megaloblastic) anemia, 346, *350, 351t*
Macrominerals. See Major minerals
MADD (Mothers Against Drunk Driving), 254
Magnesium, **434**-435, B-2t, B-5t, H
amount in body, *418,* 434
blood, 552t
in bone, 434
calcium interactions with, 369, 446t
deficiency, 434t, 435
dolomite and, 447t
extracellular concentration, 413t
food sources, 434t, *436*
hypertension and, 435, 893
intracellular concentration, 413t
ion, 413t
recommendations, 368t, 434t, 435
roles in body, 434, 434t
toxicity, 434t
vitamin B$_6$ interactions with, 354
in water, 435
Magnesium carbonate, 5n
calcium supplements with, 446
Magnesium hydroxide, 446t, 447t
Major minerals, 10, 409, **418**-437. *See also*
Mineral(s); *specific minerals*
Malabsorption, 98, 727-731, *728, 729t*
bacterial overgrowth causing, 738-739, *739*
cancer and, 939
celiac disease and, 741-742
Crohn's disease and, 736-738
cystic fibrosis and, 733-736
fat, 559, 709, 727-731
fat-restricted diets for, 728-729, 729t, 730
after gastric surgery, 709-710
intestinal surgery causing, 739-741, *740, 746*
laboratory tests, 749t
pancreatitis and, 731-733, *734*
syndromes, 731-742, 732t
ulcerative colitis and, 744-745
Maleficence principle, 797
Malignant, **934**
Malnutrition, **20**

acute, 807, 808t
alcohol and, 251-252, 253t
behavior and, 640-641, 643t
BMR and, 263t
in children, 481-482, 640-642, 643t
chronic, 807, 808t
congestive heart failure and, 896
diagnosis. *See* Nutrition assessment
drugs and, 526
early pregnancy and, 597-598
fertility and, 597
fetal development and, 598
lead toxicity and, 481-482, 642
mixed, 807, 808t
nephrotic syndrome and, 911
in older adults, 675, 675t
physical findings, 537t
pregnancy and, 597-598
protein-energy. *See* Protein-energy malnutrition (PEM)
protein quality and, 199
risk factors in older adults, 675t, 681
stress response and, 807, *808,* 808t
symptoms, 20
zinc, 466
see also Hunger; Malabsorption; Nutrition status
Malt sugar. *See* Maltose
Maltase, **113**
Maltitol, **135,** 138t
Maltodextrin, 176
Maltose, **106**
formation, *106*
hydrolysis, *106,* 113
Managed care, **959**-960
Manganese, 450, 473, 474t, B-2t
amount in body, *418*
deficiency, 473, 474t
environmental contamination with, 473
food sources, 473, 474t
RDI, 55t
recommendations, 474t
roles in body, 473, 474t
toxicity, 473, 474t
Mango
vitamin A in, *386*
vitamin C in, *363*
Mannitol, **135,** 138t
Mannose, 109n
MAO inhibitors. *See* Monoamine oxidase inhibitors
Maple sugar, **122,** 129
Maple syrup, 129
Marasmus, **200**-201, 808t
kwashiorkor vs., 199-200, 200t
see also Protein-energy malnutrition (PEM)
Marasmus-kwashiorkor mix, 201
Margarine, 147, H
butter vs., 165
Margin of safety (additives), **504**
Marijuana
adolescent use, 652-654
alternative therapy using, 690
pregnancy and, 604
Marinating, safety, 490
"Market Basket Survey," 500-501
Massage therapy, **689**
Mastication, **695**
difficulties, 695t-697
Matrix, **188**
Maturity-onset diabetes of the young (MODY),

847. *See also* Diabetes mellitus
Mayonnaise, H
safety, 491, 494t
MCH. See Mean corpuscular hemoglobin
MCHC. See Mean corpuscular hemoglobin concentration
MCT oil, fat-restricted diets and, 729-730
MCV. See Mean corpuscular volume
MDI (multiple daily injections), **860**
Meal(s)/mealtime
Alzheimer's disease and, 679
before and after athletic competition, 285-286
child eating habits and, 639, 645-648, 647t
childhood diabetes and, 865
congregate sites, 681, 683
diabetic diet and, 854-856, 857t, 866-867
digestive process and, 92
exchange lists and, 57t, 575
glycemic effect and, 120-121
grazing, 120, 154
hypoglycemia after, 871-872
hypoglycemia before, 864
with infants, 637-638
iron absorbed from, 454
missed in IDDM, 853
planning. *See* Diet planning
school, 648t
for singles, 681-684
very-low-kcalorie diets and, 299
weight gain and, 310
in weight-loss plans, 301-303, 302t
Meals on Wheels, 683
Mean corpuscular hemoglobin (MCH), tests, 552t
Mean corpuscular hemoglobin concentration (MCHC), tests, 552t
Mean corpuscular volume (MCV), E-30t
tests, 552t
Measles, vitamin A and, 380-381
Measurements, D-1 to D-3, inside front cover (right)
anthropometric. *See* Anthropometric measurements
household, 54t
metric, 6-7, 54t
protein quality, J-1 to J-3, J-2t
Meat(s), H
alternates, *42, 44, 46, 47*
bovine growth hormone in, 509, 510
calcium in, *431*
choices, 50-51
cholesterol in, 152, 153t
in exchange lists, 570-571, 571t, *572*-573, G-11t
fat in, 50, 168, 169
folate in, *348*
in food group plans, 41, *42, 46, 47*
iron in, *462*
irradiated, 510
magnesium in, *436*
MFP factor in, 453, 454
niacin in, *338*
nitrites in, 505, 506
potassium in, *425*
recommendations based on Mediterranean diet, 215-216
riboflavin in, *335*
safe refrigerator storage, 494t
safety, 490, *490,* 492, *492*
selenium in, *472*

smoked, 421
thiamin in, 330, *330*, 330t, *332*
tyramine-containing, 529t
unsafe handling, 492
vitamin A in, 386
vitamin B$_6$ in, 344
vitamin C in, 363
vitamin E in, 395
zinc in, 469
Meat replacement, **210**
vitamin B$_{12}$ and, 350
Meat-restricted foodways, 209-216. *See also*
Vegetarian diets
Mechanical soft diet, **696**-697, 698
Mechanical ventilator, **899**
Medical approach (to dietary recommendations), **26**
Medical conditions. *See* Illness
Medical family tree, *543*
Medical food, 779, 780
Medical history. *See* Health history
Medical insurance, 959-961
Medical nutrition therapy, 519, **519,** 565-567
for anorexia nervosa, 318
in bulimia nervosa, 320, 321t
in cancer, 244
education about. *See* Nutrition education
for PEM, 202
for PKU, 135
planning. *See* Diet planning
rationale, 565-566
see also Diet(s); Diet therapy; Nutrition support; *specific type of diet*
Medical procedures, effects on nutrition status,
810
Medical record, **578**-579
tube feeding and, 775
Medical schools, nutrition education in, 29
Medical treatments, right to refuse, 798-799
Medicare, 959
Medication(s). *See* Drug(s)
Medicine, alternative, 688-693
Meditation, **689**
Mediterranean diets, 213-216
criticisms, 215
heart health and, 64-65
implications, 215-216
pyramid, 213-215, *215,* 216
Mediterranean peoples, lactose intolerance in,
115
Medium-chain fatty acids, 158
Medium-chain triglycerides
digestion and absorption, 730
fat-restricted diets and, 729-730
Medulla, brain stem, *250*
Megaloblastic anemia. *See* Macrocytic (mega-
loblastic) anemia
Melanin, 194
Melanocyte, **A-3**
Melanocyte-stimulating hormone (MSH), A-3
Melanomas, **934**
Melatonin, **689**
Men
BMR estimation in, 265t, 267
body fat, 271, 272
bone mass and hormones, 442-443
daily iron losses in, 455n
eating disorders among, 315
ideal body weight, 547
iron RDA for, 460
waist-to-hip ratio, 273

see also Gender differences
Menadione, **396,** 397t. *See also* Vitamin K
Menaquinone, 397t. *See also* Vitamin K
Mendelevium, B-2t
Menopause
calcium needs after, 674-675
calcium recommendations after, 445
calcium supplements after, 445
osteoporosis after, 440, 440t, 442. *See also*
Osteoporosis
see also Older adults
Menstruation/menstrual period
anorexia nervosa and, 317
iron loss during, 455n, 456
PMS and, 341
water retention and, 295n
see also Amenorrhea
Mental disturbances
in hepatic coma, 830
illness effects on nutrition status, 524-525
see also Emotions
Menus
diabetic diet, 858
fat-restricted diet, 730
high-fiber diet, 744
in hospital, *821-822, 821-823*
for one-year-old child, 632
phenylalanine-restricted, 841
postgastrectomy diet, 709
for pregnant and lactating women, 593
protein-restricted, sodium-restricted, 834
renal diet, 925
MEOS (microsomal ethanol-oxidizing system),
246, 249
mEq. *See* Milliequivalents
Mercury, 477, B-2t
in breast milk, 610
calcium supplements and, 446t, 447t
in drinking water, 516
fish contaminated with, 496-497, 498
maternal levels during pregnancy, 605
Messenger RNA, protein synthesis and, 186,
187
Metabolic alkalosis, 423n
Metabolic rate, basal. *See* Basal metabolic rate
(BMR)
Metabolism, **9,** 219-244
aerobic, 226, 282, *282*
alcohol, 247-249, *248*
aspartame, 135-136, *136*
B vitamin coenzymes in, 352, *353*
basal, **262**-263
cancer and, 940
carbohydrate, 116-121, 148
chemical reactions in, 219-223
drug-nutrient interactions and, 527t,
528-529
energy. *See* Energy metabolism
fasting vs. stress responses, 806, *806*
fat, 160-163, *161, 162,* 282-283
fat cell, 290
HIV-related alterations, 953
illness effects on, 524
inborn error of, **839**-844, *840, 843*
infant vs. adult, 623
iron, *452,* 452-455, *453, 455,* 472
liver in, 222, 223t
oxidative, 402, 472
protein, 148, 193-195
slowing during starvation, 243
stress response effects on, 804-807, 805t, 806

very-low-kcalorie diet and, 300t
water generation during, 410
zinc, 464-466, *465*
zinc and, 467t
see also specific substance
Metalloenzyme(s), **463**
manganese and, 473
molybdenum and, 476
Metallothionein, **464**
copper and, 465-466
Metamucil, 727
Metastasize, **934**
Metastatic calcification, **918**
Meters (m), 7
Methane, B-4
colon cancer and, 98
Methionine, 181t, 196, 347n
sulfur in, 435
vitamin B$_{12}$ and, 347
Methotrexate, folate and, *528*
Methyl alcohol (methanol), aspartame metabo-
lism and, *136*
Methylcellulose, 296
Methylcobalamin, 347
Methylene chloride, decaffeination using, 508
Methylmercury. *See* Mercury
Metric measures, 6-7, 54t, D-3
Mexican cuisine, 66-67. *See also* Hispanics
MFP factor, **453**
iron absorption and, 453, 454, *455,* 461
mg (milligram), 6, 7
MI (myocardial infarction). *See* Heart attacks
Micelles, *156,* **158**
Microalbuminuria, **853**
Microangiopathies, **848**
in diabetes, 850
Microcytic anemia, 342t, 360t
hypochromic, **456**
Microgram, 6
Microminerals. *See* Trace minerals
Microsomal ethanol-oxidizing system (MEOS),
246, 249
Microsomes, **246**
Microvillus/microvilli, **83,** *84,* 85
Microwave ovens
additives from packaging of foods for,
507-508
meat or poultry cooking in, 490
safety of containers for, 508
Microwaves, 510n
Midarm circumferences, 548, 549, E-23 to
E-24, E-26t, *E-27*
Midbrain, *250*
Middle East, zinc deficiency in, 466
MIH (MSH-inhibiting hormone), A-3
Milk alkali syndrome, 446t
Milk allergy, lactose intolerance vs., 115
Milk and milk products, H
"beverages" or "drinks," 40
bovine growth hormone in, 509-510
breast. *See* Lactation
breast milk. *See* Breast milk
calcium-fortified, 432
calcium in, 429, 430, *431,* 432
in choice system, I-7t
choices, 51
cholesterol in, 153t
comparison of nutrients in, 632t
Crohn's disease and, 737
in exchange lists, 571t, *573,* G-7t
fat in, 168, 169

folate in, *348*
in food group plans, 40, *43, 46, 47*
goat's, 346
health claims on labels and, 61
introduction in children, 634, 637
iodine in, 470, 471
iron absorption and, 455
iron in, *462*
low-fat options, 430
magnesium in, *436*
niacin in, *338*
nutrients in, 124t
pasteurization, 487
PBB contamination of, 497
potassium in, *425*
powdered, 432
processing for room-temperature storage, 510, 683
protein in, 198, 198t
recommended daily servings, 430
riboflavin in, *333,* 334t, *335*
safety, 491
soy "milk" as alternate, 44. *See also* Soy "milk"
thiamin in, *332*
vitamin A in, *385, 386*
vitamin B$_6$ in, *344*
vitamin C in, *363*
vitamin D in, *333, 390*
vitamin E in, *395*
weight gain and, 311
zinc absorption and, 464
zinc in, *469*
Milk anemia, **637**
Milk chocolate, 164
Milk sugar. *See* Lactose
Millet, magnesium in, *436*
Milliequivalents (mEq), **413**
electrolyte concentrations, 413t
Milligrams (mg), 6, 7
Milliliter (mL), 6
Millimeters (mm), 7
Mineral(s), 4, 5, *5,* **10, 418**
absorption, *82,* 92-93. *See also* Absorption
additives, 507
amounts in body, *418*
body's handling of, 418
in breast milk, 627t, 629
cancer and, 944
chronic renal failure and, 920t, 921-922, 923
in cirrhosis, 832
in cow's milk, 627t
in cystic fibrosis, 735
dietary balance and, 37-38
in infant formula, 627t
lactation and, 607-608
major, 409, **418-437**
needs during infancy, 621, *623*
needs during stress, 815
older adults and, 674-675
physical activity and, 284
phytic acid and, 111
pregnancy and, 594-595
requirements, 16-17, *17*
requirements during illness, 562
supplements, 284, 366-372, 368t
trace, **418,** 450-477
water and body fluids and, 409-417
see also Deficiency(ies); Electrolyte(s); Food(s); RDA; Toxicity(ies); *specific minerals*

Mineral oil, 97
Mineral water, **516**
Mineralization, **388**
Miscellaneous foods, in food group plans, 40-41, *43, 47*
Misinformation, **30.** *See also* Food myths; Quackery
Mitochondria, *222,* **A-0** to **A-1**
pyruvate in, 225n
Mixed malnutrition, 807, 808t
Mixed salads, safety, 491
Mixed triglyceride, *145*
mL (milliliter), 6
mm (millimeter), 7
Moderate exercise, 282
Moderation (dietary), 38
alcohol, **246-247**
in childhood, 663
Modified diet, **567,** 568t-569t. *See also* Medical nutrition therapy
Modular formulas, 758
Modules, **758**
Molasses, **122,** 129
calcium in, *431*
nutrients in, 124t
Mole, B-7n
Molecule, **5**
polar, B-7
Molybdenum, 450, **476,** 476t, B-2t
food sources, 476, 476t
RDI, 55t
recommendations, 476t
role in body, 476, 476t
toxicity, 476, 476t
Monoamine oxidase (MAO) inhibitors, E-2t
tyramine interactions with, 528-529
Monoglutamate, 342, 343
Monoglyceride(s), **154**
micelles and, 158
Monomeric formula, **758**
Monosaccharides, 102t, 102-105, *103, 104, 105*
absorption, 114, *114*
condensation to form disaccharide, 105, *106*
structure, C-1
Monosodium glutamate (MSG), 54, 67, 420, 507
Monounsaturated fatty acid, *143,* **144,** H
effects on blood lipids, 164
Morbid obesity, **298**
More (on labels), 60t
Morning sickness, 595
Mortality. *See* Death
Mothers Against Drunk Driving (MADD), 254
Motility, **76**
fat digestion and, 92
stress effects on, 807-808
Mouth, **74**
cancer, 403, 945t
in carbohydrate digestion, *112,* 113
in digestive process, 73, 76, *82*
disorders, 695t-697
in fat digestion, 154, *155*
folate deficiency and, 347t
HIV-related infections, 951-952
niacin deficiency and, 336t
in nutrition assessment, 537t
riboflavin deficiency and, 334t
ulcers, **697**
vitamin B$_6$ deficiency and, 342t
vitamin C deficiency and, 360t

see also Tongue
MSG (monosodium glutamate), 54, 67, 420, 507
MSH (melanocyte-stimulating hormone), A-3
MSH-inhibiting hormone (MIH), A-3
Mucilages, 110
Mucopolysaccharides, structure, C-3
Mucosal ferritin, **452**
Mucosal transferrin, **452**
Mucous, **78**
Mucous membranes, **78, 379**
vitamin A and integrity of, *379, 379*
Mucus, **78**
cystic fibrosis and, 734
vitamin A and, 379, 383
Multiple daily injections (MDI), **860**
Multiple organ systems
bacterial translocation and failure of, 810
modified diet for conditions affecting, 569t
"Munchies," 654
Muscle endurance, **282**
Muscle(s)/muscular system
atrophy, **282**
bone strength and, 443
building, 283, 311
calcium and, 429
in childhood malnutrition, 643t
in digestion, 76-78, *77*
glucose and glycogen in, 107, 240n
iron and, 457t
magnesium and, 434
midarm circumference, 548, 549, E-23, E-26t, *E-27*
in nutrition assessment, 537t
oxygen needs, 226
protein used in building, 283
strength training and, 311
thiamin and, 330t
triglycerides and, 160
vitamin A and, 383t
vitamin B$_6$ and, 342t
vitamin C and, 360t
vitamin D and, 389t
vitamin E deficiency and, 392t, 393
zinc and, 467t
Muscle-stimulating devices, 296
Muscle strength, **282**
Muscular dystrophy, **393**
Mushrooms
niacin in, 338
riboflavin in, 335
Mustard greens, calcium in, *432*
Mutation, **839**
Mutual supplementation, **196-197**
Myocardial infarction. *See* Heart attacks
Myoglobin, **192,** 451
iron in, 451
Myristic acid, 164, C-4t
Myrrh, 691
Myths. *See* Food myths

NAD (nicotinamide-adenine dinucleotide), **246,** 334
in alcohol metabolism, 248
in glucose metabolism, 352
NADH, **246,** 248, 249
NADP (nicotinamide adenine dinucleotide phosphate), 334
Nails
in childhood malnutrition, 643t
in nutrition assessment, 537t

Naloxone, in bulimia nervosa, 321
Naltrexone, 297n
Naphthoquinone, 397t. *See also* Vitamin K
Naproxen
    peptic ulcer due to, 99n
    peptic ulcers due to, 705
Narcotic, **246**
NAS. *See* National Academy of Sciences
Nasoduodenal (ND), **764,** 765t
Nasoenteric, **764**
Nasogastric (NG), **764,** 765
Nasojejunal (NJ), **764,** 765t
National Academy of Sciences (NAS), 14, 15, F-4
    sustainable agriculture and, 502
    see also National Research Council
National Agricultural Library, F-2
National Association of Anorexia Nervosa and Associated Disorders, 319
National Association to Advance Fat Acceptance, *293*
National Center for Nutrition and Dietetics hotline, 61n
National Health and Nutrition Examination Survey (NHANES), 23
National Institute of Nutrition, F-4
National Institutes of Health
    on alternative therapies, 690
    on bovine growth hormone, 509
National Lead Information Center hotlines, 484n
National Nutrition Monitoring and Related Research Act, 23
National Pesticide Hotline, 502n
National Research Council (NRC), 14, F-4
    on cyclamate, 136
    on fluoridation, 474-475
    see also Food and Nutrition Board
National School Lunch Program, 648, 649, 651
Nationwide Food Consumption Survey (NFCS), 23
Native Americans
    ethnic diet of, 66
    lactose intolerance in, 115
Natural pesticides, 502
Natural toxicants, 498-499
Natural vitamins, 355
Natural water, **516**
Naturopathic medicine, **689**
Nausea, 94-96, 702-704, **703**
    control in cancer, 946
    in hepatitis, 828
    during pregnancy, 595
    tube feeding and, 773t
    see also Vomiting
Navy beans
    folate in, *348*
    magnesium in, *436*
ND (nasoduodenal), **764,** 765t
Needle catheter jejunostomy, 771
Negative feedback, **A-3**
Negative nitrogen balance, **194**
"Negligible-risk" standard, 504
Neodymium, B-2t
Neon, B-2t
Neoplasm, **934.** *See also* Cancer
Nepal, vitamin A supplements in, 380
Nephritis, **916**
Nephrons, 88, **911**
Nephropathy, **848, 916**
Nephrosclerosis, **916**

Nephrotic syndrome, **910**-913
Neptunium, B-2t
Nerves/nervous system, A-6 to A-8, *A-7*
    alcohol and, 249-251, *250,* 251t, 253t
    in digestion and absorption, 90-92
    folate deficiency and, 347t
    iron and, 457t
    magnesium deficiency and, 435
    niacin and, 336t, 354
    pantothenic acid and, 340t
    PKU and, 842
    riboflavin and, 334t
    solanine poisoning and, 498
    thiamin and, 330t
    vitamin A and, 383t
    vitamin B_6 and, 342t
    vitamin B_{12} and, 349, 351t
    vitamin C and, 360t
    vitamin D and, 389t
    vitamin E deficiency and, 392t, 393
    zinc and, 467t
    see also Brain
NET (nutrition education and training) program, 649-650
Net protein utilization (NPU), **198,** J-3
Neural tube defects, 586-587
    folate and, 345-346, 587-588
Neuron, **678**
Neuropathy, **848**
    diabetic, 850-851
Neurotransmitters, **194**
    Alzheimer's disease and, 678-679
    hepatic coma and, 830
Nevirapine, 950
Newborn. *See* Infant(s)
NFCS (Nationwide Food Consumption Survey), 23
NG (nasogastric), **764,** 765
NHANES (National Health and Nutrition Examination Survey), 23
Niacin, **334,** H
    blood cholesterol and, 336, 663
    in children, 663
    deficiency, **334,** 336, 336t, *337,* 354
    determination of intake, 337
    food sources, 336t, 337, *338*
    pregnancy and, 592
    RDI, 55t
    recommendations, 334, 336t, 368t
    toxicity, 336, 336t
    use as ergogenic aid, 371t
    see also B vitamins
Niacin equivalents, **334,** 337
"Niacin flush," 336
Niacinamide. *See* Niacin
Nickel, 450, 477, B-2t
Nicotinamide. *See* Niacin
Nicotinamide-adenine dinucleotide. *See* NAD
Nicotinamide-adenine dinucleotide phosphate (NADP), 334
Nicotine
    foods affecting absorption of, 527-528
    see also Smoking
Nicotinic acid. *See* Niacin
NIDDM. *See* Noninsulin-dependent diabetes mellitus
Night blindness, **378**
    vitamin A deficiency and, 381, *381*
    see also Blindness
Niobium, B-2t
Nitrates, **505**

Nitric oxide, 400n
Nitrites, **505**-506
Nitrogen, 5, *5,* B-2t, B-3, B-5t
    biological value of protein and, 197-198
    net protein utilization and, 198
    number of bonds formed by, 102, *103*
Nitrogen balance, **194**
Nitrogen-containing waste products
    accumulation in renal failure, 914, 917
Nitrogen equilibrium, **194**
Nitrosamines, **505**-506
    cancer and, 937
NJ (nasojejunal), **764,** 765t
No (on labels), 60t
Nobelium, B-2t
Nocturnal hypoglycemia, **864**
Noncommunicable diseases, chronic, **24**
Nonfat milk, powdered, 432
Nonfat milk/milk products, H
Nonfood sources of nutrients
    copper, 473
    manganese, 473
    vitamin D, 390-391, 441
    vitamin K, 394, 397
Nonfood substances, craving for. *See* Pica
Noninsulin-dependent diabetes mellitus (NIDDM), **120,** 846t, **847**
    drug therapy in, 867-868
    nonketotic coma in, 849
    in obesity, 275
    risk factors, 851
    treatment, 865-868
    see also Diabetes mellitus
Nonjudgmental responses, judgmental responses vs., 531
Nonketotic coma, hyperosmolar hyperglycemic, **848,** 849
Nonnutrients, **5, 402**
    in disease prevention, 405, 406t
Nonnutritive sweeteners. *See* Artificial sweeteners
Nonstarch polysaccharides, 108-109. *See also* Fiber(s)
Nonsteroidal anti-inflammatory drugs, peptic ulcer due to, 99n
Norepinephrine, 194, A-4
Northern European(s)
    cuisine, 63-64
    lactose intolerance in, 115
NPO, **566**
NPU (net protein utilization), **198,** J-3
NRC. *See* National Research Council
Nucleotides, **815**
    immune function and, 815
Nucleus, **A-0**
    cell, A-0
Nurse
    in nutrition education, 565
    on nutrition support team, 582, 583
Nursing bottle tooth decay, **633,** *633*
Nursing care plans, 579
Nutraceuticals, **372,** 405
Nutrient(s), **4**-11
    absorption. *See* Absorption
    additives, **505,** 507
    AIDS-related losses, 952-953
    antioxidant, 402-403. *See also* Antioxidant(s)
    in bread, *51*
    breaking down for energy, 224-238. *See also* Energy metabolism

in breast milk, 629, 629-630
cancer-induced losses, 939
chemical composition, 5
childhood needs, 638-639
classes, 4
in Daily Food Guide, 40
deficiency. *See* Deficiency; Deficiency(ies)
delivery during stress, 816-817
digestion. *See* Digestion
energy-yielding, **6**-10. *See also* Energy-
    yielding nutrients
in enteral formulas, 758-759
essential, **5**, 149
indispensable, **5**
infant needs, 626-627, 628
intakes vs. standards, 533
interactions. *See* Drug-nutrient interactions;
    Nutrient interactions
intravenous solutions, 784
on labels, 54-55. *See also* Labeling
naive vs. accurate view of needs, 17, *18*
needs and formula selection, 760
needs during pregnancy, 591-595, *592*
needs during severe stress, 811-816
needs in chronic renal failure, 920t
needs in cystic fibrosis, 734-735
needs of older adults, 671-676, 676t
nutrition care plan and needs, 562
overdose. *See* Toxicity(ies)
physiological vs. pharmacological effects of,
    336
recommendations, 14-20
recommended intakes, G-1 to G-4t, G-14,
    I-0t to I-2t
research on, 11-14
in sugars vs. other foods, 124t
supplementation for increased needs, 367
supplements. *See* Supplement(s)
toxicity. *See* Toxicity
transport. *See* Transport
see also Food(s); RDA; *specific nutrients*
Nutrient density, **38,** 41, *42*, 123-124, 302
of specific foods, 331. *See also specific foods;*
    specific nutrients
Nutrient interactions
    B vitamin, 354
    beta-carotene and vitamin E, 369
    calcium, 369, 434
    calcium and fiber, 429
    calcium and iron, 37-38, 369, 446t
    calcium and magnesium, 369, 446t
    calcium and manganese, 473
    calcium and protein, 444-445
    calcium and vitamin B$_6$, 354
    calcium and vitamin D, 387-388, 390, 428,
        429, 441, 446t
    calcium and zinc, 369
    cobalt and vitamin B$_{12}$, 477, 477
    copper and vitamin C, 451
    copper and zinc, 369, 465-466, 468, 473
    with drugs. *See* Drug-nutrient interactions
    effects on absorption, 92-93, 113
    fiber and calcium, 429
    fiber and iron, 453, 455
    folate and vitamin B$_{12}$, 346, 349, 354
    iodine and selenium, 451
    iron and calcium, 37-38, 369, 446t
    iron and fiber, 453, 455
    iron and LDL cholesterol, 459
    iron and lead, 451
    iron and magnesium, 369

iron and manganese, 451, 473
iron and vitamin C, 86, 451, 453, 454, *455,*
    459
iron and zinc, 369, 465
magnesium, 369
magnesium and calcium, 369, 434, 446t
magnesium and iron, 369
magnesium and vitamin B$_6$, 354
manganese and calcium, 473
manganese and iron, 451, 473
phosphorus and vitamin D, 387-388
phytic acid and minerals, 111, 453
protein and calcium, 444-445
protein and vitamin B$_6$, 341
riboflavin and vitamin B$_6$, 354
selenium and iodine, 451
trace minerals, 451
vitamin A and zinc, 466
vitamin B$_6$ and calcium, 354
vitamin B$_6$ and magnesium, 354
vitamin B$_6$ and protein, 341
vitamin B$_6$ and riboflavin, 354
vitamin B$_{12}$ and cobalt, 477, 477
vitamin B$_{12}$ and folate, 346, 349, 354
vitamin C and copper, 451
vitamin C and iron, 86, 451, 453, 454, *455,*
    459
vitamin C and vitamin E, 402, 403
vitamin D and minerals, 387-388, 390, 428,
    429, 441, 446t
vitamin E, 369
vitamin E and vitamin C, 402, 403-404
vitamin K and vitamin E, 369
zinc, 464
zinc and calcium, 369
zinc and copper, 369, 465-466, 468, 473
zinc and iron, 369, 465
zinc and vitamin A, 466
Nutrition
    enteral. *See* Enteral nutrition
    food choices and, 3-4
    life cycle, 585-610, 626-655, 666-684. *See*
        also specific life cycle stages
    parenteral. *See* Parenteral nutrition
    science of, **11**-14
Nutrition assessment, 20, **21, 520**-536, 537t,
    E-12 to E-31
    anthropometric measurements in, 544-550
    biochemical analyses in, 550-555
    cancer and, 956
    cardiovascular disease and, 901
    chewing and swallowing disorders and, 700
    data analysis, 562-563
    diabetes and, 873
    feeding disabilities and, 717, 718t
    historical information in, 21, 520t-536
    HIV infection and, 956
    hypoglycemia and, 873
    of individuals, 21-23
    intravenous feedings and, 792
    iron deficiency and, 456
    kidney disease and, 927
    laboratory tests in, 22
    liver disorders and, 836-837
    lower GI tract disorders and, 748
    nutrition education needs and, 562-563
    physical examination in, 22, 536, 536t, 537t
    of populations, 23-24
    summary, *564*
    tube feedings and, 776
    upper GI tract disorders and, 700, 713

Nutrition care plan, **519,** 564
    development, 563-579
    evaluation, 565
    implementation, 563-565
    records, 579
    summary, *564*
    see also Medical nutrition therapy
Nutrition care process, **519,** 562
Nutrition education, 575-578
    application of, 576
    counseling checklist, 577t
    limitations, 578
    in medical schools, 29
    planning for, 562-563
Nutrition education and training (NET) pro-
    gram, 649-650
Nutrition Facts, on labels, 54-55
Nutrition formulas
    for weight gain, 311
    see also Enteral formulas; Formulas; Infant
        formulas
Nutrition Foundation, Inc., F-4
Nutrition information
    on labels, 52, 54-55. *See also* Labeling
    life-threatening misinformation about sup-
        plements, 367-369
    in medical record, 579
    reliable, sources of, *34,* 35
    valid, distinguishing from misinformation,
        29-35
Nutrition Information Service, F-4
Nutrition intervention
    in anorexia nervosa, 318t
    see also Diet therapy; *specific disorders or inter-*
        ventions
Nutrition Labeling and Education Act of 1990,
    51. *See also* Labeling
Nutrition problem list, 562
Nutrition Program for Older Americans (Title
    III), 683
Nutrition Recommendations for Canadians, 26,
    27t
Nutrition research, 11-14. *See also* Research
Nutrition resources, F-1 to F-7
Nutrition Reviews, 34
Nutrition screening, **555**-556
    for older adults, 681, 682t
Nutrition Screening Initiative, 681, 682t
Nutrition status
    alcohol and, 245-254, *248, 250,* 251t-254t
    biochemical tests and, 552t, E-26 to E-31t
    in celiac disease, 742
    chronic obstructive pulmonary disease and,
        900
    in Crohn's disease, 737
    dietary factors affecting, 531t
    drugs affecting, 525-530, 526t, 527t, 528,
        529t
    health factors affecting, 521-525, 524t
    in malabsorption syndromes, 732t
    secondary effects of stress and illness on,
        810-811
    severe stress and, 807-808, *808,* 808t
    socioeconomic factors affecting, 530-531
    supplements and, 366-367
    weight as indicator of, 548t
    see also Nutrition assessment
Nutrition status survey, **23**
Nutrition support
    before bone marrow transplant, 945, 948
    in cancer, 943-948, 945t

in Crohn's disease, 737
in diverticular disease, 743-744
ethical issues, 797-802, *800, 801*
in HIV infection, 953-955
after intestinal surgery, 746-747
for ostomates, 746-747
specialized home support, 736, 793-795
during stress, 811-817
in ulcerative colitis, 745
Nutrition support team, 581-583, *582*
Nutrition therapy. *See* Diet therapy; Medical
nutrition therapy
Nutritional adequacy. *See* Dietary adequacy
Nutritional health, fitness and, 279-280
Nutritional yeast, **333.** *See also* Yeast
Nutritionist, **30**
Nutritive sweeteners, **135**
Nuts, H
in exchange lists, 570
iron absorption and, 455
see also Legumes; *specific type*

OA (Overeaters Anonymous), 307
Oatrim, 176, 177t
Oats, H
Obese gene, 290
Obesity
"android" vs. "gynoid," 272
binge eating in, 321
cancer and, 275
cardiovascular disease and, 275, 884t, 891
causes of, 288-292, *289*
central, **272,** 275
childhood, 658-663
cholesterol and, 660
clinically severe, **298**
defined by BMI, 270
development in children, 660-661
diabetes and, 275
fat intake and, 166-167
good choices for treatment, 301-308
health risks, 274-275, 293, 540, 884t
hyperplastic vs. hypertrophic, 288
hypertension and, 275, 891, 892
management in children, 645
morbid, **298**
poor choices for treatment, 294-301
pregnancy and, 589
prevalence, 288, *288*
prevention in children, 645, 661
sugar and, 125
surgical treatment of, *706,* 711-712
television and, 292, 644, 660-661
treatment controversies, 292-294
see also Diet(s); Overweight; Weight; Weight
loss
Obligatory water excretion, **411**
Obstructive pulmonary disease, chronic,
900-901
Occupational therapists, feeding disabilities
and, 717, 720
Octacosanol, 371t
Odors
food safety and, 493
ostomates' concerns about, 747-748
Office of Alternative Medicine, 690
Oils, 141, H
tropical, 146
see also Fat; *specific oils*
Okra, folate in, *348*
Older adults

aging process and, 668-670
arthritis in, 677
brain function in, 678-680, 679t
calcium absorption in, 441
calcium recommendations for, 430
calcium supplements in, 446t
cataracts in, 676-677
chromium deficiency in, 476
diabetes management in, 870-871
energy needs, 671-673
exercise and, 672-673
food assistance programs for, 681, 683
food choices and eating habits of, 681-684
malnutrition in, 675, 675t
mineral needs, 674-675
nutrient needs, 671-676, 676t
osteoporosis in, 440, 440t. *See also* Osteoporosis
population trends, 666, *666, 667*
strategies for, 680t
supplements for, 675
vitamin needs, 673-674
water requirements, 671
Olean. *See* Olestra
Oleic acid, *143,* 144t, *147,* C-4t
Olestra, 177t, 177-178
Oligopeptide, **182**
Oliguria, **921**
in acute renal failure, 915, 916
Oliguric phase (acute renal failure), **914**
Olive oil, 65, *146,* H
Olives, H
in exchange lists, 570
Omega, **148**
Omega-3 fatty acid, 141, 148-**149,** *149*
cancer and, 165
food sources, 149, 150t
health benefits from, 165
heart disease and, 906
recommendations, 149, 169
Omega-6 fatty acid, 141, **148,** *149*
cancer and, 165-166
food sources, 149-150, 150t
recommendations, 169
Omnivores, **210**
Onions, H
phytochemicals in, 406t
Opiates, fetal effects, 604
Opportunistic infections, **949**
Opsin, 193, 376, 377, **378**
Oral antidiabetic agents, **867**
Oral cavity. *See* Mouth
Oral contraceptives, E-12t
breast milk and, 609
folate and, 346
weight and, 295n
Oral diets. *See* Diet(s); Food(s)
Oral formulas, 761
helping clients to accept, 762
Oral hypoglycemic agents, E-2t
Oral-motor abilities, feeding disabilities and,
717, 720, 720t
Oral rehydration therapy (ORT), **416**
Oral rehydration therapy formulas, 725
Orange juice, calcium-fortified, 432
Oranges, vitamin C in, *363*
Oregano, flavonoids in, 405, 406t
Organ meats
cholesterol in, 152, 153t
see also Meat(s)
Organelles, **A-0**

Organic, **5**
Organic compounds, 5
in drinking water, 516
Organic halogen, **495**
Organic nutrients, elements in, 5
Ornithine, 180n
Orogastric, **764**
Orthomolecular medicine, **689**
Oryzanol, 371t
Osmium, B-2t
Osmolality, **759**
Osmotic diarrhea, **724**
Osmotic pressure, 412, **414,** *415*
Osteitis fibrosis, **918**
Osteoblasts, **379,** 382t, *428*
Osteoclasts, **379,** 382t, *428*
Osteodystrophy, renal, **918,** *919*
Osteomalacia, **388,** 389t, 711, **918**
pregnancy and, 594
Osteopenia, **634, 918**
Osteoporosis, **433,** 439-447
in athletes, 317, *317,* 442
body weight and, 443-444
boron and, 477
calcium and, 59, 367, 675
fluoride and, 445, 475
genetics and, 443
physical activity and, 443
prevalence, 439
protective factors, 444t
protein and, 203, 444-445
race and, 443
risk factors, 203, 442-444, 444t
stress fractures and, 316
type I, **439**
type II, **439**
Ostomate, **747**
Ounces (oz), 7
Outcome-oriented care, 959
Ovarian cancer, 936t
Ovary, hormones, A-5, A-6
Overeaters Anonymous (OA), 307
Overeating, obesity due to, 291
Overfat, **257.** *See also* Overweight
Overnutrition, **20.** *See also* Feasting; Obesity
Overpopulation, poverty and hunger and, 620
Overt, **22**
Overweight, **268, 288n**
arthritis and, 677
defined by BMI, 270, 288n
health risks, 274-275, 540
overfat vs., 257
pregnancy and, 589
societal attitudes toward, 293
see also Obesity; Weight
Ovum, **585**
Oxalate. *See* Oxalic acid
Oxalic acid, **419**
calcium and, 429
dietary restriction, 931
fat malabsorption and, 728, 730
vitamin C and, 361n
Oxidant, **402**
Oxidation, **146,** B-10
cataracts and, 677
of fats, 146, *230,* **230**-231, 238
Oxidation-reduction equilibrium, 357
iron and, 451
Oxidative metabolism
copper in, 472
riboflavin in, 402

Oxidative stress, **402**
Oxygen, 5, 5, B-2t, B-3, B-5t
　Alzheimer's disease and, 678
　energy metabolism and, 9
　exchange in vascular system, 86
　muscles' needs for, 226
　number of bonds formed by, 102, *103*
　reactive species, 400n
　singlet, 400n
Oxygen-derived free radicals, 400n. *See also*
　　Free radical(s)
Oxytocin, **A-4**
Oyster shell, 446, **447t**
Oysters, H
　calcium in, 432
　raw, 493
　riboflavin in, *335*
　safety, 493
　zinc in, *469*
oz (ounce), 7
Ozone
　bottled water and, 517
　hunger and, 618
Ozone therapy, **689**

PABA (para-aminobenzoic acid), 351
Packaging
　additives from microwave packaging, 507-
　　508
　labels and. *See* Labeling
　safety, 489, 491
Pagophagia, **458**
Pain
　"acid indigestion," 99
　bloating with, 98
　heartburn, 98
Palatability, **259**
Palladium, B-2t
Palm oil, 146, *146*
Palmitic acid, 164, C-4t
Palmitoleic acid, C-4t
Pancreas, *74*, **75**, 81t
　in blood glucose regulation, 118-119, *119*
　cancer, 936t, 945t
　cystic fibrosis and, 734
　hormones, A-4
　modified diet for conditions affecting, 569t
　transplant, 860-861
Pancreatic amylase, *112*
Pancreatic duct, *74*
Pancreatic enzymes, replacements in chronic
　　pancreatitis, 733
Pancreatic juice, **78**, 80, 81t
　regulation of, 91
Pancreatic lipase, **79**
　in fat digestion, 156, 157
Pancreatitis, 731-733, **732**, 734
Pangamic acid, 351, 371t
Pantothenic acid, **339-340**
　deficiency, 339, 340t
　food sources, 340
　RDI, 55t
　recommendations, 339, 340t, 368t
　toxicity, 340t
　see also CoA (coenzyme A)
Para-aminobenzoic acid (PABA), 351
Paraguay tea, 691
Parasympathetic (nervous system), **A-7** to A-8
Parathormone (PTH), 191t, **428**, 441n, **918**,
　　A-5
　calcium and, 428

　in chronic renal failure, 918
　vitamin D and, 389t
Parathyroid, **A-5**
Parathyroid hormone. *See* Parathormone
　　(PTH)
Parenteral nutrition, **783-795**
　in bone marrow transplant recipients, 945,
　　948
　in chronic renal failure, 923
　cyclic, **791**
　in cystic fibrosis, 736
　in diabetes, 853
　ethical issues, 797-802, *800*, *801*
　formulas, 727
　home, 736
　peripheral, **786**
　in respiratory failure, 900
　in severe diarrhea, 725
　transitional feedings after, 791
　see also Intravenous (IV) nutrition; Total
　　parenteral nutrition (TPN)
Parents
　as role models for children, 647-648
　see also Family; Genetics/genes
Parsley, iron in, *462*
Partial gastrectomy, **706**
Partial vegetarians, **210**
Passive exercise, 296
Pasta, 65
Paste, appetite for. *See* Pica
Pasteurization, **487**
Pathogens, **494**
　in drinking water, 516
　see also specific diseases or pathogens
PBB (polybrominated biphenyl), 497
PCBs (polychlorinated biphenyls)
　in breast milk, 610
　in food supply, 498
PCM (protein-kcalorie malnutrition). *See*
　　Protein-energy malnutrition (PEM)
PDCAAS (protein-digestibility-corrected
　　amino acid score), **198**, 198t, J-1, J-2t
Peak bone mass, **432**
　osteoporosis and age at, *442*
Peanut(s), 65, 152, H
　aflatoxin in, 201
　butter, H
　oil, H
Peanut butter, fat in, 170
Peanut oil, *146*
"Pear" vs. "apple" body-fat distribution, 272
Peas. *See* Black-eyed peas; Green peas; Legumes
Pectins, 109
　blood cholesterol and, 157
Peer review, 12
PEG (percutaneous endoscopic gastrostomy),
　　764
PEJ (percutaneous endoscopic jejunostomy),
　　764
Pellagra, **334**, 336, 336t, *337*, 354
Pelvis, 88
PEM. *See* Protein-energy malnutrition
Peppers, vitamin C in, *363*
Pepsin, **184**
　in protein digestion, *185*
Peptic ulcer, **96**, 99, **705-706**
　alcohol and, 252
　iron loss and, 455
Peptidase, **184**
Peptide bond, **182**. *See also* Protein/amino
　　acids (in body)

PER (protein efficiency ratio), **198**, J-3
Percent Daily Value
　for fat, 171, 172
　on labels, 56-57
　for protein, 198
Percent fat-free (on labels), 60t
Percent ideal body weight (%IBW), 547, 548t,
　　549
Percent usual body weight (%UBW), 547,
　　548t, 549
Percentages, calculation, D-2
Percutaneous endoscopic gastrostomy (PEG),
　　764
Percutaneous endoscopic jejunostomy (PEJ),
　　764
Perfringens food poisoning, 488t
Peripheral nervous system, **A-6**
Peripheral parenteral nutrition (PPN), **786**
　administration, 790
Peripheral resistance, **890**
Peripheral veins, **785**
Peripherally inserted central catheter (PICC),
　　787
Peristalsis, **76**, *77*
　reverse, 99
Peritoneal dialysis, **916**, 920t
Pernicious anemia, **349-350**, *350*, 351t
Peroxidation, **402**
　lipid, 400, 402, 473
Peroxides, B-10
Persistence (contaminants), **495**
Persistent vegetative state, **797**
　ethical issues, 798-802
Personal attitude, weight loss and, 307
Pesticides, **499**
　alternatives to, 501-502
　consumer concerns about, 501
　hazards of, 499
　hotlines, 502n
　monitoring in diet, 500-501
　monitoring in fields, 500
　natural, 502
　from other countries, 500
　regulation of, 499-501
　residues in foods, 499-502
　risk minimization, 501, 502
　tolerance level, 499
PGA (pteroylglutamic acid). *See* Folate
pH, **80**, **416**, B-7
　gastrointestinal hormones and, 91
　scale, 79, 80, *417*, B-8
　see also Acid-base balance
Pharmacist, on nutrition support team, 582,
　　583
Pharmacological effect, **336**
Phenols, 406t
Phenoxybenzamine, 297n
Phenylalanine, 134t, 135, *136*, 181t
　chemical structure, *181*
　classic PKU and, 840-842
Phenylalanine hydroxylase, classic PKU and,
　　840
Phenylketonuria (PKU), 134t, 135
　aspartame and, 135
　classic, 840, 840-843
　diet therapy for, 135
　inheritance, 843
　maternal, 842-843
　screening, 839, 840
Phenylpropanolamine, weight loss and, 297
Phenytoin, enteral nutrition and, 771

Phosphate
extracellular concentration, 413t
intracellular concentration, 413t
ion, 413t
Phosphate binders, E-12t
Phosphate pills, 371t
Phospholipids, 141, **151**, 158, 433
chemistry of, *151*, 151-152, *152*
digestion, 157
in foods, 152
roles, 152
Phosphoproteins, 433
Phosphorus, 433t, **433**-434, B-2t, B-5t, H
amount in body, *418*
blood, 552t
chronic renal failure and, 918, 920t, 922
deficiency, 433t
food sources, 433t
preterm infants and, 634
recommendations, 368t, 433t, 434
roles in body, 433, 433t
toxicity, 433t
vitamin D and, 387-388
Photon, **378**
Photophobia, 334t
Photosynthesis, **219**
Phylloquinone, 397t. *See also* Vitamin K
Physical activity
appetite control and, 304
basal metabolic rate and, 304
body fat and, 291-292
bone strength and, 443
choices for weight loss, 304-305
constipation and, 97
coronary heart disease risk and, 888-889
diabetes and, 856-858, 859t, 867
diet recommendations for, 285-286
digestion and, 92
duration and glycogen use, 281
energy expenditure and, 263-265, 264t, 266t, 267, 304
energy needs and, 812t
energy needs with aging and, 671-673
energy systems and fuels to support, 279-284, *280*, 281t
factors influencing protein use during, 283
fat use during, 282-283
fitness and, 278t, 278-279
fluids to support, 284-285, 285t
fuel mixture during, 279-280
glucose use during, 280-282
health and, 278, 278t
hydration schedule for, 285t
hypertension and, 892
insulin and, 860
intensity and glycogen use, 280
iron deficiency and, 458
longevity and, 667
obesity in children and, 660-661
protein use during, 283-284
recommendations, 278t, 283
type and intensity based on goals, 283
vitamins and minerals to support, 284
voluntary, **263**-265, 264t, 267
weight and, 291-292, 660-661
weight gain and, 311
weight loss and, 282, 283, 303-305, *305*
see also Exercise
Physical endurance
aerobic activity and, 279
diet effect on, 280, *280*

Physical examinations, in nutrition assessment, 22, 536, 536t, 537t, 550
Physical fitness. *See* Fitness
Physical therapists, 581
Physicians
diet orders prescribed by, 566-567
nutrition information from, 29-30
on nutrition support team, 581-582, 583
Physiological age, **667**
Physiological effect, **336**
Physiological fuel value, **258**
Phytate. *See* Phytic acid
Phytic acid, **111**, 406t, **419**
calcium and, 429
iron and, 453
Phytochemicals, **375**, **402**
actions, 406t
in disease prevention, 405, 406t
food sources, 406t
supplements, 405
Phytoestrogens, 406n
Phytosterols, 406t
Phytotherapy, **689**
Pica, **458**, 596
iron deficiency and, 458-459
PICC (peripherally inserted central catheter), **787**
Pickwickian syndrome, 274
Picnic foods, safety, 491
Pico waves, 510
Pigeon breast, 389t
Pigment (retina), **378**
Pigment, bile, 396
PIH. *See* Pregnancy-induced hypertension; Prolactin-inhibiting hormone
Pima Indians, 66. *See also* Native Americans
Pinto beans
calcium in, *432*
folate in, *348*
magnesium in, *436*
Pituitary, **A-3**
hormones, A-3 to A-4
PKU. *See* Phenylketonuria (PKU)
Placebo, **12**, 13
Placebo effect, **12**, 13
alternative therapies and, 690
Placenta, **585**, 586
Plant foods
in food group plans, 44
in Mediterranean diet, 214-215
phytochemicals in, 402
proteins, 196
see also Vegetables
Plaque, dental, **124**
Plaques, **883**
formation in atherosclerosis, 658, 659, 883
Plasma, 164n, 551
Platelets, **883**
Platinum, B-2t
PLP (pyridoxal phosphate), 340, 352, *353*. *See also* Vitamin B$_6$
Plumbing, water contamination via, 481, 483, 515
Plutonium, B-2t
PMS (premenstrual syndrome), 341
Pneumonia, aspiration, 698, 773t
PO, **566**
Point of unsaturation, **142**
Poisoning. *See* Food poisoning; Toxicity(ies); *specific toxins*
Polar, **413**, B-7

Polar molecules, water, 413-414, *414*
Political views, food choices and, 3
Pollution
hunger and, 618
seafood and, 493
see also Contaminant(s)
Polonium, B-2t
Polybrominated biphenyl (PBB), 497
Polychlorinated biphenyls (PCBs). *See* PCBs
Polydipsia, **848**
Polyglutamate, 342, 343
Polymeric formula, **758**
Polyols, **135**
Polypeptide, **182**
digestion in small intestine, 184
shapes of chains, 183
see also Protein/amino acids (in body)
Polyphagia, **848**, 849
Polysaccharides, 102, **107**-111
glucose and, 104
structure, C-2 to C-3
Polyunsaturated fat, **144**
cancer and, 165-166
consistency at room temperature, *145*, 145-146
effects on blood lipids, 164
food sources, 149-150, 150t
Polyunsaturated fatty acid (PUFA), 141, *144*, **144**
deficiencies, 150
vitamin E and, 393
see also Linoleic acid; Linolenic acid; Omega-3 fatty acid; Omega-6 fatty acid
Polyuria, **848**
POMR (problem-oriented medical record), 578
Pons, **250**
Population(s)
dietary recommendations for health, 26, 27t, 539-540
nutrition assessment of, 23-24
overpopulation, poverty, and hunger, 620
Population approach (to dietary recommendations), **26**, 27t
Pork, thiamin in, 332
Portal hypertension, **829**
cirrhosis and, 829
Portal systemic encephalopathy, **830**
Portal vein, **87**, *87*, 829
Portion size
in exchange lists, 571t, 571-575, *572-574*
see also Serving size
Positive nitrogen balance, **194**
Posterior, **A-3**
Postgastrectomy diet, **708**-709, 710t
Postgastrectomy hypoglycemia, **708**
Postmenopausal osteoporosis, 440t. *See also* Osteoporosis
Postmenopausal women
calcium recommendations, 445
see also Older adults
Postnecrotic cirrhosis, **828**
Postprandial hypoglycemia, **871**
Postrenal, **914**
Post-term infant, **589**
Potable (water), **516**
Potassium, **424**-426, B-2t, H
in acute renal failure, 914
amount in body, *418*
in chronic renal failure, 920t, 922
Daily Reference Value, 56t
deficiency, 424, 426, 426t

diuretics and, 426n, 894
extracellular concentration, 413t
food sources, 424, 425, 426t
hypertension and, 424, 893
intracellular concentration, 413t
ion, 413t
in processed foods, 421, *422, 424*
recommendations, 424, 426t
roles in body, 424, 426t
tests, 552t
toxicity, 426, 426t
Potatoes, H
  solanine in, 498
  sweet, *386, 395,* 406t
  vitamin C in, *362, 363*
Poultry, H
  choices, 50-51
  fat in, *50,* 168
  in food group plans, *42*
  MFP factor in, 453, 454
  niacin in, *338*
  safety, *490, 492,* 494t
  vitamin B$_6$ in, *344*
  see also Meat(s)
Pounds, 7
Poverty
  birthweight and, 598
  childhood malnutrition and, 640
  hunger and, 614, 615-616, 620
  infant formula and, 631, 633
  iron deficiency and, 457-458
  overpopulation and, 620
  PEM and, 199
  WIC program and. *See* WIC (Special Sup-
    plemental Food Program for Women,
    Infants, and Children)
Powdered bone, 446, **447t**
Powdered milk, 432
Power of attorney, 797, *801,* 801-802
PPN (peripheral parenteral nutrition), **786**
PPO (preferred provider organization), **959**
Praseodymium, B-2t
Prealbumin
  blood, 552t
  protein-energy malnutrition and, 553t
Precursors (vitamin), **326, 375**
Preeclampsia, **599**-600
Preferred provider organization (PPO), **959**
Preformed vitamin A, **375**
Pregnancy
  adolescent, 600
  alcohol during, 253, 253t, 601-604
  anorexia nervosa and, 317
  caffeine during, 605
  calcium absorption in, 429, 594
  constipation during, 595
  diabetes management in, 868-870
  drugs during, 604
  early, 586-588, 597-598
  energy needs during, 591
  exercise during, 590t, 590-591
  folate in, 345-346, 587-588, 593
  food assistance programs during, 597
  food choices during, 591, 593t, 596
  growth and development during, 585-588,
    587, 588
  heartburn during, 595-596
  hemorrhoids during, 595
  high-risk, 596t, **596**-605
  hypertension in, 599-600
  iodine deficiency in, 470

iron in, 455, 456, 594-595
lead exposure during, 480
lead poisoning during, 605
low-risk, **597**
malnutrition and, 597-598
maternal PKU and, 842-843
milk intake recommendations, 430
mineral needs during, 594-595
nausea during, 595
nutrition care plan and, 565
nutrition during, 591-596
nutrition prior to conception and, 587-588,
  597
in older women, 601
preparation for, 588-589
protein needs during, 591-592
protein RDI during, 198n
relaxin and, A-5
resources, F-5
smoking during, 604-605
supplements during, 587-588, 595t, 605
supplements in, 367, 384. *See also specific*
  nutrients
transient hypertension of, 599
vegetarian diet and, 592, 594
vitamin A in, 384
vitamin needs during, 592-594
weight and, 548
weight-gain components, 589, 590t
weight-gain recommendations, 589, *E-23*
weight loss after, 589-590
weight-loss dieting during, 605
see also Fertility; Infant(s)
Pregnancy-induced hypertension (PIH), **599,**
869
Premature infant. *See* Preterm infant
Premenstrual syndrome (PMS), 341
Prerenal, **914**
Preservatives, **505**-506
President's Council on Physical Fitness and
  Sports, F-5
Pressure sores, **810**
Preterm infant, **588**
  birthweight of, 598
  special formulas for, 634
  special needs of, 633-634
Preventive approach (to dietary recommenda-
  tions), **26**
Primary amenorrhea, **316**
Primary deficiency, **22**
Primary degenerative dementia of senile onset,
  678
Primary hypertension, **889**
Problem list, 562
Problem-oriented medical record (POMR), 578
Processed fat, 146
Processed foods
  phosphorus in, 434
  potassium in, 421, *422,* 424
  sodium in, 421, *422,* 424
  see also Food(s)
Proenzyme, **184**
Professional(s). *See* Health care professionals;
  specific type
Professional communications, 578-579
  team approach and, 579, 581-583
Professional concerns, ethical, 802
Professional nutrition organizations, F-4
Professional responsibility, enteral formulas
  and, 780-781
Progesterone, **A-6**

Prognosis, **578**
Projectile vomiting, 96
Prolactin, **A-3** to A-4
  aging and, 669n
Prolactin-inhibiting hormone (PIH), A-3
  to A-4
Proline, 180n, 181t
Promethium, B-2t
Promoters (cancer), **936,** 937
Proof (alcohol), **246**
Prooxidant(s), **402,** 404
  vitamin C as, 459
Propionic acid, 113n
Prostaglandins, 148, A-6
Prostate cancer, 403, 936t
  dietary fat and, 166
Protactinium, B-2t
Protease, **79,** 184
Protease inhibitors, 406t
Protein (dietary), 195-199, H
  acute renal failure and, 915
  biological value, 197-198
  breast milk, 629
  cancer and, 203, 244, 944, 947
  chemical composition, 5
  in choice system, I-9t to I-10t
  chronic renal failure and, 920t, 921
  cirrhosis and, 831-832
  complementary, **196**-197
  complete, **196**
  Daily Reference Value, 56t
  in diabetic diet, 853
  digestibility, **197**
  excess of, 240
  in exchange lists, 570-571, 571t, *572-573*
  fat metabolism and, 162
  health effects, 202-203
  heart disease and, 202
  high-quality, **197**
  kcalories in, 7-8, 258
  kilojoules in, 8n
  labeling regulations, 198-199
  in legumes, 44
  needs during illness, 562
  nephrotic syndrome and, 912
  niacin and, 337
  osteoporosis and, 203, 444-445
  overconsumption, 204-205
  phosphorus-containing, 433
  physical activity and, 283
  pregnancy and, 591-592
  quality, 196-198, J-1 to J-3, J-2t
  RDI, 55t, 198n
  recommendations, 15, 27t, 55t, 56t,
    203t-205, 233
  recommendations for athletes, 284
  recommendations for older adults, 673
  sources, 44, 196
  stress and, 813
  supplements, 205-206
  vegetable, 210
  in vegetarian diets, 196-197, 212
  vitamin B$_6$ and, 341
  and vitamin B$_6$ in pregnancy, 593
  in weight-loss formulas, 243-244
Protein/amino acids (in body), **180**-206, 181t
  biochemical tests of status, 551, 553t,
    553-555
  chemistry of, *180-182,* 180-183, 181t
  conditions affecting status, 553-554
  denaturation, 183

digestion, absorption, and transport, *82*, 184-186, *185. See also* Absorption; Digestion; Transport
extracellular concentration, 413t
in fluid and electrolyte regulation, 414
functions, 183, 188-193, *189-192*, 193t
in gluconeogenesis, 117
hydrophilic vs. hydrophobic, 183
inborn errors of metabolism, 839-844
intracellular concentration, 413t
iron storage, 455
liver and, 223t
metabolism. *See* Protein metabolism
nephrotic syndrome and, 911, *912*
structure, C-4 to C-5
synthesis, 186-188, *187*, *188*, 839-844
total, 552t
transport, 192, *192*
used as fuel, 283
see also Amino acid(s); *specific proteins or amino acids*
Protein-based fat replacements, 176-177, 177t
Protein deficiency. *See* Protein-energy malnutrition (PEM)
Protein-digestibility-corrected amino acid score (PDCAAS), **198**, 198t, J-1, J-2t
Protein efficiency ratio (PER), **198**, J-3
Protein-energy malnutrition (PEM), **199-202**
anorexia nervosa and, 316, 318
assessment, 553, 553t, *554*
in children, 640
classification, 199-200, 200t, 808t
congestive heart failure and, 896
head circumference and, 545
indicators of, 318n, 537t
infections in, 202
kwashiorkor, 199, 200, 200t
marasmus, 199-201, **200,** 200t
marasmus-kwashiorkor mix, 201
nephrotic syndrome and, 911
rehabilitation, 202
severe stress and, 807-808, *808*, 808t
Protein isolate, **758**
Protein-kcalorie malnutrition (PCM). *See* Protein-energy malnutrition (PEM)
Protein-losing enteropathy, **737**
Protein metabolism, 148, 193-195
alcohol and, 249
fasting and, 241
feasting and, 240
physical activity and, 283-284
Protein modules, K-8t
Protein-restricted diet
Simplesse and, 177
sodium-restricted, 834
Protein-sparing action, **117,** 195, 240
Protein-sparing fasting, **243-244**
Protein turnover, **194**
Proteinuria, **910**
Prothrombin, 394
Prothrombin time, **832**
Protoporphyrin, erythrocyte, **456**
Provitamins, **326**
Prozac (fluoxetine), in bulimia nervosa, 321
Prune juice, constipation and, 97
Prunes, 97, H
caffeic acid in, 406t
Psychological problems
alcohol and, 253t
weight cycling and, 295, *295*
see also Behavior; Emotions

Psychological stress
activity effects on, 304
aging-related, 670
HIV infection and, 951
nutrition status and, 524
overeating behaviors related to, 307
see also Stress
Psyllium, 110
Pteroylglutamic acid (PGA). *See* Folate
PTH (parathyroid hormone). *See* Parathormone
Puberty, 650-**651**
bone density in men and, 442-443
zinc deficiency and, 466, 467t
see also Adolescents/adolescence
Public health nutritionist, **30,** 30-31
Public Health Service, F-3
Public schools. *See* School
Public water, *515,* 515-517, **516,** *517. See also* Water
PUFA. *See* Polyunsaturated fatty acid
Pulmonary, **896**
Pulmonary disease, chronic obstructive, **900-901**
Pulmonary edema, in respiratory failure, 899
Pumpkin
carotenoids in, 406t
vitamin A in, 386
Pure vegetarians, **210,** 211
Pureed foods, **696,** 697, 698
Purgative, **356**
Purified water, **516**
Purine, 221
Purine-restricted diet, 932
Pyelonephritis, **916**
Pyloric sphincter, 73, *74,* **75,** 77-78
process of chyme release, 91
Pylorus, **75**
Pyramids
Mediterranean diet, 213-215, *215,* 216
USDA, 40, 41, *43, 44, 215*
Pyridoxal phosphate (PLP), 340, 352. *See also* Vitamin B_6
Pyridoxamine. *See* Vitamin B_6
Pyridoxine. *See* Vitamin B_6
Pyruvate, **224**
in alcohol metabolism, 249
extracellular concentration, 413t
intracellular concentration, 413t
in metabolism, 224-226, *225, 226,* 229-230
Pyruvic acid, **224**

Quackery/quacks, 29, **30,** 31-32, 33-34
unsound weight-loss schemes, recognizing, 296
Quality of life, weight-loss plan and, 303
Quarts, 6

Race/ethnicity
calcium nutrition and, 445
food choices and, 2
lactose intolerance and, 115
osteoporosis and, 443
see also Ethnic diets
Rachitic rosary, 389t
Radiation, **505**
foods treated with, 510-511, *511*
vitamins in milk and, 333
see also Ultraviolet radiation
Radiation enteritis, **941**
Radiation therapy, **941**

wasting and, 940t, 941
Radicals, free. *See* Free radical(s)
Radiolytic products, **510**
Radium, B-2t
Radon, B-2t
Rainforests, deforestation and hunger, 618
Randomization (in research), **12**
Rangelands, deteriorating, 618-619
Rapid weight loss, 294t
Rapport, nutrition education and, 576
Ratchet effect, **295**
Ratios, calculation, D-2
Raw sugar, **122**
RBP. *See* Retinol-binding protein
RD. *See* Registered dietitian
RDA (Recommended Dietary Allowance), **15,** G-2t to G-4t, inside front cover (left)
cystic fibrosis and, 734
energy, 15, 17, *18,* 266t, 591, 607
establishment, 16-17, *17*
folate, 347t, 587
infant, 628
intended use, 18-19
iodine, 471, 471t
iron, 457t, 460, 461
lactation and, 607
minerals, 16-17, *17*
niacin, 334, 336t
nutrient vs. energy, 17, *18*
other recommendations vs., 20
pregnancy and, 591-595, *592*
protein, 15, 203t, 203-204
revision, 19-20
riboflavin, 330, 333, 334t
selenium, 472t
thiamin, 329, 330t
use, 18-20
vitamin A, 382t
vitamin B_6, 341, 342t
vitamin B_{12}, 349, 351t
vitamin C, 359, 360t
vitamin E, 392t
vitamin K, 397t
vitamins, 16-17, *17*
zinc, 467t, 468
see also DRI (Dietary Reference Intake); *specific nutrients*
RDI (Reference Daily Intakes), **55,** 55t, 56, inside front cover (right)
protein, 198n
RE (retinol equivalents), **381**
Reactive hypoglycemia, **871-872,** 872t
Reactive oxygen species, 400n
Rebound hyperglycemia, **862**
Rebound scurvy, **362**
Recessive gene, **839**
Recombinant DNA technology, **512**
Recommended Dietary Allowance. *See* RDA
Recommended Nutrient Intakes. *See* RNI
Records. *See* Medical record
Recovery (stress response), 668
Recovery phase (acute renal failure), **914**
Rectum, 73, *74,* **75,** 78
Red bell peppers, vitamin C in, *363*
Red blood cells
anemic, *349, 350,* 456, *458*
normal, *350, 458*
normal vs. sickle cells, *188*
vitamin E and, 393
Red wine, 63-64. *See also* Alcohol; Wine
Redox state, 357

Reduced (on labels), 60t
Reduced kcalorie (on labels), 60t
REE (resting energy expenditure), **262**
Refeeding syndrome, **811**
Reference Daily Intakes (RDI), **55**, 55t, inside front cover (right)
Reference protein, **197**
    protein quality evaluation using, 197
Refined, **45**
Reflux, **77**
Reflux esophagitis, **700**-702, *701, 702t*, 703
    hiatal hernia and, 700-701
Refrigeration, safe food storage times and temperatures in, 490, 494t
Regional ileitis, **736**
Registered dietitian (RD), **21, 30,** 961
    ADA hotline for finding, 30n
Registration, **30**
Regular diets, 567
Rehabilitation, PEM and, 202
Rehydration
    oral, 416
    oral formulas, 725
Relaxin, **A-5**
Religious dietary traditions, 3, 69
Remodeling (bone), **379**
Renal, **911**
Renal artery, 88
Renal colic, **930**
Renal failure, **910**
    acute, 913-916
    chronic, 916-927
    zinc and, 467t
    see also Kidney(s)
Renal insufficiency, **920**, 920t
Renal osteodystrophy, **918**, *919*
Renal reserve, **917**
Renal threshold, **848**
Renal vein, 88
Renin, **411, 911, A-5**
    blood pressure and, 411
    salt sensitivity and, 420n
Rennin, **511**
Replication (research), **12**
Reproductive system
    zinc and, 467t
    see also Pregnancy
Requirement, **16**
Research, 11-14
    on alcohol dehydrogenase in women, 247
    on artificial sweeteners, 133, 136
    identifying valid information from, 32-33, 33t
    on obesity, 288-292
    population surveys in, 23-24
    reports on U.S. nutrition status, 24n
    rumors vs., 14
    on vitamin B$_6$ toxicity, 341
    on vitamin C, 11-13
Research articles, 32-33, 33t
Resection. *See* Surgery; specific site
Residual, gastric, **768**
Residue (in colon), **759**
Residues (pesticide), **499**-502
Resistance
    peripheral, **890**
    in stress response, 668
Resistance activity. *See* Strength training
Resistant starch, **113**
Resource use, sustainable, **616,** 620-621
Resources, F-1 to F-7

Respiratory acidosis, **788**
Respiratory distress, **869**
Respiratory failure, **898**-900
Respiratory quotient (RQ), **899**
Respiratory system
    HIV infection and, 952
    very-low-kcalorie diet side effects in, 300t
    vitamin C in infections, 358-359
    see also Lung(s)
Respiratory therapists, 581
Resting energy expenditure (REE), **262**
Retin-A, 384
Retina, **378**
Retinal, **375**
    chemical structure, *376*
    see also Vitamin A
Retinoic acid, **375**
    chemical structure, *376*
    see also Vitamin A
Retinoids, **375**
Retinol, **375**
    alcohol and, 252
    chemical structure, *376*
    food sources, 382t
    see also Vitamin A
Retinol-binding protein (RBP), **375**
    protein-energy malnutrition and, 553t
Retinol equivalent (RE), **381**
Retinopathy, **848**
Reverse peristalsis, 99
Review journals, *34*
Rhamnose, 109n
Rhenium, B-2t
Rheumatic heart disease, **894**
Rheumatoid arthritis, 677
Rhodium, B-2t
Rhodopsin, **378**
Riboflavin, **330,** H
    deficiency, 333, 334t
    food sources, 333, 334t, *335*
    in oxidative metabolism, 402
    pregnancy and, 592
    RDI, 55t
    recommendations, 330, 333, 334t, 368t
    vitamin B$_6$ and, 354
    see also B vitamins
Ribonucleic acid. *See* RNA
Ribose, 221
Ribosomes, *187,* **A-0**
Rice, H
    beriberi and, 329
Rice bran, 110
Rich in (on labels), 60t
Rickets, **388,** *388,* 389t
    of prematurity, **634**
    see also Vitamin D
Ricotta cheese, zinc in, *469*
Rights, individual, 798-799
Rigor, calcium, **429**
Risk, **486**
Risk factors, 24-26
    cancer, 165, 404
    cardiovascular disease, 164, 883-886, 884t, 891
    chronic diseases, 24-26
    diabetes, 851
    health status and, 539-540, *540,* 541t, *542*
    hypertension, 891
    malnutrition in older adults, 675t, 681
    osteoporosis, 203, 442-444, 444t
Ritonavir, 950

RNA
    protein synthesis and, 186, *187*
    use as ergogenic aid, 371t
RNA polymerase, 463n
RNI (Recommended Nutrient Intakes), 15, I-0t to I-2t
    age and, 671n
    lactation and, 607
    omega-3 fatty acids, 169n
    omega-6 fatty acids, 169n
    pregnancy and, 591-595
    vitamin C, 359, *359*
Rods (of retina), **378**
Rolaids, 447t
Rough endoplasmic reticulum, **A-1**
Rounds, professional communication and, 579, 583
Royal jelly, 371t
RQ (respiratory quotient), **899**
Rubidium, B-2t
Rutabaga, calcium in, *432*
Ruthenium, B-2t

Saccharin, 133, 134t, **135,** 421
    exception to Delaney Clause, 503-504
Safety, **501**
    of artificial sweeteners, 133-136
    consumer concerns about foods, 486-513
    consumer concerns about public water, 515-516
    defense against lead contamination and, 483-484
    margin of, **504**
    resources, F-3
    see also Contaminant(s)
Safflower oil, *146*
Salad, safety, 491
Salad bars
    fat in, 170
    sulfites in, 506
Salad dressing, 170
Saline, in intravenous solutions, 785
Saliva, **78,** 81t
    in digestion, 79
    reduced flow in chewing difficulties, 697
Salivary glands, *74,* **78,** *79,* 81t
    amylase and, *112,* 113
    in fat digestion, 154, *155*
Salmonella, 487, 488, 488t
    radiation and, 510
Salmonellosis, 488t
Salt(s), **412**
    aluminum, 446
    blood pressure and, 420
    cell, 370t
    dissociation in water, 412-413
    iodized, 471
    limitation in hypertension, 892
    recommendations, 27t
    sodium in, 420
    strategies for reducing intake, 421
    tablets, 423
    vomiting and body balance of, 96
    water in dissolution of, *414*
    see also Potassium; Sodium
Salt-free (on labels), 60t
Salt sensitivity, hypertension and, 420, 892
Samarium, B-2t
Sample size, in research, 13
Saponins, 406t
Saquinavir, 950

Sarcomas, **934**
  Kaposi's, **952**
Sardines, calcium in, *431, 432*
Satiety, **259**-261
  overriding signals of, 261
  weight loss and, 303
Saturated fat, **144,** *145*
  atherosclerosis and, 888
  Daily Reference Value, 56t
  health risks of, 59, 61, 164
  recommendations, 167
Saturated fat-free (on labels), 60t
Saturated fatty acids, 27t, **144**
  structure, 142, C-4t
  see also Saturated fat
Sauna baths, 298
Sauna belts, 296
Scandium, B-2t
School
  nutrition at, 648t, 648-650
  nutrition education at, 649-650
School Breakfast Program, 640, 648, 649
School Lunch Program, 648, 649
Science of nutrition, *11*-14
Scientific method, *11*
Sclera, 457t
Scorbutic gums, *361*
"Scorbutic pose," *361*
Scurvy, **356,** 360t, 360-361, *361*
  rebound, **362**
  see also Vitamin C
SDA (specific dynamic activity), **265**
SDAT (senile dementia of the Alzheimer's
    type), **678**-679
SDE (specific dynamic effect), **265**
Seafood
  cholesterol in, 152, 153t
  iodine in, 471
  raw, 493
  safety, 490, 493
  in voluntary labeling program, 52, 53t
  see also Fish; *specific type*
Seaweeds, calcium in, 432
Secondary amenorrhea, 316
Secondary deficiency, **22**
Secondary hypertension, **889**
Secretin, 90n, **91,** A-6
  malabsorption and, 709
Secretory diarrhea, **724**
Sedentary (behavior), 278-279, **282.** *See also*
    Physical activity; Television watching
Seeds. *See* Legumes; *specific type*
Segmentation, intestinal, **76,** *77*
Selectively permeable (cell membrane), **412**
Selenium, 450, **471**-472, 472t, B-2t
  amount in body, *418*
  cancer and, 471-472
  deficiency, 471, 472t
  food sources, 472t
  RDI, 55t
  recommendations, 472t
  roles in body, 471, 472t
  toxicity, 472, 472t
Self-esteem, weight loss and, 306, 307
Self-help groups, weight loss and, 307
Semivegetarians, **210**
Senile cataracts, 677
Senile dementia, **678**
Senile dementia of the Alzheimer's type
    (SDAT), **678**-679
Senile osteoporosis, 440t. *See also* Osteoporosis

Senna leaves, 691
Sepsis, **788, 804**
  bacterial translocation and, 810
Septicemia, **804**
Serine, 181t
Serotonergic agents, 297n
Serotonin, 194, **340**
  foods containing, 559-560
  vitamin B$_6$ and, 340
Serum, 164n, **551**
Serum albumin, protein-energy malnutrition
    and, 553t
Serum amylase, 552t
  pancreatitis and, 732
Serum creatinine, 552t
Serum enzymes, 552t
Serum ferritin, E-31t
Serum iron, E-31t
Serum lipase, 552t
Serum transferrin, protein-energy malnutrition
    and, 553, 553t
Serving size
  for children, 646
  in Daily Food Guide, 41, *42-43*
  in diet history, 535
  in exchange system, 574
  on labels, 54, 54t
  of meats, 51
  for weight gain, 310
  for weight loss, 302
Sesame seeds, calcium in, *310*
Set-point theory, 290-**291**
Seventh-Day Adventists, 69, 210
Severe diarrhea, 724-725
Severe hyperglycemia, and ketoacidosis, 865
Severe hypoglycemia, 864-865
Severe stress, **804**-817. *See also* Stress
Sewage treatment, 516
Sex. *See* Gender differences; Men; Women
Sex hormones, 153, A-6. *See also* Estrogen
Sexual maturation. *See* Puberty
SGA (small for gestational age), **598**
Shellfish. *See* Seafood
Shock, **811**
Shopper's Guide to Low-Lead China, 483n
Shopping
  dietary guidelines and, 45, 48-51
  environmentally conscious, 623t
  food labels and. *See* Labeling
  singles and, 682-684
Short-bowel syndrome, **739**-741
  intestinal adaptation in, 753-754
Short-chain fatty acids, 113n, 158
  intestinal adaptation and, 752-753
Short-gut syndrome, **739**
Shrimp
  iron in, *462*
  niacin in, *338*
  vitamin E in, *395*
  zinc in, *469*
  see also Seafood
Shunts, 829-**830**
SI (International System of Units), 6
Sickle-cell anemia, **188**
SIDS (sudden infant death syndrome),
    604-**605**
  botulism and, 635n
Sigmoid, **75**
Silent heart attack, **850**
Silicon, 450, 477, B-2t
Silver, 477, B-2t

Simple carbohydrates, **102**-107
Simple goiter, **470**
Simple sugars, **102**
Simplesse, 176-177, 177t
Simultaneous multiple analysis (SMA), **551**
Singles, meals for, 681-684
Singlet oxygen, 400n. *See also* Oxygen
Sioux Indians, 66
Sirloin steak, zinc in, *469*
SIRS (systemic inflammatory response syn-
    drome), **805**
Sitophobia, **699**
Skin
  in acute renal failure, 915
  antigen testing, 550
  B vitamins and, 355
  in childhood malnutrition, 643t
  in chronic renal failure, 917
  induration, **550**
  iron and, 457, 457t
  niacin and, 336, 336t, *337*, 354
  in nutrition assessment, 537t, 550
  pressure sores, 810
  protein and, 189
  tube feeding and, 773t
  vitamin A and, 382t
  vitamin B$_6$ deficiency and, 342t
  vitamin C and, 360t
  water loss from, 411
  zinc deficiency and, 467t
Sleep
  BMR and, 263t
  digestion and, 92
  vitamin B$_6$ and, 341
Sleep apnea, 274
Sliding hiatal hernia, *701*
SMA (simultaneous multiple analysis), **551**
Small-for-date babies, **598**
Small for gestational age (SGA), **598**
Small intestine, *74, 75*
  in absorption, 83, *84, 85,* 114, *114*
  adaptation after resection, 752-754
  blind loop syndrome, 710
  in carbohydrate digestion, *112,* 113
  in digestive process, 73, 80, *82*
  in fat digestion, 155-157, *156-157*
  in protein digestion, 184, *185*
  resection causing malabsorption, 739-741,
    740
Smoked fish, 421
Smoked meats, 421
Smoking, 25
  in adolescence, 654-655
  BMR and, 263t
  childhood education about, 663
  folate and, 346
  infant exposure to, 604-605
  lactation and, 609
  lung cancer and, 404
  nitrosamines from, 506
  osteoporosis and, 444
  pregnancy and, 604-605
  vitamin C and, 359, *359*, 360t
Smooth endoplasmic reticulum, **A-1**
Snacks
  for adolescents, 652, 653t
  for children, 647
  sodium intake and, 421
  for weight gain, 310-311
Snow peas, vitamin C in, *363*
Social interactions

aging and, 670
food choices and, 2
Social workers, 581
Societal attitudes, eating disorders and, 315, 321-322
Society for Nutrition Education, F-4
Socioeconomic history, 21, 520t, *521*, **530**-531
Socioeconomic status
aging and, 670
factors affecting food choices, 530t
iron deficiency and, 457-458
PEM and, 199
see also Poverty
SOD. *See* Superoxide dismutase
Soda, carbonated, 129. *See also* Cola beverages
Sodium, **419**-423, B-2t, B-5t, H
aldosterone and retention of, 411
amount in body, *418*
in breast milk, 630
chloride deficiency and, 423
chronic renal failure and, 920t, 924
cirrhosis and, 832, 833t
congestive heart failure and, 896
Daily Reference Value, 56t
deficiency, 420t, 422-423
diabetes and, 853
drugs containing, 529-530
extracellular concentration, 413t
food sources, 420t, 421-422
health risks, 541t
hypertension and, 59, 420, 423, 892
imbalance, 416
infants with cystic fibrosis and, 735
intake surveys, 420-421
intracellular concentration, 413t
ion, 412-413, 413t
ions, *B-5* to *B-6*
nephrotic syndrome and, 912
in processed foods, 421, *422*, 424
recommendations, 27t, 56t, 419-420, 420t
roles in body, 419, 420t
in salt, 420
tests, 552t
toxicity, 420t, 423
see also Salt(s)
Sodium bicarbonate, 421
Sodium chloride. *See* Salt; Sodium
Sodium cyanide, 5n
Sodium cyclamate, 134t
Sodium fluoride, 475
Sodium-free (on labels), 60t
Sodium polystyrene sulfate, E-12t
Sodium-potassium ATPase, **414**
Sodium-potassium pump, **414**
Sodium-restricted diet
kidney stones and, 931
protein-restricted, 834
Sodium saccharin, 421. *See also* Saccharin
Soft diet, mechanical, **696**-697, 698
Soft drinks, aspartame content, 137t
Soft water, **516**
Soil
contaminants, *497*
hunger and, 618
iodine in, 470
Solanine, **498**
Solid foods, introduction, 634-637, 635t
Soluble fibers, 110, 111t
Solutes, **414**
loss by different routes, 416

Somatic nervous system, **A-7**
Somatomedin-C, 554
Somatostatin (GIH), **A-3**
Somatotropin (GH), **A-3**. *See also* Growth hormone
Somogyi effect, **862**
Sorbitol, **135**, 138t
drugs containing, 529
South Americans. *See* Hispanics
Southern cuisine, 65-66
Southern European cuisine, 64-65
Soy
infant formulas based on, 633
iron absorption and, 455
phytochemicals in, 406t
Soy "milk," 44
calcium in, *432*
thiamin in, *332*
Soy sauce, 420
Soybean(s), 152, H
caffeic acid in, 406t
oil, H
Soybean curd. *See* Tofu
Soybean oil, *146*
vitamin E in, 394, *395*
Spastic constipation, 97
Special feeding devices, *719*, 720
Special formulas
enteral, 780
infant, 633, 634
Special nutrition support. *See* Nutrition support
Special Supplemental Food Program for Women, Infants, and Children. *See* WIC
Specific dynamic activity (SDA), **265**
Specific dynamic effect (SDE), **265**
Sperm, **585**
Sphincter, **75**
cardiac, 73, *74*, **75**, 77, 98, **701**, 702t
ileocecal, *74*, **75**, 78
pyloric, 73, *74*, **75**, 77-78, 91
Spices
mouth ulcers and, 697
in pureed foods, 697
sodium-free, 421
see also Flavor enhancers
Spina bifida, **345**. *See also* Neural tube defects
Spinach
calcium in, *431, 432*
carotenoids in, 406t
folate in, *348*
iron in, *462*
magnesium in, *436*
niacin in, *338*
potassium in, *425*
riboflavin in, *335*
thiamin in, *332*
vitamin A in, *386*
vitamin B$_6$ in, *344*
vitamin C in, *363*
vitamin E in, *395*
zinc in, *469*
Spirits, distilled, **246**, 252t
Spirulina, 296, 371t
Spleen
vitamin A and, 383t
zinc deficiency and, 467t
Sport Medicine and Science Council of Canada, F-5
Spot reducing, 305
Spring water, **516**

Sprue, celiac, **741**-742, 743t
Squash
potassium in, *425*
thiamin in, *332*
vitamin A in, *386*
vitamin B$_6$ in, *344*
Standard diets, **567**
Standard enteral formulas, 779-780
Standard formula, **758**
Staphylococcal food poisoning, 489t
Staphylococcus aureus, 489t
Starch, **108, C-2**
blockers, 296
in choice system, I-3t to G-4t
digestion and absorption, 82, 111-114, *112*, *114*. *See also* Absorption; Digestion
in exchange lists, 570, 571t, *572*, G-6t
glucose and, 104
health effects of, 126-127
molecular structure, *108, 109*
recommendations, 128
resistant, **113**
Starvation
BMR and, 263t
metabolic effects, 195, 240-244, *241, 242*
symptoms, 243
see also Anorexia nervosa; Fasting; Malnutrition
Stavudine (d4T), 950
Steam baths, 298
Stearic acid, 142, *142*, 144t, 164, C-4t
food sources, 164
Steatorrhea, **727**, *739*
Steatosis, hepatic, **827**
Sterile, **396**
Steroids
herbal, 371t
potassium and, 426
Sterols, 141, **152**
chemistry of, *152*, 152-154
roles, 153-154
see also Cholesterol
Stimulants
child behavior and, 643-644
for hyperactivity, 643
see also Amphetamines; Caffeine
Stoma, 746, **746**
Stomach, *74*, **75**
alcohol in, 247
cancer, 403, 936t, 945t
in carbohydrate digestion, *112*, 113
in digestive process, 73, *74*, 76, 79-80, *82*
disorders, 699-713
in fat digestion, 154, *155*
gastrin and, A-6
gastritis, 349
nerve receptors in, 91
pH, 91
pressure effect on reflux, *701*
in protein digestion, 184, *185*
surgery, 706-712
surgery in obesity treatment, *298*, 298-299
see also Digestion
Stools, **81**
fiber and, 113, 127
tests for GI bleeding, 559
see also Constipation; Diarrhea
Strawberries
potassium in, *425*
vitamin C in, *363*

Strength training, 311
  aging and, 672, 673
  recommendations for fitness, 278t
Stress, **668,** 804
  activity effects on, 304
  BMR and, 263t
  body's response to, 804-811
  energy needs and, 812t, 812-815
  enteral nutrition in, 780, 815
  fluids and electrolytes in, 811
  GI tract immune function and, 808-810,
    809t
  hormonal changes during, 805t, 805-806
  longevity and, 668-669
  metabolic responses to, 804-807, 805t, 806
  nutrient delivery during, 816-817
  nutrient needs during, 811-816
  nutrition status during, 807-808, 808, 808t
  nutrition support during, 811-817
  oxidative, **402**
  protein needs during, 813-815
  secondary effects on nutrition status,
    810-811
  severe, **804**-817
  supplements and, 367
  supplements claiming to relieve, 372
  vitamin C and, 358
  see also Emotions; Illness; *specific stresses*
Stress eating, **261**
Stress fractures, **316**
Stress response, **668,** 804
  phases, 806
Stressor, **668,** 804
Strict vegetarians, **210,** 211
Stroke, **897**-898
  potassium intake and, 424
  see also Cardiovascular disease (CVD); Feed-
    ing disabilities
Stroke Belt (U.S.), 66
Strontium, B-2t
Struvite, **930**
  kidney stones composed of, 930, 932
Stunting, chronic PEM and, 199
Subclavian vein, **90**
Subclinical deficiency, **23**
Subcutaneous fat, 272
Subjective Global Assessment, 555
Substitute food, **51**
Subtotal gastrectomy, **706**
Succinate, 371t
Sucralose, 133, 134t, **135,** 136
Sucrase, **113**
Sucrose, **106**
  hydrolysis, 113
Sucrose polyester (olestra), 177t, 177-178
Suction lipectomy, 299
Sudan, vitamin A supplements in, 380
Sudden infant death syndrome (SIDS),
  604-**605**
  botulism and, 635n
Sugar(s), 102t, 102-107, 121-126
  alternatives, 133-138
  behavior and, 125
  dental caries and, 124-125
  digestion and absorption, 82. *See also*
    Absorption; Digestion
  drugs containing, 529
  energy and, 114
  estimated intake, 122
  fruit vs., 123

health effects of, 122-125
  heart disease and, 125
  honey vs., 103, 123
  hyperactivity and, 643
  nutrients in, 123-124, 124t
  obesity and, 125
  recommendations, 103, 114, 125-126,
    129-130
  see also Carbohydrate(s); Sweeteners
Sugar alcohols, **135,** 138, 138t
Sugar-free (on labels), 60t
Sulfate
  extracellular concentration, 413t
  intracellular concentration, 413t
  ion, 413t
Sulfites, **506**
Sulfonylureas, **867**
Sulforaphane, 406t
Sulfur, **435,** B-2t, B-5t
  amount in body, *418*
  food sources, 437t
  roles in body, 435, 437t
  toxicity, 437t
Sunflower oil, *146*
Sunflower seeds
  magnesium in, 314t, *436*
  thiamin in, *255, 332*
Sunlight, vitamin D from, 390-391, 441
Superoxide dismutase (SOD), 472n
  use as ergogenic aid, 371t
Superoxide radical, 400n
Supplement(s), **372**
  amino acid, 184, 205-206, 296
  anorexia nervosa and, 318
  antioxidant, 404, 405
  B vitamin, 354-355
  beta-carotene, 404
  bioavailability and antagonistic actions,
    368-369
  body's defenses and, 367
  calcium, 367, 445-447, 446t, 447t, 922
  contents, 370-371
  cost, 372
  in cystic fibrosis, 735
  disease risks and, 367
  false sense of security with, 368
  fish oil, 169, 907
  fluoride, 445
  folate, 345, 367, 587-588
  forms, 369-370
  for infants, 367, 630, 630t
  invalid reasons for taking, 368
  iron, 463
  during lactation, 608
  lecithin, 152, 679
  life-threatening misinformation about,
    367-368
  misleading claims about, 371-372
  nutrient needs and, 367
  nutrition status and, 366-367
  for older adults, 675
  overt deficiencies and, 366
  physical activity and, 284
  phytochemical, 405
  in pregnancy, 367, 587-588, 595t, 605
  protein, 205-206
  recommendations, 27t
  regulation, 372
  salt, 423
  selection, 369-372

toxicity from, 367
  trace minerals, 450
  unknown needs and, 368
  used by athletes, 205, 369, 370t-371t
  very-low-kcalorie diets and, 299
  vitamin A, 380-381
  vitamin C, 11-13, 404
  vitamin D, 441
  vitamin E, 404
  vitamin/mineral, 284, 366-372, 368t
  zinc, 468
Supplementation, mutual, **196**
Support groups, weight loss and, 307
Surface water, 515
Surgeon General's Report on Nutrition and
  Health, 541
Surgery
  in cancer treatment, 941t, 942
  coronary, 887
  gastric, 706-712
  intestinal adaptation after, 752-754
  large intestine resections, 745-749, 746
  malabsorption caused by, 739-741, *740, 746*
  in obesity treatment, 298, 298-299
  organ transplants, 834-837
  in ulcerative colitis, 745
Sushi, 68, **493**
Sustainable (resource use), **614**
  pesticide alternatives and, 502
  worldwide development, 620-621
Swallowing, *94*
  alleviation of problems in cancer, 947
  belching and, 98
  difficulties, 697-699, 717
Sweat, fluid losses via, 284
Sweet potatoes
  carotenoids in, 406t
  vitamin A in, 386
  vitamin E in, *395*
Sweeteners/sweets
  artificial, 133-138, **135,** 503-504, 605
  children and, 639
  in Daily Food Guide, 39, *43*
  diabetic diet and, 852-853
  infants and, 636
  on labels, 53
  nutritive, **135**
  per capita use, *121,* 121-122
  postgastrectomy, 708
  recommendations, 129-130
  weight loss and, 303
  see also specific sweeteners
Swelling. *See* Edema
Swiss cheese
  calcium in, *431*
  zinc in, *469*
Sympathetic (nervous system), **A-7** to A-8
Symptomatic allergy, **645**
Synergism, vitamin C and vitamin E, 403
Synthetase, **189**
Systemic inflammatory response syndrome
  (SIRS), **805**

T_3 (triiodothyronine), 470
T_4. *See* Thyroxin
T-lymphocyte, CD4+, **949**
Table sugar, 106. *See also* Sucrose; White sugar
Tachycardia, **896**
Tacrine, 678
Take Off Pounds Sensibly (TOPS), 307

Tannic acid, iron absorption and, 455
Tanning lamps, vitamin D and, 391
Tantalum, B-2t
Taste perceptions
    aging and, 670
    improvement in cancer, 946
Taste preferences, 2
Taurine, 180n
TCA (Krebs) cycle, 226-**227**, *227*, 235, C-14
    to C-16
    in alcohol metabolism, 248, *248*
    biotin and, 337
    cell and, A-1n
    fatty acid oxidation and, 231
    manganese and, 473
    riboflavin coenzyme and, *333*
TE (tocopherol equivalents), **393**
Tea
    flavonoids in, 405, 406t
    iron absorption and, 455
    see also Caffeine
Team approach, 581-583, *582*
    diabetes and, 877
Technetium, B-2t
Teenagers. *See* Adolescents
Teeth
    absence of, 696
    in childhood malnutrition, 643t
    fetal development, 594
    fluoride and, 427, 474-475, *475*
    formation, 427, *427*
    loss with aging, 669
    nursing bottle decay, 633, *633*
    in nutrition assessment, 537t
    sugar and, 124-125
    vitamin A and, 382t
    vitamin D and, 389t
    see also Dental caries
Telephone hotlines. *See* Hotlines
Television watching
    child behavior and, 644
    obesity and, 292, 660-661
Tellurium, B-2t
Tempeh, **210**
Temperature
    measurement, D-3
    safety of hot and cold foods, 490, 492, *492*
    see also Body temperature; Environmental
        temperature
Tension-fatigue syndrome, **642**
    television and, 644
Teratogenic, **604**
Terbium, B-2t
Term infant, **588**
Terminal illness, **797**
    ethical issues, 797-802
Testes, male bone density and, 442
Testosterone, **A-6**
Tetany
    calcium, **429**
    magnesium and, 435
Tetracycline
    calcium supplements and, 446t
    food interactions with, 527
Tetrahydrofolate (THF), 342, 352, *353*
Tetrahydrolipostatin, weight loss and, 297
Tetraiodothyronine, 470. *See also* Thyroxin
    (T$_4$)
Textured vegetable protein, **210**
Thallium, B-2t

Thawing, safety, 490
THC (delta-9-tetrahydrocannabinol), 653n
Therapeutic diet, **567**. *See also* Medical nutri-
    tion therapy
Thermic effect of food, 261, **265**
Thermogenesis, **261**
    adaptive, **265**
Thermogenic agents, 297n
THF. *See* Tetrahydrofolate
Thiamin, **329**-330, 330t, H
    deficiency, 329-330, 330t
    food sources, 330, *330*, 330t, *332*
    pregnancy and, 592
    RDI, 55t
    recommendations, 329, 330t, 368t
    sulfites and, 506
    sulfur in, 435
    see also B vitamins
Thiamin pyrophosphate (TPP), 329, 352, *353*
Thirst, **410**
    alcohol and, 250
    sodium and, 419
Thoracic duct, **90**
Thorium, B-2t
3-in-1 admixtures, **790**
3TC (lamivudine), 950
Threonine, 181t, 196
Thrombin, 394
Thrombosis, **883**
Thromboxanes, 148
Thrush, **952**
Thulium, B-2t
Thyroid gland
    goiter and, 470
    goitrogens and, 470, 498
    iodide and, 470
Thyroid-stimulating hormone (TSH), A-3
    iodine and, 470
Thyroxin, A-4
Thyroxin (T$_4$), 191t, 194, 470
    BMR and, 263t
Thyroxin-binding prealbumin. *See* Prealbumin
TIA (transient ischemic attack), **897**
Tin, 477, B-2t
Titanium, B-2t
Title III (Nutrition Program for Older Ameri-
    cans), 683
Tobacco
    pregnancy and, 604-605
    see also Smoking
Tocopherol, **391**. *See also* Vitamin E
Tocopherol equivalents (TE), **393**
Tocotrienols, 391n, 393n
Tofu, **210**, 213n
    calcium in, *431, 432*
    iron in, *462*
    magnesium in, *436*
    zinc in, *469*
Tolerance level, **499**
Tomato juice
    folate in, *348*
    iron in, *462*
    magnesium in, *436*
    niacin in, *338*
    potassium in, *425*
    thiamin in, *332*
    vitamin A in, *386*
    vitamin B$_6$ in, *344*
    vitamin C in, *363*
    vitamin E in, *395*

zinc in, *469*
Tomatoes, carotenoids in, 406t
Tongue
    B vitamin deficiencies and, 355, *355*
    in childhood malnutrition, 643t
    folate deficiency and, 347t
    niacin deficiency and, 336t
    in nutrition assessment, 537t
    riboflavin deficiency and, 334t
    vitamin B$_6$ deficiency and, 342t
    vitamin B$_{12}$ deficiency and, 351t
Tooth. *See* Teeth
TOPS (Take Off Pounds Sensibly), 307
Tortillas, 67
Total Diet Study, 500-501
Total gastrectomy, **706**
Total lymphocyte count, protein-energy malnu-
    trition and, 554
Total nutrient admixtures, **790**
Total parenteral nutrition (TPN)
    in acute renal failure, 916
    in cancer, 944
    catheter insertion and care, 788
    central, 786, **786-787**, 787t
    central veins used for, 786
    in cirrhosis, 834
    complications, 789t
    composition of solutions, 787-788
    in Crohn's disease, 737
    cyclic infusion, 791
    in HIV infection, 954-955
    home, 793-795
    after intestinal surgery, 752, 753-754
    monitoring, 790t
    peripheral, 786
    solution administration, 789-791
    transition to enteral feedings from, 791-792
    in ulcerative colitis, 745
    see also Parenteral nutrition
Total protein, 552t
    in breast milk, 629
Total vegetarians, **210**, 211
Toxic goiter, **470**
Toxicity(ies), 17, *18*, 20, **486**
    artificial sweeteners, 133, 136
    B vitamin, 356
    calcium, 427t, 429, 446t
    chloride, 423, 424t
    choline, 351
    chromium, 476t
    copper, 473, 473t
    dose levels and, 341, *343*
    fluoride, 474t, 475, *475*
    folate, 347t
    food-borne illnesses, 487-494
    iodine, 470, 471t
    iron, 367, 457t, 459-460
    lead. *See* Lead
    lecithin, 351
    magnesium, 434t
    manganese, 473, 474t
    molybdenum, 476, 476t
    natural toxicants in foods, 498-499
    niacin, 336, 336t
    pantothenic acid, 340t
    phosphorus, 433t
    physical examination and, 22
    phytochemical, 405
    potassium, 426, 426t
    selenium, 472, 472t

sodium, 420t, 423
sulfur, 437t
supplements causing, 367
trace minerals, 450
vitamin A, 367, *380*, 382t, 383-384
vitamin B₆, 341, 342t
vitamin C, 360t, 361-362
vitamin D, 388, 389t, 390, 446t
vitamin E, 392t, 393
vitamin K, 396, 397t
water, 410
zinc, 466-468, 467t
see also Contaminant(s); Food poisoning
Toxins
bioaccumulation in food chain, *495*, *496*
see also Toxicity(ies); *specific toxins*
TPN. *See* Total parenteral nutrition
TPP (thiamin pyrophosphate), 329, 353
Trabecular bone, **439**, *439*-440
osteoporosis and, 440, *440*, 440t. *See also*
Osteoporosis
Trace minerals, 10, **418**, 450-477. *See also* Mineral(s); *specific minerals*
Trachea, *74*, *75*
food lodged in. *See* Choking
Trade organizations, F-5
Training
effect on fat use, 282
effect on glycogen use, 282
effect on protein use, 284
see also Physical activity
Trans-fatty acids, *147*, **147**
food labels and, 170
formation, 147
health risks from, 164-165
sources, 147
Transamination, **233**-234, *234*
Transfer RNA, protein synthesis and, 186, *187*
Transferrin, **192**
blood, 452, 455, 552t
mucosal, **452**
protein-energy malnutrition and, 553, 553t
saturation in iron deficiency, E-31t
zinc and, 465
Transgenic organism, **512**
Transient ischemic attack (TIA), **897**
Translocation (bacteria), 809t, **809**-810
Transnasal, **764**
Transnasal feeding tube, **764**, 765-766
Transplants
bone marrow, **942**-943, 945, 948
kidney, 925t, *925*-926
liver, 834-837
pancreas, 860-861
Transport (nutrient), 86-90, *87*-89
active, 83, *85*
iron, 455
lipid, 158, *159*-160
nutrient preparation for, 86
vitamin, 327
see also Circulatory system(s); Digestion
Transport proteins, 192, *192*
Transthyretin. *See* Prealbumin
Trauma, **804**
hip fractures, 439. *See also* Osteoporosis
see also Stress; *specific type*
Travel, food safety during, 494
Traveler's diarrhea, 489t, 494
Tremor, flapping, **830**
TRH (TSH-releasing hormone), A-3

Triacylglycerols, **141**. *See also* Triglycerides
Tricarboxylic acid cycle. *See* TCA (Krebs) cycle
Triceps fatfold. *See* Fatfold measures
Trichinella spiralis, 489t
radiation and, 510
Trichinosis, 489t
Triglycerides, **141**, 158
alcohol and, 887
in blood, 160, 559
carbons, *231*
chemistry of, 141-151
coronary heart disease risk and, 884t, 885
desirable blood level, 164
fatty liver and, 827
formation of, 142, *143*
hydrolysis, 157, *157*
medium-chain, 729-730
mixed, *145*
roles in nutrition, 148
stress and, 815
see also Atherosclerosis; Cardiovascular disease (CVD); Fat; Fatty acid(s); Glycerol; Heart disease
Triiodothyronine (T₃), 470
Tripeptidases, **184**
in protein digestion, *185*
Tripeptide, **182**. *See also* Protein/amino acids (in body)
Tropical oils, 146, *146*
Trypsin, in protein digestion, *185*
Tryptophan, 181t, 194, 196
niacin and, 334
supplements, 206
TSH. *See* Thyroid-stimulating hormone
TSH-releasing hormone (TRH), A-3
Tube feedings, 761-775
in acute renal failure, 916
advantages, 761-762
in cancer, 944
candidates, 761, 763t
in cirrhosis, 834
complications, 771-774, 773t
continuous, 768-769
in cystic fibrosis, 736
documentation, 775
drug administration and, 769-771
in dysphagia, 699
gastric, 765
in HIV infection, 954
intermittent, 768
intestinal, 765
mechanical problems, 771, 773t
monitoring, 772t
schedule, 768-769
supplemental water in, 769
transition from IV feeding to, 791-792
transition to table foods from, 775
volume progression, 768
see also Enteral nutrition; Feeding tubes
Tuberculosis, treatment and vitamin B₆, 340-341
Tubule, **911**
Tumor, **934**. *See also* Cancer
Tums, 447t, 529-530
Tuna, niacin in, 338
Tungsten, B-2t
Turbinado sugar, **122**
Turkey (food)
zinc in, 469

see also Poultry
Turkey (country), zinc deficiency in, 466
Turnip greens
calcium in, *432*
folate in, *348*
vitamin A in, 386
24-hour recall, diet history, **531**, *532*
"2—40—140" rule, 492
Type I diabetes. *See* Insulin-dependent diabetes mellitus (IDDM)
Type I osteoporosis, **439**. *See also* Osteoporosis
Type II diabetes. *See* Noninsulin-dependent diabetes mellitus (NIDDM)
Type II osteoporosis, **439**. *See also* Osteoporosis
Tyramine, MAO inhibitors and, 528-529
Tyramine-controlled diet, 529t
Tyrosine, 181t, 194
classic PKU and, 840

Ubiquinone (coenzyme Q₁₀), 351, 370t
UHT treatment. *See* Ultrahigh temperature treatment
Ulcer(s), **96**, 99
decubitus, **810**
esophageal, **700**
mouth, **697**
peptic, **96**, 99, 252, 455, **705**-706
Ulcerative colitis, 736, **744**-745
Ultrahigh temperature (UHT) treatment, **510**, 683
Ultraviolet radiation
ozone and, 618
vitamin D and, 391
see also Sunlight
Umbilical cord, **585**
Umbilicus, **585**
Unavailable carbohydrates, **108**
Unbleached flour, 45
UNCED (United Nations Conference on Environment and Development), 621n
Unconventional therapies, **689**
Undernutrition, 20
serum proteins and, 553t, 553-554
Underwater weighing, 273, *273*, 548
Underweight, **268**, 308-311
causes of, 309-310
defined by BMI, 270
health risks, 274
pregnancy and, 588, 589
see also Weight
UNICEF (United Nations International Children's Emergency Fund), vitamin A deficiency and, 380
United Nations, Food and Agricultural Organization. *See* FAO (Food and Agricultural Organization)
United Nations Conference on Environment and Development (UNCED), 621n
United States
aging population in, 666, *666*, 667
causes of death and illness in, *25*, 25t, 539t
hunger in, 614-616, 621-622
iodine intake in, 470-471
iron deficiency in, 457
organizations providing nutrition resources, F-2 to F-3
population nutrition assessment in, 23-24
sodium consumption in, 420
zinc intake in, 468
see also U.S. *entries*

Unleavened bread, 466n
Unorthodox therapies, **689**
Unsaturated fat, **144,** *145*
Unsaturated fatty acid, *143,* **144**
    structure, C-4t
    see also Unsaturated fat
Unsaturation, point of, **142**
Unspecified eating disorders, 315, 321, 322t.
    See also Eating disorders
Upper-body fat, **272**
Upper gastrointestinal tract, 696
    disorders, 695-713
Upper safe (nutrient level), **17**
Uranium, B-2t
Urea, 195, **234**
    excretion, 234, *235*
    manganese and, 473
    synthesis, *234*
Urea cycle, C-18 to C-19
Urea kinetic modeling, **921**
Urea nitrogen, blood, 552t, 914, 917
Uremia, **914.** *See also* Renal failure
Uremic frost, **917**
Uremic syndrome, 914-**915,** 917, 918
Ureter, 88
Urethra, **379**
Uric acid, 249
    accumulation in renal failure, 914, 917
    blood, 552t
    kidney stones composed of, 930, 932
Urinary tract. *See specific parts*
Urinary urea nitrogen (UUN), 554
Urine, 86, 88
    5-HIAA in, 559-560
    alcohol in, 249
    amount excreted daily, 411
    creatinine excretion, 554-555
    drug-nutrient interactions affecting excre-
        tion, 529
    laboratory tests. *See* Laboratory tests
    protein losses in nephrotic syndrome, 911, *912*
U.S. Department of Education (DOE), 31
U.S. exchange system, G-6t to G-14t
U.S. government (nutrition resources), F-2 to
    F-3
U.S. Pharmacopoeia (USP), 370n
    on purified water, 516
    on supplement forms, 370
U.S. RDA. *See* RDA (Recommended Dietary
    Allowance)
USDA (U.S. Department of Agriculture), **486**
    aflatoxin and, 201
    Daily Food Guide, 40-44, 41t, *42-43. See
        also* Daily Food Guide
    Extension Service, 491, 493
    Food Guide Pyramid, 40, 41, *43,* 44
    food labels and, 51, 52
    Food Stamp Program, **614,** 616
    Meat and Poultry Hotline, 490
    meat safety and, 490, 492
    national nutrition assessment and, 23
    nutrition resources from, F-2
    pesticides and, 499
    School Lunch and School Breakfast Pro-
        grams, 640, 648, 649
    WIC program. *See* WIC
USP. *See* U.S. Pharmacopoeia
Usual intake, diet history, 532, *532*
Uterus, **585**
UUN (urinary urea nitrogen), 554

Vagotomy, **706,** *706*
Valerian, 691
Validity (research), **12,** 14
Valine, 181t
Values, food choices and, 3
Vanadium, 477, B-2t
Variable (research), **12**
Varices, esophageal, 829-**830,** 834
Variety (dietary), **38-39**
    nutrient absorption and, 92-93
Vascular system
    in nutrient transport, 86-89, *87-89*
    see also Cardiovascular system
Vasoconstrictor, **411**
    angiotensin as, 411
Vasopressin, **411, A-4.** *See also* ADH (antidi-
    uretic hormone)
Vegan, **210**
    inadequacy of diet, 211
    vitamin B$_{12}$ and, 350
    vitamin D in, 594
Vegetable oil, 145-146, *146*
    vitamin E in, 394, 395
    see also specific type
Vegetable protein, textured, **210**
Vegetables, H
    calcium in, *431, 432, 432*
    cancer and, 61, 127, 403, 404-405
    for children, 646
    in choice system, I-5t to I-7t
    choices, 50
    in exchange lists, 571t, *572,* G-9t
    fat intake and, 168, 169-170
    fiber in, 129t
    folate in, 347, *348*
    in food group plans, 41, *42,* 46, 47
    goitrogens in, 498
    health claims on labels and, 61
    iron in, *462*
    irradiated, 510
    lignin in, 110
    magnesium in, 435, *436*
    natural toxicants in, 498
    niacin in, 337, *338*
    nonnutrient compounds in, 405, 406t
    oils, H
    oxalates in, 429
    pesticide residues on, *499. See also* Pesticides
    phytochemicals in, 406t
    potassium in, *425*
    proteins in, 196, 197
    riboflavin in, 333, *335*
    specific nutrients in, 331. *See also specific
        nutrients*
    thiamin in, *332*
    tyramine-containing, 529t
    vitamin A in, 385, *386*
    vitamin B$_6$ in, *344*
    vitamin C in, 362, *363*
    vitamin E in, 395
    vitamin K in, 397
    in voluntary labeling program, 52, 53t
    weight loss and, 302
    zinc in, 468, *469*
    see also Plant foods
Vegetarian(s), **210**
Vegetarian diets, 209-213
    adequacy, 211
    Daily Food Guide, 44
    health benefits, 209-211

    inadequacy of strict diet, 211
    planning, 211-213, 212t
    in pregnancy, 592, 594
    problems associated with, 211
    protein in, 196-197
    riboflavin in, 333
Vein(s), **86-88**
    central, **786**
    feeding through. *See* Intravenous (IV) nutri-
        tion
    hepatic, 829
    peripheral, **785**
    portal, 829
    see also specific veins
Ventilator, mechanical, **899**
Verbal communication, with professionals, 579,
    583
Very-low-density lipoprotein (VLDL), **159,** *161*
Very-low-kcalorie diets (VLCD), 299-301
    recommended criteria for, 299
    side effects of, 300t
Very low sodium (on labels), 60t
Villus/villi, **83,** *84,* 85
Viruses, 487n
    proteins in defense against, 192-193
    see also specific viruses
Viscosity, fibers and, 110
Visible fat, **170**
Vision
    vitamin A in, 376-378, *377*
    see also Eyes
Vitamin(s), 4, 5, **10, 326-364**
    absorption, 327. *See also* Absorption
    additives, 507
    in breast milk, 627t, 629
    cancer and, 944
    chronic renal failure and, 920t, 922-923
    in cirrhosis, 832
    in cow's milk, 627t
    in cystic fibrosis, 735
    elements in, 5
    function, 326
    impostors, 350-351
    in infant formula, 627t
    lactation and, 607-608
    measurement in foods, 326
    megadoses during pregnancy, 605
    natural, 355
    needs during childhood, 639
    needs during illness, 562
    needs during infancy, 621, 623
    needs during stress, 815
    organic nature of, 327
    physical activity and, 284
    precursors, **326**
    requirements, 16-17, *17*
    solubility, 327
    structure, 326
    structures, C-6 to C-11
    supplements, 284, 366-372, 368t, 404
    water-miscible, **730,** 735
    see also Deficiency(ies); Food(s); RDA; Toxi-
        city; *specific vitamins*
Vitamin A, 328t, 375-387, H
    activity, **385**
    alcohol and, 252
    cancer and, 403
    in cell differentiation, 378-379, *379*
    childhood deficiency, 640
    cirrhosis and, 832

colors of foods containing, 385, *385*
conversion of compounds, 375, *376*
deficiency, 380, 380-383, *381*, 382t-383t, *384*
food sources, 382t, 384-387, *385, 386*
forms, 375, *376*
in growth, 379
in immunity, 379
infectious diseases and, 380-381
older adults and, 673-674
olestra and, 178
preformed, **375**
RDI, 55t
recommendations, 368t, 380, 382t
roles in body, 375-379, *377, 379*
supplements, 380-381
in tooth formation, *427*
toxicity, 367, 380, 382t, 383-384
in vision, 376-378, *377*
zinc deficiency and, 466
see also Beta-carotene
Vitamin B$_1$. *See* Thiamin
Vitamin B$_2$. *See* Riboflavin
Vitamin B$_3$. *See* Niacin
"Vitamin B$_5$." *See* Pantothenic acid
Vitamin B$_6$, **340**-342, 342t, H
calcium and, 354
chronic renal failure and, 920t, 922
deficiency, 341, 342t
food sources, 341-342, 342t, *344*
magnesium and, 354
pregnancy and, 593
RDI, 55t
recommendations, 341, 342t, 368t
recommendations for older adults, 674
riboflavin and, 354
toxicity, 341, 342t
see also B vitamins
Vitamin B$_{12}$, **347,** 349
absorption, 349
anemia after gastrectomy and, 711
blind loop syndrome and, 710
chronic gastritis and, 705
cobalt and, 477, *477*
deficiency, 349-350, *350*, 351t
folate and, 346, 349, 354
food sources, 350, 351t
nervous system and, 349, 351t
pregnancy and, 594
RDI, 55t
recommendations, 349, 351t, 368t
recommendations for older adults, 674
in vegetarian diet, 213
see also B vitamins
"Vitamin B$_{15}$," 351
"Vitamin B$_{17}$," 351
"Vitamin B$_T$." *See* Carnitine
Vitamin C, 328t, 356-362, H
active forms, *357*
anticoagulant interactions with, 361n
as antioxidant, 357, *357*, 402, 506, 677
aspirin and, 529
cancer and, 403
chronic renal failure and, 922
in collagen formation, 357-358, *358*
in common cold and respiratory infections, 11-13, 358-359
deficiency, 356, 359-361, 360t
in disease prevention, 359
food sources, 360t, 362, *363*

foods providing for infants, 636
GI bleeding and, 559
heart disease and, 403-404
iron absorption and, 86, 453, 454, *455*, 459
preservation in foods, 362
as prooxidant, 459
RDI, 55t
recommendations, 359, *359*, 360t, 368t
research on effects of, 11-13
smoking and, 655
in stress reaction, 358
supplements, 404
in tooth formation, *427*
toxicity, 360t, 361-362
vitamin E and, 402, 403-404
Vitamin D, 153, 328t, 387-391
active, **911**
in bone growth, 387-388
breast milk and, 629
calcium and, 428, 429, 441, A-5
calcium supplements with, 446, 446t
cholesterol and, *152*
chronic renal failure and, 918, 920t, 922-923
cirrhosis and, 832
deficiency, 388, *388*, 389t
food sources, 389t, 390
infant deficiency, 629
infant supplements, 630t
milk fortification with, 333
older adults and, 674
olestra and, 178
during pregnancy, 594
RDI, 55t
recommendations, 368t, 390-391
riboflavin in milk and, 333
roles in body, 387-388
from sunlight, 390-391, 441
supplements and osteoporosis, 441
synthesis and activation, 387, *387*
target tissues, 388
toxicity, 388, 389t, 390, 446t
in vegetarian diet, 213
Vitamin D-refractory rickets, **388**
Vitamin D$_2$, **387**
Vitamin D$_3$, **387**
Vitamin E, 328t, 391-394
as antioxidant, 391-392, 402, 506, 677
beta-carotene interactions with, 369
cancer and, 403, 404
cardiovascular disease and, 403, 905
deficiency, 392t, 393
diabetes and, 402
food sources, 392t, 394, *395*
glutathione peroxidase and, 471
nutrient interactions, 369
olestra and, 178
RDI, 55t
recommendations, 368t, 392t, 393
supplements, 404
toxicity, 392t, 393
vitamin C and, 402, 403-404
vitamin K and, 369
Vitamin K, 328t, 394, 396-397
anticoagulants and, 396
cirrhosis and, 832
deficiency, 394, 396, 397t
food sources, 397
intestinal flora and, 80, 394, 396
intravenous solutions and, 784
newborns and, 367, 396

olestra and, 178
RDI, 55t
toxicity, 396, 397t
vitamin E and, 369
warfarin interactions with, 528
Vitamin P, 351
VLCD. *See* Very-low-kcalorie diets
VLDL (very-low-density lipoprotein), **159,** *161*
Volume measurement, 6, D-3
Voluntary activities, energy expenditures and, **263**-265, 264t, 267
Voluntary labeling, 51-52, 53t
Vomiting, 94-**96,** 702-704
cancer and, 946
hydrochloric acid and, 423
self-induced. *See* Bulimia nervosa
tube feeding and, 773t

Waist-to-hip ratio, 273
Warfarin (Coumadin)
vitamin K interactions with, 528
see also Anticoagulants
Waste products, accumulation in acute renal failure, 914, 917
Wasting
causes in malabsorption syndromes, 734t
chronic PEM and, 199, 201
chronic renal failure and, 918-919, 919t
underweight and, 274
Wasting disorders, 934-956. *See also* Cancer; Human immunodeficiency virus (HIV)
Water, 5, *5,* 10, H
ADH and retention of, 411
artesian, **516**
attraction by electrolytes, 413-414, *414*
balance, **409**-411, 410t
blood pressure and, 411-412, *412*
blood volume and, 411-412, *412*
body fluids and, 409-417
body weight and, 258
bottled, 517
calcium in, 435
cleansing process, 515-516
constipation and, 97
contaminants, 481, 483, 516, 517
copper in, 473
distilled, **516**
energy metabolism and, 9
in enteral formulas, 769
excretion, 410t, 411
excretion regulation, 411-412, *412*
fibers and, 110
fluids delivering, 411
fluoridated, 474-475, **516**
following electrolytes, 414, *415*
food sources, 410, 410t
hard, 435, **516**
home treatments, 517
infant needs, 626-627, 635
insensible losses, 411n
intoxication, **410**
lactation and, 608
lead in, 481
magnesium in, 435
metabolic, 410, 410t
molecule, *B-5, B-7*
natural, **516**
in older adults, 671
purified, **516**
recommendations, 16, 411

recommendations for physical activity, 284-285, 285t
safety concerns, 515-516
safety while traveling, 494
salt dissociation in, 412-413
scarcity, 618
soft, **516**
sources, *515*, 515-516
supplemental in tube feeding, 769
supply, *515*, 515-517, 618
systems and regulations, 516-517
urea excretion and, 234
weight loss and, 303
see also Fluid(s)
Water-miscible vitamins, **730,** 735
"Water pills." *See* Diuretic(s)
Water retention, 295-297
Water-soluble vitamins, 10, 326t, 326-364
fat-soluble vitamins vs., 328t
see also Vitamin(s); *specific vitamins*
Watercress, calcium in, *432*
Watermelon, H
thiamin in, *332*
vitamin B$_6$ in, *344*
Wean, **631**
Weight (body), 27t
alcohol effects on, 253t
artificial sweeteners and, 137-138
blood alcohol concentration and, 251n, 251t
BMR estimation from, 265t, 267
body composition and, 266, 268
carbohydrate intake and, 102, 126
changing standards, 268, 269t
cystic fibrosis and, 735-736
Diet and Health recommendations for control, 26, 27t
disagreements over standards, 268-270
fiber and, 126
genetics and, 289-290
healthy, 268, 269t
and height ranges based on BMI, inside back cover
and height tables/charts, 268-270, 269t, 546, 547, E-21t to E-23
hydrodensitometry, 273, *273*, 548
ideal, 547, 548t, 549
kcalories for weight loss based on, 302
measurement, 545, 547-548, 548
monitoring in upper GI tract disorders, 713
as nutrition status indicator, 548t
osteoporosis and, 443-444
before pregnancy, 588-589
protein intake and, 203
protein RDA and, 15n
recommendations, 268-271, 269t
set-point theory of, 290-291
smoking and, 655
usual, 547, 548t, 549
vegetarian diet and, 209
water and, 258
water percentage, 409
see also Obesity; Weight gain; Weight loss; Underweight
Weight control resources, F-4 to F-5
Weight cycling, **295**
Weight gain
anorexia nervosa treatment and, 318
in breastfed infants, 629
drug effects on food intake and, 526

energy needs for, 812t
during first five years of life, 626
genetic tendency toward, 290
lecithin supplements and, 152
overly rapid, 258
pointers for, 310-311
during pregnancy, 548, 589, 590t, E-23
regain after weight loss, 290
repeated cycle of weight loss and, 295
strategies for, 310-311
after very-low-kcalorie diet, 300-301
Weight loss
alternative strategies used in, 295-299, 298
anorexia nervosa and. *See* Anorexia nervosa
in atherosclerosis prevention, 887
behavior modification in, 305-309, 306
benefits of, 301
consumer bill of rights, 294t
controversies, 292-294
dangers of, 294t, 294-295, 295
energy intake for, 257-258
fat loss vs., 243
features of unsound schemes and diets for, 296
fiber and, 126
after gastrectomy, 709
good choices, 301-308, 302t, 304-306
in hypertension treatment, 892
in IDDM, 849
low-carbohydrate diet for, 243
maintenance of, 301, 306
in NIDDM treatment, 867
nutrition care plan for, 563
overly rapid, 257-258
physical activity and, 282, 283, 303-305, 305
pointers for, 301-303
poor choices, 294t, 294-301, 295, 298, 300t
after pregnancy, 589-590, 607
during pregnancy, 605
protein-sparing fast for, 243-244
rapid, 294t
regained weight after, 290
repeated cycle of weight gain and, 295
very-low-kcalorie diets for, 299-301, 300t
Weight Watchers (WW), 307
Weights and measures, D-3. *See also* Measurements
Well water, 515, **516**
Wernicke-Korsakoff syndrome, **329**
West African cuisine, 65-66
Wheat, 48
Wheat bread
calcium in, *432*
see also Breads
Wheat flour, **45**
Wheat germ, 152
Wheat germ oil, 371t
vitamin E in, 394, 395
Whey, 116
White Americans, lactose intolerance in, 115
White blood cells, tests, 552t
White fat, brown fat vs., 289
White flour, **45**
White sugar, 106, **122,** 129
nutrients in, 124t
WHO (World Health Organization), 20, **486,** F-3
calcium recommendations, 430
nutrition recommendations, G-14
pesticides and, 501

protein-digestibility-corrected amino acid score, 198
reference protein standard, 197
rehydration formula, 727
vitamin A deficiency and, 380
Whole grain, **45,** 49
Whole wheat bread
nutrients in, 124t
see also Breads
Whole-wheat flour, **45**
WIC (Special Supplemental Food Program for Women, Infants, and Children)
iron deficiency and, 457-458
pregnancy and, 597
Wine, 63-64, **246,** 252t
flavonoids in, 405, 406t
lead in foil seals, 483
see also Alcohol
Withdrawal reaction, **362**
Without (on labels), 60t
Women
alcohol dehydrogenase, production of, 247
athletes, 316-317, *317. See also* Athletes
BMR estimation in, 265t, 267
body fat, 271, 272
calcium requirements, 430, 445
cancer in obesity, 275
daily iron losses in, 455n
eating disorders and, 322-323
fluoride supplements in, 445
folate requirements, 345-346
ideal body weight, 547
iron deficiency in, 456
iron RDA for, 460, 461
osteoporosis in, 439, *442,* 442-443, 675. *See also* Osteoporosis
pregnant. *See* Pregnancy
premenstrual syndrome in, 341
waist-to-hip ratio, 273
see also Gender differences
Women, Infants, and Children Supplemental Food program. *See* WIC
World Health Organization. *See* WHO
World hunger, 616-621
resources, F-6
Wrist circumference, frame size and, E-20
WW (Weight Watchers), 307

Xanthophylls, **385**
Xenon, B-2t
Xerophthalmia, **382,** 382t
Xerosis, **382,** 382t
Xylitol, **135,** 138t
Xylose, 109n

Yeast, 333, H
vitamin B$_{12}$ in, 350
see also Brewer's yeast
Yo-yo effect, **295**
Yogurt, H
aspartame content, 137t
calcium in, *431*
in food group plans, 40, *43*
lactose intolerance and, 115
riboflavin in, *335*
zinc in, *469*
see also Milk and milk products
Yohimbe, 371t
Ytterbium, B-2t
Yttrium, B-2t

Zalcitabine (ddC), 950
Zeaxanthin, 406n
Zero (on labels), 60t
Zero nitrogen balance, **194**
"Zero risk" standard, 504
Zidovudine (AZT), 950
Zinc, 450, 463-468, B-2t, H
  absorption, 464
  amount in body, *418*
  in breast milk, 630
  calcium and, 369
  childhood deficiency, 640

contamination, 468
copper and, 369, 465-466, 468, 473
deficiency, 466, 467t
enteropancreatic circulation, 464, *465*
enzymes assisted by, 463
food sources, 467t, 468, *468*, *469*
losses, 466
metabolism, 464-466, *465*
metallothionein and, 464
nutrient interactions, 369, 464, 465-466, 468
in older adults, 674
pregnancy and, 595

RDI, 55t
recommendations, 368t, 467t, 468
roles in body, 463-464, 467t
supplements, 468
toxicity, 466-468, 467t
transport by albumin, 464-465
in vegetarian diet, 212-213
Zinc malnutrition, 466
Zirconium, B-2t
Zollinger-Ellison syndrome, **705**
  treatment, 706
Zygote, **585**

CHAPTER OPENING ELECTRON MICROGRAPHS © Michael Davidson

1 carrot; 36 spinach; 71 green pepper; 101 fructose; 146 olecic acid; 179 hemoglobin; 218 acetyl coA; 256 adenosine triphosphate; 287 litesse; 325 vitamin C; 374 beta carotene; 408 calcium; 449 selenium; 485 capsaicin; 518 leptin; 543 vitamin A; 561 thiamine; 584 folate; 625 growth hormone; 665 serotonin; 694 vitamin B 12; 722 vitamin D; 755 glutamine; 782 arginine; 803 epinephrine; 825 ammonia; 845 glucose; 881 prostaglandin; 909 urea; 933 AZT; 963 vitamin E.

PHOTO CREDITS

Acceptable Weight for Height Based on Body Mass Index (BMI)

To determine your acceptable weight range, find your height in the top line. Look down the column below it and find the range represented by the color blue. Look to the left column to see what weights are acceptable for you.

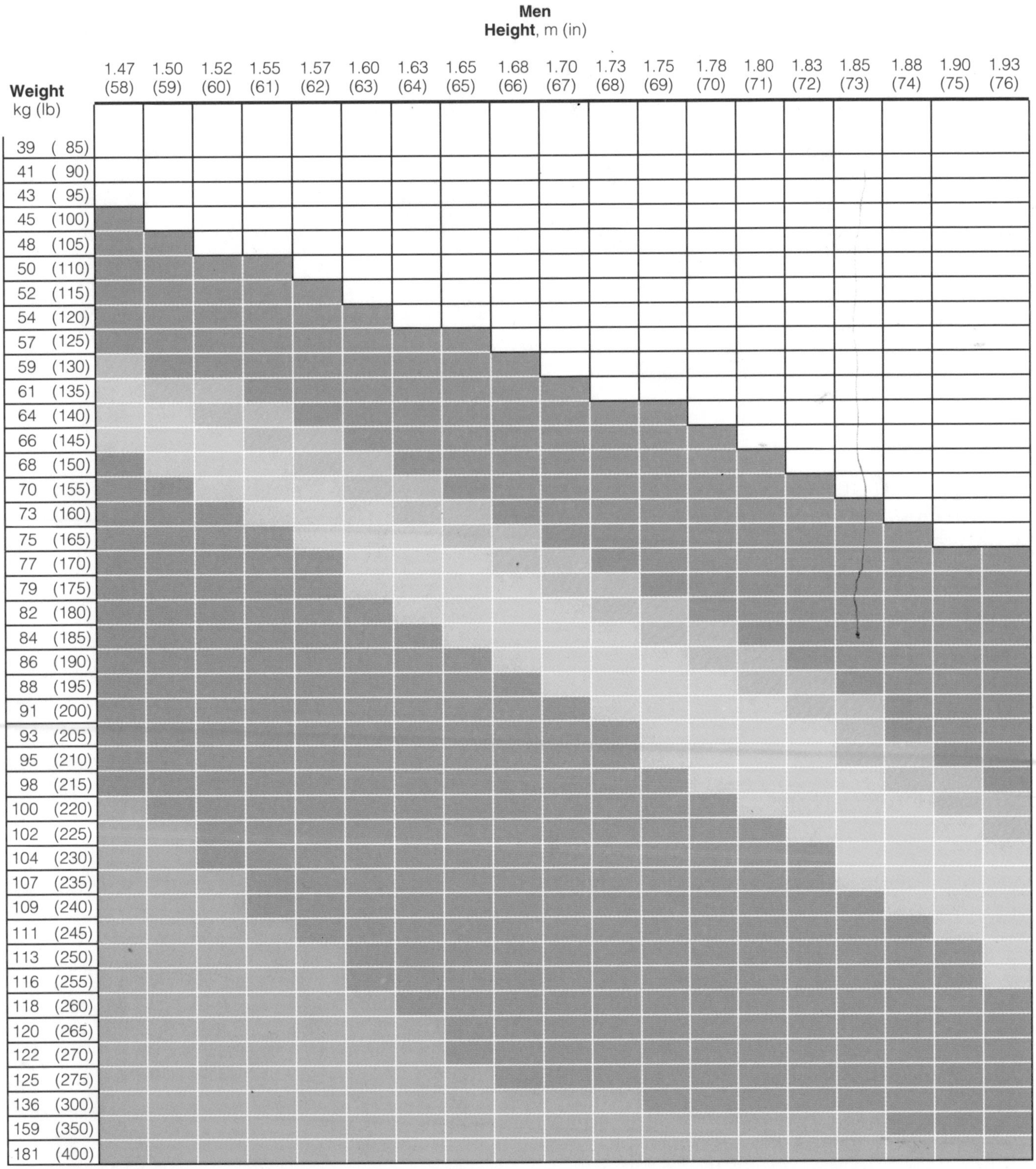

Men
Height, m (in)

Weight kg (lb)	1.47 (58)	1.50 (59)	1.52 (60)	1.55 (61)	1.57 (62)	1.60 (63)	1.63 (64)	1.65 (65)	1.68 (66)	1.70 (67)	1.73 (68)	1.75 (69)	1.78 (70)	1.80 (71)	1.83 (72)	1.85 (73)	1.88 (74)	1.90 (75)	1.93 (76)
39 (85)
41 (90)
43 (95)
45 (100)
48 (105)
50 (110)
52 (115)
54 (120)
57 (125)
59 (130)
61 (135)
64 (140)
66 (145)
68 (150)
70 (155)
73 (160)
75 (165)
77 (170)
79 (175)
82 (180)
84 (185)
86 (190)
88 (195)
91 (200)
93 (205)
95 (210)
98 (215)
100 (220)
102 (225)
104 (230)
107 (235)
109 (240)
111 (245)
113 (250)
116 (255)
118 (260)
120 (265)
122 (270)
125 (275)
136 (300)
159 (350)
181 (400)

Key:
- ☐ Underweight (BMI = < 20.7 for men and < 19.1 for women)
- Acceptable weight (BMI = 20.7 to 26.4 for men and 19.1 to 25.8 for women)
- Marginal overweight (BMI = 26.4 to 27.8 for men and 25.8 to 27.3 for women)
- Overweight (BMI = 27.8 to 31.1 for men and 27.3 to 32.2 for women)
- Severe overweight (BMI = 31.1 to 45.4 for men and 32.3 to 44.8 for women)
- Morbid obesity (BMI = > 45.4 for men and > 44.8 for women)

Note: For more information on the body mass index, see Chapter 8 and Appendix E.

Source: Adapted from M. I. Rowland, A nomogram for computing body index, *Dietetic Currents* 16 (1989): 8–9, used with permission from Ross Laboratories, Columbus, OH 43216. Copyright 1989 Ross Laboratories.